MW00845424

# Pediatric Gastrointestinal Disease

# Pediatric Gastrointestinal Disease

## Pathophysiology
## Diagnosis
## Management

SECOND EDITION

**ROBERT WYLLIE, M.D.**
Head, Department of Pediatric Gastroenterology and Nutrition
Chair, Department of Medical Subspecialties, Pediatrics
The Cleveland Clinic Foundation
Cleveland, Ohio

**JEFFREY S. HYAMS, M.D.**
Professor, Department of Pediatrics
University of Connecticut School of Medicine
Farmington, Connecticut

Head, Division of Digestive Diseases and Nutrition
Connecticut Children's Medical Center
Hartford, Connecticut

**W.B. SAUNDERS COMPANY**
***A Division of Harcourt Brace & Company***
Philadelphia London Toronto Montreal Sydney Tokyo

**W.B. SAUNDERS COMPANY**
*A Division of Harcourt Brace & Company*

The Curtis Center
Independence Square West
Philadelphia, Pennsylvania 19106

**Library of Congress Cataloging-in-Publication Data**

Pediatric gastrointestinal disease / [edited by] Robert Wyllie, Jeffrey S. Hyams.—2nd ed.

p. cm.

Includes bibliographical references and index.

ISBN 0–7216–7461–5

1. Pediatric gastroenterology. I. Wyllie, R. (Robert) II. Hyams, Jeffrey S. [DNLM: 1. Digestive System Diseases—in infancy & childhood. 2. Digestive System Diseases—in adolescence. WS 310 P37145 1999]

RJ446.P364 1999 618.92′33—dc21

DNLM/DLC 98–28621

PEDIATRIC GASTROINTESTINAL DISEASE: Pathophysiology, Diagnosis, Management ISBN 0–7216–7461–5



Printed in the United States of America.

Last digit is the print number: 9 8 7 6 5 4 3 2 1

*To our patients*
*and their families*

# Contributors

**Frederick Alexander, M.D.**
Associate Clinical Professor of Surgery, Ohio State University, Columbus, Ohio; Staff Surgeon and Chairman, Department of Pediatric Surgery, The Cleveland Clinic Foundation, Cleveland, Ohio
*Pyloric Stenosis and Congenital Anomalies of the Stomach and Duodenum; Inguinal Hernia and Hydrocele*

**Joel M. Andres, M.D.**
Pediatric Gastroenterologist, Arnold Palmer Children's Hospital, Orlando, Florida
*Polyps and Polyposis Syndromes*

**Dean L. Antonson, M.D.**
Associate Professor of Pediatrics, University of Nebraska Medical Center, Omaha, Nebraska
*Eating Disorders and Obesity*

**Salvatore Auricchio, M.D., Ph.D.**
Professor of Pediatrics, Department of Pediatrics, University Federico II, Naples, Italy
*Celiac Disease*

**Dorsey M. Bass, M.D.**
Assistant Professor of Pediatrics, Stanford University, Stanford, California; Attending Gastroenterologist, Lucile Packard Children's Hospital, Palo Alto, California
*Enteric Parasites*

**Steven K. Bergstrom, M.D.**
Assistant Professor of Pediatrics, University of Connecticut School of Medicine, Farmington, Connecticut; Staff Oncologist, Connecticut Children's Medical Center, Hartford, Connecticut
*Neoplasms of the Gastrointestinal Tract*

**Uwe Blecker, M.D.**
Associate Professor of Pediatrics, Jefferson Medical College, Thomas Jefferson University, Philadelphia, Pennsylvania; Director, Nutrition Support Services, and Attending Physician, Division of Gastroenterology and Nutrition, Alfred I. duPont Hospital for Children, Wilmington, Delaware
*Gastritis and Ulcers in Children*

**Athos Bousvaros, M.D.**
Instructor in Pediatrics, Harvard Medical School; Assistant in Gastroenterology, Children's Hospital, Boston, Massachusetts
*Gastrointestinal Manifestations of Primary Immunodeficiencies*

**Randall S. Burd, M.D., Ph.D.**
Assistant Professor of Surgery, Division of Pediatric Surgery, University of Missouri–Columbia School of Medicine, Columbia, Missouri
*Hirschsprung's Disease*

**William J. Byrne, M.D.**
Clinical Professor of Pediatrics, University of California School of Medicine, San Francisco, California; Medical Director and Senior Vice President for Medical Affairs, Children's Hospital Oakland, Oakland, California
*Caustic Ingestion and Foreign Bodies*

**Mitchell B. Cohen, M.D.**
Professor of Pediatrics, University of Cincinnati College of Medicine; Attending Physician, Children's Hospital Medical Center, Cincinnati, Ohio
*Infectious Diarrhea*

**Richard B. Colletti, M.D.**
Associate Professor of Pediatrics, University of Vermont College of Medicine, Burlington, Vermont
*Ascites*

**Claudia A. Conkin, M.S., R.D.**
Director, Food and Nutrition Services, Texas Children's Hospital, Houston, Texas
*Nutritional Assessment*

**Fernando del Rosario, M.D.**
Assistant Professor of Pediatrics, University of Pittsburgh School of Medicine; Faculty, Children's Hospital of Pittsburgh, Pittsburgh, Pennsylvania
*Achalasia and Other Motor Disorders*

**Carlo Di Lorenzo, M.D.**
Associate Professor of Pediatrics, University of Pittsburgh School of Medicine; Faculty, Children's Hospital of Pittsburgh, Pittsburgh, Pennsylvania
*Achalasia and Other Motor Disorders*

**Sigmund H. Ein, M.D.C.M., F.R.C.S.(C), F.A.C.S., F.A.A.P.**
Associate Professor, Department of Surgery, Faculty of Medicine, University of Toronto; Staff Surgeon, Division of General Surgery, The Hospital for Sick Children; Consultant Staff, Department of Newborn and Developmental Paediatrics, Women's College Hospital; Associate Staff, Department of Surgery, Mount Sinai Hospital; Provisional Staff, Department of Obstetrics, Gynecology and Pediatrics, Wellesley Hospital, Toronto, Ontario, Canada
*Congenital Malformations of the Esophagus*

**Jonathan S. Evans, M.D.**
Assistant Professor of Pediatrics, Mayo Medical School, Rochester, Minnesota; Nemours Children's Clinic, Jacksonville, Florida
*Acute and Chronic Hepatitis*

**Mark A. Gilger, M.D.**
Associate Professor of Pediatrics, Baylor College of Medicine; Medical Director, Gastrointestinal Procedures Suite, Texas Children's Hospital, Houston, Texas
*Diseases of the Gallbladder*

**Wallace A. Gleason, Jr., M.D.**
Professor of Pediatrics, and Director, Division of Gastroenterology, Hepatology and Nutrition, Assistant Dean for Admissions, University of Texas–Houston Health Science Center; Chief, Pediatric Gastroenterology, Hepatology and Nutrition, Hermann Children's Hospital, Houston, Texas
*Protein-Losing Enteropathy*

**Benjamin D. Gold, M.D.**
Assistant Professor of Pediatrics and Microbiology, and Attending Physician, Division of Pediatric Gastroenterology and Nutrition, Emory University School of Medicine; Director, Helicobacter Laboratory, Foodborne and Diarrheal Diseases Branch, National Center for Infectious Diseases, Centers for Disease Control and Prevention, Atlanta, Georgia
*Gastritis and Ulcers in Children*

**Regino P. González-Peralta, M.D.**
Assistant Professor, Division of Gastroenterology and Hepatology, Department of Pediatrics and Section of Hepatobiliary Diseases, College of Medicine, University of Florida; Attending Physician, Shands Children's Hospital, Gainesville, Florida
*Polyps and Polyposis Syndromes*

**John R. Gosche, M.D., Ph.D.**
Assistant Professor of Surgery and Pediatrics, Yale University School of Medicine; Attending Staff, Yale-New Haven Children's Hospital, New Haven, Connecticut
*Congenital Anomalies of the Midgut*

**Glenn R. Gourley, M.D.**
Professor, Department of Pediatrics, University of Wisconsin–Madison, School of Medicine, and Waisman Center on Mental Retardation and Human Development; Director, Pediatric Gastroenterology Training Program, University of Wisconsin Hospital and Clinics, Madison, Wisconsin
*Jaundice*

**Jay L. Grosfeld, M.D.**
Lafayette Page Professor and Chairman, Department of Surgery, Indiana University School of Medicine; Surgeon-in-Chief, James Whitcomb Riley Hospital for Children, Indianapolis, Indiana
*Intussusception in Infants and Children*

**Leo A. Heitlinger, M.D.**
Associate Professor of Pediatrics, College of Medicine and Public Health, Ohio State University; Director, Specialty Clinics, Medical Director, Gastrointestinal Procedures, Children's Hospital, Columbus, Ohio
*Gastrointestinal Hemorrhage*

**Donald W. Hight, M.D.**
Associate Professor of Surgery, and Director, Department of Pediatric Surgery, Department of Surgery, University of Connecticut School of Medicine, Farmington, Connecticut; Director, Department of Pediatric Surgery, and Associate Director, Surgical Service, Connecticut Children's Medical Center, Hartford, Connecticut
*Abdominal Masses in Pediatric Patients*

**Jeffrey S. Hyams, M.D.**
Professor, Department of Pediatrics, University of Connecticut School of Medicine, Farmington, Connecticut; Head, Division of Digestive Diseases and Nutrition, Connecticut Children's Medical Center, Hartford, Connecticut
*Crohn's Disease*

**Paul E. Hyman, M.D.**
Associate Clinical Professor of Pediatrics, University of California, Los Angeles, Los Angeles, California; Director, Pediatric Gastrointestinal Motility Center, Children's Hospital of Orange County, Orange, California
*Gastric Motility Disorders; Chronic Intestinal Pseudo-obstruction*

**Maureen M. Jonas, M.D.**
Associate Professor of Pediatrics, Harvard Medical School; Associate in Gastroenterology, Children's Hospital, Boston, Massachusetts
*Neonatal Hepatitis*

**Nicola L. Jones, M.D., F.R.C.P.C.**
Departments of Molecular Microbiology and Medical Genetics and Pediatrics, University of Toronto; Fellow, Division of Gastroenterology/Nutrition, The Hospital for Sick Children, Toronto, Ontario, Canada
*Gastropathies: Pathophysiology and Clinical Features*

**Christopher Justinich, M.D.**
Assistant Professor, University of Connecticut School of Medicine, Farmington, Connecticut; Pediatric Gastroenterologist, Division of Digestive Diseases and Nutrition, Connecticut Children's Medical Center, Hartford, Connecticut
*Allergic Bowel Disease and Eosinophilic Gastroenteritis*

**Marsha H. Kay, M.D.**
Staff Physician, Division of Pediatrics, Section of Pediatric Gastroenterology and Nutrition, The Cleveland Clinic Foundation, Cleveland, Ohio
*Liver Failure and Transplantation*

**Michael D. Klein, M.D.**
Professor of Surgery, Wayne State University School of Medicine; Surgeon-in-Chief, Children's Hospital of Michigan, Detroit, Michigan
*Hirschsprung's Disease*

**Robert M. Kliegman, M.D.**
Professor and Chairman, Department of Pediatrics, Medical College of Wisconsin; Pediatrician-in-Chief, Children's Hospital of Wisconsin, Milwaukee, Wisconsin
*Neonatal Necrotizing Enterocolitis*

**Samuel A. Kocoshis, M.D.**
Professor of Pediatrics, University of Pittsburgh School of Medicine; Director of Pediatric Gastroenterology, Children's Hospital of Pittsburgh, Pittsburgh, Pennsylvania
*Other Diseases of the Small Intestine and Colon*

**Edward L. Krawitt, M.D.**
Professor of Medicine, University of Vermont College of Medicine, Burlington, Vermont
*Ascites*

**D. Wayne Laney, Jr., M.D.**
Assistant Professor of Pediatric and Nutrition Services, University of Alabama School of Medicine, Birmingham, Alabama
*Infectious Diarrhea*

**B U.K. Li, M.D.**
Associate Professor of Pediatrics, Ohio State University; Attending Gastroenterologist, Columbus Children's Hospital, Columbus, Ohio
*Vomiting*

**Vera Loening-Baucke, M.D.**
Professor, Division of General Pediatrics, The University of Iowa Hospitals and Clinics, Iowa City, Iowa
*Constipation and Encopresis*

**James K. Madison, Ph.D.**
Assistant Professor of Pediatrics, University of Nebraska; Research and Program Development Coordinator, Eating Disorders Program, Nebraska Health System, Omaha, Nebraska
*Eating Disorders and Obesity*

**Lori A. Mahajan, M.D.**
Chief, Pediatric Gastroenterology, Wright Patterson Air Force Base, WPAFB, Ohio
*Chronic Abdominal Pain of Childhood and Adolescence*

**Elizabeth E. Mannick, M.D.**
Assistant Professor of Pediatrics, Department of Pediatrics, Division of Gastroenterology and Nutrition, University of Rochester School of Medicine and Dentistry, Rochester, New York
*Maldigestion and Malabsorption*

**James F. Markowitz, M.D.**
Associate Professor, New York University School of Medicine, New York, New York; Associate Director, The Center for Pediatric Ileitis and Colitis, Division of Pediatric Gastroenterology, North Shore University Hospital, Manhasset, New York
*Ulcerative Colitis*

**Maria R. Mascarenhas, M.B.B.S.**
Assistant Professor of Pediatrics, University of Pennsylvania School of Medicine; Director, Nutrition Support Service, Children's Hospital of Philadelphia, Philadelphia, Pennsylvania
*Parenteral and Enteral Nutrition*

**Peter A. Mattei, M.D.**
Pediatric Surgeon, Alfred I. duPont Hospital for Children, Wilmington, Delaware
*Appendicitis*

**H. Juhling McClung, M.D.**
Professor of Pediatrics, College of Medicine and Public Health, Ohio State University; Chief, Section of Gastroenterology, Children's Hospital, Columbus, Ohio
*Gastrointestinal Hemorrhage*

**Suzanne V. McDiarmid, M.D.**
Associate Professor of Pediatrics and Surgery, University of California, Los Angeles, School of Medicine; Director, Pediatric Liver Transplantation, UCLA Medical Center, Los Angeles, California
*Liver Failure and Transplantation*

**Adam G. Mezoff, M.D.**
Associate Professor of Pediatrics and Medicine, Wright State University; Director of Gastroenterology/Nutritional Support, Children's Medical Center, Dayton, Ohio
*Bezoars*

**Tracie L. Miller, M.D.**
Associate Professor of Pediatrics, University of Rochester School of Medicine; Co-Chief, Division of Pediatric Gastroenterology and Nutrition, University of Rochester Medical Center, Children's Hospital at Strong Memorial Hospital, Rochester, New York
*Gastrointestinal Complications of Secondary Immunodeficiency Syndromes*

**Kathleen J. Motil, M.D., Ph.D.**
Assistant Professor of Pediatrics, Baylor College of Medicine; Active Staff, Section of Pediatric Gastroenterology and Nutrition, Texas Children's Hospital, Houston, Texas
*Nutritional Assessment*

**Hillel Naon, M.D.**
Assistant Professor of Pediatrics, University of Southern California School of Medicine, Los Angeles, California
*Secretory Neoplasms of the Pancreas*

**Susan R. Orenstein, M.D.**
Professor of Pediatrics, Pediatric Gastroenterology, University of Pittsburgh School of Medicine; Children's Hospital of Pittsburgh, Pittsburgh, Pennsylvania
*Gastroesophageal Reflux*

**Alberto Peña, M.D.**
Professor of Surgery, Albert Einstein College of Medicine, Bronx, New York; Chief, Pediatric Surgery, Schneider Children's Hospital, Long Island Jewish Medical Center, New Hyde Park, New York
*Imperforate Anus*

**David H. Perlmutter, M.D.**
Donald B. Strominger Professor of Pediatrics, and Professor of Cell Biology and Physiology, Washington University School of Medicine; Director, Division of Gastroenterology and Nutrition, St. Louis Children's Hospital, St. Louis, Missouri
*Metabolic Disorders of the Liver*

**J. Duncan Phillips, M.D.**
Assistant Professor of Surgery, School of Medicine, University of Southern California; Attending Surgeon, Children's Hospital, Los Angeles, California
*Abdominal Surgical Emergencies*

**Sarah M. Phillips, M.S., R.D.**
Manager, Nutrition Support Team, Texas Children's Hospital, Houston, Texas
*Nutritional Assessment*

**Daniel L. Preud'Homme, M.D.**
Assistant Professor, Department of Pediatrics, Wright State University; Associate Director of Gastroenterology/Nutritional Support, Children's Medical Center, Dayton, Ohio
*Bezoars*

**Roy Proujansky, M.D.**
Associate Professor of Pediatrics, Vice Chairman for Research, Department of Pediatrics, Jefferson Medical College, Thomas Jefferson University, Philadelphia, Pennsylvania; Chief, Division of Gastroenterology and Nutrition, Alfred I. duPont Hospital for Children, Wilmington, Delaware
*Protracted Diarrhea*

**Philip Rosenthal, M.D.**
Professor of Pediatrics and Surgery, Medical Director, Pediatric Liver Transplant Program, and Director, Pediatric Hepatology, University of California, San Francisco, San Francisco, California
*Biliary Atresia and Neonatal Disorders of the Bile Ducts*

**Howard Ross, M.D.**
Surgical Resident and Clinical Fellow, Department of Surgery, University of Connecticut School of Medicine, Farmington, Connecticut
*Abdominal Masses in Pediatric Patients*

**Robert J. Rothbaum, M.D.**
Associate Professor of Pediatrics, Washington University School of Medicine; St. Louis Children's Hospital, St. Louis, Missouri
*Cystic Fibrosis and Congenital Anomalies of the Exocrine Pancreas*

**Marshall Z. Schwartz, M.D.**
Professor of Surgery and Pediatrics, Vice Chairman, Department of Surgery, Jefferson Medical College, Thomas Jefferson University, Philadelphia, Pennsylvania; Associate Medical Director, and Vice Chairman, Department of Surgery, Alfred I. duPont Hospital for Children, Wilmington, Delaware
*Meckel's Diverticulum and Other Omphalomesenteric Duct Remnants*

**Thomas J. Sferra, M.D.**
Assistant Professor of Pediatrics, College of Medicine and Public Health, Ohio State University; Attending Gastroenterologist, Columbus Children's Hospital, Columbus, Ohio
*Vomiting*

**Philip M. Sherman, M.D., F.R.C.P.C.**
Professor of Pediatrics and Microbiology, University of Toronto; Senior Scientist, Research Institute, The Hospital for Sick Children, Toronto, Ontario, Canada
*Gastropathies: Pathophysiology and Clinical Features*

**Benjamin L. Shneider, M.D.**
Associate Professor of Pediatrics, Mount Sinai School of Medicine; Pediatric Gastroenterologist, Mount Sinai Medical Center, New York, New York
*Portal Hypertension*

**Constantinos G. Siafakas, M.D.**
Visiting Consultant, Aghia Sophia Children's Hospital, Athens, Greece; formerly Research Fellow in Gastroenterology, Children's Hospital, Boston, Massachusetts
*Neonatal Hepatitis*

**Robert H. Squires, Jr., M.D.**
Associate Professor of Pediatrics, University of Texas Southwestern Medical Center; Attending Physician, Children's Medical Center, Dallas, Texas
*Management of Diarrhea*

**Virginia A. Stallings, M.D.**
Professor of Pediatrics, University of Pennsylvania School of Medicine; Chief, Nutrition Section, Children's Hospital of Philadelphia, Philadelphia, Pennsylvania
*Parenteral and Enteral Nutrition*

**Rita Steffen, M.D.**
Staff, Pediatric Gastroenterology and Nutrition, Division of Pediatrics, Cleveland Clinic Foundation, Cleveland, Ohio
*Constipation and Encopresis*

**Richard J. Stevenson, M.D.**
Assistant Professor of Surgery, Department of Pediatric Surgery, Children's Hospital Medical Center, Cincinnati, Ohio
*Appendicitis*

**Francisco A. Sylvester, M.D.**
Assistant Professor of Pediatrics, University of Connecticut School of Medicine; Pediatric Gastroenterologist, St. Louis Children's Hospital, Farmington, Connecticut; Pediatric Gastroenterologist, Connecticut Children's Medical Center, Hartford, Connecticut
*Other Diseases of the Esophagus*

**Jeffrey H. Teckman, M.D.**
Assistant Professor of Pediatrics, Washington University School of Medicine; Pediatric Gastroenterologist, St. Louis Children's Hospital, St. Louis, Missouri
*Metabolic Disorders of the Liver*

**Andrew M. Tershakovec, M.D.**
Associate Professor, Department of Pediatrics, University of Pennsylvania School of Medicine; Associate Physician, Division of Gastroenterology and Nutrition, The Children's Hospital of Philadelphia, Philadelphia, Pennsylvania
*Parenteral and Enteral Nutrition*

**Daniel W. Thomas, M.D.**
Associate Professor of Pediatrics, University of Southern California School of Medicine; Head, Gastroenterology and Nutrition, Children's Hospital, Los Angeles, California
*Secretory Neoplasms of the Pancreas*

**Vasundhara Tolia, M.D.**
Professor of Pediatrics, Wayne State University; Director of Gastroenterology, Children's Hospital of Michigan, Detroit, Michigan
*Failure to Thrive*

**Robert J. Touloukian, M.D.**
Professor of Surgery and Pediatrics, Yale University School of Medicine; Chief, Pediatric Surgery, Yale–New Haven Children's Hospital, New Haven, Connecticut
*Congenital Anomalies of the Midgut*

**William R. Treem, M.D.**
Professor of Pediatrics, Duke University School of Medicine; Chief, Division of Pediatric Gastroenterology, Hepatology, and Nutrition, Duke Children's Hospital, Durham, North Carolina
*Short Bowel Syndrome*

**Riccardo Troncone, M.D.**
Researcher, Department of Pediatrics, University Federico II, Naples, Italy
*Celiac Disease*

**William P. Tunell, M.D.**
Emeritus Professor of Surgery, University of Oklahoma College of Medicine, Oklahoma City, Oklahoma
*Anterior Abdominal Wall Defects*

**Aliye Uc, M.D.**
Fellow, University of Iowa Hospitals and Clinics, Iowa City, Iowa
*Gastric Motility Disorders*

**John N. Udall, Jr., M.D., Ph.D.**
Professor of Pediatric Gastroenterology and Nutrition, Louisiana State University Medical Center; Chief, Pediatric Gastroenterology and Nutrition, Children's Hospital, New Orleans, Louisiana
*Maldigestion and Malabsorption*

**Jon A. Vanderhoof, M.D.**
Professor of Pediatrics, and Director, Joint Section of Pediatric Gastroenterology and Nutrition, University of Nebraska/Creighton University, Omaha, Nebraska
*Diarrhea*

**Richard G. Weiss, M.D.**
Assistant Professor of Clinical Surgery, Pediatrics, and Emergency Medicine, University of Connecticut School of Medicine, Farmington, Connecticut; Associate Director, Department of Pediatric Surgery, Connecticut Children's Medical Center, Hartford, Connecticut
*Abdominal Masses in Pediatric Patients*

**Steven L. Werlin, M.D.**
Professor of Pediatrics, Medical College of Wisconsin; Director of Gastroenterology, Children's Hospital of Wisconsin, Milwaukee, Wisconsin
*Pancreatitis*

**Karen W. West, M.D.**
Associate Professor of Pediatric Surgery, Indiana University School of Medicine; Attending Surgeon, James Whitcomb Riley Hospital for Children, Indianapolis, Indiana
*Intussusception in Infants and Children*

**Robert Wyllie, M.D.**
Head, Department of Pediatric Gastroenterology and Nutrition, and Chair, Department of Medical Subspecialties, Pediatrics, The Cleveland Clinic Foundation, Cleveland, Ohio
*Chronic Abdominal Pain of Childhood and Adolescence*

**Donna K. Zeiter, M.D.**
Assistant Professor of Pediatrics, University of Connecticut School of Medicine; Pediatric Gastroenterologist, Connecticut Children's Medical Center, Hartford, Connecticut
*Infant and Toddler Nutrition*

**Moritz M. Ziegler, M.D.**
Professor of Surgery, Harvard Medical School; Chairman, Department of Surgery, and Surgeon-in-Chief, Children's Hospital, Boston, Massachusetts
*Appendicitis*

# Preface to the Second Edition

Pediatric gastroenterology has continued to undergo a dramatic evolution since the publication of the first edition of this textbook in 1993. Newer methods of diagnosis and the burgeoning number of pharmaceutical alternatives have given us many more alternatives in evaluating and treating children with gastrointestinal disease. The second edition was written in response to these changes.

We have tried to broaden the scope of the textbook to include all facets of clinical pediatric gastrointestinal disease. New chapters were added covering the basic aspects of pediatric liver disease. To keep the book a manageable size, we have sharpened our clinical focus and incorporated the basic aspects of anatomy and physiology into the relevant clinical chapters and eliminated chapters on specific pediatric procedures that are better covered in more comprehensive textbooks dedicated to those topics. The book is organized into distinct sections, starting with common clinical problems and followed by organ-specific diseases. Sections on diseases of the esophagus, stomach, and the small and large bowel are followed by chapters reviewing the clinical facets of pediatric liver disease. The last two sections review diseases of the pancreas and basic nutrition in children.

We would like to thank the staff at W.B. Saunders for their support and encouragement. Donna Morrissey, Denise LeMelledo, and Arlene Chappelle all provided assistance. Our senior editor, Judith Fletcher, cajoled and encouraged us to make changes for this edition of the text. Most importantly, we want to thank our families for their patience and understanding as we edited the second edition of the text while maintaining busy clinical practices.

The greatest reward for editing the first edition of *Pediatric Gastrointestinal Disease: Pathophysiology, Diagnosis, Management* was to learn that it was helpful to students and our colleagues in the management of their clinical practices. Producing the book is a team effort, and we would like to thank the authors who gave time from their busy schedules to contribute to the book, demonstrating their continued commitment and dedication to the care of children with gastrointestinal disorders.

ROBERT WYLLIE, M.D.
JEFFREY S. HYAMS, M.D.

## NOTICE

Gastroenterology is an ever-changing field. Standard safety precautions must be followed, but as new research and clinical experience broaden our knowledge, changes in treatment and drug therapy become necessary or appropriate. Readers are advised to check the product information currently provided by the manufacturer of each drug to be administered to verify the recommended dose, the method and duration of administration, and the contraindications. It is the responsibility of the treating physician, relying on experience and knowledge of the patient, to determine dosages and the best treatment for the patient. Neither the publisher nor the editor assumes any responsibility for any injury and/or damage to persons or property.

THE PUBLISHER

# Contents

# SECTION ONE

# CLINICAL PROBLEMS

# Chapter 1

# Chronic Abdominal Pain of Childhood and Adolescence

*Lori Mahajan and Robert Wyllie*

Chronic abdominal pain is a common, yet often enigmatic affliction of childhood and adolescence. The generally accepted definition of chronic abdominal pain is derived from Apley's pioneering study of 1,000 school children in the late 1950s.[1] He characterized abdominal pain as chronic or recurrent if at least one episode of pain occurs per month for 3 consecutive months and is severe enough to interfere with routine functioning. Initial studies indicated that chronic abdominal pain affects 10% to 15% of school-age children; however, more recent data suggest that approximately 20% of middle school and high school students experience abdominal pain on a daily to weekly basis.[1–3]

Chronic abdominal pain can be classified as either organic or nonorganic, depending on whether a discrete cause is identified. Nonorganic chronic abdominal pain, or "functional" abdominal pain, refers to abdominal pain that cannot be explained on the basis of structural or biochemical abnormalities. Functional abdominal pain is not synonymous with *psychogenic* or *imaginary* abdominal pain, but it is generally accepted to represent genuine pain. Such pain can be further classified by location as epigastric, periumbilical, or infraumbilical.[4] The periumbilical form is the most common and thus is the focus of this chapter. The epigastric form is associated with episodic or persistent pain in the upper abdomen as well as early satiety, bloating, belching, nausea, or vomiting. It is commonly referred to as non-ulcer dyspepsia.[5] The infraumbilical form is accompanied by cramps, abdominal distention or bloating, and altered consistency or frequency of stooling. The latter is thought to be equivalent to the commonly recognized functional gastrointestinal disorder of adults, irritable bowel syndrome (IBS).[6]

Early investigators found an organic cause for recurrent abdominal pain (RAP) in only 5% to 10% of patients.[1] Progressive refinement of endoscopic techniques and radiologic imaging modalities and the advent of breath hydrogen analysis have greatly enhanced our ability to identify organic causes of RAP. As a result, the percentage of patients with functional abdominal pain appears to be decreasing. A study by Hyams and associates examined 227 children with RAP. Seventy-six patients (33%) were found to have definable causes of RAP such as inflammatory bowel disease, carbohydrate malabsorption, peptic inflammation, or celiac disease.[6]

The possibility of overlooking a serious organic condition is of most concern to the physician. This chapter reviews the neurophysiology of abdominal pain and the distinguishing characteristics of functional abdominal pain versus common organic causes of recurrent abdominal pain. The diagnostic and therapeutic approaches to the child who presents with RAP are also reviewed.

## NEUROPHYSIOLOGY OF ABDOMINAL PAIN

Neuroreceptors capable of responding to noxious stimuli, known as nociceptors, are located throughout the abdominal viscera and the supporting structures. Pain originating from abdominal viscera (visceral pain) is less well characterized and poorly localized in comparison to pain originating from more superficial structures such as the peritoneum (parietal pain). A basic understanding of the differences between these two forms of pain is important for determining the cause of a patient's complaint.

Visceral pain originates from afferent nerve fibers located within the walls or tissue of abdominal viscera. The pain impulse, once generated, is carried primarily by small, unmyelinated, slow conducting C fibers.[7–9] The termination of these fibers within the spinal column occurs over four to five spinal segments. This results in pain that is sensed by the individual as a poorly localized soreness. In addition, visceral pain is often perceived in the midline and accompanied by symptoms of autonomic disturbance such as nausea, emesis, diaphoresis, and pallor. Parietal pain is conducted by both the small, unmyelinated C fibers and by the large, thinly myelinated, rapid conducting A-delta fibers. The A-delta fibers respond to tactile, thermal, and chemical stimulation and convey discriminative information, including the location and intensity of stimuli.[7, 8] Because the nociceptors

**TABLE 1–1. Development, Innervation, and Pain Perception Associated with Abdominal Structures**

| PRIMITIVE STRUCTURE | DIFFERENTIATED STRUCTURE | SPINAL SEGMENT INNERVATION | LOCATION OF PERCEIVED PAIN |
|---|---|---|---|
| Foregut | Distal esophagus, stomach, duodenum, liver, biliary tree, pancreas | T5-T9 | Midline: xiphoid–umbilicus |
| Midgut | Remainder of small intestine, appendix, ascending colon, proximal two thirds of transverse colon | T8-L1 | Periumbilical |
| Hindgut | Distal third of transverse colon, descending and rectosigmoid colon | T11-L1 | Midline: umbilicus–symphysis pubis |
| Nephrogenic cord | Kidneys, ureters, ovaries, fallopian tubes | T10-L1 | Lateralized |

associated with somatic pain are located in the parietal peritoneum and supporting tissues, pain is often aggravated by movement. Therefore, a patient experiencing parietal pain is likely to lie still, whereas a patient with visceral pain is often described as restless.[8] Knowledge of these basic principles enables us to appreciate how the location of pain changes with the course of the illness. For example, the patient with cholecystitis or appendicitis may initially complain of dull, mid-abdominal pain (visceral pain) that subsequently becomes localized to the right upper or right lower quadrant as the inflammatory process proceeds to involve the adjacent peritoneum (parietal pain).

Another differentiating factor between visceral and parietal nociceptors relates to the recognition of particular forms of noxious stimuli. Visceral nociceptors usually do not generate impulses secondary to stimuli that would excite parietal receptors. For example, the intact mucosa of the gastrointestinal tract is relatively insensitive to pricking, cutting, or crushing stimuli that would cause intense pain if applied to the skin or more superficial structures.[8] This explains why endoscopic biopsy, polypectomy, and application of electrocautery are not associated with perceived pain by the patient.

The perception of pain also has a strong embryologic basis.[7–10] Because most abdominal viscera begin embryologically as midline structures, they have bilateral, symmetric innervation. The location of abdominal pain is determined by the level at which the afferent nerves from abdominal viscera enter the spinal cord. Abdominal structures derived from the embryonic foregut, including the distal esophagus, stomach, duodenum, liver, biliary tree, and pancreas, are innervated by nerves that enter the spinal cord from segments T5 to T9. Clinically, pain from these organs is perceived in the midline, from the xiphoid to the umbilicus. Structures arising from the primitive midgut include the majority of the small intestine, appendix, ascending colon, and proximal two thirds of the transverse colon. The afferent nerves innervating these structures enter the spinal cord from segments T8 to L1, with associated pain perceived in the periumbilical region. Structures derived from the embryonic hindgut include the distal one third of the transverse colon, the descending colon, and the rectosigmoid. These structures are innervated by spinal segments T11 to L1, with resultant pain from the structures experienced between the umbilicus and symphysis pubis. The genitourinary system develops from a mass of mesoderm located on each side of the primitive aorta in the trunk region, known as the nephrogenic cord.[11] The kidneys, ureters, ovaries, and fallopian tubes receive unilateral innervation from spinal segments T10 to L1. As a result, pain originating from these structures may be lateralized (Table 1–1).

Another important feature of abdominal pain is its tendency to be associated with well-localized pain in an area remote from the abdominal pathology, known as referred pain. Referred pain is associated with skin hyperalgesia over the cutaneous dermatome supplied by the same neural segment as the injured organ. Understanding the typical patterns of pain referral can be helpful in making a correct diagnosis. For example, the pancreas is innervated by visceral nerves that enter the spinal cord between segments T5 and T9. Pain from a pancreatic lesion is referred to cutaneous dermatomes with T5 to T9 innervation located in the midback and interscapular regions. Pain of hepatic or biliary origin is often referred to the right subscapular region.[8–10]

Thus, abdominal pain may comprise visceral pain, parietal pain, referred pain, or a combination of these components. Visceral pain is often accompanied by nausea, emesis, or diaphoresis and is perceived as a poorly localized midline discomfort. In sharp contrast, parietal pain is more intense, well localized, and often aggravated by movement. Pain can be referred to the cutaneous dermatome whose afferent nerve enters the same spinal cord segment as the affected abdominal organ. An understanding of the interrelation of the gastrointestinal tract and nervous system is important in the evaluation and accurate diagnosis of the patient with abdominal pain.

## FUNCTIONAL ABDOMINAL PAIN

### Epidemiology

Although there is general agreement that the pain of functional RAP is genuine and not imaginary, the pathogenesis remains unclear. Many have, therefore, turned to epidemiology for insight. In Apley's original survey of 1,000 unselected children in primary and secondary modern schools, 10.8% of children were found to have RAP. Girls were more commonly affected than boys, 12.3% versus 9.5%.[1] There were no complaints of pain in children younger than 5 years of age. Between 10% and 12% of males ages 5 to 10 years had RAP, followed by a decline in incidence with a later peak at age 14 years. In contrast, however, females had a sharp rise in the incidence of RAP after age 8 years, with more than 25% of all females affected at age 9 years, followed by a steady decline. A more recent study of RAP in 6-year-olds by Faull and Nicol showed that at least an equal number of children experience chronic abdominal pain that does not interfere with normal daily activity; thus, they are rarely brought to the attention of the health care provider.[12] In addition, Hyams and colleagues studied 507 adolescents in a suburban town in the United States. The investigators found that abdominal pain occurred at least weekly in 13% to 17% of adolescents, but that only half of these individuals had sought medical attention within the preceding year.[3]

## Psychosocial Factors

Particular personality traits and family psychosocial dynamics have been identified in association with functional RAP of childhood. Children with functional abdominal pain are frequently timid, nervous, or anxious and are often described as perfectionists or overachievers.[4] Measures of intelligence in these children have not been found to differ significantly from those of controls. Birth order is thought to possibly contribute to development of symptoms, because children with RAP are typically the first- or last-born in the family.[2, 4]

Studies show that children with functional abdominal pain, like behaviorally disordered children, experience more life stressors than healthy controls.[13] Mother, teacher, and child self-report questionnaires indicate that children with RAP have higher levels of emotional distress and internalize problems more often than well children.[14] Despite this, children with functional RAP have not been found to have an increased incidence of depression or other psychological disorders when compared with children with abdominal pain of organic origin.[15, 16] Raymer and colleagues found that psychological distress accompanies both organic and nonorganic abdominal pain in children and that psychological evaluation may not readily distinguish organic from nonorganic pain.[16]

Absence from school is relatively common among children with functional RAP.[2, 4, 17] Liebman observed school absenteeism of more than 1 day in 10 in 28% of these children.[4] Regular school attendance was observed in only 9%. Physical education was the school activity most commonly associated with development of abdominal pain.

The child's home environment is thought to greatly influence the child's RAP. Parents relate the onset of pain to significant events (excitement, punishment, or family disturbance) almost 70% of the time. Marital discord with excessive arguing and/or violence, separation, or divorce is found in almost 40% of affected families. In addition, extreme parenting techniques such as parental oversubmissiveness or excessive punishment have also commonly been found in these families.[2, 17]

## Family History

A significantly higher proportion of children with RAP have relatives with alcoholism, antisocial or conduct disorder, attention deficit disorder, or somatization disorder when compared with children with organically based abdominal pain.[18] The patient often comes from a "painful family" (i.e., family members have a high frequency of medical complaints).[1, 2] The parents and siblings of patients with functional RAP have an increased incidence of RAP, nervous breakdown, and migraines when compared with controls. Stone and Barbero found that 56% of mothers and 44% of fathers of patients with RAP had medical illnesses.[2] Approximately half of the mothers had gastrointestinal complaints diagnosed as "functional" by their physician, and 10% carried the diagnosis of migraine headaches. Similarly, 46% of fathers with medical conditions had gastrointestinal illness and 10% had migraines. In addition, almost 25% of the mothers with a child with RAP have a mild level of psychiatric depression. It is unclear whether the mother's feelings result from having a child with RAP or whether the mother's emotional state contributes to the child's development of pain.[15]

## Perinatal and Past Medical History

Mothers of patients with RAP report that their pregnancies were characterized by excessive nausea, emesis, fatigue, or headaches. Difficult labor and delivery with breech presentation or cesarean section is reported in 20% to 31%. Neonatal difficulty, including respiratory distress, infection, or colic, is reported in 20%. The child's past history may also reveal recurrent nightmares, toilet training difficulties, and enuresis.[2, 4]

## Pathophysiology

Investigations into the etiology of functional RAP have primarily focused on two mechanisms: autonomic nervous system function and intestinal motility. The autonomic nervous system (ANS) is considered the biologic anlage for internal emotional responses. Because emotion is thought to play a possible role in functional RAP, studies of autonomic function in these individuals have been conducted. Rubin and coworkers conducted a controlled study of 13 children with RAP using pupillary reactivity as a measure of ANS responsivity.[19] No sigificant difference between children with RAP and healthy controls was noted at rest or while under stress; however, a significant difference was noted following the stressful condition. This was manifested as a small initial decrement of pupillary dilatation in the children with RAP. The authors concluded that the mechanism of drive reduction after stress is aberrant in children with RAP. Apley and colleagues did not replicate the finding of increased recovery time following a stressor; however, they did note that children with RAP were more likely to have an "unstable recovery."[20] Kopel and colleagues found increased rectosigmoid motility after subcutaneous injection of prostigmine methylsulfate in children with RAP when compared with controls.[21] The authors concluded that patients with RAP have increased sensitivity to parasympathetic stimulation and, therefore, have a generalized autonomic imbalance. Feuerstein and associates, using cold pressor stress, found no differences in physiology, behavior, or self-report in the stress or recovery phases of children with RAP as compared with healthy controls.[22] Thus, data regarding autonomic function in children with RAP are contradictory, and a clear etiologic role for ANS instability has not been established.

**TABLE 1–2. Characteristic Presentation of Functional RAP**

- Patient age: >5 years
- Paroxysmal abdominal pain
- Pain location: epigastric, periumbilical, infraumbilical
- Pain characterization: dull, sharp or cramping, non-radiating
- Symptom duration: three or more episodes in 3 months
- Symptom-free intervals
- No temporal correlation of pain with activity, meals, or bowel pattern
- Pain interferes with normal activity
- Normal physical examination
- Normal laboratory studies

Although the etiology of functional abdominal pain remains uncertain, manometric studies indicate that underlying altered gastrointestinal motility in combination with heightened awareness in certain individuals may contribute to its pathogenesis.[23, 24] Pineiro-Carrero and colleagues[23] demonstrated that patients with functional RAP had more frequent migrating motor complexes with slower propagation velocities as compared with healthy controls. In addition, these patients also had high pressure duodenal contractions that were associated with abdominal pain during the study period.[23] Subsequently, Hyman and coworkers identified manometric abnormalities in 89% of patients with functional RAP undergoing antroduodenal manometry.[24]

More recent investigations have focused on the structural integrity of the small intestine. Van der Meer and associates studied small bowel permeability in 87 children with RAP by measuring 24-hour urinary excretion of orally administered 51Cr-EDTA.[25] The mean urinary excretion of this compound was significantly higher in children with RAP. The authors concluded that this increased small bowel permeability in children with RAP may indicate an intestinal etiology for patient complaints. In a subsequent study, of 39 children with RAP, microscopic findings on duodenal biopsy were compared with intestinal permeability to 51Cr-EDTA. The authors identified a significant association between microscopic duodenal inflammation and abnormal permeability.[26]

## Conceptual Model

Children have a limited ability to differentiate between emotional stress and somatic pain. Children may use abdominal pain to indicate fear or anxiety, hunger, nausea, or the urge to defecate.[27] In addition, children from "painful families" in which frequent physical complaints predominate may perceive illness as a way of life.[1]

A comprehensive conceptual model of functional RAP in children was proposed by Levine and Rappaport to attempt to explain the multifactorial basis and differing manifestations.[28] In this model, four primary forces are proposed to mediate RAP in childhood: (1) somatic predisposition, dysfunction, or disorder; (2) lifestyle and habit; (3) milieu and critical events; and (4) temperament and learned response patterns. This model suggests that a somatic propensity toward abdominal pain localized to the abdomen occurs in a living milieu that itself is affected in part by critical life events. The milieu may or may not trigger or intensify the pain. The child's own lifestyle and habits also serve as influential forces to promote or counteract symptom development. Finally, the child has a variety of temperamental traits and learned responses that influence appreciation of pain. These four forces interact to mediate functional RAP and can serve as targets for evaluation and therapy.

## Presentation

The characteristic features of functional RAP are summarized in Table 1–2. The associated abdominal pain is visceral in nature. The pain may last from a few minutes to several hours. The pain is characteristically in the midline, located from the epigastrium to the infraumbilical region. Pain is described as a cramping or aching sensation, but is often difficult for the child to describe. The pain intensity ranges from mild to severe enough to cause the child to halt normal activity and lie down. Pain may be associated with pallor or diaphoresis. The abdominal pain may occur at any time during the day and is commonly reported in the morning, prior to school, around dinner, and at bedtime. In addition, functional RAP typically does not awaken the patient from sleep, and the child feels well between episodes.[1, 2, 4, 6, 17]

Children with functional RAP have normal growth parameters and appear healthy on physical examination. Mild abdominal tenderness without rebound or guarding may be found on examination, most often in one or both lower quadrants.[4] Results of laboratory investigation, including complete blood count, liver enzyme assay, sedimentation rate, and urinalysis, are characteristically normal. Imaging studies, if performed, are also normal.[1, 2, 4, 6] When evaluating a child with RAP, it is crucial to recognize signs or symptoms suggestive of more serious underlying organic illness. These are listed in Table 1–3.

# EVALUATION OF THE CHILD WITH CHRONIC ABDOMINAL PAIN

The initial evaluation of the child with RAP should include a comprehensive interview with the child and parents, a thorough physical examination, and specific screening laboratory studies. In addition to performing the evaluation, the physician must also convey genuine concern and establish a trusting and supportive environment. Ensure that adequate time is allotted for this process.

**TABLE 1–3. Findings Suggestive of Organic Etiology in a Child with RAP**

- Patient age: <5 years
- Constitutional symptoms: fever, weight loss or growth deceleration, joint symptoms
- Emesis, particularly if bile- or blood-stained
- Pain that awakens the child from sleep
- Pain well localized away from the umbilicus
- Referred pain to the back, shoulders, or extremities
- Dysuria, hematuria, or flank pain
- Family medical history of inflammatory bowel disease, peptic ulcer disease, etc.
- Perianal disease (tags, fissures, fistulas)
- Occult or gross blood in the stool
- Abnormal screening laboratory studies (elevated white blood count or erythrocyte sedimentation rate, hypoalbuminemia, anemia)

## History

As with many other conditions, a thorough and detailed history is the most important component of the patient's assessment and often leads to the correct diagnosis. Initial questions should be directed at the patient. It is important to hear the patient's complaints in his or her own words and to minimize parental influence on patient response to questions. Ask the patient to indicate with his or her own hand the location of the pain. It is not helpful when the entire hand is swept diffusely across the abdomen, but it may be helpful when one finger is used to localize an area of pain.

Information should be sought regarding the quality, intensity, duration, and timing of the pain. Sharp pain suggests a cutaneous or more superficial structural origin; poorly localized pain is more characteristic of visceral or functional etiology.[9] Inquire how well the patient sleeps at night. Pain that awakens the patient from sleep usually indicates organic disease. Temporal correlation of the abdominal pain and other symptoms such as nausea, emesis, diarrhea, constipation, or fever are also suggestive of organic disease. In addition, ask whether there is any relationship between the pain and food consumption, activity, or posture.

Medications, including prescription and over-the-counter products, should be accurately recorded. Ask whether the child starting taking such products prior to the onset of the abdominal pain. This is of particular importance in patients with conditions such as jeuvenile rheumatoid arthritis or recurrent headaches who regularly use nonsteroidal anti-inflammatory medications for pain relief, because these medications are known to cause both gastritis and mucosal ulceration.[29] Also ask whether medications have been taken in an attempt to relieve the child's abdominal pain, and if so, how efficacious they were. Transient improvement following a laxative may indicate chronic constipation as the cause of the RAP; and temporary relief following antacids may indicate peptic inflammation.

When the history does not identify any temporal relationship of the abdominal pain to food, activity, or stressors, it is often helpful to have the patient and/or parents maintain an abdominal pain diary detailing the time, location, intensity, and character of the pain, time and content of meals, daily activities, and stooling pattern. This may allow for the identification of physical or emotional stressors that contribute to the abdominal pain.

## Physical Examination

The physical examination should begin during the history gathering process. The physician should carefully note the patient's facial expressions, respiratory pattern, body positioning, and movements. Also, it is important to carefully note how the child interacts with family members during the interview and how he or she climbs onto and down from the examination table. It is usually reassuring when the patient energetically jumps from the table following examination.

The importance of performing a meticulous physical examination cannot be overemphasized. To facilitate a thorough examination, all clothing should be removed and the patient placed in a patient gown. It is important for the examiner to carefully cover the patient to maintain modesty and prevent embarrassment. The physical examination should be performed with the parents present. This often makes the child more comfortable and allows the parents to appreciate the thoroughness of the examination. The older child or adolescent may prefer that only the parent of the same sex remain in the room during the examination. It is usually best to ask the patient what would make him or her the most comfortable.

A careful review of the child's growth parameters using standard charts should be made. Normal growth is reassuring and is a consistent finding in children with functional RAP. In contrast, growth failure or weight loss is suggestive of an organic etiology. Particular attention should be given to the abdominal examination. It is essential to an adequate examination that the patient is as relaxed as possible, lighting is adequate, and the abdomen is fully exposed from the xiphoid to the symphysis pubis. Before laying hands on the abdomen, carefully inspect the abdomen for the presence of distention, peristaltic waves, striae, dilated vessels, or scars indicative of previous surgery. Next, the character of the bowel sounds should be noted. High-pitched, frequent bowel sounds may indicate a partial bowel obstruction; hypoactive bowel sounds are consistent with ileus. Detailed palpation of the entire abdomen should then be performed to evaluate organ size, presence or absence of masses, or any areas of tenderness. Because the most frequently identified organic causes of RAP are localized to the urinary tract, careful attention must be given to each flank in an attempt to detect hydronephrosis and to the costovertebral angle to assess for tenderness. Hernial orifices should be carefully examined. The perianal region must be thoroughly inspected for fissures, fistulas, or skin tags. Digital rectal examination is mandatory to assess external anal sphincter tone, the size of the rectal vault, volume and consistency of stool present in the rectal vault, and Hemoccult status of the stool. Because the child is often free of abdominal pain at the time of the initial examination, it is important to reexamine the child during an episode of abdominal pain.

## Laboratory and Imaging Studies

Laboratory, radiologic, and endoscopic evaluation of the patient with chronic abdominal pain should be individualized according to the information obtained during the history and physical examination. Most authors, however, recommend the following studies as an initial screen for all patients with RAP: complete blood count, urinalysis with culture, serum aminotransferases, erythrocyte sedimentation rate, and fecal examination for ova and parasites.[30–32] It has been suggested that these screening studies, in addition to a normal physical examination, effectively rule out an organic cause in 95% of cases.[30] Other noninvasive studies such as lactose breath hydrogen testing and abdominal ultrasound should be performed if indicated. Ultrasound has gained a prominent role over the past several years because it is painless and does not involve radiation. Three separate studies to investigate the diagnostic value of routine abdominal ultrasound in children with RAP, however, have failed to demonstrate its utility in this clinical setting.[33–35] In these studies, a total of 217 patients were evaluated. Sixteen patients were found to have abnormalities identified by abdominal ultrasound, but

**TABLE 1–4. ORGANIC CAUSES OF CHRONIC ABDOMINAL PAIN**

| | |
|---|---|
| **Gastrointestinal** | **Respiratory** |
| Esophagitis | Infection, inflammation, or tumor near diaphragm |
| Gastritis | **Genitourinary** |
| Peptic ulcer | Ureteropelvic junction obstruction/hydronephrosis |
| Malrotation (with Ladd's bands or intermittent volvulus) | Nephrolithiasis |
| Duplications | Recurrent pyelonephritis/cystitis |
| Polyps | Hematocolpos |
| Hernias (diaphragmatic, internal, umbilical, inguinal) | Mittelschmerz |
| Inflammatory bowel disease | Endometriosis |
| Constipation | **Metabolic/Hematologic** |
| Parasitic infection (e.g., *Giardia*) | Porphyria |
| Bezoar or foreign body | Hereditary angioedema |
| Carbohydrate malabsorption | Diabetes mellitus |
| Intussusception | Lead poisoning |
| Tumor (e.g., lymphoma) | Sickle cell disease |
| **Hepatobiliary/Pancreatic** | Collagen vascular disease |
| Chronic hepatitis | **Musculoskeletal** |
| Cholelithiasis | Trauma, tumor, infection of vertebral column (e.g., leukemia, herpes zoster, discitis) |
| Cholecystitis | |
| Choledochal cyst | |
| Chronic pancreatitis | |
| Pancreatic pseudocyst | |

in no case could the pain be attributed to the abnormality. Thus, the ultrasound did not influence management. In addition, one author suggested that the ultrasound may have even been detrimental when findings such as an accessory uterine horn, a uterus small for age, and absence of an ovary were identified, because these caused anxiety and prompted further unnecessary consultation.[34]

## DIFFERENTIAL DIAGNOSIS

More than 100 causes of abdominal pain have been identified in children and adolescents.[31] Table 1–4 lists many of these causes by organ system. The following discussion briefly reviews two additional recognized patterns of functional RAP, non-ulcer dyspepsia and irritable bowel syndrome, as well as the more commonly identified organic causes of RAP of childhood.

### Non-ulcer Dyspepsia

Non-ulcer dyspepsia refers to intermittent upper abdominal pain or discomfort, early satiety, fullness, bloating, nausea, or vomiting in the absence of demonstrable structural abnormalities of the gastrointestinal tract.[36] Although non-ulcer dyspepsia is a well-established diagnosis in the adult population, it has been recognized as a cause of RAP in children only since the early 1990s.[37] Suggested etiologic agents include psychological stress, environmental factors, gastric secretory abnormalities, and disordered antroduodenal motility.[37–40] *Helicobacter pylori* colonization of the gastric antrum has been found to strongly correlate with duodenal ulcer disease in both children and adults; however, in the absence of active peptic ulcer disease, it is not clear whether this microorganism produces clinical symptoms. Several studies of pediatric patients have indicated that epigastric abdominal discomfort is more common in children with *H. pylori* infection compared with those without antral colonization.[41, 42] In contrast, other pediatric studies show that specific symptomatology is not related to *H. pylori* infection in children.[43, 44] Gormally and associates[45] studied 19 children with *H. pylori* infection of the gastric antrum and RAP. The authors found that following eradication of *H. pylori*, symptoms consistently resolved only in those patients who had duodenal ulceration associated with antral gastritis. They concluded that *H. pylori* gastritis does not cause symptoms in children in the absence of duodenal ulcer disease.[45] Thus, the precise role of *H. pylori* colonization of the gastric antrum as a cause of non-ulcer dyspepsia remains controversial. Until this is clarified, it should be emphasized to the patient and parents that the cause of non-ulcer dyspepsia is likely multifactorial and that medication to eradicate *H. pylori* is administered to eliminate one possible contributing factor to the symptom complex.

### Irritable Bowel Syndrome

Irritable bowel syndrome (IBS) is the most common disorder encountered by gastroenterologists caring for adult patients and is emerging as a common cause of RAP in the pediatric population.[3, 46] One study showed that 14% of high school students and 6% of middle school students have RAP and defecation patterns consistent with the diagnosis of IBS. Unlike in the adult population, where females are affected two times more often than males, there is an equal sex distribution of IBS in childhood and adolescence.[3]

IBS is classified as a functional gastrointestinal disorder. Physical examination is typically normal, and laboratory studies in these patients have failed to identify any biochemical, microbiologic, or histologic abnormalities. As with other forms of functional RAP, symptoms should be continuous or recurrent for a minimum of 3 months prior to establishing the diagnosis. Diagnosis also relies on finding a variable defecation pattern at least 25% of the time with three or more of the following: bloating or abdominal distention, altered stool consistency, altered stool frequency, altered stool passage (straining, urgency, feeling of incomplete stool evacuation), passage of mucus. Abdominal pain is typically relieved by defecation or associated with a change in the frequency or consistency of stool.[47] Affected children, like adults, may have a diarrhea-predominant form, a constipation-predominant form, or a variable pattern of defecation.[3]

As with other forms of functional RAP, the precise cause of IBS is unclear. IBS is generally considered to be a multifactorial disorder with contributing motor, psychological, and autonomic factors. Patients with diarrhea-predominant IBS have been found to have sympathetic adrenergic dysfunction, whereas those with constipation-predominant IBS have vagal cholinergic dysfunction.[48] Essential components of therapy are education and reassurance. The efficacy of specific interventions such as dietary fiber supplementation and anticholinergic agents remains controversial. Psychological consultation should be made when appropriate.

### Chronic Constipation

Chronic constipation is a common condition in children, accounting for up to 25% of all referrals to the pediatric gastroenterologist.[49] It leads to colonic distention, gas formation, and painful defecation. There are both functional and organic (myogenic, neurologic, mechanical) forms of chronic constipation.[50] In patients with functional constipation, there is typically voluntary withholding of stool. This may be secondary to such factors as the previous passage of a painful stool or refusal to use a public restroom. Such withholding behavior, if prolonged, results in rectal and colonic accumulation of stool, overstretching of anal sphincters, and resultant fecal soiling. Thus, both physical and psychological factors perpetuate this cycle.[51] Diagnosis is often readily made through history and physical examination. A flat plate radiograph of the abdomen is sometimes helpful, especially if the patient's body habitus precludes deep palpation of the abdomen.

Therapy is directed at prevention of withholding, establishment of a regular stooling pattern, and return of normal anorectal sensation. Effective therapy integrates medical with behavioral management techniques. A variety of medications have been found effective, including mineral oil, osmotic agents (lactulose), and prokinetic agents (cisapride), as well as increased dietary fiber. If psychosocial or emotional issues predominate, referral to a specialist may be indicated. Patients who are compliant with therapy but continue to have symptoms may benefit from evaluation of anorectal dynamics and use of biofeedback training.[52, 53] Those patients with an organic etiology, such as Hirschsprung's or Chagas' disease, may require surgical intervention.

## Peptic Disease

Peptic disease refers not only to ulcer formation in the stomach and duodenum but also to gastroesophageal reflux and gastritis. Ulcers are typically associated with underlying systemic illness in children younger than the age of 10 years. Gastric ulcers may occur in association with extensive burns, head trauma, and ingestion of nonsteroidal anti-inflammatory medications or corticosteroids. Such ulcers usually do not recur, and there is typically no family history of ulcer disease. In contrast, ulcers in older children usually occur in the absence of underlying illness or medication ingestion. A positive family history can often be elicited. Such ulcers are often recurrent and have been associated with antral colonization with *H. pylori*.[54, 55] Epidemiologic studies show that the rate of acquisition of *H. pylori* increases with age, is higher in blacks than whites, and is inversely proportional to socioeconomic status.[56, 57] Intrafamilial clustering of *H. pylori* infection has been found, suggesting person-to-person spread of the bacteria.[58] There is a lack of correlation between endoscopic and histologic findings in patients with *H. pylori*; therefore, antral biopsy is recommended to exclude the diagnosis even when endoscopic findings are normal.[55]

The vast majority of pediatric patients with peptic ulcer disease present with abdominal pain. Abdominal pain secondary to peptic ulceration in adults is considered classic if it is located in the epigastric region, occurs following meals, and awakens the patient in the early morning hours. Pain experienced by children younger than age 12 years is atypical and occurs anywhere in the middle to upper abdomen, is unrelated to meals, and had no periodicity. Peptic ulcer disease in children older than 12 years is similar to the classic adult pattern.[59, 60] Endoscopy is the procedure of choice when mucosal abnormalities are suspected, because contrast radiography of the upper gastrointestinal tract has been found to be unreliable for establishing the diagnosis of peptic ulcer disease in children.[61]

## Carbohydrate Intolerance

Dietary carbohydrates that are malabsorbed serve as substrates for bacterial fermentation in the colon.[62] By-products of bacterial fermentation include hydrogen, carbon dioxide, and volatile fatty acids such as acetate, propionate, and butyrate. The resultant clinical symptoms include abdominal cramping, bloating with abdominal distention, diarrhea, and excessive flatulence.[63]

Malabsorption of lactose is widely recognized as a cause of gastrointestinal distress. The prevalence of lactose malabsorption varies widely among different races, with the lowest prevalence found in Scandinavia and Northwest Europe. In sharp contrast, between 70% to 100% of North American Indians, Australian aboriginal populations, and inhabitants of Southeast Asia are lactose intolerant. There is also a high prevalence in those of Italian, Turkish, and African descent.[64, 65] Historical information regarding the temporal relationship of lactose consumption to clinical symptoms has been found to be a poor predictor of the presence of lactose intolerance.[66] The least invasive means to establish the diagnosis of lactose malabsorption is breath hydrogen testing.[67] If the test is positive, a strict lactose elimination diet for 2 weeks and maintenance of an abdominal pain diary is advised. Resolution of the abdominal complaints confirms lactase deficiency as the cause. Subsequently, lactose can be introduced back into the diet and the patient supplemented with lactase during periods of lactose consumption to minimize symptoms.[63]

Fructose and sorbitol are common dietary carbohydrates that also may be malabsorbed. Fructose-containing foods include fruits, fruit juices, and honey.[68] The fruits highest in fructose include apples (5 g/100 g of apple) and pears (5–6.5 g/100 g of pear). The fructose content of apple and pear juice are comparable, with 6 g/100 mL of juice. Excessive intake of these products may lead to abdominal pain in susceptible individuals and should be discouraged.[69] Sorbitol is a polyalcohol sugar commonly found in "sugar-free" gums and confections. It is poorly absorbed by the small intestinal mucosa and has been shown to cause chronic abdominal pain in children.[70]

## Inflammatory Bowel Disease

Chronic abdominal pain is a common finding in children with inflammatory bowel disease (IBD). The presenting symptoms in patients with Crohn's disease are variable and include abdominal pain, anorexia, weight loss, growth failure, and diarrhea. The associated abdominal pain is usually intense and frequently awakens the child from sleep.[71] Perianal disease develops in 30% to 50% of children with Crohn's disease, emphasizing the importance of careful inspection of the perianal region during physical examination.[72] More than 80% of children with ulcerative colitis present with hematochezia, diarrhea, and abdominal cramping.[73] Laboratory findings suggestive of IBD include anemia, elevated erythrocyte sedimentation rate, thrombocytosis, hypoalbuminemia, and heme-positive stool.[74] Accurate diagnosis relies on a combination of clinical, laboratory, endoscopic, histologic, and radiologic findings.

## Pancreatitis

Chronic pancreatitis is characterized by recurrent episodes of abdominal pain with eventual development of pancreatic insufficiency in some individuals.[75] The associated epigastric pain is often initiated by a large meal or stress. Nausea and vomiting are frequently present. Resolution of symptoms usually occurs over 4 to 8 days, and patients are clinically well between attacks. Some patients experience no abdominal symptoms and have diabetes mellitus or evidence of pancreatic insufficiency at the time of their initial presentation.

The cause of chronic pancreatitis in children often remains unclear. Hereditary pancreatitis has been identified as the cause in more than 600 individuals, with symptom onset in the first two decades of life occurring in 80%.[76] Other conditions associated with chronic pancreatitis include congenital or acquired ductal anomalies, cystic fibrosis, hypercalcemia, organic acidemias, and hyperlipidemia types I, IIA, and V.[77, 78]

Serum amylase and lipase levels may be elevated or normal during a painful episode.[75] Plain radiographs of the abdomen may show evidence of pancreatic calcification. Ultrasound and computed tomography scan may be useful for assessing glandular size or pseudocyst formation. Endoscopic retrograde cholangiopancreatography has become a valuable tool for the diagnosis of ductal abnormalities and is a valuable therapeutic modality for stricture dilation, stone removal, and sphincterotomy.[79]

## Genitourinary Disorders

Ureteropelvic junction (UPJ) obstruction is an established cause of renal damage in children, which if diagnosed early, allows salvage of renal tissue and function. It occurs more commonly in males and is most often left-sided.[80, 81] Nonspecific RAP may be the only presenting complaint in a child with UPJ obstruction. It has been shown that a normal urinalysis and physical examination do not always exclude a genitourinary abnormality as a cause of the pain.[82] RAP is the presenting symptom in 59% of children older than 1 year of age with UPJ obstruction.[83] The diagnosis of UPJ obstruction in infancy is rarely delayed, because patients usually manifest with an abdominal mass or urinary tract infection. As children become older, the diagnosis becomes more difficult to make because the presenting complaint is often RAP. Studies show that 35% to 58% of all children with UPJ obstruction present with RAP; however, 70% of patients older than 6 years of age present with RAP.[80, 81, 84] It is especially important to consider UPJ obstruction when the pain is referred to the groin or flank. Additional clues to the diagnosis include abdominal mass to the right or left of midline and hematuria on urinalysis.

Nephrolithiasis is another diagnostic consideration in the child with RAP. In a study of 216 children with nephrolithiasis, Bensman and coworkers found that 20% presented with recurrent episodes of abdominal pain.[85] Ultrasound has become a valuable tool for the evaluation of these genitourinary abnormalities and should be performed when such disorders are suspected.

## Parasitic Infections

Giardiasis is an infection of the small intestines with the protozoan parasite *Giardia lamblia*. This organism is found throughout temperate and tropical regions worldwide and is the most common human protozoal enteropathogen.[86] Infection typically follows ingestion of fresh water contaminated with the cysts.[87] Although infection is self-limited in the majority of cases, 30% of patients develop chronic symptoms with abdominal pain, nausea, flatulence, diarrhea, and weight loss secondary to malabsorption.[86] Diagnosis is made through identification of the cysts or trophozoites on light microscopy of fresh stool specimens. Trophozoites may also be identified in duodenal aspirates or endoscopic biopsy specimens of the proximal small intestine. Immunodiagnostic approaches including detection of *Giardia* antigen in serum and fecal specimens are not universally available and remain under investigation.[88–90]

Individuals infected with parasitic helminths such as *Ascaris lumbricoides* (roundworm) and *Trichuris trichiura* (whipworm) are often asymptomatic; however, heavy infestations may produce chronic abdominal pain, anorexia, diarrhea, rectal prolapse, or even bowel obstruction.[91, 92] Ova and parasite screening should be performed when infection is suspected.

## Congenital Anomalies

Malrotation is defined as incomplete or abnormal rotation of the intestine about the superior mesenteric artery.[93] The diagnosis is straightforward in the setting of acute duodenal obstruction. Most cases present in infancy, and the diagnosis is readily made by the presence of the "double bubble" on plain radiographs of the abdomen or malpositioned bowel on upper gastrointestinal series or barium enema.[94] In the older child, the diagnosis may not be readily apparent because the presentation is not typically duodenal obstruction. Fifty percent of older children with intestinal malrotation present with chronic abdominal pain with or without emesis. The associated abdominal pain is usually transient and diffuse and is not associated with physical findings. The pain is most often postprandial and may be accompanied by bilious emesis, diarrhea, or evidence of malabsorption.[95]

Alimentary tract duplications are cystic or tubular structures, attached to the intestine, often sharing a common muscular wall and vascular supply.[96] The most commonly involved site is the ileum. Abdominal pain, gastrointestinal hemorrhage, and obstruction due to mass effect have been identified as the most common presenting signs and symptoms of duplications in children.[97]

## THERAPY OF FUNCTIONAL CHRONIC ABDOMINAL PAIN

Because functional abdominal pain in a child or adolescent often affects the entire family, therapy must be directed at the family as a unit. Successful therapy depends on education, reassurance, and ongoing support for the patient and family members. It is of utmost importance, therefore, for the physician to gain the trust of the child and parents and establish a supportive and caring environment.

Once the diagnosis of functional abdominal pain has been made, it is important to clearly review with the child and parents how the diagnosis was reached. It is often helpful to show the child's growth parameters on the growth chart to emphasize that normal growth and development are present. Detail how the constellation of symptoms fits the diagnostic criteria of a functional condition (i.e., periumbilical location of the pain, no associated fever or weight loss, and so forth). Reassure the family by reviewing the normal physical examination and screening laboratory studies. Also stress to the family that this is a common condition affecting up to 20% of all school-age children. Knowing that other families are similarly afflicted and are successfully coping with the condition may provide reassurance and a sense of confidence for the family.

The goal of therapy is to decrease stress or tension for the child while promoting normal patterns of activity and school attendance. The first step is to acknowledge that the pain the child is experiencing is genuine and not imagined. It is often helpful to explain the pain and the term *functional* so the patient and parents have a better understanding of the situation. Several authors recommend using an analogy such as the almost universally experienced headache.[30, 98, 99] Most will understand that headaches cause genuine pain and do not necessarily represent underlying organic pathology. It is also helpful to explain that research indicates that abdominal pain may result from specific patterns of intestinal motility and that the contractions of the gastrointestinal tract are often related to our emotional state through hormonal and neural pathways. Thus, emotional upset or stress may result in such symptoms as abdominal cramping, constipation, diarrhea, diaphoresis, or pallor in susceptible individuals.

The family and physician should work together to identify any source of stress that could be contributing to development or perpetuation of the child's symptoms. Additional history may be necessary to identify personality traits or sociocultural factors that may contribute to the child's condition. If a stressor is apparent and unavoidable, such as a chronically ill family member or the loss of a loved one, referral to a consultant who can provide coping mechanisms and ongoing counseling may be indicated. Referral to a specialist is also warranted when it is evident that a somatization disorder is present or when a child is modeling the pain behavior of a parent.

Rapid return to school with alteration of specifically aversive elements should be advised. The importance of acknowledging the abdominal pain without encouraging it should be emphasized to the parents. If the pain is not acknowledged, the child may exhibit extreme pain behavior in order to convince the parent that the pain exists. Therefore, some authors recommend designating a certain time of the day for the child to discuss the pain with the parent.[100, 101] Also, discuss with the parents the possibility that secondary gain may play a role in the continued pain behavior of the child. Assess how often pain behavior has resulted in the child remaining home from school or being exempt from participation in physical education class at school or performance of household duties. If pain appears to be maintained by secondary gain, specific rules need to be established. For example, if the child is in enough distress to stay home from school, he or she is then considered ill enough to remain in bed without any television, toys, or other special privileges.

Pharmacologic therapy with antispasmodics, sedatives, or analgesic agents is seldom efficacious and may potentially be harmful. Research indicates that there is a potential role for dietary manipulation with an increase in dietary fiber. Feldman and colleagues[102] conducted a double-blind, placebo-controlled, randomized study of 52 children with RAP. The authors demonstrated that the addition of 10 g of fiber daily for 6 weeks resulted in a decrease in the number of pain episodes in almost 50% of patients.[102]

## PROGNOSIS

Long-term follow-up of individuals who had been admitted to the hospital as children for RAP indicates that between 35% and 50% will have complete resolution of their symptoms.[103–105] Abdominal pain continues into adulthood in approximately 25%, and the remaining individuals develop other complaints such as headaches. Apley and Hale demonstrated that those patients who received therapy consisting of an explanation of the RAP and reassurance developed fewer nonabdominal complaints in later life and were less likely to relapse than individuals who had received no such therapy.[103]

Prognostic indicators of RAP have also been identified and are summarized in Table 1–5. Apley found that factors predictive of a good outcome included female sex, age of onset after age 6 years, treatment started within 6 months of symptom onset, and a "normal family." Poor prognostic indicators included male sex, onset of symptoms before age 6 years, symptoms of greater than 6 months duration prior to therapy and a "painful family."[103] In addition, Magni and colleagues identified a painful family, many surgical

**TABLE 1–5. Factors Influencing Long-Term Prognosis of Functional Abdominal Pain**

| FACTOR | PROGNOSIS BETTER | PROGNOSIS WORSE |
|---|---|---|
| Sex | Female | Male |
| Age of onset | >6 years | <6 years |
| Family | Normal | "Painful" |
| Duration of symptoms | <6 months | > 6 months |
| Education level completed | ≥ High school | < High school |
| Socioeconomic class | Middle-upper | Lower |
| Operations (appendectomy, tonsillectomy) | Infrequent | Frequent |

Data from Apley J, Hale B: Children with recurrent abdominal pain: how do they grow up? BMJ 1973;3:7–9; and Magni G, Pierri M, Donzelli F: Recurrent abdominal pain in children: a long term follow-up. Eur J Pediatr 1987;146:72–74.

procedures, a low educational level, and low socioeconomic status as poor prognostic indicators in children with RAP.[105]

Long-term studies also indicate that once the diagnosis of functional RAP is made, an organic disorder is rarely identified. The longest follow-up study was performed by Christensen and Mortensen, who evaluated 34 individuals 28 to 30 years after their initial diagnosis of RAP.[104] Discrete evidence of organic disease was found in only two patients, both identified as having duodenal ulcers.

## PREVENTION

Prevention of functional abdominal pain begins with the primary care physician at the well-child visits. Parents should be advised against excessive anxiety with minor illnesses and provision of secondary gain with minor injuries.[98] Parents should also be advised against oversubmissiveness or rigid parenting styles with excessive use of punishment. Open communication between family members as the child grows should be encouraged. Stress the importance of a supportive, loving environment and recommend that the family members work together to find solutions early for stressful situations the child encounters. Any individual, health care provider or family member, who has encountered a child with functional abdominal pain must realize that the old adage "an ounce of prevention is worth a pound of cure" was surely directed at this affliction.

### REFERENCES


1. Apley J, Naish N: Recurrent abdominal pains: a field survey of 1,000 school children. Arch Dis Child 1958;33:165–170.
2. Stone RT, Barbero GJ: Recurrent abdominal pain in childhood. Pediatrics 1970;45:732–738.
3. Hyams JS, Burke G, Davis PM, et al: Abdominal pain and irritable bowel syndrome in adolescents: a community-based study. J Pediatr 1996;129:220–226.
4. Liebman W: Recurrent abdominal pain in children: a retrospective survey of 119 patients. Clin Pediatr 1978;17:149–153.
5. Drossman DA, Thompson WG, Talley NJ, et al: Identification of sub-groups of functional gastrointestinal disorders. Gastroenterol Int 1990;3:159–172.
6. Hyams JS, Treem WR, Justinich CJ, et al: Characterization of symptoms in children with recurrent abdominal pain: resemblance to irritable bowel syndrome. J Pediatr Gastroenterol Nutr 1995;20:209–214.
7. Currie DJ: Abdominal Pain. New York, Hemisphere Publishing Corporation, 1979.
8. Haubrich W: Gastrointestinal Symptoms: Clinical Interpretation. Philadelphia, BC Decker, 1991.
9. Ness TJ, Gebhart GF: Visceral pain: a review of experimental studies. Pain 1990;41:167–234.
10. Antonson D: Abdominal pain. Gastrointest Endosc Clin N Am 1994;4:1–21.
11. Moore K: The Developing Human, 3rd ed. Philadelphia, WB Saunders, 1982.
12. Faull C, Nicol AR: Abdominal pain in six-year-olds: an epidemiological study in a new town. J Child Psychol Psychiatry 1986;27:251–260.
13. Hodges K, Kline J, Barbero G, et al: Life events occurring in families of children with recurrent abdominal pain. J Psychosom Res 1984;28:185–188.
14. Walker L, Garber J, Greene J: Psychosocial correlates of recurrent childhood pain: a comparison of pediatric patients with recurrent abdominal pain, organic illness and psychiatric disorders. J Abnorm Psychol 1993;102:248–258.
15. Hodges K, Kline J, Barbero G, Flanery R: Depressive symptoms in children with recurrent abdominal pain and in their families. J Pediatr 1985;107:622–626.
16. Raymer D, Weininger O, Hamilton JR: Psychological problems in children with abdominal pain. Lancet 1984;1:439–440.
17. Oster J: Recurrent abdominal pain, headache and limb pains in children and adolescents. Pediatrics 1972;50:429–436.
18. Routh DK, Ernst AR: Somatization disorder in relatives of children and adolescents with functional abdominal pain. J Pediatr Psychol 1984;9:427–437.
19. Rubin LS, Barbero GJ, Sibinga MS: Pupillary reactivity in children with recurrent abdominal pain. Psychosom Med 1967;29:111–120.
20. Apley J, Haslam DR, Tulloch G: Pupillary reaction in children with recurrent abdominal pain. Arch Dis Child 1971;46:337–340.
21. Kopel FB, Kim IC, Barbero GJ: Comparison of rectosigmoid motility in normal children, children with recurrent abdominal pain, and children with ulcerative colitis. Pediatrics 1967;39:539–545.
22. Feuerstein M, Barr RG, Francoeur TE, et al: Potential biobehavioral mechanisms of recurrent abdominal pain in children. Pain 1982;13:287–298.
23. Pineiro-Carrero VM, Andres JM, Davis RH, et al: Abnormal gastroduodenal motility in children and adolescents with recurrent functional abdominal pain. J Pediatr 1988;113:820–825.
24. Hyman PE, Napolitano JA, Diego A, et al: Antroduodenal manometry in the evaluation of chronic functional gastrointestinal symptoms. Pediatrics 1990;86:39–44.
25. van der Meer SB, Forget PP, Heidendal GA: Small bowel permeability to 51Cr-EDTA in children with recurrent abdominal pain. Acta Paediatr Scand 1990;79:422–426.
26. van der Meer SB, Forget PP, Arends JW: Abnormal small bowel permeability and duodenitis in recurrent abdominal pain. Arch Dis Child 1990;65:1311–1314.
27. Fleisher DR, Hyman PE: Recurrent abdominal pain in children. Semin Gastrointest Dis 1994;5:15–19.
28. Levine M, Rappaport L: Recurrent abdominal pain in school children: the loneliness of the long-distance physician. Pediatr Clin North Am 1984;31:969–991.
29. Soll AH, Kurata J, McGuigan JE: Ulcers, nonsteroidal antiinflammatory drugs and related matters. Gastroenterology 1989;96:561–568.
30. Bain HW: Chronic vague abdominal pain in children. Pediatr Clin North Am 1974;21:991–1000.
31. Oberlander TF, Rappaport LA: Recurrent abdominal pain during childhood. Pediatr Rev 1993;14:313–319.
32. Dodge JA: Recurrent abdominal pain in children. BMJ 1976;1:385–387.
33. Van der Meer SB, Forget PP, Arends JW, et al: Diagnostic value of ultrasound in children with recurrent abdominal pain. Pediatr Radiol 1990;20:501–503.
34. Shanon A, Martin DJ, Feldman W: Ultrasonographic studies in the management of recurrent abdominal pain. Pediatrics 1990;86:35–38.
35. Schmidt RE, Babcock DS, Farrell MK: Use of abdominal and pelvic ultrasound in the evaluation of chronic abdominal pain. Clin Pediatr 1993;32:147–150.
36. Talley NJ, Philips SF: Non-ulcer dyspepsia. Potential causes and pathophysiology. Ann Intern Med 1988;108:865–879.
37. Cucchiara S, Bortolotti M, Colombo C, et al: Abnormalities of gastrointestinal motility in children with non-ulcer dyspepsia and in children with gastroesophageal reflux disease. Dig Dis Sci 1991;36:1066–1073.
38. Richter JE: Stress and psychologic and environmental factors in functional dyspepsia. Scand J Gastroenterol Suppl 1991;182:40–46.
39. Nyren O: Secretory abnormalities in functional dyspepsia. Scand J Gastroenterol Suppl 1991;182:25–28.
40. Di Lorenzo C, Hyman PE, Flores AF, et al: Antroduodenal manometry in children and adults with severe nonulcer dyspepsia. Scand J Gastroenterol 1994;29:799–806.
41. Hardikar W, Davidson PM, Cameron DJS, et al: *Helicobacter pylori* infection in children. J Gastroenterol Hepatol 1991;6:450–454.
42. Mahoney MJ, Wyatt JI, Littlewood JM: Management and response to treatment of *Helicobacter pylori* gastritis. Arch Dis Child 1992;67:940–943.
43. Glassman MS, Schwartz SM, Medow MS, et al: *Campylobacter pylori* related gastrointestinal disease in children. Incidence and clinical findings. Dig Dis Sci 1989;34:1501–1504.
44. Reifen R, Rasooly I, Drumm B, et al: *Helicobacter pylori* infection in children. Is there specific symptomatology? Dig Dis Sci 1994;39:1488–1492.
45. Gormally SM, Prakash N, Durnin MT, et al: Association of symptoms with *Helicobacter pylori* infection in children. J Pediatr 1995;126:753–756.

46. Mitchell CM, Drossman DA: Survey of the AGA membership relating to patients with functional GI disorders. Gastroenterology 1987;92:1282–1284.
47. Thompson WG, Dotevall G, Drossman DA, et al: Irritable bowel syndrome: guidelines for the diagnosis. Gastroenterol Int 1989;2:92–95.
48. Aggarwal A, Cutts T, Abell T, et al: Predominant symptoms in irritable bowel syndrome correlate with specific autonomic nervous system abnormalities. Gastroenterology 1994;106:945–950.
49. Fleisher DR: Diagnosis and treatment of disorders of defecation in children. Pediatr Ann 1976;5:71–101.
50. Miglioli M: Constipation: physiopathology and classification. Ital J Gastroenterol 1991;23:10–12.
51. Swanwick T: Encopresis in children: a cyclical model of constipation and faecal retention. Br J Gen Pract 1991;41:514–516.
52. Loening-Baucke V: Modulation of abnormal defecation dynamics by biofeedback treatment in chronically constipated children with encopresis. J Pediatr 1990;116:214–222.
53. Dahl J, Lindquist BL, Tysk C, et al: Behavioral medicine treatment in chronic constipation with paradoxical anal sphincter contraction. Dis Colon Rectum 1991;34:769–776.
54. Yeung CK, Fu KH, Yeun KY, et al: *Helicobacter pylori* and associated duodenal ulcer. Arch Dis Child 1990;65:1212–1216.
55. Drumm B, Sherman P, Cutz E, et al: Association of *Campylobacter pylori* on the gastric mucosa with gastritis in children. N Engl J Med 1987;316:1557–1561.
56. Fiedorek S, Malaty H, Evans D, et al: Factors influencing the epidemiology of *Helicobacter pylori* infection in children. Pediatrics 1991;88:578–82.
57. Kosunen TU, Hook J, Rautelin HI, et al: Age-dependent increase of *Campylobacter pylori* antibodies in blood donors. Scand J Gastroenterol 1989;24:110–114.
58. Drumm B, Perez-Perez GI, Blaser MJ, et al: Intrafamilial clustering of *Helicobacter pylori* infection. N Engl J Med 1990;322:359–363.
59. Tolia V, Dubois R: Peptic ulcer disease in children and adolescents: a ten-year experience. J Clin Pediatr 1983;22:665–669.
60. Deckelbaum RJ, Roy CC, Luissier-Lazaroff J, et al: Peptic ulcer disease: a clinical study in 73 children. Can Med Assoc J 1974;111:225–228.
61. Drumm B, Rhoades JM, Stringer DA, et al: Peptic ulcer disease in children: etiology, clinical findings and clinical course. Pediatrics 1988;82:410–414.
62. Ruppin H, Bar-Meir S, Soergel KH, et al: Absorption of short chain fatty acids by the colon. Gastroenterology 1980;78:1500–1507.
63. Hyams JS: Recurrent abdominal pain in children. Curr Opin Pediatr 1995;7:529–532.
64. Simoons FJ: The geographic hypothesis and lactose malabsorption: a weighing of the evidence. Am J Dig Dis 1978;23:963–980.
65. Gudmand-Hoyer E: The clinical significance of disaccharide maldigestion. Am J Clin Nutr 1994;59(suppl):735S–741S.
66. Barr RG, Levine MD, Watkins JB: Recurrent abdominal pain of childhood due to lactose intolerance. N Engl J Med 1979;300:1449–1452.
67. Liebman W: Recurrent abdominal pain in children: lactose and sucrose intolerance, a prospective study. Pediatrics 1979;64:43–45.
68. Hardinge MG, Swarner JB, Crooks H: Carbohydrates in foods. J Am Diet Assoc 1965;46:197–204.
69. Kneepkens CM, Vonk RJ, Fernandes J: Incomplete intestinal absorption of fructose. Arch Dis Child 1984;59:735–738.
70. Hyams JS: Chronic abdominal pain caused by sorbitol malabsorption. J Pediatr 1982;100:772–773.
71. Justinich CJ, Hyams JS: Inflammatory bowel disease in children and adolescents. Gastrointest Endosc Clin N Am 1994;4:39–54.
72. Markowitz J, Daum F, Aiges H, et al: Perianal disease in children and adolescents with Crohn's disease. Gastroenterology 1984;86:829–833.
73. Michener WM: Ulcerative colitis in children. Problems in management. Pediatr Clin North Am 1967;14:159–163.
74. Thomas DW, Sinatra FR: Screening laboratory tests for Crohn's disease. West J Med 1989;150:163–164.
75. Grendell JH, Cello JP: Chronic pancreatitis. In Sleisenger MH, Fordtran JS (eds): Gastrointestinal Disease, 4th ed. Philadelphia, WB Saunders, 1989, pp 1842–1872.
76. Wyllie R: Hereditary pancreatitis. Am J Gastroenterol 1997;92:1079–1080.
77. Mathew P, Wyllie R, Caufield M, et al: Chronic pancreatitis in late childhood and adolescence. Clin Pediatr 1994;33:88–94.
78. Cameron JL, Capuzzi DM, Zuidema GD, et al: Acute pancreatitis with hyperlipidemia: evidence of a persistent defect in lipid metabolism. Am J Med 1974;56:482–487.
79. Steffen R, Guelrud M, Sivak MV Jr: Endoscopic retrograde cholangiopancreatography. In Wyllie R, Hyams J (eds): Pediatric Gastrointestinal Disease. Philadelphia, WB Saunders, pp 999–1015.
80. Drake DP, Stevens PS, Eckstein HB: Hydronephrosis secondary to ureteropelvic junction obstruction in children: a review of 14 years of experience. J Urol 1978;119:649–651.
81. Kelalis PP, Culp OS, Stickter GB, et al: Ureteropelvic junctions obstruction in children: experiences with 109 cases. J Urol 1971;106:418–422.
82. Byrne WJ, Arnold WC, Stannard MW: Ureteropelvic junction obstruction presenting with recurrent abdominal pain: diagnosis by ultrasound. Pediatrics 1985;76:934–937.
83. Johnston JH, Evans JP, Glassberg KI, et al: Pelvic hydronephrosis in children: a review of 219 personal cases. J Urol 1977;117:97–101.
84. White J: Ureteropelvic junction obstruction in children. Am Fam Physician 1984;29:211–216.
85. Bensman A, Roubach L, Allouch G, et al: Urolithiasis in children. Acta Paediatr Scand 1983;72:879–883.
86. Farthing M: Giardiasis. Gastroenterol Clin North Am 1996;25:493–514.
87. Jephcott AE, Begg NT, Baker IA: Outbreak of giardiasis associated with mains water in the United Kingdom. Lancet 1986;1:730–732.
88. Farthing MJG: Immunopathology of giardiasis. Springer Semin Immunopathol 1990;12:269–282.
89. Ungar BLP, Yolken RH, Nash TE, et al: Enzyme-linked immunosorbent assay for detection of Giardia lamblia in fecal specimens. J Infect Dis 1984;149:90–97.
90. Wiencka J, Olding-Stenkvist E, Schroder H, et al: Detection of Giardia antigen in stool samples by a semi-quantitative enzyme immunoassay test. Scand J Infect Dis 1989;21:443–448.
91. Salas SD, Heifetz R, Barrett-Connor E: Intestinal parasites in Central American immigrants in the United States. Arch Intern Med 1990;150:1514–1516.
92. Gilman RH, Chong YH, Davis C, et al: The adverse consequences of heavy *Trichuris* infection. Trans R Soc Trop Med Hyg 1983;77:432–438.
93. Wang C, Welch GE: Anomalies of intestinal rotation in adolescents and adults. Surgery 1963;54:839–855.
94. Louw JH, Cywes S: Embryology and anomalies of the intestine. In Berk JE, Haubrich WS, Kalser MH (eds): Bockus Gastroenterology, 4th ed. Philadelphia, WB Saunders, 1985, pp 1439–1473.
95. Janik JS, Ein SH: Normal intestinal rotation with nonfixation: a cause of chronic abdominal pain. J Pediatr Surg 1979;14:670–674.
96. Smith JR: Accessory enteric formations: a classification and nomenclature. Arch Dis Child 1960;35:87–89.
97. Bissler JJ, Klein RL: Alimentary tract duplications in children. Clin Pediatr 1988;27:152–157.
98. Farrell MK: Abdominal pain. Pediatrics 1984;74(suppl):955–957.
99. Scott RB: Recurrent abdominal pain during childhood. Can Fam Physician 1994;40:539–547.
100. McGrath PJ, Feldman W: Clinical approach to recurrent abdominal pain in children. J Dev Behav Pediatr 1986;7:56–61.
101. Zeltzer LK, Barr RG, McGrath PA, et al: Pediatric pain: interacting behavioral and physical factors. Pediatrics 1992;90:816–821.
102. Feldman W, McGrath P, Hodgson C, et al: The use of dietary fiber in the management of simple, childhood, idiopathic, recurrent abdominal pain. Am J Dis Child 1985;139:1216–1218.
103. Apley J, Hale B: Children with recurrent abdominal pain: how do they grow up? BMJ 1973;3:7–9.
104. Christensen MF, Mortensen O: Long-term prognosis in children with recurrent abdominal pain. Arch Dis Child 1975;50:110–114.
105. Magni G, Pierri M, Donzelli F: Recurrent abdominal pain in children: a long term follow-up. Eur J Pediatr 1987;146:72–74.

# Chapter 2

# Vomiting

B U.K. Li and Thomas J. Sferra

It has been suggested that the ability to vomit developed as a protective mechanism to rid the body of ingested toxins.[1] Unfortunately, vomiting also frequently occurs unrelated to the ingestion of noxious agents, a circumstance that produces several clinical challenges. First, vomiting is a sign of many diseases that affect different organ systems. Therefore, determining the cause of a vomiting episode can be difficult. Second, vomiting can produce several complications (e.g., electrolyte derangement, Mallory-Weiss syndrome) that demand diagnosis and treatment. Third, vomiting is a frequent complication of medical therapy (surgical procedures, cancer chemotherapy). Finally, selection of appropriate therapies for this distressing problem is necessary to improve patient comfort and avoid additional medical complications of the vomiting.

## THE VOMITING EVENT

### Definition

Vomiting (emesis) is a complex reflex behavioral response to a variety of stimuli (see below). The emetic reflex has three phases: (1) a prodromal period consisting of the sensation of nausea and signs of autonomic nervous system stimulation; (2) retching; and (3) vomiting, or forceful expulsion of the stomach contents through the oral cavity.[2–5] Although the overall sequence of these three phases is stereotypical, each can occur independently of the others. For example, nausea does not always progress to vomiting, and pharyngeal stimulation can induce vomiting without a prodrome of nausea. It is important to note that *vomiting* and *regurgitation* (defined as effortless reflux of the intragastric contents into the esophagus) are not synonymous. Clinically, vomiting can clearly be distinguished from regurgitation as regurgitation is not preceded by prodromal events, retching does not occur, and gastric contents are not forcibly expelled. The differentiation between vomiting and regurgitation is critical, as each has different causes and is produced by distinctive physiologic mechanisms.

### Physical Description

The events that herald the onset of the act of vomiting are nausea and several autonomic manifestations.[2, 5, 6] *Nausea* is a subjective experience difficult to define. It is usually described as an unpleasant, but painless, sensation localized to the epigastrium. Associated with this sensation is the feeling that vomiting is imminent. The autonomic signs of the prodrome include cutaneous vasoconstriction, sweating, dilation of pupils, increased salivation, and tachycardia. Several autonomic gastrointestinal (GI) motor events characterize the emetic prodrome.[6–9] There is inhibition of spontaneous contractions within the GI tract and dilatation of the proximal stomach. The esophageal skeletal muscle contracts longitudinally, pulling the relaxed proximal stomach (hiatus and cardia) into the thoracic cavity, with subsequent loss of the abdominal segment of the esophagus. These changes result in an anatomic position that allows free flow of gastric contents into the esophagus.[10] Soon after the onset of inhibition of contractile activity, a single large-amplitude contraction is initiated in the jejunum that propagates toward the stomach at 8 to 10 cm per second.[8, 11] This retropulsive event is termed the *retrograde giant contraction* (RGC). It serve to propel the duodenal contents into the stomach before the onset of retching.[10, 12] The RGC is followed in turn by a brief period of moderate-amplitude contractions in the distal small intestine and a second period of inhibition that can last several minutes.[7]

The two major somatic motor components of vomiting (retching and expulsion) are produced by the coordinated activity of the respiratory, pharyngeal, and abdominal muscles, resulting in rhythmic changes in intrathoracic and intra-abdominal pressures.[4, 13] During each cycle of retching, the glottis closes and the diaphragm, external intercostal muscles, and abdominal muscles contract,[14, 15] producing large negative intrathoracic and positive intra-abdominal pressure spikes. The esophagus dilates, and the atonic proximal stomach continues to be displaced into the thoracic cavity. The antireflux mechanisms are overcome, and the gastric contents move into and out of the esophagus with each cycle of retching.[10]

Sometime after the onset of retching, expulsion, or vomiting, occurs. During this event the external intercostal muscles and the hiatal region of the diaphragm relax and the abdominal muscles and costal diaphragm contract violently,[14, 15] producing positive pressures in both abdomen and thorax, resulting in oral propulsion of the gastric contents. Retrograde contraction of the cervical esophagus assists in oral expulsion.[9] After expulsion, antegrade peristalsis in the

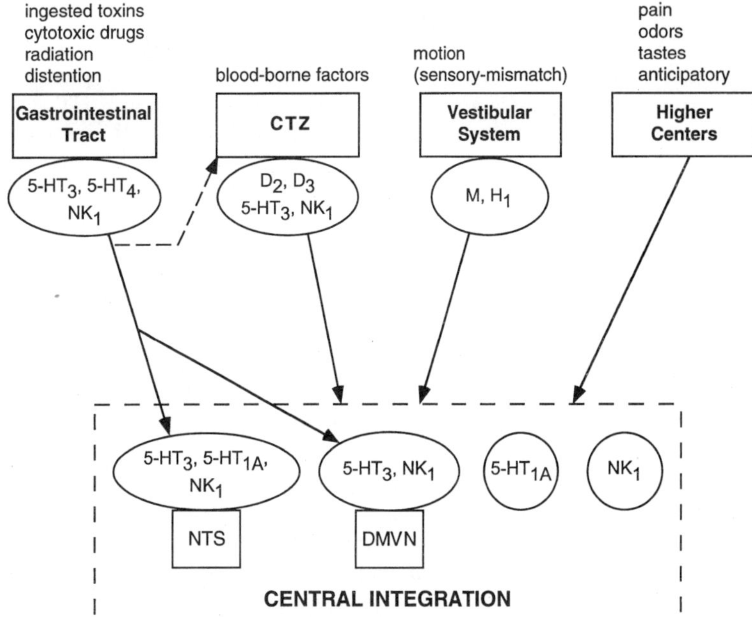


**FIGURE 2–1.** Schematic representation of the afferent limb and central integration of the emetic reflex. Receptors known to be involved in each pathway are listed within ovals. The region of central integration is designated by a dashed box to indicate that no single central locus exists as a "vomiting center." The nucleus of the solitary tract (NTS) and the dorsal motor vagal nucleus (DMVN) may each play a role in central integration. 5-HT, 5-hydroxytryptamine (serotonin); D, dopamine; M, acetylcholine muscarinic; H, histamine; NK, neurokinin.

esophagus clears the lumen of residual material[3]; the proximal stomach returns to its normal intra-abdominal position, restoring the normal antireflux anatomy.

## Gastrointestinal Motor Activity During Nausea and Vomiting

GI motor activity during the emetic reflex is mediated by the vagus nerve.[7–9] Vagal preganglionic parasympathetic fibers can activate both inhibitory and excitatory pathways in the enteric nervous system. These GI motor correlates follow a wide range of stimuli that induce nausea and vomiting[8]; however, these motor events do not appear to be the cause of the sensation of nausea. Moreover, the stereotypical somatic pattern of retching and vomiting continues even when the GI motor correlates of vomiting are prevented by disruption of the vagal efferents.[8, 9]

Although GI motor activity is not necessary for retching and vomiting, the motor changes that do occur may serve a significant role. As a defense against noxious ingested agents,[1] relaxation of the stomach can confine a toxin before it is expelled, and the RCG can move toxins and alkaline duodenal secretions to the stomach to buffer and dilute gastric irritants (e.g., vinegar, hypertonic saline) in preparation for expulsion. The buffering of the gastic contents can also serve to protect the esophagus from acid injury. Finally, changes in the position of the stomach can place it in an advantageous position for compression by the abdominal musculature.[10]

A different pattern of GI motor activity is observed in circumstances in which nausea is induced by motion.[16, 17] Before the onset of nausea, an increase occurs in the gastric slow-wave from 3 to 9 cycles per minute.[18] This phenomena, known as *tachygastria,* is controlled by central cholinergic and α-adrenergic pathways.[19] In motion-induced nausea, the GI motor activity appears to play a role in the induction of symptoms.[18]

## The Emetic Reflex

The emetic reflex consists of an afferent limb (receptor and pathway), central integration and control, and an efferent limb (pathway and effector) (Fig. 2–1).[20, 21] This reflex can be induced by visceral pain and inflammation, toxins, motion, pregnancy, radiation exposure, postoperative states, and unpleasant emotions. The diverse afferent receptors and pathways may originate within the gut, oropharynx, heart, vestibular system, or central nervous system (e.g., area postrema, hypothalamus, and cortical regions). These multiple afferent pathways are integrated within the central nervous system, and the emetic reflex is completed through a common integrated efferent limb consisting of multiple pathways and effectors.

Within the GI tract multiple receptors are capable of initiating the emetic reflex.[5, 22] Mechanoreceptors present within the muscularis are activated by changes in tension and may be stimulated by passive distention or active contraction of the bowel wall. These conditions are present in bowel obstruction, a clinical state of which vomiting is frequently an associated sign. Chemoreceptors within the mucosa of the stomach and proximal small bowel respond to a wide range of chemical irritants (hydrochloric acid [HCl], copper sulfate, vinegar, hypertonic saline, syrup of ipecac) and are involved in the emetic reflex induced by radiation and chemotherapeutic agents. The afferent pathways from the GI tract are mediated principally via the vagus nerves; the splanchnic nerves play a minor role.[22] Vagal afferent fibers project centrad, principally to the dorsomedial portion of the nucleus of the solitary tract (NTS) and to a lesser extent to the area postrema and the dorsal motor vagal nucleus.[22–24]

Circulating toxins can trigger the emetic reflex. The major detector of blood-borne noxious agents is the chemoreceptor trigger zone (CTZ),[25–27] which is located within the area postrema on the floor of the fourth ventricle, outside the blood-brain barrier. Substances in the cerebrospinal fluid and blood stream can be detected by the cells of this region. Several types of receptors for endogenous neurotransmitters and neuropeptides have been localized to the CTZ.[26, 28] Intravenous infusion or direct application to the CTZ of these neuroactive agents (dopamine, acetylcholine, enkephalin, peptide YY, substance P) can induce vomiting.[29, 30] Stimulation of the CTZ is essential for the induction of vomiting by these and other agents (apomorphine, cisplatin) but not for that induced by the stimulation of abdominal vagal afferents or motion. In addition to playing a role in vomiting, the area postrema is involved in taste aversion, the control of food intake, and fluid homeostasis.[27]

Activation of the afferent limb of the vomiting reflex may also occur through real or apparent motion of the body. Motion-induced vomiting is the result of a sensory mismatch involving the visual, vestibular, and proprioceptive systems,[31] although an intact vestibular system is a necessary component.[32] Histamine ($H_1$) and cholinergic muscarinic receptors are involved in the afferent limb of this pathway.[33] In addition to the above afferent pathways, stimulated by unpleasant situations or in instances of conditioned vomiting (e.g., anticipatory vomiting in chemotherapy), higher cortical centers can activate the emetic reflex.

After activation, the afferent systems project centrad. Although no single central locus has been identified as a "vomiting center," two models of central coordination of the emetic reflex have been proposed: (1) a group of nuclei (paraventricular system of nuclei, defined by their connection to the area postrema) form a linked neural system whose activation can account for all of the phenomena associated with vomiting[34, 35]; (2) vomiting is produced by the sequential activation of a series of discrete effector (motor) nuclei[1] as opposed to being activated in parallel by a single locus. Furthermore, the concept of a localized "vomiting center" has been refuted by recent anatomic studies implicating a widely distributed area within the medulla as being involved in the organization and control of the emetic reflex.[36, 37]

### Neurochemical Basis

A wide variety of neurotransmitters, neuroactive peptides, and hormones are involved in the emetic reflex. As investigations proceed into the physiology of vomiting and the pharmacology of antiemetic agents, the role of these and other mediators will continue to be defined.

Dopaminergic pathways have long been known to participate in the emetic reflex. Apomorphine, a commonly used experimental emetic agent, acts through the dopamine ($D_2$ subtype) receptor.[38] Furthermore, several clinically effective antiemetic agents (e.g., domperidone) are $D_2$ receptor antagonists. The site of action of these agents (agonists and antagonists) is the CTZ,[25, 27] where $D_2$ receptors are present in high density.[28] These receptors participate in the emetic reflex induced by several, but not all, noxious agents acting through the CTZ. In addition to this subclass of receptors, recent evidence has implicated $D_3$ receptors within the area postrema as having a role in the emetic reflex.[39]

The importance of serotonin (5-hydroxytryptamine or 5-HT) and serotonin receptors[40] in the emetic reflex has been demonstrated by the observation that cisplatin-induced vomiting can be prevented by blockade of 5-$HT_3$ receptors.[41, 42] In addition to its involvement in mediating the emetic response to several chemotherapeutic agents, 5-$HT_3$ receptors play an important role in vomiting induced by radiation therapy[43] and noxious substances in the GI tract.[44, 45] The 5-$HT_3$ receptors are present on vagal afferent fibers in the GI tract and the presynaptic vagal afferent terminals within the central nervous system, specifically in the NTS and CTZ in the area postrema.[46, 47] Current evidence indicates that chemotherapeutic agents, irradiation, and various noxious substances act directly on the GI mucosa, inducing release of serotonin from enterochromaffin cells.[42, 48] Vagal afferents terminating near these cells are stimulated, producing afferent activation of the emetic reflex. The precise role of the 5-$HT_3$ receptors on the presynaptic vagal afferents within the central nervous system has not been fully elucidated, but they appear to facilitate the emetic reflex induced by some afferent pathways (e.g., cranial irradiation, chemotherapeutic agents within the cerebrospinal fluid).[43, 49] Other members of the 5-HT receptor family also may be involved in the emetic reflex. The 5-$HT_4$ receptor has been shown to be necessary in the afferent limb of the emetic reflex induced by at least one GI irritant.[50] Blockade of central 5-$HT_{1A}$ receptors, located primarily in the NTS, prevents emesis induced by a broad range of stimuli.[51, 52]

Substance P (a member of the neurokinin family of peptides) and its receptor neurokinin $NK_1$ are widely distributed in the central nervous system and peripheral neural and extraneural tissues.[53, 54] Evidence in animal models of vomiting has demonstrated that this ligand and receptor are critical to the emetic response produced by a wide range of stimuli.[55–57] $NK_1$ receptor antagonists prevent vomiting produced by intravenous (morphine) and intragastric toxins (ipecac, copper sulfate), chemotherapeutic agents (cisplatin), and motion. The site of action of these antagonists is believed to be the $NK_1$ receptors located in the central nervous system (NTS, dorsal motor vagal nucleus).[56–58] Since blockade of this receptor prevents emesis induced by both peripheral- and central-acting agents, it has been suggested that $NK_1$ receptors are critical elements in the central integration or effector pathway common to all emesis-inducing stimuli.[56] Further study of the $NK_1$ receptor may result in the development of a new class of antiemetic agent possessing a broad spectrum of activity.

## CLINICAL ASPECTS OF VOMITING

### Temporal Patterns

There are three temporal patterns of vomiting, one *acute* and two recurrent, *chronic* and *cyclic* (Fig. 2–2). Because of its frequent association with infections of childhood such as viral gastroenteritis, the acute form is the most common and is characterized by a discrete episode of vomiting of moderate to high intensity. Recurrent vomiting is also a common problem encountered by pediatric gastroenterologists. Over a 5-year period we evaluated 106 consecutive cases that could be further subclassified: two thirds as chronic, a low-grade, daily pattern, and one third as cyclic, an intensive but intermittent one (Table 2–1).[59] Those with the chronic pattern were mildly ill, whereas those with the cyclic pattern tended to have stereotypic bouts associated with pallor, lethargy, and dehydration. Because both the acute and cyclic patterns can produce violent vomiting, until the repetitive nature

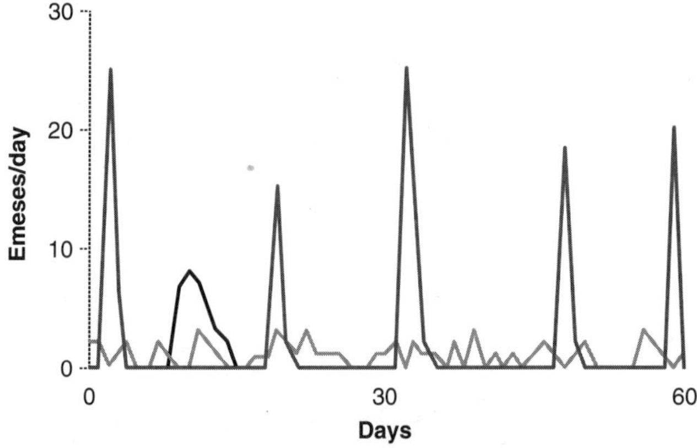


**FIGURE 2–2.** Representation of acute, chronic and cyclic patterns of vomiting. Three temporal patterns of vomiting are depicted: *acute, chronic,* and *cyclic.* The number of emeses per day is plotted on the vertical axis over a 2-month period. The *acute* pattern is represented by a single episode of moderate vomiting intensity; the *chronic* one by a recurrent low-grade vomiting pattern that occurs on a daily basis; and the *cyclic* one by recurrent, discrete episodes of high-intensity vomiting that occur once every several weeks with normal health in between.

(> 3 episodes) becomes evident, the cyclic pattern is understandably misclassified as an acute one and thus is misdiagnosed as a viral gastroenteritis.

## Differential Diagnosis

The epidemiology of underlying causes varies with the temporal pattern of vomiting (Table 2–2).[59–61] The acute pattern is dominated by infections both in the GI tract and outside. Other causes include obstruction of the GI tract, increased intracranial pressure resulting from neurologic injury, and poisoning. Among those with the chronic pattern, GI disorders outnumbered extraintestinal ones by a ratio of 7:1; the most common ones were peptic and infectious (*Helicobacter pylori*–induced) inflammation of the upper GI tract.[59] In contrast, the diagnostic profile in those with the cyclic pattern was reversed: extraintestinal disorders, including abdominal migraine, exceeded GI ones by a ratio of 5:1. Although the hallmark of idiopathic *cyclic vomiting syndrome* is the cyclic pattern of vomiting, episodic vomiting is the central manifestation of a number of neurologic (e.g., secondary to subtentorial neoplasm), endocrine (e.g., Addison's disease), and metabolic disorders (e.g., disorders of fatty acid oxidation).

Causes of vomiting also vary with the age of the child (Table 2–3). Although most congenital anomalies of the GI tract present in the neonatal period, webs and duplications can be found throughout childhood.[63, 64] Malrotation or nonfixation of the small intestine compounded by intermittent volvulus can cause cyclic vomiting at any age.[66, 67] Duodenal obstruction from superior mesenteric artery syndrome is associated with acute weight loss of anorexia nervosa, extensive burns, and immobilization in a body cast in children and adolescents.[70] Duodenal hematoma typically follows accidental trauma to the abdomen in bicycling children but can result from abuse of toddlers.

Although peptic and infectious injuries of the upper gastrointestinal tract are most common, allergic and inflammatory (Crohn's disease) ones also occur. Two unusual forms that affect toddlers include chronic granulomatous disease–induced antral obstruction[71] and cytomegalovirus-associated gastropathy of Ménétrier associated with hypoalbuminemia and anasarca.[72] Typhilitis, a necrotizing inflammation of the cecum, principally affects children with acute lymphocytic leukemia during chemotherapy-induced neutropenia.[73] Besides the congenital form of intestinal dysmotility, acquired viral and diabetes-induced gastroparesis can begin during adolescence.[74] Gallbladder dyskinesia, a cause of nausea, vomiting, and right upper quadrant pain, is in adolescents a newly recognized entity.[77]

Addison's disease can mimic cyclic vomiting syndrome at all ages, manifesting itself with recurring bouts of vomiting and hyponatremic dehydration until the hyperpigmentation appears.[78] Pheochromocytoma, as part of a multiple endo-

**TABLE 2–1. Differentiating Acute, Chronic, and Cyclic Patterns of Vomiting**

| | EPIDEMIOLOGY | | |
|---|---|---|---|
| CLINICAL FEATURE | Acute | Chronic Recurrent | Cyclic Recurrent |
| Acuity | Most common<br>Moderate–severe, ± dehydration | ⅔ of recurrent vomiting<br>Not acutely ill | ⅓ of recurrent vomiting<br>Severe, dehydrated |
| Intensity | Moderate to high | Low, ≤4 emeses/hr at peak | High, ≥4 emeses/hr at peak |
| Recurrence | No | Frequent, 2 episodes/wk | Infrequent, ≤ 2 episodes/wk |
| Stereotypy | Unique: *If child has had 3 similar episodes, consider cyclic pattern* | No | Yes |
| Onset | Variable | Daytime | Early morning |
| Symptoms | Fever, abdominal pain, diarrhea | Abdominal pain, diarrhea | Pallor, lethargy, nausea, abdominal pain |
| Household contacts affected | Usually | No | No |
| Family history of migraine headache | | 14% positive | 72% positive |
| Causes | Most often infection | Ratio of GI to extra-GI causes 7:1; upper GI tract mucosal injury most common | Ratio of extra-GI to GI causes 5:1; abdominal migraine and cyclic vomiting syndrome most common |

**TABLE 2–2. Causes of Vomiting by Temporal Pattern**

| CATEGORY | ACUTE | CHRONIC | CYCLIC |
|---|---|---|---|
| Infectious | Gastroenteritis*<br>Otitis media*<br>Streptococcal pharyngitis<br>Acute sinusitis<br>Hepatitis<br>Pyelonephritis<br>Meningitis | *H. pylori**<br>Giardiasis<br>Chronic sinusitis* | Chronic sinusitis* |
| Gastrointestinal | Inguinal hernia<br>Meconium ileus equivalent<br>Intussusception<br>Malrotation with volvulus<br>Appendicitis<br>Cholecystitis<br>Pancreatitis | Anatomic obstruction<br>GERD ± esophagitis*<br>Gastritis*<br>Peptic ulcer or duodenitis<br>Achalasia<br>SMA syndrome | GERD ± esophagitis<br>Malrotation with volvulus |
| Genitourinary | Pyelonephritis<br>UPJ obstruction | Pyelonephritis<br>Pregnancy<br>Uremia | Acute hydronephrosis secondary to ureteral stenosis |
| Endocrine, Metabolic | Diabetic ketoacidosis | Adrenal hyperplasia | Diabetic ketoacidosis<br>Addison's disease<br>MCAD deficiency<br>Partial OTC deficiency<br>MELAS syndrome<br>Acute intermittent porphyria |
| Neurologic | Concussion<br>Subdural hematoma<br>Reye's syndrome | Arnold-Chiari malformation<br>Subtentorial neoplasm | Abdominal migraine*<br>Migraine headaches*<br>Arnold-Chiari malformation<br>Subtentorial neoplasm<br>Reye's syndrome |
| Other | Toxic ingestion<br>Food poisoning | Rumination<br>Psychogenic<br>Bulimia | Cyclic vomiting syndrome*<br>Munchausen by proxy (e.g., ipecac poisoning) |

*Most common disorders.

GERD, gastroesophageal reflux disease; MCAD, medium-chain acyl-CoA dehydrogenase deficiency; MELAS, mitochondrial myopathy, encephalopathy, lactic acidosis, and stroke-like episodes; OTC, ornithine transcarbamylase deficiency; SMA, superior mesenteric artery; UPJ, ureteropelvic junction.

Data from references 59, 60, and 61.

**TABLE 2–3. Causes of Vomiting by Organ System and Age at Presentation**

| CAUSE | NEONATE (≤1 mo) | INFANT 1–12 (mo) | CHILD 1–11 (yr) | ADOLESCENT >11 (yr) | REFERENCE |
|---|---|---|---|---|---|
| **Extra-GI Infections** | | | | | |
| Otitis media | | ——— | ——— | ····· | |
| Acute or chronic sinusitis | | | ——— | ——— | |
| Streptococcal pharyngitis | | | ——— | ——— | |
| Pneumonitis | | ——— | ——— | ····· | |
| Pyelonephritis | ——— | ——— | ——— | ——— | |
| Meningitis | ——— | ——— | ——— | ——— | |
| **GI Infections** | | | | | |
| Gastroenteritis | | ——— | ——— | ——— | |
| Infectious colitis | | ····· | ——— | ——— | |
| Parasitic infections | | | ——— | ——— | |
| *H. pylori* gastritis | | | ——— | ——— | |
| Giardiasis | | | ——— | ——— | |
| Hepatitis | | | ——— | ——— | |
| Hepatic abscess | | | ——— | ····· | |
| **Anatomic Insults** | | | | | |
| Congenital atresias and stenoses, tracheoesophageal fistula, webs, duplications, imperforate anus | ——— | ——— | ····· | ····· | 62–64 |
| Meconium ileus or equivalent | ——— | ——— | ——— | ——— | 65 |
| Inguinal hernia | ——— | ——— | ——— | ——— | |
| Malrotation with volvulus | ——— | ——— | ——— | ——— | 66, 67 |
| Intussusception | | ——— | ——— | ····· | 68 |
| Appendicitis | | | ——— | ——— | 69 |
| SMA syndrome | | | | ——— | 70 |
| Bezoar | | ——— | ——— | | |
| Duodenal hematoma | | ——— | ——— | ——— | |
| Surgical adhesions | ——— | ——— | ——— | ——— | |
| **Mucosal Injuries** | | | | | |
| GERD ± esophagitis, stricture | ——— | ——— | ——— | ——— | |
| Gastritis ± *H. pylori* | | | ——— | ——— | |

**TABLE 2–3. Causes of Vomiting by Organ System and Age at Presentation** *Continued*

| CAUSE | NEONATE (≤1 mo) | INFANT 1–12 (mo) | CHILD 1–11 (yr) | ADOLESCENT >11 (yr) | REFERENCE |
|---|---|---|---|---|---|
| Peptic ulcer or duodenitis | | | ——— | ——— | |
| Cow or soy protein sensitivity | ——— | ——— | ——— | | |
| Celiac disease | | …… | ——— | ——— | |
| Chronic granulomatous disease | | | ——— | …… | 71 |
| Ménétrier's disease | | | ——— | …… | 72 |
| Crohn's disease | | …… | ——— | ——— | |
| Ulcerative colitis | | | ——— | ——— | |
| Typhilitis | | | ——— | …… | 73 |
| **GI Motility Disorders** | | | | | |
| Oropharyngeal discoordination | ——— | ——— | ——— | …… | |
| Achalasia | | | …… | ——— | |
| Gastroparesis | | | …… | ——— | 74 |
| Paralytic ileus | ——— | ——— | ——— | ——— | |
| Hirschsprung's disease | ——— | ——— | …… | …… | |
| Pseudo-obstruction | ——— | ——— | …… | …… | 75 |
| Familial dysautonomia | | ——— | ——— | ——— | 76 |
| **Visceral GI Disorders** | | | | | |
| Cholecystitis | | | …… | ——— | |
| Cholelithiasis | | | …… | ——— | |
| Gallbladder dyskinesia | | | | ——— | 77 |
| Choledochal cyst | ——— | ——— | …… | | |
| Pancreatitis | | | ——— | ——— | |
| **Endocrine Derangements** | | | | | |
| Adrenal hyperplasia | ——— | ——— | | | |
| Addison's disease | ——— | ——— | ——— | ——— | 78 |
| Diabetic ketoacidosis | …… | …… | ——— | ——— | |
| Pheochromocytoma | | | …… | …… | 79 |
| Carcinoid syndrome | | | …… | …… | 80 |
| Zollinger-Ellison syndrome | | | …… | …… | 81 |
| **Metabolic Derangements** | | | | | |
| Organic acidemias | ——— | ——— | …… | …… | |
| Disorders of fatty acid oxidation | …… | ——— | ——— | …… | 82 |
| Amino acidemias | ——— | ——— | …… | …… | |
| Urea cycle defects | ——— | ——— | …… | …… | 83 |
| Hereditary fructose intolerance | …… | ——— | | | |
| Mitochondriopathies | …… | ——— | ——— | | 84 |
| Storage diseases | ——— | ——— | …… | …… | |
| Acute intermittent porphyria | | | …… | ——— | 85 |
| **Genitourinary Disorders** | | | | | |
| Ureteropelvic obstruction | | ——— | ——— | …… | |
| Hydronephrosis secondary to ureteral obstruction | | …… | ——— | …… | 86 |
| Renal stones | | …… | ——— | ——— | |
| Uremia | …… | ——— | ——— | ——— | |
| Hydrometrocolpos | …… | ——— | ——— | ——— | |
| Pregnancy | | | | ——— | |
| **Neurologic Disorders** | | | | | |
| Hydrocephalus with shunt dysfunction | ——— | ——— | ——— | ——— | |
| Arnold-Chiari malformation | ——— | ——— | ——— | ——— | |
| Pseudotumor cerebri | | | …… | ——— | 87 |
| Concussion | ——— | ——— | ——— | ——— | 88 |
| Subdural hematoma | ——— | ——— | ——— | ——— | |
| Subarachnoid hemorrhage | | | ——— | ——— | |
| Intracranial neoplasm | | | ——— | ——— | 89 |
| Reye's syndrome | | | ——— | …… | |
| Migraine headaches | | | ——— | ——— | |
| Abdominal migraine | | | ——— | ——— | 90, 91 |
| Epilepsy | | | …… | | 92 |
| **Other Causes** | | | | | |
| Overfeeding | | ——— | | | |
| Rumination | | | ——— | ——— | |
| Toxic ingestion | | | ——— | ——— | |
| Lead poisoning | | | ——— | …… | |
| Food poisoning | | | ——— | ——— | |
| Psychogenic vomiting | | | ——— | ——— | |
| Bulimia | | | | ——— | |
| Cyclic vomiting syndrome | | ——— | ——— | ——— | 59, 61, 93 |
| Munchausen by proxy (ipecac poisoning) | | | ——— | | 94 |

GERD, gastroesophageal reflux disease; SMA, superior mesenteric artery.
———, typically presents in this age group; ……, occasionally or rarely presents in this age group.

**TABLE 2–4. Clinical Clues to Diagnosis**

| ASSOCIATED SYMPTOM OR SIGN | DIAGNOSTIC CONSIDERATION | ASSOCIATED SYMPTOM OR SIGN | DIAGNOSTIC CONSIDERATION |
|---|---|---|---|
| **Systemic Manifestations** | | **Gastrointestinal Symptoms** | |
| Acute illness, dehydration | Infection, ingestion, cyclic vomiting, surgical emergency | Nausea | Absence of nausea suggests increased intracranial pressure |
| Chronic malnutrition | Malabsorption syndrome | Abdominal pain | Substernal, esophagitis; epigastric, upper GI tract, pancreas; right upper quadrant, gallbladder |
| **Temporal Pattern** | | | |
| Low-grade, daily | Chronic vomiting pattern (e.g., upper GI tract disease) | Diarrhea | Enteric infection |
| Postprandial | Upper GI tract disease (e.g., gastritis), biliary and pancreatic disorders | Constipation | Hirschsprung's disease, pseudo-obstruction, hypercalcemia |
| Relationship to diet | Fat, cholecystitis, pancreatitis; protein, allergy; fructose, hereditary fructose intolerance | Dysphagia | Achalasia, esophageal stricture |
| | | Visible peristalsis | Gastric outlet obstruction |
| | | Surgical scars | Postoperative surgical adhesions, surgical vagotomy |
| Early morning onset | Sinusitis, subtentorial neoplasm, cyclic vomiting syndrome | Succussion splash | Gastric outlet obstruction with gastric distention |
| High intensity | Cyclic vomiting syndrome, bowel obstruction | Bowel sounds | Decreased: paralytic ileus, atony; increased: mechanical obstruction |
| Stereotypical (well episodes between) | Cyclic vomiting syndrome (see differential diagnosis in Table 2–2) | Severe abdominal tenderness with rebound | Perforated viscera, peritonitis |
| Rapid onset and subsidence | Cyclic vomiting syndrome | Abdominal mass | Pyloric stenosis, congenital malformations, ovarian cyst, pregnancy, abdominal neoplasm |
| **Character of Emesis** | | | |
| Effortless | Gastroesophageal reflux, regurgitation, rumination | **Neurologic Symptoms** | |
| Projectile | Upper GI tract obstruction | Headache | Allergy, chronic sinusitis, migraine, increased intracranial pressure |
| Mucous | Allergy, chronic sinusitis | | |
| Bilious | Postampullary obstruction, cyclic vomiting syndrome | Postnasal drip, congestion | Allergy, chronic sinusitis |
| Bloody | Esophagitis, Mallory-Weiss injury, allergic gastroenteropathy, bleeding diathesis | Vertigo | Migraine, Meniere's disease |
| | | Seizures | Epilepsy |
| Undigested food | Achalasia | Abnormal muscle tone | Cerebral palsy, metabolic disorder, mitochondriopathy |
| Clear, large volume | Ménétrier's disease, Zollinger-Ellison syndrome | Abnormal fundoscopic examination or bulging fontanelle | Increased intracranial pressure |
| Malodorous | *H. pylori*, giardiasis, small bowel bacterial overgrowth, colonic obstruction | | |
| | | **Family History and Epidemiology** | |
| | | Peptic ulcer disease | Peptic ulcer disease, *H. pylori* gastritis |
| | | Migraine headaches | Abdominal migraine, cyclic vomiting syndrome |
| | | Contaminated water | *Giardia, Cryptosporidium,* other parasites |
| | | Travel | Traveler's *(Escherichia coli)* diarrhea, giardiasis |

crine neoplasia type 2b,[79] carcinoid syndrome,[80] and gastrinoma[81] are rare in children and adolescents. Although metabolic disorders usually present in infancy with vomiting and failure to thrive, medium-chain acyl-CoA dehydrogenase deficiency,[82] partial ornithine transcarbamylase deficiency,[83] and acute intermittent porphyria[85] can present with episodic vomiting in older children and adolescents.

Acute hydronephrosis resulting from ureteral stenosis can appear as either an acute or a cyclic vomiting pattern, so-called Dietl's crisis.[86] Increased intracranial pressure can result not only from structural lesions but also from pseudotumor cerebri associated with obesity, corticosteroid taper, vitamin A deficit or excess, tetracycline use, and hypophosphatasia.[87] Both migraine headache and abdominal migraine are associated with a high prevalence of vomiting in 40% of affected patients.[95] Epilepsy as a cause of recurrent abdominal pain and vomiting without evident seizure activity remains a controversial entity.[96]

Psychogenic vomiting and Munchausen by proxy (ipecac poisoning) have to be considered when the clinical pattern does not fit known disorders, laboratory testing is negative, and psychosocial stresses are evident (see Psychogenic Vomiting). Because of its lipid solubility, ipecac can be detected on a toxicology screen as much as 2 months after administration.[94]

## Clinical Clues to Diagnosis

Clinical clues to aid in differential diagnosis are presented in Table 2–4. Hematemesis commonly results from peptic esophagitis and Mallory-Weiss injury, and less often from allergic gastroenteropathy, Crohn's disease, and vasculitis involving the upper GI tract. In the face of nonspecific gastric petechaie, vomiting occasionally originates from a bleeding diathesis such as that of von Willebrand's disease. The most worrisome cause of early morning vomiting is a neoplasm of the posterior fossa. The absence of nausea also supports increased intracranial pressure as the potential cause of emesis; however, the early morning pattern of nausea and vomiting associated with a history of congestion, postnasal drainage, and cough-and-vomit sequence most often results from environmental allergies and chronic sinusitis. Vertigo is commonly associated with a migraine headache or middle ear dysfunction (e.g, Meniere's syndrome).

Unlike adults, for whom eating often provides pain relief, children more often experience exacerbation of their abdominal pain and vomiting from eating. Malodorous breath is associated with chronic sinusitis, *Helicobacter pylori* gastritis, giardiasis, and small bowel bacterial overgrowth. Although seen infrequently, visible peristalsis in infants and a succussion splash in children are indications of a gastric outlet obstruction that is causing gastric distention. Abdominal masses can be seen in congenital (e.g., mesenteric cyst) or acquired non-neoplastic (e.g., ovarian cysts) and neoplastic (e.g., Burkitt's lymphoma) lesions. In a female teenager, pregnancy should always be considered as a cause of an abdominal mass and excluded.

Repetitive, stereotypic, intense bouts of vomiting that begin suddenly in the early morning hours and resolve rapidly are characteristic of cyclic vomiting syndrome and abdominal migraine (see Cyclic Vomiting Syndrome and Abdominal Migraine). Vomiting associated with hypo- or hypertonia suggests the possibility of either oropharyngeal discoordination and aspiration or intractable gastroesophageal reflux disease associated with cerebral palsy or a metabolic disorder that affects muscle tone (e.g., mitochondrial respiratory chain defect).[84]

## Evaluation

Evaluation and treatment of acute vomiting is the purview of the primary care or emergency room physician. The clinical assessment of dehydration without laboratory assessment is usually sufficient basis to begin intravenous rehydration (Table 2–5).[60, 97] Stool virus testing and bacterial cultures in presumed enteritis or colitis can aid in assessing the infectious risk to others. Abdominal radiographs and surgical consultation are indicated when the physical examination reveals acute abdominal signs. When emesis is voluminous and frequent, empiric antiemetic therapy (e.g., promethazine suppositories) may forestall development of dehydration and avoid the need for intravenous therapy.

Recent development of clinical pathways in the managed care environment has given rise to a schema in which screening tests and empiric treatment precede definitive testing and treatment: chronic vomiting may be assessed by screening laboratory tests (e.g., *H. pylori* antibody) and treated empirically with $H_2$ antagonists before definitive testing and specific therapy. If the condition does not improve, the following definitive tests are then considered: an esophagogastroduodenoscopy to detect peptic, infectious, inflammatory, and allergic mucosal injuries; small bowel radiography to evaluate possible anatomic lesions and Crohn's disease; abdominal ultrasound to assess suspected cholelithiasis, pancreatic pseudocyst, or hydronephrosis; and sinus films (or computed tomography [CT]) to document chronic sinusitis. Sinus evaluation has a 10% yield in chronic vomiting.[59]

Because these are episodic disorders, test results are typically abnormal only during a symptomatic bout of cyclic vomiting, so blood and urine screening for metabolic disorders must be obtained *during the episode.*[60] The serum chemistry profile can detect hyperglycemia in diabetes mellitus or hypoglycemia in disorders of fatty acid oxidation, hyponatremia in Addison's disease, an anion gap and low bicarbonate in organic acidosis, elevated hepatic transaminases in hepatobiliary disorders, and elevated amylase and lipase in pancreatic disorders. Serum is analyzed for elevations of ammonia in urea cycle defects, lactic acid in lactic acidosis, amino acids in specific aminoacidemias, and deficiency of carnitine in disorders of fatty acid oxidation. After screening

**TABLE 2–5. Initial Diagnostic Evaluation by Temporal Pattern of Vomiting**

| | STUDIES | | |
|---|---|---|---|
| | **Acute** | **Chronic** | **Cyclic** |
| Screening testing | Electrolytes<br>BUN<br>Creatinine | CBC, ESR<br>Chemistry profile<br>Urinalysis<br>*H. pylori* antibody<br>Stool *Giardia* antigen | *(Test during the episode!)*<br>Blood<br>CBC<br>Chemistry (including amylase, lipase)<br>Ammonia<br>Lactate<br>Carnitine<br>Amino acids<br>Urine<br>Urinalysis<br>Organic acids<br>δ-ALA<br>Porphobilinogen<br>Carnitine |
| Definitive testing | Rotavirus ELISA<br>Stool cultures<br>*Giardia* antigen<br>Abdominal radiographs<br>Surgical consult | Endoscopy with biopsies<br>Sinus films<br>UGI/SBFT series<br>Abdominal ultrasound | UGI/SBFT series<br>Endoscopy with biopsies<br>Sinus radiography<br>Head CT/MRI<br>Abdominal ultrasound<br>Definitive metabolic testing |

ALA, aminolevulinic acid; BUN, blood urea nitrogen; CBC, complete blood count; ESR, erythrocyte sedimentation rate; ELISA, enzyme-linked immunosorbent assay; UGI/SBFT, upper GI with small bowel follow-through.

Data from references 60 and 97.

**TABLE 2–6. Antinausea and Antiemetic Medications**

| DRUG CLASS/GENERIC | BRAND NAME | DOSAGES* | MECHANISMS | SIDE EFFECTS | INDICATIONS | POTENTIAL APPLICATIONS |
|---|---|---|---|---|---|---|
| **Antihistamines (minimal antiemetic activity)** | | | | | | |
| Diphenhydramine | Benadryl, Benylin | 1.25 mg/kg q 6 hr PO or IV | Vestibular suppression, anti-ACh effect, and $H_1$ antagonist | Sedation, anticholinergic effects† | Motion sickness, mild chemotherapy-induced vomiting | Contraindicated with MAO inhibitors, GI obstruction |
| Hydroxyzine | Atarax, Vistaril | 0.5–0.6 mg/kg q 6 hr PO | | | | |
| Dimenhydrinate | Dramamine | 1.25 mg/kg q 6 hr PO or IM | | Sedation | | |
| Cyclizine | Marezine | 1 mg/kg q 8 hr PO or IM<br>$>$ 10 yr of age: 50 mg q 4–6 hr PO or IM | Vestibular suppression, anti-ACh effect | | | |
| Meclizine | Antivert | $>$ 12 yr of age: 25–100 mg/24 hr PO divided tid–qid | | | | |
| **Phenothiazines (mild to moderate antiemetic activity)** | | | | | | |
| Promethazine | Phenergan | 0.25–0.5 mg/kg/dose q 4–6 hr PR or IM | $D_2$ receptor antagonist at CTZ and $H_1$ antagonist | Anticholinergic effects,† extrapyramidal reactions | Chemotherapy-induced vomiting | |
| Prochlorperazine | Compazine | $>$ 10 kg: 0.1–0.15 mg/kg/dose IM<br>$>$ 10 kg: 0.4 mg/kg/24 hr divided tid–qid PO or PR<br>Maximum 10 mg/dose | $D_2$ receptor antagonist at CTZ | | | |
| Chlorpromazine | Thorazine | $>$ 6 mo of age: 0.5–1 mg/kg/dose IV or PO q 6–8 hr | | | | |
| **Substituted Benzamides (much antiemetic activity)** | | | | | | |
| Cisapride | Propulsid | –0.2–0.3 mg/kg tid–qid PO<br>Adults: 10 mg tid–qid PO | 5-$HT_4$ agonist with ACh release in gut | Diarrhea, abdominal pain, headache | Gastroesophageal reflux, gastroparesis | Arrhythmias with antifungal and macrolide antibiotics, cyclic vomiting |
| Metoclopramide | Reglan | 0.1 mg/kg/dose IM, IV, or PO up to qid. The total daily dose should not exceed 0.5 mg/kg.<br>Adults: 10 mg IM, IV, or PO 30 min before each meal and at bedtime | $D_2$ antagonist at CTZ and gut, 5-$HT_4$ agonist in gut | Irritability and extrapyramidal reactions | Gastroesophageal reflux, gastroparesis, chemotherapy-induced vomiting | |
| Trimethobenzamide | Tigan | Children $<$ 14 kg: 100 mg/dose PR tid–qid<br>Children 14–40 kg: 100–200 mg/dose PO or PR tid–qid<br>Not recommended for neonates or premature infants. | $D_2$ antagonist at CTZ | | | |

| | | | | | | |
|---|---|---|---|---|---|---|
| **5-$HT_3$ Receptor Antagonists (much antiemetic activity)** | | | | | | |
| Ondansetron | Zofran | 0.15 mg/kg IV q 8 hr or<br>Surface area < 0.3 $m^2$: 1 mg/dose PO<br>Surface area 0.3–0.6 $m^2$: 2 mg/dose PO<br>Surface area 0.6–1.0 $m^2$: 3 mg/dose PO<br>Surface area > 1 $m^2$: 4 mg/dose PO | 5-$HT_3$ antagonist at CTZ and vagal afferents in gut | Headache | Chemotherapy, postoperative | Cyclic vomiting |
| Granisetron | Kytril | Age 2–16 years: 10 μg/kg IV q 6 hr | | | | Cyclic vomiting |
| Tropisetron | Navoban | No dose recommendations available. | | | | |
| **Anticholinergics (minimal antiemetic activity)** | | | | | | |
| Scopolamine | Transderm Scōp | Not recommended for pediatric use.<br>1 patch is 1 mg scopolamine q 3 days | Vestibular suppression, anti-ACh effect on central pattern generator | Sedation, anticholinergic effects† | Prophylaxis of motion sickness | |
| **Benzimidazole Derivative (mild to moderate antiemetic activity)** | | | | | | |
| Domperidone | Motilium | 0.6 mg/kg/dose tid–qid PO or Age < 2 yr: 10 mg PR bid–qid<br>2–4 yr: 15 mg PR qid<br>4–6 yr: 23 mg PR qid<br>> 6 yr: 30 mg PR qid | $D_2$ antagonist in gut | Headaches | Gastroparesis, chemotherapy | Not available in United States |
| **Butyrophenone (mild to moderate antiemetic activity)** | | | | | | |
| Droperidol | Inapsine | 0.05–0.075 mg/kg/dose IM or IV for one dose | $D_2$ antagonist at CTZ, anxiolytic action and sedation | Hypotension, sedation, extrapyramidal effects | Chemotherapy, post-operative | |
| **Benzodiazepines (minimal antiemetic activity)** | | | | | | |
| Lorazepam | Ativan | 0.03–0.1 mg/kg/dose IV | Enhanced central GABA-ergic inhibition inducing anxiolysis, sedation, and amnesia | Sedation, respiratory depression | Chemotherapy adjunct | Cyclic vomiting adjunct |
| Diazepam | Valium | 0.1–0.3 mg/kg IV prn<br>Maximum: < 0.6 mg/kg/24 hr | | | | |
| **Corticosteroids (mild to moderate antiemetic activity)** | | | | | | |
| Dexamethasone | Decadron | Initial dose: 10 mg/$m^2$ IV, maximum 20 mg, then 5 mg/$m^2$ q 6 hr IV | Unknown | Adrenal suppression | Chemotherapy | |
| **Cannabinoids (mild to moderate antiemetic activity)** | | | | | | |
| Dronabinol | Marinol | > 12 yr: 5 mg/$m^2$/dose q 4–6 hr PO<br>Maximum: 15 mg/$m^2$/dose | Unknown | Disorientation, vertigo, hallucinations | Chemotherapy | |
| Nabilone | Cesamet | < 18 kg: 0.5 mg PO bid<br>18–30 kg: 1 mg PO bid<br>> 30 kg: 1 mg PO tid | | | | |

*These doses are used for antiemetic effect rather than other indications.
†Anticholinergic effects: blurred vision, dry mouth, hypotension, palpitations, urine retention.
ACh, acetylcholine; CTZ, chemotrigger zone; D, dopamine; H, histamine; 5-HT, 5-hydroxytryptamine; GABA, γ-aminobutyric acid.
Within the same drug class, in the blank space, the same attributes apply from the medication above.
Data from references 99, 100, and 101.

children with pyelonephritis for pyuria and those with hematuria for nephrolithiasis (idiopathic hypercalciuria), the urine is analyzed for elevations in organic acids, carnitine esters, and δ-aminolevulinic acid and porphobilinogen in organic acidurias, disorders of fatty acid oxidation, and acute intermittent porphyria, respectively. Positive screening results necessitate appropriate definitive testing. For example, the absence of ketones, presence of dicarboxylic aciduria, and elevated urinary esterified–free carnitine ratio of greater than 4:1 implicate a disorder of fatty acid oxidation, and diagnosis entails definitive plasma acylcarnitine and urinary acylglycine profiles. Evaluation of GI involvement includes small bowel radiography for malrotation, an esophagogastroduodenoscopy for mucosal inflammation, and abdominal ultrasonography for hydronephrosis, cholelithiasis, and pancreatic pseudocyst. With a history suggestive of increased intracranial pressure (e.g., headache, early morning onset), CT scan or magnetic resonance imaging (MRI) of the brain is indicated. In the absence of a definitive diagnosis, a trial of prophylactic antimigraine or intestinal prokinetic therapy may be instituted to treat suspected abdominal migraine or GI dysmotility as causes of the cyclic vomiting.

## Complications

The two principal complications of acute or cyclic vomiting (during the episode) include dehydration with electrolyte derangement and hematemesis from a Mallory-Weiss injury. The electrolyte disturbance resulting from varying proportions of losses of gastric HCl, pancreatic bicarbonate ($HCO_3$), and gastric and intestinal sodium chloride (NaCl) is generally corrected with standard intravenous replacement. Hypochloremic, hypokalemic alkalosis results from high-grade gastric outlet obstruction and predominant loss of gastric $H^+$ and $Cl^-$. In pyloric stenosis, risk factors for development of this electrolyte profile include female gender, black race, longer duration of illness, and more severe dehydration.[98] Preoperative correction of electrolyte imbalance has reduced the perioperative morbidity of pyloromyotomy.

The Mallory-Weiss injury in our experience has less often been the classic mucosal tear at the gastroesophageal junction and more often a discrete hemorrhagic bruise in the gastric cardia visualized on the retroflex endoscopic view just below the gastroesophageal junction. This injury presumably results from traumatization of that gastric tissue by repeated herniation through the gastroesophageal junction during retching and vomiting. If the bleeding is not hemodynamically significant, short-term use of $H_2$ antagonists and sucralfate is sufficient.

Complications of peptic injury to the esophagus (e.g., stricture formation and Barrett's metaplasia) and bronchopulmonary aspiration are more likely to occur with long-standing chronic (rather than acute or cyclic) vomiting associated with gastroesophageal reflux disease in which the esophageal mucosa is exposed to acid for prolonged periods. Failure to thrive as a complication of chronic vomiting can occur by three mechanisms, including loss of calories, inflammatory burden, and protein-losing enteropathy. Besides nutritional assessment and anthropometric monitoring, aggressive nutritional supplementation may include continuous nasogastric or transpyloric feedings.

## Pharmacologic Treatment

Although the therapy should be directed toward the cause, empiric therapy of the vomiting symptom may be indicated when the severity of the acute or cyclic vomiting places the child at risk of dehydration and other complications. When diagnostic confirmation of cyclic vomiting syndrome is not possible, a positive response to the antimigraine therapy can support the diagnosis of abdominal migraine. A comprehensive listing of therapeutic agents by pharmacologic category is presented in Table 2–6.[99–101]

Antihistamines (e.g., meclizine) are minimally active antiemetics but have efficacy in motion sickness because of their effects on vestibular function of the middle ear. As a result of $D_2$ receptor antagonist activity, phenothiazines (e.g., promethazine) have mild to moderate activity in chemotherapy-induced vomiting but carry a substantial risk of extrapyramidal reactions. Substituted benzamides (e.g., cisapride) are effective prokinetic agents in gastroparesis and other motility disorders. Butyrophenones (e.g., droperidol) have mild to moderate efficacy when used in chemotherapy and postoperative settings but also carry risk of extrapyramidal side effects. Benzodiazepines have minimal antiemetic effectiveness but can be effective adjuncts to other antiemetics. Cannabinoids have mild to moderate potency but are associated with psychiatric side effects.

The newer serotoninergic agonists and antagonists have demonstrated marked antiemetic potential. The $5\text{-}HT_3$ antagonists (e.g., ondansetron) have demonstrated greater antiemetic efficacy in postoperative and chemotherapeutic settings than did previous combination regimens. The $5\text{-}HT_{1D}$ agonists (e.g., sumatriptan) have recently shown promise for aborting pediatric migraine headaches[102] and treating cyclic vomiting.[103, 104] Because $5\text{-}HT_3$ and $5\text{-}HT_{1D}$ agents have both central and peripheral effects, the antiemetic effects may result from a combination of actions. $5\text{-}HT_3$ antagonists act both at the chemotrigger zone and on peripheral vagal afferents, possibly inhibiting serotonin release by enterochromaffin cells in the intestine. The $5\text{-}HT_{1D}$ agents constrict cerebral blood vessels but relax the gastric fundus.

# SPECIFIC VOMITING DISORDERS

## Cyclic Vomiting Syndrome and Abdominal Migraine

Although cyclic vomiting syndrome is now increasingly recognized, it remains a poorly understood disorder.[59–61] On the basis of its 1.9% prevalence among 5- to 15-year-olds in Aberdeen, Scotland, cyclic vomiting appears to be common rather than rare.[105] Both its original description by Samuel Gee[106] in 1882 and the current consensus on diagnostic criteria for cyclic vomiting syndrome[107] reached in 1994 reflect the same emphasis on intermittent, intense, stereotypical episodes of vomiting with normal health between (Table 2–7).[90, 91, 107] Although the cyclic *pattern* of vomiting is the key diagnostic feature of cyclic vomiting *syndrome,* the pattern represents a starting point for diagnostic testing and the syndrome refers to those idiopathic cases for which diagnostic testing is negative; within those, a secondary diagnosis of abdominal migraine may be made.[108]

Although cyclic vomiting has been variously considered to be a migraine or epileptic variant, metabolic disorder, or psychiatric disturbance, the cause and pathogenesis remain elusive.[109] Because of similarities in clinical features, a relationship to abdominal migraine has been proposed (see Table 2–7).[110, 111] The historical criteria for abdominal migraine proposed by Lundberg[90] and Symon and Russell[91] overlap with the consensus criteria for cyclic vomiting syndrome, especially the discrete episodes with interval wellness, the stereotypy, and the associated symptoms of pallor, lethargy, abdominal pain, and vomiting.[107] Based on electroencephalographic and autonomic function data demonstrating similar visual evoked and autonomic responses, there is support for a pathophysiologic overlap between cyclic vomiting and abdominal migraine.[112, 113] Until a definitive marker becomes available for migraines, the relationship between these two entities remains unproven. Other possible pathogenic mechanisms include a hypothalamic discharge with release of adrenocorticotropin (ACTH), prostaglandin $E_2$ ($PGE_2$), vasopressin, and peripheral catecholamines as described by Wolff and Sato and others[114–116] and GI dysmotility.[117]

In our series of 180 children who presented with the cyclic vomiting syndrome and abdominal migraine, the typical patient is a 5- to 8-year-old girl or boy who has stereotypical, severe (15 emeses) episodes once every 2 to 4 weeks and is completely healthy between episodes. Although the term *cyclic* has been applied to the condition, only 47% have regular intervals, and *episodic* would be more precise. The attacks most frequently begin at 3:00 to 6:00 AM, are preceded by a short prodrome (half hour or less), last 24 hours, require intravenous (IV) hydration (51%), and cause 15 days of school absence per year. Because the vomiting usually results in prostration and dehydration, the condition is most often misdiagnosed as repeated bouts of gastroenteritis. Besides the intense vomiting, common symptoms (in more than 70% of children) include pallor, lethargy, anorexia, nausea, retching, and abdominal pain. In many instances the parents can identify a proximate event—psychological stress (e.g., birthday, travel), a common infection (e.g., sinusitis, streptococcal pharyngitis), or a food (e.g., chocolate, cheese); however, typical migraine *symptoms* of headaches and photophobia affect only 30% to 40% of children. This vomiting pattern resolves during the teenage years but may be replaced by recurrent migraine headaches.

Because the cyclic pattern of vomiting is sensitive but not specific for the cyclic vomiting *syndrome,* the syndrome remains a diagnosis of exclusion with normal results of laboratory, radiographic, and endoscopic testing (see Table 2–5). Underscoring the need for the thorough testing, in one series of 31 children with migraine headaches associated with nausea, vomiting, and abdominal pain, 29 (94%) were found to have esophagitis, gastritis, or duodenitis.[118] The diagnosis of abdominal migraine can be made by the historical criteria of stereotypic episodes of abdominal pain with vomiting associated with pallor and lethargy, and a family history of migraine headaches (see Table 2–7).[90, 91] Although vomiting can occur in the ictal phase,[92] abdominal epilepsy[119] accompanied by electroencephalographic changes[120] now appears to be a rare cause of vomiting and abdominal pain.[96]

**TABLE 2–7. Diagnostic Criteria for Cyclic Vomiting and Abdominal Migraine**[90, 91, 107]

| VARIABLE | CYCLIC VOMITING SYNDROME | ABDOMINAL MIGRAINE |
|---|---|---|
| Temporal pattern | Recurrent stereotypic episodes of *vomiting* lasting hours | Recurrent stereotypic episodes of midline *abdominal pain* lasting > 6 hours |
| Associated symptoms | Pallor, lethargy, anorexia, nausea, retching, *abdominal pain* | Pallor, lethargy, anorexia, nausea, *vomiting* |
| Family history | No family history of migraine | Family history of migraine |
| Laboratory testing | Negative laboratory, radiographic, and endoscopic tests | Negative laboratory, radiographic and endoscopic tests |
| Therapeutic response | May or may not respond to antimigraine therapy | Positive response to antimigraine therapy |

In the absence of known disease, treatment remains empiric and includes supportive therapy, antiemetics, antimigraine agents, prokinetic agents, and neuroleptic medications (Table 2–8).[121] Promising therapies include newer serotoninergic agents, both $5\text{-HT}_3$ antiemetics (e.g., ondansetron) and the $5\text{-HT}_{1D}$ (e.g., sumatriptan) antimigraine agent. In the absence of rigorous therapeutic trials, no definitive recommendations can be made. Supportive therapy, especially intravenous fluids containing dextrose, can attenuate the episode, perhaps by terminating the ketosis.[59] Potent $5\text{-HT}_3$ antagonist antiemetics (e.g., ondansetron) have been used as abortive agents, with encouraging results.[122] Antimigraine agents have been used successfully both as prophylactic (e.g., low-dose propranolol) and abortive agents, including (e.g., sumatriptan), further supporting the putative relationship to migraine phenomena.[59, 103, 104] Blunting the estrogen decline with low-estrogen birth control pills has been helpful for catamenial (menstrual) migraines in teenage girls.[124, 125] Low-dose erythromycin used as a gastric prokinetic agent appears effective both as a prophylactic and an abortive agent.[123] In this frustrating illness, with its disruptive, unpredictable occurrence, high level of morbidity, lack of definitive diagnosis and established therapy, parental support from the physician may by itself serve to relieve family stress and reduce the frequency of episodes.[97]

## Postoperative Nausea and Vomiting

The incidence of postoperative nausea and vomiting in children is 20% to 24% after elective operations, including strabismus repair, tonsillectomy, dental surgery, and inguinal herniorraphy.[126, 127] Although the mechanisms have not been elucidated, there appear to be a number of risk factors for the development of postoperative vomiting. These include age greater than 2 years, female gender, certain operations (tonsillectomies, strabismus repair, otoplasties, and ureter surgery have greater risk than endoscopy and appendectomy), anesthetic used (cyclopropane has greater risk than

**TABLE 2–8. Medications Used to Treat Cyclic Vomiting Syndrome and Abdominal Migraine**[59–61, 99–101, 121–123]

| DRUG CLASS | BRAND NAME | DOSAGE | MECHANISMS OF ACTION | SIDE EFFECTS | COMMENTS |
|---|---|---|---|---|---|
| **ABORTIFACIENT** | | | | | |
| ***Supportive*** | | | | | |
| IV hydration | | | Stops ketosis, replaces $Na^+$, $K^+$, and lost volume | | Glucose may be most effective component by terminating ketosis |
| Lorazepam | Ativan | 0.05–0.1 mg/kg IV or PO q 6 hr | Central enhanced GABA-ergic inhibition inducing sedation, anxiolysis, and amnesia | Sedation, respiratory depression | Adjunct to allow child to sleep |
| ***Antimigraine*** | | | | | |
| Isometheptene | Midrin | Age $>$12 yr, 1 capsule/hr PO but $\leq$5 capsules q 24 hr | Sympathomimetic vasoconstrictor | Dizziness | Not effective in vomiting child |
| Sumatriptan | Imitrex | Age $>$12 yr; 6 mg SC, may repeat in 1 hr (maximum dose: 2 injections/24 hr) | 5-$HT_{1D}$ agonist induces cerebral vasoconstriction, relaxes gastric fundus | Transient burning in neck and chest, headache | Use SC form if child is vomiting<br>Contraindicated with coronary vasospasm or hemiplegic or basilar artery migraine |
| Ketorolac | Toradol | 0.5–1.0 mg/kg IV/IM $\times$ 1, then 0.2–0.5 mg/kg q 6–8 hr | Cyclooxygenase inhibitor of prostaglandin synthesis | GI bleeding, contraindicated in ASA sensitivity | Can be given intravenously<br>Contraindicated with ASA sensitivity |
| ***Antiemetic*** | | | | | |
| Ondansetron | Zofran | 0.15 mg/kg IV q 8 hr | 5-$HT_3$ antagonist in CTZ and vagal afferents in gut | Headache | Use IV form if child is vomiting |
| Granisetron | Kytril | 10 μg/kg IV q 6–8 hr | | | |
| Tropisetron | | | | | |
| **PROPHYLACTIC** | | | | | |
| ***Antimigraine*** | | | | | |
| Propranolol | Inderal | 0.5–1 mg/kg/day maximum PO divided bid or tid; 10–20 mg tid | $\beta_1$-, $\beta_2$-adrenergic antagonist | Hypotension, bradycardia, fatigability | Use in small doses<br>Contraindicated in asthma, heart block<br>Withdraw gradually, monitor pulse |
| Atenolol | Tenormin | 0.7–1.4 mg/kg/day PO divided bid or tid | $\beta_1$-adrenergic antagonist | | |

| | | | | | |
|---|---|---|---|---|---|
| Cyproheptadine | Periactin | 0.25 mg/kg/day PO divided bid or tid | $H_1$ antagonist and 5-$HT_2$ antagonist | Sedation, anticholinergic effects,* weight gain due to appetite stimulation | Contraindicated with asthma, MAO inhibitors, GI obstruction |
| Pizotyline | Sandomigran | 1.5 mg/day divided qd or tid | | | Not available in U.S. |
| Amitriptyline | Elavil | 1.5–3 mg/kg/day PO divided qd or tid<br>Age <6 yr, 10–30 mg/day<br>6–12 yr, 50–100 mg/day<br>>12 yr, 100–200 mg/day | Tricyclic antidepressant, increases synaptic norepinephrine, 5-$HT_2$ antagonist | Sedation, anticholinergic effects* | Contraindicated with SVT, MAO inhibitor, GI obstruction<br>Monitor therapeutic levels |
| Nortriptyline | Pamelor | 1–3 mg/kg/day PO divided qd or tid | | | |
| ***Neuroleptic*** | | | | | |
| Phenobarbital | Luminal | 2–3 mg/kg/day PO divided qd or bid | $GABA_A$ potentiation of synaptic inhibition | Sedation | Contraindicated with acute intermittent porphyria, abdominal epilepsy |
| Phenytoin | Dilantin | 4–8 mg/kg/day PO divided bid or tid | Slows $Na^+$ and $Ca^{2+}$ channel activation | Gingival hyperplasia | Abdominal epilepsy |
| Carbamazepine | Tegretol | Age <6 yr, 10–20 mg/kg/day PO divided bid or tid<br>6–12 yr, 400–800 mg/day PO divided bid or tid<br>>12 yr, 600–1200 mg/day PO divided bid or tid | Slows $Na^+$ channel activation | Sedation, anticholinergic effects* | Contraindicated with MAO inhibitors |
| ***Prokinetic*** | | | | | |
| Erythromycin | Erythromycin Pediamycin, E-mycin | 20 mg/kg/day PO divided qid | Motilin agonist stimulates gastric motility | Gastric cramps in larger doses | Use in small, prokinetic doses 5–20 mg/kg/day, gastroparesis |
| Cisapride | Propulsid | 0.1–0.3 mg/kg dose PO tid or qid | 5-$HT_4$ agonist with ACh release in gut | Diarrhea, abdominal pain, headache | Can cause arrhythmias with imidazole antifungals and macrolide antibiotics, gastroparesis |
| ***Birth Control*** | | | | | |
| Norethindrone/ ethinyl estradiol | Loestrin | | Attenuates estrogen drop before onset of menses | Estrogen effects | Catamenial migraines |

*Anticholinergic effects include blurred vision, dry mouth, hypotension, palpitations, and urinary retention.
ACh, acetylcholine; ASA, acetylsalicylic acid; CTZ, chemotrigger zone; GABA, γ-aminobutyric acid; 5-HT, 5-hydroxytryptamine; MAO, monamine oxidase inhibitor; SVT, supraventricular tachycardia.

isoflurane, enflurane, and halothane), postoperative opioid analgesia, prior postoperative vomiting, and a history of motion sickness.[126, 128]

A number of recent randomized, double-blind, placebo-controlled trials have established that 5-$HT_3$ antagonists reduce postoperative emesis after general anesthesia in preadolescent children undergoing strabismus correction,[129] tonsillectomy,[130] and other elective operations[131] with the exception of craniotomy.[132] Head-to-head comparisons have established the superior efficacy of 5-$HT_3$ antagonists to those commonly used medications, including droperidol[130, 133, 134] and metoclopramide.[130] Although single intravenous intraoperative doses of either ondansetron (0.15 mg/kg)[135] and granisetron (0.4 μg/kg) appear equally effective during the first 4 hours,[135, 136] some studies detect a prolonged effect lasting 24 hours.[129] In the ambulatory surgery setting, the time to discharge was reduced by the use of serotoninergic agents.[134, 137] Ketorolac used for postoperative analgesia provided equivalent pain relief to morphine but with significantly less vomiting.[138]

## Chemotherapy-Induced Emesis

The current theories by which chemotherapy induces emesis include injury to the GI tract with release of mediators, direct action on the vomiting center and chemotrigger zone, and learned (anticipatory) responses.[139] Factors known to increase the incidence of vomiting in response to chemotherapy include young age (toddlers), female gender, emetogenicity of the agent (high, cisplatin; moderate, cyclophosphamide; mild, methotrexate), dose and rate of administration (slow infusion is less emetogenic). In one study of children, chemotherapy increased urinary serotonin and hydroxyindole acetic acid (5-HIAA) excretion, whereas serotonin antagonists diminished the vomiting and 5-HIAA excretion, thus implicating serotonin in the pathophysiologic cascade.[140]

The new 5-$HT_3$ antagonists are more efficacious than former regimens that included metoclopramide-dexamethasone and chlorpromazine-dexamethasone combinations.[141, 142] All three 5-$HT_3$ antagonists—ondansetron,[143] 3 mg/m$^2$; granisetron 10 μg/kg,[144, 145] and tropisetron 0.2 mg/kg[146]—have similar rates (75% to 96%) of complete or major control of chemotherapy-induced vomiting. Many subjects had failed standard regimens that included metoclopramide.[147] Few side effects were noted except for headache (ondansetron) and constipation (tropisetron). These 5-$HT_3$ agents appear to be more effective on the emesis that occurs within the first 24 hours than 1 to 2 weeks after administration of chemotherapy.[141] These 5-$HT_3$ agents were effective on repeated cycles of chemotherapy without loss of efficacy, could be potentiated by dexamethasone,[148] and were more effective in larger than standard doses with no additional adverse effects.[149] The 5-$HT_3$ agents also appear to be effective in controlling radiotherapy-induced emesis.[150]

## Psychogenic Vomiting

Although the term *psychogenic vomiting* has been used as a diagnosis of exclusion when no organic cause can be found, the term is not ideal—for several reasons. First, one study demonstrated that all children initially labeled as having psychogenic vomiting were found during endoscopic evaluation to have mucosal injuries of the upper GI tract.[151] Although the percentage may be high, that study illustrates the diagnostic challenge. That is, the use of more sensitive diagnostic modalities such as endoscopic biopsy and GI motility studies appear to enable more of those suspected to have psychogenic vomiting to be diagnosed with organic disease.[152] Second, careful case studies indicate that both organic and psychological factors coexist (e.g., *H. pylori* gastritis associated with anxiety-induced vomiting); thus, individual patients cannot easily be classified into either organic or psychogenic categories.[153]

Studies of psychogenic vomiting patients reveal some common predisposing factors, including a symbiotic relationship between parent and affected child, a family history of vomiting, and exogenous depression or conversion reaction secondary to the loss of a parent. To make a positive diagnosis of psychogenic vomiting, Gonzalez-Heydrich and coworkers have suggested that, in addition to the absence of positive test results one of the following psychological criteria be included: (1) vomiting as a somatic expression of anxiety; (2) cultural or family conflict or specific traumatic event with primary or secondary gain; and (3) vomiting as manipulative behavior act, including malingering or Munchausen by proxy.[153] Although one group has suggested that varying temporal patterns of vomiting may reflect different underlying psychopathologies—a cyclic pattern is associated with a higher incidence of conversion reactions and the postprandial pattern is more typical of depression—these associations remain to be confirmed in other studies.[154]

***Acknowledgments***

The authors gratefully acknowledge Jennifer Robbins and Michelle Burd for their help in organizing the cyclic vomiting patient database and references, respectively.

**REFERENCES**

1. Davis CJ, Harding RK, Leslie RA, et al: The organisation of vomiting as a protective reflex: a commentary on the first day's discussions. In Davis CJ, Lake-Bakaar GV, Grahame-Smith DG (eds): Nausea and Vomiting: Mechanisms and Treatment. Berlin, Springer-Verlag, 1986, p 65.
2. Borison HL, Wang SC: Physiology and pharmacology of vomiting. Pharmacol Rev 1953;5:193.
3. Lumsden K, Holden WS: The act of vomiting in man. Gut 1969;10:173.
4. Brizzee KR: Mechanics of vomiting: a minireview. Can J Physiol Pharmacol 1990;68:221.
5. Grundy D, Reid K: The physiology of nausea and vomiting. In Johnson LR (ed): Physiology of the Gastrointestinal Tract. New York, Raven Press, 1994, pp 879–901.
6. Lang IM: Digestive tract motor correlates of vomiting and nausea. Can J Physiol Pharmacol 1990;68:242.
7. Lang IM, Marvig J, Sarna SK, et al: Gastrointestinal myoelectric correlates of vomiting in the dog. Am J Physiol 1986;251:G830.
8. Lang IM, Sarna SK, Condon RE: Gastrointestinal motor correlates of vomiting in the dog: quantification and characterization as an independent phenomenon. Gastroenterology 1986;90:40.
9. Lang IM, Sarna SK, Dodds WJ: Pharyngeal, esophageal, and proximal gastric responses associated with vomiting. Am J Physiol 1993;265:G963.
10. Smith CC, Brizzee KR: Cineradiographic analysis of vomiting in the

cat. I. Lower esophagus, stomach, and small intestine. Gastroenterology 1961;40:654.
11. Thompson DG, Malagelada J-R: Vomiting and the small intestine. Dig Dis Sci 1982;27:1121.
12. Ehrlein H-J: Retroperistaltis and duodenogastric reflux in dogs. Scand J Gastroenterol 1981;67(suppl):29.
13. McCarthy LE, Borison HL: Respiratory mechanics of vomiting in decerebrate cats. Am J Physiol 1974;226:738.
14. Abe T, Kusuhara N, Katagiri H, et al: Differential function of the costal and crucal diaphragm during emesis in canines. Respiration Physiol 1993;91:183.
15. Abe T, Kieser TM, Tomita T, et al: Respiratory muscle function during emesis in awake canines. J Appl Physiol 1994;76:2552.
16. Koch KL: Motion sickness. In Sleisenger MH (ed): The Handbook of Nausea and Vomiting. Pawling, NY, Caduceus, 1993, p 43.
17. Miller AD: Motion-induced nausea and vomiting. In Kucharczyk J, Stewart DJ, Miller AD (ed): Nausea and Vomiting: Recent Research and Clinical Advances. Boca Raton, FL, CRC Press, 1991, p 13.
18. Stern RM, Koch KL, Stewart WR, et al: Spectral analysis of tachygastria recorded during motion sickness. Gastroenterology 1987;92:92.
19. Hasler WL, Kim MS, Chey WD, et al: Central cholinergic and α-adrenergic mediation of gastric slow wave dysrhythmias evoked during motion sickness. Am J Physiol 1995;268:G539.
20. Kucharczyk J, Stewart DJ, Miller AD (ed): Nausea and Vomiting: Recent Research and Clinical Advances. Boca Raton, FL, CRC, 1991, p 1.
21. Sleisenger MH (ed): The Handbook of Nausea and Vomiting. Pawling, NY, Caduceus, 1993, p 1.
22. Andrews PLR, Davis CJ, Bingham S, et al: The abdominal visceral innervation and the emetic reflex: pathways, pharmacology, and plasticity. Can J Physiol Pharmacol 1990;68:325.
23. Kalia M, Mesulam MM: Brain stem projections of sensory and motor components of the vagus complex in the cat: II. Laryngeal, tracheobronchial, pulmonary, cardiac, and gastrointestinal branches. J Comp Neurol 1980;193:467.
24. Gwyn DG, Leslie RA, Hopkins DA: Observations on the afferent and efferent organization of the vagus nerve and the innervation of the stomach in the squirrel monkey. J Comp Neurol 1985;239:163.
25. Wang SC, Borison HL: A new concept of organization of the central emetic mechanism: recent studies on the sites of action of apomorphine, copper sulfate and cardiac glycosides. Gastroenterology 1952;22:1.
26. Miller AD, Leslie RA: The area postrema and vomiting. Frontiers Neuroendocrinol 1994;15:301.
27. Borison HL: Area postrema: chemoreceptor circumventricular organ of the medulla oblongata. Prog Neurobiol 1989;32:351.
28. Schwartz J-C, Agid Y, Bouthenet M-L, et al: Neurochemical investigations into the human area postrema. In Davis CJ, Lake-Bakaar GV, Grahame-Smith DG (eds): Nausea and Vomiting: Mechanisms and Treatment. Berlin, Springer-Verlag, 1986, p 18.
29. Carpenter DO: Neural mechanisms of emesis. Can J Physiol Pharmacol 1990;68:230.
30. Jovanovic-Micic D, Samardzic R, Beleslin DB: The role of α-adrenergic mechanisms within the area postrema in dopamine-induced emesis. Eur J Pharmacol 1995;272:21.
31. Oman CM: Motion sickness: a synthesis and evaluation of the sensory conflict theory. Can J Physiol Pharmacol 1990;68:294.
32. Money KE: Motion sickness. Physiological Rev 1970;50:1.
33. Takeda N, Morita M, Hasegawa S, et al: Neuropharmacology of motion sickness and emesis. Acta Otolaryngol(Stockh) 1993; 501(suppl):10.
34. Lawes INC: The origin of the vomiting response: a neuroanatomical hypothesis. Can J Physiol Pharmacol 1990;68:254.
35. Lawes INC: The central connections of area postrema define the paraventricular system involved in antinoxious behaviors. In Kucharczyk J, Stewart DJ, Miller AD (ed): Nausea and Vomiting: Recent Research and Clinical Advances. Boca Raton, FL, CRC, 1991, p 77.
36. Miller AD, Nonaka S, Jakus J: Brain areas essential or non-essential for emesis. Brain Res 1994;647:255.
37. Miller AD, Ruggiero DA: Emetic reflex arc revealed by expression of the immediate-early gene *c-fos* in the cat. J Neurosci 1994:14;871.
38. Stefanini E, Clement-Cormier Y: Detection of dopamine receptors in the area postrema. Eur J Pharmacol 1981;74:257.
39. Yoshikawa T, Yoshida N, Hosoki K: Involvement of dopamine $D_3$ receptors in the area postrema in R(+)-7-OH-DPAT-induced emesis in the ferret. Eur J Pharmacol 1996;301:143.
40. Launay JM, Callebert J, Bondoux D, et al: Serotonin receptors and therapeutics. Cell Molec Biol 1994;40:327.
41. Cubeddu LX, Hoffmann IS, Fuenmayor NT, et al: Efficacy of ondansetron (GR 38032F) and the role of serotonin in cisplatin-induced nausea and vomiting. N Engl J Med 1990;322:810.
42. Cubeddu LX: Serotonin mechanisms in chemotherapy-induced emesis in cancer patients. Oncology 1996;53(suppl 1):18.
43. Naylor RJ, Rudd JA: Mechanisms of chemotherapy/radiotherapy-induced emesis in animal models. Oncology 1996;53(suppl 1):8.
44. Fukui H, Yamamoto M, Sasaki S, et al: Involvement of 5-$HT_3$ receptors and vagal afferents in copper sulfate– and cisplatin-induced emesis in monkeys. Eur J Pharmacol 1993;249:13.
45. Schwartz SM, Goldberg MJ, Gidda JS, et al: Effect of zatosetron on ipecac-induced emesis in dogs and healthy men. J Clin Pharmacol 1994;34:250.
46. Leslie RA, Reynolds DJM, Andrews PLR, et al: Evidence for presynaptic 5-hydroxytryptamine$_3$ recognition sites on vagal afferent terminals in the brainstem of the ferret. Neuroscience 1990;38:667.
47. Ohuoha DC, Knable MB, Wolf SS, et al: The subnuclear distribution of 5-$HT_3$ receptors in the human nucleus of the solitary tract and other structures of the caudal medulla. Brain Res 1994;637:222.
48. Fukui H, Yamamoto M, Ando T, et al: Increase in serotonin levels in the dog ileum and blood by cisplatin as measured by microdialysis. Neuropharmacology 1993;32:959.
49. Gale JD: Serotonergic mediation of vomiting. J Pediatr Gastroenterol Nutr 1995;21(suppl 1):S22.
50. Fukui H, Yamamoto M, Sasaki S, et al: Possible involvement of peripheral 5-$HT_4$ receptors in copper sulfate–induced vomiting in dogs. Eur J Pharmacol 1994;257:47.
51. Lucot JB, Crampton GH: Buspirone blocks motion sickness and xylazine-induced emesis in the cat. Aviat Space Environ Med 1987;58:989.
52. Lucot JB, Crampton GH: Buspirone blocks cisplatin-induced emesis in cats. J Clin Pharmacol 1987;27:817.
53. Regoli D, Boudon A, Fauchere JL: Receptors and antagonists for substance P and related peptides. Pharmacol Rev 1994;46:551.
54. Sundler F, Alumets J, Hkanson R: 5-Hydroxytryptamine–containing enterochromaffin cells: Storage site of substance P. Acta Physiol Scand Suppl 1977;452:121.
55. Gardner CJ, Twissell DJ, Dale TJ, et al: The broad-spectrum antiemetic activity of the novel non-peptide tachykinin $NK_1$ receptor antagonist GR203040. Br J Pharmacol 1995;116:3158.
56. Bountra C, Gale JD, Gardner CJ, et al: Toward understanding the aetiology and pathophysiology of the emetic reflex: novel approaches to antiemetic drugs. Oncology 1996;53(suppl 1):102.
57. Lucot JB, Obach RS, McLean S, et al: The effect of CP-99994 on the responses to provocative motion in the cat. Br J Pharmacol 1997;120:116.
58. Tattersall FD, Rycroft W, Francis B, et al: Tachykinin $NK_1$ receptor antagonists act centrally to inhibit emesis induced by the chemotherapeutic agent cisplatin in ferrets. Neuropharmacology 1996;35:1121.
59. Pfau BT, Li BUK, Murray RD, et al: Differentiating cyclic vomiting from chronic vomiting patterns in children: quantitative criteria and diagnostic implications. Pediatrics 1996;97:364.
60. Li BUK: Cyclic vomiting: new understanding of an old disorder. Contemp Pediatr 1996;13:48.
61. Fleisher DR, Matar M: The cyclic vomiting syndrome: a report of 71 cases and literature review. J Pediatr Gastroenterol Nutr 1993;17:361.
62. Nixon HH, Tawes R: Etiology and treatment of small intestinal atresia: analysis of a series of 127 jejunoileal atresias and comparison with 62 duodenal atresias. Surgery 1971;69:45.
63. Brown RA, Millar AJ, Linegar A, et al: Fenestrated duodenal membranes: an analysis of symptoms, signs, diagnosis, and treatment. J Pediatr Surg 1994;29:429.
64. Favara BE, Franciosi RA, Akers DR: Enteric duplications, 37 cases: a vascular theory of pathogenesis. Am J Dis Child 1971;122, 501.
65. Park RW, Grand RJ: Gastrointestinal manifestations of cystic fibrosis: a review. Gastroenterology 1981;81:1143.
66. Brandt ML, Pokorny WJ, McGill CW, et al: Late presentations of midgut malrotation in children. Am J Surg 1985;150:767.
67. Kealey WD, McCallion WA, Brown S, et al: Midgut volvulus in children. Br J Surg 1996;83:105.
68. Reijnen JA, Festen C, Van Roosmalen RP: Intussusception: factors related to treatment. Arch Dis Child 1990;65:871.
69. Holgersen LO, Stanley-Brown EG: Acute appendicitis with perforation. Am J Dis Child 1971;122:288.

70. Hines JR, Gore RM, Ballantyne GH: Superior mesenteric artery syndrome: diagnostic criteria and therapeutic approaches. Am J Surg 1984;148:630.
71. Dickerman JD, Colletti RB, Tampas JP: Gastric outlet obstruction in chronic granulomatous disease of childhood. Am J Dis Child 1986;140:567.
72. Sferra TJ, Pawel BR, Qualman SJ, et al: Ménétrier disease of childhood: role of cytomegalovirus and transforming growth factor α. J Pediatr 1996;128:213.
73. Meyerovitz MF, Fellows KE: Typhlitis: a cause of gastrointestinal hemorrhage in children. Am J Radiol 1984;143:833.
74. Jaehoon JO, Chung HK: Gastroparesis after a presumed viral illness: clinical and laboratory features and natural history. Mayo Clin Proc 1990;65:636.
75. Schuffler MD: Chronic intestinal pseudo-obstruction: progress and problems. J Pediatr Gastroenterol Nutr 1990;10:157.
76. Axelrod FB, Gouge TH, Ginsberg HB, et al: Fundoplication and gastrostomy in familial dysautonomia. J Pediatr 1990;118:388.
77. Lugo-Vicente HL: Gallbladder dyskinesia in children. J Soc Laparoendosc Surg 1997;1:61.
78. Woods M, Greenes D: An 11-year-old boy with vomiting, dehydration, and a tan complexion. Curr Opin Pediatr 1995;7:472.
79. Carney JA, Hayles AB: Alimentary tract manifestations of multiple endocrine neoplasia, type 2b. Mayo Clin Proc 1977;52:543.
80. Chow CW, Sudha S, Campbell PE, et al: Malignant carcinoid tumors in children. Cancer 1982;49:802.
81. Buchta RM, Kaplan JM: Zollinger-Ellison syndrome in a nine year old child: case report and review of this entity in childhood. Pediatrics 1971;47:594.
82. Hale DE, Bennett MJ: Fatty acid oxidation disorders: a new class of metabolic diseases. J Pediatr 1992;121:1.
83. Rowe PC, Newman SL, Brusilow SW: Natural history of symptomatic partial ornithine transcarbamylase deficiency. N Engl J Med 1986;314:541.
84. Hirano M, Pavlakis SG: Mitochondrial myopathy, encephalopathy, lactic acidosis, and stroke-like episodes (MELAS): current concepts. J Child Neurol 1993;9:4.
85. Stein JA, Tschudy DP: Acute intermittent porphyria: a clinical and biochemical study of 46 patients. Medicine 1970;49:1.
86. Swischuk LE: Nausea, vomiting, and diarrhea in an older child. Pediatr Emerg Care 1993;9:307.
87. Baker RS, Baumann RJ, Buncie JR: Idiopathic intracranial hypertension (pseudotumor cerebri) in pediatric patients. Pediatr Neurol 1989;5:5.
88. Jan MM, Camfield PR, Grodon K, et al: Vomiting after mild head injury is related to migraine. J Pediatr 1997;130:134.
89. Edgeworth J, Bullock P, Bailey A, et al: Why are brain tumours still being missed? Arch Dis Child 1995;74:148.
90. Lundberg PO: Abdominal migraine—diagnosis and therapy. Headache 1975;15:122.
91. Symon DNK, Russell G: Abdominal migraine: a childhood syndrome defined. Cephalalgia 1986;6:223.
92. Panayiotopoulos CP: Vomiting as an ictal manifestation of epileptic seizures and syndromes. J Neurol Neurosurg Psychiatr 1988;51:1448.
93. Hoyt CS, Stickler GB: A study of 44 children with the syndrome of recurrent vomiting. Pediatrics 1960;25:775.
94. McClung HJ, Murray RD, Braden NJ, et al: Intentional ipecac poisoning of children. Am J Dis Child 1988;142:637.
95. Lanzi G, Ballotin U, Ottolini A, et al: Cyclic vomiting and recurrent abdominal pains as migraine or epileptic equivalents. Cephalalgia 1983;3:115.
96. Papatheophilou R, Jeavons PM, Disney ME: Recurrent abdominal pain: A clinical and EEG study. Dev Med Child Neurol 1972;14:31.
97. Fleisher DR: Cyclic vomiting. In Hyman PE, DiLorenzo C (eds): Pediatric Gastroenterology Motility Disorders. New York, Academy Professional Information Services, 1994, pp 89–103.
98. Breaux CW, Hood JS, Georgeson KE: The significance of alkalosis and hypochloremia in hypertrophic pyloric stenosis. J Pediatr Surg 1989;24:1250.
99. Benitz WE: The Pediatric Drug Handbook. Chicago: Mosby–Year Book, 1995.
100. Pagliaro LA, Pagliaro AM: Problems in Pediatric Drug Therapy. Hamilton, Ill, Drug Intelligence Publications, 1995.
101. US Pharmacopeial Convention: Drug Information for the Health Care Professional. Rockville, MD, US Pharmacopeial Convention, Inc, 1997.
102. Linder SL: Subcutaneous sumatriptan in the clinical setting: the first 50 consecutive patients with acute migraine in a pediatric neurology office practice. Headache J 1996;36:419.
103. Benson J, Zorn S, Book L: Sumatriptan [Imitrex] in the treatment of cyclic vomiting. Ann Pharmacol 1995;29:997.
104. Huang S, Lavine JE: Efficacy of sumatriptan in aborting attacks of cyclic vomiting syndrome. Gastroenterology 1997;112:A751.
105. Abu-Arafeh I, Russell G: Cyclical vomiting syndrome in children: a population based study. J Pediatr Gastroenterol Nutr 1995;21:454.
106. Gee S: On fitful or recurrent vomiting. St Bart Hosp Rep 1882;18:1.
107. Li BUK (ed): Cyclic vomiting syndrome: Proceedings of the International Scientific Symposium. J Pediatr Gastroenterol Nutr 1995; 21(suppl):Svi.
108. Li BUK: Cyclic vomiting: The pattern and syndrome paradigm. In Li BUK (ed): Cyclic Vomiting Syndrome: Proceedings of the International Scientific Symposium. J Pediatr Gastroenterol Nutr 1995; 21(suppl):S6.
109. Li BUK: Cyclic vomiting syndrome: a pediatric Rorschach test. J Pediatr Gastroenterol Nutr 1993;17:351.
110. Smith CH: Recurrent vomiting in children: its etiology and treatment. J Pediatr 1937;10:719.
111. Pfau BT, Li BUK, Murray RD, et al: Cyclic vomiting in children: a migraine equivalent? Gastroenterology 1992;102:A23.
112. Mortimer MJ, Good PA: The VER as a diagnostic marker for childhood abdominal migraine. Headache 1990;30:642.
113. Rashed H, Abell TL, Cardoso J: Cyclic vomiting syndrome is associated with a distinct adrenergic abnormality. Gastroenterology 1997;112:A901.
114. Wolff SM, Adler R: A syndrome of periodic hypothalamic discharge. Am J Med 1964;36:956.
115. Sato T, Igarashi M, Minami S, et al: Recurrent attacks of vomiting, hypertension, and psychotic depression: a syndrome of periodic catecholamine and prostaglandin discharge. Acta Endocrinol 1988; 117:189.
116. Pasricha P, Schuster M, Saudek C, et al: Cyclic vomiting: association with multiple homeostatic abnormalities and response to ketorolac. Am J Gastroenterol 1996;91:2228–2232.
117. Chong SKF, Nowak TV, Goddard M, et al: Abnormal gastric emptying and myoelectrical activity in cyclic vomiting syndrome. Gastroenterology 1997;112:A712.
118. Mavromichalis I, Zaramboukas T, Giala MM: Migraine of gastrointestinal origin. Eur J Pediatr 1995;154:406.
119. Douglas EF, White PT: Abdominal epilepsy—a reappraisal. J Pediatr 1971;78:59.
120. Millichap JH, Lombroso CT, Lennox MD: Cyclic vomiting as a form of epilepsy in children. Pediatrics 1955;15:705.
121. Igarashi M, May WN, Golden GS: Pharmacological treatment of childhood migraine. J Pediatr 1992;120:653.
122. Fleisher DR: Management of cyclic vomiting syndrome. In Li BUK (ed): Cyclic vomiting syndrome: Proceedings of the International Scientific Symposium. J Pediatr Gastroenterol Nutr 1995:21(suppl 1):S52.
123. Vanderhoof JA, Young R, Kaufmann SS, et al: Treatment of cyclic vomiting syndrome in childhood with erythromycin. J Pediatr Gastroenterol Nutr 1993;17:387.
124. Edelson RN: Menstrual migraine and other hormonal aspects of migraine. Headache 1985;25:376.
125. Welch KMA, Darnley D, Simkins RT: The role of estrogen in migraine: a review and hypothesis. Cephalalgia 1984;4:227.
126. Kermode J, Walker S, Webb I: Postoperative vomiting in children. Anaesth Intens Care 1995;23:196.
127. Sossai R, Johr M, Kistler W, et al: Postoperative vomiting in children. A persisting unsolved problem. Eur J Pediatr Surg 1993;3:206.
128. Kenny GN: Risk factors for postoperative nausea and vomiting. Anaesthesia 1994;49:6.
129. Rose JB, Martin TM, Corddry DH, et al: Ondansetron reduces the incidence and severity of poststrabismus repair vomiting in children. Anesth Analg 1994;79:489.
130. Furst SR, Rodarte A: Prophylactic antiemetic treatment with ondansetron in children undergoing tonsillectomy. Anesthesiology 1994;81:799.
131. Rust M, Cohen LA: Single oral dose ondansetron in the prevention of postoperative nausea and emesis. The European and US study groups. Anaesthesia 1994;49:16.
132. Furst SR, Sullivan LJ, Soriano SG, et al: Effects of ondansetron on

emesis in the first 24 hours after craniotomy in children. Anesth Analg 1996;83:325.
133. Splinter WM, Rhine EJ, Roberts DW, et al: Ondansetron is a better prophylactic antiemetic than droperidol for tonsillectomy in children. Can J Anaesth 1995;42:848.
134. Davis PJ, McGowan FX Jr, Lansman I, et al: Effect of antiemetic therapy on recovery and hospital discharge time. A double-blind assessment of ondansetron, droperidol, and placebo in pediatric patients undergoing ambulatory surgery. Anesthesiology 1995;83:956.
135. Rose JB, Brenn BR, Corddry DH, et al: Preoperative oral ondansetron for pediatric tonsillectomy. Anesth Analg 1996;82:558.
136. Ummenhofer W, Frei FJ, Urwyler A, et al: Effects of ondansetron in the prevention of postoperative nausea and vomiting in children. Anesthesiology 1994;81:804.
137. Khalil S, Rodarte A, Weldon BC, et al: Intravenous ondansetron in established postoperative emesis in children. Anesthesiology 1996;85:270.
138. Purday JP, Reichert CC, Merrick PM: Comparative effects of three doses of intravenous ketorolac or morphine on emesis and analgesia for restorative dental surgery in children. Can J Anaesth 1996;43:221.
139. Grunberg SM, Hesketh PJ: Control of chemotherapy-induced emesis. N Engl J Med 1993;329:1790.
140. Matera MG, DiTullio M, Lucarelli C, et al: Ondansetron, an antagonist of 5-$HT_3$ receptors, in the treatment of antineoplastic drug-induced nausea and vomiting in children. J Med 1993;24:161.
141. Dick GS, Meller ST, Pinkerton CR: Randomized comparison of ondansetron and metoclopramide plus dexamethasone for chemotherapy induced emesis. Arch Dis Child 1995;71:243.
142. Miyajima Y, Numata S, Katayama I, et al: Prevention of chemotherapy-induced emesis with granisetron in children with malignant diseases. Am J Pediatr Hematol-Oncol 1994;16:236.
143. Pinkerton CR, Williams D, Wootton C, et al: 5-$HT_3$ antagonist ondansetron—an effective outpatient antiemetic in cancer treatment. Arch Dis Child 1990;65:822.
144. Craft AW, Price L, Eden OB, et al: Granisetron and antiemetic therapy in children with cancer. Med Pediatr Oncol 1995;25:28.
145. Lemerle J, Amaral D, Southall DP, et al: Efficacy and safety of granisetron in the prevention of chemotherapy-induced emesis in paediatric patients. Eur J Cancer 1991;27:1081.
146. Benoit Y, Hulstaert F, Vermylen C, et al: Tropisetron in the prevention of nausea and vomiting in 131 children receiving cytotoxic chemotherapy. Med Pediatr Oncol 1995;25:457.
147. Jacobson SJ, Shore RW, Greenberg M, et al: The efficacy and safety of granisetron in pediatric cancer patients who had failed standard antiemetic therapy during anticancer chemotherapy. Am J Pediatr Hematol-Oncol 1994;16:231.
148. Alvarez O, Freeman A, Bedros A, et al: Randomized double-blind crossover ondansetron-dexamethasone versus ondansetron-placebo study for the treatment of chemotherapy-induced nausea and vomiting in pediatric patients with malignancies. J Pediatr Hematol Oncol 1995;17:145.
149. Brock P, Brichard B, Rechnitzer C, et al: An increased loading dose of ondansetron: a North European, double-blind randomized study in children, comparing 5 $mg/m^2$ with 10 $mg/m^2$. Eur J Cancer 1996;32:1744.
150. Miralbell R, Coucke P, Behrouz F, et al: Nausea and vomiting in fractionated radiotherapy: a prospective on-demand trial of tropisetron rescue for non-responders to metoclopramide. Eur J Cancer 1995;31:1461.
151. Stacher G: Differentialdiagnose psychosomatischer Schluckstörungen. Wien Klin Wochenschr 1986;98:648.
152. Abell TL, Kim CJ, Malagelada JR: Idiopathic cyclic nausea and vomiting: a disorder of gastrointestinal motility? Mayo Clin Proc 1988;63:1169.
153. Gonzalez-Heydrich J, Kerner JA, Steiner H: Testing the psychogenic vomiting diagnosis: four pediatric patients. Am J Dis Child 1991;145:913.
154. Muraoka M, Mine K, Matsumoto K, Nakai Y: Psychogenic vomiting: the relation between patterns of vomiting and psychiatric diagnoses. Gut 1990;31:526.

# Chapter 3

# Diarrhea

*Jon A. Vanderhoof*

Diarrhea is a common complaint in pediatrics. Evaluation of an infant or child with diarrhea requires an understanding of the pathophysiology of diarrhea as well as a basic understanding of fluid absorption. After a discussion of these topics, this chapter presents an approach to the differential diagnosis of both acute and chronic diarrhea in infants and children of various ages, with most specific entities discussed in greater detail elsewhere in the text. The division of diarrhea into acute and chronic is arbitrary, but most physicians accept a minimum duration of 3 weeks before labeling symptoms as chronic.

Diarrhea is most commonly defined as either an increase in the frequency or decrease in consistency of stool. Because there is considerable variation in stool number, volume, and consistency between individuals or in the same individual, the definition is somewhat imprecise. In adults, the stool volume averages approximately 100 g/day, the primary stool constituent being water.[1, 2] Increased fiber intake markedly increases daily stool volume.[3] Normal infants pass 5 to 10 g/kg/day, and stool volume in excess of 10 g/kg/day in infants is often considered diarrhea.[4] By age 3 years, stool volumes reach adult levels. Stool losses of more than 200 g/day are defined as diarrhea in both children and adults.

## FLUID ABSORPTION

Stool consistency is determined by many factors, including such dietary factors as fiber intake. In addition, fluid and electrolyte transport has a major role in determining stool consistency and volume. Fluid and electrolyte transport is a complex process, involving both transmembrane transport and transport through the paracellular pathway, the space between the epithelial cells.[5–7] A very high percentage of fluid and electrolytes is transported through the paracellular pathway in the proximal small intestine, because the "pores" or tight junctions between cells are large, allowing rapid osmotic flow both into and out of the upper gastrointestinal tract. It is this mechanism that rapidly renders the contents of the small intestine isotonic regardless of the osmolality on entering the small bowel. Distally in the small intestine and in the colon, there is less back diffusion of sodium and water, because the paracellular pathway is much less permeable and water and electrolytes are conserved to a much greater extent.

Sodium is absorbed either coupled with chloride or, in the case of the ileum and colon, by a sodium-hydrogen exchange process co-linked with the chloride-bicarbonate exchange process.[8, 9] Water is absorbed totally by passive diffusion, following an osmotic gradient created primarily by sodium. The sodium pump, sodium potassium adenosinetriphosphatase (ATPase), is located on the basolateral membrane of the enterocyte. It is this mechanism that is responsible for maintaining a low intracellular sodium content and creating a sodium gradient across the cell membrane. Sodium, therefore, enters the enterocyte through the brush border membrane and exits through the basolateral membrane. Sodium can likely enter through a number of mechanisms, including passive diffusion, specific sodium channels, and protein carriers linked with chloride. Glucocorticoids and mineralocorticoids may influence sodium transport through alterations in the sodium channel mechanism.[10] The relative importance of these different entry mechanisms may vary from the proximal to the distal small intestine and colon. Sodium also enters the cell through a coupled mechanism with monosaccharides and amino acids.[11, 12] These mechanisms serve as driving forces for glucose and amino acid absorption as well as electrolyte and fluid absorption.

All water movement in the intestine is determined by osmotic gradients created by solute transport.[13] When sodium is transported into the intracellular space adjacent to the epithelial cell, the high osmotic gradient in this compartment draws fluid through the intercellular space at the tight junctional end. Water and sodium then diffuse inward through the basement membrane into the interstitium and enter lymphatics and capillaries. A perijunctional actin-myosin complex appears to regulate the permeability of the paracellular pathway, permitting opening of the tight junctions and allowing absorption of additional nutrients and electrolytes from lumen to blood through the paracellular route.[14]

In addition to sodium, other electrolytes play a significant, albeit lesser, role in fluid absorption. In some instances, chloride may be actively secreted into the small intestine, acting as a major stimulant of fluid secretion.[15] Chloride conduction channels appear to be present in the apical membrane of the crypt cell, acting as a major mechanism for chloride secretion in response to a positive intracellular chloride gradient or changes in a number of intracellular messengers. In the small intestine, potassium is absorbed primarily through the paracellular pathway in response to fluid fluxes, that is, solvent drag and osmotic gradients. Active absorption of potassium through energy-dependent potassium hydrogen exchange in the apical membrane may be important in the more distal small intestine and colon, where the paracellular pathway is less permeable and transcellular absorption becomes the predominant force.[16] Bicarbonate absorption is accomplished through hydrogen secretion with resultant formation of carbon dioxide and water, which subsequently diffuse back into the blood. Active secretion of bicarbonate in the ileum occurs as part of the chloride absorption process through the chloride bicarbonate exchange mechanism.[17]

Regulation of fluid and electrolyte transport in the small intestine is a complex process. It appears to be under the control of a variety of regulatory mechanisms including endocrine factors and the enteric nervous system.[17–19] Gut flora, changes in the immune system, and dietary factors are also important. Gastrointestinal peptides and neurotransmitters, as well as exogenous agents including bacterial endotoxins, all alter cyclic adenosine monophosphate (AMP) in the intestinal epithelial cell, which markedly influences electrolyte transport.[20–23]

In addition to changes in fluid and electrolyte secretion, gut motility may also influence stool volume and consistency.[24, 25] Several factors influence motility. Motility is primarily under the control of the enteric nervous system, an intrinsic nervous system modulated to some degree through the autonomic nervous system. In addition, a variety of gastrointestinal hormones and neuropeptides may alter gut motility in response to numerous stimuli, including various dietary factors. This complex interrelationship is important in several pathophysiologic states that commonly affect infants and children.

Through the processes of absorption, secretion, and motility, a volume of fluid several times that of fluid consumption and stool output is commonly handled by the small intestine and colon. Approximately 9 L of fluid each day in the older child or adult traverses the ligament of Treitz.[25, 26] This fluid includes not only ingested food, but also secretions from the stomach, liver, pancreas, and duodenum, all of which must be reabsorbed along with the nutrients in the remainder of the gastrointestinal tract. This 9 L of fluid will be reduced to 1 L by the time it reaches the ileocecal valve and enters the colon.[27] The adult colon, with a normal absorptive capacity of 3 to 4 L/day, is quite capable of absorbing this volume of fluid in the non-pathologic state. However, once this capacity is exceeded, diarrhea results.[27]

## PATHOPHYSIOLOGY

Diarrhea is often subdivided based on pathophysiology (Table 3–1). Osmotic or secretory diarrhea, motility disorders, and inflammation and/or exudation are common categories, although overlap exists. In many disease states, more than one mechanism may be responsible for the diarrhea.

**TABLE 3–1. Mechanisms of Diarrhea**

| | |
|---|---|
| Osmotic | Motility |
| Secretory | Inflammatory |

### Osmotic Diarrhea

Osmotic diarrhea is a term applied when malabsorption of an absorbable solute creates an osmotic load in the distal small intestine and colon resulting in increased fluid losses.[28] This commonly occurs when carbohydrates, relatively small osmotically active particles, are malabsorbed.[29] If an ingested material is hypertonic, rapid flux of fluid across the duodenal epithelium results in isotonicity by the time the solution reaches the ligament of Treitz. In this process, significant amounts of fluid are secreted into the small intestine and must be reabsorbed more distally. The proximal small bowel is highly permeable to water and ions, and sodium and chloride are continually secreted in the upper small intestine across a concentration gradient. In the more distal small intestine and colon, permeability tightens and the osmotic pressure created by the malabsorbed carbohydrate resists the reabsorption of water normally driven by active transport of sodium and chloride. Active reabsorption of these ions in the distal small bowel in the absence of reabsorption of the malabsorbed carbohydrate results in enteric sodium concentrations much lower than that in plasma. Further metabolism of malabsorbed carbohydrate to short-chain fatty acids such as propionate and butyrate as well as hydrogen, $CO_2$, and methane may occur.[30] Although some of these short-chain fatty acids are reabsorbed in the colon, they exert an additional osmotic load further exacerbating osmotic diarrhea. A major characteristic of osmotic diarrhea is that it stops when feeding is discontinued. Secondly, it is characterized by a sizable gap in osmolality (usually greater that 50). The "osmotic gap" is calculated by the equation: ($Na^+$ in mEq/L) + ($K^+$ in mEq/L) × 2 = measured fecal osmolality in mOsm/kg. In the absence of osmotically active malabsorbed substances, two times the sum of the sodium and potassium concentrations should equal about 290. The lower electrolyte concentrations in osmotic diarrhea suggest that some other osmotic substance is contributing to the isotonic osmotic load in the fluid expelled from the colon. In infants, bacterial metabolism of the malabsorbed carbohydrate commonly results in a stool pH of less than 5.5, another characteristic feature of many types of osmotic diarrhea.

Malabsorption of carbohydrates in infants is usually caused by diffuse mucosal injury.[31, 32] There are some conditions in which carbohydrates are selectively malabsorbed, such as congenital sucrase isomaltase deficiency, or in the older child or adult, primary acquired lactase deficiency. In addition, laxative preparations such as lactulose or milk of magnesia may produce osmotic diarrhea. Excess carbohydrate malabsorption may occur in combination with hypermotility disorders such as irritable colon of infancy, in which large volumes of hypertonic juices rapidly traverse the small intestine, further exacerbating motility-induced diarrhea. In other instances, high carbohydrate feedings may exacerbate diarrhea in children recovering from acute viral enteritis whose absorptive process may be impaired. Juices containing large quantities of carbohydrates, such as apple juice, are a common culprit, and rapid cessation of diarrhea results on withdrawal of the offending substance.[33]

### Secretory Diarrhea

Intestinal absorption of water and electrolytes is the net difference between the fluid and electrolytes secreted and fluid and electrolytes absorbed.[34] Total net absorption may be much smaller than either of the two unidirectional processes. Therefore, a change in the balance between these two unidirectional processes can markedly alter total intestinal fluid absorption and may result in secretory diarrhea.

Some investigators conceptually believe that all enterocytes are involved in both absorption and secretion, whereas others consider crypt cells the primary anatomic site of secretion. Certainly, disorders that result in villus destruction are associated with diarrhea, a component of which is often secretory. However, many secretory diarrheas occur in morphologically normal intestines.

Secretory diarrhea in the classic sense is not related to food in the gastrointestinal tract, and as a consequence, persists if the patient has fasted for an extended period of time.[25] In patients with pure secretory diarrhea, eating does not increase stool volume significantly. Pure secretory diarrheas typically do not exhibit evidence of inflammation, in that occult blood and white blood cells are absent from the stool. Because the diarrhea is not related to dietary constituents, the osmolality of the stool can be accounted for by normal ionic constituents. Therefore, doubling the sum of sodium and potassium concentrations should equal the fecal osmolality.

There is a pitfall in applying these definitive terms to secretory diarrhea. The majority of patients with gastrointestinal disease who exhibit features of secretory diarrhea may have other mechanistic processes involved.[35] Although certain inflammatory diarrheas have a secretory component, they may also have an exudative component as well as an osmotic component during feeding.

Secretory diarrhea occurs under a number of conditions. Classically, secretory diarrheas are mediated by gastrointestinal peptides such as vasoactive intestinal polypeptide (VIP) and associated with tumors such as ganglioneuroblastoma or Zollinger-Ellison syndrome.[36–38] However, other substances may induce fluid secretion, including bile acids, fatty acids, and laxatives.[39–41] Congenital disorders of fluid transport such as congenital chloridorrhea may also produce secretory diarrhea.[17]

### Motility Disorders

Although motility is not often a major cause of malabsorption, changes in motility can definitely influence absorption. Slowing intestinal transit pharmacologically or nutritionally through increased ileal fat increases absorption.[24, 25] Severe impairment of intestinal motility results in intestinal stasis with subsequent inflammation, bile acid deconjugation, and malabsorption. Hypermotility is an uncommon cause of malabsorption. However, watery diarrhea may result from rapid transit in irritable colon of infancy. Malabsorption is not significant, and growth is normal. Deranged motility may be a component in diarrhea of other causes including thyrotoxicosis, bile acid malabsorption, and a variety of other disorders.[42, 43] Documentation of hypermotility as a cause of the diarrhea is difficult, however, and pharmacologic therapy is often unrewarding.

### Inflammatory Diarrhea

Inflammation in the small intestine or colon may cause diarrhea in a number of conditions.[44–50] Exudation of mucus, protein, and blood into the gastrointestinal lumen may contribute to fecal water, electrolyte, and protein loss, but usually this occurs in association with other types of diarrhea, such as osmotic or secretory. Examples include inflammatory bowel disease, infectious disorders in the distal small bowel and colon, and celiac disease in the upper small intestine.

## DIFFERENTIAL DIAGNOSIS OF DIARRHEA

### Acute Diarrhea

In formulating a differential diagnosis in a child with diarrhea, one must first differentiate acute from chronic diarrhea. The duration of acute diarrhea is short, usually less than 2 weeks. It is most often caused by an enteric infection. Differential diagnosis varies somewhat with age, but not to the extent of chronic diarrhea.

In general, viral pathogens produce injury to the proximal small intestine, and bacterial pathogens usually involve colonic inflammation. As a consequence, viral pathogens typically produce watery diarrhea and vomiting; bacterial pathogens, bloody stools, mucus, and crampy abdominal pain. Many bacterial infections, however, have a toxin-producing component causing watery diarrhea. This may be the sole presentation of a bacterial infection.

Because infectious diarrhea typically presents with either vomiting and watery stools or bloody, mucousy diarrhea, it is often valuable to consider the differential diagnosis of these two clinical presentations separately. As mentioned previously, vomiting and watery stools are often caused by viral organisms. Rotavirus is the most common and is frequently seen in infants and small children, especially during the winter.[51, 52] Other viral pathogens, including the Norwalk agent and enterovirus, may produce a similar clinical syndrome. The disease is often abrupt in onset, with 24 to 48 hours of vomiting followed by 3 to 5 days of diarrhea. Dehydration is a relatively common complication. Although standard therapy for years has included intravenous fluid replacement to correct the dehydration, recent evidence suggests that judicious use of oral rehydration therapy will correct most cases of mild to moderate dehydration without difficulty.

Protozoal pathogens may cause proximal small bowel mucosal injury as well. Giardiasis, discussed later as a chronic pathogen (see Chapter 29), may produce an acute diarrheal syndrome. *Cryptosporidium* is a newly recognized protozoal pathogen that causes severe chronic diarrhea and malnutrition in immunocompromised patients but also produces an acute self-limited diarrheal disorder in immunocompetent patients.[53–55] This disorder may be spread through person-to-person contact, although it is highly associated with exposure to farm animals. Patients develop nausea, vomiting, abdominal cramps, low-grade fever, and profuse watery diarrhea. The disorder is self-limited, usually lasting about 2 weeks, and no specific antimicrobial therapy exists. The organism may occasionally be found in the stool but is frequently diagnosed only on intestinal biopsy.

Certain bacterial pathogens may produce a watery diarrhea. In most instances, this results through the production of toxins that induce fluid secretion in the small intestine.[56]

Cholera is a classic example. Certain species of *Aeromonas hydrophila* and *Plesiomonas shigelloides* may produce secretory watery diarrhea.[57–60] Both, however, have also been demonstrated to produce a colitis picture with crampy abdominal pain, mucus, and blood.

Acute self-limited bloody diarrhea is usually caused by a bacterial pathogen. *Shigella* and *Salmonella* are typical examples. Enteroinvasive *Escherichia coli* may also produce such a clinical picture. Enterohemorrhagic *E. coli*, type 0157H7, is recognized as one of the more common causes of bloody diarrhea in children and frequently produces hemolytic uremic syndrome and thrombotic thrombocytopenic purpura.[61] Hemolytic uremic syndrome appears to follow approximately 10% of such infections. *Clostridium difficile* may grow in large quantities after antibiotic administration and produce a colitis syndrome.[61–64] This disorder should be considered whenever a patient develops bloody diarrhea after antibiotic therapy, especially if pseudomembranes are visualized at sigmoidoscopy.

In most instances, the sigmoidoscopic appearance of infectious diarrheas are nonspecific. Histologic changes are likewise nonspecific. Through the sigmoidoscope, one visualizes the presence of spontaneous and induced friability, granularity, and loss of ramifying vessels. These findings are quite similar to those observed in ulcerative colitis. More proximal colon disease with distal spearing should suggest the possibility of other organisms such as *Yersinia enterocolitica* or the protozoal pathogen *Entamoeba histolytica*. If symptoms of cramping and bloody diarrhea and sigmoidoscopic evidence of colitis exist beyond 2 weeks in the face of negative cultures, inflammatory bowel disease should be considered a strong possibility.

## Chronic Diarrhea

Differential diagnosis of chronic diarrhea changes markedly with age, much more so than acute diarrhea. In the small infant, perhaps the most common cause of chronic diarrhea is a disorder commonly known as intractable diarrhea of infancy (Table 3–2). This term is usually used to describe diarrhea associated with diffuse mucosal injury beginning prior to 6 months of age, lasting longer than 2 weeks, and associated with malabsorption and malnutrition.[65–67] More recently, the term *protracted diarrhea of infancy* has been used, because the prognosis for this disorder has been markedly improved through the use of parenteral nutrition and newer elemental diets.[68]

The term *intractable diarrhea of infancy* implies that a distinct disease entity exists. However, there are several different disease processes that may produce histologically similar mucosal lesions resulting in a common symptom complex and similar consequences. Post-infectious diarrheal syndromes, intestinal protein intolerance syndromes, and a few other disorders all may produce similar findings.

**TABLE 3–2. Major Causes of Chronic Diarrhea in Small Infants**

| | |
|---|---|
| Intractable diarrhea of infancy | Hirschsprung's disease |
| Milk and soy protein intolerance | Munchausen syndrome by proxy |
| Protracted infectious enteritis | Congenital transport defects |
| Microvillus inclusion disease | Nutrient malabsorption |
| Autoimmune enteropathy | |

Perhaps the major cause of intractable diarrhea of infancy in most areas of the United States is cow's milk and soy protein intolerance.[69, 70] These infants commonly develop enterocolitis, with inflammation in both the small bowel and colon, a few days to weeks after initially ingesting cow's milk protein. Although inflammation may occur in any part of the gastrointestinal tract, it may also be limited to the colon. These children present during the first 3 months of life with a constellation of vomiting, irritability, poor feeding, diarrhea, and bloody stools. Stools commonly test positive for reducing substances, suggesting small bowel mucosal injury with carbohydrate malabsorption. Stool pH is usually below 5.5 for the same reason, and stool leukocytes are often present, suggestive of colitis. When cow's milk is withdrawn, symptoms resolve in a majority of milk-intolerant infants. Many relapse after a short withdrawal of cow's milk if placed on a soy formula, because a high percentage of cow's milk protein–intolerant infants are also soy intolerant. Use of a casein hydrolysate formula is often more effective in ameliorating symptoms. There are some infants who do not respond to protein hydrolysate formulas. In these instances, amino acid formulas may be helpful and deserve a trial.[71] When rechallenged with cow's milk or soy protein, children may relapse abruptly, the majority of reactions occurring within 24 to 48 hours. However, occasionally the reaction is delayed for several days. Life-threatening anaphylaxis may occur in a small minority of infants.

A small percentage of patients do not respond to withdrawal of cow's milk and soy protein from the diet and continue to have diarrhea and malabsorption while on a casein hydrolysate or amino acid formula. It is these infants who are often classified as having intractable diarrhea or protracted diarrhea of infancy.[72] A variety of histologic abnormalities are seen in the small intestine, including blunting and flattening of the villi, increased mononuclear cells with occasional polymorphonuclear infiltrates, cuboidalization of the surface epithelium, and a mild to moderate increase in mitotic activity in the crypts. These histologic lesions vary substantially and are poorly predictive of the need for long-term parenteral nutrition.[68] It is quite likely they are patchy in their distribution, and this may well account for their unpredictability. A significant percentage of patients with intractable diarrhea of infancy start out with infectious injury. A variety of enteropathogenic microorganisms may produce small bowel mucosal injury, including adherent *E. coli*, rotavirus, *Giardia*, and others. Alteration of permeability of the mucosal membrane is often thought to produce secondary cow's milk or soy protein sensitivity, which may further aggravate mucosal injury and exacerbate the intractable diarrhea state. This phenomenon may actually represent the unmasking of pre-existing subclinical milk protein intolerance. Breast feeding may offer some protection to the development of intractable diarrhea because of the anti-infectious factors present in human milk. Histologically, intractable diarrhea produced by cow's milk protein intolerance and protracted infectious enteritis have a similar appearance.

Chronic postenteritis diarrhea following infection may also occur in older infants. Zoppi and associates reviewed

48 such patients, 18 younger than 12 months of age and 30 between the ages of 12 and 30 months.[73] All had mild malabsorption and impairment of growth and chronic low-grade inflammation on intestinal biopsy. Diets were hypocaloric and high in carbohydrate, possibly a participating factor in malabsorption and poor growth. Iyngkaran and colleagues described several infants younger than 2 months of age who were challenged with cow's milk protein 6 weeks after recovery from an infectious enteritis, all of whom had been previously exposed to cow's milk.[74] Biopsies before and after milk challenge demonstrated significant mucosal injury following milk challenge, and milk challenge was significantly associated with diarrhea, vomiting, and weight loss.

Other less common causes of chronic diarrhea and mucosal injury occur in infancy. Congenital microvillus atrophy, otherwise known as microvillus inclusion disease, manifests with severe diarrhea shortly after birth and is characterized by hypoplastic atrophy of the villi.[75–78] Electron microscopy reveals ultrastructural abnormalities of the microvillus membrane consisting of shortening and depletion of the microvilli and inclusions and involutions of the brush border membrane containing microvilli. This particular lesion is considered the hallmark of congenital microvillus atrophy, and microvillus inclusions may also be seen in the colon. The disorder becomes clinically apparent a few days after birth and results in intractable diarrhea. Although long-term survival with home total parenteral nutrition (TPN) is possible, the disorder is usually fatal and does not respond to corticosteroids. Intestinal transplantation has been efficacious in the treatment of some of these patients.[79] Another disorder that can be diagnosed by electron microscopy is known as tufting enteropathy. In this disorder, microvilli are present, but their attachment to the underlying structure is abnormal. These patients likewise present with secretory diarrhea and intractable malabsorption unresponsive to medical therapy.[80, 81] Syndromatic enteropathy is another rare condition characterized by mild villus abnormality on light microscopy in association with brittle, unmanageable hair, characteristic facies, and a subtle defect in antibody production. The severity of the diarrhea and malabsorption appears variable in these cases, and some require long-term parenteral nutrition.[82]

Autoimmune enteropathy is another rare disorder characterized by severe proximal intestinal mucosal injury.[83, 84] Autoantibodies against gut epithelium are typically found, and the histologic lesion in the small intestine is usually quite severe with marked polymorphonuclear infiltration and total flattening of the mucosa resembling celiac disease. This disorder usually begins somewhat later in life than either intractable diarrhea or congenital microvillus atrophy, typically around 6 months of age. Although some patients respond to an elemental diet, immunosuppressive drugs are usually more helpful. Most respond, at least partially, to corticosteroids. Addition of 6-mercaptopurine or azathioprine may also be helpful, and reports have documented response to cyclosporine in a limited number of cases. Evidence of multi-organ autoimmune disease such as diabetes and renal involvement is not uncommon.

Treatment of intractable diarrhea, regardless of the cause, is heavily based on supplemental parenteral nutrition and continuous enteral infusion of an elemental diet. Evidence suggests that enteral feedings hasten the recovery from mucosal injury and that parenteral nutrition can often be avoided through aggressive use of continuous enteral infusion of an elemental diet.

Hirschsprung's disease should remain in the differential diagnosis of any infant who presents with intractable diarrhea. This diagnosis should be suggested if the child has had delayed passage of meconium during the first 24 hours of life or if constipation preceded the diarrhea. Predisposing factors for Hirschsprung's disease, such as a strong family history or the presence of Down syndrome, likewise should caution the clinician to consider this possibility. Although only a small percentage, around 10%, of infants with Hirschsprung's disease develop enterocolitis, the disorder carries a very high mortality rate, up to 50%. Prompt decompression of the colon proximal to the aganglionic segment either through the use of a tube or by surgical placement of an ostomy is indicated. The diagnosis of Hirschsprung's disease may be established through the use of rectal suction biopsy, provided the clinician and pathologist are skilled in obtaining and processing the specimen.

Another cause of chronic diarrhea in infants is Munchausen syndrome by proxy. A small number of cases have been reported in which administration of laxatives to small infants has produced an intractable diarrhea-like syndrome.[85, 86] The histologic changes typically seen in the small intestinal biopsy in intractable diarrhea of infancy are not present, however, and separation of the child from the caretaker results in abrupt cessation of symptoms. Parents of these infants are often overly concerned about the infant and are in constant attendance. Like Hirschsprung's disease, Munchausen's syndrome by proxy needs to be considered in the differential diagnosis of intractable diarrhea.

Congenital transport defects may result in chronic diarrhea from birth. One classic cause of congenital secretory diarrhea is congenital chloridorrhea.[87, 88] In this disorder, the chloride bicarbonate exchange mechanism in the ileum and colon is reversed and chloride is actively secreted. Excess bicarbonate absorption results in alkalosis, and chloride malabsorption results in secretory diarrhea because of the osmotic load of the secreted chloride in the colon. Marked hypokalemia occurs. Patients present in infancy with severe diarrhea and extremely watery stools containing no blood, no white blood cells, and no reducing substances. Small intestine and colon biopsy results are normal. Because of the tremendous active chloride secretion, stool chloride content exceeds that of the sum of the sodium and potassium, and the diagnosis can be strongly suspected after stool electrolyte measurement in correlation with clinical presentation.

Nutrient malabsorption may cause chronic diarrhea. Congenital glucose galactose malabsorption is a defect in monosaccharide transport in which the active transport carrier protein for glucose and galactose is absent. On ingestion of any formula containing glucose or galactose, which includes all complete infant formulas, chronic severe watery diarrhea ensues, resulting in failure to thrive, stools testing positive for reducing substances, and severe watery diarrhea. As in congenital chloridorrhea, small intestinal and colonic biopsy results are normal. Fructose can be transported in these patients and may be utilized as a therapeutic source of carbohydrates. This condition is extremely rare.

An equally rare disorder is congenital lactase deficiency, a congenital absence of lactase. This should be differentiated from primary acquired lactase deficiency, where lactase levels drop throughout late childhood. In congenital lactase deficiency, severe watery diarrhea is present from birth but resolves on treatment with a lactose-free formula. Results of small intestinal biopsies are normal, and stools are positive for reducing substances but negative for occult blood and white blood cells. Again, this condition is extremely rare and must be differentiated from the much more common milk protein enterocolitis, in which diarrhea may also resolve after milk withdrawal but in which intestinal or colonic biopsies are abnormal and stools frequently contain occult blood or white blood cells. Congenital sucrase isomaltase deficiency is a more common congenital disaccharidase deficiency state, but it is still quite rare. Because sucrose is not a common dietary carbohydrate during the first 6 months of life, these children do not develop watery stools until sucrose is administered. Again, watery diarrhea and low fecal pH are common and suggestive of carbohydrate malabsorption, but because sucrose is a nonreducing sugar, stool tests for reducing substances may be either normal or only slightly positive.

## Chronic Diarrhea in the Toddler

The differential diagnosis of chronic diarrhea changes rather markedly during the latter part of the first year and into the second year of life (Table 3–3). The most common cause of chronic diarrhea in this age group is irritable colon of infancy, also known as chronic nonspecific diarrhea.[89, 90] This disorder is often thought to be a variant of irritable bowel syndrome, and it is not uncommon to find a family history of irritable bowel syndrome, especially in parents or siblings. Infants with this disorder typically have intermittent loose watery stools. Stools vary from two to three mushy stools on some days to six to 10 watery stools on others. They are frequently forcefully expelled and are quite foul-smelling. The odor, however, is not at all characteristic of steatorrhea, but rather is more typical of fluid from the ileum, not surprising as the disorder is one of rapid transit and stools frequently spend very little time in the colon.

There are several characteristics of the clinical presentation of this disorder that help differentiate it from other causes of chronic diarrhea simply by obtaining a careful history and physical examination. The first is the intermittent nature of the diarrhea. These children often oscillate between normal and watery stools, even between diarrhea and constipation. Stools are usually not expelled at night, although it is not uncommon for children to have a very watery stool immediately on awakening in the morning. Children with chronic nonspecific diarrhea typically manifest normal growth. The exception is the child who is placed on a hypocaloric diet in an attempt to control the diarrhea.

Because of the intermittent nature of the diarrhea, the children are often misdiagnosed as having food allergies or recurrent episodes of viral enteritis. The assumption of food allergy is strengthened in the mind of the parents by the common presence of vegetable particles or other food particles in the stool, which are simply the manifestation of rapid transit. The intermittent nature of the diarrhea also suggests recurrent bouts of viral enteritis. This frequently results in institution of a hypocaloric diet, which, in turn, impairs the child's growth and weight gain.

**TABLE 3–3. Major Causes of Chronic Diarrhea in Toddlers**

| | |
|---|---|
| Irritable colon of infancy (chronic nonspecific diarrhea) | Sucrase-isomaltase deficiency |
| Protracted viral enteritis | Tumors (secretory diarrhea) |
| Giardiasis | Ulcerative colitis |
| | Celiac disease |

The mechanism for the diarrhea in this disorder appears to be altered gastrointestinal motility. Despite relatively rapid transit, absorption is reasonably intact and the child will grow well if fed adequately. Institution of high-fat, low-carbohydrate diet is often helpful both because of reduced dietary osmolality and because of the effects of ileal fat on retarding gastrointestinal motility.[91–93] When fat reaches the ileum, secretion of gastrointestinal hormones from that region slow gastric emptying and small bowel transit, thereby providing some improvement in the child's diarrhea. Occasional bouts of watery stools will still occur, but significant improvement is to be anticipated.

Another disorder seen in toddlers that closely mimics chronic nonspecific diarrhea is referred to as protracted enteritis.[90, 94–97] The disorder starts with a viral infection such as rotavirus. The institution of high-carbohydrate, low-fat feedings results in chronic hypocaloric hyperosmotic feedings, which may further exacerbate diarrhea. Low-grade mucosal injury persists, and the primarily osmotic diarrhea continues. Mild weight loss may occur, both because of the hypocaloric feedings and perhaps as a result of the low-grade malabsorption. Frequently, children with this disorder consume large quantities of apple juice or other high-carbohydrate beverages. These patients respond quite dramatically to the institution of a high-fat, low-carbohydrate diet. A small percentage, mostly those younger than 1 year of age, may be milk protein intolerant and will relapse when milk feedings are restored. Lactase deficiency is usually not a problem this late in the course of the illness. Milk protein intolerance is usually a transient condition in this setting and resolves in 2 to 4 months.

One other disorder that closely mimics chronic nonspecific diarrhea is giardiasis. *Giardia* is a proximal small intestinal protozoal pathogen that causes mucosal injury resulting in malabsorption and watery diarrhea.[98] Although it is commonly thought of as a pathogen contracted from contaminated food or water, in pediatrics it is more commonly passed from individual to individual, especially in day care centers or other crowded situations. The diarrhea in giardiasis tends to be much less intermittent than in chronic nonspecific diarrhea, and because of the proximal small bowel mucosal injury, malabsorption and weight loss are more common. Diagnosis is often difficult, because pathogens are not always recovered in the stool. In fact, stool examinations may be normal in up to 50% of patients with giardiasis. Newly developed tests for *Giardia* antigen in the stool appear to be somewhat more sensitive.[99, 100] Small intestinal biopsy with careful examination for the presence of the *Giardia* organisms or aspiration of duodenal or jejunal contents is a more sensitive means of diagnosis.

Two less common causes of watery diarrhea that can present like chronic nonspecific diarrhea are congenital sucrase isomaltase deficiency and secretory diarrhea from tumors. Sucrase isomaltase deficiency is a defect in carbohydrate digestion in which the enzyme required for hydrolysis of sucrose and alpha limit dextrins is not present in the small intestine. As a consequence, these children have watery stools from osmotic diarrhea when sucrose is introduced into the diet. This usually corresponds with the time that infants with toddler diarrhea or chronic nonspecific diarrhea develop symptoms, and as a consequence, it must be considered in the differential diagnosis even though it is quite rare. It should be suspected when screening studies indicate a chronically low stool pH (<5.5). Bacterial breakdown of the malabsorbed carbohydrates in the stool to organic acids decreases the stool pH and serves as a reasonably good screening test for this disorder. Stools are often negative for reducing substances, because sucrose is a nonreducing sugar. However, hydrolyzing the stool with hydrochloric acid prior to measuring reducing substances will result in a positive test. In performing these assays, it is important to obtain measurements while the child is ingesting sucrose.

There are a few tumors that cause secretory diarrhea in children. Although an uncommon cause of chronic diarrhea in toddlers, these do occasionally occur and must be also be considered in the differential diagnosis. Neuroblastomas, ganglioneuroblastomas, and pancreatic tumors that secrete vasoactive intestinal polypeptide are the primary ones to exclude. Twenty-four-hour urine vanillylmandelic acid (VMA) determinations as well as serum VIP determinations will adequately screen for most of them. They should be considered primarily in children who have continuous rather than intermittent diarrhea and in whom diarrhea continues even when feeding is stopped.

There are some other causes of chronic diarrhea that occur in toddlers but that vary substantially from the clinical presentation of chronic nonspecific diarrhea. These include early presentations of inflammatory bowel disease and primary malabsorptive disorders such as celiac sprue and cystic fibrosis.

Crohn's disease is very rare in children younger than the age of 5, and as a consequence, most inflammatory bowel disease seen in toddlers is ulcerative colitis. This disorder is discussed elsewhere in the text (see Chapters 32 and 33).

Celiac sprue, otherwise known as celiac disease or gluten enteropathy, has been considered to be a relatively uncommon disorder in North America. Recent evidence suggests that many cases in North America are missed. Screening studies for celiac disease are positive as frequently in North America as in Europe, and it is quite likely that a number of patients who do not present with classic signs and symptoms of celiac disease have been overlooked or misdiagnosed in North America. This disorder results in chronic proximal small intestinal inflammation following ingestion of gluten, a protein constituent in wheat, oats, barley, and rye.[101] The alpha-gliadin fraction of gluten appears to induce a hypersensitivity reaction in the small intestine, resulting in complete flattening of the villi, deepening of the crypts, and a marked increase in mitotic activity. Patients present with failure to thrive, abdominal distention, chronic diarrhea, and weight loss. Because of the mucosal injury, they are often poor eaters. Diarrhea usually develops as a later manifestation of the disease after significant failure to thrive and anorexia have already appeared. In this way, this disorder is different from chronic nonspecific diarrhea. New screening studies are now available to help determine the need for intestinal biopsies; however, biopsy diagnosis is still considered essential in establishing the diagnosis of celiac disease. Clinical response to withdrawing gluten is usually slow and inconsistent, and for this reason, symptomatic response to gluten withdrawal and challenge is not adequate for establishing the presence or absence of celiac disease.

Over the years, many have advocated three biopsies to diagnose celiac disease, one at the time of diagnosis, one several months to years after gluten withdrawal, and a third biopsy to demonstrate reoccurrence of injury after gluten challenge. In patients with classic clinical presentations who present later than the first year of life, when other common causes of mucosal injury occur less frequently, one biopsy at the time of diagnosis is probably adequate, provided the histologic features are totally consistent with celiac disease. The antibody screening tests, anti-gliadin IgA and IgG, antireticulin, and anti-endomysium have made it much easier to screen for the presence of this disease.[102–104] These are typically useful in children with growth failure in whom celiac disease is considered to be a minor consideration in differential diagnosis. An observation of high incidence of positive endomysial antibodies in North American patients suggests that increased screening for celiac disease should be considered in patients with a variety of gastrointestinal complaints. Studies vary, but approximately 95% sensitivity can be anticipated. All, however, can be abnormal in children with nonspecific mucosal injury.

Children with chronic diarrhea should be evaluated for celiac disease if they manifest the clinical characteristics of failure to thrive, abdominal distention, muscle wasting, and anorexia in association with their diarrhea, if screening studies suggest malabsorption such as low serum carotene or the presence of large quantities of fat in the stool, or if they do not respond to conservative therapy for the other more common causes of chronic diarrhea. In no instance should a child be placed on a therapeutic trial of a gluten-free diet without adequate evaluation. Children with chronic nonspecific diarrhea occasionally improve on this diet because it is typically lower in carbohydrate, and this response can make the whole picture terribly confusing.

Cystic fibrosis is often considered in the differential diagnosis of chronic diarrhea. However, these children have fat malabsorption from pancreatic insufficiency, and their carbohydrate and protein absorption are usually quite adequate. As a consequence, the stools are primarily steatorrhea and not diarrhea. Large, frequently passed foul-smelling stools that are not watery in consistency occur in the presence of failure to thrive, often with a history of recurrent respiratory infections. Ten percent of patients may present at birth with bowel obstruction secondary to meconium ileus. As these children do not have watery diarrhea, sweat chloride determination to exclude cystic fibrosis is not part of the routine evaluation of the child with chronic watery diarrhea. In the context of malabsorption and failure to thrive with large quantities of fat in the stool and a low serum carotene, sweat chloride determination should be obtained to exclude cystic fibrosis.

### *Chronic Diarrhea in School-Age Children*

The differential diagnosis again changes as the child progresses into school age (Table 3–4). Inflammatory bowel

**TABLE 3–4. Additional Causes of Chronic Diarrhea in School-Age Children**

| | |
|---|---|
| Inflammatory bowel disease | Primary acquired lactase deficiency |
| Appendiceal abscess | Constipation with encopresis? |

disease becomes more common, disorders such as chronic nonspecific diarrhea and protracted viral enteritis disappear, and other possibilities enter the differential diagnosis.

In the school-age child with chronic diarrhea, inflammatory bowel disease is important in the differential diagnosis. After age 5 years, both Crohn's disease and ulcerative colitis are relatively common, and Crohn's disease appears to be increasing in frequency. These children typically present with blood and mucus in the stool and often with abdominal pain and cramping. Growth failure is common, especially in Crohn's disease. Likewise in Crohn's disease, perianal abnormalities are often present on physical examination, which also frequently reveals some right lower quadrant tenderness, because ileal and proximal colonic involvement are most common. In such patients, colonoscopic evaluation of the colon is much more definitive in making the diagnosis than radiographic studies, and it permits histologic sampling, which improves diagnostic capabilities. These disorders are discussed extensively elsewhere in the text (see Chapters 32 and 33).

Appendicitis may cause chronic diarrhea in infants and children. Unlike in adults, appendicitis frequently results in perforation in children. Localized inflammation in the region of the cecum results in chronic diarrhea, often associated with chronic low-grade fever and some abdominal tenderness that may or may not be impressive on physical examination.

Primary acquired lactase deficiency begins to present in the school-age child. Lactase levels begin to drop between ages 3 and 5 years in such children. A gradual decrease in lactase levels results in subtle chronic increases in lactose malabsorption after ingestion of milk. The child gradually develops flatulence, abdominal pain, and loose stools after milk ingestion. In the older child, flatulence and abdominal pain may be more prominent than diarrhea. The diagnosis is easily made through the use of breath hydrogen testing, in which an oral lactose load is given and breath sampled for hydrogen content at frequent intervals thereafter. It should be pointed out that a small number of cases of milk protein intolerance have now been observed in older children, and even in adults, in which ingestion of milk protein is followed by a sudden onset of diarrhea, abdominal pain, and occasionally vomiting. In these patients, the lactose breath hydrogen test is normal, and histologic injury of the bowel after milk protein ingestion can often be demonstrated.

Finally, a number of patients with constipation may be brought to the physician by their parents for evaluation of chronic diarrhea. In this instance, the children develop a fecal impaction with overflow incontinence known as encopresis. Chronic soiling of the pants, often with loose stool, leads the parents to believe that the child has diarrhea. This disorder is quickly differentiated from diarrhea in most instances by demonstration of impaction on rectal examination. Most school-age children, even when they have diarrhea, can usually make it to the toilet to pass their stools unless the diarrhea is unusually severe. In children with encopresis, chronic soiling occurs frequently, making it fairly easy to differentiate the two by history alone.

## DIAGNOSTIC STUDIES IN DIARRHEA

Evaluation of the patient with diarrhea should start with certain screening studies (Table 3–5). Many of these are appropriate in children with either acute or chronic diarrhea. Stools positive for occult blood generally indicate inflammation. This test is most commonly positive in patients with colitis. In the case of acute diarrhea, this usually suggests a bacterial infection, whereas in chronic diarrhea, inflammatory bowel disease such as ulcerative colitis or Crohn's disease is more likely. The same is true for patients with stools positive for white blood cells. Stools positive for reducing substances or stools with a pH of less than 5.5 usually indicate carbohydrate malabsorption. The carbohydrates are fermented by colonic bacteria that produce lactic acid, and this reduces the stool pH. Although these studies are abnormal in patients with congenital defects of carbohydrate malabsorption, they usually indicate small bowel injury. In the case of acute diarrhea, viral enteritis is the most common cause. In chronic diarrhea, infants with intractable diarrhea of infancy or any other chronic enteropathy commonly have stools positive for Clinitest and/or low pH. One must remember, however, that these tests are only valid when the child is being fed adequate quantities of formula containing carbohydrates. Sucrose is a nonreducing sugar, and the presence of sucrose in the stool will not result in a stool positive for reducing substances unless bacterial action on the carbohydrate has split the disaccharide, producing some reducing sugar. Fortunately, enough bacterial action is usually present to produce some indication of increased reducing sugars in these patients. Stools positive for Sudan stain for fat indicate gross steatorrhea. This may be of either small bowel, pancreatic, or biliary origin. Because the test is not sensitive, it is not done frequently. Many have advocated the use of the 1-hour blood xylose determination as an indicator of small bowel mucosal injury, especially in patients with chronic diarrhea or suspected malabsorption syndromes. This test is neither specific nor sensitive and is currently done less frequently, given the recent introduction

**TABLE 3–5. Screening Tests in Diarrhea**

| TEST | INTERPRETATION |
|---|---|
| Stool for occult blood + | Inflammation, usually colonic |
| Stool Clinitest + | Carbohydrate malabsorption—usually proximal small bowel injury |
| Stool pH < 5.5 | Carbohydrate malabsorption—usually proximal small bowel injury |
| 1-hr blood xylose | Diffuse small bowel injury |
| Sudan stain for fat | Gross steatorrhea—small bowel, pancreatic, or biliary |
| Stool for white blood cells | Inflammation, usually colonic |

of antibody screening tests for celiac disease and the increased use of endoscopic small intestinal biopsies.

Screening studies help the clinician decide what further studies are indicated. In the case of acute diarrhea, stool studies positive for occult blood or white blood cells suggest the need for stool cultures. Stool cultures are often quite expensive, and using the screening studies to help dictate their use is often cost-effective. In acute diarrhea, low-pH stools positive for reducing substances suggest a viral pathogen and may suggest the need for viral antigen studies for common viruses such as rotavirus. Most commonly, viral diarrheas in children are self-limited, and such tests are usually not helpful in the management of the patient.

In the case of chronic diarrhea, studies indicating small bowel mucosal injury may suggest the need for looking for *Giardia* in the stool or obtaining further screening studies for celiac disease, such as anti-gliadin, anti-reticulin, and anti-endomysial antibodies. In addition, the screening studies may dictate the appropriate use of endoscopic procedures. Patients with hematest-positive stools containing white blood cells may benefit from colonoscopic examination and colon biopsies.

Traditionally, small intestinal biopsies have been of great usefulness in diagnosing the cause of chronic diarrhea. Certain diseases can be diagnosed from biopsies because of characteristic histologic features. These include intestinal lymphangicctasia, giardiasis, cryptosporidiosis, and abetalipoproteinemia. The presence of severe inflammation reactions raises the question of autoimmune enteropathy. Electron microscopic examination of the biopsy specimens can be useful in detecting microvillus inclusion disease. Disorders such as intractable diarrhea of infancy, protracted viral enteritis, milk or soy protein intolerance, malnutrition, certain immunodeficiency disorders, and even celiac disease have a fairly nonspecific inflammatory process, and it may be difficult to differentiate one from another. However, the small bowel biopsy will help assess the exact nature of the disease and document the mucosal injury.

There is some controversy about how small intestinal biopsies should be performed. Traditionally, biopsy specimens have been obtained with a suction biopsy tube. The Rubin tube, the Crosby and Carey capsules, the Watson capsule, and more recently the MediTech directable biopsy apparatus all have been used with great success in obtaining histologic specimens from infants and children. The procedure is low-risk but requires substantial expertise. Because of the time involved in obtaining samples and the skill necessary in placing the biopsy capsule, endoscopic biopsies of the small intestine have become more common. The procedure is easy, requires little time, and allows sampling from multiple sites. Using this technique, it is more difficult to perform a biopsy more distally into the small intestine. Biopsy samples are much smaller in size and susceptible to crush artifact. Mounting endoscopic biopsy specimens on small slices of cucumber fixed in alcohol, which can be subsequently imbedded, sectioned, and stained along with the biopsy sample, allow improved orientation and improved interpretation of endoscopic small intestinal biopsies. We have found this technique extremely helpful when using endoscopic biopsies for the detection of small bowel mucosal disease.

## Summary

Diarrhea in the pediatric age group may arise from many different causes. Different etiologic factors may produce diarrheal stools through one or more different mechanisms. As in most cases in pediatrics, the differential diagnosis of diarrhea varies markedly with age, especially in the case of chronic diarrhea, and the clinician must correlate the age of the patient, the nature of the stools, the chronicity of the problem, and other relevant historical factors in order to formulate an adequate differential diagnosis on which to base the evaluation.

### REFERENCES

1. Schiller LR, Hogan RB, Morawski SG, et al: The incidence and significance of bile acid malabsorption in patients with chronic idiopathic diarrhea. Gastroenterology 1987;92:151.
2. Goy JAE, Eastwood MA, Mitchell WD, et al: Fecal characteristics contrasted in the irritable bowel syndrome and diverticular disease. Am J Clin Nutr 1976;29:1480.
3. Tucker DM, Sandstead HH, Logan GM, et al: Dietary fiber and personality factors as determinants of stool output. Gastroenterology 1981;81:879.
4. Weaver LT: Bowel habit from birth to old age. J Pediatr Gastroenterol Nutr 1988;7:637–640.
5. Powell DW: Ion and water transport in the intestine. In Andreoli TE, Hoffman JF, Fanestil DD, Schultz SG (eds): Physiology of Membrane Disorders. New York, Plenum, 1986, p 559.
6. Shepherd RW, Hamilton JR, Gall DG: The postnatal development of sodium transport in the proximal small intestine of the rabbit. Pediatr Res 1980;14:250–253.
7. Phillips SF: Diarrhea: a current view of the pathophysiology. Gastroenterology 1972;63:495–518.
8. Turnberg LA, Fordtran JS, Carter NW, Rector FC: Mechanism of bicarbonate absorption and its relationship to sodium transport in the human jejunum. J Clin Invest 1970;49:548.
9. Turnberg LA, Bieberdorf FA, Morawski SG, Fordtran JS: Interrelationship of chloride, bicarbonate, sodium, and hydrogen transport in the human ileum. J Clin Invest 1970;49:557.
10. Powell DW: Barrier function of epithelia. Am J Physiol 1981;241:G275–G278.
11. Ghishan FK, Wilson FA: Developmental maturation of D-glucose transport by rat jejunal brush-border membrane vesicles. In: Am J Physiol (1985 Jan) 248(1 Pt 1):G87–92.
12. Fordtran J: Stimulation of active and passive sodium absorption by sugars in the human jejunum. J Clin Invest 1975;55:728–737.
13. Diamond JM: Solute-linked water transport in epithelia. In Hoffman FJ (ed): Membrane Transport Processes. New York, Raven Press, 1978, p 257.
14. Pappenheimer JR: Physiological regulation of transepithelial impedance in the intestinal mucosa of rats and hamsters. J Membr Biol 1987;100:137–148.
15. Field M: Intracellular mediators of secretion in the small intestine. In Binder HJ (ed): Mechanisms of Intestinal Secretion. New York, Alan R. Liss, 1979, p 83.
16. Smith PL, McCabe RD: Mechanism and regulation of transcellular potassium transport by the colon. In: Am J Physiol (1984 Nov) 247 (5 Pt 1):G445–56.
17. Bieberdorf FA, Gorden P, Fordtran JS: Pathogenesis of congenital alkalosis with diarrhea. Implications for the physiology of normal ileal electrolyte absorption and secretion. J Clin Invest 1972;51:1958–1968.
18. Cooke HJ: Neural and humoral regulation of small intestinal electrolyte transport. In Johnson LR (ed): Physiology of the Gastrointestinal Tract, 2nd ed. New York, Raven Press, 1987, p 1307.
19. Castro GA: Immunological regulation of epithelial function. Am J Physiol (Gastrointest Liver Physiol 6) 1982;243:G321–G329.
20. Bern MJ, Sturbaum CW, Karayalcin SS, et al: Immune system control

of rat and rabbit colonic electrolyte transport: role of prostaglandins ad enteric nervous system. J Clin Invest 1989;83:1810–1820.
21. Shlatz LJ, Kimberg DV, Cattieu KA: Phosphorylation of specific rat intestinal microvillus and basal-lateral membrane proteins by cyclic nucleotides. Gastroenterology 1979;76:293–299.
22. Field M, Graf LH, Laird WJ, Smith PL: Heat-stable enterotoxin of Escherichia coli: in vitro effects on guanylate cyclase activity, cyclic GMP concentration, and ion transport in small intestine. Proc Natl Acad Sci USA 1978;75:2800–2804.
23. Hughes JM, Murad F, Chang B, Guerrant RL: Role of cyclic GMP in the action of heat-stable enterotoxin of Escherichia coli. Nature 1978;271:766–756.
24. Schiller LR, Davis GR, Santa Ana CA, et al: Studies of the mechanism of the antidiarrhea effect of codeine. J Clin Invest 1982;70:999.
25. Fordtran JS: Speculations on the pathogenesis of diarrhea. Fed Proc 1967;26:1405.
26. Fordtran JS, Locklear TW: Ionic constituents and osmolality of gastric and small intestinal fluids after eating. Am J Dig Dis 1966;11:503.
27. Phillips SF, Giller J: The contribution of the colon to electrolyte and water conservation in man. J Lab Clin Med 1973;81:733.
28. Fordtran JS, Rector FC, Ewton MF, et al: Permeability characteristics of the human small intestine. J Clin Invest 1965;44:1935.
29. Christopher NL, Bayless TM: Role of the small bowel and colon in lactose-induced diarrhea. Gastroenterology 1971;60:845.
30. Bond JH, Currier BE, Buchwald H, Levitt MD: Colonic conservation of malabsorbed carbohydrate. Gastroenterology 1980;78:444.
31. Butler DG, Gall DG, Kelly MN, Hamilton JR: Transmissible gastroenteritis. Mechanisms responsible for diarrhea in an acute viral enteritis in piglets. J Clin Invest 1974;53:1335–1342.
32. Keljo DJ, MacLeod RJ, Purdue MH, et al: D-Glucose transport in piglet jejunal brush-border membranes: insights from a disease model. Am J Physiol (Gastrointest Liver Physiol 12) 1985;249:G751–G760.
33. Hyams JS, Etienne NL, Leichtner AM, Theuer RC: Carbohydrate malabsorption following fruit juice ingestion in young children. Pediatrics 1988;82:64–68.
34. Powell DW: Intestinal water and electrolyte transport. In Johnson LR (ed): Physiology of the Gastrointestinal Tract, 2nd ed. New York, Raven Press, 1987, p 1267.
35. Fordtran JS, Santa Ana CA, Morawski SG, et al: Pathophysiology of chronic diarrhoea: insights derived from intestinal perfusion studies in 31 patients. Clin Gastroenterol 1986;15:529.
36. Krejs GJ: VIPoma syndrome. Am J Med 1987;82:37–47.
37. Levine MM, Edelman R: Enteropathogenic Escherichia coli of classic serotypes associated with infant diarrhea: epidemiology and pathogenesis. Epidemiol Rev 1987;6:31–50.
38. Scheibel E, Rechnitzer C, Fahrenkrug J, Hertz H: Vasoactive intestinal polypeptide (VIP) in children with neural crest tumours. Acta Paediatr Scand 1982;71:721–725.
39. Balistreri WF, Partin JC, Schubert WK: Bile acid malabsorption—a consequence of terminal ileal dysfunction in protracted diarrhea of infancy. J Pediatr 1977;89:21.
40. Thaysen EH: Idiopathic bile acid diarrhoea reconsidered. Scand J Gastroenterol 1985;20:452.
41. Cummings JH, Sladen GE, James OFW, et al: Laxative-induced diarrhoea: a continuing clinical problem. BMJ 1974;1:537.
42. Cassuto J, Jodal M, Tuttle R, Lundgren O: On the role of intramural nerves in the pathogenesis of cholera toxin-induced intestinal secretion. Scand J Gastroenterol 1981;16:377–384.
43. Eklund S, Jodal M, Lundgren O: The enteric nervous system participates in the secretory response to the heat stable enterotoxins of Escherichia coli in rats and cats. Neuroscience 1985;14:673–681.
44. Kerzner B, Kelly MH, Gall DG, et al: Transmissible gastroenteritis. Mechanisms responsible for diarrhea in an acute viral enteritis in piglets. Gastroenterology 1979;76:20–24.
45. Shepherd RW, Gall DG, Butler DG, Hamilton JR: Transmissible gastroenteritis: sodium transport and the intestinal epithelium during the course of viral enteritis. Gastroenterology 1977;72:457–561.
46. Granger DN, Hernandez LA, Grisham MB: Reactive oxygen metabolites: mediators of cell injury in the digestive system. Viewpoints Dig Dis 1986;18:13–16.
47. Purdue MH, Gall DG: Intestinal anaphylaxis in the rat: jejunal response to in vitro antigen exposure. Am J Physiol (Gastrointest Liver Physiol 13) 1986;250:G427–G431.
48. Rothbaum R, McAdams AJ, Giannella R, Partin JC: A clinicopathologic study of enterocyte-adherent Escherichia coli: a cause of protracted diarrhea in infants. Gastroenterology 1982;83:441–454.
49. Harris J, Shields R: Absorption and secretion of water and electrolytes by the intact human colon in diffuse untreated proctocolitis. Gut 1970;11:27.
50. Gooptu D, Truelove SC, Warner GT: Absorption of electrolytes from the colon in cases of ulcerative colitis and in control subjects. Gut 1969;10:555.
51. DuPont HL: Rotaviral gastroenteritis—some recent developments. J Infect Dis 1984;149:663–666.
52. Sack DA, Rhoads M, Molla A, et al: Carbohydrate malabsorption in infants with rotavirus diarrhea. Am J Clin Nutr 1982;36:1112–1118.
53. Sallon S, Deckelbaum RJ, Schmid II, et al: Cryptosporidium, malnutrition, and chronic diarrhea in children. Am J Dis Child 1988;142:312–315.
54. Kocoshis SA, Cibull ML, Davis TE, et al: Intestinal and pulmonary cryptosporidiosis in an infant with severe combined immune deficiency. J Pediatr Gastroenterol Nutr 1984;3:149–157.
55. Soave R, Johnson WD: Cryptosporidium and Isopora Belli infections. J Infect Dis 1988;157:225–229.
56. Moriarty KJ, Turnberg LA: Bacterial toxins and diarrhoea. Clin Gastroenterol 1986;15:529.
57. Gracey M, Burke V, Robinson J: Aeromonas-associated gastroenteritis. Lancet 1982;2:1304–1306.
58. Burke V, Gracey M, Robinson J, et al: The microbiology of childhood gastroenteritis: Aeromonas species and other infective agents. J Infect Dis 1983;148:68–74.
59. Nime FA, Burek JK, Page DL, et al: Acute enterocolitis in a human being infected with the protozoan Cryptosporidium. Gastroenterology 1976;70:592–598.
60. Stephen S, Rao KNA, Kumar MS, et al: Human infection with Aeromonas species: varied clinical manifestations. Ann Intern Med 1975;83:368–369.
61. Whitington PF, Friedman AL, Chesney RW: Gastrointestinal disease in the hemolytic-uremic syndrome. Gastroenterology 1979;76:728–733.
62. Gransden WR, Damm MA, Anderson JD, et al: Further evidence associating hemolytic-uremic syndrome with infection by vero-toxin producing Escherichia coli O157:H7. J Infect Dis 1986;154:522–523.
63. Richardson SE, Karmali MA, Becker LE, et al: The histopathology of hemolytic-uremic syndrome associated with verocytotoxin-producing Escherichia coli infections. Hum Pathol 1988;19:1102–1108.
64. Pai CH, Gordon R, Sims HV, et al: Sporadic cases of hemorrhagic colitis associated with Escherichia coli O157:H7: clinical, epidemiologic, and bacteriologic features. Ann Intern Med 1984;101:738–742.
65. Avery GB, Villavicencio O, Lilly JR, et al: Intractable diarrhea in early infancy. Pediatrics 1968;41:712.
66. Larcher VF, Shepherd R, Francis DEM, et al: Protracted diarrhea of infancy. Arch Dis Child 1977;52:597.
67. Lo CW, Walker WA: Chronic protracted diarrhea of infancy: a nutritional disease. Pediatrics 1983;72:786.
68. Goldgar CM, Vanderhoof JA: Lack of correlation of small bowel biopsy and clinical course of patients with intractable diarrhea of infancy. Gastroenterology 1986;90:527–532.
69. Hill DJ, Davidson FP, Cameron DJS, et al: The spectrum of cow's milk allergy in childhood. Acta Paediatr Scand 1979;68:847.
70. Iyngkaran N, Robinson MH, Prathap K, et al: Cow's milk protein-sensitive enteropathy: combined clinical and histological criteria for diagnosis. Arch Dis Child 1978;53:20.
71. Vanderhoof JA, Murray ND, Kaufman SS, et al: Intolerance to protein hydrolysate infant formulas, an under-recognized cause of gastrointestinal symptoms in infants. J Pediatr 1997;131:741.
72. Mirakian R, Richardson A, Milla PJ, et al: Protracted diarrhoea of infancy: evidence in support of an autoimmune variant. BMJ 1986;193:113–116.
73. Zoppi G, Deganello A, Gaburro D: Persistent post-enteritis diarrhoea. Eur J Pediatr 1977;126:225.
74. Iyngkaran N, Robinson MH, Sumithran E, et al: Cow's milk protein-sensitive enteropathy: an important factor in prolonging diarrhoea of acute infective enteritis in early infancy. Arch Dis Child 1978;53:150.
75. Davidson GP, Cutz E, Hamilton JR, et al: Familiar enteropathy: a syndrome of protracted diarrhea from birth, failure to thrive, and hypoplastic villous atrophy. Gastroenterology 1978;75:783.
76. Goutet JM, Boccon-Gibod L, Chatelet F, et al: Familiar protracted diarrhoea with hypoplastic villous atrophy: report of two cases. Pediatr Res 1982;16:1045.
77. Phillips AD, Jenkins P, Raafat F, et al: Congenital microvillous atrophy specific diagnostic features. Arch Dis Child 1985;60:730.

78. Schmitz J, Ginies JL, Arnaud-Battandier F, et al: Congenital microvillous atrophy, a rare cause of neonatal intractable diarrhoea. Pediatr Res 1982;16:1014.
79. Randak C, Langnas AN, Kaufman SS, et al: Successful treatment of an infant with microvillous inclusion disease including liver/small bowel transplantation. J Pediatr Gastroenterol Nutr 1998;27:333–337.
80. Reifen RM, Cutz E, Griffiths AM, et al: Tufting enteropathy: a newly recognized clinicopathological entity associated with refractory diarrhea in infants. J Pediatr Gastroenterol Nutr 1994;18:379–385.
81. Goulet O, Kedinger M, Brousse N, et al: Intractable diarrhea of infancy with epithelial and basement membrane abnormalities. J Pediatr 1995;127:212–219.
82. Girault D, Goulet O, LeDeist F, et al: Intractable infant diarrhea associated with phenotypic abnormalities and immunodeficiencies. J Pediatr 1994;125:36–42.
83. Mirakian R, Richardson A, Milla PJ, et al: Protracted diarrhoea of infancy: evidence in support of an autoimmune variant. BMJ 1986;293:1132.
84. Unsworth J, Hutchins P, Mitchell J, et al: Flat small intestinal mucosa and autoantibodies against the gut epithelium. J Pediatr Gastroenterol Nutr 1982;1:503.
85. Ackerman NB, Strobel CT: Polle syndrome: chronic diarrhea in Munchausen's child. Gastroenterology 1981;81:1140.
86. Pickering LK, Kohl S: Munchausen syndrome by proxy. Am J Dis Child 1981;135:288.
87. Holmberg C: Congenital chloride diarrhoea. Clin Gastroenterol 1986;15:583.
88. Clark EB, Vanderhoof JA: Effects of acetazolamide on electrolyte balance in congenital chloridorrhea. J Pediatr 1977;91:148–149.
89. Davidson M, Wasserman R: The irritable colon of childhood (chronic nonspecific diarrhea syndrome). J Pediatr 1966;69:1027–1038.
90. Davidson M: Functional problems associated with colonic dysfunction. The irritable bowel syndrome. Pediatr Ann 1987;16:776–795.
91. Greene HL, Ghishan FK: Excessive fluid intake as a cause of chronic diarrhea in young children. J Pediatr 1982;102:836–840.
92. Cohen SA, Hendrics KM, Mathis RK, et al: Chronic nonspecific diarrhea: dietary relationships. Pediatrics 1979;64:402–407.
93. Lloyd-Still JD: Chronic diarrhea of childhood and the misuse of elimination diets. J Pediatr 1979;95:10–13.
94. Groothuis JR, Berman S, Chapman J: Effect of carbohydrate ingested on outcome in infants with mild gastroenteritis. J Pediatr 1986;25:85–88.
95. Klish WJ, Udall JN, Rodriguez JT, et al: Intestinal surface area in infants with acquired monosaccharide intolerance. J Pediatr 1978;92:566–571.
96. Trounce JQ, Walker-Smith JA: Sugar intolerance complicating acute gastroenteritis. Arch Dis Child 1985;60:986–990.
97. Phillips AD, Walker-Smith JA: Delayed recovery in childhood. In Walker-Smith JA, McNeish AS (eds): Diarrhoea and Malnutrition in Childhood. London, Butterworths, 1986, pp 107–112.
98. Farthing MJG, Mata LJ, Urutia JJ, Kronmal RA: Natural history of Giardia infection of infants and children in rural Guatemala and its impact on physical growth. Am J Clin Nutr 1986;43:393–403.
99. Goka AKJ, Rolston DDK, Mathan VI, Farthing MJG: Diagnosis of giardiasis by specific IgM antibody enzyme-linked immunosorbent assay. Lancet 1986;2:184–186.
100. Ungar BLP, Yolken RH, Nash TE, Quinn TC: Enzyme-linked immunosorbent assay for detection of Giardia lamblia in fecal specimens. J Infect Dis 1984;149:90–97.
101. Fasano A: Where have all the American celiacs gone? Acta Paediatr Suppl 1996;412:20–24.
102. Maki M, Hallstrom O, Vesikari T, Visakorpi JK: Evaluation of serum IgA-class reticulin antibody test for the detection of childhood celiac disease. J Pediatr 1984;105:901–905.
103. Eade DE, Lloyd RS, Lang C, Wright R: IgA and IgG reticulin antibodies in celiac and non-celiac patients. Gut 1977;18:991–993.
104. Burgin-Wolff A, Bertele RM, Berger R, et al: A reliable screening test for childhood celiac disease: fluorescent immunosorbent test for gliadin antibodies. J Pediatr 1963;102:655–660.

Chapter 4

# Constipation and Encopresis

*Rita Steffen and Vera Loening-Baucke*

Constipation is a common problem in pediatric patients, with chronic constipation accounting for at least 3% of the office visits to general pediatric practices[1] and 10% to 25%[2] of referrals to pediatric gastroenterologists. *Constipation* is defined as the passage of fewer than three stools per week or a history of painful passage of large, hard stools in children with fecal retention and withholding who may or may not be soiling.[3] A patient can be constipated in spite of passing more than three stools per week. The child can have fecal impaction with frequent small bowel movements into the toilet and fecal soiling in the underwear around this impaction.

*Encopresis* is defined as chronic fecal incontinence or soiling in a child with a developmental age of 4 years or older who has normal colon and rectal anatomy. Encopresis is the involuntary leakage of stool from a chronically dilated rectum, which often contains a central mass of retained hard stool. This phenomenon is also known as overflow incontinence; a normal stool frequency or even diarrhea may be present.

Knowledge of normal stool patterns by age and an appreciation for the variety of meanings that constipation has for pediatric patients and their parents will help the practitioner to define their expectations and to provide appropriate service in diagnosis, treatment, and referral when needed. Illness, injury, postoperative state, sudden change to a sedentary condition, and change in routines with travel and accommodations can be associated with constipation, but the problem is usually transient, unless these are additive factors in a child with chronic constipation.

## ETIOLOGY AND PATHOPHYSIOLOGY

In adults, defecation occurs normally from three times per day to three times per week.[4] Stool frequency varies with age in pediatric patients. Breast-fed infants may initially have more frequent stools than formula-fed infants, but by 4 months of age most infants, regardless of feeding source, pass, on average, two stools a day. One to seven bowel movements per day was the range reported in 93% of the infants in this study.[5] By 2 years of age, the mean frequency of bowel movements decreases to two per day. In a preschool cohort of 350 children, the frequency of bowel movements approximated 1.2 per day by 4 years of age and 96% had established the equivalent of the adult bowel pattern just noted.[6] Soiling has been reported to occur in 1% to as high as 7.5% of elementary school-age children.[7]

The normal process of defecation starts with fecal filling of the rectum, a process that initiates a reflex relaxation of the tonically contracted internal anal sphincter and is sensed by the individual, who responds by voluntarily contracting the external anal sphincter. Fecal continence is maintained in this manner until a toilet can be reached. For defecation, the external anal sphincter and puborectalis muscles relax to a point that the angle formed by the anal canal and rectum opens, making a straighter path for expulsion of stool.[8] Straining (Valsalva maneuver), through increase of intra-abdominal pressure and rectal contractions, helps to propel the bolus outside the body. Normally, the sensory epithelium within the anorectal area informs the individual by a process of anal "sampling" of the physical properties of the contents, that is, whether it is solid, liquid, or gas, or a combination of these.

The colon stores and desiccates liquid stool received from the ileum. Eating is the main stimulus for colonic propulsive contractions by means of the gastrocolic reflex, which is mediated probably by neuropeptides in the enteric nervous system and visceral nerve connections. The nutritional content supplied to the colon influences stool consistency and frequency. Inadequate dietary fiber as a stool bulking agent, decreased intake of liquids, and increased net fluid losses are constipating conditions. Stool weight is related to the amount of fiber ingested. Larger stools are evacuated more frequently. Transit through the gastrointestinal tract is faster with fiber ingestion.[9, 10] The transit time for infants, aged 1 to 3 months, is approximately 8.5 hours. Transit time increases with age, and is 30 to 48 hours in adults.[7] Decreased activity from surgery, illness, injury, and sedentary lifestyles predisposes to constipation in previously active individuals. Stress and functional changes in routine daily life can alter stool frequency; for example, vacations, camping, going back to school, access to toilet areas, and privacy have an effect on the ability to defecate successfully.

The most common cause for constipation in children is withholding of stool because of prior painful bowel movements, commonly accompanied by an anal fissure. Parents often give a history of blood on the stool or diaper or in the toilet. This painful experience is believed to initiate withholding of stool when the urge to defecate occurs. A habit cycle of stool retention results that stretches the rectum and later the sigmoid colon to accommodate the unevacuated feces and the new stool arriving behind it in the colon. The bolus remaining the longest is subject to reabsorption of fluid and electrolytes and forms the nidus for a fecal impaction. The whole process is self-perpetuating in that larger and harder stools become more difficult to pass through the anal canal, resulting in reinforcement of the painful experience and thus further withholding.

When constipation is chronic, the fecal mass can occupy the rectum, sigmoid colon, and the descending colon and even the whole colon. Encopresis or involuntary leakage of liquid or semiformed stool around this fecal mass is usually the event that causes parents to seek medical attention for the problem. Chronic rectal distention secondary to withholding and fecal retention causes decreased ability to sense stool volumes, which formerly caused a call to stool or urge to defecate.[11] The most common manometric finding in these patients is an increased threshold for rectal sensation. With long-term treatment, rectal sensation can return to normal, but it remains abnormal in some recovered children, which may explain their vulnerability to recurrent constipation and soiling.[12] Prolonged latencies are recorded in children with chronic constipation and encopresis compared with controls when the afferent pathway from the rectum is studied after mechanical distention of the rectum. This suggests a possible defect in sensation,[13] but the area needs further study.

*Paradoxical puborectalis contraction*, a term that has several different synonyms, such as abnormal defecation dynamics or anismus,[14] is a common finding on anorectal manometry of chronically constipated children[15] and adults.[14] Paradoxical contraction is defined as the inappropriate contraction of the external anal sphincter and puborectalis muscles during attempts to defecate stool, instead of relaxing these muscles. Children with abnormal contraction of the external anal sphincter and puborectalis during training for defecation also have difficulty defecating water-filled balloons and have a higher chance of treatment failure.[16] In a smaller group of infants and children (less than 5% to 10%), constipation has anatomic, neurologic, or other causes, which are discussed in the section on differential diagnosis.

## AGENTS OR MEDICATIONS ASSOCIATED WITH CONSTIPATION IN CHILDREN

Most of the major agents or medications that can cause constipation are grouped by functional class in Table 4–1, with individual agents noted as examples. This shortened list is provided as a general reference. Some liquid antacid preparations are constipating. An anticholinergic agent used in the treatment of urinary incontinence secondary to neurogenic bladder found in patients with spinal cord abnormalities, such as meningomyelocele, is oxybutynin chloride (Ditropan). Most often the bladder medication can be continued, and the constipation in this subset of children is treated successfully with softeners, suppositories, and/or enemas.

**TABLE 4–1. Agents or Medications Associated with Constipation in Children**

| |
|---|
| Anesthetics, narcotic analgesics, opiates |
| Anticholinergics and sympathomimetic agents |
| Anticonvulsants and the ketogenic diet treatment for intractable seizures |
| Antimotility agents |
| Antipsychotics, antidepressants (including tricyclics) |
| Barium from roentgenographic studies of the bowel |
| Calcium channel blockers (e.g., verapamil), antidysrhythmic agents |
| Minerals: aluminum, calcium, iron, lead, mercury, arsenic, bismuth |
| Nonsteroidal anti-inflammatory agents |

Constipation may be a significant side effect in children treated for cardiac dysrhythmias, depression, seizure disorders, and a number of other common and uncommon disorders. In most cases these medications can be continued with treatment for constipation. The exception are children on a ketogenic diet for intractable seizures. Here, consultation with the dietitian responsible for the diet may be helpful.

## CLINICAL SIGNS AND SYMPTOMS OF CHRONIC CONSTIPATION

Decreased frequency of stools should be sought in the history. When constipation becomes chronic, the number of bowel actions per day or per week may not be a reliable indicator for constipation in an individual child. Usually, an infrequent stool pattern is present at the beginning of the process, which may have been several months or years before the patient's contact with the physician. With stool retention, other signs and symptoms of constipation gradually appear and may include abdominal distention and pain, often relieved with defecation. Significant to note in the history is passage of hard and/or very large stools that may block the toilet. Soiling from seepage of liquid stool around a large fecal mass or impaction may paradoxically be diagnosed as diarrhea. A constipated child commonly will have a cycle of appetite blunting and may have periods with little or no weight gain, followed by a remarkable improvement with therapy. Efforts to withhold stool may be misinterpreted as attempts to strain or defecate. Posturing, scissoring of the legs, and dancing back and forth from one leg to another are common withholding maneuvers, and sometimes the withholding behavior may resemble a seizure.

Urinary incontinence and urinary tract infection are frequently associated with chronic constipation in childhood. Occasionally, urinary retention, megacystis, and vesicoureteral reflux can be found during urinary tract evaluation. In a study of 234 children with chronic constipation and encopresis, 29% had diurnal enuresis and 34% had nocturnal enuresis. Urinary tract infection was found in 11%. Twelve months after starting treatment for constipation, 52% had resolution of the constipation, 89% of this group had disappearance of daytime urinary incontinence, 63% were now able to stay dry at night, and all children with normal urinary tract anatomy demonstrated disappearance of recurrent urinary tract infections.[17]

Signs of constipation on the physical examination may

include abdominal distention with normal, increased, or decreased bowel sounds. Abdominal masses should be gently sought by palpation in the left and right lower quadrants and suprapubic areas. The stool mass may in severe cases extend to the epigastric area and even simulate a pregnancy in size. In school-age children soiled underpants may be noted. The lower lumbar and sacral spine areas are inspected for dimpling, surgical scars, hair tufting, or asymmetry. Anal tone and position with respect to other anatomic landmarks on the perineum are noted. The anocutaneous or "wink" reflex is elicited. Anal fissures and the size and content of the rectal ampulla are the most helpful markers of constipation. Occasionally, if the rectal examination cannot be done because the patient is too frightened, then therapy can be started on the basis of the clinical history. Deep tendon reflexes in the lower extremities are elicited and reflect spinal integrity.

## DIFFERENTIAL DIAGNOSIS

Over 90% of pediatric patients with constipation have the functional retentive type. In some children, the etiology is multifactorial, when dietary habits change to blunt the appetite and decrease intake of fluids and bulk. A dietary change from breast milk to cow's milk formula or from infant formula to cow's milk at the age of 12 months is a constipating event for some infants. When a reasonable therapeutic plan is not effective or when constipation occurs in the neonatal period or infancy, exploration of other causes is indicated. Although overlap may occur in the ages of presentation of some causes of constipation, groupings of causes to consider by age of most likely presentation are presented in Table 4–2. Importantly, the most likely time of presentation for these disorders certainly does not exclude atypical presentation. Delayed diagnosis of an underlying cause of constipation may occur with chronic use of laxatives, because some patients and their parents may perceive the bowel pattern to be tolerable and therefore not seek medical attention.

Congenital anatomic or structural defects that may result in a complete obstruction of the distal colon are recognized in the newborn period to be anorectal anomalies, with a spectrum of defects ranging from imperforate anus to the anteriorly displaced anus,[18] meconium plug syndrome, and Hirschsprung's disease. A stenotic zone in the colon after necrotizing enterocolitis may present as constipation in early infancy. Cutaneous abnormalities in the lower back may be present at birth and should raise concerns about a spinal abnormality. With growth, constipation, fecal and urinary incontinence, and urinary tract infections may appear due to tethering of the spinal cord.

Metabolic and endocrine disturbances may cause secondary constipation, including dehydration states, diabetes insipidus, hypercalcemia, and renal tubular acidosis. In the United States, newborns are screened for hypothyroidism. However, onset of hypothyroidism can occur at any age. Connective tissue diseases are associated with constipation, but usually the process needs to be present for years for bowel dysfunction to appear and therefore would be more likely to appear in adolescence or adulthood.

Anterior location of the anus, chronic intestinal pseudo-obstruction, and ultra-short segment Hirschsprung's disease are entities that may escape detection in the first year of life with breast feeding and use of softeners. Intestinal pseudo-obstruction and Hirschsprung's disease that involve a large extent of small and large intestine will present in infancy,[19] but if the disease involves only a short segment, then signs and symptoms may be intermittent and investigation could be delayed until childhood or later. Generally, the more bowel involved with the disease, the more likely the presentation will be earlier in life.

Neurologic causes of constipation can be damage to the spinal cord disrupting sacral outflow (e.g., meningomyelocele, trauma, prior surgery, some tumors and cysts, cauda equina syndrome, and tethered cord). Central and peripheral nervous system disorders that can be associated with constipation include cerebral palsy, infectious polyneuritis, amyotonia congenita, the muscular dystrophies, and degenerative disorders.

**TABLE 4–2. Causes of Constipation by Most Likely Age of Presentation**

| |
|---|
| **Newborn/Infancy** |
| Meconium plug |
| Hirschsprung's disease |
| Cystic fibrosis |
| A spectrum of congenital anorectal malformations, including imperforate anus, anal stenosis, anterior ectopic anus, and fibrous bands within the anal canal (anal band) |
| Chronic idiopathic intestinal pseudo-obstruction |
| Endocrine: hypothyroidism |
| Metabolic: diabetes insipidus, renal tubular acidosis |
| Withholding |
| Dietary changes |
| **Toddlers and Ages 2 to 4 Years** |
| Anal fissures, withholding, functional stool retention |
| Toilet refusal |
| Short segment Hirschsprung's disease |
| Neurologic disorders: central or muscular with hypotonia |
| Spinal cord: meningomyelocele, tumors, tethered cord |
| **School Age** |
| Withholding |
| Toilet or bathroom access limited/unavailable |
| Limited ability to recognize physiologic cues, and preoccupation with other activities |
| Tethered cord |
| **Adolescent** |
| Irritable bowel syndrome, constipation-predominant type |
| Spinal cord injury (accidents, trauma) |
| Dieting |
| Anorexia |
| Pregnancy |
| Idiopathic slow transit constipation, primarily seen in females |
| Laxative abuse |
| **Any Age** |
| Medication side effect, dietary, postoperative state |
| Previous anorectal surgery |
| Withholding, and overflow from chronic rectal distention |
| Relatively rapid change to sedentary state, dehydration |
| Hypothyroidism |

## EVALUATION

Age of the patient at presentation is one of the clues to the differential diagnosis (see Table 4–2). Constipation in the first year of life, specifically in the newborn period, calls for the clinician to work with the radiologist and pediatric surgeon to rule out congenital anorectal malformations, Hirschsprung's disease, small left colon syndrome, cystic fibrosis, and meconium plug syndrome. Failure to pass meconium within the first 24 hours of life, and certainly within the first 48 hours of life, suggests a distal obstruction and is an indication for abdominal radiographs and further work-up.

The history focuses on frequency of bowel movements, stool consistency, toileting habits, toileting history and attempts, and episodes of encopresis. Between visits a stool chart can sharpen the details of the history and document response to therapy and compliance by the child and the parents. The medications that may have constipation as a side effect and any systemic illness or surgery that may contribute to constipation need to be reviewed. It is helpful to briefly review dietary habits for total volume and types of fluids consumed in a typical day; alternatively, it can be done prospectively with the daily diary brought in for follow-up. For patients who have a history of encopresis, passage of large stools that may block the toilet is not uncommon.

Observation of the child in the office while doing the history is helpful, because withholding behavior or posturing can often be noted and the parent-child interaction can be observed. Inspection of the abdomen for distention and palpation for stool masses in the region of the sigmoid colon and rectum is done. The lumbosacral spine area is inspected for defects. If the child is cooperative, the anocutaneous "wink reflex" is elicited. The rectal examination gives information on the location or position of the anal opening on the perineum with respect to the other structures. The tone of the sphincter muscles is assessed, and any stenotic areas or bands can be detected. A digital sweep around the rectal vault gives information about rectal dilation, presence or absence of fecal impaction, and stool consistency. Some children may be able to "squeeze" or "push" when asked, and information about defecatory dynamics is obtained. It is possible to detect paradoxical contraction with this maneuver in some patients. In the case of the uncooperative frightened child, we never force a rectal examination and will rely on the history to initiate therapy.

## INVESTIGATIONS

If the digital rectal examination does not reveal rectal distention with stool, or could not be performed, then the plain abdominal roentgenogram can be used to assess the colonic caliber and contents in chronically constipated children and encopretics.[20]

Anorectal manometry is indicated for the pediatric patient who presents with constipation very early in life and children who have had a prolonged course of treatment or are refractory to a reasonable treatment program that has been instituted for an adequate duration. An enema is usually given as preparation, and the child lies in the left lateral position. The procedure is explained to the patient and caregivers. Conscious sedation is indicated in a few selected patients and can be given orally or intravenously.

Several technical systems are available to record pressures. At the Cleveland Clinic we use a manometry catheter with tiny water-perfused channels located in the tip around the central port to measure the pressure within the rectal balloon. Four water-perfused ports have pressure transducers radially arranged at 90 degrees from each other at the same level to measure pressures within the anal canal. A schematic drawing of the anorectal region with the manometry catheter and anal surface electrodes is shown in Figure 4–1.

Anorectal manometry is used to assess the pressures in the anal sphincter muscles at rest, during squeezing and straining (Fig. 4–2). A pressure tracing demonstrating a normal voluntary squeeze response is shown in Figure 4–2*A*: an abrupt rise above the baseline pressure is present in the three tracings measuring anal canal pressure, and this falls back to baseline at the end of the squeeze. Simultaneously, the uppermost channel provides the myoelectrical recruitment pattern of the external anal sphincter before, during, and after the squeeze. The rectal pressure does not rise during the squeeze. A normal strain for defecation is shown in Figure 4–2*B*: during attempted defecation, rectal pressure increases while the anal canal pressure decreases, creating the normal gradient that will favor defecation of the fecal bolus. The external anal sphincter electromyogram is inhibited after an initial short increase in activity. A second increase is seen at the end of the defecation attempt, corresponding to anal canal closure. By contrast, Figure 4–2*C* demonstrates what is recorded during a paradoxical strain: pressures in the anal canal and rectum and electromyographic activity increase, leading to a pattern of "obstructed defecation" or a functional pelvic outlet obstruction. This pattern is not uncommon in both pediatric and adult patients with constipation.

The anal resting pressure is created chiefly by the internal anal sphincter. When a rectal balloon is inflated, the anal pressure normally decreases and then returns to the resting anal canal pressure (Fig. 4–3*A*). This rectoanal inhibitory reflex is possible because the ganglion cells located in the submucosal layer and between the muscle layers of the

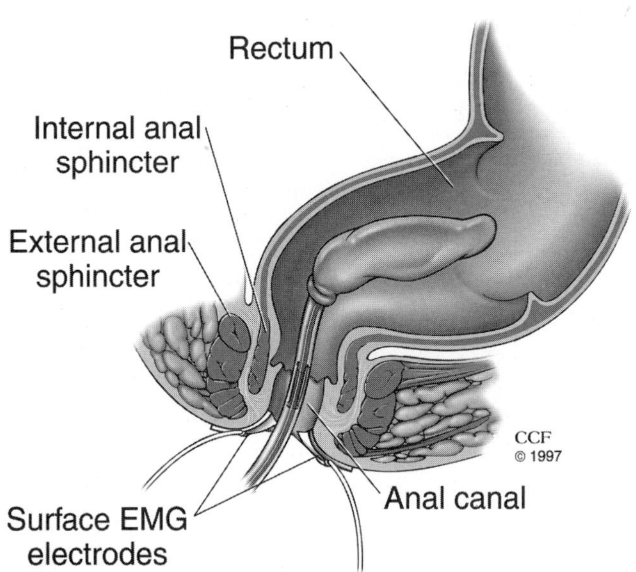


**FIGURE 4–1.** Schematic drawing of the anorectal region with the manometry catheter and anal surface electrodes. (Copyright 1997, Cleveland Clinic Foundation.)

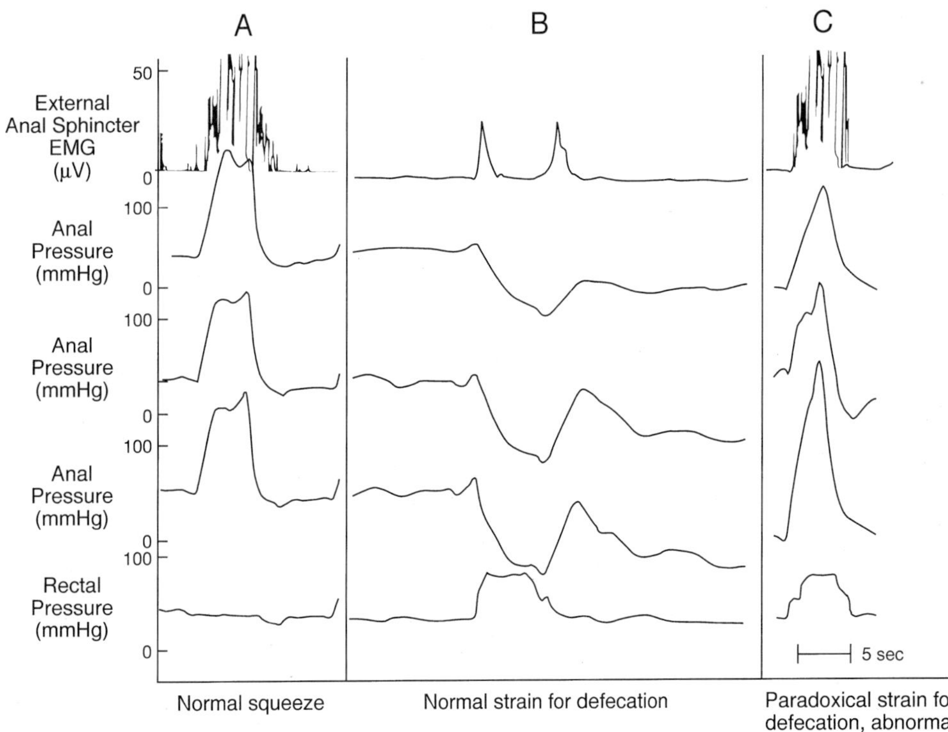


**FIGURE 4–2.** Patterns of anorectal manometry and surface electromyography for a normal squeeze *(A)*, during straining *(B)*, and paradoxical straining *(C)*.

bowel mediate the information from the rectum to the internal anal sphincter to inhibit the resting pressure. This reflex relaxation is not seen in patients with Hirschsprung's disease (see Fig. 4–3*B*). The absence of ganglion cells can extend from the distal rectum to a variable distance proximal, most commonly to the rectosigmoid region. With balloon distention, the anal pressure of patients with Hirschsprung's disease will not relax but, instead, will stay at the same level or show a paradoxical increase (see Fig. 4–3*B*). When this reflex is not seen, a rectal biopsy is indicated.

Electromyography of the external anal sphincter can be recorded with surface electrodes adherent to the skin on the anal verge (see Fig. 4–1).[21] When combined with anorectal manometry,[22] the electromyogram provides additional information and is helpful in defining the defecation dynamics.[23] Electromyography combined with anorectal manometry is

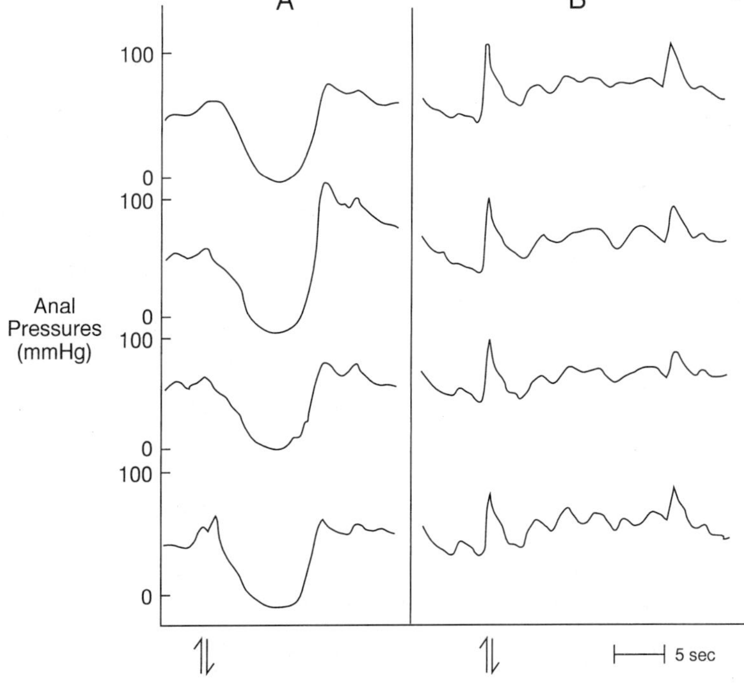


**FIGURE 4–3.** Anorectal manometry. Recordings from four radially arranged transducers at the same level within the anal canal. The arrows indicate the point at which the rectal balloon is rapidly inflated and deflated with 25 mL of air. *A*, The anal pressure tracings demonstrate a normal reflex relaxation of the internal sphincter, a normal "rectoanal inhibitory reflex." The majority of the "drop" in anal pressure is produced by relaxation of the tonically contracted internal anal sphincter. *B*, Tracings from a patient with Hirschsprung's disease: the rectoanal inhibitory reflex is absent.

used to provide biofeedback to selected children with abnormal defecation dynamics (e.g., pelvic floor dyssynergia, paradoxical puborectalis contraction).

The unprepped barium enema is helpful in demonstrating the so-called transition zone between the narrow aganglionic segment and the dilated ganglionated bowel proximal to it (Fig. 4–4). To the left in Figure 4–4*A* is an unprepped barium enema examination from a 5-year-old boy with functional, chronic retentive constipation and encopresis. The rectum is dilated with stool, but there is a smooth contour funneling upward from the anal canal and continuing into the sigmoid colon. This patient demonstrated a normal rectoanal inhibitory reflex on anorectal manometry, excluding Hirschsprung's disease. In contrast, Figure 4–4*B* shows an unprepped barium enema examination of a 10-year-old boy with distal short-segment Hirschsprung's disease. The rectum is massively dilated with retained stool. The aganglionic segment is limited to the lower rectum, which will not relax, creating a functional obstruction. The ganglionated bowel is dilated to accommodate the fecal contents. The black arrows show the narrow rectum, which was aganglionic on biopsy; this area should be as large or larger than the dilated rectum proximal to it. The child was referred to the pediatric surgeon for resection and a "pull-through" procedure. Further discussion on surgery for Hirschsprung's disease is found in Chapter 41.

Other studies available for evaluating patients with constipation are ingestion of radiopaque markers to measure intestinal transit time[24, 25] and colonic manometry.[26] Colonic manometry requires colonoscopic placement of the catheter with the motility recordings done the following day before and after a meal and bisacodyl administration. This test is time consuming and invasive and is usually reserved for children with intractable constipation. Di Lorenzo and coworkers have differentiated children with functional fecal retention from those with neuropathy or myopathy of the colon with this technique.[26] Others have used an electronic barostat to measure transit and motility in the colon.[27] This technique helps in the localization of an abnormal segment of bowel that can be missed by the colonic manometry technique.[27] A dynamic proctogram or defecography can provide further information about the anus and rectum during rest, squeeze, and straining.

## TREATMENT

Disimpaction is the first step in treating chronic constipation and encopresis. The initial "clean out" can be accomplished with enemas, oral electrolyte solutions, or a variety of softening agents. When the fecal impaction is high in the descending colon, a trial of a higher-volume enema (600 to 1000 mL saline or milk of molasses mixture of 1 part molasses and 1 part milk) may be more effective than the small, 2¼-ounce pediatric Fleet phosphate enema. Caution is in order regarding phosphate enemas because of potential electrolyte disturbances with hypocalcemia, hyperphosphatemia, and hypernatremia, which may result in tetany, coma, and death.[28, 29] For some children, disimpaction may take several days.

The maintenance phase follows and consists of softener or lubricant therapy and regular, timed toilet sitting, which is best done after meals. The treatment is tailored to the patient and parents' abilities to reinforce and comply with a program that needs to be maintained for several months to years. Most often, daily defecation is maintained by daily administration of softeners or laxatives. These medications are used according to age, body weight, and severity of the constipation. The actual choice of medication—mineral oil, lactulose, sorbitol, or milk of magnesia—is determined by the child's taste preference and is not as important as an adequate dosage and the child's and parent's compliance with the treatment regimen. Mineral oil is an emollient agent for treating functional stool retention. It will make

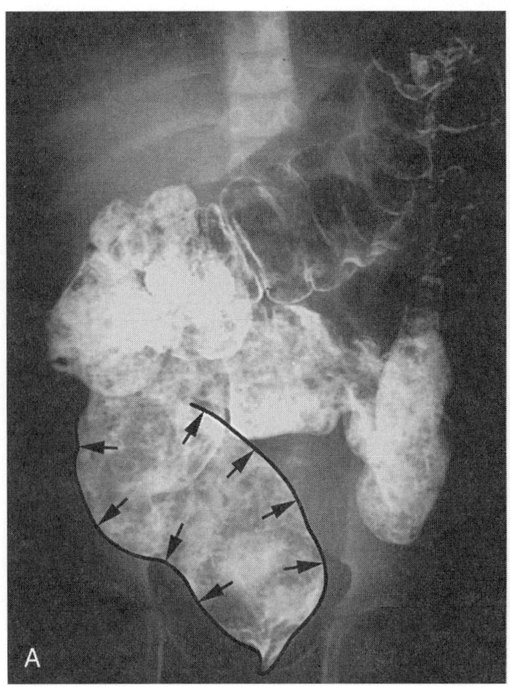


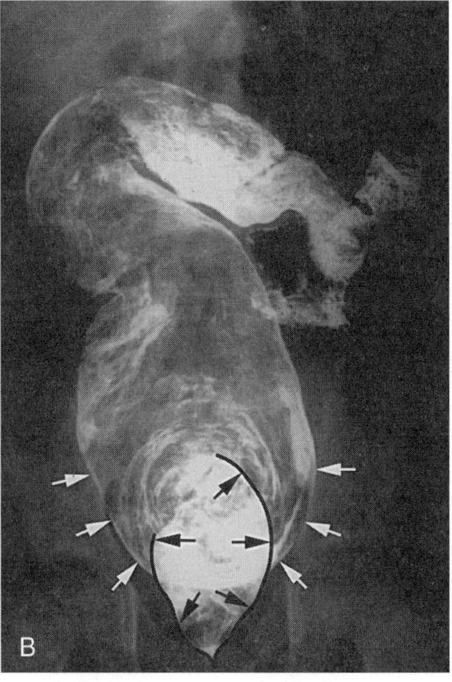


**FIGURE 4–4.** Unprepped barium enema. *A*, Acquired megarectum and megasigmoid in a 5-year-old boy with long-standing retentive constipation, refusal to sit on the toilet, and encopresis. The arrows point to the uniformly dilated rectum and sigmoid colon. *B*, A 10-year-old boy with distal short-segment Hirschsprung's disease. The zone affected by aganglionosis is marked with the black arrows, and the white arrows indicate the normally innervated dilated colon above it. The area between the aganglionic and ganglionated bowel is referred to as "transition zone."

withholding difficult to impossible because it lubricates passage of stool through the anal canal. Anal oil seepage is an undesirable side effect. It eventually will break the child's association of pain with stooling. A starting dose can be 1 to 3 mL/kg/day in one or two doses. Mineral oil can be mixed with milk or juice and chilled. In a series of 25 chronically constipated children on mineral oil, at 4 months serum levels of retinol and α-tocopherol were normal, whereas levels of β-carotene were decreased. Continuation of mineral oil therapy was recommended without concern for fat-soluble vitamin deficiencies.[30]

Mineral oil poses a risk of aspiration and pneumonia for patients with cerebral palsy, seizure disorders, and dysphagia. In these patients, we prefer to use 1 to 3 mL/kg/day of the pentose sugar lactulose. Lactulose is an essentially nonabsorbable carbohydrate that osmotically drags fluid into the feces, making the stools soft and easier to pass. Milk of magnesia is successful owing to the relative nonabsorption of magnesium and the resultant increase in luminal osmolality. In children who have fecal retention of mostly soft-formed stools, a dosage of 1 mL/kg/day is usually adequate. In the child who has severe constipation with rock-hard stools or very infrequent bowel movements, the starting dosage is 3 mL/kg/day given with the evening meal or divided up. Often stool softeners and laxatives are ineffective in the initial treatment of the megarectum/megacolon of patients who have disease states that place limitations on the act of defecation such as hypotonia, cerebral palsy, severe mental retardation, spina bifida, patients who still suffer from constipation with rectal atony. In them, daily Senokot (1 to 3 teaspoonfuls or tablets/day) will stimulate defecation.

A bulking agent, dissolved in water and flavored, can be successfully used in many patients.[31] For younger children, pear nectar has a relatively high fiber content and is well tolerated in the diet. Changing from the regular cow's milk formula to a protein hydrolysate-based formula usually relieves the constipation in infants, although initially the change in taste may decrease the amount of formula taken.

The laxative and behavioral approach has been described in 1963. Since then, only a few new treatment approaches have been suggested and explored. A prokinetic agent, cisapride, which is chemically related to metoclopramide, is free of the side effect of acute dystonic reaction. It is available in a suspension and is well tolerated by pediatric patients. Recommended dosage is 0.2 mg/kg of body weight three times daily. However, the medication must not be taken simultaneously with erythromycin-related antibiotics and antifungal agents because of the small but potential risk of cardiac dysrhythmias. The action of cisapride appears to involve the facilitation of acetylcholine release in the intramural plexuses. Experiments suggest that cisapride induces gastrointestinal peristalsis by stimulation of 5-$HT_4$ receptors in the myenteric plexus and antagonizing 5-$HT_3$ receptors. Four publications report the results of cisapride treatment in constipated children.[32–35] Two randomized controlled studies using cisapride by Staiano and coworkers[32] from Italy and Odeka and associates[34] from England were published. Staiano and coworkers[32] showed significantly increased stool frequency and decreased laxative and suppository use after 12 weeks of cisapride treatment in nine children with functional constipation, defined as fewer than four bowel movements/week and/or a total gastrointestinal transit time of more than 33 hours. Placebo significantly decreased laxative or suppository use but had no significant effect on stool frequency. Total gastrointestinal transit time decreased significantly but did not normalize after 12 weeks of cisapride treatment. Odeka and associates[34] defined constipation as pain and difficulty or delay in defecation. Their study did not show a significant effect on stool frequency and showed a decrease, but not a significant decrease, in total gastrointestinal transit time after 8 weeks of cisapride treatment and placebo. The two open label studies showed significant improvement in encopresis,[33, 35] whereas a significant increase in stool frequency was only noted in one of the two studies.[3] Double-blind, placebo-controlled trials should help to further define the role of cisapride in treating childhood constipation.[36]

A stool chart with information on medication taken, stool frequency, consistency, volume, soiling accidents, and willingness to sit on the toilet is helpful in follow-up for assessing compliance with the bowel program and for making recommendations on dosage, time to taper off softeners, and when to add adjunctive therapy. Education of the parents and patient regarding the process of constipation, encopresis and treatment is provided and may help in compliance and recovery. Follow-up is essential, because chronic constipation persists for many years in one third of patients and reinforcement is needed for patients who have relapsed while off therapy.[37] Stool toileting refusal in children aged 2 to 5 years who have achieved bladder control is not uncommon. If these children have hard painful bowel movements or are withholding stool, then stool softeners need to be given. For those children who pass a normal soft bowel movement daily into their underwear, toilet training should be interrupted and the child should be put back into diapers. This resulted in 89% of the children spontaneously using the toilet for bowel movements within 3 months.[38] Consultation with the pediatric psychologist is sometimes needed to develop a behavioral approach for a particular child and family.

Biofeedback with electromyography and/or manometry is an option for training a subset of children with abnormal defecation maneuvers. It was thought that teaching normal defecation dynamics with biofeedback would improve recovery rates. Biofeedback treatment in children with chronic constipation and encopresis was mainly directed toward relaxing the external anal sphincter and pelvic floor during defecation attempts. Many uncontrolled studies suggest that biofeedback training is an effective therapy for children with constipation and encopresis; recovery rates ranged from 37% to 100%. But no significant benefit of biofeedback was observed in four of five randomized controlled studies[39–43] and in two nonrandomized controlled studies.[44, 45]

## PROGNOSIS AND CONCLUSIONS

For fecal retention or withholding the prognosis is good to excellent, as long as compliance with the bowel program, including stool softeners, scheduled toilet sitting, and other individualized components appropriate for a particular child, are maintained. The rectum can and will return to a normal caliber slowly over several months, and rectal sensation will improve to normal ranges again. The prognosis for full recovery, defined as no soiling and no constipation while off medication, was 48% at 5-year follow-up.[46]

Urinary incontinence and recurrent urinary tract infections have a good prognosis for resolution with treatment for the underlying chronic constipation. Stool and behavioral charting can provide valuable information at follow-up, because it guides the clinician in adjusting the softener or laxative and helps monitor compliance. A frequent error made by parents, physicians, and patients is stopping the stool softener or laxatives too soon after an initial response is noted. Medication needs to be restarted when a setback to the previous pattern of soiling or painful or infrequent passage of large or hard stools occurs.

## REFERENCES


1. Loening-Baucke V: Chronic constipation in children. Gastroenterol 1993;105:1557–1564.
2. Taitz LS, Water JKH, Urwin OM, Molnar D: Factors associated with outcome in management of defecation disorders. Arch Dis Child 1986;61:472–477.
3. Croffie JM, Fitzgerald JF, Walker WA, et al (eds): Pediatric Gastrointestinal Disease: Pathophysiology, Diagnosis, Management, 2nd ed. St. Louis, Mosby–Year Book, 1996, pp 984–997.
4. Drossman DA, Sandler RS, McKee DC, Lovitz AJ: Bowel patterns among subjects not seeking health care. Gastroenterology 1982;83:529–534.
5. Weaver LT, Ewing G, Taylor LC: The bowel habit of milk-fed infants. J Pediatr Gastroenterol Nutr 1988;7:568–571.
6. Weaver LT, Steiner H: The bowel habit of young children. Arch Dis Child 1984;59:649–652.
7. Rosenberg AJ, Wyllie R, Hyams JS (eds): Pediatric Gastrointestinal Disease: Pathophysiology, Diagnosis, Management. Philadelphia: WB Saunders, 1993, pp 198–208.
8. Whitehead WE, Schuster MM: Anorectal physiology and pathophysiology. Am J Gastroenterol 1987;82:487–497.
9. Burkitt DP, Walker ARP, Painter NS: Effect of dietary fibre on stools and transit-times, and its role in the causation of disease. Lancet 1972;2:1408–1412.
10. Müller-Lissner SA: Effect of wheat bran on weight of stool and gastrointestinal transit time: a meta analysis. BMJ 1988;296:615–617.
11. Meunier P, Marechal JM, De Beaujeu MJ: Rectoanal pressures and rectal sensitivity studies in chronic childhood constipation. Gastroenterol 1979;77:330–336.
12. Loening-Baucke V: Sensitivity of the sigmoid colon and rectum in children treated for chronic constipation. J Pediatr Gastroenterol Nutr 1984;3:454–459.
13. Loening-Baucke V, Yamada T: Is the afferent pathway from the rectum impaired in children with chronic constipation and encopresis? Gastroenterol 1995;109:397–403.
14. Preston DM, Lennard-Jones JE: Anismus in chronic constipation. Dig Dis Sci 1985;30:413–418.
15. Steffen R, Schroeder TK: Paradoxical puborectalis contraction in children (letter; comment). Dis Colon Rectum 1992;35:1193–1194.
16. Loening-Baucke V: Factors determining outcome in children with chronic constipation and faecal soiling. Gut 1989;30:999–1006.
17. Loening-Baucke V: Urinary incontinence and urinary tract infection and their resolution with treatment of chronic constipation of childhood. Pediatrics 1997;100:228–232.
18. Ishitani MB, Rodgers BM: Anteriorly displaced anus: an under-recognized cause of chronic constipation. Pediatr Surg Int 1991;6:217–220.
19. Rudolph CD, Hyman PE, Altschuler SM, et al: Diagnosis and treatment of chronic intestinal pseudo-obstruction in children: report of consensus workshop. J Pediatr Gastroenterol Nutr 1997;24:102–112.
20. Rockney RM, McQuade WH, Days AL: The plain abdominal roentgenogram in the management of encopresis. Arch Pediatr Adolesc Med 1995;149:623–627.
21. O'Donnell P, Beck C, Doyle R, Eubanks C: Surface electrodes in perineal electromyography. Urology 1988;32:375–379.
22. Pescatori M, Ravo B: Diagnostic anorectal functional studies. Tech Colorectal Surg 1997;68:1231–1248.
23. Steffen R, Schroeder TK, Wyllie R, et al: Mechanisms of constipation in pediatric patients demonstrated by rectal motility and EMG (abstract). Am J Gastroenterol 1994;89:1698.
24. Hinton JM, Lennard-Jones JE, Young AC: A new method for studying gut transit times using radioopaque markers. Gut 1969;10:842–847.
25. Metcalf AM, Phillips SF, Zinsmeister AR, et al: Simplified assessment of segmental colonic transit. Gastroenterol 1987;92:40–47.
26. Di Lorenzo C, Flores AF, Reddy SN, Hyman PE: Use of colonic manometry to differentiate causes of intractable constipation in children. J Pediatr 1992;120:690–695.
27. von der Ohe MR, Camilleri M, Carryer PW: A patient with localized megacolon and intractable constipation: evidence for impairment of colonic muscle tone. Am J Gastroenterol 1994;89:1867–1870.
28. Martin RR, Lisehora GR, Braxton M Jr, Barcia PJ: Fatal poisoning from sodium phosphate enema: case report and experimental study. JAMA 1987;257:2190–2192.
29. Sotos JF, Cutler EA, Finkel MA, Doody D: Hypocalcemic coma following two pediatric phosphate enemas. Pediatrics 1977;60:305–307.
30. Clark JH, Russell GJ, Fitzgerald JF, Nagamori KE: Serum beta-carotene, retinol, and alpha-tocopherol levels during mineral oil therapy for constipation. Am J Dis Child 1987;141:1210–1212.
31. Hamilton JW, Wagner J, Burdick BB, Bass P: Clinical evaluation of methylcellulose as a bulk laxative. Dig Dis Sci 1988;33:993–998.
32. Staiano A, Cucchiara S, Andreotti MR, et al: Effect of cisapride on chronic idiopathic constipation in children. Dig Dis Sci 1991;36:733–736.
33. Nurko S, Garcia-Aranda JA, Guerrero VY, Worona LB: Treatment of intractable constipation in children: experience with cisapride. J Pediatr Gastroenterol Nutr 1996;22:38–44.
34. Odeka EB, Sagher F, Miller V, Doig C: Use of cisapride in treatment of constipation in children. J Pediatr Gastroenterol Nutr 1997;25:199–203.
35. Murray RD, Li BU, McClung HJ, et al: Cisapride for intractable constipation in children: observations from an open trial. J Pediatr Gastroenterol Nutr 1990;11:503–508.
36. Loening-Baucke V: Cisapride for children with intractable constipation: an interim verdict! J Pediatr Gastroenterol Nutr 1996;22:3–5.
37. Loening-Baucke V: Constipation in early childhood: patient characteristics, treatment, and long-term follow up. Gut 1993;34:1400–1404.
38. Taubman B: Toilet training and toilet refusal for stool only: a prospective study. Pediatrics 1997;99:54–58.
39. Wald A, Chandra R, Gabel S, Chiponis D: Evaluation of biofeedback in childhood encopresis. J Pediatr Gastroenterol Nutr 1987;6:554–558.
40. Loening-Baucke V: Modulation of abnormal defecation dynamics by biofeedback treatment in chronically constipated children with encopresis. J Pediatr 1990;116:214–222.
41. Nolan T, Catto-Smith A, Coffey C, Wells J: EMG biofeedback training in anismus-related encopresis does not produce sustained continence. Arch Pediatr Adolesc Med 1995;149:48A.
42. van der Plas RN, Benninga MA, Buller HA, et al: Biofeedback training in treatment of childhood constipation: a randomized, controlled study. Lancet 1996;348:776–780.
43. van der Plas RN, Benninga MA, Redekop WK, et al: Randomised trial of biofeedback training for encopresis. Arch Dis Child 1996;75:367–374.
44. Loening-Baucke V: Biofeedback treatment for chronic constipation and encopresis in childhood: long-term outcome. Pediatrics 1995;96:105–110.
45. Cox DJ, Sutphen J, Borowitz S, et al: Simple electromyographic biofeedback treatment for chronic pediatric constipation/encopresis: preliminary report. Biofeedback Self Regul 1994;19:41–50.
46. Staiano A, Andreotti MR, Greco L, et al: Long-term follow-up of children with chronic constipation. Dig Dis Sci 1994;39:561–564.

Chapter 5

# Failure to Thrive

Vasundhara Tolia

Normal growth is an important marker of health. Growth is a continuous process that begins with conception and ends when the epiphyses fuse after puberty. Normal growth can be defined as a pattern of progression in height and weight that is consistent with the established standards for age in accordance with the genetic potential of the individual. Growth monitoring is one of the primary concerns of the pediatrician, because deviation from normal may be the first obvious sign of lack of well-being. Early diagnosis and aggressive intervention in such cases are essential to prevent or minimize permanent effects on the child's physical and mental health.[1, 2]

Failure to thrive (FTT) is a term used to describe physical growth failure in infants and young children that may be accompanied by retarded social and motor achievements. It is a descriptive symptom rather than a specific disease entity. Other terms, such as growth failure, failure to gain weight, and growth faltering, have been suggested to replace FTT.[3] FTT is a commonly used term in industrialized countries for the past 60 years,[4] but it should not be considered a separate entity from protein-energy malnutrition. Although the latter occurs more commonly in developing nations, both conditions represent parts of the spectrum of a common entity, childhood undernutrition.

Definition and classification of FTT has plagued both clinicians and researchers because of the diversity and ambiguity in the literature. Wilcox and colleagues[5] described FTT as an entity with a continuing problem of definition, with no consensus of indices and no quantitative terms used for diagnosis. It is a term applied to a child younger than 3 years of age who is disproportionately failing to gain weight in comparison to height and suggests sustained deviation for at least 6 months from the child's growth trajectory. Traditionally, FTT was described as a weight persistently below the third or fifth percentile for age on a standard growth chart in the absence of constitutional delay, or as a deceleration of growth velocity in which at least two major percentile lines are crossed or the child weighs less than 80% of ideal weight for age, based on standardized growth charts.[6, 7] It is necessary to consider genetic and other factors that limit a child's growth potential when interpreting such data.

The causes of malnutrition have been used to categorize FTT as organic, nonorganic, or mixed.[8] A schema of classification is presented in Figure 5–1. Organic causes of FTT include natal or perinatal insults and gastrointestinal, neurologic, and other systemic diseases with either insufficient caloric intake and excessive calorie utilization or losses.[9] Nonorganic FTT (NOFTT) is a major cause of FTT referrals to tertiary care centers in the United States. It results from environmental or multiple psychosocial factors and most frequently is associated with parental deprivation or impaired interaction between infant and caregiver.[9–11] Specific categories of FTT and NOFTT are not separate entities but a spectrum of growth failure with significant overlap. Mixed FTT can potentially occur in any chronic organic disease in which secondary aberrant behavior and appetite suppression occur. Anthropologic classification of FTT by all three growth parameters—weight, height, and head circumference—divides the diagnosis into three major categories. The disease groups associated with each type are shown in Table 5–1. NOFTT is usually associated with the type I category, but other types of growth failure may occur rarely with long-standing malnutrition. Table 5–2 lists various diseases in which FTT can occur.

## NORMAL RANGE OF GROWTH

Quetelet initially started the study of growth measurements in Europe.[12] Bowditch created the first growth charts for children in the 19th century,[13] and an evolution of data on growth of children followed during the next 100 years. The charts from the National Center for Health Statistics now are the most frequently used growth standards.[14] The World Health Organization has recommended that these charts be used as an international standard for all children, regardless of race.

Infants vary widely in their growth patterns, and growth does not always proceed in a smooth curve as the charts might indicate. Familiarity with norms of weight gain and height increase for different ages allows the physician to discern subtle changes in a child's development. Published data on the expected incremental gains in weight and length during the first 2 years of life, shown in Tables 5–3 and 5–4, are helpful for monitoring the growth of children.[15, 16] The crucial measurement of growth is length and not always weight gain. There are many pediatric diseases, such as cardiac, renal, and thyroid disease, in which stature is affected rather than weight. In general, a low weight for age

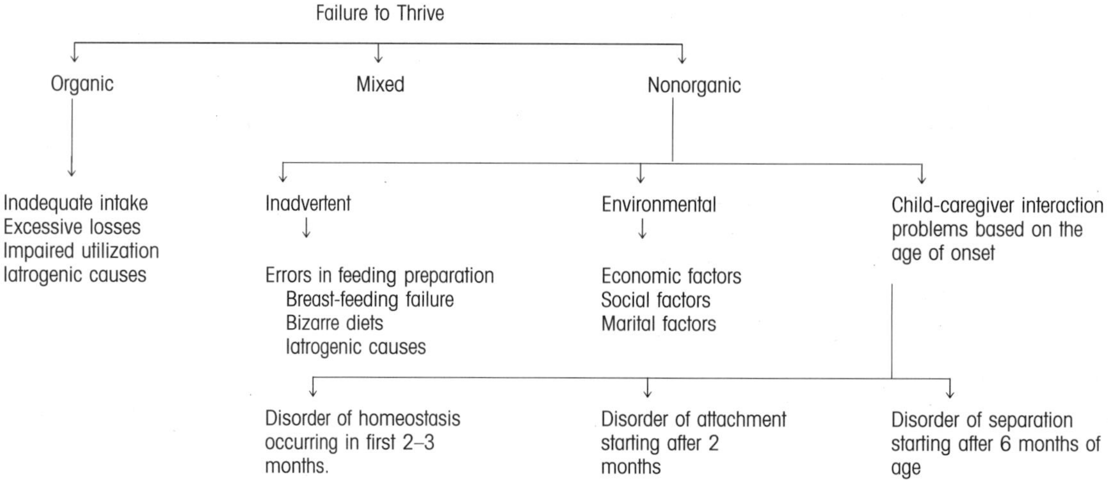


**FIGURE 5–1.** Etiologic classification of failure to thrive.

alone suggests acute malnutrition, whereas depressed height for age indicates more chronic malnutrition.

A series of observations of the anthropometric parameters is necessary to determine the pattern of growth; a single plot on the standard growth chart is much less meaningful. An infant who stays within a given percentile rating month after month is likely to be manifesting satisfactory progress, and a small, temporary deviation into another percentile is not a serious event. On the other hand, an infant who deviates from the usual percentile to a lower channel, and remains there, may require identification of the cause and its differentiation from "catch-down" weight. In the pattern of "catch-down" weight, an infant deviates to a lower percentile than the birth percentile. Such a phenomenon may be an early signal for FTT or simply a variation of normal, whereby the child settles between the intrauterine and genetic growth potential.[17]

Premature birth by 4 or more weeks should be age adjusted until catch-up growth occurs or until 2 years of age. The weight percentile of an infant between 4 and 8 weeks of age has been found to be better than the birth percentile as a predictor of the percentile at 1 year of age.[7] Birth weight is affected by maternal weight, parity, smoking, and alcohol consumption, whereas later growth is influenced by the environment and the genetic endowment.[18]

## MEDIATORS OF GROWTH

Growth is not always continuously linear but instead occurs in steps between periods of saltation and stasis. The growth rate varies in different seasons, generally being fastest in spring and summer.[19] Growth, including the ability to catch up, is governed by a complex chain of hormonal interactions. Growth hormone is secreted in a pulsatile fashion, with a frequency of one pulse approximately every 3 hours.[20] Large-amplitude pulses of growth hormone secretion occur at night with the onset of sleep and are not strictly related to stage IV sleep.[21] Growth is regulated by the growth hormone of the pituitary gland; by its regulatory factors (somatostatin and growth-releasing factor) and mediating agents (somatomedins and insulin-like growth factors), which act mostly on chondrogenesis[22]; and by other hormones (thyroid hormones[23, 24] and gonadal steroids), which exert a positive effect on bone maturation and osteogenesis.

The role of cortisol in the physiologic regulation of growth is not clear.[25] However, a slightly increased cortisol level with spontaneous or induced hypercorticism can inhibit or arrest growth and maturation. Other factors, such as insulin-like growth factor-1, erythropoietin, and nerve, epidermal, fibroblastic, and platelet growth factors, also have an important role in this extremely complex continuum.[26]

Linear growth during the period from birth to 21 years has been analyzed with the use of a mathematic model derived by Karlberg and associates.[27] Phases of growth have been divided into infancy, childhood, and pubertal components. The infancy component, extending up to 6 months after birth, appears to be largely nutritionally determined. This period of growth is less influenced by growth hormone than is the childhood growth period, which begins after 6 months of age. The childhood growth phase has two components of basic growth: the growth hormone–independent and

**TABLE 5–1. Three Major Anthropologic Categories of Failure to Thrive**

| TYPE | WEIGHT | HEIGHT | HEAD CIRCUMFERENCE | ASSOCIATED DISEASES |
|---|---|---|---|---|
| Type I | Decreased | Decreased/Normal | Normal | Malnutrition of organic or non-organic origin, usually secondary to intestinal, pancreatic, or liver disease systemic illness, or psychosocial factors. |
| Type II | Decreased | Decreased | Normal | Endocrinopathies, bony dystrophy, constitutional short stature |
| Type III | Decreased | Decreased | Decreased | Chromosomal-metabolic disease, intrauterine and perinatal insults |

the growth hormone–dependent phases. The pubertal portion of growth is regulated by both growth and gonadal hormones.

Children with psychosocial dwarfism usually have hypopituitarism, in which the most common endocrine deficiency is that of growth hormone, although other hormones may be involved.[28] Removal from the adverse environment is associated with catch-up growth and reversal of hypopituitarism. Skuse and associates[29] described a new stress-related syndrome of growth failure and hyperphagia in children associated with reversible growth hormone insufficiency.

**TABLE 5–2. Causes of Failure To Thrive**

**Decreased Calorie Intake**

Neurologic disorders with impaired swallowing
Injury to mouth and esophagus–trauma, infections, neoplasms
Congenital anomalies affecting oronasopharyngeal or upper gastrointestinal tract
Chromosomal abnormalities
Metabolic diseases
Diseases leading to anorexia
- Malignancy
- Renal disease
- Cardiac disease
- Liver disease
- Inflammatory bowel disease
- Psychologic
- Neglect or abuse
- Acquired immunodeficiency syndrome
- Gastroesophageal reflux disease with esophagitis

Accidental or inadvertent reduction in caloric intake—decreased breast milk, improper formula preparation, bizarre diet
Psychosocial–maternal- or infant-related factors
Iatrogenic—food allergy diets, special diets from misdiagnosis

**Increased Requirements**

Sepsis
Trauma
Burns
Chronic respiratory disease
Hyperthyroidism
Congenital heart disease
Diencephalic syndrome
Hyperactivity
Chronic infection

**Impaired Utilization**

Inborn errors of metabolism

**Excessive Caloric Losses**

Persistent vomiting
- Pyloric stenosis
- Gastroesophageal reflux

Malabsorptive states
- Pancreatic insufficiency
- Celiac disease
- Enzyme deficiency
- Short bowel
- Anatomic gut lesions
- Microvillus inclusion disease
- Protein-losing enteropathy
- Chronic inflammatory bowel disease
- Chronic immunodeficiency
- Allergic gastroenteropathy
- Parasite infestation
- Chronic enteric infection
- Postenteritis syndrome
- Chronic cholestasis

Diabetes mellitus

**TABLE 5–3. Weight Gain per Day from Birth to 24 Months of Age in 3-Month Increments**

| BOYS | | GIRLS | |
|---|---|---|---|
| Age (mo) | Weight Gain (g/day) | Age (mo) | Weight Gain (g/day) |
| Birth to 3 | 31 ± 5.9 | Birth to 3 | 26 ± 5.5 |
| 1–4 | 27 ± 5.1 | 1–3 | 24 ± 5.1 |
| 2–5 | 21 ± 4.3 | 2–5 | 20 ± 3.9 |
| 3–6 | 18 ± 2.9 | 3–6 | 17 ± 4.6 |
| 4–7 | 16 ± 2.4 | 4–7 | 15 ± 4.8 |
| 5–8 | 14 ± 2.4 | 5–8 | 14 ± 4.7 |
| 6–9 | 13 ± 2.4 | 6–9 | 13 ± 4.6 |
| 7–10 | 12 ± 2.4 | 7–10 | 12 ± 4.5 |
| 8–11 | 11 ± 2.4 | 8–11 | 11 ± 4.4 |
| 9–12 | 11 ± 2.3 | 9–12 | 11 ± 4.3 |
| 10–13 | 10 ± 2.3 | 10–13 | 10 ± 4.2 |
| 11–14 | 10 ± 2.3 | 11–14 | 10 ± 4.2 |
| 12–15 | 9 ± 2.3 | 12–15 | 9 ± 4.1 |
| 13–16 | 9 ± 2.3 | 13–16 | 9 ± 4.0 |
| 14–17 | 8 ± 2.2 | 14–17 | 9 ± 3.9 |
| 15–18 | 8 ± 2.2 | 15–18 | 8 ± 3.9 |
| 16–19 | 8 ± 2.2 | 16–19 | 8 ± 3.8 |
| 17–20 | 8 ± 2.2 | 17–20 | 8 ± 3.8 |
| 18–21 | 7 ± 2.2 | 18–21 | 8 ± 3.7 |
| 19–22 | 7 ± 2.1 | 19–22 | 7 ± 3.6 |
| 20–23 | 7 ± 2.1 | 20–23 | 7 ± 3.6 |
| 21–24 | 7 ± 2.1 | 21–24 | 7 ± 3.5 |

From birth through 3 months of age, based on data from studies of infant growth and nutrition conducted at the University of Iowa; from 3 through 6 months of age, based on data from both the University of Iowa and the Fels longitudinal study; from 6 through 12 months of age, based on data from the Fels longitudinal study. Values are expressed as means ± standard deviation.

Adapted from Guo SM, Roche AF, Fomon SJ, et al: Reference data on gains in weight and length during the first two years of life. J Pediatr 1991;119:355–362; and Leung AK, Robson WM, Fagan JE: Assessment of the child with failure to thrive. Am Fam Physician 1993;48:1432–1438, with permission.

Hormonally, the hyperphagic children showed poor physiologic (nocturnal) and pharmacologically stimulated growth hormone release and marked improvement on retesting 2 to 3 weeks after removal from the stressful environment. The authors make a strong case that the behavioral and growth characteristics of these children point to a new syndrome, but nothing more is understood about the interactions between psychology, hypothalamic function, and nutritional status that bring about this symptom cluster in some stressed, short children.

## HISTORICAL PERSPECTIVE OF FAILURE TO THRIVE

It is difficult to ascertain when and by whom the term *failure to thrive* was invented. The first noted reference by Frederick II, dates back to the 13th century. He wanted to investigate the spontaneous evolution of the primary language of mankind in the absence of other extraneous influences.[30] He sent a group of newborn infants to an island with a wet nurse who was forbidden to interact in any way with these infants except to feed them. None of the infants lived. Frederick's interest in human language probably was the first experiment to demonstrate severe effects on infants

**TABLE 5–4. Gain in Length per Day from Birth to 24 Months of Age in 3-Month Increments**

| BOYS | | GIRLS | |
|---|---|---|---|
| **Age (mo)** | **Length Gain (mm/day)** | **Age (mo)** | **Length Gain (mm/day)** |
| Birth to 3 | 1.07 ± 0.11 | Birth to 3 | 0.99 ± 0.10 |
| 1–4 | 1.00 ± 0.08 | 1–3 | 0.95 ± 0.10 |
| 2–5 | 0.84 ± 0.09 | 2–5 | 0.80 ± 0.10 |
| 3–6 | 0.69 ± 0.08 | 3–6 | 0.67 ± 0.08 |
| 4–7 | 0.62 ± 0.06 | 4–7 | 0.60 ± 0.06 |
| 5–8 | 0.56 ± 0.05 | 5–8 | 0.56 ± 0.05 |
| 6–9 | 0.52 ± 0.05 | 6–9 | 0.52 ± 0.05 |
| 7–10 | 0.48 ± 0.05 | 7–10 | 0.48 ± 0.04 |
| 8–11 | 0.45 ± 0.04 | 8–11 | 0.46 ± 0.04 |
| 9–12 | 0.43 ± 0.04 | 9–12 | 0.44 ± 0.04 |
| 10–13 | 0.41 ± 0.04 | 10–13 | 0.42 ± 0.04 |
| 11–14 | 0.39 ± 0.04 | 11–14 | 0.40 ± 0.04 |
| 12–15 | 0.37 ± 0.04 | 12–15 | 0.38 ± 0.04 |
| 13–16 | 0.36 ± 0.04 | 13–16 | 0.37 ± 0.04 |
| 14–17 | 0.35 ± 0.04 | 14–17 | 0.36 ± 0.04 |
| 15–18 | 0.33 ± 0.04 | 15–18 | 0.34 ± 0.04 |
| 16–19 | 0.32 ± 0.04 | 16–19 | 0.33 ± 0.04 |
| 17–20 | 0.31 ± 0.04 | 17–20 | 0.32 ± 0.04 |
| 18–21 | 0.03 ± 0.04 | 18–21 | 0.32 ± 0.04 |
| 19–22 | 0.03 ± 0.04 | 19–22 | 0.31 ± 0.04 |
| 20–23 | 0.29 ± 0.04 | 20–23 | 0.30 ± 0.04 |
| 21–24 | 0.28 ± 0.04 | 21–24 | 0.29 ± 0.04 |

From birth through 3 months of age, based on data from studies of infant growth and nutrition conducted at the University of Iowa; from 3 through 6 months of age, based on data from both the University of Iowa and the Fels longitudinal study; from 6 through 12 months of age, based on data from the Fels longitudinal study. Values are expressed as means ± standard deviation.

Adapted from Guo SM, Roche AF, Fomon SJ, et al: Reference data on gains in weight and length during the first two years of life. J Pediatr 1991;119:355–362; and Leung AKC, Robson LM, Fagan JE. Assessment of the child with failure to thrive. Am Fam Physician 1993;48:1432–1438, with permission.

who were not nurtured with love and is a classic example of NOFTT.

In 1915, Chapin observed that infants younger than 1 year of age had a high mortality rate during hospitalization and urged early discharge after resolution of acute symptoms.[31] Chapin's concerns for atrophic infants did not attract a great deal of attention, and many years passed before Bakwin presented a very astute and graphic description of the effect of loneliness on hospitalized infants kept in isolation.[32] These infants were denied regular visitation by their families because of cross-infection leading to high mortality. Bakwin also observed that isolation during the first 2 postnatal weeks did not affect the infants as much. He believed that the receptive senses develop quickly after 2 weeks of age, so that by 8 to 12 weeks the infant interacts with smiles and animation. Such a response was not observed in infants who were isolated for prolonged periods. These observations have been corroborated by others and suggest that the first few postnatal months constitute a sensitive period for the relation between growth and mental development.[33] Widdowson[34] reported that children receiving tender loving care but fewer calories gained weight better than children living in an adverse emotional environment but receiving more calories.

Spitz[35] coined the term *anaclitic depression* for the effects of psychosocial deprivation on children in institutions in 1945 and applied the term *hospitalism* to this syndrome. In the ensuing years it was recognized that some infants living in their own homes failed to thrive and exhibited signs and symptoms of failure of physical growth, motor retardation, and malnutrition.[36] A majority of these infants were cared for by their mothers inadequately. Powell and coworkers[28] described 3- to 11-year-old children with "deprivation dwarfism" who had short stature, abnormal home situations, and bizarre eating habits. It was believed that this baffling starvation which occurs in children who are maternally deprived resulted solely from the lack of tender loving care, social stimulation, physical handling, and sensory stimulation. Such beliefs were refuted by Whitten and colleagues,[37] who demonstrated that the lack of mothering by itself does not cause physical stunting and growth failure unless adequate amounts of food are withheld or, less frequently, the child's appetite fails. They further observed that when infants with sustained maternal deprivation in their own homes were fed ad libitum in the hospital, most gained weight at an accelerated rate.[38] Weight increased in those not receiving increased mothering at the same rate as in children receiving both increased mothering and increased calories.

Subtle variations of this theme leading to growth failure continue to be described. Lifshitz and Moses[39] reported on eight children who developed growth failure due to overzealous application of a cholesterol-lowering diet by the parent. Parents have inadvertently or knowingly restricted calories for fear of obesity[40] or because of religious and cultural attitudes.[41] Careful monitoring of these children with diet correction normalized growth. Excess fruit juice consumption leading to low intake of calorie-dense foods has also been noted to contribute to NOFTT.[42] Devastating consequences resulting from unguided parental feeding practices such as vegetarianism or high-protein diets have also been described in children.[43]

The ultimate cause of FTT, despite other circumstantial and emotional attributes, is inadequate caloric intake leading to malnutrition. Keys and associates[44] demonstrated in adults that an intake at least 50% higher than the individual's usual daily intake is necessary after prolonged starvation for nutritional and psychological recovery. Such supernormal energy requirements for recovery are necessary in infants with growth failure as well. Furthermore, it is the total calories rather than the dietary composition that is important. When proper nutritional therapy of growth retardation is instituted, after an initial period of inertia, there is an excessive increase of growth rate, leading to "catch-up" growth. After the period of growth catch-up, the growth rate becomes normal for the child's age and genetic endowment.

## PATHOGENESIS OF FAILURE TO THRIVE

Vietze and colleagues[45] used a transactional approach in a prospective, longitudinal study of mothers and infants who were later diagnosed with NOFTT and a control group of mothers and infants without NOFTT. They evaluated maternal history, including social and developmental aspects and attitudes toward child-rearing. The infant's biologic and temperamental aptitudes were measured and maternal-infant interaction was observed early during hospitalization. This study showed no significant differences in infant behavior or in any of the maternal characteristics between the two groups. It was, however, obvious that infants with significantly lower birth weights and shorter gestational ages developed NOFTT later on. The mothers of these infants spent a significantly shorter time gazing at their infants, compared with the control group of mothers. The authors speculated that a combination of adverse environmental conditions, such as poverty, lack of support, and absence of the father, can jeopardize mother-infant bonding when the baby is born small or prematurely. These observations were confirmed in another retrospective study.[46]

A subsequent prospective study suggested that NOFTT correlates significantly with turmoil during the mother's childhood and parental conflict.[47] Difficult pregnancy, prematurity, and residual minor medical problems in infants at discharge from the nursery also predispose to an aberrant mother-infant relationship. A prospective study on the risk factors and outcomes for FTT in low-birth-weight, preterm infants showed that only young maternal age and advanced maternal education predicted the occurrence of FTT.[48] Identification of advanced maternal education as a predictor of future nutritional problems is unique in the literature on FTT and needs further corroboration.

Frequently, the diagnosis of NOFTT is made by exclusion after an initial evaluation has revealed no organic disorder. Suspicion of NOFTT is confirmed if the child gains weight in the hospital. Initially, the condition was believed to be secondary to lack of adequate mothering and was labeled "maternal deprivation syndrome." Now, however, a broader view of the syndrome utilizing the transactional or interactional hypothesis, encompasses the multifaceted nature of the problem. This view takes into account parental problems (lack of nurturing in childhood, illnesses, emotional state) and those of the child (temperament, development) as well as their interaction and the environment (family support, poverty, stresses).[49] Tables 5–5 and 5–6 list parental and infant characteristics that predispose to the occurrence of growth failure.

## EPIDEMIOLOGY AND INCIDENCE

National data are not available regarding the exact prevalence of FTT. Although growth deficiency occurs in all socioeconomic strata, its prevalence is highest in poor families. FTT has been reported to affect up to 10% of children seen in outpatient clinics[50] and may account for 1% to 5% of all hospitalizations of children younger than 2 years of age in the United States.[49, 50] We determined the incidence of the diagnosis of FTT at Children's Hospital of Michigan for the years 1995 and 1996 for both outpatients and inpatients using the International Classification of Diseases code 783.4, which encompasses the broad category of FTT. The primary diagnosis of FTT was present in only 3% and 3.1% of outpatients in 1995 and 1996, respectively, excluding the primary gastrointestinal, neurologic, cardiac, or other system diseases in which FTT would be a secondary diagnosis. These figures suggest either an increased awareness or early intervention in NOFTT cases, or both. The inpatient diagnosis of NOFTT was prevalent in only 0.47% and 0.41% of cases for 1995 and 1996, respectively. This may reflect the current major shift toward outpatient care and earlier outpatient intervention.

**TABLE 5–5. Characteristics of Parents of Infants with Nonorganic Failure to Thrive**

| | |
|---|---|
| Lack of social support | Burn out |
| Depression | Family crises |
| Alcoholism | Conflict with spouse |
| Drug abuse | Separation from spouse |
| Less education | Absent spouse |
| Unplanned pregnancy | Loss of employment |
| Disturbed childhood for parent | Advanced maternal education |
| Excessive stress | Young mother |

**TABLE 5–6. Characteristics of Infants with Nonorganic Failure to Thrive**

| | |
|---|---|
| Temperament | "Funny looking" or with abnormalities |
| Irritable | |
| Fussy | Feeding difficulties |
| Jittery | Resists food |
| Colicky | Poor suck |
| Difficulty with handling | Gags, chokes or coughs during feeding |
| Overactive | Spitting and vomiting |
| Passive | Arches with feeding |
| Nonvocalizing | Irritable after feeding |
| Nonresponsive | |

## EVALUATION

The causes of organic FTT are legion. Major categories are listed in Table 5–2. The single best tool for differentiating among the various types of FTT is a comprehensive history and physical examination.

Regardless of the underlying cause of FTT (organic or nonorganic), the onset usually is gradual and the presentation very subtle, so that the parents may not realize that their child has a growth problem. It is often the pediatrician who begins to note the pattern of deceleration of growth over a few consecutive visits and suspects the diagnosis. The value of growth charts for longitudinal monitoring of the progress of a particular child for weight, height, and head circumference cannot be overemphasized. The parents may register disbelief or shock at being informed of the condition, because the child may be totally asymptomatic and apparently developing normally. The approach to a child with FTT requires patience and sensitivity. It is important to understand the parents' perspective regarding their child's growth, not to be accusatory, and to know whether the issue has been addressed previously. It is not unusual to be evaluating such patients for a second opinion, so winning the confidence of the parents and making them feel comfortable facilitates further communication and management.

A proper and extensive dietary, social, developmental, family, and medical history is the most important initial step. During this interview, the physician should be observing the parent-infant interaction and the infant's activity and behavior. Prenatal and perinatal data regarding infections during pregnancy; use of drugs, alcohol, and tobacco; difficult pregnancy or labor, or both; full-term versus premature labor; birth weight; gestational age; Apgar scores; medical problems; and any difficulties during feeding should be elicited in detail. The past medical history should include a review of frequent illnesses, medications, accidents, hospitalizations, and any history of pica or lead ingestion. Family history should be elicited regarding the growth patterns of parents and siblings and the presence of any congenital or familial diseases or other medical problems.

Developmental history includes a review of the ages at which different milestones were achieved by the infant. The perception of the parents as to how the child compares with peers is helpful. Careful questioning of the parents concerning the child's intake is very important. Specific questions regarding the type of feeding (i.e., formula versus nursing), changes in formula, exact recipe for formula preparation, volume of intake per feeding, and total number of feedings should be asked. The child's food likes and dislikes, time taken over a feeding, and intake of solids should also be determined. Other factors to consider are the position of the infant during feeding, who administers the feeding, and the emotional state of the caregiver. A 3-day diet diary to assess nutritional adequacy should be obtained. It is helpful to actually observe the parent-child interaction during a feeding to determine whether the parent responds appropriately to the child's cues and whether the child finishes the bottle or fatigues easily. Maladaptive feeding behaviors such as gagging, choking, refusing feeding, or vomiting during feeding should be noted.

The nursing pattern of a breast-fed infant should be assessed. Severe complications have occasionally been reported in the absence of any obvious symptoms in nursed infants. The progress of a nursing infant should be assessed initially at about 2 weeks of age. Studies suggest that breast milk supplies alone may not be sufficient to cover all of the infant's energy needs beyond 3 to 4 months of age.[53] The potential risk factors for accidental FTT in a breast-fed infant include infrequent or brief feedings, maternal ingestion of a milk suppressant (e.g., alcohol, diuretics), inadequate milk supply, nipple problems, inadequate let-down reflex, and poor sucking. Breast-fed infants who are not receiving adequate calories may respond in two distinct ways, either with excessive crying or with excessive sleeping.[54–56] The milk supply may be inadequate secondary to maternal malnutrition, exhaustion, or depression. Many other variables contribute to successful nursing, including the size of the infant, the volume of milk the mother can produce, the mother's need to rejoin the workforce, and the quantity and degree of maternal-infant interaction. Prospective studies of dietary intake and growth in infants who were exclusively nursed revealed that breast-fed infants consumed approximately 20 Kcal/kg per day less than formula-fed control infants.[57] However, they gained weight at a faster rate for the first 2 months and at a slightly decreased rate up to 6 months.

If early growth is faltering (i.e., growth changes in the first few months of life are detected), intervention is required.[58] A few simple questions can help exclude early faltering among breast-fed infants. If the infant is satisfied after 15 minutes at each breast, has normal stools (golden and soft) of moderate volume, and has eight or more wet diapers per day in the absence of growth deviation, the physician can reassure the parent. Most mothers who discontinue breast-feeding or begin supplements are under a mistaken assumption that their milk supply is insufficient. By evaluating the growth velocity of the infant, the physician can determine the appropriate advice (i.e., reassurance versus adding supplement). However, if there is any uncertainty, the infant can be weighed before and after feeding while the duration of the feeding is timed and the feeding technique is observed.

It is always necessary to exclude associated chronic systemic diseases. The primary disease is not always suspected or diagnosed until the child is evaluated for poor height and weight percentiles. Chronic renal diseases leading to metabolic acidosis, chronic malnutrition, and recurrent infections, along with interference with bone growth and mineralization, can cause growth failure.[59–61] Significant congenital cardiac abnormalities commonly cause growth failure that is more profound in infancy.[62] The presence of heart failure appears to be a major determinant of decreased growth, rather than the presence or absence of cyanosis. Surgical correction of these anomalies diminishes the frequency of growth impairment.[63]

Moderate growth retardation was reported in a group of untreated asthmatic children and appeared to be directly correlated with the severity of asthma.[64] Steroid use accentuates the poor growth retardation by disturbing the sleep pattern and by secondary interference with nocturnal growth hormone secretion.[65] Obstructive sleep apnea has been shown to cause delayed growth secondary to increased caloric expenditure caused by increased work of breathing during sleep.[66] Chronic lung infections and pancreatic insufficiency both contribute to decreased growth in cystic fibrosis.[67, 68]

Hematologic diseases such as hemoglobinopathies and red blood cell enzymatic deficiencies may cause growth retardation.[69, 70] Chronic anemia by itself can cause growth delay and interfere with learning ability.[71, 72] Chronic infections of the middle ear or of the urinary tract, tuberculosis, and human immunodeficiency virus infection lead to striking impairment of growth.[73] Defective skeletal development, as in chondrodystrophic bone diseases and chronic rickets, causes decreased linear growth. Chromosomal and genetic abnormalities such as Down syndrome and Turner's syndrome are invariably associated with decreased growth. Neurologically handicapped children have a significantly decreased growth rate.[74, 75] A myriad of gastrointestinal disorders are associated with growth failure due to increased losses from vomiting or stooling. Excessive vomiting, as in intestinal malrotation, pyloric stenosis, and severe gastroesophageal reflux disease, causes decreased weight gain. Dysphagia or anorexia from esophageal inflammation in gastroesophageal reflux disease can lead to decreased caloric intake.[76] Celiac disease,[77] allergic gastroenteropathies, chronic diarrhea of infancy, and chronic inflammatory bowel disease[78] can all result in inadequate weight gain. Stools may be described as watery, oily, foul-smelling, and excessive. Weight is more compromised than height in most of these diseases. A history of jaundice may suggest chronic liver disease with multiple nutritional deficiencies, especially of fat-soluble vitamins.[79] Chronic immunologic diseases, neurologic diseases, and rheumatologic conditions also can cause FTT.[80]

A review of family dynamics is usually minimized in a busy practitioner's office, but it is of importance in the evaluation of infants with growth delay. Mothers of infants diagnosed with FTT display behaviors which are not seen in mothers of normal infants. These mothers are less responsive to their infants, have less verbal interaction, and do not accept their infants as well.[81] It has also been observed that the homes of infants with growth failure are more disorganized. In infants with NOFTT, reduced vocalization of mother-infant dyads, in comparison with control pairs, was reported by Berkowitz and Senter.[82] Mathisen and associates[83] compared the feeding situations in the homes of affected infants with those in a matched comparison group and noted that the infants with FTT had more delays in oral-motor coordination, had less ability to communicate needs during meal times, and were more difficult to handle because of temperament. In addition, these infants were more likely to be fed in inappropriate positions for age and were surrounded by more distractions during feedings.

Fosson and Wilson[84] observed feeding sessions after an interview in the presence of all family members and noted that the mothers of children with NOFTT responded less to their infants' cues. Other factors affecting the feeding situation were sibling rivalry, displaced maternal anger, low self-esteem, and chaotic family life. Although interactions between mother and child may be very different during observation in the office than at home, still it should be possible from such observations to assess whether the relationship is strained or relaxed. If the parent fails to attend to the infant or ignores or responds negatively to the child, then obviously the relationship is strained. The child who is friendly with office staff and turns to strangers to be comforted may be emotionally rejected at home, suggesting social deprivation.

A note should be made of who else is in the home, the involvement of the father, the interparental relationship, whether the child was born out of wedlock, whether the pregnancy was planned, the financial situation of the family, the parental level of education and comprehension, and any mental illnesses.[85] Many parents of children with FTT experience feelings of guilt, anger, and inadequacy when psychosocial problems are uncovered. They perceive efforts to intercede with hostility and as a criticism of their parenting abilities. Reinforcement of the goal of enhancing the parent-child relationship so as to improve the child's health helps diffuse such a situation.[86]

Finally, there are perfectly normal infants with very caring parents who refuse to eat enough from a very early age. They just show disinterest in feeding or have very limited appetites and have no organic diseases. This category of NOFTT also needs to be recognized.[87] The cause of this very-early-onset infantile anorexia is unclear, because these families are different from usual NOFTT families in that they are very focused on the infant's eating patterns and have no other predisposing factors for NOFTT. Feeding is a reciprocal process that develops based on the quality of interactions between the caregiver and the infant. Maladaptive interactions may occur throughout the three stages of development: homeostasis, attachment, and separation or individuation. Specific feeding disorders causing growth failure can arise during any of these stages.

The physical examination of a child who is growing poorly should focus on identifying the signs of underlying organic disease, the severity of malnutrition, and any important concomitant findings such as evidence of physical abuse, neglect, or the presence of deprivation behaviors. A psychomotor developmental assessment should also be obtained. A thin child with wasted limbs, protuberant abdomen, flattened buttocks, hair and skin changes, yet relatively well-preserved buccal fat should be carefully assessed for organic diseases. When height and head circumference are also declining, a chronic nutritional problem or a metabolic, chromosomal, genetic, or neurologic disease is suggested. The latter diseases are usually associated with developmental delay, in which case other deformities such as microcephaly or spasticity are obvious. An infant with significant reflux may spit and vomit continuously during the session, arch during feeding, and refuse the bottle.

A child with chronic diarrheal disease may have significant diaper rash. Stool in the diaper or from a sample can be examined for presence of oil droplets, volume, consistency, and presence of blood. Parents should be asked whether the stool floats in the toilet. Rash at the mucocutaneous junction and brittle, thin hair may suggest zinc deficiency, as in acrodermatitis enteropathica.[88] Furthermore, association of zinc deficiency with dwarfism has been reported.[89] Iodine deficiency interferes with growth through the absence of thyroid hormone synthesis.[90] Every organ system should be checked thoroughly. Fatigue during feeding may be present with heart disease, and unexplained fevers and night sweats may suggest an infectious process such as tuberculosis. Joint swellings, clubbing, cyanosis, signs of itching, and xanthomas should be noted. The abdomen should be palpated thoroughly for liver or spleen enlargement and percussed if distended to evaluate for ascites. A palpable liver does not necessarily mean an enlarged liver, as decreased abdominal muscle tone in otherwise normal infants may allow the liver to dip below the costal margin. Limbs should be examined for deformities and muscle tone, and a complete neurologic examination should be performed. The presence of cleft lip or palate or of sucking and swallowing difficulties should be noted, because some of these problems contribute significantly to feeding difficulties. The presence of cheilosis, glossitis, or any other mucosal lesions may signify vitamin deficiencies or infectious processes. More commonly, infants with NOFTT are jittery, irritable, and fussy. Older infants appear apathetic, withdrawn, and apprehensive and do not vocalize much.[47] Powell and coworkers[85] observed that flexed hips and knees, expressionless face, general inactivity, abnormal gaze, and lack of response to stimuli were seen more frequently among infants diagnosed with FTT.

Accurate measurements are very important. Experienced personnel should use similar techniques for height, weight, and head circumference measurements at each visit. Any previous such measurements should be plotted to assess the growth pattern. Usually, weight alone is affected and is seen to be decelerating over longer than 3 to 6 months. Height-for-weight and weight-for-height should be calculated. When weight or height is below the 5th to 10th percentiles, growth retardation is suspected, mandating careful follow-up of these infants. All measurements should be corrected for prematurity until the child's second birthday. Preterm infants with both symmetric and asymmetric intrauterine growth retardation have been reported to demonstrate limited catch-up growth when observed for up to 3 years of corrected age.[91]

Hokken-Koelega and colleagues[92] performed a longitudinal study to assess postnatal growth of small-for-gestational-age infants and to find predictive factors for catch-up growth in excess of the third percentile for length during the first 2 years of life. Catch-up growth to this height was noted in 85% of healthy small infants, with no significant difference between premature and full-term small-for-gestational-age infants by 2 years. In premature small infants, the standard deviation score for birth length was a better predictor of catch-up in length at 2 years, but in full-term small infants the score for birth weight was more reliable. Nutritional assessment, as determined by midarm circumference and triceps skinfold thickness and compared with established standards, can help to assess for depletion of fat and muscle protein stores.[93] Various methods have been used to categorize the degree of undernutrition by comparing a child's weight and height with reference standards, but there is a lack of consistency in how anthropometric indices are used to define this condition.[5] Several established methods to categorize nutritional status[94–96] are shown in Table 5–7. A broad variation between the number of children classified as malnourished and the degree of undernutrition was detected by these methods.[97] Based on these results, it was recommended that these systems be used only to define a child as having a risk of possible adverse effects of undernutrition, and not as being malnourished.

## LABORATORY INVESTIGATIONS

Considerable controversy exists regarding the usefulness of laboratory tests in the evaluation of FTT. Basic laboratory screening studies may include a urinalysis, urine culture, a complete blood count, erythrocyte sedimentation rate, blood urea nitrogen, creatinine, calcium, phosphorus, total protein, albumin, and electrolyte levels. The serum lead concentration should be checked, since pica may be more prevalent in this population.[98] Stool examination for occult blood and ova or parasites is helpful in screening for unsuspected parasitic infestations. A skin test for tuberculosis should be done. The need for more extensive laboratory investigations should be individualized based on the history and physical examination, as well as the results of initial screening tests, because an undirected, shotgun approach with multiple laboratory tests has an extremely low yield.[47, 99] An algorithm for evaluating the cause of growth failure is shown in Figure 5–2. Table 5–8 lists various other tests that can be performed, based on individualized judgment, to obtain the proper diagnosis.

**TABLE 5–7. Three Methods to Categorize Undernutrition in Children**

| DEGREE OF UNDER-NUTRITION | METHOD 1 (GOMEZ ET AL)[94]: % MEDIAN WEIGHT-FOR-AGE | METHOD 2 (WATERLOW)[95]: % MEDIAN WEIGHT-FOR-HEIGHT | METHOD 3 (McLAREN ET AL)[96]: % MEDIAN WEIGHT/HEIGHT-FOR-AGE RATIO |
|---|---|---|---|
| None | >90 | >90 | >90 |
| Mild | 76–90 | 80–90 | 85–90 |
| Moderate | 60–74 | 70–79 | 75–84 |
| Severe | <60 | <70 | <75 |

From Wright JA, Ashenburg GA, Whitaker RC: Comparison of methods to categorize undernutrition in children. J Pediatr 1994;124:944–946, with permission.

**TABLE 5–8. Optional Investigations for Organic Failure to Thrive**

Quantitative immunoglobulins, *Helicobacter pylori,* immunoglobulin G
Antigliadin, anti-reticulin, and anti-endomysial antibodies
Serum vasoactive intestinal peptide
Urine organic acids, catecholamines, amino acids
Chromosomal studies, growth hormone levels
Human immunodeficiency virus antibody, liver function tests, thyroid studies
Stool cultures, ova and parasites, alpha$_1$-antitrypsin in stool
Barium contrast studies
Abdominal ultrasound
Head CT/MRI
Sweat chloride, breath testing
Extended intraesophageal pH monitoring
Small intestinal biopsy and upper endoscopy
Electrocardiogram chest radiograph, bone age, skeletal survey
Other specific tests as indicated

## MANAGEMENT

The goals of nutritional management of the child with FTT include the following:

1. Provision of adequate calories, protein, and other nutrients for catch-up growth
2. Nutritional counseling to the family regarding exact amounts, types, and preparation of formula and foods
3. Ongoing monitoring of nutritional status and rate of growth
4. Specific treatment of complications or deficiencies
5. Long-term monitoring and follow-up
6. Education of the family on social and nurturing techniques and how to recognize the infant's distress and hunger cues
7. Supportive economic assistance for supplies and other needs

In most cases, early intervention can be managed by the primary care provider in an ambulatory setting.[18, 100] Since many of these families have economic problems and travel for frequent follow-ups can be problematic, regular home visits by a nurse can provide relevant information regarding family dynamics and the progress of the child. Hospitalization should be avoided whenever possible in mild cases, because it further impairs the parent-child relationship and decreases the morale of parents. An interdisciplinary team approach is essential for the management of more complex cases, including the involvement of a nutritionist, social worker, occupational therapist, and psychologist as well as the pediatric gastroenterologist.[101] Each member of the team investigates appropriate parameters so that a unified treatment plan can be devised. Deficiency of digestive enzymes and reversible endocrinopathy can be a consequence of prolonged malnutrition in infants and young children. Both these secondary phenomena further compound growth failure. Proper understanding of the pathophysiology of their occurrence and rapid correction with appropriate nutritional rehabilitation are essential. Observation in a hospital setting for such complex cases is more effective.

For children with organic FTT, the underlying medical condition should be treated. The type of caloric supplementation must be based on the severity of malnutrition and the underlying disease. For example, a child with celiac disease

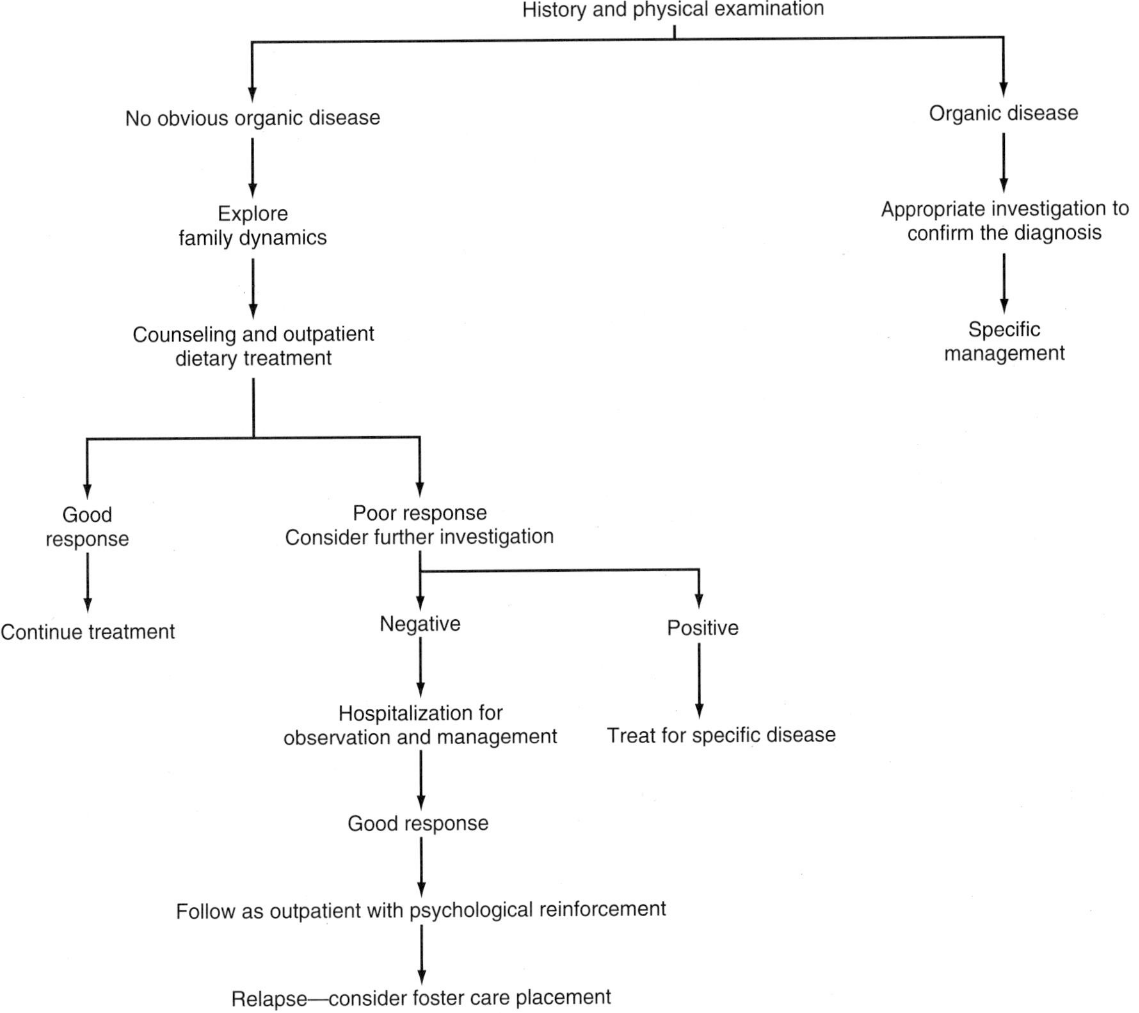


**FIGURE 5–2.** Algorithm for approach to a child with failure to thrive.

needs a gluten-free, low-lactose diet in the beginning; after some time, lactose may be reintroduced slowly, because with regeneration of the villi lactase activity returns. In a patient with renal failure or liver disease with encephalopathy, protein intake must be monitored. In cases of severe malnutrition, a brief phase of peripheral hyperalimentation during rehabilitation of the gut with dilute formula may enhance recovery. Occasionally, restricted diets are imposed by physicians for allergies or misdiagnoses, and iatrogenic malnutrition can result from misguided feeding practices.[102] Indications for hospitalization include severe malnutrition, medically instability with associated organic disease, dehydration with electrolyte abnormalities, high risk of or evidence of physical abuse in a child with psychological FTT, failure of outpatient therapy, or need to confirm the diagnosis and observe caregiver-child interactions.

When calories and protein are provided for normal age-specific requirements, the growth of the child with undernutrition will proceed only along the low percentile to which the child has fallen. Excess calories and protein must be provided to restore deficits in weight and height and to promote compensatory catch-up growth.[103, 104] Nutritional requirements can be assessed with the use of a formula for calories and protein:[105]

$$\text{Catch-up growth requirement (Kcal/kg/day)} = \frac{\text{Calories required for weight age (Kcal/kg/day)} \times \text{Ideal weight for age (kg)}}{\text{Actual weight (kg)}}$$

When protein (in g/kg/day) is substituted for kilocalories, the same formula also determines protein requirements. Besides lacking in energy and protein, these children usually are deficient in micronutrients such as iron, zinc, and vitamin D. Accordingly, a multivitamin supplement with additional specific nutrients is recommended. The volume of food necessary for rehabilitation is large, so the use of fortified foods to increase nutrient density is helpful while the medical condition, renal solute load, and gastrointestinal tolerance are considered. Infants often drink better than they eat, so drinks with 27 to 30 cal/oz can be used. Refeeding should proceed cautiously, because significantly undernourished children may develop diarrhea, vomiting, and circulatory decompensation.[100] Furthermore, accelerated growth must be maintained for 4 to 9 months to restore a child's weight for appropriate height. Catch-up height will lag several months behind catch-up weight; nutritional intervention needs to be continued until appropriate height for age is reached.

If the infant has food aversion, vomiting, rumination, or hostility during refeeding, tube feeding should be implemented to bypass these barriers. Feeding problems and misconceptions of parents about the proper amounts and types of foods should be corrected. The family should receive help and information regarding resources available from public welfare agencies, support groups for parents, and transportation services. When infants repeatedly show good progress in hospital with relapses and lack of weight gain at home, foster placement should be considered.[103]

Growth faltering in breast-fed infants can be managed by increasing the maternal milk supply while meeting the requirement for calories with the use of banked human milk or a formula supplement. The mother can continue to nurse and can use an electric pump to stimulate further milk secretion. If the milk supply does not appear to be adequate despite these measures, supplemental feedings must be continued while the mother decides whether to continue nursing or to wean the infant from the breast. Management of infants with behavioral feeding disorders is best accomplished by attempting to make the eating process enjoyable and nutritionally adequate.[106]

An algorithm for the approach to an infant with NOFTT who has no obvious psychosocial problems is depicted in Figure 5–3.

## PREVENTION

If the population at risk for development of NOFTT can be identified early, then prevention techniques can be implemented before its onset. The parental and infant characteristics listed in Tables 5–5 and 5–6 are helpful for preselecting families at risk who could benefit by learning nurturing techniques, how to interpret the child's behavior, and how to assess developmental milestones. If a home health nurse monitors such a maternal-infant dyad and educates the mother, she may realize how her actions affect her child and subsequently seek further help.[47]

## DEVELOPMENTAL INTERVENTION

Several studies have demonstrated the beneficial effects of a combination of nutritional rehabilitation and developmental intervention guided by the results of the Denver Development and Feeding Skills Assessment. Murray and Glassman[107] reported significantly better development scores in malnourished children who received focused and sustained developmental intervention for 3 years beginning before 2 years of age, compared with the untreated malnourished group. Similar results have been reported from developing countries.[49, 108] A prospective, randomized trial of multifaceted intervention, as used in the Infant Health and Development Program in preterm infants with low birth

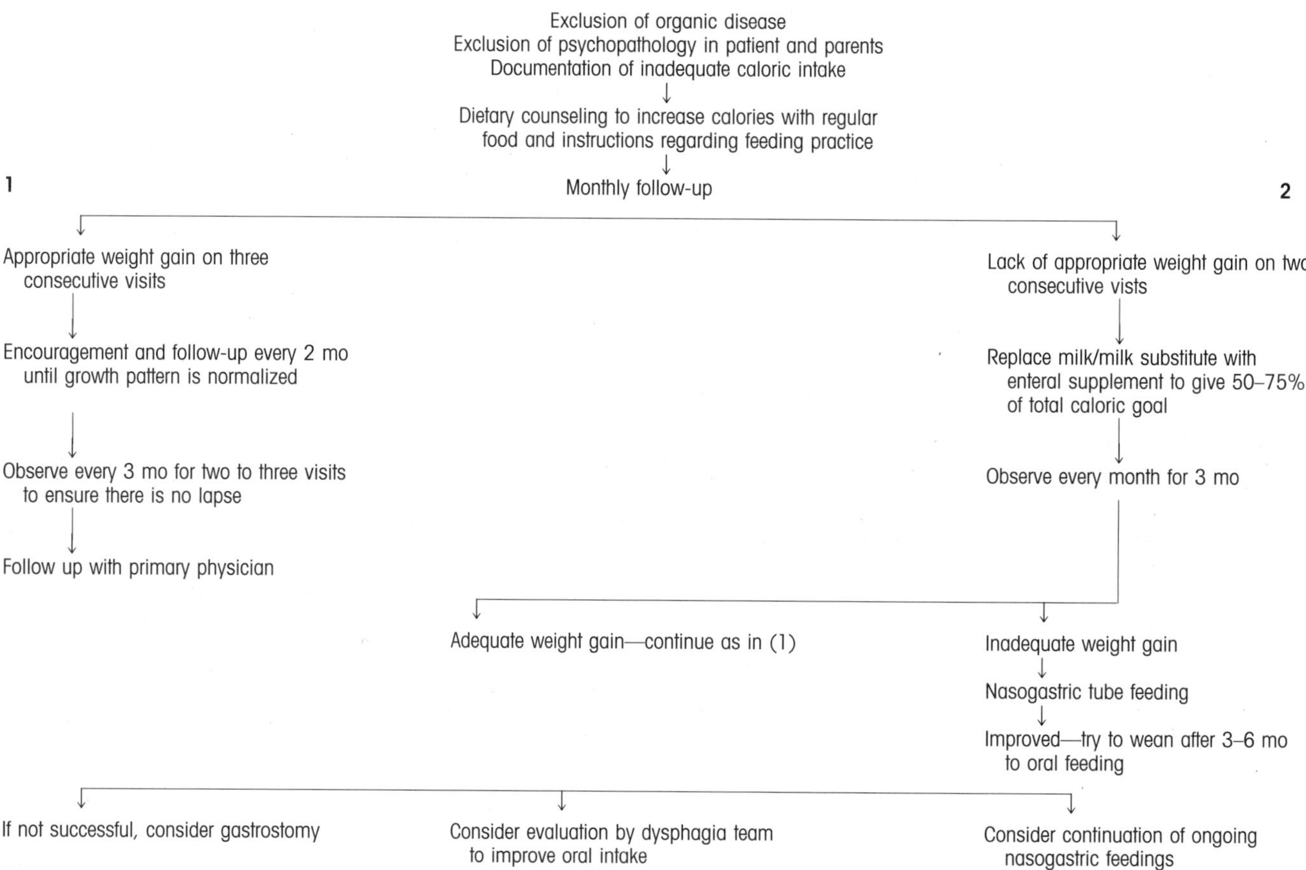


**FIGURE 5–3.** Algorithm for management of patients with nonorganic failure to thrive. (From Tolia V: Very early onset non-organic failure to thrive in infants. J Pediatr Gastroenterol Nutr 1995;20:73–80, with permission.)

weight, showed beneficial effects on IQ at 3 years but no effect on the incidence of FTT.[109] This ongoing trial also demonstrated that these beneficial effects were directly proportional to compliance. Black and coworkers[110] studied the efficacy of a 1-year, home-based early intervention program on the growth and development of children with NOFTT. Subjects were randomly assigned to receive intervention services in a multidisciplinary growth and nutrition clinic or similar therapy plus weekly home visits. Regardless of the grouping, children's nutrition improved; children with the dual intervention had better receptive language over time, without any effect on motor development. The impact on intervention was dependent on the child's age at the time of recruitment to the trial, with younger children faring better.

## LONG-TERM EFFECTS AND PROGNOSIS

NOFTT may be multifactorial in origin, and the outcome depends on the timing, duration, and intensity of the nutritional insult, so the prognosis is unpredictable. In industrialized countries, the prognosis is good with early intervention in mild to moderate undernutrition. Uncontrolled long-term follow-up studies of children with NOFTT treated with hospitalization as the therapeutic modality have shown poor prognosis.[111] Even though hospitalization increases the probability of sustained catch-up growth, it affects psychosocial development only moderately.[112, 113] The sequelae of FTT can be serious. Severe malnutrition in infancy not only influences growth and stature but interferes with normal development of the central nervous system, causing cognitive and developmental impairment. Early malnutrition correlates with persistent fine and gross motor dysfunction seen in later life.[114] When the brain is deprived of an optimal supply of nutrients, generalized morphologic distortion occurs, affecting areas of brain that are maturing at the time of the nutritional insult.[100]

Kessel and associates[115] described an 11-month-old infant with microcephaly, developmental delay, severe growth failure, and marked cortical atrophy on brain CT. Appropriate dietary intervention transformed this infant into a normally developing infant in 2 months, with normalization of body weight and head circumference and impressive improvement in CT findings. This is an exception, because most of the effects, such as decreased ability to maintain attention, increased emotional outbursts, less interaction with people, and slow language development, have been reported to persist for years after the phase of undernutrition.[116] The most striking effects of early malnutrition are behavioral and mental (Table 5–9).[117] Malnutrition and subsequent poor growth and development in a young child appear to be accentuated by family contexts of impoverishment, dysfunctional relationships, inadequate education, and lack of developmentally enriching experiences.[118] Aylward[119] reported that a child whose developmental status is optimal at the end of the first year and is in an optimal environment has a good prognosis, but that the outcome is poor if both factors are suboptimal.

**TABLE 5–9. Long-Term Behavioral Effects of Early Malnutrition**

| |
|---|
| Impaired school performance |
| Attention deficits |
| Emotional outbursts |
| Deficits in cognitive development |
| Intellectual delays (IQ) |
| Low self-esteem |
| Impaired intersensory integration |

Traditionally, the broadly defined disorder FTT has been dichotomized into the categories of organic FTT and NOFTT. A multitude of biologic and environmental variables have been recognized that contribute to the poor weight gain patterns of infants and toddlers. Therefore, a third category, mixed FTT, has been added to the traditional nosology. Disturbed parent-child interaction is the most common cause of NOFTT, which poses a dilemma: Is the infant temperamentally difficult or easily disorganized and cannot offer clear signals to the mother, or is the mother at fault? The assessment and management of FTT should be interdisciplinary, because serious growth problems in infancy place a child at significant risk for developmental disabilities in the future.


*Acknowledgments*

The author wishes to thank Kirit, Vinay, and Sanjay for their patience and Sonja C. Battle for her expert secretarial assistance.


## REFERENCES


1. Kristiansson B, Fallstom SP: Growth at the age of 4 years subsequent to early failure to thrive. Child Abuse Negl 1987;11:35–40.
2. Singer L: Long term hospitalization of failure to thrive infants: developmental outcome at 3 years. Child Abuse Negl 1986;10:479–486.
3. Bithoney WG, Dubowitz H, Egan H: Failure to thrive/growth deficiency. Pediatr Rev 1992;13:453–460.
4. Holt LE, McIntosh R: Holt's diseases of infancy and childhood, 10th ed. New York: Appleton-Century, 1933.
5. Wilcox WD, Nieburg P, Miller DS: Failure to thrive: a continuing problem of definition. Clin Pediatr 1989;28:391–394.
6. Porter B, Skuse D: When does slow weight gain become "failure to thrive"? Arch Dis Child 1991;66:905–906.
7. Edwards AGK, Halse PC, Parkin JM, et al: Recognizing failure to thrive in early childhood. Arch Dis Child 1990;65:1263–1265.
8. Homer C. Ludwig S: Categorization of etiology of failure to thrive. Am J Dis Child 1981;135:848–851.
9. Frank D, Silva M, Needlman R: Failure to thrive: mystery, myth and method. Contemp Pediatr 1993;10:114–133.
10. Sills RH, Sills IN: Don't overlook environmental causes of failure to thrive. Contemp Pediatr 1986;3:25–42.
11. Chatoor I: Infantile anorexia nervosa a development disorder of separation and individuation J Am Acad Psychoanal 1989;17:43–64.
12. Promerance HH: Growth and its assessment. Adv Pediatr 1995;42:545–574.
13. Bowditch HP: The growth of children. Eighth annual report of the Massachusetts State Board of Health. Boston, 1877, pp 273–323.
14. Hamill PVV, Drizd TA, Johnson CL, et al: 1976 National Center for Health Statistics growth charts. Monthly Vital Statistics Report 25, no. 3 (suppl). DHEW publication HRA 76. Washington, DC, US Department of Health and Human Services, 1976.
15. Guo SM, Roche AF, Fomon SJ, et al: Reference data on gains in weight and length during the first two years of life. J Pediatr 1991;119:355–362.
16. Leung AK, Robson WM, Fagan JE. Assessment of the child with failure to thrive. Am Fam Physician 1993;48:1432–1438.
17. Smith DW, Teung W, Rogers JE, et al: Shifting linear growth during infancy: illustration of genetic factors in growth from fetal life through infancy. J Pediatr 1976;89:225–230.
18. Marcovitch H: Failure to thrive. BMJ 1994;308:35–38.

19. Brook CGD, Hindmarsh P, Stanhope R: Growth and growth hormone secretion. Endocrinology 1988;119:179–184.
20. Miller JD, Tannenbaum GS, Colle E, et al: Daytime pulsatile growth hormone secretion during childhood and adolescence. J Clin Endocrinol Metab 1982;55:989–994.
21. Adlar P, Buzi F, Jones J, et al: Physiological growth hormone secretion during slow-wave sleep in short prepubertal children. Clin Endocrinol 1987;12:355–435.
22. Isaksson OG, Lindahl A, Nilsson A, et al: Mechanism on the stimulatory affect of growth hormone on longitudinal bone growth. Endocr Rev 1987;8:426–438.
23. Fisher DA, Hoath S, Lakshmanan J: The thyroid hormone effects on growth and development may be mediated by growth factors. Endocrinol Exp 1982;16:259–271.
24. O'Brian JT: Thyroid hormone homeostasis in states of relative caloric deprivation. Metabolism 1980;29:721–729.
25. Evans RM: The steroid and thyroid hormone receptor superfamily. Science 1988;240:889–895.
26. Hill DJ, Milner RDG: Insulin as a growth factor. Pediatr Res 1985;19:879–886.
27. Karlberg J, Engstrom I, Karlberg P, et al: Analysis of linear growth using a mathematical model. Acta Pediatr Scand 1987;76:478–488.
28. Powell GT, Brasel JA, Raiti S, et al: Emotional deprivation and grown retardation simulating idiopathic hypopituitarism: II. Clinical evaluation of the syndrome. N Engl J Med 1967;276:1279–1283.
29. Skuse D, Albanese A, Stanhope R, et al: A new stress-related syndrome of a growth failure and hyperphagia in children associated with reversibility of growth hormone insufficiency. Lancet 1996;348:353–358.
30. Cupoli JM, Hallock JA, Barness LA: Failure to thrive. Curr Probl Pediatr 1980;10:1–43.
31. Chapin HD: Are institutions for infants necessary? JAMA 1915;64:1–3.
32. Bakwin H: Loneliness in infants. Am J Dis Child 1942;63:30–40.
33. Skuse D, Pickles A, Wolke D, et al: Postnatal growth and mental development: evidence for a "sensitive period." J Child Psychol Psychiatry 1994;35:521–545.
34. Widdowson E: Metal contentment and physical growth. Lancet 1951;1:1316–1318.
35. Spitz RA: Hospitalism. Psychoanal Study Child 1945;1:53–74.
36. Talbot N, Sobel E, Burke B, et al: Dwarfism in healthy children: its possible relation to emotional, nutritional and endocrine disturbances. N Engl J. Med 1947;236:783–793.
37. Whitten C, Pettit MG, Fischoff J: Evidence that growth failure from maternal deprivation is secondary to under eating. JAMA 1969;209:1675–1682.
38. Fischoff J, Whitten C, Pettit MG. A psychiatric study of mothers of infants with growth failure secondary to maternal deprivation. J Pediatr 1971;79:209–215.
39. Lifshitz F, Moses N: Growth failure: a complication of dietary treatment of hypercholesterolemia. Am J Dis Child 1989;143:537–542.
40. Pugliese MT, Lifshitz F, Grad G, et al: Fear of obesity: a cause of short stature and delayed puberty. N Engl J Med 1983;309:513–518.
41. Pugliese MT, Weyman-Dawn M, Moses N, et al: Parental health beliefs as a cause of non-organic failure to thrive. Pediatrics 1987;80:175–182.
42. Smith MM, Lifshitz F: Excess fruit juice consumption as a contributing factor in nonorganic failure to thrive. Pediatrics 1994;93:438–443.
43. Hanning RH, Zlotkin SH: Unconventional eating practices and their health implications. Pediatr Clin North Am 1985;32:429–455.
44. Keys A, Brozek J, Herschel A, et al: The Biology of Human Starvation. Minneapolis, University of Minnesota Press, 1956.
45. Vietze PM, Falsey S, O'Conner S, et al (eds): High risk infants and children: adult and peer interactions. New York, Academic Press, 1980.
46. Hergenroeder AC, Taylor PM, Rogers KD, et al: Neonatal characteristics of maltreated infants and children. Am J Dis Child 1985;139:295–298.
47. Altermeier WA III, O'Conner SM, Sherrod KB, et al: Prospective study of antecedents for non-organic failure to thrive. J Pediatr 1985;106:360–365.
48. Kellcher KJ, Casey PH, Bradley RH, et al: Risk factors and outcomes for failure to thrive in low birth weight preterm infants. Pediatrics 1993;91:941–948.
49. Skuse DH: Nonorganic failure to thrive: a reappraisal. Arch Dis Child 1985;60:173–178.
50. Berwick DM: Non-organic failure to thrive. Pediatr Rev 1980;1:265–270.
51. Drotar D: Research and practice in failure to thrive: the state of art zero to three. Bulletin of the National Center for Clinical Infant Programs 1985;5:1–4.
52. Mitchell WG, Gorrell RW, Greenberg RA: Failure to thrive: a study in a primary care setting. Epidemiology and follow-up. Pediatrics 1980;65:971–977.
53. Whitehead RG: For how long is exclusive breast feeding adequate to satisfy the dietary energy needs of the average young baby? Pediatr Res 1995;37:239–243.
54. Davies DP, Evans TJ: Failure to thrive at the breast. Lancet 1976;2:1994–1195.
55. Weston JA, Stage AF, Hathaway P, et al: Prolonged breast feeding and nonorganic failure to thrive. Am J Dis Child 1987;141:242–243.
56. Habbick BF, Gerrard JW: Failure to thrive in the contented breast-fed baby. Can Med Assoc J 1984;131:765–768.
57. Stuff JE, Nichols BL: Nutrient intake and growth performance of older infants fed human milk. J Pediatr 1989;15:959–968.
58. Gilmore HE, Rowland TW: Critical malnutrition in breast-fed infants. Am J Dis Child 1978;132:885–887.
59. Chan JCM, McEnery PT, Chinchalli VM: Growth failure in children with renal diseases: a clinical trial in pediatric nephrology. Growth Failure in Renal Diseases (GFRD) study. J Pediatr 1990;116:S1–S62.
60. Warady BA, Kriley M, Lovell H, et al: Growth and development of infants with end stage renal disease receiving long-term peritoneal dialysis. J Pediatr 1988;112:714–719.
61. Tejani A, Fine R, Alexander S, et al: Factors predictive of sustained growth in children after renal transplantation. J Pediatr 1993;122:397–402.
62. Salzer HR, Haschlee F, Wimmer M, et al: Growth and nutritional intake of infant with congenital heart disease. Pediatr Cardiol 1989;10:17–23.
63. Posekitt EM: Food, growth and congenital heart disease. Nutr Health 1987;5:153–161.
64. Russell G: Asthma and growth. Arch Dis Child 1993;69:695–698.
65. Thomas BC, Stanhope R, Grant DB: Impaired growth in children with asthma during treatment with conventional doses of inhaled corticosteroids. Arch Dis Child 1994;83:193–199.
66. Marcus CL, Carroll JL, Koerner CB, et al: Determinants of growth in children with obstructive sleep apnea syndrome. J Pediatr 1994;125:556–562.
67. Buchdath RM, Felleylov C, Marchant JL, et al: Energy and nutrient intakes in cystic fibrosis. Arch Dis Child 1989;64:373–378.
68. Gerson WT, Swan T, Walker WWA: Nutrition support in cystic fibrosis. Nutr Rev 1987;45:353–360.
69. Borgana-Pignatti C, De Stefano P, Zonta L, et al: Growth and sexual maturation in thalassemia major. J Pediatr 1985;106:150–155.
70. Finan AC, Elmer MA, Sasanaw SR, et al: Nutritional factors and growth in children with sickle cell disease. Am J Dis Child 1988;142:237–240.
71. Lazoff B, Jimenez E, Wolf AW: Long-term developmental outcome in infants with iron deficiency. N Engl J Med 1991;325:687–694.
72. Palti H. Maijer A, Adler B: Learning achievement and behavior at school of anemic and non-anemic infants. Early Hum Dev 1985;10:217–223.
73. McKinney RE, Robertson JWR, Duke Pediatric AIDS Clinical Trials Unit. Effect on human immunodeficiency virus infection on the growth of young children. J Pediatr 1993;123:579–582.
74. Shapiro BK, Green P, Krick J, et al: Growth of severely impaired children: neurological versus nutritional factors. Dev Med Child Neurol 1986;28:729–733.
75. Gisel EG, Patrick J: Identification of children with cerebral palsy unable to maintain a normal nutritional state. Lancet 1988;1:283–286.
76. Hyman PE: Gastroesophageal reflux: one reason why baby won't eat. J Pediatr 1994;125:S103–109.
77. Seidman E, Lelieko N, Ament A, et al: Nutritional issues in pediatric inflammatory bowel disease. J Pediatr Gastroenterol Nutr 1991;12:424–438.
78. Cacciara E, Salardi S, Lazzasri, R, et al: Short stature and celiac disease: a relationship to consider even in patients with no gastrointestinal tract symptoms. J Pediatr 1983;103:708–711.
79. Kleinman R, Warman KY: Nutrition in liver disease. In Baker S, Baker R, Davis A (eds): Pediatric Enteral Nutrition. New York, Chapman & Hall, 1994, pp 261–279.

80. Amundson J, Sherbondy A, Van Dyke D, et al: Early identification and treatment necessary to prevent malnutrition in children and adolescent with severe disabilities. J Am Diet Assoc 1994;94:880–883.
81. Casey PH, Bradley R, Wortham B: Social and nonsocial home environments of infants with non-organic failure to thrive. Pediatrics 1984;73:348–353.
82. Berkowitz CD, Senter SA: Characteristics of mother-infant interactions in nonorganic failure to thrive. J Fam Pract 1987;25:377–383.
83. Mathisen B, Skuse D, Wolke D, et al: Oral-motor dysfunction and failure to thrive among inner city infants. Dev Med Child Neurol 1989;31:293–302.
84. Fosson A, Wilson J: Family interactions surrounding feeding of infants with nonorganic failure to thrive. Clin Pediatr 1987;26:518–523.
85. Powell GF, Low JF, Speers MA: Behavior as a diagnostic aid in failure to thrive. J Dev Behav Pediatr 1987;8:18–24.
86. Casey PH. Failure to thrive: transitional perspective. J Dev Behav Pediatr 1987;8:37–38.
87. Tolia V: Very early onset nonorganic failure to thrive in infants. J Pediatr Gastroenterol Nutr 1995;20:73–80.
88. Neldner KH, Hambidge KM: Zinc therapy of acrodermatitis enteropathica N Engl J Med 1975;292:879–882.
89. Prasad AS, Miale A, Farid Z, et al: Zinc metabolism in normals and patients with the syndrome of iron deficiency anemia, hypogonadism and dwarfism. J Clin Lab Med 1963;61:537–549.
90. Ingenbleck Y, Beckers C: Triiodothyromine and thyroid stimulating hormone in protein-calorie malnutrition in infants. Lancet 1975;2:845–847.
91. Strauss RS, Dietz WH: Effects of intrauterine growth retardation to premature infants on early childhood growth. J Pediatr 1997;130:95–102.
92. Hokken-Koelega ACS, DeRidder MAJ, Lemmen RJ, et al: Children born small for gestational age: do they catch up? Pediatr Res 1995;38:267–271.
93. Freisancho AR: New norms of upper limb fat and muscle areas for assessment of nutritional status. Am J Clin Nutr 1981;34:2540–2545.
94. Gomez F, Galvan RR, Cravioto J, et al: Malnutrition in infancy and childhood with special reference to kwashiorkor. Adv Pediatr 1955;7:131–169.
95. Waterlow JC: Classification and definition of protein calorie malnutrition. BMJ 1972;3:566–569.
96. McLaren DS, Read WWC: Weight/length classification of nutritional status. Lancet 1975;2:219–220.
97. Wright JA, Ashenburg CA, Whitaker RC: Comparison of methods to categorize undernutrition in children. J Pediatr 1994;124:944–946.
98. Leung AK: Pica. Can J Pediatr 1989;1:4–7.
99. Berwick DM, Levey JC, Kleinerman R: Failure to thrive: diagnostic yield of hospitalization. Arch Dis Child 1982;57:347–351.
100. Frank DA, Zeisel SH: Failure to thrive. Pediatr Clin North Am 1988;35:1187–1206.
101. Showers J, Mandelkorn R, Coury DL, et al: Non-organic failure to thrive; identification and intervention. J Pediatr Nurs 1986;1:240–246.
102. Chase HP, Kumar V, Caldwell RT, et al: Kwashiorkor in the United States. Pediatrics 1980;66:972–976.
103. Pipes PL, Trahms CM: Nutrition: Growth and development. In Pipes PL, Trahms CM (eds): Nutrition in Infancy and Childhood, 5th ed. St. Louis, Mosby, 1993, pp 1–29.
104. Pipes PL, Trahms CM: Nutrient needs of infants and children. In Pipes PL, Trahms CM (eds): Nutrition in Infancy and Childhood, 5th ed. St. Louis, Mosby, 1993, pp 30–58.
105. Rathbun JM, Peterson KE: Nutrition in failure to thrive. In Grand RJ, Sutphen JL, Dietz WH (eds): Pediatric Nutrition. Boston, Butterworths, 1987, pp 629–643.
106. Arvedson JC: Behavioral issues and implications with pediatric feeding disorders. Semin Speech Lang 1997;18:51–69.
107. Murray C, Glassman M: Nutrient requirements during growth and recovery from failure to thrive. In Accaredo PJ (ed): Failure to Thrive in Infancy and Early Childhood. Baltimore, MD, University Park Press, 1981.
108. Granthan-McGregor S, Schofield W, Powell C: Development of severely malnourished children who receive psychosocial stimulation: Six year follow-up Pediatrics 1987;79:247–254.
109. Casey PH, Kellcher KJ, Bradley RH, et al: A multifaceted intervention for infants with failure to thrive. Arch Pediatr Adolesc Med 1994;148:1071–1077.
110. Black MM, Dubowitz H, Hutcheson J, et al: A randomized clinical trial of home intervention for children with failure to thrive. Pediatrics 1995;95:807–814.
111. Oates RK, Peacock A, Forrest D: Long-term effects of non-organic failure to thrive. Pediatrics 1985;7536–7540.
112. Casey PH, Wortham B, Nelson JY: Management of children with failure to thrive in a rural ambulatory setting. Clin Pediatr 1985;23:325–330.
113. Fryer GE: The efficacy of hospitalization of non-organic failure to thrive children: a meta-analysis. International Journal of Child Abuse and Neglect 1988;12:375–381.
114. Henry JJ: Routine growth monitoring and assessment of growth disorders. J Pediatr Health Care 1992;6:291–301.
115. Kessel A, Tal Y, Jaffe M, et al: Reversible brain atrophy and reversible developmental retardation in a malnourished infant. Isr J Med Sci 1996;32:306–308.
116. Barrett DE, Radke-Yarrow M, Klein RE: Chronic malnutrition and child behaviour: effects of early caloric supplementation on social and emotional functioning at school age. Dev Psychol 1982;18:541–556.
117. Galler JR, Ross RN: Malnutrition and mental development. In Suskind RM, Lewinter-Suskind L, eds: Textbook of Pediatric Nutrition, 2nd ed. New York, Raven Press, 1993, pp 173–179.
118. Drotar D, Sturn L: Influences on the home environment of preschool children with early histories of non-organic failure to thrive. J Dev Behav Pediatr 1989;10:229–239.
119. Aylward GP: The relationship between environmental risk and developmental outcome. J Dev Behav Pediatr 1992;13:222–229.

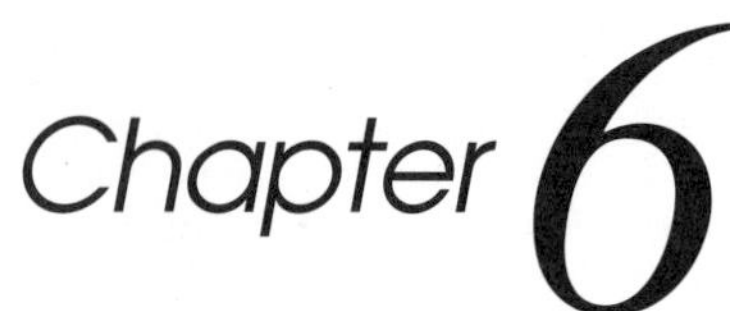

# Chapter 6

# Gastrointestinal Hemorrhage

*Leo A. Heitlinger and H. Juhling McClung*

In the eyes of the parent, the presence of blood in stool or vomitus is an indication of severe disease. Because this is an uncommon event in infants and children, the primary care physician frequently calls on the specialist for assistance. It is both difficult and imperative that the gastroenterologist, surgeon, or emergency room physician rapidly assess and triage patients with gastrointestinal bleeding. Patients who are seriously ill require timely, focused, and appropriate assessment and treatment. In contrast, patients with trivial bleeding who are not seriously ill may require patience, limited assessment, and little if any treatment. Balancing these extremes can challenge the gastroenterologist, surgeon, or emergency room physician who cares for the patient while meeting the expectations of the family and the primary physician.[1]

This review describes an approach to the patient with gastrointestinal bleeding that will assist the physician in determining the urgency with which to proceed with an evaluation and reviewing the utility of diagnostic tests, the differential diagnosis, and therapeutic modalities available for use. It does not detail the pathophysiology of the disorders associated with gastrointestinal blood loss which are reviewed elsewhere, but key studies are cited to direct the interested reader to more comprehensive sources.

## DEFINITIONS

*Melena* is the passage of black, tarry stools. *Hematochezia* is the passage of bright or dark red blood per rectum. *Hematemesis* is the passage of vomited material that is black ("coffee grounds") or contains frank blood.

## TELEPHONE INTAKE

The challenge in the assessment of the patient with gastrointestinal blood loss is determining whether the patient is seriously ill and should undergo immediate examination and perhaps endoscopic studies.[2] This challenge typically is addressed at several levels. First, the initial contact by telephone requires discipline and experience; the quality of information gathered determines the appropriate course of action. If office personnel are those who collect the initial intake information, it is imperative that they be well trained and adhere to clearly defined standards for the physician's practice. The information must be relayed to the physician in a timely fashion for appropriate action; intakes of patients who may be critically ill cannot wait to be relayed at the end of the day.

The initial triage call must contain the following information to determine whether the patient is seriously or critically ill (Table 6–1). First, the source, magnitude, and duration of bleeding must be documented. If a parent is relaying the history, it must be determined whether the parent has witnessed the symptoms firsthand. If not, the parent should question the caregiver who witnessed the symptoms; if the child is of sufficient age, the parent should solicit information from the child as well. Second, the interviewer must determine whether other gastrointestinal symptoms (e.g., diarrhea, cramping, abdominal pain, constipation, vomiting) are present. Third, the presence of other systemic symptoms (e.g., fever, rash, dizziness, shortness of breath, pallor, palpitations, cool extremities) should be recorded. Fourth, an abbreviated review of systems and family history that includes gastrointestinal disorders, liver disease, bleeding diatheses, and medication use must be obtained. If symptoms of impending shock are present, instructions should be given to access local emergency services.

Phone intake from patients known to the physician's practice who are chronically ill represent a special case.[3] A patient with long-standing ulcerative colitis who describes tenesmus and small-volume, liquid stools that are almost all blood requires a different approach from a new patient with painless, intermittent rectal bleeding. The approach to this group of patients must be individualized based on diagnosis, the family's knowledge of the illness, current medications, previous response to medications, distance from the medical center, and availability and interest of local primary care physicians. The decision-making for this group of patients is difficult but is best addressed on an individual basis rather than by generalization.

Contacts from other physicians, particularly if the patient is in their office, can be handled somewhat differently. First,

**TABLE 6–1. Historical Information**

**Present Illness**

Source of bleeding
Magnitude of bleeding
Duration of bleeding
Associated gastrointestinal symptoms (vomiting, diarrhea, pain)
Associated systemic symptoms (fever, rash, joint pains)

**Review of Systems**

Gastrointestinal disorders
Liver disease
Bleeding diatheses
Anesthesia reactions
Medications (NSAIDs, warfarin, hepatotoxins)

**Family History**

Gastrointestinal disorders (polyps, ulcers, colitis)
Liver disease
Bleeding diatheses
Anesthesia reactions

NSAIDs, nonsteroidal anti-inflammatory drugs.

the signs that can be observed by the physician augment the symptoms addressed in the contact with the caregiver. Second, the physician can go beyond the usual examination to elicit signs that the consultant may require (e.g., spider hemangiomata in a child with hematemesis). Third, if signs of shock or impending shock are present, stabilization can begin before the patient is transported for diagnostic studies.

## PHYSICIAN ASSESSMENT

A telephone call from the family or a referring physician or a review of information collected by office personnel typically begins the process of assessment. The questions that must be addressed are (1) Has the child been bleeding? (2) Has the child had bleeding of sufficient magnitude to result in actual or impending circulatory compromise? (3) Is the child bleeding now? and (4) What actions are required?

Foods and medications can alter the color of stool or vomitus[4–6] and initiate a series of events that can be uncomfortable and expensive and may entail some risk (Table 6–2). Red foods and medications and deeply pigmented foods such as blueberries can all result in stools and vomitus that can fool even the experienced observer into believing that blood is present. Although it is reassuring to find that a child with black stools recently ingested a bismuth preparation, it is imperative to determine whether the stools are guaiac-positive. If the test is rapidly positive, the child has been passing blood until proved otherwise. If a single test is negative and the stools have been only intermittently dark, then serial stool examinations, determination of the blood count, and observation may be indicated. In the case of vomitus, a test kit for gastric fluid (e.g., Gastroccult) should be used rather than the routine stool kits, because they are more reliable at acid pH.[7]

The questions of duration and magnitude of bleeding are more difficult to answer. First, children beyond the age of toilet training do not routinely share their bowel habits with their parents. In addition, they do not know the range of normal or what is abnormal. Frank blood makes children alarmed regardless of the source, but melena may be ignored for some time. Second, lay persons routinely overestimate the amount of blood passed in the stool or in vomited material. In practice, comparison with the first day of a menstrual period provides a useful guide to the amount of blood passed. If the water of the commode is opacified with blood, the bleeding is likely to be significant.

On physical examination (Table 6–3), the presence or absence of signs of anemia (e.g., pallor) is useful to confirm whether a significant amount of blood has been lost. Typically, gradual blood loss is better tolerated than rapid blood loss, and has a lower likelihood of cardiovascular decompensation. In both acute and chronic blood loss, decompensation eventually occurs. The presence of resting tachycardia or orthostatic changes in blood pressure and heart rate indicates actual or impending decompensation of circulatory status regardless of the duration of bleeding.

Laboratory studies can assist the physician in assessing the magnitude and duration of blood loss. For chronic loss, reductions in the red blood cell (RBC) count, hemoglobin, and hematocrit are the most useful indices of the magnitude of loss. With acute bleeding, values must be interpreted in light of the hydration status. The presence of anemia with normal RBC volume is indicative of rapid loss of circulating volume; conversely, the presence of anemia with reduced RBC volume is suggestive of chronic loss. Caveats to these last points include folate or vitamin $B_{12}$ deficiency in the former case, and hemoglobinopathies in the latter.

The question of whether the child is actively bleeding at the time of the examination can be difficult to answer. Placement of a nasogastric tube is often employed to evalu-

**TABLE 6–2. Substances that Commonly Color Emesis or Stools**

| Red | Black |
|---|---|
| Candies | Bismuth |
| Fruit punch | Activated charcoal |
| Beets | Iron |
| Laxatives | Spinach |
| Phenytoin | Blueberries |
| Rifampin | Licorice |

**TABLE 6–3. Physical Examination**

**Skin**

Pallor
Jaundice
Ecchymoses
Abnormal blood vessels
Hydration

**Head, Eyes, Ears, Nose, and Throat**

Nasopharyngeal injection, oozing
Tonsillar enlargement, bleeding

**Cardiovascular**

Heart rate, lying and sitting
Pulse pressure, lying and sitting
Gallop rhythm
Capillary filling

**Abdomen**

Organomegaly
Tenderness

**Perineum**

Fissure
Fistula
Induration

**Rectum**

Gross blood
Melena
Tenderness

ate complaints of hematemesis and melena, symptoms most often associated with sources of bleeding in the upper gastrointestinal tract. If the lavage aspirate is clear and contains neither coffee grounds nor fresh blood, bleeding proximal to the ligament of Treitz is less likely.[8] If the aspirate contains coffee grounds and then rapidly clears, the bleeding probably originated in the upper intestinal tract but has ceased. If the aspirate contains fresh blood or a mixture of fresh and old blood that does not rapidly clear, the bleeding probably originated in the proximal gastrointestinal tract and continues to be active. Regarding more distal sources, the best assessment of active bleeding is observation of stool output and character combined with serial RBC, hemoglobin, or hematocrit measurements.

The actions to be taken are dictated by the history and the findings on physical examination. The history begins with a review of the data collected at telephone triage or during the contact with another physician. The initial focus should be to identify the patient at risk for circulatory compromise. The questions should initially be brief and should be asked while the initial physical assessment proceeds. The initial physical assessment must include the following: vital signs, including the orthostatic maneuvers; examination of the skin for signs of pallor, jaundice, pruritus, spider hemangiomata, ecchymoses, and prominent vessels on the abdomen; examination of the abdomen for organomegaly, masses, and tenderness; examination of the oropharynx for signs of bleeding from the nasopharynx or tonsils; examination of the perineum for fissures, fistulas, or indurations; rectal examination for tenderness and blood; and, in the case of hematemesis, consideration of nasogastric aspiration. If the patient has signs of actual or impending circulatory compromise, resuscitation should be prompt and thorough. Resuscitation should be completed before radiographic or endoscopic studies are considered.

If the initial physical examination does not demonstrate the presence of actual or impending circulatory compromise, then a complete history of the present illness, along with a review of systems, a family history, and the physical examination should be completed as would be appropriate for any consultation.

## LABORATORY ASSESSMENT

The history and physical examination should guide the use of laboratory tests in patients with gastrointestinal bleeding. In general, laboratory tests should be limited to those that are appropriate to the clinical setting. For some patients, testing may be extensive, but for most the indicated studies are decidedly fewer (Table 6–4).

Patients with hematemesis, melena, or both, require limited laboratory testing if they do not show signs of cardiovascular compromise, systemic disease, or portal hypertension. A complete blood count with platelet quantification and possibly prothrombin and partial thromboplastin times may be indicated in this setting. Patients with signs and symptoms suggestive of isolated portal hypertension or chronic liver disease with cirrhosis require an extensive evaluation to assess the magnitude of altered hepatic synthetic, metabolic, and excretory function. In addition, studies are needed to identify the cause of liver disease. Imaging studies leading to later elective liver biopsy are also a part of the evaluation for almost all patients in this situation. Patients with signs and symptoms of other chronic diseases, such as decreased muscle mass, subcutaneous tissue mass, fever, or fatigue, may require more extensive testing appropriate to the age of the patient.

**TABLE 6–4. Laboratory Studies**

| Signs of Shock—Systemic or Liver Disease Absent | Signs of Shock—Systemic or Liver Disease Present |
|---|---|
| Complete blood count | Complete blood count |
| Erythrocyte sedimentation rate | Erythrocyte sedimentation rate |
| BUN | Prothrombin time |
| Prothrombin time | Partial thromboplastin time |
| Partial thromboplastin time | Guaiac stool, emesis |
| Guaiac stool, emesis | Blood typing and crossmatch |
| | Aspartate aminotransferase |
| | Alanine aminotransferase |
| | $\gamma$-Glutamyl transpeptidase |
| | BUN |
| | Creatinine |
| | Albumin |
| | Total protein |

Patients who present with hematochezia also may require a variable number of tests.[9] Children with painless rectal bleeding consistent with polyps should have a complete blood count. Children with massive, paroxysmal, painless rectal bleeding require a blood count but no studies other than a nuclear medicine scan to rule out the presence of a Meckel's diverticulum. Infants with a history and physical examination consistent with functional constipation, anal fissure, or allergic colitis require little if any laboratory testing. In contrast, children with signs of an acute illness including fever and joint pains require a complete blood count, erythrocyte sedimentation rate, stool examination for culture for enteric pathogens, ova and parasite examination, and *Clostridium difficile* toxin assay. If there is concern that the patient is dehydrated or that hemolytic-uremic syndrome is present, or if it is unclear whether the bleeding is occurring in the upper or the lower portion of the intestinal tract, serum bicarbonate, blood urea nitrogen, (BUN) and creatinine should be measured and urine output must be monitored. The BUN/creatinine ratio may be useful in assessing whether the blood is arising high or low in the intestinal tract.[10] Children who appear chronically ill and present with rectal bleeding and for whom inflammatory bowel disease is a consideration should have a complete blood count, erythrocyte sedimentation rate, liver function tests, and determinations of total protein and albumin. In brief, the laboratory tests should be appropriate to the clinical setting.

## IMAGING STUDIES

The utility of imaging studies as an initial test in the evaluation of patients with gastrointestinal bleeding has been limited because of advances in endoscopic equipment and techniques.[11] Imaging studies continue to be useful in the evaluation of areas not accessible to the endoscopist and in the evaluation of patients with significant bleeding, the cause of which has eluded the endoscopist (Table 6–5).

**TABLE 6–5. Imaging Studies**

| TEST | INDICATION |
|---|---|
| Upper gastrointestinal series | Dysphagia<br>Odynophagia<br>Drooling |
| Barium enema | Suspected intussusception<br>Stricture found at colonoscopy |
| Abdominal ultrasound | Suspected portal hypertension |
| Meckel's scan | Suspected Meckel's diverticulum |
| Sulfur colloid scan | Obscure gastrointestinal bleeding |
| Labeled RBC scan | Obscure gastrointestinal bleeding |
| Angiography | Obscure gastrointestinal bleeding |

In patients in whom the source of bleeding is thought to be the nasopharynx or sinuses,[12] computed tomography of the sinuses, rather than plain sinus radiographs, should be considered. As nasopharyngoscopy continues to advance, endoscopic examinations of these areas by otolaryngologists may well become the standard of care within the next few years.

Particularly in younger children, it is often difficult to distinguish hemoptysis from hematemesis.[13] Plain radiographs of the chest may be helpful in eliminating cystic fibrosis, bronchiectasis, and other chronic lung diseases from the differential diagnosis.

Contrast radiography may be indicated before endoscopy in patients with dysphagia, odynophagia, and an inability to control secretions who present with melena or hematemesis.[14] This approach avoids a separate initial endoscopic diagnostic study in favor of performance of both diagnostic and therapeutic endoscopy at the same session (i.e., diagnosis and dilatation of an esophageal stricture in a single session). Contrast radiographs should not be performed as the initial study to rule out the presence of esophagitis, gastritis, or peptic ulcers, because endoscopy is a more sensitive examination.

Sonography of the esophagus or porta hepatis is useful to assess for the presence or absence of varices. These studies typically are used in the patient who is not actively bleeding.

The evaluation of patients with hematochezia typically does not rely on contrast radiographic studies as the initial examination. Flexible proctoscopy, sigmoidoscopy, or colonoscopy usually is the initial examination when the anatomy or mucosa should be visualized.[15] These examinations are more sensitive in regard to mucosal detail and polyps; in addition, mucosal biopsies can be obtained from areas of interest. Contrast radiography is indicated if an examination was incomplete or a stricture was encountered that limited the insertion of the instrument. Exceptions to this paradigm include bleeding associated with severe pain compatible with intussception, in which case an air or barium enema is indicated for reduction, and massive painless bleeding of a suspected Meckel's diverticulum, for which a nuclear medicine examination is the procedure of choice.

For obscure bleeding in either the upper or lower gastrointestinal tract, imaging studies can be particularly useful. Nuclear medicine studies (technetium-labeled sulfur colloid or RBCs) are often attempted to identify the source of bleeding within the actively bleeding gastrointestinal tract.[16, 17] The labeled RBC scan is approximately one order of magnitude more sensitive than sulfur colloid or angiography in identifying the site of bleeding. Angiography is technically challenging but offers not only the possibility of identification of the bleeding source but also a means of treatment (e.g., embolization,[18] vasopressin infusion). The selection of study should be made in consultation with a radiologist; the field continues to change rapidly, and local expertise varies widely.

## ENDOSCOPY

The purposes of endoscopic examinations in the patient with gastrointestinal bleeding are to provide insight into the diagnosis and potentially to treat the bleeding site (Table 6–6). During diagnostic endoscopy, a segment of the gastrointestinal mucosa can be visually examined and biopsies and cultures can be obtained. When lesions are visualized, they can be photographed for later consultation with colleagues. If possible, an attempt to identify markers of likelihood of subsequent bleeding, such as a visible vessel in an ulcer crater, should be made. During therapeutic endoscopy, specific lesions are identified and treatments such as variceal ablation are administered.

As in all of medicine, a diagnostic or therapeutic procedure should not be performed unless the practitioner has adequate training, expertise, and knowledge to perform the procedure. In 1995, the American Society for Gastrointestinal Endoscopy published guidelines for training programs regarding the minimum number of procedures required before a physician has attained sufficient competence to perform diagnostic and therapeutic endoscopy.[19] The North American Society for Pediatric Gastroenterology and Nutrition subsequently provided guidelines for procedures to be performed in infants and children.[20] Neither set of guidelines specifically addressed the evaluation of the patient with gastrointestinal blood loss. The evaluation of the actively bleeding child is among the most complex and challenging of all problems. It is imperative that the goals, risks, and precautions required for the evaluation of infants and children with such complaints be well understood by the practitioner; these examinations should not be performed by well-intentioned but inexperienced personnel. One must strive for safely performed examinations that meet their objectives and provide guidance to therapy of the child.

Selection of patients for endoscopic examination is usually straightforward. Infants and children with anemia and guaiac-positive stools, even in the absence of melena, hema-

**TABLE 6–6. Endoscopy**

| TEST | INDICATION |
|---|---|
| Esophagogastroduodenoscopy | Hematemesis<br>Melena |
| Flexible sigmoidoscopy | Hematochezia |
| Colonoscopy | Hematochezia |
| Enteroscopy | Obscure gastrointestinal blood loss |

tochezia, or hematemesis, often need upper endoscopic examinations. In adults older than 50 years of age, or younger if they belong to a high-risk group for colorectal cancer, flexible sigmoidoscopy or colonoscopy is the examination of choice if no signs or symptoms are present to suggest proximal disease.[21] In childhood, the yield of examinations for colorectal cancer is not likely to be fruitful. In contrast, occult esophagitis or peptic disease and early inflammatory bowel disease are more likely considerations in children. A thorough knowledge of the age-specific differential diagnosis is required to make appropriate judgments regarding the selection of endoscopic examinations.

Preparation of the patient is also critically important if safe, effective examinations are to be performed. In emergency situations, resuscitation of the patient has higher priority than a hastily performed examination in an unstable patient. The assistance of an intensivist or anesthesiologist can provide reassurance that the patient is adequately resuscitated and will be maintained in homeostasis during the examination. In the critically ill, the choice of sedation or anesthetic regimen is of paramount importance for the performance of a safe and effective examination.

The patient must also be adequately prepared for the endoscopist to visualize the mucosa to an appropriate degree. For example, a patient with painless hematochezia who has a negative Meckel's scan but has not had laxatives, enemas, or suppositories, alone or in combination, is not a suitable candidate for a successful examination of the colonic mucosa. Waiting for adequate preparation while providing supportive care in this setting is preferred over examination of the inadequately prepared colon. In patients who require rapid preparation of the colon, polyethylene glycol solutions have become the standard of care. These solutions can be administered either orally or via a nasogastric tube (≥50 mL/kg). In our experience, children younger than 10 years of age are unlikely to ingest sufficient volume at a rate adequate to evacuate the colon. In patients who do not require preparation for an urgent examination, several options are available. First, a combination of oral stimulants (e.g., magnesium citrate, senna, bisacodyl) with enemas or suppositories can be given. Second, a clear liquid diet can be imposed for several days, followed by enemas until clear fluid is produced. In contrast, a patient with signs and symptoms compatible with ulcerative colitis often needs minimal preparation to remove stool before the examination can proceed.

In the case of upper intestinal bleeding, newer guidelines suggest that a patient requires only 2 hours of fasting after a clear liquid meal before sedation or anesthesia.[22, 23] Longer times are often required to clear solid foods, barium, antacids, or sucralfate so as to allow adequate visualization of the mucosa. Unless there is an emergency situation, it is better to allow adequate time to clear the stomach before examination. In an emergency, gastric lavage with large-bore tubes is often helpful to provide clearance of the stomach contents to a degree sufficient to allow adequate examination of the mucosa. Use of smaller-bore tubes in young patients is often insufficient to provide adequate clearance of the stomach for a complete examination of the gastric mucosa.

The concept of urgent versus elective endoscopy has been one of considerable debate. Urgent endoscopy allows prompt diagnosis and the ability to guide or perform therapy to hasten cessation of bleeding. On the other hand, urgent endoscopy carries the risk of rapid decompensation in an unstable patient and poor visualization of the field due to inadequate preparation. Therefore, the trend has been to perform urgent endoscopy only on patients who cannot be stabilized and in whom surgery to provide emergency therapy is contemplated. In this setting, the increased risks become appropriate; one will either attempt to stop the bleeding with endoscopic treatment or provide guidance to the surgeon who will do so by other operative means.

The question of whether diagnostic or therapeutic endoscopy should be performed in the actively bleeding patient has also engendered considerable debate. In the adult, the standard of care has evolved in favor of therapeutic endoscopy; that is, the endoscopist should be prepared to proceed with therapy if a bleeding lesion such as a varix is encountered. The problem with this approach in infants and children is that, because of the relative rarity of such patients, it is difficult for the pediatric gastroenterologist to obtain sufficient experience to become proficient with the therapeutic techniques required to treat a bleeding lesion. At many centers, an attempt has been made to have a limited number of practitioners perform therapeutic endoscopy so that they can accumulate the necessary experience.[24, 25] At other centers, surgeons or adult gastroenterologists are asked to assist with such patients. In the latter setting, it is critical that the pediatric gastroenterologist collaborate with other practitioners to ensure that lesions are interpreted in the appropriate context. Furthermore, although the surgeon or adult gastroenterologist may be expert with the techniques required to achieve hemostasis, he or she is not likely to be expert in pediatric endoscopy. These issues remain controversial and will undoubtedly evolve in the coming years.

The selection of the endoscopic examination to be performed is relatively standard. For patients with melena or hematemesis in whom the source of bleeding is likely to be proximal to the ligament of Treitz, the first examination is typically esophagogastroduodenoscopy. In patients with hematochezia, flexible sigmoidoscopy is considered the first examination by most practitioners. Many practitioners prefer to use colonoscopy as the first examination, because a significant number of polyps are found proximal to the splenic flexure.[26] In addition, in patients with inflammatory bowel disease it is often helpful to assess the extent of involvement at initial endoscopy. One study showed that the two approaches were of equal cost-effectiveness in pediatric patients.[27] In patients with blood loss and anemia, when esophagogastroduodenoscopy and colonoscopy fail to identify the cause or site of bleeding, endoscopy of the small bowel (enteroscopy) has proved useful at some centers.[28] The procedure is time-consuming, and some instruments are limited to visualization only. This technique, as yet in its infancy, will probably come into greater use as the instruments and techniques evolve. The alternative of intraoperative endoscopy is also an imperfect technique with described risks.[29] The coming years should see refinements in the approach to this group of patients.

## THERAPY

The first tenet in the treatment of patients with gastrointestinal hemorrhage is supportive care: fluids, blood products,

**TABLE 6–7. Therapy**

**Supportive Care**

- Intravenous fluids (normal saline, Ringer's lactate)
- Blood products (whole blood, packed RBCs, fresh-frozen plasma)
- Pressors

**Specific Care**

- Barrier agents (sucralfate)
- $H_2$ antagonists (cimetidine, ranitidine, famotidine, nizatidine)
- Proton pump inhibitors (omeprazole, lansoprazole)
- Somatostatin analogue

**Endoscopic Therapy**

- Coagulation (cautery, heater probe, laser)
- Variceal injection or ligation
- Polypectomy

and drugs used in resuscitation.[30] For patients who are not critically ill, these approaches are not required. In the patient who has signs of cardiovascular compromise, appropriate supportive treatment and monitoring must be provided. In many cases, this requires the assistance of intensivists. When the patient has been adequately stabilized, diagnostic and therapeutic studies can proceed to allow more specific therapy to begin (Table 6–7).

Patients with stress ulcers, varices, and diffuse gastritis as the cause of significant upper gastrointestinal hemorrhage have traditionally been treated with lavage and vasopressin. In more recent years, lavage has not been used as a treatment but rather as a means to prepare the patient for endoscopy or to assess whether the patient is continuing to bleed. The literature is replete with multiple citations but few controlled studies that support the efficacy of iced lavage with or without epinephrine; these techniques are not without risks and are probably of little benefit,[31] and they have ceased to be standard practice. Vasopressin is an effective agent to decrease splanchnic blood flow and thereby decrease gastrointestinal bleeding; it is also known to have significant side effects that have limited its use. Since the long-acting somatostatin analogue became available, vasopressin use has steadily declined. Somatostatin is at least as effective as vasopressin and has a reduced frequency and severity of side effects compared with vasopressin.[32, 33]

Techniques available during therapeutic endoscopy are numerous but can be grouped for the purposes of this discussion.[34] The merits of each technique are beyond the scope of this review but can be obtained elsewhere. Heat can be used to cauterize a bleeding site.[35] Methods include monopolar cautery, bipolar cautery, heater probe, and several laser techniques.[36] Pressure can be used to tamponade a bleeding site.[37] Techniques include paravariceal injection of varices or bleeding vessels with saline, saline with epinephrine, or a sclerosant (paravariceal injection only). Direct injection of vessels[38] can also be used; varices can be injected with ethanol, detergent, or fatty acids.[39] Vessels can also be ligated. Varices can be banded with rubber bands.[40] Bleeding sites can be oversewn with ligatures through the endoscope. Finally, polyps can be removed with electrocautery using monopolar or bipolar snares. The merits of each technique can be found in the appropriate citations.

## DIFFERENTIAL DIAGNOSIS

The diagnosis of gastrointestinal bleeding in the newborn (Table 6–8) presents special challenges. First, significant bleeding in the newborn is not common. Second, when significant bleeding does occur, the limited reserve of neonates makes them prone to decompensate quickly.

The most common cause of blood in the stool or emesis of newborns is swallowed blood, either from amniotic fluid or from a fissure in the nipple of the breast-feeding mother. The Apt test[41, 42] can be used to determine whether the blood is of maternal origin. Sensitivity to dietary proteins, most commonly cow milk or soy milk, can manifest in the neonate as streaks of blood and mucus in the stool even in the absence of other symptoms such as rash, wheezing, diarrhea, vomiting, or anaphylaxis.[43] Necrotizing enterocolitis is an important cause of bleeding because, if it is not rapidly diagnosed and treated, the condition can rapidly progress.[44] Typically, feeding intolerance and abdominal distention in the preterm infant occur before the onset of bleeding. Much less commonly, bleeding is the presenting symptom or the complex occurs in the full-term newborn. Stress ulcers or gastritis can manifest in the neonatal period; when present, they occur in critically ill newborns in the first several days of life.[45]

Coagulopathy should not be missed in the newborn. Potential causes include vitamin K deficiency due to lack of prophylaxis, maternal idiopathic thrombocytopenic purpura or use of nonsteroidal anti-inflammatory drugs, hemophilia, or von Willebrand's disease.[46] Vitamin K and the platelet defects most often do not cause gastrointestinal blood loss. Von Willebrand's disease, in contrast, relatively frequently manifests with mucosal bleeding.[47]

Infections with enteric organisms can cause bleeding in the newborn period. However, the *Clostridium* toxin assays must be interpreted cautiously, since the organism may not be a pathogen in this age group.[48]

**TABLE 6–8. Differential Diagnosis: Neonates**

**Hematemesis, Melena**

- Swallowed maternal blood
- Stress ulcers, gastritis
- Duplication cyst
- Vascular malformations
- Vitamin K deficiency
- Hemophilia
- Maternal idiopathic thrombocytopenic purpura
- Maternal NSAID use

**Hematochezia**

- Swallowed maternal blood
- Dietary protein intolerance
- Infectious colitis
- Necrotizing enterocolitis
- Hirschsprung's disease with enterocolitis
- Duplication cyst
- Vascular malformations
- Vitamin K deficiency
- Hemophilia
- Maternal idiopathic thrombocytopenic purpura
- Maternal NSAID use

NSAID, nonsteroidal anti-inflammatory drug.

**TABLE 6–9. Differential Diagnosis: Infants**

| Hematemesis, Melena | Hematochezia |
|---|---|
| Esophagitis | Anal fissures |
| Gastritis | Intussusception |
| | Infectious colitis |
| | Dietary protein intolerance |
| | Meckel's diverticulum |
| | Duplication cyst |
| | Vascular malformations |

Bleeding in an infant more than 1 month of age includes many of the items listed previously as well as other conditions (Table 6–9). Infections with enteric organisms are more common in infants than in neonates. Dietary protein intolerance can occur up to the age of several months; the presentation typically is delayed in the breast-fed infant until formula is introduced. Less commonly, antigens from the maternal diet are implicated.

Peptic disease (e.g., esophagitis, gastritis) is relatively common in the irritable infant.[49] Bleeding is usually occult but may be of sufficient magnitude to be associated with anemia. Bleeding is rarely the sole symptom; vomiting, regurgitation, and irritability, alone or in combination, are common.

Anal fissures, intussusception, and Meckel's diverticulum are important causes of blood loss in this age group. Anal fissures most often occur in patients with obvious constipation. Occasionally, the parents describe normal stools in a patient with anal fissure; when this is the case, irritability or abdominal pain is frequently described. Intussusception typically manifests with colicky pain, currant-jelly stools, and an abdominal mass.[50] In this age group, most patients are unlikely to have an identified lead point, in sharp contrast to the older child, in whom duplication cysts, polyps, and lymphoma must be sought. Meckel's diverticulum typically causes painless bright or dark rectal bleeding that is usually paroxysmal in onset and massive in quantity.[51]

Preschool and school-aged children share many disorders with neonates and infants (Table 6–10). Peptic disease, infections with enteric organisms, anal fissures, intussusception, and Meckel's diverticulum all occur in this age group. As in the infant, primary peptic ulcer is very uncommon; almost all ulcers are secondary to multisystem disease, head trauma, or serious infection with shock.[52, 53] Infections, intussusception, and Meckel's diverticulum manifest as described previously, except that a search for a lead point is required in the older child with intussusception.

**TABLE 6–10. Differential Diagnosis: Children**

| Hematemesis, Melena | Hematochezia |
|---|---|
| Esophagitis | Anal fissures |
| Gastritis | Infectious colitis |
| Peptic ulcer disease | Polyps |
| Mallory-Weiss tears | Lymphoid nodular hyperplasia |
| Esophageal varices | Inflammatory bowel disease |
| Pill ulcers | Henoch-Schönlein purpura |
| | Intussusception |
| | Meckel's diverticulum |
| | Hemolytic-uremic syndrome |

In this age group several other disorders must be considered. In the patient with vomiting and retching who develops hematemesis, Mallory-Weiss tears of the esophageal mucosa and bleeding from esophageal varices are considerations. In both situations, the patient may describe very little or no pain and yet have massive bleeding. Painless rectal bleeding in children may be caused by polyps.[54] Most often, the complaint is painless bleeding, but in some patients the polyp may be a lead point for intussusception. The bleeding is bright and coats the stool if the polyp is in the rectum; it may be darker and mixed with stool if the lesion is more proximal. Lymphoid nodular hyperplasia of the colon is common in children.[55] When bleeding occurs, it typically is of minor consequence in terms of volume or symptoms.

In children who are acutely or chronically ill, other considerations come into play. Henoch-Schönlein purpura can manifest with variable amounts of bleeding, usually associated with crampy abdominal pain.[56] Uncommonly, the bleeding occurs before the rash. Hemolytic-uremic syndrome is most common in this age group. The typical presentation is an acute gastroenteritis, with or without rectal bleeding, in which, as the diarrhea abates, urine output declines and the child becomes pale and edematous. Other systemic vasculitides[57] should be considered if the more common Henoch-Schönlein purpura and hemolytic-uremic syndrome are excluded. Inflammatory bowel disease, discussed in more detail later, can occur in this age group. A significant percentage of patients with inflammatory bowel disease present with either occult or obvious blood loss, most commonly in association with other symptoms.

Adolescents with gastrointestinal blood loss may have some of the disorders listed previously. However, in most cases the differential diagnosis approximates that of the young adult (Table 6–11).

Melena is most commonly caused by peptic disease in this age group (e.g., esophagitis, gastritis, gastric or duodenal ulcer). In ambulatory, previously healthy adolescents, melena is rarely an isolated symptom if peptic disease is present; each of these conditions is commonly associated with abdominal pain. Esophageal disease may also be associated with chest pain, dysphagia, odynophagia, and halitosis. Gastritis and primary duodenal ulcers are most often associated with *Helicobacter pylori* infection in this population, as in adults. The dramatic, unrestricted use of nonsteroidal anti-inflammatory drugs in this age group leads to increased gastric bleeding.[58]

Hematemesis in the previously well adolescent may be caused by varices associated with previously unrecognized liver disease or portal vein thrombosis.[59] Although symptoms may be denied, signs of chronic liver disease (e.g., splenomegaly, ascites, icterus) may well be present. Mallory-Weiss

**TABLE 6–11. Differential Diagnosis: Adolescents**

| Hematemesis, Melena | Hematochezia |
|---|---|
| Esophagitis | Infectious colitis |
| Gastritis | Inflammatory bowel disease |
| Peptic ulcer disease | Anal fissures |
| Mallory-Weiss tears | Polyps |
| Esophageal varices | |
| Pill ulcers | |

tears[60] and peptic disease may manifest with hematemesis; like melena, this is rarely an isolated symptom in this population.

Rectal bleeding in this age group is most commonly caused by colitis. Infectious colitis is considerably more common than colitis caused by Crohn's disease or ulcerative colitis. Typically, infectious colitides are of shorter duration and are associated with signs of acute illness such as fever.[61] Ulcerative colitis and infectious colitides may be extremely difficult to distinguish from one another, particularly early in the course of ulcerative colitis. Often, signs of chronicity on biopsy are required to distinguish chronic idiopathic inflammatory bowel disease from infectious colitis. Crohn's disease, when it involves only the colon, may manifest in a similar fashion. The more common ileocolonic form of Crohn's disease is more insidious, with weight loss, cramping, and diarrhea preceding the onset of bleeding.

Polyps can occur in the adolescent. Juvenile polyps are uncommon after puberty. Therefore, a more aggressive approach of surveillance is required than in younger children, particularly if a family history of early colon cancer or polyposis is present.[62]

## REFERENCES


1. Helfand M, Marton KI, Zimmer-Gembeck MJ, Sox HC Jr: History of visible rectal bleeding in a primary care population: initial assessment and a 10-year follow-up. JAMA 1997;277:44–48.
2. Kollef MH, Canfield DA, Zuckerman GR: Triage considerations for patients with acute gastrointestinal hemorrhage admitted to a medical intensive care unit. Crit Care Med 1995;23:1048–1054.
3. Bitton A, Peppercorn MA: Emergencies in inflammatory bowel disease. Crit Care Clin 1995;11:513–529.
4. Knoben JE: Drug-induced discoloration of feces and urine. In Anderson PO, Knoben JE, Troutman WG, Davis LJ (eds): Handbook of Clinical Drug Data 1997–1998, 8th ed. Stamford, CT, Appleton & Lange, 1997, pp 734–736.
5. Anonymous: Fecal discoloration induced by drugs, chemicals and disease states. In DRUGDEX [database online], Vol 93, Denver, CO, Rocky Mountain Drug Consultation Center, July 1997. Available from: Drug consults, Micromedix.
6. Anonymous: Causes of urine discoloration. In DRUGDEX [database online], Vol 93, Denver, CO, Rocky Mountain Drug Consultation Center, July 1997. Available from: Drug consults, Micromedix.
7. Tunget CL, Clark RF, Manoguerra AS, Turchen SG: Iron overdose and detection of gastrointestinal bleeding with the hemoccult and gastroccult assays. Ann Emerg Med 1995;26:54–57.
8. Cuellar RE, Gavaler JS, Alexander JA, et al: Gastrointestinal tract hemorrhage: the value of a nasogastric aspirate. Arch Intern Med 1990;150:1381–1384.
9. Teach SJ, Fleisher GR: Rectal Bleeding in the pediatric emergency department. Ann Emerg Med 1994;23:1252–1258.
10. Mortensen PB, Nohr M, Moller-Petersen JF, Balslev I: The diagnostic value of serum urea/creatinine ratio in distinguishing between upper and lower gastrointestinal bleeding: a prospective study. Dan Med Bull 1994;41:237–240.
11. Treem WR: Gastrointestinal bleeding in children. Gastrointest Endosc Clin North Am 1994;4:75–97.
12. Wolf M, Roth Y, Leventon G: Epistaxis mimicking upper gastrointestinal bleeding. J Fam Pract 1990;30:95–97.
13. Pianosi P, Al-Sadoon H: Hemoptysis in children. Pediatr Rev 1996;17:344–348.
14. Ackert JJ, Sherman A, Lustbader IJ, McCauley DI: Spontaneous intramural hematoma of the esophagus. Am J Gastroenterol 1989;84:1325–1328.
15. Richter JM, Christensen MR, Kaplan LM, Nishioka NS: Effectiveness of current technology in the diagnosis and management of lower gastrointestinal hemorrhage. Gastrointest Endosc 1995;41:93–98.
16. Emslie JT, Zarnegar K, Siegel ME, Beart RW Jr: Technetium-99m-labeled red blood cell scans in the investigation of gastrointestinal bleeding. Dis Colon Rectum 1996;39:750–754.
17. Miller JH: The role of radionuclide-labeled cells in the diagnosis of abdominal disease in children. Semin Nucl Med 1993;23:219–230.
18. Sharma VS, Valji K, Bookstein JJ: Gastrointestinal hemorrhage in AIDS: arteriographic diagnosis and transcatheter treatment. Radiology 1992;185:447–451.
19. American Society for Gastrointestinal Endoscopy Position statement. Maintaining competency in endoscopic skills. Gastrointest Endosc 1995;42:620–621.
20. Hassall E: Requirements for training to ensure competence of endoscopists performing invasive procedures in children. J Pediatr Gastroenterol Nutr 1997;24:345–347.
21. Korkis AM, McCougall CJ: Rectal bleeding in patients less than 50 years of age. Dig Dis Sci 1995;40:1520–1523.
22. Cote CJ: NPO after midnight for children: a reappraisal. Anesthesiology 1990;72:589–592.
23. Ingebo KR, Rayhorn NJ, Hecht RM, et al: Sedation in children: adequacy of two-hour fasting. J Pediatr 1997;131:155–158.
24. Freeman ML: Training endoscopists to recognize the stigmata of hemorrhage in bleeding ulcers. Endoscopy 1995;27:90–92.
25. Willie R, Kay MH: Therapeutic intervention for nonvariceal gastrointestinal hemorrhage. J Pediatr Gastroenterol Nutr 1996;22:123–133.
26. Mestre JR: The changing pattern of juvenile polyps. Am J Gastroenterol 1986;81:312–314.
27. Deutsch DE, Olson AD: Colonoscopy or sigmoidoscopy as the initial evaluation of pediatric patients with colitis: a survey of physician behavior and a cost analysis. J Pediatr Gastroenterol Nutr 1997;25:26–31.
28. Vakil N, Huilgol V, Kahn I: Effect of push enteroscopy on transfusion requirements and quality of life in patients with unexplained gastrointestinal bleeding. Am J Gastroenterol 1997;92:425–428.
29. Scott-Conner CE, Subramony C: Localization of small intestinal bleeding: the role of intraoperative endoscopy. Surg Endosc 1994;8:915–917.
30. Tobin JR, Wetzel RC: Shock and multi-organ system failure. In Rogers MC (ed): Textbook of Pediatric Intensive Care. Baltimore, Williams & Wilkins, 1996, pp 555–605.
31. Andrus CH: The effect of irrigant temperature in upper gastrointestinal hemorrhage: a requiem for iced saline lavage. Am J Gastroenterol 1987;82:1062–1064.
32. Baxter JN, Jenkins SA: Somatostatin: an alternative to sclerotherapy? Scand J Gastroenterol 1994;207(suppl):17–22.
33. Chan LY, Sung JJY: The role of pharmaco-therapy for acute variceal haemorrhage in the era of endoscopic haemostasis. Aliment Pharmacol Ther 1997;11:45–50.
34. Steffes CP, Sugawa C: Endoscopic management of nonvariceal gastrointestinal bleeding. World J Surg 1992;16:1025–1033.
35. Sanowski RA: Thermal application for gastrointestinal bleeding. J Clin Gastroenterol 1986;8:239–244.
36. Gupta PK, Fleisher DE: Nonvariceal upper gastrointestinal bleeding. Med Clin North Am 1993;77:973–992.
37. Hunt PS, Korman MG, Hansky J, Parkin WG: An 8-year prospective experience with balloon tamponade in emergency control of bleeding esophageal varices. Dig Dis Sci 1982;27:413–416.
38. Llach J, Bordas JM, Salmeron JM, et al: A prospective randomized trial of heater probe thermocoagulation versus injection therapy in peptic ulcer hemorrhage. Gastrointest Endosc 1996;43:117–120.
39. Hassal E: Sclerotherapy for extrahepatic portal hypertension in childhood. J Pediatr 1989;115:69–74.
40. Price MR, Sartorelli KH, Karrer FM, et al: Management of esophageal varices in children by endoscopic variceal ligation. J Pediatr Surg 1996;31:1056–1059.
41. Apt L, Downey W: Melena neonatorum: the swallowed blood syndrome. A simple test for the differentiation of adult and fetal hemoglobin in bloody stools. J Pediatr 1955;47:6–12.
42. Guritzky RP, Rudnitsky G: Bloody neonatal diaper. Ann Emerg Med 1996;27:662–664.
43. Machida HM: Allergic colitis in infancy: clinical and pathologic aspects. J Pediatr Gastroenterol Nutr 1994;19:22–26.
44. Grosfeld JL, Molinari F, Chaet M, et al: Gastrointestinal perforation and peritonitis in infants and children: experience with 179 cases over ten years. Surgery 1996;120:650–655.
45. Liebman WM, Thaler MM, Bujanover Y: Endoscopic evaluation of upper gastrointestinal bleeding in the newborn. Am J Gastroenterol 1978;69:607–608.

46. Hathaway WE: The bleeding newborn. Semin Hematol 1975;12:175–188.
47. Gill FM: Congenital bleeding disorders: hemophilia and von Willebrand's disease. Med Clin North Am 1984;68:601–615.
48. Sheretz RJ, Sarubbi FA: The prevalence of *Clostridium difficile* and toxin in a nursery population: a comparison between patients with necrotizing enterocolitis and an asymptomatic group. J Pediatr 1982;100:435–439.
49. Heine RG, Jaquiery A, Lubitz L, et al: Role of gastro-oesophageal reflux in infant irritability. Arch Dis Child 1995;73:121–125.
50. Silber G: Lower gastrointestinal bleeding. Pediatr Rev 1990;12:85–93.
51. StVil D, Brandt ML, Panic S, et al: Meckel's diverticulum in children: a 20-year review. J Pediatr Surg 1991;26:1289–1292.
52. Lacroix J, Nadeau D, Laberge S, et al: Frequency of upper gastrointestinal bleeding in a pediatric intensive care unit. Crit Care Med 1992;20:35–42.
53. Cochran EB, Phelps SJ, Tolley EA, Stidham GL: Prevalence of, and risk factors for, upper gastrointestinal tract bleeding in critically ill pediatric patients. Crit Care Med 1992;20:1519–1523.
54. Euler A, Siebert J: The role of sigmoidoscopy, radiographs, and colonoscopy in the diagnostic evaluation of pediatric age patients with suspected juvenile polyps. J Pediatr Surg 1981;16:500–502.
55. Ng WT, Wong MK, Kong CK, Yuen WF: Lymphoid nodular hyperplasia: an unusual finding at laparoscopic surgery for a suspected bleeding Meckel's diverticulum. Gastrointest Endosc 1993;39:833–836.
56. Causey AL, Woodall BN, Wahl NG, et al: Henoch-Schonlein purpura: four cases and a review. J Emerg Med 1994;12:331–341.
57. Griffin P, Olmstead L, Petras R: *Escherichia coli* 0157:H7-associated colitis: a clinical and histological study of 11 cases. Gastroenterology 1990;99:142–149.
58. LiVoti G, Acierno C, Tulone V, Cataliotti F: Relationship between upper gastrointestinal bleeding and non-steroidal anti-inflammatory drugs in children. Pediatr Surg Int 1997;12:264–265.
59. Ando H, Kaneko K, Ito F, et al: Anatomy and etiology of extrahepatic portal vein obstruction in children leading to bleeding esophageal varices. J Am Coll Surg 1996;183:643–647.
60. Paquet KJ, Mercado-Diaz M, Kalk JF: Frequency, significance and therapy of the Mallory-Weiss syndrome in patients with portal hypertension. Hepatology 1990;11:879–883.
61. Schumacher G, Sandstedt B, Mollby R, Kollberg B: Clinical and histologic features differentiating non-relapsing colitis from first attacks of inflammatory bowel disease. Scand J Gastroenterol 1991;26:151–161.
62. Mougenot J, Baldassarre M, Mashako L, et al: Rectocolic polyps in the child: analysis of 183 cases. Arch Fr Pediatr 1989;46:245–248.

# Chapter 7

# Eating Disorders and Obesity

Dean L. Antonson and James K. Madison

## ANOREXIA NERVOSA

### Historical Perspective

The first clinical description of anorexia nervosa in the medical literature was published by Richard Morton, physician to James II, in his textbook of medicine in 1689.[1] Significant time then elapsed before further descriptions of anorexia nervosa were noted in the literature, with Robert Whytt reporting a case in 1767 and Dr. Louis-Victor Marce of Paris reporting his observations in 1859.[2] In 1914, Simmonds described a case of cachexia associated with pituitary infarction and suggested that the common cause for anorexia nervosa may well be pituitary insufficiency.[3] However, in 1949 Sheehan clearly established that pituitary insufficiency was rare, concluding that the majority of patients with anorexia nervosa did not have this dysfunction.[4] It was not until the 20th century that significant advancements in the understanding of anorexia nervosa occurred. More recent contributions have been added by the extensive work of Gerald Russell, who also was the first to describe and define bulimia nervosa.[5]

### Epidemiology

Five well-controlled, multinational studies have examined the incidence of anorexia nervosa over sequential decades in a single population.[5] In Sweden, the incidence increased from 0.08 to 0.45 per 100,000 population from 1940 to 1960; in Monroe County, New York, it increased from 0.37 to 0.64 per 100,000 population from 1960 to 1976; and in Rochester, Minnesota, it increased from 4.63 to 14.2 per 100,000 population from 1950 to 1984.[5] Several investigators have normalized these rates to look at the specific at-risk population of young women between 15 and 25 years of age. They reported incidences ranging from 30 to as high as 156 per 100,000 population, making anorexia nervosa the third most common illness in female adolescents and young adults, after obesity and asthma.[6] Because patients with eating disorders are often very secretive about their behaviors and significant underreporting can be anticipated, the higher incidence rate may be more accurate. Several additional surveys indicate that anorexia nervosa may occur in as many as 1% to 5% of high school and college-age women.[7, 8] The incidence for males with anorexia nervosa is 5% to 10% of that for females.

The most commonly quoted prevalence rates for anorexia nervosa are between 0.5% and 1%, including the rates identified by the American Psychiatric Association in 1994.[9] A 1996 study from Sweden determined the prevalence rates for 15-year-olds to be 0.84% for girls and 0.09% for boys.[6]

Individuals who are significantly involved in abnormal eating behaviors and are undergoing significant weight loss, yet who fail to meet all the criteria for anorexia nervosa, are considered to have a partial syndrome. Prevalence rates for the partial syndrome have been calculated to be between 5% and 10% for young women aged 16 to 25 years.[6, 10]

More common is the pervasive presence of dieting behaviors in Western societies and the simultaneous presence of a distorted body image. A survey from Canada found that, by the age of 18 years, 50% of adolescent girls perceived themselves as being too fat, even though 80% of this group had normal body weights. Eighty percent of this same female population desired to lose weight.[11] In a similar U.S. study, one half of all underweight female adolescents desired to lose weight, and 80% claimed that they were unhappy with their present weights.[11] In a study from the Centers for Disease Control and Prevention, 44% of all adolescent girls were involved with dieting, whereas only 15% of boys were similarly concerned.[9] Forty percent of the adolescent girls felt very negatively about their body image, with their greatest displeasure being focused on their hips, waist, and thighs.[9]

Although most early reports described anorexia nervosa as occurring primarily in white, middle- to upper-class females, more recent studies have demonstrated that anorexia nervosa is present at all socioeconomic levels and is seen in minority as well as white populations.[6, 10, 12] Anorexia nervosa is especially prominent in appearance-related sports and occupations such as acting, modeling, ballet dancing, and gymnastics. Interestingly, there also appears to be a high risk among graduate students studying nutrition.[13] Additional factors that place adolescent girls at risk for anorexia nervosa include the onset of dieting behavior, the presence of a physical illness that results in weight loss, and the presence of characteristic personality factors such as low self-esteem, obsessive-compulsive personality traits, body image distortion, and body image dissatisfaction.[6] Genetic factors are also important, with numerous studies documenting an increased incidence of anorexia among first-degree relatives of patients with the disorder.[6] There is also a higher incidence of anorexia nervosa in urban as opposed to rural areas.[14]

## Clinical Presentation and Development

Anorexia nervosa generally begins with an attempt to diet, primarily because of a perception of being fat and overweight. The majority of individuals developing anorexia nervosa are at a normal weight when dieting begins, generally set a moderate goal of weight loss of approximately 10 to 15 pounds, and initially simply reduce overall calorie intake. Often, many rituals develop with food, such as eating the same specific food for months at a time, eating food prepared in an identical manner each day, or eating foods in a specified sequence. To further enhance their weight loss, most of these individuals also significantly increase their exercise activity. The initial moderate effort to diet then evolves into a marked preoccupation with food, calorie restriction, pursuit of thinness, and body image distortion.

Typically, patients develop an intense fear of fat, often limiting their fat intake to less than 5 to 10 g/day. There is a marked distortion of body image, with perception of being overweight despite emaciation. The ability to sense hunger and satiety is ablated. Weight loss continues to progress, with the combination of severe caloric restriction and increased exercise activity leading to a progressive weight loss and the development of anorexia nervosa.

## Etiology

The etiology and pathogenesis of anorexia nervosa are unknown. All current theories agree that the onset, development, and progression of anorexia nervosa represent a multifactorial process.[11] There are familial, developmental, social, cultural, physiologic, and genetic factors that combine to predispose the susceptible female patient to the development of this disorder. As described by Garner and Garfinkel,[15] for anorexia nervosa to develop, a succession of factors must be involved: predisposing factors (individual, familial, and sociocultural), precipitating factors (stressors, diet, illness, and weight loss), and perpetuating factors (cognitive reinforcement and effects of starvation). Predisposing individual factors include cognitive deficits in ego development, misperception of external stimuli, psychic instability, anxiety, and insecurity during adolescence.[16] Predisposing familial factors include family patterns of enmeshment, rigidity, overprotectiveness, lack of conflict resolution, and perhaps inattentive nurturing in infancy. Sociocultural values placed on thinness play a prominent role. The significant biologic effects of starvation also play an important role in the progression of the disorder. Precipitating factors include low self-esteem and the omnipresent stresses of adolescent life, with a heightened focus on criticisms and negative self-perceptions. Perpetuating factors include the early cognitive reinforcement and praise that uniformly accompany initial weight loss and the physiologic effects of progressive starvation. Recent investigations have proposed that changing levels of neurotransmitters and polypeptides within the central nervous system are involved in the perpetuation of anorexia nervosa.[17–19] Both serotonergic and adrenergic activities are reduced in patients with anorexia nervosa, and levels do not fully return to normal even after full weight recovery has been achieved, at least not in the early follow-up periods.[17, 18]

Several theories have been proposed that combine these factors and events to explain the development and progression of anorexia nervosa.[11] Conflicts, stresses, and failure result in low self-esteem and dissatisfaction, and the perfectionistic tendencies of these individuals then funnel the need to control some aspect of life toward dieting and weight loss (thinness being equated with success). A spiral of weight loss, fear of weight gain, intensified dieting, body image dissatisfaction, and the effects of starvation then leads to uncontrolled progressive weight loss and an increasing feeling of success and control.

## Clinical and Laboratory Features

The rather typical appearance of marked starvation and cachexia, along with noted muscle wasting, marked decrease in subcutaneous tissue stores, and prepubescent body habitus, is easily identified. Vital signs frequently demonstrate hypothermia, bradycardia, and hypotension. Body temperatures are often 1° to 2°F below normal, the resting pulse may be as low as 40 beats/min, and blood pressure may be reduced to as low as 90/60 mm Hg. Moderate to marked acrocyanosis and peripheral edema are frequently seen. Skin and hair changes occur, including dry, pale, atrophic skin, a yellow discoloration to the skin secondary to carotenemia, thinning of the scalp hair, and the development of lanugo hair, particularly over the face, upper arms, and back. Deep tendon reflexes are decreased on neurologic examination. Despite the cachectic appearance, individuals with anorexia nervosa often appear energetic, only rarely being described as lethargic. Lethargy occurring in a patient with anorexia nervosa is worrisome and may be the harbinger of early organ failure.

Despite the profound starvation and emaciation, serum laboratory values generally remain normal. Most patients have normal serum electrolyte and chemistry profiles, which rarely reflect the level of starvation. When present, the most common electrolyte abnormalities are hypokalemia, hyponatremia, and mild metabolic alkalosis. A summary of chemical, hematologic, endocrinologic, and immunologic abnormalities is shown in Table 7–1.

It is uncommon for patients with anorexia nervosa to present to the physician complaining of the physical changes that occur with starvation. Rather, they are likely to complain of menstrual irregularity, depression, lethargy, or repeated sports injury. Additionally, complaints may include weakness, palpitations, intermittent chest pain, abdominal pain, or frequent headaches.

An extensive array of clinical complications results from

**TABLE 7–1. Medical Complications of Anorexia Nervosa**

| | |
|---|---|
| **Central Nervous System** | |
| Widened sulci | Decreased libido |
| Enlarged ventricles | Decreased concentration |
| Decreased pituitary size | Decreased short-term memory |
| Altered serotonergic pathways | Decreased visuospatial analysis |
| Reduced nonadrenergic activity | Decreased learning |
| Psychomotor retardation | Decreased problem-solving |
| Depression | Decreased perception |
| Labile mood | Decreased attention (focusing/ execution) |
| Sleep disorders | |
| **Dermatologic** | |
| Lanugo hair | Thin scalp hair |
| Carotenemia | Pruritus |
| Brittle nails | Pale skin |
| Acrocyanosis | Dry skin |
| **Musculoskeletal** | |
| Decreased muscle mass, weakness | Proximal myopathy |
| | Osteopenia |
| Collagen loss | Pathologic fractures |
| **Pulmonary** | |
| Aspiration pneumonia | Pneumomediastinum |
| Ventilatory failure | |
| **Gastrointestinal** | |
| Gastroparesis, early satiety | Pancreatitis |
| Constipation | Esophagitis, esophageal tears |
| Abdominal pain | Peptic ulcers |
| Decreased motility | Hepatitis |
| Superior mesenteric artery syndrome | Malabsorption |
| | Reduced taste |
| Postprandial fullness, bloating | |
| **Hematologic** | |
| Leukopenia | Anemia |
| Decreased erythrocyte sedimentation rate | Thrombocytopenia |
| Leukemia | |
| **Cardiovascular** | |
| Arrhythmias | Sudden death |
| Bradycardia | Electrocardiographic changes |
| Hypotension | Decreased QRS amplitude |
| Mitral valve prolapse | Changes in ST/T waves |
| Left ventricular dysfunction | Prolonged PR interval |
| Refeeding myocardiopathy | Junctional rhythm |
| **Fluid and Electrolyte** | |
| Dehydration | Metabolic acidosis |
| Hypokalemia | Hypomagnesemia |
| Hyponatremia | Rebound edema |
| Hypochloremia | Hypophosphatemia |
| Metabolic alkalosis | |
| **Metabolic** | |
| Hypercholesterolemia | Hypoproteinemia |
| Decreased metabolic rate | Decreased zinc levels |
| Increased $\beta$-hydroxybutyric fatty acids | Impaired temperature regulation |
| **Endocrine** | |
| Amenorrhea | Diabetes insipidus |
| Sick euthyroid state | Decreased luteinizing hormone |
| Insensitivity to cold, hypothermia | Decreased follicle-stimulating hormone |
| Increased cortisol levels | |
| Osteopenia | Decreased luteinizing hormone–releasing hormone release |
| Hypothalamic-pituitary-adrenal dysfunction | |
| Hypoglycemia | Increased growth hormone |
| Decreased insulin production | Multifollicular ovaries |
| | Impaired release of vasopressin |
| | Decreased reproductive function |
| **Immunologic** | |
| Decreased cell-mediated immunity | Reduced serum complement |
| Reduced CD4- and CD8-positive cells | Decreased cytokines ($\alpha$-interferon, interleukin-2) |
| Decreased bactericidal capacity of granulocytes | Increased interleukin-6 and transforming growth factor-$\beta$ |
| Reduced granulocyte adherence | |
| **Renal** | |
| Prerenal azotemia | Mesangial sclerosis |
| Impaired renal concentration | Stones |

anorexia nervosa (see Table 7–1). By and large, all of these changes are attributable to progressive starvation and emaciation. During starvation, organ mass decreases at a rate slightly faster than that of skeletal muscle mass. As can be inferred by the relatively normal serum laboratory values in these patients, organ function, although decreasing, remains relatively preserved, with organ failure occurring only as a terminal event.

After suicide, the most common cause of death in patients with anorexia nervosa results from cardiac arrhythmias.[11, 20, 21] It is uncertain whether these effects are caused primarily by the inherent nutritional deficits induced within the conduction fibers themselves or by the loss of supporting tissue separating the conduction fibers, which have been catabolized to provide protein and energy in the face of starvation. Woodside[11] stated that arrhythmias occurring in the face of profound bradycardia are most worrisome and carry a significant risk for tachyarrhythmias and sudden death. Additionally, significant prolongation of the QT interval has been stated to be an ominous sign, predicting a significant risk for sudden death.[21] Equally worrisome are the profound cardiotoxic effects seen when syrup of ipecac has been used as a means of purging by the anorexic.

There are both acute and long-term consequences of starvation on bone mineralization and development. Malnutrition results in poor bone growth and reduced bone turnover.[21] Delayed puberty often leads to decreased bone density[21] and osteoporosis, resulting in an increased rate of fractures. Severe malnutrition and osteoporosis in early adolescence may lead to a stunting of linear growth, particularly when it occurs in association with primary amenorrhea.[22] Studies in older adolescents and young adults suggest that the osteoporosis is reversible.[10, 21]

Menstruation and reproductive function are significantly affected by anorexia nervosa. Impaired gonadal hormonal secretion is decreased by the effects of starvation on the hypothalamic-pituitary axis, with lowered levels of follicle-stimulating hormone and luteinizing hormone resembling those seen in prepubertal girls. Additional changes include loss of positive feedback to estrogen and multifollicular changes within the ovaries.[21] Ten percent of a large sample of women who had anorexia nervosa demonstrated infertility problems.[21] In addition, the rate of infant prematurity was increased by twofold, and perinatal mortality was increased by sixfold.[21]

Structural changes within the brain are commonly seen in patients with anorexia nervosa and again are thought to be secondary to the profound effects of starvation.[23] Computed tomography and magnetic resonance imaging scans of the brain have demonstrated widening of the sulci and an increase in ventricular size.[23] The known psychological changes that occur with starvation include a decrease in the ability to concentrate, a decrease in short-term memory, depression, a decrease in learning, a decrease in problem solving, a decrease in perception, and a decrease in attention, particularly focusing and execution.[21]

The two most common gastrointestinal problems that occur with starvation are a decrease in gastrointestinal motility and constipation. Constipation is present in most patients with anorexia nervosa. Although difficulties associated with gastroparesis generally self-resolve in 3 to 4 weeks with improved nutrition, the use of cisapride for 1 to 2 months is often quite helpful in diminishing the symptoms of bloating and postprandial fullness. Metabolic alkalosis, which is the most prominent electrolyte abnormality in anorexia nervosa, may be seen in up to 25% of patients, particularly in those who are vomiting or using laxatives.[21]

## Diagnostic Criteria

Presented in Table 7–2 are the revised diagnostic criteria for anorexia nervosa as listed in the *Diagnostic and Statistical Manual of Mental Disorders,* fourth edition (DSM-4).[24] These criteria were revised in an attempt to resolve the difficulties occurring in earlier editions of this manual, which did not adequately define and separate those patients who have features of both anorexia and bulimia. There are now two subcategories for anorexia nervosa: the restricting type, in which binge-eating or purging behavior does not occur, and the binge-eating/purging type, in which it does.

**TABLE 7–2. Diagnostic Criteria for Anorexia Nervosa**

1. Refusal to maintain body weight over a minimally normal weight for age and height (e.g., weight loss leading to a maintenance of body weight <85% of that expected; or failure to make expected weight gain during period of growth leading to body weight <85% of that expected).
2. Intense fear of gaining weight or becoming fat, even though underweight.
3. Disturbance in the way in which body weight or shape is experienced, undue influence of body weight or shape on self-evaluation, or denial of the seriousness of the current low body weight.
4. In postmenarcheal females, amenorrhea (i.e., the absence of at least three consecutive menstrual cycles). (A woman is considered to have amenorrhea if her periods occur only after administration of hormone, such as estrogen).

**Restricting type:** During the current episode of anorexia nervosa, the person has not regularly engaged in binge eating or purging behavior (i.e., self-induced vomiting or the misuse of laxatives, diuretics, or enemas).

**Binge-Eating/Purging type:** During the current episode of anorexia nervosa, the person has regularly engaged in binge eating or purging behavior (i.e., self-induced vomiting or the misuse of laxatives, diuretics, or enemas).

Adapted from American Psychiatric Association: Diagnostic and Statistical Manual of Mental Disorders, 4th ed. Washington, DC, American Psychiatric Association, 1994. 

## Treatment

Because of the complexity and interweaving of the psychological, nutritional, and medical problems present in anorexia nervosa, treatment must be structured to incorporate all three of these areas. The most urgent aspect of the early rehabilitation period is reversal of the significant starvation that is present. The goal of reestablishing feeding is achieved by initiating a calorie intake of approximately 200 to 250 calories above the intake level at the time of presentation. The caloric intake is then sequentially increased by 250 to 300 calories every 4 to 5 days to achieve a steady weight gain of approximately 1.5 kg/wk for the hospitalized patient, or 0.75 to 1.0 kg/wk for the outpatient. Meals need to be supervised closely and supplemented with liquid enteral products for food items not consumed. A slow, steady weight gain to 100% of ideal body weight for patients younger than 16 years of age, or to 90% to 100% of ideal body weight for older patients, is set as the goal.

In supervising nutritional intake and weight gain, the nutritionist plays an integral role in addressing and resolving the patient's unusual thoughts concerning food, eliminating food rituals and food fears, and removing misconceptions about food and calories. The nutritionist also is a key resource in addressing issues of body image distortion and body dissatisfaction. As the recovery process progresses, further nutritional advice is necessary, particularly with condensing calories, because individuals recovering from starvation often require up to 4,000 or 5,000 calories/day to maintain weight gain. This occurs as a result of alterations in the metabolic rate. During the early refeeding period, as the metabolic rate changes, significant calories are expended as heat, resulting in the need for progressively higher calorie intakes. As the metabolic rate readjusts, caloric intake requirements slowly return toward normal over a period of 4 to 6 months.

Medical treatment focuses primarily on nutritional rehabilitation in conjunction with the dietitian. In the first several days of treatment, any electrolyte abnormalities that have been noted need to be corrected. Hypoglycemia is particularly common in patients with anorexia who are purging by vomiting or using laxatives. Potassium supplementation may be required if potassium levels are below 3 mEq/L. Constipation is managed with the use of psyllium and the occasional use of milk of magnesia. Stimulant cathartics should be avoided. Most of the changes associated with starvation self-correct with slow refeeding. Hospitalization may be required if the patient presents initially at or below 70% to 75% of ideal body weight, with signs of hemodynamic compromise, significant electrocardiographic (ECG) abnormalities, dehydration, electrolyte abnormalities, profound weakness, mental confusion, or failure to progress with intensive outpatient management. Because of earlier recognition, only rarely is enteral tube feeding or hyperalimentation necessary. Caution and surveillance in the early refeeding phase are prudent. The psychotherapeutic and pharmacotherapeutic approach to treatment for both anorexia nervosa and bulimia nervosa is discussed later in this chapter.

## Prognosis: Morbidity and Mortality

The morbidity and mortality from anorexia nervosa remain significant. As this disorder was increasing in frequency since the 1970s, mortality rates were generally reported in the 5% to 10% range. More recent studies have demonstrated that, although early mortality remains at about 5%, late mortality may be as high as 13% to 20%.[11] Suicide remains the primary cause of death, followed by cardiac arrhythmias, infections, gastrointestinal complications, and emaciation.[21] Morbidity rates are estimated to be 25%, with morbidity reflecting the multi-organ system dysfunctions associated with starvation.[14] The most common problems are osteoporosis, renal insufficiency, and infections.[21]

Numerous studies are now also appearing to better define the long-term prognosis for patients with anorexia nervosa. Rates for full recovery are widely variable, ranging from 32% to 71% after 20 years.[11] A 5-year outcome study demonstrated 68% of patients to be well, with 10% persisting in having problems with anorexia nervosa, 4% with anorexia nervosa and bulimia nervosa, 14% with partial anorexia, and 4% with partial bulimia.[11] Comorbidity with other psychiatric disorders continues to be recognized. Follow-up studies of adolescents have demonstrated that 30% continue to have problems with affective disorders and 43% with anxiety disorders.[11]

## BULIMIA NERVOSA

### Historical Perspective

The first clinical description of bulimia nervosa was provided by Gerald Russell in 1979.[25] The condition was further defined when it was included in the DSM-3 in 1980. The term *bulimia,* however, was first used by Trevisa in 1398 to mean an immoderate appetite.[26] Slowly, the term *bulimia* gradually came to be associated with gluttonous overeating and induced vomiting, and this condition was included as a disorder by Janet in his classic work on neuroses in 1903.[26, 27] The psychiatric disorder of bulimia nervosa, however, should be distinguished from the gluttony and induced vomiting (bulimia) of these early reports. Bulimia nervosa has been a recognized clinical disorder only since 1979, when it was given that title by Russell.[25]

### Epidemiology

Like anorexia nervosa, bulimia nervosa is a disorder that occurs primarily in adolescent or young adult women. The male-to-female ratio is between 1:10 and 1:20, similar to that for anorexia nervosa. The overall incidence of bulimia nervosa is significantly higher than that of anorexia nervosa—between 3% to 10% for high school and college-age women, with some series reporting incidences as high as 20%.[28, 29] The lifetime risk rates for bulimia nervosa were calculated by Fombonne to be 1.9% for women and 0.2% for men.[30] Fifty percent of patients develop bulimia nervosa before the age of 18 years.[11]

Prevalence rates for bulimia nervosa range from 3% to 10% in most studies.[9, 11, 28] The American Psychiatric Association places the prevalence of bulimia nervosa at 1% to 3% of the general population.[9]

The incidence of the partial syndrome of bulimia nervosa, in which the patient manifests many but not all of the symptoms of bulimia, is further increased, with many studies reporting that 17% to 19% of college-age women engage in bulimic behaviors.[20, 31]

### Development and Clinical Presentation

Bulimia nervosa generally begins with initiation of a diet by a teenager or young adult, again in reaction to the perception of being fat and overweight. After a relatively short period, dieting is deemed unsuccessful and too difficult to maintain. A means of short-circuiting the process to achieve a more rapid weight loss is then sought. The patient experiments with various means of purging, such as vomiting, use of diuretics, or use of laxatives to eliminate the calories ingested. The loss of calories resulting from the purging behavior (or from restricted caloric intake after a binge) produces increasing hunger. The patient developing bulimia is unable to control her desire for food and initiates a binge-eating episode. The average intake of a binge episode has been estimated to be 4,000 calories.[11] Severe guilt, resulting from the consumption of large amounts of food and superimposed on an impulsive behavioral pattern with poor self-control, culminates in an intense desire to eliminate the food, and purging then recurs. An initial sense of relief often follows the purging episode, and some patients with bulimia transfer this feeling to situations of stress. Purging may then become a mechanism of stress relief as well. While this process is developing, the bulimic individual remains very secretive about her behaviors, often concealing them from friends and family for years. Unlike the patient with anorexia nervosa, the bulimic patient ultimately perceives her difficulties as problematic and often seeks help or assistance, particularly when the disorder progresses to the point that most of her daily thoughts and actions are controlled by this process.

Early in the process, bulimic individuals may seek medical attention, but not because of the difficulties or guilt associated with bingeing and purging. Rather, they present with requests for information on weight loss and dieting or requests for diuretics and treatment of fluid retention.

### Etiology

The pathogenesis of bulimia nervosa, like that of anorexia nervosa, is multifactorial and encompasses familial, developmental, social, cultural, physiologic, and genetic factors. Familial factors are supported by the strong association of bulimia with affective disorders (depression and dysthymia) and a strong family history of affective disorders in first-degree relatives. Depression has been reported to be present in as many as 50% of first-degree family members of bulimics.[32] Additionally, alcoholism and drug addiction are prevalent, alcoholism being reported in 50% to 60% of first- and second-degree family members.[33] Common behavioral patterns within families include high levels of family conflict, unstructured and ambivalent lines of authority, high achievement orientation, and low expressivity.[34] Affective instability and low self-esteem are the hallmark personality features of bulimia nervosa.[34] Marked ineffectiveness, significant self-criticism, learned helplessness, and a high achievement orientation all are significant predisposing factors. Significant body dissatisfaction, body image distortion, and difficulties with sexual identification are also present. Studies have shown that the incidence of sexual abuse in bulimia nervosa is no higher than that seen in adolescents presenting with other psychiatric disorders.[35]

Dieting in the bulimic individual rarely progresses to the point of fully disrupting hunger and satiety. The poorly self-controlled, impulsive individual developing bulimia cannot override the strong urge of hunger, loses control, and binges on food. The subsequent sense of loss of control resulting from this behavior further intensifies the desire to diet. When rapid results are not achieved by dieting, a means to short-circuit the process by purging is sought. Although initially this is followed by relief, the bulimic individual begins to loathe once again the loss of self-control resulting from the purging and attempts to intensify dieting, thereby establishing a positive reinforcing loop that results in repetitive cycles of bingeing and purging.

## Clinical and Laboratory Features of Bulimia Nervosa

Most bulimic individuals are of normal weight, and their behavior remains quite secretive until their difficulties with loss of control lead to their desire to confront it. Before this, however, it is not uncommon for the bulimic individual to seek medical care for one of the many associated signs or symptoms of this disorder, including fluid retention, abdominal fullness, frequent headaches, chest pain, constipation, hematemesis, and dental problems (Table 7–3). On physical examination, three distinct abnormalities may be recognized that are pathognomonic for bulimia nervosa. These are calluses or scarring over the dorsum of the hand or fingers used to induce vomiting (Russell's sign), hypertrophy of the salivary glands (sialoadenitis), and erosion of the dental enamel (perimolysis). Up to 70% of bulimics have dental caries, and an even greater percentage demonstrate perimolysis on careful examination.[36] A chronic sore throat is frequently reported, and on physical examination the posterior pharyngeal areas are erythematous. Occasionally, Mallory-Weiss tears and esophageal rupture occur with persistent and frequent vomiting. Esophageal rupture (Boerhaave's tear) continues to carry a mortality rate of 20%.[28] Although amenorrhea is uncommon, menstrual irregularities are frequently noted.[21]

On laboratory testing, the bulimic individual is often found to have electrolyte abnormalities, most commonly hypokalemia, hyponatremia, and hypochloremic alkalosis.[37] Profound electrolyte abnormalities, with potassium levels lower than 3.0 mEq/L, can occur with laxative or diuretic abuse. Chronic dehydration is frequently present as well (see Table 7–3).

## Medical Complications

Table 7–3 lists the common medical complications seen in association with bulimia nervosa. The majority of these complications are caused by the abnormal bingeing and

**TABLE 7–3. Clinical and Laboratory Complications of Bulimia Nervosa**

| | |
|---|---|
| **Gastrointestinal** | |
| Constipation | Dyspepsia |
| Cathartic colon | Barrett's esophagus |
| Esophagitis | Gastroparesis |
| Esophageal ulcer, stricture, rupture | Pancreatitis |
| Mallory-Weiss tear | Gastric rupture |
| Dysphagia | Abdominal pain |
| **Oral/Dental** | |
| Perimolysis—lingual and occlusal surfaces | Cheilosis |
| Dental caries | Sialadenosis 10–50% |
| Pharyngeal erythema/soreness | Salivary hypermylasemia |
| **Dermatologic** | |
| Russell's sign (calluses over fingers) | |
| **Cardiovascular** | |
| Arrhythmias | Ipecac toxicity |
| Hypotension | Palpitations |
| Mitral valve prolapse | |
| **Pulmonary** | |
| Aspiration pneumonia | Pneumothorax |
| Pneumomediastinum | |
| **Neurologic** | |
| Seizures (diet pill toxicity) | Increased ventricular size |
| Neuromyopathy (ipecac toxicity) | Widened sulci |
| **Renal** | |
| Failure | Proteinuria |
| Hematuria | Azotemia |
| Dehydration | |
| **Fluid and Electrolyte** | |
| Dehydration | Metabolic alkalosis |
| Hypokalemia | Metabolic acidosis |
| Hyponatremia | Pseudo-Bartter's syndrome |
| Hypochloremia | Hypomagnesemia |
| **Endocrinologic** | |
| Increased cortisol | Irregular menses |
| Hypoglycemia | Increased miscarriage rates |
| Increased birth complications | |

purging behaviors used by the patient. Gastrointestinal side effects remain the most common, including abdominal and epigastric pain, hematemesis, persistent sore throat, and constipation. Gastrointestinal and electrolyte abnormalities are frequently seen with laxative abuse and may be quite prominent. Over-the-counter laxatives containing phenolphthalein are usually used. The amount of laxatives taken varies from 3 to 4 doses per day up to 150 per day. Long-term chronic use of stimulant cathartics may ultimately result in a cathartic colon requiring extensive medical and possibly surgical management.

ECG abnormalities are again common in patients with bulimia nervosa. Particularly worrisome are the ECG abnormalities occurring in association with profound hypokalemia, which can result in arrhythmias and sudden death. Cardiac arrhythmias are the leading cause of death among patients with bulimia nervosa.[11] As with anorexia nervosa, central nervous system changes, with an increase in sulcal spaces and ventricular size, have been noted for bulimia nervosa.[21] Again, these structural changes appear to be only partially reversible after treatment of the disorder. Erosion of the dental enamel, particularly involving the lingual and occlusal surfaces, may be severe. Complete loss of teeth may occur as early as the third decade.

## Diagnostic Criteria

Table 7–4 details the revised diagnostic criteria for bulimia nervosa as listed in the DSM-4.[24] Again, two subtypes are described for bulimia nervosa to help clarify the diagnosis in those patients who have mixed features of both anorexia and bulimia nervosa. The purging type of bulimic patient uses laxatives, diuretics, enemas, or vomiting, whereas the nonpurging type uses other compensatory behaviors, such as fasting or excessive exercise.

## Treatment

If electrolyte abnormalities are severe and particularly if potassium levels are below 3.0 mEq/L, potassium supplementation may be required during the first few days of treatment. Dental consultation should be obtained for the majority of individuals who have used vomiting as a means of purging. The most troublesome medical problem is pseudo-Bartter's syndrome, which can occur after the abrupt discontinuation of diet pills or laxatives in patients who have had significant abuse of these medications.[38] Chronic laxative and diuretic abuse leads to a chronic state of dehydration, activating the renin-angiotensin-aldosterone system and resulting in hyperaldosteronism. Significant fluid retention and peripheral edema can occur within 2 to 7 days after cessation of the use of laxatives or diuretics in these patients. Diuretic therapy is frequently required for fluid mobilization, after which a slow tapering of diuretic medication can be achieved over the course of 4 to 12 weeks, while aldosterone levels slowly normalize. Potassium supplementation is frequently required during this period. Nutritional rehabilitation of the patient with bulimia nervosa focuses on stopping the purging behaviors; dispelling the myths and inaccuracies regarding food, calories, and fat; and improving the body image distortion.

**TABLE 7–4. Diagnostic Criteria for Bulimia Nervosa**

1. Recurrent episodes of binge-eating. An episode of binge-eating is characterized by both of the following: (1) eating, in a discrete period of time (e.g., within any 2-hour period), an amount of food that is definitely larger than most people would eat in a similar period of time and under similar circumstances, and (2) a sense of lack of control over eating during the episode (e.g., a feeling that one cannot stop eating or cannot control what or how much one is eating).
2. Recurrent inappropriate compensatory behavior to prevent weight gain, such as self-induced vomiting; misuse of laxatives, diuretics, enemas, or other medications; fasting; or excessive exercise.
3. These behaviors both occur, on average, at least twice a week for 3 months.
4. Self-evaluation is unduly influenced by body shape and weight.
5. The disturbance does not occur exclusively during episodes of anorexia nervosa.

**Purging type:** During the current episode of bulimia nervosa, the person has regularly engaged in self-induced vomiting or the misuse of laxatives, diuretics, or enemas.

**Nonpurging type:** During the current episode of bulimia nervosa, the person has engaged in other inappropriate compensatory behaviors, such as fasting or excessive exercise.

Adapted from American Psychiatric Association: Diagnostic and Statistical Manual of Mental Disorders, 4th ed. Washington, DC, American Psychiatric Association, 1994. Copyright 1994 American Psychiatric Association.

## Prognosis: Morbidity and Mortality

Mortality rates for bulimia nervosa within 2 to 5 years of diagnosis continue to remain at 5%.[11] Fifty percent to 60% of patients demonstrate recovery over this same period, with a relapse rate of 30% to 50%.[11] A review summarized by Woodside[11] of four follow-up studies in patients 2 years after treatment demonstrated that 20% to 25% were well, 10% to 15% had minor slips, 15% had major slips, 15% were ill most of the time, and another 20% to 25% were ill continuously. The most prominent factor resulting in failure to remain well was comorbidity with alcohol or drug use.[11]

# PSYCHOTHERAPY AND PSYCHOTROPIC MEDICATIONS FOR ANOREXIA NERVOSA AND BULIMIA NERVOSA

## Pretreatment Assessment Issues

A careful evaluation of the patient's psychological status is warranted. Goals include excluding other explanations of the eating disturbance, assessing for the presence of other psychopathology, and developing clinical hypotheses about the psychological processes that initiated and maintain the disorder. Some of the most common psychological causes for disturbed eating, aside from anorexia and bulimia and related disorders, are depression, somatoform disorders, conditioned aversion, and obsessive-compulsive disorder. These disorders can produce patterns of behavior very similar to those seen in eating disorders. All of these conditions can coexist with an eating disorder and may interact with symptoms of eating disorders in complex ways.

Failure to identify and treat concomitant psychological disorders results in poorer long-term adaptation and decreased likelihood of successful treatment for the eating disorder. Malnutrition is known to produce depressive symptoms. Because rates of depression are high among people with eating disorders (69% in a University of Nebraska clinical sample), this is a particularly important diagnostic category of which the treatment team must be aware. Rates of obsessive-compulsive disorder as high as 69% have been found in a sample of anorexia patients.[39] The differential for this disorder again becomes important in that many patients with eating disorders have obsessions and compulsions regarding food or weight. These do not justify the additional diagnosis of obsessive-compulsive disorder unless there is evidence of manifestations that are not part of the typical patterns of thought and action seen in patients with eating disorders. When both disorders are present, the treatment plan must be modified to account for this great complexity. Anxiety disorders and addictive behaviors also are highly prevalent among patients with eating disorders and warrant careful attention during the evaluation. The frequent presence of a history of sexual abuse among such patients also indicates the need for screening for post-traumatic stress disorders.

Treatment should begin with consideration of why this particular person developed an eating disorder at this particular time in her life. Issues that have been identified as common among people with eating disorders, such as perfectionism, mistrust, poor awareness of internal cues, and ineffectiveness, should be addressed. Additionally, the specific forms of eating-related thoughts and beliefs to which the patient subscribes should be identified. General patterns of behavior and attitudes toward self and others also are relevant, with particular attention to significant personality disorders, impulsivity, and deficits in self-concept. Sources of stress should be identified. Family factors such as adaptability, cohesiveness, conflict resolution, openness to expressed emotion, and emotional support are particularly relevant to treatment planning for children and adolescents.

## Hospitalization

The most fundamental decision when treating a patient with a newly diagnosed eating disorder is whether hospitalization is necessary. One factor in this decision is the body weight of the patient. Anorexic patients who are at less than 70% to 75% of their ideal body weight are typically too compromised physically and psychologically to effectively engage in outpatient care. We have found that some long-term anorexic patients who are ready to commit to treatment are stable enough to make use of partial hospital programs rather than requiring full hospitalization. Conversely, younger patients with more recent onset tend to show signs of medical instability at higher weights than do older patients with more chronic conditions. Combined with the stronger denial that is common among young patients, they become poor candidates for outpatient approaches at higher weights. Because these younger patients also have the greatest opportunity to recover from such potential long-range problems as osteoporosis, we advocate more aggressive treatment, often considering hospitalization at 80% of ideal body weight.

For patients with bulimia, medical stability is a key issue in determining hospitalization. However, a very intense symptom such as vomiting six or more times per day also leads to consideration of hospitalization. Among both anorexic and bulimic patients, failure to achieve appropriate eating patterns and weight on an outpatient basis should be regarded as grounds to move the patient to more intensive care, such as partial hospital, residential, or inpatient treatment. The presence of suicidal thoughts or serious self-injurious behavior also favors inpatient treatment, as it would for any patient. Finally, the coexistence of other significant mental health disorders (e.g., major depression, substance abuse or dependency) also indicates that outpatient care will be very difficult or not practical.

## Treatment Modalities

### *Psychopharmacology*

At this time, no psychotropic medication has been shown to effectively treat the core symptoms of anorexia. Clinically, some anorexic patients do improve with administration of an antidepressant or other medication. Unpublished observations have suggested that the use of antidepressant medications may affect the rate of relapse among anorexics, but these data remain rather preliminary at this time.

Antidepressant medications have demonstrated effectiveness with bulimia. Significant reductions in frequency of bingeing and purging and a variety of other measures of bulimic behavior have been shown with the use of imipramine,[40] desipramine,[41] and fluoxetine.[42] Goldbloom and Olmsted[43] showed that 8 weeks of treatment with a dose of 60 mg/day of fluoxetine (Prozac) was more effective than either placebo or a 20-mg dose. Agras and colleagues[44] showed that 24 weeks of treatment with desipramine was more effective than 16 weeks. Other studies have demonstrated decreasing effectiveness with single medications over time, necessitating multiple sequential medication trials.[45] The proportion of patients showing complete symptom remission tends to be lower with medication alone than when medication is combined with other treatments (see later discussion). Mitchell and coworkers noted that few studies of antidepressants show more than one third of patients in remission at the end of the medication trial.[40] Goldstein and associates reported only 19% complete symptom remission among their patients treated with Prozac.[42]

### *Family Therapy*

Minuchen and colleagues emphasized family processes of enmeshment, poor conflict resolution, and difficulty adapting to change in their seminal volume on family therapy for patients with eating disorders.[46] They were able to demonstrate the effectiveness of structural family therapy for patients with anorexia. Systemic[47] and behavioral[48] methods also have been prominent in the treatment of eating disorders. Shugar and Krueger demonstrated significant correlation between family communication of aggression and improvement in patients' symptoms using systemic interventions.[49] Their findings particularly implicate covert expression of aggression as a factor that may maintain anorexic behavior and thought patterns. VanFurth and coworkers found that maternal hostility correlated with improvement in anorexic patients during treatment.[50] Humphrey studied ratings of parent behavior and found that parents of anorexic patients tended to engage more in passive forms of hostility such as negating and ignoring their children, whereas parents of bulimics were more blaming and belittling than parents of adolescents without eating disorders.[51]

There are two major caveats regarding family therapy for patients with eating disorders. First, it is important that the family understand that the recommendation is made to help them aid in the recovery of their family member, not because the treatment team believes that the family caused the eating disorder. Second, there has been little research comparing the effectiveness of family therapy with that of other forms of intervention. Robin and colleagues did not find any significant difference in results between 16 months of ego-oriented individual psychotherapy and 16 months of behavioral family systems therapy.[48] More concerning are the results of Russell and associates comparing family therapy and individual psychotherapy for the treatment of anorexia and bulimia.[52] They found that family therapy was significantly better than individual therapy for patients with anorexia who were younger than 18 years of age and had a duration of their disorder of less than 3 years. Older patients with anorexia did significantly better with individual therapy. Patients with bulimia did not show differential effects and did not show much improvement with either therapy method.[52]

## *Cognitive Behavioral Therapy*

Cognitive behavioral therapy (CBT) seeks to alter behavioral patterns, distortions in beliefs, and dysfunctional self-perceptions that promote eating-disorder behaviors. The therapist assumes that the patient's beliefs about weight and body size trigger and maintain such behaviors. Initially, the therapist helps the patient challenge the dysfunctional beliefs by using corrective information, logic, and experiential tests that the patient conducts as a form of homework. Ultimately, the patient learns to challenge mistaken beliefs and to correct other distortions such as negative self-evaluation, black-and-white thinking, and perfectionistic attitudes. Fairburn and coworkers provided a detailed explanation of the treatment model and methods for treating bulimia.[53] Garner and Bemis described modifications applicable to anorexia, but most of the research continues to focus on bulimia.[54]

At this time, CBT has the strongest research support of any intervention for eating disorders. Fairburn demonstrated that this approach can produce success rates as high as 70% in outpatient treatment of bulimia.[55] Fairburn and colleagues monitored a group of patients who had received 18 weeks of treatment and found that almost 66% had no eating disorder after a mean follow-up period of 5.8 years.[56] Wilson and Fairburn pooled data from 19 comparable controlled trials of CBT and demonstrated an 84% reduction in purging and a 79% reduction in binge-eating.[57] The average complete abstinence rates were 48% and 62% for purging and binge-eating, respectively. Mitchell and his colleagues demonstrated similarly impressive results using group CBT. CBT was shown to be superior to either behavioral therapy or placebo.[58] Mitchell and coworkers also presented evidence that twice-weekly therapy sessions may be more effective than traditional once-weekly schedules, at least in the context of group CBT.[59]

CBT typically is superior to antidepressants alone. There seems little advantage in treating bulimic symptoms with antidepressants plus CBT rather than CBT alone.[60] Herzog and Sacks found some indications that the combined treatment is more effective in earlier phases of therapy.[61] Mitchell and associates also noted that depressive symptoms improved more with combined CBT and imipramine treatment than with CBT alone, even though symptoms of the eating disorder were equally improved with either intervention.[58] Walsh and his colleagues demonstrated some advantage in controlling binge-eating and depressive symptoms with a two-step antidepressant intervention that was used for patients who did not respond to an initial intervention with desipramine.[62]

## *Interpersonal Therapy*

Interpersonal therapy (IPT) was originally developed as a treatment for depression and has had well-documented success in that context.[63] Fairburn and coworkers included IPT as a treatment control in a study of the effectiveness of CBT.[64] The therapist helps the patient evaluate interpersonal skills, conflicts with significant people, difficulty in role transitions, and resolution of any significant loss. The emphasis is on solving interpersonal problems and patterns of relating to others rather than on changing thoughts.

Although initial assessment indicated that IPT did not affect patients' concerns about weight and preoccupation with dieting, at 12 and 24 months of follow-up patients treated with IPT could not be differentiated from those treated with CBT.[64] Even on early post-treatment assessment, overt behavioral symptoms were not significantly different between the two groups of patients, although results in both cases were superior to those in untreated controls. The care with which these studies were conducted and the clarity of the results suggest that IPT should be given serious consideration in the treatment of bulimia, even though more research must be conducted. Wilfley modified IPT for administration in a group format and reported good initial success in reducing binge-eating with this method.[65]

## *Psychodynamic Psychotherapy*

Although the American Psychiatric Association practice guidelines[66] imply that psychodynamic therapy is appropriate for treating eating disorders and may be particularly useful with patients who are refractory to other treatments, there is sparse evidence to support this viewpoint. Garner and associates demonstrated a 62% reduction in purging with the use of an 18-week psychodynamically oriented treatment.[67] CBT produced reductions of 81.9% in their study. More significant was the discrepancy in abstinence rate: 12% for the dynamically treated group compared with 36% for those treated with CBT. Walsh and colleagues evaluated the effectiveness of a supportive, psychodynamically based treatment for bulimia in a double-blind, placebo-controlled study including medications and CBT.[62] CBT produced results superior to those achieved with supportive therapy or antidepressants alone. Supportive therapy combined with antidepressants was no more effective than antidepressants alone.

# PEDIATRIC OBESITY

## Historical Perspective

Obesity has been present in Western societies since recorded time. Captured in the writings, paintings, and sculptures of these early periods, the human body was commonly portrayed as mildly obese. This was especially true for women; the rotund female body was often considered more healthy, fertile, and prosperous.[68] In classical Greek and Roman cultures, attempts to define the ideal female form included a round head, broad shoulders, stocky torso, wide hips, and short legs.[68] Since the early 1900s, two major factors have reversed the historical trend of equating obesity with wealth and prosperity: the striving of suffragists to end male dominance[68] and, more importantly, the increasing medical knowledge of nutrition and the adverse consequences of obesity.

## Definition

There is as yet no absolute or clear-cut definition of obesity in childhood or adolescence. In pragmatic terms, obesity can be considered to be present whenever there is an excess accumulation of body fat stores that exceeds an average or healthy range. The methods most commonly used to estimate body fat are obtained from anthropometric data and include the body mass index (BMI) and either triceps or subscapular skinfold thicknesses. BMI is calculated by dividing the weight in kilograms by the height in meters squared. Other parameters used to estimate body fat stores include mean body weight for height, current weight for height, and the ponderal index, which is obtained by dividing the weight in kilograms by the height in meters cubed. On the basis of these parameters, suggested guidelines for defining obesity in children include an actual weight for height that is 20% or more above the mean, a BMI above the 85th percentile (some authors use the 90th percentile), and a triceps skinfold thickness 85% greater than the mean.[69, 70] Superobesity has been suggested to be present if the mean weight for height is 40% or more above the mean or if the BMI or the triceps skinfold thickness is above the 95th percentile.[70]

All techniques used to determine lean body mass and obtain body fat measurements indirectly (by subtracting lean body mass from body weight) are cumbersome and too expensive to be used in the routine clinical setting. They are, however, quite important as research tools, and they provide more accurate information than body measurements do. These research methods include measurement of total body water (with the use of radioisotope labeling), total body potassium, electrical conductivity, bioelectrical impedance, photon absorptiometry, and bone density and the development of predictive equations. All of these methods are based on the fact that the composition and biochemical properties of fat differ from those of all other tissues (constituting the lean body mass) and that if the proportion of total body weight of one of these two compartments is known, that of the other can be obtained. Further information on these various research methods and their applications is available in several reviews.[71, 72]

## Prevalence

The prevalence of child and adolescent obesity has increased dramatically since the 1960s, as documented in five national surveys extending from 1963 to 1991.[73] In these surveys, between 3,000 and 14,000 youths, aged 6 through 17 years, were examined. Obesity was defined as a BMI exceeding the 85th percentile, marked obesity as a BMI exceeding the 95th percentile.

For all race and ethnic groups combined, the prevalence of obesity was 22% and that of marked obesity was 10.9%. Among 6- to 11-year-old boys, the prevalence of obesity was 20.5% for non-Hispanic whites, 26.5% for non-Hispanic blacks, and 33.3% for Mexican Americans. Among girls of a similar age, the rates were 21.5% for non-Hispanic whites, 31.4% for non-Hispanic blacks, and 29% for Mexican Americans. Among boys in the older age group (12 to 17 years), obesity was present in 23.1% of non-Hispanic whites, 21.1% of non-Hispanic blacks, and 26.7% of Mexican Americans. Among the older girls, the prevalence was 20.3% for non-Hispanic whites, 29.9% for non-Hispanic blacks, and 23.4% for Mexican Americans. Among girls in both age groups, non-Hispanic blacks had the highest prevalence of obesity and non-Hispanic whites had the lowest. For boys in both age categories, Mexican Americans had the highest prevalence of obesity; the lowest prevalence for the younger boys was found in non-Hispanic whites, and for the older boys in non-Hispanic blacks.[73]

Regarding trends in the increased prevalence of obesity, the greatest increases occurred between the period 1976 to 1980 and the period 1988 to 1991. Among all age and sex groups, the increase in prevalence of obesity was greatest (9 percentage points) for blacks. However, the greatest increase in marked obesity occurred among white male adolescents (9 percentage points), with the increase in all other race, sex, and age groups being more moderate (2.5 to 5.5 percentage points).[73]

## Epidemiology

Numerous risk factors have been associated with the development of childhood and adolescent obesity, including environmental, familial, genetic, cultural, ethnic, and behavioral factors. The two most important risk factors appear to be parental obesity and ethnic background.[69, 74] In examining the weight of children of obese and nonobese parents, investigators noted that if both parents were obese, 80% of the children developed obesity; if one parent was obese, about 50% of the children developed obesity; and if neither parent was obese, only 10% of the children became obese.[74]

Ethnic differences are also important, with higher levels of obesity being present among African Americans, Mexican Americans, Cubans, and Native Americans.[75] One of the highest prevalence rates for obesity occurs in the Pima Indian tribe of the southwestern United States, where, by adulthood, more than 75% of tribal members are obese and more than 45% have type II diabetes.[74]

Additional familial factors associated with a higher prevalence of obesity include higher socioeconomic class, increased parental education, and small family size.[69] Patterns of activity and inactivity along with family lifestyle are important. Children whose parents are actively involved in exercise programs are leaner than children whose parents are not.[69] Environmental factors are contributory, with obesity being more prevalent in the northeastern United States.[69] As is true for the eating disorders, obesity is more prominent in major metropolitan areas than in rural areas.[69]

## Heredity and Genetics

Although the combination of increased energy intake and decreased physical activity is probably responsible for most child and adolescent obesity, a strong body of evidence suggests that genetic factors are also contributory. In studies within families, including studies of monozygotic and dizygotic twins, the degree and distribution of fat, fat-free mass, and the rate of fat accumulation were all similar.[69] Furthermore, the similarity of these factors increased among related family members as their degree of genetic similarity increased.[69]

Research in the area of genetic susceptibility has increased since the discovery of a specific *OB* gene in mice that results in inherited obesity. The mouse *OB* gene, expressed exclusively in adipose tissue, is responsible for the production of a protein (leptin) that, when released through the circulation, affects central nervous system control to reduce appetite and increase satiety. Obesity in humans, however, appears to be much more complex, since leptin levels in obese humans are increased.[76]

The following is a summary of the studies to date, both in animal models and in humans, that have shown an association between gene abnormalities and obesity.[77] There are now 12 known loci linked to mendelian disorders exhibiting obesity as a clinical feature. Eight chromosomal regions with quantitative trait loci for obesity have been identified in mice, and 10 proposed candidate genes have been identified in human subjects that demonstrate a statistical association with BMI or body fat. Nine loci are linked to a relevant phenotype, and in four cases the evidence for linkage is strong. These markers are mapped to the chromosomal locations 2p25, 6p21.3, 7q33, and 20q12–13.11. Under continuing investigation are additional regions that may be related to obesity, including 1p, 3p, 11p, 15q, and Xq.[77] The current hypothesis proposes that these gene candidates act as "susceptibility" genes rather than necessary genes.[78] Susceptibility for developing obesity occurs in the presence of these genes, with the precipitating behavioral and environmental factors remaining primarily responsible.

## Energy Intake

Data supporting the concept that obese individuals become overweight at least in part because of an increase in caloric intake have not been clearly established. A number of surveys have examined the macronutrient intake of children and adolescents longitudinally over several years.[73, 79] In all of these studies, the total caloric intake of obese and nonobese children did not differ. However, these studies had a major methodologic problem in that both obese and nonobese persons under-report nutrient intake.

Although overall calorie intake is not dissimilar, obese children tend to derive a greater percentage of their dietary calories from fat. A study determined that children at risk for obesity or who developed obesity consumed 34.4% of their calories from fat, compared with 32% for the low-risk group.[79] The National Heart, Lung, and Blood Institute Growth and Health Study (NGHS) study also demonstrated that as the percentages of energy derived from total fat and saturated fat increased, so did obesity.[79]

Although a strong association between increased fat intake and obesity has not been determined, the metabolic consequences of such consumption favor fat deposition and decreased thermic expenditure. Thirty percent of the total calories available from carbohydrate are used to convert carbohydrate to fat, whereas only 3% of the energy available from fat is required to convert dietary fat to its storage form.[69] Furthermore, only small amounts of excessive fat intake are necessary to produce weight gain. As stated by Dietz and Robinson, 5 lb of weight gain can accrue in a year with an excess intake of only 50 Kcal/day, which can be achieved by consuming 16 oz of 2% rather than 1% milk or placing an extra teaspoon of butter on a dinner roll.[69] In summary, although total caloric intake of obese and non-obese children may not differ significantly, it is likely that small excesses of fat intake consumed daily over an extended period result in a slow accumulation of excess body fat.

## Energy Expenditure

Energy expenditure is composed of three parts: the resting metabolic rate, the thermic effect of food, and physical activity. The resting metabolic rate accounts for 65% to 70% of total energy expenditure, the thermic effect of food for 10%, and physical activity for 20%. Although the results of prospective studies are somewhat mixed, data are accumulating to suggest that small variances in total energy expenditure are involved in the development of obesity in children. Roberts examined energy intake in infants born to lean and to overweight mothers, measuring total energy expenditure, resting metabolic rate, and energy intake at 12 weeks of age and subsequently throughout the first year of life by the double water-labeled technique.[80] None of the infants of lean mothers developed obesity, whereas 50% of those at risk for obesity (i.e., those born to mothers who were overweight) became obese. No differences were noted in body composition or resting metabolic rate between lean and obese infants. Total energy expenditure was 20.7% lower in infants who developed obesity than in the normal infants.[80] Other investigators examined energy expenditure in children at 4 to 5 years of age, and again at 15 to 16 years of age.[80] Both total energy expenditure and resting metabolic rate of the children at risk for obesity (i.e., those with at least one obese parent) were low. On average, there was a 22% reduction in total energy expenditure in this group over the period of 10 years, which resulted in substantially more weight gain than in the normal children.[80]

Other investigators have found somewhat variable results. Wells et al[81] examined 30 infants at 12 weeks of age and again at 2.5 to 3.5 years of age and found no relation between total energy expenditure and later fatness. Goran and colleagues[82] examined 101 prepubertal children at 5 years of age and reexamined 68 of them a year later. Although no correlation was found between body fat mass and physical activity level, a small portion of the variance in body fat mass in obese children resulted from a decrease in recreational activity time.[82] This finding was previously supported by numerous other studies confirming that the prevalence of obesity increases with time spent on activities associated with the more sedentary lifestyle of today's society (e.g., television watching, computer games).[83]

## Differential Diagnosis

For most obese children and adolescents, the cause is primary and not associated with a clinical syndrome. However, a few of these patients (approximately 1%) present with rare disorders of which obesity is a component. In general, syndromatic obesity is associated with short stature, delayed bone age, and delayed development of secondary sexual characteristics, whereas primary obesity is associated with increased height, advanced bone age, and early puberty.[69] The disorders associated with obesity are listed in Table 7–5.

**TABLE 7–5. Disorders Associated with Obesity**

| | |
|---|---|
| **Genetic** | |
| Alström-Hallgren syndrome | Carpenter's syndrome |
| Cohen's syndrome | Laurence-Moon-Biedl syndrome |
| Stein-Leventhal syndrome | Prader-Willi syndrome |
| Turner's syndrome | X-Linked obesity |
| **Endocrine** | |
| Cushing's syndrome | Growth hormone deficiency |
| Hyperinsulinemia | Hypothyroidism |
| Panhypopituitarism | Pseudo-hypoparathyroidism (type I) |

## Medical and Psychological Consequences of Obesity

There are profound physical and psychological consequences that occur as a result of child and adolescent obesity. As in adults, obesity in children and adolescents contributes to the development of progressive disease states, including cardiovascular disease, hypertension, increased risk for coronary artery disease, diabetes mellitus, insulin resistance, hepatic and gallbladder disease, and musculoskeletal problems (Table 7–6).

Genetically determined fat distribution is similar in children and adolescents and in adults. In adults, abdominal fat, also referred to as upper body fat, is associated with increased rates of diabetes, hypertension, breast cancer, and coronary artery disease.[84] Visceral fat is associated with impaired glucose and lipid metabolism.[84] Excessive fat deposition on the buttocks or thighs, also called lower body fat, appears to carry less serious medical consequences but is noted to cause joint problems, varicose veins, skin ulcers, and rashes.[84] Children whose fat distribution is primarily abdominal develop problems with hypertension, adverse lipid profiles, and insulin resistance.[85] Gluteofemoral obesity is associated with Blount's disease and slipped capital femoral epiphysis.[69]

Hypertension is two times as prevalent in adolescents who are overweight than in the normal population.[86] Obese adolescents have an increased and redistributed cardiac output, increased sodium retention, structural abnormalities in resistant vessels, myocardial hypertrophy, and myocardial dysfunction, a component of which is related to insulin resistance.[86] Increased insulin resistance, along with the obesity-associated changes of central body fatness, hypertension, and dyslipidemia, results in an increased risk for the development of coronary artery disease in adulthood.

Additional medical consequences of childhood obesity include hepatic steatosis and gallbladder disease. Cholesterol gallstones are reported more frequently in obese children. Pseudotumor cerebri and complications of decreased pulmonary function, obstructive sleep apnea, primary alveolar hypoventilation, and pickwickian syndrome can occur. Both adolescents and children have been noted to have impaired cell-mediated immunity,[87] and such alterations may contribute in part to the increased incidence of cancer known to occur in adults with obesity.

The psychosocial consequences of child and adolescent obesity are significant and profound. Even as early as 6 years of age, children have developed a negative association and negative stereotypes with the presentation of pictures of obese children.[69] Overweight children are rejected by their peers and consistently rated more poorly than other children, even those with disabilities. College acceptance rates are decreased, psychosocial involvement at work is altered, and obese persons are generally associated with a lower social class status.[69] It has been reported that the negative perception of obesity is so powerful that other negative characteristics have no added effect.[88]

**TABLE 7–6. Medical Complications of Obesity**

| | |
|---|---|
| **Cardiovascular** | |
| Hypertension | Hypercholesterolemia |
| Hypertriglyceridemia | Increased low-density lipoproteins |
| Increased very-low-density lipoproteins | Decreased high-density lipoproteins |
| Myocardial hypertrophy | Structural changes in resistant vessels |
| **Dermatologic** | |
| Acanthosis nigricans | Varicose veins |
| Skin irritation, maceration | Stretch marks |
| **Endocrine** | |
| Early puberty | Hyperinsulinemia |
| Insulin resistance | Sodium retention |
| **Gastrointestinal** | |
| Cholelithiasis | Gallbladder disease |
| Hepatic steatosis | |
| **Immunologic** | |
| Impaired cell-mediated immunity | Reversed CD4-CD8 ratio |
| Decreased tumor necrosis factor | |
| **Musculoskeletal** | |
| Blount's disease (tibia vara) | Slipped capital femoral epiphysis |
| **Neurologic** | |
| Pseudotumor cerebri | |
| **Pulmonary** | |
| Pickwickian syndrome | Primary alveolar hypoventilation |
| Obstructive sleep apnea | |
| **Eating Disorders** | |

## Prevention and Treatment

Childhood obesity remains a very serious problem, with 25% to 50% of obese children ultimately becoming obese adults.[69] In some series, up to 74% of obese adolescents have difficulties extending into adulthood.[69] In addition, obese adults who were obese as children have more profound and severe difficulties than those who became obese after adolescence. Fifty-year follow-up studies of obese adolescents have demonstrated increased morbidity and mortality, even independent of ultimate adult body weight status.[89]

Until recently, treatment programs for childhood obesity yielded only marginal and disappointing results, similar to the experience in adults. As reported by Dietz and Robinson,[69] treatment of 5- to 12-year-old obese children decreased the percentage who were overweight by only 25% at 1 year, 14% at 5 years, and 7% at 10 years in selected follow-up samples. The implementation of strong, family-based programs using a multidisciplinary team approach is now beginning to show more encouraging results.

The major components of all obesity programs are education, calorie restriction, increased physical activity, and behavioral changes. In studies summarized by Epstein,[89] 43% of children involved in family-based behavioral programs were able to maintain weight decreases of 20% over 5- and 10-year follow-up periods. Additionally, 58% and 64% of children were able to maintain a weight 20% less than their initial weight after implementation of aerobic and lifestyle exercise programs, respectively, compared with 20% of children using calisthenics alone. Suskind and associates[90] demonstrated similar improvements in children with the use of a family-based behavioral therapeutic approach.

Nutrition education is an important component of all behaviorally-oriented weight reduction programs. Many misconceptions about food, calories, and nutrition exist in obese children and adolescents. Moderate calorie restriction is one of the two most important aspects of any weight reduction program. Although food and dietary records are often inaccurate, they can be used as a basis for establishing the eating behaviors of each patient, serving then as guidelines for diet modifications. As outlined by the American Heart Association, the general principles of calorie restriction include providing a diet in which fat comprises 25% to 30% of calories, allowing first helpings but not second helpings, allowing healthy snack foods such as fruits and vegetables, avoiding the use of food as a reward, and including favorite foods, which should not be forbidden.[91, 92] Food intake should be reduced gradually. Just as a small increase in caloric intake is all that is required to establish progressive weight gain over an extended period, a similarly small reduction in calories, perhaps 40 to 100 calories/day, is all that is necessary to achieve slow, progressive weight loss. A pragmatic goal is to have the child lose approximately 1 lb/wk.

Highly restrictive diets should be reserved for those children and adolescents who are massively obese and have concomitant problems with hypertension, sleep apnea, diabetes, or pseudotumor cerebri.[69] These diets should contain a minimum of 2 g of protein per kilogram of ideal body weight and should probably be supplemented with potassium, calcium, other minerals, and multivitamins.[69] Careful dietary and medical supervision is important during the weight loss period. In both minimally restrictive and highly restrictive dietary approaches, adequate calories and protein must be maintained to protect the coexisting processes of continuing growth and maturation.

In addition to calorie restriction, increased activity levels, especially maintenance of increased physical activity over a prolonged period, is the second key component for long-term success.[93, 94] For young children, no formal exercise program is required. Simply limiting the amount of time spent in sedentary activities and encouraging outside activities that normally result in increased exercise (e.g., playing, running) usually suffices. In older children and adolescents, a formal exercise program should be employed, but it should be tailored to the structure of the family. Most exercise programs should be part of a larger, family-oriented approach and incorporate family lifestyle changes, including involvement of one or both parents in the exercise program.[94]

Behavioral modification techniques employed to change eating behaviors should include self-monitoring, contingency training, positive reinforcement, and cognitive restructuring of the child and adolescent within the context of the family.[69] In contingency training, the families need to be alert for when inappropriate food intake is occurring and provide alternative means of behaviors. Positive reinforcement should be prompt and consistent.[69] Cognitive restructuring assists in placing diet and food in a more appropriate perspective within the overall lifestyle of the family.[69]

Several new drugs have been employed for the treatment of morbid obesity in adults, including phentermine and fenfluramine, although fenfluramine has been recalled by the Food and Drug Administration. A third agent, sibutramine, which inhibits reuptake of both noradrenaline and 5-hydroxytryptamine, has been studied and was recently approved for use.[95] Because of their significant and potentially serious side effects and their unknown effects on growth, use of these medications in children cannot be recommended at this time.

The key to prevention of childhood obesity is anticipation and recognition. As stated previously, if one or both parents are obese, the likelihood of a child's developing obesity is significantly increased. Additional risk factors that can lead to childhood obesity were reviewed by Epstein.[89] These include a ninefold increase in risk for children who were neglected, a sevenfold increase for those from nonsupportive home environments, and a 4.5% increase for those from homes where the parents were unaware of their child's sweet-eating habits.[89] Furthermore, a child's individual psychosocial problems, including peer relations, learning problems, and behavioral problems, may be associated with rapid increases in weight.[89] In children with these or other previously mentioned risk factors, body weight should be monitored twice yearly, and intervention should be begun promptly if weight increases significantly. Early recognition, a careful family and dietary history, early intervention with simple dietary changes, limitation of television watching, and an increase in physical activities are the best preventive approaches to reverse early-developing childhood obesity.

## REFERENCES


1. Bemporad JR: Self-starvation through the ages: reflections on the prehistory of anorexia nervosa. Int J Eat Disord 1996;19:217–237.
2. Blinder BE, Chad K: Eating disorders: a historical perspective. In Alexander-Mott L, Lumsden DB (eds): Understanding Eating Disorders: Anorexia Nervosa, Bulimia Nervosa, and Obesity. Washington, DC, Taylor & Francis, 1994, pp 3–35.
3. Lucas AR: Anorexia nervosa: historical background and biopsychosocial determinants. Semin Adolesc Med 1986;2:1–9.
4. Slaby AE, Dwenger R: History of anorexia nervosa. In Giannini AJ, Slaby AE (eds): The Eating Disorders. New York, Springer-Verlag, 1993, pp 1–17.
5. Russell GFM: Anorexia nervosa through time. In Szmukler G, Dare C, Treasure J (eds): Handbook of Eating Disorders. New York, John Wiley & Sons, 1995, pp 5–17.
6. Wakeling A: Epidemiology of anorexia nervosa. Psychiatr Res 1996;62:3–9.
7. Hill OW: Epidemiologic aspects of anorexia nervosa. Adv Pschysom Med 1977;9:45–62.
8. Kurtzman FD, Yaher J, Landsverk J, et al: Eating disorders among selected female student populations at UCLA. J Am Diet Assoc 1989;39:45–53.
9. Thompson JK: Introduction. Body image, eating disorders, and obesity: an emerging synthesis. In Thompson JK (ed): Body Image, Eating Disorders, and Obesity. Washington, DC, American Psychological Association, 1996, pp 1–20.
10. Mehler PS: Eating disorders: 1. Anorexia nervosa. Hosp Pract 1996;31:109–117.
11. Woodside DB: A review of anorexia nervosa and bulimia nervosa. Curr Probl Pediatr 1995;25:67–89.
12. Crago M, Shisslak CM, Estes LS: Eating disturbances among American minority groups: a review. Int J Eat Disord 1996;19:239–248.

13. Drake MA: Symptoms of anorexia nervosa in female university dietetic majors. J Am Diet Assoc 1989;39:97–98.
14. Kuboki T, Nomura S, Ide M, et al: Epidemiological data on anorexia nervosa in Japan. Psychiatr Res 1996;62:11–16.
15. Garner DM, Garfinkel PE: Socio-cultural factors in the development of anorexia nervosa. Psychol Med 1980;10:647–656.
16. Vandereycken W, Meerman R: What are the causes? In Anorexia Nervosa. A Clinician's Guide to Treatment. Berlin, Walter deGruyter, 1984, pp 43–64.
17. Brewerton TD, Jimerson DC: Studies of serotonin function in anorexia nervosa. Psychiatr Res 1996;62:31–42.
18. Pirke KM: Central and peripheral noradrenalin regulation in eating disorders. Psychiatr Res 1996;62:43–49.
19. Kaye WH: Neuropeptide abnormalities in anorexia nervosa. Psychiatr Res 1996;62:65–74.
20. Zerbe KJ: Anorexia nervosa and bulimia nervosa: when the pursuit of bodily perfection becomes a killer. Postgrad Med 1996;99:161–189.
21. Treasure J, Szmukler G: Medical complications of chronic anorexia nervosa. In Szmukler G, Dare C, Treasure J (eds): Handbook of Eating Disorders. New York, John Wiley & Sons, 1995, pp 197–220.
22. Russell GFM: Premenarchal anorexia nervosa and its sequelae. J Psychiatr Res 1985;19:363–369.
23. Herholz K: Neuroimaging in anorexia nervosa. Psychiatr Res 1996;62:105–110.
24. Eating disorders. In American Psychiatric Association: Diagnostic and Statistical Manual of Mental Disorders, 4th ed. Washington, DC, American Psychiatric Association, 1994, pp 539–550.
25. Russell GFM: Bulimia nervosa: an ominous variant of anorexia nervosa. Psychol Med 1979;9:429–448.
26. Giannini AJ: A history of bulimia. In Giannini AJ, Slaby AE (eds): The Eating Disorders. New York, Springer-Verlag, 1993, pp 18–21.
27. Ziolko HU: Bulimia: a historical outline. Int J Eat Disord 1996;20:345–358.
28. Mehler PS: Eating disorders: 2. Bulimia nervosa. Hosp Pract 1996;31:107–126.
29. Crowther JH, Wolf EM, Sherwood NE: Epidemiology of bulimia nervosa. In Crowther JH, Tennenbaum DL, HobFoll SE, Stephens MA (eds): The Etiology of Bulimia Nervosa. Washington, DC, Hemisphere Publishing, 1992, pp 1–26.
30. Fombonne E: Is bulimia nervosa increasing in frequency? Int J Eat Disord 1996;19:287–296.
31. Heatherton TF, Nichols P, Mahamedi F, Keel P: Body weight, dieting, and eating disorder symptoms among college students, 1982 to 1992. Am J Psychiatr 1995;152:1623–1629.
32. Laessle RG: Affective disorders and bulimic syndromes. In Fichter MM (ed): Bulimia Nervosa: Basic Research, Diagnosis, and Therapy. New York, John Wiley & Sons, 1990, pp 112–125.
33. Bulik CM: Drug and alcohol abuse by bulimic women and their families. Am J Psychiatry 1987;144:1604–1606.
34. Wonderlich S: Relationship of family and personality factors in bulimia. In Crowther JH, Tennenbaum DL, HobFoll SE, Stephens MA (eds): The Etiology of Bulimia Nervosa. Washington, DC, Hemisphere Publishing, 1992, pp 103–126.
35. Pope HG, Hudson JI: Is childhood sexual abuse a risk factor for bulimia nervosa? Am J Psychiatry 1992;149:455–463.
36. McComb RJ: Dental aspects of anorexia nervosa and bulimia nervosa. In Kaplan AS, Garfinkel PE (eds): Medical Issues and the Eating Disorders: The Interface. New York, Brunner/Mazel, 1993, pp 101–122.
37. Mitchell JE, Pyle RL, Eckert ED, et al: Electrolyte and other physiological abnormalities in patients with bulimia. Psychol Med 1983;13:273–278.
38. Mitchell JE, Pomeroy C, Seppala M, Huber M: Pseudo-Bartter's syndrome, diuretic abuse, idiopathic edema, and eating disorders. Int J Eat Disord 1988;7:225–237.
39. Thiel A, Brooks A, Ohlmeier M, et al: Obsessive-compulsive disorder among patients with anorexia nervosa and bulimia nervosa. Am J Psychiatry 1995;152:72–75.
40. Mitchell JE, Pyle RL, Eckert E, et al: A comparison study of antidepressants and structured intensive group psychotherapy in the treatment of bulimia nervosa. Arch Gen Psychiatry 1990;47:149–157.
41. Walsh BT, Wilson GT, Loeb KL, et al: Medication and psychotherapy in the treatment of bulimia nervosa. Am J Psychiatry 1997;154:523–531.
42. Goldstein DJ, Wilson MG, Thompson VL, et al: Long-term fluoxetine treatment of bulimia nervosa. Br J Psychiatry 1995;166:660–666.
43. Goldbloom DS, Olmsted MP: Pharmacotherapy of bulimia nervosa with fluoxetine: assessment of clinically significant attitudinal change. Am J Psychiatry 1993;150:770–774.
44. Agras WS, Rossiter EM, Arnow B, et al: One year follow-up of psychosocial and pharmacologic treatments for bulimia nervosa. J Clin Psychiatry 1994;55:179–183.
45. Pope HG, Hudson JI: Biological treatment of eating disorders. In Emmett SW (ed): Theory and Treatment of Anorexia Nervosa and Bulimia. New York, Brunner/Mazel, 1985, pp 73–92.
46. Minuchen S, Roseman BL, Baker L: Psychosomatic Families: Anorexia Nervosa in Context. Cambridge, Harvard University Press, 1978.
47. Selvini-Palazzoli M: Self-starvation: From Individual to Family Therapy in Treatment of Anorexia Nervosa, 2nd ed. New York, Jason Aronson, 1978.
48. Robin AL, Siegel PT, Moye A: Family versus individual therapy for anorexia: impact on family conflict. Int J Eat Disord 1995;17:313–322.
49. Shugar G, Krueger S: Aggressive family communication, weight gain, and improved eating attitudes during systemic family therapy for anorexia nervosa. Int J Eat Disord 1995;17:23–31.
50. VanFurth EF, VanStrein DC, Martina LM, et al: Expressed emotion and the prediction of outcome in adolescent eating disorders. Int J Eat Disord 1996;20:19–31.
51. Humphrey LL: Family process in anorexia and bulimia. Address to the Thirteenth National Conference on Eating Disorders, Columbus, Ohio, October 1994.
52. Russell GF, Szmulker GI, Dare C, Eisler I: An evaluation of family therapy in anorexia nervosa and bulimia nervosa. Arch Gen Psychiatry 1987;44:1047–1056.
53. Fairburn CG, Marcus MD, Wilson GT: Cognitive behaviour therapy for binge eating and bulimia nervosa: a comprehensive treatment manual. In Fairburn G, Wilson GT (eds). Binge Eating: Nature, Assessment and Treatment. New York, Guilford Press, 1993, pp 361–404.
54. Garner DM, Bemis KM: Cognitive therapy for anorexia nervosa. In Garner DM, Garfinkel PE (eds): Handbook of Psychotherapy for Anorexia Nervosa and Bulimia. New York, Guilford Press, 1985, pp 107–146.
55. Fairburn CG: Cognitive behavioral treatment for bulimia. In Garner DM, Garfinkel PE (eds). Handbook of Psychotherapy for Anorexia Nervosa and Bulimia. New York, Guilford Press, 1985, pp 160–192.
56. Fairburn CG, Norman PA, Welch SL, et al: A prospective study of outcome in bulimia nervosa and the long-term effects of three psychosocial treatments. Arch Gen Psychiatry 1995;52:304–312.
57. Wilson GT, Fairburn CG: Treatment of eating disorders. In Nathan PE, Gorman JM (eds). Psychotherapies and Drugs That Work: A Review of the Outcome Studies. New York, Oxford University Press (in press).
58. Mitchell JE, Pyle RL, Eckert ED, et al: Antidepressant vs. group therapy in the treatment of bulimia. Psychopharmacol Bull 1987;23:41–44.
59. Mitchell JE, Pyle RL, Pomeroy C, et al: Cognitive behavioral group psychotherapy of bulimia nervosa: importance of logistical variables. Int J Eat Disord 1993;14:277–287.
60. Wilson GT: Cognitive behavioral treatment of bulimia nervosa. Clin Psychol 1997;50:10–12.
61. Herzog DB, Sacks NR: Bulimia nervosa: comparison of treatment responders vs. nonresponders. Psychopharmacol Bull 1993;29:121–125.
62. Walsh BT, Wilson GT, Loeb KL, et al: Medication and psychotherapy in the treatment of bulimia nervosa. Am J Psychiatry 1997;154:523–531.
63. Klerman GL, Weissman MM, Rounsaville BJ, Chevron ES: Interpersonal Therapy of Depression. New York, Basic Books, 1984.
64. Fairburn CG, Peveler RC, Jones R, et al: Predictors of 12-month outcome in bulimia nervosa and the influences of attitudes to shape and weight. J Consult Clin Psychol 1993;61:696–698.
65. Wilfley DE: Interpersonal psychotherapy adapted for group and for the treatment of binge eating disorder. Presented at the Thirteenth National Conference on Eating Disorders, Columbus, Ohio, October 1994.
66. Yager J, Andersen A, Devlin M, et al: Practice guidelines for eating disorders. Am J Psychiatry 1993;150:207–223.
67. Garner DM, Rockert W, Davis R, et al: Comparison between cognitive behavioral and supportive-expressive therapy for bulimia nervosa. Am J Psychiatry 1993;150:37–46.
68. Kocjan DK, Giannini AJ: The history of obesity. In Giannini AJ, Slaby AE (eds): The Eating Disorders. New York, Springer-Verlag, 1993, pp 22–28.
69. Dietz WH, Robinson TN: Assessment and treatment of childhood obesity. Pediatr Rev 1993;14:337–344.

70. Williams CL, Bollella M, Carter BJ: Treatment of childhood obesity in pediatric practice. (Williams CL, Kimm SYS, eds: Prevention and Treatment of Childhood Obesity.) Ann N Y Acad Sci 1993;699:207–219.
71. Roche AF: Methodological considerations in the assessment of childhood obesity. (Williams CL, Kimm SYS, eds: Prevention and Treatment of Childhood Obesity.) Ann N Y Acad Sci 1993;699:6–17.
72. Ellis KJ: Measuring body fatness in children and young adults: comparison of bioelectric impedance analysis, total body electrical conductivity, and dual-energy x-ray absorptiometry. Int J Obes 1996;20:866–873.
73. Troiano RP, Flegal KM, Kuczmarski RJ, et al: Overweight prevalence and trends for children and adolescents: The National Health and Examinations Surveys, 1963 to 1991. Arch Pediatr Adolesc Med 1995;149:1085–1091.
74. Rea WS, Extein IL: Biological factors in obesity. In Giannini AJ, Slaby AE (eds): The Eating Disorders. New York, Springer-Verlag, 1993, pp 63–75.
75. Kumanyika S: Ethnicity and obesity development in children. (Williams CL, Kimm SYS, eds: Prevention and Treatment of Childhood Obesity.) Ann N Y Acad Sci 1993;699:81–92.
76. Arner P: The role of genes for obesity and its complications in man. Int J Obes 1996;20(suppl 4):17–20.
77. Bouchard C: The genetics of obesity: promising advances and failures. Int J Obes 1996;20(suppl 4):11–14.
78. Bouchard C, Pérusse L: Genetic aspects of obesity. (Williams CL, Kimm SYS, eds: Prevention and Treatment of Childhood Obesity.) Ann N Y Acad Sci 1993;699:26–35.
79. Kimm SYS: Obesity prevention and macronutrient intakes of children in the United States. (Williams CL, Kimm SYS, eds: Prevention and Treatment of Childhood Obesity.) Ann N Y Acad Sci 1993;699:70–80.
80. Roberts SB: Energy expenditure and the development of early obesity. (Williams CL, Kimm SYS, eds: Prevention and Treatment of Childhood Obesity.) Ann N Y Acad Sci 1993;699:18–25.
81. Wells JCK, Stanley M, Laidlaw AS, et al: The relationship between components of infant energy expenditure and childhood body fatness. Int J Obes 1996;20:848–853.
82. Goran MI, Hunter G, Nagy TR, Johnson R: Physical activity related energy expenditure and fat mass in young children. Int J Obes 1997;21:171–178.
83. Dietz WH: Therapeutic strategies in childhood obesity. Horm Res 1993;39(suppl 3):86–90.
84. Rand CSW: Obesity: definition, diagnostic criteria, and associated health problems. In Alexander-Mott L, Lumsden DB (eds): Understanding Eating Disorders. Washington, DC, Taylor & Francis, 1994, pp 221–241.
85. Berenson GS, Srinivasan SR, Wattigney WA, Harsha DW: Obesity and cardiovascular risk in children. (Williams CL, Kimm SYS, eds: Prevention and Treatment of Childhood Obesity.) Ann N Y Acad Sci 1993;699:93–103.
86. Rocchini AP: Hemodynamic and cardiac consequences of childhood obesity. (Williams CL, Kimm SYS, eds: Prevention and Treatment of Childhood Obesity.) Ann N Y Acad Sci 1993;699:46–56.
87. Boeck MA, Chen C, Cunningham-Rundles S: Altered immune function in a morbidly obese pediatric population. (Williams CL, Kimm SYS, eds: Prevention and Treatment of Childhood Obesity.) Ann N Y Acad Sci 1993;699:253–256.
88. Yuker HE, Allison DB: Obesity: sociocultural perspectives. In Alexander-Mott L, Lumsden DB (eds): Understanding Eating Disorders. Washington, DC, Taylor & Francis, 1994, pp 243–270.
89. Epstein LH: Family-based behavioral intervention for obese children. Int J Obes 1996;20(suppl 1):514–521.
90. Suskind RM, Sothern MS, Farris RP, et al: Recent advances in the treatment of childhood obesity. (Williams CL, Kimm SYS, eds: Prevention and Treatment of Childhood Obesity.) Ann N Y Acad Sci 1993;699:181–199.
91. Strong WB, et al: In Integrated Cardiovascular Health Promotion in Childhood. Dallas, TX, American Heart Association, 1992.
92. McCarty B, Mellin L: Obesity. In Rickert VI (ed): Adolescent Nutrition. New York, Chapman & Hall, 1996, pp 199–219.
93. Dietz WH: Therapeutic strategies in childhood obesity. Horm Res 1993;39(suppl 3):86–90.
94. Epstein LH: Methodological issues and ten-year outcomes for obese children. (Williams CL, Kimm SYS, eds: Prevention and Treatment of Childhood Obesity.) Ann N Y Acad Sci 1993;699:237–249.
95. Stock MJ: Sibutramine: a review of the pharmacology of a novel anti-obesity agent. Int J Obes 1997;21(suppl 1):525–529.

# Chapter 8

# Jaundice

Glenn R. Gourley

The term *jaundice* originated from the French *jaune,* which means "yellow." Jaundice, or icterus (from the Greek *ikteros*), refers to the yellow discoloration of the skin, sclerae, and other tissues caused by deposition of the bile pigment bilirubin. Jaundice is a sign that the serum bilirubin concentration has risen above normal levels (approximately 1.4 mg/dL after 6 months of age; 1 mg/dL = 17 mmol/L). The intensity of the yellow color is directly related to the level of serum bilirubin and the related degree of deposition of bilirubin into the extravascular tissues.

## BILIRUBIN METABOLISM

The term *bilirubin* is derived from Latin (*bilis,* bile; *ruber,* red) and was used in 1864 by Städeler[1] to describe the red-colored bile pigment. Bilirubin is formed from the degradation of heme-containing compounds (Fig. 8–1). The largest source for the production of bilirubin is hemoglobin. However, other heme-containing proteins are also degraded to bilirubin, including the cytochromes, catalases, tryptophan pyrrolase, and muscle myoglobin.[2]

The formation of bilirubin is accomplished by cleavage of the tetrapyrrole ring of protoheme (protoporphyrin IX), which results in a linear tetrapyrrole. The first enzyme system involved in the formation of bilirubin is microsomal heme oxygenase. It is located primarily in the reticuloendothelial tissues[3] and to a lesser degree in tissue macrophages and intestinal epithelium.[4] This enzyme system results in reduction of the porphyrin iron ($Fe^{3+}$ to $Fe^{2+}$) and hydroxylation of the α methine (=C–) carbon. This α-carbon is then oxidatively excised from the tetrapyrrole ring, yielding carbon monoxide. This excision opens the ring structure and is associated with oxygenation of the two carbons adjacent to the site of cleavage. The cleaved α-carbon is excreted as carbon monoxide, and the released iron can be reused by the body. The resultant linear tetrapyrrole is biliverdin IXα. The *IX* designation is a result of Fischer's grouping of the protoporphyrin isomers, group IX being the physiologic source of bilirubin.[5]

The stereospecificity of the enzyme produces cleavage almost exclusively at the α-carbon of the tetrapyrrole. This is unlike in vitro chemical oxidation, which results in cleavage at any of the four carbons (α, β, γ, and δ) linking the four pyrrole rings and produces equimolar amount of the α, β, γ, and δ isomers.[6] The central (C10) carbon on biliverdin IXα is then reduced from a methine to a methylene group ($-CH_2-$), thus forming bilirubin IXα. This is accomplished by the cytosolic enzyme biliverdin reductase.[7] The proximity of this enzyme results in very little biliverdin ever being present in the circulation.

Bilirubin formation can be assessed by measurement of carbon monoxide production. Such assessments indicate that the daily production rate of bilirubin is 6 to 8 mg/kg per 24 hours in healthy, full-term infants and 3 to 4 mg/kg per 24 hours in healthy adults.[8, 9] In mammals, approximately 80% of bilirubin produced daily originates from hemoglobin.[10–13] Degradation of hepatic and renal heme appears to account for most of the remaining 20%, reflecting the very rapid turnover of certain of these heme proteins. Although the precise fate of myoglobin heme is unknown, its turnover appears to be so slow as to be relatively insignificant.[14]

Catabolism of hemoglobin occurs very largely from the sequestration of erythrocytes at the end of their life span (120 days in adult humans, 90 days in newborns, 50–60 days in rats). A small fraction of newly synthesized hemoglobin is degraded in the bone marrow. This process, termed *ineffective erythropoiesis,* normally represents less than 3% of daily bilirubin production but may be substantially increased in persons with hemoglobinopathies, vitamin deficiencies, or heavy metal intoxication.[15–17] Infants produce more bilirubin per unit body weight because their red blood cell (RBC) mass is greater and their RBC life span is shorter. Additionally, hepatic heme proteins represent a larger fraction of total body weight in infants.

Bilirubin requires biotransformation to more water-soluble derivatives before excretion from the body.[18] Bilirubin is not linear but rather has extensive internal hydrogen bonding, as shown in Figure 8–2. The internal hydrogen bonding of bilirubin makes the molecule extremely hydrophobic and insoluble in aqueous media. Knowledge of this stereochemistry is important for understanding phototherapy.

When bilirubin is transported from its sites of production to the liver for excretion, a carrier molecule is necessary. Albumin serves this purpose[19] and has very high affinity for bilirubin.[20]

Bilirubin is taken up into the hepatocyte from the hepatic sinusoids by a carrier molecule in the plasma membrane,[21, 22] which also transports other organic anions such as bromsulfophthalein.[23] This carrier protein is competitively

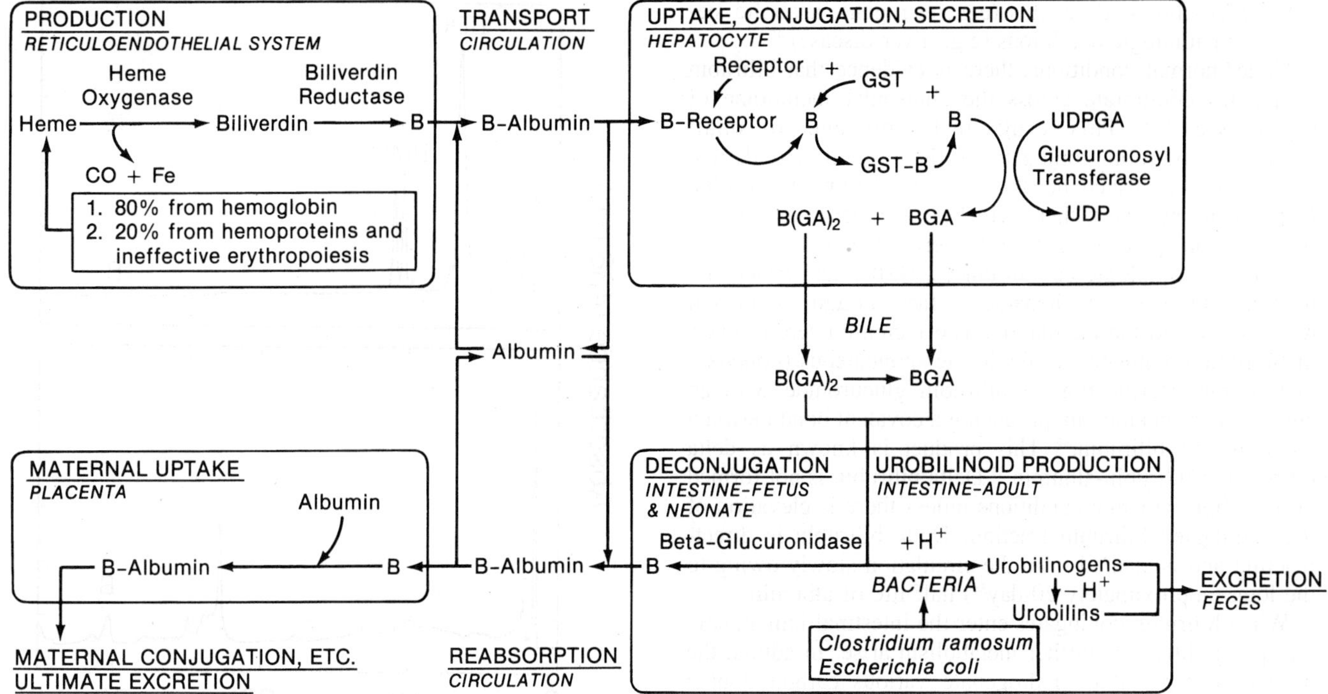


**FIGURE 8–1.** Metabolism of bilirubin (B) in the fetus, neonate, and adult. GA, glucuronic acid; UDP, uridine diphosphate; GST, glutathione-S-transferase.

inhibited by simultaneous exposure to bromsulfophthalein or indocyanine green. Some refer to this liver plasma membrane carrier as bilitranslocase.[24] Review of this uptake mechanism has shown it to meet the necessary kinetic criteria for carrier-mediated transport in a number of experimental models ranging from intact patients to isolated hepatocytes and sinusoidal membrane vesicles.[25]

Once within the aqueous environment of the hepatocyte, bilirubin is again bound by a protein carrier, glutathione *S*-transferase, traditionally referred to as ligandin.[26] This is a family of cytosolic proteins that have enzymatic activity and also bind nonsubstrate ligands. Although the affinity of purified glutathione *S*-transferase for bilirubin (acid dissociation constant = $10^6$) is less than that of albumin,[27] this compound is believed to be of importance in preventing bilirubin and its conjugates from refluxing back into the circulation.[28]

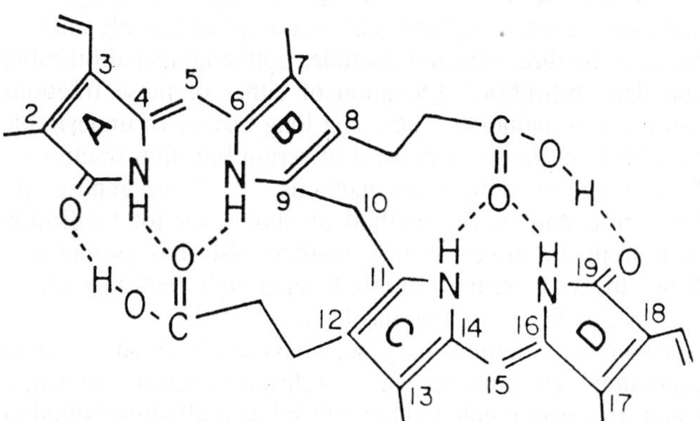


**FIGURE 8–2.** 4Z,15Z-Bilirubin IXα. The internal hydrogen bonding which shields the polar propionic acid groups is responsible for the hydrophobic nature of bilirubin.

Bilirubin is conjugated with glucuronic acid within the endoplasmic reticulum of the hepatocyte. The glucuronic acid donor is uridine diphosphate glucuronic acid (UDP-glucuronic acid). The enzyme responsible for this conjugation is bilirubin glucuronosyltransferase (BGT). Several different classes of glucuronosyltransferases, with different substrate specificity, have been described.[29–31] Catalysis of bilirubin by BGT results in both monoglucuronides and diglucuronides of bilirubin (BMGs and BDGs, respectively).[32] Depletion of hepatic UDP-glucuronic acid results in decreased BDGs and increased BMGs.[33] BGT activity for bilirubin can be induced by narcotics, anticonvulsants, contraceptive steroids, and bilirubin itself.[34] Alternatively, BGT activity can be decreased by caloric and protein restriction.[35] The isolation and characterization of cDNA clones which encode functional BGT have been reported in human liver.[36]

After bilirubin conjugation, the BMGs and BDGs are excreted through the hepatocyte canalicular membrane into the bile canaliculi. In normal adult duodenal bile, 70% to 90% of the bile pigments are BDGs, and 7% to 27% are BMGs.[37–39] Smaller amounts of other bilirubin conjugates are also seen. However, in normal infants there is decreased BGT activity in the liver,[40] and duodenal bile contains less BDG and more BMG than in the adult.[41, 42] After the first week of life, the rate-limiting step in bilirubin clearance is secretion of bilirubin conjugates by the hepatocyte.[43, 44] Canalicular secretion of bilirubin conjugates can be increased by choleretic agents (e.g., phenobarbital) and decreased by cholestatic agents (e.g., estrogens, anabolic steroids) or pathologic conditions (e.g., liver disease).[45]

Under normal conditions, there is evidence that bilirubin conjugates equilibrate across the sinusoidal membrane of hepatocytes.[46–48] This results in the presence of small amounts of bilirubin conjugates in the systemic circulation. If there is diminished hepatic glucuronidation of bilirubin (e.g., in the neonate), there will be a decreased amount of bilirubin conjugates present in the serum.[46, 47, 49–51]

In many pathologic circumstances, BMGs and BDGs are not excreted from the hepatocyte fast enough to prevent reflux back into the circulation. The increased serum levels of bilirubin conjugates results in the spontaneous (nonenzymatic) transesterification of bilirubin glucuronide with an amino group on albumin, producing a covalent bond between albumin and bilirubin.[52] This product is known as delta bilirubin or bilirubin-albumin.[53] Delta bilirubin is not formed in hyperbilirubinemic conditions unless there is elevation of the conjugated bilirubin fraction. Delta bilirubin is direct-reacting and is cleared from the circulation slowly owing to the long (approximately 20-day[54]) half-life of albumin.

When bilirubin conjugates enter the intestinal lumen, several possibilities for further metabolism arise. In adults, the normal bacterial flora hydrogenate various carbon double bonds in bilirubin to produce assorted urobilinogens. Subsequent oxidation produces the related urobilins. The large number of unsaturated bonds in bilirubin results in a large family of related reduction-oxidation products known as urobilinoids,[55] which are excreted in the feces. The conversion of bilirubin conjugates to urobilinoids is important because it blocks the intestinal absorption of bilirubin, known as the enterohepatic circulation.[56] Neonates lack an intestinal bacterial flora and are more likely to absorb bilirubin from the intestine. This difference in bile pigment excretion between adults and neonates is demonstrated in Figures 8–3 and 8–4. Bilirubin conjugates in the intestine can also act as substrate for either bacterial[57–59] or endogenous tissue[60] β-glucuronidase. This enzyme hydrolyzes glucuronic acid from bilirubin glucuronides. The unconjugated bilirubin produced is more rapidly absorbed from the intestine.[61] After birth, increased intestinal β-glucuronidase can increase the neonate's likelihood of experiencing higher serum bilirubin levels.[62] The ability of endogenous tissue β-glucuronidase to deconjugate bilirubin glucuronides has been demonstrated in germ-free animals.[63]

Neonates are at risk for the intestinal absorption of bilirubin because (1) their bile contains increased levels of BMG, which allows easier conversion to bilirubin; (2) they have within the intestinal lumen significant amounts of β-glucuronidase, which hydrolyzes bilirubin conjugates to bilirubin, which is more easily absorbed from the intestine; (3) they lack an intestinal flora to convert bilirubin conjugates to urobilinoids; and (4) meconium, the intestinal contents accumulated during gestation, contains significant amounts of bilirubin and β-glucuronidase.[64] Conditions that prolong meconium passage (e.g., Hirschsprung's disease, meconium ileus, meconium plug syndrome) are associated with hyperbilirubinemia.[65, 66] Earlier passage of meconium has been shown to be associated with lower serum bilirubin levels.[67–69] The enterohepatic circulation of bilirubin can be blocked by the enteral administration of compounds that bind bilirubin, such as agar,[70, 71] charcoal,[72] and cholestyramine.[73]

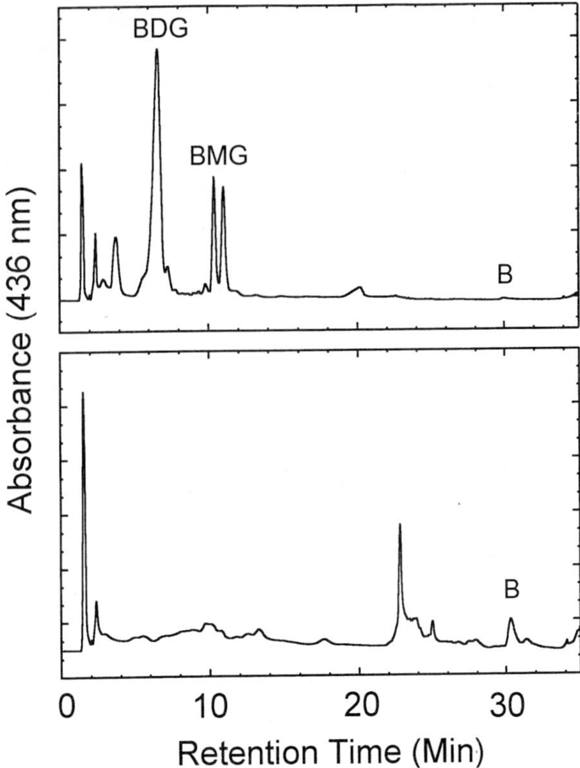


**FIGURE 8–3.** Bile pigment excretion in an adult as assessed by HPLC. *Top chromatogram*, duodenal bile (20 μL) from a normal man (GG). *Bottom chromatogram*, fecal extract equivalent to 50 mg of wet stool from the same normal man (GG). The BDGs and BMGs which predominate in adult bile are not present in adult stool because they are converted to urobilinoids by intestinal bacteria. Small amounts of bilirubin (B) are present in adult feces. (From Gourley GR: Bilirubin metabolism and kernicterus. Adv Pediatr 1997;44:173–229, with permission).

## ASSESSMENT OF JAUNDICE

Measurements of serum bilirubin are very common in the newborn nursery and in one study were made at least once in 61% of full-term newborn infants.[74] Two components of total serum bilirubin can be measured routinely in the clinical laboratory: conjugated bilirubin (direct fraction) and unconjugated bilirubin (indirect fraction). Although the terms *direct* and *indirect* are used equivalently with conjugated and unconjugated bilirubin, this is not quantitatively correct, because the direct fraction includes both conjugated bilirubin and delta bilirubin.[75] Elevation of either of these fractions can result in jaundice. There is a long history of undesirable variability in the measurement of serum bilirubin fractions.[76] Of the various laboratory methods,[75, 77, 78] the Jendrassik-Grof procedure is the method of choice for total bilirubin measurement, although this method also has problems.[79] When the total serum bilirubin level is high, factitious elevation of the direct fraction has been reported.[80]

Two newer methods have been developed which can more accurately determine the various bilirubin fractions (unconjugated, monoconjugated, diconjugated, and albumin-bound or delta): high-performance liquid chromatography (HPLC)[81] and multilayered slides (Ektachem).[82, 83] HPLC analysis is superior but too expensive and time-consuming for the clini-

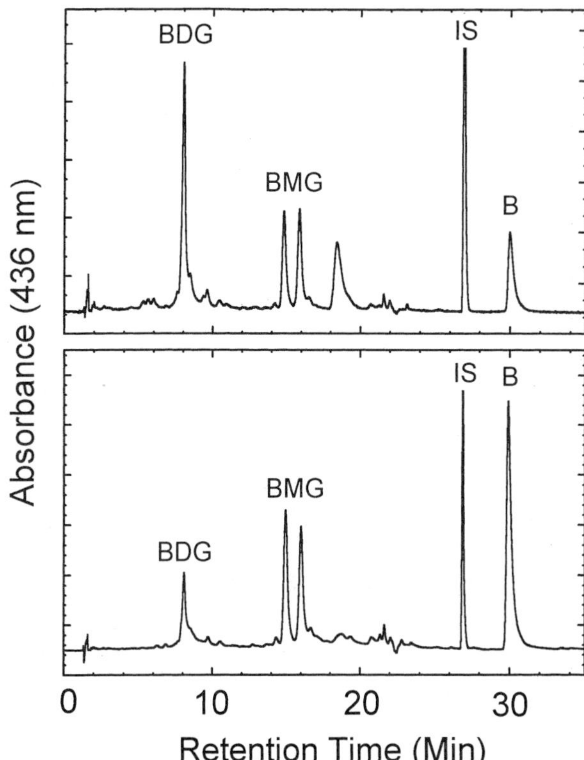


**FIGURE 8–4.** The top chromatogram shows the analysis of a sample of duodenal bile (20 μL) from a full-term, jaundiced, 6-day-old infant. The bottom chromatogram shows the analysis of a sample of fecal extract equivalent to 4 mg wet stool from the same infant. Neonates lack an intestinal bacterial flora, and hence large quantities of BDGs, BMGs, and bilirubin (B) are present in feces. The deglucuronidation action of intestinal β-glucuronidase is evident from the relatively decreased amounts of BDG and the increased amounts of BMG and B. IS, internal standard. (From Gourley GR: Bilirubin metabolism and kernicterus. Adv Pediatr 1997;44:173–229, with permission.)

cal laboratory.[75] HPLC analysis of serum from normal human neonates in the first 4 days of life[84] showed that unconjugated and conjugated bilirubin levels rise in parallel, with the conjugated fraction making up only 1.2% to 1.6% of total pigment (compared with 3.6% in adults). Because of the long half-life of delta bilirubin, the conjugated bilirubin measurement indicates relief from biliary cholestasis earlier than the direct bilirubin measurement does.[85]

There are conflicting data regarding the relative accuracy of measurements of capillary and venous serum bilirubin.[86, 87] However, as Maisels[88] pointed out, the literature regarding kernicterus, phototherapy, and exchange transfusion is based on bilirubin measurements in capillary samples.

Noninvasive methods to measure jaundice levels also exist and have been shown to be particularly useful in neonates. One method involves the use of a handheld "jaundice meter" which utilizes reflectance spectrophotometry to measure skin color (Minolta/Air-Shields Jaundice Meter,[90] Air-Shields Vickers, Hatboro, PA) and develop a "jaundice index." Numerous studies have shown a high correlation ($r > 0.9$) between the jaundice index and serum bilirubin levels.[89] Both the jaundice index at 24 hours of age and the ratio of increase in jaundice index during the first 24 hours per kilogram of birth weight were shown in one study to be useful in predicting the development of hyperbilirubinemia.[90] A less technical method to quantitate jaundice, which utilizes a Plexiglas color chart that is pressed against the infant's nose (Ingram Icterometer, Thomas A. Ingram, Birmingham, England), has been found to be useful in assessing jaundice.[91, 92]

## NEONATAL JAUNDICE

Infants usually are not jaundiced at the moment of birth, because the placenta has the ability to clear bilirubin from the fetal circulation. However, during the first week of life, most if not all infants have elevated serum bilirubin concentrations (>1.4 mg/dL). As the serum bilirubin rises, the skin becomes more jaundiced in a cephalopedal manner. Icterus is first appreciated in the head and progresses caudally to the palms and soles. Kramer[93] found the following serum indirect bilirubin levels as jaundice progressed: head and neck, 4 to 8 mg/dL; upper trunk, 5 to 12 mg/dL; lower trunk and thighs, 8 to 16 mg/dL; arms and lower legs, 11 to 18 mg/dL; palms and soles, more than 15 mg/dL. When the bilirubin was higher than 15 mg/dL, the entire body was icteric. Jaundice is best appreciated by blanching the skin with gentle digital pressure under well-illuminated (white light) conditions. In at least one third of infants, visible jaundice is apparent. Moderate jaundice (>12 mg/dL) occurs in at least 12% of breast-fed infants and 4% of formula-fed infants, and severe jaundice (>15 mg/dL) occurs in 2% and 0.3% of these respective feeding groups.[94]

Fundamentally, jaundice has only two causes: increased production or decreased excretion of bilirubin. These mechanisms are not mutually exclusive; specific examples are listed in Table 8–1. One possible clinical approach to arrive at these diagnoses is presented in Figure 8–5.

The high incidence of jaundice in otherwise completely normal neonates has resulted in the term physiologic jaundice. However, physiologic jaundice is merely the result of

**TABLE 8–1. Causes of Neonatal Hyperbilirubinemia**

| |
|---|
| **Increased Production of Bilirubin** |
| Fetal-maternal blood group incompatibilities |
| Extravascular blood in body tissues |
| Polycythemia |
| Red blood cell abnormalities (hemoglobinopathies, membrane and enzyme defects) |
| Induction of labor |
| **Decreased Excretion of Bilirubin** |
| Increased enterohepatic circulation of bilirubin |
| Breast feeding |
| Inborn errors of metabolism |
| Hormones and drugs |
| Prematurity |
| Hepatic hypoperfusion |
| Cholestatic syndromes |
| Obstruction of the biliary tree |
| **Combined Increased Production and Decreased Excretion of Bilirubin** |
| Sepsis |
| Intrauterine infection |
| Congenital cirrhosis |

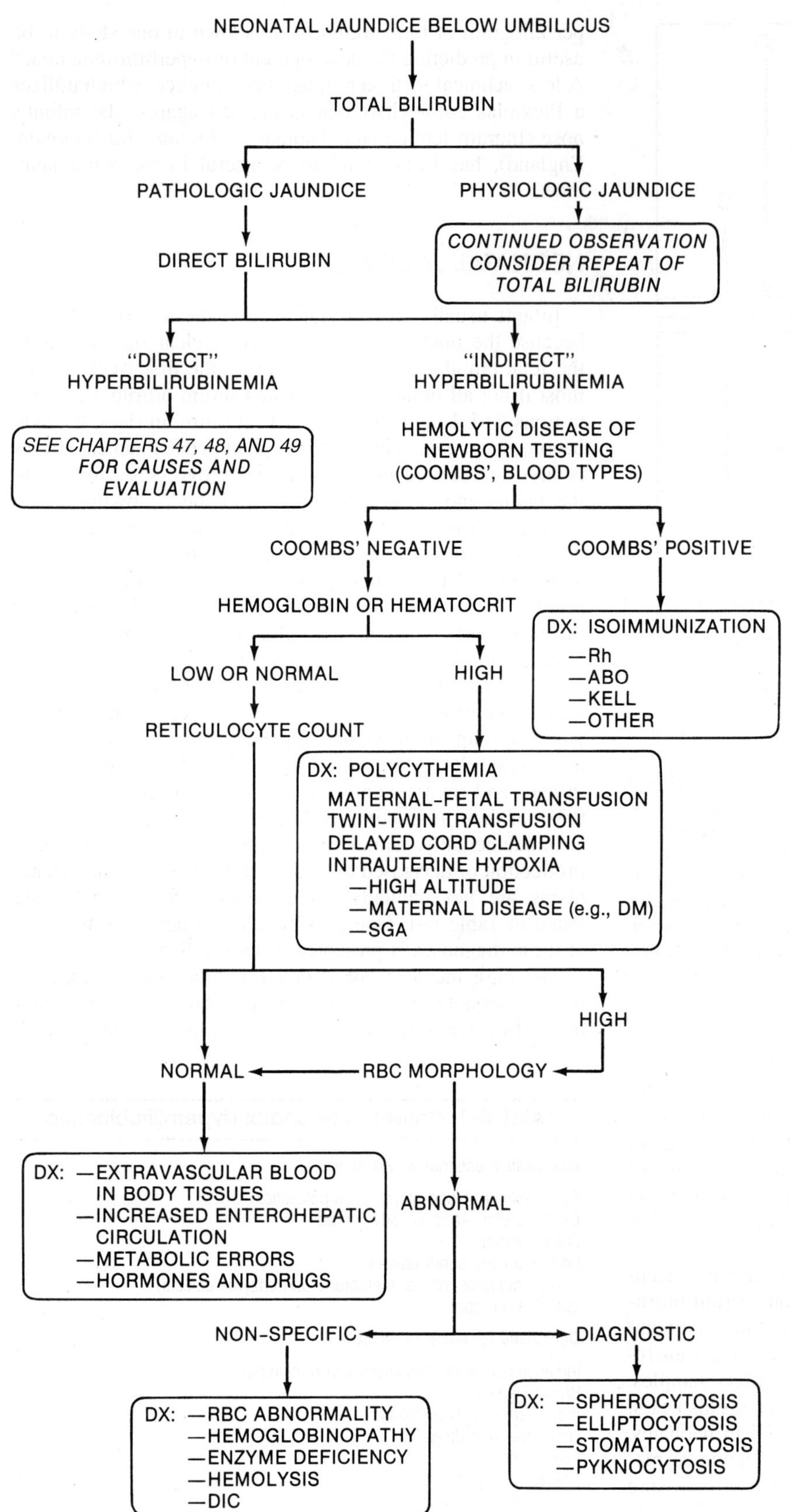


**FIGURE 8–5.** A clinical approach to the diagnosis of neonatal jaundice.

a number of factors involving increased bilirubin production and decreased excretion. Jaundice should always be considered to be a sign of possible disease and not routinely explained as physiologic. Specific characteristics of neonatal jaundice to be considered abnormal until proved otherwise include (1) development of jaundice before 36 hours of age; (2) persistence of jaundice beyond 10 days of age, (3) a serum bilirubin concentration higher than 12 mg/dL at any time, and (4) elevation of the direct-reacting fraction of bilirubin to more than 2 mg/dL at any time.

Factors associated with increased neonatal bilirubin levels are low birth weight; certain races (Oriental, Native American, Greek); maternal medications (e.g., oxytocin); premature rupture of the membranes; increased weight loss after birth; delayed meconium passage; breast-feeding; and neonatal infection.[95, 96] Factors associated with decreased neonatal bilirubin levels include maternal smoking, black race, and certain drugs given to the mother (e.g., phenobarbital).

## Neonatal Jaundice Caused by Increased Production of Bilirubin

The most common cause of severe early jaundice is fetal-maternal blood group incompatibility with resulting isoimmunization. Maternal immunization develops because of leakage of erythrocytes from the fetal to the maternal circulation. When the fetal erythrocytes carry different antigens, they are recognized as foreign by the maternal immune system, which forms antibodies against them (maternal sensitization). These antibodies (immunoglobulin G) cross the placental barrier into the fetal circulation and bind to fetal erythrocytes. In Rh incompatibility, sequestration and destruction of the antibody-coated erythrocytes takes place in the reticuloendothelial system of the fetus. In ABO incompatibility, hemolysis is intravascular, complement-mediated, and usually not as severe as in Rh disease.[97] Significant hemolysis can also result from incompatibilities between minor blood group antigens (e.g., Kell).[98] These conditions are associated predominately with elevation of unconjugated bilirubin, but occasionally the conjugated fraction is also increased.

Rh incompatibility usually does not develop until the second pregnancy. Therefore, prenatal blood typing and serial testing of Rh-negative mothers for the development of Rh antibodies provide important information to guide possible intrauterine care. If maternal Rh antibodies develop during pregnancy, potentially helpful measures include serial amniocentesis (with bilirubin measurement),[99, 100] ultrasound assessment of the fetus,[101, 102] intrauterine transfusion,[103, 104] and premature delivery. The prophylactic administration of anti-D gammaglobulin[105] has been most helpful in preventing Rh sensitization. The newborn infant with Rh incompatibility presents with pallor, hepatosplenomegaly, and a rapidly developing jaundice in the first hours of life. If the problem is severe, the infant may be born with generalized edema (fetal hydrops). Laboratory findings in the neonate's blood include reticulocytosis, anemia, a positive direct Coombs' test and a rapidly rising serum bilirubin level. Exchange transfusion continues to be an important therapy for seriously affected infants.[106]

ABO incompatibility usually manifests clinically with the first pregnancy. ABO hemolytic disease is largely limited to infants with blood group A or B who are born to group O mothers. ABO hemolytic disease is relatively rare in type A or B mothers. Development of jaundice is not as rapid as with Rh disease; a serum bilirubin concentration higher than 12 mg/dL on day 3 of life would be typical. Laboratory abnormalities include reticulocytosis (>10%) and a weakly positive direct Coombs' test, although this is sometimes negative. Spherocytes are the most prominent feature seen in the peripheral blood smear of neonates with ABO incompatibility.

When extravascular blood is present within the body, the hemoglobin can be rapidly converted to bilirubin by tissue macrophages. Examples of this type of increased bilirubin production include cephalohematoma; ecchymoses; petechiae; occult intracranial, intestinal, or pulmonary hemorrhage; and swallowed maternal blood. The Apt test can be used to distinguish blood of maternal or infant origin because of differences in alkali resistance between fetal and adult hemoglobin.[107, 108]

Polycythemia (venipuncture hematocrit >65%) can cause hyperbilirubinemia because the absolute increase in RBC mass results in elevated bilirubin production through normal rates of erythrocyte breakdown. A number of mechanisms can result in neonatal polycythemia,[109] including maternal-fetal transfusion, a delay in cord clamping,[110] twin-twin transfusions, intrauterine hypoxia, and maternal diseases (e.g., diabetes mellitus[111]). Therapy for symptomatic polycythemia is partial exchange transfusion; therapy for asymptomatic polycythemia remains controversial.[110]

A number of specific abnormalities related to the RBC can result in neonatal jaundice, including hemoglobinopathies and RBC membrane or enzyme defects. Hereditary spherocytosis is not usually a neonatal problem, but hemolytic crises can occur and can manifest with a rising bilirubin level and a falling hematocrit. The characteristic spherocytes seen in the peripheral blood smear may be impossible to distinguish from those seen with ABO hemolytic disease. Other hemolytic anemias associated with neonatal jaundice include drug-induced hemolysis, deficiencies of the erythrocyte enzymes (e.g., glucose-6-phosphate dehydrogenase deficiency, pyruvate kinase deficiency), and hemolysis induced by vitamin K or bacteria. α-Thalassemia can result in severe hemolysis and lethal hydrops fetalis.[112] γ β-Thalassemia may also occur, with hemolysis and severe neonatal hyperbilirubinemia.[113] Drugs or other substances responsible for hemolysis can be passed to the fetus or neonate across the placenta or via the breast milk.

Induction of labor with oxytocin has been shown to be associated with neonatal jaundice. There is a significant association between hyponatremia and jaundice in infants of mothers who received oxytocin to induce labor.[114, 115] The explanation for this observation is not clear.

## Neonatal Jaundice Caused by Decreased Excretion of Bilirubin

Increased enterohepatic circulation of bilirubin is believed to be an important factor in neonatal jaundice. As previously reviewed, neonates are at risk for the intestinal absorption of bilirubin because they lack an intestinal flora, they have significant amounts of β-glucuronidase within the intestinal lumen, and their meconium contains significant amounts of bilirubin.[64] Conditions which prolong meconium passage (e.g., Hirschsprung's disease, meconium ileus, meconium plug syndrome) are associated with hyperbilirubinemia.[65, 66] Earlier passage of meconium has been shown to be associated with lower serum bilirubin levels.[67, 68] Earlier passage of meconium may be facilitated by rectal temperature measurement during the neonatal period.[69] The enterohepatic circulation of bilirubin can be blocked by enteral administration of compounds that bind bilirubin, such as agar[56, 70, 116] charcoal,[72] and cholestyramine.[73]

Breast feeding has been clearly identified as a factor related to neonatal jaundice,[94, 117] and this subject has been reviewed elsewhere.[118, 119] Breast-fed infants have significantly higher serum bilirubin levels than formula-fed infants on each of the first 5 days of life,[120] and this unconjugated hyperbilirubinemia can persist for weeks[121] to months.[122, 123] Research has shown that bilirubin is a significant antioxidant which is possibly of physiologic benefit in protecting against cellular damage by free radicals.[124, 125] During the first week of life some distinguish this early jaundice as "breast-feeding jaundice" to differentiate it from the later breast milk jaundice syndrome, which occurs after the first week of life.[126–128] There is probably overlap between these conditions and physiologic jaundice. Early reports linking breast milk and jaundice with a steroid (pregnane-3α,20β-diol) in some milk samples[129] have not been confirmed by more recent, larger studies employing more sensitive methods.[130] There are also conflicting data regarding the association of this jaundice with increased lipase activity in the breast milk, which results in increased levels of free fatty acids that could inhibit hepatic BGT.[131–134] The enterohepatic circulation of bilirubin might be facilitated by the presence of β-glucuronidase[62, 135] or some other substance in human milk.[136] Other factors possibly related to jaundice in breast-fed infants include caloric intake, fluid intake, weight loss, delayed meconium passage, intestinal bacterial flora, and inhibition of BGT by an unidentified factor in the milk.[118] It has been suggested that a healthy, breast-fed infant with unconjugated hyperbilirubinemia, normal hemoglobin concentration, normal reticulocyte count, normal blood smear, no blood group incompatibility, and no other abnormality on physical examination may be presumed to have early breast-feeding jaundice.[119]

Because there is no specific laboratory test to confirm a diagnosis of breast milk jaundice, it is important to rule out treatable causes of jaundice before ascribing the hyperbilirubinemia to breast milk. The American Academy of Pediatrics Practice Parameter provides recommendations for the evaluation and treatment of neonatal jaundice.[137] The age of the infant is important in assessing the severity of neonatal jaundice and the need for evaluation and treatment (Table 8–2). If the bilirubin level is rising, published recommendations support encouraging mothers to breast feed more frequently,[119, 138] with an average suggested interval between feeds of 2 hours and no feeding supplements.[138] More frequent nursing may not increase intake, but it has been suggested to increase peristalsis and stool frequency, thus promoting bilirubin excretion.[139] However, one study comparing "frequent" (9 feedings per day) versus "demand" (6.5 feedings per day) feeding schedules during the first 3 days of life showed no significant relation between the frequency of breast feeding and infant serum bilirubin levels in 275 infants.[140] The point at which breast feeding should be discontinued is controversial; recommendations include total bilirubin levels of 14,[141] 15,[127] 16 to 17,[138] and 18 to 20 mg/dL.[95, 138] When breast feeding is interrupted, formula feeding may be initiated for 24 to 48 hours, or breast and formula feeding can be alternated with each feeding. A fall in the serum bilirubin level of 2 to 5 mg/dL[139] is consistent with a diagnosis of breast milk jaundice. Breast feeding may then be resumed; although the serum bilirubin levels may rise for several days, they will gradually level off and decline.[119, 127] In one study, interruption of breast feeding for approximately 50 hours (during which time a formula was given) was shown to have the same bilirubin-lowering effect as a similar duration of phototherapy.[142]

**TABLE 8–2. Management of Hyperbilirubinemia in the Healthy Term Newborn***

| | TSB LEVEL (mg/dL [mmol/L]) | | | |
|---|---|---|---|---|
| AGE (hr) | Consider Phototherapy† | Phototherapy | Exchange Transfusion if Intensive Phototherapy Fails‡ | Exchange Transfusion and Intensive Phototherapy |
| 25–48 | ≥12(170) | ≥15(260) | ≥20(340) | ≥25(430) |
| 49–72 | ≥15(260) | ≥18(310) | ≥25(430) | ≥30(510) |
| >72 | ≥17(290) | ≥20(340) | ≥25(430) | ≥30(510) |

TSB, total serum bilirubin

*Full-term infants who are clinically jaundiced at ≤24 hours old are not considered healthy and require further evaluation.

†Phototherapy at these TSB levels is a clinical option, meaning that the intervention is available and may be used on the basis of individual clinical judgment.

‡Intensive phototherapy should produce a decline in TSB of 1 to 2 mg/dL within 4 to 6 hours, and the TSB level should continue to fall and remain below the threshold level for exchange transfusion. If this does not occur, it is considered a failure of phototherapy.

From Provisional Committee for Quality Improvement and Subcommittee on Hyperbilirubinemia. Practice parameter: management of hyperbilirubinemia in the healthy term newborn. Pediatrics 1994;94:558–565. Used with permission of the American Academy of Pediatrics.

There is much controversy about the potential dangers of hyperbilirubinemia in full-term newborns who do not have isoimmune or other types of hemolytic disease.[143–146] Regardless of whether hyperbilirubinemia in these infants causes mild neurodevelopmental or intellectual handicaps, there is no doubt that frank kernicterus in this population is rare. Few pediatricians have ever seen a case, and there is a widespread belief that kernicterus does not occur in otherwise healthy, breast-fed infants, although some cases have been described.[147] Maisels and Newman[148] documented the occurrence of classic kernicterus in full-term, otherwise healthy, breast-fed infants. They reviewed 22 cases referred for litigation, looking for infants who had 37 weeks or more gestation, showed signs of acute bilirubin encephalopathy, and had typical neurologic sequelae. During the period from 1979 to 1991, six infants met the criteria. They had peak serum bilirubin levels of 39.0 to 49.7 mg/dL at 4 to 10 days of life. No cause for hyperbilirubinemia other than breast feeding could be determined. It was concluded that, although rare, kernicterus can occur in apparently healthy, full-term, breast-fed newborns who do not have hemolytic disease or any other discernible cause for their jaundice.[148]

Several inborn errors of metabolism can cause neonatal hyperbilirubinemia. Crigler-Najjar syndrome (CN), or congenital nonhemolytic jaundice,[149–151] is characterized by a hereditary deficiency of hepatic BGT.[152, 153] This syndrome may be divided into CN1 and CN2 (Arias' syndrome[154]) according to the response to phenobarbital—a significant decrease of serum bilirubin in CN2 and no response in CN1. In CN1, serum bilirubin levels typically range from approximately 15 to 45 mg/dL and there is a risk of both neonatal and later kernicterus.[152, 155] Hyperbilirubinemia is less severe in CN2 patients, varying from approximately 8 to 25 mg/dL. CN2 is associated with a much lower incidence of kernicterus, although such damage has been documented.[156, 157] Bile pigment analysis has been reported to aid in the differentiation of CN1 from CN2 [158] and in the differential diagnosis of unconjugated hyperbilirubinemia.[47, 159] In both forms of CN, traces of monoconjugates can be detected in serum and bile, but no diconjugates are present.[160] Whereas phenobarbital can increase the level of serum monoconjugated bilirubin even in patients with CN1,[161] the diagnosis of CN1 versus CN2 is based on finding a substantial decrease of unconjugated bilirubin in the serum after administration of phenobarbital in CN2. In the first months of life, a phenobarbital trial can still be unsuccessful in the presence of CN2.[160] Therapy for CN1 has included lifelong phototherapy,[162, 163] bilirubin binders (agar, cholestyramine,[70, 73] calcium phosphate[164]) to interrupt the enterohepatic circulation, plasmapheresis for acute episodes of severe hyperbilirubinemia related to intercurrent illness,[152, 165] and, rarely, heme oxygenase inhibition to prevent bilirubin production.[166, 167] In CN1, orthotopic liver transplantation has been performed,[168–171] even though liver function is otherwise normal, because of concern about kernicterus. Several mutations in the bilirubin UDP-glucuronosyltransferase (UGT 1) gene of CN1 and CN2 patients have been identified[172] which result in complete inactivation of this enzyme in CN1 patients and markedly reduced glucuronidation in CN2 patients. A third type of CN has also been reported[173]; it resembles CN1 in that there is no biliary excretion of bilirubin glucuronide. However, patients with CN3 do excrete monoglucoside and diglucoside conjugates of bilirubin. It has been speculated that CN3 patients lack the long-proposed permease,[174] which has been hypothesized to transport UDP-glucuronic acid to the luminal side of the endoplasmic reticulum, where glucuronosyltransferase is located. This absence forces utilization of a very inefficient substrate for conjugation to bilirubin, UDP-glucose.

Various hormones and drugs may cause development of neonatal unconjugated hyperbilirubinemia. Congenital hypothyroidism can manifest with serum bilirubin higher than 12 mg/dL before the development of other clinical findings.[175] Similarly, hypopituitarism and anencephaly may be associated with jaundice caused by inadequate thyroxine, which is necessary for hepatic clearance of bilirubin.

Infants of diabetic mothers have prolonged and higher serum bilirubin levels than control patients.[176] Explanations include prematurity, polycythemia, substrate deficiency for glucuronidation (secondary to hypoglycemia), and poor hepatic perfusion (secondary to either respiratory distress, persistent fetal circulation, or cardiomyopathy).

The Lucey-Driscoll syndrome[177] consists of neonatal hyperbilirubinemia within families in whom there is in vitro inhibition of BGT by both maternal and infant serum. It is presumed that this is caused by gestational hormones.

Drugs may interfere with the metabolism of bilirubin and result in hyperbilirubinemia or displacement of bilirubin from albumin.[178] Such displacement increases the risk of kernicterus and can be caused by sulfonamides,[179] moxalactam,[180] or ceftriaxone[181] (independent of its sludge-producing effect[182]). The popular Chinese herb, Chuen-Lin, given to 28% to 51% of Chinese newborn infants, has been shown to have a significant effect in displacing bilirubin from albumin.[183] Pancuronium bromide[184] and chloral hydrate[185] have been suggested as causes of neonatal hyperbilirubinemia. Jaundice may result from drug-induced liver disease.[186]

Prematurity is frequently associated with unconjugated hyperbilirubinemia in the neonatal period. Hepatic UDP-glucuronosyltransferase activity is markedly decreased in premature infants and rises steadily from 30 weeks' gestation until reaching adult levels at 14 weeks after birth.[40] In addition there may be deficiencies for both uptake[187] and secretion.[188] Bilirubin clearance improves rapidly after birth.[189]

Metabolic diseases including galactosemia, hereditary fructose intolerance, tyrosinemia, alpha$_1$-antitrypsin deficiency, and others can manifest with jaundice and are described elsewhere in this textbook (see Chapter 49).

Hepatic hypoperfusion can result in neonatal jaundice. Inadequate perfusion of the hepatic sinusoids may not allow sufficient hepatocyte uptake and metabolism of bilirubin. Causes include patent ductus venosus (e.g., with respiratory distress syndrome), congestive heart failure, and portal venous thrombosis. Obstruction of the biliary tree can cause neonatal jaundice; its causes, including such entities as biliary atresia, choledochal cyst, cholelithiasis, and cholangitis, are discussed elsewhere in this text (see Chapter 48). Gallbladder sludge produced by ceftriaxone,[190] total parenteral nutrition,[191] or postsurgical fasting[192] can potentially develop into symptomatic gallstones.[193]

Other cholestatic syndromes can result in jaundice owing to decreased excretion of bilirubin. These syndromes manifest with elevation of the direct (conjugated) bilirubin fraction. They are reviewed elsewhere in this text (see Chapter 47).

## Neonatal Jaundice Caused by Both Increased Production and Decreased Excretion of Bilirubin

In neonatal diseases with jaundice caused by decreased excretion and increased production of bilirubin, both conjugated and unconjugated bilirubin fractions can be elevated. Bacterial sepsis increases bilirubin production by producing erythrocyte hemolysis as a result of hemolysins released by bacteria. Endotoxins released by bacteria can also decrease canalicular bile formation.

Intrauterine infection is an important cause of neonatal hepatitis and jaundice and is reviewed elsewhere in this text (see Chapter 47). Congenital cirrhosis and hepatic fibrosis have also been reported as causes of jaundice in newborn infants. Abnormal erythrocytes may contribute to bilirubin production. Diagnosis usually is made with liver biopsy.

## Toxicity of Neonatal Jaundice

Reviews of both neonatal bilirubin toxicity[178, 194, 195] and the mechanisms of bilirubin cytotoxicity[178, 194, 196] have been published elsewhere. Yellow staining of brain nuclei in a severely jaundiced baby was first reported by Hervieux in 1847.[197] The term *kernikterus* (from the German *kern*, "nuclei," and the Greek *ikterus*, "jaundice" or "yellow") was first used by Schmorl[198] in 1903, when he described similar yellow staining of certain brain nuclei in six infants who died with severe neonatal jaundice. It has been suggested that the term *kernicterus* should be reserved for cases exhibiting classic symptoms and findings (Table 8–3), with *bilirubin encephalopathy* used for all the other conditions of brain damage thought to be related to jaundice.[199] Although kernicterus was originally a pathologic term, it has also been used to describe the acute and chronic clinical conditions shown in Table 8–3. Historically, the most common setting in which kernicterus has occurred is maternal–infant Rh blood group incompatibility. Infants with hemolytic jaundice are more vulnerable to bilirubin toxicity than are newborns with nonhemolytic uncomplicated jaundice.[200–202] However, hemolysis is not necessary for kernicterus. This is strikingly exemplified by CN,[149, 203] a disorder in which deficient hepatic bilirubin glucuronidation results in decreased bilirubin excretion with severe hyperbilirubinemia and, potentially, kernicterus. Kernicterus also has been identified in otherwise healthy breast-fed, full-term newborn infants with no evidence of hemolysis.[148] Though the neonatal period is the most common time for bilirubin-related brain damage, the neurotoxicity of bilirubin has also been documented in adults with CN.[204]

The acute and chronic clinical findings associated with kernicterus (see Table 8–3) are seen in severely jaundiced infants after the first 48 hours of life. Early in the course, the symptoms may be subtle, mimicking those of sepsis, asphyxia, or hypoglycemia.[205] Bilirubin encephalopathy can manifest in a more subtle fashion, with lowered IQ[206] and abnormal cognitive function[207, 208] yet no associated spasticity or athetosis.

**TABLE 8–3. Clinical Features of Bilirubin Encephalopathy (Kernicterus)**

| ACUTE | CHRONIC |
|---|---|
| Poor feeding with feeble suck | Motor delay |
| Lethargy | Choreoathetosis |
| High-pitched cry | Asymmetric spasticity |
| Hypertonia/hypotonia | Paresis of upward gaze |
| Decerebrate/opisthotonic posturing | Dental dysplasia |
| Seizures | Mental retardation |
| Sensorineural hearing loss | Cognitive dysfunction |
| Incomplete Moro reflex | Sensorineural hearing loss |
| Thermal instability (hypothermia/hyperthermia) | |
| Eye findings (setting sun, oculogyric crises) | |
| Fever | |
| Death | |

From Gourley GR: Bilirubin metabolism and kernicterus. Adv Pediatr 1997;44:173–229. See also references 148, 194, and 199.

Pathologic findings in kernicterus have classically been described as preferential bilirubin (icteric) discoloration of the basal ganglia, with relative sparing of the cerebral cortex and white matter.[194, 209–211] Brain stem involvement affects mainly cranial nerve nuclei of the tegmentum, particularly the oculomotor and dentate nuclei, and the cerebellar flocculi. Associated destructive lesions in the white matter, such as periventricular infarcts, have also been reported.[205] The staining of specific brain nuclei (kernicterus) must be distinguished from the nonspecific staining which results from damage to the blood-brain barrier and is associated with diffuse staining of the brain.[210, 212]

The absolute level of serum bilirubin has not been a good predictor of the risk of severe neonatal jaundice. However, it has long been known that kernicterus is likely when serum unconjugated bilirubin levels are higher than 30 mg/dL and unlikely when they are lower than 20 mg/dL.[143, 201, 213] In one study, 90% of the patients with bilirubin levels greater than 35 mg/dL either died or had cerebral palsy or physical retardation.[213] On the other hand, no developmental retardation was found in infants with bilirubin levels lower than 20 mg/dL.[129] Albumin concentration is an important variable because of its high affinity for binding with bilirubin. Drugs and organic anions also bind to albumin and can displace bilirubin, thereby increasing the level of free bilirubin, which can diffuse into cells and cause toxicity.[214, 215] The most notable example of this is the kernicterus which occurred with low bilirubin levels when sulfisoxazole was given to premature infants.[216]

## Management of Neonatal Jaundice

The management of neonatal jaundice has been reviewed elsewhere,[139] including a practice parameter developed by the American Academy of Pediatrics[137] (see Table 8–2). In both conjugated and unconjugated hyperbilirubinemia, initial therapy should be directed at the primary cause of the jaundice. In addition, elevation of the unconjugated bilirubin fraction should prompt concern about possible kernicterus independent of the cause of the jaundice.[195] Medication usage must be monitored. Newer drugs such as ceftriaxone are also strong bilirubin displacers with a potential for inducing bilirubin encephalopathy.[181, 217] Therapeutic options to lower the unconjugated bilirubin concentration include phototherapy, exchange transfusion, enzyme induction, interruption of the enterohepatic circulation, and interruption of breast feeding.

Phototherapy consists of irradiation of the jaundiced infant with light and has been reviewed elsewhere.[218, 219] The photon energy of light changes the structure of the bilirubin molecule in two ways, both of which interrupt the internal hydrogen bonding and make the bilirubin more water-soluble, so that it can be excreted into bile or urine without glucuronidation. One change involves a 180-degree rotation around the double bonds between either the A and B or the C and D rings,[220] converting the normal Z configuration to the E configuration. 4Z,15E-Bilirubin is preferentially formed and can spontaneously reisomerize to native bilirubin. More importantly, a new, seven-membered ring structure can be formed between rings A and B, resulting in "lumirubin"[221] or "cyclobilirubin."[222] Lumirubin appears to be the major route to explain the success of phototherapy.[223] Phototherapy devices employing woven fiberoptic pads are now available.[224] Proposed guidelines for phototherapy have been published elsewhere.[137, 139, 225–227] In general, phototherapy is used to prevent serum bilirubin concentrations from reaching levels that would necessitate exchange transfusion. Phototherapy is now frequently done at home,[228, 229] as endorsed by the American Academy of Pediatrics.[230] Despite documented complications,[231–233] phototherapy is widely used and is generally safe. Phototherapy should not be employed without prior diagnostic evaluation of the cause of the jaundice. Optimal positioning and irradiance are important.[227]

Exchange transfusion is the most rapid method to acutely lower the serum bilirubin concentration. Indications for exchange transfusion vary and have been published elsewhere[137, 139, 231, 234–236] (see Table 8–2). Although there are many well-described risks with exchange transfusion, mortality should be low (<0.6%) if it is performed properly.[189, 237, 238]

There are a number of pharmacologic approaches to the prevention and treatment of neonatal hyperbilirubinemia.[239] The enterohepatic circulation can be interrupted by enteral administration of agents that bind bilirubin in the intestine and prevent reabsorption, such as agar,[56, 70, 71] cholestyramine,[73] and activated charcoal.[72] Increased intestinal peristalsis would be expected to allow less time for bilirubin absorption. Frequent feedings[240] and rectal stimulation[69] are associated with lower serum bilirubin levels. Enteral feedings of bilirubin oxidase, an enzyme that degrades bilirubin,[241, 242] is another approach that remains experimental at present.[243] Another experimental approach utilized intravenous bilirubin oxidase.[242, 244]

Because neonatal hepatic UDP-glucuronosyltransferase activity is low,[40] it is not surprising that induction of hepatic UDP-glucuronosyltransferase results in lower serum bilirubin levels. Such induction in the neonate can be accomplished with prenatal maternal use of phenobarbital or diphenylhydantoin.[245–247] In the postnatal period, use of phenobarbital by the neonate has the same bilirubin-lowering effect.[248] Clofibrate is advocated by some as a simple, nontoxic pharmacologic treatment that induces BGT.[249]

An alternative approach to treat neonatal hyperbilirubinemia is to block the first enzyme responsible for the production of bilirubin, heme oxygenase. This can be accomplished by several different metalloporphyrins, as previously reviewed.[250, 251] Tin-protoporphyrin has been used successfully in the experimental management of jaundice in neonates with ABO incompatibility.[252] In addition to inhibiting bilirubin production, metalloporphyrins are photosensitizers which can accelerate the destruction of bilirubin by light but can cause unwanted side effects.[253] Kappas and colleagues[254] compared tin-mesoporphyrin (SnMP, 6 μmol per kilogram of birth weight) versus phototherapy given to paired infants according to strict criteria determined by plasma bilirubin levels and age and concluded that a single dose of SnMP entirely supplanted the need for phototherapy and significantly reduced medical resources used to monitor hyperbilirubinemia. Other clinical trials showed that one dose of SnMP given shortly after birth decreased the development of jaundice in preterm Greek newborns and reduced the need for phototherapy.[255, 256] Treatment of neonatal jaundice with heme oxygenase inhibition remains experimental at this time.

Another experimental therapy for neonatal hyperbilirubinemia is hemoperfusion. Research into this method has employed hemoperfusion with ion exchange,[257] bilirubin oxidase,[258] and sorbents.[259]

## JAUNDICE IN INFANTS AND OLDER CHILDREN

A brief list of the causes of jaundice in infants and older children is presented in Table 8–4. Several hereditary hyperbilirubinemia syndromes may manifest in infants or older children. These include Gilbert's syndrome, Dubin-Johnson syndrome, and Rotor's syndrome.

Gilbert's syndrome usually is not recognized until after puberty. It is characterized by a hereditary, chronic, mild, unconjugated hyperbilirubinemia with otherwise normal liver function test results.[151, 260, 261] Gilbert's syndrome appears to be a heterogeneous group of disorders that share a decrease in hepatic BGT activity of at least 50%.[262–264] Based on plasma clearance of other organic anions (bromsulfophthalein and indocyanine green), there appear to be at least four subtypes of Gilbert's syndrome.[265, 266] Mild hemolysis can be seen. Patients with this disorder show a pronounced increase of serum bilirubin concentration in response to fasting.[267] The clinical manifestations of Gilbert's syndrome are commonly associated with a DNA polymorphism in the promoter region of *UGT1A*, the gene that encodes bilirubin UDP-glucuronosyltransferase,[268, 269] although more rare heterozygous missense mutations in the coding region of *UGT1A* have also been reported.[270, 271] Odell[272] speculated that some infants with neonatal jaundice are manifesting Gilbert's syndrome because of the transient hormonal milieu (estrogenization) of the fetus. Recent data show that infants homozygous for this DNA polymorphism have a more rapid rise in jaundice during the first 2 days of life.[273] Although

**TABLE 8–4. Causes of Jaundice in Infants and Older Children**

Metabolic disorders
- Hereditary hyperbilirubinemias—Gilbert's syndrome, Dubin-Johnson syndrome, Rotor's syndrome, Crigler-Najjar syndrome
- Wilson's disease
- Alpha$_1$-antitrypsin deficiency
- Cystic fibrosis

Viral hepatitis—hepatitis A, B, C, D, E; Epstein-Barr virus; cytomegalovirus
Chronic active hepatitis
Biliary tract disease—cholecystitis, cholelithiasis, Caroli's disease, choledochal cyst
Tumor—hepatic, biliary, pancreatic, peritoneal, duodenal
Red blood cell abnormalities
- Sickle cell disease
- Thalassemia
- Hemolysis

Drugs/toxins—acetaminophen, valproate, chlorpromazine, Amanita toxin, sepsis, others
Sclerosing cholangitis—primary, secondary to inflammatory bowel disease
Veno-occlusive disease—pyrrolidizine alkaloids, bone marrow transplantation
Impaired delivery of bilirubin to liver—congestive heart failure, cirrhosis

Gilbert's syndrome is usually associated with no negative implications for health or longevity, some patients complain of fatigue or abdominal pain.

Dubin-Johnson syndrome and Rotor's syndrome are two distinct but similar hyperbilirubinemia syndromes[274] with autosomal recessive inheritance. In both syndromes the direct and indirect fractions of bilirubin are elevated but the results of other liver function tests, including serum bile acid concentrations, are normal.[275–277] Rotor's syndrome can be seen in early childhood,[278] whereas Dubin-Johnson syndrome manifests from birth to 40 years of age. In both conditions total serum bilirubin levels usually range from approximately 2 to 7 mg/dL, with at least half present as conjugated bilirubin,[277, 279] but can reach 20 mg/dL under certain conditions (e.g., intercurrent illness).[279, 280]

Dubin-Johnson syndrome is more common than Rotor's syndrome, and the hyperbilirubinemia is often exacerbated by pregnancy and the use of oral contraceptives.[281] Liver histology is completely normal in Rotor's syndrome. In Dubin-Johnson syndrome, liver examination may reveal a distinctive brown-black pigmentation that is visible grossly, with storage located in the lysosomes microscopically.[282] This pigment is believed to originate from melanin[283, 284] or from metabolites of epinephrine.[285] Dubin-Johnson syndrome is more common in males, but there is no male predominance in Rotor's syndrome. Oral cholecystography is normal in Rotor's syndrome but often fails to visualize the gallbladder in Dubin-Johnson syndrome.

An important pathophysiologic finding in Rotor's syndrome is the marked reduction in hepatic anion storage.[286, 287] This is consistent with the finding of deficient glutathione *S*-transferase activity in a patient with Rotor'syndrome.[288] Decreased storage allows both direct and indirect bilirubin fractions to reflux back into the circulation, explaining the elevation of both in serum. Hepatic anion storage is normal in Dubin-Johnson syndrome, but there is a marked decrease in secretion by the biliary canaliculus,[281, 289] allowing reflux of conjugated bilirubin back into the circulation.

Also useful in differentiating these two syndromes is the difference in total urinary excretion of coproporphyrins I and III. Urinary coproporphyrin excretion is 2.5 to 5 times higher than normal in Rotor's syndrome[290] but is usually normal or slightly elevated in Dubin-Johnson syndrome. Further, there are significant differences in the distribution of total urinary coproporphyrins I and III, with isomer I less than 80% of the total in Rotor's syndrome[291] and more than 80% of the total in Dubin-Johnson syndrome (normal, 25%).[292, 293]

Patients with Rotor's syndrome are asymptomatic and require no therapy. Although jaundice is life-long, there is no associated morbidity or mortality. Although Dubin-Johnson syndrome is also associated with normal health and longevity, a significant number of patients have nonspecific abdominal complaints and hepatomegaly. Diagnosis can be made by confirming conjugated hyperbilirubinemia and otherwise normal liver function tests. Coproporphyrin excretion in the urine or hepatic scintigraphy[294, 295] allows differentiation of the two syndromes.

The other causes of jaundice listed in Table 8–4 are described elsewhere in this textbook.

***Acknowledgments***

This work was supported in part by National Institutes of Health Grants HD 28619 and HD 03352.The author gratefully acknowledges the assistance of Bill Kreamer and Brenda Egan.

## REFERENCES

1. Städeler G: Ueber die farbstoffe der galle. Justus Liebigs Ann Chem 1864;132:323–354.
2. Schmid R, McDonagh AF: The enzymatic formation of bilirubin. Ann N Y Acad Sci 1975;244:533–552.
3. Tenhunen R, Marver HS, Schmid R: Microsomal heme oxygenase: characterization of the enzyme. J Biol Chem 1969;244:6388–6394.
4. Raffin SB, Woo CH, Roost KT, et al: Intestinal absorption of hemoglobin iron-heme cleavage by mucosal heme oxygenase. J Clin Invest 1974;54:1344–1352.
5. Fischer H, Orth H: Die Chemie des Pyrrols. Leipzig, Akademische Verlagsgesellschaft M.B.H., 1937, p 626.
6. O'Carra P, Colleran E: Methine bridge selectivity in haem-cleavage reactions: relevance to the mechanism of haem catabolism. Biochem Soc Trans 1976;4:209–214.
7. Colleran E, O'Carra P: Enzymology and comparative physiology of biliverdin reduction. In Berk PD, Berlin NE (eds): International Symposium on Chemistry and Physiology of Bile Pigments. Washington, DC, US Government Printing Office, 1977, p 69.
8. Maisels MJ, Pathak A, Nelson NM, et al: Endogenous production of carbon monoxide in normal and erythroblastotic infants. J Clin Invest 1971;50:1–8.
9. Bloomer JR, Berk PD, Howe RB, et al: Comparison of fecal urobilinogen excretion with bilirubin production in normal volunteers and patients with increased bilirubin production. Clin Chim Acta 1970;29:463.
10. Whipple GH, Hooper CW: Bile pigment metabolism: VII. Bile pigment output influenced by hemoglobin injections, anemia and blood regeneration. Am J Physiol 1917;43:258–274.
11. London IM: Conversion of hematin to bile pigment. J Biol Chem 1950;184:373–376.
12. Ostrow JD, Jandle JG, Schmid R: The formation of bilirubin from hemoglobin in vivo. J Clin Invest 1962;41:1628–1637.
13. Coburn RF, Kane PB: Maximal erythrocyte and hemoglobin catabolism. J Clin Invest 1968;47:1435–1446.
14. Daly JS, Little JM, Troxler RF, et al: Metabolism of 3H-myoglobin. Nature 1967;216:1030–1031.
15. London IM, West R: The formation of bile pigment in pernicious anemia. J Biol Chem 1950;184:359–364.
16. Gray CH, Scott JJ: The effect of haemorrhage on the incorporation [α-$C^{14}$] glycine into stercobilin. J Biochem 1959;71:38–42.
17. Robinson SH, Tsong M, Brown BW, et al: The sources of bile pigment in the rat: studies of early labeled fraction. J Clin Invest 1966;45:1569–1586.
18. Bonnett R, Davies JE, Hursthouse MB: Structure of bilirubin. Nature 1976;262:327–328.
19. Bennhold H: Uber die vehikelfunktion der serumeiweisskorper. Ergeb Inn Med Kinderheilkd 1932;42:273–375.
20. Jacobsen J: Binding of bilirubin to human serum albumin—determination of the dissociation constants. FEBS Lett 1969;5:112–114.
21. Berk PD, Potter BJ, Stremmel W: Role of plasma membrane ligand-binding proteins in the hepatocellular uptake of albumin-bound organic anions. Hepatology 1987;7:165–176.
22. Scharschmidt BF, Waggoner JG, Berk PD: Hepatic organic anion uptake in the rat. J Clin Invest 1975;56:1280–1292.
23. Stremmel W, Gerber M, Glezerov V, et al: Physiochemical and immunohistological studies of a sulfobromophthalein- and bilirubin-binding protein from rat liver plasma membranes. J Clin Invest 1983;71:1796–1805.
24. Lunazzi GC, Tiribelli C, Gazzin B, et al: Further studies on bilitranslocase, a plasma membrane protein involved in organic anion hepatic uptake. Biochim Biophys Acta 1982;685:117–122.
25. Berk PD, Stremmel W: Hepatocellular uptake of organic anions. In

Popper H, Schaffner F (eds): Progress in Liver Diseases, vol VIII. New York: Grune & Stratton, 1986, pp 125–144.
26. Boyer TD: The glutathione *S*-transferases: an update. Hepatology 1989;9:486–496.
27. Kamisaka K, Listowsky I, Arias IM: Circular dichroism studies of Y protein (ligandin), a major organic anion binding protein in liver, kidney and small intestine. Ann N Y Acad Sci 1973;226:148–153.
28. Wolkoff AW, Goresky CA, Sellin J, et al: Role of ligandin in transfer of bilirubin from plasma into liver. Am J Physiol 1979;236:E638–648.
29. Mackenzie PI, Joffe MM, Munson PJ, et al: Separation of different UDP glucuronosyltransferase activities according to charge heterogeneity by chromatofocusing using mouse liver microsomes: three major types of aglycones. Biochem Pharmacol 1985;34:737–746.
30. Koster AS, Schirmer G, Bock KW: Immunochemical and functional characterization of UDP-glucuronosyltransferases from rat liver, intestine and kidney. Biochem Pharmacol 1986;35:3971–3975.
31. Burchell B, Coughtrie WH: UDP-glucuronosyltransferases. Pharmacol Ther 1989;43:261–289.
32. Hauser SC, Ziurys JC, Gollan JL: Regulation of bilirubin glucuronide synthesis in primate (macaca fascicularis) liver—kinetic analysis of microsomal bilirubin uridine diphosphate glucuronyltransferase. Gastroenterology 1986;91:287–296.
33. Kamisako T, Adachi Y, Yamamoto T: Effect of UDP-glucuronic acid depletion by salicylamide on biliary bilirubin excretion in the rat. J Pharmacol Exp Ther 1990;254:380–382.
34. Maddrey WC, Cukier JO, Maglalang AC, et al: Hepatic bilirubin UDP-glucuronyltransferase in patients with sickle cell anemia. Gastroenterology 1978;74:193–195.
35. Duvaldestin P, Mahu JL, Berthelot P: Effect of fasting on substrate specificity of rat liver UDP-glucuronylsyltransferase. Biochim Biophys Acta 1976;384:81–86.
36. Ritter JK, Crawford JM, Owens IS: Cloning of two human liver bilirubin UDP-glucuronosyltransferase cDNAs with expression in COS-1 cells. J Biol Chem 1991;266:1043–1047.
37. Gourley GR, Siegel FL, Odell GB: A rapid method for collection and analysis of bile pigments in humans. Gastroenterology 1984;86:1322A.
38. Fevery J, Blanckaert N, Heirwegh KPM, et al: Unconjugated bilirubin and an increased proportion of bilirubin monoconjugates in the bile of patients with Gilbert's syndrome and Crigler-Najjar disease. J Clin Invest 1977;60:970–979.
39. Goresky CA, Gordon ER, Shaffer EA, et al: Definition of a conjugation dysfunction in Gilbert's syndrome: studies of the handling of bilirubin loads and of the pattern of bilirubin conjugates secreted in bile. Clin Sci (Colch) 1978;55:63–71.
40. Kawade N, Onishi S: The prenatal and postnatal development of UDP-glucuronyltransferase activity towards bilirubin and the effect of premature birth on this activity in the human liver. Biochem J 1981;196:257–260.
41. Fevery J, Blanckaert N, Berthelot P, et al: Bilirubin metabolism in neonatal life. In Javitt BN (ed): Neonatal Hepatitis and Biliary Atresia. Washington, DC, US Government Printing Office, 1979 , pp 251–266.
42. Blumenthal SG, Taggart DB, Rasmusseen RD, et al: Conjugated and unconjugated bilirubins in humans and Rhesus monkeys: structural identity of bilirubins from biles and meconiums of newborn humans and Rhesus monkeys. Biochem J 1979;179:537–547.
43. Natzschka JC, Odell GB: The influence of albumin on the distribution and excretion of bilirubin in jaundiced rats. Pediatrics 1966;37:51–61.
44. Arias IM, Johnson L, Wolfson S: Biliary excretion of injected conjugated and unconjugated bilirubin by normal and Gunn rats. Am J Physiol 1961;200:1091–1094.
45. Zimmerman HJ: Hormonal derivatives and other drugs used to treat endocrine disease. In Hepatotoxicity: The Adverse Effects of Drugs and Other Chemicals on the Liver. New York, Appleton, Crofts, 1978, pp 436–467.
46. Fevery J, Blanckaert N: Review: what can we learn from analysis of serum bilirubin? J Hepatol 1986;2:113–121.
47. Muraca M, Fevery J, Blanckaert N: Relationships between serum bilirubins and production and conjugation of bilirubin: studies in Gilbert's syndrome, Crigler-Najjar disease, hemolytic disorders, and rat models. Gastroenterology 1987;92:309–317.
48. Van Steenbergen W, Fevery J: Effects of uridine diphosphate glucuronosyltransferase activity on the maximal secretion rate of bilirubin conjugates in the rat. Gastroenterology 1990;99:488–499.
49. Sieg A, Stiehl A, Raedsch R, et al: Gilbert's syndrome diagnosis by typical serum bilirubin pattern. Clin Chim Acta 1986;154:41–48.
50. Rubaltelli FF, Muraca M, Vilei MT, et al. Unconjugated and conjugated bilirubin pigments during perinatal development: III. Studies on serum of breast-fed and formula-fed neonates. Biol Neonate 1991;60:144–147.
51. Ullrich D, Fevery J, Sieg A, et al: The influence of gestational age on bilirubin conjugation in newborns. Eur J Clin Invest 1991;21:83–89.
52. Weiss JS, Guatam A, Lauff JJ, et al: The clinical importance of a protein-bound fraction of serum bilirubin in patients with hyperbilirubinemia. N Engl J Med 1983;309:147–150.
53. Brett EM, Hicks JM, Powers DM, et al: Delta bilirubin in serum of pediatric patients: correlations with age and disease. Clin Chem 1984;30:1561–1564.
54. Berson SA, Yalow RS, Schreiber SS: Tracer experiments with $I^{131}$ labeled human serum albumin: distribution and degradation studies. J Clin Invest 1953;32:746–768.
55. Billing BH: Intestinal and renal metabolism of bilirubin including enterohepatic circulation. In Ostrow JD (ed): Bile Pigments and Jaundice. New York, Marcel Dekker, 1986, 255–269.
56. Poland RL, Odell GB: Physiologic jaundice: the enterohepatic circulation of bilirubin. N Engl J Med 1971;284:1–6.
57. Hawksworth G, Drasar BS, Hill MJ: Intestinal bacteria and the hydrolysis of glycosidic bonds. J Med Microbiol 1971;4:451–459.
58. Kent TH, Fischer LJ, Marr R: Glucuronidase activity in intestinal contents of rat and man and relationship to bacterial flora. Proc Soc Exp Biol Med 1972;140:590–594.
59. Nanno M, Morotomi M, Takayama H, et al: Mutagenic activation of biliary metabolites of benzo(α)pyrene by beta-glucuronidase-positive bacteria in human faeces. J Med Microbiol 1986;22:351–355.
60. Musa BU, Doe RP, Seal US: Purification and properties of human liver β-glucuronidase. J Biol Chem 1965;240:2811–2816.
61. Lester R, Schmid R: Intestinal absorption of bile pigments: I. The enterohepatic circulation of bilirubin in the cat. J Clin Invest 1963;42:736–746.
62. Gourley GR, Arend RA: β-glucuronidase and hyperbilirubinemia in breast-fed and formula-fed babies. Lancet 1986;1:644–646.
63. Saxerholt H, Skar V, Midtvedt T: HPLC separation and quantification of bilirubin and its glucuronide conjugates in faeces and intestinal contents of germ-free rats. Scand J Clin Lab Invest 1990;50:487–495.
64. Odell GB: Normal metabolism of bilirubin during neonatal life. In Neonatal Hyperbilirubinemia. New York, Grune & Stratton, 1980, pp 35–49.
65. Boggs TR Jr, Bishop H: Neonatal hyperbilirubinemia associated with high obstruction of the small bowel. J Pediatr 1965;66:349–356.
66. Porto SO: Jaundice in congenital malrotation of the intestine. Am J Dis Child 1969;117:684–688.
67. Clarkson JE, Cowan JO, Herbison GP: Jaundice in full-term healthy neonates: a population study. Aust Paediatr J 1984;20:303–308.
68. Rosta J, Makoi Z, Kertesz A: Delayed meconium passage and hyperbilirubinemia. Lancet 1986;2:1138.
69. Cottrell BH, Anderson GC: Rectal or axillary temperature measurement: effect on plasma bilirubin and intestinal transit of meconium. J Pediatr Gastroenterol Nutr 1984;3:734–739.
70. Odell GB, Gutcher GR, Whitington PF, et al: Enteral administration of agar as an effective adjunct to phototherapy of neonatal hyperbilirubinemia. Pediatr Res 1983;17:810–814.
71. Kemper K, Horwitz RI, McCarthy P: Decreased neonatal serum bilirubin with plain agar: a meta-analysis. Pediatrics 1988;82:631–638.
72. Ulstrom RA, Eisenblam E: The enterohepatic shunting of bilirubin in the newborn infant: I. Use of oral activated charcoal to reduce normal serum bilirubin values. J Pediatr 1964;65:27–37.
73. Arrowsmith WA, Payne RB, Littlewood JM: Comparison of treatments for congenital nonobstructive nonhaemolytic hyperbilirubinemia. Arch Dis Child 1975;50:197–201.
74. Newman TB, Easterling MJ, Goldman ES, et al: Laboratory evaluation of jaundice in newborns: frequency, cost and yield. Am J Dis Child 1990;144:364–368.
75. Rutledge JC, Ou CN: Bilirubin and the laboratory: advances in the 1980's, considerations for the 1990's. Pediatr Clin North Am 1989;36:189–197.
76. Schreiner RL, Glick MR: Interlaboratory bilirubin variability. Pediatrics 1982;69:277–281.
77. Rosenthal P, Keefe MT, Henton D, et al: Total and direct-reacting bilirubin values by automated methods compared with liquid chromatography and with manual methods for determining delta bilirubin [see comments]. Clin Chem 1990;36:788–791.

78. Westwood A: The analysis of bilirubin in serum. Ann Clin Biochem 1991;28:119–130.
79. Schlebusch H, Axer K, Schneider C, et al: Comparison of five routine methods with the candidate reference method for the determination of bilirubin in neonatal serum. J Clin Chem Clin Biochem 1990;28:203–210.
80. Mair B, Klempner LB: Abnormally high values for direct bilirubin in the serum of newborns as measured with the DuPont aca. Am J Clin Pathol 1987;87:642–644.
81. Blanckaert N, Kabra PM, Farina FA: Measurement of bilirubin and its monoconjugates and diconjugates in human serum by alkaline methanolysis and high-performance liquid chromatography. J Lab Clin Med 1980;96:198–212.
82. Wu TW, Dappen GM, Powers DM: The Kodak EKTACHEM Clinical Chemisty slide for measurement of bilirubin in newborns: principles and performance. Clin Chem 1982;28:2366–2372.
83. Wu TW, Dappen GM, Spayd RW: The EKTACHEM Clinical Chemistry slide for simultaneous determination of unconjugated and sugar-conjugated bilirubin. Clin Chem 1984;30:1304–1309.
84. Muraca M, Rubaltelli FF, Blanckaert N, et al: Unconjugated and conjugated bilirubin pigments during perinatal development: II. Studies on serum of healthy newborns and of neonates with erythroblastosis fetalis. Biol Neonate 1990;57:1–9.
85. Arvan D, Shirey TL: Conjugated bilirubin: a better indicator of impaired hepatobiliary excretion than direct bilirubin. Ann Clin Lab Sci 1985;15:252–259.
86. Leslie GI, Phillips JB, Cassady G: Capillary and venous bilirubin values: are they really different? Am J Dis Child 1987;141:1199–1200.
87. Eidelman AI, Schimmel MS: Capillary and venous bilirubin values: they are different—and how! Am J Dis Child 1989;143:642.
88. Maisels MJ: Capillary vs venous bilirubin values letter. Am J Dis Child 1990;144:521–522.
89. Schumacher RE: Noninvasive measurements of bilirubin in the newborn. Clin Perinatol 1990;17:417–435.
90. Yamauchi Y, Yamanouchi I: Clinical application of transcutaneous bilirubin measurement. Acta Paediatr Scand 1990;79:385–390.
91. Schumacher RE, Thornbery JM, Gutcher GR: Transcutaneous bilirubinometry: a comparison of old and new methods. Pediatrics 1985;76:10–14.
92. Gossett IH, Oxon BM: A Perspex icterometer for neonates. Lancet 1960;1:87–88.
93. Kramer LI: Advancement of dermal icterus in the jaundiced newborn. Am J Dis Child 1969;118:454–458.
94. Schneider AP: Breast milk jaundice in the newborn: a real entity. JAMA 1986;255:3270–3274.
95. Maisels MJ: Neonatal jaundice. In Avery GB (ed): Neonatology: Pathophysiology and Management of the Newborn. Philadelphia, JB Lippincott, 1987, pp 534–629.
96. Linn S, Schoenbaum SC, Monson RR, et al: Epidemiology of neonatal hyperbilirubinemia. Pediatrics 1985;75:770–774.
97. Zipursky A: Mechanisms of hemolysis. Mead Johnson Symp Perinat Dev Med 1982;17–24.
98. Wenk RE, Goldstein P, Felix JK: Kell alloimmunization, hemolytic disease of the newborn, and perinatal management. Obstet Gynecol 1985;66:473–476.
99. Bevis DCA: The antenatal prediction of hemolytic disease of the newborn. Lancet 1952;1:395–398.
100. Odell GB: Evaluation of fetal hemolysis. N Engl J Med 1970;282:1204–1205.
101. Frigoletto FD, Greene MF, Benacerraf BR, et al: Ultrasonographic fetal surveillance in the management of the isoimmunized pregnancy. N Engl J Med 1986;315:430–432.
102. Vintzileos AM, Campbell WA, Storlazzi E, et al: Fetal liver ultrasound measurements in isoimmunized pregnancies. Obstet Gynecol 1986;62:162–167.
103. Grannum PA, Copel JA, Plaxe SC, et al: In utero exchange transfusion by direct intravascular injection in severe erythroblastosis fetalis. N Engl J Med 1986;314:1431–1434.
104. Queenan JT: Erythroblastosis fetalis: closing the circle. N Engl J Med 1986;314:1448–1449.
105. Clarke CA: Prevention of Rh-hemolytic disease. Br Med J 1967;4:484–485.
106. Allen FH Jr, Diamond LK: Erythroblastosis Fetalis, Including Exchange Transfusion Technique. Boston, Little, Brown, 1958, pp 1–155.
107. Apt L, Downey WS: Melena neonatorum: the "swallowed blood syndrome." J Pediatr 1955;47:6–12.
108. Jacobs DS, Kasten BL, Demott WR, et al: Apt test. In Laboratory Test Handbook with DRG Index. St. Louis, Mosby/Lexi-Comp, 1984, p 277.
109. Danish EH: Neonatal polycythemia. In Brown EB (ed): Progress in Hematology, vol 14. New York, Grune & Stratton, 1986, pp 55–98.
110. Oh W: Neonatal polycythemia and hyperviscosity. Pediatr Clin North Am 1986;33:523–532.
111. Mimouni F, Miodovnik M, Siddiqi TA, et al: Neonatal polycythemia in infants of insulin-dependent diabetic mothers. Obstet Gynecol 1986;68:370–372.
112. Liang ST, Wong VCW, So WWK, et al: Homozygous α-thalassemia: clinical presentation, diagnosis and management. A review of 46 cases. Br J Obstet Gynaecol 1985;92:680–684.
113. Kan YW, Forget BG, Nathan DG: Gamma-beta thalassemia: a cause of hemolytic disease of the newborn. N Engl J Med 1972;286:129–134.
114. Singhi S, Chookang E, Hall JSE: Intrapartum infusion of aqueous glucose solution, transplacental hyponatraemia, and risk of neonatal jaundice. Br J Obstet Gynaecol 1984;99:1014–1018.
115. D'Souza SW, Lieberman B, Cadman J, et al: Oxytocin induction of labour: hyponatraemia and neonatal jaundice. Eur J Obstet Gynecol Reprod Biol 1986;22:309–317.
116. Poland RL, Odell GB: The binding of bilirubin to agar. Proc Soc Exp Biol Med 1974;146:1114–1118.
117. Gourley GR, Kreamer B, Arend R: Effect of diet on fecal excretion and jaundice during the first three weeks of life. Gastroenterology 1992;103:660–667.
118. Gourley GR: The pathophysiology of breast milk jaundice. In Polin RA, Fox WW (eds): Fetal and Neonatal Physiology. Philadelphia, WB Saunders, 1992, pp 1173–1179.
119. Gartner LM, Auerbach KG: Breast milk and breastfeeding jaundice. In Barness LA (ed): Advances in Pediatrics, vol 34. Chicago, Year Book Medical Publishers, 1987, pp 249–274.
120. Saigal S, Lunyk O, Bennett KJ, et al: Serum bilirubin levels in breast- and formula-fed infants in the first 5 days of life. Can Med Assoc J 1982;127:985–989.
121. Kivlahan C, James EJP: The natural history of neonatal jaundice. Pediatrics 1984;74:364–370.
122. Gartner LM, Arias IM: Studies of prolonged neonatal jaundice in the breast-fed infant. J Pediatr 1966;68:54–66.
123. Grunebaum E, Amir J, Merlob P, et al: Breast milk jaundice: natural history, familial incidence and late neurodevelopmental outcome of the infant. Eur J Pediatr 1991;150:267–270.
124. McDonagh AF: Is bilirubin good for you? Clin Perinatol 1990;17:359–369.
125. Schwertner HA, Jackson WG, Tolan G: Association of low serum concentration of bilirubin with increased risk of coronary artery disease. Clin Chem 1994;40:18–23.
126. Behrman RE, Kliegman JM: Jaundice and hyperbilirubinemia in the newborn. In Behrman RE, Vaughan VCI, Nelson WE (eds): Nelson Textbook of Pediatrics, 12th ed. Philadelphia, WB Saunders, 1983, pp 378–381.
127. Lascari AD: "Early" breast-feeding jaundice: clinical significance. J Pediatr 1986;108:156–158.
128. Orlowski JP: Breast milk jaundice: early and late. Cleve Clin Q 1983;50:339.
129. Arias IM, Gartner LM, Seifter S, et al: Prolonged neonatal unconjugated hyperbilirubinemia associated with breast feeding and a steroid, pregnane-3(alpha), 20(beta)-diol in maternal milk that inhibits glucuronide formation in vitro. J Clin Invest 1964;43:2037–2047.
130. Murphy JF, Hughs I, Verrier Jones ER, et al: Pregnanediols and breast-milk jaundice. Arch Dis Child 1981;56:474–476.
131. Bevan BR, Holton JB: Inhibition of bilirubin conjugation in rat liver slices by free fatty acids, with relevance to the problem of breast-milk jaundice. Clin Chim Acta 1972;41:101–107.
132. Poland RL, Schultz GE, Gayatri G: High milk lipase activity associated with breast-milk jaundice. Pediatr Res 1980;14:1328–1331.
133. Hernell O: Breast-milk jaundice. J Pediatr 1982;99:311–314.
134. Constantopoulos A, Messaritakis J, Matsanoitis N: Breast-milk jaundice: the role of lipoprotein lipase and the free fatty acids. Eur J Pediatr 1980;134:35–38.
135. Gaffney PT, Buttenshaw RL, Ward M, et al: Breast milk β-glucuronidase and neonatal jaundice. Lancet 1986;1:1161–1162.
136. Alonso EM, Whitington PF, Whitington SH, et al: Enterohepatic circulation of nonconjugated bilirubin in rats fed with human milk. J Pediatr 1991;118:425–430.

137. Anonymous: Practice parameter: management of hyperbilirubinemia in the healthy term newborn. American Academy of Pediatrics Provisional Committee for Quality Improvement and Subcommittee on Hyperbilirubinemia [published erratum appears in Pediatrics 1995 95:458–461]. Pediatrics 1994;94:558–565.
138. Gartner LM: Breast milk jaundice. In Levine RL, Maisels MJ (eds): Hyperbilirubinemia in the Newborn: report of the 85th Ross Conference on Pediatric Research. Columbus, OH, Ross Laboratories, 1983, pp 75–86.
139. Cashore WJ, Stern L: The management of hyperbilirubinemia. Clin Perinatol 1984;11:339–357.
140. Maisels MJ, Vain N, Acquavita AM, et al: The effect of breast-feeding frequency on serum bilirubin levels. Am J Obstet Gynecol 1994;170:880–883.
141. Osborn LM, Bolus R: Breast feeding and jaundice in the first week of life. J Fam Pract 1985;20:475.
142. Amato M, Howald H, von Muralt G: Interruption of breast-feeding versus phototherapy as treatment of hyperbilirubinemia in full-term infants. Helv Paediatr Acta 1985;40:127–131.
143. Newman TB, Maisels MJ: Does hyperbilirubinemia damage the brain of healthy full-term infants? Clin Perinatol 1990;17:331–358.
144. Newman TB, Klebanoff MA: Neonatal hyperbilirubinemia and long-term outcome: another look at the Collaborative Perinatal Project [see comments]. Pediatrics 1993;92:651–657.
145. Valaes T: Bilirubin toxicity: the problem was solved a generation ago. Pediatrics 1992;89:819–821.
146. Newman TB, Maisels MJ: Response to commentaries re: Evaluation and treatment of jaundice in the term newborn: a kinder, gentler approach. Pediatrics 1992;89:831–833.
147. Johnson L: Hyperbilirubinemia in the term infant: when to worry, when to treat. N Y State J Med 1991;91:483–487.
148. Maisels MJ, Newman TB: Kernicterus in otherwise healthy, breast-fed term newborns. Pediatrics 1995;96:730–733.
149. Crigler JF, Najjar VA: Congenital familial nonhemolytic jaundice with kernicterus. Pediatrics 1952;10:169–180.
150. Crigler JF, Gold NI: Effect of phenobarbital on bilirubin metabolism in an infant with congenital, nonhemolytic, unconjugated hyperbilirubinemia, and kernicterus. J Clin Invest 1969;48:42–55.
151. Anonymous: The familial unconjugated hyperbilirubinemias. Semin Liver Dis 1994;14:356–385.
152. Blaschke TF, Berke PD, Scharschmidt BF, et al: Crigler-Najjar syndrome: an unusual course with development of neurological damage at age eighteen. Pediatr Res 1974;8:573–590.
153. Duhamel G, Blanckaert N, Metreau JM, et al: An unusual case of Crigler-Najjar disease in the adult: classification of types I and II revisited. J Hepatol 1985;1:47–53.
154. Arias IM, Gartner LM, Cohen M, et al: Chronic nonhemolytic unconjugated hyperbilirubinemia with glucuronyl transferase deficiency. Am J Med 1969;47:395–409.
155. Blumenschein SD, Kallen RJ, Storey B, et al: Familial nonhemolytic jaundice with late onset of neurologic damage. Pediatrics 1968;42:786–792.
156. Gollan JL, Huang SM, Billing B, et al: Prolonged survival in 3 brothers with severe type II Crigler-Najjar syndrome: ultrastructural and metabolic studies. Gastroenterology 1975;68:1543–1555.
157. Gordon ER, Shaffer EA, Sass-Kortsak A: Bilirubin secretion and conjugation in the Crigler-Najjar syndrome type II. Gastroenterology 1976;70:761–765.
158. Sinaasappel M, Jansen PL: The differential diagnosis of Crigler-Najjar disease, types 1 and 2, by bile pigment analysis. Gastroenterology 1991;100:783–789.
159. Muraca M, Blanckaert N: Liquid chromatography assay and identification of mono- and diesterconjugates of bilirubin in normal serum. Clin Chem 1983;29:1767–1771.
160. Rubaltelli FF, Novello A, Zancan L, et al: Serum and bile bilirubin pigments in the differential diagnosis of Crigler-Najjar disease. Pediatrics 1994;94:553–556.
161. Persico M, Romano M, Muraca M, et al: Responsiveness to phenobarbital in an adult with Crigler-Najjar disease associated with neurological involvement and skin hyperextensibility. Hepatology 1991;13:213–215.
162. Gorodischer R, Levy G, Krasner J, et al: Congenital nonobstructive, nonhemolytic jaundice: effect of phototherapy. N Engl J Med 1970;282:375–380.
163. Job H, Hart G, Lealman G: Improvements in long term phototherapy for patients with Crigler-Najjar syndrome type I. Phys Med Biol 1996;41:2549–2556.
164. van der Veere CN, Jansen PL, Sinaasappel M, et al: Oral calcium phosphate: a new therapy for Crigler-Najjar disease? Gastroenterology 1997;112:455–462.
165. Sherker AH, Heathcote J: Acute hepatitis in Crigler-Najjar syndrome. Am J Gastroenterol 1987;82:883–885.
166. Rubaltelli FF, Guerrini P, Reddi E, et al: Tin-protoporphyrin in the management of children with Crigler-Najjar disease. Pediatrics 1989;84:728–731.
167. Rubaltelli FF, Dario C, Zancan L: Congenital nonobstructive, nonhemolytic jaundice: effect of tin-mesoporphyrin. Pediatrics 1995;95:942–944.
168. Kaufman SS, Wood RP, Shaw BW, et al: Orthotopic liver transplantation for type 1 Crigler-Najjar syndrome. Hepatology 1986;6:1259–1262.
169. Shevell MI, Bernard B, Adelson JW, et al: Crigler-Najjar syndrome type I: treatment by home phototherapy followed by orthotopic hepatic transplantation. J Pediatr 1987;110:429–431.
170. van der Veere CN, Sinaasappel M, McDonagh AF, et al: Current therapy for Crigler-Najjar syndrome type 1: report of a world registry. Hepatology 1996;24:311–315.
171. Sokal EM, Silva ES, Hermans D, et al: Orthotopic liver transplantation for Crigler-Najjar type I disease in six children. Transplantation 1995;60:1095–1098.
172. Seppen J, Bosma PJ, Goldhoorn BG, et al: Discrimination between Crigler-Najjar type I and II by expression of mutant bilirubin uridine diphosphate-glucuronosyltransferase. J Clin Invest 1994;94:2385–2391.
173. Odell GB, Whitington PF: Crigler-Najjar syndrome, type III: a new variant of hereditary non-hemolytic, non-conjugated hyperbilirubinemia. Hepatology 1990;12:871.
174. Berry C, Hallinan T: Summary of a novel, three-component regulatory model for uridine diphosphate glucuronyltransferase. Biochem Soc Trans 1976;4:650–652.
175. Thompson GN, McCrossin RB, Penfold JL, et al: Management and outcome of children with congenital hypothyroidism detected on neonatal screening in South Australia. Med J Aust 1986;145:18–22.
176. Jahrig D, Jahrig K, Stiete S, et al: Neonatal jaundice in infants of diabetic mothers. Acta Paediatr Scand 1989;360(suppl):101–107.
177. Arias IM, Wolfson S, Lucey JF, et al: Transient familial neonatal hyperbilirubinemia. J Clin Invest 1956;44:1442–1450.
178. Walker PC: Neonatal bilirubin toxicity: a review of kernicterus and the implications of drug-induced bilirubin displacement. Clin Pharmacokinet 1987;13:26–50.
179. Odell GB: Studies in kernicterus: I. Protein binding of bilirubin. J Clin Invest 1959;38:823.
180. Stutman HR, Parker KM, Marks MI: Potential of moxalactam and other new antimicrobial agents for bilirubin-albumin displacement in neonates. Pediatrics 1985;75:294–298.
181. Brodersen R, Robertson A: Ceftriaxone binding to human serum albumin: competition with bilirubin. Mol Pharmacol 1989;36:478–483.
182. Park HZ, Lee SP, Schy AL: Ceftriaxone-associated gallbladder sludge: identification of calcium-ceftriaxone salt as a major component of gallbladder precipitate. Gastroenterology 1991;100:1665–1670.
183. Yeung CY, Lee FT, Wong HN: Effect of a popular Chinese herb on neonatal bilirubin protein binding. Biol Neonate 1990;58:98–103.
184. Freeman J, Lesko SM, Mitchell AA, et al: Hyperbilirubinemia following exposure to pancuronium bromide in newborns. Dev Pharmacol Ther 1990;14:209–215.
185. Lambert GH, Muraskas J, Anderson CL, et al: Direct hyperbilirubinemia associated with chloral hydrate administration in the newborn. Pediatrics 1990;86:277–281.
186. Farrell GC: Drug-Induced Liver Disease. New York, Churchill Livingstone, 1994.
187. Obrinsky W, Denley ML, Brauer RW: Sulfobromophthalein sodium excretion test as a measure of liver function in premature infants. Pediatrics 1952;9:421–438.
188. Vest M, Rossier R: Detoxification in the newborn: the ability of the newborn infant to form conjugates with glucuronic acid, glycine, acetate and glutathione. Ann N Y Acad Sci 1963;111:183–198.
189. Boggs TR Jr, Westphal MD Jr: Mortality of exchange transfusions. Pediatrics 1960;26:745–755.
190. Lee SP, Lipsky BA, Teefey SA: Gallbladder sludge and antibiotics. Pediatr Infect Dis J 1990;9:422–423.

191. Messing B, Bories C, Kunstlinger F, et al: Does total parenteral nutrition induce gallbladder sludge formation in lithiasis? Gastroenterology 1983;84:1012–1019.
192. Bolondi L, Gaiani S, Testa S, et al: Gallbladder sludge formation during fasting after gastrointestinal tract surgery. Gut 1985;26:734–738.
193. Lee SP, Maher K, Nicholls JF: Origin and fate of biliary sludge. Gastroenterology 1988;94:170–176.
194. Odell GB, Schutta HS: Bilirubin encephalopathy. In McCandless DW (ed): Cerebral Energy Metabolism and Metabolic Encephalopathy. New York, Plenum, 1985, pp 229–261.
195. Gourley GR: Bilirubin metabolism and kernicterus. Adv Pediatr 1997;44:173–229.
196. Brodersen R, Stern L: Deposition of bilirubin acid in the central nervous system: a hypothesis for the development of kernicterus. Acta Paediatr Scand 1990;79:12–19.
197. Hansen TWR, Sagvolden T, Bratlid D: Open-field behavior of rats previously subjected to short-term hyperbilirubinemia with or without blood-brain barrier manipulations. Brain Res 1987;424:26.
198. Schmorl G: Zur kenntnis des ikterus neonatorum, insbesondere der dabei auftretenden gehirnveranderungen. Verh Dtsch Ges Pathol 1903;6:109
199. Bratlid D: How bilirubin gets into the brain. Clin Perinatol 1990;17:449–465.
200. Newman TB, Maisels MJ: Evaluation and treatment of jaundice in the term newborn: a kinder, gentler approach (review) [see comments]. Pediatrics 1992;89:809–818.
201. Hsia DY-Y, Allen FH Jr, Gellis SS, et al: Erythroblastosis fetalis: VIII. Studies of serum bilirubin in relation to kernicterus. N Engl J Med 1952;247:668–671.
202. Mollison PL, Cutbush M: Haemolytic disease of the newborn. In Gairdner D (ed): Recent Advances in Pediatrics. New York, Blakiston & Son, 1954, p 110.
203. Gourley G: Disorders of bilirubin metabolism. In Suchy FJ (ed): Liver Disease in Children. St. Louis, Mosby, 1994, pp 401–413.
204. Gardner WA Jr, Konigsmark BW: Familial nonhemolytic jaundice: bilirubinosis and encephalopathy. Pediatrics 1969;43:365–376.
205. Friede RL: Developmental Neuropathy, 2nd ed. New York, Springer-Verlag, 1989, pp 115–124.
206. Seidman DS, Paz I, Laor A, et al: Apgar scores and cognitive performance at 17 years of age. Obstet Gynecol 1991;77:875–878.
207. Odell GB, Storey GNB, Rosenberg LA: Studies in kernicterus: III. The saturation of serum proteins with bilirubin during neonatal life and its relationship to brain damage at five years. J Pediatr 1970;76:12–21.
208. Johnson L, Boggs TR Jr: Bilirubin-dependent brain damage: incidence and indication for treatment. In Odell GB, Schaffer R, Simopoulous AP (eds): Phototherapy in the Newborn: An Overview. Washington, DC, National Academy of Sciences, 1974, pp 122–149.
209. Turkel SB, Miller CA, Guttenberg ME, et al: A clinical pathologic reappraisal of kernicterus. Pediatrics 1982;69:267–272.
210. Ahdab-Barmada M, Moossy J: The neuropathology of kernicterus in the premature neonate: diagnostic problems. J Neuropathol Exp Neurol 1984;43:45–56.
211. Haymaker W, Margoles C, Pentschew A, et al: Pathology of kernicterus and posticteric encephalopathy. In Kernicterus and its Importance in Cerebral Palsy: 11th Annual Meeting, New Orleans. Springfield, IL: Charles C Thomas, 1961, p 21–228.
212. Odell GB: Free bilirubin is of importance. Pediatrics 1982;70:659.
213. Ose T, Tsuruhara T, Araki M, et al: Follow-up study of exchange transfusion for hyperbilirubinemia in infants in Japan. Pediatrics 1967;40:196–201.
214. Odell GB: The dissociation of bilirubin from albumin and its clinical implications. J Pediatr 1959;55:268–279.
215. Wadsworth SJ, Suh B: In vitro displacement of bilirubin by antibiotics and 2-hydroxybenzoylglycine in newborns. Antimicrob Agents Chemother 1988;32:1571–1575.
216. Harris RC, Lucey JF, MacLean JR: Kernicterus in premature infants associated with low concentrations of bilirubin in the plasma. Pediatrics 1958;21:875–884.
217. Martin E, Fanconi S, Kalin P, et al: Ceftriaxone–bilirubin-albumin interactions in the neonate: an in vivo study. Eur J Pediatr 1993;152:530–534.
218. Ennever JF: Blue light, green light, white light, more light: treatment of neonatal jaundice. Clin Perinatol 1990;17:467–481.
219. Pratesi R, Agati G, Fusi F: Phototherapy for neonatal hyperbilirubinemia. Photodermatology 1989;6:244–257.
220. McDonagh AF, Lightner DA: "Like a shrivelled blood orange": bilirubin, jaundice and phototherapy. Pediatrics 1985;75:443–445.
221. McDonagh AF, Palma LA, Lightner DA: Phototherapy for neonatal jaundice: stereospecific and regioselective photoisomerization of bilirubin bound to human serum albumin and NMR characterization of intramolecular cyclized photoproducts. J Am Chem Soc 1982;104:6867–6869.
222. Itoh S, Onishi S, Manabe M, et al: Wavelength dependence of the geometric and structural photoisomerization of bilirubin bound to human serum albumin. Biol Neonate 1987;51:10–17.
223. Onishi S, Isobe K, Itoh S, et al: Metabolism of bilirubin and its photoisomers in newborn infants during phototherapy. J Biochem (Toyko) 1986;100:789–795.
224. Rosenfeld W, Twist P, Concepcion L: A new device for phototherapy. Pediatr Res 1989;25:227A.
225. Fetus and Newborn Committee, Canadian Paediatric Society: Use of phototherapy for neonatal hyperbilirubinemia. Can Med Assoc J 1986;134:1237–1245.
226. Polin RA: Management of neonatal hyperbilirubinemia: rational use of phototherapy. Biol Neonate 1990;58(suppl 1):32–43.
227. Maisels MJ: Why use homeopathic doses of phototherapy. Pediatrics 1996;98:283–287.
228. Grabert BE, Wardwell C, Harburg SK: Home phototherapy: an alternative to prolonged hospitalization of the full-term, well newborn. Clin Pediatr 1986;25:291–294.
229. Ludwig MA: Phototherapy in the home setting. J Pediatr Health Care 1990;4:304–308.
230. Greenwald JL: Hyperbilirubinemia in otherwise healthy infants. Am Fam Physician 1988;38:151–158.
231. Gourley GR, Odell GB: Bilirubin metabolism in the fetus and neonate. In Lebenthal E (ed): Human Gastrointestinal Development. New York, Raven Press, 1989, pp 581–621.
232. De Curtis M, Guandalini S, Fasano A, et al: Diarrhea in jaundiced neonates treated with phototherapy: a role of intestinal secretion. Arch Dis Child 1989;64:1161–1164.
233. Drew JH, Marriage KJ, Bayle V: Phototherapy: short and long-term complications. Arch Dis Child 1976;51:454–458.
234. Odell GB: Treatment of neonatal hyperbilirubinemia. In Neonatal Hyperbilirubinemia. New York, Grune & Stratton, 1980, p 117.
235. Gartner LM, Lee K: Jaundice and liver disease: part I. Unconjugated hyperbilirubinemia. In Fanaroff AA, Martin RJ (eds): Behrman's Neonatal-Perinatal Medicine, 3rd ed. St. Louis, CV Mosby, 1983, pp 754–770.
236. Maisels MJ: Neonatal jaundice. In Avery GB (ed): Neonatology, 2nd ed. Philadelphia, JB Lippincott, 1981, pp 473–544.
237. Shapiro M: Safer exchange transfusions with ACD blood. Bibliotheca Haematologica 1965; Fasc 23:883–886.
238. Weldon VV, Odell GB: Mortality risk of exchange transfusion. Pediatrics 1968;41:797–801.
239. Valaes TN, Harvey-Wilkes K: Pharmacologic approaches to the prevention and treatment of neonatal hyperbilirubinemia. Clin Perinatol 1990;17:245–273.
240. De Carvalho M, Klaus MH, Merkatz RB: Frequency of breast-feeding and serum bilirubin concentration. Am J Dis Child 1982;136:737–738.
241. Wu T-W, Li GS: A new bilirubin-degrading enzyme from orange peels. Biochem Cell Biol 1988;66:1248.
242. Johnson L, Gourley G, Kreamer W, et al: Bilirubin oxidase (box) feedings to delay or eliminate the need for exchange transfusion (ex) in a full term G6PD deficient infant. Pediatr Res 1996;39:219A.
243. Johnson L, Dworanczyk R, Jenkins D: Bilirubin oxidase (BOX) feedings at varying time intervals and enzyme concentrations in infant Gunn rats. Pediatr Res 1989;25:116A
244. Kimura M, Matsumura Y, Miyauchi Y, et al: A new tactic for the treatment of jaundice: an injectable polymer-conjugated bilirubin oxidase. Proc Soc Exp Biol Med 1988;188:364–369.
245. Gartner LM, Lee KS, Vaisman L, et al: Development of bilirubin transport and metabolism in the newborn rhesus monkey. J Pediatr 1977;90:513–531.
246. Waltman R, Nigrin G, Bonura F, et al: Ethanol in prevention of hyperbilirubinaemia in the newborn. Lancet 1969;2:1265–1267.
247. Rayburn W, Donn S, Piehl E, et al: Antenatal phenobarbital and bilirubin metabolism in the very low birth weight infant. Am J Obstet Gynecol 1988;159:1491–1493.

248. Stern L, Khanna NN, Levy G, et al: Effect of phenobarbital on hyperbilirubinemia and glucuronide formation in newborns. Am J Dis Child 1970;120:26–31.
249. Gabilan JC, Benattar C, Lindenbaum A: Clofibrate treatment of neonatal jaundice. Pediatrics 1990;86:647–648.
250. Stevenson DK, Rodgers PA, Vreman HJ: The use of metalloporphyrins for the chemoprevention of neonatal jaundice. Am J Dis Child 1989;143:353–356.
251. Rodgers PA, Stevenson DK: Developmental biology of heme oxygenase. Clin Perinatol 1990;17:275–291.
252. Kappas A, Drummond GS, Manola T, et al: Sn-protoporphyrin use in the management of hyperbilirubinemia in term newborns with direct Coombs-positive ABO-imcompatibility. Pediatrics 1988;81:485–497.
253. Vreman HJ, Stevenson DK: Metalloporphyrin-enhanced photodegradation of bilirubin in vitro. Am J Dis Child 1990;144:590–594.
254. Kappas A, Drummond GS, Henschke C, et al: Direct comparison of Sn-mesoporphyrin, an inhibitor of bilirubin production, and phototherapy in controlling hyperbilirubinemia in term and near-term newborns. Pediatrics 1995;95:468–474.
255. Valaes T, Petmezaki S, Henschke C, et al: Control of jaundice in preterm newborns by an inhibitor of bilirubin production: studies with tin-mesoporphyrin. Pediatrics 1994;93:1–11.
256. Kappas A, Drummond GS, Henschke C, et al: Control of hyperbilirubinemia in preterm and term newborns by an inhibitor of bilirubin production. In Cosmi EV, DiRenzo GC (eds): Current Progress in Perinatal Medicine. Proceedings of the Second World Congress of Perinatal Medicine, Rome, Italy. London, Parthenon Publishing Group, 1994, pp 623–629.
257. Mor L, Thaler I, Brandes JM, et al: In vivo hemoperfusion studies of bilirubin removal from jaundiced dogs. Int J Artif Organs 1981;4:192–198.
258. Mullon CJ, Tosone CM, Langer R: Simulation of bilirubin detoxification in the newborn using an extracorporeal bilirubin oxidase reactor. Pediatr Res 1989;26:452–457.
259. Brian BF, Dorson WJ, Pizziconi VB: Augmented hemoperfusion for hyperbilirubinemia. Trans Am Soc Artif Intern Organs 1988;34:585–589.
260. Odell GB, Gourley GR: Hereditary hyperbilirubinemia. In Lebenthal E (ed): Textbook of Gastroenterology and Nutrition in Infancy, 2nd ed. New York, Raven Press, 1989, pp 949–967.
261. Watson KJ, Gollan JL: Gilbert's syndrome. Baillieres Clin Gastroenterol 1989;3:337–355.
262. Black M, Billing BH: Hepatic bilirubin UDP-glucuronyl transferase activity in liver disease. N Engl J Med 1969;280:1266–1271.
263. Felsher BF, Craig JR, Carpio N: Hepatic bilirubin glucuronidation in Gilbert's syndrome. J Lab Clin Med 1973;81:829–837.
264. Auclair C, Hakim J, Boivin H, et al: Bilirubin and paranitrophenol glucuronyl transferase activities of the liver in patients with Gilbert's syndrome. Enzyme 1976;21:97–107.
265. Martin JF, Vierling JM, Wolkoff AW, et al: Abnormal hepatic transport of indocyanine green in Gilbert's syndrome. Gastroenterology 1976;70:385–391.
266. Ohkubo H, Okuda K, Jida S: A constitutional unconjugated hyperbilirubinemia combined with indocyanine green intolerance: a new functional disorder. Hepatology 1981;1:319–324.
267. Felsher BF, Richard D, Redeker AG: The reciprocal relation between caloric intake and the degree of hyperbilirubinemia in Gilbert's syndrome. N Engl J Med 1970;283:170–172.
268. Bosma PJ, Chowdhury JR, Bakker C, et al: The genetic basis of the reduced expression of bilirubin UDP-glucuronosyltransferase 1 in Gilbert's syndrome. N Engl J Med 1995;333:1171–1175.
269. Monaghan G, Ryan M, Seddon R, et al: Genetic variation in bilirubin UDP-glucuronosyltransferase gene promoter and Gilbert's syndrome [see comments]. Lancet 1996;347:578–581.
270. Aono S, Adachi Y, Uyama E, et al: Analysis of genes for bilirubin UDP-glucuronosyltransferase in Gilbert's syndrome [see comments]. Lancet 1995;345:958–959.
271. Sato H, Adachi Y, Koiwai O: The genetic basis of Gilbert's syndrome. Lancet 1996;347:557–558.
272. Odell GB: The estrogenation of the newborn. In Neonatal Hyperbilirubinemia. New York, Grune & Stratton, 1980, pp 39–41.
273. Bancroft JD, Kreamer B, Gourley GR: Neonatal jaundice and Gilbert syndrome. J Pediatr 1998;132:656–660.
274. Zimniak P: Dubin-Johnson and Rotor syndromes: molecular basis and pathogenesis (review). Semin Liver Dis 1993;13:248–260.
275. Rotor AB, Manahan L, Florentin A: Familial nonhemolytic jaundice with direct van den Bergh reaction. Acta Med Phil 1948;5:37–49.
276. Namihisa T, Yamaguchi K: The constitutional hyperbilirubinemia in Japan: studies on 139 cases reported during the period 1963–1969. Gastroenterol Jpn 1973;8:311–321.
277. Javitt NB, Kondo T, Kuchiba K: Bile acid excretion in Dubin-Johnson syndrome. Gastroenterology 1978;75:931–932.
278. Vest MF, Kaufmann JH, Fritz E: Chronic nonhaemolytic jaundice with conjugated bilirubin in the serum and normal histology: a case study. Arch Dis Child 1960;36:600–604.
279. Wolkoff AW: Inheritable disorders manifested by conjugated hyperbilirubinemia. Semin Liver Dis 1983;3:65–72.
280. Gustein SL, Alpert L, Arias IM: Studies of hepatic excretory function: IV. Biliary excretion of sulfobromophthalein sodium in a patient with Dubin-Johnson syndrome and a biliary fistula. Isr J Med Sci 1968;4:36–40.
281. Cohen L, Lewis C, Arias IM: Pregnancy, oral contraceptives and chronic familial jaundice with predominantly conjugated hyperbilirubinemia (Dubin-Johnson syndrome). Gastroenterology 1972;62:1182–1190.
282. Muscatello U, Mussini I, Agnolucci MT: Dubin-Johnson syndrome: an electron microscopic study of the liver cell. Acta Hepatosplenol 1967;14:162–170.
283. Ehrlich JC, Novikoff AB, Platt R, et al: Hepatocellular lipofuscin and the pigment of chronic idiopathic jaundice. Bull N Y Acad Med 1960;36:488–491.
284. Swartz HM, Sarna T, Varma RR: On the nature and excretion of the hepatic pigment in the Dubin-Johnson syndrome. Gastroenterology 1979;76:958–964.
285. Arias IM, Blumberg W: The pigment in Dubin-Johnson syndrome. Gastroenterology 1979;77:820–821.
286. Wolpert E, Pascasio FM, Wolkoff AW: Abnormal sulfobromophthalein metabolism in Rotor's syndrome and obligate heterozygotes. N Engl J Med 1977;296:1099–1101.
287. Dhumeaux D, Berthelot P: Chronic hyperbilirubinemia associated with hepatic uptake and storage impairment. Gastroenterology 1975;69:988–993.
288. Adachi Y, Yamamoto T: Partial defect in hepatic glutathione *S*-transferase activity in a case of Rotor's syndrome. Gastroenterology 1987;22:34–38.
289. Shani M, Gilon E, Ben-Ezzer J, et al: Sulfobromophthalein tolerance test in patients with Dubin-Johnson syndrome and their relatives. Gastroenterology 1970;59:842–847.
290. Wolkoff AW, Wolpert E, Pascasio FN, et al: Rotor's syndrome: a distinct inheritable pathophysiologic entity. Am J Med 1976;60:173–179.
291. Shimizu Y, Naruto H, Ida S, et al: Urinary coproporphyrin isomers in Rotor's syndrome: a study of eight families. Hepatology 1981;1:173–178.
292. Ben-Ezzer J, Blonder J, Shani M, et al: Dubin-Johnson syndrome: abnormal excretion of the isomers of urinary coproporphyrin by patients with Dubin-Johnson syndrome in Israel. Clin Sci (Colch) 1971;40:17–30.
293. Kondo T, Kuchiba K, Shimizu Y: Coporporphyrin isomers in Dubin-Johnson syndrome. Gastroenterology 1976;70:1117–1120.
294. Bar-Meir S, Baron J, Seligson U, et al: 99mTc-HIDA cholescintigraphy in Dubin-Johnson and Rotor syndromes. Nucl Med 1982;142:743–746.
295. LeBouthillier G, Morais J, Picard M, et al: Scintigraphic aspect of Rotor's disease with technetium-99m-mebrofenin. J Nucl Med 1992;33:1550–1552.

Chapter 9

# Ascites

Richard B. Colletti and Edward L. Krawitt

Ascites is defined as the pathologic accumulation of fluid within the peritoneal cavity. The word *ascites* is derived from the Greek *askites* and *askos*, meaning "bag," "bladder," or "belly." Ascites can occur in utero or at any age. In children it is usually the result of liver or renal disease. Heart disease, pancreatitis, disruption of the urinary tract, spread of cancer to the mesentery, and abdominal trauma are other causes.

## ETIOLOGY

The cause of ascites varies considerably according to the age of the patient. Different hepatic and nonhepatic causes have been reported in the fetus, the neonate, the infant and child, and the adult.

### Fetal Ascites

Isolated ascites, in the absence of hydrops, occurs uncommonly in the fetus. There have been only a small number of reported cases of fetal ascites (Fig. 9–1). It appears that many cases resolve spontaneously before birth and are not associated with fetal wastage or chronic illness.[1] A list of some of the causes of fetal ascites is presented in Table 9–1.

Cytomegalovirus, the most common congenital infection of the fetus and neonate, can cause fetal ascites and liver disease.[2, 3] Although the pathogenesis of ascites in these cases may be uncertain, hepatocellular degeneration with extensive bridging fibrosis of the liver was present in utero in one case, and in another case intrahepatic calcifications were seen.[4] The presence of ascites in utero does not necessarily indicate severe infection or a poor prognosis,[5] but most of the reported cases have been fatal. Toxoplasmosis and hepatosplenomegaly were present at birth in an infant who had fetal ascites.[6] Niemann-Pick disease type C[7, 8] and neonatal hemochromatosis[9] are other hepatic disorders that rarely cause fetal ascites.

Intrauterine meconium peritonitis, a sterile peritonitis caused by fetal bowel perforation, can cause ascites. Meconium ileus diagnosed by fetal ultrasound is often milder and has a better prognosis than symptomatic cases diagnosed after birth. However, the presence of ascites in utero indicates a more complicated course that may require surgery.[10] Fetal ascites has also been reported in a case of malrotation of the intestines with compression of the superior mesenteric vessels[11] and in two cases of intrauterine intussusception.[12] Other gastrointestinal causes of fetal ascites include cystic fibrosis and jejunal atresia.[13]

Genitourinary causes of fetal ascites include hydronephrosis, multicystic kidney, and ruptured kidney or bladder caused by obstruction of the lower urinary tract. Chylous ascites was detected in utero in a case of Turner's syndrome, consistent with generalized lymphatic hypoplasia.[14] Ovarian, cardiac, neoplastic, and other chromosomal abnormalities are also associated with fetal ascites.[15–19]

### Neonatal Ascites

Ascites in the neonate is caused by many of the same disorders that can cause fetal ascites (Table 9–2). Neonatal

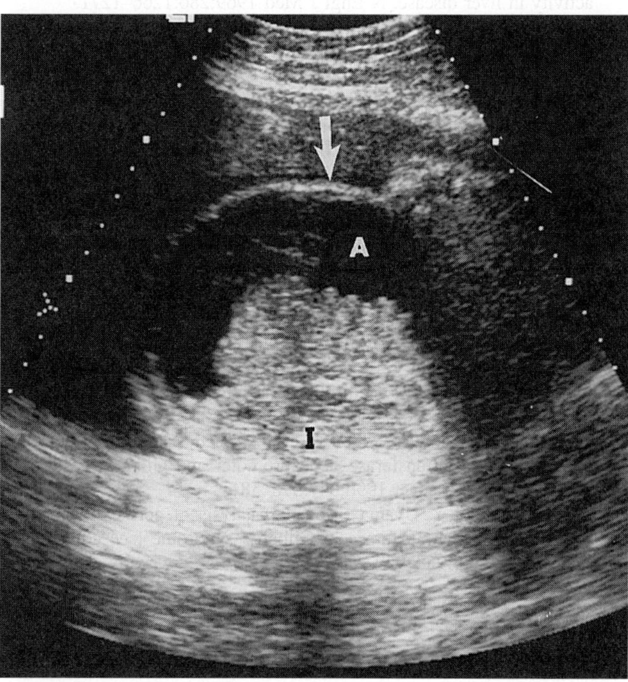


**FIGURE 9–1.** Fetal ascites (A) is seen on ultrasound as surrounding the intestines (I). The anterior abdominal wall of the fetus is also seen *(arrow)*.

liver diseases, such as alpha$_1$-antitrypsin deficiency, biliary atresia, congenital hepatic fibrosis, and hepatitis, infrequently produce ascites in the first month of life.[20–22] Ascites was a presenting sign in two newborns with Budd-Chiari syndrome; in one it was idiopathic, and in the other a right diaphragmatic hernia with hepatic vein obstruction was present.[23, 24] Perforation of the common bile duct and a ruptured cystic mesenchymal hamartoma are other hepatobiliary causes of neonatal ascites.[25]

Malrotation of the small intestine with malposition of the portal vein, intestinal perforation, and acute appendicitis are gastrointestinal causes of neonatal ascites.[26] Extravasation of parenteral nutrition from a catheter inserted into the femoral vein has resulted in neonatal ascites.[27] Insertion of an umbilical artery catheter in a newborn can cause perforation of the bladder or urachal remnant with extravasation of urine into the peritoneal cavity.[28, 29] Most cases of uroascites in the newborn result from obstructive uropathy caused by posterior urethral valves.[30] Ureterocele, lower ureteral stenosis, and ureteral atresia can also lead to rupture of the bladder or kidney. Rarely, neonatal rupture of the bladder occurs in the absence of a demonstrable anatomic urinary tract obstruction.[31, 32] Lysosomal storage disease in a patient presenting with neonatal ascites has been reported.[33]

Neonatal ascites has also been reported in cases of a ruptured corpus luteum ovarian cyst[34] and cutis marmorata telangiectatica congenita with hepatosplenomegaly.[35] An intravenous vitamin E preparation, E-Ferol, caused liver injury with ascites in clusters of premature infants.[36] Pseudo-ascites was present in a neonate who was thought to have ascites but instead had long tubular duplication of the small bowel.[37]

**TABLE 9–1. Causes of Ascites in the Fetus**

| Hepatic Disorders | Nonhepatic Disorders |
|---|---|
| Cytomegalovirus infection | Gastrointestinal disorders |
| Niemann-Pick disease type C | Meconium peritonitis |
| Biliary atresia | Malrotation of the intestines |
| Neonatal hemochromatosis | Intussusception |
| | Jejunal atresia |
| | Cystic fibrosis |
| | Infection |
| | Parvovirus |
| | Syphilis |
| | Cytomegalovirus |
| | Toxoplasmosis |
| | Genitourinary tract disorders |
| | Hydronephrosis |
| | Multicystic kidney |
| | Urinary tract obstruction |
| | Ruptured bladder |
| | Perirenal extravasation |
| | Ovarian cyst |
| | Chylous ascites |
| | Cardiac disorders |
| | Arrhythmia |
| | Heart failure |
| | Chromosomal abnormalities |
| | Trisomy |
| | Turner's syndrome |
| | Other |
| | Neoplasm |
| | Other |
| | Inborn error of metabolism |
| | Hemolytic anemia |
| | Generalized hydrops |
| | Idiopathic |
| | Other |

**TABLE 9–2. Causes of Ascites in the Neonate**

| Hepatobiliary Disorders | Nonhepatic Disorders |
|---|---|
| Cirrhosis | Gastrointestinal |
| Alpha$_1$-antitrypsin deficiency | Malrotation of the intestines |
| Congenital hepatic fibrosis | Intestinal perforation |
| Hepatitis | Acute appendicitis |
| Budd-Chiari syndrome caused by diaphragmatic hernia | Jejunal atresia |
| Perforated common bile duct | Pancreatitis |
| Ruptured cystic mesenchymal hamartoma | Chylous ascites |
| | Central venous hyperalimentation |
| | Metabolic storage diseases |
| | Lysosomal storage diseases |
| | Wolman's disease |
| | Urinary tract |
| | Obstructive uropathy |
| | Bladder rupture |
| | Renal rupture or extravasation |
| | Spontaneous bladder rupture |
| | Bladder injury from umbilical artery catheterization |
| | Nephrotic syndrome |
| | Cardiac |
| | Arrhythmia |
| | Heart failure |
| | Other |
| | Cutis marmorata telangiectatica congenita |
| | Intravenous vitamin E preparation, E-Ferol |
| | Pseudo-ascites |
| | Duplication of the small bowel |
| | Other |

## Ascites in Infants and Children

Cirrhosis is the most common hepatic cause of ascites in infants and children (Table 9–3). Ascites has been observed in infants with congenital hepatic fibrosis[38] and in school-age children with acute hepatitis A virus infection that resolved without complication.[39] Recurrent ascites has been reported in an infant with perinatally acquired cytomegalovirus infection.[40] Budd-Chiari syndrome occurring after hepatic trauma can cause ascites.[41] Ascites can also be a presenting manifestation of idiopathic perforation of an extrahepatic bile duct in infancy.[42–44]

Pancreatic ascites occurs rarely in children.[45] One third of cases occur in infants younger than 1 year of age.[46] Serum amylase may be normal; the diagnosis may be missed unless the amylase concentration of the ascitic fluid is measured. Ascites appears to be an accurate and independent predictor of severity of pancreatitis and pseudocyst formation.[47]

Chylous ascites in infants and children occurs in intestinal lymphangiectasia, in lymphatic duct obstruction, and after traumatic injury to the mesenteric lymphatic ducts.[48] Intractable ascites was reported in a child undergoing peritoneal dialysis.[49] Overtransfusion can cause ascites and pulmonary edema.[50] Ventriculoperitoneal shunts can rarely cause ascites as a result of a subclinical low-grade bacterial peritonitis[51] or poor absorption of cerebrospinal fluid with an elevated protein concentration, as is seen in some cases of optic glioma.[52] Neoplastic lesions in the abdomen that are associated with ascites include Wilms' tumor, clear cell sarcoma of the kidney, lymphoma, and germ cell and ovarian tumors.[53] Ascites has been a presenting feature of mesenteric fibromatosis[54] and malignant peritoneal mesothelioma[55] and has been produced by peritoneal seeding of neuroblastoma.[53]

Intraperitoneal fluid collections occur after liver transplantation in the pediatric population;[56] massive ascitic fluid loss with coagulation disturbances has also been reported.[57,58] A patient with vitamin A intoxication presented with ascites and a normal serum vitamin concentration.[59] Another patient with vitamin A intoxication presented with ascites and a pleural effusion.[60] Ascites can also be a presenting sign of peritonitis in chronic granulomatous disease of childhood.[61] An infant with pyloric duplication presented with hemorrhagic ascites.[62] Ascites occurred as a complication of parenteral feeding through a catheter in the inferior vena cava.[63] Pseudo-ascites has been reported in cases of celiac disease (with dilated small intestinal loops filled with copious fluid),[64] omental cyst,[65] and cystic mesothelioma of the peritoneum.[66]

### Ascites in Adults

The most common cause of ascites in adults is parenchymal liver disease. Cirrhosis and alcoholic hepatitis account for more than three quarters of cases[67] (Table 9–4). Malignancy is the next most common cause, predominantly from liver metastasis, ovarian cancer, and lymphoma.[68] Heart failure, pancreatitis, and tuberculosis account for most of the other cases.[69] Henoch-Schönlein purpura, a disorder more common in children than adults, can cause hemorrhagic ascites.[70]

**TABLE 9–3. Causes of Ascites in the Infant and Child**

| Hepatobiliary Disorders | Nonhepatic Disorders |
|---|---|
| Cirrhosis | Pancreatitis |
| Congenital hepatic fibrosis | Chylous ascites |
| Infection | Post-traumatic |
| Hepatitis A virus | Nontraumatic |
| Cytomegalovirus | Urinary tract |
| Budd-Chiari syndrome | Nephrotic syndrome |
| Perforated common bile duct | Peritoneal dialysis |
| | Heart failure |
| | Overtransfusion |
| | Ventriculoperitoneal shunts |
| | Neoplasm |
| | Neurofibromatosis |
| | Mesenteric fibromatosis |
| | Malignant mesothelioma |
| | Liver transplantation |
| | Serositis |
| | Eosinophilic gastroenteritis |
| | Henoch-Schönlein purpura |
| | Other |
| | Vitamin A intoxication |
| | Chronic granulomatous disease |
| | Congenital diaphragmatic hernia |
| | Pyloric duplication |
| | Inferior vena cava hyperalimentation |
| | Pseudo-ascites |
| | Celiac disease |
| | Cystic mesothelioma of the peritoneum |
| | Omental cyst |
| | Other |

**TABLE 9–4. Causes of Ascites in the Adult**

| Causes |
|---|
| **Hepatobiliary Disorders** |
| Cirrhosis |
| Alcoholic hepatitis |
| Massive liver metastasis |
| Budd-Chiari syndrome |
| Portal vein thrombosis |
| Biliary ascites |
| **Nonhepatic Disorders** |
| Heart failure |
| Peritoneal carcinomatosis |
| Tuberculous peritonitis |
| Pancreatic ascites |
| Serositis from connective tissue disease |
| Nephrotic syndrome |
| Other |

## PATHOPHYSIOLOGY

### Anatomy and Physiology

Ascites occurs when hydrostatic and osmotic pressures of hepatic and mesenteric capillaries produce a net transfer of fluid from blood vessels to lymphatic vessels at a rate that exceeds the drainage capacity of the lymphatics. In the normal liver, blood flow from the hepatic artery and portal vein perfuses the hepatic sinusoids; it then leaves the liver through hepatic veins that lead to the inferior vena cava (Fig. 9–2). Pressure in the sinusoids is normally low, about 2 mm Hg, because precapillary resistance is considerably greater than postcapillary resistance. The space of Disse is defined by the hepatocytes on one side and by the sinusoidal lining cells on the other side.[71] Hepatic lymph is formed by filtration of sinusoidal plasma into the space of Disse; it drains from the liver via the transdiaphragmatic lymphatic vessels to the thoracic duct, which empties into the left subclavian vein. The sinusoidal endothelium is highly permeable to albumin; the concentration of protein in hepatic lymph is very close to that of plasma, so there is normally no significant osmotic gradient across the sinusoidal membrane. The amount of fluid in the peritoneal cavity of a normal adult is less than 150 mL (Table 9–5).

In the intestines, blood from the mesenteric capillaries drains via the mesenteric veins into the portal vein (see Fig. 9–2). The mean pressure of the mesenteric capillary is normally about 20 mm Hg. Intestinal lymph drains from regional lymphatics into the thoracic duct. The mesenteric capillary membrane is relatively impermeable to albumin; the concentration of protein in mesenteric lymph is only about one fifth that of plasma, so there is a significant osmotic gradient that promotes the return of interstitial fluid into the capillary. In the normal adult the flow of lymph in the thoracic duct is about 800 to 1,000 mL per day.[72]

### Cirrhotic Ascites

Portal hypertension precedes the development of cirrhotic ascites. Increased sinusoidal pressure caused by cirrhosis

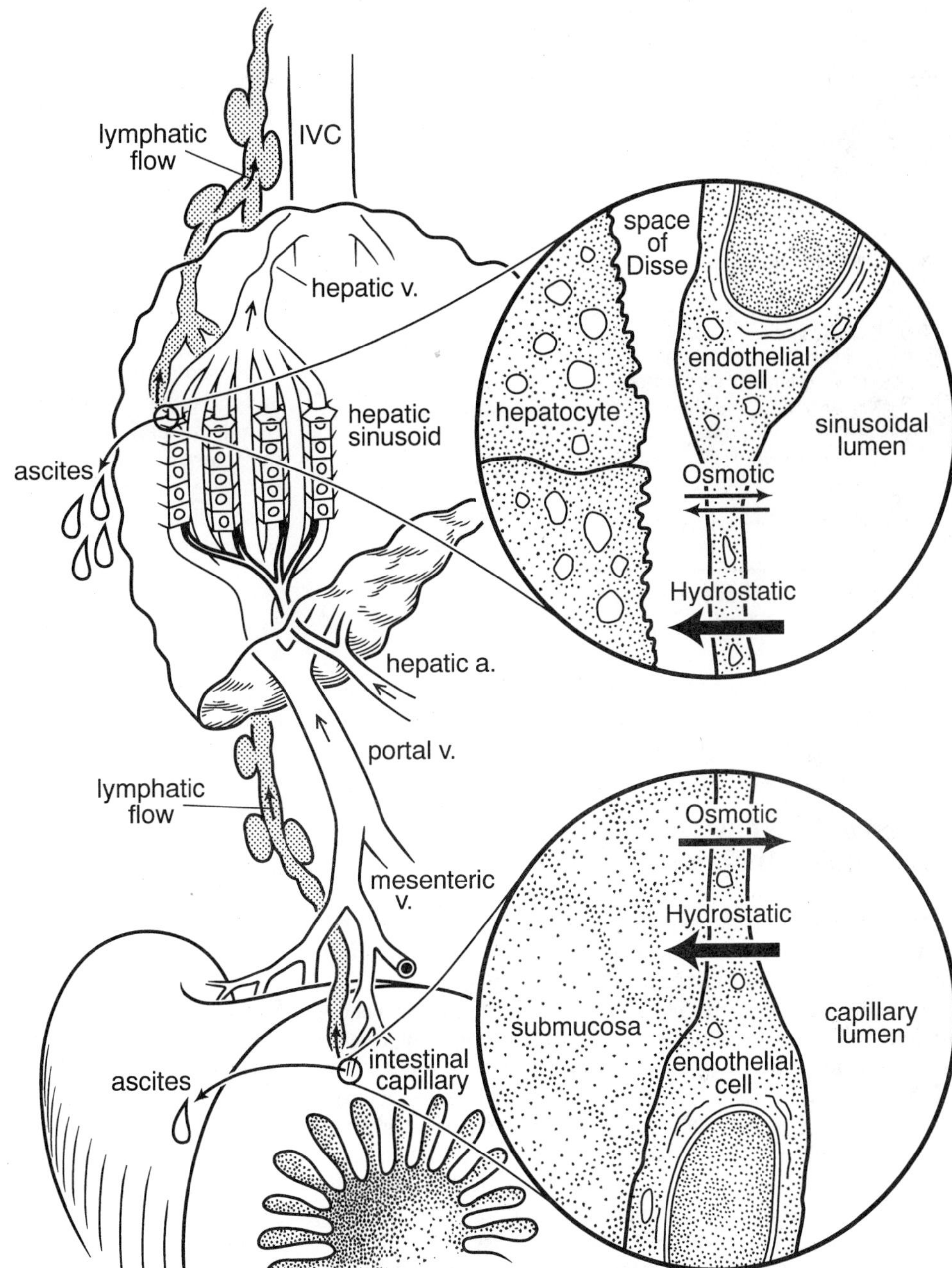


**FIGURE 9–2.** Hepatic lymph is formed by filtration of sinusoidal plasma into the space of Disse; it drains from the liver via the transdiaphragmatic lymphatic vessels to the thoracic duct. The sinusoidal endothelium is highly permeable to albumin; there is normally no significant osmotic gradient across the sinusoidal membrane. Intestinal lymph drains from regional lymphatics into the thoracic duct. The mesenteric capillary membrane is relatively impermeable to albumin; there is a significant osmotic gradient that promotes the return of interstitial fluid into the capillary lumen. Ascites occurs when the net transfer of fluid from blood vessels to lymphatic vessels exceeds the drainage capacity of the lymphatics; fluid seeps through the hepatic capsule and, to a lesser extent, the intestine. (Adapted from Dudley FJ: Pathophysiology of ascites formation. Gastroenterol Clin North Am 1992;21:215–235, with permission.)

increases the hydrostatic pressure gradient across the sinusoidal membrane and results in increased lymph formation. When hepatic lymphatic drainage cannot keep up with the increased lymph formation, lymph seeps through the hepatic capsule into the peritoneal cavity. In severe cirrhosis, capillarization of the sinusoidal membrane slows lymph production; capillarization is the formation of a basement membrane, defenestration, and deposition of collagen in the space of Disse. As a result, the permeability to protein of the sinusoidal membrane decreases; the lower protein concentration of the lymph decreases the osmotic gradient. The permeability to protein of the hepatic capsule also decreases, with a concomitant counteracting effect on ascites formation.[72, 73]

The mesenteric capillaries respond to sinusoidal and portal hypertension with several mechanisms that oppose mesenteric lymph formation. Precapillary resistance increases as a result of arteriolar contraction; the surface area available for transudation is reduced; the permeability of the capillary membrane is reduced; hydrostatic pressure in the interstitium increases as fluid accumulates there. Up to 900 mL of ascitic fluid can be reabsorbed daily through intestinal or diaphragmatic lymphatics or mesenteric capillaries.[72]

It is not known whether ascitic fluid is formed predominantly in the liver or in the mesentery. Animal experiments suggest that the liver is the source. When the liver of a dog with portal hypertension is placed within the thorax, pleural fluid accumulates instead of ascites; when it is placed within a bag, fluid accumulates in the bag.[74, 75] In contrast, the protein concentration of ascites more closely resembles intestinal lymph than hepatic lymph. However, as cirrhosis

**TABLE 9–5. Ascites: A Quantitative Perspective***

| | |
|---|---|
| Sinusoidal pressure | |
| Normal | 2 mm Hg |
| Cirrhosis | 5–30 mm Hg |
| Mesenteric capillary pressure | 20 mm Hg |
| Lymphatic flow (thoracic duct) | |
| Normal | 0.8–1.0 L/day |
| Cirrhosis with ascites | 8–10 L/day |
| Peritoneum | |
| Normal fluid volume | <150 mL |
| Volume capacity | 20 L |
| Compliance | 10 mL/kg per mm Hg |
| Reabsorptive capacity | 0.9 L/day |
| Minimum volume of ascites required | |
| For detection by physical examination | |
| Shifting dullness | 1.5–3.0 L |
| For detection by X-ray | |
| Hepatic angle, flank stripe | 0.8 L |
| For detection by ultrasound | |
| Adult | <100 mL |
| Morison's pouch or pelvic cul-de-sac | <10 mL |
| Infant | 10–20 mL |

*For adults unless otherwise indicated.

worsens, the protein concentration of hepatic lymph eventually becomes as low as that of intestinal lymph owing to capillarization of the sinusoids.[76]

## Underfill, Overflow, and Peripheral Vasodilation Theories

In addition to portal hypertension, abnormal retention of sodium and water is a feature of ascites. Several theories have been proposed to explain the sequence of events leading to the development of ascites and sodium and water retention. The *underfill* theory proposed that portal hypertension leads to ascites formation, which results in a contracted blood volume, decreased renal perfusion, and secondary renal sodium and water retention.[77, 78] Such patients would be expected to have intravascular hypovolemia and low cardiac output. However, patients with ascites typically have an expanded blood volume and high cardiac output. To explain this discrepancy, the *overflow* theory proposed that an unknown hepatorenal reflex causes sodium and water retention first, followed by increasing blood volume which, combined with portal hypertension, leads to ascites.[79, 80]

The *peripheral vasodilation* theory proposed that vasodilation of peripheral vessels is the first step, leading to systemic hypotension and a decrease in cardiac output, followed by renal retention of sodium and water, plasma volume expansion, and finally ascites.[81] It is proposed that the process is initiated by an excess of endogenous vasodilators resulting from either abnormal liver production or impaired liver catabolism.[73, 82]

The response to the decreased effective arterial blood volume is mediated by afferent glossopharyngeal nerves from the baroreceptors to the central nervous system, leading to an increase in efferent sympathetic nervous adrenergic tone. The efferent arm consists of sympathetic constriction of arterioles, stimulation of renin release from the juxtaglomerular process with activation of the renin-angiotensin-aldosterone system, and increased cardiac output. Baroreceptor input to the supraoptic and paraventricular nuclei in the hypothalamus produces increased secretion of arginine vasopressin. These changes lead to increased sodium and water retention and expansion of the plasma volume.[82] With progressive worsening of cirrhosis, there is further expansion of plasma volume, increased formation of lymph, overloading of lymphatic ducts, and spillage of fluid into the peritoneal cavity. There is some evidence that contradicts the peripheral vasodilation hypothesis, but at this time it appears to be the best explanation for the development of ascites.[83, 84]

The patient with decompensated cirrhosis has a hyperdynamic circulatory state with an expanded blood volume, increased cardiac output, tachycardia, a wide pulse pressure, and peripheral vasodilation. Hypoalbuminemia exacerbates lymph formation by decreasing the osmotic gradient, drawing interstitial fluid into the vascular space. Peripheral edema results when increased abdominal pressure from ascites raises the pressure of the inferior vena cava, producing an increase in hydrostatic pressure in the capillaries of the legs.

## Noncirrhotic Ascites

Evidence suggests that ascites caused by heart failure or the nephrotic syndrome results from decreased effective arterial blood volume with secondary activation of the central nervous sympathetic adrenergic system, the renin-angiotensin-aldosterone system, and vasopressin, leading to renal sodium and water retention.[85] In patients with heart failure, hepatic congestion increases portal venous pressure. In the nephrotic syndrome, hypoalbuminemia potentiates the movement of plasma into the interstitium.

# DIAGNOSIS

## History and Physical Examination

Patients who develop ascites often have a history of increased abdominal girth and recent weight gain.[86] There may be a history of chronic liver disease or hepatitis. The physical examination may reveal a protuberant abdomen, bulging flanks, and dullness to percussion in the flanks. Jaundice, spider angiomas, umbilical collateral veins, clubbing, and palmar erythema are signs suggestive of liver disease.

The presence of bulging flanks can be caused by free fluid in the peritoneum, organomegaly, or obesity. The abdomen can be percussed to distinguish ascites from obesity. In a supine patient with ascites, gas-filled loops of small intestine float to the top of the mid-abdomen. The percussion note of the mid-abdomen is tympanitic, and the ascites-filled flanks exhibit dullness to percussion. If the patient is then placed in a lateral position, dullness to percussion shifts to the dependent side. The test for shifting dullness has a sensitivity of 60% to 88% and a specificity of 56% to 90%.[87] It has been estimated that the minimum volume of ascitic fluid required to detect shifting dullness is 1.5 to 3.0 L.[82]

The test for a fluid wave requires two examiners, four hands, and a cooperative, supine patient. The sides of the hands of one examiner press down the midline of the patient's abdomen, while the other examiner taps one flank with one hand and senses a fluid wave in the other flank with the other hand. The test for a fluid wave has a sensitivity of 50% to 80% and a specificity of 82% to 92%.[87]

## Body Imaging Studies

Abdominal plain radiographs detect ascites indirectly, by changes in the hepatic angle or by the presence of a flank stripe sign. The most sensitive technique is ultrasound, which can detect as little as 100 mL of free abdominal fluid in the adult. Minimal ascites is seen in the most dependent spaces, the hepatorenal recess (Morison's pouch) and the pelvic cul-de-sac; real-time sonography can detect less than 10 mL there[87] (Fig. 9–3). It has been estimated that in supine infants 10 to 20 mL can be detected by ultrasound in the perivesical area.[88] Intraperitoneal fluid-debris levels and ascites have been demonstrated in neonates with abdominal distention who at surgery were found to have necrotizing enterocolitis and intestinal perforation.[89] Ultrasound has also been used successfully to detect free intraperitoneal fluid after blunt abdominal trauma.[90] Sonography of intestinal lymphangiectasia in children demonstrates diffuse bowel wall thickening, mesenteric edema, and dilated mesenteric lymphatics, as well as ascites.[91]

Ascites can also be detected by computed tomography (CT) or magnetic resonance imaging[92] (Figs. 9–4 and 9–5). CT demonstrates extrapancreatic fluid collections in children with acute pancreatitis.[93] High-density ascites and other features of tuberculous peritonitis have been demonstrated in children by CT.[94] Chylous ascitic fluid has been shown by both CT and ultrasound to develop a unique biphasic fat-fluid level when the patient remains recumbent.[95]

## Diagnostic Abdominal Paracentesis

Analysis of a sample of ascitic fluid can help determine the cause of ascites at initial presentation, and paracentesis is necessary to diagnose bacterial peritonitis. Abdominal paracentesis is recommended to detect bacterial peritonitis

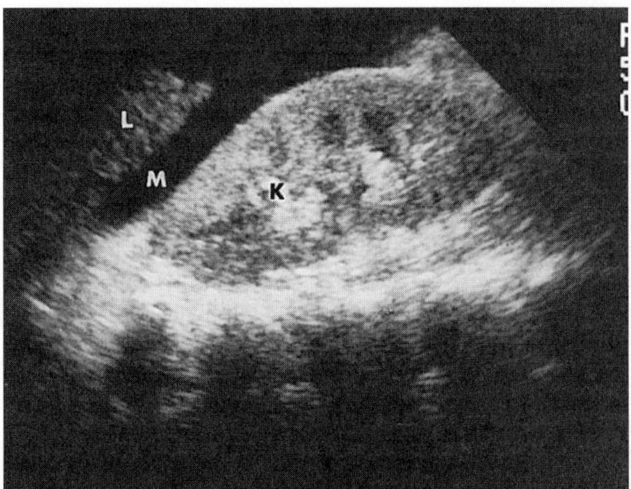


**FIGURE 9–3.** Ascites is seen on ultrasound in Morison's pouch (M) between a tip of the liver (L) and the right kidney (K) of a 12-year-old with cryptogenic cirrhosis.

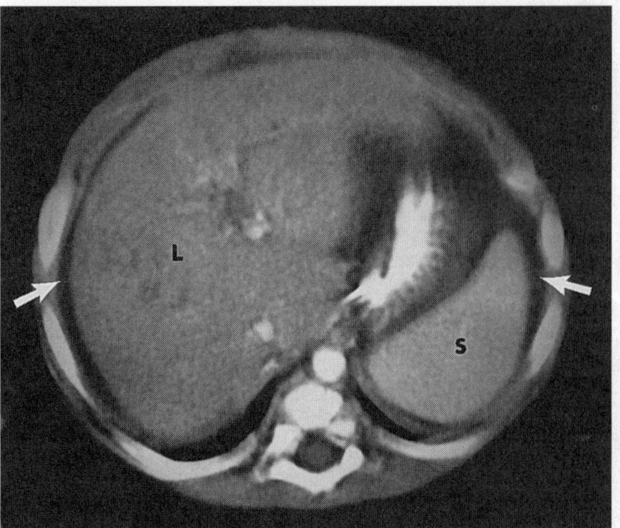


**FIGURE 9–4.** A small amount of ascites *(arrows)* is detected by CT as a rim around the liver (L) and spleen (S) of this infant with biliary atresia after a Kasai procedure. Radiopaque intestine lies between the two organs.

when ascites first appears, when patients are hospitalized, and when there is clinical deterioration, particularly fever or abdominal pain.[96]

If the cause of ascites is not apparent, examination of ascitic fluid can aid in identification of the cause. Elevation of the ascitic fluid amylase concentration indicates pancreatitis or intestinal perforation; polymicrobial infection indicates intestinal perforation. Uroascites is present when the concentrations of urea and creatinine are higher in ascitic fluid than in serum. Elevated bilirubin indicates perforation of the biliary tree or upper intestine. Chylous ascites is indicated by a milky appearance and a concentration of triglycerides in ascitic fluid higher than in serum.

The difference in the concentration of albumin in serum and in ascitic fluid, called the *serum-ascites albumin concentration gradient,* can reliably separate ascites into two categories, the high-gradient (>1.1 g/dL) and the low-gradient (<1.1 g/dL) types. High-gradient ascites is present when there is portal hypertension, in conditions such as cirrhosis, alcoholic ascites, heart failure, massive liver metastases, fulminant hepatic failure, Budd-Chiari syndrome, portal vein thrombosis, veno-occlusive disease, and myxedema. Low-gradient ascites occurs in the absence of portal hypertension in conditions such as peritoneal carcinomatosis, tuberculous peritonitis, pancreatic ascites, biliary ascites, nephrotic syndrome, and serositis caused by connective tissue disease.[97, 98]

It is now recognized that the exudate-transudate concept, based on the concentration of total protein in ascitic fluid, is unreliable and outmoded.[99] In a study of 901 paracenteses, measurement of the ascitic fluid total protein correctly classified the cause of ascites only 56% of the time, whereas the serum-ascites albumin concentration gradient differentiated the cause of ascites resulting from portal hypertension 97% of the time.[100]

The technique of paracentesis has been described in detail.[68, 101] A midline site is preferred because of less vascularity there. Scars should be avoided, because bowel may be adherent to them. If a midline scar is present or if the level

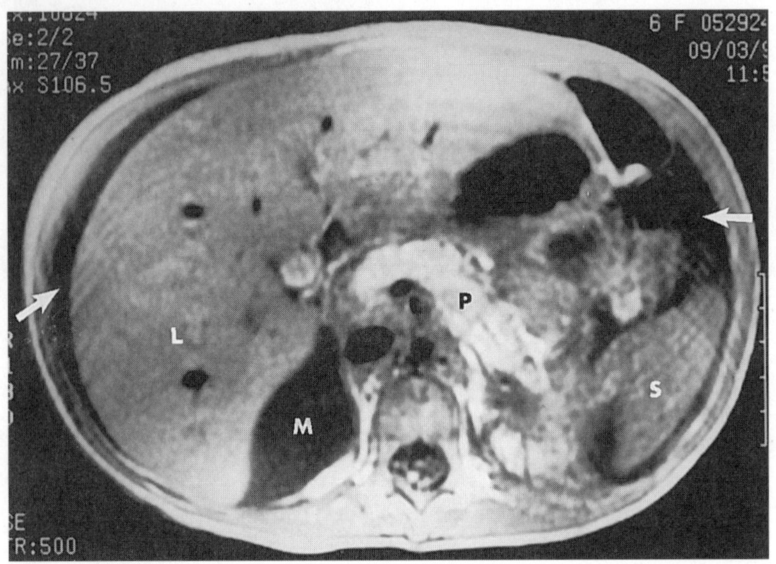


**FIGURE 9–5.** Ascites *(arrows)* is seen by magnetic resonance imaging as a rim around the liver (L), in Morison's pouch (M), and anterior to the spleen (S). The pancreas (P) is also visualized.

of dullness to percussion cannot be determined, then the flank with greater dullness is selected. Ultrasound localization of fluid is an accurate and safe method for selecting a paracentesis site.

Ascitic fluid is submitted to the laboratory in an anticoagulant tube for a leukocyte count and differential. Bedside inoculation of blood culture bottles with ascitic fluid should also be performed. In addition, at the time of the first paracentesis, measurement of the albumin concentration is performed. If there is not sufficient fluid to perform all three tests, then the leukocyte count and differential is performed first, because of its value in deciding whether to treat with antibiotics for possible bacterial peritonitis, as described later. Performance of additional tests is optional and depends on the clinical situation.

Complications of paracentesis are uncommon although bleeding is seen occasionally. In one prospective study of 125 adults with 229 paracenteses, there were no deaths attributable to paracentesis.[102] Except for frank diffuse intravascular coagulopathy, paracentesis can be performed despite prolongation of the prothrombin time.

## TREATMENT

Treatment of ascites is indicated in most, but not all, patients. Small amounts of ascitic fluid that do not produce symptoms or appear to have clinical sequelae may require little or no treatment. Tense ascites causing respiratory embarrassment, severe pain, or other major clinical problems should be treated promptly.

Mobilization of ascitic fluid is accomplished by creating a negative sodium balance until ascites has diminished or resolved; then the sodium balance is maintained so that ascites does not recur. In most patients treatment of ascites consists of restriction of dietary sodium and administration of diuretics. On occasion, fluid restriction is also employed. Ascites that does not respond to diuretics can be treated with large-volume paracentesis, peritoneovenous shunting, or transjugular intrahepatic portosystemic stent shunting. Ultimately, orthotopic liver transplantation may be required.

### Restriction of Sodium and Fluids

It is recommended that dietary sodium be limited to 44 to 88 mEq (1–2 g) per day in the adult, or approximately 17 to 35 mEq (0.4–0.8 g) per 1,000 calories. Most pediatric hepatologists recommend restriction of sodium intake; either a diet with no added sodium or approximately 2 mEq sodium per kilogram of body weight per day is advised. Restriction of dietary sodium by itself is sufficient for only a small minority of patients; treatment with diuretics usually is required. Many patients require sodium restriction even when they are treated with diuretics.

Increased levels of vasopressin cause water retention, but most patients with ascites do not have clinically significant hyponatremia. Restriction of water intake usually is not recommended until serum sodium decreases to 125 or 130 mEq/L or less.

### Diuretics

Spironolactone is the most effective diuretic because of its ability to block the marked hyperaldosteronism that is characteristic of cirrhotic ascites. Metabolites of spironolactone act on the cortical and medullary collecting tubules by inhibiting the binding of aldosterone to a specific receptor protein there (Fig. 9–6). Because it acts distally, spironolactone can normally inhibit the reabsorption of only 2% of the filtered sodium. In patients with cirrhosis, the bioactive metabolites of spironolactone have prolonged half-lives, ranging from 24 to 58 hours; as a result, more than 5 days is required to achieve steady-state conditions, and administration of medication more than once daily is unnecessary.[103]

A randomized comparative study demonstrated that 95% of nonazotemic cirrhotic patients with avid sodium retention responded to spironolactone treatment, but only 52% responded to furosemide. The patients who did not respond to furosemide had higher levels of renin and aldosterone; they were subsequently treated with spironolactone, and 90% of them responded to it.[104] Cirrhotic patients with ascites who do not respond to spironolactone treatment have a lower

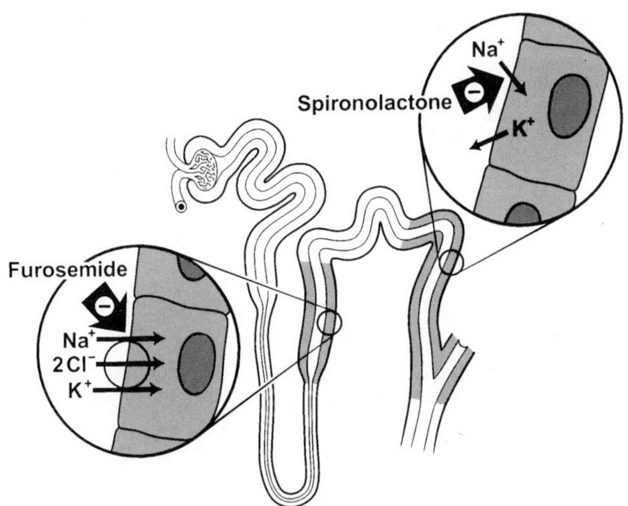


**FIGURE 9–6.** Furosemide acts on the renal epithelial cells of the thick ascending loop of Henle by inhibiting the sodium-chloride-potassium carrier cotransport system. Metabolites of spironolactone act on the cortical and medullary collecting tubules by inhibiting the binding of aldosterone to a specific receptor protein there, resulting in impairment of $Na^+$ absorption and $K^+$ excretion.

fractional sodium delivery to the distal renal tubule as a result of enhanced sodium reabsorption in the proximal tubule.[105]

Furosemide is a loop diuretic that acts on the thick ascending limb of the loop of Henle; it has no effect on the distal and collecting tubules (see Fig. 9–6). Furosemide can increase sodium excretion by as much as 30% of filtered sodium. After oral administration, furosemide is absorbed rapidly, has an onset of effect within 30 minutes, a peak effect in 1 to 2 hours, and a duration of action of 3 to 4 hours.[106] Intravenous furosemide can cause a potentially hazardous sudden decrease in glomerular filtration rate.[97]

Diuretic treatment is begun with spironolactone, either alone or, in more severe cases, in combination with furosemide (Table 9–6).[102, 107] One approach is to begin treatment with spironolactone, 2 to 3 mg per kilogram of body weight (up to 100 mg) as a single morning dose; if there is no response, the dose is increased by 2 mg/kg (up to 100 mg) every 5 to 7 days until a maximum dose of 4 to 6 mg/kg (up to 400 mg) is reached. If there is still no response, oral furosemide 1 mg/kg (up to 40 mg) daily is added, and the dose is increased by 1 mg/kg (up to 40 mg) every 5 to 7 days if necessary until a maximum dose of 2 to 4 mg/kg (up to 160 mg) is reached. An alternative approach that may hasten the onset of diuresis is to begin treatment with both spironolactone, 2 mg/kg (up to 100 mg), and furosemide, 1 mg/kg (up to 40 mg), as a single morning dose. If necessary, the dosages of both spironolactone and furosemide can be increased every 5 to 7 days until maximum doses of 4 to 6 mg/kg (up to 400 mg) and 2 to 4 mg/kg (up to 160 mg), respectively, are reached.

**TABLE 9–6. Diuretic Treatment**

| DRUG | SPIRONOLACTONE | FUROSEMIDE |
|---|---|---|
| Starting dose | 2–3 mg/kg, up to 100 mg | 1 mg/kg, up to 40 mg |
| Incremental dose | 2 mg/kg, up to 100 mg | 1 mg/kg, up to 40 mg |
| Maximum dose | 4–6 mg/kg, up to 400 mg | 2–4 mg/kg, up to 160 mg |

A gradual approach to diuretic therapy that avoids adverse effects is preferred. The goal of therapy is to reduce the body weight by approximately 0.5% to 1% (up to 300–500 g) each day until ascites is gone, and then to prevent the reaccumulation of ascites (Table 9–7). No more than 900 mL of ascites can be reabsorbed in 1 day in an adult, so weight loss of more than 900 g/day is associated with contraction of plasma volume.[108] However, peripheral edema can be mobilized more rapidly; adult patients with peripheral edema can safely lose 1.5 kg daily.[109]

Spironolactone treatment can lead to hyperkalemic acidosis; furosemide treatment can lead to hypokalemic alkalosis. When both drugs are used together, disturbances of potassium and pH occur less commonly. Complications of diuretic therapy also include renal failure secondary to intravascular volume depletion, hyponatremia, hepatic encephalopathy, antiandrogenic effects, and muscle cramps. Use of nonsteroidal anti-inflammatory agents reduces the diuretic effect of furosemide.[110]

## Therapeutic Paracentesis

Therapeutic paracentesis of diuretic-resistant tense ascites has been shown to be a safe, rapid, and effective treatment.[111, 112] Repeated removal of 4 to 6 L/day of ascitic fluid has become a standard treatment in adults. With total paracentesis, in which all the ascitic fluid is mobilized in one paracentesis session, on average 10.7 L was removed in 1 hour, and 22 L was removed from one patient.[113] Repeated large-volume paracentesis can lead to protein and complement depletion. When more than 4 to 6 L is removed, or when repeated large-volume paracentesis is performed, there is a significant increase in blood urea nitrogen, elevation of plasma renin activity and plasma aldosterone concentration, and reduction of serum sodium. These changes, which indicate a physiologic response to the contraction of blood volume, are not usually manifested clinically by symptoms or signs. These hemodynamic alterations can be prevented by the intravenous infusion of 40 g of albumin after each paracentesis.[113–115]

The need for intravenous albumin after paracentesis is a controversial subject.[116] Albumin infusions can produce downregulation of the albumin synthesis gene. Parenteral albumin is costly; other, less expensive plasma expanders that have been studied, including dextran 70 and polygeline,

**TABLE 9–7. Goal of Diuretic Treatment**

| PRETREATMENT WEIGHT (kg) | DESIRED DAILY WEIGHT LOSS (g)* |
|---|---|
| 5–10 | 25–100 |
| 11–20 | 50–200 |
| 21–30 | 100–300 |
| 31–40 | 150–400 |
| 41–50 | 200–500 |
| >50 | 300–500 |

*0.5–1.0% of body weight per day.

have not proved to be as effective as albumin in the prevention of postparacentesis circulatory dysfunction. Patients who received albumin after total paracentesis had a longer time before rehospitalization and a longer survival time than patients who received other plasma expanders.[117]

Infants and young children can develop ascites rapidly, without gradual stretching of the abdominal wall; they are subject to respiratory distress and other sequelae of rapidly increased intra-abdominal pressure. In such situations paracentesis is performed to provide symptomatic relief.[118] Intravenous albumin is generally administered after therapeutic paracentesis in children.

### Peritoneovenous Shunting

The peritoneovenous shunt was invented to create a conduit for ascites in the peritoneum to return to the vascular space in the superior vena cava.[119] The LeVeen shunt consists of a perforated tube in the abdomen that is connected with a one-way pressure-sensitive valve to a silicone catheter that extends subcutaneously into a jugular vein. Ascitic fluid flows to the vascular compartment when there is a pressure gradient of 3 cm $H_2O$ or more between the abdomen and the superior vena cava. The Denver shunt has a pumping mechanism as well. Peritoneovenous shunting often results in reduction or elimination of ascites, with restoration of effective blood volume; reductions in the concentrations of renin, angiotensin, aldosterone, and vasopressin; and an increase in atrial natriuretic factor responsiveness.[107, 120] Peritoneovenous shunting was more rapidly effective than medical management in alleviating disabling intractable ascites caused by alcoholic cirrhosis, although the survival rates were similar.[121]

Complications include coagulopathy, shunt obstruction, superior vena caval thrombosis and obstruction, pulmonary embolization, and *Staphylococcus* sepsis. Technical modifications have not been able to prevent these complications.[122]

A reversed ventriculoperitoneal shunt was adapted as a peritoneovenous shunt in a premature neonate with idiopathic Budd-Chiari syndrome; ascites resolved, and the patient recovered.[123] A 15-month-old infant with post-traumatic Budd-Chiari syndrome was effectively treated with a LeVeen shunt, and the ascites subsequently resolved.[41] A modified Denver shunt was used successfully to treat severe ascites in a newborn.[124] The LeVeen shunt has been used in older children as well.

### Transjugular Intrahepatic Portosystemic Stent Shunting

Transjugular intrahepatic portosystemic stent shunting lowers portal pressure and prevents rebleeding from esophageal varices[125] (see Chapter 51). It also effectively alleviates cirrhotic ascites.[126] It induces a delayed natriuresis and improves proximal renal tubular reabsorption of sodium, renin-angiotensin-aldosterone activity, and central blood volume despite continued arterial vasodilation.[85, 127] However, the survival rate is lower in patients treated with this stent than in those who receive large-volume paracentesis.[128]

### Other Treatments

Attempts to develop techniques to ultrafilter ascites and reinfuse it, either into blood or into the peritoneum, have not been successful in supplanting other approaches, either in adults[129, 130] or in children.[131–133] In some patients, orthotopic liver transplantation may be the only effective therapy.

## SPONTANEOUS BACTERIAL PERITONITIS

Spontaneous bacterial peritonitis (SBP) is defined as an infection of ascitic fluid without evidence of an abdominal source. Secondary bacterial peritonitis is defined as an intra-abdominal infection caused by a problem that requires surgical treatment, such as intestinal perforation, a perirenal abscess, or gallbladder empyema.

The incidence of SBP in children is not known.[134] In a report of 321 children with chronic liver disease, there were 12 episodes of SBP in 11 patients; all 11 had ascites.[135] The patients presented with abdominal distention, fever, malaise, and abdominal pain; some patients also had vomiting, diarrhea, and worsening jaundice. Diffuse abdominal tenderness and rebound tenderness were present; encephalopathy had developed or worsened in most of the patients. Cultures of ascitic fluid detected a single organism in 11 of the episodes. *Streptococcus pneumoniae* was isolated in 73%, *Klebsiella pneumoniae* in 18%, and *Haemophilus influenzae* in 9%. Blood cultures were also positive in 9 of the 11 episodes. Despite treatment with antibiotics, 64% of these patients died. Opsinization and serum complement levels (C3 and C4) were low in almost all of the patients who were tested.

In a second report, four children with cirrhotic ascites and hematemesis also had abdominal pain, fever, and peritonitis.[136] Cultures of ascites were positive for *S. pneumoniae*; blood cultures were also positive. One patient, who had complicated variceal bleeding, died.

Studies in adults indicate that SBP may be present even when symptoms suggestive of peritonitis are absent.[68] It is recommended that diagnostic paracentesis be performed when ascites first appears, at the time of a hospitalization, or if clinical deterioration, unexplained fever, abdominal pain, or other suspicious symptoms are present. About two thirds of the organisms identified in ascitic fluid were *Escherichia coli, K. pneumoniae*, or miscellaneous gram-negative bacteria. *Pneumococcus* accounted for only 12%. Anaerobic organisms accounted for only 1% of cases; fungi were not detected.

Bedside inoculation of blood culture bottles with ascitic fluid is more sensitive than the conventional method for detecting bacterial peritonitis.[137] The conventional method of culture consists of transporting ascitic fluid to the laboratory, where several drops of fluid are cultured in agar plates. However, the median concentration of bacteria in infected ascites is only one organism per milliliter. When 2 mL of ascitic fluid is placed in a blood culture bottle at the bedside, sensitivity improves from 43% to 93%. A Gram stain of ascitic fluid is only about 10% sensitive; however, it can rapidly identify polymicrobial infection caused by intestinal perforation in some cases.

The leukocyte count of ascitic fluid is normally less than

500 cells/mm$^3$, and the polymorphonuclear cell (PMN) count is less than 250 cells/mm$^3$. Samples of ascitic fluid that contain a predominance of neutrophils and an absolute PMN count greater than 250 cells/mm$^3$ are assumed to be infected.[97] In SBP, the PMN count is elevated and the ascites culture is positive. When the PMN count is elevated but the ascites culture is negative, it probably means that the culture is falsely negative and an infection is present. When the PMN count is normal but the culture is positive, it most likely represents transient bacterascites, which resolves in most cases without antibiotics; it could also represent early SBP.

If SBP is diagnosed by paracentesis or culture, antibiotic treatment should be initiated. A non-nephrotoxic broad-spectrum antibiotic with gram-negative coverage, such as cefotaxime, is recommended for treatment of SBP in adults. In children it is also necessary to provide adequate coverage of *S. pneumoniae*.

Prophylaxis for primary or recurrent SBP has been recommended in certain clinical situations. Use of ciprofloxacin, norfloxacin, and trimethoprim-sulfamethoxazole has been reported in adults but not in children. Once-weekly dosage may be adequate.[138]

## REFERENCES


1. Zelop C, Benacerraf BR: The causes and natural history of fetal ascites. Prenat Diagn 1994;14:941–946.
2. Sun CJ, Greene CL, Nagey DA: Hepatic fibrosis in congenital cytomegalovirus infection with fetal ascites and pulmonary hypoplasia. Pediatr Pathol 1990;10:641–646.
3. Stocker T: Congenital cytomegalovirus infection presenting as massive ascites with secondary pulmonary hypoplasia. Hum Pathol 1985;16:1173–1175.
4. Yamashita Y, Iwanaga R, Goto A, et al: Congenital cytomegalovirus infection associated with fetal ascites and intrahepatic calcifications. Acta Paediatr Scand 1989;78:965–967.
5. Binder ND, Buckmaster JW, Benda GI: Outcome for fetus with ascites and cytomegalovirus infection. Pediatrics 1988;82:100–103.
6. Blaakaer J: Ultrasonic diagnosis of fetal ascites and toxoplasmosis. Acta Obstet Gynecol Scand 1986;65:653–654.
7. Maconochie IK, Chong S, Mieli-Vergani G, et al: Fetal ascites: an unusual presentation of Niemann-Pick disease type C. Arch Dis Child 1989;64:1391–1393.
8. Manning DJ, Price WIJ, Pearse RG: Fetal ascites: an unusual presentation of Niemann-Pick disease type C. Arch Dis Child 1990;65:335–336.
9. Singh S, Sills JH, Waffarn F: Interesting case presentation: neonatal hemachromatosis as a cause of ascites. J Perinatol 1990;10:214–216.
10. Dirkes K, Crombeholme TM, Craigo SD, et al: The natural history of meconium peritonitis diagnosed in utero. J Pediatr Surg 1995;30:979–982.
11. Hertel J, Volsted Pedersen P: Congenital ascites due to mesenteric vessel constriction caused by malrotation of the intestines. Acta Paediatr Scand 1979;68:281–283.
12. Woodall DL, Birken GA, Williamson K, Lobe TE: Isolated fetal-neonatal abdominal ascites: a sign of intrauterine intussusception. J Pediatr Surg 1987;22:506–507.
13. Voss LM, Hadden W, Pease PW, Clarkson PM: Neonatal ascites due to congenital jejunal obstruction. Aust Paediatr J 1988;24:260–261.
14. Wax JR, Blakemore KJ, Baser I, Stetten G: Isolated fetal ascites detected by sonography: an unusual presentation of Turner syndrome. Obstet Gynecol 1992;79:862–863.
15. Greenberg F, Stein F, Gresik MV, et al: The Perlman familial nephroblastomatosis syndrome. Am J Med Genet 1986;24:101–110.
16. Heaton FC, Vaughan R: Intrauterine supraventricular tachycardia: cardioversion with maternal digoxin. Obstet Gynecol 1982;60:749–752.
17. Griscom NT, Colodny AH, Rosenberg HK, et al: Diagnostic aspects of neonatal ascites: report of 27 cases. AJR Am J Roentgenol 1977;128:961–970.
18. Machin GA. Diseases causing fetal and neonatal ascites. Pediatr Pathol 1985;4:195–211.
19. Shweni PM, Kambaran SR, Ramdial K: Fetal ascites. S Afr Med J 1984;66:616–618.
20. Ghishan FK, Nau S, Younoszai MK: Portal hypertension in a neonate with congenital hepatic fibrosis. South Med J 1981;74:243–244.
21. Ghishan FK, Gray GF, Greene HL: Alpha-1 antitrypsin deficiency presenting with ascites and cirrhosis in the neonatal period. Gastroenterology 1983;85:435–438.
22. Deckelbaum RJ, Weizman CMZ, Bauer CR: Ascites in the newborn associated with hepatitis. Clin Pediatr 1980;19:374–376.
23. Gilsanz V, Emons D, Hansmann M, et al: Hydrothorax, ascites, and right diaphragmatic hernia. Radiology 986;158:243–246.
24. Jaffe R, Yunis EJ: Congenital Budd-Chiari syndrome. Pediatr Pathol 1983;1:187–192.
25. George JC, Cohen MD, Tarver RD, Rosales RN: Ruptured cystic mesenchymal hamartoma: an unusual cause of neonatal ascites. Pediatr Radiol 1994;24:304–305.
26. Puvabanditsin S, Garrow E, Vizarra R: An unusual cause of congenital ascites. Acta Paediatr 1995;84:829–830.
27. Spriggs DW, Brantley RE: Thoracic and abdominal extravasation: a complication of hyperalimentation in infants. AJR Am J Roentgenol 1977;128:419–422.
28. Dmochowski RR, Crandell SS, Corriere JN: Bladder injury and uroascites from umbilical artery catheterization. Pediatrics 1986;77:421–422.
29. Hepworth RC, Milstein JM: The transected urachus: an unusual cause of neonatal ascites. Pediatrics 1984;73:397–400.
30. Garrett RA, Franken EA: Neonatal ascites: perirenal urinary extravasation with bladder outlet obstruction. J Urol 1969;102:627–632.
31. Murphy D, Simmons M, Guiney EJ: Neonatal urinary ascites in the absence of urinary tract obstruction. J Pediatr Surg 1978;13:529–531.
32. Morrell P, Coulthard MG, Hey EN: Neonatal urinary ascites. Arch Dis Child 1985;60:676–678.
33. Gillan JE, Lowden JA, Gaskin K, Cutz E: Congenital ascites as a presenting sign of lysosomal storage disease. J Pediatr 1984;104:225–231.
34. Vyas ID, Variend S, Dickson JAS: Ruptured ovarian cyst as a cause of ascites in a newborn infant. Z Kinderchir 1984;39:143–144.
35. Schultz RB, Kocoshis S: Cutis marmorata telangiectatica congenita and neonatal ascites. J Pediatr 1979;95:157.
36. Martone WJ, Williams WW, Mortensen ML, et al: Illness with fatalities in premature infants: association with an intravenous vitamin E preparation, E-Ferol. Pediatrics 1986;78:591–600.
37. Purohit DM, Lakin CA, Othersen HB: Neonatal pseudoascites: an unusual presentation of long tubular duplication of small bowel. J Pediatr Surg 1979;14:193–194.
38. Caine Y, Deckelbaum RJ, Weizman Z, et al: Congenital hepatic fibrosis: unusual presentations. Arch Dis Child 1984;59:1094–1096.
39. Cohen HA, Amir J, Frydman M, et al: Infection with the hepatitis A virus associated with ascites in children. Am J Dis Child 1992;146:1014–1016.
40. Levy I, Shohat M, Levy Y, et al: Recurrent ascites in an infant with perinatally acquired cytomegalovirus infection. Eur J Pediatr 1989;148:531–532.
41. Klein MD, Philippart AI: Posttraumatic Budd-Chiari syndrome with late reversibility of hepatic venous obstruction. J Pediatr Surg 1979;14:661–663.
42. Abbas Banani S, Bahador A, Nezakatgoo N: Idiopathic perforation of the extrahepatic bile duct in infancy: pathogenesis, diagnosis, and management. J Pediatr Surg 1993;28:950–952.
43. Stringel G, Mercer S: Idiopathic perforation of the biliary tract in infancy. J Pediatr Surg 1983;18:546–550.
44. So SKS, Lindahl JA, Sharp HL, et al: Bile ascites during infancy: diagnosis using disofenin Tc 99m sequential scintiphotography. Pediatrics 1983;71:402–405.
45. D'Cruz AJ, Kamath PS, Ramachandra C, Jalihal A: Pancreatic ascites in children. Acta Paediatr Jpn 1995;37:630–633.
46. Athow AC, Wilkinson ML, Saunders AJS, Drake DP: Pancreatic ascites presenting in infancy, with review of the literature. Dig Dis Sci 1991;36:245–250.
47. Maringhini A, Ciambra M, Patti R, et al: Ascites, pleural and pericardial effusions in acute pancreatitis. Dig Dis Sci 1996;41:848–852.

48. Chase GJ, O'Shea PA, Collins E, Brem AS: Protein-losing enteropathy in systemic lupus erythematosus. Hum Pathol 1982;13:1053–1055.
49. Moore ES, Chung EE, Cevallos EE: Intractable ascites in a child during peritoneal dialysis. J Pediatr 1977;91:949–951.
50. Eldor J, Olsha O, Farkas A: Over-transfusion ascites. Resuscitation 1991;21:289–291.
51. Goodman GM, Gourley GR: Ascites complicating ventriculoperitoneal shunts. J Pediatr Gastroenterol Nutr 1988;7:780–782.
52. West GA, Berger MS, Geyer JR: Childhood optic pathway tumors associated with ascites following ventriculoperitoneal shunt placement. Pediatr Neurosurg 1994;21:254–259.
53. Fernbach SK: Ascites produced by peritoneal seeding of neuroblastoma. Pediatr Radiol 1993;23:569.
54. Mecrow IK, Miller V, Lendon M, Doig CM: Mesenteric fibromatosis presenting with ascites in childhood. J Pediatr Gastroenterol Nutr 1990;11:118–122.
55. Berry PJ, Favara BE, Odom LF: Malignant peritoneal mesothelioma in a child. Pediatr Pathol 1986;5:397–409.
56. Duncan KA, King SE, Ratcliffe JF: Intraperitoneal fluid collections following liver transplantation in a paediatric population. Clin Radiol 1995;50:40–43.
57. Gane E, Langley P, Williams R: Massive ascitic fluid loss and coagulation disturbances after liver transplantation. Gastroenterology 1995;109:1631–1638.
58. John TG, Plevris JN, Redhead DN, et al: Massive ascitic fluid loss after liver transplantation. Gastroenterology 1996;111:564–565.
59. Mendoza FS, Johnson F, Kerner JA, et al: Vitamin A intoxication presenting with ascites and a normal vitamin A level. West J Med 1988;148:88–90.
60. Rosenberg HK, Berezin S, Heyman S, et al: Pleural effusion and ascites: unusual presenting features in a pediatric patient with vitamin A intoxication. Clin Pediatr 1982;21:435–440.
61. Rossi TM, Cumella J, Baswell D, Park B: Case report: ascites as a presenting sign of peritonitis in chronic granulomatous disease of childhood. Clin Pediatr 1987;26:544–545.
62. Novak RW, Boeckman CR: Pyloric duplication presenting with hemorrhagic ascites. Clin Pediatr 1983;22:386–388.
63. Axelsson CK, Knudsen FU: Catheter-induced ascites: an unusual complication of parenteral feeding. Intensive Care Med 1978;4:91–92.
64. Granot E, Deckelbaum RJ: "Pseudoascites" as a presenting physical sign of celiac disease. Am J Gastroenterol 1983;778:730–731.
65. Gyves-Ray K, Hernandez RJ, Hillemeier AC: Pseudoascites: unusual presentation of omental cyst. Pediatr Radiol 1990;20:560–561.
66. McCullagh M, Keen C, Dykes E: Cystic mesothelioma of the peritoneum: a rare cause of "ascites" in children. J Pediatr Surg 1994;29:1205–1207.
67. Runyon BA: Ascites and bacterial peritonitis. In Sleisenger MH, Fordtran JS (eds): Gastrointestinal Disease: Pathophysiology, Diagnosis, Management. Philadelphia, WB Saunders, 1993.
68. Runyon BA: Ascites. In Schiff L, Schiff ER (eds): Diseases of the Liver. Philadelphia, JB Lippincott, 1993.
69. Aiza I, Perez GO, Schiff ER: Management of ascites in patients with chronic liver disease. Am J Gastroenterol 1994;89:1949–1956.
70. Archimandritis A, Kalos A, Pantzos A, et al: Hemorrhagic ascites in a patient with anaphylactoid purpura. J Clin Gastroenterol 1994;18:257–258.
71. Millward-Sadler GH, Jezequel AM: Normal histology and ultrastructure. In Wright R, Alberti KGMM, Karran S, Millward-Sadler GH (eds): Liver and Biliary Disease. London, WB Saunders, 1979.
72. Dudley FJ: Pathophysiology of ascites formation. Gastroenterol Clin North Am 1992;21:215–236.
73. Henriksen JH: Cirrhosis: ascites and hepatorenal syndrome. Recent advances in pathogenesis. J Hepatol 1995;23(suppl 1):25–30.
74. Freeman S: Recent progress in the physiology and biochemistry of the liver. Med Clin North Am 1953;37:109–124.
75. Hyatt RE, Smith JR: The mechanism of ascites: a physiologic appraisal. Am J Med 1954;16:434–448.
76. Arroyo V, Gines P: Mechanism of sodium retention and ascites formation in cirrhosis. J Hepatol 1993;17(suppl 2):S24–S28.
77. Atkinson M, Losowsky MS: The mechanism of ascites formation in chronic liver disease. Q J Med 1961;30:153–166.
78. Sherlock S, Shaldon S: The aetiology and management of ascites in patients with hepatic cirrhosis: a review. Gut 1963;4:95–105.
79. Lieberman FL, Ito S, Reynolds TB: Effective plasma volume in cirrhosis with ascites. J Clin Invest 1969;48:975–981.
80. Lieberman FL, Denison EK, Reynolds TB: Relationship of plasma volume, portal hypertension, ascites, and renal sodium retention in cirrhosis: the overflow theory of ascites formation. Ann N Y Acad Sci 1970;170:202–212.
81. Schrier RW, Arroyo V, Bernardi M, et al: Peripheral arterial vasodilation hypothesis: a proposal for the initiation of renal sodium and water retention in cirrhosis. Hepatology 1988;8:1151–1157.
82. Bichet D, Szatalowicz V, Chaimovitz C, Schrier RW: Role of vasopressin in abnormal water excretion in cirrhotic patients. Ann Intern Med 1982;96:413–417.
83. Jimenez W, Arroyo V: Pathogenesis of sodium retention in cirrhosis. J Hepatol 1993;18:147–150.
84. Wong F, Sniderman K, Liu P, Blendis L: The mechanism of the initial natriuresis after transjugular intrahepatic portosystemic shunt. Gastroenterology 1997;112:899–907.
85. Schrier RW: Pathogenesis of sodium and water retention in high-output and low-output cardiac failure, nephrotic syndrome, cirrhosis, and pregnancy. N Engl J Med 1988;319:1065–1072.
86. Williams JW, Simel DL: Does this patient have ascites? How to divine fluid in the abdomen. JAMA 1992;267:2645–2648.
87. Nguyen KT, Sauerbrei EE, Nolan RL: The peritoneum and the diaphragm. In Rumack CM, Wilson SR, Charboneau JW (eds): Diagnostic Ultrasound. St. Louis, Mosby–Year Book, 1991.
88. Dinkel E, Lehnart R, Troger J, et al: Sonographic evidence of intraperitoneal fluid. Pediatr Radiol 1984;14:299–303.
89. Miller SF, Seibert JJ, Kinder DL, Wilson AR: Use of ultrasound in the detection of occult bowel perforation in neonates. J Ultrasound Med 1993;12:531–535.
90. Akgur FM, Tanyel FC, Akhan O, et al: The place of ultrasonographic examination in the initial evaluation of children sustaining blunt abdominal trauma. J Pediatr Surg 1993;28:78–81.
91. Dorne HL, Jequier S: Sonography of intestinal lymphangiectasia. J Ultrasound Med 1986;5:13–16.
92. Heiken JP: Abdominal wall and peritoneal cavity. In Lee JKT, Sagel SS, Stanley RJ (eds): Computed Body Tomography. New York, Raven Press, 1989.
93. King LR, Siegel MJ, Balfe DM: Acute pancreatitis in children: CT findings of intra- and extrapancreatic fluid collections. Radiology 1995;195:196–200.
94. Epstein BM, Mann JH: CT of abdominal tuberculosis. AJR Am J Roentgenol 1982;139:861–866.
95. Hibbeln JF, Wehmueller MD, Wilbur AC: Chylous ascites: CT and ultrasound appearance. Abdom Imaging 1995;20:138–140.
96. Runyon BA: Care of patients with ascites. N Engl J Med 1994;330:337–342.
97. Pare P, Talbot J, Hoefs JC: Serum ascites albumin concentration gradient: a physiologic approach to the differential diagnosis of ascites. Gastroenterology 1983;85:240–244.
98. Harjai KJ, Kamble MS, Ashar VJ, et al: Portal venous pressure and the serum-ascites albumin concentration gradient. Cleve Clin J Med 1995;62:62–67.
99. Rector WG, Reynolds TB: Superiority of the serum-ascites albumin difference over the ascites total protein concentration in separation of "transudative" and "exudative" ascites. Am J Med 1984;77:83–85.
100. Runyon BA, Montano AA, Akriviadis EA, et al: The serum-ascites albumin gradient is superior to the exudate-transudate concept in the differential diagnosis of ascites. Ann Intern Med 1992;117:215–220.
101. Wyllie R, Arasu TS, Fitzgerald JF: Ascites: pathophysiology and management. J Pediatr 1980;97:167–176.
102. Runyon BA: Paracentesis of ascitic fluid: a safe procedure. Arch Intern Med 1986;146:2259–2261.
103. Sungaila I, Bartle WR, Walker SE, et al: Spironolactone pharmacokinetics and pharmacodynamics in patients with cirrhotic ascites. Gastroenterology 1992;102:1680–1685.
104. Perez-Ayuso RM, Arroyo V, Planas R, et al: Randomized comparative study of efficacy of furosemide versus spironolactone in nonazotemic cirrhosis with ascites. Gastroenterology 1983;84:961–968.
105. Gatta A, Angeli P, Caregaro L, et al: A pathophysiological interpretation of unresponsiveness to spironolactone in a stepped-care approach to the diuretic treatment of ascites in nonazotemic cirrhotic patients. Hepatology 1991;14:231–236.
106. Arroyo V, Gines P, Planas R: Treatment of ascites in cirrhosis: diuretics, peritoneovenous shunt, and large-volume paracentesis. Gastroenterol Clin North Am 1992;21:237–256.
107. Arroyo V, Gines P, Gerbes AL, et al: Definition and diagnostic

criteria of refractory ascites and hepatorenal syndrome in cirrhosis. Hepatology 1996;23:164–176.
108. Shear L, Ching S, Gabuzda GJ: Compartmentalization of ascites and edema in patients with hepatic cirrhosis. N Engl J Med 1970;282:1391–1396.
109. Pockros PJ, Reynolds TB: Rapid diuresis in patients with ascites from chronic liver disease: the importance of peripheral edema. Gastroenterology 1986;90:1827–1833.
110. Planas R, Arroyo V, Rimola A, et al: Acetylsalicylic acid suppresses the renal hemodynamic effect and reduces the diuretic action of furosemide in cirrhosis with ascites. Gastroenterology 1983;84:247–252.
111. Gines P, Arroyo V, Quintero E, et al: Comparison of paracentesis and diuretics in the treatment of cirrhotics with tense ascites. Gastroenterology 1987;93:234–241.
112. Salerno F, Badalamenti S, Incerti P, et al: Repeated paracentesis and i.v. albumin infusion to treat "tense" ascites in cirrhotic patients. J Hepatol 1987;5:102–108.
113. Gines P, Tito L, Arroyo V, et al: Randomized comparative study of therapeutic paracentesis with and without intravenous albumin in cirrhosis. Gastroenterology 1988;94:1493–1502.
114. Simon DM, McCain JR, Bonkovsky HL, et al: Effects of therapeutic paracentesis on systemic and hepatic hemodynamics and on renal and hormonal function. Hepatology 1987;7:423–429.
115. Luca A, Garcia-Pagan JC, Bosch J, et al: Beneficial effects of intravenous albumin infusion on the hemodynamic and humoral changes after total paracentesis. Hepatology 1995;22:753–758.
116. Forouzandeh B, Konicek F, Sheagren JN: Large-volume paracentesis in the treatment of cirrhotic patients with refractory ascites. J Clin Gastroenterol 1996;22:207–210.
117. Gines A, Fernandez G, Monescillo A, et al: Randomized trial comparing albumin, dextran 70, and polygeline in cirrhotic patients with ascites treated by paracentesis. Gastroenterology 1996;111:1002–1010.
118. Baden HP, Morray JP: Drainage of tense ascites in children after cardiac surgery. J Cardiothorac Vasc Anesth 1995;9:720–721.
119. Leveen HH, Christoudias G, Ip M, et al: Peritoneo-venous shunting for ascites. Ann Surg 1974;180:580–591.
120. Tobe SW, Morali GA, Greig PD, et al: Peritoneovenous shunting restores atrial natriuretic factor responsiveness in refractory hepatic ascites. Gastroenterology 1993;105:202–207.
121. Stanley MM, Ochi S, Lee KK, et al: Peritoneovenous shunting as compared with medical treatment in patients with alcoholic cirrhosis and massive ascites. N Engl J Med 1989;1632–1638.
122. Gines A, Planas R, Paolo A, et al: Treatment of patients with cirrhosis and refractory ascites using LeVeen shunt with titanium tip: comparison with therapeutic paracentesis. Hepatology 1995;22:124–131.
123. Garcia VF, Howell CG, Barbot D, Ziegler MM: Small tube peritoneovenous shunting for the management of neonatal intractable ascites. Surg Obstet Gynecol 1985;160:273–274.
124. Pettitt BJ: Use of a modified Denver peritoneovenous shunt in a newborn with intractable ascites. J Pediatr Surg 1992;27:108–109.
125. Conn HO: Transjugular intrahepatic portal-systemic shunts: the state of the art. Hepatology 1993;17:148–158.
126. Ochs A, Rossle M, Haag K, et al: The transjugular intrahepatic portosystemic stent-shunt procedure for refractory ascites. N Engl J Med 1995;332:1192–1197.
127. Wong F, Sniderman K, Liu P, et al: Transjugular intrahepatic portosystemic stent shunt: effects on hemodynamics and sodium homeostasis in cirrhosis and refractory ascites. Ann Intern Med 1995;122:816–822.
128. Grace ND: TIPS: the long and the short of it. Gastroenterology 1997;112:1040–1043.
129. Lai KN, Leung JWC, Vallance-Owen J: Dialytic ultrafiltration by hemofilter in treatment of patients with refractory ascites and renal insufficiency. Am J Gastroenterol 1987;82:665–668.
130. Rossaro L, Graziotto A, Bonato S, et al: Concentrated ascitic fluid reinfusion after cascade filtration in tense ascites. Dig Dis Sci 1993;38:903–908.
131. Assadi FK, Gordon D, Kecskes SA, John E: Treatment of refractory ascites by ultrafiltration-reinfusion of ascitic fluid peritoneally. J Pediatr 1985;106:943–946.
132. Noble-Jamieson G, Jamieson N, Barnes ND: Ultrafiltration for intractable ascites after liver transplantation. Arch Dis Child 1991;66:988–989.
133. Rector FE, Whittlesey G: Effective control of chylous ascites: an alternative approach. J Pediatr Surg 1993;28:76–77.
134. Clark JH, Fitzgerald JF, Kleiman MB: Spontaneous bacterial peritonitis. J Pediatr 1984;104:495–500.
135. Larcher VF, Manolaki N, Vegnente A, et al: Spontaneous bacterial peritonitis in children with chronic liver disease: clinical features and etiologic factors. J Pediatr 1985;106:907–912.
136. Glassman MS, Berezin S, Boyle JT: Bacterial peritonitis and sepsis presenting as acute gastrointestinal bleeding in patients with portal hypertension. Pediatr Emerg Care 1993;9:19–22.
137. Runyon BA, Canawati HN, Akriviadis EA: Optimization of ascitic fluid culture technique. Gastroenterology 1988;95:1351–1355.
138. Rolachon A, Cordier L, Bacq Y, et al: Ciprofloxacin and long term prevention of spontaneous bacterial peritonitis: results of a prospective controlled trial. Hepatology 1995;22:1171–1174.

Chapter 10

# Caustic Ingestion and Foreign Bodies

William J. Byrne

## CAUSTIC INGESTION

The ingestion of caustic substances remains a health hazard for infants and children. Despite the Poison Prevention Packaging Act of 1970, which limited the concentration of caustic agents in household products to 10% and required these products to be sold in child-resistant containers, the incidence of exposures has increased. The Poison Control Centers National Data Bank reported in 1990 that caustic ingestions numbered 11,516 for alkaline agents and 4,748 for acidic agents.[1] At the top of the list were household bleaches, automatic dishwasher detergents, laundry detergents, swimming pool or aquarium products, and toilet bowl and oven cleaners. Table 10–1 lists the caustic ingredients found in common household products.

**TABLE 10–1. Caustic Ingredients Found in Common Household Products**

| PRODUCT | INGREDIENT |
|---|---|
| **Alkalis** | |
| Liquid Plumber | Sodium hydroxide |
| Drano | Sodium hydroxide |
| Clinitest tablets | Sodium hydroxide |
| Oven cleaner | Sodium hydroxide |
| **Detergents** | |
| Dishwashing liquids | Sodium phosphates |
| Laundry detergent | Sodium carbonates, sodium phosphates |
| Cleaner | Sodium phosphates |
| **Acids** | |
| Mister Plumber | Sulfuric acid |
| Lysol Toilet Bowl Cleaner | Hydrochloric acid |
| Saniflush Toilet Bowl Cleaner | Sodium bisulfate |
| Vanish Toilet Bowl Cleaner | Sodium bisulfate |
| Metal cleaners | Hydrofluoric acid |
| **Bleach** | |
| Clorox | Sodium hypochlorite |
| Peroxide | Hydrogen peroxide |
| Tile cleaners | Sodium hypochlorite, sodium hydroxide |

The extent and severity of the injury to the esophagus or stomach depends on the type of agent, its physical state, concentration, pH, and quantity ingested. Solid agents in the form of pellets, powder, or granules cause immediate pain and are quickly extruded. Acidic solutions also cause immediate pain and have a bitter taste; unless the ingestion was intentional, they are also expelled quickly. Alkaline solutions are often odorless and tasteless and do not produce discomfort even after several swallows. The result is extensive contiguous circumferential damage along the entire esophagus.

Alkaline substances produce liquefaction necrosis, with intense inflammation and saponification of the mucosal, submucosal, and muscular layers of both the esophagus and the stomach. Krey demonstrated in an animal model that a 3.8% solution of sodium hydroxide in contact with the esophageal mucosa for 10 seconds caused necrosis of the mucosa and submucosa extending into the muscle layer.[1] A 10.7% solution resulted in damage that extended to the outer muscle layer, and a 22.5% solution produced a full-thickness burn. Vancura and colleagues demonstrated that the pH of a solution may be a more useful clinical indicator of risk for damage.[2] A pH of 12.5 or greater, regardless of the concentration, results in some degree of ulceration.

Acidic substances cause injury by coagulation necrosis with eschar formation. Because of the eschar formation, the pH of the esophagus, and the resistance of squamous epithelium to acid injury, the esophagus is spared in many acid ingestions.[3] The prepyloric area of the stomach usually is the site of the acute injury. Nonetheless, the esophagus should be evaluated carefully. Because acids have a low ratio of viscosity to specific gravity their transit time is rapid, and skip areas are frequently seen on endoscopy.

Household bleach contains sodium hypochlorite in concentrations of less than 10%. With a pH of about 6.5, the risk of esophageal injury is low. Swimming pool cleaners, on the other hand, contain up to 20% sodium hypochlorite and should be considered to pose a high risk for tissue damage.[4] Dishwashing detergents contain balance builders, sodium salts of carbonates, phosphates, and silicates that increase the pH to between 11.8 and 12.7. The granular forms are more likely to cause caustic burns than their liquid counterparts. The caustic agent in drain or oven cleaners is usually sodium or potassium hydroxide. Although the concentration is usually less than 10%, the pH of 11.5 or higher makes them capable of producing severe injury. Dilute solutions of ammonia found in commercial window cleaners are considered to be nontoxic. Strong acids, usually hydrochloric, sulfuric, or phosphoric, are commonly found in toilet bowl cleaners, swimming pool cleaners, battery fluids, and antirust compounds. Hydrofluoric acid, used in pottery glazing, photography, and metal cleaning, is extremely toxic. Fluoride ions produce not only local tissue destruction but also systemic symptoms. Various members of the pepper family can cause esophageal burns. If you can't pick it up without burning your fingers, don't eat it.

## Evaluation and Management

The evaluation begins with a good clinical history, including the type and volume of the ingested substance. Having the container is very helpful. After the ingestion the child is usually frightened, crying, and spitting. Burns may be seen on the lips or in the oropharynx. With alkalis the oral burns are usually yellow or brown, whereas with acids the oral injury is characterized by whitish-gray necrotic areas. Thirty percent to 50% of patients with oral burns also have esophageal burns.[5] However, the absence of oral burns does not exclude the possibility of an esophageal or gastric burn.[6] Crain and associates reported that children who present with two or more symptoms, including drooling, vomiting, dysphagia, abdominal pain, or stridor, have a 50% chance of having esophageal burns.[7] Others have not been able to substantiate this finding.

Vomiting should not be induced because of the risks of increasing the esophageal injury and of aspiration. The symptomatic child should be admitted to the hospital, given nothing by mouth, and started on intravenous fluids. Endoscopy is the only reliable way to evaluate the upper gastrointestinal tract. A contrast study should not be performed. Whether all patients with a history of caustic ingestion need to undergo endoscopy is controversial. Proponents of endoscopy suggest that the procedure influences the decision of whether therapy (i.e., antibiotics, steroids, string placement, stenting, or gastrostomy) is necessary. If the procedure is done too early, within 4 to 6 hours, the severity of the esophageal damage may be underestimated. Opponents of universal endoscopy refer to the rare, almost reportable, case of esophageal stricture in the absence of oral burns or other symptoms. A "middle-of-the-road" approach is to perform endoscopy only for those children with oral burns or other symptoms suggesting caustic ingestion. Exceptions are made if the ingestion was intentional or if the history is unequivocal for the ingestion of a true acid or alkali (pH $<3$ or $>11.5$).

Endoscopy should be done 12 to 24 hours after the ingestion. General anesthesia reduces the risk of perforation and allows for careful evaluation of the oral cavity and hypopharynx. Holinger devised a classification for esophageal burns[8] (Table 10–2). Once a third-degree burn is seen, the instrument should not be advanced further, and the procedure should be terminated. Any further endoscopic procedures should be delayed for a minimum of 3 weeks. The esophageal wall is weakest between 7 and 21 days after ingestion, during which time collagen is being deposited to repair tissue.[9]

**TABLE 10–2. Clinical Staging of Esophageal Burns**

| BURN | CHARACTERISTICS |
|---|---|
| First-degree | Hyperemia and edema of the mucosa<br>Damage limited to the mucosa |
| Second-degree | Exudate, erosions, shallow ulcers<br>Destruction of the mucosa and submucosa with penetration of the injury to the muscle layers |
| Third-degree | Deep ulceration, circumferential necrosis, often the presence of a black coagulum<br>Full-thickness injury with extension into the pleura and mediastinum |

Children with first-degree burns require no specific therapy. Usually within 24 to 48 hours oral intake is reestablished and the patient may be discharged. Patients with second- and third-degree burns should be given intravenous antibiotics. Ampicillin, 100 mg/kg per day for 10 to 14 days, is the drug of choice. Alternatives include erythromycin or a third-generation cephalosporin. Antibiotics, by preventing infection, may hasten tissue repair but do not prevent stricture formation. The use of steroids is controversial. Three studies involving 165 patients suggested that steroids were harmful.[4] Anderson and coworkers, in a study conducted over 18 years involving 60 children, concluded that steroids did not protect against stricture formation.[5] No data exist regarding the potential benefit of early steroid use (i.e., within the first 6 hours).

The management of extensive second- or third-degree burns requires an aggressive approach. If the esophageal tissue appears viable, a surgical gastrostomy is performed and a stent is placed to reduce the morbidity related to stricture formation. If the viability of the esophagus is in question, surgical exploration is delayed for 24 to 36 hours. At that time a decision can be made regarding the need for esophagectomy.

Esophageal stricture formation may be evident as early as 21 days after ingestion. At this time an esophagogram should be done on all patients with previously documented second- or third-degree burns. Dilation can be accomplished with Tucker's dilators if a string was placed at the initial endoscopy, or under direct vision with the Puestow wire technique or inflatable dilators. Although some have advocated early dilation, the effect on outcome does not justify the risk.[10] Very long, tight structures may necessitate esophageal replacement.

The risk of squamous cell carcinoma after lye ingestion is approximately 1,000-fold greater than for the general population.[11] The latency period is long—41 years in one series.[11] Most of the carcinomas were found in the area of the tracheal bifurcation. Later in life periodic surveillance of these patients is necessary.

## FOREIGN BODIES

Toddlers and young children frequently evaluate their surroundings by tasting and swallowing new and unusual objects. The peak incidence of foreign body ingestion occurs between 6 months and 3 years of age.[12] Older children and adolescents with mental retardation or psychiatric disturbances may swallow virtually anything. These patients present the clinician with the unique challenge of deciding on the appropriate application of expectant management, endoscopy, or surgery.

Because the management of foreign bodies is based on collected experience rather than controlled studies, each case must be approached on an individual basis. The type of foreign object, its location in the gastrointestinal tract, and whether the patient is symptomatic are all important variables in the application of treatment guidelines. Table 10–3 lists the more commonly swallowed objects. Of all foreign bodies that reach the stomach, 80% to 90% pass spontaneously, 10% to 20% require endoscopic removal, and 1% require surgery.[13] Objects that may not pass include those with a diameter of more than 20 mm and those that are more than 5 cm in length (Fig. 10–1).[14, 15] Because of the risk of perforation, sharp objects, such as chicken or fish bones, long pins, and toothpicks, should be removed endoscopically rather than allowed to pass spontaneously.[16]

Infants and children most often ingest coins, buttons, batteries, and toys, whereas adults experience more problems with bones and meat. The possibility of a second foreign body should always be considered. Recurrent ingestion is not uncommon, particularly among the mentally retarded and adolescents with psychiatric disorders. Over time, a total of 2,533 objects was retrieved from the stomach of one patient.[17]

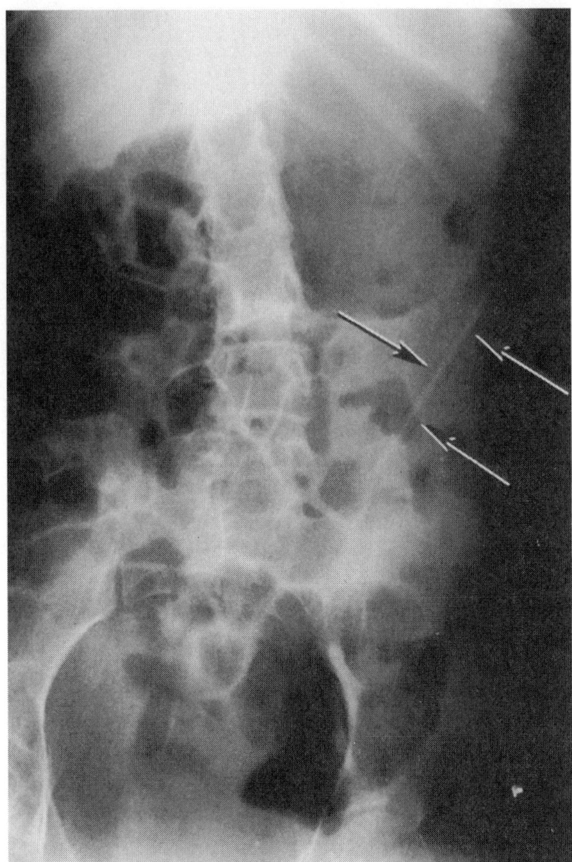

**FIGURE 10–1.** This 13-year-old girl was being monitored for scoliosis. An abdominal film showed a long, thin foreign body in the descending colon *(arrows)*. The patient admitted to having swallowed a pencil several weeks before.

## Specific Types of Foreign Bodies

### *Coins*

Coins are the most frequently swallowed foreign objects and account for the majority of esophageal foreign bodies in children. More than 2,800 cases were reported by the American Association of Poison Control Centers Database in 1987.[18] Half of the patients were younger than 2 years of age, and 29% were younger than 1 year of age.[19] Coins lodged in the esophagus may not produce symptoms. Hodge and associates[20] reviewed radiographs from 80 children with a history of having swallowed a coin. In 25 (31%) the coin was stuck in the esophagus. Eleven of the patients (44%) were asymptomatic. Schunk and colleagues reported a similar experience in 52 patients.[21] In this series the coin was found in the esophagus in 30 patients (58%), 9 of whom (30%) were asymptomatic. The authors of both studies concluded that all children who swallow coins should undergo prompt roentgenographic evaluation. Although this recommendation seems prudent, it is not without controversy.[22, 23] In the esophagus the flat surface of the coin is seen on an anteroposterior view and the edge on lateral views (Fig. 10–2). The opposite is true for coins in the trachea: The anteroposterior view reveals the edge and the lateral view the flat surface.

**TABLE 10–3. Foreign Bodies Commonly Ingested by Infants, Children, and Adolescents**

| | |
|---|---|
| Coins | Glass fragments |
| Disk (button) batteries | Pop tabs |
| Straight pins | Broken dental retainers |
| Hat pins | Ballpoint pen tops |
| Chicken or fish bones | Keys |
| Toothpicks | Marbles |
| Screws | Crayons |
| Nails | Silverware |
| Thumbtacks | Erasers |
| Safety pins | Bottle caps |
| Razor blades | Seashells |
| Meat | |

Esophageal foreign bodies, whether symptomatic or not, should be removed. In the symptomatic patient this needs to be done as soon as possible. In the asymptomatic patient a temporizing approach should be taken. Experience indicates that the foreign body usually passes into the stomach within 24 hours, either spontaneously or after the ingestion of liquids.[20–23] When passage does not occur, the child is at risk for complications such as esophageal perforation,[24] tracheoesophageal fistula,[25] and esophagoaortic fistula.[26] These severe complications occurred after 4 months,[24] 8 years,[25] and 1 week,[26] respectively. Chaikhouni and coworkers,[27] in a review of 88 patients with esophageal foreign bodies, found that the only consistent risk factor for a major complication was the presence of the coin in the esophagus for more than 24 hours. From Schunk and associates' series,[21] two

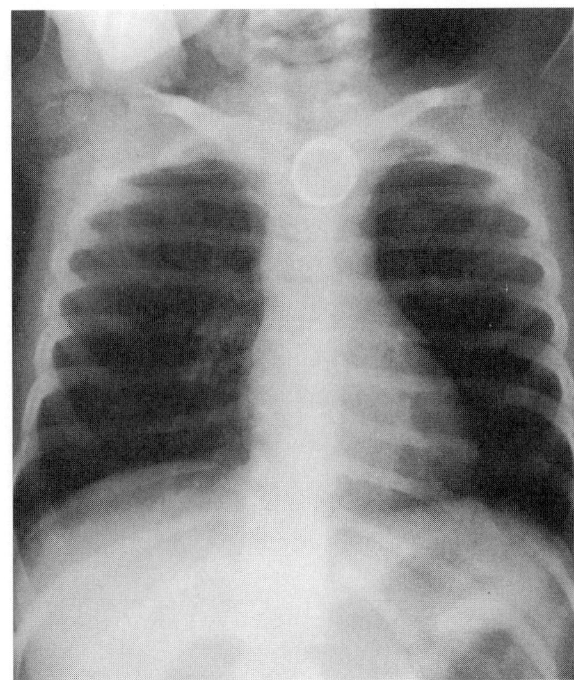

**FIGURE 10–2.** Anteroposterior (AP) view of the chest showing a bottle cap lodged in the cervical esophagus. The flat surface, as with coins, is present on the AP view.

asymptomatic patients had coins removed after impactions of 5 days. Mucosal erosion was present in one case, and in the other the coin was embedded in the mucosa. The type of coin may be important. The new zinc penny (97.6% zinc, 2.4% copper), which replaced the copper penny (95% copper, 5% zinc) in 1982, is more corrosive in the esophagus. Although 24 hours appears to be a safe waiting period, if the coin has not passed into the stomach by then, it should be removed. A number of techniques may be employed. There are advocates for the use of rigid endoscopy,[28] flexible endoscopy,[29, 30] Foley catheters,[20, 21, 31] and bougie dilator advancement.[32] Which technique is best is controversial.

As a general rule, coins 20 mm or less in diameter in the stomach may be expected to pass spontaneously through the gastrointestinal tract. The diameters of U.S. coins are pennies, 18 mm; nickels, 21 mm; dimes, 17 mm; quarters, 24 mm; half-dollars, 30 mm; and dollars, 26 and 38 mm. Once it has been determined that the coin is in the stomach, the parents should be instructed to examine the stools for passage of the coin. Unless symptoms of gastric outlet obstruction occur (i.e., abdominal pain, vomiting, or both), endoscopic removal should be delayed. If the parents do not report passage of the coin, an abdominal film should be taken 1 week after ingestion. Subsequent films taken every 7 to 10 days may be used to monitor passage of the coin. If after 4 weeks the coin remains in the stomach, it should be removed endoscopically.

## Disk (Button) Batteries

Before 1982, only six cases of disk (button) battery ingestion had been reported in the medical literature. Two of the children died,[33, 34] and two experienced serious morbidity.[35, 36] With their more widespread use in hearing aids, watches, calculators, cameras, and toys, battery ingestion has increased substantially.[37–42] According to data reported from the National Poison Center Network, between 510 and 850 disk battery ingestions occur annually in the United States.[43] Litovitz initially reported 119 button battery ingestions occurring over an 11-month period.[37] Seventy-one percent of the patients were younger than 5 years of age. Forty-eight percent of the ingested batteries were either loose or had been discarded, 34.4% were in the product, and 3.4% were in the manufacturer's packaging. The prevalence of ingested batteries that had been left out underscores the need for parental and public education regarding prompt disposal or safe storage of these items out of the sight and reach of children. Hearing-aid batteries were the most common type swallowed (33.9%). Of the 18 swallowed hearing-aid batteries, 14 were swallowed by hearing-impaired children who had removed the batteries from their own hearing aids. An update of the registry analyzing 2,382 cases of cylindrical and button battery ingestion reported similar trends.[38]

Disk batteries are composed of four systems: (1) the mercuric oxide system with mercuric oxide cathode and zinc anode; (2) the silver oxide system with a silver oxide cathode and zinc anode; (3) a manganese oxide system with a manganese dioxide cathode and zinc anode; and (4) a lithium system. All four systems contain a 20% to 45% solution of either potassium or sodium hydroxide. Batteries cause tissue injury by any one or a combination of the following mechanisms: pressure necrosis, low-voltage burns, or corrosive injury due to liquefaction necrosis induced by leakage of the alkaline solution. Mercury toxicity is more of a theoretical concern. In contrast to mercuric oxide, elemental mercury is readily absorbed. Elemental mercury is produced when mercuric oxide is reduced in the presence of gastric acid and iron from the corroding steel casing of the battery. To date, only one case of mild mercury poisoning has been documented.[44] Ninety percent of all disk batteries pass spontaneously through the gastrointestinal tract.[37] Eighty-five percent of these do so within 72 hours.

Management of a disk battery ingestion depends on its location. The child should be given nothing by mouth. Emetics have not been helpful and are not indicated.[33, 37, 38] Urgent roentgenographic examination, visualizing the gut from mouth to anus, must be performed. When the object is lodged in the esophagus, the radiologist should be able to distinguish between a disk battery and a coin.[45] In the anteroposterior projection, disk batteries demonstrate a double-density shadow owing to the bilaminar structure of the battery. On lateral view, the edges of most disk batteries are round and present a step-off at the junction of the anode and cathode. Disk batteries lodged in the esophagus demand urgent removal. Contact time of as little as 1 hour may result in mucosal injury, and within 4 hours all layers of the esophagus may be involved. Endoscopic retrieval under general anesthesia is the procedure of choice. Advantages over the Foley catheter technique include the ability to assess directly the esophageal mucosa and the avoidance of aspiration into the respiratory tree during withdrawal. The battery may be removed from the esophagus with the through-the-scope balloon or carefully pushed into the stomach and "netted" with a polyp retrieval net or snared with a polyp snare. The presence of significant tissue damage in the esophagus warrants a follow-up barium study in 10 to 14 days to rule out stricture formation or a fistula.

Once the battery is in the stomach, a more conservative course may be taken. All but the largest batteries (i.e., those greater than 20 mm in diameter) should pass. In a series of 119 button battery ingestions, 68.8% passed within 48 hours and 85.4% passed within 72 hours, with a range of 12 hours to 14 days.[37] Cathartics, such as magnesium sulfate or magnesium citrate, or a prokinetic agent, such as metoclopramide, may be given to hasten transit time. Although of no proven efficacy, antacids or histamine $H_2$ blockers may be given to reduce acid secretion and thereby theoretically reduce the risk of mercury poisoning. The child may be monitored as an outpatient, and the parents should be instructed to strain the stools. If after 48 hours the battery has not passed, a repeat abdominal film should be taken. Continued presence of the battery in the stomach necessitates endoscopic removal. Although the battery may temporarily "hang up" in the ileum, cecum, or ascending colon, there has been only one reported complication involving the intestine. In this patient the disk battery lodged in a Meckel's diverticulum and resulted in a fatal perforation.[36] Abdominal films should be repeated until the battery's elimination can be documented. Surgical removal becomes necessary when the battery fails to move over a period of 5 days or the patient develops symptoms of abdominal pain or peritoneal irritation.

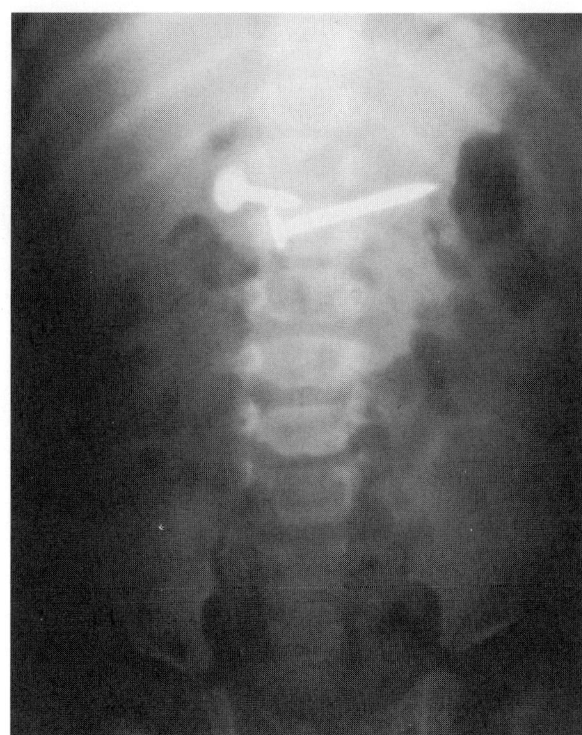

**FIGURE 10–3.** Plain radiograph of the abdomen shows two nails in the stomach of a 15-month-old infant. These were removed endoscopically.

## *Sharp or Elongated Foreign Bodies*

Sharp or pointed foreign bodies, as well as elongated foreign bodies, can sometimes be difficult to manage (Fig. 10–3). As a group, sharp or pointed objects, particularly fish or chicken bones, long straight pins, and toothpicks, carry a higher risk for significant morbidity.[46–51] Fifteen percent to 35% of perforations from foreign body ingestion are caused by sharp or pointed objects. Perforations are particularly likely to occur in the C loop of the duodenum, at the ligament of Trietz, in the terminal ileum or ileocecal region, and in the sigmoid colon. Certain objects such as bones, long straight pins, and toothpicks carry a significantly higher risk.[50, 51] As a general guideline, in adolescents or older children, an object longer than 5 cm or wider than 2 cm is not likely to pass. For infants and young children, the limit is 3 cm in length. High-risk objects and those exceeding these dimensions require urgent endoscopic removal from the stomach or proximal duodenum. Small nails, screws, pins, and thumbtacks may be managed conservatively.

Animal studies have shown that the bowel dilates locally in response to mucosal contact with a sharp object.[52] This reflex relaxation of the muscle wall, combined with axial flow in the lumen, tends to turn sharp objects around, preventing perforation. When possible, a high-roughage diet should be started. Serial abdominal films should be obtained at 4- to 5-day intervals. If a pin or other sharp object stays in place for 5 days or longer or the patient develops abdominal symptoms, it is likely that the object has penetrated the bowel wall or is lodged in a Meckel's diverticulum or the appendix.[53] Surgical intervention is then necessary.

Open safety pins present a major problem. If the pin is lodged in the esophagus with the open end proximal and the spring distal, the patient should undergo endoscopy; the pin should be carefully pushed into the stomach and then retrieved using an overtube. When the orientation is reversed, the pin should be grasped, pulled into an overtube, and withdrawn. Closed safety pins, once in the stomach, will pass and require only careful follow-up.

Razor blades in the esophagus may be removed either through the rigid esophagoscope or with a large endoscope using an overtube. Although once it is in the stomach, a razor blade may pass, it should be removed endoscopically.

## *Meat*

Meat impaction in the esophagus is uncommon in children. When it does occur, it is usually secondary to an esophageal abnormality such as a stricture or motility disorder.[54] Hot dogs and meat are the most common offenders and usually lodge in the distal esophagus.[55] Management depends on the symptoms. If the child is having difficulty handling secretions, an urgent endoscopy for removal should be done. Because of the high risk of stricture, the object should not be pushed into the stomach unless it is known that there is no distal pathology. If there are no problems with handling secretions, endoscopy may be delayed for 12 hours. Unless the object passes, further postponement is unwise because of the increasing risk of complications.[27] Sedation or glucagon, or both, may be helpful in facilitating passage.[56–58]

Glucagon is particularly effective with objects in the distal one third of the esophagus because of its ability to decrease lower esophageal sphincter pressure.[58] Disruption of a meat impaction with papain (Adolph's Meat Tenderizer) is thought to be effective, but its use cannot be recommended.[59, 60] It is

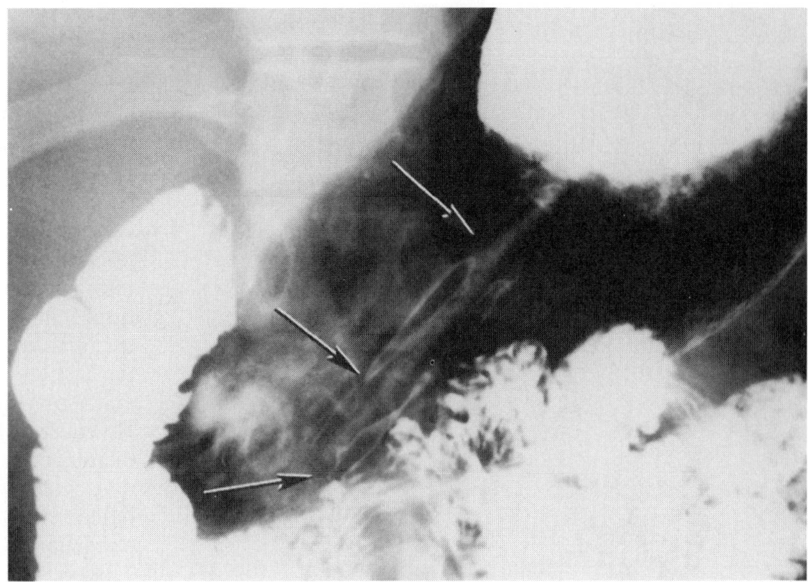

**FIGURE 10–4.** Contrast study outlining the handle *(arrows)* of a plastic fork in the stomach.

debatable whether enzymatic digestion of the meat actually occurs, and injury to the esophageal wall is a potential risk. Two deaths from perforation have been attributed to the administration of this agent.[61] Once the meat passes, an esophagogram or an upper endoscopy should be done to exclude esophageal pathology.

### *Radiolucent Foreign Bodies*

Glass, plastic, wood, and aluminum can pop tabs may be difficult to see on routine radiographs, particularly if the object is lodged in the hypopharynx or cervical esophagus. Thin barium may be used to try to outline the object (Fig. 10–4). If it is identified in the esophagus, it should be removed endoscopically. Endoscopy is also indicated if the patient is symptomatic. Failure to identify the object in an asymptomatic patient or the presence of the object in the stomach warrants only careful follow-up by the parents for its passage in the stool.

## Technical Aspects of Foreign Body Management

The technique used to remove a foreign body depends on its type, its location in the gastrointestinal tract, and the age of the patient. Objects may hang up anywhere, increasing the risk of perforation. Common sites are areas of angulation or narrowing of the lumen (Fig. 10–5). Before any foreign body is extracted, the object should be duplicated, the procedure carefully preplanned, and a dry run carried out. A number of devices are available to grasp the object (Fig. 10–6). Which device to use is an individual preference. Coins are best retrieved with a basket, polyp retrieval net, polyp snare, or rat-tooth jaw if the rim is present. Screws, pins, nails, and other long objects may be grasped with the alligator jaws or rubber-tipped jaws. The rat-tooth jaws are useful for removing food from the esophagus. Large objects or those with no edges, such as marbles or seeds, are best trapped in the basket or netted with the polyp retrieval net. Remember Jackson's axiom when removing sharp or pointed objects: "Advancing points puncture, trailing do not."[62] Regardless of whether the procedure is done under conscious sedation or general anesthesia, a Kelly or McGill forceps and laryngoscope must be available in case the object is lost in the hypopharynx. Surgical removal of a foreign body is sometimes necessary.

### *Esophagus*

Most esophageal foreign bodies lodge at one of three primary sites: the level of the cricopharyngeal muscle, the

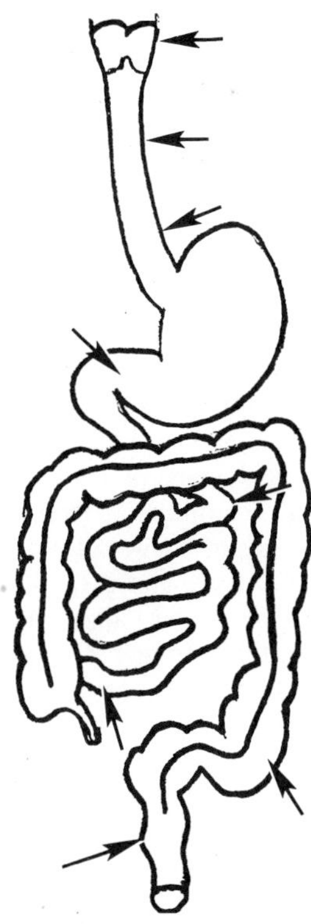

**FIGURE 10–5.** Sites *(arrows)* in the gastrointestinal tract where foreign bodies may arrest after ingestion.

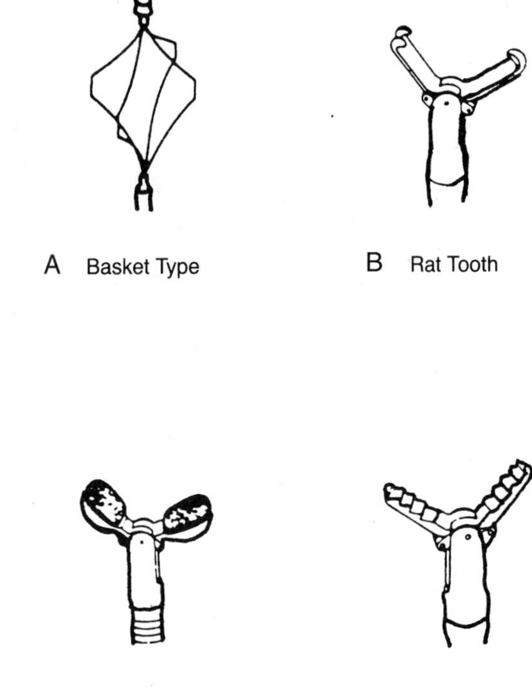


**FIGURE 10–6.** Devices available for the removal of foreign bodies. *A*, Basket for trapping coins, marbles and other rounded objects. *B*, Rat-tooth jaws for grasping food and other soft materials. *C* and *D,* Alligator jaws and rubber-tipped jaws for grasping screws, nails, and pins.

level of the aortic arch, or the gastroesophageal junction. It also must be kept in mind that pathologic narrowing may be responsible for an object's failure to progress. Coins lodged in the esophagus may be given up to 24 hours to pass, but disk button batteries require urgent removal. Sharp objects may cause penetrating esophageal injury and should be removed immediately.

**CLINICAL MANIFESTATIONS.** Although most patients present with symptoms of chest pain and salivation, some are asymptomatic. Therefore, the history of an ingestion must be taken seriously. Patients may initially choke or cough and then gag in an effort to regurgitate the object. Pain may be perceived at the level of the obstruction or referred to the sternal notch. Pain may be severe, and the patient may be in considerable distress.

**DIAGNOSIS.** The history of a foreign body ingestion warrants radiographic examination from the mouth to the anus. Plain anteroposterior views of the neck, chest, and abdomen, as well as lateral views of the neck and chest, should be done. Failure to visualize the object does not preclude its presence. Objects such as plastic, wood, aluminum, glass, and bones are radiolucent and difficult to detect. In the symptomatic patient, failure to visualize the object warrants urgent endoscopy. Contrast radiography may be useful in the asymptomatic patient (see Fig. 10–4). Barium-coated cotton pledgets should not be used because they add another foreign body and may make subsequent endoscopic examination and retrieval more difficult.

**MANAGEMENT.** With the exception of coins, all esophageal foreign bodies should be removed under direct vision. This allows evaluation of the mucosa for underlying pathology before the object's extraction. Coins may be removed with a Foley catheter.[31] The procedure is relatively simple but should be attempted only by experienced personnel. It is done under fluoroscopy after the patient has been immobilized on a papoose board or wrapped securely in a sheet. A Foley catheter is passed orally. Once the tip of the catheter passes beyond the foreign body, the balloon is inflated with contrast material. The patient is then placed into a prone oblique position, and the fluoroscopic table is turned into a head-down position. Then, applying a steady traction, the Foley catheter is withdrawn, its balloon pulling the foreign body ahead of it. Once out of the esophagus, aided by gravity, the object should fall out of the mouth. However, a laryngoscope and forceps must be available. If the object cannot be dislodged with steady traction, intravenous glucagon, 0.05 mg/kg, may be given in an effort to induce sufficient esophageal relaxation to permit successful extraction. Failure after glucagon warrants endoscopic intervention. The Foley catheter technique should not be used to remove disk button batteries.

If the foreign body is in the cervical esophagus or its exact location is unknown, insertion of the endoscope should be done under direct vision. Before removal of the object, the esophageal mucosa should be carefully inspected for signs of injury. Foreign bodies should never be extracted forcibly. Adequate insufflation of air to distend the esophagus, parenteral glucagon to induce relaxation, and orientation of the object into the frontal plane facilitate successful removal. Trauma to the esophagus from sharp objects may be avoided by using an overtube (Fig. 10–7). Open safety pins, with the spring end oriented distally, should be carefully pushed into the stomach, turned, grasped securely with the spring end oriented proximally, and removed using an overtube. Severe mucosal disruption and bleeding, or the presence of chest pain after the procedure, suggests esophageal perforation. A contrast study of the esophagus should be done.

## *Stomach and Duodenum*

Objects may fail to pass through the pylorus, or they may become lodged there or in the duodenal sweep. For coins,

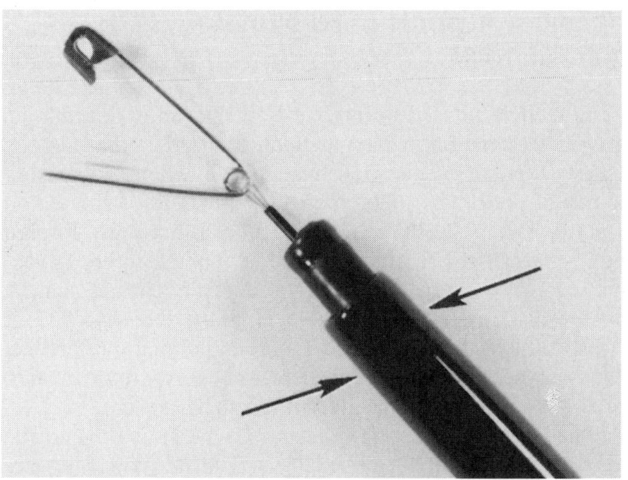

**FIGURE 10–7.** Sharp objects should be securely grasped and pulled into the overtube *(arrows)*, which has been passed over the endoscope. The entire apparatus is then withdrawn.

disk batteries, and other blunt objects, observation is appropriate, because those smaller than 20 mm in diameter are likely to pass through the pylorus and subsequently through the entire digestive tract. Failure of a disk battery to pass within 48 hours warrants removal of the object. Four weeks may be allowed for coins. Sharp objects greater than 5 cm in length should be removed endoscopically because of the risk of perforation.

**CLINICAL MANIFESTATIONS.** Most patients are asymptomatic. Vomiting and pain suggest pyloric obstruction; if coupled with fever and peritoneal signs, they suggest perforation. Duodenal perforation from a sharp object such as a pin or toothpick may produce only minimal symptoms. The diagnosis requires a high index of suspicion.

**MANAGEMENT.** Endoscopic retrieval of a gastric foreign body requires planning and practice with the correct accessory before the procedure is begun. Just before the procedure, an abdominal film should be done to be sure the object has not moved into the intestine. Retrieval is often facilitated by positioning the object along the greater curvature in the body of the stomach before attempting to grasp it. Sharp objects should be removed with an overtube to prevent trauma to the esophagus during withdrawal.

### Colon and Rectum

Children occasionally place objects in the rectum. Small, blunt objects are passed spontaneously. Large or sharp objects require retrieval. This can be done through a sigmoidoscope or with the use of a vaginal speculum and Kocher clamp. Adequate sedation with local or general anesthesia is essential to relax the anal sphincter. A long foreign object should be oriented in the vertical plane before an attempt is made to remove it. If the object is beyond the reach of the sigmoidoscope, observation for 12 to 24 hours will allow the object to descend. The other alternative is to use an upper endoscope, a retrieval forceps, and an overtube. After removal of the object, the sigmoidoscopy should be repeated to look for mucosal injury.[63]

## Bezoars

Bezoars are a rare and unique form of gastrointestinal foreign body that have held a certain mystic fascination through the ages.[64] The term *bezoar* is derived from the Arabic *badzehr* or the Persian *padzahr,* both of which mean "antidote to poison." From antiquity until the late 18th century, a bezoar from an animal's stomach was highly revered because of its magical powers. Taken internally, it neutralized poisons, destroyed venoms, and counteracted attacks of epilepsy, dysentery, plague, and leprosy. Worn as a charm, it provided protection from evil spirits. Today the term *bezoar* refers to the accumulation of exogenous matter in the stomach and small intestine.

In an early extensive review of bezoars, DeBakey and Ochsner noted that 90% of all patients were female, and that the peak age group was between 10 and 19 years.[64] Bezoars are classified on the basis of their composition. Trichobezoars are composed primarily of the patient's own hair. Trichotillomania with trichophagia may result in bezoar formation and is indicative of a personality disorder. McGehee and Buchanan,[65] reporting on two children with trichobezoars and iron deficiency, suggested that trichophagia was a form of pica. Other sources of the fibers for bezoar formation include carpets, blankets, animal hair, and doll's hair. Trichobezoars may become quite large and can form a cast of the stomach if they have been present for many years. A "tail" may extend from the gastric portion of the bezoar into the small intestine, resulting in obstructive jaundice[66] and pancreatitis.[67] Protein-losing gastroenteropathy and steatorrhea have been reported in association with trichobezoars.[68, 69] In one report,[69] the microscopic appearance of the gastric mucosa showed hyperplasia similar to that seen with chronic hypertrophic gastritis, which was suggested as the cause of the protein loss.

Phytobezoars are composed of a heterogeneity of plant and vegetable material. Among adults this is the most common form of bezoar. In DeBakey and Ochsner's review of bezoars,[64] 92 (73%) of 126 phytobezoars were caused by the ingestion of persimmons. Persimmon bezoar (diospyrobezoar) occurs after the ingestion of large amounts of the unripe fruit. The pulp, which contains phlobatannin, coagulates in the stomach on contact with acid.[70] Fortunately, persimmons are not a favorite of children because of their tart taste. Other substances that may form phytobezoars when ingested in excessive amounts include celery, pumpkin, grape skins, prunes, raisins, leeks, wild beets, and grass. Hypochlorhydria, decreased antral motility, and poor chewing of food are predisposing factors in phytobezoar formation. They have been described in patients with muscular dystrophy,[71] diabetic gastroparesis,[72] and $H_2$ receptor antagonist use.[73]

Although initially described in full-term infants, most lactobezoars are found in premature low-birth-weight infants.[74, 75] Early reports hypothesized that lactobezoars were caused by improperly prepared hypertonic formulas or by dehydration. In the early 1980s there was an apparent increase in the incidence of lactobezoars in low-birth-weight infants, which now seems to have waned. This rise in the number of cases was attributed to specialized premature infant formulas and, in particular, to their high casein content. Schreiner and coworkers[76] found no lactobezoars during a 14-month period in 223 infants weighing less than 2,000 g who were fed whey-predominant formulas, whereas they found a 6.6% incidence in a similar group fed casein-predominant formulas. However, Ross Laboratories, a major manufacturer of casein-predominant formulas, used its market share and Schreiner and coworkers' 6.6% incidence figure and concluded that 1,300 cases should occur yearly if casein is solely responsible.[77] This expected number of cases far exceeded the actual number of reported cases. Further, lactobezoars have been reported in exclusively breast-fed infants.[78] Although the firmer curds formed by casein are important contributors, other factors are involved in lactobezoar formation, including (1) a trend to earlier and more rapid advancement of feedings in very small or very ill premature infants; (2) the use of high-caloric-density formulas; (3) the higher calcium and protein content of special formulas for premature infants; (4) continuous drip feedings; and (5) the unique physiology of gastric secretion and gastric emptying in low-birth-weight infants.

Concretions of dehydrated antacid—antacid bezoars—may form in patients with poor gastric motility. Premature infants or patients in the intensive care unit receiving high-dose antacid therapy for acid peptic disease or for prophylaxis against stress-related bleeding are especially at risk.[79]

**CLINICAL MANIFESTATIONS.** Trichobezoars present with symptoms suggesting gastric outlet or intestinal obstruction, or both, including anorexia, vomiting, and weight loss. In 70% of cases there are complaints of abdominal pain, and abdominal distention is frequently noted.[69] Patchy baldness from hair pulling may be a useful clue.[65] Abdominal palpation usually reveals a firm mass in the left upper quadrant. Abdominal crepitus may also be noted. Frequently, severe halitosis is present owing to the putrefying material in the stomach. Laboratory evaluation may show iron-deficiency anemia, hypoproteinemia, or steatorrhea.

Phytobezoars result in a similar presentation, although in only half of cases is a mass palpable. Peptic ulceration is also more common, owing to phytobezoars' more abrasive nature.

Symptoms suggestive of the presence of a lactobezoar in a premature infant include abdominal distention, vomiting, and increasing gastric residual volumes. A mass may be palpable in the left upper quadrant. Some cases may be clinically silent, with the lactobezoar found incidentally on a radiographic study. Gastric perforation as a presenting manifestation has been described.[74, 80]

**DIAGNOSIS.** Plain abdominal films may reveal amorphous, granular, calcified configurations of solid-like material within the stomach, suggesting the presence of a bezoar. An upper gastrointestinal series shows a movable mass within the barium field, and on a postevacuation film the mass is often outlined by a thin barium shell. On ultrasound, an echogenic arc of air between the bezoar and the gastric wall is strongly suggestive of the diagnosis. Computed tomography with contrast is the radiographic study of choice because it not only demonstrates the bezoar as a free-floating filling defect within the stomach but also provides quantitative information about size. The latter is particularly useful in the management of trichobezoars, which, unless they are very small, require surgical removal. Endoscopy provides definitive evidence of the bezoar's presence and type and may also be a means for therapeutic dissolution.

**MANAGEMENT.** The treatment of all but the smallest trichobezoars is surgical (Fig. 10–8). Endoscopic fragmentation and retrieval can be technically challenging because of the density of the bezoar and the need to make multiple passes with the endoscope or to use an overtube. Novel approaches that have been described include extracorporeal shock wave lithotripsy,[81] endoscopic removal with a gallstone lithotripter,[82] and removal with laparoscope.[83] Some phytobezoars may be physically disrupted or dissolved. Therefore, a trial of medical therapy is warranted before gastrotomy is performed. Techniques include a clear liquid lavage plus metoclopramide[84] and endoscopic fragmentation with a biopsy forceps or polyp snare.[85] Madsen and associates[86] reported the successful use of a Teledyne Water Pik (Fort Collins, CO) in five patients. Dissolving of phytobezoars with papain[87] or acetylcysteine[88] has been reported, but the use of enzyme cellulase has met with the most success.[89, 90] Lactobezoars are treated by withholding feedings for 48 hours and maintaining hydration with intravenous fluids. Resolution is usually prompt, and endoscopic disruption is rarely necessary.

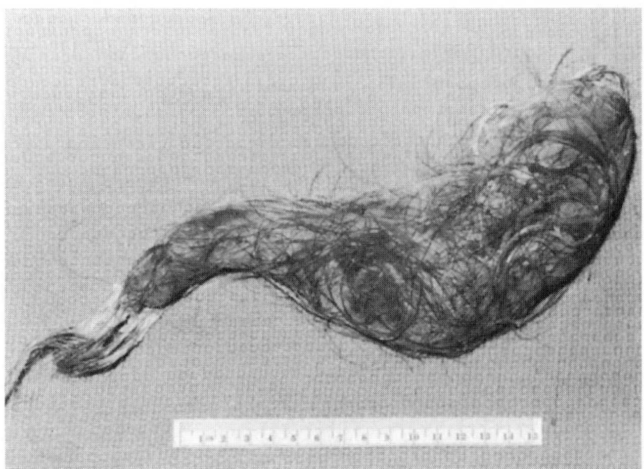

**FIGURE 10–8.** Trichobezoar removed surgically from the stomach of a 2½-year-old boy who presented with vomiting and failure to thrive.

## REFERENCES


1. Krey H: On the treatment of corrosive lesions in the esophagus: an experimental study. Acta Otolaryngol 1952;102:1–11.
2. Vancura EM, Clinton JE, Ruiz E, et al: Toxicity of alkaline solutions. Ann Emerg Med 1980;9:118–124.
3. Maull KI, Scher LA, Greenfield LJ: Surgical implications of acid ingestion. Surg Gynecol Obstet 1979;148:895–901.
4. Nelson R, Watson P, Kelly M: Caustic ingestion. Ann Emerg Med 1983;12:559–563.
5. Anderson KD, Rouse TM, Randolph JG: A controlled trial of corticosteroids in children with corrosive injury of the esophagus. N Engl J Med 1990;323:637–640.
6. Gaudreault P, Parent M, McGuigan MA, et al: Predictability of esophageal injury from signs and symptoms: a study of caustic ingestion in 378 children. Pediatrics 1983;71:767–775.
7. Crain EF, Gershel JC, Mezey AP: Caustic ingestions: symptoms as predictors of esophageal injury. Am J Dis Child 1984;38:863–865.
8. Holinger P. Management of lesions caused by chemical burns. Ann Otol Rhinol Laryngol 1968;71:819–824.
9. Waserman RL, Ginsburg CM: Caustic substances injuries. J Pediatr 1985;107:169–174.
10. Ferguson MK, Migliore M, Staszak VM, et al: Early evaluation and therapy for caustic esophageal injury. Am J Surg 1989;157:116–120.
11. Appelgvist P: Lye corrosion carcinoma of the esophagus: a review of 63 cases. Gut 1988;29:157–160.
12. Alexander W, Kadish JA, Dunbar JS: Ingested foreign bodies in children. In Kaufmann HJ (ed): Progress in Pediatric Radiology. 2nd ed. Chicago, Year Book Medical Publishers, 1969, pp 256–285.
13. Schwartz GF, Polsky HS: Ingested foreign bodies of the gastrointestinal tract. Am Surg 1985;51:173–179.
14. Waye JD: Removal of foreign bodies from the upper intestinal tract with fiberoptic instruments. Am J Gastroenterol 1976;65:557–560.
15. Koch H: Operative endoscopy. Gastrointest Endosc 1977;24:65–68.
16. Maleki M, Evans WE: Foreign body perforation of the intestinal tract. Arch Surg 1970;101:475–477.
17. Chalk SG, Faucer H: Foreign bodies in the stomach. Arch Surg 1928;16:494–500.
18. Litovitz TL, Schmitz BF, Matyumas N, et al: 1987 annual report of the American Association of Poison Control Centers National Data Collection System. Am J Emerg Med 1988;6:479–515.
19. Jackson RM, Hawkins DB: Coins in the esophagus. What is the best management? Int J Pediatr Otorhinolaryngol 1986;12:127–135.
20. Hodge D, Tecklenburg F, Fleisher G: Coin ingestion: does every child need a radiograph? Ann Emerg Med 1985;14:443–446.

21. Schunk JE, Cornele H, Bolte R: Pediatric coin ingestions. Am J Dis Child 1989;143:546–548.
22. Caravati EM, Bennett DL, McElwee NE: Pediatric coin ingestion. Am J Dis Child 1989;143:549–551.
23. Fulginiti VA: Is standard practice in pediatrics "standard"? A potential lesson for experts and practitioners. Am J Dis Child 1989;143:529–530.
24. Nahmah BJ, Mueller C: Asymptomatic esophageal perforation by a coin in a child. Ann Emerg Med 1984;13:627–629.
25. Obiako MN: Tracheoesophageal fistula: a complication of foreign body. Ann Otol Rhinol Laryngol 1982;91:325–327.
26. Vella EE, Booth PJ: Foreign body in the esophagus. Br Med J 1965;2:1042.
27. Chaikhouni A, Kratz JM, Crawford FA: Foreign bodies of the esophagus. Ann Surg 1985;51:173–179.
28. Gracia C, Frey CF, Balaz IB: Diagnosis and management of ingested foreign bodies: A ten-year experience. Ann Emerg Med 1984;13:30–34.
29. Christie DL, Ament ME: Removal of foreign bodies from esophagus and stomach with flexible fiberoptic panendoscopes. Pediatrics 1976;57:931–936.
30. Bendig DW: Removal of blunt esophageal foreign bodies by flexible endoscopy without general anesthesia. Am J Dis Child 1986;140:789–790.
31. Campbell JB, Quattromani FL, Foley LC: Foley catheter removal of blunt esophageal foreign bodies: experience with 100 consecutive children. Pediatr Radiol 1983;13:116–119.
32. Bonadio WA, Jona JZ, Glicklich M, et al: Esophageal bougienage technique for coin ingestion in children. J Pediatr Surg 1988;23:917–918.
33. Litovitz TL: Button battery ingestions: A review of 56 cases. JAMA 1983;249:2495–2500.
34. Temple DM, McNeese MC: Hazards of battery ingestion. Pediatrics 1983;71:100–103.
35. Vottler TP, Nash JC, Rudledge JC: The hazard of ingested alkaline disk batteries in children. JAMA 1983;249:2504–2506.
36. Maves MD, Carithers JS, Birck KG: Esophageal burns secondary to disk battery ingestion. Ann Otol Rhinol Laryngol 1984;93:364–369.
37. Litovitz TL: Battery ingestions: Product accessibility and clinical course. Pediatrics 1985;75:469–476.
38. Litovitz TL, Schmitz BF: Ingestion of cylindrical and button batteries: an analysis of 2382 cases. Pediatrics 1992;89:747–757.
39. National Poison Center Network Computer System for Documenting Data in Poison Exposures. Pittsburgh, 1981.
40. Blatnik BS, Toohill RJ, Lehman RH: Fatal complications from an alkaline battery foreign body in the esophagus. Ann Otol 1977;86:611–615.
41. Shabino CL, Feinberg AN: Esophageal perforation secondary to alkaline battery ingestion. J Am Coll Emerg Pract 1979;8:360–362.
42. Votteler TP: Warning: Ingested disk batteries. Tex Med J 1981;77:7.
43. Willis GA, Ho WC: Perforation of Meckel's diverticulum by an alkaline hearing aid battery. Can Med Assoc J 1982;126:497–498.
44. Kulig K, Rumack CM, Rumack BH, et al: Disk battery ingestion: elevated urine mercury levels and enema removal of battery fragments. JAMA 1983;249:2502–2504.
45. Maves MD, Lloyd TV, Carithers JS: Radiographic identification of ingested disk batteries. Pediatr Radiol 1986;16:154–156.
46. Abel RM, Fischer JE, Henderson HH: Penetration of the alimentary tract by a foreign body with migration to the liver. Arch Surg 1971;102:227–229.
47. Grosfeld JL, Eng K: Right iliac artery-duodenal fistula in infancy due to a "whisk-broom" bristle perforation. Ann Surg 1972;176:761–762.
48. Rosch W, Classen M: Fiberendoscopic foreign body removal from the upper gastrointestinal tract. Endoscopy 1972;4:193–197.
49. Esposito G: Left empyema and pneumothorax after perforation of the stomach, diaphragm, and pleura by an intragastric foreign body. Ann Chir Infant 1973;14:413–416.
50. Maleki M, Evans WE: Foreign body perforation of the intestinal tract. Arch Surg 1970;101:475–477.
51. Schwartz JT, Graham DY: Toothpick perforation of the intestines. Ann Surg 1977;185:64–66.
52. Carp L: Foreign bodies in the intestine. Ann Surg 1927;85:575–585.
53. Kassner EG, Mutchler RW, Klotz DH, et al: Uncomplicated foreign bodies of appendix in children: radiologic observations. J Pediatr Surg 1974;9:207–209.
54. Buchin PJ: Foreign bodies of the esophagus. N Y State J Med 1981;81:1057–1059.
55. Vizcarrondo FJ, Brady PG, Nord H: Foreign bodies of the upper gastrointestinal tract. Gastrointest Endosc 1983;29:208–210.
56. Ferrucci JR, Long JA: Radiologic treatment of esophageal food impaction using intravenous glucagon. Radiology 1977;127:25–28.
57. Trenkner SW, Maglinte DT, Lehman G, et al: Esophageal food impaction: treatment with glucagon. Radiology 1983;149:401–403.
58. Friedland GW: The treatment of acute esophageal food impaction. Radiology 1983;149:601–602.
59. Andersen HA, Bernatz PE, Grindlay JH: Perforation of the esophagus after use of a digestive agent: report of a case and experimental study. Ann Otol Rhinol Laryngol 1959;68:890–896.
60. Holsinger JW, Frison RL, Sealy WC: Esophageal perforation following meat impaction and papain ingestion. JAMA 1968;204:188–189.
61. Goldmer F, Danley D: Enzymatic digestion of esophageal meat impaction. Dig Dis Sci 1985;30:546–550.
62. Jackson C, Jackson CL: Disease of the Air and Food Passages of Foreign Body Origin. Philadelphia, WB Saunders, 1937.
63. Barone JE, Sohn M, Nealon TF: Perforations and foreign bodies of the rectum: report of 28 cases. Ann Surg 1976;184:601–606.
64. DeBakey M, Ochsner A: Bezoars and concretions: comprehensive review of the literature with an analysis of 303 collected cases and a presentation of 8 additional cases. Surgery 1938;4:934–963; Surgery 1939;5:132–160.
65. McGehee FT Jr, Buchanan GR: Trichophagia and trichobezoar: etiologic role of iron deficiency. J Pediatr 1980;97:946–948.
66. Schreiber H, Filston HC: Obstructive jaundice due to gastric trichobezoar. J Pediatr Surg 1976;11:103–104.
67. Shawis RN, Doig CM: Gastric trichobezoar associated with transient pancreatitis. Arch Dis Child 1984;59:994–995.
68. Hossenbocus A, Colin-Jones DG: Trichobezoar, gastric polyposis, protein-losing gastroenteropathy and steatorrhea. Gut 1973;14:730–732.
69. Valberg LS, McCorriston JR, Partington MW: Bezoar: an unusual cause of protein-losing gastroenteropathy. Can Med Assoc J 1966;94:388–391.
70. Izumi S, Isida K, Iwamoto M: Mechanism of formation of phytobezoars with special reference to persimmon ball. Jpn J Med Sci Trans II Biochem 1933;2:21–33.
71. Kuiper D: Gastric bezoar in a patient with myotonic dystrophy. Am J Dis Child 1971;16:529–531.
72. Brady P: Gastric phytobezoars consequent to delayed gastric emptying. Gastrointest Endosc 1978;24:159–161.
73. Nichols T: Phytobezoar formation: a new complication of cimetidine therapy. Ann Intern Med 1981;95:70–72.
74. Erenberg A, Shaw RD, Yousefzadeh D: Lactobezoar in the low-birth-weight infant. Pediatrics 1979;63:642–646.
75. Schreiner RL, Brady MS, Franken EA: Increased incidence of lactobezoars in low birth weight infants. Am J Dis Child 1979;133:936–940.
76. Schreiner RL, Brady MS, Ernst JA, et al: Lack of lactobezoars in infants given predominantly whey protein formulas. Am J Dis Child 1982;136:437–439.
77. Kashyap S: Lactobezoar risk. Pediatrics 1988;81:177–178.
78. Yoss BS: Human milk lactobezoars. J Pediatr 1984;105:819–822.
79. Portugeuz-Malavasi A, Aranda JV: Antacid bezoars in a newborn. Pediatrics 1979;63:679–680.
80. Levkoff AH, Gadsden RH, Hennigar GR: Lactobezoar and gastric perforation in a neonate. J Pediatr 1970;77:875–877.
81. Benes J, Chmel J, Jodl J: Treatment of gastric bezoar by extracorporeal shock wave lithotripsy. Endoscopy 1991;23:346–348.
82. Lubke HJ, Winklemann RS, Berges W, et al: Gastric phytobezoar: endoscopic removal using the gallstone lithotripter. Z Gastroenterol 1988;26:393–396.
83. Filipi CJ, Perdikis G, Hender RA: An intraluminal surgical approach to the management of gastric bezoars. Surg Endosc 1995;9:831–833.
84. Delpre G, Glanz I, Neeman A: New therapeutic approach in postoperative phytobezoars. J Clin Gastroenterol 1984;6:231–233.
85. Diettrich N, Gaw F: Postgastrectomy phytobezoars: endoscopic diagnosis and treatment. Arch Surg 1985;120:432–437.
86. Madsen R, Skibba R, Galvan A: Gastric bezoars. A technique of endoscopic removal. Dig Dis Sci 1978;23:717–720.
87. Sparberg M, Nielsen A, Andruczak R: Bezoar following gastrostomy. Am J Dig Dis 1968;13:579–581.
88. Schlang H: Acetylcysteine in removal of bezoar. JAMA 1970;214:1329.
89. Deal D, Vitale P, Raffin S: Dissolution of a postgastrectomy bezoar by cellulase. Gastroenterology 1973;64:467–469.
90. Stanten A, Peters H: Enzymatic dissolution of phytobezoars. Am J Surg 1975;130:259–261.

Chapter 11

# Abdominal Masses in Pediatric Patients

*Howard Ross, Donald W. Hight, and Richard G. Weiss*

Few other clinical disorders evoke more concern from pediatricians and families than the discovery of an abdominal mass in a child. Despite the observation that more than half of palpable masses in the neonate are related to hepatosplenomegaly and are of a nonsurgical nature, the threat of incurable cancer and extensive surgery remain a preoccupation of both family and physician until a diagnosis is established. Although a thorough physical examination is an essential starting point, a detailed account of familial disorders, maternal age, lost pregnancies, consanguinity, and age of the presenting child plays a crucial role in determining the differential diagnosis and extent of disease. The use of accurately performed noninvasive imaging studies remains the essential element in the prompt diagnosis and treatment of an abdominal mass.

Age remains the critical variable in the evaluation of a pediatric patient with an abdominal mass. In neonates (<3 months), 85% of masses are benign and are located in the retroperitoneum (Fig. 11–1). More than 50% involve obstructive uropathies of the upper tracts and renal pelvis.[1] Malignant conditions include neuroblastoma and sacrococcygeal teratoma with extension into the pelvis. The gastrointestinal tract is rarely a source of solid tumor growth in the neonatal period. With advancing age, the incidence of malignant abdominal masses manifesting as retroperitoneal tumors (Wilms' tumor, neuroblastoma) increases (Fig. 11–2).

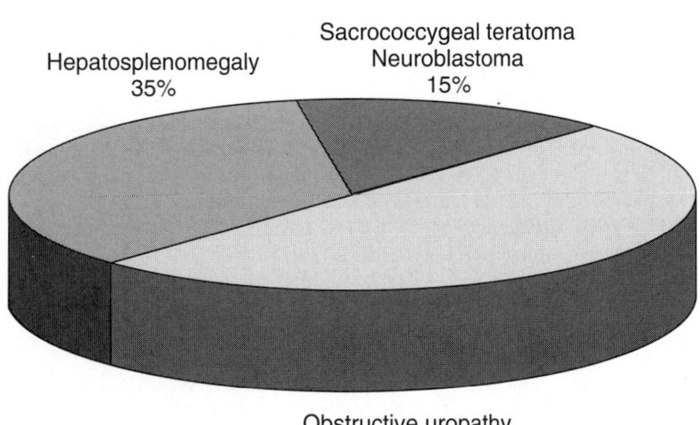


**FIGURE 11–1.** Abdominal masses in neonates.

## DIAGNOSTIC METHODS

The diagnostic evaluation of an abdominal mass begins with a history and physical examination and proceeds to the selection of an imaging modality. The techniques chosen should provide a diagnosis in the most expeditious manner.[2] Examinations which generate results that do not alter or affect treatment should be avoided. The age and clinical presentation of the patient influence the likelihood that a particular test will add valuable information. Appropriate examination selection facilitates rapid patient treatment, reduces exposure to potential comorbidities (radiation, intravenous contrast medium, sedating medication), minimizes patient discomfort, and is cost-effective.

### Abdominal Radiography

The plain abdominal radiograph is a valuable examination in the child with symptoms of intestinal obstruction and a palpable abdominal mass. The ability of an abdominal radiograph to demonstrate dilated bowel, air-fluid levels, bowel wall thickening, and intestinal gas patterns makes it a tool that can guide initial operative management. Patterns of

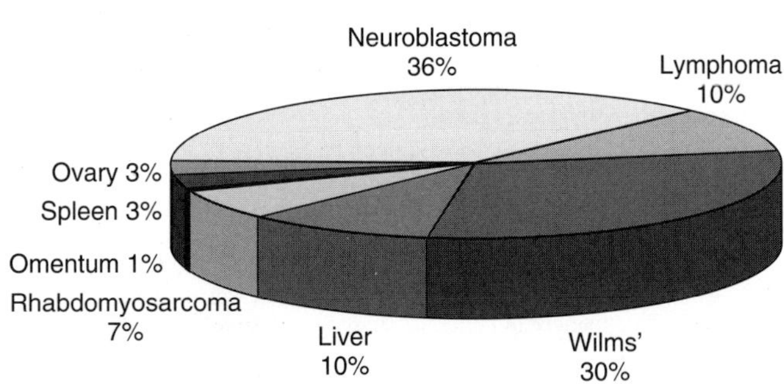


**FIGURE 11–2.** Abdominal masses in infants and children.

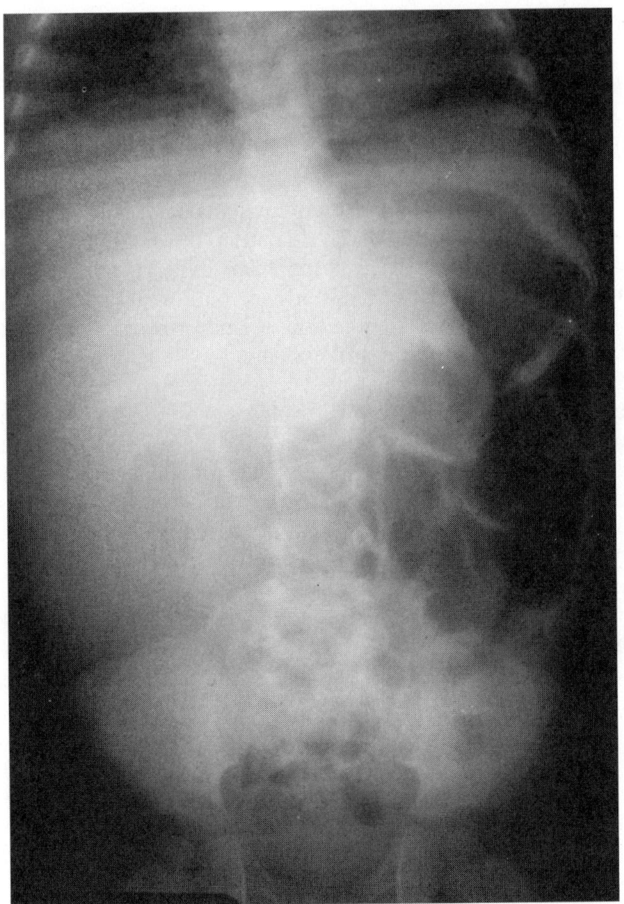

**FIGURE 11–3.** Plain radiograph of the abdomen showing a large right flank mass with visceral displacement.

calcification are depicted on radiographs. In comparison to computed tomography (CT), the abdominal radiograph has less value in the evaluation of palpable lesions that are not causing obstructive symptoms (Fig. 11–3).

## Ultrasonography

Ultrasonography is an ideal method to both define a mass as being cystic or solid and describe its size and shape. Doppler ultrasound permits evaluation of flow velocities in blood vessels and can document the presence of thrombus or tumor in a blood vessel lumen. This is the preferred evaluation for neonates, whose masses are often cystic or multiloculated. Ovarian cysts and solid lesions are well visualized. Ultrasound is not an appropriate examination to evaluate more than a small portion of the abdomen. Significant gaseous distention hampers evaluation. Size and spatial relationships between organs are better evaluated by CT and magnetic resonance imaging (MRI).

## Computed Tomography

CT is today's gold standard for the evaluation of an abdominal mass. CT acts as a noninvasive scalpel by which organs and blood vessels are examined in two or three dimensions. Spatial relationships between adjacent organs are clearly defined. Infants and children have a greater frequency of solid masses than do neonates, making CT an important tool in this older age group. The utility of the CT scan is exemplified in the evaluation of a Wilms' tumor: the precise tumor location, size, local involvement, nodal spread, and vascular invasion are revealed (Fig. 11–4). In the same scanning session, metastases to the liver and lung can be evaluated. High-speed CT scanning methods often make the use of sedation or general anesthesia unnecessary.

## Magnetic Resonance Imaging

Like the CT scan, MRI provides exquisite two-dimensional imaging of the pediatric abdomen and soft tissue planes. The advantage of MRI over CT in the pediatric patient is its superior ability to delineate planes between tissues.[3] Tissue invasion by tumor is best revealed by MRI. In the particular instance of neuroblastoma, spinal canal and great vessel invasion can be well demonstrated (Fig. 11–5). Important anatomic information can help determine operability and therefore directly affects the initial management of the patient. MRI is generally less accessible and frequently requires the use of sedation to ensure clarity and detailed examination in the pediatric patient. The use of contrast enhancement is seldom required because of the ability to assess tissue characteristics by magnetic frequency modulation.

## Excretory Urography

Renal and urinary tract disorders constitute a large percentage of abdominal masses in both the neonate and the older child. CT has made the excretory urogram largely obsolete in the evaluation of a pediatric abdominal mass. CT reveals renal concentrating ability, structure, renal artery and vein position, ureteral size, and two-dimensional views of the bladder. Excretory urography is best used to assess the

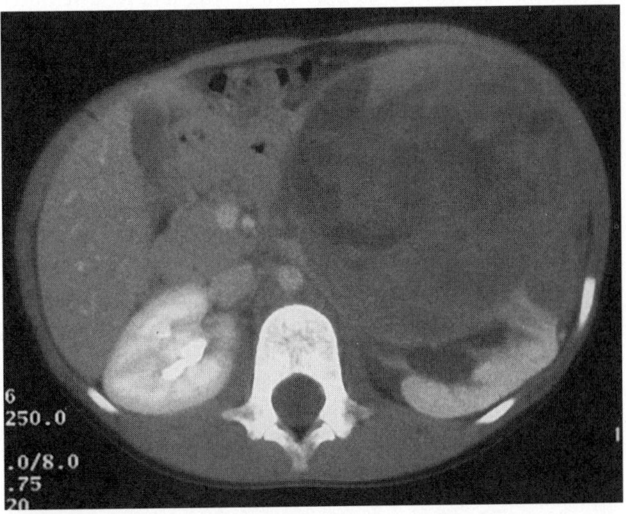


**FIGURE 11–4.** CT image showing a renal mass with compression of the midline vasculature structures.

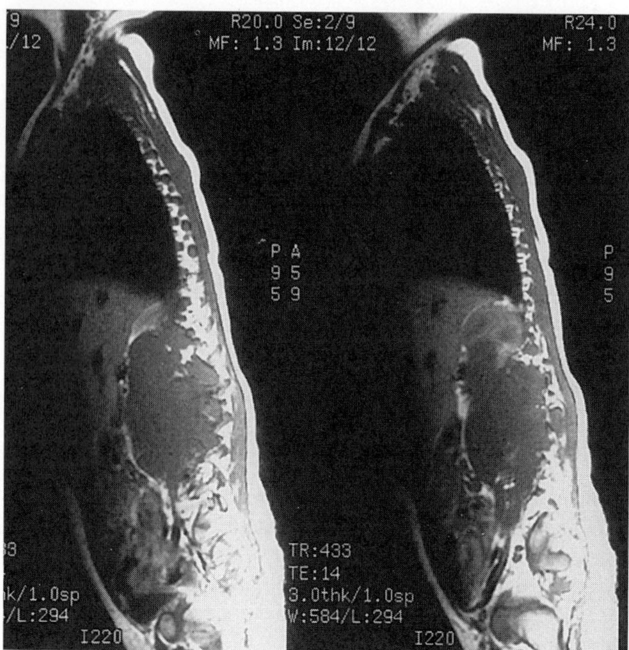


**FIGURE 11–5.** Sagittal view of a neuroblastoma with displacement of the spinal cord.

level of obstruction in congenital strictures of the ureteropelvic junction or distal ureter or in obstruction caused by stone formation.[4]

## Arteriography

The role of arteriography has diminished with the increased use of contrast-enhanced CT scans and magnetic resonance angiography. Percutaneous arteriography is specifically suited for the study of vascular anatomy of the liver in the assessment of the resectability of hepatic tumors. Selected vascular studies have proved helpful in isolating small lesions of the pancreas, such as adenomas and islet cell tumors. Although angiography provides exquisite details of vascular anatomy, it is time-consuming and requires high levels of exposure to radiation.

## Prenatal Ultrasound

The ability to detect in utero fetal abnormalities, including abdominal masses, has improved markedly in the past decade. Beginning at 20 weeks of gestational age, the fetus can be screened for growth and structural abnormalities. Obstructive uropathies, intestinal anomalies, and cardiac malformations can be accurately diagnosed and suitable postnatal treatment planned. In utero fetal surgery, either percutaneous decompression of obstructed genitourinary systems or direct intervention and repair of diaphragmatic hernias, is still restricted to specialized investigational centers. Early discovery of an abdominal mass and preparation of the parents for postnatal surgery may enable the surgeon to remove a localized tumor such as a neuroblastoma before metastatic spread occurs.

# ABDOMINAL MASSES IN THE NEONATE

## Kidney

### *Hydronephrosis*

Hydronephrosis, the most common cause of an abdominal mass in the neonate, is a dilatation of the renal pelvis and collecting system resulting from either mechanical or functional obstruction of the urinary outflow tract. Obstruction of the ureteropelvic junction often causes massive dilatation of the renal pelvis and collecting system. The obstruction may result from extrinsic compression by an aberrant accessory artery to the lower pole of the kidney or from a dysfunctional segment of the ureter. Chronic vesicoureteral reflux causes an elevated hydrostatic pressure and a functional obstruction of the ureter, leading to hydronephrosis and hydroureter. The inflammation caused by pyelonephritis may lead to ureteral strictures and progressive hydronephrosis.

Bilateral hydronephrosis is found in 15% of infants with hydronephrosis and is associated with megaureters and massive distention of the urinary bladder. In the male neonate, this condition is most commonly caused by posterior urethral valves (Fig. 11–6). The infant presents with a distended abdomen, overflow incontinence, and bilateral flank masses. Prolonged in utero renal obstruction may lead to loss of renal parenchyma and urinary ascites. An ultrasound examination demonstrates a dilated collecting system and renal pelvis with a residual rim of renal parenchyma.

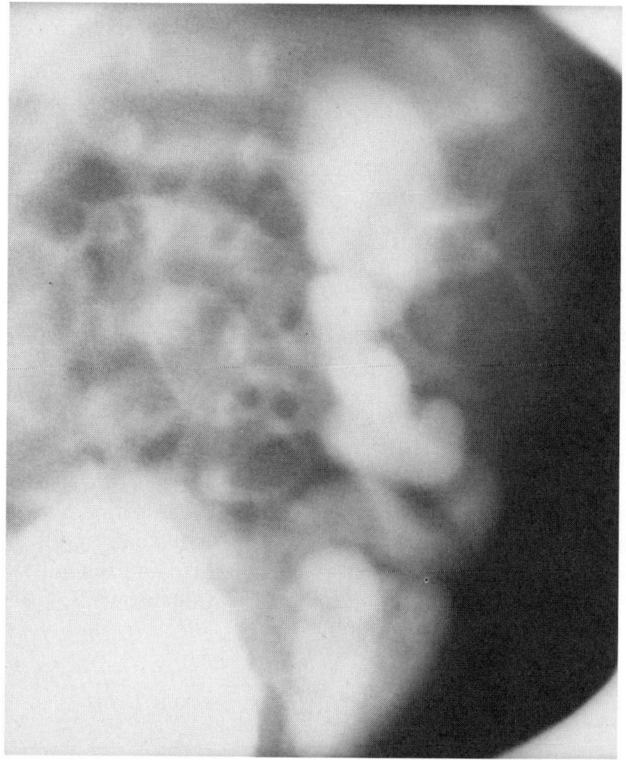

**FIGURE 11–6.** Voiding cystourethrogram showing severe ureteral reflux and enlarged bladder associated with posterior urethral valves.

## Multicystic Dysplastic Kidney

Multicystic dysplastic kidney is the most common cystic renal disease in newborns,[5] with 60% of cases discovered incidentally by the age of 1 year. It produces multiloculated cysts and must be distinguished from polycystic kidney disease. The dysplastic collecting tubules become distended with urine after nephron formation is complete by the 20th week of gestation. A cycle of elevated hydrostatic pressure, tissue ischemia, and hypoxia leads to necrosis and diminished renal function. A gradual involution of cysts then occurs. Macroscopically, the proximal ureter is usually absent or atretic and the renal artery is hypoplastic. Multicystic dysplastic kidney is frequently unilateral, but 15% to 20% of cases are bilateral, with no sex or familial predilection.[6] Plain roentgenograms show eggshell calcification in older patients. Renal ultrasound, the procedure of choice, demonstrates grape-like clusters of multiloculated cysts. An intravenous pyelogram or renal scan shows little, if any, functional excretion. Retrograde pyelography is necessary to document an atretic or obstructed collecting system.

In utero diagnosis may be made by 28 weeks of gestation using prenatal ultrasound. Involution of renal cysts in the developing fetus is not a reliable predictor of improved renal function.[7] Although nonoperative management has been suggested, nephrectomy in the neonate is recommended at 6 to 12 months of age because of the likelihood of the subsequent onset of pain, infection, hypertension, or the chance of malignant tumor degeneration.[5] Hydronephrosis or ureteropelvic obstruction has been reported in the contralateral kidney in as many as 20% of patients. Preoperative ultrasonographic imaging and careful exploration at the time of surgery should be performed to exclude coexisting anomalies in the opposite kidney.

## Infantile Polycystic Kidney Disease

Infantile polycystic kidney disease, an autosomal recessive disease, is usually discovered incidentally in the first few days of life. The excretory urogram outlines a cyst-filled kidney with a spongelike appearance. Diffuse bilateral renal enlargement and increased echogenicity due to multiple small cysts is seen on ultrasound. The condition is typically bilateral and may be associated with both cystic and fibrotic disease of the liver. Renal parenchymal cysts develop as a result of tubular ectasia. The clinical spectrum of infantile polycystic kidney disease may range from severe renal tubular disease with minimal hepatic involvement to scant renal disease with extensive hepatic fibrosis. A perfusion scan confirms nephromegaly with scant renal blood flow. Treatment is supportive and nonoperative in the neonatal period. Renal transplantation remains the only option as renal function deteriorates.

## Renal Vein Thrombosis

Neonates presenting with a firm, smooth flank mass, abdominal distention, hypernatremia, and hematuria after stress or a septic episode may have developed renal vein thrombosis. This entity occurs after hypoperfusion of the kidney due to shock, sepsis, or hemoconcentration. Antecedent gastrointestinal disease or perinatal sepsis may also produce this condition. Unless hemodynamic instability is rapidly corrected, venous thrombosis may progress to renal arterial compromise and parenchymal infarction. Renal vein thrombosis has been associated with steroid and thiazide use during pregnancy, maternal diabetes, and hypoglycemic seizures in the neonate.

Findings on ultrasound show a diffusely enlarged, edematous kidney with increased echogenicity. Presence of thrombus in the inferior vena cava or encroachment of the contralateral renal vein may also be seen. The renal perfusion scan findings may range from nonvisualization to normal function, depending on the contralateral blood flow and the acuteness of the venous thrombosis. Treatment should be supportive, with attention directed to underlying hypovolemia and management of transient renal insufficiency. Anticoagulation is indicated in high-risk patients with nephrotic syndrome if there is clinical evidence of pulmonary embolism or evidence of bilateral involvement.[8] Renal function generally improves with supportive measures, although nephrectomy may be necessary if uncontrollable sepsis or hypertension develops. Thrombectomy of the renal vein is seldom indicated owing to the high rate of recurrent occlusion.

## Mesoblastic Nephroma

Mesoblastic nephroma is the most common renal tumor in the neonate.[9] This benign neoplasm is a solid, encapsulated mass of disordered renal parenchyma. Bundles of connective tissue growing between intact nephrons may exhibit an infiltrative growth pattern at the interface of normal renal parenchyma. This has formally been referred to as a fetal hamartoma or benign congenital Wilms' tumor. Recent studies have suggested a pathologic spectrum of disease, with classic benign nodular mesoblastic nephroma at one end and spindle cell sarcoma at the other. Between the two extremes of histopathology are cell types of indeterminate biologic activity.[10] Beckwith[11] identified cellular types that warrant adjuvant chemotherapy because of the high risk of local recurrence or metastatic spread. Distention of the pelvicaliceal system, as demonstrated by intravenous pyelography, makes this condition indistinguishable from Wilms' tumor. Long-term survival exceeds 95% when nephrectomy includes all residual tumor.[12]

## Nephroblastomatosis

A rare lesion of the neonatal kidney, nephroblastomatosis is characterized by small, localized nodules along with the bilateral subcapsular aggregates of persistent renal blastoma. This tissue is believed to be a precursor to subcapsular Wilms' tumor. Multifocal nephroblastomatosis has been reported in 25% of patients with Wilms' tumor.[13] Ultrasound demonstrates solid echogenic or subcortical nodules and bilateral renal enlargement. Intravenous pyelography may show nephromegaly with pelvicaliceal distention resembling Wilms' tumor or adult polycystic kidney disease. The treatment is controversial and requires a biopsy of renal parenchyma and a careful evaluation of bilateral renal function. Continued close observation with frequent imaging studies is required because of the risk of developing Wilms' tumor.

## Adrenal Gland

Spontaneous hemorrhage produces an adrenal mass in the neonatal period. The incidence in neonates is 1.7 per 1,000; hemorrhage involves the right adrenal gland in 70% of cases and is bilateral in 8 to 10%.[9] The cause is related to sepsis, stress, birth trauma, asphyxia, or anoxic encephalopathy. The neonate appears acutely ill, with an associated epigastric or flank mass. Spontaneous hemorrhage occurs within the gland, and ultrasound demonstrates an echoic suprarenal mass with variable compression and displacement of the kidney. Subsequent follow-up imaging may show a mixed echogenic pattern as the formed clot and calcification appear. Differentiation between hemorrhagic neuroblastoma and other associated benign masses may be difficult. Measurements of urinary catecholamines should be performed to rule out neuroblastoma. Once the diagnosis is established, treatment is generally supportive, nonoperative, and directed at correction of the underlying illness. Adrenal hemorrhage usually is resorbed with expectant management. Exploration is necessary only if the diagnosis is in doubt, the hematoma continues to expand, or the clot liquifies, creating a large retroperitoneal cyst.

### *Sacrococcygeal Teratoma*

Sacrococcygeal teratoma often manifests at birth as an external mass posterior to the anus (Fig. 11–7). It may also occur primarily as an abdominal or pelvic mass palpable by bimanual rectal examination. Intraspinal extension can produce symptomatic neurologic sequelae. The tumor is thought to arise from the coccyx, although the precise site of origin may vary. It is frequently detectable in utero by prenatal ultrasound. Ninety percent of teratomas diagnosed at birth are benign, whereas more than 70% of those found at 4 months or later contain malignant neural elements.[14] Favorable features include the presence of calcification or large cystic elements. Malignant tumors have a higher proportion of solid tissue, with infiltrative elements and numerous areas of hemorrhage. Plain abdominal radiographs may show calcification. Ultrasound is helpful in defining the intrapelvic extent of the mass. CT scanning may further determine the extent of the mass by demonstrating adjacent tissue invasion and the size of solid and cystic components within the tumor mass. Treatment is complete surgical excision, including the removal of the coccyx. Fewer than 10% of these tumors require adjuvant chemotherapy if surgical excision is complete. Frequent postoperative follow-up examinations for 2 to 3 years should include rectal examination to look for recurrent presacral tumor. Rectal incontinence after tumor excision may occur in a small percentage of patients.

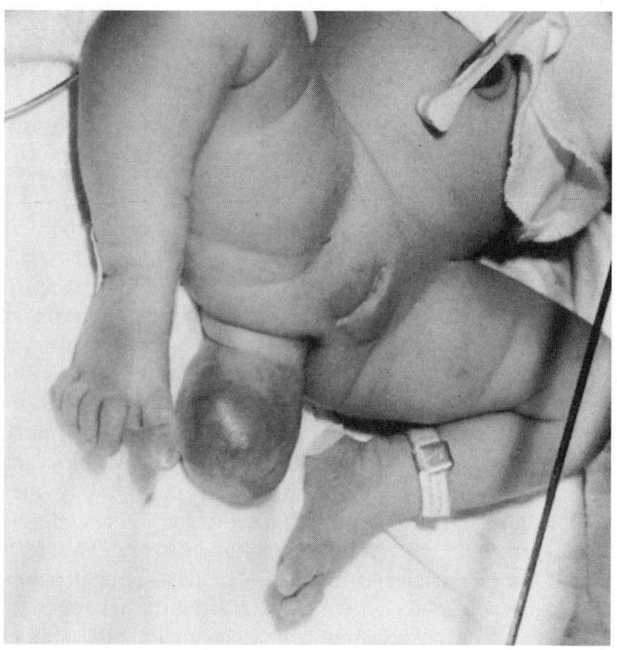

**FIGURE 11–7.** Neonate with sacrococcygeal teratoma.

## Uterus

Hydrometrocolpos manifests as a large, lower midline mass arising from the pelvis of a female infant. The distended uterus or vagina is caused by an imperforate hymen or congenital cervical or vaginal stenosis or atresia. Transplacental maternal estrogen stimulates increased production of mucus from the cervix and uterus, resulting in distention of the vagina or uterus. Physical examination of the abdomen and lower perineum may reveal a bulging hymen or large suprapubic mass. Ultrasound and retrograde contrast studies of the genitourinary system should be performed to exclude renal anomalies. Treatment includes surgical incision and decompression of the obstructed uterus or vagina. Preservation of reproductive function and normal uterine anatomy should be of the highest priority.[15]

If the vaginal introitus is patent on physical examination, associated anomalies including ectopic ureters, imperforate anus, and rectovaginal fistula should be excluded. Diagnostic work-up using ultrasound, barium enema, cystography, and cystoscopy may be necessary to complete the evaluation. Treatment remains surgical and is directed at correction of the anatomic defects.

The female patient may go undiagnosed until puberty, when a clinical history of developing secondary sexual characteristics, pelvic cramps, and primary amenorrhea emerges. Simple hymenotomy is curative for imperforate hymen. A high incidence of endometriosis and secondary peritonitis with adhesions may result from reflux of endometrial secretions through the fallopian tubes.

# ABDOMINAL MASSES IN INFANTS AND CHILDREN

Approximately 20% of abdominal masses in infants arise from the gastrointestinal tract (15%) or the hepatobiliary system (5%).[16] Plain films may suggest a mass effect with bowel gas displacement or an obstructive pattern. Contrast studies usually are required to better define the site of the lesion. Bowel obstruction manifests with distension, vomiting, and episodes of abdominal pain. Cancers of the gastrointestinal tract are rare, comprising less than 1% of pediatric malignancies. Lymphoma and sarcoma of the intestine frequently manifest in the older patient.[16]

## Stomach

The typical presentation of hypertrophic pyloric stenosis is that of nonbilious projectile vomiting after each feeding in an infant between 3 and 7 weeks of age. The exact cause of pyloric hypertrophy is unknown, but the pathophysiology is that of progressive thickening of the circumferential muscle of the pyloric sphincter. The pyloric channel becomes narrowed and elongated. After repeated vomiting episodes, the infant becomes dehydrated, with electrolytes demonstrating a hypochloremic, hypokalemic metabolic alkalosis. A 1- to 2-cm mobile mass may be palpable in the epigastrium. This mass is referred to as an "olive" because of its similarities to an olive in size and feel. Palpation is facilitated by examining a relaxed infant whose stomach has been emptied by a nasogastric tube. Operative treatment may be based on history and physical examination alone. In equivocal cases, ultrasound can identify a thickened pyloric channel wall and increased channel length.[17] Postoperative morbidity of pyloromyotomy results from unsuspected mucosal perforations; long-term results indicate normal pyloric function[18] (see Chapter 17).

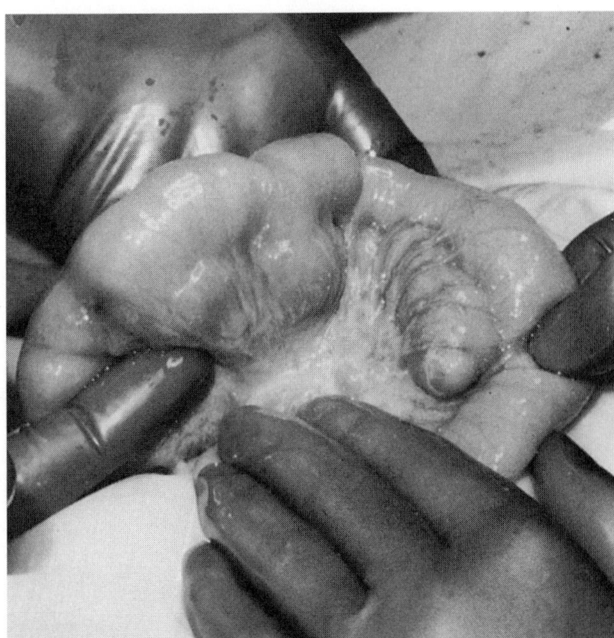

**FIGURE 11–8.** Ileal duplication located along the mesenteric border of the intestine.

## Intestine

### Intestinal Duplication

Duplication cysts of the intestinal tract are developmental abnormalities which can occur anywhere from the mouth to the anus. Intra-abdominal duplications are most common, with 50% of all duplications located in the jejunum and ileum. Gastric and duodenal duplications occur in 6% of all cases, and colorectal cysts occur in 17%. Duplication cysts are found in the bowel mesentery and are lined with gastric mucosa in 30% of cases. The cysts share both a common blood supply with the adjacent intestinal segment and a common muscular wall (Fig. 11–8). The lumens of duplications do not commonly communicate with the attached bowel. Multiple sites occur in 20% of cases. Painful symptoms caused by the presence of a duplication cyst result from obstruction, torsion, and volvulus of the involved bowel. Gastric acid secretion from the cyst lining may produce bleeding and bowel perforation due to mucosal ulceration. The diagnosis of a duplication can be difficult, with correct identification made only at operation. Ultrasound is helpful in the evaluation of a duplication because it can readily differentiate cystic from solid structures. Ultrasound may identify a three-layered image representing the duplication cyst, common wall, and outer bowel wall. Abdominal radiography may show partially obstructed bowel resulting from mass effect or volvulus. Technetium nuclear scanning may identify gastric mucosal uptake and may be helpful in locating smaller duplications as sources of gastrointestinal bleeding. Treatment consists of surgical resection of the duplication cyst and involved segment.

### Intestinal Obstruction

Midgut volvulus and intussusception are two disease states whose presentation can be accompanied by abdominal mass on physical examination. Midgut volvulus most commonly manifests after the neonatal period, but it can occur at any age as a result of abnormal intestinal fixation. The diagnosis is suggested by the acute onset of bilious vomiting. Abdominal examination may reveal peritonitis accompanied by dehydration and signs of septic shock. Midgut volvulus is a surgical emergency, because the twisting of the superior mesenteric artery limits blood flow and precipitates intestinal necrosis. Abdominal radiography may reveal small bowel obstruction, a "double bubble," a dislocated bowel gas pattern, or a dilated stomach. An upper gastrointestinal contrast radiography series is the gold standard used to diagnose malrotation. The clinical presentation of an acute abdomen, however, necessitates immediate laparotomy after volume resuscitation (see Chapter 12).

Intussusception is the telescoping of proximal intestine into the lumen of more distal bowel. The classic presentation is that of a child from 6 to 24 months of age with episodes of crampy abdominal pain separated by pain-free, quiet periods. Delayed identification of the problem can result in a child's passing hemorrhagic clots mixed with fecal material; this mixture is referred to as "currant-jelly" stool. A firm mass in the right upper quadrant may be palpable between episodes of pain. A contrast enema of Gastrografin, air, or barium can be both diagnostic and therapeutic.[19] Attempts at closed hydrostatic reduction should be aborted after three attempts. Excessive intraluminal pressures can perforate the bowel, resulting in a potentially fatal outcome[20] (see Chapter 38).

### Intestinal Tumors

Non-Hodgkin's lymphoma represents the most common tumor of the small intestine in children. One third of non-Hodgkin's lymphomas begin in the abdomen, and half of these originate in the intestine. Most are B cell lymphomas. The child may present with an asymptomatic abdominal

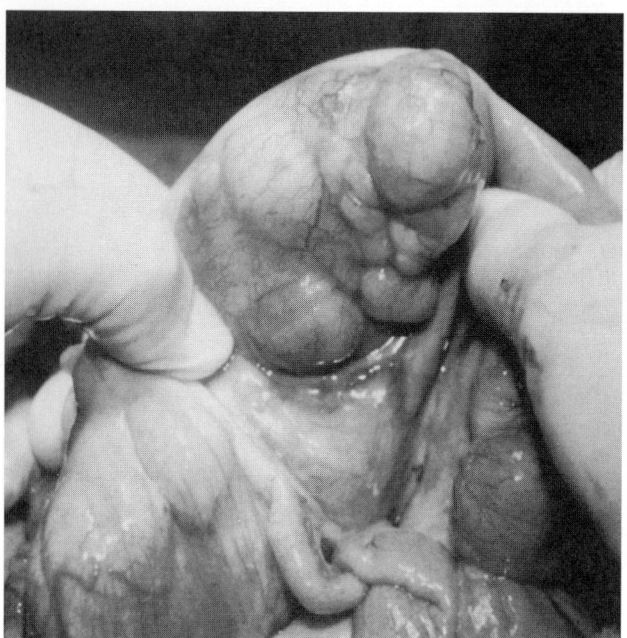

**FIGURE 11–9.** Burkitt's lymphoma of the terminal ileum.

mass or with acute abdominal pain due to intestinal perforation or obstruction (Fig. 11–9). The treatment of non-Hodgkin's lymphoma is chemotherapy, but surgical staging plays an important role in optimization of therapy. Isolated small bowel lymphoma that can be resected primarily is associated with a favorable prognosis. Carcinoids, leiomyosarcomas, adenocarcinomas, and sarcomas can occur but are rare in children.

### *Mesenteric Cysts*

Cysts of the mesentery can occur anywhere along the length of the gastrointestinal tract. Most cysts (75%) appear in persons 10 years of age or older, with the incidence peaking in the fourth decade in life.[21] Roughly 30% of cysts are asymptomatic and are discovered as incidental findings. Cysts cause gradual abdominal distention, chronic abdominal pain, or other nonspecific gastrointestinal complaints. Acute findings of hemorrhage, infection, or rupture develop in 60% of pediatric patients.

An ultrasound examination demonstrates a large, unilocular or septate, echolucent mass. If palpable on physical examination, the cyst is soft, compressible, and mobile. Colonic cyst fluid is clear and serous in character, whereas small bowel mesenteric cysts are often chylous, containing fat globules and lymphocytes. Surgical excision is the treatment of choice, although the risks of recurrent cyst formation and infection remain long-term complications.

### *Omental Cysts*

Less common than mesenteric cysts, omental cysts are thought to arise in obstructed lymphatic channels within the omentum. Whether post-traumatic or congenital, most of these cysts occur in older children, with 70% manifesting by early adult life. Most (90%) are asymptomatic, although traction on the omentum may result in compression or torsion of the small bowel and symptoms of abdominal pain or partial small bowel obstruction.[22] Omental cysts are often flaccid and usually are compressible and mobile. Once found, they should be excised with a surrounding rim of normal omentum.

### *Lymphangioma*

Multicystic lymphatic collections seen in the neck as cystic hygromas may also arise within the abdomen. Simple capillary, cavernous, and cystic lymphangiomas have been described in the small bowel mesentery, mesocolon, omentum, retroperitoneum, pancreas, and spleen. Usually asymptomatic and incidentally discovered, lymphangiomas may cause pain, occult infection, intestinal obstruction, ascites, or hemorrhage into dilated lymphatics. Ultrasound demonstrates multiloculated, cystic masses with thin walls and variable echogenicity. Complete excision is often difficult, and the chance of recurrent cyst formation is high.

## Liver

The differential diagnosis of a hepatic mass includes hepatoblastoma, hepatocellular carcinoma, hepatic adenoma, hamartoma, sarcoma, focal nodular hyperplasia, vascular lesions, cysts, and abscesses. Approximately two thirds of hepatic tumors are malignant. Hepatoblastoma and hepatocellular carcinoma represent 90% of these hepatic malignancies. The most common presentation for hepatoblastoma and hepatocellular carcinoma is that of an asymptomatic palpable mass. Abdominal pain, nausea, vomiting, and anorexia are common additional symptoms. Hepatic abscess occurs in the context of fever and right upper quadrant pain.

Evaluation of a hepatic mass begins with abdominal ultrasound. Ultrasonography differentiates cystic masses from solid lesions and identifies hepatic ductal dilation and vascular distortion. CT with intravenous contrast allows description of the lesion within hepatic segments, defines the relationship to vascular structures, and helps determine resectability. Angiography may be required to provide a map of vascular inflow to hepatic tumors. Digital magnetic resonance angiography can be complementary to CT and is easier to perform in smaller patients.

### *Malignant Tumors*

Hepatoblastoma and hepatocellular carcinoma are epithelial tumors.[23] Hepatoblastoma usually occurs before 2 years of age, whereas hepatocellular carcinoma occurs frequently in the teenage years. Hepatoblastoma has been associated with Beckwith-Wiedemann syndrome and familial adenomatous polyposis. Hepatocellular carcinoma develops both spontaneously and in the context of chronic liver diseases. Elevation of alpha-fetoprotein is noted in up to 90% of children with hepatoblastoma and in 50% of those with hepatocellular carcinoma. Alpha-fetoprotein levels can be monitored to indicate postoperative recurrence. If the mass is located within anatomic boundaries of the liver, the treatment of either hepatoblastoma or hepatocellular carcinoma includes surgical resection. Resection may be curative, but fewer than one third of hepatoblastomas and hepatocellular carcinomas are resectable at presentation. Preoperative chemotherapy has been effective in downstaging hepatoblastoma, enabling subsequent resection.

Sarcomas of the liver include malignant mesenchymoma, rhabdomyosarcoma, and angiosarcoma. The treatment of these tumors includes surgery, chemotherapy, and radiotherapy. Long-term survival is poor.

### Benign Liver Masses

Hemangiomas are lesions composed of dilated vascular spaces. Cavernous hemangiomas occur in children and are largely asymptomatic. Hemangiomas may first appear in infancy and spontaneously involute. The characteristic CT picture is that of a rim-enhancing lesion with delayed central filling after administration of an intravenous contrast agent. Complications of hemangioma are rare but include congestive heart failure, thrombocytopenia, and rupture. Arterial embolization can be used to occlude inflow and steroids to diminish thrombocytopenia. Surgical resection can be performed for solitary lesions amenable to lobectomy if medical treatment proves ineffective.[24]

Adenoma, focal nodular hyperplasia, and hamartoma are benign lesions that occur as solitary lesions. Adenomas commonly originate in the right hepatic lobe and may be quite large at the time of discovery. Differentiation from hepatocellular carcinoma can be difficult. Surgical resection is curative. Focal nodular hyperplasia is found in children younger than 15 years of age and has been associated with oral contraceptive use. Definitive diagnosis of focal nodular hyperplasia through biopsy allows for nonoperative observation. Hamartomas of the liver occur in the infant and younger child. A combination of ultrasound, CT, and nuclear scanning yields a definitive diagnosis of hamartoma as a characteristic mixed solid and cystic lesion with diminished blood supply. Surgical resection is curative in large lesions.

Cysts can be congenital or caused by echinococcal infection. Most congenital cysts can be managed with marsupialization or resection. The Casoni intradermal test is used to identify hydatid disease. Therapy consists of ultrasound-guided aspiration of echinococcal cysts combined with appropriate antimicrobial administration. Hepatic abscesses are often caused by *Staphylococcus aureus, Streptococcus pyogenes,* or *Escherichia coli.* Treatment for large abscesses includes percutaneous drainage and antibiotic therapy. Antibiotic therapy alone is indicated for multiple small abscesses. The mortality rate for hepatic abscesses remains high.

### Choledochal Cysts

Choledochal cysts are localized dilatations of the biliary tree and are generally discovered in older infants and children. Dilatation may be focal or fusiform, may involve intrahepatic or extrahepatic bile ducts, and often produces a palpable abdominal mass. Twenty to 30% of these cysts manifest before the age of 1 year, and 60% by age 10. Females outnumber males 4:1.[25] The classic triad of abdominal pain, jaundice, and a palpable epigastric mass is seen in only a minority of patients. More detailed discussion can be found in Chapter 48.

## Adrenal

### Pheochromocytoma

Vasoactive secreting tumors of the adrenal gland occur in fewer than 50% of children developing an adrenal mass. Children, however, have a high incidence of bilateral tumors that arise in multiple extra-adrenal locations. Malignant transformation occurs in fewer than 2% of pheochromocytomas but is most common when the tumor arises in an extra-adrenal location. The majority of patients present with hypertension and associated disorders such as multiple endocrine adenopathy, von Hippel-Lindau disease, or neurofibromatosis. A CT scan is excellent for staging the disease, and a metaiodobenzylguanidine (MIBG) scan is useful for follow-up evaluation demonstrating recurrent adrenal or metastatic disease.[26]

### Adrenal Cortical Neoplasms

Although they comprise fewer than 1% of pediatric neoplasms, adrenal cortical tumors often produce symptoms of hyperadrenalism. Females outnumber males 5:1, with androgenic effects, virilization, and pseudoprecocious puberty suggestive of hyperfunctioning adrenal cortical secretion. Cushing's syndrome, feminization, and hyperaldosteronism are rare. Ultrasound demonstrates a solid adrenal mass with variable echogenicity within the tumor. Hemorrhage, necrosis, and calcifications are frequently noted. CT or MRI accurately assesses the extent of local disease and reveals metastatic disease in the liver, retroperitoneum, or inferior vena cava. Because invasion is present in 50% of patients, an evaluation for metastatic disease is mandatory. Surgery is the primary treatment when disease is localized. Chemotherapy may be required preoperatively for large tumors to improve resectability and reduce regional extension and lymph node involvement. After incomplete surgical removal, adjuvant treatment is required.

## Spleen

A palpable mass in the left upper quadrant of a child may be caused by an enlarged spleen. In diseases such as idiopathic thrombocytopenic purpura, sickle cell anemia, and the thalassemias, accelerated removal of platelets and red blood cells results in splenic enlargement. The abnormal production of or infiltration by cellular elements in lymphoma and leukemia can cause splenomegaly. The spleen can become enlarged as a response to viral infection. Primary tumors of the spleen and splenic artery aneurysms are rare causes of increased splenic size in children.

Cystic abnormalities of the splenic parenchyma may be congenital and may be lined with a squamous epithelium. Secondary cysts are acquired subsequent to trauma. They may not have an epithelial lining, and they are filled with a characteristic brown liquid. Infectious cysts resulting from parasitic involvement occur rarely in the United States. Percutaneous drainage of cysts is associated with a high recurrence rate. Surgical unroofing and partial splenectomy are surgical options.[27]

The evaluation of an enlarged spleen is guided by the

concurrent signs and symptoms observed in the child. Diagnostic imaging of the spleen should begin with ultrasound, by which the size and consistency are well demonstrated and vascular abnormalities are identified. CT scanning can add additional valuable information.

## Pancreas

Pancreatic masses are uncommon in children and rare in neonates. Benign processes include pseudocyst, duplication cyst, and focal phlegmonous areas of inflammation. Carcinomas are more common than sarcomas. Clinically, the patient presents with abdominal or epigastric pain and fullness, weight loss, diarrhea, or evidence of endocrine abnormalities. Jaundice is less common.

Von Hippel-Lindau disease, consisting of multiple pancreatic and renal cysts with associated angiomas of the retina and cerebellum, is rare. Diagnostic imaging by ultrasound or CT usually demonstrates a pancreatic or peripancreatic mass of homogeneous echogenicity.

## Appendix

Appendiceal abscess can be the cause of an abdominal mass in older children. A small, localized perforation with periappendicitis and abscess formation occurs after a protracted period of abdominal pain or undiagnosed acute appendicitis. A right lower quadrant mass may be found on abdominal examination, and plain roentgenograms often demonstrate an appendicolith. Interval appendectomy may be performed by the open or laparoscopic method 6 to 8 weeks after antibiotic therapy is started. The risk of subsequent appendicitis and the need for prophylactic appendectomy after medical therapy of appendiceal abscess are controversial[28, 29] (see Chapter 37).

## Ovary

Follicular and theca lutein cysts stimulated by maternal estrogen or placental chorionic gonadotropins account for 3% to 5% of neonatal abdominal masses.[9] Small ovarian cysts are easily visualized on ultrasound. Most cysts spontaneously involute before or shortly after delivery. Bilateral cysts are found 10% of the time and may be associated with a history of maternal diabetes.

Tumors or cysts of the ovary can develop at any age, although they occur frequently at puberty. Abdominal or pelvic pain secondary to torsion, adhesions, hemorrhage, or rupture may occur. A palpable lower abdominal mass is noted 50% to 80% of the time (Fig. 11–10). The majority of pelvic masses (85%) are benign and cystic. Solid masses have a higher incidence of malignancy. Ultrasound is an excellent imaging technique to demonstrate the solid or cystic nature of the ovary. Complex mixed echogenic masses, loss of definition of adjacent organs, ascites, and lymphadenopathy suggest malignancy. CT is most sensitive in identifying hemorrhage and necrosis and in determining the extent of disease if malignancy is suspected.

Enlarging symptomatic or "complex" cysts secondary to hemorrhage, torsion, or adhesions to adjacent organs should be surgically excised with preservation of residual ovarian tissue. Simple cysts smaller than 4 cm in diameter may be observed.[30] Simple ovarian cysts are treated with laparoscopic fenestration if they are larger than 5 cm. Dermoid cysts may be excised by either laparoscopic technique or laparotomy.[31]

Tumors of the ovary represent 2% of childhood tumors, and more than 30% are malignant. The majority (75% to 80%) are germ cell tumors, including teratomas, dysgerminomas, and choriocarcinomas. Mesenchymal tumors and granulosa-theca cell tumors may produce estrogen and result in a clinical presentation with precocious puberty and feminization. Androblastoma causes virilization and secondary androgen secretion. Epithelial cell tumors—cystadenocarcinoma, serous, or mucous—are rare prior to puberty. Yolk sac tumors (endodermal sinus tumor) secrete alphafetoprotein; choriocarcinomas and embryonal tumors secrete human chorionic gonadotropin; and germinomas express alkaline phosphatase.

Epithelioid cancers are rare in childhood. Surgery is the primary treatment and includes salpingo-oophorectomy of the involved side along with careful inspection of the contra-

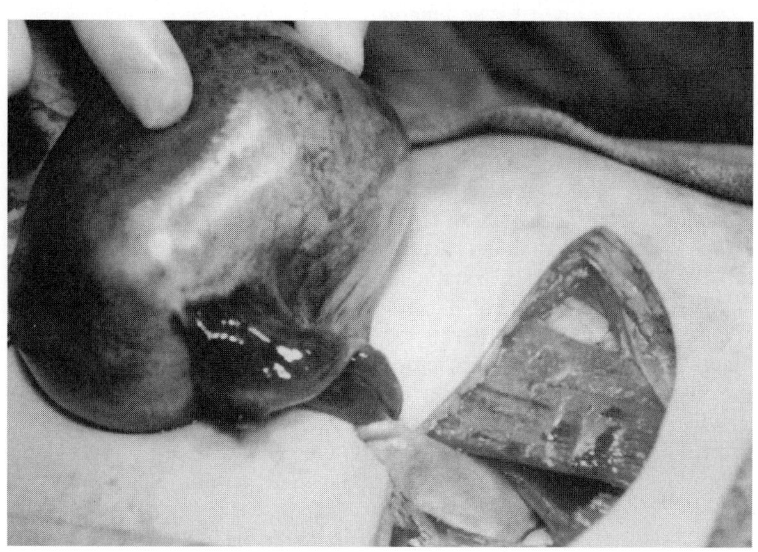

**FIGURE 11–10.** Torsion of the ovary with infarction.

lateral ovary, since 10% to 15% of cases are bilateral. Tumor extension beyond the ovary dictates total abdominal hysterectomy and bilateral salpingo-oophorectomy. Adjuvant chemotherapy and hormone replacement may be necessary.

## Retroperitoneum

### Neuroblastoma

Neuroblastoma and Wilms' tumor are the two most common intra-abdominal tumors in childhood.[32] Neuroblastomas originate from sympathetic nervous system tissue. The most common clinical presentation is that of an abdominal mass (50% to 70% of cases). Adrenal neuroblastoma is centered in the medulla in 50% of cases, in the paraspinal ganglia in 25%, and in the pelvis in 5%. Neuroblastomas can also originate in the posterior mediastinum and in the cervical region.

The initial evaluation of a patient with suspected neuroblastoma involves radiologic examination and laboratory testing. Abdominal radiography and ultrasonography are complementary. The abdominal radiograph reveals fine microcalcifications in approximately 50% of patients. Ultrasonography provides information about adjacent organ involvement and possible vascular invasion. CT and MRI are useful for their abilities to determine organ involvement, local invasion, distant metastasis, and detailed spatial relationships (Fig. 11–11).

The serum levels of neuron-specific enolase, ferritin, and lactate dehydrogenase can be used as prognostic markers and to monitor tumor recurrence. Increased levels of each of these markers preoperatively has been associated with poor prognosis and recurrence. The urinary catecholamine metabolite vanillylmandelic acid can also be used for prognostication and to indicate recurrence.

The Evans classification system describes tumor spread from disease limited to the organ of origin (stage 1) through metastatic spread to skeletal, organ, soft tissue, or distant lymph nodes (stage 4).[33] Stage 4S describes tumors with disease confined to the organ of origin and one metastatic site (either skin, liver, or bone marrow). Other staging systems evaluate the clinicopathologic findings at operation and provide an international staging system which describes both tumor spread and resectability. More than half of patients with neuroblastoma present with advanced disease (Evans stage 3 or 4)[33] (Fig. 11–12).

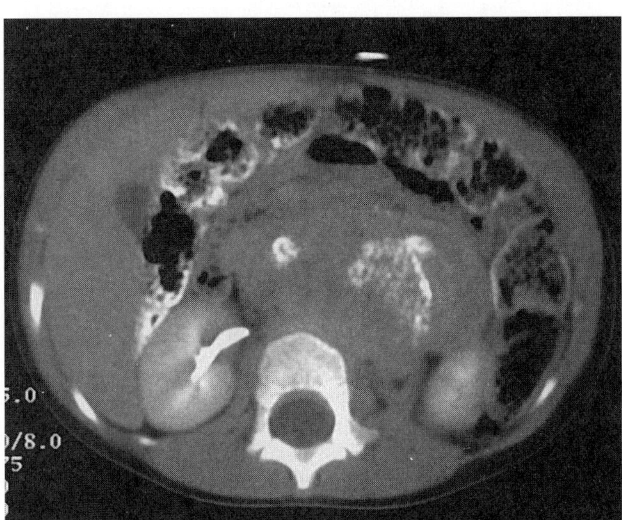

**FIGURE 11–11.** CT image showing a calcified tumor surrounding the central vessels.

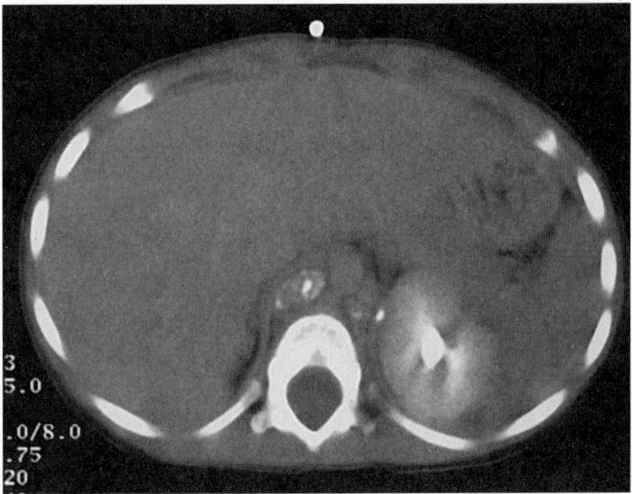

**FIGURE 11–12.** Extension of calcified neuroblastoma in mediastinal lymph nodes.

The treatment of neuroblastoma consists of combinations of surgical resection with adjuvant chemotherapy and radiotherapy. Factors affecting treatment regimens include age (older or younger than 1 year), amplification of the *MYCN* oncogene, serum ferritin and lactate dehydrogenase levels, and histology. Patients presenting before 1 year of age have the highest rate of disease-free survival.[34] *MYCN* oncogene amplification indicates a poor prognosis. The 10-year survival rates diminish from 88% for patients with Evans stage 1 disease to 21% for patients with stage 4 disease. Those with stage 4S have a 10-year survival rate of 81%.[34] The isolated metastases of the stage 4S neuroblastoma often spontaneously resolve.

### Wilms' Tumor

Approximately 400 new cases of Wilms' tumor occur in the United States each year. Wilms' tumor arises in the renal parenchyma. The most common presentation is that of an asymptomatic abdominal mass. Elevated blood pressure is seen in 25% of patients. Hematuria, fatigue, or pain is evident in 25% of cases. An association exists with Beckwith-Wiedemann syndrome, hemihypertrophy, and aniridia.[35]

A Wilms' tumor discovered as a left-sided mass must be differentiated from an enlarged spleen. Although it is more common for a neuroblastoma to cross the abdominal midline, a large Wilms' tumor may extend into the contralateral renal fossa. Ultrasound is useful as a first diagnostic study in the evaluation of a Wilms' tumor. Ultrasound can determine whether the mass originates in the kidney or is extrarenal, and whether it is cystic or solid. It is essential to determine whether there is tumor thrombus in the renal vein or inferior vena cava. CT provides a detailed view of tumor spread to adjacent tissue planes. The contralateral kidney must be evaluated for both tumor involvement and the ability to

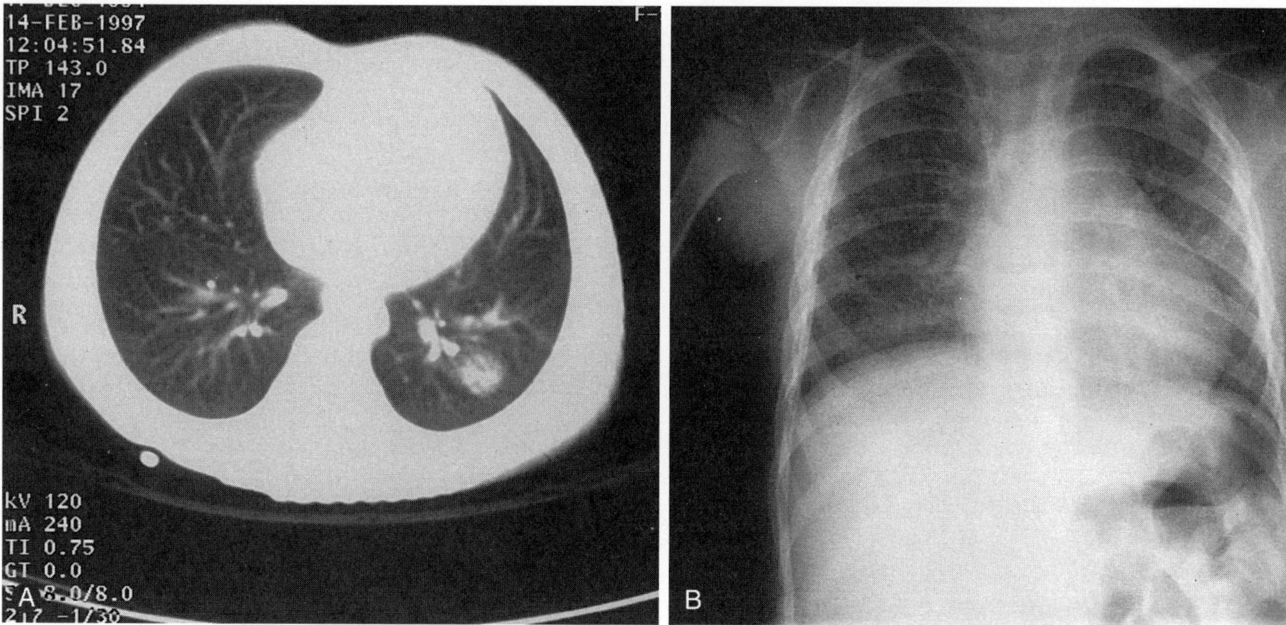


**FIGURE 11–13.** Chest CT scan identifying pulmonary metastasis not readily noted on the plain radiograph in a patient with Wilms' tumor.

concentrate radiographic contrast dye. A small percentage of contralateral Wilms' tumors may be identified by CT. CT radiography is used to identify pulmonary metastases (Fig. 11–13).

The staging of a Wilms' tumor depends on operative findings. Staging progresses from localized intrarenal tumor (stage 1), to extrarenal spread (stage 2), to locally advanced intra-abdominal spread (stage 3), to distant hematogenous disease (stage 4). Stage 5 classification indicates tumors in both kidneys. The treatment of a Wilms' tumor usually begins with surgical excision. The abdomen is inspected for disease extension outside the renal capsule and for extrarenal spread to periaortic and inferior vena caval lymph nodes, the peritoneum, and the liver. Adjuvant therapy includes chemotherapy and radiotherapy, depending on tumor stage and histology.

## *Rhabdomyosarcoma*

Sarcomas are malignancies arising from mesenchymal tissues; they are found in multiple sites throughout thc body. Rhabdomyosarcomas originate from a striated muscle precursor and represent approximately two thirds of all nonosseous sarcomas. The remaining one third of sarcomas originate from more than ten different cell types. Rhabdomyosarcomas manifesting after infancy originate in the trunk and extremities, whereas head and neck, bladder, and vaginal tumors occur predominantly in the youngest age group.[36] Sarcomas invade local structures and metastasize predominantly to the lung. Other sites of metastasis include the liver, bone marrow, and lymph nodes. Presenting signs and symptoms relate to the site of origin and structures involved with tumor. Patients with retroperitoneal sarcoma present with a palpable abdominal mass, intestinal obstruction, obstructive uropathy, hematuria, and pain. Treatment of rhabdomyosarcoma consists of resection of the tumor and involved organs in combination with adjuvant chemotherapy and irradiation.[37] The overall survival rate of patients with rhabdomyosarcoma after surgery and chemotherapy is 50%.

## REFERENCES


1. Stevenson RJ: Abdominal masses. Surg Clin North Am 1985;65:1481–1504.
2. Teele RL, Share JC: The abdominal mass in the neonate. Semin Roentgenol 1988;23:175–184.
3. Boechat MI, Kangarloo H: Magnetic resonance imaging of the abdomen in children. AJR Am J Radiol 1989;152:1245–1250.
4. Hensle TW, Reng KS: Urinary tract reconstruction. In Ashcraft H (ed): Pediatric Surgery, 2nd ed. Philadelphia, WB Saunders, 1993, pp 648–663.
5. Snyder HM III: Cystic disease of the kidney, dysplasia, and agenesis. In Welch KJ, Randolph JG, Ravitch MM, et al (eds): Pediatric Surgery, 4th ed. Chicago, Year Book Medical Publishers, 1986, pp 1126–1134.
6. Avni EF, Thoria Y, Lalmand B, et al: Multicystic dysplastic kidney: natural history from in utero diagnosis and postnatal follow-up. J Urol 1987;138:1420–1424.
7. Guez S, Assael BM, Melzi ML, et al: Shortcomings in predicting postnatal renal function using prenatal urine biochemistry in fetuses with congenital hydronephrosis. J Pediatr Surg 1996;31:1401–1404.
8. Duncan RE, Evans AT, Martin LW: Natural history and treatment of renal vein thrombosis in children. J Pediatr Surg 1977;12:639–645.
9. Hartman GE, Shochat SJ: Abdominal mass lesions in the newborn: diagnosis and treatment. Clin Perinatol 1989;16:123–135.
10. Altman AJ, Quinn JJ: Management of malignant solid tumors. In Nathan D, Orkin S (eds): Nathan and Oski's Hematology of Infancy and Childhood, 5th ed. Philadelphia, WB Saunders, 1998, pp 1381–1458.
11. Beckwith JB: Wilms' tumor and other renal tumors of childhood: an update. J Urol 1986;136:320–324.
12. Howell CG, Otherson HB, Kiviat NE, et al: Therapy and outcome in 51 children with mesoblastic nephroma: a report of the national Wilms' tumor study. J Pediatr Surg 1982;17:826–831.
13. Mertin DF, Kirks DR: Diagnostic imaging of pediatric abdominal masses. Pediatr Clin North Am 1985;32:1397–1425.
14. Gilcrease MZ, Brandt ML, Hawkins EP: Yolk sac tumor identified at autopsy after surgical excision of immature sacrococcygeal teratoma. J Pediatr Surg 1995;30:875–877.
15. Tran AT, Arensman RM, Falterman KW: Diagnosis and management of hydrohematometrocolpos syndromes. Am J Dis Child 1987;141:632–634.

16. Sty JR, Wells RG: Other abdominal and pelvic masses in children. Semin Roentgenol 1988;23:216–231.
17. Godpole P, Sprigg A, Dickson JA, Lin PC: Ultrasound compared with clinical examination in infantile hypertrophic pyloric stenosis. Arch Dis Child 1996;75:335–337.
18. Hight DW, Benson CD, Philippart AI, Hertzler JH: Management of mucosal perforations during pyloromyotomy for infantile pyloric stenosis. Surgery 1981;90:85–86.
19. Daneman A, Alton DJ: Intussusception, issues and controversies related to diagnosis and reduction. Radiol Clin North Am 1996;34:743–56.
20. Daneman A, Alton DJ, Ein S, et al: Perforation during attempted intussusception reduction in children: a comparison of perforation with barium and air. Pediatr Radiol 1995;25:81–88.
21. Vanck VN, Phillips AK: Retroperitoneal mesenteric and omental cysts. Arch Surg 1984;119:838–842.
22. Molander ML, Mortensson W, Uden R: Omental and mesenteric cysts in children. Acta Paediatr Scand 1982;71:272–279.
23. Wheatley JM, LaQuaglia MP: Management of hepatic epithelial malignancy in childhood and adolescence. Semin Surg Oncol 1993;9:532–540.
24. Iyer CP, Stanley P, Mahour GH: Hepatic hemangiomas in infants and children: a review of thirty cases. Am Surg 1996;62:356–360.
25. Oldham KT, Hart MJ, White TT: Choledochal cysts presenting in late childhood and adulthood. Am J Surg 1981;141:568–571.
26. Daneman A: Adrenal neoplasms in children. Semin Roentgenol 1988;23:205–215.
27. Tsakayannis DE, Mitchell K, Kozakewich HP, Shamberger RC: Splenic preservation in the management of splenic epidermoid cysts in children. J Pediatr Surg 1995;30:1468–1470.
28. Ein SH, Shandling B: Is interval appendectomy necessary after rupture of an appendiceal mass? J Pediatr Surg 1996;31:849–850.
29. Price MR, Haase GM, Sartorelli KH, Meagher DP: Recurrent appendicitis after initial conservative management of appendiceal abscess. J Pediatr Surg 1996;31:291–294.
30. Brandt ML, Luks FI, Filiatrault D, et al: Surgical indications in antenatally diagnosed ovarian cysts. J Pediatr Surg 1991;26:276–282.
31. Silva PD, Ripple J: Outpatient mini laparotomy ovarian cystectomy for benign teratomas in teenagers. J Pediatr Surg 1996;31:1383–1386.
32. Bernstein ML, Leclerc JM, Bunin G, et al: A population-based study of neuroblastoma incidence, survival and mortality in North America. J Clin Oncol 1992;10:323–327.
33. Evans AE, D'Angio GJ, Randolf J: A proposed staging for children with neuroblastoma: Children's Cancer Study Group A. Cancer 1971;27:374–378.
34. DeCou JM, Bowman LC, Rao BN, et al: Infants with neuroblastoma have improved survival with resection of the primary tumor. J Pediatr Surg 1995;30:937–941.
35. Green DM, D'Angio GJ, Beckwith JB, et al: Wilms' tumor. CA Cancer J Clin 1996;46:46–63.
36. LaQuaglia MP: Extremity rhabdomyosarcoma: biological principles, staging, and treatment. Semin Surg Oncol 1993;9:510–519.
37. Corpron CA, Andrassy RJ: Surgical management of rhabdomyosarcoma in children. Curr Opin Pediatr 1996;83:283–286.

# Chapter 12

# Abdominal Surgical Emergencies

J. Duncan Phillips

A number of abdominal conditions requiring urgent surgical intervention can manifest in infants and children. Age is the single most important piece of data in the patient's history, since many of these conditions occur almost exclusively in newborns (e.g., necrotizing enterocolitis [NEC]) and others almost always occur later in childhood (e.g., appendicitis, which is rare in children younger than 1 year of age). Other important aspects of the patient history are listed in Table 12–1. A thorough physical examination should include vital signs (temperature, pulse, blood pressure, and respiratory rate), examination of the skin (to assess for jaundice), auscultation of the heart and lungs, a thorough abdominal examination, examination of the genitalia, and (except in preterm infants) a digital rectal examination. The choice of laboratory and radiographic tests should be individualized. Prompt surgical evaluation should not be delayed while awaiting the results of a laboratory test that may turn out to be unhelpful. If an abdominal surgical condition is suspected, consultation with a pediatric surgeon or with a general surgeon with special training in the care of children should be obtained expeditiously.

## PATIENT PREPARATION

Except in extremely rare cases, the dictum *REO* (resuscitate, evaluate, then operate) should be followed. Because all pediatric abdominal operations require general anesthesia, intravenous access should be obtained and an appropriate blood specimen should be sent to the blood bank in case intraoperative transfusion is necessary. The parent or legal guardian, if not present, should be contacted immediately and informed of the possible need for urgent operation.

**TABLE 12–1. Components of the Patient's History**

- Age
- Sex
- Symptoms
  - Duration
  - Quality
  - Associated symptoms
  - History of similar symptoms in the past
- Past medical history, including the following:
  - History of prematurity
  - History of previous abdominal operations
- Family history, specifically the following:
  - Childhood illnesses
  - Familial syndromes
  - Similar illnesses in other family members

## NECROTIZING ENTEROCOLITIS

NEC is an intestinal illness that usually affects premature infants and is characterized by ischemia, reperfusion, infection, and possible necrosis (see Chapter 36). NEC affects approximately 2 per 1,000 newborns and affects approximately 2% of all infants in neonatal intensive care units.[1] Ninety percent to 95% of patients with NEC are premature, with a mean gestational age of 30 weeks and a mean birth weight of 1.5 kg.[2] Risk factors are listed in Table 12–2.

It is believed that some systemic stress triggers the onset of the disease with a transient episode of gut ischemia. Because of relative stasis of blood flow, thrombi form in the intestinal capillaries, with resultant damage to the capillary membranes. With reperfusion there is a disruption of cellular integrity, with bacterial invasion into the wall of the intestine with a subsequent severe inflammatory response.[3] Clinical findings are listed in Table 12–3.

Diagnosis can frequently be confirmed with simple radio-

**TABLE 12–2. Risk Factors for Necrotizing Enterocolitis**

- Hypoxia or asphyxia
- Apnea or pulmonary disease
- Hypotension or shock
- Early feedings
- Umbilical artery or umbilical vein catheters
- Other
  - Breech presentation
  - Twins
  - Jaundice
  - Heart disease
  - Anemia
  - Drugs

**TABLE 12–3. Clinical Findings in Necrotizing Enterocolitis**

| |
|---|
| Abdominal distention |
| High gastric residual volumes (check with orogastric or nasogastric tube) |
| Vomiting |
| Diarrhea |
| Hematochezia |
| Systemic findings: apnea, lethargy, pallor |

graphs obtained at the bedside: a "flat-plate" anteroposterior view of the abdomen (kidney, ureter, and bladder [KUB]) and a cross-table lateral view. The finding that is diagnostic of NEC is pneumatosis intestinalis, with gas bubbles in the wall of the intestine (Fig. 12–1). Other findings suggestive of NEC include dilated loops of intestine, a "fixed loop" seen on serial radiographs taken 6 to 12 hours apart, disappearance of all bowel gas, the appearance of ascites, gas in the portal vein, and pneumoperitoneum.[2]

Although fewer than half of all babies with NEC require surgical intervention, a pediatric surgery consultation should be obtained to assist with evaluation and resuscitation of the patient. Treatment is designed to support intestinal perfusion and oxygenation, decrease bacterial translocation, and provide nutrition for healing. The child should be given nothing by mouth, an orogastric (OG) or nasogastric (NG) tube should be inserted for gastric decompression, broad-spectrum intravenous antibiotics should be begun, and nutrition should be provided with total parenteral nutrition. Because NEC is a disease in evolution, the child should be continuously monitored and new data should be obtained serially. Repeat radiographs and complete blood counts should be done every 6 to 12 hours, and physical examinations should be performed frequently.

Laparotomy is indicated for NEC if there is suspicion or evidence for a segment of necrotic intestine in the abdomen. Although pneumoperitoneum (free air) on a lateral abdominal radiograph is highly suggestive, other findings suggestive of intestinal necrosis include inflammatory changes in the abdominal wall (so-called red abdomen), a palpable inflammatory mass on physical examination, a fixed loop or obstructive pattern on serial radiographs, bedside paracentesis results positive for intestinal contents, and unremitting sepsis unresponsive to maximal nonoperative therapy.[2] The laparotomy typically is done with the use of general anesthesia through a generous transverse incision. Dead segments of intestine should be resected, with the liberal use of stomas in unstable patients. Primary anastomosis can be accomplished in a few selected stable patients. Because NEC is a disease in evolution, areas of intestine may be somewhat ischemic but not frankly necrotic; a second-look laparotomy 24 to 48 hours later may be necessary to reassess areas of intestine that have questionable viability. Bedside peritoneal drainage, with avoidance of formal laparotomy, has been advocated in unstable, extremely premature infants.[4, 5]

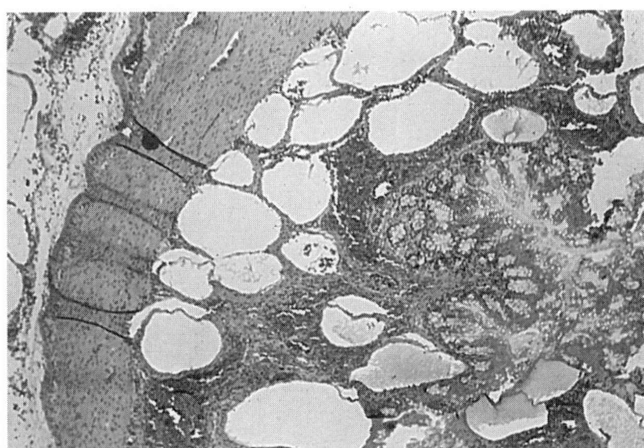

**FIGURE 12–1.** Necrotizing enterocolitis. Photomicrograph of cross-section of resected segment of colon wall, demonstrating severe inflammation of all layers, with large gas bubbles in submucosa. (Courtesy of Kathryn D. Anderson, MD, Children's Hospital, Los Angeles, CA.)

Overall, 20% to 60% of infants with NEC require surgical intervention, and 50% to 85% of those survive.[6] Patients who heal from NEC without surgical intervention run a 20% risk of subsequent stricture formation; therefore, any infant affected by NEC should be watched closely for the development of obstructive symptoms.

## ISOLATED INTESTINAL PERFORATION

Isolated intestinal perforation (also called idiopathic intestinal perforation or localized intestinal perforation) affects premature infants. This condition can be present at any location throughout the small and large intestine, and in multiple sites simultaneously, but it most commonly occurs in the distal ileum.[7] Perforation sites are usually located on the antimesenteric border of the intestine, and surrounding intestine is almost always histologically normal.[8] The origin of this condition has been attributed to intestinal ischemia resulting from diminished splanchnic blood flow, which can occur with in utero cocaine exposure, postnatal treatment with indomethacin,[9] or the use of umbilical artery catheters. Diagnosis usually is made at the time of laparotomy, after detection of pneumoperitoneum by abdominal radiography. Treatment involves prompt laparotomy with resection of the involved intestinal segment, with either primary end-to-end repair or creation of a temporary intestinal stoma, to be followed by stoma closure at a later date. Survival rates are high.

## GASTRIC PERFORATION

Neonatal gastric perforation is a distinct clinical entity which can cause massive pneumoperitoneum in premature infants. Although it was previously thought to be caused by peptic ulceration,[10] a number of more recent studies have suggested that this condition is iatrogenic and occurs after either inadvertent esophageal intubation with an endotracheal tube or vigorous respiratory resuscitation using a mask.[11] After fluid resuscitation, prompt laparotomy is indicated, with primary repair. The survival rate is high.[12]

## CONGENITAL INTESTINAL OBSTRUCTION

### Atresias and Stenoses

Intestinal atresia is the most common cause of intestinal obstruction in neonates, occurring with an incidence of ap-

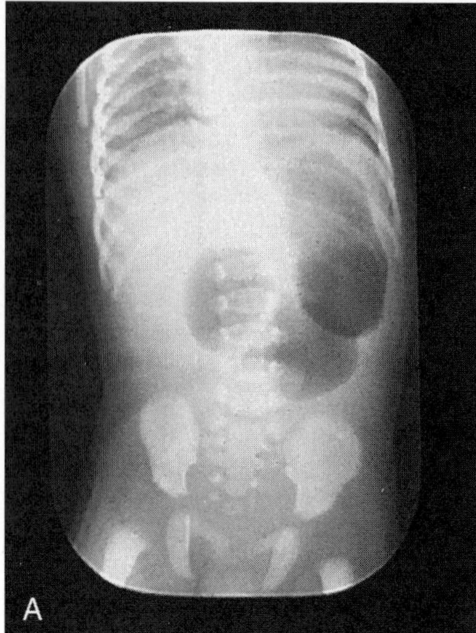


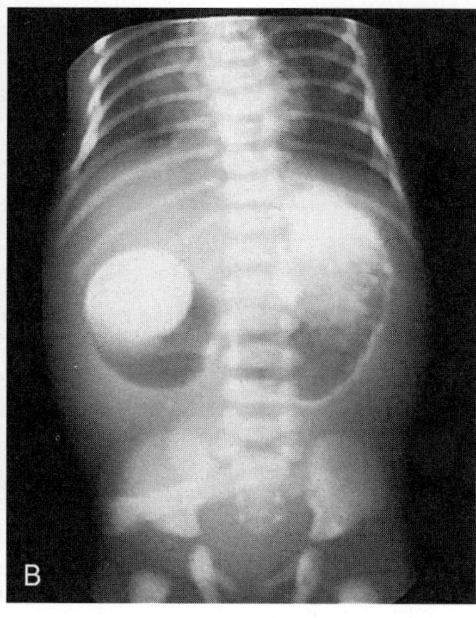


**FIGURE 12–2.** Duodenal atresia. *A,* "Double-bubble" sign, strongly suggestive of congenital duodenal obstruction. *B,* A small amount of contrast material, infused via OG tube, confirms the diagnosis. (Courtesy of Kathryn D. Anderson, MD, Children's Hospital, Los Angeles, CA.)

proximately 1 in 2,700 live births. It is almost always surgically correctable, with an overall survival rate of more than 90%.[13]

Duodenal atresia occurs because of failure of luminal recanalization during the solid cord stage of duodenal development (third to seventh week of gestation). Thirty percent of affected babies have other major congenital anomalies, and 30% have trisomy 21 (Down syndrome). It is occasionally associated with the VATER constellation of anomalies (*v*ertebral defects, imperforate *a*nus, *t*racheo*e*sophageal fistula, and *r*adial and *r*enal dysplasia). The most common presenting sign is bilious emesis. In 80% of affected infants, the obstruction is postampullary with consequent bilious emesis, and in 20% it is preampullary. Seventy percent of affected infants have delayed passage of meconium, 40% present with jaundice, and a variable number have abdominal distention. Work-up includes bedside abdominal radiography, looking for the "double-bubble" sign (Fig. 12–2*A*). The differential diagnosis includes malrotation (see later discussion); therefore, if the "double bubble" is unclear, a small amount of contrast material can be infused through an OG or NG tube to clarify the diagnosis (see Fig. 12–2*B*). With OG or NG decompression, perforation of the blind-ending duodenal segment is extremely rare. Surgery can be delayed for days or even weeks if necessary. Repair usually is performed through a right supraumbilical transverse incision with primary repair (i.e., duodenoduodenostomy or duodenojejunostomy). Because 3% to 5% of infants with duodenal atresia have multiple sites of obstruction, a Silastic or rubber catheter is usually passed proximally and distally to check for other sites of obstruction. Gastrostomy tube insertion is used at the discretion of the operating surgeon. Transanastomotic gastroduodenal feeding tubes have not been shown to shorten hospitalization or the time to full enteral feedings.[14]

Jejunal or ileal atresia is thought to be caused by an in utero ischemic event with thrombosis of a feeding mesenteric blood vessel. The site of obstruction is jejunal 50% of the time and ileal 50% of the time. Other anomalies are rare. These infants are usually small for gestational age, with evidence of in utero growth retardation. Infants typically present with abdominal distention and vomiting. Abdominal radiographs typically show evidence of small bowel obstruction. Treatment involves intestinal decompression with an NG or OG tube. Once hemodynamic stability has been achieved, repair should be performed promptly because of the risk of perforation of the proximal dilated segment. Primary repair with end-to-end anastomosis can usually be achieved without the need for a diverting stoma. Because the proximal bulbous tip has diminished numbers of ganglion cells, it may never regain normal peristaltic activity and should therefore be resected or tapered with a stapling device before anastomosis (Fig. 12–3).

## Hirschsprung's Disease

Hirschsprung's disease (see Chapter 41) results from the failure of in utero migration and development of neuroblasts. These cells normally migrate caudally in the bowel during weeks 6 through 12 of gestation to form the ganglion cells of Meissner's (submucosal) and Auerbach's (muscular) plex-

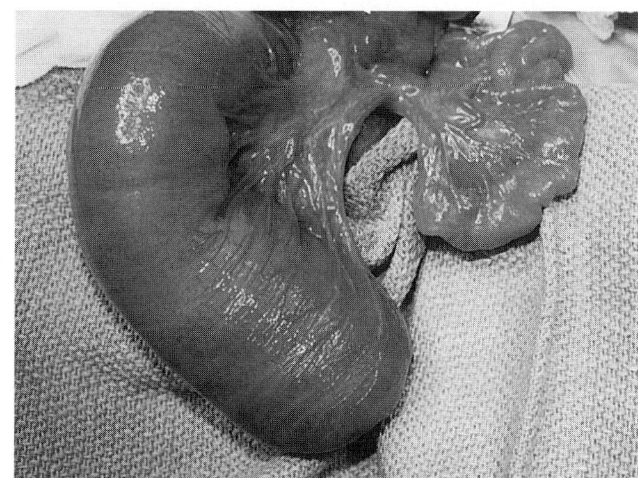

**FIGURE 12–3.** Ileal atresia. Proximal blind-ending segment *(left)* should undergo resection of bulbous tip, or tapering, before anastomosis to distal ("downstream") ileum *(right).*

uses. Absence of these cells causes a lack of progression of the normal intestinal peristaltic waves through the affected segment. Although the typical transition zone (from normally-innervated bowel proximally to abnormal intestine distally) is at the rectosigmoid,[15, 16] some affected infants have transition zones that are more proximal (distal ileum or right colon) or more distal (so-called short-segment Hirsch sprung's disease, with a transition zone distal to the peritoneal reflection).[17] The diagnosis is suggested by contrast enema showing an intestinal transition zone and confirmed by suction rectal biopsy showing the absence of ganglion cells and nerve trunk hypertrophy.

Hirschpsrung's enterocolitis is an inflammatory condition affecting approximately 20% to 30% of Hirschsprung's patients; it can occur in the newborn period, after creation of a diverting colostomy, or even after definitive resection of affected bowel.[16] Intestine proximal and/or distal to the transition zone becomes edematous and inflamed. This process can quickly become full-thickness and cause intestinal ischemia and even perforation. Symptoms, which can develop and progress over a time course as short as 6 to 8 hours, include fever, irritability, abdominal distention, vomiting, and diarrhea. The stool is classically light tan to gray and foul-smelling. Contrast enema may reveal a saw-toothed appearance of the bowel wall.

Numerous organisms have been implicated in the pathogenesis of Hirschpsrung's enterocolitis, including viruses, staphylococci, gram-negative enterics, and anaerobes. Some authors have detected *Clostridium difficile* toxin in the stool of affected children.

Treatment involves immediate hospitalization and surgical consultation with the institution of intravenous hydration and broad-spectrum intravenous antibiotics. A typical regimen, covering the bacteria mentioned, would consist of vancomycin, a third-generation cephalosporin, and metronidazole. Perhaps most importantly, frequent saline irrigations through a rubber or silicone catheter, designed to flush out potentially toxic bacteria or bacterial toxins, should be instituted immediately. In patients without stomas, these irrigations are done per rectum. In patients with a previous diversion, irrigations are done via the stoma.

Treatment should be continued for 5 to 10 days. If clinical improvement does not occur, or if evidence of intestinal necrosis or perforation appears, urgent laparotomy may be necessary. Perforated segments of bowel and severely affected segments distal to the transition zone should be resected, with establishment of a proximal diverting intestinal stoma. Intestinal segments with mild or moderate inflammation which are located proximal to the transition zone may recover and therefore should not be resected, if possible.

## Imperforate Anus

This anomaly affects approximately 1 in 5,000 newborns (see Chapter 42). It is one manifestation of a variety of pelvic conditions known as anorectal malformations. These anomalies occur because of failure of fusion of the urorectal septum to the cloacal membrane during the first 8 weeks of gestation. Affected infants have either "high" anomalies, with fistulas to the genitourinary system (usually to the urethra in boys and to the vagina or posterior fourchette in girls), or "low" anomalies, with fistulas to the perineum. Immediate management includes NG or OG decompression, intravenous hydration, and work-up for other anomalies, which frequently are present. Low anomalies are treated with perineal anoplasty. High anomalies typically require creation of a divided sigmoid colostomy in the newborn period, followed by perineal reconstruction at the age of 4 to 12 months.[18]

## Abdominal Wall Defects

Abdominal wall defects, gastroschisis and omphalocele, occur in approximately 1 out of 4,000 newborns. Gastroschisis is thought to develop from a failure of vascularization of the abdominal wall, most likely from complete reabsorption of the right umbilical vein in utero.[19] The defect is almost always just to the right of the umbilicus, allowing intestinal evisceration in utero (Fig. 12–4). The intestine, exposed to amniotic fluid, becomes thickened and inflamed.[20] Ten percent of affected infants have associated anomalies—most often intestinal atresia, presumably from occlusion of the affected intestinal segment at the fascial edge. At delivery, the exposed viscera should immediately be covered with saline-moistened sterile gauze and an impermeable barrier (e.g., Saran Wrap). An NG or OG tube should be inserted for decompression, followed by prompt surgical closure, usually within 4 hours. Because "third-space" losses can be dramatic (equivalent to an extensive skin burn), aggressive fluid resuscitation is indicated. Repair is either with primary closure, if technically feasible, or with the placement of a prosthetic "chimney" (Fig. 12–5), with gradual staged reduction over a 3- to 10-day period and subsequent fascial closure.[21, 22] The survival rate of patients with this anomaly now approaches 95%.[21] However, because of the intestinal inflammation, return of intestinal function may take 30 to

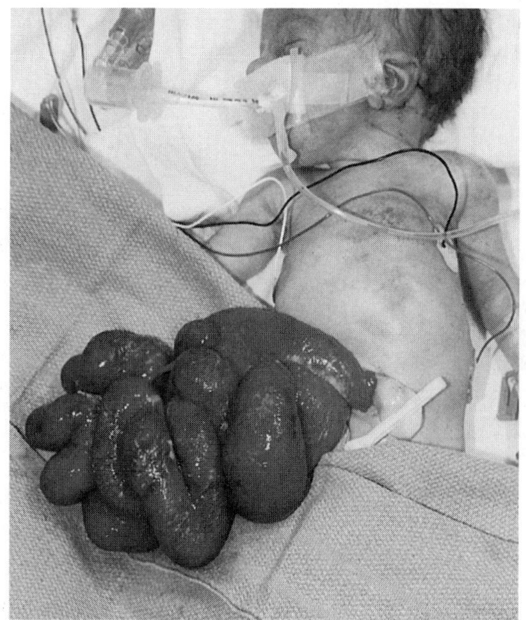

**FIGURE 12–4.** Gastroschisis. Eviscerated intestine, to the right of the umbilicus, is thickened, edematous, and covered with a hemorrhagic serosal "peel" of fibrinous exudate.

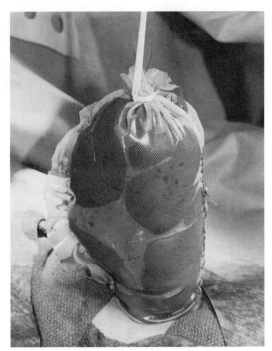

**FIGURE 12–5.** Gastroschisis, after placement of prosthetic "chimney."

40 days. Therefore, all of these infants require central venous access and total parenteral nutrition.[23]

Omphalocele (Fig. 12–6) can be considered a failure of formation of the midportion of the abdominal wall. The defect is covered by a membrane.[19] Approximately 50% of infants with this defect have other major congenital anomalies.[24] Small defects can be closed primarily, but large defects may require the placement of a prosthetic "chimney" with gradual staged reduction, or skin coverage only with the development of a large ventral hernia, or placement of a prosthetic material such as Gortex at the fascial level with skin coverage over it.[25] Occasionally, premature infants and those who are otherwise unstable have the defect painted with silver sulfadiazine or another topical agent, allowing the exposed area to gradually epithelialize, with delayed fascial closure at a later date.[24]

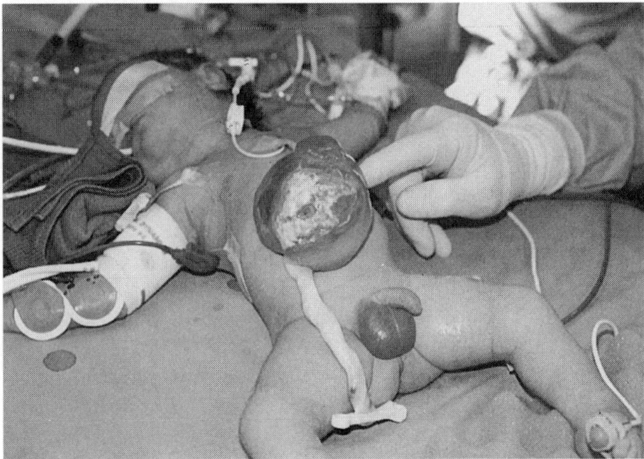

**FIGURE 12–6.** Omphalocele. Midline abdominal wall defect, covered by membrane.

## Malrotation and Midgut Volvulus

The congenital anomaly of midgut fixation occurs in approximately 1 in 500 live births and results from a failure of normal 270-degree rotation of the midgut around the superior mesenteric artery in utero. Affected infants lack the normal broad base of the small bowel mesentery, which usually extends from the ligament of Treitz lateral to the spine in the left upper quadrant down to the ileocecal junction in the right lower quadrant. Symptoms usually develop when the midgut begins to twist around its superior mesenteric artery pedicle, which can eventually occlude the vascular supply (Fig. 12–7). Symptoms may be intermittent and chronic or acute and catastrophic. Approximately half of affected infants develop symptoms in the first month of life, 90% within the first year of life.

Vomiting is the most common presenting sign.[26] Although the vomitus is classically described as bilious, it is initially bilious in only 80% of affected infants and progressively becomes bilious in only half of the remaining infants. Affected infants become irritable and cry frequently. Approximately 10% pass blood per rectum. The abdominal physical examination has been reported to be normal in two thirds of affected infants, and abdominal tenderness and/or distention is found in only about one fifth. Plain radiographs (KUB) are frequently not helpful, because the results are nonspecific in 50% of affected infants and reportedly normal in 20%.[27] Although a contrast enema may demonstrate the malrotation, it is normal in up to 20% of infants. The diagnostic test of choice is an upper gastrointestinal series (UGI), which has a diagnostic accuracy of approximately 95%. Because malrotation, with the subsequent development of midgut volvulus, can rapidly lead to intestinal ischemia and death, every child in which this anomaly is suspected requires an *immediate* UGI.

If the malrotation has led to midgut volvulus, emergency

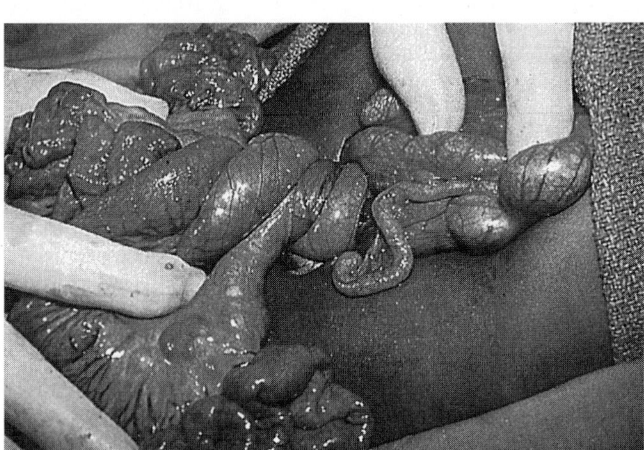

**FIGURE 12–7.** Malrotation with midgut volvulus. The midgut has twisted around the superior mesenteric artery pedicle, causing vascular compression and intestinal ischemia. (From Nakayama DK: Pediatric Surgery: A Color Atlas. New York, Gower Medical Publishing, 1991.)

laparotomy is indicated. The intestine must be untwisted as quickly as possible, and the child should be taken immediately to the operating room for this procedure. Resuscitation is carried out in the operating room. In this case, the REO rule (described previously) should be broken. The operation (the so-called Ladd's procedure) is done through a generous right upper quadrant transverse incision and involves untwisting the volvulus in a counterclockwise direction, dividing the Ladd's bands (congenital bands extending from the cecum to the right upper quadrant, which partially obstruct the duodenum), performing an appendectomy, and positioning the small intestine to the right side of the abdomen and the large intestine to the left. The procedure works by lengthening the distance between the duodenojejunal junction and the ileocecal junction. The development of postoperative adhesions helps prevent recurrence of the volvulus, which is extremely rare. Infarcted areas of intestine are resected, with the generous use of stomas. Because some areas of intestine may have questionable viability, a second-look laparotomy done 24 to 48 hours later may be necessary. If the entire midgut has become infarcted, long-term survival is rare, and serious consideration may be given to withdrawing support after obtaining input from the surgeon, gastroenterologist, and family. Overall, 20% of affected infants die, and a variable percentage develop short-bowel syndrome. Although the treatment of patients with asymptomatic malrotation is somewhat controversial, most pediatric surgeons recommend elective correction to prevent the catastrophic complication of midgut volvulus.

## ACQUIRED AND INFLAMMATORY CONDITIONS

### Hypertrophic Pyloric Stenosis

Hypertrophic pyloric stenosis is a common entity that occurs in approximately 3 per 1,000 live births, with a 4.5:1 male-to-female predominance.[28] It typically develops in infants between 2 and 5 weeks of age. It is thought to be acquired postnatally and therefore not to be a true congenital obstruction (see Chapter 17). Symptoms include nonbilious projectile vomiting 30 to 60 minutes after feedings. The vomitus may eventually become brownish or bloody as a result of gastric irritation. On examination, a pyloric "olive" may be palpable (in 70%); if so, no further diagnostic tests need be done. If the stenosis is not palpable, useful tests include a UGI series (string sign) or an abdominal ultrasound examination. Ultrasound measurement criteria include a pyloric diameter greater than 14 mm, length greater than 16 mm, or thickness greater than 4 mm.

The differential diagnosis includes gastroesophageal reflux, malrotation, other congenital obstructions (antral web or gastric duplication), central nervous system lesions with subsequent vomiting, and "pylorospasm" (a condition seen more commonly in extremely premature infants).

Treatment involves fluid resuscitation to correct the inevitable hypokalemic, hypochloremic metabolic alkalosis; this may take 12 to 24 hours, or even longer if the child has had symptoms for several days. Treatment is by Ramstedt's pyloromyotomy with longitudinal disruption of the thickened fibers of the pylorus. This can be done through a right upper quadrant incision, through a transumbilical incision,[29] or laparoscopically.[30] Feedings usually can be started postoperatively within 6 to 8 hours, with gradual advancement of the feedings and discharge within 24 to 36 hours. Recurrence is extremely rare.

### Meckel's Diverticulitis

The Meckel's diverticulum (see Chapter 40), a remnant of the omphalomesenteric duct, has been called the "organ of two's" since its incidence is approximately 2% of the population, it is typically located (in adults) 2 feet proximal to the ileocecal valve, and it is, on average, 2 inches long.[31] Eighty percent of symptomatic diverticula have ectopic gastric mucosa within them. If symptoms develop, 50% of affected patients become symptomatic in the first 2 years of life. One fourth to one half of symptomatic patients develop lower gastrointestinal hemorrhage from ulceration produced by the ectopic gastric mucosa. About one third of symptomatic infants develop intestinal obstruction, since the tip of the Meckel's diverticulum can still be attached to the undersurface of the umbilicus. Approximately one fourth of affected infants develop Meckel's diverticulitis with pain from peptic ulceration. Diagnosis is made by a "Meckel's scan," in which a radioisotope (technetium) is used to identify ectopic gastric mucosa.[32] The scan has a reported sensitivity of 80% to 90%. Meckel's diverticulitis can also mimic appendicitis, with right lower quadrant abdominal pain, tenderness, fever, and leukocytosis. Treatment involves Meckel's diverticulectomy through a right lower quadrant transverse incision. If the patient has presented with gastrointestinal hemorrhage the ileal lumen should be inspected, because peptic ulceration may be found on the ileal wall opposite the diverticulum.

### Intussusception

Infants with intussusception typically present between the ages of 5 and 12 months (see Chapter 38). The cause is probably hypertrophied Peyer's patches within the wall of the distal ileum which have become inflamed from an antecedent viral infection. Although intussusceptions can involve only the small bowel or only the large intestine, the most common type is the ileocolic intussusception.[33] An affected infant typically presents with dramatic attacks of abdominal pain and screaming that occur in cycles, approximately every 10 to 15 minutes. Eventually, with mucosal ischemia and subsequent sloughing, the infant may pass a "currant-jelly" stool. Progressive vomiting develops. Initially infants vomit their food, and then the vomitus gradually becomes bilious. If symptoms persist, the child becomes dehydrated or bacteremic, or both, with eventual lethargy and somnolence. Between 40% and 70% of affected infants have a palpable mass (the intussusception) in the right upper quadrant. Treatment involves intravenous hydration and the institution of intravenous antibiotics. Fifty percent to 70% of intussusceptions can be reduced in a retrograde fashion with the use of contrast enema (either barium or air, depending on the institution).[34, 35] The "rule of three's" should be used: the barium container is raised 3 feet above the patient and at least three attempts at reduction should be made, with each attempt lasting for at least 3 minutes. If nonoperative reduction is unsuccessful, urgent laparotomy is indicated to prevent infarction of the intussuscepted bowel segment. The approach usually is through a right lower quadrant incision. If the intussusception cannot be reduced manually, resection may be required, with either primary anastomosis or creation of stomas. A lead point, such as a Meckel's diverticulum or the rare abdominal tumor, is sought and, if present, resected as well. The appendix typically is removed so that later examining physicians are not confused by the right lower quadrant incision.

## Appendicitis

There are approximately 60,000 pediatric cases of acute appendicitis in the United States each year. Rupture occurs in approximately one third of cases, and some children still die annually from this disease.[36, 37] Mortality approaches 5% in complicated perforated cases, yet appendicitis is easily treated with surgery and intravenous antibiotics (see Chapter 37).

Left untreated, acute appendicitis can progress to suppuration, with a fibrinous exudate on the surface of the appendix and early evidence of walling off by the omentum. Further progression can lead to gangrene and eventually to free rupture into the peritoneal cavity, with the development of thick purulent peritoneal fluid, partial or complete ileal obstruction from inflammation, and diffuse peritonitis. Although this progression to perforation typically takes about 24 hours, some patients progress much more slowly (48 to 72 hours) or more quickly (8 hours) to perforation.

The typical appendicitis patient complains initially of abdominal pain, usually beginning before other symptoms.[38] The pain classically begins periumbilically and then localizes to the right lower quadrant over a 6- to 8-hour period. The pain is usually gradual in onset and steady, but it continues to increase in intensity and is worsened by movement. Children usually develop anorexia as well as nausea, vomiting, and low-grade fever. On examination, the child appears ill; that is, the child walks slowly, appears apprehensive, climbs slowly onto the examining table, and lies very still. It is unusual for a child with appendicitis to run around the examining room.

The cardinal sign is point tenderness at McBurney's point, located midway between the right anterior superior iliac spine and the umbilicus. The patient develops guarding, muscle spasm, and diminished bowel sounds. With perforation, an abdominal mass may be felt on palpation of the abdomen or on digital rectal examination. The conventional test for rebound tenderness, in which the physician presses down on the child's abdomen and then abruptly lets go, can be brutally painful to a small child and therefore is not recommended. Gentle percussion and/or palpation usually is sufficient to diagnose appendicitis. Laboratory tests usually reveal leukocytosis with the development of premature forms (bands). Occasionally, a child with acute appendicitis has a completely normal leukocyte count. Mild pyuria may develop as a result of irritation of the right ureter or bladder by appendiceal inflammation.

Plain abdominal radiographs show a calcified fecalith in 20% of affected patients.[39] Expensive, sophisticated tests such as ultrasound, barium enema, and computed tomography scans usually are indicated only in unusual cases in which the diagnosis is unclear.[40, 41]

Inflammation of a retrocecal appendix, which may be present in approximately 15% of the general population, can be difficult to diagnose. This may cause flank or back pain and/or dysuria. The child may present with minimal abdominal findings and may be referred to several different physicians or other specialists because of the difficult diagnosis. A digital rectal examination, with palpation of an inflamed, tender area in the right lower quadrant, may be quite helpful. The differential diagnosis of acute appendicitis is broad (Table 12–4).

Treatment begins with resuscitation. The child should be given nothing by mouth, and intravenous hydration should be started. A surgical consultation should be obtained. If the appendix is perforated, the child may require NG decompression, placement of a Foley catheter to guide fluid resuscitation, and even preoperative stabilization in an intensive care unit. This may take from 2 to 12 hours. Once the diagnosis of acute or perforated appendicitis is made, broad-spectrum intravenous antibiotics should be started. Treatment involves laparotomy and appendectomy through a right lower quadrant incision (open laparotomy) or laparoscopically.[42] If perforation has occurred, the abdomen and pelvis typically are irrigated with sterile saline and/or antibiotic solution. Some pediatric surgeons drain the abdomen postoperatively with either Jackson-Pratt or Penrose drains.[43] Children with missed appendicitis (i.e., appendix perforated and walled off by omentum, without diffuse peritonitis) can often be successfully managed with a 7- to 10-day course of intravenous antibiotics followed by discharge from the hospital, with a subsequent interval appendectomy 6 to 8 weeks later.[44] Recuperation after appendectomy varies depending on the severity of the illness. With acute appendicitis, the hospital stay may be as short as 24 hours, with return to normal activity in a few days. However, with perforated appendicitis and diffuse peritonitis, there is a fairly high morbidity rate and a number of possible postoperative complications, including wound infection, abscess, and bowel obstruction.[45]

**TABLE 12–4. Differential Diagnosis of Appendicitis**

| |
|---|
| Gastroenteritis |
| Mesenteric adenitis |
| Constipation |
| Urinary tract infection |
| Salpingitis or pelvic inflammatory disease |
| Meckel's diverticulitis |
| Pneumonia—right lower lobe |
| Primary peritonitis |
| Intussusception |
| Regional enteritis or Crohn's disease |
| Cholecystitis |
| Ovarian cyst or torsion |
| Sickle cell crisis |
| Omental infarction |
| Mittelschmerz |
| Other |

## Intestinal Obstruction

### Adhesions

Adhesions, bands or strings of fibrinous connective tissue, can form after any abdominal or pelvic operation or diffuse intra-abdominal inflammatory process (e.g., peritonitis from perforated appendicitis).[46] Although poorly understood, adhesions are believed to be more likely to form after procedures that involve prolonged, extensive dissection and bleeding. No surgical technique or medication has been shown to prevent their formation. Adhesive intestinal obstruction, which occurs after approximately 3% of all laparotomies,[47] is caused when an intestinal segment twists around an adhesion and becomes occluded. If left untreated, obstructed segments can become edematous, inflamed, and even gangrenous.[48]

Patients with a history of abdominal surgery may develop adhesive obstruction days to years later. They typically present with vomiting and crampy abdominal pain that is colicky in nature, coming in cycles every 10 to 15 minutes. During pain attacks, auscultation may reveal high-pitched, "tinkling" bowel sounds. Diagnosis is usually made with standard abdominal radiographs (KUB and upright), which demonstrate dilated small bowel loops with multiple air-fluid levels.

In the absence of peritoneal signs, partial obstructions often resolve spontaneously as the obstructed intestinal segment untwists itself. Treatment involves hospitalization for NG decompression and intravenous hydration. Complete obstructions (i.e., obstructions in patients no longer passing stool or flatus) require surgical repair (enterolysis), since bowel may become infarcted. Infarcted segments usually can be removed with primary anastomosis.

### Tumors

Intestinal obstruction can develop proximal to intra-abdominal or pelvic tumors, such as lymphomas, carcinoids, carcinomas, and sarcomas.[49] Treatment involves urgent laparotomy and resection (if technically feasible) with primary anastomosis (small bowel) or creation of a proximal diverting stoma (large bowel).

## REFERENCES


1. Snyder CL, Gittes GK, Murphy, JP, et al: Survival after necrotizing enterocolitis in infants weighing less than 1,000 g: 25 years' experience at a single institution. J Pediatr Surg 1997;32:434–437.
2. Grosfeld JL, Cheu H, Schlatter M, et al: Changing trends in necrotizing enterocolitis: experience with 302 cases in two decades. Ann Surg 1991;214:300–307.
3. Nowicki PT, Nankervis CA: The role of the circulation in the pathogenesis of necrotizing enterocolitis. Clin Perinatal 1994;21:219–234.
4. Ein SH, Shandling B, Wesson D, et al: A 13-year experience with peritoneal drainage under local anesthesia for necrotizing enterocolitis perforation. J Pediatr Surg 1990;25:1034–1037.
5. Morgan LJ, Shochat SJ, Hartman GE: Peritoneal drainage as primary management of perforated NEC in the very low birth weight infant. J Pediatr Surg 1994;29:310–315.
6. Rowe MI, Reblock KK, Kurkchubasche AG, et al: Necrotizing enterocolitis in the extremely low birth weight infant. J Pediatr Surg 1994;29:987–991.
7. Buchheit JQ, Stewart DL: Clinical comparison of localized intestinal perforation and necrotizing enterocolitis in neonates. Pediatrics 1994;93:32–36.
8. Weinberg G, Kleinhaus S, Boley SJ: Idiopathic intestinal perforations in the newborn: an increasingly common entity. J Pediatr Surg 1989;1007–1008.
9. Wolf WM, Snover DC, Leonard AS: Localized intestinal perforation following intravenous indomethacin in premature infants. J Pediatr Surg 1989;4:409–410.
10. Kiesewetter WB: Spontaneous rupture of the stomach in the newborn. Am J Dis Child 1956;91:162–167.
11. Houck WS, Griffin JA: Spontaneous linear tears of the stomach in the newborn infant. Ann Surg 1981;193:763–768.
12. Rosser SB, Clark CH, Elechi EN: Spontaneous neonatal gastric perforation. J Pediatr Surg 1982;17:390–394.
13. Mooney D, Lewis JE, Connors RH, et al: Newborn duodenal atresia: an improving outlook. Am J Surg 1987;153:347–349.
14. Gavopoulos S, Limas CH, Avtzoglou P, et al: Operative and postoperative management of congenital duodenal obstruction: a 10-year experience. Pediatr Surg Int 1993;8:122–124.
15. Rescorla FJ, Morrison AM, Engles D, et al: Hirschsprung's disease: evaluation of mortality and long-term function in 260 cases. Arch Surg 1992;127:934–942.
16. Foster P, Cowan G, Wrenn EL: Twenty-five years' experience with Hirschsprung's disease. J Pediatr Surg 1990;25:531–534.
17. Sawin R, Hatch E, Schaller R, et al: Limited surgery for lower-segment Hirschsprung's disease. Arch Surg 1994;129:920–925.
18. deVries PA, Pẽna A: Posterior sagittal anorectoplasty. J Pediatr Surg 1982;17:638–643.
19. deVries PA: The pathogenesis of gastroschisis and omphalocele. J Pediatr Surg 1982;15:245–251.
20. Tibboel D, Vermey-Keers C, Kluck P, et al: The natural history of gastroschisis during fetal life: development of the fibrous coating on the bowel loops. Teratology 1986;33:267–272.
21. Fonkalsrud EW: Selective repair of neonatal gastroschisis based on degree of visceroabdominal disproportion. Ann Surg 1980;191:139–144.
22. Schwartz MZ, Tyson KRT, Milliorn K, et al: Staged reduction using a Silastic sac is the treatment of choice for large congenital abdominal wall defects. J Pediatr Surg 1983;18:713–719.
23. Tunell WP, Puffinbarger NK, Tuggle DW: Abdominal wall defects in infants: survival and implications for adult life. Ann Surg 1995;221:525–530.
24. Nuchtern JG, Baxter R, Hatch EI: Nonoperative initial management versus Silon chimney for treatment of giant omphalocele. J Pediatr Surg 1995;30:771–776.
25. Bauer JJ, Salky BA, Gelernt IM: Repair of large abdominal wall defects with expanded polytetrafluoroethylene (PTFE). Ann Surg 1987;206:765–769.
26. Millar AJW, Rode H, Brown RA: The deadly vomit: malrotation and midgut volvulus. A review of 137 cases. Pediatr Surg Int 1987;2:172–176.
27. Ford EG, Senas MO, Srikanth MS: Malrotation of the intestine in children. Ann Surg 1992;215:172–178.
28. Poon SCT, Zhang AL, Cartmill T, et al: Changing patterns of diagnosis and treatment of infantile hypertrophic pyloric stenosis: a clinical audit of 303 patients. J Pediatr Surg 1996;31:1611–1615.
29. Huddard SN, Bianchi A, Kumar V, et al: Ramstedt's pyloromyotomy: circumumbilical versus transverse approach. Pediatr Surg 1993;8:395–396.
30. Ford WDA, Crameri JA, Holland AJA: The learning curve for laparoscopic pyloromyotomy. J Pediatr Surg 1997;32:552–554.
31. Cullen JJ, Kelly KA, Moir CR, et al: Surgical management of Meckel's diverticulum. Ann Surg 1994;220:564–569.
32. Dutro JA, Santanello SA, Unger F, et al: Rectal bleeding in a 4-month-old boy. JAMA 1986;256:2239–2240.
33. Grant HW, Buccimazza I, Hadley GP: A comparison of colo-colic and ileo-colic intussusception. J Pediatr Surg 1996;31:1607-1610.
34. Skipper RP, Boeckman CR, Klein RL: Childhood intussusception. Surg Gynecol Obstet 1990;171:151–153.
35. Ein SH, Palder SB, Alton DJ, et al: Intussusception: toward less surgery? J Pediatr Surg 1994;29:433–435.
36. Hunter IC, Paterson JG, Davidson AI: Deaths from acute appendicitis: a review of twenty-one cases in Scotland from 1974 to 1979. J R Coll Surg Edinb 1986;31:161–163.
37. Pledger HG, Fahy LT, Van Mourik GA, et al: Deaths in children with

a diagnosis of acute appendicitis in England and Wales 1980–1984. Br Med J 1987;295:1233–1235.
38. Wagner JM, McKinney WP, Carpenter JL: Does this patient have appendicitis? JAMA 1996;276:1589–1594.
39. Nitecki S, Karmeli R, Israel H, et al: Appendiceal calculi and fecaliths as indications for appendectomy. Surg Gynecol Obstet 1990;171:185–188.
40. Kang WM, Lee CH, Chou YH, et al: A clinical evaluation of ultrasonagraphy in the diagnosis of acute appendicitis. Surgery 1989;105:154–159.
41. Schwerk WB, Wichtrup B, Rothmund M, et al: Ultrasonography in the diagnosis of acute appendicitis: a prospective study. Gastroenterology 1989;97:630–639.
42. Ghoneimi AE, Valla JS, Limonne B, et al: Laparoscopic appendectomy in children: report of 1,379 cases. J Pediatr Surg 1994;29:786–789.
43. Johnson DA, Kosloske AM, Macarthur C: Perforated appendicitis in children: to drain or not drain? Pediatr Surg Int 1993;8:402–405.
44. Elmore JR, Dibbins AW, Curci MR: The treatment of complicated appendicitis in children. Arch Surg 1987;122:424–427.
45. Samelson SL, Reyes HM: Management of perforated appendicitis in children—revisited. Arch Surg 1987;122:691–696.
46. O'Leary JP, Wickbom G, Cha SO, et al: The role of feces, necrotic tissue, and various blocking agents in the prevention of adhesions. Ann Surg 1988;207:693–698.
47. Weigelt JA, Kingman RG: Complications of negative laparotomy for trauma. Am J Surg 1988;156:544–547.
48. Frazee RC, Mucha P, Farnell MB, Van Heerden JA: Volvulus of the small intestine. Ann Surg 1988;208;565–568.
49. Bethel CAI, Bhattacharyya NB, Hutchinson C: Alimentary tract malignancies in children. J Pediatr Surg 1997;32:1004–1009.

# SECTION TWO

# THE ESOPHAGUS

# Chapter 13

# Congenital Malformations of the Esophagus

Sigmund H. Ein

The story of esophageal atresia (EA) and tracheoesophageal fistula (TEF) repairs reads like the gradual mastery of most other surgical problems.[1–5] Durston first described an infant with EA in 1670,[6] but not until the time of Vogt[7] (1929) and then Gross[8] (1953) was a classification of EA varieties developed. Various surgical attempts were made from the late 1800s until 1943, when Haight and Towsley[9] were the first to successfully repair EA and TEF. Before that event, all patients (including 32 reported by Lanman[10]) who were primarily repaired had died. Two years before the first success of Haight and Towsley,[9] Leven[11] and Ladd[12] each had had a survivor but had not achieved a primary repair.

## EMBRYOLOGY AND PATHOGENESIS

EA and TEF occur in 1 in 3,000 to 5,000 live births[13–15] and are equally distributed according to sex. Embryologically, the esophagus, stomach, trachea, and lungs all are derived from the foregut.[16, 17] The foregut is partitioned by a septum into two separate tubes (Fig. 13–1): (1) the trachea anteriorly, which then continues to develop cartilaginous rings and lung buds; and (2) the esophagus posteriorly, which stretches from the pharynx to the stomach. This process is complete by the fourth fetal week (when the embryo is 8-mm long). For unknown reasons, there is an incomplete tubular separation of the esophagus from top to bottom, causing an atresia,[18] and in most instances the posterior esophagus fails to separate completely from the trachea, creating a variety of TEFs or clefts, or both. Tracheal anomalies (atresias, stenoses, and clefts) may also occur in conjunction with esophageal defects.[19, 20]

Between the third and fourth fetal weeks (when embryos are between 3–4 and 8-mm long), the laryngotracheal sulcus is completed along with the segmentation of the parietal mesoderm on each side of the notochord with the formation of sclerotomes, myotomes, and vertebrae. Segmentation of the embryo, therefore, happens at the same time that the tracheobronchial tree and the esophagus separate.[21, 22]

Half of the mothers of a fetus with an EA have polyhydramnios,[23] an association that may increase the chances for prenatal diagnosis. Neonates who have an EA with or without a TEF vary in weight from 800 to 4,000 g (averaging 2,500 g); 50% weigh more than 2,500 g, and the remaining 50% are considered premature (weighing <2,500 g). About 50% have other anomalies,[24–26] with more than 40% having from one to four other defects[27]: cardiovascular,[28, 29] 25% (most common are patent ductus arteriosus and ventricular and atrial septal defects); gastrointestinal, 15% (imperforate anus and duodenal atresia); skeletal,[30] 10% (digital and vertebral); genitourinary,[31, 32] 5% (hypospadias and undescended testis); and other congenital lesions, 15% (trisomy or lung agenesis or hypoplasia). As the number of systems with defects increases, the weight of the neonate decreases; 10% have defects incompatible with life (i.e., trisomy or complex

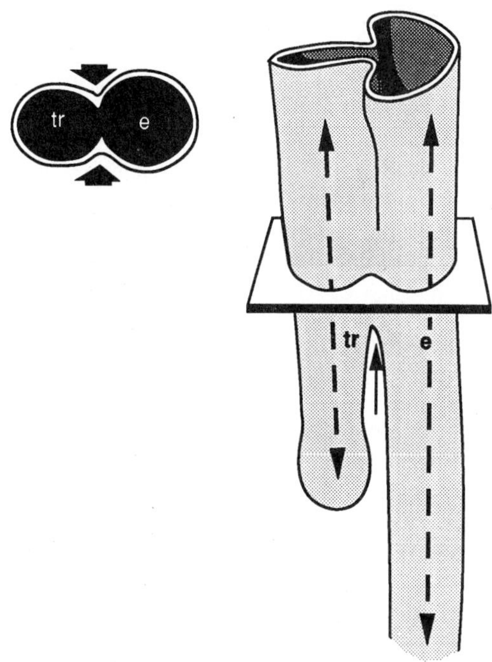


**FIGURE 13–1.** By the fourth fetal week (8-mm-long embryo), the foregut is partitioned into trachea anteriorly and esophagus posteriorly by a transverse septum; the septum also moves cephalad and caudally.

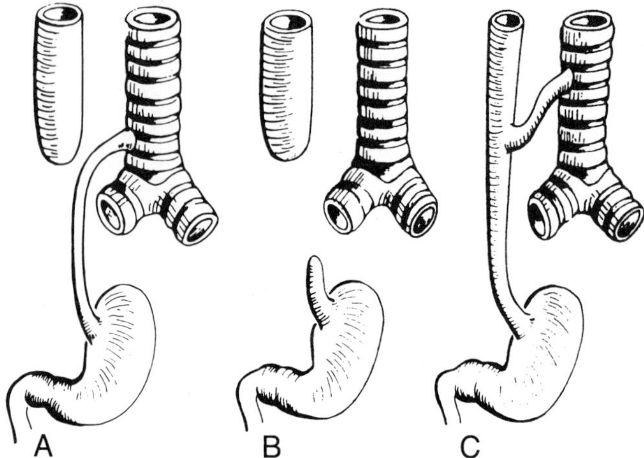


**FIGURE 13–2.** The three most common types of EA and TEF, accounting for 98% of cases. *A,* Proximal atresia and distal TEF (85%). *B,* Pure atresia (10%). *C,* H-TEF (3%).

cardiac defects).[21, 33, 34] Aside from these groups of anomalies, the variety and complexity of abnormalities associated with EA and TEF mean that no specific combination will occur frequently, even in a large sample of patients. However, several syndromes are recognized in which there appears to be a common denominator, including those defects referred to as *VATER,**[35, 36] *VACTERL,*†[37, 38] and *CHARGE.*‡[39, 40] The occurrence of an extracardiac malformation should increase the suspicion that a child who has an EA with TEF also has a cardiac lesion (32%), and this likelihood increases twofold when there are two or more extracardiac abnormalities.[41] As with most common birth defects, the pathogenesis of an EA with or without TEF may be related to both genetic and environmental factors.[42, 43] Most authors[6, 44] have reported normal karyotypes in infants with VATER syndrome.[35] It is likely that this malformation occurs early within the first trimester, when there is organ differentiation and septation (division). This possibility has led others to speculate that the developmental cause of EA and TEF may also affect other organ systems at the same time.[45] The fact that multiple anomalies and low birth weight often coexist suggests that these anomalies cause intrauterine growth retardation.[46] Families with these congenital esophageal defects have been reported.[47, 48]

## CLASSIFICATION

Although there are many varieties and combinations of EA with and without TEF, the three most common are proximal EA and distal TEF (85%), pure EA (10%), and H-TEF (3%; see later discussion); the rest are rare (2%[49–51]; Fig. 13–2). Acquired TEF in the pediatric patient is not common and is usually caused by a foreign body.[52, 53] Early recognition and treatment of the disease and its associated anomalies have greatly improved the survival rate.[27, 54, 55]

*VATER, *v*ertebral defects, imperforate *a*nus, *t*racheo*e*sophageal fistula with esophageal atresia, *r*adial and *r*enal dysplasia.

†VACTERL, *v*ertebral, *a*nal, *c*ardiac, *t*racheal, *e*sophageal, *r*enal, *l*imb.

‡CHARGE, *c*oloboma, *h*eart disease, choanal *a*tresia, *r*etarded growth and development, *g*enital hypoplasia, *e*ar anomalies and deafness.

### Esophageal Atresia with Distal Tracheoesophageal Fistula

Infants with EA and distal TEF (Fig. 13–2*A*) constitute about 85% of the total number of patients with congenital esophageal defects; one half are premature, and one half have other anomalies. The esophageal gap is usually 1 to 2 cm, and the distal TEF most commonly joins the trachea at the carina. Variations can exist in these defects; the atretic gap can be millimeters to inches wide, and the fistula can join higher on the trachea or lower on the right main bronchus.

#### *Diagnosis*

An EA and distal TEF should be diagnosed, as soon as the infant is delivered, by passage of a nasoesophageal radiopaque tube that stops 3 to 4 inches (6.25–10 cm) into the blind upper esophageal pouch (Fig. 13–3)[56]; the tube should be left in place on suction, with hourly instillations of air, and a chest radiograph should be obtained. A tube smaller than 10-Fr will coil in the blind upper pouch and give a false sense of being in the stomach. If nasal obstruction (choanal atresia) exists, the tube can then be passed by

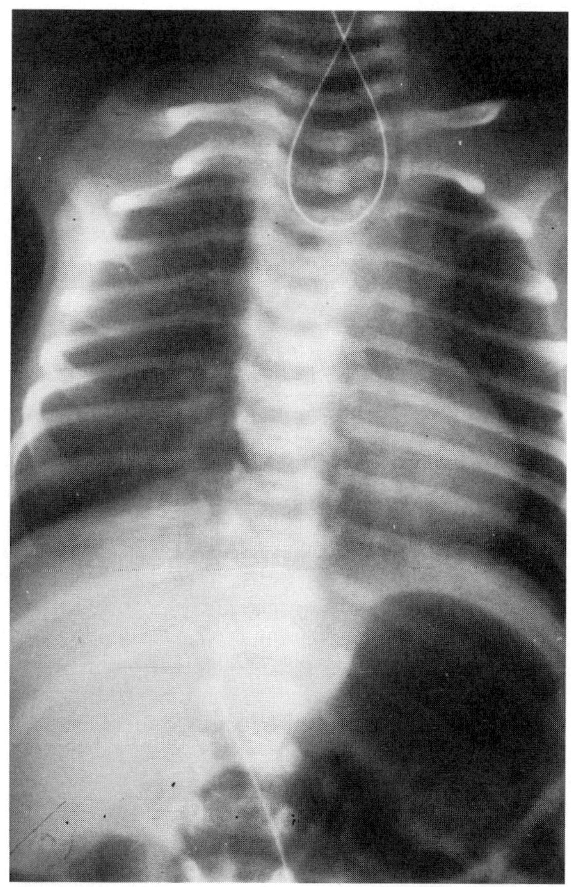

**FIGURE 13–3.** Coiled radiopaque nasogastric tube in blind upper pouch, giving a false impression of being in the stomach. Note the air in the gastrointestinal tract, indicating a distal TEF. Rarely, the TEF is so big that a large amount of air enters the stomach, and preliminary gastrostomy will be necessary to avoid gastric perforation.

mouth. If this simple, easy step is not carried out soon after birth, then the neonate will cough, choke, sputter, or turn blue on its saliva or with the first feeds. The latter situation is not rare but it should never occur. A false passage from the nasoesophageal tube occasionally happens; this possibility is signaled by a difficult tube passage and the presence of bloody mucus in the tube and the oropharyngeal area. A radiopaque water-soluble esophagram is then indicated. The treatment is the same as for an esophageal anastomotic leak.

The chest radiograph also shows the state of the lung fields. The commonest area of lung involvement from aspiration is the right upper lobe, and the prompt treatment of aspiration pneumonia with oxygen and antibiotics and the prevention of reaspiration are indicated. There is rarely any need to put contrast material into the upper pouch.[49, 57] The chest radiograph usually reveals enough of the abdomen to determine whether any gas is present within the gastrointestinal tract, indicating a lower (distal) TEF (see Fig. 13–3). Rarely (in 15% of instances), the distal TEF is obliterated (without a long gap between the EA ends) so that there will be no gas in the bowel below the diaphragm.[58] Vertebral body defects (extra vertebrae or hemivertebrae; Fig. 13–4) and rib anomalies (extra ribs or hypoplastic ribs) raise the suspicion of an EA with TEF. The incidence of these skeletal anomalies can be as high as 45%.[21, 22, 59] Heart size and the side of the descending aorta can be noted on chest radiograph. Cardiovascular abnormalities are diagnosed in 40% of patients by clinical examination, and in 60% by catheterization, autopsy, or both.[41] When the aorta is on the ipsilateral side, the repair of an EA is said to be more difficult; however, this occurrence is so unusual that it is often not even looked for, especially if there is no initial evidence of a congenital heart defect.[60] Dextrocardia usually signals that other congenital anomalies are present.

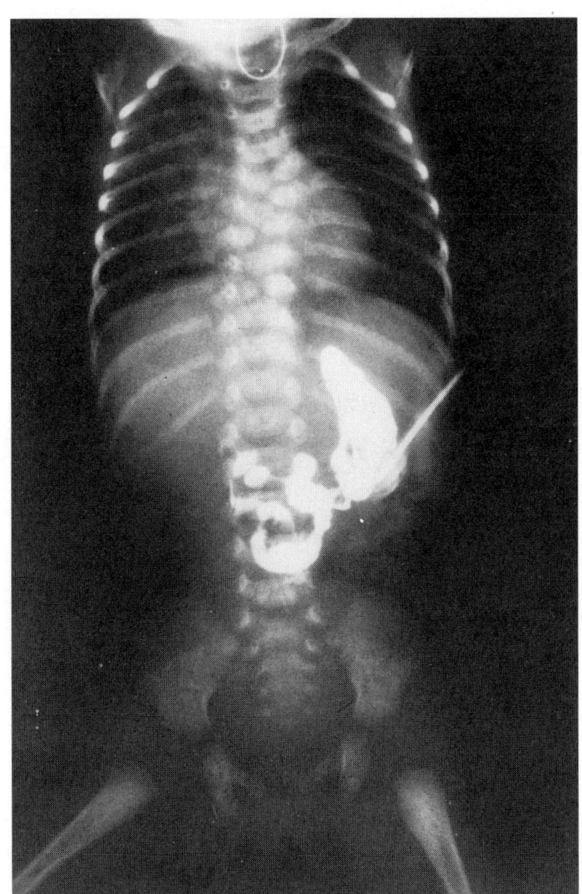

**FIGURE 13–4.** Thoracic vertebral body defects that often accompany the EA and TEF anomaly.

Most major associated defects, except for renal agenesis, require some form of surgical intervention early in the child's life. Surgery may not be indicated for the minor defects; the procedures that are performed are probably minimal and can be scheduled for a later date.[27] The commonest associated congenital anomalies are found in the cardiovascular system and include patent ductus arteriosus, ventricular and atrial defects, tetralogy of Fallot, and coarctation of the aorta. There is no known association between extracardiac malformation and the type of cardiac lesion (if any) that a neonate with EA and TEF may have.[41]

Most gastrointestinal anomalies require fairly urgent surgery and may seriously affect the treatment of EA and TEF.[27] In spite of the frequent coexistence of gastrointestinal lesions with cardiac abnormalities (with the former type often requiring several operations), endocarditis is not a problem[44] with appropriate antibiotic prophylaxis.[27] None of the skeletal defects requires immediate repair; therefore, routine screening of the spine in these neonates is unnecessary.[22, 61] Almost none of the genitourinary abnormalities requires immediate surgical intervention, although early identification is important.

### *Initial Management*

The patient with EA and TEF must always be transported in the upright position to avoid gastroesophageal reflux of the highly acidic gastric juices. Intravenous fluids, electrolytes, and antibiotics are given.[62–64] Intensive care nursing on a one-to-one basis is critical,[65] and the oropharynx is suctioned frequently in spite of a properly functioning nasoesophageal tube in the upper pouch. By the next day, the neonate is usually well enough to be taken to the operating room for the definitive repair. If there is a delay for any reason, no harm will come from the wait as long as the stomach is not overdistended, or no gastroduodenal contents are refluxing into the distal esophagus, through the TEF and into the tracheobronchial tree.

### *Surgical Approach*

The usual anastomotic gap is about 1 to 2 cm, and any gap greater than that size increases the technical difficulty and the associated postoperative morbidity. The anastomosis is usually between an upper esophageal pouch, which is the size of an adult's small finger, and the lower esophagus, which is usually smaller than a lead pencil. There are two types of anastomoses currently done (Fig. 13–5): (1) end-to-end, one layer and two layers,[9] and (2) end-to-side, after the distal TEF is ligated in continuity.[66, 67] The first type is the commonest anastomosis performed by most pediatric surgeons. There are more leaks with a one-layer anastomosis but more strictures with a two-layer anastomosis,[68] and recurrent fistulas are commoner with an end-to-side anastomosis.[69, 70] If a rare (2%) proximal fistula is present

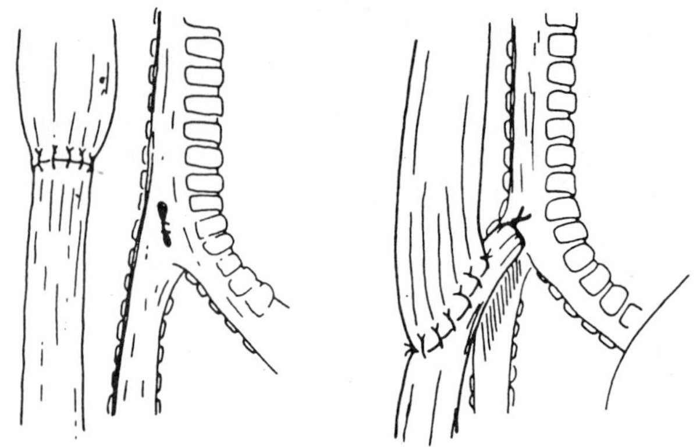

**FIGURE 13–5.** The two types of esophageal anastomoses: end-to-end and end-to-side.

(Fig. 13–6), it will be found (and divided) when the upper pouch is being mobilized.[49, 57]

Although Waterston and coworkers' 1962 classification[71] of the group of EA with the poorest prognosis (birth weight <2,500 g, pneumonia, or other congenital anomalies) has been updated, there are some instances that preclude a primary anastomosis after the TEF has been ligated and divided. These include significant respiratory problems or a number of gross associated anomalies in severely ill premature infants[72, 73]; a thin upper esophageal pouch usually found in the infant with cleft palate who is unable to swallow in utero; and an upper esophageal pouch that barely enters the chest. Corrective methods range from not performing a primary repair (staging)[74] to attempting to elongate the upper esophageal segment or committing the infant to an immediate neck esophagostomy and a later esophageal replacement. Staging does not preclude an anastomosis.[75] The most popular method of elongation is the circular myotomy,[76] which adds about 1 cm of length per myotomy. Other methods of upper and lower pouch elongation other than waiting a few months with repeated swallowing and gastroesophageal reflux are upper pouch bougienage,[77] electromagnetic bougienage,[78] the suture fistula technique,[79, 80] and an esophageal flap esophagoplasty.[81] When the anastomosis is completed, some surgeons place a small trans anastomotic (nasogastric) feeding tube down the repaired esophagus into the stomach.[82] This is done so that if an anastomotic leak occurs, the nasogastric tube can be used for enteral feeding for the 1 or 2 weeks needed for the leak to heal; otherwise, the infant would require a feeding gastrostomy or total parenteral nutrition (TPN).[83] Most often a chest tube is placed because of the thoracotomy and in the event of an anastomotic leak.

### Early Postoperative Management

Weaning from ventilatory support occasionally may be prolonged.[84] Gastrostomy or nasogastric tube feeds can usually be started on the fourth postoperative day if there is no clinical evidence of an anastomotic leak.[85] Any feeds put into the stomach by a gastrostomy or a feeding tube run the risk of refluxing into the repaired esophagus and threatening the integrity of the new anastomosis. Therefore, within the first week after esophageal surgery, only small amounts of

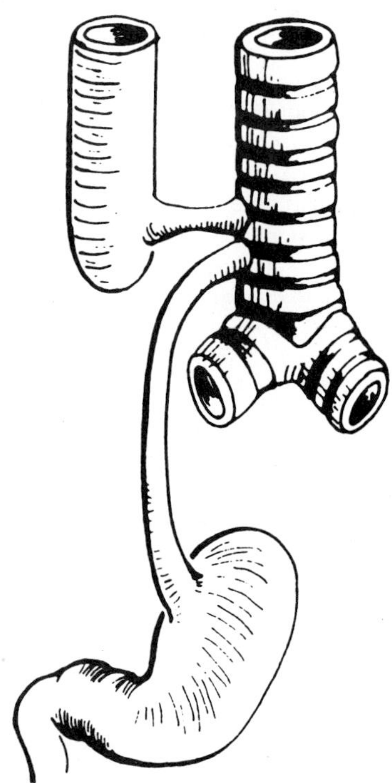

**FIGURE 13–6.** Rare proximal TEFs will be found when the upper pouch is mobilized.

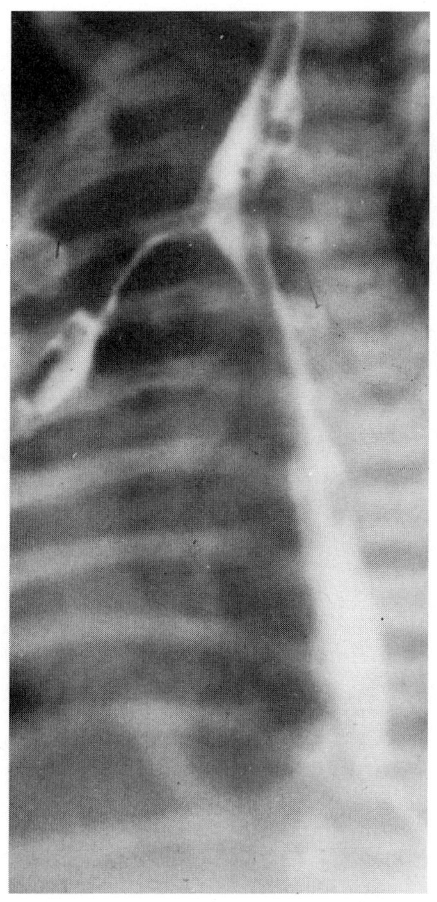

**FIGURE 13–7.** Anastomotic leak (seen on esophagram) usually occurs on the third or fourth postoperative day.

feeds should be given slowly and in hourly drips. If no complications develop during the first postoperative week, a water-soluble radiopaque contrast esophagram is obtained; if there is no leak, all tubes are removed, and the infant is started on oral feeds. About 50% of the infants with a repaired EA do quite well and go home feeding normally within a few weeks after surgery.[72]

The major worry about the neonatal esophageal anastomosis is a leak (Fig. 13–7). At least 50% of these EA anastomoses leak to some degree; the clinical manifestations depend on the size of the leak. Most leaks are asymptomatic and only seen on the esophagram. The typical symptomatic anastomotic leak presents on the third or fourth postoperative day with some respiratory distress in an infant who becomes tachypneic, cyanotic, and septic; the chest radiograph typically shows a right pyopneumothorax. Ventilation may be necessary if the infant is seriously ill. Antibiotics and possibly another chest tube are required. The leak should be reassessed with an esophagram weekly until it heals, which will occur in several weeks. Nutrition can be maintained by tube feeds (provided that they do not reflux into the esophagus and out the anastomotic leak) or even TPN. Once the leak has closed, as determined both clinically and radiologically, the infant can be fed by mouth.

Many EA anastomotic leaks produce strictures,[68] and 30% to 40% of these strictures are symptomatic with coughing, regurgitation, aspiration, and failure to gain weight (Fig. 13–8). The stricture may progress remarkably before the infant (on a fluid diet) becomes symptomatic. The diagnosis is confirmed by esophagram or esophagoscopy, or both. Most strictures will respond to one or more dilatations[69, 86, 87]; however, these dilatations should not begin until 3 or 4 weeks after the anastomosis. If the stricture fails to respond to dilatations, or if the response is transient, the presence of gastroesophageal reflux must be ruled out.[88, 89] If the latter problem is not corrected, little permanent response to dilatations can be expected. Abnormal distal esophageal motility is evident on fluoroscopic examination of the repaired esophagus.[90, 91] It is unusual that dilatations are required in patients older than 1 or 2 years of age. It is rare to have to resect a persistent strictured EA anastomosis. In rare instances, a long-term temporary esophageal stent may be required (Fig. 13–9).[92, 93]

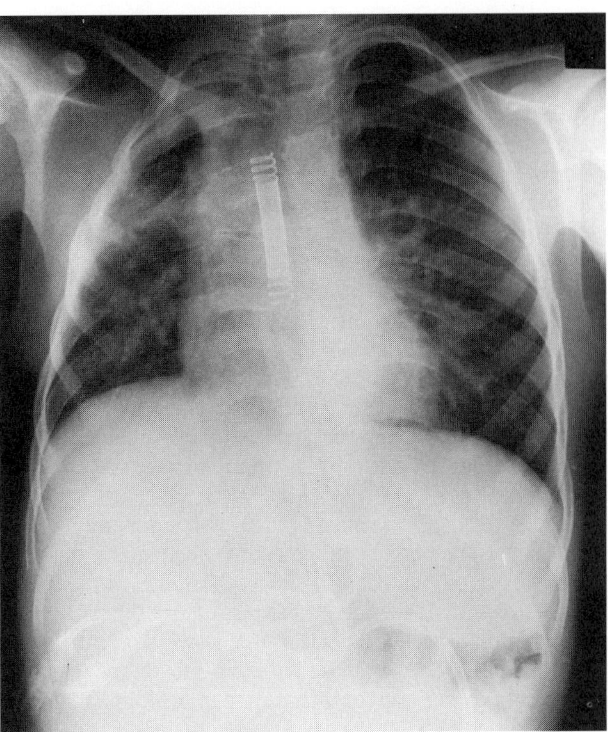

**FIGURE 13–9.** Five-year-old child with repaired pure EA (six thoracotomies and three antireflux procedures) with persistent anastomotic stricture. The stent is employed on a long-term temporary basis.

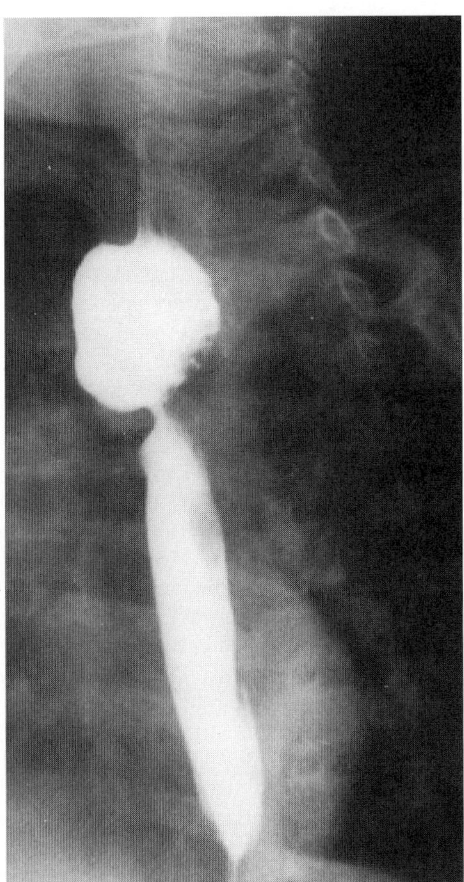

**FIGURE 13–8.** Symptomatic anastomotic stricture that occurs in 30% to 40% of EA repairs. Most strictures require and respond to several dilatations.

## *Late Postoperative Management*

For the first 3 months after surgical correction of an EA and distal TEF in an infant, there are usually no problems with swallowing because the newly joined esophagus does not have to handle more than fluids. Thereafter, the parents must slowly advance both the quantity and the quality of foods given until the anastomosis has matured and reached its maximum width and until the child can understand that he or she will always have to chew food well, eat slowly, and drink frequently during the meal. When baby foods are added, some dysphagia may become evident, and this warrants immediate investigation. A routine chest radiograph will show whether pneumonia is present, and a contrast study of the esophagus and stomach will detect any upper gastrointestinal tract disorder. The best method to demonstrate a recurrent TEF (10%) or a missed H-TEF (Fig. 13–10) is a tube esophagram.[94] After the search for the fistula, the infant should be given some contrast solution to swallow to reveal the presence of aspiration due to muscular incoordination (pharyngoesophageal dyskinesia) or fatigue, tracheomalacia, anastomotic stricture, gastroesophageal reflux, or pyloric stenosis.[95, 96] Gastroesophageal reflux is a significant problem in infants after EA and TEF surgical repair. Twenty percent of these patients will have severe enough anastomotic, respiratory, or gastrointestinal disturbances to require antireflux surgery.[97, 98] Even then, recurrent reflux may be a problem owing to the abnormal distal esophageal swallowing mechanism, short esophagus, or the surgeon's fear of wrapping the lower esophagus too tightly.[96, 99–101]

There is well-documented evidence that squamous metaplasia[102] and tracheomalacia[103] due to inadequately formed and missing cartilage occur in the tracheal area of the TEF.[104] Because of squamous metaplasia, respiratory ciliated columnar epithelium needed to clear the airway of mucus and secretions is absent in the TEF, leading to frequent respiratory infections during the first few years of life.[105, 106] The more easily collapsible trachea (tracheomalacia) adds to this problem and also accounts for the brassy, ducklike cough in these infants that is exacerbated by upper respiratory tract infections, especially during their early years. It is estimated that 25% to 50% of infants with EA and TEF will have tracheomalacia; 10%[107] of these infants (weeks or months after their repair) will have definite sudden respiratory symptoms ("dying spells") always associated with feeds. The cause of these arrests is said to be an obstructed or flattened trachea between the innominate artery and aortic arch anteriorly and the distended upper esophageal pouch posteriorly during feeds (Fig. 13–11). The telltale radiograph sign is a narrow upper trachea just below the clavicles seen on a lateral chest radiograph (see Fig. 13–11). At bronchoscopy, the trachea is narrowed anteroposteriorly to a slitlike aperture that may completely obliterate with coughing, straining, or eating. Tracheostomy will keep the trachea open, but suspension of the innominate artery and aortic arch to the back of the sternum is easier and more successful, with no long-term side effects.[108–110] However, since the mid 1990s, long-term temporary airway stents have been used with satisfactory results (Fig. 13–12).[111–113]

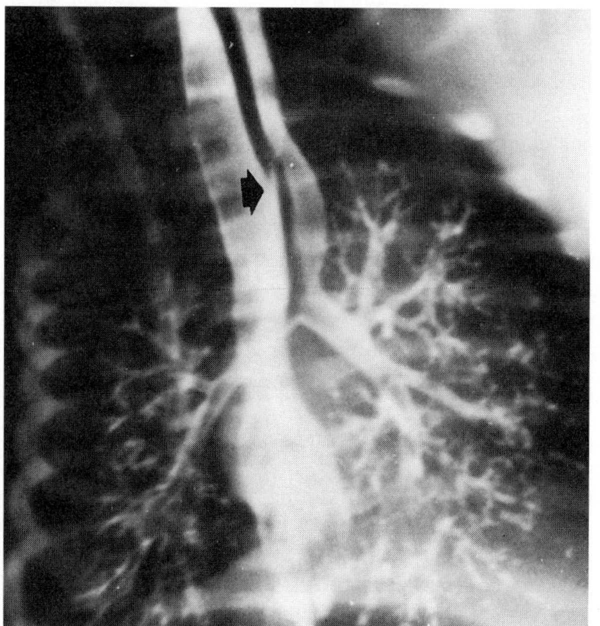

**FIGURE 13–10.** H-TEF *(arrow)* is best demonstrated by a prone pull-back esophagram using water-soluble radiopaque contrast solution. Note that the fistula is located just below the clavicles and runs upward from the esophagus to the trachea. A recurrent TEF is always seen at the anastomotic level.

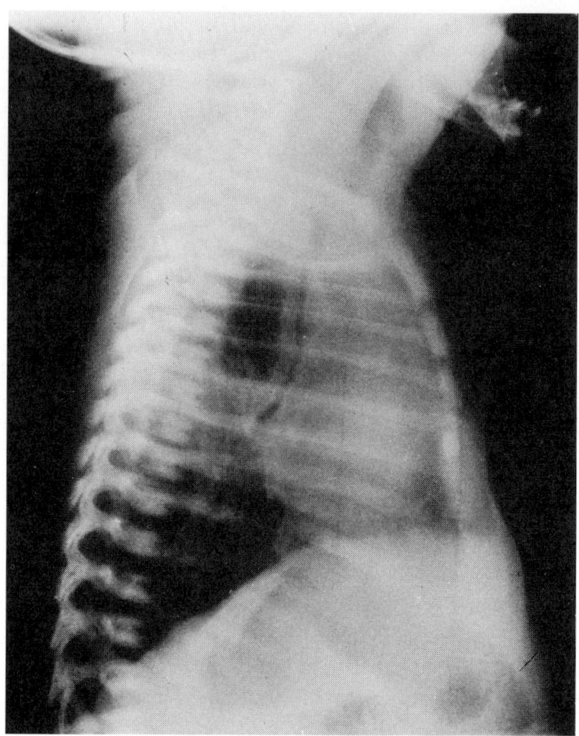

**FIGURE 13–11.** Tracheomalacia becomes symptomatic when the trachea is flattened between the aortic arch anteriorly and the distended proximal esophagus posteriorly (usually during feeds). If it is severe, suspending the aortic arch to the back of the sternum or placing a tracheal stent provides immediate relief.

It may require several years before some of these children can consume a normal unrestricted diet. During the toddler years, impacted foreign bodies (especially lumps of food) are frequently seen, because this is an age group in which food is often not well chewed; even a minor narrowing associated with a poorly coordinated distal esophagus will result in an impaction at the anastomosis.[91]

Skeletal deformities (thoracic flattening and protrusion [Fig. 13–13], shoulder elevation, and scoliosis) are abnormalities that originate with the thoracotomy incision and any postoperative problems within the pleural cavity; however, they are not obvious until the child is into the toddler age range and older. Their incidence may range from about 5% to as high as 50%. Appropriate orthopedic management is required.[114, 115]

### Prognosis

In the past, much prognostic emphasis was placed on the weight of the neonate with EA and TEF; Waterston[71] and

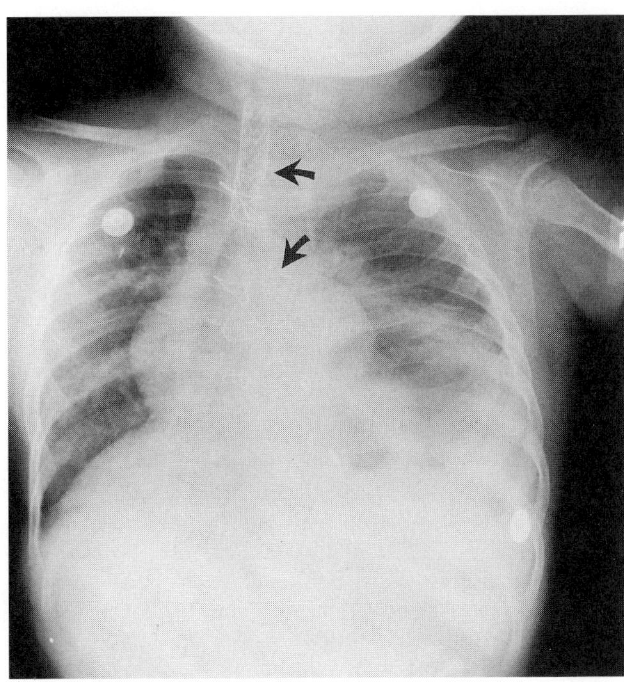

**FIGURE 13–12.** Infant with severe tracheobronchomalacia with tracheal and left bronchial stents *(arrows).*

others[46, 54, 55, 68] believed that low birth weight alone (<2,500 g) lowered the survival rate significantly. This correlation continues to exist,[27] but it is not nearly as strong as earlier. The consensus is that the surgeon should proceed with a primary anastomosis regardless of the patient's weight unless there are other complications.[116–118] The lungs are the determining factor. Staging is now reserved for mitigating circumstances such as severe lung disease (respiratory distress syndrome, pneumonia) and other severe congenital anomalies.[54, 55]

About half the infants with an EA and distal TEF have no other anomalies, and they survive.[119–123] However, the problems begin when other anomalies are added in the other 50% of neonates with EA and TEF.[54, 55, 119] The survival rates decrease proportionately with the presence of additional defects: 75% survival with one additional anomaly, and 60% survival with more than one.[27] Prematurity coincides with an increase in the number of associated anomalies. The cardiovascular defects seem to be the most important in affecting the survival of these babies.[124, 125]

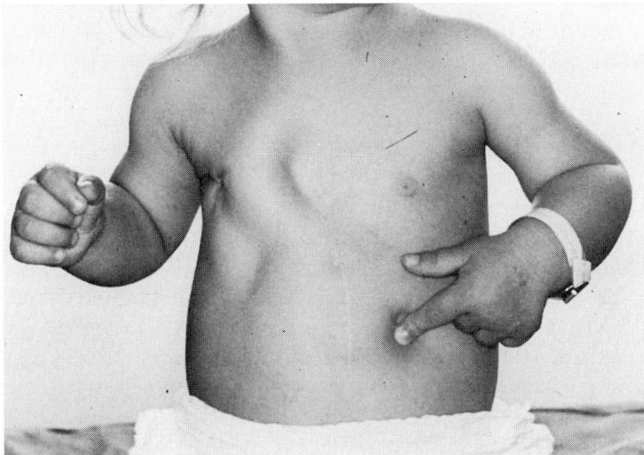

**FIGURE 13–13.** Thoracic flattening and protrusion that originate occasionally from the neonatal right thoracotomy incision to repair the EA and TEF.

## Pure Esophageal Atresia

Pure EA (see Fig. 13–2*B*) is much less common than the previously discussed EA with distal TEF. Forty percent of the patients are premature, and 50% have other anomalies.[126] Infants with this esophageal defect have their own set of problems, not so much with the immediate neonatal course but with surgical attempts to bridge the usual wide gap between esophageal ends, significantly wider than in infants with an EA and distal TEF.[123]

The presentation of an infant with pure EA is usually not much different from that of an infant with both an EA and a distal TEF, so that the diagnosis should be made immediately after delivery when a nasogastric tube will not pass into the stomach. The same risk of a false passage made by the tube exists (as in the infant with EA and TEF).[127] The major difference in these infants, however, is that the threat of reflux aspiration of gastric acid into the distal esophagus and into the respiratory tract is nonexistent (because there is no TEF); the only concern is aspiration of saliva into the airway. The lack of a distal TEF can be diagnosed radiologically by noting the absence of gas within the gastrointestinal tract in the abdomen (Fig. 13–14); this is not a foolproof method, because about 15% of such atresias have an obliterated distal TEF without a long gap between the EA ends.[58] The lack of gastrointestinal air prohibits the demonstration of other distal intestinal atresias (e.g., duodenal atresia).

Although fewer neonates with pure EA are premature than in the group with a proximal EA and distal TEF, at least half have other anomalies in the same systems as the infants with EA and TEF; one difference is that 20% have Down syndrome.[126, 128] There are fewer cardiac anomalies than in the EA and TEF group but more gastrointestinal and skeletal defects.

There is no urgency to perform the esophageal reconstruction, which is seldom feasible in the newborn, since the two blind esophageal ends are many centimeters apart initially. Therefore, the immediate focus of surgical attention (after the initial evaluation and stabilization) is on the feeding gastrostomy. There is an increased chance of associated duodenal atresia[129]; the surgeon must check for this anomaly when making the gastrostomy by injecting some fluid into the stomach and watching it enter the jejunum past the ligament of Treitz. All of the above can be more easily accomplished via the percutaneous route in the hands of a skilled interventional radiologist.[130] Feeds through the new gastrostomy in the infant with pure EA can be started in a few days, with small hourly amounts dripped slowly into the stomach rather than larger bolus feeds pushed in rapidly. After a few weeks, the feeds can be safely increased in volume and spaced over 3 or 4 hours to stretch the stomach and to allow reflux into the lower esophageal segment to distend it.

The blind upper pouch must remain on constant suction.

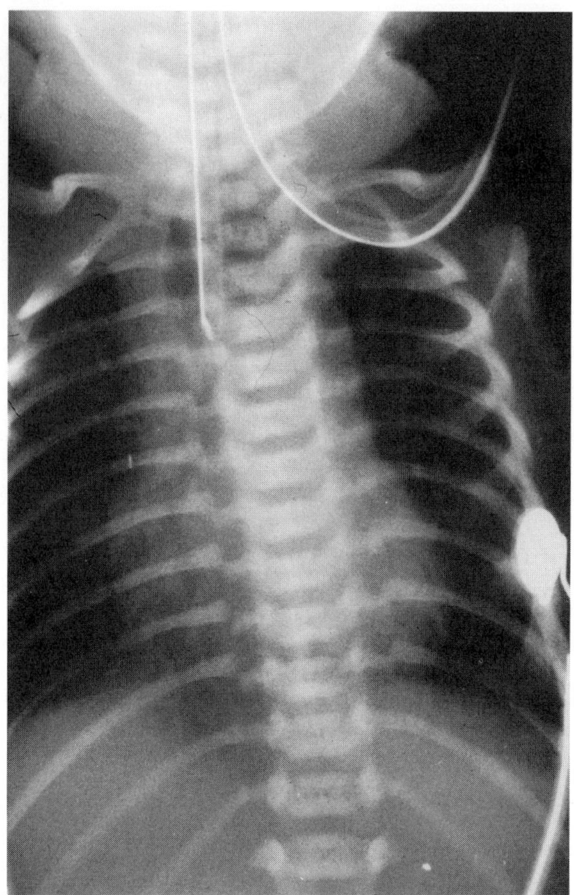

**FIGURE 13–14.** Pure EA. The lack of a distal TEF can be identified radiologically by noting the absence of gas within the gastrointestinal tract.

Ten to 20 mL of saliva (with its high salt content) is removed every 8 hours and should be returned to the infant in the form of normal saline and potassium to avoid salt depletion and hypokalemia. At monthly intervals, the two esophageal pouches are assessed radiologically to see how close they are. If the gap is 3 cm or less (three vertebral bodies), a primary repair is possible with the same technical aids used for bridging a wide gap for the infant with EA and distal TEF. Seventy-five percent of pure esophageal atresias can be primarily repaired if one waits for 3 months and/or for the baby's weight to double.[100] The principle is the same as that with the common EA defect: the child's own esophagus (no matter what has to be safely done to bring it together) is infinitely better than any replacement that can be constructed.[131–133]

The immediate postoperative concerns for the infant with pure EA are related to the anastomosis (as with the EA and TEF group), except that there are no TEF problems; the anastomotic problems, however, are more significant because the tension and pull, between the two esophageal pouches is greater in the pure EA group. After the repair has healed, there is the same dysfunction observed on radiograph of the lower esophageal segment.[90, 126] If dysphagia develops after a few months, investigations must be undertaken to rule out the same problems outlined for the EA with distal TEF group, except for a recurrent TEF. In spite of the unaffected trachea, tracheomalacia may still occur. Gastroesophageal reflux is a significant problem in infants with pure EA, possibly because of the greater pull upward on the lower esophageal pouch (including mobilization of the stomach).[128] It is estimated that as many as one third of these infants will require antireflux surgery within 3 months of their primary anastomosis, with a 30% recurrence rate.[100, 134]

## Esophageal Replacement

If the gap between the two esophageal pouches is wider than 3 or 4 cm, the esophagus cannot be united for a primary anastomosis, and the infant will require an esophageal replacement.[135, 136] At a weight of 6 kg (15 lb), the time, age, and size are appropriate for the construction of a conduit to connect the two esophageal pouches.[137] Options include colon,[138–141] gastric tube replacement,[142–145] gastric transposition (pull-up),[128, 146–150] elongation of the lesser gastric curvature,[151] jejunal free graft,[152–154] and other ingenious techniques.[155] Regardless of which procedure is used, the staged procedure and the neck anastomosis are safer for obvious reasons. All of these operative techniques require the suspension of oral feeds for at least 1 week, and they require gastrostomy, gastrojejunostomy, or jejunostomy tube feeds until the anastomoses heal; the alternative is TPN.

The survival rate in infants with pure EA parallels the rate in the EA and TEF group in that associated anomalies and prematurity tend to lower survival, but, as medical and nursing expertise improves, so do the results. Prior to the 1970s, the survival rate was as low as 40%,[126] but in the 1990s this rate has more than doubled.[100] Colon and gastric tube replacements have been performed for at least 30 years, and both have stood the test of time.[138, 143, 147, 156] Most of the serious complications occur within 3 years after surgery. Almost all the children with no other significant anomalies are within two standard deviations of the mean in height and weight. Sixty to 70% are without symptoms; the others have only minor complaints (dysphagia with lumpy foods, nightly regurgitation, or thoracic skeletal deformity). All of the children are satisfied with their new esophagus. The newer gastric interposition (pull-up) procedure has a similar spectrum of early and late complications. All three replacements have a mortality rate of less than 10%, with long-term overall results of 70% very good, 25% good, and 5% fair to poor.[138, 143, 147, 156]

## H-Tracheoesophageal Fistula

H-TEF (see Fig. 13–2*C*) is the third most common type of all the congenital esophageal problems and yet has an incidence of only about 3% to 5%. It has also been referred to as an *N-fistula.*[157, 158] The infants with this anomaly are usually of normal size and seldom have other anomalies.

It is unusual to make this diagnosis before several weeks of life or even months have passed, during which time there have been repeated episodes of pneumonia. The esophagus and trachea are quite normal, except that there is a short fistula between the two (an "H") that runs from the esophagus upward to the trachea. Because of this upward course (an "N"), not every swallow is aspirated into the trachea.

These neonates often cough, choke, sputter, and turn blue with fluids more than they do with solids. In a similar fashion, air gets into the gastrointestinal tract, and these infants tend to have a gas-filled and bloated abdomen. The most important aspects of establishing the diagnosis are to remember that this type of fistula can and does exist and to exclude the presence of the defect in any infant with chronic chest problems. The diagnosis must be made by esophagram using water-soluble radiopaque contrast material, cinefluorography, and the same technique as that for a recurrent TEF[159] (see Fig. 13–10). More than one such study may be necessary to identify the H-fistula, which is usually singular and located just below the level of the clavicles. Endoscopic examination is another option to identify the H-TEF from within using dye or a ureteral catheter[160]; this method is not as popular as the radiologic technique.[6, 157] Once the diagnosis has been made, the emergency is over; antibiotics will clear up the chest infection, and the feeds can be delivered by nasogastric tube prior to division of the fistula(s).

The operative repair of an H-TEF must not be undertaken based only on suspicion; there must be absolute confirmation that the fistula is indeed present. It is most often corrected by a cervical (neck) operation; the much rarer lower H-TEF requires the usual right third or fourth intercostal space thoracotomy. Regardless of the surgical approach, the operative technique is the same for any H-TEF (and recurrent TEF)[161]: isolation, division, and closure of the side hole in both the trachea and the esophagus. The two resultant suture lines must not be left touching or else a recurrent TEF may develop between them.[6, 157] An easier and equally successful method of closing an H-TEF and/or a recurrent TEF has been with glue using the talents of a skilled pediatric endoscopist and/or interventional radiologist.[162–164]

The postoperative course is related initially to the trachea and how much trauma it suffered during the fistula repair. Hopefully, the recurrent laryngeal nerves are not affected, but in some of these infants there is still the necessity for postoperative intubation with or without ventilation for a few days. The same method of tube feedings that was used preoperatively is continued. At 1 week after surgery, a repeat esophagram is carried out, and if all the sites are well healed, the feeding tube is removed and the infant is bottle-fed. The occurrence of leaks and recurrent fistulas is unusual. A number of these infants exhibit a temporary form of pharyngoesophageal dyskinesia with bouts of aspiration pneumonia, this time over the top rather than through the fistula.[126]

## Rare Variants of Tracheoesophageal Fistula

Rare forms of TEF (Fig. 13–15) constitute no more than 2% of all the EA and TEFs.[49, 57, 165] The major problem is that most are not recognized early. They may be associated with an EA and, if so, may be from the blind upper esophageal pouch, the blind lower esophageal pouch, or both. Because there is frequently a gasless abdomen on radiograph, one may not expect that one or both of the blind esophageal segments have a TEF. Therefore, a gasless abdomen on radiograph does not necessarily exclude a proximal esophageal pouch TEF because this fistula may be obliterated (20%),[49] just as the distal TEF can be (15%).[58] Infants

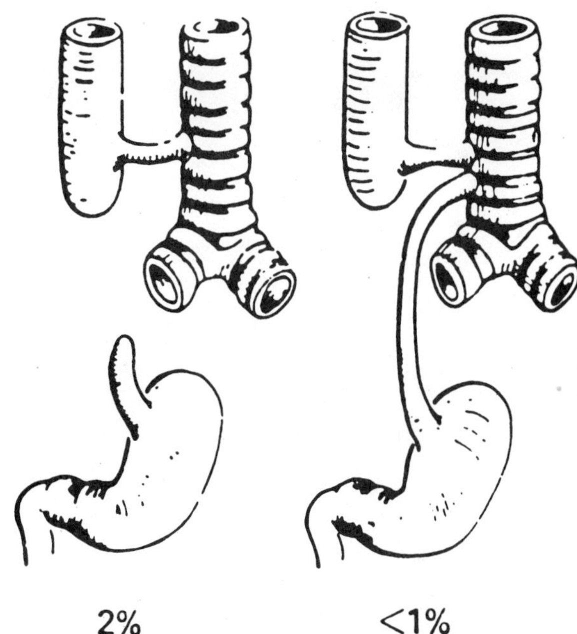


**FIGURE 13–15.** The major problem with the rare TEFs is that they are not recognized early. They may or may not be associated with an EA and may be single or multiple.

with this disorder have the same collection of anomalies involving other systems. Their presenting symptoms are both from the EA and, more severely (60%),[49] from tracheobronchial soiling through the fistula(s). For obvious reasons, most of the upper pouch fistulas may be overlooked during the work-up.[166, 167]

If there is no clinical or radiologic evidence of a TEF, the surgical approach for the rare EA types should be the same as that for a pure EA (i.e., gastrostomy first). When the TEFs become clinically evident, radiologic proof can then be obtained, and the appropriate surgical closure of the TEF accomplished through the neck or pleural cavity, or both. The use of endoscopic glue may also be considered (see previous discussion). The postoperative course, complications, and results are similar to the other types of EA and TEF.

*Congenital esophagopulmonary fistulas* are unusual in that many (24%) are not discovered until adult life,[168] when most of the patients have chronic irreversible pulmonary disease (Fig. 13–16). The same association with other congenital anomalies is seen as in the more common EA with TEF group. The right bronchial tree is involved more than twice as often as the left (as in other types of bronchopulmonary anomalies). Patient age at diagnosis is older than that of TEFs, probably because the esophagopulmonary fistulas are smaller and more localized to smaller segments of the lung. The fistulous tract is lined by stratified squamous epithelium and becomes junctional with respiratory epithelium when it reaches the respiratory tract. Mucous glands, smooth muscle, and rudimentary tracheal rings all have been found in the fistulous tract. In 1954, the first esophagocystic pulmonary fistula was identified[168]; it is a rare variant of an esophagopulmonary fistula. In some instances numerous cysts are present throughout the lung, some of which are connected with bronchi; the cysts are lined by ciliated pseudostratified co-

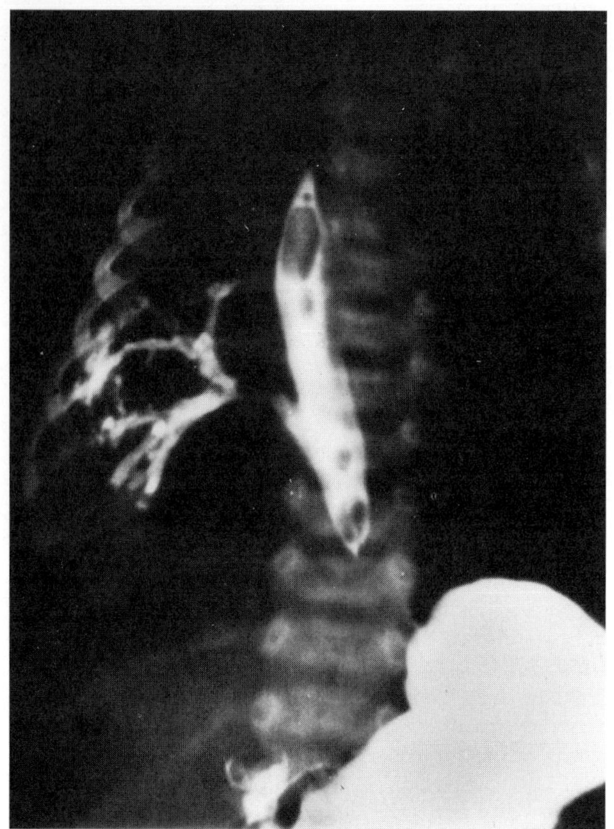

**FIGURE 13–16.** Congenital esophagopulmonary fistula is usually right-sided. Occasionally, the communication resembles a bronchus and leads to a lobar sequestration.

lumnar epithelium. This entity is similar to the "ciliated epithelial cyst of the esophagus" that arises via a fistula from the lower esophagus also on the right side. In a few cases of aberrant lower lobes (extralobar and intralobar sequestration), there is a communication with the esophagus; occasionally, this communication is similar to a bronchus.[169] It has been proposed that "extralobar pulmonary sequestrations are derived from independent evaginations of cells with respiratory potential displaced on the esophagus."[170] Investigations must include radiology (the esophagram is positive in at least two thirds of cases)[171] and endoscopy. The surgical approach involves dividing the fistula and resecting the diseased lung; results are quite successful.

A *laryngotracheoesophageal cleft* is another rare variant of EA and TEF, except that the TEF runs more or less from the larynx all the way down to the carina.[172, 173] Three types are currently described: type 1, a laryngeal cleft; type 2, a partial cleft of the esophagus and the trachea; and type 3, a complete cleft from the larynx to the carina.[174] Richter first described this defect in 1792, but no further reports appeared in the literature until 1949.[6, 175] The first successful repair of a type 1 defect was in 1955.[174] The original foregut somehow fails to separate into two separate tubes by the fourth week, and it ends up as trachea in the anterior half and as esophagus in the posterior segment. It has been suggested that this cleft results from an arrest of the cephalad development of the tracheoesophageal septum.[176] Interruption of the septum formation extends the cleft upward into the larynx.[177] Twenty percent of infants with a laryngotracheoesophageal cleft also have an associated EA and TEF.[172]

The clinical symptoms depend on the size of the cleft; they usually occur shortly after birth without feeds and include weak cry, coughing, choking, cyanosis, aspiration, pneumonia, apnea, and respiratory distress. Emergency intubation may be necessary.

Establishing the diagnosis is not always easy—the key is a high degree of suspicion. Swallow of water-soluble radiopaque contrast material shows an immediate massive aspiration from the pharyngoesophageal area into the trachea, so that the cleft cannot be seen easily.[178, 179] Even direct laryngoscopy and bronchoscopy may look normal until it is recognized that the bronchoscope or endotracheal tube can slip backward into the esophagus quite easily, creating an immediate moment of inadequate ventilation.[180]

Gastrostomy is necessary early in the treatment plan. Operative repair is not easy, nor is it often successful. All these infants end up intubated or with a tracheostomy, or both, usually for a long time. Recurrent TEFs are common; the repair effort is prolonged; and the results are fair. The first survivor of a complete laryngotracheoesophageal cleft (type 3) repair was reported only in 1984.[181]

## Esophageal Stenosis and Web (Diaphragm)

Esophageal stenosis and web (diaphragm), variants of EA, are even rarer than those described in the previous section, occurring in 1:25,000 to 50,000 live births.[182] They were originally thought to be acquired inflammatory lesions due to gastroesophageal reflux[6] but have since been reclassified as true congenital lesions. There are different varieties of stenoses, including web (diaphragm) and fibromuscular stenosis.[182–185] Tracheobronchial remnants in the wall of the esophagus were first reported in 1936.[186, 187] After the tracheoesophageal septum forms, and both the esophagus and the tracheobronchial tree elongate, mesenchymal cells of the respiratory diverticulum become embedded in the esophageal wall in the form of respiratory epithelium, glands, and cartilage (Fig. 13–17). This ectopic focus can cause a stenosis that does not stretch. The development of an esophageal web (diaphragm) is similar to other gastrointestinal webs; it is a failure of the temporarily solid 10-week intestine to recanalize. The web may be associated with EA[186] or TEF,[188] or both (Fig. 13–18). Fibromuscular stenosis has been compared with pyloric stenosis in that the lower esophagus (with[189, 190] or without[191–193] an accompanying EA, TEF, or both) has a localized segmental hypertrophy. Whether it is caused by a remnant of a perforated membrane (web) or a failure of the lumen to recanalize after being a temporary solid core is open to speculation. Microscopically, both the web and the segmental area have similar mucosal and submucosal components. Whereas the more common types of EA and TEF are associated with other anomalies in 50% of patients, this group has less than half of that association (imperforate anus or Down syndrome).[183, 186] The stenoses become apparent in infancy when the feeds are advanced to more solid components, and the resulting dysphagia leads to vomiting, failure to thrive, and aspiration. Esophageal webs (membranes) and their variations all present in neonates with

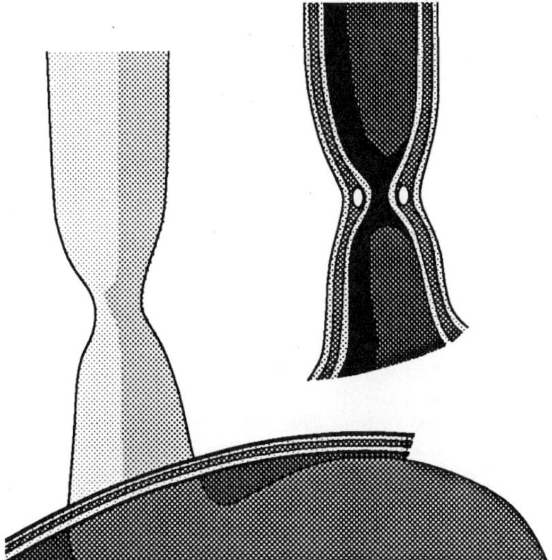

**FIGURE 13–17.** Most esophageal stenoses occur in the lower esophagus. Some stenoses may have an ectopic focus of respiratory tissue in the esophageal wall.

symptoms and signs of EA.[186, 194, 195] All three of these pathologic entities require prompt radiologic or endoscopic evaluation, or both (Fig. 13–19). Gastroesophageal reflux for any reason (duodenal obstruction or malrotation) can be ruled out as a cause of this type of lesion by an upper gastrointestinal radiopaque contrast study. The exact location of the defect within the esophagus should be identified—most of the tracheobronchial remnant stenoses are in the distal part of the esophagus, whereas the webs (diaphragms) are in the middle. Endoscopy shows that the stenosis (due to tracheobronchial remnants) is more irregular and much firmer than the fibromuscular type[124]; the web (diaphragm) has a typical shelflike appearance. Repair of the

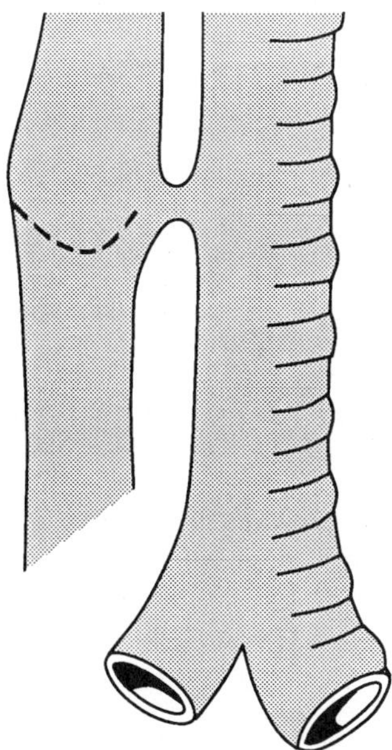

**FIGURE 13–18.** Most esophageal webs (diaphragms) are found in the mid-esophagus. They may or may not be associated with an EA or a TEF, or both.

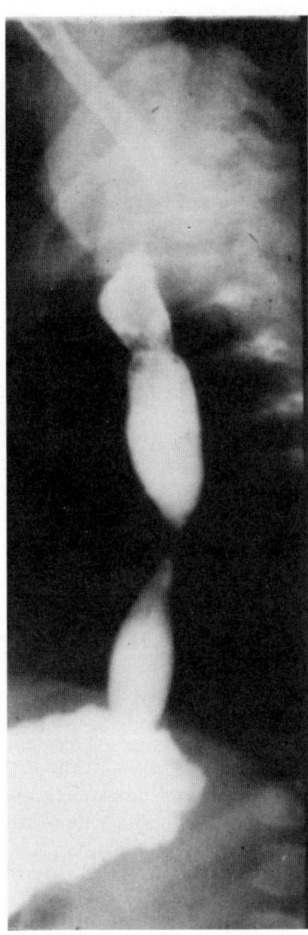

**FIGURE 13–19.** Lower esophageal congenital stenosis in an infant with a repaired EA and TEF. Gastroesophageal reflux has been ruled out.

tracheobronchial remnant stenosis is best accomplished by thoracotomy and esophageal resection, since these stiff remnants make dilatation of the esophagus difficult and dangerous. The web (diaphragm) may be successfully treated by skilled endoscopy[196] or by resection; the softer, more pliable fibromuscular stenosis can usually be successfully dilated. If esophageal resection is required for a low stenosis, and if it can be done through the abdomen, consideration should be given to an antireflux procedure to avoid iatrogenic gastroesophageal reflux.[183] The results of treatment are good.

## REFERENCES


1. Ashcraft KW, Holder TM: The story of esophageal atresia and tracheoesophageal fistula. Surgery 1969;65:332–340.
2. Myers NA: Evolution of the management of oesophageal atresia from 1948–1988. Pediatr Surg Int 1991;6:407–411.
3. Myers NA: The early history of esophageal atresia and tracheoesophageal fistula. In Beasley SW, Myers NA, Auldist AW (eds): Oesophageal Atresia. London, Chapman & Hall, 1991, pp 1–16.
4. Myers NA: The history of esophageal surgery: pediatric aspects. Pediatr Surg Int 1997;12:101–107.
5. Spitz L: Esophageal atresia: past, present, and future. J Pediatr Surg 1996;31:19–25.
6. Randolph JG: Esophageal atresia and congenital stenosis. In Welch KJ, Randolph JG, Ravitch MM, et al (eds): Pediatric Surgery. Chicago, Year Book Medical, 1986, pp 682–697.
7. Vogt EC: Congenital esophageal atresia. Am J Roentgenol 1929; 22:463–465.

8. Gross RE: The Surgery of Infancy and Childhood. Philadelphia, WB Saunders, 1953, pp 75–102.
9. Haight C, Towsley HA: Congenital atresia of the esophagus with tracheoesophageal fistula: extrapleural ligation of fistula and end-to-end anastomosis of esophageal segments. Surg Gynecol Obstet 1943;76:672–688.
10. Lanman TH: Congenital atresia of the esophagus: a study of 32 cases. Arch Surg 1940;41:1060–1083.
11. Leven NL: Congenital atresia of the esophagus with tracheoesophageal fistula: report of successful extrapleural ligation of fistulous communication and cervical esophagostomy. J Thorac Surg 1941;10:648–657.
12. Ladd WE: The surgical treatment of esophageal atresia and tracheoesophageal fistulas. N Engl J Med 1944;230:625–637.
13. Haight C: Some observations on esophageal atresias and tracheoesophageal fistulas of congenital origin. J Thorac Surg 1959;34:141–172.
14. Myers NA: Oesophageal atresia with distal tracheoesophageal fistulas: a long-term follow-up. Prog Pediatr Surg 1977;10:5–18.
15. Sulamaa M, Gripenberg L, Alvenainen EK: Prognosis and treatment of congenital atresia of the esophagus. Acta Chir Scand 1951;102:141–157.
16. Gray SW, Skandalakis JE: Embryology for Surgeons. Philadelphia, WB Saunders, 1972, pp 63–100.
17. Beasley SW: Embryology. In Beasley SW, Myers NA, Auldist AW (eds): Oesophageal Atresia. London, Chapman & Hall, 1991, pp 31–43.
18. Amoury RA: Structure and function of the esophagus in infancy and early childhood. In Ashcraft KW, Holder TM (eds): Pediatric Esophageal Surgery. Orlando, Grune & Stratton, 1986, pp 1–28.
19. Sankaran K, Bhagirath CP, Bingham WT, et al: Tracheal atresia, proximal esophageal atresia, and distal tracheoesophageal fistula: report of two cases and review of the literature. Pediatrics 1983;71:821–823.
20. Peison B, Levitsky E, Sprowls JJ: Tracheoesophageal fistula associated with tracheal atresia and malformation of the larynx. J Pediatr Surg 1970;5:464–467.
21. Bond-Taylor W, Starer F, Atwell JD: Vertebral anomalies associated with esophageal atresia and tracheoesophageal fistula with reference to the initial operative mortality. J Pediatr Surg 1973;8:9–13.
22. Dickens DRV, Myers NA: Oesophageal atresia and vertebral anomalies. Pediatr Surg Int 1987;2:278–281.
23. Scott JS, Wilson JK: Hydramnios as an early sign of esophageal atresia. Lancet 1957;2:569–572.
24. Myers NA, Beasley SW, Auldist AW: Oesophageal atresia and associated anomalies: a plea for uniform documentation. Pediatr Surg Int 1992;2:97–100.
25. Myers NA, Beasley SW, Auldist AW: Associated anomalies. In Beasley SW, Myers NA, Auldist AW (eds): Oesophageal Atresia. London, Chapman & Hall, 1991, pp 211–228.
26. Sapin E, Berg A, Raynaud P, et al: Coexisting left congenital diaphragmatic hernia and esophageal atresia with tracheoesophageal fistula: successful management in a premature infant. J Pediatr Surg 1996;31:989–991.
27. Ein SH, Shandling B, Wesson D, et al: Esophageal atresia with distal tracheoesophageal fistula: associated anomalies and prognosis in the 1980's. J Pediatr Surg 1989;24:1055–1059.
28. Mee RBB, Beasley SW, Auldist AW, et al: Influence of congenital heart disease on management of oesophageal atresia. Pediatr Surg Int 1992;2:90–93.
29. Mee RBB, Congenital heart disease. In Beasley SW, Myers NA, Auldist AW (eds): Oesophageal Atresia. London, Chapman & Hall, 1991, pp 229–239.
30. Beasley SW, Phelan E, Kelly JH, et al: Urinary tract abnormalities in association with oesophageal atresia: frequency, significance, and influence on management. Pediatr Surg Int 1992;2:94–96.
31. Phelan E, Kelly JH, Beasley SW: Urinary tract anomalies. In Beasley SW, Myers NA, Auldist AW (eds): Oesophageal Atresia. London, Chapman & Hall, 1991, pp 241–248.
32. Dickens DRV: Orthopaedic abnormalities. In Beasley SW, Myers NA, Auldist AW (eds): Oesophageal Atresia. London, Chapman & Hall, 1991, pp 249–262.
33. Atwell JD, Beard RC: Congenital anomalies of the upper urinary tract associated with esophageal atresia and tracheoesophageal fistula. J Pediatr Surg 1974;9:825–831.
34. Campbell N: Case selection. In Beasley SW, Myers NA, Auldist AW (eds): Oesophageal Atresia. London, Chapman & Hall, 1991, pp 287–301.
35. Quan L, Smith DW: The VATER association—vertebral defects, anal atresia, T-E fistula with esophageal atresia, radial and renal dysplasia: a spectrum of associated defects. J Pediatr 1973;82:104–107.
36. Fabris S, Cavazzana A, Gamba P: VATER syndrome and esophageal foregut duplication: a new association. Pediatr Surg Int 1995;10:252–254.
37. Khoury MJ, Cordero JF, Greenberg F, et al: A population study of VACTERL association: evidence for its etiologic heterogeneity. Pediatrics 1983;71:815–820.
38. Temtanry SA, Miller JD: Extending the scope of the VATER association: definition of the VATER syndrome. J Pediatr 1974;85:345–349.
39. Valente A, Brereton RJ: Oesophageal atresia and the CHARGE association. Pediatr Surg Int 1987;2:93–94.
40. Kutiyanawala M, Wise RKH, Brereton L, et al: CHARGE and esophageal atresia. J Pediatr Surg 1992;5:558–560.
41. Ein SH, Izukawa T, Su WJ, et al: The influence of cardiovascular malformations on the prognosis of esophageal atresia and distal tracheoesophageal fistula. Pediatr Surg Int 1989;4:318–321.
42. Kluth D, Habenicht R: The embryology of usual and unusual types of esophageal atresia. Pediatr Surg Int 1987;2:223–227.
43. Bankier A, Brady J, Myers NA: Epidemiology and genetics. In Beasley SW, Myers NA, Auldist AW (eds): Oesophageal Atresia. London, Chapman & Hall, 1991, pp 17–29.
44. Weber TR, Smith W, Grosfeld JL: Surgical experience in infants with the VATER association. J Pediatr Surg 1980;15:849–854.
45. Holder TM, Ashcraft KW: Cardiac disease. In Welch KJ, Randolph JG, Ravitch MM, et al (eds): Pediatric Surgery, 4th ed. Chicago, Year Book, 1986, pp 1385–1389.
46. German JC, Mahour GH, Woolley MM: Esophageal atresia and associated anomalies. J Pediatr Surg 1976;11:299–306.
47. Schimle RN, Leape LL, Holder TM: Familial occurrence of esophageal atresia: a preliminary report. In Birth Defects: Original Article Series. Vol 8. 1972, pp 22–23.
48. McIntosh D, Wright JE: Tracheoesophageal fistula in siblings. Pediatr Surg Int 1986;1:246–248.
49. Cass D, Auldist A: Oesophageal atresia with proximal tracheoesophageal fistula. Pediatr Surg Int 1987;2:212–215.
50. Ashcraft KW, Holder TM: Esophageal atresia and tracheoesophageal malformations. In Holder TM, Ashcraft KW (eds): Pediatric Surgery. Philadelphia, WB Saunders, 1980, pp 266–283.
51. Beasley SW: Anatomy. In Beasley SW, Myers NA, Auldist AW (eds): Oesophageal Atresia. London, Chapman & Hall, 1991, pp 45–58.
52. Szold A, Udassin R, Seror D, et al: Acquired tracheoesophageal fistula in infancy and childhood. J Pediatr Surg 1991;26:672–675.
53. Al-Arfah AL, Khwaja MS, El-Mouzan M: Acquired tracheoesophageal fistula. Pediatr Surg Int 1991;6:125–127.
54. Pohlson EC, Schaller RT, Tapper D: Improved survival with primary anastomosis in the low-birth-weight neonate with esophageal atresia and tracheoesophageal fistula. J Pediatr Surg 1988;23:418–421.
55. Louhimo I, Lindahl H: Esophageal atresia: primary results of 500 consecutively treated patients. J Pediatr Surg 1983;18:217–229.
56. Myers NA, Beasley SW: Diagnosis. In Beasley SW, Myers NA, Auldist AW (eds): Oesophageal Atresia. London, Chapman & Hall, 1991, pp 77–92.
57. Van der Zee DC, Van der Staak FHT, Severijnen RSUM, et al: Proximal fistula in esophageal atresia: pitfall in a routine procedure. Pediatr Surg Int 1988;3:23–26.
58. Goh DW, Brereton RJ, Spitz L: Esophageal atresia with obstructed tracheoesophageal fistula and gasless abdomen. J Pediatr Surg 1991;26:160–162.
59. Weigel W, Kaufman HJ: The frequency and types of other congenital anomalies in association with tracheoesophageal malformation. Clin Pediatr 1976;15:819–834.
60. Stringel G, Coln D, Guertin L: Esophageal atresia and right aortic arch. Pediatr Surg Int 1990;5:103–105.
61. Knight PJ, Clatworthy HW: Screening for latent malformations: cost effectiveness in neonates with correctable anomalies. J Pediatr Surg 1982;17:123–129.
62. Antimicrobial prophylaxis in surgery. Med Lett 1987;29:91–94.
63. Bell MJ, Kosloske AM, Martin L, et al: Antimicrobial prophylaxis in pediatric surgical patients. Presented at the Meeting of the Surgical Section of the American Academy of Pediatrics, San Francisco, October 1983.

64. Roy RND: Transport of the neonate with oesophageal atresia. In Beasley SW, Myers NA, Auldist AW (eds): Oesophageal Atresia. London, Chapman & Hall, 1991, pp 93–102.
65. Telfer HM, McDonnell GE: Nursing care. In Beasley SW, Myers NA, Auldist AW (eds): Oesophageal Atresia. London, Chapman & Hall, 1991, pp 265–274.
66. Ty TC, Brunet C, Beardmore HE: A variation in the operative technique for the treatment of esophageal atresia and tracheoesophageal fistula. J Pediatr Surg 1967;2:118–125.
67. Touloukian RJ, Pickett LK, Spackman T: Repair of esophageal atresia by end-to-side anastomosis and ligation of the tracheoesophageal fistula: a critical review of 18 cases. J Pediatr Surg 1974;9:305–310.
68. Holder TM, Cloud DT, Lewis JE Jr, et al: Esophageal atresia and tracheoesophageal fistula: a survey of its members by the surgical section of the American Academy of Pediatrics. Pediatrics 1964;34:542–549.
69. Ein SH, Theman TE: A comparison of the results of primary repair of esophageal atresia with tracheoesophageal fistula using end-to-side and end-to-end anastomoses. J Pediatr Surg 1973;8:641–645.
70. Poenaru D, Laberge J-M, Neilson IR, et al: A more than 25-year experience with end-to-end versus end-to-side repair for esophageal atresia. J Pediatr Surg 1991;4:472–477.
71. Waterston DJ, Bonham-Carter RE, Aberdeen E: Oesophageal atresia: tracheoesophageal fistula. A study of survival in 218 infants. Lancet 1962;1:819–822.
72. Beasley SW, Auldist AW: Oesophageal atresia with distal tracheoesophageal fistula. In Beasley SW, Myers NA, Auldist AW (eds): Oesophageal Atresia. London, Chapman & Hall, 1991, pp 119–135.
73. Abrahamson J, Shandling B: Esophageal atresia in the underweight baby: a challenge. J Pediatr Surg 1972;7:608–613.
74. Koop CE, Hamilton JP: Atresia of the esophagus: increased survival with staged procedures in the poor-risk infant. Ann Surg 1965;162:389–401.
75. Alexander F, Johanningman AJ, Martin LW: Staged repair improves outcome of high-risk premature infants with esophageal atresia and tracheoesophageal atresia. J Pediatr Surg 1993;28:151–154.
76. Livaditis A: Esophageal atresia: a method of overriding large segmental gaps. Z Kinderchir 1973;13:298–306.
77. Howard R, Myers NA: Esophageal atresia: a technique for elongating the upper pouch. Surgery 1965;58:725–727.
78. Hendren WH, Hale JR: Electromagnetic bougienage to lengthen esophageal segments in congenital esophageal atresia. N Engl J Med 1975;293:428–432.
79. Rehbein F, Schweden N: Reconstruction of the esophagus without colon transplantation in cases of atresia. J Pediatr Surg 1971;6:746–751.
80. Shafer AD, David TE: Suture fistula as a means of connecting upper and lower segments in esophageal atresia. J Pediatr Surg 1974;9:669–673.
81. Davenport M, Bianchi A: Early experience with oesophageal flap oesophagoplasty for repair of oesophageal atresia. Pediatr Surg Int 1990;5:332–335.
82. Moriarty KP, Jacir NN, Harris BH, et al: Transanastomotic feeding tubes in repair of esophageal atresia. J Pediatr Surg 1996;31:53–55.
83. Kiely E, Satz L: is routine gastrostomy necessary in the management of oesophageal atresia? Pediatr Surg Int 1987;2:6–9.
84. Davics MRQ, Beale PG: Protection of oesophageal anastomosis following uncomplicated repair of common-type oesophageal atresia by non-reversal of anaesthesia and graded withdrawal of respiratory support. Pediatr Surg Int 1991;6:98–100.
85. Auldist AW, Beasley SE: Oesophageal complications. In Beasley SW, Myers NA, Auldist AW (eds): Oesophageal Atresia. London, Chapman & Hall, 1991, pp 305–329.
86. Chittmittrapap S, Spitz L, Kiely EM, et al: Anastomotic stricture following repair of esophageal atresia. J Pediatr Surg 1990;25:508–511.
87. Allmendinger N, Hallisey MJ, Markowitz SK, et al: Balloon dilatation of esophageal strictures in children. J Pediatr Surg 1996;31:334–336.
88. Pieretti R, Shandling B, Stephens CA: Resistant esophageal stenosis associated with reflux after repair of esophageal atresia: a therapeutic approach. J Pediatr Surg 1974;9:355–357.
89. Gutierrez-Samroman C, Vila-Carbo J, Segarra-Llido V, et al: Long-term nutritional evaluation of 70 patients operated on for esophageal atresia. Pediatr Surg Int 1988;3:123–127.
90. Desjardins JG, Stephens CA, Moes CAF: Results of surgical treatment of congenital tracheoesophageal fistula, with a note on cine-fluorographic findings. Ann Surg 1964;160:141–145.
91. Stokes KB: Pathophysiology. In Beasley SW, Myers NA, Auldist AW (eds): Oesophageal Atresia. London, Chapman & Hall, 1991, pp 59–73.
92. DePeppo F, Rivosecchi M, Federici G, et al: Conservative treatment of corrosive esophageal strictures: a comparative study of endoscopic dilatations and esophageal stenting. Pediatr Surg Int 1993;8:3–7.
93. Mutaf O: Treatment of corrosive esophageal strictures by long-term stenting. J Pediatr Surg 1996;31:681–685.
94. Vos A, Ekkelkamp S: Congenital tracheoesophageal fistula: preventing recurrence. J Pediatr Surg 1996;31:936–938.
95. Glasson MJ, Bandrevics V, Cohen DH: Hypertrophic pyloric stenosis complicating esophageal atresia. Surgery 1973;74:530–535.
96. Jolly SG, Johnson DG, Roberts CC, et al: Patterns of gastroesophageal reflux in children following repair of esophageal atresia and distal tracheoesophageal fistula. J Pediatr Surg 1980;15:857–862.
97. Wheatley MJ, Coran AG, Wesley JR: Efficacy of the Nissen fundoplication in the management of gastroesophageal reflux following esophageal atresia repair. J Pediatr Surg 1993;28:53–55.
98. Lindahl H, Rintala R, Sariola H: Chronic esophagitis and gastric metaplasia are frequent late complications of esophageal atresia. J Pediatr Surg 1993;28:1178–1180.
99. Caniano D, Ginn-Pease E, King DR: The failed antireflux procedure: analysis of risk factors and morbidity. J Pediatr Surg 1990;25:1022–1026.
100. Ein SH, Shandling B, Heiss K: Pure esophageal atresia: outlook in the 1990s. J Pediatr Surg 1993;28:1147–1150.
101. Lindahl H, Rintala R, Sariola H, et al: Cervical Barrett's esophagus: a common complication of gastric tube reconstruction. J Pediatr Surg 1990;25:446–448.
102. Emery JL, Halladin J: Squamous epithelium in respiratory tract of children with tracheoesophageal fistula. Arch Dis Child 1971;46:236–242.
103. Spitz L, Phelan PD: Tracheomalacia. In Beasley SW, Myers NA, Auldist AW (eds): Oesophageal Atresia. London, Chapman & Hall, 1991, pp 331–340.
104. Usui N, Kamata S, Ishikawa S, et al: Anomalies of the tracheobronchial tree in patients with esophageal atresia. J Pediatr Surg 1996;31:258–262.
105. Milligan DWA, Levison H: Lung function in children following repair of tracheoesophageal fistula. J Pediatr Surg 1979;95:24–27.
106. Dudley NE, Phelan PD: Respiratory complications in long-term survivors of esophageal atresia. Arch Dis Child 1976;51:279–282.
107. Schwartz MZ, Filler RM: Tracheal compression as a cause of apnea following repair of tracheoesophageal fistula: treatment by aortopexy. J Pediatr Surg 1980;15:842–848.
108. Filler RM, Rossello PJ, Lebowitz RL: Life-threatening anoxic spells caused by tracheal compression after repair of esophageal atresia: correction by surgery. J Pediatr Surg 1976;11:738–748.
109. Mustard WT, Bayliss CD, Fearon B, et al: Tracheal compression by the innominate artery in children. Ann Thorac Surg 1969;8:312–319.
110. Gross RE, Neuhauser EB: compression of the trachea by an anomolous innominate artery: an operation for its relief. Am J Dis Child 1948;75:570–574.
111. Lochbihler H, Hoelzl J, Dietz HG: Tissue compatability and biodegradation of new absorbable stents for tracheal stabilization: an experimental study. J Pediatr Surg 1997;32:717–720.
112. Filler RM, Forte V, Chait PG: Tracheobronchial stenting for airway obstruction. Presented at 28th Annual Meeting, American Pediatric Surgical Association, Naples, Florida, May 18–21, 1997.
113. Tsugawa C, Nishijima E, Muraji T, et al: A shape-memory airway stent for tracheobronchomalacia in children: an experimental and clinical study. J Pediatr Surg 1997;32:50–53.
114. Freeman NV, Walkden J: Previously unreported shoulder deformity following right lateral thoracotomy for esophageal atresia. J Pediatr Surg 1969;4:627–636.
115. Durning RP, Scoles PV, Fox OD: Scoliosis after thoractomy in tracheoesophageal fistula patients. J Bone Joint Surg 1980;62:1156–1159.
116. Holder TM: Esophageal atresia and tracheoesophageal fistula. In Ashcraft KW, Holder TM (eds): Pediatric Esophageal Surgery. Philadelphia, Grune & Stratton, 1986, pp 29–52.
117. Randolph JG, Altman RP, Anderson KD: Selective surgical management based upon clinical status in infants with esophageal atresia. J Thorac Cardiovasc Surg 1977;74:335–342.

118. Raffensperger JG: Discussion. In Randolph JG, Altman RP, Anderson KD: Selective surgical management based upon clinical status in infants with esophageal atresia. J Thorac Cardiovasc Surg 1977;74:342.
119. Myers NA: Oesophageal atresia and/or tracheo-oesophageal fistula: a study of mortality. Prog Pediatr Surg 1979;13:141–165.
120. Beasley SW, Myers NA: Trends in mortality in oesophageal atresia. Pediatr Surg Int 1992;2:86–89.
121. Beasley SW, Myers NA: Trends in mortality. In Beasley SW, Myers NA, Auldist AW (eds): Oesophageal Atresia. London, Chapman & Hall, 1991, pp 361–367.
122. Beasley SW, Phelan PD, Chetcuti PAJ: Late results following repair of oesophageal atresia. In Beasley SW, Myers NA, Auldist AW (eds): Oesophageal Atresia. London, Chapman & Hall, 1991, pp 369–394.
123. Beasley SW: Oesophageal atresia without fistula. In Beasley SW, Myers NA, Auldist AW (eds): Oesophageal Atresia. London, Chapman & Hall, 1991, pp 137–159.
124. Montgomery M, Frenckner B, Freyschuss U, et al: Esophageal atresia: long-term-follow-up of respiratory function, maximal working capacity, and esophageal function. Pediatr Surg Int 1995;10:519–522.
125. Zaccara A, Felici F, Turchetta A, et al: Physical fitness testing in children operated on for tracheoesophageal fistula. J Pediatr Surg 1995;30:1334–1337.
126. Cumming WA: Esophageal atresia and tracheoesophageal fistula. Radiol Clin North Am 1975;13:277–295.
127. Blair GK, Filler RM, Theodarescu D: Neonatal pharyngo-esophageal perforation mimicking esophageal atresia: clues to diagnosis. J Pediatr Surg 1987;22:770–774.
128. Myers NA, Beasley SW, Auldist AW, et al: Oesophageal atresia without fistula: anastomosis or replacement? Pediatr Surg Int 1987;2:216–222.
129. Sinha CK, Gangopadhyay AN, Sahoo SP, et al: A new variant of esophageal atresia with tracheoesophageal fistula and duodenal atresia: a diagnostic dilemma. Pediatr Surg Int 1997;12:186–187.
130. Croaker GDH, Najmaldin AS: Laparoscopically assisted percutaneous endoscopic gastrostomy. Pediatr Surg Int 1997;12:130–131.
131. Chavin K, Field G, Chandler J, et al: Save the child's esophagus: management of major disruption after repair of esophageal atresia. J Pediatr Surg 1996;31:48–52.
132. dela Hunt MN, Fleet MS, Wagget J: Delayed primary anastomosis for wide-defect esophageal atresia: a 17-year experience. Pediatr Surg Int 1994;9:21–23.
133. Ein SH, Shandling B: Pure esophageal atresia: a 50-year review. J Pediatr Surg 1994;29:1208–1211.
134. Lindahl H, Rintala R, Louhimo I: Failure of Nissen fundoplication to control gastroesophageal reflux in esophageal atresia patients. J Pediatr Surg 1989;24:985–987.
135. Myers NA, Beasley SW, Auldist AW: Oesophageal replacement. In Beasley SW, Myers NA, Auldist AW (eds): Oesophageal Atresia. London, Chapman & Hall, 1991, pp 171–191.
136. Stinger MD: Oesophageal substitution [Editorial comment]. Pediatr Surg Int 1996;11:213.
137. Gomez MV: Esophageal replacement in patients under 3 months of age. J Pediatr Surg 1994;29:487–491.
138. German JC, Waterston DI: Colon interposition for the replacement of the esophagus in children. J Pediatr Surg 1976;11:227–234.
139. Dickson JAS: Esophageal substitution with colon: the Waterston operation. Pediatr Surg Int 1996;11:224–226.
140. Raffensperger JG, Luck SR, Reynolds M, et al: Intestinal bypass of the esophagus. J Pediatr Surg 1996;31:38–47.
141. Ahmad SA, Sylvester KG, Hebra A, et al: Esophageal replacement using the colon: is it a good choice? J Pediatr Surg 1996;31:1026–1031.
142. Ein SH, Shandling B, Simpson JS, et al: A further look at the gastric tube as an esophageal replacement in infants and children. J Pediatr Surg 1973;8:859–868.
143. Ein SH, Shandling B, Stephens CA: Twenty-one-year experience with the pediatric gastric tube. J Pediatr Surg 1987;22:77–81.
144. Anderson KD, Randolph JG: The gastric tube for esophageal replacement in children. J Thorac Cardiovasc Surg 1973;6:333–342.
145. Randolph JG: The reversed gastric tube for esophageal replacement in children. Pediatr Surg Int 1996;11:221–223.
146. Spitz L: Gastric transposition via the mediastinal route for infants with long-gap esophageal atresia. J Pediatr Surg 1984;19:149–154.
147. Spitz L: Gastric transposition for oesophageal substitution in children. J Pediatr Surg 1992;27:252–259.
148. Schärli AF: Esophageal reconstruction in very long atresias by elongation of the lesser curvature. Pediatr Surg Int 1992;2:101–105.
149. Spitz L: Gastric transposition for oesophageal replacement. Pediatr Surg Int 1996;11:218–220.
150. Davenport M, Hosie GP, Tasker RC, et al: Long-term effects of gastric transposition in children: a physiologic study. J Pediatr Surg 1996;31:588–593.
151. Scharli AF: Esophageal reconstruction by elongation of the lesser gastric curvature. Pediatr Surg Int 1996;11:214–217.
152. Spicer RD, Cusick EL: Oesophageal substitution by jejunal free graft: follow-up data and an evaluation. Pediatr Surg Int 1996;11:227–229.
153. Bax NMA, Rövekamp MH, Pull Tergunne AJ, et al: Early one-stage orthotopic jejunal pedicle-graft interposition in long-gap esophageal atresia. Pediatr Surg Int 1994;9:483–485.
154. Cusick EL, Batchelor AAG, Spicer RD: Development of a technique for jejunal interposition in long-gap esophageal atresia. J Pediatr Surg 1993;28:990–994.
155. Evans M: Application of Collis gastroplasty to the management of esophageal atresia. J Pediatr Surg 1995;30:1232–1235.
156. Lindahl H, Louhimo I, Virkola K: Colon interposition or gastric tube? Follow-up study of colon-esophagus and gastric tube–esophagus patients. J Pediatr Surg 1983;18:58–63.
157. Myers NA, Egami K: Congenital tracheo-oesophageal fistula: "H" or "N" fistula. Pediatr Surg Int 1987;2:198–211.
158. Kent M, Myers NA, Beasley SW: Tracheo-oesophageal fistula: the "H" fistula. In Beasley SW, Myers NA, Auldist AW (eds): Oesophageal Atresia. London, Chapman & Hall, 1991, pp 193–207.
159. Stringer DA, Ein SH: Recurrent tracheoesophageal fistula: a protocol for investigation. Radiology 1984;151:637–641.
160. Gans SL, Berci G: Inside tracheoesophageal fistula: new endoscopic approaches. J Pediatr Surg 1973;8:205–211.
161. Ein SH, Stringer DA, Stephens CA, et al: Recurrent tracheoesophageal fistulas: seventeen-year review. J Pediatr Surg 1983;18:436–441.
162. Wiseman N: Endoscopic closure of recurrent tracheoesophageal fistula using Tisseel. J Pediatr Surg 1995;30:1236–1237.
163. Wood RE, Lacey SR, Azizkhan RG: Endoscopic management of large postresection bronchopleural fistulae with methocrylate adhesive (SuperGlue). J Pediatr Surg 1992;27:201–202.
164. Gutierrez C, Barrios JE, Lluna J, et al: Recurrent tracheoesophageal fistula treated with fibrin glue. J Pediatr Surg 1994;29:1567–1569.
165. Hays DM, Woolley MW, Snyder WH Jr: Esophageal atresia and tracheoesophageal fistula: management of the uncommon types. J Pediatr Surg 1966;1:240–252.
166. Rodgers BM, Johnson AM, Minor GR, et al: Esophageal atresia with double fistula: the missed anomaly. Ann Thorac Surg 1984;38:195–200.
167. Auldist AW: Oesophageal atresia with proximal tracheo-oesophageal fistula. In Beasley SW, Myers, NA, Auldist AW (eds): Oesophageal Atresia. London, Chapman & Hall, 1991, pp 161–170.
168. Blackburn WR, Amoury RA: Congenital esophago-pulmonary fistulas without esophageal atresia: an analysis of 260 fistulas in infants, children, and adults. Rev Surg 1966;23:153–175.
169. Hanna E: Broncho-esophageal fistula with total sequestration of the right lung. Ann Surg 1963;159:599–603.
170. Moscarella AA, Wyllie RH: Congenital communication between the esophagus and isolated ectopic pulmonary tissue. J Thorac Cardiovas Surg 1967;55:672–676.
171. Paulin R, Longtin L: Congenital bronchoesophageal fistula in an adult. Can Med Assoc J 1970;102:964–966.
172. Mahour GH, Cohen SR, Woolley MD: Laryngotracheo-esophageal cleft associated with esophageal atresia and multiple tracheoesophageal fistulas in a twin. J Thorac Cardiovasc Surg 1973;65:223–226.
173. Zachary RB, Emery JL: Failure of separation of larynx and trachea from the esophagus: persistent esophagotrachea. Surgery 1961; 49:525–529.
174. Petterson G: Laryngo-tracheo-esophageal cleft. Z Kinderchir 1969; 7:43–49.
175. Finlay HVL: Familial congenital stridor. Arch Dis Child 1949;24:219–223.
176. Blumberg JB, Stevenson JK, Lemire RJ, et al: Laryngo-tracheoesophageal cleft, the embryologic complications: review of the literature. Surgery 1965;57:559–566.
177. Delahunty JE, Cherry J: Congenital laryngeal cleft. Ann Otolaryngol 1969;78:96–106.
178. Frates RE: Roentgen signs in laryngotracheoesophageal cleft. Radiology 1967;88:484–486.

179. Griscom NT: Persistent esophagotrachea: the most severe degree of laryngotracheoesophageal cleft. Am J Roentgenol 1966;97:211–215.
180. Burroughs N, Leape LL: Laryngotracheoesophageal cleft: report of a case successfully treated and review of the literature. Pediatrics 1974;53:516–522.
181. Donahoe PK, Gee PE: Complete laryngotracheal cleft: management and repair. J Pediatr Surg 1984;19:143–147.
182. Wright VM: The esophagus: congenital anomalies. In Walker WA, Durie PR, Hamilton JR (eds): Pediatric Gastrointestinal Disease. Philadelphia, Decker, 1991, p 369.
183. Nihoul-Fekete C, DeBacker A, Lortat-Jacob S, et al: Congenital esophageal stenosis: a review of 20 cases. Pediatr Surg Int 1987;2:86–92.
184. Gopal SC, Gangopadhyay AN, Pandit SK, et al: Membranous atresia of the lower esophagus. Pediatr Surg Int 1993;8:140–141.
185. Murphy, SG, Yazbeck S, Russo P: Isolated congenital esophageal stenosis. J Pediatr Surg 1995;30:1238–1241.
186. Scherer LR, Grosfeld JL: Congenital esophageal stenosis, esophageal duplication, neurenteric cyst, and esophageal diverticulum. In Ashcraft KW, Holder TM (eds): Pediatric Esophageal Surgery. Orlando, Grune & Stratton, 1986, pp 53–71.
187. Karaguzel G, Tanyel FC, Akcoren Z, et al: Intramural tracheobronchial remnants associated with esophageal atresia: diagnostic aids. Pediatr Surg Int 1993;8:138–139.
188. Touloukian JR: Membranous esophageal obstruction simulating atresia with a double tracheoesophageal fistula in a neonate. J Thorac Cardiovas Surg 1972;65:191–194.
189. Deiraniya AK: Congenital oesophageal stenosis due to tracheobronchial remnants. Thorax 1974;29:720–725.
190. Margarit J, Castonon M, Ribo JM, et al: Congenital esophageal stenosis associated with tracheoesophageal fistula. Pediatr Surg Int 1994; 9:577–578.
191. Paulino F, Roselli A, Aprigliano F: Congenital esophageal stricture due to tracheobronchial remnants. Surgery 1962;53:547–550.
192. Ishida M, Tsuchida Y, Saito S, et al: Congenital esophageal stenosis due to tracheobronchial remnants. J Pediatr Surg 1969;4:339–345.
193. Heyman MB, Berquist WE, Fonkalsrud EW, et al: Esophageal muscular ring and VACTERL association: a case report. Pediatrics 1981;67:683–686.
194. Minnis JF Jr, Burko H, Brevetti G: Segmental duplication of the esophagus associated with esophageal atresia and tracheoesophageal fistula. Ann Surg 1961;156:271–275.
195. Yahr WZ, Azzoni AA, Santulli TV: Congenital atresia of the esophagus with tracheoesophageal fistula: an unusual variant. Surgery 1962;52:937–941.
196. Roy GT, Cohen RC, Williams SJ: Endoscopic laser division of an esophageal web in a child. J Pediatr Surg 1996;31:439–440.

# Chapter 14

# Gastroesophageal Reflux

*Susan R. Orenstein*

Gastroesophageal reflux (GER) is one of the most common gastrointestinal problems in children. It produces a wide variety of symptoms and ranges in severity from physiologic regurgitation of infancy to a life-threatening disorder. This chapter touches on its pathophysiology and reviews in more detail its clinical manifestations, differential diagnosis, evaluation, and therapy.

## PATHOPHYSIOLOGY

Episodes of GER occur in normal children and adults, in whom brief episodes happen about five times hourly after meals. Physiologic episodes are infrequent while awake but fasting and virtually never occur during sleep. These normal GER episodes must be differentiated from gastroesophageal reflux disease (GERD), in which GER produces pathologic effects. GERD results from increased frequency or duration of GER episodes, from increased noxiousness of the refluxate, or from refluxate reaching hazardous locations beyond the esophagus, such as the airway, or producing dangerous responses, such as apnea (Table 14–1).

### Increased Frequency or Duration of Reflux

Lower esophageal sphincter (LES) tone is the main barrier to the retrograde movement of gastric contents; it is bolstered by the crural diaphragm and by other minor factors historically stressed in the surgical literature—the cardioesophageal angle of His, the phrenoesophageal ligament, and the "mucosal rosette" at the gastroesophageal junction.

Reflux episodes occur only when LES tone is near zero, certainly less than 5 mm Hg.[1] Most often, this absent LES tone is due to "transient LES relaxations" (TLESRs) (Fig. 14–1).[2–4] Persistent LES hypotonia was previously considered the major mechanism for GER episodes, but it is currently understood to be responsible for only a minority of GER episodes, usually in the context of chronic GERD and esophagitis, when long-standing inflammation makes the LES dysfunctional.[5] All of the factors responsible for maintaining LES tone are not yet determined, but nitric oxide likely plays an important role.[6, 7]

Increased intragastric pressure provokes reflux, particularly in the context of low LES pressure.[8–10] Contraction of the diaphragmatic hiatus during Valsalva, cough, or exercise defends against reflux when increased intra-abdominal pressure would otherwise provoke it,[11, 12] and this active increase in pressure around the sphincter is complemented by passive transmission of increased intra-abdominal pressure to the intra-abdominal LES.[13] The importance of diaphragmatic factors is underscored by the increased reflux observed in patients with congenital or acquired diaphragmatic (hiatal)

**TABLE 14–1. Pathophysiology of Reflux**

I. Increased Frequency of Reflux Episodes
   A. LES hypotonia
   B. TLESRs
      1. Increased in reflux disease?
         a. Primarily (e.g., lack of supine suppression)?
         b. Secondarily (e.g., secondary to increased sleep arousals)?
      2. Result in reflux episodes more often in reflux disease?
         a. Because of provocative positioning, delayed gastric emptying, etc.?
   C. Defective perisphincteric support
      1. Non-intra-abdominal LES (hiatal hernia)
      2. Crural sphincteric dysfunction
      3. Other—"mucosal rosette," cardioesophageal angle, phrenoesophageal ligament
   D. Increased gastric pressure
      1. Decreased gastric compliance
      2. Delayed gastric emptying
      3. Externally applied increased abdominal pressure
   E. Increased gastric volume
      1. Large meal
      2. Gastric hypersecretion
      3. Delayed gastric emptying
II. Decreased Esophageal Clearance of Refluxate
   A. Gravity effects—supine position
   B. Peristaltic dysfunction or infrequent swallowing
   C. Defective salivation
III. Increased Noxiousness of Refluxate
   A. Acid
   B. Pepsin
   C. Bile acids
   D. Trypsin
IV. Defective Mucosal Resistance to Refluxate
V. Effects of Upper Esophageal Dysfunction
VI. Effects of Sleep
   A. Gravity—noxious material at cardia & to pharynx, decreased clearance
   B. Decreased salivation & swallowing
   C. UES hypotonia

hernias or in iron lungs.[14, 15] Thus, hiatal hernia has regained the notoriety it had temporarily lost as a culprit in long-term GERD.[16] Intragastric pressure is affected by multiple factors in addition to intra-abdominal pressure, including gastric compliance (lower in infants than adults[17]), the volume of gastric secretion, meal size in relation to gastric volume (higher in infants), gastric emptying,[18–20] and body position (particularly in infants, whose limited torso tone makes "sitting" provocative[21]).

Patients with reflux disease often manifest prolonged reflux episodes, indicating dysfunction of esophageal clearance, which may be both a cause and a result of GERD.[22, 23] Mechanisms that promote clearance, and thus reduce damage to the esophageal mucosa, are bulk clearance of refluxate (by gravity and peristalsis) and neutralization of the residual (by salivary bicarbonate) (Fig. 14–2).[24]

## Increased Noxiousness of Refluxate

The degree of esophagitis correlates best with acid exposure.[25, 26] This aspect of GERD is favorable to infants,

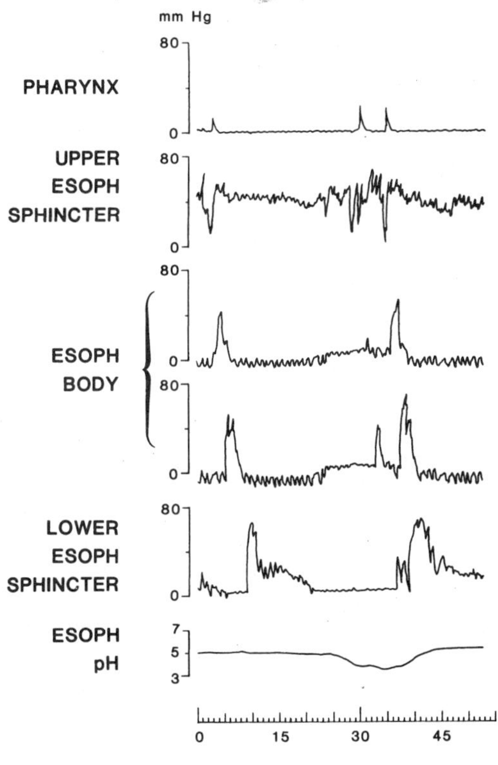


**FIGURE 14–1.** Transient lower esophageal sphincter relaxation (TLESR). A pH probe in the distal esophagus (bottom channel) records an episode of reflux due to a transient relaxation of the LES ("lower esoph sphincter" channel) unassociated with a swallow. The reflux causes a small pressure rise in the esophageal body, which is termed a *common cavity*, and is followed by two swallows that clear the refluxate. (From Orenstein SR: Gastroesophageal reflux. Curr Prob Pediatr 1991;21:195, with permission.)

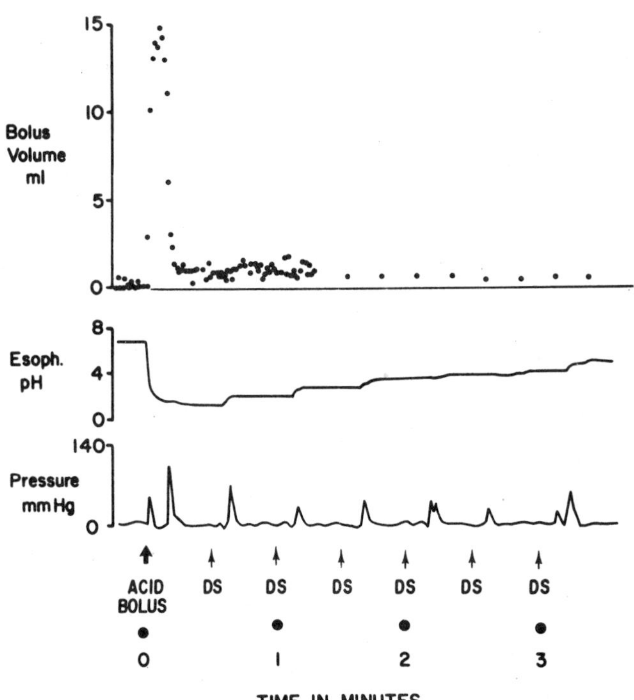


**FIGURE 14–2.** Relations among esophageal acid clearance, motor activity, and emptying of fluid volume. Top channel shows, in a supine normal adult, the volume of acid in the esophagus (quantified scintigraphically) following injection of a 15-mL bolus of 0.1N hydrochloric acid (pH 1.2) labeled with 100 μCi of $^{99m}$Tc sulfur colloid into the esophageal lumen. The second channel shows distal esophageal pH. The bottom channel shows distal esophageal pressures. Despite clearance of the injected bolus volume to less than 1 mL by the secondary (nonswallow) peristaltic sequence, esophageal pH did not begin to rise until the first primary peristaltic dry swallow (DS—without ingested material) wave. (Reprinted with permission from Helm JF, Dodds WJ, Pelc LR, et al: Effect of esophageal emptying and saliva on clearance of acid from the esophagus. N Engl J Med 1984;310:284–288.)

whose gastric pH remains high for much of the day because of buffering by frequent milk feedings,[27] despite acid secretory function at adult levels by several months of age. Other components contributing to the noxiousness of refluxate are pepsin, bile acids, and trypsin. The latter two depend on duodenogastric reflux preceding gastroesophageal reflux and are implicated in the genesis of strictures and Barrett's esophagus.

Just as esophageal clearance modulates the effects of reflux frequency, mucosal resistance modulates the noxiousness of the components of refluxate. Exploration of this aspect of GERD is limited currently,[28] but it can be postulated to explain the relative resistance of esophageal mucosa compared with airway mucosa.[29]

## Nonesophageal Reflux Destinations and Effects

Although esophagitis and its sequelae are the most common consequences of GERD, regurgitation (particularly in infants) and airway manifestations (due to aspiration or esophago-respiratory reflexes) are important nonesophageal consequences. The upper esophageal sphincter (UES)[30, 31] and reflex arcs[32] between the esophagus and airway are important pathophysiologically in these manifestations.

## Sleep State

Normal individuals rarely experience TLESRs or reflux episodes during sleep, but sleep is particularly hazardous in GERD.[33] Supine recumbency removes all the beneficial gravitational effects of the erect position. Noxious materials, rather than air, are positioned at the cardia, available to move into the esophagus during TLESRs. A given volume of refluxate is also more likely to reach the pharynx in this position, and clearance of refluxate may be impaired, particularly in patients with infrequent swallowing or peristaltic dysfunction. Both salivation and swallowing frequency are markedly reduced during sleep, further impairing clearance.[34] The UES is atonic during sleep, allowing reflux access to the airway.

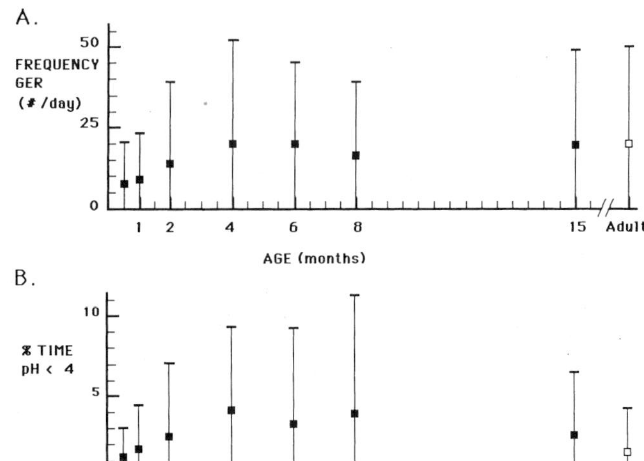


**FIGURE 14–3.** Physiologic reflux: range of normal values during development. Graphic representation of normal ranges (mean ± 2 SD) for reflux in children of various ages (n = 285) and in adults (n = 15). *Top panel* depicts frequency of reflux episodes; *bottom panel* depicts total duration of esophageal acidification throughout the day, during normal activities and diet. (From Orenstein SR: Gastroesophageal reflux. Curr Prob Pediatr 1991;21:202, with permission.)

# CLINICAL PRESENTATIONS

## GER Disease in Infants Versus Children and Adults

Older children and adults manifest GER disease similarly, but infants exhibit considerable differences from older children. These differences include both the temporal course of reflux and its specific manifestations.

Reflux disease tends to persist in older children and adults, 50% of whom have a chronic relapsing course.[35] In infants, however, GERD usually resolves during the first 1 or 2 years.[36, 37] This is true for both the physiologic "spitting" of normal infants and for pathologic infant reflux, which is responsible for considerable morbidity and occasional mortality while it persists.

Also in contrast to adults, symptoms of esophagitis are not the major manifestations of reflux in infants, although histologic esophagitis is common.[38–40] Prominent clinical manifestations in infants include malnutrition due to regurgitation, nonspecific irritability, and apnea. Rumination, stridor, lower respiratory disease, and neurobehavioral symptoms also may bring infants and young children to medical attention.

The fact that reflux differs in infants and adults suggests underlying developmental differences in the pathophysiology of reflux. These differences are only beginning to be explored.

## Epidemiology

Normal infants and adults manifest similar amounts of acid reflux, as demonstrated by esophageal pH probe (Fig. 14–3),[41, 42] but it must be remembered that the frequent infant formula feedings buffer gastric contents much of the day. Premature infants may reflux more, owing to developmental immaturity.[43, 44] Although infants regurgitate considerably more than older children or adults, and parents of many infants perceive this regurgitation as a problem, this symptom seems to correspond in frequency and importance to the occasional minor heartburn experienced by normal adults.[45] Annual physician visits (about 7%) and complicated GERD requiring subspecialist referral (about 2%) occur at similar frequencies in infants and adults.[46–48] The natural history of GERD has been explored in children[49] and adults.[50–52] The large majority of infants with GERD outgrow its manifestations by a year or so of age. This is in contrast to older children and adults with GERD, half of whom experience a chronic, relapsing course. These patterns have implications for management, including the issues of empirical therapy, maintenance pharmacotherapy, and the more definitive surgical approaches.

## Regurgitation and Its Consequences

Because regurgitant reflux is evident without diagnostic testing, this type of reflux received the earliest attention in children. In infants with reflux, less than 20% of scintigraphically or pH probe–detected reflux episodes produce emesis.[53–55] Abdominal muscle contraction may play a role in regurgitant reflux.[54]

Usually little more than a nuisance, regurgitation produces caloric insufficiency and malnutrition in an important minority of infants. Regurgitant reflux in infants may consist of a small amount of material effortlessly drooling from the mouth or may be projectile and voluminous. (Poor intake, as well as regurgitation, may contribute to failure to thrive and may be due to the discomfort of esophagitis.[56])

## Esophagitis and Its Consequences

Esophagitis, identified histologically, occurs in 61% to 83% of infants with clinically important reflux.[38–40] Factors that increase the exposure of the esophagus to noxious material, particularly acid, make esophagitis more likely. Although esophagitis may present as pain, it can also be asymptomatic.

### Chest Pain, Dysphagia, Blood Loss

Typical substernal burning pain *("heartburn," pyrosis)* occurs in many children suffering from esophagitis. Its exacerbation by acid drinks[57] and its relief by liquid antacids help diagnostically. It should be distinguished from the epigastric pain that is more likely to represent gastric peptic disease and from vaguer dyspeptic symptoms. *Odynophagia*, which is pain on swallowing, usually represents esophageal inflammation; a subgroup of patients with odynophagia have reflux esophagitis. In nonverbal infants, behaviors suggesting esophagitis include crying, irritability, sleep disturbance, "colic," and even pushing fingers into the back of the mouth.[56, 58, 59] Infants may also appear avidly hungry for the bottle until their first swallows and then become irritable and refuse to drink.[60, 61]

Dysphagia, the sensation of food "sticking" or "not going down right," is an important symptom of reflux.[62] Dysphagia has been linked to esophagitis, to peristaltic dysfunction accompanying reflux disease, and to peptic stricture.[23, 63] The response of dysphagia to therapy for reflux esophagitis has been variable.[64–66]

Hematemesis or iron-deficiency anemia may be the first symptom of severe esophagitis in children who do not feel, or cannot express, the discomfort of pyrosis.

### Asymptomatic Esophagitis

Patients whose esophagitis is asymptomatic are in some ways more problematic.[67] Even severe esophagitis may remain asymptomatic, as demonstrated by children who present with peptic strictures without having experienced any discomfort attributable to esophagitis. The *completely* asymptomatic person will evade diagnosis, but there should be a high index of suspicion of esophagitis in patients with any symptoms suggesting reflux disease.

### Complicated Esophagitis

Complications of esophagitis include acute hematemesis and chronic anemia, but the two most important long-term complications are stricture and Barrett's esophagus.

**PEPTIC STRICTURE.** Peptic strictures (Fig. 14–4) represent an undesirable endpoint of reflux esophagitis.[68, 69] In a French series of 59 cases, 50% of the children were younger than 2 years of age, 25% were between ages 2 and 5, and the remainder were between ages 5 and 15,[70] although it is possible that the infant preponderance was caused by inclusion of some cases of congenital stenosis.

Peptic strictures may be preceded by chronic heartburn or by asymptomatic esophagitis, but the primary symptom of the stricture itself is dysphagia. An esophageal food impaction always prompts consideration of a stricture. Infants taking a liquid diet may present late; regurgitation of undigested liquids and drooling of saliva suggest severe narrowing.

Diagnosis of a stricture is clearest radiographically. Pressure injection of barium delineates the narrowed area better than simple swallowing of barium, particularly in uncooperative children resisting swallowing because of the dysphagia. Peptic strictures are usually about one third of the esophageal length above the diaphragm, between T6 and T10. It is best to follow radiography with endoscopy to diagnose the type of stenosis and to treat with balloon dilation. If the stricture permits endoscopic passage, biopsy samples are taken just below it to confirm esophagitis and to evaluate for Barrett's epithelium. (Such sampling can be done after dilation if the stricture is initially too narrow.) Most stenotic lesions in the esophagus are reflux related, but if esophagitis is absent, other causes must be considered.

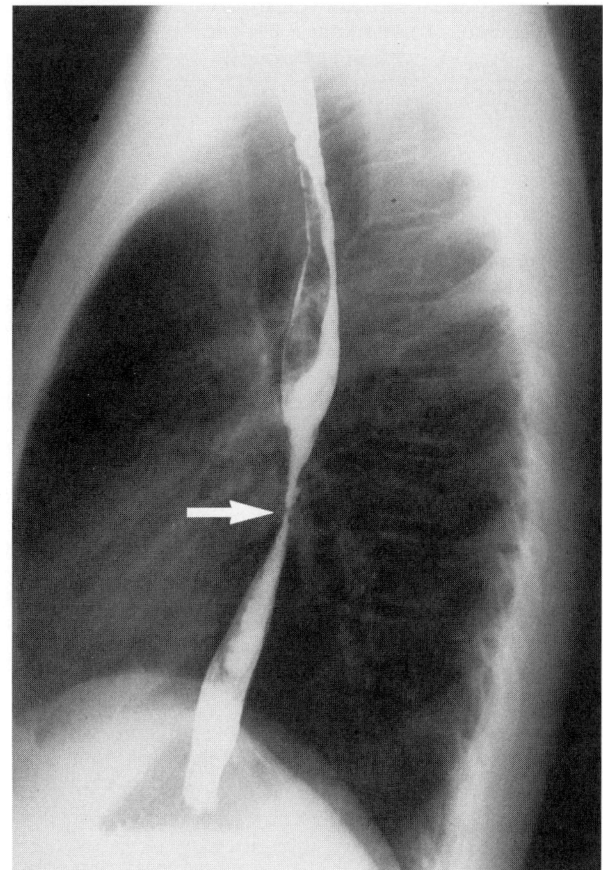

**FIGURE 14–4.** Barium esophagram demonstrating an esophageal stricture due to reflux *(arrow)*.

Treatment of peptic strictures has two goals: dilating the stricture and arresting the reflux. Transendoscopic balloon dilators have the advantages of endoscopic visualization and safer radial forces, but, at a given diameter, mercury-weighted bougies may dilate more effectively.[71–73] A single dilation is usually inadequate for resolution of the stricture, and repeat dilations usually are required, particularly before obliteration of the reflux.[74, 75] Occasionally, refractory strictures will benefit from injection of corticosteroids during endoscopic dilation.[76] Recurrent dilations have been performed in children under general anesthesia, during sedation, and even while awake; the optimal method for each case depends on the patient, the physician, and the setting.[71] Perforation and significant hemorrhage are the most common complications. Fundoplication eliminates the reflux most de-

**TABLE 14–2. Prevention of Respiratory Sequelae During Swallow**

| STRUCTURES | PROTECTIVE FUNCTIONS |
|---|---|
| Mouth | Palate rise |
| Pharynx | Epiglottic tilt |
| Larynx | Cord closure |
| Esophagus | |
| Upper esophageal sphincter | Complete relaxation, coordinated with pharynx |
| Esophageal body | Primary peristalsis |
| Lower esophageal sphincter | Early, complete, prolonged relaxation |

From Putnam PE, Ricker DH, Orenstein SR: Gastroesophageal reflux. In Beckerman R, Brouillette R, Hunt C (eds): Respiratory Control Disorders in Infants and Children. Baltimore, Williams & Wilkins, 1992, p 323; © 1992, the Williams & Wilkins Company, with permission.

finitively and is usually performed following one or several dilations. In the absence of fundoplication, nearly half of patients with chronic peptic strictures develop Barrett's esophagus.[77]

**BARRETT'S ESOPHAGUS.** Barrett's epithelium is defined as metaplastic columnar epithelium replacing the normal squamous epithelium in the esophagus. Whereas any columnar epithelium was designated Barrett's epithelium formerly, currently intestinal metaplasia with goblet cells is considered the only transformation with premalignant significance.[78, 79] Its prevalence is 2% to 20% in adults with peptic esophagitis and as high as 44% in those with a stricture.[77, 80] More than 170 cases have been reported in children,[81] and Barrett's esophagus was found in 13% of children undergoing endoscopy for esophagitis symptoms,[82] although the earliest reports did not distinguish gastric from intestinal metaplasia.[79, 83–85] A male preponderance has been suggested.[86]

Predisposing associations are total gastrectomy, gastric tube replacements of the lower esophagus, and chemotherapy; these associations are likely due to esophageal epithelial injury by bile, trypsin, acid, pepsin, or the chemotherapy.[87–91] Thus, duodenogastric reflux has frequently been implicated.[92–95] *Helicobacter pylori* has been described on the metaplastic gastric epithelium.[96]

Barrett's esophagus does not produce unique symptoms. It is suggested endoscopically by the unusual red of the metaplastic areas and confirmed histologically. Radiographic signs of Barrett's esophagus are due to the complications: deep ulcers and midesophageal strictures.[97]

The esophageal ulcers, strictures, and adenocarcinoma that indicate complicated Barrett's esophagus occur more often in adults but can affect children. Barrett's ulcers are often deep, sometimes even leading to esophagotracheal fistulization, but they heal completely with aggressive antireflux therapy.[98, 99] More than 50% of 24 children in two studies reported with Barrett's esophagus demonstrated strictures.[82, 86] Esophageal adenocarcinoma has a grim prognosis. At diagnosis of Barrett's esophagus in adults, its prevalence is 7% to 22%, and Barrett's-associated adenocarcinoma has been described in children.[100] The incidence of adenocarcinoma is 1 per 52 to 441 patient years of follow-up in Barrett's esophagus patients, 30 to 125 times higher than the rate in the general population.[101, 102] These numbers are particularly ominous when pediatric patients are considered, because of the many anticipated years of increased susceptibility. Adenocarcinoma is particularly likely to arise in smokers and in patients with dysplasia.

Although regression of Barrett's esophagus with rigorous antireflux therapy is controversial,[103–106] vigorous antireflux therapy using fundoplication is recommended in the hope of arresting the transformation through dysplasia to adenocarcinoma.[107] Some attempts have been made at actual ablation of the abnormal epithelium.[108, 109] Annual endoscopic and histologic surveillance is performed indefinitely, to try to diagnose dysplasia before it progresses to adenocarcinoma.

## Respiratory Symptoms and Consequences

As techniques to document nonregurgitant reflux were applied more widely to infants, it became evident that respiratory sequelae were among the most important and most complex manifestations of reflux in children.[110, 111] Although aspiration causes some of these manifestations, particularly aspiration pneumonitis, it has become clear that reflex respiratory responses to refluxate that may remain intraesophageal are actually more common mechanisms. Both lower and upper respiratory tract symptoms may be caused by reflux, and otolaryngologic symptoms have received the most recent attention.

**TABLE 14–3. Prevention of Respiratory Sequelae Due to Reflux**

| STRUCTURES | PROTECTIVE FUNCTIONS | DYSFUNCTIONS |
|---|---|---|
| Stomach | Antegrade emptying | Delayed gastric emptying |
| Esophagus | | |
| Associated structures | Diaphragmatic hiatal tone | Hiatal hernia |
| LES | LES tone | Hypotensive LES |
| | Distinction of gas vs. liquid | Transient LES relaxations to liquid |
| Body | Secondary peristalsis | Impaired esophageal clearance |
| UES | UES tone | Hypotensive UES |
| Larynx, pharynx, mouth | Distinction of gas vs. liquid | Transient UES relaxations to liquid |
| | Swallow reflex | Impaired swallow reflex |
| | Cord closure | Impaired cord closure |
| | Arytenoid-epiglottic approximation | Impaired arytenoid-epiglottic approximation |

From Putnam PE, Ricker DH, Orenstein SR: Gastroesophageal reflux. In Beckerman R, Brouillette R, Hunt C (eds): Respiratory Control Disorders in Infants and Children. Baltimore, Williams & Wilkins, 1992, p 323; © 1992, the Williams & Wilkins Company, with permission.

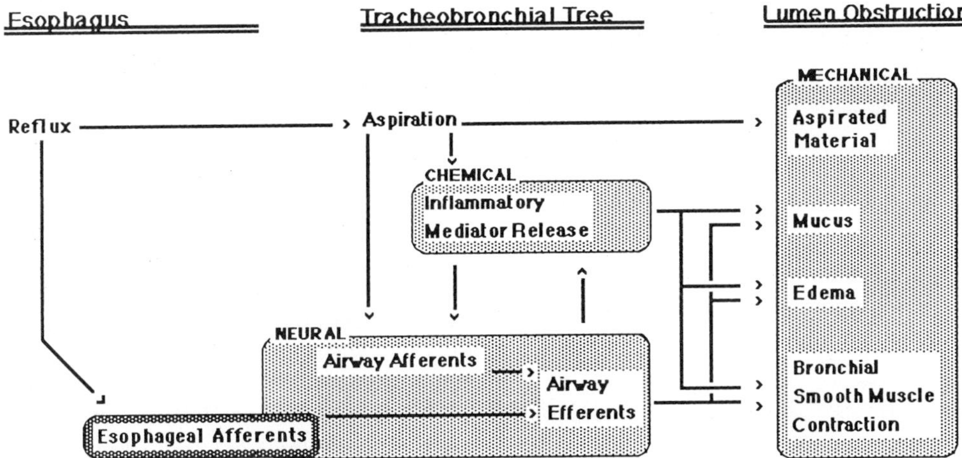


**FIGURE 14–5.** Mechanisms for reflux-associated respiratory dysfunction. Reflux may produce respiratory disease directly, by mechanical occlusion of the lumen with aspirated material, or indirectly. Reflux narrows the airway indirectly via neural or chemical induction of mucus secretion, edema, or muscle contraction. The neural mechanism can have local (airway) or distal (esophageal) afferents. (From Putnam PE, Ricker DH, Orenstein SR: Gastroesophageal reflux. In Beckerman R, Brouilette R, Hunt C [eds]: Respiratory Control Disorders in Infants and Children. Baltimore, Williams & Wilkins, 1992, p 324. © 1992, the William & Wilkins Company, with permission.)

## *Pathophysiology*

The routes of food and air intersect in the pharynx, mandating exquisite controls to prevent food or gastric contents entering the respiratory tract above or below this intersection. Coordination of respiration with swallowing and protections against aspiration are listed in Tables 14–2 and 14–3.[32, 112]

When the physiologic protections fail, reflux causes respiratory disease, by mechanisms diagrammed in Figure 14–5.[32] When any of the three mechanisms (mechanical, neural, or chemical) involve the lower airway, bronchial obstruction results; when they involve the upper airway, laryngeal (or nasal, sinus, or eustacean) obstruction results. Bronchial obstruction, manifest as wheezing, for example, may have as its immediate cause aspirated material, locally produced secretions, mucosal edema, or smooth muscle contraction (Fig. 14–6). The latter three immediate causes may be the end result of either airway stimulation by aspirated material or esophageal stimulation by refluxed material.

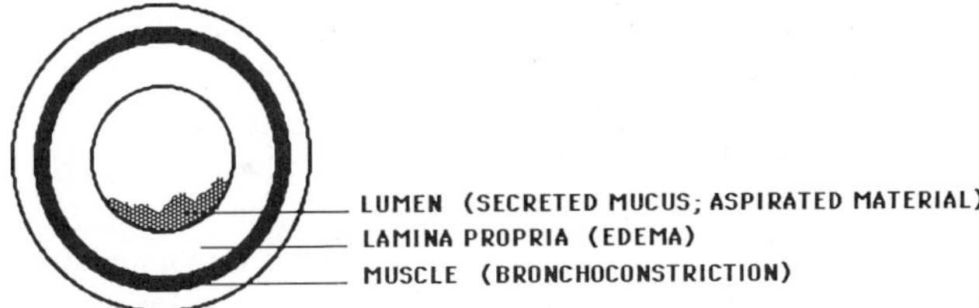


**FIGURE 14–6.** Four potential components of bronchial obstruction. Concentric loci of airway obstruction are the lumen, which can be narrowed by material from extrapulmonary or intrapulmonary sources; the lamina propria, which can be expanded at the expense of the lumen by edema; and the bronchial musculature, which can narrow the lumen by contracting. (From Putnam PE, Ricker DH, Orenstein SR: Gastroesophageal reflux. In Beckerman R, Brouilette R, Hunt C [eds]: Respiratory Control Disorders in Infants and Children. Baltimore, Williams & Wilkins, 1992, p 325. © 1992, the Williams & Wilkins Company, with permission.)

"Macroaspiration" of a large quantity of gastric material may lead to mechanical luminal obstruction and chemical pneumonitis. Reflux rarely results in such severe aspiration except in patients with depressed consciousness. "Microaspiration" insufficient to cause radiographic changes may nevertheless stimulate upper airway neural elements or the release of inflammatory mediators, thereby resulting in laryngospasm or bronchospasm.

Activation of vagal bronchoconstrictive reflexes with acid-sensitive afferents in the esophagus may require both labile bronchial musculature and esophagitis (to "uncover" vagal afferent receptors).

Respiratory disease provoked by reflux can, in turn, contribute to the perpetuation of a vicious circle by exacerbating reflux (Table 14–4). Thus, reflux may be exacerbated by elevated abdominal pressure during coughing and wheezing[110]; reduced intrathoracic pressure during stridor and hiccups[113–116]; pharmacologic lowering of LES pressure by beta-adrenergic agonists, xanthines, or nicotine[117–121]; mechanical disruption of LES competence by nasogastric intubation[122]; diminution of crural support of the LES during mechanical ventilation[15]; increased gastric volume during nutritional rehabilitation with bolus tube feedings[123, 124]; or provocative positioning for chest physiotherapy or mechanical ventilation.[125]

## *Respiratory Disorders Caused or Exacerbated by Reflux*

Reflux results in respiratory disease when the protective mechanisms fail (see Table 14–3).[126]

**PNEUMONIA AND OTHER RESULTS OF ASPIRATION.** Pulmonary aspiration of gastric contents during reflux clearly causes some acute cases of pneumonia and has

**TABLE 14–4. Reflux and Respiratory Disease: Interactions**

**Reflux Causing Respiratory Disorders**

- With aspiration (mechanical obstruction; local neural and chemical mediators)
  - Macroaspiration (aspiration pneumonia)
  - Microaspiration (chronic nonspecific lower respiratory disease? apnea?)
- Without aspiration (neural mediation from esophageal afferents)
  - Reflex bronchospasm
  - Reflex laryngospasm (obstructive apnea; stridor)
  - Reflex central responses (central apnea; bradycardia)

**Respiratory Disorders (Activities/Therapies) Causing Reflux**

- Thoracoabdominal pressure relationships
  - Forced expiration (cough, wheeze)
  - Forced inspiration (stridor, hiccups)
- Lower esophageal sphincter incompetence
  - Reflexive
  - Smoking
  - Drugs
  - Nasogastric tube
- Volume and noxiousness of gastric contents—due to drugs
- Gravity—during chest physiotherapy, mechanical ventilation

also been implicated in some instances of granulomatous pneumonia, lung abscess, obliterative bronchiolitis, pulmonary fibrosis, and chronic bronchitis.[127] Diagnosis of aspiration pneumonia remains problematic in individual cases, because aspiration during reflux is infrequent and is difficult to distinguish from aspiration during swallowing or even from hematogenously acquired pneumonitis. The attempt should be made, however, because the long-term management differs significantly.

**ASTHMA, BRONCHIAL OBSTRUCTION.** Reflux is quantitatively abnormal in 25% to 80% of children with asthma and correlates with measures of respiratory symptoms.[128–132] In some asthmatics, individual reflux episodes show a temporal relationship to wheezing and bronchospastic symptoms improve after therapy for reflux.[133–136] Esophageal acidification induces or potentiates bronchospasm by a vagal reflex, most reliably in asthmatics who manifest esophagitis.[118, 137–144]

Underlying reflux is especially suggested in those asthmatics with nocturnal symptoms, including cough, because esophagitis is more likely to be stimulated at night, microaspiration is less likely to be defended against during sleep, and most other causes of asthmatic symptoms (allergens, stress, viral illnesses) are not increased nocturnally.[132, 139] Reflux-related disease should also be considered in any child whose asthma is resistant to medical management. The modified Bernstein test with associated pulmonary function testing is the most rigorous test to diagnose reflux-related bronchospasm. Alternatively, if abnormal reflux is documented by pH probe or endoscopic esophagitis, for example, response of the asthma to medical management of the reflux may be considered supporting evidence for this mechanism. Although empirical therapy could be considered, the aggressiveness and chronicity of antireflux therapy required in reflux-associated asthma makes definitive diagnosis preferable.[145]

**APNEA, LARYNGEAL OBSTRUCTION.** Symptomatic laryngospasm as a response to reflux generally occurs in younger children than does bronchospasm. This may be because of the relatively small cross-sectional area of the upper airway, because of a tendency toward greater laxity of upper airway structures, or because of an immaturity of nervous control of the respiratory system.

Apnea is among the most serious effects of reflux and may be responsible for a proportion of the infant mortality designated sudden infant death syndrome (SIDS) and a larger proportion of apparent life-threatening events.[146] It is characterized as obstructive (owing to obstruction of the airway, as from laryngospasm) or central (owing to cessation of respiratory efforts); both types may be elaborations of protective reflexes preventing aspiration of pharyngeal material. Reflex laryngospasm is the more common type of reflux-associated apnea and may involve afferents in the esophagus or larynx.[147–150] A temporal relationship between spontaneous reflux and apnea can be documented using a nasal thermistor and thoracic impedance to identify obstructive apnea.[149–151] Some infants with recurrent respiratory arrest become free of such episodes after medical or surgical treatment of reflux.[148, 152, 153]

Reflux-related apnea in infants has been associated with a characteristic symptom complex that should suggest the diagnosis, particularly in the first 6 months of life: a recently fed, supine or seated infant with a prior history of regurgitation becomes rigid, apneic, staring, and plethoric, and then cyanotic or pale.[154] There may be no coughing, choking, or gagging. Parents may remember seeing respiratory efforts, suggesting obstructive apnea. Diagnosis may be achieved by pH probe with polysomnography but requires that episodes be frequent enough for detection during 24 hours of monitoring.

Most infants displaying this worrisome symptom of reflux will outgrow both their reflux and the propensity toward apnea during the first year of life, so the interim management becomes an essential issue. Some authors have advocated fundoplication for all such infants, but, even in infants with life-threatening apnea, rigorous medical therapy, sometimes supplemented with cardiopulmonary monitoring, has proved adequate in most instances.

**STRIDOR, PARTIAL LARYNGEAL OBSTRUCTION.** An interesting analogy to the association of reflux and obstructive apnea is the association of reflux and stridor in a few scattered reports, in which stridor may be seen as a manifestation of incomplete laryngeal obstruction.[113, 114, 155] Reflex laryngospasm manifest as stridor may require the presence of esophagitis, laryngitis, or an abnormal upper respiratory tract. Stridor due to reflux-associated laryngospasm must be distinguished from stridor due to laryngomalacia, laryngeal lesions such as cysts, or laryngitis (which may in turn be due to reflux); this distinction is best accomplished laryngoscopically. Further evaluation may include either the modified Bernstein test or careful documentation of stridor during the pH probe test.

**CENTRAL APNEA AND BRADYCARDIA.** Pathologic central apnea usually occurs during sleep, and its association with reflux is unclear.[156, 157] Laryngeal and nasopharyngeal receptors adjacent to the oropharynx may mediate swallowing-associated and reflux-associated central apnea, which may reach pathologic durations in some infants.[158–160]

Bradycardia unrelated to apnea occurs during or after feeding in some preterm infants; whether this is due to

GERD or to a vagal response to feeding is often unclear.[156, 161]

### Complex Respiratory Diseases and Reflux

In addition to the simple unidirectional causality between reflux and respiratory symptoms discussed earlier, bidirectional interactions may also play a role in more complex pulmonary disorders, several of which have received particular attention.

**BRONCHOPULMONARY DYSPLASIA.** Gastroesophageal reflux may prolong the course of bronchopulmonary dysplasia (BPD)[162–164]; an improvement in pulmonary status has been reported after fundoplication. Although a better understanding of the association of BPD and reflux is needed, the overinflation, wheezing, and airway reactivity that characterize BPD mandate consideration of reflux in patient management.

**CYSTIC FIBROSIS.** Hyperinflation and chronic cough may predispose to reflux in cystic fibrosis (CF).[165–169] Studies have found a greater incidence of reflux in patients with CF than in asymptomatic siblings, an association between reflux and reduced pulmonary function, and a positive response to medical or surgical management of reflux.

As is the case for BPD, further work is needed before the role of reflux in CF is fully understood. In the meantime, reflux should be considered not only as a possible cause of the pulmonary disease in CF but also as a consequence of the pulmonary disease or its treatment.

**ESOPHAGEAL ATRESIA AND TRACHEOESOPHAGEAL FISTULA.**[170–172] Esophageal atresia occurs with tracheoesophageal fistula more than 90% of the time. Chronic respiratory disease often follows repair of esophageal atresia. It has been attributed to aspiration both during and between meals, the former due to anastomotic stricture and the latter due to hypotensive LES with resultant reflux. Both the former and latter are exacerbated by abnormal distal esophageal peristalsis. These abnormalities of esophageal motility appear to be congenital, perhaps the result of morphologic abnormalities of Auerbach's plexus in the distal esophagus.

### Miscellaneous Respiratory Symptoms Related to Reflux

**BELCHING (ERUCTATION).** Belching occurs during transient relaxations of the LES and is an important method of venting air from the stomach.[173] When a fundoplication prevents the normal occurrence of TLESRs, the discomfort of "gas bloat" is the result. Belching requires not only TLESRs but also relaxation of the crural diaphragm and the UES. The UES relaxes in response to esophageal body distention by gas, in contrast to its contractile response to esophageal body distention by fluid. Like the gas bloat that occurs when LES relaxation to gastric distention is prevented, severe chest pain has been described in a patient whose UES failed to relax when gas was refluxed from her stomach into her esophagus.[174]

**HICCUPS (SINGULTUS).** Hiccups are an involuntary reflex contraction of the diaphragm followed by laryngeal closure.[115, 116] Hiccups have been temporally associated with spontaneous and induced esophageal acidification in both adults and infants. Those that occur with reflux may represent an involuntary reflex in the setting of esophagitis. Conversely, the increased gastroesophageal pressure gradient generated by the hiccups may produce the acid reflux. The response of hiccups to therapy for reflux has been variable.

**COUGH.** Cough was the sole presenting manifestation of reflux in some adults, correlated with distal rather than proximal esophageal acidification, and responded to antireflux therapy.[10, 175, 176] Coughing has also been associated with acid reflux in infants. Reflux may cause cough (representing bronchospasm or reflex clearance of microaspiration); on the other hand, coughing may cause reflux by its effect on thoracoabdominal pressure relationships. Care is thus needed in interpretation when cough and reflux coexist (Fig. 14–7).

**HOARSENESS.** Hoarseness has received attention as a possible consequence of reflux in adults and children.[177–179] The described characteristics of the reflux, response to therapy, and postulated mechanisms have varied.[180, 181] Laryngoscopic findings have included normal mucosa; chronic arytenoid or vocal cord inflammation (edema, erythema), granulomas, or contact ulcers; and scarring, stenosis, or cancer. As with other forms of reflux-related respiratory symptoms, postulated mechanisms have included direct acid injury and an indirect path mediated by reflexive chronic coughing and throat clearing in response to reflux. Reflux should be considered in the occasional hoarse patient when evaluation, including laryngoscopy, suggests that reflux is responsible and eliminates other causes.

**PHARYNGONASAL REGURGITATION.** The regurgitation of material into the nasopharynx or nose, either during swallowing or during reflux, is a little-explored phenomenon occurring largely in infants. A description of the findings in 57 infants and children who demonstrated pharyngonasal reflux during barium swallow has been published, as have occasional case reports.[182] Although it represents a failure of the normal airway protections, pharyngonasal regurgitation usually resolves without long-term consequence. It is most frequent in the first 3 months of life and may be associated with prematurity or with neuromuscular disease. It may produce apnea, because it may occlude the nose of infants who are obligate nose-breathers. It may also be responsible for chronic nasal congestion.

**OTHER SUPRAESOPHAGEAL MANIFESTATIONS OF REFLUX.** Chronic subglottic stenosis, sinusitis, otitis, and dental erosions[183] have been compellingly linked to reflux, and data supporting these links are accumulating.[184]

## Neurobehavioral Symptoms

### Sandifer's Syndrome

Neurobehavioral manifestations of reflux are exemplified by the posturing of Sandifer's syndrome:

> The movements are of varying type and severity, involving the head and neck and sometimes the upper part of the trunk, but not the limbs. They usually consist primarily of a sudden extension of the head and neck into the position of opisthotonus. The head may be twisted continuously from side to side. The upper part of the trunk may become bent acutely to one side so

A

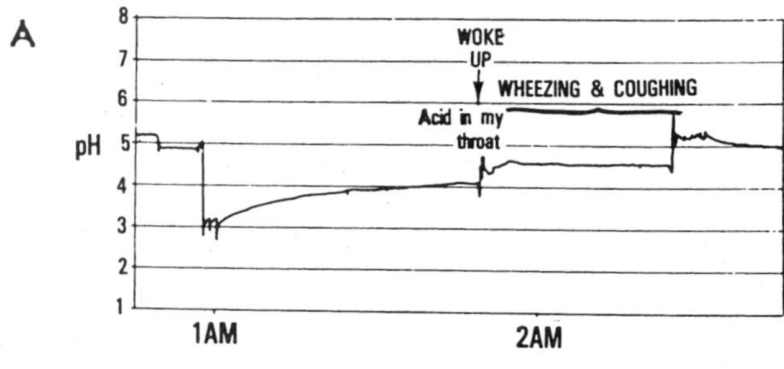


B

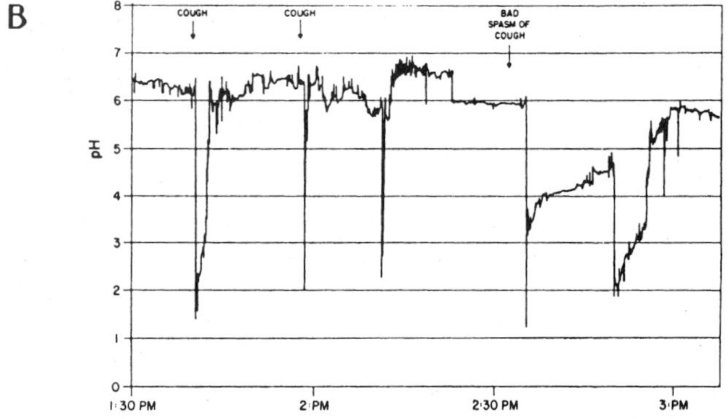


C

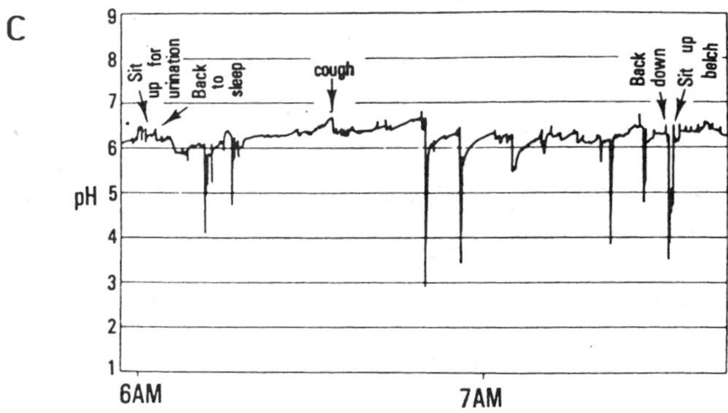


**FIGURE 14–7.** Three relationships between cough and reflux. pH probe tracings from three adults, showing *(A)* nocturnal supine reflux preceding cough in a patient with pathologic reflux, *(B)* cough preceding reflux in a patient with primary respiratory disease, and *(C)* no temporal relationship between cough and reflux in a third patient. These temporal relationships suggest causal ones. (Adapted from Pellegrini CA, DeMeester TR, Johnson LF, et al: Gastroesophageal reflux and pulmonary aspiration: incidence, functional abnormality, and results of surgical therapy. Surgery 1979;86:110–119, with permission.)

that the head is pointing to the floor. The child may seem to be trying to turn himself upside down. A habitual position in some of the children has been lying supine on a bed with the head and neck hyper-extended over the side of the bed pointing to the floor. The head may be held inclined to one side for prolonged periods so that the abnormality might be described as an abnormal posture rather than movement. The movements sometimes continue no matter what other activity the child is engaged in. They may be accentuated during and immediately after meals. They cease during sleep.[185]

Interestingly, manometric evaluation of one child suggested that esophageal clearance may be improved by the posturing.[186]

### Less Specific Neurobehavioral Manifestations

In infants, behaviors that seem to be attenuated versions of Sandifer's syndrome may suggest reflux. These include arching and staring associated with obstructive apnea, periods of cyanosis suggesting neonatal seizures, and irritable stretching or neck extension.

### Rumination

The gagging, regurgitation, mouthing, and swallowing of refluxed material identified as rumination[187] may be either a cause of, or a response to, reflux. In individual infants, it may be difficult to determine whether a primary psychosocial cause exists for the behaviors, which have then resulted in reflux, or whether the reflux is primary and the behaviors are merely a response to esophagitis. In either instance, vicious cycles may be initiated, and diagnosis and treatment of reflux and esophagitis may be important to resolution of the symptoms.

## DIAGNOSIS

### General Principles

Diagnostic evaluation begins with detailed history taking, which may be simplified by use of a structured questionnaire for this exceedingly common disorder.[45, 188, 189] The physical examination is most useful in distinguishing abnormalities that suggest nonreflux disorders causing the symptoms. Formal diagnostic testing is undertaken only in patients suspected of having pathologic effects from reflux. Thus, infants with regurgitation but without nutritional or other sequelae are simply managed with the conservative antireflux measures described later. Even when nutritional effects (such as a drop in weight-for-length percentiles) are manifest, infants whose regurgitation does not suggest anatomic or metabolic disease may also have a trial of such nonpharmacologic therapy without further diagnostic measures if they are closely monitored for improvement during the early stages of therapy. Atypical emesis and emesis that does not clear during initial therapy should usually be evaluated radiographically. Infants with symptoms other than emesis should usually have a diagnostic evaluation tailored to their presentation before being considered for pharmacologic therapy. The role of empirical therapy for this often chronic disorder is unclear in infants and children, as well as in adults.[190] It is probably optimal to limit empirical therapy to a 2-month period.

For pediatric patients whose symptoms suggest esophagitis, the most efficient evaluation is probably esophageal biopsy, with or without endoscopy; endoscopy is useful (especially in older children) to exclude peptic ulcer disease elsewhere in the upper gastrointestinal tract. Evaluation for reflux in patients presenting with respiratory or neurobehavioral symptoms may begin with pH probe, with attention to documentation of synchrony of reflux episodes and discrete symptoms. Such documentation may include concurrent pneumogram or pulmonary function testing. Intraluminal acid infusion may be used in difficult cases and to sort out cause-and-effect relationships. Scintigraphy is useful, perhaps even in place of pH probe testing, in centers at which it has been refined to demonstrate even extremely brief episodes, and especially in patients in whom evaluation for aspiration or delayed gastric emptying is desirable, or in those in whom it is important to detect reflux of neutralized postprandial gastric contents.

Algorithms directed at cost-effective evaluation have been proposed, but a great deal more work is required in this area.[191, 192]

## Radiology

In the pediatric age range, fluoroscopic evaluation is most useful in those children with emesis or feeding problems, to eliminate other diagnoses from consideration. Barium fluoroscopy can identify congenital or acquired structural causes for emesis, such as webs, stenoses, or malrotation of the upper gastrointestinal tract. Dysmotility of the esophagus causing feeding problems in the absence of pathologic reflux can also be suggested by the esophagogram. Severe esophagitis or peptic strictures are reflux-related problems that are amenable to radiographic diagnosis (see Fig. 14–4). Air-contrast (double-contrast) radiography of the esophagus, a fairly specialized procedure, can delineate mucosal detail to a degree that is impossible with routine barium fluoroscopy, but it is not as sensitive as endoscopy.

## Scintigraphy

Technetium scintigraphy produces an image that is less sharp than barium fluoroscopy, but it has several advantages over fluoroscopy for evaluation of reflux. It can monitor for reflux after physiologic, nonacid, meals; the monitoring can be prolonged for an hour or so (until the radionuclide has emptied from the stomach) or even overnight (to evaluate for aspiration) without augmentation of the radiation exposure; and the radiation exposure is typically severalfold less than that from a routine barium study, an important consideration for young children. Its sensitivity for detection of reflux is reported to be 59% to 93%[193–195]; differences in sensitivity are likely to result from differences in technique, and regurgitant reflux is frequently missed.[196] Aspiration and quantitative gastric emptying may be evaluated scintigraphically; however, scintigraphy's sensitivity for aspiration is low and scintigraphic evaluation of gastric emptying may be affected artifactually by superimposition of the distal duodenal image over that of the stomach. Bulk esophageal clearance is also amenable to scintigraphic evaluation. Optimal use of scintigraphy for evaluation of reflux demands that the radiologist take advantage of computer capabilities for continual monitoring in very brief time intervals, rather than merely acquiring an occasional image on the gamma camera (Fig. 14–8).[197–199] This technique is underused, and its capability is undeveloped in most institutions.

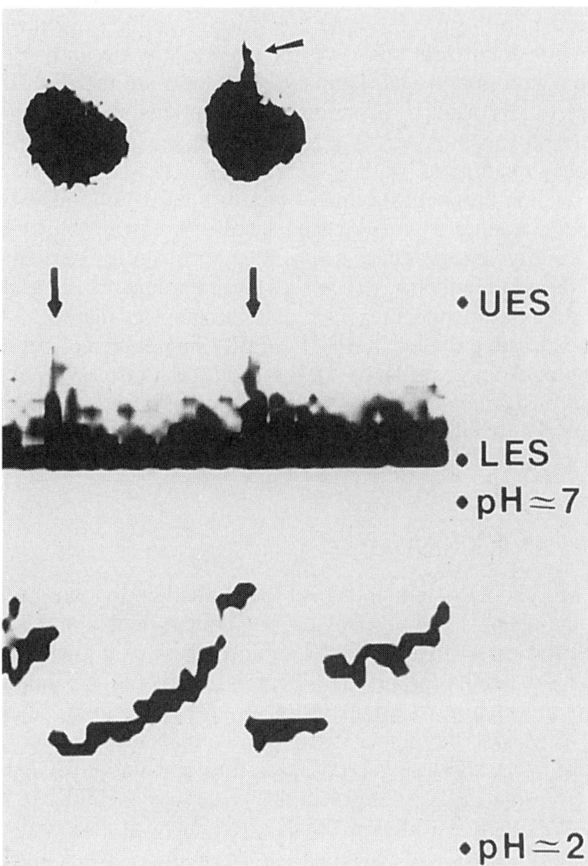


**FIGURE 14–8.** Scintigraphic respresentations of reflux. The top panel shows a posterior view of an infant's stomach filled with $^{99m}$Tc sulfur colloid-labeled apple juice before *(left image)* and during *(right image)* gastroesophageal reflux *(arrow)*. The middle panel shows, on a different occasion, a scintigraphic "condensed dynamic image" representation of two episodes of reflux *(arrows)* over a 10-minute period, depicted essentially continuously; the abscissa is time and the ordinate shows the spatial location of the refluxate in the esophagus, with markers for the upper (UES) and lower (LES) esophageal sphincters. The bottom panel is a pH probe recording from the distal esophagus at the same time as the scintigraphic representation above it; the abscissa is time and the ordinate shows the degree of acidification at one point in the distal esophagus, with markers indicating pH of 7 and 2. (Adapted from Rosenthal MS, Klein HA, Orenstein SR: Simultaneous acquisition of physiological data and nuclear medicine images. J Nucl Med 1988;29:1848–1852, with permission.)

## Endoscopy, Biopsy, and Histology

### *Endoscopy and Biopsy*

Endoscopy is useful to evaluate symptoms of pain, dysphagia, vomiting, or hematemesis to differentiate between reflux disease and other gastrointestinal disease with similar symptoms. Scoring systems for peptic esophagitis recognize a range of endoscopic signs, from erythema and hyperemia (which may be unreliable), through erosions and ulcerations, to strictures and Barrett's esophagus.[200] Such endoscopic evidence should always be supported by histologic evidence from biopsies to identify nonreflux causes for the changes.

Because of the necessarily brief chronology of reflux in infants, reliable endoscopic manifestations of esophagitis are uncommon (despite the frequency of histologic esophagitis).[38, 201] In addition, other lesions of the upper gastrointestinal tract that may mimic inflammatory sequelae of reflux, such as peptic ulcers, are less frequent in infants than in adults. The small size of pediatric endoscopes may make histologic assessment of biopsy samples obtained through them less sensitive for esophagitis, because basal layer hyperplasia and papillary elongation are usually difficult to evaluate.[110] Therefore, some infants may be most efficiently evaluated for peptic esophagitis using a suction biopsy instrument.[192, 202]

Suction esophageal biopsy requires no sedation, takes less than a minute in experienced hands, results in negligible morbidity, and produces a specimen adequate for evaluation of the morphometric as well as the inflammatory measures of reflux esophagopathy.[203, 204] Suction biopsies may be done by estimating the location of the LES using published regression equations (Table 14–5),[205] but they can also be done by rigorously identifying the manometric LES through the biopsy port, so that the false-positive results from distal esophageal mucosa are avoided.[206]

### *Histopathology*

Morphometric parameters of the epithelium that are useful in the diagnosis of esophagitis are papillary height and basal cell thickness (Fig. 14–9).[40] Useful markers of inflammation include lamina propria eosinophils, epithelial eosinophils and neutrophils, "squiggle cells," and telangiectasia.[40] Table 14–6 shows the upper limits of normal for the various parameters signifying esophagitis. Documentation of histologic esophagitis is useful in that it defines a child's reflux as pathologic and thus warranting treatment. It also prompts specific use of acid-reducing therapeutic measures.

Diagnosis of Barrett's esophagus requires histologic evaluation of specimens diligently identified as being of esophageal, rather than gastric, origin. The three types of metaplastic columnar epithelium found in Barrett's esophagus are cardiac ("junctional"—containing gastric mucous cells, but no parietal or chief cells), fundic (containing gastric mucous cells with parietal or chief cells), and intestinal ("specialized columnar"—containing goblet cells and often villi with brush borders; see Fig. 14–9). An "intermediate type," without any parietal, chief, goblet, or brush border cells and no cardiac glands, has also been described.[102] The cardiac epithelium, in particular, and the intermediate type may be extremely difficult to distinguish from normal epithelium from the stomach adjacent to the esophagus, especially in the presence of a hiatal hernia. It seems that dysplasia and carcinoma occur almost exclusively in the intestinal and intermediate epithelium.[102]

A visually recognizable patch of gastric mucosa in the upper third of the esophagus (an "inlet patch") is considered to be a congenital lesion with an incidence of 4%. Usually asymptomatic, it has also been reported to cause upper esophageal stricture. Its presence in the upper esophagus and clear separation from normal gastric epithelium help to distinguish it from Barrett's esophagus.

**TABLE 14–5. Esophageal Length Regression Equations**

| NOSE TO DIAPHRAGM (LES)* | MOUTH TO DIAPHRAGM (LES)* |
|---|---|
| .252 (height in cm) + 5 (*r* = .93)† | .226 (height in cm) + 6.7 (*r* = .97)† |
| .24 (height in cm) + 5.2 (*r* = .96)‡ | |
| .47 (crown-rump in cm) + .57 (*r* = .93)‡ | |

*pH probes and esophageal biopsies are generally performed at 87% of this distance.

†Data from Strobel CT, Byrne WJ, Ament ME, et al: Correlation of esophageal lengths in children with height: application to the Tuttle test without prior esophageal manometry. J Pediatr 1979;103:215–218.

‡Data from Putman PE, Orenstein SR: Determining esophageal length from crown-rump length. Pediatr Res 1991;29:111A.

## Esophageal Manometry

The role of manometry is limited to those children with symptoms suggestive of esophageal dysmotility or those for whom antireflux surgery is contemplated. Infants with repaired esophageal atresia, for example, are a special group in whom reflux is common and often severe, but in whom the frequent peristaltic dysfunction of the distal esophageal segment makes a tight fundoplication potentially hazardous.

## Intraluminal Esophageal Acid Perfusion

Intraluminal esophageal acid perfusion using chest pain (the Bernstein test) or other end points (the modified Bernstein test) has found expanded use recently, both in clinical practice and in research. It permits causal linkage of particular symptoms with esophageal acidification. In contrast to the spontaneous acidification accessible to pH probe, the timing and duration of acidification can be controlled, and complex observations can be precisely timed to periods of acidification and neutralization. This technique has been applied to respiratory symptoms (such as bronchospasm,[138, 143] apnea,[207] stridor,[114] and hiccups[116]), to chest pain in children,[137, 207] and to Sandifer's syndrome (unpublished data).

## Esophageal pH Monitoring

Twenty-four-hour monitoring of intraluminal esophageal pH is regarded in children, as in adults, as the gold standard for diagnosing reflux; and indications and methods for its use have been published.[208–211]

Because children can mimic their usual activities fairly well while hospitalized, and because they need close monitoring to ensure that they neither remove the probe nor destroy the equipment, pediatric pH probe studies are performed more often on inpatients than on outpatients. The probe placement is determined by regression equations linking esophageal length to height,[205] radiographically, or manometrically. Studies of whether monitoring periods briefer than 24 hours are valid measures of reflux have produced conflicting results; most centers still monitor for 24 hours. Although the pH probe can quantify frequency and duration of acid reflux, it cannot detect the more neutral reflux that occurs as long as 2 hours after infant formula feedings. Whether to use less physiologic feedings of acidic liquids (such as apple juice) to preserve the ability to detect postprandial reflux is an unresolved issue. The amount of reflux detected will vary greatly depending on technical points such

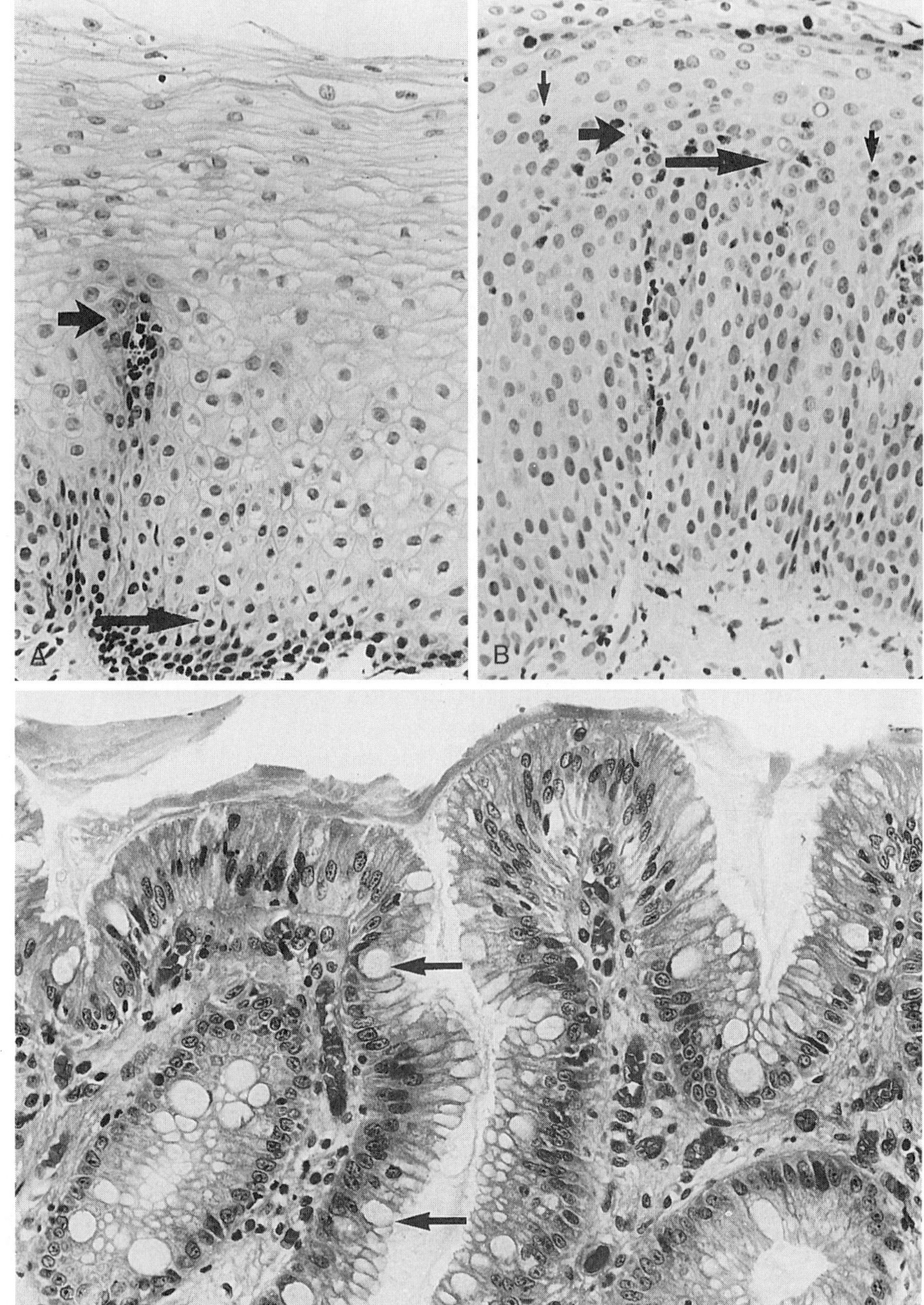


**FIGURE 14–9.** Histologic sequelae of reflux. *A*, Normal esophageal squamous epithelium: the basal layer *(below long arrow)* is about 10% of the epithelial thickness, and papillae *(below short arrow)* are about 50%. Inflammatory cells are absent. *B*, Histologic esophagitis: the basal zone *(below long horizontal arrow)* is expanded to 70% of the epithelial thickness, and papillae *(below short horizontal arrow)* are elongated to 75% of the epithelial thickness. Degranulating eosinophils *(vertical arrows)* infiltrate the epithelium. *C*, Barrett's epithelium: intestinal columnar epithelium with goblet cells *(arrows)* has replaced the normal squamous epithelium in this esophageal specimen. (Adapted from Orenstein SR: Gastroesophageal reflux. Curr Prob Pediatr 1991;21:218, with permission.)

**TABLE 14–6. Histologic Markers for Esophagitis**

| HISTOLOGIC MARKER | NORMAL RANGE | SENSITIVITY (%) | NEGATIVE PREDICTIVE VALUE (%) |
|---|---|---|---|
| Basal cell thickness | <25%* | 89 | 73 |
| Papillary height | <53%* | 30 | 30 |
| Epithelial eosinophils | 0/mm† | 26 | 29 |
| Lamina propria eosinophils | <0.8/mm† | 41 | 33 |
| Epithelial neutrophils | 0/mm† | 15 | 26 |

*Expressed as percentage of total epithelial thickness.

†Expressed as number of cells per millimeter of muscularis mucosae length.

Adapted from Black DD, Haggitt RC, Orenstein SR, Whitington P: Esophagitis in infants: morphometric histologic diagnosis and correlation with measures of gastroesophageal reflux. Gastroenterology 1990;98:1408–1414, with permission.

as feeding type and position in which an infant is placed (Fig. 14–10), details that contribute to the large day-to-day variability in pH probe results.[212, 213]

In addition to identifying patterns of normal or abnormal reflux (Fig. 14–11), pH probe studies are scored to define reflux as quantitatively normal or abnormal. Scoring of pH probe studies generally includes quantification of the number of acid reflux episodes, of the average duration of such episodes, and of the total proportion of time during which the esophagus is acidified (Fig. 14–12). The number of reflux episodes lasting longer than 5 minutes, the duration of the longest episode, and the mean duration of reflux during sleep[214] are other measures reflecting clearance. Age-related normal values for these parameters have been defined (see Fig. 14–3).[27, 42, 215] Derived scores are used by some investigators to define reflux as pathologic or not[216–220]; such derived scores have the disadvantage of obscuring the data on which they are based, and they tend to reduce the information sought from the test to the simple identification of the child as "normal" or "abnormal." A computerized scoring system that quantifies the degree of acidification as well as its temporal aspects is intriguing but has not yet been completely evaluated.[25, 221] Dual and multiple probes have been used to explore the relationship of abnormal proximal reflux to respiratory symptoms.[222, 223]

Perhaps more important than the quantity of reflux is the association of reflux episodes with the symptoms that prompted evaluation (see Fig. 14–7).[224, 225] This can be done during pH probe evaluation, but it requires careful monitoring, particularly in children. Apneic episodes, for instance, can be sought during concurrent pH probe and pneumocardiography, but the pneumocardiographic data must be temporally linked to the pH probe data with precision and must include nasal thermistor or end-tidal carbon dioxide measurements to document obstructive apnea.

Esophageal pH probe monitoring can be used to evaluate response to therapy.[226] Antacids and other acid-reducing therapy should usually be stopped during such repeat pH probe studies, but whether to discontinue prokinetic agents depends on the question being addressed.

## Ultrasound and Esophageal Bilirubin Monitoring

Ultrasound has been proposed as useful in the evaluation of GERD, but experience is quite limited.[227] The same may

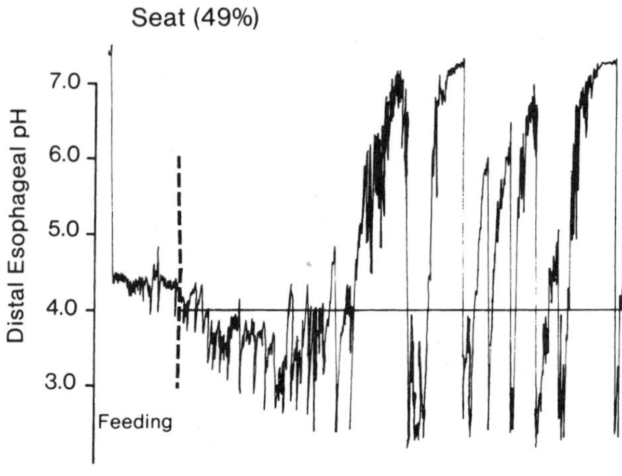


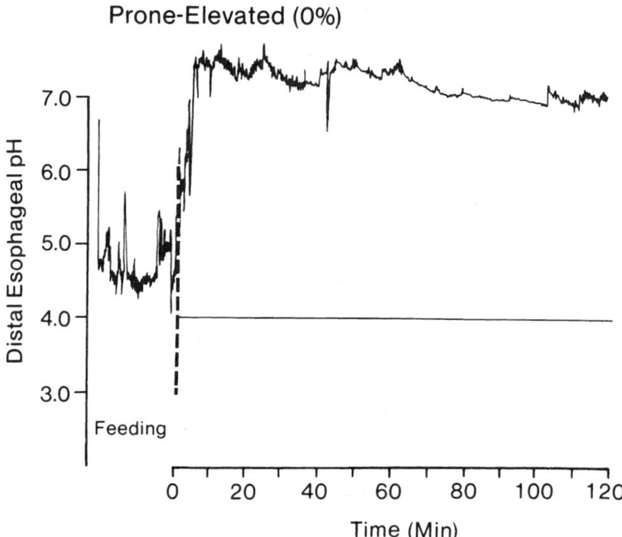


**FIGURE 14–10.** Effect of position on reflux quantity. An infant monitored in two different positions during two otherwise identical postprandial periods. In the seated position, the distal esophageal pH was below 4 for 49% of the time; in the prone, head-elevated position, the pH was never below 4.

be said for a spectrophotometric esophageal probe designed to detect bilirubin and thus to document duodenogastroesophageal reflux.[93]

## Miscellaneous Tests to Diagnose Aspiration

In a patient with an abnormal chest radiograph, the diagnosis of recurrent aspiration during reflux is suggested by impairment of protective mechanisms by neurologic debility or depressed consciousness (see Table 14–3) or by choking and coughing during regurgitation.

Identification of children with aspiration due to disordered swallowing, rather than to reflux, may be achieved by swallowing studies involving videofluoroscopy. (These children often aspirate silently, without airway protection by coughing, so may be difficult to diagnose otherwise.)

Methods to document aspiration of stomach contents include direct sampling of tracheobronchial secretions for de-

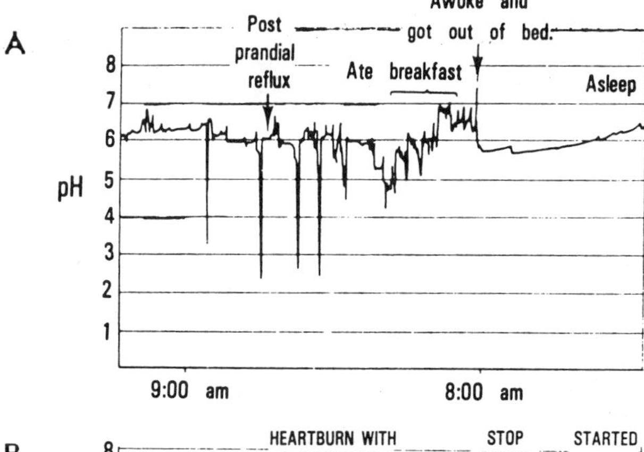


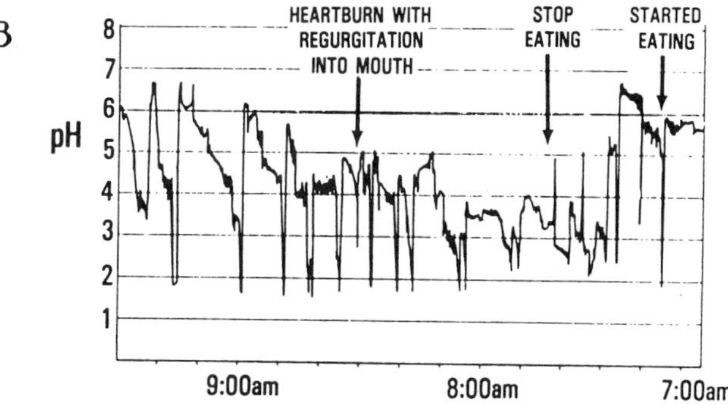


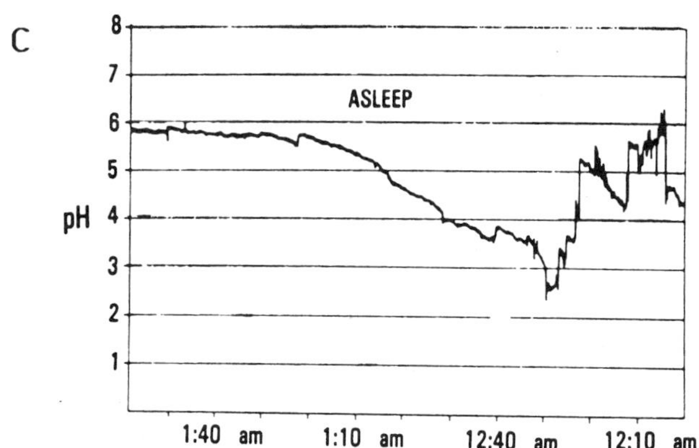


**FIGURE 14–11.** Patterns of reflux detected by pH probe. *A*, Occasional episodes of brief postprandial reflux are normal. *B*, Abnormal postprandial reflux may consist of more frequent episodes, which are nonetheless brief. *C*, Reflux during sleep is generally abnormal; even if infrequent, it may produce pathologic effects because it is poorly cleared during sleep. (Note that time is read from right to left on these tracings.) (Adapted from Johnson LF: New concepts and methods in the study and treatment of gastroesophageal reflux disease. Med Clin North Am 1981;65:1195–1222, with permission.)

tection of lipid-laden macrophages, lactose, or dyes administered intragastrically.[228–231] These methods are invasive, requiring tracheal intubation or bronchoscopy, and are thus most suitable for patients requiring such instrumentation for other reasons. The intubation itself may affect the results. Finally, a high incidence of false-positive results may limit the clinical utility of these tests.

Methods that do not require tracheal intubation or bronchoscopy are the upper gastrointestinal series and the more sensitive gastroesophageal scintigraphy[232]; these methods involve radiation exposure, however, and are fairly insensitive because of the limited duration of monitoring possible. The radionuclide salivagram is another scintigraphic method directed at aspiration.[233] Variability of technique (including positioning, provocative maneuvers, radionuclide dose, and timing of imaging) is probably responsible for the marked variation in the frequency with which aspiration is detected by these methods.

The bronchoscopic and microscopic characteristics of aspiration have been described and suggest the possibility of implicating aspiration by retrospective evaluation soon after a suggestive episode[234, 235]; they may, however, be insensitive for microaspiration.

## Summary of Diagnostic Evaluation

The approach to an individual patient may also be guided by the questions being asked.

### *Is There Pathologic Reflux?*

The presence of pathologic reflux can be defined endoscopically, histologically, by pH probe, radiographically, or scintigraphically. Reflux that produces endoscopic or (more sensitively) histologic esophagitis is certainly pathologic; thus many clinicians use endoscopy with grasp biopsies or blind esophageal suction biopsies to diagnose pathologic reflux.

Reflux that may be pathologic in quantity or effect does not always produce esophagitis, so quantification of reflux and documentation of its temporal relationship to symptoms are often accomplished with intraluminal esophageal pH monitoring. Documentation of reflux in pathologic quantities, even if pathologic effects have not been demonstrated with certainty, may be used to justify treatment of reflux. If the symptoms that prompted therapy resolve during treatment, the resolution is evidence that reflux may have been responsible. The pH probe also may be used to define a temporal association between acid reflux episodes and intermittent symptoms (e.g., respiratory or neurobehavioral). The pH probe does not detect reflux of nonacid material and thus may not detect reflux occurrence after neutral-pH feedings.

Barium esophagography has often been used to diagnose reflux, but its lack of sensitivity (owing to the brief monitoring time) and specificity (owing to the presence of physiologic reflux in normal people) frequently makes it a poor choice for this purpose. It is best used to observe anatomy and function and to eliminate other gastrointestinal disorders from consideration.

Gastroesophageal scintigraphy produces less sharply detailed images than do barium contrast studies, but continuous monitoring throughout an entire postprandial period is possible. It is therefore likely that, with improved software and establishment of normal values, such nuclear medicine studies will be able to define pathologic quantities of reflux with a sensitivity between that of the barium esophagogram and that of the pH probe and to avoid some of the nonphysiologic aspects of the pH probe. Both scintigraphy and barium esophagography can also confirm pulmonary aspiration, although the false-negative result rate may be high.

## GASTROESOPHAGEAL ACID – REFLUX MONITORING

FILE NUMBER

| PATIENT NAME | UNIT NO. | DATE | REFERRING PHYSICIAN |
|---|---|---|---|
| | | / / | |

**HISTORY**

| PATIENT WEIGHT | PATIENT HEIGHT | DISTANCE FROM NARES/INCISORS | BY RADIOGRAPHY / MANOMETRY / CALCULATION |
|---|---|---|---|
| | | | .87 [5 + 0.252 (HT.) ] = |

**pH PROBE STUDY**

| FEEDING NO. TYPE/VOL. CONDITIONS ★ | TIME | TIME pH <4 (%) | #pH<4 | #>5 MIN. | LONGEST | OTHER ★★ |
|---|---|---|---|---|---|---|
| 1. | | | | | | |
| 2. | | | | | | |
| 3. | | | | | | |
| 4. | | | | | | |
| 5. | | | | | | |
| 6. | | | | | | |
| 7. | | | | | | |
| 8. | | | | | | |

**OVERALL STUDY**

| TOTAL | | | | | | |
|---|---|---|---|---|---|---|

| | NORMAL | PATIENT |
|---|---|---|
| **FASTING** | | |
| % TIME pH < 4 | UP TO 2.2 | |
| NO. EPISODES / HR. | UP TO 1 | |
| LONGEST EPISODE (MIN.) | UP TO 12 | |
| **2 HOUR POST PRANDIAL** | **NORMAL** | **PATIENT** |
| % TIME pH < 4 | UP TO 10 | |
| NO. EPISODES / HR. | UP TO 5 | |
| LONGEST EPISODE (MIN.) | UP TO 12 | |

**OVERALL REFLUX SCORE**

| # / d + 4 ( # > 5′ / d ) = | UP TO 50 | |
|---|---|---|

**INTERPRETATION**

★POSITION, MEDICATION, WAKEFULNESS, OTHER ★★VOMIT, WHEEZE, COUGH, APNEA, OTHER ASSOCIATED SX.

| PHYSICIAN'S SIGNATURE | DATE |
|---|---|
| | |

**FIGURE 14–12.** pH probe scoring form. Form used at Children's Hospital of Pittsburgh for scoring pH probe studies. The calculation for insertion distance is near the top of the page. (From Strobel CT, Byrne WJ, Ament ME, et al: Correlation of esophageal lengths in children with height: application to the Tuttle test without prior esophageal manometry. J Pediatr 1979;103:215–218, with permission.) The composite score is found lower on the page. (From Euler AR, Byrne WJ: Twenty-four-hour esophageal intraluminal pH probe testing: a comparative analysis. Gastroenterology 1981;80:957–961, with permission.) (Previously published in Orenstein SR: Gastroesophageal reflux. Curr Prob Pediatr 1991;21:221, with permission.)

### Is There a Temporal Relationship Between Reflux and a Particular Symptom?

Documentation of a temporal association more reliably indicates causality. Therefore, intermittent symptoms and reflux episodes may be tested for temporal association by observing for the symptom (e.g., bronchospasm, apnea) during pH probe monitoring. The association may be documented by video recording, cutaneous oxygen monitoring, pulmonary function tests, pneumocardiogram, nasal thermistor monitoring, or esophageal motility testing.

### Is Reflux Causing the Symptom?

A temporal association between intermittent symptoms and reflux episodes suggests causality, this is more conclusively demonstrated when simulation of reflux by esophageal acid infusion (modified Bernstein test) produces the symptom. Again, observation of the symptom may be supplemented by objective measurements such as those discussed earlier.

## DIFFERENTIAL DIAGNOSIS

Because symptoms of pediatric GERD vary considerably, and because their histories are brief and often secondhand, the differential diagnostic considerations are broad (Table 14–7). Emesis may represent metabolic or structural defects; irritability may represent other causes of discomfort; respiratory symptoms may represent primary respiratory disease; and neurobehavioral signs may represent primary neurologic or metabolic disease. These considerations prompt a broader evaluation than simply evaluating for reflux.

Allergic, or eosinophilic, esophagogastroenteropathy has been recognized to mimic GERD.[236, 237] It may present as emesis and irritability in the infant or as esophageal pain or emesis in the older child. Esophageal biopsy samples often contain copious eosinophils, which in the past were interpreted as due to reflux.[238, 239] There is often a family history of allergy or a positive response to food antigens (or positive radioallergosorbent test), but some children have neither. A 2-week trial of an elemental formula is a cost-effective initial diagnostic test in the infant; finding gastric or duodenal, as well as esophageal, eosinophils is suggestive in the older child.

**TABLE 14–7. Differential Diagnosis of Reflux Symptoms**

| |
|---|
| **Regurgitation, Vomiting (see Tables 2–1, 2–2, and 2–3)** |
| **Pain, Esophagitis Symptoms** |
| Cardiac pain |
| Pulmonary or mediastinal pain; chest wall pain (e.g., costochondritis) |
| Nonesophagitis upper gastrointestinal inflammation (e.g., peptic ulcer disease) |
| Nonesophagitis dysphagia |
| Many possible causes of nonspecific irritability in infants |
| Functional; malingering |
| **Respiratory Symptoms (e.g., wheeze, stridor, cough)** |
| Extrinsic compression (e.g., vascular ring) |
| Intrinsic obstruction (e.g., malformation, foreign body, cyst, tumor) |
| Airways reactive to other stimuli (e.g., allergens, infection) |
| Infection, inflammation, cystic fibrosis, pertussis, asthma, other "central" events (e.g., central apnea; "cough tic") |
| **Neurobehavioral Symptoms (Sandifer's syndrome, seizure-like spells)** |
| Seizures |
| Dystonic reaction to drugs |
| Vestibular disorders |
| Early pertussis |

Adapted from Orenstein SR: Gastroesophageal reflux. Curr Prob Pediatr 1991;21:223, with permission.

## THERAPY

### General Principles

In contrast to adults and older children, most infants with symptomatic reflux will be free of pathologic reflux within a year. Thus, antireflux measures and pharmacotherapy when required will often result in the gratifying resolution of disease in these younger patients.

Stepwise augmentation of therapeutic intensity begins with conservative antireflux measures, continuing with a prokinetic agent if pathologic reflux is present. Acid-reducing therapy is added in that majority of patients in whom esophagitis is present. Surgical management is reserved for serious manifestations unresponsive to maximal nonsurgical therapy or for intractable disease persisting beyond 18 to 24 months of age (Table 14–8).

The issues related to long-term management of this chronic, relapsing disease in older children and adults are complex and include the use of intermittent, low-dose, or nocturnal maintenance pharmacotherapy.[240]

### Conservative Antireflux Measures

Initial treatment of reflux typically involves body positioning and dietary measures.

#### Positioning

**INFANTS.** In the past, the recommendation for infants, as for older patients, was to be seated ("upright") to minimize reflux. However, it has been established that the poor truncal tone of infants actually makes seated positioning detrimental[21]; thus, prone positioning is desirable whenever infants with reflux are not being held strictly vertical by their caretakers. Although elevation of the head of the bed has been recommended for infants in the prone position, a large controlled study failed to show a significant benefit of such head elevation when compared with the simple flat prone position.[241] In addition to decreasing reflux, the prone position improves gastric emptying, decreases aspiration, decreases energy expenditure,[2] decreases crying time, and has numerous beneficial effects on respiratory disease. The right-side-down lateral position has theoretical advantages, such as augmentation of gastric emptying as well as separating gastric contents from the gastroesophageal junction, but this position has not been definitively compared with the prone position. The American Academy of Pediatrics' recommendation—that normal infants be placed supine (or side-lying) to sleep to minimize risk of SIDS—specifically

**TABLE 14–8. Therapy for Reflux**

I. Conservative
  A. Position: prone or completely upright (avoid supine, semi-seated)
  B. Thicken infant feedings: 1 Tbsp dry rice cereal/oz formula (= 30 cal/oz, if original formula is 20 cal/oz)
  C. Fast before bedtime
  D. Avoid large meals, obesity, tight clothing
  E. Avoid foods and medications that lower LES tone or increase gastric acidity:
    Fatty foods, citrus, tomato, carbonated or acid beverages, coffee, alcohol, smoke exposure
    Anticholinergics, adrenergics, xanthines (theophylline, caffeine), calcium channel blockers, prostaglandins
II. Pharmacologic*
  A. Prokinetic:
    Metoclopramide (0.1 mg/kg/dose qid: AC, HS)
      {restlessness, drowsiness, dystonic reactions—antidote: diphenhydramine}
      {{gastrointestinal obstruction, perforation, hemorrhage; pheochromocytoma; extrapyramidal risk}}
    Bethanechol (0.1–0.3 mg/kg/dose tid or qid: AC, HS)
      {cholinergic: hypotension, flushing, headache, bronchospasm, salivation, abdominal cramping}
      {{urinary or gastrointestinal obstruction, perforation, hemorrhage, recent surgery, peritonitis, hypotension, bradycardia, epilepsy, asthma, hyperthyroidism, peptic ulcer}}
    Cisapride (0.2 mg/kg/dose qid AC, HS)
      {cramping, arrhythmias}
      {{concurrent use of macrolide or antifungal antibiotics: ketoconazole, itraconazole, miconazole, troleandomycin, erythromycin, clarithromycin}}
  B. Anti-Acid:
    Cimetidine (5–10 mg/kg/dose qid AC, HS) {headache, confusion, pancytopenia, gynecomastia, cholestasis}
    Ranitidine (4–5 mg/kg/day divided bid to tid) {similar to cimetidine, less gynecomastia, more hepatitis}
    Famotidine (0.5 mg/kg/dose bid or tid; adult 40 mg HS)
    Omeprazole (0.7–3.3 mg/kg/dose qd or divide bid; adult 20 mg HS or bid)
    Antacids (0.5–1 mL/kg/dose, 3–8 times a day: 1–2 hr PC, HS) {diarrhea, constipation, rickets, aluminum or magnesium toxicity}
  C. Barrier or miscellaneous mechanism
    Sucralfate slurry (1 g in 5 to 15-mL solution, qid PC, HS)—protects against bile salts, trypsin, acid
      {constipation, gastric concretions, potential binding of other medications}
    Alginate-antacid (0.2–0.5 mL/kg/dose 3–8 times a day PC)
III. Surgical
    Fundoplication (complete vs. loose wrap; ± gastrostomy, ± pyloroplasty)

*Usual course is 8 weeks.
( ) = Common doses.
{ } = Partial list of side effects.
{{ }} = Partial list of contraindications.

exempts infants with GERD; virtually all of the additional risk of SIDS from prone positioning can be eliminated by avoidance of puffy, potentially suffocating bedding.[242, 243]

**CHILDREN.** For older children, optimal positioning probably comprises standing or sitting upright while awake and sleeping prone, possibly with the head of the bed elevated. At any age, the prone position is preferable to the supine during recumbency; supine positions, including supine-seated positions, worsen reflux, as do head-down positions. Thus, chest physiotherapy that requires provocative positions is probably best performed fasting and perhaps with antacid pretreatment. Chronically ventilated patients may benefit from prone in preference to supine positioning, in spite of the technical difficulties with head positioning in such patients.

### Diet

**THICKENING OF INFANT FORMULA.** Thickening of formula has been recommended for years as therapy for infants with reflux. Usually this thickening is achieved by adding rice cereal to milk formula in a concentration that requires enlarging the nipple to allow adequate flow. Although this therapy has not been shown by pH probe or by scintigraphic evaluation to decrease reflux, it does decrease the number and total volume of emeses.[55] Because such thickening also diminishes crying (and therefore probably energy expenditure) and increases the caloric density of the formula, it is ideal therapy for infants with nutritional deficits due to regurgitant reflux. Although infants are unable to retain all of the extra energy and nitrogen in the cereal, infants with regurgitation improve their weight accretion during such therapy. Whether it should also be used for nonregurgitant reflux is not yet resolved. Although not observed in a very short-term study, the main side effect is constipation.

**SMALL AND FREQUENT FEEDINGS.** Small, frequent meals are recommended because of the probable correlation between gastric volume and reflux quantity. It is possible, however, that the frequency of feedings might counteract the benefits of the small feedings by converting more time to the postprandial period, in which most reflux occurs. This is a complex issue, with no clear answers at present. A reasonable approach is to recommend smaller, more frequent feedings for those infants who are being given unusually large volumes at infrequent feedings.

Fasting several hours before bedtime in the older child is relatively simple to implement and is uncontroversial, except perhaps in children with very poor nutrition.

**OTHER DIETARY MEASURES.** In older pediatric patients, weight reduction in the obese and avoidance of foods known to have detrimental effects on LES tone or on gastric acidity are frequently suggested. These foods include fatty foods, acid foods (such as many citrus juices, carbonated beverages, and tomato products[57]), coffee, and alcohol. Compliance with these recommendations is probably limited.

### Other Conservative Measures

Additional measures that can be used in infants and children, as in adults, are avoidance of tight clothing, slow infusion of intragastric tube feedings,[244] and elimination of exposure to secondhand smoke[245, 246] and to unnecessary drugs that are known to exacerbate reflux.

## Pharmacotherapy

Medications are usually not added to the treatment regimen unless pathologic reflux has been demonstrated. Reasonable exceptions are prophylactic pharmacotherapy during exacerbations of severe respiratory disease, during short-term mechanical ventilation, or in other provocative situations such as aggressive nutritional rehabilitation with intragastric feedings.

These drugs consist of prokinetic agents, which augment sphincter pressure and may also increase gastric emptying, and acid-reducing agents, which counteract the major known injurious component of gastric contents. Several maintenance protocols have been compared in adults,[247] but the optimal algorithm for the use of these agents in children is not established. Using a prokinetic agent for reflux without esophagitis, and adding acid suppression for esophagitis, sucralfate for severe erosions and ulceration, and antacids for undiagnosed or breakthrough symptoms is logical. Cost-effectiveness strategies are in initial stages of exploration.[248]

### Prokinetic Agents

For children in whom pathologic gastroesophageal reflux has been demonstrated, the use of a prokinetic agent has theoretical support for its ability to raise tonic LES pressure, improve esophageal clearance, and speed gastric emptying.[249] However, all prokinetic agents have had mixed clinical results, and none decreases the frequency of LES relaxations.

Experience with cisapride, a noncholinergic, non-antidopaminergic agent that enhances postganglionic acetylcholine release, has been favorable in children; and it has superseded other prokinetic agents in the management of pediatric GERD.[250–252] Because of rare reports of serious arrhythmias during concurrent use with some antibiotics, we provide a list of the implicated antibiotics to the parents with each new prescription.[253, 254]

Other prokinetics are used when cisapride is contraindicated or ineffective. Bethanechol, a cholinergic drug that augments LES pressure, esophageal peristaltic amplitude and duration, and salivary flow, has had mixed clinical results; and its potential for exacerbating bronchospasm limits its use in children with respiratory symptoms. Metoclopramide, a dopamine antagonist, raises LES pressure and improves gastric emptying and esophageal peristalsis, but the narrow margin of error between therapeutic effect and central nervous system side effects mandates caution in its use.[255, 256] Published experience with domperidone, a peripheral dopamine antagonist, is even more limited in children than in adults.[257] Erythromycin increases gastric emptying but may have no significant effect on esophageal motility.

### Acid-Reducing and Mucosal-Protecting Agents

Because a relationship has been demonstrated between esophageal acid exposure and esophagitis, even in infants, it is reasonable to treat children who have esophagitis with acid-reducing therapies. Such therapies include antisecretory and acid-neutralizing drugs.

**ANTISECRETORY.** Histamine-receptor ($H_2$) antagonists have been used successfully in children.[258] The most extensive experience is with cimetidine, but ranitidine, famotidine, and nizatidine have also been used. Currently, cimetidine has several advantages in the child already being treated with a four-times-daily prokinetic agent: an identical dosing schedule, more clearly defined dosing requirements,[259] and lower (generic) cost.

Agents such as omeprazole and lansoprazole that block the parietal cell proton pump reduce acid secretion more completely than do the histamine-receptor antagonists, which leave the gastrin receptors and cholinergic input unaffected. They are effective in otherwise intractable esophagitis, but problems of rapid relapse on withdrawal and concerns about safety limit their use in children to those requiring particularly aggressive therapy.[260–263]

**ACID-NEUTRALIZING.** It has been suggested that antacids are as efficacious as $H_2$ antagonists for treatment of esophagitis in young children,[264] but the frequency of administration (more than six doses per day) makes compliance unlikely, and the large dose raises concern about potential side effects. A very few infants have developed craniosynostosis and rickets after chronic antacid therapy. They may have had other environmental, dietary, or inherited causes, but it is probably wise to limit chronic antacid use and to avoid using it in formula feedings, because of a potential to bind calcium or produce aluminum or magnesium toxicity.[265–267]

A good strategy is to use $H_2$ blockade for children with proven esophagitis who are already being treated with a prokinetic. Antacids can be used as supplemental therapy for pain, as limited primary therapy for children who would benefit from their constipating (aluminum) or stool-softening (magnesium) features, or as short-term empirical therapy when esophagitis has not been documented.

**MUSCOSAL PROTECTIVE.** In tablet or suspension, sucralfate has been shown in one study involving children to be comparable in efficacy to cimetidine, although the dose of the latter was low.[268] Sucralfate is a particularly useful agent in children with severe esophagitis encompassing erosions or ulcerations.[269]

Explorations of the efficacy of alginate-antacid compounds in children are similarly scarce, as well as contradictory.

## Surgical Therapy

Surgical therapy is used in children with severe or intractable symptoms and is considered the most definitive antireflux therapy.[270, 271] The recent expansion of management options not requiring laparotomy (proton pump inhibitors, gastrojejunostomy feedings,[272, 273] and laparoscopic fundoplication[274, 275]) has somewhat reduced the need for standard Nissen fundoplication (Fig. 14–13).[276, 277]

### Fundoplication

**INDICATIONS.** There are several groups of children with reflux disease who are more likely to require fundoplication. These include children with peptic strictures, Barrett's esophagus, neurologic deficits, gastrostomy tube feedings, or respiratory disease associated with intractable reflux (e.g., repaired esophageal atresia or BPD).

Neurologically devastated children with reflux often are chronically supine, have increased abdominal pressure due to spasticity, and have poor oropharyngeal handling of food. They are thus susceptible to respiratory compromise from aspiration during feeding as well as from reflux. Although percutaneous gastrostomy feedings have been used for nutrition in such patients, a gastrostomy tube combined with fundoplication is often optimal treatment. Infants with BPD

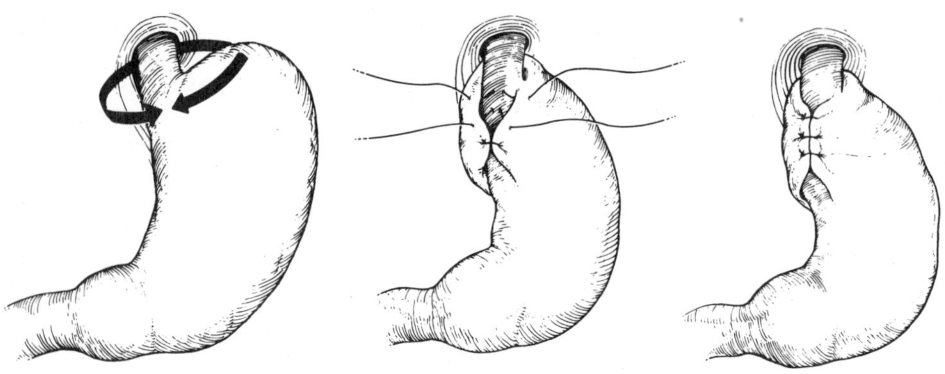

**FIGURE 14–13.** Diagram of a Nissen fundoplication. (From Schatzlein MH, Ballantine TVN, Thirunavukkarasu S, et al: Gastroesophageal reflux in infants and children. Arch Surg 1979; 114:505–510. Copyright 1979, American Medical Association, with permission.)

may require fundoplication because their provocative positioning, chronic ventilator dependency, need for nasogastric feedings, disturbed thoracoabdominal pressure relationships, and aggravating medications make them resistant to medical management of reflux.

In neurologically normal older children with reflux-related respiratory symptoms or esophagitis, medical treatment of the reflux is usually effective, but the symptoms often recur when such therapy is discontinued. For such patients the alternatives of chronic medical therapy and surgical fundoplication can be weighed with the families.

**SUCCESS RATE.** Fundoplication is the most reliable way to prevent reflux, the efficacy being related to the function of the wrap as a valve as well as to its known augmentation of LES pressure.[278, 279] Most pediatric series report the reduction or elimination of reflux in more than 90% of patients. Accurate preoperative identification of reflux as the cause of the symptoms is crucial: some failures of surgical therapy have resulted from an incorrect assumption that reflux was the source of the symptoms in need of therapy. An important, but unresolved, issue is the long-term efficacy of the wrap, which may gradually become incompetent.[280, 281]

**COMPLICATIONS.** Although surgical success rates are high, both short- and long-term complications are frequent, and are more common in those children most likely to require surgical therapy: those with neurologic deficits or strictures.[282] Complications include herniation of the wrap through the hiatus, small bowel obstruction due to adhesions, and intraperitoneal leakage through an associated gastrostomy. Long-term problems include "gas bloat," inability to burp or vomit when necessary, and dysphagia. Problems related to gastric emptying include "dumping" (rapid emptying) and retching due to delayed emptying.[283]

Preventive strategies for these complications include the use of an intraluminal bougie during surgery; attention to crural closure and fixation of the wrap to the crura and diaphragm; pyloromyotomy in patients with preoperative gastric stasis[284]; and avoidance of trauma to intestinal serosa or liver capsule.

"Loose" or Thal fundoplications are applicable in patients with esophageal dysmotility, such as esophageal atresia, but the reduced efficacy makes them of limited benefit if complete prevention of reflux is desired, and they may not be useful in children with neurologic disability or feeding gastrostomies. A gastrostomy for feeding and venting is useful in those children in whom dysfunctional swallow contributes to respiratory disease and for those in whom gas bloat may be a problem; a gastrostomy is often performed in infants to protect the wrap postoperatively, even if its later closure is anticipated.

### *Crural Repair*

Hiatal hernia is not repaired unless it is associated with complications, with intractable reflux being the most common. Thus, crural repair is undertaken as part of an antireflux procedure, generally fundoplication.

## REFERENCES


1. Dent J, Dodds W, Hogan W, et al: Factors that influence induction of gastroesophageal reflux in normal human subjects. Dig Dis Sci 1988;33:270–275.
2. Kawahara H, Dent J, Davidson G: Mechanisms responsible for gastroesophageal reflux in children. Gastroenterology 1997;113:399–408.
3. Mittal R, Holloway R, Penagini R, et al: Transient lower esophageal sphincter relaxation. Gastroenterology 1995;109:601–610.
4. Omari T, Miki K, Davidson G, et al: Characterisation of relaxation of the lower oesophageal sphincter in healthy premature infants. Gut 1997;40:370–375.
5. Dent J, Holloway R, Toouli J, et al: Mechanisms of lower oesophageal sphincter incompetence in patients with symptomatic gastrooesophageal reflux. Gut 1988;29:1020–1028.
6. Preiksaitis H, Tremblay L, Diamant N: Nitric oxide mediates inhibitory nerve effects in human esophagus and lower esophageal sphincter. Dig Dis Sci 1994;39:770–775.
7. Mittal RK, Smith TK: Is nitric oxide the noncholinergic, nonadrenergic neurotransmitter responsible for lower esophageal sphincter relaxation? Gastroenterology 1993;104:656–658.
8. Dodds W, Dent J, Hogan W, et al: Mechanisms of gastroesophageal reflux in patients with reflux esophagitis. N Engl J Med 1982;307:1547–1552.
9. Werlin S, Dodds W, Hogan W, et al: Mechanisms of gastroesophageal reflux in children. J Pediatr 1980;97:244–249.
10. Feranchak A, Orenstein S, Cohn J: Behaviors associated with onset of gastroesophageal reflux episodes in infants: prospective study using split-screen video and pH probe. Clin Pediatr 1994;33:654–662.
11. Mittal R, Rochester D, McCallum R: Effect of the diaphragmatic contraction on lower oesophageal sphincter pressure in man. Gut 1987;28:1564–1568.
12. Kraus B, Sinclair J, Castell D: Gastroesophageal reflux in runners: characteristics and treatment. Ann Intern Med 1990;112:429–433.
13. Altorki N, Skinner D: Pathophysiology of gastroesophageal reflux. Am J Med 1989;86:685–689.
14. Stolar CJ, Levy JP, Dillon PW, et al: Anatomic and functional abnormalities of the esophagus in infants surviving congenital diaphragmatic hernia. Am J Surg 1990;159:204–207.
15. Marino W, Jain N, Pitchumoni C: Induction of lower esophageal sphincter (LES) dysfunction during use of the negative pressure body ventilator. Am J Gastroenterol 1988;83:1376–1380.
16. Santos G: Is hiatus hernia responsible for reflux? Chest 1983;84:242–244.

17. DiLorenzo C, Mertz H, Rehm D, et al: Postnatal maturation of gastric response to distension in newborn infants. Gastroenterology 1994;107:1222.
18. Hillemeier A, Lange R, McCallum R, et al: Delayed gastric emptying in infants with gastroesophageal reflux. J Pediatr 1981;98:190–193.
19. Lin C-H, Tolia V, Kuhns L, et al: Role of gastric emptying in infants with complicated gastroesophageal reflux. Pediatr Res 1989;25:118A.
20. Cannon R, Stadalnik R: Postprandial gastric motility in infants with gastroesophageal reflux and delayed gastric emptying. J Nucl Med 1993;34:2120–2123.
21. Orenstein S, Whitington P, Orenstein D: The infant seat as treatment for gastroesophageal reflux. N Engl J Med 1983;309:760–763.
22. Howard J, Reynolds R, Frei J, et al: Macroscopic healing of esophagitis does not improve esophageal motility. Dig Dis Sci 1994;39:648–654.
23. Cucchiara S, Staiano A, DiLorenzo C, et al: Esophageal motor abnormalities in children with gastroesophageal reflux and peptic esophagitis. J Pediatr 1986;108:907–910.
24. Helm J, Dodds W, Pelc L, et al: Effect of esophageal emptying and saliva on clearance of acid from the esophagus. N Engl J Med 1984;310:284–288.
25. Vandenplas Y, Franckx-Goossens A, Pipeleers-Marichal M: Area under pH 4: advantages of a new parameter in the interpretation of esophageal pH monitoring data. J Pediatr Gastroenterol Nutr 1989;9:34–39.
26. Collen M, Lewis J, Benjamin S: Gastric acid hypersecretion in refractory gastroesophageal reflux disease. Gastroenterology 1990;98:654–661.
27. Sutphen J, Dillard V: Effects of maturation and gastric acidity on gastroesophageal reflux in infants. Am J Dis Child 1986;140:1062–1064.
28. Orlando R: The pathogenesis of gastroesophageal reflux disease: the relationship between epithelial defense, dysmotility, and acid exposure. Am J Gastroenterol 1997;92:3S–7S.
29. Little F, Kohut R, Koufman J, Marshall R: Effect of gastric acid on the pathogenesis of subglottic stenosis. Ann Otol Rhinol Laryngol 1985;94:516–519.
30. Davidson G, Dent J, Willing J: Monitoring of upper oesophageal sphincter pressure in children. Gut 1991;32:607–611.
31. Sondheimer J: Upper esophageal sphincter and pharyngoesophageal motor function in infants with and without gastroesophageal reflux. Gastroenterology 1983;85:301–305.
32. Putnam PE, Ricker DH, Orenstein SR: Gastroesophageal reflux. In Beckerman R, Brouilette R, Hunt C (eds): Respiratory Control Disorders in Infants and Children. Baltimore, Williams & Wilkins, 1992, pp 322–341.
33. Jeffery H, Heacock H: Impact of sleep and movement on gastro-oesophageal reflux in healthy, newborn infants. Arch Dis Child 1991;66:1136–1139.
34. Sondheimer J: Clearance of spontaneous gastroesophageal reflux in awake and sleeping infants. Gastroenterology 1989;97:821–826.
35. Treem W, Davis P, Hyams J: Gastroesophageal reflux in the older child: presentation, response to treatment and long-term follow-up. Clin Pediatr 1991;30:435–440.
36. Carre I: A historical review of the clinical consequences of hiatal hernia (partial thoracic stomach) and gastroesophageal reflux. In Gellis S (ed): Gastroesophageal Reflux: Report of the 76th Ross Conference on Pediatric Research. Columbus, OH, Ross Laboratories, 1979, pp 1–12.
37. Shepherd R, Wren J, Evans S, et al: Gastroesophageal reflux in children: clinical profile, course and outcome with active therapy in 126 cases. Clin Pediatr 1987;26:55–60.
38. Shub M, Ulshen M, Hargrove C, et al: Esophagitis: a frequent consequence of gastroesophageal reflux in infancy. J Pediatr 1985;107:881–884.
39. Hyams J, Ricci A Jr, Leichtner A: Clinical and laboratory correlates of esophagitis in young children. J Pediatr Gastroenterol Nutr 1988;7:52–56.
40. Black D, Haggitt R, Orenstein S, Whitington P: Esophagitis in infants: morphometric histologic diagnosis and correlation with measures of gastroesophageal reflux. Gastroenterology 1990;98:1408–1414.
41. Johnson L, DeMeester T: Twenty-four-hour pH monitoring of the distal esophagus: a quantitative measure of gastroesophageal reflux. Am J Gastroenterol 1974;62:325–332.
42. Vandenplas Y, Sacre-Smits L: Continuous 24-hour esophageal pH monitoring in 285 asymptomatic infants 0–15 months old. J Pediatr Gastroenterol Nutr 1987;6:220–224.
43. Jeffery J, Page M: Developmental maturation of gastro-oesophageal reflux in preterm infants. Acta Paediatr 1995;84:245–250.
44. Campfield J, Shah B, Angelides A, Hirsch B: Incidence of gastroesophageal reflux (GER) in VLBW. Pediatr Res 1992;31:106A.
45. Nelson S, Chen E, Syniar G, Christoffel K: Prevalence of symptoms of gastroesophageal reflux during infancy. Arch Pediatr Adolesc Med 1997;151:569–572.
46. Castell D: Introduction to pathophysiology of gastroesophageal reflux. In Castell D, Wu W, Ott D (eds): Gastro-Esophageal Reflux Disease: Pathogenesis, Diagnosis, Therapy. Mount Kisco, NY, Futura, 1985, pp 3–9.
47. Orenstein S: Gastroesophageal reflux. In Hyman P, DiLorenzo C (eds): Pediatric Gastrointestinal Motility Disorders. New York, Academy Professional Information Services, 1994, pp 55–88.
48. Locke GI, Talley N, Fett S, et al: Prevalence and clinical spectrum of gastroesophageal reflux: a population-based study in Olmsted County, Minnesota. Gastroenterology 1997;112:1448–1456.
49. Carre I: The natural history of the partial thoracic stomach (hiatus hernia) in children. Arch Dis Child 1959;34:344–353.
50. Isolauri J, Luostarinen M, Isolauri E, et al: Natural course of gastroesophageal reflux disease: 17–22 year follow-up of 60 patients. Am J Gastroenterol 1997;92:37–41.
51. Kuster E, Ros E, Toledo-Pimentel V, et al: Predictive factors of the long term outcome in gastro-oesophageal reflux disease: Six year follow up of 107 patients. Gut 1994;35:8–14.
52. Pace F, Santalucia F, Bianchi Porro G: Natural history of gastro-oesophageal reflux disease with oesophagitis. Gut 1991;32:845–848.
53. Paton J, Nanayakkhara C, Simpson H: Vomiting and gastro-oesophageal reflux. Arch Dis Child 1988;63:837–838.
54. Orenstein S, Dent J, Deneault L, et al: Regurgitant reflux, vs. non-regurgitant reflux, is preceded by rectus abdominus contraction in infants. Neurogastroenterol Mot 1994;6:271–277.
55. Orenstein S, Magill H, Brooks P: Thickening of infant feedings for therapy of gastroesophageal reflux. J Pediatr 1987;110:181–186.
56. Ryan P, Lander M, Ong T, Shepherd R: When does reflux oesophagitis occur with gastro-oesophageal reflux in infants? A clinical and endoscopic study, and correlation with outcome. Aust Paediatr J 1983;19:90–93.
57. Feldman M, Barnett C: Relationships between the acidity and osmolality of popular beverages and reported heartburn. Gastroenterology 1995;108:125–131.
58. Heine R, Jaquiery A, Lubitz L, et al: Role of gastro-oesophageal reflux in infant irritability. Arch Dis Child 1995;73:121–125.
59. Vandenplas Y, de Pont S, Devreker T, et al: Gastroesophageal reflux (GER) as a cause for excessive crying in infants. J Pediatr Gastroenterol Nutr 1995;21:333.
60. Dellert S, Hyams J, Treem W, Geertsma M: Feeding resistance and gastroesophageal reflux in infancy. J Pediatr Gastroenterol Nutr 1993;17:66–71.
61. Hyman P: Gastroesophageal reflux: one reason why baby won't eat. J Pediatr 1994;125:S103–S109.
62. Catto-Smith A, Machida H, Butzner J, et al: The role of gastroesophageal reflux in pediatric dysphagia. J Pediatr Gastroenterol Nutr 1991;12:159–165.
63. Triadafilopoulos G: Nonobstructive dysphagia in reflux esophagitis. Am J Gastroenterol 1989;84:614–618.
64. Allen M, McIntosh D, Robinson M: Healing or amelioration of esophagitis does not result in increased lower esophageal sphincter or esophageal contractile pressure. Am J Gastroenterol 1990;85:1331–1334.
65. Gill R, Bowes K, Murphy P, Kingma Y: Esophageal motor abnormalities in gastroesophageal reflux and the effects of fundoplication. Gastroenterology 1986;91:364–369.
66. Marshall J, Gerhardt D: Improvement in esophageal motor dysfunction with treatment of reflux esophagitis: a report of two cases. Am J Gastroenterol 1982;77:351–353.
67. Booth IW: Silent gastro-oesophageal reflux: how much do we miss? Arch Dis Child 1992;67:1325–1327.
68. Ben Rejeb M, Bouche O, Zeitoun P: Study of 47 consecutive patients with peptic esophageal stricture compared with 3880 cases of reflux esophagitis. Dig Dis Sci 1992;37:733–736.
69. Rode H, Millar AJW, Brown RA, Cywes S: Reflux strictures of the esophagus in children. J Pediatr Surg 1992;27:462–465.

70. Nihoul-Fekete C, Mitrofanoff P, Lortat-Jacob S: Les stenoses peptiques de L'oesophage chez l'enfant. Ann Pediatr 1979;26:692–698.
71. Orenstein S, Whitington P: Esophageal stricture dilatation in awake children. J Pediatr Gastroenterol Nutr 1985;4:557–562.
72. Johnsen A, Jensen L, Mauritzen K: Balloon-dilatation of esophageal strictures in children. Pediatr Radiol 1986;16:388–391.
73. Dalzell AM, Shepherd RW, Cleghorn GJ, Patrick MK: Esophageal stricture in children: fiberoptic endoscopy and dilation under fluoroscopic control. J Pediatr Gastroenterol Nutr 1992;15:426–430.
74. Glick M: Clinical course of esophageal stricture managed by bougienage. Dig Dis Sci 1982;27:884–888.
75. Patterson D, Graham D, Lacey Smith J, et al: Natural history of benign esophageal stricture treated by dilatation. Gastroenterology 1983;85:346–350.
76. Berenson G, Wyllie R, Caulfield M, Steffen R: Intralesional steroids in the treatment of refractory esophageal strictures. J Pediatr Gastroenterol Nutr 1994;18:250–252.
77. Spechler S, Sperber H, Doos W, Schimmel E: The prevalence of Barrett's esophagus in patients with chronic peptic esophageal strictures. Dig Dis Sci 1983;28:769–774.
78. Barrett N: The lower esophagus lined by columnar epithelium. Surgery 1957;41:881–894.
79. Kim S, Waring J, Spechler S, et al: Diagnostic inconsistencies in Barrett's esophagus. Gastroenterology 1994;107:945–949.
80. Cameron AJ, Lomboy CT: Barrett's esophagus: age, prevalence, and extent of columnar epithelium. Gastroenterology 1992;103:1241–1245.
81. Tudor R: Barrett's esophagus in children: 170 cases. Q & R Clinic, 1988.
82. Dahms B, Rothstein F: Barrett's esophagus in children: a consequence of chronic gastroesophageal reflux. Gastroenterology 1984;86:318–323.
83. Hassall E: Barrett's esophagus: new definitions and approaches in children (invited review). J Pediatr Gastroenterol Nutr 1993;16:345–364.
84. Othersen H, Ocampo R, Parker E, et al: Barrett's esophagus in children: diagnosis and management. Ann Surg 1993;217:676–681.
85. Qualman S, Murray R, McClung J, Lucas J: Intestinal metaplasia is age related in Barrett's esophagus. Arch Pathol Lab Med 1990; 114:1236–1240.
86. Hassall E, Weinstein W, Ament M: Barrett's esophagus in childhood. Gastroenterology 1985;89:1331–1337.
87. Lindahl H, Rintala R, Sariola H, Louhimo I: Cervical Barrett's esophagus: a common complication of gastric tube reconstruction. J Pediatr Surg 1990;25:446–448.
88. Dahms B, Greco M, Strandjord S, Rothstein F: Barrett's esophagus in three children after antileukemia chemotherapy. Cancer 1987;60:2896–2900.
89. Saul S: The myths and realities of Barrett's esophagus. Endosc Rev September/October 1987:21–37.
90. Richter J: Barrett's esophagus: Too much acid, alkali, or both? Gastroenterology 1990;98:798–799.
91. Vaezi M, Richter J: Synergism of acid and duodenogastroesophageal reflux in complicated Barrett's esophagus. Surgery 1995;117:699–704.
92. Attwood SEA, Ball CS, Barlow AP, et al: Role of intragastric and intraoesophageal alkalinisation in the genesis of complications in Barrett's columnar lined lower oesophagus. Gut 1993;34:11–15.
93. Caldwell M, Caulon P, Byrne M, et al: Ambulatory esophageal bile reflux monitoring in Barrett's oesophagus. Br J Surg 1995;82:657–660.
94. Champion G, Richter J, Vaezi M, et al: Duodenogastroesophageal reflux: relationship to pH and importance in Barrett's esophagus. Gastroenterology 1994;107:747–754.
95. Liron R, Parrilla P, Martinez de Haro L, et al: Quantification of duodenogastric reflux in Barrett's esophagus. Am J Gastroenterol 1997;92:32–36.
96. DeGiacomo C, Fiocca R, Villani L, et al: Barrett's ulcer and *Campylobacter*-like organisms infection in a child. J Pediatr Gastroenterol Nutr 1988;7:766–768.
97. Yulish B, Rothstein F, Halpin T: Radiographic findings in children and young adults with Barrett's esophagus. AJR 1987;148:353–357.
98. Diehl J, Thomas L, Bloom M, et al: Tracheoesophageal fistula associated with Barrett's ulcer: the importance of reflux control. Ann Thorac Surg 1988;45:449–450.
99. Komorowski R, Hogan W, Chausow D: Barrett's ulcer: the clinical significance today. Am J Gastroenterol 1996;91:2310–2313.
100. Hoeffel J, Nihoul-Fekete C, Schmitt M: Esophageal adenocarcinoma after gastroesophageal reflux in children. J Pediatr 1989;115:259–261.
101. Drewitz D, Sampliner R, Garewal H: The incidence of adenocarcinoma in Barrett's esophagus: A prospective study of 170 patients followed 4.8 years. Am J Gastroenterol 1997;92:212.
102. Hameeteman W, Tytgat G, Houthoff H, vandenTweel J: Barrett's esophagus: development of dysplasia and adenocarcinoma. Gastroenterology 1989;96:1249–1256.
103. Cheu HW, Grosfeld JL, Heifetz SA, et al: Persistence of Barrett's esophagus in children after antireflux surgery: influence on follow-up care. J Pediatr Surg 1992;27:260–266.
104. Chow W-H, Finkle W, McLaughlin J, et al: The relation of gastroesophageal reflux disease and its treatment to adenocarcinomas of the esophagus and gastric cardia. JAMA 1995;274:474–477.
105. Sagar P, Ackroyd R, Hosie K, et al: Regression and progression of Barrett's oesophagus after antireflux surgery. Br J Surg 1995;82:806–810.
106. Williamson W, Ellis F Jr, Gibb S, et al: Effect of antireflux operation on Barrett's mucosa. Ann Thorac Surg 1990;49:537–542.
107. Katzka D, Castell D: Successful elimination of reflux symptoms does not insure adequate control of acid reflux in patients with Barrett's esophagus. Am J Gastroenterol 1994;89:989–991.
108. Berenson M, Johnson T, Markowitz N, et al: Restoration of squamous mucosa after ablation of Barrett's esophageal epithelium. Gastroenterology 1993;104:1686–1691.
109. Overholt B, Panjehpour M: Photodynamic therapy for Barrett's esophagus: clinical update. Am J Gastroenterol 1996;91:1719–1723.
110. Orenstein S, Orenstein D: Gastroesophageal reflux and respiratory disease in children. J Pediatr 1988;112:847–858.
111. Kenna M: The effect of gastroesophageal reflux on the pediatric airway. Int Anesthesiol Clin 1992;30:83–91.
112. Shaker R: Airway protective mechanisms: current concepts. Dysphagia 1995;10:216–227.
113. Orenstein S, Orenstein D, Whitington P: Gastroesophageal reflux causing stridor. Chest 1983;84:301–302.
114. Orenstein S, Kocoshis S, Orenstein D, Proujansky R: Stridor and gastroesophageal reflux: diagnostic use of intraluminal esophageal acid perfusion (Bernstein test). Pediatr Pulmonol 1987;3:420–424.
115. Shay S, Myers R, Johnson L: Hiccups associated with reflux esophagitis. Gastroenterology 1984;87:204–207.
116. Gluck M, Pope C II: Chronic hiccups and gastroesophageal reflux disease: the acid perfusion test as a provocative maneuver. Ann Intern Med 1986;105:219–220.
117. Ruzkowski C, Sanowski R, Austin J, et al: The effects of inhaled albuterol and oral theophylline on gastroesophageal reflux in patients with gastroesophageal reflux disease and obstructive lung disease. Arch Intern Med 1992;152:783–785.
118. Stein M, Towner T, Weber R, et al: The effect of theophylline on the lower esophageal sphincter pressure. Ann Allergy 1980;45:238–241.
119. Berquist WE, Rachelefsky GS, Kadden M, et al: Effect of theophylline on gastroesophageal reflux in normal adults. J Allergy Clin Immunol 1981;67:407–411.
120. DiMarino A, Cohen S: Effect of an oral beta$_2$-adrenergic agonist on lower esophageal sphincter pressure in normals and in patients with achalasia. Dig Dis Sci 1982;27:1063–1066.
121. Rattan S, Goyal R: Effect of nicotine on the lower esophageal sphincter. Gastroenterology 1975;69:154–159.
122. Spiliopoulos A, Megevand R: Oesophagite peptique stenosante après sondage oeso-gastrique. Helv Chir Acta 1980;47:527–532.
123. Berezin S, Schwarz SM, Halata MS, Newman LJ: Gastroesophageal reflux secondary to gastrostomy tube placement. Am J Dis Child 1986;140:699–701.
124. Jolley SG, Tunell WP, Hoelzer DJ, et al: Lower esophageal pressure changes with tube gastrostomy: a causative factor of gastroesophageal reflux in children? J Pediatr Surg 1986;21:624–627.
125. Vandenplas Y, Diericx A, Blecker U, et al: Esophageal pH monitoring data during chest physiotherapy. J Pediatr Gastroenterol Nutr 1991;13:23–26.
126. Hampton FJ, MacFadyen UM, Beardsmore CS, Simpson H: Gastro-oesophageal reflux and respiratory function in infants with respiratory symptoms. Arch Dis Child 1991;66:848–853.
127. Chen P-H, Chang M-H, Hsu S-C: Gastroesophageal reflux in children with chronic recurrent bronchopulmonary infection. J Pediatr Gastroenterol Nutr 1991;13:16–22.
128. Gustafsson PM, Kjellman N-IM, Tibbling L: Bronchial asthma and

acid reflux into the distal and proximal oesophagus. Arch Dis Child 1990;65:1255–1258.
129. Tucci F, Resti M, Fontana R, et al: Gastroesophageal reflux and bronchial asthma: prevalence and effect of cisapride therapy. J Pediatr Gastroenterol Nutr 1993;17:265–270.
130. Berquist W, Rachelefsky G, Kadden M, et al: Gastroesophageal reflux–associated recurrent pneumonia and chronic asthma in children. Pediatrics 1981;68:29–35.
131. Shapiro G, Christie D: Gastroesophageal reflux in steroid-dependent asthmatic youths. Pediatrics 1979;63:207–212.
132. Martin M, Grunstein M, Larsen G: The relationship of gastroesophageal reflux to nocturnal wheezing in children with asthma. Ann Allergy 1982;49:318–322.
133. Eid N, Shepherd R, Thomson M: Persistent wheezing and gastroesophageal reflux in infants. Pediatr Pulmonol 1994;18:39–44.
134. Gustafsson P, Kjellman N-I, Tibbling L: A trial of ranitidine in asthmatic children and adolescents with or without pathologic gastro-oesophageal reflux. Eur Respir J 1992;5:201–206.
135. Harding S, Richter J, Guzzo M, et al: Asthma and gastroesophageal reflux: acid suppressive therapy improves asthma outcome. Am J Med 1996;100:395–405.
136. Harding S, Richter J: The role of gastroesophageal reflux in chronic cough and asthma. Chest 1997;111:1389–1402.
137. Berezin S, Medow MS, Glassman MS, Newman LJ: Esophageal chest pain in children with asthma. J Pediatr Gastroenterol Nutr 1991;12:52–55.
138. Davis R, Larsen G, Grunstein M: Respiratory response to intraesophageal acid infusion in asthmatic children during sleep. J Allergy Clin Immunol 1983;72:393–398.
139. Spaulding H, Mansfield L, Stein M, et al: Further investigation of the association between gastroesophageal reflux and bronchoconstriction. J Allergy Clin Immunol 1982;69:516–521.
140. Mansfield L, Hameister H, Spaulding H, et al: The role of the vagus nerve in airway narrowing caused by intraesophageal hydrochloric acid provocation and esophageal distention. Ann Allergy 1981; 47:431–434.
141. Mansfield L, Stein M: Gastroesophageal reflux and asthma: a possible reflex mechanism. Ann Allergy 1978;41:224–226.
142. Mansfield L: Gastroesophageal reflux and respiratory disorders: a review. Ann Allergy 1989;62:158–163.
143. Denjean A, Herve P, Simonneau G, et al: Effects of acid infusion into the esophagus on airflow obstruction and bronchial hyperreactivity in adult asthmatic patients. Chest 1985;5:201S–S202.
144. Herve P, Denjean A, Jian R, et al: Intraesophageal perfusion of acid increases the bronchomotor response to methacholine and to isocapnic hyperventilation in asthmatic subjects. Am Rev Respir Dis 1986; 134:986–989.
145. Larrain A, Carrasco E, Galleguillos F, et al: Medical and surgical treatment of non-allergic asthma associated with gastroesophageal reflux. Chest 1991;99:1330–1336.
146. Kahn A, Rebuffat E, Franco P, et al: Apparent life-threatening events and apnea of infancy. In Beckerman R, Brouilette R, Hunt C (eds): Respiratory Control Disorders in Infants and Children. Baltimore, Williams & Wilkins, 1992, pp 178–189.
147. Bauman N, Sandler A, Schmidt C, et al: Reflex laryngospasm induced by stimulation of distal esophageal afferents. Laryngoscope 1994;104:209–214.
148. Herbst J, Minton S, Book L: Gastroesophageal reflux causing respiratory distress and apnea in newborn infants. J Pediatr 1979;95:763–768.
149. Menon A, Schefft G, Thach B: Apnea associated with regurgitation in infants. J Pediatr 1985;106:625–629.
150. Menon A, Schefft G, Thach B: Frequency and significance of swallowing during prolonged apnea in infants. Am Rev Respir Dis 1984;130:969–973.
151. Herbst J, Book L, Bray P: Gastroesophageal reflux in the "near miss" sudden infant death syndrome. J Pediatr 1978;92:73–75.
152. Leape L, Ramenofsky M: Surgical treatment of gastroesophageal reflux in children. Am J Dis Child 1980;134:935–938.
153. Ramenofsky M, Leape L: Continuous upper esophageal pH monitoring in infants and children with gastroesophageal reflux, pneumonia, and apneic spells. J Pediatr Surg 1981;16:374–378.
154. Spitzer A, Boyle J, Tuchman D, Fox W: Awake apnea associated with gastroesophageal reflux: a specific clinical syndrome. J Pediatr 1984;104:200–205.
155. Nielson D, Heldt G, Tooley W: Stridor and gastroesophageal reflux in infants. Pediatrics 1990;85:1034–1039.
156. Guilleminault C, Coons S: Apnea and bradycardia during feeding in infants weighing >2000 gm. J Pediatr 1984;104:932–935.
157. Kenigsberg K, Griswold P, Buckley B, et al: Cardiac effects of esophageal stimulation: possible relationship between gastroesophageal reflux (GER) and sudden infant death syndrome (SIDS). J Pediatr Surg 1983;18:542–545.
158. Downing S, Lee J: Laryngeal chemosensitivity: a possible mechanism for sudden infant death. Pediatrics 1975;55:640–649.
159. Plaxico D, Loughlin G: Nasopharyngeal reflux and neonatal apnea. Am J Dis Child 1981;135:793–794.
160. Perkett E, Vaughan R: Evidence for a laryngeal chemoreflex in some human preterm infants. Acta Paediatr Scand 1982;71:969–972.
161. Suys B, De Wolf D, Hauser B, et al: Bradycardia and gastroesophageal reflux in term and preterm infants: is there any relation? J Pediatr Gastroenterol Nutr 1994;19:187–190.
162. Hrabovsky EE, Mullett MD: Gastroesophageal reflux and the premature infant. J Pediatr Surg 1986;21:583–587.
163. Lew C, Keens T, O'Neal M, et al: Gastroesophageal reflux prevents recovery from bronchopulmonary dysplasia. Clin Res 1981;29:149A.
164. Sindel B, Maisels M, Ballantine T, Karl S: The effect of a Nissen fundoplication on infants with chronic lung disease. Pediatr Res 1985;19:365A.
165. Cucchiara S, Santamaria F, Andreotti MR, et al: Mechanisms of gastro-oesophageal reflux in cystic fibrosis. Arch Dis Child 1991;66:617–622.
166. Bendig DW, Seilheimer DK, Wagner ML, et al: Complications of gastroesophageal reflux in patients with cystic fibrosis. J Pediatr 1982;100:536–540.
167. Scott RB, OLoughlin EV, Gall DG: Gastroesophageal reflux in patients with cystic fibrosis. J Pediatr 1985;106:223–227.
168. Vinocur CD, Marmon L, Schidlow DV, Weintraub WH: Gastroesophageal reflux in the infant with cystic fibrosis. Am J Surg 1985;149:182–186.
169. Stringer D, Sprigg A, Juodis E, et al: The association of cystic fibrosis, gastroesophageal reflux, and reduced pulmonary function. Can Assoc Radiol 1988;39:100–102.
170. Romeo G, Zuccarello B, Proietto F, Romeo C: Disorders of the esophageal motor activity in atresia of the esophagus. J Pediatr Surg 1987;22:120–124.
171. Nakazato Y, Landing BH, Wells TR: Abnormal Auerbach plexus in the esophagus and stomach of patients with esophageal atresia and tracheoesophageal fistula. J Pediatr Surg 1986;21:831–837.
172. Nakazato Y, Wells T, Landing B: Abnormal tracheal innervation in patients with esophageal atresia and tracheo-esophageal fistula: study of the intrinsic tracheal nerve plexuses by a microdissection technique. J Pediatr Surg 1986;21:838–844.
173. Wyman J, Dent J, Heddle R, et al: Control of belching by the lower oesophageal sphincter. Gut 1990;31:639–646.
174. Kahrilas P, Dodds W, Hogan W: Dysfunction of the belch reflex: a cause of incapacitating chest pain. Gastroenterology 1987;93:818–822.
175. Ing A, Ngu M, Breslin A: Pathogenesis of chronic persistent cough associated with gastroesophageal reflux. Am J Respir Crit Care Med 1994;149:160–167.
176. Irwin R, French C: Chronic cough due to gastroesophageal reflux: clinical diagnostic and pathogenic aspects. Chest 1993;104:1511–1517.
177. Katz P: Ambulatory esophageal and hypopharyngeal pH monitoring in patients with hoarseness. Am J Gastroenterol 1990;85:35–40.
178. Putnam PE, Orenstein SR: Hoarseness in a child with gastroesophageal reflux. Acta Pediatr Scand 1992;81:635–636.
179. Richter J: Hoarseness and gastroesophageal reflux: what is the relationship (selected summary). Gastroenterology 1990;98:1717–1719.
180. Jacob P, Kahrilas PJ, Herzon G: Proximal esophageal pH-metry in patients with "reflux laryngitis." Gastroenterology 1991;100:305–310.
181. Kamel P, Kahrilas P, Hanson D, et al: Prospective trial of omeprazole in the treatment of "reflux laryngitis." Gastroenterology 1992; 102:A93.
182. Oestreich A, Dunbar J: Pharyngonasal reflux: spectrum and significance in early childhood. AJR 1984;141:923–925.
183. Aine L, Baer M, Maki M: Dental erosions caused by gastroesophageal reflux disease in children. J Dent Child 1993;60(3):210–214.
184. Gaynor EB: Otolaryngologic manifestations of gastroesophageal reflux. Am J Gastroenterol 1991;86:801–808.
185. Sutcliffe J: Torsion spasms and abnormal postures in children with hiatus hernia: Sandifer's syndrome. Progr Pediat Radiol 1969;2:190–197.

186. Puntis J, Smith H, Buick R, Booth I: Effect of dystonic movements on oesophageal peristalsis in Sandifer's syndrome. Arch Dis Child 1989;64:1311–1313.
187. Amarnath RP, Perrault JF: Rumination in normal children: diagnosis and clinical considerations (abstract). Gastroenterology 1991;100:A25.
188. Orenstein SR, Cohn JF, Shalaby TM, Kartan R: Reliability and validity of an infant gastroesophageal reflux questionnaire. Clin Pediatr 1993;32:472–484.
189. Orenstein S, Shalaby T, Cohn J: Reflux symptoms in 100 normal infants: diagnostic validity of the Infant Gastroesophageal Reflux Questionnaire. Clin Pediatr 1996;35:607–614.
190. Schindlbeck N, Klauser A, Voderholzer W, Muller-Lissner S: Empiric therapy for gastroesophageal reflux disease. Arch Intern Med 1995; 155:1808–1812.
191. Provenzale D, Lipscomb J: Cost-effectiveness: definitions and use in the gastroenterology literature. Am J Gastroenterol 1996;91:1488–1493.
192. Bern E, Mobassaleh M: Cost-effectiveness analysis of diagnostic procedures to detect esophagitis in infancy. J Pediatr Gastroenterol Nutr 1995;21:334.
193. Seibert J, Byrne W, Euler A, et al: Gastroesophageal reflux—the acid test: scintigraphy or pH probe? AJR 1983;140:1087–1090.
194. Rudd T, Christie D: Demonstration of gastroesophageal reflux in children by radionuclide gastroesophagography. Radiol 1979;131:483–486.
195. Heyman S, Kirkpatrick J, Winter H, Treves S: An improved radionuclide method for the diagnosis of gastroesophageal reflux and aspiration in children (milk scan). Radiology 1979;131:479–482.
196. Paton J, Cosgriff P, Nanayakkara C: The analytical sensitivity of Tc99m radionuclide "milk" scanning in the detection of gastro-oesophageal reflux. Pediatr Radiol 1985;15:381–383.
197. Rosenthal M, Klein H, Orenstein S: Simultaneous acquisition of physiological data and nuclear medicine images. J Nucl Med 1988;29:1848–1852.
198. Klein H: Esophageal and other condensed dynamic images. Clin Nucl Med 1985;10:530–531.
199. Orenstein SR, Klein HA, Rosenthal MS: Simultaneous comparison of pH probe and scintigraphy for gastroesophageal reflux (GER). Gastroenterology 1987;92:1561.
200. Armstrong D, Bennett R, Blum A, et al: The endoscopic assessment of esophagitis: a progress report on observer agreement. Gastroenterology 1996;111:85–92.
201. Biller J, Winter H, Grand R, Allred E: Are endoscopic changes predictive of histologic esophagitis in children. J Pediatr 1983; 103:215–218.
202. Casteel H, Fiedorek S, Kiel E: Arterial blood oxygen desaturation in infants and children during upper gastrointestinal endoscopy. Gastrointest Endosc 1990;36:489–493.
203. Putnam PE, Orenstein SR: Blind esophageal suction biopsy in children less than 2 years of age. Gastroenterology 1992;102:A149.
204. Friesen C, Zwick D, Streed C, et al: Grasp biopsy, suction biopsy, and clinical history in the evaluation of esophagitis in infants 0–6 months of age. J Pediatr Gastroenterol Nutr 1995;20:300–304.
205. Putnam PE, Orenstein SR: Crown-rump length and pH probe length (author's reply). J Pediatr Gastroenterol Nutr 1992;15:222–223.
206. Whitington P, Orenstein S: Manometric guidance in suction biopsy of the esophagus in children. J Pediatr Gastroenterol Nutr 1984;3:535–538.
207. Friesen C, Streed C, Carney L, et al: Esophagitis and modified Bernstein tests in infants with apparent life-threatening events. Pediatrics 1994;94:541–544.
208. Cucchiara S, Staiano A, Gobio CL, et al: Value of the 24 hour intraoesophageal pH monitoring in children. Gut 1990;31:129–133.
209. Colletti R, Christie D, Orenstein S: Indications for pediatric esophageal pH monitoring: Statement of the North American Society for Pediatric Gastroenterology and Nutrition (NASPGN). J Pediatr Gastroenterol Nutr 1995;21:253–262.
210. Vandenplas Y, Loeb H: The interpretation of oesophageal pH monitoring data. Eur J Pediatr 1990;149:598–602.
211. Vandenplas Y, Goyvaerts H, Helven R, Sacre L: Gastroesophageal reflux, as measured by 24-hour pH monitoring, in 509 healthy infants screened for risk of sudden infant death syndrome. Pediatrics 1991;88:834–840.
212. Hampton F, MacFadyen U, Simpson H: Reproducibility of 24 hour oesophageal pH studies in infants. Arch Dis Child 1990;65:1249–1254.
213. Hampton FJ, MacFadyen UM, Mayberry JF: Variations in results of simultaneous ambulatory pH monitoring. Dig Dis Sci 1992;37:506–512.
214. Halpern LM, Jolley SG, Tunnell WP, et al: The mean duration of gastroesophageal reflux during sleep as an indicator of respiratory symptoms from gastroesophageal reflux in children. J Pediatr Surg 1991;26:686–690.
215. Dreizzen E, Escourrou P, Odievre M, et al: Esophageal reflux in symptomatic and asymptomatic infants: postprandial and circadian variations. J Pediatr Gastroenterol Nutr 1990;10:316–321.
216. Barabino A: Comparison among three different methods of analysis of oesophageal pH monitoring. J Pediatr Gastroenterol Nutr 1991;13:314–315.
217. Friesen CA, Hayes R, Hodge C, Roberts CC: Comparison of methods of assessing 24-hour intraesophageal pH recordings in children. J Pediatr Gastroenterol Nutr 1992;14:252–255.
218. Grill BB: Twenty-four-hour esophageal pH monitoring: what's the score? J Pediatr Gastroenterol Nutr 1992;14:249–251.
219. Jolley S, Johnson D, Herbst J, et al: An assessment of gastroesophageal reflux in children by extended monitoring of the distal esophagus. Surgery 1978;84:16–22.
220. Euler A, Byrne W: Twenty-four-hour esophageal intraluminal pH probe testing: a comparative analysis. Gastroenterology 1981;80:957–961.
221. Tovar J, Izquierdo M, Eizaguirre I: The area under pH curve: a single-figure parameter representative of esophageal acid exposure. J Pediatr Surg 1991;26:163–167.
222. Dobhan R, Castell D: Normal and abnormal proximal esophageal acid exposure: results of ambulatory dual-probe pH monitoring. Am J Gastroenterol 1993;88:25–29.
223. Vaezi M, Schroeder P, Richter J: Reproducibility of proximal probe pH parameters in 24-hour ambulatory esophageal pH monitoring. Am J Gastroenterol 1997;92:825–829.
224. Breumelhof R, Smout AJPM: The symptom sensitivity index: a valuable additional parameter in 24-hour esophageal pH recording. Am J Gastroenterol 1991;86:160–164.
225. Johnston B, Collins J, McFarland R, Love A: Are esophageal symptoms reflux-related? A study of different scoring systems in a cohort of patients with heartburn. Am J Gastroenterol 1994;89:497–502.
226. Katzka D, Paoletti V, Leite L, Castell D: Prolonged ambulatory pH monitoring in patients with persistent gastroesophageal reflux disease symptoms: testing while on therapy identifies the need for more aggressive anti-reflux therapy. Am J Gastroenterol 1996;91:2110–2113.
227. Westra S, Derkx H, Taminiau J: Symptomatic gastroesophageal reflux: diagnosis with ultrasound. J Pediatr Gastroenterol Nutr 1994;19:58–64.
228. Williams H, Freeman M: Milk inhalation pneumonia: the significance of fat filled macrophages in tracheal secretions. Aust Paediatr J 1973;9:286–288.
229. Brand J, Brodsky N, Hurt H: No evidence of aspiration in intubated infants fed by orogastric (OG) or oroduodenal (OD) routes. Pediatr Res 1986;20:405A.
230. Nussbaum E, Maggi J, Galant S: Association of lipid-laden alveolar macrophages and gastroesophageal reflux in children. Pediatr Res 1986;20:475A.
231. Hopper A, LK K, Stevenson D, et al: Detection of gastric contents in tracheal fluid of infants by lactose assay. J Pediatr 1983;102:415–418.
232. McVeagh P, Howman-Giles R, Kemp A: Pulmonary aspiration studied by radionuclide milk scanning and barium swallow roentgenography. Am J Dis Child 1987;141:917–921.
233. Bar-Sever Z, Connolly L, Treves S: The radionuclide salivagram in children with pulmonary disease and a high risk of aspiration. Pediatr Radiol 1995;25:S180–S183.
234. Wolfe J, Bone R, Ruth W: Diagnosis of gastric aspiration by fiberoptic bronchoscopy. Chest 1976;70:458–459.
235. Wynne J, Ramphal R, Hood C: Tracheal mucosal damage after aspiration: a scanning electron microscope study. Am Rev Respir Dis 1981;124:728–732.
236. Cavataio F, Iacono G, Montalto G, et al: Gastroesophageal reflux associated with cow's milk allergy in infants: which diagnostic examinations are useful? Am J Gastroenterol 1996;91:1215–1220.
237. Kelly K, Lazenby A, Rowe P, et al: Eosinophilic esophagitis attributed to gastroesophageal reflux: improvement with an amino acid-based formula. Gastroenterology 1995;109:1503–1512.

238. Justinich C, Kalafus D, Esposito P, et al: Mucosal mast cells distinguish allergic from gastroesophageal reflux-induced esophagitis (abstract). J Pediatr Gastroenterol Nutr 1996;23:342.
239. Winter H, Madara J, Stafford R, et al: Intraepithelial eosinophils: a new diagnostic criterion for reflux esophagitis. Gastroenterology 1982;83:818–823.
240. Richter J: Long-term management of gastroesophageal reflux disease and its complications. Am J Gastroenterol 1997;92:30S–35S.
241. Orenstein S: Prone positioning in infant gastroesophageal reflux: is elevation of the head worth the trouble? J Pediatr 1990;117:184–187.
242. Orenstein SR, Mitchell AA, Davidson Ward S: Concerning the American Academy of Pediatrics Recommendation on Sleep Position for Infants. Pediatrics 1993;91:497–499.
243. Orenstein S: The prone alternative (commentary). Pediatrics 1994; 94:104–105.
244. Abe T, Hata Y, Sasaki F, et al: The effect of tube feeding on postprandial gastroesophageal reflux. J Pediatr Surg 1993;28:56–58.
245. Kadakia S, Kikendall J, Maydonovitch C, Johnson L: Effect of cigarette smoking on gastroesophageal reflux measured by 24-h ambulatory esophageal pH monitoring. Am J Gastroenterol 1995;90:1785–1790.
246. Shabib S, Cutz E, Sherman P: Passive smoking is a risk factor for esophagitis in children. J Pediatr 1995;127:435–437.
247. Vigneri S, Termini R, Leandro G, et al: A comparison of five maintenance therapies for reflux esophagitis. N Engl J Med 1995;333:1106–1110.
248. Hillman AL, Bloom BS, Fendrick AM, Schwarz JS: Cost and quality effects of alternative treatments for persistent gastroesophageal reflux disease. Arch Intern Med 1992;152:1467–1472.
249. Reynolds J, Putnam P: Prokinetic agents. Gastroenterol Clin North Am 1992;21:567–596.
250. Cucchiara S, Staiano A, Boccieri A, et al: Effects of cisapride on parameters of oesophageal motility and on the prolonged intraoesophageal pH test in infants with gastro-oesophageal reflux disease. Gut 1990;31:21–25.
251. Booth I: Treatment of gastro-oesophageal reflux in infancy with cisapride. In Cadranal S (ed): Gastro-oesophageal Reflux in Childhood. Amsterdam: Excerpta Medica, 1990, pp 13–21.
252. McCallum RW: Cisapride: a new class of prokinetic agent. The ACG Committee on FDA-related matters. American College of Gastroenterology. Am J Gastroenterol 1991;86:135–149.
253. Shulman R: Report from the NASPGN Therapeutics Subcommittee (Medical Position Paper): Cisapride and the attack of the P-450s. J Pediatr Gastroenterol Nutr 1996;23:395–397.
254. Lewin M, Bryant R, Fenrich A, Grifka R: Cisapride-induced long QT interval. J Pediatr 1996;128:279–281.
255. Hyams J, Leichtner A, Zamett L, Walters J: Effect of metoclopramide on prolonged intraesophageal pH testing in infants with gastroesophageal reflux. J Pediatr Gastroenterol Nutr 1986;5:716–720.
256. Putnam PE, Orenstein SR, Wessel HB, Stowe RM: Tardive dyskinesia associated with metoclopramide use in a child. J Pediatr 1992; 121:983–985.
257. Bines JE, Quinlan J-E, Treves S, et al: Efficacy of domperidone in infants and children with gastroesophageal reflux. J Pediatr Gastroenterol Nutr 1992;14:400–405.
258. Kelly D: Do $H_2$ receptor antagonists have a therapeutic role in childhood? J Pediatr Gastroenterol Nutr 1994;19:270–276.
259. Lambert J, Mobassaleh M, Grand R: Efficacy of cimetidine for gastric acid suppression in pediatric patients. J Pediatr 1992;120:474–478.
260. Cucchiara S, Minella R, Iervolino C, et al: Omeprazole and high dose ranitidine in the treatment of refractory reflux oesophagitis. Arch Dis Child 1993;69:655–659.
261. Gunasekaran T, Hassall E: Efficacy and safety of omeprazole for severe gastroesophageal reflux in children. J Pediatr 1993;123:148–154.
262. Marcuard S, Albernaz L, Khazanie P: Omeprazole therapy causes malabsorption of cyanocobalamin (vitamin $B_{12}$). Ann Intern Med 1994;120:211–215.
263. Maton P: Omeprazole. N Engl J Med 1991;324:965–975.
264. Cucchiara S, Staiano A, Romaniello G, et al: Antacids and cimetidine treatment for gastro-oesophageal reflux and peptic oesophagitis. Arch Dis Child 1984;59:842–847.
265. Pivnick E, Kerr N, Kaufman R, et al: Rickets secondary to phosphate depletion: a sequela of antacid use in infancy. Clin Pediatr 1995;34(2): 73–78.
266. Brand J, Greer F: Hypermagnesemia and intestinal perforation following antacid administration in a premature infant. Pediatrics 1990;85:121–124.
267. Tsou V, Young R, Hart M, Vanderhoof J: Elevated plasma aluminum levels in normal infants receiving antacids containing aluminum. Pediatrics 1991;87:148–151.
268. Herrera JL, Shay SS, McCabe M, et al: Sucralfate used as adjunctive therapy in patients with severe erosive peptic esophagitis resulting from gastroesophageal reflux. Am J Gastroenterol 1990;85:1335–1338.
269. McCarthy D: Sucralfate. N Engl J Med 1991;325:1017–1025.
270. Hoffman M, Ross A: Surgical management of gastroesophageal reflux in children. In Rosenthal S, Sheppard J, Lotze M (eds): Dysphagia and the Child with Developmental Disabilities. San Diego, Singular Publishing Group, 1995, pp 283–304.
271. Spechler S, Department of Veterans Affairs Gastroesophageal Reflux Disease Study Group: Comparison of medical and surgical therapy for complicated gastroesophageal reflux disease in veterans. N Engl J Med 1992;326:786–792.
272. Albanese C, Towbin R, Ulman I, et al: Percutaneous gastrojejunostomy versus Nissen fundoplication for enteral feeding of the neurologically impaired child with gastroesophageal reflux. J Pediatr 1993;123:371–375.
273. Stringel G: Gastrostomy with antireflux properties. J Pediatr Surg 1990;25:1019–1021.
274. Gotley D, Smithers B, Rhodes M, et al: Laparoscopic Nissen fundoplication—200 consecutive cases. Gut 1996;38:487–491.
275. Waring J, Hunter J, Oddsdottir M, et al: The preoperative evaluation of patients considered for laparoscopic antireflux surgery. Am J Gastroenterol 1995;90:35–38.
276. Hassall E: Wrap session: is the Nissen slipping? Can medical treatment replace surgery for severe gastroesophageal reflux disease in children? Am J Gastroenterol 1995;90:1212–1220.
277. deHaro LM, Paricio PP, Escandell MAO, et al: Antireflux mechanism of Nissen fundoplication: a manometric study. Scand J Gastroenterol 1992;27:417–420.
278. Ireland A, Holloway R, Toouli J, Dent J: Mechanism underlying the antireflux action of fundoplication. Gut 1993;34:303–308.
279. Kazerooni N, VanCamp J, Hirschl R, et al: Fundoplication in 160 children under 2 years of age. J Pediatr Surg 1994;29:677–681.
280. Johansson J, Johansson F, Joelsson B, et al: Outcome 5 years after 360° fundoplication for gastro-oesophageal reflux disease. Br J Surg 1993;80:46–49.
281. Luostarinen M, Isolauri J, Laitinen J, et al: Fate of Nissen fundoplication after 20 years: a clinical, endoscopical, and functional analysis. Gut 1993;34:1015–1020.
282. Pearl R, Robie D, Ein S, et al: Complications of gastroesophageal antireflux surgery in neurologically impaired versus neurologically normal children. J Pediatr Surg 1990;25:1169–1173.
283. DiLorenzo C, Flores A, Hyman PE: Intestinal motility in symptomatic children with fundoplication. J Pediatr Gastroenterol Nutr 1991; 12:169–173.
284. Maxson R, Harp S, Jackson R, et al: Delayed gastric emptying in neurologically impaired children with gastroesophageal reflux: the role of pyloroplasty. J Pediatr Surg 1994;29:726–729.

Chapter 15

# Achalasia and Other Motor Disorders

Fernando del Rosario and Carlo Di Lorenzo

The esophagus is a muscular tube with sphincters at both ends. Its main goal is to stay empty in spite of numerous intrusions from above or below. Functionally, the esophagus may be divided into three areas: the upper esophageal sphincter (UES), the esophageal body, and the lower esophageal sphincter (LES). The UES contracts during inspiration to prevent air from entering the esophagus and protects the airways from gastric content during episodes of gastroesophageal reflux (GER). The esophageal body uses primary peristalsis to clear the esophagus from pharyngeal contents during swallowing and secondary peristalsis to eliminate gastric content during episodes of GER. The LES is the main barrier against GER. The most common motor disorder of the esophagus is an impaired LES function leading to GER, a condition discussed in Chapter 14. In this chapter the focus is on less common esophageal motor disorders, with special emphasis on entities that have been described in children.

## UPPER ESOPHAGEAL SPHINCTER DYSFUNCTION

The UES is a zone of intraluminal high pressure, formed primarily by the horizontal fibers of the cricopharyngeal muscle. It is likely that fibers of the pharyngeal constrictor muscle and the highest muscle fibers of the esophagus also contribute to forming the UES. This striated muscle segment is maintained in a state of constant contraction and relaxes momentarily in response to a swallow. Normal deglutition occurs when the pharyngeal contraction occurs simultaneously with the complete relaxation of the UES. When this sequence of events is uncoordinated or the UES relaxation is incomplete the bolus is mishandled. Symptoms of UES dysfunction include choking, tracheal aspirations with repetitive coughing episodes, nasopharyngeal regurgitation, drooling, and dysphagia. The dysphagia associated with UES dysfunction is called *transfer dysphagia*, which describes the difficulty to initiate the act of swallowing. The term *globus hystericus* or *globus sensation* is used when there is a sensation of a "lump in the throat" or a constant cervical fullness. In children, dysfunctions of the UES are often accompanied by other evidence of neurologic or muscle disease. Diffuse central nervous system dysfunctions, as seen in cerebral palsy, might affect the swallowing center in the brain stem or the cranial nerves involved in the swallowing process. Type I and type II Chiari malformations have been associated with dysphagia in young children. Surgical decompression of the malformation led to complete clinical and manometric resolution of the UES dysfunction.[1] Other conditions associated with abnormal UES function include Silver-Russell syndrome, $5p^-$ (cri-du-chat) syndrome, and minimal change myopathy.[2] UES dysfunction may also result from cervical inflammatory or constrictive processes limiting the laryngeal or hyoid bone movement and altering the UES function. The onset of symptoms related to UES dysfunction is usually during infancy. When the swallowing difficulty is due to a motor disorder, it usually occurs with both liquids and solids. Difficulty with only solids is more suggestive of a mechanical obstruction. The diagnostic assessment of a child with transfer dysphagia begins with a complete examination of mouth, neck, and cranial nerves. A modified barium swallow with different-consistency boluses allows a careful assessment of the pharyngeal and esophageal portion of the swallowing process. Esophageal manometry provides information complementary to the radiologic study.[3] Videoradiography is a qualitative test aimed at studying the bolus transit and the movement of tongue, soft palate, epiglottis, and larynx. It may also detect aspiration. Manometry quantitates pharyngeal and UES pressures, coordination between pharyngeal contraction and UES relaxation, and degree of UES relaxation. Such information is more reliably obtained by using either perfused sleeve sensors or solid-state circumferentially recording transducers.[4] The most commonly diagnosed UES abnormality is the cricopharyngeal spasm or *cricopharyngeal achalasia*. This term has been used to indicate all forms of UES dysfunctions and has its radiologic correlate in a prominent cricopharyngeal muscle ("bar"). Up to 5% of adults and many normal infants have a radiologic horizontal esophageal bar,[5] and at times patients with radiographic bars do not have elevated UES pressures.[6] Abnormal coordination between pharyngeal contraction and UES relaxation has also been described. There may be premature cricopharyngeal closure[7] or delayed cricopharyngeal relaxation.[8] The latter has been associated with administration of nitrazepam, causing drooling.[9] Treatment of UES dysfunction should be aimed at correcting the primary neurologic abnormality.[10] Conservative treatment may be indicated in young infants because spontaneous improvement may occur. In older children, resolution of symptoms has been achieved with either bougie dilatation or cricopharyngeal myotomy.[2,7]

## ACHALASIA

Achalasia is a primary esophageal motor disorder that is characterized by (1) increased LES pressure, (2) absent or incomplete LES relaxation in response to a swallow, (3) loss of esophageal peristalsis, and (4) elevated intraesophageal pressure. It presents as an obstruction at the level of the gastroesophageal junction with subsequent dilatation of the lower esophagus due to absence of esophageal peristalsis. *Vigorous achalasia* is a term used to describe the rare patient with high-pressure tertiary contractions.[11] The incidence of achalasia has been estimated as 1 in 10,000.[12] The most recent epidemiologic study of achalasia by Mayberry and Mayell determined an incidence rate of 0.1 to 0.3 cases per 100,000 children per year in 129 English children.[13]

### Genetics

The role of genetic factors in achalasia has yet to be fully elucidated. Nihoul-Fekete and coworkers suggested that childhood achalasia in certain cases represented a congenital problem based on the occurrence of achalasia in the first 6 months of life.[14] Achalasia has been associated with a variety of syndromes (familial dysautonomia, glucocorticoid insufficiency, Rozycki's syndrome, adrenal insufficiency/alacrima/achalasia syndrome), suggesting that genetic factors may play a role in the etiology of the disease.[14–16] Although Mayberry and Mayell found no familial distribution in their study population,[13] others have reported concordance in monozygotic twins,[17] siblings, and close relatives.[12,18,19] There was a male preponderance among familial cases.[20] Some suggested that there may be an autosomal recessive inheritance pattern based on findings that a third of published familial cases were products of consanguineous parents.[18,19]

### Pathophysiology

The esophageal smooth muscle is predominantly affected in achalasia (Table 15–1).[21] Most cases of achalasia are idiopathic. Theories on the pathogenesis of achalasia have included neurogenic, myogenic, and hormonal processes.[22] One report even suggests that varicella-zoster may have some etiologic importance after investigators found a significantly high presence of the virus in tissue obtained at cardiomyotomy in three patients with achalasia by using DNA hybridization.[23]

Consistent, but not constant, pathologic findings include degeneration of ganglion cells in the myenteric plexus (Auerbach's plexus) and loss of nerves innervating the smooth muscle cells of the LES.[24,25] Other neuropathologic findings that have been described include chronic inflammatory infiltrates in the myenteric plexus and degenerative changes in the smooth muscle or nerve fibers.[24] Many reports have found absent ganglion cells in the distal esophagus of children with achalasia.[26] Others have found sufficient numbers of ganglion cells but extensive perineural fibrosis.[22,27] It is believed that the incomplete relaxation of the LES is due to absence, functional impairment, or lack of central connections of postganglionic inhibitory nerves.[28] These abnormalities, which appear to be localized in the inner circular muscle layer, result in supersensitivity of the LES muscles to cholinergic agonists and a paradoxical contractile LES response to cholecystokinin.[28,29] Ultrastructural studies have also demonstrated abnormality of the vagal innervation of the LES.[30]

**TABLE 15–1. Disorders of the Esophageal Smooth Muscle**

| |
|---|
| **Primary Esophageal Motility Disorders** |
| Achalasia |
| Diffuse esophageal spasm |
| Nutcracker esophagus |
| Nonspecific esophageal motility disorders |
| **Secondary Esophageal Motility Disorders** |
| Gastroesophageal reflux |
| Chronic intestinal pseudo-obstruction |
| Esophageal atresia |
| Tracheoesophageal fistula |
| Collagen vascular diseases (e.g., scleroderma, dermatomyositis, systemic lupus erythematosus) |
| Metabolic disorders (diabetes mellitus, thyroid disorders) |
| Neuromuscular disorders (e.g., muscular dystrophies, myasthenia gravis) |
| Chagas' disease |
| Iatrogenic (e.g., sclerotherapy, caustic ingestion, surgery) |
| Exogenous factors (drugs, silicone breast implants) |
| Psychiatric disorders (bulimia, anorexia nervosa, depression) |
| Graft-versus-host disease |

A hormonal cause for achalasia has been considered because of the finding that vasoactive intestinal polypeptide (VIP) is reduced or completely absent in patients with achalasia.[31] VIP has been postulated as a major inhibitory transmitter released at the intramural postganglionic neurons of the LES.[32,33] It inhibits nonadrenergic, noncholinergic pathways, resulting in LES relaxation,[34] and is abundant in gut sphincters.[33]

Nitric oxide (NO) has also been found to be a mediator for the nonadrenergic, noncholinergic effects in the esophagus and LES.[35–38] It is not known whether NO is the final mediator. Animal studies have shown that loss of NO inhibitory myenteric neurons resulted in decreased or absence of LES relaxation and in decreased amplitude of swallow-induced esophageal contractions.[36,37] Human studies have demonstrated (1) absence of NO synthase in the LES of patients with achalasia and (2) LES relaxation when NO was added to the muscle strips of patients with achalasia.[35,38]

### Clinical Presentation

Fewer than 5% of children with achalasia manifested symptoms before 15 years of age.[12] A worldwide survey of achalasia in childhood conducted by Myers and associates showed that 6% of 175 affected children were identified as having achalasia during infancy.[20] The mean age at the time of diagnosis in pediatric patients was 8.8 years according to a review of all the pediatric series available.[21] The youngest

**TABLE 15–2. Clinical Symptoms in Children with Achalasia**

| SYMPTOMS | % OF CHILDREN |
|---|---|
| Vomiting | 84.1 |
| Dysphagia | 83.7 |
| Weight loss | 76.5 |
| Failure to thrive | 54.4 |
| Nocturnal regurgitation | 40.8 |
| Substernal pain | 38.2 |
| Nocturnal cough | 28.8 |
| Recurrent pneumonias | 20.9 |
| Odynophagia | 11.0 |

From Nurko S: Other motor disorders. In Walker WA, Durie PR, Hamilton JR, et al (eds): Pediatric Gastrointestinal Disease, Pathophysiology, Diagnosis, Management, Vol 1, 2nd ed. St. Louis, Mosby–Year Book, 1996, p 477, with permission.

patient reported to have achalasia was a 900-g, 14-day-old premature infant.[39, 40] The review of all pediatric series available shows a female-to-male ratio of 1.1:1.

The development of symptoms is often gradual, with a mean duration of symptoms of 23 months before diagnosis (range: 1 month to 8 years). The most common symptom is vomiting, progressive dysphagia, weight loss, and failure to thrive (Table 15–2). Infants and toddlers tend to have feeding aversion, failure to thrive, or gastroesophageal reflux (GER). Respiratory symptoms, such as recurrent pneumonias and nocturnal cough, predominate. Older children have dysphagia, regurgitation, and retrosternal pain. Dysphagia on ingestion of solids occurs initially, but dysphagia with liquids subsequently develops with worsening of the disease.[41] Patients describe the sensation of food getting stuck in the middle of the chest.[42] Some swallow repeatedly to get the food into their stomach.[42] Vomited material is undigested and not mixed with gastric juice.[43] There may be the perception of food matter sloshing around in the dilated esophagus. Sudden death from aspiration of esophageal contents is a serious complication.[41]

## Diagnosis

### Radiography

A plain chest radiograph showing a widened mediastinum, esophageal air-fluid level, or absence of gastric air may be suggestive of achalasia (Fig. 15–1). A barium swallow may show variable degrees of esophageal dilatation with tapering at the esophageal junction—"bird's beak" deformity (Fig. 15–2).[44, 45] Esophageal dilatation may be so severe that the esophagus takes on an S shape—"sigmoid esophagus." One may also see absence of peristalsis, tertiary contractions, and failure of LES relaxation.[45]

### Manometry

Manometry is the preferred method of diagnosis. It provides quantitative information about the severity of the disease and response to treatment.[46] Characteristic manometric findings include (1) increased LES pressure, (2) absence of peristalsis, (3) incomplete or abnormal LES relaxation, and (4) elevated intraesophageal pressure.

The LES pressure may be normal to twice normal.[46, 47] Absence of peristalsis is the hallmark of the disease and often involves the entire length of the esophagus.[47] Tertiary contractions have been described; and if pressures are greater

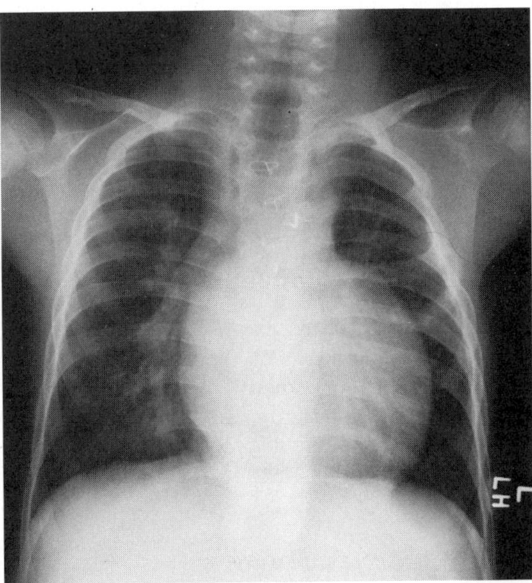


**FIGURE 15–1.** Anteroposterior chest film of a 5-year-old boy with achalasia. There is no air-fluid level in the esophagus, but there is a widened mediastinum.

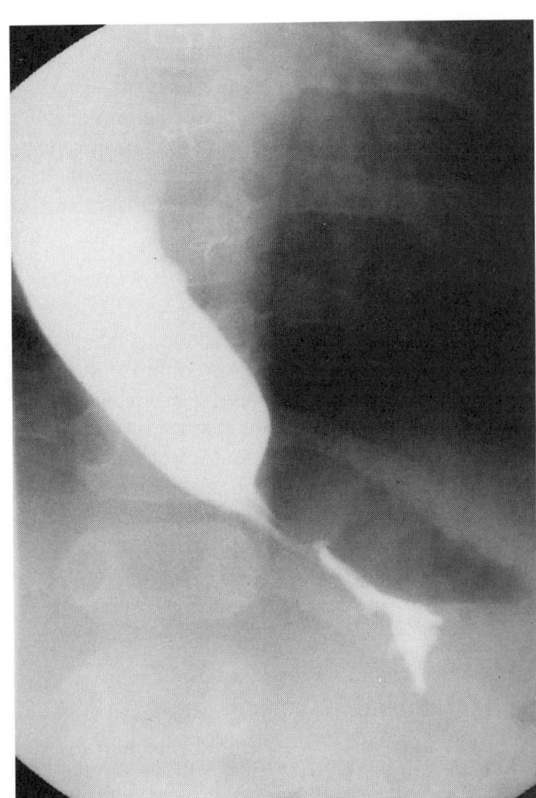

**FIGURE 15–2.** Barium swallow of a 5-year-old boy with achalasia demonstrating distal esophageal dilatation and narrowing at the LES ("bird's beak" or "rat's tail" deformity).

than 50 to 60 mm Hg or if more than three pressure waves appear in response to a swallow, the condition is referred to as vigorous achalasia.[11] Abnormal LES relaxation occurs in more than 70% of patients with achalasia.[47] Elevated intraesophageal pressures result from the functional obstruction at the LES. A study of 50 patients with achalasia show esophageal pressures that were 6.1 ± 0.7 mm higher than fundic pressures in 80% of cases, and there is no correlation between LES and intraesophageal pressures.[48] Manometric abnormalities are found even in infants, as demonstrated by Asch and colleagues in a 2-week-old who was found to have no esophageal peristalsis and had an LES pressure up to 40 mm Hg.[49]

Data on UES function in patients with achalasia are few. There have been reports of acute airway obstruction in patients with achalasia, prompting speculation that pharyngeal and UES abnormalities are present in achalasia.[50] A study of 19 patients with achalasia found increased UES residual pressure, shorter duration of UES relaxation with swallowing, and more rapid onset of pharyngeal contractions after UES relaxation; all of which did not correlate with the degree and duration of symptoms.[50] It is not clear whether these abnormalities lead to impaired pharyngeal function or whether delayed esophageal emptying secondary to a hypertonic LES result in regurgitation and possible aspiration of esophageal contents.

Repeat manometry is not usually necessary after therapy if symptoms disappear. Post-treatment manometry can be expected to show low LES pressure but persistently incomplete LES relaxation. Return of peristalsis after treatment remains controversial.[51, 52]

### *Endoscopy*

Endoscopy is primarily used to assess the presence of inflammation, infection, carcinoma, or leiomyoma in the esophagus and to insert a guidewire for positioning of a balloon for LES dilatation. The esophagus appears patulous, and there may be esophagitis secondary to food stasis. The LES does not dilate with insufflation of air.

### *Radionuclide Tests*

The most commonly used radionuclide to label a solid or liquid meal is technetium-99m sulfur colloid.[53] Radionuclide tests have primarily been used to assess esophageal emptying before and after therapy. They are also useful in differentiating achalasia from other conditions, such as scleroderma, because of differing retention patterns. Patients with achalasia tend to retain the tracer even in an upright position.[54] However, these tests provide no predictive information on the eventual success of a particular therapy or a patient's response to therapy.

### *Provocative Tests*

Subcutaneous administration of acetyl-β-methacholine (mecholyl) produces a rise in the esophageal baseline pressure and the appearance of repetitive high-amplitude contractions in the esophagus. However, it is a painful test and contraindicated in those with asthma or heart disease. This test is considered abnormal if there is a rise in esophageal pressure greater than 25 mm Hg lasting for at least 30 seconds within 8 minutes after 5 to 10 mg of mecholyl has been administered.[55]

## Differential Diagnosis

Achalasia has to be differentiated from other causes of esophageal obstruction, as enumerated in Table 15–1. There have been reports of children diagnosed with achalasia who after surgical exploration were found to have leiomyomas of the distal esophagus.[56] In adults, a variety of carcinomas (adenocarcinoma of the stomach, oat cell carcinoma of the lung, pancreatic carcinoma) have been reported to present with manometric features similar to achalasia.[57, 58] In Latin America where infection with *Trypanosoma cruzi* is common, Chagas' disease needs to be considered in anyone suspected of having achalasia.[59] The trypanosome causes neuronal destruction of the myenteric plexus, resulting in clinical and manometric findings similar to primary achalasia. Some patients have also been erroneously diagnosed to have anorexia nervosa and were later discovered to have achalasia.[42, 60]

## Treatment

The cornerstone of therapy is relief of the functional LES obstruction. However, nutritional rehabilitation cannot be ignored, especially in patients who have suffered extreme weight loss. Elevation of the head of the bed helps improve esophageal emptying and decrease nocturnal regurgitation.

### *Pharmacologic Therapy*

Isosorbide dinitrate, a smooth muscle relaxant, has been shown to cause a significant LES relaxation in 15 adult patients with achalasia.[61] This has been confirmed manometrically and with radionuclide esophageal emptying scans. However, as many as 50% of the patients had long-term side effects, primarily headaches and hypotension, or became drug resistant.

Nifedipine, a calcium channel blocker, has also been shown to decrease LES pressure in patients with achalasia at doses of 10 to 20 mg,[61–63] and to decrease the amplitude of esophageal contractions.[64] The experience in children is limited.[22, 62, 63] In the largest report, in which four adolescents were given 10 mg of nifedipine, there was good clinical response and a manometrically documented fall in LES pressure.[62] Excellent long-term response was demonstrated in two thirds of patients in one study, and side effects were rare.[65] A comparison between isosorbide and nifedipine in adults showed that whereas nifedipine was not as effective as isosorbide, patients on nifedipine had fewer side effects.[61] As a result, nifedipine has been the drug of choice to treat achalasia. The major concerns of pharmacotherapy are patient compliance and long-term effects. Its major role is to provide relief of symptoms until more definitive therapy can be performed[61, 62] or if pneumatic dilatation or surgery is contraindicated.[65]

### *Nonpharmacologic Therapy*

The two most successful modalities to relieve the functional obstruction in achalasia are pneumatic dilatation and esophageal myotomy.

**DILATATION.** Pneumatic dilatation is accomplished by placing a dilating device at the level of the LES and inflating it to stretch the esophageal muscle and the LES.[22, 66] It is unclear whether pneumatic dilatation actually tears the LES as well. Animal studies fail to demonstrate that muscle fibers actually tear.[51] Proper placement of the dilator is aided by an endoscopically placed guidewire and fluoroscopy. The midportion of the balloon must be in the LES before inflation of the balloon. The balloon may be inflated up to three times, followed by repeat endoscopy. The pressure and duration of distention used vary from center to center, with minimum pressures of 300 mm Hg and inflation periods of 15 seconds up to several minutes.[47, 56] Young children and individuals who do not sedate well with conscious sedation should have their procedure performed under general anesthesia. A variety of balloon dilators (Mosher bag, Browne-McHardy dilators, Rigiflex dilators) are available. Latex balloon dilators have no predetermined diameters so their size depends on the pressures used. The Browne-McHardy dilator has a net over the balloon to control maximum diameter. Rigiflex dilators, which we prefer to use, are nonelastic plastic balloons with predetermined diameters that have been used with high success rates and low complications.[67, 68]

The success rate of pneumatic dilatation in adults varies from 60% to 90% after a single dilatation.[69] The relapse rate is 25.8% according to one study.[70] If the first dilatation is unsuccessful, 38% and 19% improve after a second or third dilatation, respectively.[71] Those who have a poor response initially generally respond less well to repeated dilatations.[71] One prospective study on adult patients report a worse outcome in younger patients and that postdilatation LES pressure is a valuable factor for predicting long-term clinical response.[46]

Pneumatic dilatation for children with achalasia has resulted in an overall improvement rate of 50% (76/151) based on data from the available pediatric series.[21, 72] The rate of improvement has ranged from 35% to 100%.[12, 43] Twenty-five percent may require surgery.[21] Some authors suggested that children older than 9 years of age responded best to dilatation.[12] It was also suggested that if symptoms recurred within 6 months after initial dilatation, surgery would likely be eventually required.[73]

The morbidity and mortality rates for pneumatic diltation are 5% and 0.7%, respectively, according to one published report.[70] The main complications include esophageal perforation,[69, 74, 75] fever, and pleural effusions.[74] The incidence of fever and pleural effusions is approximately 4%.[74] Rare complications include persistent esophageal pain,[76] aspiration pneumonia,[12] oropharyngeal hematoma,[12] and bleeding. GER can be a late complication of pneumatic dilatation in 1% to 9% of adults and 12% of children with achalasia.[73, 77]

The incidence of esophageal perforation after pneumatic dilatation in adults is 1% to 5%.[69, 74] The perforation usually occurs at the anterolateral esophageal wall and is usually accompanied by severe chest pain, fever, and sometimes dysphagia; mediastinal or subcutaneous emphysema; or a pleural effusion.[78] A plain radiograph may demonstrate emphysematous changes or effusions.[78] Definitive diagnosis of perforation is made with a water-soluble contrast esophagogram. In fact, many clinicians advocate the routine use of postdilatation esophagograms because of reports of deaths resulting from missed esophageal perforations due to paucity of symptoms.[21, 75, 79] Delayed perforations of the esophagus after pneumatic dilatation have been described, underscoring the importance of close observation after pneumatic dilatation and repeat contrast studies if symptoms should develop.[79] Risk factors for perforation include prior pneumatic dilatation and the use of a Browne-McHardy dilator at pressures greater than 11 psi.[80] Mortality after perforation can be as high as 50%.[75, 78] Most clinicians would treat small perforations with intravenous antibiotics and parenteral nutrition.[77] Others advocate aggressive surgical intervention in the form of suturing the perforation followed by a modified Heller procedure.[78] The risk of perforation can be minimized by careful attention to the placement of the balloon dilator under fluroscopy and inflation pressures used.

Successful dilatation of two children with achalasia older than 8 years of age using a transendoscopic method has been reported.[81] Dilatation using bougies has typically been associated with a high incidence of esophageal perforation and only temporary relief, so this mode of therapy is no longer advocated.[12, 45, 46]

**SURGERY.** The most common surgical procedure used for achalasia is the Heller myotomy and its variants.[82, 83] The different variations depend on the type of approach (thoracic versus abdominal) or length of the myotomy (the vertical incision of the esophagus extending along the serosal surface of the distal esophagus and transecting the circular muscle fibers of the LES).[82] An adequate myotomy is one that is long enough to relieve obstruction but not so long as to permit excessive GER. Most patients require only a short myotomy.[84] Satisfactory results has been reported in 64% to 94% of adult patients.[63, 75, 85] Compared with pneumatic dilatation, myotomy had better long-term results (85% vs. 65%).[75] Myotomies after pneumatic dilatation have usually been successful despite the failure of the dilatation.[45, 75]

In children, the overall improvement rate was 84% in those who underwent myotomy.[21] Long-term results in more recent series have been excellent, leading their authors to suggest that primary treatment of achalasia in children should be surgical.[14, 76]

Late complications of esophagomyotomy are the need for reoperation, due to persistence of obstructive symptoms, and GER.[21, 75] Death after myotomy has not been reported, but the morbidity rate is 3% to 7%, including perforation in 1.4% to 3.2% of cases.[21, 75] Other complications include phrenic nerve paralysis, excessive hemorrhage, and esophageal and gastric herniation, resulting in necrosis. Significant persistent dysphagia after myotomy has been reported in 1% to 9% of patients.[44, 86] It is most frequently due to an inadequate myotomy[44] or an incompetent LES causing stricture and peptic esophagitis.[86] It is the most frequent indication for reoperation in up to 58% of patients.[86] Manometry and endoscopy are important in differentiating between an inadequate myotomy and a complication from the operation.

Persistence of obstructive symptoms, one of the main long-term complications after surgery, is usually due to an inadequate myotomy.[44, 86] Therefore, some authors recommend that the myotomy should extend 1 to 1.5 cm onto the gastric cardia to ensure that the entire length of the gastroesophageal junction is transected.[44] However, excessive encroachment onto the stomach may result in the development of GER, the other major long-term postmyotomy complication. The incidence of postmyotomy GER ranges from 3% to 60% (10–36% in children).[73, 75, 86–88] Its incidence appears to increase with time.[88] The presence of a stricture (3–6%) or severe esophagitis is indicative of postmyotomy GER.[73, 75, 87] A study of 70 postmyotomy patients detected asymptomatic GER in 14.3% and Barrett's esophagus in 4.5%.[87]

Some authors have suggested that an antireflux procedure be routinely performed at the time of myotomy to prevent GER.[89, 90] Others suggest that an antireflux procedure should only be done if esophagitis, pathologic GER, hiatal hernia, or diverticulum is present.[90, 91] Esophageal pH monitoring may not be helpful in establishing the frequency of GER in some cases because lactic acid from food residue in the distal esophagus can result in false-positive results.[92] Proponents for no antireflux procedure at the time of myotomy argue that there is only a small percentage of patients who develop postmyotomy GER.[85] Therefore, it is not necessary to subject all patients to a longer and more difficult procedure, especially if persistence of esophageal dysmotility due to achalasia combined with delayed esophageal emptying secondary to an antireflux procedure can lead to obstructive symptoms.[89]

#### *Botulinum Toxin*

Botulinum toxin is a neurotoxin that binds to presynaptic cholinergic terminals causing inhibition of acetylcholine release at the neuromuscular junction.[93] It is thought that botulinum toxin reduces LES pressure in patients with achalasia by decreasing the excitatory cholinergic innervation to the sphincter.[94]

Intrasphincteric injection of botulinum toxin has been found to be effective and safe in treating adults with achalasia.[94–96] The first experience with botulinum toxin in the treatment of children with achalasia was reported by Khoshoo and colleagues.[97] All three children experienced immediate resolution of symptoms. Unfortunately, the response was short-lived. Thus, repeated injections may be necessary. Obviously, more information needs to be collected regarding this modality's efficacy and long-term safety and in what clinical scenario it would be most useful.


#### *Summary*

It is agreed by most that the role of pharmacologic therapy in children with achalasia is that of short-term palliation. For long-term therapy, either pneumatic dilatation or myotomy is preferred. Because pneumatic dilatation is effective and safe, requires a shorter hospital stay, and is generally less costly than surgery unless repeated dilatations are necessary, it is prudent to perform a pneumatic dilatation first. If repeated dilatations are necessary and symptom-free periods are short, then myotomy should be done. It is important that the patient be evaluated for the presence of significant GER or hiatal hernia before myotomy to decide on whether an antireflux procedure is also necessary. Once more data are available on the use of botulinum toxin, one could then consider using botulinum toxin before myotomy in those patients who have failed pneumatic dilatation.


### Prognosis

Even after successful therapy with either pneumatic dilatation or myotomy and a symptom-free period, recurrence of obstructive symptoms may develop. It may be due to slow progression of the degenerative process of the myenteric plexus or to resistance to therapy. Esophageal cancer, particularly squamous carcinoma, may be a late complication in 5% of adult patients.[98–100] The mean time from diagnosis of achalasia to the occurrence of malignancy is 17 years.[99] This complication is more likely in those patients who have had a long course without treatment or failed therapy.[100] This has resulted in some authors advocating surveillance endoscopy every 3 to 5 years.[101] There is no information about the incidence of esophageal carcinoma in patients who developed achalasia as children. With our current knowledge, it is recommended that the diagnostic work-up in treated patients depend on clinical symptoms. Children should be observed closely with a low threshold for initiating an evaluation if symptoms should develop. Surveillance endoscopy may not be cost effective, and there are no data showing that such an approach can alter outcome.[98]

## OTHER MOTOR DISORDERS

### Esophagitis

Many children with peptic esophagitis have ineffective esophageal peristalsis and clearance.[102] Abnormal esophageal motility may have a pathogenic role in GER disease by prolonging the contact time between the esophageal mucosa and the gastric refluxate. In adults, there is a correlation between degree of esophageal inflammation and severity of esophageal motor disorder.[103] It is unclear whether esophageal motility improves after healing of the esophagitis.[104, 105]

### Esophageal Spasm

There is a wide body of literature discussing entities such as diffuse esophageal spasm and nutcracker esophagus. Although these are entities commonly considered in the differential diagnosis of adults presenting with noncardiac chest pain, very little is known about their prevalence in children. Diffuse esophageal spasm is a condition affecting the esophageal smooth muscle, and manometric abnormalities are most pronounced in the segment just above the LES. Typical motility features include repetitive contractions after a single swallow, nonperistaltic, simultaneous, and multipeaked peristaltic waves. Amplitude and duration are often exaggerated, and there may be an elevation in the baseline esophageal pressure. In most cases, the abnormal contractions are interspaced with normal contractions. Many swallowing sequences or use of solid boluses during testing may be necessary to uncover the motor disorder. Glassman and coworkers have described diffuse esophageal spasm and nutcracker esophagus in nine adolescent children presenting with chest pain.[106] Only one child responded to medical treatment with calcium channel blockers. A motor disorder similar to diffuse esophageal spasm has been described in an infant presenting with apnea and bradycardia.[107]

## Tracheoesophageal Fistula

Surgical repair of esophageal atresia restores anatomic continuity but does not normalize the esophageal motor function. Many children who have survived an esophageal atresia repair continue to have dysphagia, regurgitation, heartburn, and chronic respiratory symptoms. Long-term follow-up studies of these children have demonstrated absent peristalsis, frequent tertiary contractions, low or absent LES pressure, and GER.[108] The etiology of the esophageal motor dysfunction remains unclear. It has been suggested that the motor disorder could be part of the congenital abnormality or be secondary to ischemia or damage to the esophageal branches of the vagus nerve during surgery.

## Neuromuscular Diseases

In patients with *Hirschsprung's disease*, motor abnormalities are not restricted to the aganglionic segment but may be demonstrated in the more proximal bowel. Staiano and coworkers have reported a high percentage of abnormal peristaltic sequences in the esophagus of children before and after surgical treatment of Hirschsprung's disease.[109] Children with *psychomotor retardation* often have esophageal dysmotility that persists after successful GER treatment and predisposes them to GER relapses. Motor abnormalities are found both in the striated and smooth muscle portions of the esophagus.[110] Some infants with *minimal change myopathy* may present initially with recurrent respiratory tract infections and feeding difficulties. The esophageal manometry shows no esophageal peristalsis and may lead the physician to suspect the myopathy.[111] *Chronic intestinal pseudo-obstruction* is a condition characterized by chronic symptoms of bowel obstruction in the absence of a fixed, lumen-occupying lesion. It is a rare condition that may involve any area of the gastrointestinal tract. The esophagus is less frequently affected in children than in adults. Patients with the myopathic form of the disease have low LES pressure and weak peristaltic contractions. Subjects with neuropathy may have achalasia or abnormal peristalsis with high-pressure, nonpropagating pressure waves. A careful motility study of the esophagus may obviate the need for more invasive motility studies in the minority of children with esophageal involvement. Children with *scleroderma* may present with dysphagia, heartburn, and regurgitation. Esophageal dysmotility is detected in 73% of children and adolescents with scleroderma and mixed connective tissue disease.[112] Primary neurogenic dysfunction or atrophy and sclerosis of the esophageal smooth muscle may cause the esophageal abnormalities. Typical manometric features include decreased LES pressure and low-amplitude, simultaneous contractions in the distal esophagus. There is no correlation between manometric abnormalities and disease duration or Raynaud's phenomenon.[112] The study of the esophageal manifestations of scleroderma and intestinal pseudo-obstruction constitutes one of the acceptable indications for esophageal manometry in children based on a medical position statement by the North American Society for Pediatric Gastroenterology and Nutrition.[113]

## Other Disorders

Both reduction of esophageal caliber and impairment of the esophageal motor functions play a role in causing dysphagia in children with a history of *caustic ingestion*. Esophageal transit is delayed, and there is manometric evidence of segmental aperistalsis with normal UES and LES function.[114]

Esophageal dysmotility has been reported in a group of children breast fed by a mother with *silicone breast implants*.[115] The children presented with recurrent vomiting, dysphagia, and abdominal pain and were found to have low LES pressure and a significantly impaired esophageal peristalsis with nearly absent contractions in the distal esophagus. There was no improvement in manometric findings after a 2-year follow-up. The authors hypothesized a persistent autonomic nervous system dysfunction not related to humoral autoimmune responses.[116]

**REFERENCES**


1. Putnam PE, Orenstein SR, Pang D, et al: Cricopharyngeal dysfunction associated with Chiari malformation. Pediatrics 1992;89:871–876.
2. Staiano AM, Cucchiara S, De Vizia B, et al: Disorders of upper esophageal sphincter motility in children. J Pediatr Gastroenterol Nutr 1987;6:892–898.
3. Castell JA, Castell DO: Upper esophageal sphincter and pharyngeal function and oropharyngeal (transfer dysphagia). Gastroenterol Clin North Am 1996;25:35–50.
4. Castell JA, Dalton CB, Castell DO: Pharyngeal and upper esophageal sphincter manometry in humans. Am J Physiol 1990;258;G173.
5. Gideon A, Nolte K: The non-obstructive pharyngoesophageal cross roll. Ann Radiol 1973;16:129–135.
6. Kilman WJ, Goyal RK: Disorders of pharyngeal and upper esophageal sphincter motor function. Arch Intern Med 1976;36:592–601.
7. Dinari G, Danziger Y, Mimouni M, et al: Cricopharyngeal dysfunction in childhood: treatment by dilatations. J Pediatr Gastroenterol Nutr 1987;6:212–216.
8. Margulies SE, Brunt PW, Donner MW: Familial dysautonomia, a cineradiographic study of the swallowing mechanism. Radiology 1968;90:107–112.
9. Wyllie E, Wyllie R, Cruse RP, et al: The mechanisms of nitrazepam-induced drooling and aspiration. N Engl J Med 1986;314:35–38.
10. Reichert TJ, Bluestone CD, Stool SE, et al: Congenital cricopharyngeal achalasia. Ann Otol Rhinol Laryngol 1977;86:603–610.
11. Sanderson DR, Ellis FH Jr, Schlegel JF, et al: Syndrome of vigorous achalasia: clinical and physiologic observations. Dis Chest 1967;52:508–517.
12. Azizkhan RG, Tapper D, Eraklis A: Achalasia in childhood: a 20-year experience. Pediatr Surg 1980;15:452–456.
13. Mayberry JB, Mayell MJ: Epidemiological study of achalasia in children. Gut 1988;29:90–93.
14. Nihoul-Fekete C, Bawab F, Lortat-Jacob S, et al: Achalasia of the esophagus in childhood: surgical treatment in 35 cases, with special reference to familial cases and glucocorticoid defiency association. Hepatogastroenterology 1991;38:510–513.
15. Grant DB, Barnes ND, Dumic M, et al: Neurological and adrenal dysfunction in the adrenal insufficiency/alacrima/achalasia (3A) syndrome. Arch Dis Child 1993;68:779–782.
16. Rozycki DL, Rube RJ, Rapin I, et al: Autosomal recessive deafness associated with short stature, vitiligo, muscle wasting and achalasia. Arch Otolaryngol 1971;93:194–197.
17. Stein DT, Knauer M: Achalasia in monozygotic twins. Dig Dis Sci 1982;27:636–640.
18. Westely CR, Herbst JJ, Goldman S, et al: Infantile achalasia: inherited as an autosomal recessive disorder. J Pediatr 1975;87:243–246.
19. Kaar TK, Waldron R, Ashraf MS, et al: Familial infantile esophageal achalasia. Arch Dis Child 1991;66:1353–1354.
20. Myers NA, Jolley SG, Taylor R: Achalasia of the cardia in children: a world-wide survey. J Pediatr Surg 1994;29:1375–1379.
21. Nurko S: Other motor disorders: In Walker WA, Durie PR, Hamilton

JR, et al (eds): Pediatric Gastrointestinal Disease, Pathophysiology, Diagnosis, Management, 2nd ed. St. Louis, CV Mosby, 1996, vol 1, pp 469–502.
22. Buick RG, Spitz L: Achalasia of the cardia in children. Br J Surg 1985;72:341–343.
23. Robertson CS, Martin BA, Atkinson M: Varicella-zoster virus DNA in the esophageal myenteric plexus in achalasia. Gut 1993;34:299–302.
24. Qualman SJ, Haupt HM, Yange P, et al: Esophageal Lewy bodies associated with ganglion cell loss in achalasia. Gastroenterology 1984;87:848–856.
25. Cassella RR, Brown AL Jr, Sayre GP, et al: Achalasia of the esophagus: pathologic and etiologic considerations. Ann Surg 1964;160:474–487.
26. Elder JB: Achalasia of the cardia in childhood. Digestion 1970;3:90–96.
27. Rickham PP, Boekman CR: Achalasia of the esophagus in young children. Clin Pediatr 1963;2:676–681.
28. Holloway RH, Dodds WJ, Helm JF, et al: Integrity of cholinergic innervation to the lower esophageal sphincter in achalasia. Gastroenterology 1986;90:924–929.
29. Dodds WJ, Dent J, Hogan WJ, et al: Paradoxical lower esophageal sphincter contraction induced by cholecystokinin-octapeptide in patients with achalasia. Gastroenterology 1981;80:327–333.
30. Cassella RR, Ellis FH, Brown AH: Fine structural changes in achalasia of the esophagus: I. Vagus nerves. Am J Pathol 1965;46:279–288.
31. Aggestrup S, Uddman R, Jensen SL, et al: Regulatory peptides in the lower esophageal sphincter of man. Regul Pept 1985;10:167–178.
32. Biancani P, Walsh JH, Behar J: Vasoactive intestinal polypeptide: a neurotransmitter for lower esophageal sphincter relaxation. J Clin Invest 1984;73:963–967.
33. Alumets J, Schaffalitzky De Muckadell O, Fahrenkrug J, et al: A rich VIP nerve supply is characteristic of sphincters. Nature 1979;280:155–156.
34. Guelrud M, Rossiter A, Souney PF, et al: The effect of vasoactive intestinal polypeptide on the lower esophageal sphincter in achalasia. Gastroenterology 1992;103:377–382.
35. Preisksaitis HG, Tremblay L, Diamant NE: Nitric oxide mediates inhibitory nerve effects in human esophagus and lower esophageal sphincter. Dig Dis Sci 1994;39:770–775.
36. Gaumnitz EA, Bass P, Osinski MA, et al: Electrophysiological and pharmacological responses of chronically denervated lower esophageal sphincter of the opossum. Gastroenterology 1995;109:789–799.
37. Murray J, Bates JN, Conklin JL: Nerve-mediated nitric oxide production by opossum lower esophageal sphincter. Dig Dis Sci 1994;39:1872–1876.
38. Anand N, Paterson WG: Role of nitric oxide in esophageal peristalsis. Am J Physiol 1994;266:123–131.
39. Polk HC, Burford TH: Disorders of the distal esophagus in infancy and childhood. Am J Dis Child 1964;108:243–251.
40. Bosher LP, Shaw A: Achalasia in siblings. Am J Dis Child 1981;135:709–710.
41. Singh H, Gupta HL, Sethi RS, et al: Cardiac achalasia in childhood. Postgrad Med J 1969;45:327–335.
42. Boyle JT, Cohen S, Watkins JB: Successful treatment of achalasia in childhood by pneumatic dilatation. J Pediatr 1981;99:35–40.
43. Moersch HJ: Cardiospasm in infancy and childhood. Am J Dis Child 1929;38:294–298.
44. Lemmer JH, Coran AG, Wesley JR: Achalasia in children: treatment by anterior esophageal myotomy (modified Heller operation). J Pediatr Surg 1985;20:333–338.
45. Nakayama DK, Shorter NA, Boyle JT, et al: Pneumatic dilatation and operative treatment of achalasia in children. J Pediatr Surg 1987;22:619–622.
46. Eckardt VF, Aignherr C, Bernhard G: Predictors of outcome in patients with achalasia treated by pneumatic dilatation. Gastroenterology 1992;103:1732–1738.
47. Cohen S: Motor disorders of the esophagus. N Engl J Med 1979;301:184–192.
48. Uribe P, Csendes A, Larrain A, et al: Motility studies in fifty patients with achalasia of the esophagus. Am J Gastroenterol 1974;62:333–336.
49. Asch MJ, Liebman W, Lechman RS, et al: Esophageal achalasia: diagnosis and cardiomyotomy in a newborn infant. J Pediatr Surg 1974;9:911–912.
50. Dudnick RS, Castell JA, Castell DO: Abnormal upper esophageal sphincter function in achalasia. Am J Gastroenterol 1992;87:1712–1715.
51. Vantrappen G, Janssens J, Hellemans J, et al: Achalasia, diffuse esophageal spasm, and related motility disorders. Gastroenterology 1979;76:450–457.
52. Coccia G, Bortolotti M, Michetti P, et al: Return of peristalsis after nifedipine therapy in patients with idiopathic esophageal achalasia. Am J Gastroenterol 1992;87:1705–1708.
53. Holloway RH, Krosin G, Lange RC: Radionuclide esophageal emptying of a solid meal to quantitate results of therapy in achalasia. Gastroenterology 1983;84:771–776.
54. Russell CO, Hill LD, Holmes ER, et al: Radionuclide transit: a sensitive screening test for esophageal dysfunction. Gastroenterology 1981;80:887–892.
55. Kramer P, Ingelfinger FJ: Esophageal sensitivity to Mecholyl in cardiospasm. Gastroenterology 1968;54:771–773.
56. Payne WS, Ellis FH, Olsen AM: Treatment of cardiospasm (achalasia of the esophagus) in children. Surgery 1961;50:731–735.
57. Tucker HJ, Snape WJ, Cohen S: Achalasia secondary to carcinoma: manometric and clinical features. Ann Intern Med 1978;89:315–318.
58. Helm J, et al: Carcinoma of the cardia masquerading as idiopathic achalasia. Gastroenterology 1982;82:1082A.
59. Betarrello A, Pinott HW: Esophageal involvement in Chagas' disease. Clin Gastroenterol 1976;5:103–109.
60. Duane PD, Magee TM, Alexander MJ, et al: Esophageal achalasia in adolescent women mistaken for anorexia nervosa. BMJ 1992;305:43.
61. Gelfond M, Rosen P, Gilat T: Isosorbide dinitrate and nifedipine treatment of achalasia: a clinical, manometric and radionuclide evaluation. Gastroenterology 1982;83:963–969.
62. Maksimak M, Perlmutter DH, Winter HS: The use of nifedipine in the treatment of achalasia in children. J Pediatr Gastroenterol Nutr 1986;5:883–886.
63. Smith H, Buick R, Booth I, et al: The use of nifedipine for treatment of achalasia in children (letter). J Pediatr Gastroenterol Nutr 1988;7:146.
64. Richter JE, Dalton CB, Buice RG: Nifedipine, a potent inhibitor of contractions in the body of the human esophagus. Gastroenterology 1985;89:549–554.
65. Thomas E, Lebow RA, Gubler RJ, et al: Nifedipine for the poor risk elderly patient with achalasia: objective response demonstrated by solid meal study. South Med J 1984;77:394–401.
66. Samarasinghe DA, Nicholson GI, Hamilton I: Dilatation of achalasia in the young: a useful alternative. Gastrointest Endosc 1991;37:568–569.
67. Stark GA, Castell DO, Richter JE, et al: Prospective randomized comparison of Browne-McHardy and microvasive balloon dilators in the treatment of achalasia. Am J Gastroenterol 1990;85:1322–1326.
68. Kadakia SC, Wong RK: Graded pneumatic dilatation using Rigiflex achalasia dilators in patients with primary esophageal achalasia. Am J Gastroenterol 1993;88:34–38.
69. Parkman H, Reynolds JC, Ouyang A, et al: Pneumatic dilatation or esophagomyotomy treatment for idiopathic achalasia: clinical outcomes and cost analysis. Dig Dis Sci 1993;38:75–85.
70. Salis GB, Chiocca JC, Perisse E, et al: Esophageal achalasia: 20 years' experience with nonsurgical treatment. Acta Gastroenterol Latinoam 1991;21:11–16.
71. Olsen AM, Harrington SW, Moersch JH, et al: The treatment of cardiospasm: analysis of a twelve year experience. J Thorac Surg 1951;22:164–187.
72. Huet F, Mougenot JF, Saleh T, et al: Esophageal dilatation in pediatrics: a study of 33 patients. Arch Pediatr 1995;2:423–430.
73. Seo JK, Winter HS: Esophageal manometric and clinical response to treatment in children with achalasia (abstract). Gastroenterology 1987;92:1634.
74. Mandelstam P, Sugawa C, Silvis SE, et al: Complications associated with esophagogastroduodenoscopy and with esophageal dilatation. Gastrointest Endosc 1976;23:16–19.
75. Okike N, Payne WS, Neufeld DM, et al: Esophagomyotomy versus forceful dilatation for achalasia of the esophagus: results in 899 patients. Ann Thorac Surg 1979;28:119–125.
76. Emblem R, Stringer MD, Hall CM, et al: Current results of surgery for achalasia of the cardia. Arch Dis Child 1993;68:749–751.
77. Dellipiani AW, Hewetson KA: Pneumatic dilatation in the management of achalasia: experience of 45 cases. Q J Med 1986;58:253–258.
78. Miller RE, Tiszenkel HI: Esophageal perforation due to pneumatic dilatation for achalasia. Surg Gynecol Obstet 1988;166:458–460.

79. Ott DJ, Richter JE, Wu WC, et al: Radiographic evaluation of esophagus immediately after pneumatic dilatation for achalasia. Dig Dis Sci 1987;32:962–967.
80. Nair LA, Reynolds JC, Parkman HP, et al: Complications during pneumatic dilatation for achalasia or diffuse esophageal spasm: analysis of risk factors, early clinical characteristics and outcome. Dig Dis Sci 1993;38:1893–1904.
81. Perisic VN: Achalasia in children. Am J Dis Child 1988;142:16.
82. Csendes A, Braghetto I, Burdiles P, et al: A prospective randomized study comparing forceful dilatation and esophagomyotomy in patients with achalasia of the esophagus. Gastroenterology 1981;80:789–795.
83. Heller E: Extramukose Cardiaplastik beim chronischen Cardiopasmus mit Dilatation des Oesophagus. Mitt Grenzgeb Med Chir 1913;27:141–149.
84. Herbst JJ: Achalasia and other motor disorders. In Wyllie R, Hyams JS (eds): Pediatric Gastrointestinal Disease: Pathophysiology, Diagnosis, Management. Philadelphia, WB Saunders, 1993, pp 391–401.
85. Ellis FH: Esophagomyotomy for achalasia: a 22-year experience. Br J Surg 1993;80:882–885.
86. Ellis FH, Gibb SP: Reoperation after esophagomyotomy for achalasia of the esophagus. Am J Surg 1975;129:407–412.
87. Agha FP, Keren DF: Barrett's esophagus complicating achalasia after esophagomyotomy. J Clin Gastroenterol 1987;9:232–237.
88. Jara FM, Toledo-Pereyra LH, Lewis JW, et al: Long-term results of esophagomyotomy for achalasia of the esophagus. Arch Surg 1979;114:935–936.
89. Nussinson LE, Hager H, Samara M: Familial achalasia with absent tear production. J Pediatr Gastroenterol Nutr 1988;7:284–287.
90. Skinner DB: Myotomy and achalasia (editorial). Ann Thorac Surg 1984;37:183–184.
91. Murray GF, Battaglini JW, Keagy BA, et al: Selective application of fundoplication in achalasia. Ann Thorac Surg 1984;37:185–188.
92. Smart HL, Foster PN, Evans DF, et al: Twenty four hour esophageal acidity in achalasia before and after pneumatic dilatation. Gut 1987;28:883–887.
93. Gooch JL, Sandell TV: Botulism toxin for spasticity and athetosis in children with cerebral palsy. Arch Phys Med Rehabil 1996;77:508–511.
94. Pasricha PJ, Rai R, Ravich WJ, et al: Botulinum toxin for achalasia: long-term outcome and predictors of response. Gastroenterology 1996;110:1410–1415.
95. Cohen S, Parkman HP: Treatment of achalasia—whalebone to botulinum toxin. N Engl J Med 1995;332:815–816.
96. Cuilliere C, Ducrotte P, Zerbib F, et al: Achalasia: outcome of patients treated with intrasphincteric injection of botulinum toxin. Gut 1997;41:87–92.
97. Khoshoo V, LaGarde DC, Udall JN: Intrasphincteric injection of botulinum toxin for treating achalasia in children (abstract). J Pediatr Gastroenterol Nutr 1995;21:335.
98. Choung JJ, Dubovik S, McCallum RW: Achalasia as a risk factor for esophageal carcinoma: a reappraisal. Dig Dis Sci 1984;29:1105–1108.
99. Norton GA, Postkehwat RW, Thompson WM: Esophageal carcinoma: a summary of populations at risk. South Med J 1980;73:23–27.
100. Aggestrup S, Holm JC, Sorenstein JR: Does achalasia predispose to cancer of the esophagus? Chest 1992;102:1013–1016.
101. Benjamin SB, Richter JE, Cordova CM, et al: Prospective manometric evaluation with pharmacological provocation of patients with suspected esophageal motility dysfunction. Gastroenterology 1984;84:893–901.
102. Hillemeier AC, Grill BB, McCallum R, et al: Esophageal and gastric motor abnormalities in gastroesophageal reflux during infancy. Gastroenterology 1983;84:741–746.
103. Kahrilas PJ, Dodds WJ, Hogan WJ, et al: Esophageal peristaltic dysfunction in peptic esophagitis. Gastroenterology 1986;91:897–904.
104. Cucchiara S, Staiano AM, Di Lorenzo C, et al: Esophageal motor abnormalities in children with gastroesophageal reflux and peptic esophagitis. J Pediatr 1986;108:907–910.
105. Allen ML, McIntosh DL, Robinson MG: Healing or amelioration of esophagitis does not result in increased lower esophageal sphincter contractile pressure. Am J Gastroenterol 1990;85:1331–1334.
106. Glassman MS, Medow MS, Berezin S, et al: Spectrum of esophageal disorders in children with chest pain. Dig Dis Sci 1992;37:663–666.
107. Fontan JP, Heldt GP, Heyman MB, et al: Esophageal spasm associated with apnea and bradycardia in an infant. Pediatrics 1984;73:52–55.
108. Werlin SL, Dodds WJ, Hogan WJ, et al: Esophageal motor function in esophageal atresia. Dig Dis Sci 1981;26:796–800.
109. Staiano A, Corazziari E, Andreotti MR, et al: Esophageal motility in children with Hirschsprung's disease. Am J Dis Child 1991;145:310–313.
110. Staiano A, Cucchiara S, Del Giudice E, et al: Disorders of oesophageal motility in children with psychomotor retardation and gastroesophageal reflux. Eur J Pediatr 1991;150:638–641.
111. Staiano A, Cucchiara S, Del Giudice E, et al: Oesophageal motor involvement in minimal change myopathy. Ital J Gastroenterol 1989;21:159–163.
112. Flick JA, Boyle JT, Tuchman DN, et al: Esophageal motor abnormalities in children and adolescents with scleroderma and mixed connective tissue disease. Pediatrics 1988;82:107–111.
113. Gilger MA, Boyle JT, Sondheimer JM, et al: Indication for pediatric esophageal manometry. J Pediatr Gastroenterol Nutr 1997;24:616–618.
114. Cadranel S, Di Lorenzo C, Rodesch P, et al: Caustic ingestion and esophageal function. J Pediatr Gastroenterol Nutr 1990;10:164–168.
115. Levine JJ, Ilowite NT: Scleroderma-like esophageal disease in children breast-fed by mothers with silicone breast implants. JAMA 1994;271:213–216.
116. Levine JJ, Trachman H, Gold DM, et al: Esophageal dysmotility in children breast-fed by mothers with silicone breast implants. Dig Dis Sci 1996;41:1600–1603.

# Chapter 16

# Other Diseases of the Esophagus

*Francisco A. Sylvester*

## ESOPHAGEAL INFECTIONS

Most patients who acquire esophageal infections have an underlying risk factor, such as primary or secondary immunodeficiencies, hypochlorhydria, antibiotic treatment, or abnormalities of esophageal structure and function (e.g., progressive systemic sclerosis, achalasia, stricture, esophageal burns).[1–11]

### Candida

*Candida albicans* is part of the normal human flora but may become pathogenic in patients who are debilitated or have local anatomic or physiologic abnormalities of the esophagus. Children with *Candida* esophagitis may present with or without concomitant oral thrush.[12–15]

In patients with acquired immunodeficiency syndrome (AIDS), *Candida* esophagitis is responsible for the majority of cases of esophageal disease.[16] The risk of fungal (or viral) infection rises in proportion to the severity of the immunodeficiency.[17, 18] Patients with severe immunodeficiency may have concurrent infections with multiple organisms, including *Candida,* herpes simplex virus (HSV), and cytomegalovirus.[13, 19–21]

Symptoms of *Candida* esophagitis may be absent or may include odynophagia, chest pain, and hematemesis. Tracheoesophageal fistula has been reported as a complication of infectious esophagitis.[22]

Endoscopy is recommended for evaluation of esophageal symptoms in patients with suspected *Candida* esophagitis.[16] The typical appearance of yellowish-white, confluent plaques can be seen in these patients (Fig. 16–1). Diagnosis is confirmed by biopsy of the affected mucosa and by culture.

Treatment of *Candida* esophagitis requires the use of systemic antifungal agents. Fluconazole (5 mg/kg per day) is usually effective.[23] Wilcox and colleagues[24] have proposed the use of empirical therapy with fluconazole as a highly efficacious, safe, and cost-effective strategy for persons infected with the human immunodeficiency virus (HIV) who have new-onset esophageal symptoms. If fluconazole fails to control the infection, amphotericin B can be used.[15] In bone marrow transplant recipients, prophylaxis with fluconazole was shown to reduce the incidence of both systemic and superficial fungal infections.[25]

### Herpes Simplex

Primary HSV infection usually results in self-limited oropharyngeal infection in healthy hosts. However, several cases of esophageal HSV infection have been reported in such persons.[26–29] It is believed that these infections are part of primary HSV infection (usually HSV1), but this has not been proved.[26, 30] In healthy persons, reactivation of HSV usually results in herpes labialis. In immunocompromised

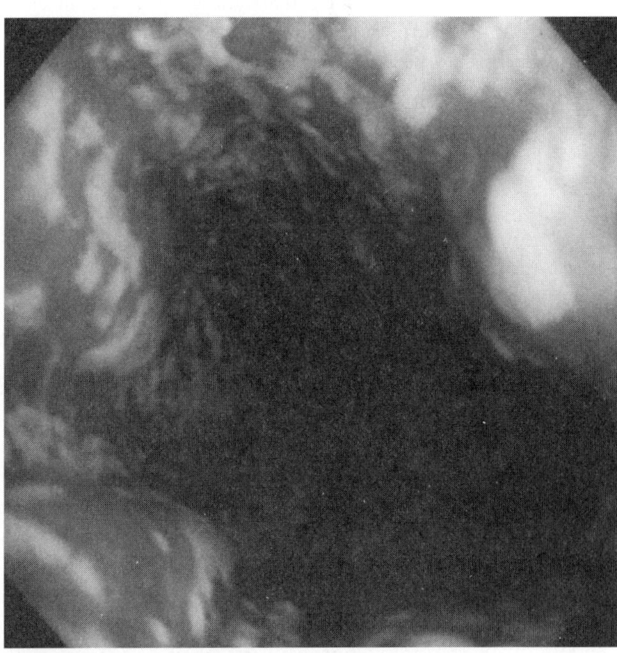

**FIGURE 16–1.** Endoscopic view of the esophagus of a healthy 8-year-old boy with dysphagia, showing erythematous esophageal mucosa overlaid with linear white confluent plaques suggestive of *Candida* esophagitis. (Courtesy of Christopher J. Justinich, MD.)

patients, reactivation of HSV may result in infection of multiple organs.[31, 32] The esophagus is the most common place for such infections to occur.[31]

Symptoms of herpes esophagitis may include a prodrome of respiratory infection, fever, myalgias, and sore throat, especially in immunocompetent individuals,[26, 30] or it can be asymptomatic.[31] This prodrome is followed by odynophagia and retrosternal pain. Nausea, vomiting, fever, and hematemesis may occur.[26, 29, 31, 33–35] Because HSV infection is usually confined to the squamous epithelium even in immunocompromised hosts, systemic and intra-abdominal symptoms are uncommon. Complications of severe HSV esophagitis may occur, including mucosal necrosis, superinfection with other organisms, hemorrhage, strictures, HSV pneumonia, tracheoesophageal fistula formation, perforation, and disseminated HSV infection.[35–38] In the normal host HSV esophagitis is a self-limited illness, but in the immunodeficient patient HSV infection can be severe and prolonged.[34, 39]

Radiographic findings of HSV esophagitis are nonspecific,[40] and endoscopic confirmation is required to make the diagnosis. The earliest lesions are small vesicles seen mostly in the middle-to-distal esophagus, which then slough to produce 1- to 3-mm ulcers. The uninvolved mucosa has a normal appearance. If the infection progresses, ulcers coalesce and an inflammatory exudate difficult to distinguish from *Candida* esophagitis may develop.[39, 41–43] Endoscopic appearance therefore is not specific, and the diagnosis of HSV esophagitis needs to be confirmed by the demonstration of HSV by histology, cytology, or culture.[20, 32] Diagnostic histologic changes of HSV infection include multinucleated giant cells, ballooning degeneration, "ground-glass" intranuclear Cowdry type A inclusion bodies, and margination of chromatin. In contrast to cytomegalovirus infection, there are no cytoplasmic inclusion bodies.[9] Biopsies of the ulcer base are usually inadequate to diagnose HSV infection, but the virus can be detected in ulcer margins and islands of squamous epithelium. Viral culture of directed brushings and biopsies is more sensitive than microscopic examination for the diagnosis of HSV esophagitis.[44]

In immunocompetent patients HSV esophagitis is a self-limited illness, requires only supportive care, and usually resolves in 10 to 17 days.[26, 30, 39] Acyclovir may shorten the duration of disease in these patients,[39] especially if it is started immediately after the onset of esophageal symptoms.[28] Immunodeficient patients are treated with acyclovir (250 mg/m$^2$ q 8 hr intravenously for 7–10 days, followed by oral acyclovir to complete 2 weeks).[9, 45] HSV strains resistant to acyclovir have been reported secondary to mutations in viral DNA polymerase and thymidine kinase.[46, 47] These strains can be treated with high-dose constant acyclovir infusion (1.5–2.0 mg/kg per hour) for 6 weeks or with foscarnet (60 mg/kg slow intravenous infusion q 8 hr for 14–21 days).[46–49] HSV isolates resistant to both foscarnet and acyclovir have been reported. Vidarabine is an alternative to treat these patients.[49]

Immunocompromised patients at risk for systemic HSV infections (HSV-seropositive transplant recipients and AIDS patients with recurrent herpetic infections) benefit from acyclovir prophylaxis. Prophylaxis has almost eliminated HSV esophagitis among solid organ and bone marrow transplant recipients.[50, 51]

## Cytomegalovirus

CMV is acquired usually perinatally or in early infancy. In adults it is acquired through sexual contact. Primary CMV infection in immunologically normal persons is frequently asymptomatic or associated with a mild mononucleosis-like syndrome.[52] Once the infection is acquired, there is a lifelong risk for intermittent reactivation.[53] Esophagitis caused by CMV occurs almost exclusively in immunosuppressed persons,[9, 53] and only rarely in normal hosts.[54] In patients with AIDS, esophagitis is the most common gastrointestinal manifestation of CMV infection.[20, 55] CMV frequently infects organ transplant recipients, in whom any part of the gastrointestinal tract can be affected, including the esophagus.[53]

Because CMV can affect other sites of the gastrointestinal tract at the same time as the esophagus, systemic symptoms may predominate, including fever, diarrhea, weight loss, nausea, and vomiting. Dysphagia, odynophagia, and retrosternal pain are less common than in HSV esophagitis.[33, 56, 57] In transplant recipients and patients with AIDS, CMV esophagitis can coexist with both HSV and *Candida.*[19, 33] CMV esophagitis may result in esophageal stricture, but perforation is rare.[58, 59] In bone marrow transplant recipients it has been reported that large mucosal lesions secondary to CMV infection can lead to persistent nausea, anorexia, and intestinal bleeding even after the virus has been successfully eradicated.[57]

The diagnosis of CMV esophagitis relies on endoscopic biopsies.[46] Serology,[60–62] cultures of blood, throat, stool or urine,[33, 60, 62–65] and double-contrast esophagograms[19, 66] may be suggestive of CMV infection but are not helpful in establishing CMV as the specific etiologic agent responsible for a particular esophageal infection. The endoscopic appearance of CMV esophagitis is highly variable, usually affecting the middle-to-distal portion of the esophagus.[67] Superficial, serpiginous erosions with nonraised borders,[68, 69] a single shallow esophageal ulcer,[65, 70] and mucosal hemorrhage[53] can be found, but no endoscopic feature is pathognomonic for CMV. Because the squamous epithelium of the esophagus is *not* infected by CMV, biopsy specimens need to be taken from the base of ulcers to obtain infected fibroblasts and endothelial cells for diagnosis.[33, 69] However, gastric and intestinal epithelium can harbor CMV, and biopsies from these areas may be helpful to diagnose enteric CMV infection.[9] Histologically, large cells (25- to 35-μm) can be found in the lamina propria, with a basophilic intranuclear inclusion surrounded by a clear halo ("owl's-eye") inclusion and clusters of small intracytoplasmatic inclusions.[63] These "cytomegalic" cells provide evidence of tissue infection with CMV.[53]

Immunohistochemical methods to detect CMV antigens and in situ hybridization techniques are also available to confirm CMV infection.[69, 71, 72] Viral culture is the most sensitive method to diagnose CMV enteric infection, and techniques using immunologic staining of centrifugation cultures can provide a diagnosis of CMV infection in less than 48 hours.[73] CMV culture results need to be interpreted with caution, because a positive culture may not correlate well with CMV disease.[13, 74, 75] Culture positivity rates in non-CMV lesions may be as high as 17% in patients with AIDS.[74]

Gastrointestinal CMV disease requires antiviral therapy in persons with sustained immunosuppression.[68] Intravenous ganciclovir (5 mg/kg q 12 hr for 2 weeks followed by maintenance with 5 mg/kg qd, 5–7 days/week in patients who have recurrent disease or are thought to be at high risk for recurrence[9, 76]) and intravenous foscarnet (60 mg/kg q 8 hr for 2 weeks followed by maintenance with 60 mg/kg qd if necessary[56, 59, 77–80]) are both effective agents in the treatment of CMV infection.[81, 82] When therapy with ganciclovir is ineffective[57] or results in significant toxicity, foscarnet can be used as an alternative first-line drug. A combination of ganciclovir and foscarnet has been used to treat AIDS patients with progressive CMV disease who failed treatment with either drug alone.[83] CMV resistant to both ganciclovir and foscarnet has been reported.[84] Prophylactic ganciclovir after solid organ or bone marrow transplantation has been reported to be highly effective in preventing both infection and disease.[85–89] In CMV-seropositive bone marrow transplant recipients, prophylaxis with acyclovir confers partial protection until the leukocyte count permits ganciclovir use.[77, 88, 89] Acyclovir prophylaxis has also been effective in reducing CMV infection and disease in cadaveric renal transplant recipients.[90]

### Other Infections of the Esophagus

**HISTOPLASMOSIS.** *Histoplasma capsulatum* is a dimorphic fungus found in the Ohio and Mississippi River valleys. Initial infection with *Histoplasma* occurs by inhalation of spores, which reach the alveoli and are ingested by macrophages. These cells can spread to the regional lymph nodes and then hematogenously.[91] After several weeks, necrotizing granulomas appear in the lymph nodes and lungs.[92] Gastrointestinal involvement by *Histoplasma* is very rare in the pediatric age group.[93–95] Esophageal histoplasmosis occurs usually as a complication of pulmonary histoplasmosis with granulomatous mediastinal lymph node involvement,[94] and the vast majority of these patients do not have any underlying conditions causing immunosuppression.[94] Primary esophageal histoplasmosis is very rare.[92] Fibrosing mediastinitis, an exaggerated host response to foci of infection with *Histoplasma,* can lead to encasement and obstruction of the esophagus with no mucosal involvement.[92] In these patients, definitive diagnosis may require thoracoscopy or thoracotomy.[94] In AIDS patients, esophageal involvement can occur in the context of disseminated histoplasmosis.[96] Complications of esophageal histoplasmosis include esophageal fistulas[97] and esophageal perforation causing back pain.[98] Symptomatic infection with *Histoplasma* responds to systemic antifungal agents (itraconazole, amphotericin B),[32] but mediastinal fibrosis may be resistant to these drugs.

**TUBERCULOSIS.** Primary tuberculosis of the esophagus is very rare.[99–102] Most cases are secondary to tuberculous infection of other organs, including mediastinal lymph nodes or lung,[103, 104] or miliary tuberculosis.[100] Because tuberculosis of the esophagus usually occurs late in the development of the disease, it is extremely rare in children.[105, 106] Esophageal tuberculosis can manifest with dysphagia, fever, and weight loss.[107] Usually the middle third of the esophagus is affected. The diagnosis can be made by a combination of purified protein derivative (PPD), imaging studies (chest films, esophagogram, chest computed tomographic scan), and endoscopic biopsies. The endoscopic lesion is ulcerative,[108] granular with miliary mucosal granulomas, or hyperplastic with fibrosis, luminal narrowing, and stricture formation,[109] and it can be confused with an esophageal tumor.[110] Complications include fatal hematemesis from esophagoaortic fistula,[107, 111] tracheoesophageal fistula,[112] and perforation.[113] Antituberculous therapy is effective in healing esophageal tuberculosis.[102, 106]

**HUMAN IMMUNODEFICIENCY VIRUS.** Idiopathic esophageal ulceration associated with HIV infection has been described in adults.[65, 114] The first case of idiopathic esophageal ulcers in a child with AIDS was recently reported.[115] This 27-month-old boy had a 2-month history of decreased oral intake due to progressive dysphagia, odynophagia, and retrosternal pain. Endoscopy revealed two large ulcers with elevated margins. Histology showed hyperplasia and chronic inflammation of the mucosa. No histologic or culture evidence was found for fungi, bacteria, CMV, HSV, or acid-fast bacilli. Immunohistochemistry was positive for HIV p24 antigen on biopsy tissue from the ulcer edges. This patient responded both clinically and endoscopically to prednisone (1 mg/kg per day),[116] which was slowly tapered over a period of 3 weeks.

**CRYPTOSPORIDIUM.** A 2-year-old child with AIDS and esophageal cryptosporidiosis has been reported.[117] The child presented with severe diarrhea, oral thrush, marked dysphagia, and vomiting. This patient had endoscopic evidence of esophagitis but no esophageal candidiasis. Esophageal biopsies showed infection with *Cryptosporidium.*

## DRUG-INDUCED ESOPHAGITIS

Drug-induced esophageal injury tends to occur at esophageal anatomic narrowings, most commonly in the middle third behind the left atrium, or in patients with strictures or motility disorders. In a review of 175 cases of drug-induced esophagitis, the agents most commonly implicated were tetracyclines, emepronium bromide, slow-release potassium chloride, quinidine, aspirin, and nonsteroidal anti-inflammatory agents.[118] Injury is more likely if pills are taken without water or while lying down. The diagnosis is suspected based on the history of drug ingestion and the symptoms of retrosternal pain, dysphagia, odynophagia, or hematemesis. Endoscopy should be performed in patients with severe, unusually persistent, or atypical symptoms.[119] Endoscopy can show "kissing" ulcers in the midesophagus (Fig. 16–2) or erosions. Treatment includes acid blockade and sucralfate. Future occurrences can be prevented by swallowing medications while upright with several ounces of fluid and avoiding the supine position immediately after taking a medication.[119]

## RADIATION ESOPHAGITIS

The esophagus is relatively radioresistant compared with the rest of the gastrointestinal tract. Several factors influence the susceptibility of the esophagus to radiation injury, including dose, fractionation, schedule, and concomitant chemotherapy.[119]

### Pathophysiology

At doses greater than 30 Gy symptoms of esophagitis appear, including retrosternal burning and dysphagia. At

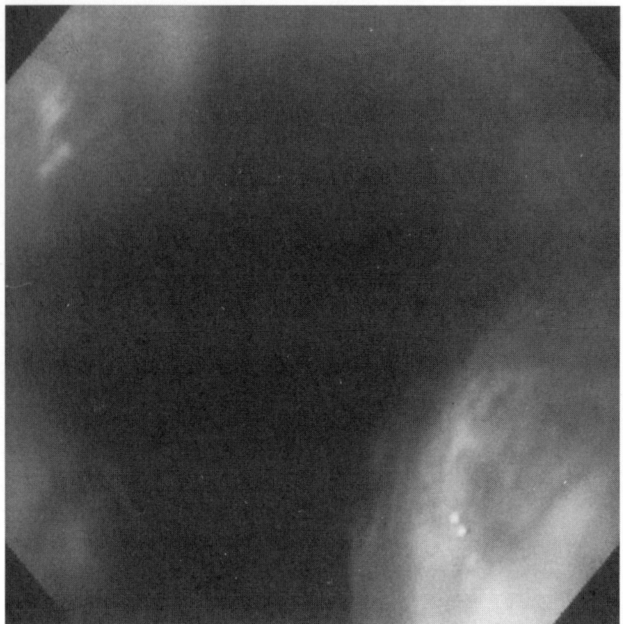

**FIGURE 16–2.** Endoscopic view of ulceration produced at opposite sides of the esophagus by a tetracycline tablet in an adolescent. (Courtesy of Christopher J. Justinich, MD.)

doses of 50 Gy severe esophagitis is produced, and at 60 Gy strictures and fistulas may occur.

Histologically, in radiation esophagitis the esophageal lining is affected first, with epithelial degeneration, followed by submucosal endothelial swelling, epithelial sloughing, and necrosis of the lamina propria.[120] The inflammatory changes usually start within 2 weeks of the initial dose and resolve within 3 to 4 weeks after administration of the last fraction.[119]

## Diagnosis and Treatment

Symptoms of radiation esophagitis can include dysphagia, odynophagia, and retrosternal chest pain. If endoscopy is needed for diagnosis, biopsies and brushings should be obtained and examined for opportunistic infections. The symptoms of radiation esophagitis can be treated with antacids, sucralfate, $H_2$ blockers, proton-pump inhibitors, and/or local anesthetics.[119] Calcium channel blockers and amifostine have been suggested to have radioprotective properties, but their clinical use in children awaits further studies.[121, 122]

## Complications

The passage of solid food is expected to improve a week after the last dose of radiation, but motility problems can persist.[123] Strictures,[124] tracheoesophageal fistula, and bleeding are complications of radiation-induced esophageal damage.[119]

### REFERENCES


1. Dudley JP, Kobayashi R, Rosenblatt HM, et al: *Candida* laryngitis in chronic mucocutaneous candidiasis: its association with *Candida* esophagitis. Ann Otol Rhinol Laryngol 1980;89:574–575.
2. Kobayashi RH, Rosenblatt HM, Carney JM, et al: *Candida* esophagitis and laryngitis in chronic mucocutaneous candidiasis. Pediatrics 1980;66:380–384.
3. Hachiya KA, Kobayashi RH, Antonson DL: *Candida* esophagitis following antibiotic usage. Pediatr Infect Dis 1982;1:168–170.
4. Naito Y, Yoshikawa T, Oyamadda H, et al: Esophageal candidiasis. Gastroenterol Jpn 1988;23:363–370.
5. Ammann AJ, Hong R: Disorders of the T cell system. In Stiehm ER (ed): Immunologic Disorders in Infants and Children. Philadelphia, WB Saunders, 1989, p 286.
6. Thapa BR, Kumar L: *Candida* esophagitis after antibiotic use. Indian J Pediatr 1989;56:296–299.
7. Vermeersch B, Rysselaere M, Dekeyser K, et al: Fungal colonization of the esophagus. Am J Gastroenterol 1989;84:1079–1083.
8. Leibovitz E, Rigaud M, Chandwani S, et al: Disseminated fungal infections in children infected with human immunodeficiency virus. Pediatr Infect Dis J 1991;10:888–894.
9. Baehr PH, McDonald GB: Esophageal infections: risk factors, presentation, diagnosis, and treatment. Gastroenterology 1994;106:509–532.
10. Sood A, Sharma M, Jain NP, et al: Esophageal candidiasis following omeprazole therapy: a report of two cases. Indian J Gastroenterol 1995;14:71–72.
11. Ganatra JV, Bostwick HE, Medow MS, et al: *Candida* esophagitis in a child with achalasia. J Pediatr Gastroenterol Nutr 1996;22:330–333.
12. Porro GB, Parente F, Cernuschi M: The diagnosis of esophageal candidiasis in patients with acquired immune deficiency syndrome: is endoscopy always necessary? Am J Gastroenterol 1989;84:143–146.
13. Bonacini M, Laine L, Gal AA, et al: Prospective evaluation of blind brushing of the esophagus for *Candida* esophagitis in patients with human immunodeficiency virus infection. Am J Gastroenterol 1990;85:385–389.
14. Young C, Chang MH, Chen JM: Fungal esophagitis in children. Acta Paediatr Sin 1993;34:436–42.
15. Braegger CP, Albisetti M, Nadal D: Extensive esophageal candidiasis in the absence of oral lesions in pediatric AIDS. J Pediatr Gastroenterol Nutr 1995;21:104–106.
16. Laine L, Bonacini M: Esophageal disease in human immunodeficiency virus infection. Arch Intern Med 1994;154:1577–1582.
17. Pedersen C, Gerstoft J, Lindhardt BO, Sindrup J: *Candida* esophagitis associated with acute human immunodeficiency virus infection. J Infect Dis 1987;156:529–530.
18. Imam N, Carpenter CC, Mayer KH, et al: Hierarchical pattern of mucosal candida infections in HIV-seropositive women. Am J Med 1990;89:142–146.
19. Connolly GM, Hawkins D, Harcourt-Webster JN, et al: Oesophageal symptoms, their causes, treatment, and prognosis in patients with the acquired immunodeficiency syndrome. Gut 1989;30:1033–1039.
20. Bonacini M, Young T, Laine L: The causes of esophageal symptoms in human immunodeficiency virus infection: a prospective study of 110 patients. Arch Intern Med 1991;151:1567–1572.
21. Laine L, Dretler RH, Conteas CN, et al: Fluconazole compared with ketoconazole for the treatment of *Candida* esophagitis in AIDS: a randomized trial. Ann Intern Med 1992;117:655–660.
22. Obrecht WF Jr, Richter JE, Olympio GA, Gelfand DW: Tracheoesophageal fistula: a serious complication of infectious esophagitis. Gastroenterology 1984;87:1174–1179.
23. Barbaro G, Barbarini G, Calderon W, et al: Fluconazole versus itraconazole for candida esophagitis in acquired immunodeficiency syndrome. Candida esophagitis. Gastroenterology 1996;111:1169–1177.
24. Wilcox CM, Alexander LN, Clark WS, Thompson SE 3rd: Fluconazole compared with endoscopy for human immunodeficiency virus-infected patients with esophageal symptoms. Gastroenterology 1996;110:1803–1809.
25. Goodman JL, Winston DJ, Greenfield RA, et al: A controlled trial of fluconazole to prevent fungal infections in patients undergoing bone marrow transplantation. N Engl J Med 1992;326:845–851.
26. Desigan G, Schneider RP: Herpes simplex esophagitis in healthy adults. South Med J 1985;78:1135–1137.
27. Lambert H, Eastham EJ: Herpes oesophagitis in a healthy 8 year-old. Arch Dis Child 1987;62:301–302.
28. Chusid MJ, Oechler HW, Werlin SL: Herpetic esophagitis in an immunocompetent boy. Wis Med J 1992;91:71–72.
29. Elliott SY, Kerns FT, Kitchen LW: Herpes esophagitis in immunocompetent adults: report of two cases and review of the literature. W V Med J 1993;89:188–190.

30. DiPalma JA, Brady CE: Herpes simplex esophagitis in a nonimmunosuppressed host with gastroesophageal reflux. Gastrointest Endosc 1984;30:24–25.
31. Buss DH, Scharyj M: Herpesvirus infection of the esophagus and other visceral organs in adults; incidence and clinical significance. Am J Med 1979;66:457–462.
32. McBane RD, Gross JB Jr: Herpes esophagitis: clinical syndrome, endoscopic appearance, and diagnosis in 23 patients. Gastrointest Endosc 1991;37:600–603.
33. McDonald GB, Sharma P, Hackman RC, et al: Esophageal infections in immunosuppressed patients after marrow transplantation. Gastroenterology 1985;88:1111–1117.
34. Ginaldi S, Burgert W Jr, Paulk HT Jr: Herpes esophagitis in immunocompetent patients. Am Fam Phys 1987;36:160–164.
35. Agha FP, Lee HH, Nostrant TT: Herpetic esophagitis: a diagnostic challenge in immunocompromised patients. Am J Gastroenterol 1986;81:246–253.
36. Marshall JB, Smart JR, Elmer C, et al: Herpes esophagitis causing an unsuspected esophageal food bolus impaction in an institutionalized patient (letter). J Clin Gastroenterol 1992;15:179–180.
37. Cronstedt JL, Bouchama A, Hainau B, et al: Spontaneous esophageal perforation in herpes simplex esophagitis. Am J Gastroenterol 1992;87:124–127.
38. Cirillo NW, Lyon DT, Schuller AM: Tracheoesophageal fistula complicating herpes esophagitis in AIDS. Am J Gastroenterol 1993;88:587–589.
39. Shortsleeve MJ, Levine MS: Herpes esophagitis in otherwise healthy patients: clinical and radiographic findings. Radiology 1992;182:859–861.
40. Levine MS, Loevner LA, Saul SH, et al: Herpes esophagitis: sensitivity of double-contrast esophagography. AJR Am J Roentgenol 1988;151:57–62.
41. Watts SJ, Alexander LC, Fawcett K, et al: Herpes simplex esophagitis in a renal transplant patient treated with cyclosporine A: a case report. Am J Gastroenterol 1986;81:185–188.
42. Byard RW, Champion MC, Orizaga M: Variability in the clinical presentation and endoscopic findings of herpetic esophagitis. Endoscopy 1987;19:153–155.
43. Jenkins D, Wicks AC: Herpes simplex esophagitis in a renal transplant patient: the need for antiviral therapy. Am J Gastroenterol 1988;83:331–332.
44. Cardillo MR, Forte F: Brush cytology in the diagnosis of herpetic esophagitis: a case report. Endoscopy 1988;20:156–157.
45. Sutton FM, Graham DY, Goodgame RW: Infectious esophagitis. Gastrointest Endosc Clin North Am 1994;4:713–729.
46. Collins P, Larder BA, Oliver NM, et al: Characterization of a DNA polymerase mutant of herpes simplex virus from a severely immunocompromised patient receiving acyclovir. J Gen Virol 1989;70:375–382.
47. Sacks SL, Wanklin RJ, Reece DE, et al: Progressive esophagitis from acyclovir-resistant herpes simplex: clinical roles for DNA polymerase mutants and viral heterogeneity? Ann Intern Med 1989;111:893–899.
48. Birch CJ, Tachedjian G, Doherty RR, et al: Altered sensitivity to antiviral drugs of herpes simplex virus isolates from a patient with the acquired immunodeficiency syndrome. J Infect Dis 1990;162:731–734.
49. Safrin S, Assaykeen T, Follansbee S, Mills J: Foscarnet therapy for acyclovir-resistant mucocutaneous herpes simplex virus infection in 26 AIDS patients: preliminary data. J Infect Dis 1990;161:1078–1084.
50. Selby PJ, Powles RL, Easton D, et al: The prophylactic role of intravenous and long-term oral acyclovir after allogeneic bone marrow transplantation. Br J Cancer 1989;59:434–438.
51. Tang IY, Maddux MS, Veremis SA, et al: Low-dose oral acyclovir for prevention of herpes simplex virus infection during OKT3 therapy. Transplant Proc 1989;21:1758–1760.
52. Ho M: Epidemiology of cytomegalovirus infections. Rev Infect Dis 1990;12:S701–S710.
53. Goodgame RW: Gastrointestinal cytomegalovirus disease. Ann Intern Med 1993;119:924–935.
54. Venkataramani A, Schlueter AJ, Spech TJ, Greenberg E: Cytomegalovirus esophagitis in an immunocompetent host. Gastrointest Endosc 1994;40:392–393.
55. Drew WL: Cytomegalovirus infection in patients with AIDS. J Infect Dis 1988;158:449–456.
56. Weber JN, Thom S, Barrison I, et al: Cytomegalovirus colitis and oesophageal ulceration in the context of AIDS: clinical manifestations and preliminary report of treatment with Foscarnet (phosphonoformate). Gut 1987;28:482–487.
57. Reed EC, Wolford JL, Kopecky KJ, et al: Ganciclovir for the treatment of cytomegalovirus gastroenteritis in bone marrow transplant patients: a randomized, placebo-controlled trial. Ann Intern Med 1990;112:505–510.
58. Goodgame RW, Ross PG, Kim HS, et al: Esophageal stricture after cytomegalovirus ulcer treated with ganciclovir. J Clin Gastroenterol 1991;13:678–681.
59. Dieterich DT, Poles MA, Dicker M, et al: Foscarnet treatment of cytomegalovirus gastrointestinal infections in acquired immunodeficiency syndrome patients who have failed ganciclovir induction. Am J Gastroenterol 1993;88:542–548.
60. Culpepper-Morgan JA, Kotler DP, Scholes JV, Tierney AR: Evaluation of diagnostic criteria for mucosal cytomegalic inclusion disease in the acquired immune deficiency syndrome. Am J Gastroenterol 1987;82:1264–1270.
61. Lazzarotto T, Dal Monte P, Boccuni MC, et al: Lack of correlation between virus detection and serologic tests for diagnosis of active cytomegalovirus infection in patients with AIDS. J Clin Microbiol 1992;30:1027–1029.
62. Quinnan GV Jr, Masur H, Rook AH, et al: Herpesvirus infections in the acquired immune deficiency syndrome. JAMA 1984;252:72–77.
63. Drew WL: Diagnosis of cytomegalovirus infection. Rev Infect Dis 1988;10:S468–S476.
64. Zurlo JJ, O'Neill D, Polis MA, et al: Lack of clinical utility of cytomegalovirus blood and urine cultures in patients with HIV infection. Ann Intern Med 1993;118:12–17.
65. Sor S, Levine MS, Kowalski TE, et al: Giant ulcers of the esophagus in patients with human immunodeficiency virus: clinical, radiographic, and pathologic findings. Radiology 1995;194:447–451.
66. Levine MS, Loercher G, Katzka DA, et al: Giant, human immunodeficiency virus-related ulcers in the esophagus. Radiology 1991;180:323–326.
67. Wilcox CM, Straub RF, Schwartz DA: Prospective endoscopic characterization of cytomegalovirus esophagitis in AIDS. Gastrointest Endosc 1994;40:481–484.
68. Balthazar EJ, Megibow AJ, Hulnick DH: Cytomegalovirus esophagitis and gastritis in AIDS. AJR Am J Roentgenol 1985;144:1201–1204.
69. Theise ND, Rotterdam H, Dieterich D: Cytomegalovirus esophagitis in AIDS: diagnosis by endoscopic biopsy. Am J Gastroenterol 1991;86:1123–1126.
70. Wilcox CM, Straub RF, Schwartz DA: Cytomegalovirus esophagitis in AIDS: a prospective evaluation of clinical response to ganciclovir therapy, relapse rate, and long-term outcome. Am J Med 1995;98:169–176.
71. Schwartz DA, Wilcox CM: Atypical cytomegalovirus inclusions in gastrointestinal biopsy specimens from patients with the acquired immunodeficiency syndrome: diagnostic role of in situ nucleic acid hybridization. Hum Pathol 1992;23:1019–1026.
72. Goodgame RW, Genta RM, Estrada R, et al: Frequency of positive tests for cytomegalovirus in AIDS patients: endoscopic lesions compared with normal mucosa. Am J Gastroenterol 1993;88:338–343.
73. Hackman RC, Wolford JL, Gleaves CA, et al: Recognition and rapid diagnosis of upper gastrointestinal cytomegalovirus infection in marrow transplant recipients: a comparison of seven virologic methods. Transplantation 1994;57:231–237.
74. Clayton F, Klein EB, Kotler DP: Correlation of in situ hybridization with histology and viral culture in patients with acquired immunodeficiency syndrome with cytomegalovirus colitis. Arch Pathol Lab Med 1989;113:1124–1126.
75. Laine L, Bonacini M, Sattler F, et al: Cytomegalovirus and *Candida* esophagitis in patients with AIDS. J Acquir Immune Defic Syndr 1992;5:605–609.
76. Wilcox CM, Diehl DL, Cello JP, et al: Cytomegalovirus esophagitis in patients with AIDS: a clinical, endoscopic, and pathologic correlation. Ann Intern Med 1990;113:589–593.
77. Meyers JD, Reed EC, Shepp DH, et al: Acyclovir for prevention of cytomegalovirus infection and disease after allogeneic marrow transplantation. N Engl J Med 1988;318:70–75.
78. Drobyski WR, Knox KK, Carrigan DR, Ash RC: Foscarnet therapy of ganciclovir-resistant cytomegalovirus in marrow transplantation. Transplantation 1991;52:155–157.
79. Nelson MR, Connolly GM, Hawkins DA, Gazzard BG: Foscarnet in the treatment of cytomegalovirus infection of the esophagus and colon

in patients with the acquired immune deficiency syndrome. Am J Gastroenterol 1991;86:876–881.
80. Blanshard C: Treatment of HIV-related cytomegalovirus disease of the gastrointestinal tract with foscarnet. J Acquir Immune Defic Syndr 1992;5:S25–S28.
81. Jacobson MA: Ganciclovir therapy for opportunistic cytomegalovirus disease in AIDS. AIDS Clin Rev 1990:149–163.
82. Meyers JD: Prevention and treatment of cytomegalovirus infection. Annu Rev Med 1991;42:179–187.
83. Dieterich DT, Poles MA, Lew EA, et al: Concurrent use of ganciclovir and foscarnet to treat cytomegalovirus infection in AIDS patients. J Infect Dis 1993;167:1184–1188.
84. Knox KK, Drobyski WR, Carrigan DR: Cytomegalovirus isolate resistant to ganciclovir and foscarnet from a marrow transplant patient. Lancet 1991;337:1292–1293.
85. Schmidt GM, Horak DA, Niland JC, et al: A randomized, controlled trial of prophylactic ganciclovir for cytomegalovirus pulmonary infection in recipients of allogeneic bone marrow transplants: The City of Hope–Stanford–Syntex CMV Study Group. N Engl J Med 1991;324:1005–1011.
86. Stratta RJ, Shaefer MS, Cushing KA, et al: Successful prophylaxis of cytomegalovirus disease after primary CMV exposure in liver transplant recipients. Transplantation 1991;51:90–97.
87. Merigan TC, Renlund DG, Keay S, et al: A controlled trial of ganciclovir to prevent cytomegalovirus disease after heart transplantation. N Engl J Med 1992;326:1182–1186.
88. Goodrich JM, Bowden RA, Fisher L, et al: Ganciclovir prophylaxis to prevent cytomegalovirus disease after allogeneic marrow transplant. Ann Intern Med 1993;118:173–178.
89. Winston DJ, Wirin D, Shaked A, Busuttil RW: Randomised comparison of ganciclovir and high-dose acyclovir for long-term cytomegalovirus prophylaxis in liver-transplant recipients. Lancet 1995;346:69–74.
90. Balfour HH Jr, Chace BA, Stapleton JT, et al: A randomized, placebo-controlled trial of oral acyclovir for the prevention of cytomegalovirus disease in recipients of renal allografts. N Engl J Med 1989;320:1381–1387.
91. Johnson PC, Sarosi GA: The endemic mycoses: surgical considerations. Semin Thorac Cardiovasc Surg 1995;7:95–103.
92. Fucci JC, Nightengale ML: Primary esophageal histoplasmosis. Am J Gastroenterol 1997;92:530–531.
93. Kirchner SG, Hernanz-Schulman M, Stein SM, et al: Imaging of pediatric mediastinal histoplasmosis. Radiographics 1991;11:365–381.
94. Marshall JB, Singh R, Demmy TL, et al: Mediastinal histoplasmosis presenting with esophageal involvement and dysphagia: case study. Dysphagia 1995;10:53–58.
95. Tu RK, Peters ME, Gourley GR, Hong R: Esophageal histoplasmosis in a child with immunodeficiency with hyper-IgM. AJR Am J Roentgenol 1991;157:381–382.
96. Forsmark CE, Wilcox CM, Darragh TM, Cello JP: Disseminated histoplasmosis in AIDS: an unusual case of esophageal involvement and gastrointestinal bleeding. Gastrointest Endosc 1990;36:604–605.
97. Coss KC, Wheat LJ, Conces DJ Jr, et al: Esophageal fistula complicating mediastinal histoplasmosis: response to amphotericin B. Am J Med 1987;83:343–346.
98. Coscia MF, Hormuth DA, Huang WL: Back pain secondary to esophageal perforation in an adolescent. Spine 1992;17:1256–1259.
99. Mir-Madjlessi SH, Tavassolie H: Primary tuberculous granulomatous esophagogastro-duodenitis: a report of a case. J Trop Med Hyg 1985;88:253–256.
100. Al-Idrissi HY, Satti MB, Al-Quorain A, et al: Granulomatous oesophagitis: a case of tuberculosis limited to the oesophagus. Ann Trop Med Parasitol 1987;81:129–133.
101. Tornero Estebanez C, Alcaniz Escandell C, Pons Espana E, Villanueva Guardia A: Tuberculosis primaria de esofago. Med Clin (Barc) 1992;98:357–358.
102. Tassios P, Ladas S, Giannopoulos G, et al: Tuberculous esophagitis: report of a case and review of modern approaches to diagnosis and treatment. Hepatogastroenterology 1995;42:185–188.
103. Damtew B, Frengley D, Wolinsky E, Spagnuolo PJ: Esophageal tuberculosis: mimicry of gastrointestinal malignancy. Rev Infect Dis 1987;9:140–146.
104. Wort SJ, Puleston JM, Hill PD, Holdstock GE: Primary tuberculosis of the oesophagus. Lancet 1997;349:1072.
105. Savage PE, Grundy A: Oesophageal tuberculosis: an unusual cause of dysphagia. Br J Radiol 1984;57:1153–1155.
106. Eng J, Sabanathan S: Tuberculosis of the esophagus. Dig Dis Sci 1991;36:536–540.
107. Mokoena T, Shama DM, Ngakane H, Bryer JV: Oesophageal tuberculosis: a review of eleven cases. Postgrad J Med 1992;68:110–115.
108. Brullet E, Font B, Rey M, et al: Esophageal tuberculosis: early diagnosis by endoscopy. Endoscopy 1993;25:485.
109. Gordon AH, Marshall JB: Esophageal tuberculosis: definitive diagnosis by endoscopy. Am J Gastroenterol 1990;85:174–177.
110. de Mas R, Lombeck G, Riemann JF: Tuberculosis of the oesophagus masquerading as ulcerated tumour. Endoscopy 1986;18:153–155.
111. Iwamoto I, Tomita Y, Takasaki M, et al: Esophagoaortic fistula caused by esophageal tuberculosis: report of a case. Surg Today 1995;25:381–384.
112. Vidyasagar B, Bhat SS, Rao HL, et al: Tracheo-oesophageal fistula in an adult. Indian J Chest Dis Allied Sci 1991;33:31–34.
113. Adkins MS, Raccuia JS, Acinapura AJ: Esophageal perforation in a patient with acquired immunodeficiency syndrome. Ann Thorac Surg 1990;50:299–300.
114. Wilcox CM, Schwartz DA: Endoscopic characterization of idiopathic esophageal ulceration associated with human immunodeficiency virus infection. J Clin Gastroenterol 1993;16:251–256.
115. Narwal S, Galeano NF, Pottenger E, et al: Idiopathic esophageal ulcers in a child with AIDS. J Pediatr Gastroenterol Nutr 1997;24:211–214.
116. Kotler DP, Reka S, Orenstein JM, Fox CH: Chronic idiopathic esophageal ulceration in the acquired immunodeficiency syndrome: characterization and treatment with corticosteroids. J Clin Gastroenterol 1992;284–290.
117. Kazlow PG, Shah K, Benkov KJ, et al: Esophageal cryptosporidiosis in a child with acquired immune deficiency syndrome. Gastroenterology 1986;91:1301–1303.
118. Eng J, Sabanathan S: Drug-induced esophagitis. Am J Gastroenterol 1991;86:1127–1133.
119. Trowers E, Thomas C Jr, Silverstein FE: Chemical-and radiation-induced esophageal injury. Gastrointest Endosc Clin North Am 1994;4:657–675.
120. Chowhan NM: Injurious effects of radiation on the esophagus. Am J Gastroenterol 1990;85:115–120.
121. Floersheim GL: Radioprotective effects of calcium antagonists used alone or with other types of radioprotectors. Radiat Res 1993;133:80–87.
122. Schuchter LM: Guidelines for the administration of amifostine. Semin Oncol 1996;23:40–43.
123. Seeman H, Gates JA, Traube M: Esophageal motor dysfunction years after radiation therapy. Dig Dis Sci 1992;37:303–306.
124. Mahboubi S, Silber JH: Radiation-induced esophageal strictures in children with cancer. Eur Radiol 1997;7:119–122.

# SECTION THREE

# THE STOMACH

Chapter 17

# Pyloric Stenosis and Congenital Anomalies of the Stomach and Duodenum

Frederick Alexander

## EMBRYOLOGY

Basic to an understanding of the congenital disorders of the stomach and duodenum is a knowledge of normal foregut embryology. The primitive foregut begins as a pharyngeal structure that elongates to form the primordia of the esophagus and the stomach.[1] The stomach first appears as a local dilatation between segments C3 and C5 at the fifth week of gestation. The next few weeks of gestation are a period of rapid elongation of the cranial foregut and intense mucosal proliferation of both the esophagus and the duodenum. At the end of the seventh week, the stomach is located at the level of T11 to L4 and there is differentiation of the greater and lesser curvature, probably related to the differential growth of the opposite sides of the stomach. In classic view, the stomach then rotates clockwise about its vertical axis to bring the left vagus nerve anterior to the stomach and the right vagus posterior. Subsequent rotation on its anteroposterior axis allows the stomach to assume its final position. Finally, by the 10th week of gestation, rugae and longitudinal muscles are apparent in the stomach, and the lumen in both the esophagus and the duodenum has been formed by recanalization.[2]

## PYLORIC STENOSIS

### History

The first description of hypertrophic pyloric stenosis was made in 1788 by Hezekiah Beardsley, who described an obstructing scirrhosity in the pylorus at autopsy in a 5-year-old child.[3] Hirschsprung provided an accurate description of the condition in 1888 and first applied the name *congenital hypertrophic pyloric stenosis*.[4] Before the first attempt at extramucous pyloroplasty by Dufour and Fredette in 1908,[5] surgical options for this disorder consisted of gastroenterostomy, pyloric resection, jejunostomy, and intraluminal dilatation of the pyloric canal. Surgical mortality exceeded 60%, whereas 10% to 46% of infants died with conservative therapy. Extramucous pyloroplasty was only partially successful and often led to massive bleeding in that sutures cut through the pyloric muscle. In 1912, Ramstedt[6] took a decisive step by limiting the operative repair to splitting of the pyloric muscle, which was subsequently proved to be curative and remains standard treatment today.

### Incidence and Heredity

Laron and Horne[7] reported an incidence of 1 in 913 live births in the Pittsburgh area. They also found the incidence to be 2.5 times greater in white infants than in black infants. Jed and associates[8] found that the incidence of pyloric stenosis in Olmsted County, Minnesota, increased in boys from 1.7 per 1,000 live births for the period 1950 to 1954, to 6.2 per 1,000 live births for the period 1980 to 1984, whereas rates for girls changed only from 0.6 to 0.9 per 1,000 live births during this period. Kerr[9] found an unprecedented rise in the incidence of pyloric stenosis in the central region of Scotland, from an average of 2.2 per 1,000 live births for the period 1970 to 1977, to 8.8 per 1,000 live births in 1979. Knox and colleagues[10] found a similar increase in the incidence of pyloric stenosis in the West Midlands Health Region between 1974 and 1980, which correlated with a 31% increase in breast feeding in Great Britain during the same period.[10, 11] It has been suggested that there may be seasonal variation in pyloric stenosis. However, there is currently no evidence to support this.

Pyloric stenosis is based on a polygenic mode of inheritance modified by sex.[12] The ratio of males to females with pyloric stenosis ranges between 4:1 and 6:1. Although believed to be more common in first-born children, pyloric stenosis has recently been shown to be more closely associated with smaller family size and higher socioeconomic class than with birth order.[13] Jed and associates[8] reported a positive family history in 13% of affected children. Other studies have shown that a mother who had pyloric stenosis has a four times greater chance of having a child with pyloric stenosis than does a similarly affected father.[14]

## Pathogenesis

The exact cause of hypertrophic pyloric stenosis is unknown. In most instances, the child presents with vomiting after 3 weeks of age; however, about 20% of patients with a classic type are symptomatic from birth.[15, 16] Rollins and colleagues[17] showed prospectively, using sonography, that pyloric muscle hypertrophy is not present during the early newborn period in infants who later develop infantile pyloric stenosis. Sonography has also been used to show that subclinical disease may cause minor degrees of vomiting, with subsequent gradual resolution.[18] Late development of hypertrophic pyloric stenosis is rare but may occur in association with transpyloric feeding tubes.[19]

Lynn[20] proposed in 1960 that milk curds propelled by gastric peristalsis against a closed pyloric canal produce edema that narrows the pyloric canal and causes work hypertrophy of the pyloric and gastric musculature. Whether the initial cause is edema or an unexplained spasm of the antropyloric muscle, it seems clear that a vicious cycle is established that progresses to high-grade obstruction of the pyloric canal. Hypergastrinemia associated with hyperacidity has been suggested as a possible cause of pyloric stenosis.[21] In addition, elevations of prostaglandins $E_2$ and $F_{2\alpha}$, both potent smooth muscle constrictors, have been found in infants with pyloric stenosis.[22] However, all these findings probably represent secondary phenomena caused by chronic gastric retention and distention. Defective cholinergic innervation of the pyloric muscle has been suggested.[23]

## Clinical Presentation

Nonbilious vomiting is the initial sign of infantile hypertrophic pyloric stenosis. The vomiting may or may not be projectile, is usually progressive, and may become brownish as a result of gastritis in later stages. Prolonged vomiting can lead to dehydration, weight loss, and failure to thrive.

The onset of vomiting may occur as early as the first week or as late as 5 months of age.[24] As vomiting continues, hydrogen ion loss leads to an elevation of the serum bicarbonate, followed by a decrease in serum chloride and the development of hypochloremic alkalosis.[25, 26] Serum potassium levels usually remain normal; however, when potassium depletion does occur, it may lead to paradoxical aciduria owing to the preferential loss of hydrogen ions across the distal renal tubules in exchange for sodium reabsorption.[26]

Jaundice occurs in association with pyloric stenosis in approximately 2% to 5% of infants.[27, 28] Approximately 50% of jaundiced infants with pyloric stenosis have a serum bilirubin level (mostly unconjugated) between 5 and 10 mg/dL.[29] Such elevations in serum unconjugated bilirubin have been seen in certain infants with neonatal bowel obstruction and have been ascribed in the past to the effects of acute starvation on an immature liver. Woolley and coworkers[30] found decreased levels of glucuronyl transferase in infants with hypertrophic pyloric stenosis. Labrune and colleagues[31] found abnormally low levels of glucuronyl transferase in several infants 4 to 5 months after pyloromyotomy, suggesting that the jaundice associated with pyloric stenosis may be an early manifestation of Gilbert's syndrome. The role of caloric deprivation remains unclear, because a reduction in bilirubin levels occurs within 6 to 24 hours postoperatively, long before adequate caloric intake resumes.

Although there is no defined relation between pyloric stenosis and other abnormalities, associated anomalies may be present in 6% to 20% of infants.[32] Many surgeons have noted a higher than expected occurrence of esophageal atresia and malrotation, which may occur in approximately 5% of infants with pyloric stenosis.[33]

## Diagnostic Evaluation

The diagnosis of pyloric stenosis is best made by physical examination with the palpation of a pyloric mass. This firm, small, movable mass is similar to the size and shape of an olive and is located in the midepigastrium. A pyloric mass is pathognomonic and is palpable by experienced examiners in 80% of cases. To optimize the physical examination, it is important first to empty the stomach of all air and fluid using a 10F Replogle oral gastric tube. The catheter may then be removed, and the infant may be comforted with 5% glucose in water given orally. Occasionally, small doses of a sedative may be given to facilitate the examination.

Imaging procedures should be reserved for infants with bilious vomiting and those with nonbilious vomiting in whom experienced examiners are unable to feel a pyloric mass. In the latter group of infants, the differential diagnosis includes gastroenteritis, gastroesophageal reflux, pylorospasm, allergic gastroenteropathy, and, rarely, antral or pyloric webs. To distinguish among these conditions, an upper gastrointestinal series (UGIS) may be performed. The characteristic findings of pyloric stenosis on UGIS are a constant elongation of the pyloric canal,[34] a double track of barium along the pyloric canal caused by the folding of compressed mucosa,[35] and a prepyloric bulge into the distal antrum, producing an appearance that resembles shoulders or an umbrella[36] (Fig. 17–1). Delay in gastric emptying may not be used as a sign of pyloric stenosis, because the pylorus can display a wide range of emptying times in normal infants.

Sonography has been advocated as the imaging procedure of choice to confirm the diagnosis of pyloric stenosis.[37, 38] Sonography displays the hypertrophic pyloric musculature as a broad ring with a low echo density and an inner layer of high echo density corresponding to the mucosa. Criteria for hypertrophic pyloric stenosis have been developed that include a muscle thickness equal to or greater than 4 mm,[39] a pyloric length greater than 16 mm,[40] or both (Fig. 17–2). Using these criteria, Gobdole and colleagues[41] found that sonography had a sensitivity of 97%, a specificity of 100%, and positive and negative predictive values of 100% and 98%, respectively. Forman and associates[42] reported that a palpable pyloric mass had a predictive value of 100%; but, in the absence of palpable mass, infants still had a 44%

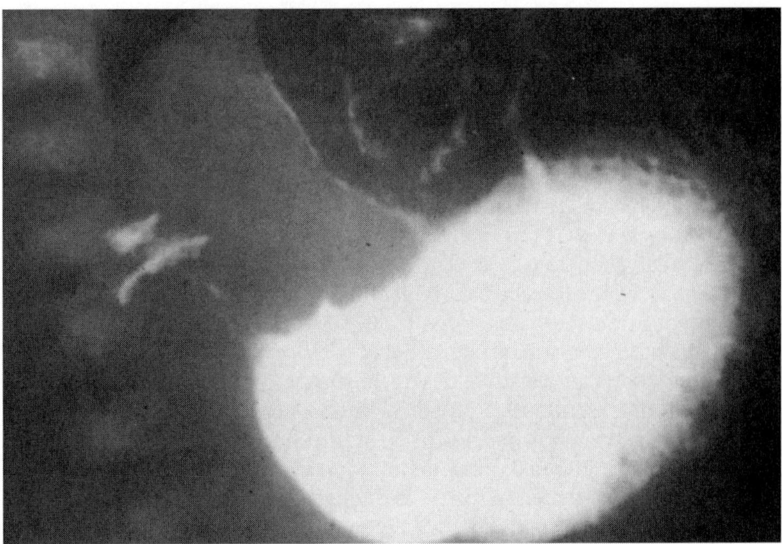

**FIGURE 17–1.** UGIS showing elongated pyloric channel and double tract sign with shouldering of antrum characteristic of hypertrophic pyloric stenosis.

chance of pyloric stenosis. A positive sonogram indicated pyloric stenosis with 100% probability, a negative sonogram left only 8% of patients undetected.

## Treatment

Initial treatment is directed toward correction of dehydration and hypochloremic alkalosis. Although serum potassium levels are usually normal, total body potassium may be markedly depleted before serum samples reflect hypokalemia. The degree of dehydration may be assessed according to the usual clinical parameters but is often reflected by the degree of hypochloremic alkalosis. Although most infants can be prepared for surgery within a 24-hour period, advanced dehydration and alkalosis may require preoperative preparation over several days.

For those infants with minimal dehydration and a normal electrolyte pattern, many surgeons advocate oral institution of a balanced electrolyte solution once the stomach has been

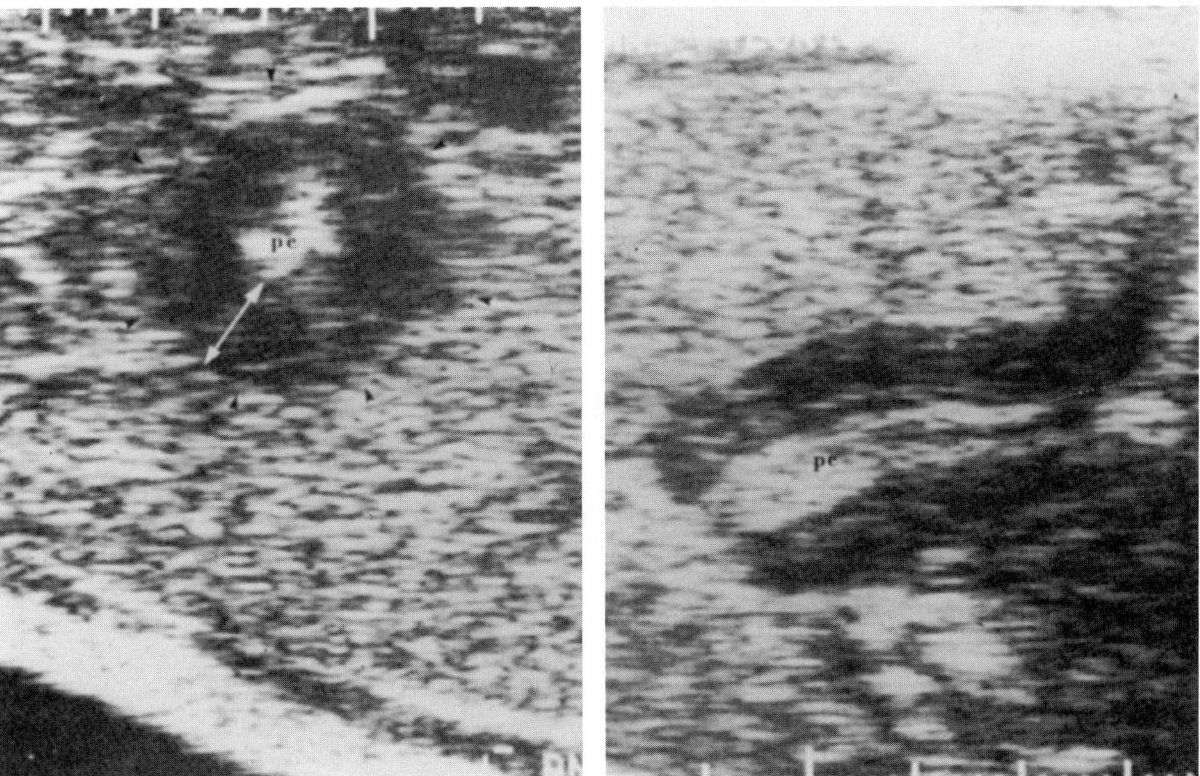


**FIGURE 17–2.** Cross-sectional *(left)* and transverse *(right)* sonograms of hypertrophic pyloric stenosis showing increased thickness and length of pyloric muscle. pc, pyloric channel.

lavaged with normal saline to remove obstructing milk curds and barium. Because vomiting may be persistent and the serum chloride and bicarbonate may be unreliable indices of the extent of the fluid and electrolytes losses, it is prudent to begin intravenous fluid, using 5% dextrose and 0.33% saline with 5 mmol of potassium chloride added to each 250-mL intravenous bottle, even for those infants with apparently minimal dehydration.

Infants with moderate to severe fluid and electrolyte disturbances, in whom serum bicarbonate may range from 25 to 60 mmol/L, are best treated with 5% dextrose in 0.45% to 0.9% saline given initially as a bolus of 10 to 20 mL/kg as required, and then at 1.5 times maintenance for as long as required, until serum electrolytes approach normal levels and total body water is judged to be sufficient. Once the stomach has been emptied, most infants stop vomiting. Only in rare cases is continued nasogastric drainage required, and then intravenous rates and electrolyte concentration must be adjusted to cover ongoing losses. Finally, after the infant has voided, it is important to add 5 to 10 mmol of potassium chloride to each 250-mL bottle to help correct the hypochloremic alkalosis.

Correction of alkalemia before surgery is essential to prevent postanesthetic apnea, which may occur as a result of alkalemic depression of the respiratory center.[43] Several reports have indicated the incidence of postoperative apnea to range between 1% and 3%.[44, 45] The stomach should be drained with an oral gastric tube before induction of anesthesia to prevent aspiration.

The Ramstedt pyloromyotomy remains the surgical procedure of choice (Fig. 17–3). It is performed through a short right transverse incision placed at the liver edge. The pyloric mass is delivered into the wound and is then serosally incised, and the underlying muscle is bluntly split, allowing the mucosa to pout up into the cleft, indicating a release of the obstructive process. Important technical features of this operation include avoidance of a mucosal tear in the region of the pyloric vein, where the risk is greatest, and extension of the pyloromyotomy to the antrum, where recurrence is most likely. Mucosal disruption is inconsequential as long as it is recognized and treated by repair with absorbable suture and decompression of the stomach for 48 hours.

Postoperative vomiting is a well-recognized phenomenon, occurring in as many as 50% of the infants. It is probably caused by persistent local edema along with inefficient gastric emptying.[46] In most cases, however, diluted feedings may be initiated within 12 to 24 hours after surgery, and most infants may be advanced to maintenance oral feedings within 36 to 48 hours after surgery. If vomiting continues, radiologic reassessment of persistent hypertrophic pyloric stenosis may be difficult. Serial sonograms taken postoperatively reveal initial swelling of the muscles with rapid involution over the next 3 weeks and attainment of normal thickness by 6 weeks.[47] Persistent hypertrophic pyloric stenosis due to an incomplete pyloromyotomy appears as persistent gastric outlet obstruction with muscle hypertrophy, but it may have a tapered appearance.[48]

## Results

The surgical treatment of pyloric stenosis is curative,[49] and the prognosis for infants with pyloric stenosis depends on the associated anomalies. Reports indicate a mortality rate of 0.5% or fewer, recurrence in 1% to 3%, and an incidence of wound infection and adhesions between 1% and 5%.[50–52] Postoperative bleeding is rare, and transfusion is almost never required.

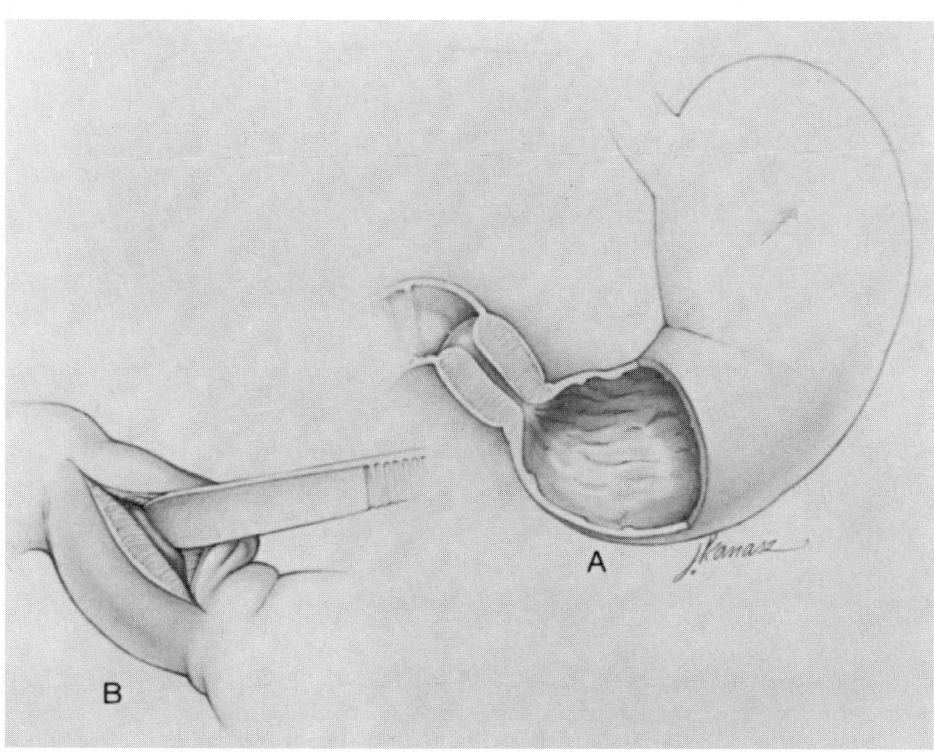


**FIGURE 17–3.** *A,* Cross-section of the elongated, narrow pyloric channel typical of pyloric stenosis. *B,* Pyloromyotomy is begun by bluntly separating muscle fibers on the anterior surface of the pylorus.

## CONGENITAL GASTRIC OUTLET OBSTRUCTION

### History

Atresia limited to the pyloric antrum was first described by Calder in 1733.[53] Subsequently, Crooks[54] described the first pyloric membrane in 1828. Laudener in 1897 reported the first incomplete prepyloric membrane.[55] The first description of an antral web in the English literature was made by Parsons and Barding[56] in 1933. Since then, approximately 127 cases of congenital outlet obstruction have been reported involving the pylorus and antrum in three general forms: complete segmental defects, fibrous cords, and webs.[57]

### Incidence

Congenital gastric outlet obstruction due to pyloric atresia or prepyloric or antral webs is rare, representing fewer than 1% of all atresias and diaphragms of the alimentary tract.[58, 59] Cook and Rickham[55] reported an incidence of 0.003% during a period of 25 years at the Liverpool Regional Neonatal Center. Pyloric webs are by far the most common of these obstructions; according to Bell and coworkers,[60] only 32 cases of antral webs were reported in children 16 years of age or younger. The rarity of these lesions notwithstanding, Tunnell and Ide Smith[61] state that the diagnosis of antral webs in infancy is being made with increasing frequency.

### Etiology and Pathology

The cause of these defects is unknown. However, because the antrum and pylorus do not undergo mucosal proliferation, the cause is not related to failure of canalization. Instead, it is speculated that discontinuation of the endodermal tube before the eighth week of gestation leads to segmentation defects, and endodermal redundancy after the eighth week leads to antral web formation. Given early fixation and excellent collateral circulation of the stomach and duodenum, it is unlikely that in utero vascular accidents are causative factors.

Reports indicate that the defects involving the antrum or pylorus are of several types[62] (Fig. 17–4). Antral defects are least common, with antral gap atresia occurring in 1% and antral membranes with partial openings occurring in 5% of patients. Pyloric gap atresias with complete or cord separation of the pylorus account for approximately 27% of the cases. Pyloric webs are most common, occurring in 67% of cases, including single and double membranes and solid atresias 1 to 2 cm in thickness.

Pyloric atresia may occur in an autosomal recessive mode in association with epidermolysis bullosa letalis.[63–65] Eighteen cases of pyloric atresia–epidermolysis bullosa syndrome have been reported since Korber and Glasson's initial report in 1977.[66] Gedde-Dahl and Lambrecht[67] showed that families with this syndrome are of two ethnic groups (American Indian and Lebanese-Turkish), evidence that favors genetic linkage between two autosomal recessive genes.

### Clinical Manifestations

Infants with antral or pyloric webs present quite differently from older children with the disorder.[57] Infants present with nonbilious vomiting, usually within the first days of life, along with feeding difficulties and distention of the stomach. Older children tend to present with epigastric pain, weight loss, nausea and vomiting, or symptoms compatible with peptic ulcer disease. Distribution by sex is almost equal.[62] Polyhydramnios is reported in 61% of neonatal cases, and there is a high percentage of infants with low birth weight.[62, 68, 69] Rupture of the stomach in pyloric atresia may occur as early as 12 hours after birth.[70]

### Diagnosis

The diagnosis of congenital outlet obstruction may be suggested by the nonspecific findings of a large, dilated stomach with a single gas bubble. Because a dilated stomach with no gas in the distal bowel may also be seen in gastric hypotonia of the newborn,[71] it is important to proceed to UGIS. Bell and coworkers[60] reported that the UGIS is 90% accurate in the diagnosis of congenital outlet obstruction. The typical UGIS findings of pyloric atresia are the absence of the beak sign (seen with pyloric stenosis or duplication) and the presence of a pyloric dimple sign (formed by the shallow pyloric cavity at the proximal point of the atresia).[72] In pyloric atresia, sonographic examination may reveal an

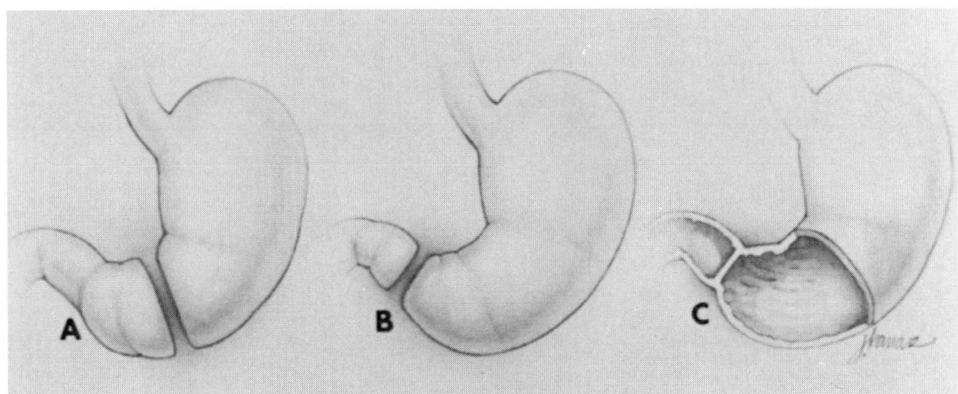


**FIGURE 17–4.** Congenital gastric outlet obstruction. *A,* Antral gap atresia: 1% of cases. *B,* Pyloric gap atresia: 27% of cases. *C,* Pyloric web: 67% of cases.

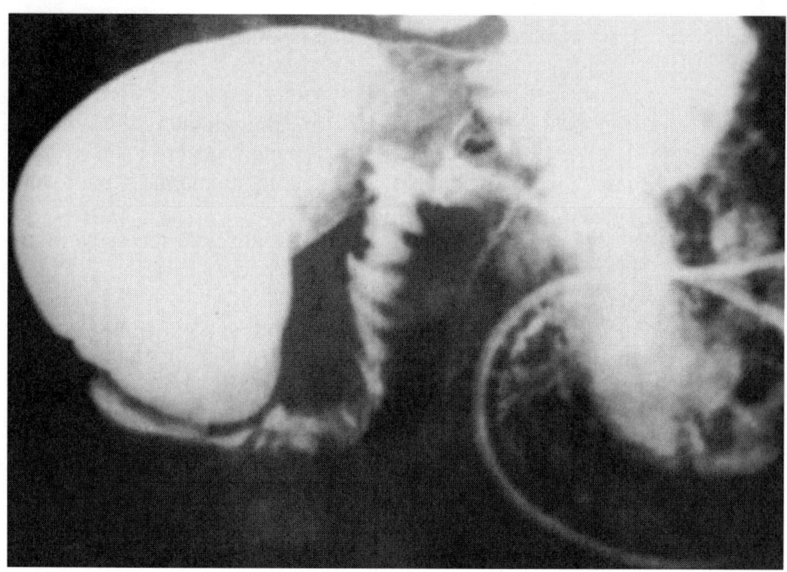

**FIGURE 17–5.** UGIS showing weblike filling defect of distal antrum and partial gastric outlet obstruction characteristic of antral web.

absence of the typical echolucent pattern of the pyloric muscle. An antral web may appear on an upper gastrointestinal radiograph as a thin septum projecting into the antral lumen, perpendicular to its longitudinal axis and several centimeters proximal to the pyloric canal (Fig. 17–5). In older infants and children, gastroscopy may be helpful when UGIS is unclear. Failure to pass the gastroscope into the duodenum is diagnostic of congenital gastric obstruction.

## Treatment

As with hypertrophic pyloric stenosis, correction of dehydration and hypochloremic alkalosis is essential. Persistent vomiting should be treated with nasogastric suction and lavage if there has been previous feeding.

Operative repair should be approached through a transverse supraumbilical incision. The stomach is opened, and a Foley catheter is passed to exclude a windsock diaphragm, which is a membranous septum that has prolapsed through the pyloric canal[73] (Fig. 17–6). Standard treatment of an antral web is simple excision. Pyloric webs or septa are best treated by Heineke-Mikulicz pyloroplasty. For gap-type atresia, gastrojejunostomy and gastroduodenostomy both have been performed; however, the latter appears to offer superior results.[64, 74]

Antral webs or membranes would seem to be ideal lesions for endoscopic management, since they consist mainly of mucosa and submucosa. A few such attempts have been reported, and one infant who underwent endoscopic resection of an antral web later developed stricture and required surgical management.[75] Endoscopic treatment should be reserved for selected older children, and radial incisions should be used to prevent stenosis.[76]

## Results

The survival rate is 95% for infants and children undergoing excision of an antral web, 85% after pyloroplasty for pyloric membrane, and 84% in infants with gap atresia after gastroduodenostomy.

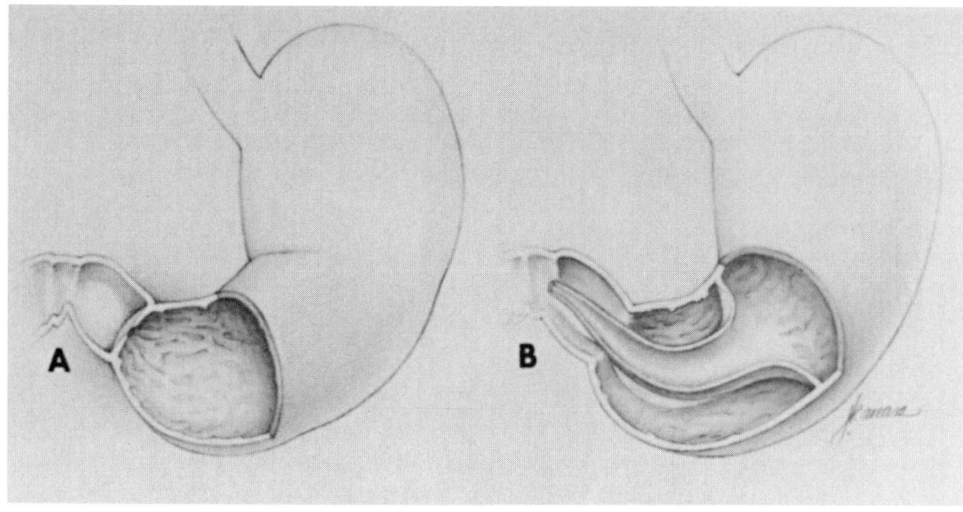


**FIGURE 17–6.** Prepyloric web *(A)* and windsock deformity *(B)*. Antral webs with partial openings account for 5% of all cases of congenital outlet obstruction.

# GASTRIC VOLVULUS

## History

Gastric volvulus was first described by Berti in 1866.[77] In 1904, Borchardt[78] described the classic triad of clinical manifestations: (1) sudden onset of violent epigastric pain, (2) intractable retching without production of vomitus, and (3) inability to pass a tube into the stomach. Gastric volvulus is rare and is encountered more frequently in adults than in children. Only five cases in children younger than 10 years of age were reported in a review of 260 cases between 1914 and 1971.[79] Gastric volvulus may be acute or chronic, but according to Cole and Dickerson,[80] it is more likely to be acute in infants and young children.

## Anatomy and Pathogenesis

The peritoneal attachments (ligaments) of the stomach are shown in Figure 17–7. For a volvulus to occur, these ligaments must be absent or stretched. In most cases there are associated mesenteric abnormalities, such as malrotation[81] and abnormal mobility at the hiatus.[82] Cole and Dickerson[80] reported eventration or herniation of the diaphragm in 65% of patients with gastric volvulus up to 10 years of age. Idowu and colleagues[83] reported an even higher incidence of diaphragmatic abnormalities in infants up to 1 month of age with gastric volvulus. Several cases of acute gastric volvulus have been reported in infants and smaller children with asplenia syndrome.[84] Approximately one third of patients with gastric volvulus have no associated abnormality, and in this group the cause may be related to gastric distention.[81, 82]

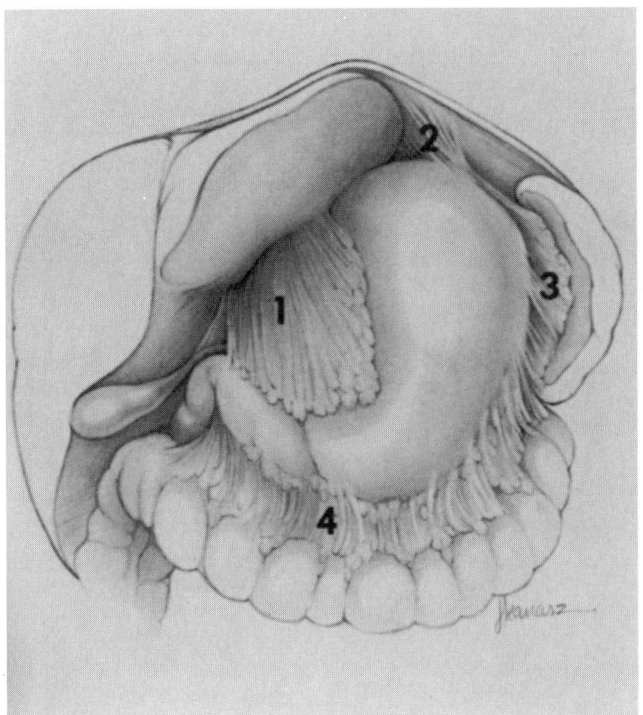


**FIGURE 17–7.** Peritoneal attachments of the stomach include (1) gastrohepatic ligament, (2) gastrophrenic ligament, (3) gastrosplenic ligament, and (4) gastrocolic ligament.

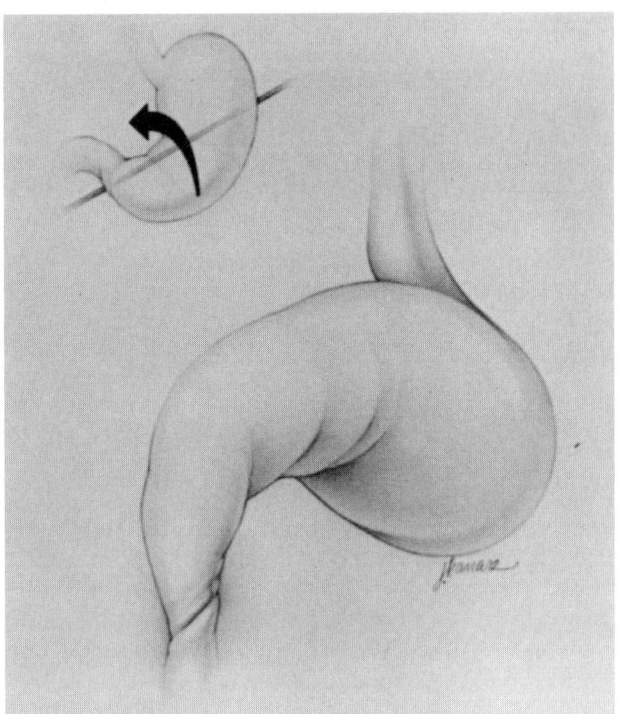

**FIGURE 17–8.** Organoaxial volvulus occurs in the longitudinal axis of the stomach.

Gastric volvulus occurs when one part of the stomach rotates abnormally around another part. Rotation may occur along the longitudinal axis of the stomach to produce organoaxial volvulus (Fig. 17–8) or along the transverse axis to produce mesenteroaxial volvulus (Fig. 17–9). Organoaxial volvulus is more common in children, occurring in approximately two thirds of the reported cases.[82] Rarely, mixed volvulus may occur if the stomach is rotated in both planes. Torsion beyond 180 degrees results in complete gastric obstruction and strangulation of the vasculature.

## Clinical Presentation

The clinical features of acute gastric volvulus are nonspecific but suggest high obstruction of the gastrointestinal tract.[85] The triad of Borchardt may not always apply in children. For example, pain in newborns is difficult to assess. Second, gastric volvulus in infants may produce bilious or nonbilious vomiting. Third, not all infants with gastric volvulus exhibit abdominal distention, and in many infants a nasogastric tube may be passed relatively easily.[80] Acute volvulus can advance rapidly to gastric strangulation, perforation, and cardiovascular collapse and should be treated as a surgical emergency. Chronic gastric volvulus, more common in older children, usually presents with postprandial pain, belching, vomiting, and early satiety. Rarely does chronic volvulus lead to vascular compromise.

Gastric volvulus may be suggested on plain radiographs by a dilated stomach. In mesenteroaxial volvulus, erect radiographic films often show a double fluid level and a

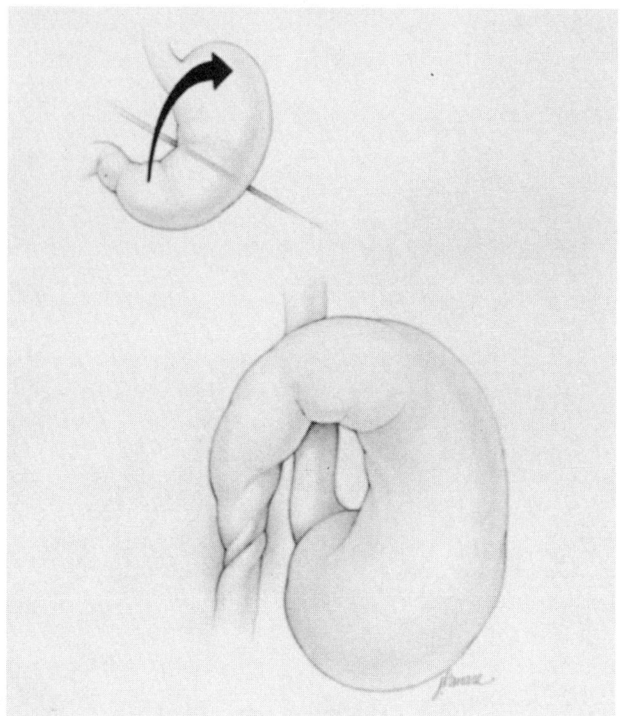

**FIGURE 17–9.** Mesenteroaxial volvulus occurs in the transverse axis of the stomach.

"beak" located near the esophagogastric junction, which is caused by gaseous distention of the inverted antrum.[81] In erect films, organoaxial volvulus shows just one air-fluid level and no characteristic beak. If a nasogastric tube is passed, the gastroesophageal junction is seen inferior to its normal position with respect to the fundus. On UGIS the gastroesophageal junction is in the normal position; the stomach is visualized upside-down and often is apparently located within the left chest when there is an associated hiatal hernia or other diaphragmatic defect (Fig. 17–10).

### Treatment

Acute gastric volvulus requires surgery as soon as adequate resuscitation has been performed. The stomach should be decompressed by nasogastric suction or, alternatively, by needle aspiration. Once the volvulus is reduced, predisposing causes should be investigated. Hiatal hernia, diaphragmatic eventration, or diaphragmatic hernia should be surgically corrected; anterior gastrostomy along with gastropexy usually is curative. A fundoplication or other antireflux procedures should be performed only if there is evidence of severe reflux.[83]

In certain cases of chronic gastric volvulus, endoscopic correction has been advocated.[86] With air insufflation at a minimum, the endoscope is turned into a loop and rotated 180 degrees in a clockwise or counterclockwise direction. Endoscopic examination after this maneuver may reveal the stomach to be in a normal position. Although dual percutaneous endoscopic gastrostomy has been used in the management of chronic gastric volvulus in adults, this technique would seem to offer little advantage in children, who usually require a general anesthetic for repair of acute gastric volvulus.

## CONGENITAL MICROGASTRIA

### History

Microgastria was first described at necropsy of an adult by Dide in 1894.[87] Blank and Chisholm[88] reported a 26-year follow-up of a patient with congenital microgastria first seen in 1947.

### Etiology

Microgastria is a rare congenital anomaly characterized by a small, tubular stomach, megaesophagus, and incomplete gastric rotation.[89] Multiple associated anomalies have been described, including malrotation, situs inversus, and asplenia.[90] Skeletal anomalies are common and include micrognathia, radial and ulnar hypoplasia, and hypoplastic nails.

### Clinical Presentation

The most frequent symptoms of microgastria are vomiting and failure to thrive.[89] These symptoms generally result from

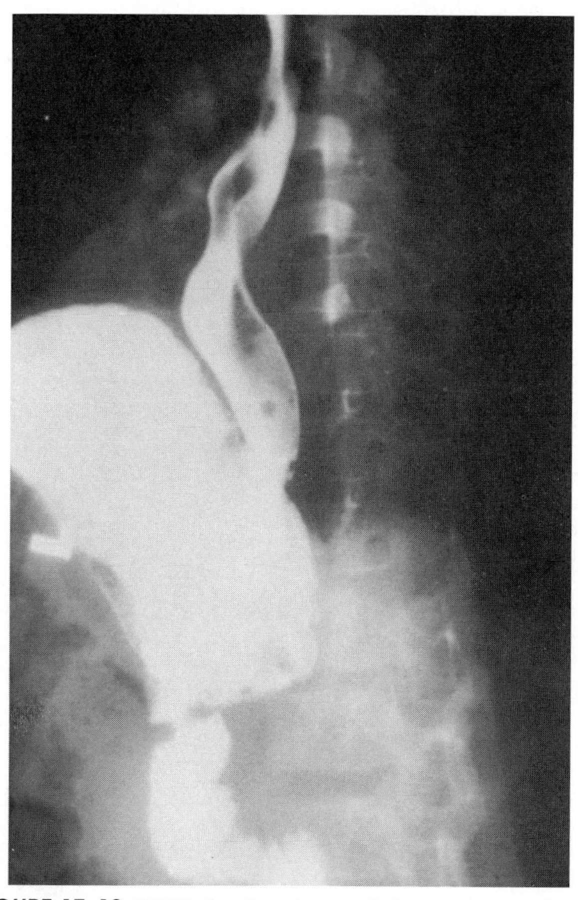

**FIGURE 17–10.** UGIS showing characteristic appearance of stomach in mesenteroaxial gastric volvulus.

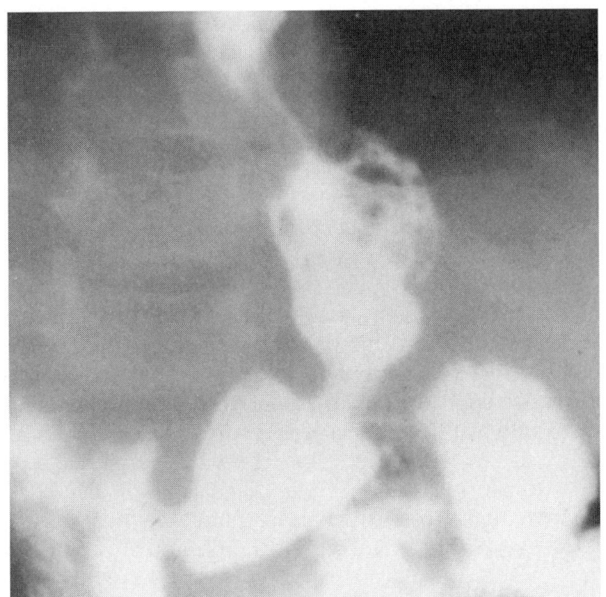

**FIGURE 17–11.** UGIS showing typical appearance of microgastria with gastroesophageal reflux.

associated gastroesophageal reflux, which may also cause aspiration, esophageal erosion, and hemorrhage as well as a dilated esophagus.

### Diagnosis

The diagnosis of microgastria is usually made by UGIS (Fig. 17–11). Endoscopy and esophageal pH studies may be helpful in the setting of severe gastroesophageal reflux.

### Treatment

Treatment is usually medical and consists of continuous gastrostomy or jejunostomy tube feedings. Gastroesophageal reflux should be treated conservatively with antacids and metoclopramide. When gastroesophageal reflux cannot be managed medically, antireflux procedures using the Hill or Thal repair may be considered. In most instances, the stomach gradually dilates to accommodate oral feedings. In certain protracted cases, construction of a jejunal reservoir has been recommended.[91]

## GASTRIC AND DUODENAL DUPLICATION

### History

Reginald Fitz[92] coined the word *duplication* to describe what he thought were cystic remnants of the omphalomesenteric duct. Various cystic abnormalities of the gastrointestinal tract were subsequently described, and in 1952 Gross and colleagues[93] suggested that the term *duplication* be used for all such anomalies, irrespective of their site, morphology, or embryologic derivation. Gastroduodenal duplications account for fewer than 10% of all alimentary tract duplications and were classified by Rowling in 1959[94] according to the following criteria: (1) the cyst wall is contiguous with the stomach wall; (2) the cyst is surrounded by smooth muscle contiguous with stomach muscle; and (3) the cyst wall is lined by alimentary epithelium. In 1979 Schwartz and coworkers[95] described a gastric duplication that was ectopic and separate from the stomach, taking issue with the requirement for continuity of the cyst wall with the stomach.

### Embryogenesis and Pathology

Bremer[96] proposed that gastroduodenal duplications result from an error of recanalization in which there is coalescence of vacuoles within the embryonic duct wall or fusion of the longitudinal epithelial folds to form a hollow tube. Although this description may apply to duodenal duplications, the embryonic stomach does not go through a stage of mucosal proliferation and recanalization. McLetchie and associates[97] proposed an alternative theory in which abnormal adhesions between the notochord and the embryonic endoderm form a traction diverticulum, disorganizing endoderm as the embryo grows. Torma[98] pointed out that this theory may explain the frequent association of gastric duplications with esophageal and pancreatic duplications. Gastric duplications are closed, spherical structures on the greater curvature of the stomach and may be associated with enterogenous cysts in the posterior mediastinum, the esophagus, or the duodenum.[99–101] Gastric duplications may be tubular or cystic, and most are smaller than 12 cm in diameter. Wieczorek and colleagues[101] found that 82% of gastric duplications are cystic and do not communicate with the stomach, whereas 18% are tubular and do communicate. Several cases have been described in which ectopic pancreatic tissue lines the cyst along with gastric mucosa.[98] Rarely, gastroduodenal duplications may be extensive tubular structures that traverse the diaphragm and are associated with anomalous upper cervical and thoracic vertebra.[102, 103]

Associated congenital anomalies occur in 35% of patients with gastric duplications.[104] The most common anomaly is another cyst, especially of the esophagus or duodenum, but vertebral anomalies and ectopic pancreas are frequently found.

### Presentation

A literature review in 1984 found a total of 109 reported gastric duplications.[101] More than half of all gastroduodenal duplications are diagnosed within the first year of life, and the female-to-male ratio is 2:1. The clinical presentation depends on the size and location of the cyst and the presence or absence of communication with the alimentary tract. The most common presentation is that of gastric outlet obstruction, but in 65% of cases there is a palpable abdominal mass.[101] In many cases there is abdominal pain, weight loss, and failure to thrive. Occasionally, a large duplication cyst may perforate secondary to ulceration caused by stasis of gastric enzymes and hydrochloric acid within the cyst.[105] Noncommunicating duplications may cause gastric irritation, leading to gastritis or peptic ulceration. Therefore, hematemesis or melena may be seen in approximately 30% of older children.[101] Finally, when there is a coexistent gastric and pancreatic duplication, pancreatitis or erosion into a contiguous viscus (e.g., the transverse colon) may occur.[106, 107]

### Diagnosis

Usually, a gastric duplication is revealed by UGIS as an extrinsic defect located on the greater curve of the stomach. A more distal cyst may distort the pyloric or duodenal channel, or both, and usually causes delayed gastric emptying. Sonography or computed tomographic scanning may be helpful in demonstrating contiguous cystic structures. Technetium 99m scanning can localize ectopic gastric mucosa but, because of overlapping uptake, is of little help in demonstrating structures adjacent to the stomach.[107]

### Treatment

In most instances, the treatment of a gastroduodenal duplication is excision of the cyst, either by dissection from a common wall or by excision of the cyst with a margin of normal stomach and primary closure.[101, 108] If there is a coexistent pancreatic duplication, the accessory pancreatic lobe can be ligated and transected at its origin.[106, 107] If the aberrant pancreatic lobe is adherent to the stomach, an attempt should be made to dissect it free before a more extensive resection is undertaken. Similarly, it may be possible to avoid an extensive resection in the region of the gastroesophageal junction or pyloric channel by performing a partial excision of the gastroduodenal duplication and stripping the mucosa along the common wall to prevent subsequent ulceration.[108] If complete resection or partial resection with mucosal stripping is not technically possible, marsupialization can be accomplished with internal drainage either into the duodenum or using a Roux-en-Y loop of jejunum.[109]

### Results

The overall mortality rate is approximately 3%.[101] In more than 10% of patients, perforation of the duplication cyst had occurred either freely into the peritoneal cavity or with fistula formation into adjacent structures. However, there has been only one reported death as a complication of cyst perforation.[110]

## DUODENAL STENOSIS AND ATRESIA

### History

Theremine[111] reported 11 cases of duodenal atresia in 1877. In 1901, Cordes[112] described the clinical manifestations of the anomaly and found 56 cases in the literature with no survivors. The first successful operation on a child with duodenal atresia was reported by Ernst[113] in 1916. By 1931 only nine survivors were located by Webb and Wangensteen,[114] who refined the techniques of surgical repair. Finally, Ladd and Gross[115] developed the techniques that are still in use today.

### Etiology and Pathology

Duodenal atresia is thought to arise from the failure of recanalization of the duodenal lumina or the persistence of epithelial proliferation that occurs between the fourth and the fifth weeks of gestation.[116] Less commonly, an annular pancreas causes external compression of the second portion of the duodenum. This may occur when the tip of the ventral pancreatic bud becomes fixed to the duodenal wall and, as rotation occurs, is drawn around the right side of the duodenum to fuse with the dorsal pancreas.[117] Duodenal stenosis usually occurs with annular pancreas but may also occur with extrinsic indentation of the duodenal wall caused by mesenteric bands or preduodenal portal veins. Duodenal atresia may exist as an intact diaphragm or membrane formed of mucosa and submucosa (type 1), as a short fibrous cord connecting two blind ends of duodenum (type 2), or a gap between blind duodenal ends (type 3).[1] Type 1 atresia is most common; it is located proximal to the ampulla of Vater in 15% to 30% of cases and at or distal to the ampulla of Vater in 70% to 85% of cases.[118, 119]

### Incidence

The incidence of congenital duodenal obstruction is about 1 in 10,000;[120] about half of these infants are born prematurely, with a female-to-male ratio of more than 2:1.[118, 120] The relative incidence of various forms of congenital duodenal obstruction is duodenal atresia in 42%, annular pancreas in 33%, and duodenal diaphragm in 23% of neonates.[119]

### Associated Anomalies

Down syndrome occurs in 10% to 30% of infants with duodenal atresia.[118, 120] Infants with duodenal atresia have a high risk of potentially life-threatening congenital anomalies, such as esophageal atresia in 10% to 20%, malrotation in 20%, congenital heart disease in 10% to 15%, and anorectal anomalies in approximately 5%.[118, 119, 121, 122] Overall, about one third of infants with congenital duodenal obstruction have a life-threatening congenital anomaly, and half of those have multiple anomalies. The combination of duodenal atresia, esophageal atresia, and anorectal anomaly is almost always associated with anomalies of other systems and is almost always fatal.[122]

### Clinical Presentation and Diagnosis

Bilious vomiting without abdominal distention is the most typical presentation of congenital duodenal obstruction. One third of patients have nonbilious vomiting as a result of supra-ampullary atresia, and almost one half have upper abdominal distention secondary to gastric dilatation. Meconium stools may be passed in the early stages; however, absence of meconium stools is not a dependable sign of

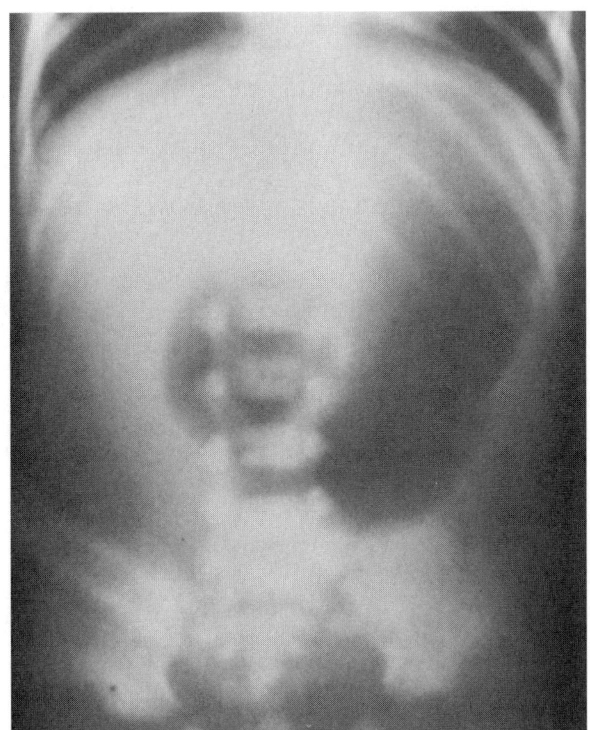

**FIGURE 17–12.** Double-bubble gas pattern characteristic of duodenal atresia.

complete intestinal obstruction in the neonate. Polyhydramnios occurs in approximately 50% of pregnancies in which there is congenital duodenal obstruction. This occurs because high intestinal obstruction prevents the normal absorption of amniotic fluid in the distal small intestine.[123]

The finding of a markedly distended stomach and first portion of duodenum without distal air on kidney, ureter, and bladder radiographic studies is known as the *double-bubble sign* and is pathognomonic of duodenal atresia (Fig. 17–12). If nasogastric suction has already been instituted, it may be useful to instill 50 mL of air by nasogastric tube to demonstrate this finding. Prenatal diagnosis of duodenal atresia has become common with the increased use of prenatal sonography, which may also be used to detect associated anomalies.[124] If sonography is not obtained prenatally, it should be performed before surgery, along with echocardiography and radiography of the chest and spine.

A UGIS usually is not necessary to diagnose duodenal atresia and may be hazardous. On the other hand, the most important differential diagnosis to make is that of malrotation and volvulus, which can cause gangrene of the entire midgut within 6 to 12 hours. Therefore, if plain films are not diagnostic, UGIS should be performed with a nasogastric tube in place and by an experienced radiologist.

## Treatment

The initial management of an infant with duodenal obstruction includes placement of a nasogastric or oral gastric tube, institution of intravenous fluids, and appropriate respiratory care. If malrotation and volvulus have been excluded, definitive surgery may be postponed to evaluate and treat life-threatening associated anomalies. In general, the repair of duodenal atresia is superseded by treatment of those life-threatening anomalies discussed previously.

The most frequently used surgical repair for all forms of intrinsic duodenal obstruction is the duodenoduodenostomy[125, 126] (Fig. 17–13). It has been recognized that anastomotic function may recover earlier when the dilated proximal duodenum is tapered.[127, 128] This allows more effective coaptation of the opposing walls of the dilated intestines, leading to improved peristalsis.[129, 130] Most surgeons prefer to leave a gastrostomy tube, because it drains more effectively and is less injurious to pulmonary status than is a nasogastric tube. Hyperalimentation is commonly used until the infant is feeding. Transanastomotic silicone tubes continue to be used by many surgeons for postoperative jejunal feedings; however, at least one study has shown that these

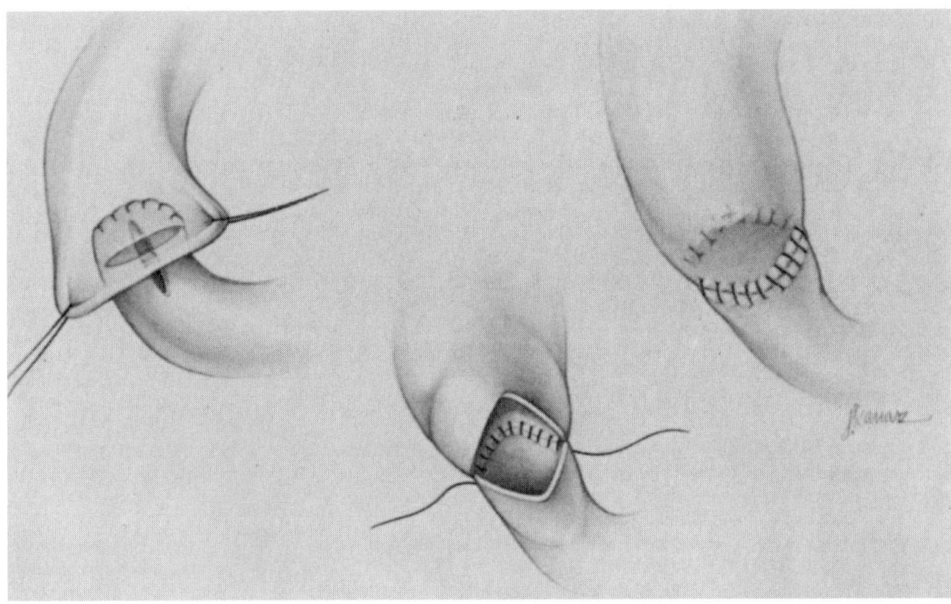

**FIGURE 17–13.** Diamond-shaped anastomosis developed by Kimura and associates,[126] which reduces time to initiation of oral feedings.

tubes prolong the time until oral diet is tolerated and increase total length of hospitalization.[118]

## Results

Survival after surgical repair of congenital duodenal obstruction ranges between 70% and 100%, depending on the incidence of prematurity and associated anomalies. In most reports, the majority of deaths were directly attributable to associated anomalies. However, a large multi-institutional survey of duodenal atresia taken in 1969 showed that anastomotic problems were responsible for 16% of the deaths.[131] This percentage is operator dependent, but today, in experienced hands, it should be less than 5%. Although prolonged intravenous hyperalimentation was formerly required in many patients with megaduodenum, most infants treated with duodenoduodenostomy now may be started on feedings within 1 week and may be discharged from the hospital within 2 or 3 weeks.[132]

Attention has been focused on the late follow-up of duodenal atresia, in which more than 25% of patients were symptomatic with abdominal pain as a result of chronic alkaline biliary reflux and blind loop syndrome secondary to a poorly emptying proximal duodenal pouch.[133] This complication may become less of an issue as more patients undergo tapering procedures. However, the importance of long-term follow-up of all patients for duodenal atresia cannot be overemphasized.

### REFERENCES


1. Gray SW, Skandalakis JE: Embryology for Surgeons. Philadelphia, WB Saunders, 1971, pp 101–105.
2. Moutsouris C: The "solid stage" and congenital intestinal atresia. J Pediatr Surg 1966;1:446–450.
3. Donovan EJ: Hezekiah Beardsley: congenital hypertrophic stenosis of the pylorus. Arch Pediatr 1958;75:359.
4. Hirschsprung H: Falle von angeborener pylorusstenose: beobachtet bie salingen. Jahrb Kinderhlk 1888;27:61.
5. Dufour H, Fredette P: La steanose hypertrophique du pylore chez le noursson et son traitement chir surgical. Rev Chir 1908;37:208.
6. Borgwardt G: Conrad Ramstedt: an appreciation. Z Kinderchir 1986;41:195–200.
7. Laron Z, Horne LM: The incidence of infantile pyloric stenosis. Am J Dis Child 1957;94:151.
8. Jed MB, Melton J, Griffin MR, et al: Factors associated with infantile hypertrophic pyloric stenosis. Am J Dis Child 1988;142:334–337.
9. Kerr AM: Unprecedented rise in incidence of infantile hypertrophic pyloric stenosis. Br Med J 1980;13:714–715.
10. Knox EG, Armstrong E, Hanes R: Changing incidence of infantile hypertrophic pyloric stenosis. Arch Dis Child 1983;58:582–585.
11. Martin J, Monk J: Infant feeding in 1980. OPCS. London, Social Survey Division, HNSO, 1982.
12. Carter CO, Evans KA: Inheritance of congenital pyloric stenosis. J Med Genet 1969;6:233–239.
13. Dodge JA: Infantile hypertrophic pyloric stenosis in Belfast. Arch Dis Child 1975;50:171–178.
14. McKeown T, MacMahon B: Infantile hypertrophic pyloric stenosis in parent and child. Arch Dis Child 1955;30:497.
15. Androssi JR, Haff RC, Larsen GL: Infantile hypertrophic pyloric stenosis during the first week of life. Clin Pediatr 1977;16:474.
16. Geer LL, Gaisie G, Mandell VS, et al: Evolution of pyloric stenosis in the first week of life. Pediatr Radiol 1985;15:205–206.
17. Rollins MD, Shields, MD, Quinn RJM, et al: Pyloric stenosis: congenital or acquired? Arch Dis Child 1989;64:137–138.
18. Stunden RJ, LeQuesne GW, Little KET: The improved ultrasound diagnosis of hypertrophic pyloric stenosis. Pediatr Radiol 1986:16:200–205.
19. Latchaw LAC, Jacir NN, Harris BH: The development of pyloric stenosis during transpyloric feeding. J Pediatr Surg 1989;24:823–824.
20. Lynn H: The mechanism of pyloric stenosis and its relationship to preoperative preparation. Arch Surg 1960;81:453.
21. Spits L, Zail SS: Serum gastrin levels in congenital hypertrophic pyloric stenosis. J Pediatr Surg 1976;11:33.
22. Laferla G, Watson J, Fyfe AHB, et al: The role of prostaglandins $E_2$ and $F_2$ alpha in infantile hypertrophic pyloric stenosis. J Pediatr Surg 1986;21:410–412.
23. Kobayashi H, Obriain DS, Puri P: Defective cholinergic innervation in pyloric muscle of patients with hypertrophic pyloric stenosis. Pediatr Surg 1994;9:338–341.
24. Rendle-Short J, Zachary RB: Congenital pyloric stenosis in older babies. Arch Dis Child 1955;30:70.
25. Touloukin RJ, Higgins E: The spectrum of serum electrolytes in hypertrophic pyloric stenosis. J Pediatr Surg 1983;18:394–397.
26. Winters RW: Metabolic Alkaloses of Pyloric Stenosis: The Body Fluid in Pediatrics. Boston, Little, Brown, 1973, pp 402–414.
27. Benson CD: Infantile hypertrophic pyloric stenosis. In Welsh KJ, Randolph JG, Ravitch MM, et al (eds): Pediatric Surgery, 4th ed. Chicago, Year Book Medical Publishers, 1986, pp 811–815.
28. Mackay AJ, Mackellar A: Infantile hypertrophic pyloric stenosis: a review of two-hundred and twenty-two cases. Aust N Z J Surg 1986;56:131–133.
29. Chaves-Carbello E, Harris LE, Lynn HB: Jaundice associated with pyloric stenosis and neonatal small bowel obstruction. Clin Pediatr 1968;7:198–202.
30. Woolley MM, Felsher BF, Asch MJ, et al: Jaundice, hypertrophic pyloric stenosis, and hepatic glucuronyl transferase. J Pediatr Surg 1974;9:359–363.
31. Labrune T, Myara A, Huguet P, et al: Jaundice with hypertrophic pyloric stenosis: a possible early manifestation of Gilbert syndrome. J Pediatr 1989;15:93–95.
32. Ahmed S: Infantile pyloric stenosis associated with major anomalies of the alimentary tract. J Pediatr Surg 1970;5:660–666.
33. Ziedan B, Wyatt J, Mackersie A, et al: Recent results of treatment of infantile hypertrophic pyloric stenosis. Arch Dis Child 1988;63:1060–1064.
34. Meuwissen T, Sloof JP: Roentgenologic diagnosis of congenital hypertrophic pyloric stenosis. Acta Pediatr 1932;14:19–48.
35. Herran PJ, Darling DB, Sciamma F: The value of the double tract sign of the differentiating factor between pyloric spasm and hypertrophic pyloric stenosis. Radiology 1966;86:723–725.
36. Shopfner CE, Kalmon EH, Coin CG: The diagnosis of hypertrophic pyloric stenosis. AJR Am J Roentgenol 1964;91:796–800.
37. Ball TI, Atkinson GO, Gay BB: Ultrasound diagnosis of hypertrophic pyloric stenosis: real-time application and demonstration of new sonographic sign. Radiology 1983;147:499–502.
38. Teele RL, Smith EH: Ultrasound and the diagnosis of idiopathic hypertrophic pyloric stenosis. N Engl J Med 1977;296:1149–1150.
39. Blumhagen JD, Nobel HG: Muscle thickness in hypertrophic pyloric stenosis: sonographic determination. AJR Am J Roentgenol 1983;140:221–223.
40. Wilson DA, VanHoutte JJ: The reliable sonographic diagnosis of hypertrophic pyloric stenosis. J Clin Ultrasound 1984;12:201–204.
41. Gobdole P, Sprigg A, Dickson JA, et al: Ultrasound compared with clinical examination in infantile hypertrophic pyloric stenosis. Arch Dis Child 1996;75:335–337.
42. Forman HP, Leonida JC, Kronfeld GD: A rational approach to diagnosis of hypertrophic pyloric stenosis: do the results match the claims? J Pediatr Surg 1990;25:262.
43. Kumar V, Bailey WC: Electrolyte and acid-base problems in hypertrophic pyloric stenosis in infancy. Indian Pediatr 1935;12:839.
44. Steven IM, Allen TH, Sweeny DB: Congenital hypertrophic pyloric stenosis: the anaesthetist's view. Anaesth Intensive Care 1973;1:544–546.
45. Conn AW: Anaesthesia for pyloromyotomy in infancy. Can Anaesth Soc J 1963;10:18–29.
46. Scharli AF, Leditschke JF: Gastric motility after pyloromyotomy in infants: a reappraisal of postoperative feeding. Surgery 1968;64:1133–1137.
47. Sauerbrei EE, Paloschi GGB: The ultrasonic features of hypertrophic pyloric stenosis, with emphasis on the postoperative appearance. Radiology 1983;147:503–506.

48. Jamroz GA, Blocker SH, McAlister WH: Radiographic findings after incomplete pyloromyotomy. Gastrointest Radiol 1986;11:139–141.
49. Scharli A, Sieber WK, Kiesewetter WB: Hypertrophic pyloric stenosis at the Children's Hospital of Pittsburgh from 1912 to 1967. J Pediatr Surg 1969;4:108–114.
50. Bell MJ: Infantile pyloric stenosis: Experience with three hundred and five cases at the Louisville Children's Hospital. Surgery 1968;64:983–989.
51. Benson CD: Infantile pyloric stenosis: historical aspects and current surgical concepts. Prog Pediatr Surg 1971;1:63–88.
52. Gibbs MK, vanHeerden JA, Lynn HB: Congenital hypertrophic pyloric stenosis: surgical experience. Mayo Clin Proc 1975;50:312–316.
53. Calder J: Two examples of children preternatural conformation of the guts. Med Essays and Obs (Edinburgh) 1733;1:205.
54. Crooks: Estomac se terminant en cude sac. Arch Gen Med 1828;17:264.
55. Cook RCM, Rickham PP: Gastric Outlet Obstruction in Neonatal Surgery, 2nd ed. London, Butterworth, 1978, pp 335–338.
56. Parsons LG, Barding S: Disease of Infancy and Childhood. London, Oxford University, 1933.
57. Moore CM: Congenital gastric outlet obstruction. J Pediatr Surg 1989;24:1242–1246.
58. Gerber BC, Aberdeen SO: Pre-pyloric diaphragm, an unusual abnormality. Arch Surg 1965;90:472–475.
59. Simstein NL: Congenital gastric anomalies. Am Surg 1986;52:264–268.
60. Bell MJ, Ternberg JL, McAlister W, et al: Antral diaphragm: a cause of gastric outlet obstruction in infants and children. J Pediatr 1977;90:196–202.
61. Tunnell WP, Ide Smith E: Antral web in infancy. J Pediatr Surg 1980;15:152–155.
62. Kume K, Ikeda K, Hayashida Y, et al: Congenital pyloric atresia: a report of three cases and review of the literature. J Pediatr Surg 1980;16:259–268.
63. El Shafie M, Stidham LG, Klippel CH, et al: Pyloric atresia epidermolysis bullosa letalis: a lethal combination in two premature newborn siblings. J Pediatr Surg 1979;14:446–449.
64. Bar-Maor JA, Nissan S, Nero S: Pyloric atresia. J Med Genet 1972;9:70–72.
65. Pearson RW, Potter B, Strauss F: Epidermolysis bullosa hereditaria letalis. Arch Dermatol 1974;109:349–355.
66. Korber JS, Glasson MJ: Pyloric atresia associated with epidermolysis bullosa. J Pediatr 1977;90:600–601.
67. Gedde-Dahl T Jr, Lambrecht IA: Principles and Practices in Medical Genetics. New York, Churchill-Livingstone, 1981.
68. Ducharme JC, Bensousson AL: Pyloric atresia. J Pediatr Surg 1975;10:149–150.
69. Sloop RD, Montagne ACW: Gastric outlet obstruction due to congenital pyloric mucosal membrane. Am Surg 1967;165:598–604.
70. Burnett HA, Halpert B: Perforation of the stomach of a newborn infant with pyloric atresias. Arch Pathol 1947;44:318.
71. Franklin EA: Gastrointestinal Imaging in Pediatrics, 2nd ed. Philadelphia, Harper & Row, 1982, pp 131–142.
72. Gruenbaum M, Kornreich L, Ziv N: The imaging diagnosis of pyloric atresia. Z Kinderchir 1985;40:308–311.
73. Bell MH, Ternberg JL, Keating JP, et al: Prepyloric gastric antral web: a puzzling epidemic. J Pediatr Surg 1978;13:307–313.
74. Talwalker VC: Pyloric atresia: a case report. J Pediatr Surg 1967;2:458–460.
75. Brandt LJ, Boley SJ, Dom F, et al: Endoscopic resection of an obstructing antral web in an infant. Dig Dis Sci 1978;5:65–85.
76. Al-Kawas FH: Endoscopic laser treatment of an obstructing antral web. Gastrointest Endosc 1988;34:349–351.
77. Berti A: Singolare attortigliamento dell' esofago duodeno sequito da rapida morte. Gass Med Ital 1866;9:139.
78. Borchardt M: Zur Patologie und terapie des magenvolvuls. Arch Klin Chir 1904;74:243.
79. Wastell C, Ellis H: Volvulus of the stomach: a review with a reported eight cases. Br J Surg 1971;58:557–562.
80. Cole BC, Dickerson SJ: Acute volvulus of the stomach in infants and children. Surgery 1971;70:707–717.
81. Ziprkowski MN, Teele RL: Gastric volvulus in childhood. AJR Am J Roentgenol 1979;132:921–925.
82. Cammeron AEP, Howard ER: Gastric volvulus in childhood. J Pediatr Surg 1987;22:944–947.
83. Idowu J, Aitken DR, Gorgeson KE: Gastric volvulus in the newborn. Arch Surg 1980;115:1046–1049.
84. Aoyama K, Tateishi K: Gastric volvulus in three children with asplenia syndrome. J Pediatr Surg 1986;21:307–310.
85. Campbell JB: Neonatal gastric volvulus. AJR Am J Roentgenol 1979;132:723–725.
86. Eckhauser ML, Ferron JP: The use of dual percutaneous endoscopic gastrostomy in the management of chronic intermittent gastric volvulus. Gastrointest Endosc 1985;31:340–342.
87. Dide M: Sur un estomac d'adulte type foetal. Bull Soc Anat Paris 1894;69:669.
88. Blank E, Chisholm AJ: Congenital microgastria: a case report with a 26-year follow-up. Pediatrics 1973;51:1037.
89. Campbell JR: Congenital microgastria. In Pediatric Surgery. Chicago, Year Book Medical Publishers, 1986, pp 827–828.
90. Kessler H, Smulevicz JJ: Microgastria associated with agenesis of the spleen. Radiology 1973;107:393.
91. Neifield JP, Berman WF, Lawrence W Jr, et al: Management of congenital microgastria with a jejunal reservoir pouch. J Pediatr Surg 1980;15:882.
92. Fitz RH: Persistent omphalo-mesenteric remains: their importance in the causation of intestinal duplication, cyst formation, and obstruction. Am J Med Sci 1884;88:30–57.
93. Gross RE, Holcomb GW Jr, Farber S: Duplications of the alimentary tract. Pediatrics 1952;9:449–468.
94. Rowling JT: Some observations of gastric cysts. Br J Surg 1959;46:441–445.
95. Schwartz DL, So HB, Becker JM: An ectopic gastric duplication arising from the pancreas and presenting with pneumoperitoneum. J Pediatr Surg 1979;14:187–188.
96. Bremer JL: Diverticula and duplications of the intestinal tract. Arch Pathol Lab Med 1944;38:132–140.
97. McLetchie NGB, Purves JK, Saunders RL: The genesis of gastric and certain intestinal diverticula and enterogenous cysts. Surg Gynecol Obstet 1954;99:135–141.
98. Torma MJ: Of double stomachs. Arch Surg 1974;109:155–157.
99. Alschibija T, Putnam TC, Yablin BA: Duplication of the stomach simulating hypertrophic pyloric stenosis. Am J Dis Child 1974;127:120–122.
100. Bowmen M, Singh MP: Pyloric duplication in a preterm neonate. J Pediatr Surg 1984;19:158–159.
101. Wieczorek RL, Seidman I, Ranson JH, et al: Congenital duplication of the stomach: case report and review of the English literature. Am J Gastroenterol 1984;79:597–602.
102. Lister J, Rickham PP: Neonatal surgery. In Rickham PP, Irving IM, (eds): Neonatal Surgery, 2nd ed. London, Butterworth, 1978, pp 401–404.
103. Fitzgivens RJ Jr, Neugent FW, Ellis FH, et al: Unusual thoracoabdominal duplication associated with pancreatopleural fistula. Gastroenterology 1980;79:344–347.
104. Bartels RJ: Duplication of the stomach: case report and review of the literature. Ann Surg 1976;33:747–752.
105. Sieunarine K, Manmohansingh E: Gastric duplication cysts presenting as an acute abdomen in a child. J Pediatr Surg 1989;24:1152.
106. Rosenlund ML, Schnaufer L: Gastric duplications presenting as cyclical abdominal pain. Clin Pediatr 1978;17:747–748.
107. Spence RK, Schnaufer L, Mahboubi S: Coexistent gastric duplication and accessory pancreas: clinical manifestations, embryogenesis, and treatment. J Pediatr Surg 1986;21:68–70.
108. Bishop HC, Koop CE: Surgical management of duplications of the alimentary tract. Am J Surg 1964;167:434–442.
109. Holcomb GW, Gheissari A, O'Neill JA, et al: Surgical management of the alimentary tract duplications. Ann Surg 1988;209:167–174.
110. Bower RJ, Silber WK, Kiesewetter WB: Alimentary tract duplication in children. Ann Surg 1978;188:669–674.
111. Theremine: Veger kongenitale occlusionen des Duenndarms. Deutsche Ztschr Chir 1877;8:34.
112. Cordes L: Congenital occlusion of the duodenum. Arch Pediatr 1901;18:401.
113. Ernst NP: A case of congenital atresia of the duodenum treated successfully by operation. Br Med J 1916;1:1644.
114. Webb CH, Wangensteen OH: Congenital intestinal atresia. Am J Dis Child 1931;41:242.
115. Ladd WE, Gross RE: Abdominal Surgery of Infancy and Childhood. Philadelphia, WB Saunders, 1941.

116. Tandler J: Zur Entwicklungsgeschichte des menschlichen Duodenoms. Morphol JG 1902;29:187.
117. Lecco TM: Zur Morphologie des Pankreas annulare Sitzungsb. Akad Wissensch Cl 1910;119:391.
118. Mooney D, Lewis JE, Connors RH, et al: Newborn duodenal atresia: improving outlook. Am J Surg 1987;153:347–349.
119. Spigland N, Yazbeck S: Complications associated with surgical treatment of congenital intrinsic duodenal obstruction. J Pediatr Surg 1990;25:1127–1130.
120. Nixon HH: Duodenal atresia. Br J Hosp Med 1989;41:134–140.
121. Wayne ER, Burrington JD: Management of 97 children with duodenal obstruction. Arch Surg 1973;107:857–861.
122. Danismend EN, Brown S, Frank JD: Morbidity and mortality in duodenal atresia. Z Kinderchir 1986;41:86–88.
123. Lloyd JR, Clatworthy HW: Hydramnios as an aid to the early diagnosis of congenital obstruction of the alimentary tract. Pediatrics 1958;21:903.
124. Hayden CK, Schwartz NZ, Davis M, et al: Combined esophageal and duodenal atresia: sonographic findings. AJR Am J Roentgenol 1983;140:224.
125. Weitzman JJ, Prennin LP: An improved technique for the correction of congenital duodenal obstruction in neonates. J Pediatr Surg 1974;9:385–388.
126. Kimura K, Mukohara N, Nishijima E, et al: Diamond-shaped anastomoses for duodenal atresia: an experience with forty-four patients over fifteen years. J Pediatr Surg 1990;25:977–979.
127. Weisgerberg G, Boreau M: Resultats immediates et secondaires duodenoduodeostomies avec modelage dans le traitement de obstructions duodenales congenitales completes du nouveau-ne. Chir Pediatr 1982;23:369–372.
128. Adzick NS, Harrison MR, deLorimier AA: Tapering duodenoplasty for megaduodenum associated with duodenal atresia. J Pediatr Surg 1986;21:311–312.
129. DeLorimier AA, Norman DA, Gooding CA, et al: Model for the cinefluoroscopic and manometric study of chronic intestinal obstruction. J Pediatr Surg 1973;8:785–791.
130. Cloutier R: Intestinal smooth muscle response to chronic obstruction: possible applications in jejunoileal atresia. J Pediatr Surg 1975;10:3–8.
131. Fonkalsrud EW, deLorimier AA, Hayes D: Congenital atresia and stenosis of the duodenum. Pediatrics 1969;43:79–83.
132. Weber TR, Lewis JE, Mooney D, et al: Duodenal atresia: a comparison of techniques of repair. J Pediatr Surg 1986;21:1133–1136.
133. Kokkonen ML, Kalima T, Jaaskelainen J, et al: Duodenal atresia: late follow-up. J Pediatr Surg 1988;23:216–220.

Chapter 18

# Gastritis and Ulcers in Children

*Benjamin D. Gold and Uwe Blecker*

Peptic ulcer disease causes significant morbidity and mortality in adults.[1–3] Although gastric and duodenal ulcers occur infrequently in children, a Canadian study estimated that these conditions accounted for roughly 1 in 2,500 pediatric hospital admissions.[4] Studies have yet to be performed that evaluate both the overall prevalence of peptic ulcer disease in large pediatric populations and the health care impact on the care of children. Gastritis, the "precursor" lesion to mucosal ulceration (i.e., peptic ulcer disease) is an important clinical entity and an important cause of abdominal pain in children.[5, 6] It appears that ulcer frequency in children is increased over previous reports, and multicenter studies may contribute to a better understanding of the prevalence and economic impact of these entities in the pediatric population.[4, 7] The overall prevalence of gastritis in children is not defined, but an understanding of the causes of pediatric gastritis and mucosal ulceration is critical for the management of children with abdominal pain.[8]

Inflammation of the gastric and duodenal mucosa is the end result of an imbalance between mucosal defensive and aggressive factors (Table 18–1). The degree of imbalance between defensive and aggressive factors can result in varying amounts of inflammation, gastritis, and/or frank mucosal ulceration. Gastritis and ulcers of the duodenum or stomach have historically been classified as either primary or secondary[9, 10] (Table 18–2). The majority of children with chronic-active or chronic gastritis and ulcers in the stomach or duodenum have secondary inflammation or mucosal ulceration. These ulcers generally occur because of a systemic condition such as head trauma or overwhelming sepsis or as a sequel of drug ingestion (i.e., nonsteroidal anti-inflammatory agents [NSAIDs]).[11, 12] Secondary gastroduodenal ulcers can also occur in specific disease conditions such as Zollinger-Ellison syndrome (ZES) or Crohn's disease.[13–15] In addition, secondary ulcers have uncommonly been reported as a sequela to other diseases such as cystic fibrosis and sickle cell disease.[16–19] Finally, careful historical information obtained from children with secondary ulcers sometimes reveals a family history of peptic ulcer disease.[20, 21]

Current evidence indicates that persons younger than 18 years of age who present with duodenal or gastric ulcers and have no other identified causes have primary gastroduodenal ulceration.[21, 22] An easily elicited family history of peptic ulcer disease is a frequent, positive finding in such cases.[23–25] In almost all of these patients, mucosal inflammation and, less frequently, ulceration is caused by a spiral-shaped, gram-negative, microaerobic rod, properly named *Helicobacter pylori*.[26, 27]

Therefore, the term *primary* seems less relevant than previously noted. Further evidence for the "familial" nature of primary gastritis and peptic ulceration occurring in children is the finding of *H. pylori* clustering among family members of affected individuals.[28, 29] *H. pylori* infects almost 50% of the world's population, but most people do not experience symptoms reportable to a physician and are unaware of their infection. *H. pylori* colonizes the gastric antrum and has satisfied Koch's postulates as a human pathogen causing primary, chronic-active gastritis in children[30, 31] as well as adults.[32–34] Many investigations provide compelling evidence that this organism is associated with a significant proportion (90–100%) of duodenal ulcers and a lesser proportion of gastric ulcers in children.[35, 36] It is also apparent that the more significant the gastroduodenal inflammation, the earlier *H. pylori* infection was acquired.[37–39] Furthermore, recent epidemiologic evidence has linked chronic *H. pylori* infec-

**TABLE 18–1. Aggressive and Defensive Factors Involved in the Gastroduodenal Mucosal Balance**

| AGGRESSIVE FACTORS | MUCOSAL DEFENSIVE FACTORS |
|---|---|
| Vascular injury—decreased microcirculation | Mucosal circulation—adequate microcirculation |
| Cancer chemotherapeutic agents | Epithelial cell turnover |
| Aspirin | Increased bicarbonate secretion |
| NSAIDs | Inhibit gastric acid secretion |
| Infectious agents: CMV, herpesvirus | Preserve vascular flow/ microcirculation |
| Systemic stress: increased catecholamines | Restore epithelial cell surface |
| Increased pepsin secretion | Mucous layer—glycoproteins, glycocalyx |
| *H. pylori* | Bicarbonate layer—pH gradient |
| | Immunoglobulins: IgG, IgA |

**TABLE 18–2. Classification and Causes of Gastritis and Ulcers in Children**

| CLASSIFICATION/CATEGORY | ETIOLOGY |
|---|---|
| **Primary** | *Helicobacter pylori* |
| **Secondary** | |
| Excessive acid production | Zollinger-Ellison syndrome<br>Antral G-cell hyperplasia<br>Antral G-cell hyperfunction<br>Systemic mastocytosis<br>Renal failure, hyperparathyroidism |
| Stress | Infants: traumatic delivery, neonatal sepsis, perinatal asphyxia<br>Children: shock, trauma, sepsis, head injury, burns |
| Other conditions | Eosinophilic gastroenteritis<br>Ménétrier's disease, hypertrophic gastritis<br>Lymphocytic (varioliform) gastritis<br>Autoimmune (atrophic) gastritis<br>Gastroduodenal Crohn's disease |
| Drug-related | NSAIDs, with or without *H. pylori*<br>Aspirin<br>Ethanol (alcohol) |

tion (probably beginning in childhood) with the development of gastric carcinoma.[40, 41]

Although many host and bacterial factors have been identified as playing a role in gastroduodenal inflammation since the "discovery" of *H. pylori* in 1983 in Perth, Australia, by Marshall and Warren,[42, 43] there are still many features of *H. pylori*-associated disease in humans that remain undefined. An understanding of *H. pylori* as an etiologic agent in gastroduodenal inflammation and neoplasia is paramount to defining the pathogenesis of gastritis and peptic ulcer disease in children.

## PATHOGENESIS

### Acid Secretion

Studies that have evaluated the natural history of gastric acid output demonstrate that by 3 to 4 years of age gastric secretion approximates adult values.[44–46] Secretions in the stomach are maintained in a delicate balance in each of the three phases of digestion; cephalic, gastric, and intestinal. The initial or cephalic phase occurs even before the ingestion of food products, simply by anticipation, sight, or smell of food. Once protein has reached the stomach milieu, there is activation of the gastric phase of secretion, with an initial increase in intragastric pH and gastric distention. Once the ingested meal protein has reached the duodenum, the intestinal phase occurs. Hydrochloric acid secretion occurs in the parietal cells, which are located primarily in the body and fundus of the stomach in the midportions of the oxyntic glands. The hydrogen ion pump, a target of many of the new therapies used for acid reduction (i.e., omeprazole, lansoprazole), works via an $H^+$,$K^+$-ATPase mechanism that exchanges potassium ions for hydrogen ions across the epithelial cell apical membrane. Chloride ions move passively with potassium ions in exchange for hydrogen ions. Stimulation of parietal cell acid secretion occurs via multiple pathways, including neuroendocrine (acetylcholine, vagus), endocrine (gastrin, pepsin), and paracrine (histamine) routes. Standard acid suppression therapy (e.g., ranitidine, famotidine) targets these paracrine mechanisms by antagonism of the histamine $H_2$ receptors.[47]

Gastric ulcers are generally associated with a lower acid secretion.[48] However, acid secretion is usually above normal in patients with duodenal ulceration.[49, 50] It has also been postulated that gastritis and duodenitis contribute in the natural history of ulcer development of both types, because of the decreased protection of the mucosal barrier lining the stomach and duodenum and the increased epithelial cell exposure to hydrochloric acid.[51–53] Although the majority of studies on acid secretion have been performed in adults, primarily for methodologic and technical reasons, the findings in pediatric studies comparing duodenal ulcer patients with controls have been consistent with adult patterns of acid secretion: higher gastric acid output in association with mucosal ulceration.[23, 24, 49, 54–56] However, there is tremendous overlap between acid output values in these children and in normal controls.[57]

One study demonstrated a difference in acid secretion between children with gastric ulcers and those with duodenal ulcers.[58] In a study of 82 subjects—10 children with gastric ulcers, 9 children with duodenal ulcers, 58 nonulcer pediatric patients, and 5 healthy adults—the authors looked at 24-hour pH measurements as a determination of acid secretion. Gastric acidity was significantly reduced in those patients with primary (i.e., *H. pylori*-associated) gastric ulcers. However, gastric acidity was increased or above adult levels in those children with duodenal ulcers.[58]

Another pediatric study demonstrated that there is a 24-hour acid output pattern that is distinct in ulcer patients compared with normal controls.[59] Each subject had intragastric pH monitoring over a 48-hour period: the first 24 hours untreated, and the second 24 hours with three doses of the acid-suppressing $H_2$ receptor antagonist, cimetidine. The authors found that children with duodenal ulcers lacked the "intragastric pH inversion" that occurs in normal subjects at about midnight and had persistent hypergastric acidity for the majority of the 24 hours. However, most adult studies demonstrate that knowledge of the maximal acid output, the acid output over a 24-hour period, or even the basal acid output does not allow one to predict the likelihood of ulcer development.

### Bicarbonate-Mucus Barrier

The pathogenesis of gastritis and gastroduodenal ulceration is also mediated, in part, by disturbances in bicarbonate secretion and the mucous layer overlying gastric and duodenal epithelium. The mucous layer serves as a barrier to luminal pepsin and hydrochloric acid, preventing access of pepsin to the apical surface of the epithelial cells and neutralizing the acid through the presence of bicarbonate secreted into the mucus layer. The mucous layer also provides protection for the epithelial cell turnover in both normal and perturbed states and protection from mechanical damage during the hypermotile state of the digestive and intestinal phases of digestion. Mucosal production of bicarbonate can be stimulated by prostaglandins but inhibited by NSAIDs.[60]

Although controversy still exists, studies show that there are impaired rates of proximal duodenal bicarbonate production in patients with duodenal ulceration.[61, 62]

It has been demonstrated in both humans and ferrets that when there is inflammation in the stomach and duodenum as a result of *Helicobacter* infection, there is a concurrent decrease in the mucosal surface hydrophobicity. This is thought to be caused in part by a disturbance in the mucous layer.[63–65] It is believed that the mucus confers the hydrophobicity to the stomach, and its decreased production and erosion leads to exposure of gastric epithelial cells to pepsin, acid, and other aggressive factors. Adult studies have demonstrated that a decreased polymerization of the component glycoproteins of mucus contributes to the deficient structure of the mucus in duodenal ulcer patients.[66] Evidence points to disturbances in the gastroduodenal mucous layer and bicarbonate secretion as factors in ulcer pathogenesis, but no studies have been done in children.

### Genetic Factors

Gastric hormones, specifically gastrin[67] and pepsinogens I and II,[68] have received a great deal of attention as potential inflammatory or ulcer-causing factors. Early studies had findings that were suggestive of an inheritable pattern of increased serum pepsinogen levels. These investigations showed that children with duodenal ulcers and their parents had increased levels of serum pepsinogen I.[69] Subsequent studies evaluating children with *H. pylori* infection demonstrated that chronic infection is associated with increased levels of serum pepsinogen.[70] Because this organism clearly clusters in families, this observation was taken as circumstantial evidence for the "inheritable" nature of peptic ulcer disease.[28] Work on inflammatory bowel disease indicates that genetic factors may contribute significantly to disease development in susceptible persons.[71, 72]

## CAUSES OF SECONDARY PEPTIC ULCER DISEASE

### Excessive Acid Secretion (Zollinger-Ellison Syndrome, Gastrinoma)

Although rare, these conditions of excessive acid production affect children and can result in multiple erosions and frank ulcers in the stomach, duodenum, and jejunum.[73] Of the secondary causes of ulcers, this is one group in which a family history of ulcers, a history of endocrine diseases, or quite commonly, a family history of hyperpepsinogenemia I is found. There are believed to be three types of disorders that result in excessive acid production: antral G-cell hyperplasia, antral G-cell hyperfunction, and Zollinger-Ellison syndrome (ZES). ZES is a condition associated with ulcers in atypical locations (i.e., jejunum) that are refractory to standard antisecretory therapy. ZES should be highly suspected if the patient has severe peptic ulceration, kidney stones, watery diarrhea, or malabsorption, particularly in the presence of gastric ulcers, hypergastrinemia, and a gastrinoma. The location of the gastrinomas is typically the pancreas, but they may also occur in the stomach and in the duodenum.[74]

Patients with multiple endocrine neoplasia type I (MEN I) and ZES often become symptomatic in childhood, and more often at an earlier age than do those with sporadic ZES. More than 50% of gastrinomas are not visualized by preoperative imaging studies; however, these tests are recommended in the diagnostic evaluation of the patient who presents with the typical symptom complex.[75] Imaging studies that are recommended for localizing the gastrinoma are computed tomography (CT), magnetic resonance imaging (MRI), radionucleotide octreotide scanning, ultrasound, and selective arterial secretin testing.[75] Although it is technically difficult to perform reproducibly in children, the safe management of these patients is not accomplished unless acid output is measured.[76] Proton pump inhibitors, in doses of 40 to 80 mg/day or more, are commonly the drug of choice for acid suppression and symptom relief before surgical ablation and, often, vagotomy and gastric resection.[77] Typically, patients with ZES have fasting serum gastrin levels higher than 125 pg/mL and basal gastric acid hypersecretion greater than 15 mEq/hr.[75]

Similar serum gastrin concentrations but no family history or other associated syndrome findings (e.g., watery diarrhea, endocrine abnormalities) are seen with antral G cell hyperplasia and hyperfunction. Antral G cell hyperplasia is described as an increase in the total density or numbers of G cells in the correct anatomic location, and G cell hyperfunction is thought to result from a normal density of G cells in their normal location but hypersecretion of gastrin.[78] Ulcers in both the G cell disorders tend to be located in the stomach and upper duodenum, a somewhat different location from those ulcers associated with ZES.[79, 80] Treatment of these disorders usually is directed at maintenance of acid suppression with doses of antisecretory agents as high as for ZES patients. Often surgical management is required, including gastrectomy and vagotomy, because these disorders can be extremely refractory and frequently do not have well-circumscribed lesions that are resectable.[80]

### Other Disorders of Acid "Hypersecretion"

Hyperparathyroidism may be found associated with the MEN syndromes. In particular, hyperparathyroidism and the hypercalcemia associated with this condition are found in patients with ZES associated with MEN I.[75] The hypersecretion of acid is thought to be caused primarily by the gastrinomas associated with MEN I and ZES.[81] Isolated hyperparathyroidism has been associated with gastric ulcers believed to be caused by excess acid secretion in response to hypercalcemia. Chronic renal disease is also found to be associated with an increased frequency of gastric and duodenal ulcers. Although "systemic stress" and circulating catecholamine-induced hypergastrinemia have been postulated in these patients, the increased incidence of peptic ulcers in patients undergoing dialysis as a result of chronic renal failure and before kidney transplantation is not well understood.[82] Excessive circulating levels of histamine and subsequent stimulation of gastric parietal cells with acid production and mucosal ulceration of the stomach and pylorus have been reported in children with systemic mastocytosis.[83] Gastrointestinal symptoms such as vomiting and nausea, abdominal pain, and diarrhea are commonly associated with systemic mastocytosis in addition to gastric and upper duodenal ulcers. Acid secretion is high in a small number of these patients, and symptom relief is found after antisecretory therapy with $H_2$ receptor antagonists. However, although serum gastrin levels are low in these patients, consistent with histamine-induced gastric acid stimulation, plasma histamine levels and the density of mucosal mast cell load do not appear to correlate with the degree of ulceration.[84, 85]

## Crohn's Disease

Gastritis and mucosal ulceration is found in 25% to 40% of children and adults with Crohn's disease (see Chapter 32). One case report has documented the stomach and duodenum as the only location of lesions in a patient with Crohn's disease on initial presentation.[86–89] Multiple mucosal biopsies at the time of endoscopy aids in the diagnosis.[90, 91]

## Other Gastritides and Ulcer-Causing Disorders

### Eosinophilic Gastroenteritis

Commonly found characteristics in eosinophilic gastroenteritis (see Chapter 27) are an eosinophilic infiltration of the gastrointestinal mucosa with associated clinical findings based on the anatomic location of the infiltrating eosinophils, such as vomiting, nausea, abdominal pain, and gastric outlet obstruction (observed with upper gastrointestinal disease).[92–94] Upper endoscopy with gastric and duodenal biopsies should be performed in all cases of suspected eosinophilic gastroenteritis and has been universally helpful in the diagnosis. Mucosal erosions can be found, but frank mucosal ulceration is rare.

### Hypertrophic Gastritis (Ménétrier's Disease)

Gastropathies are discussed in detail in Chapter 19. This disease entity commonly manifests with symptoms of upper gastrointestinal tract obstruction (e.g., vomiting and nausea) and severe protein losses. It is a rare cause of protein-losing enteropathy in infants[95] and children.[96, 97] Infectious causes for this disease have been described; in particular, there is compelling evidence for a causal link between the development of hypertrophic gastritis and cytomegalovirus (CMV) infection in both children and adults.[97–100]

More controversial is the association with *H. pylori* and Ménétrier's disease, which is based on the "disappearance" of the protein-losing gastropathy after *H. pylori* eradication.[101] Some authors contend that "classic" Ménétrier's disease is a true form of gastropathy and that there is another distinct entity with similar presenting symptoms that can be differentiated on histologic evaluation of gastric biopsies—namely, hypertrophic lymphocytic gastritis.[102]

### Autoimmune Gastritis and Varioliform Gastritis

Two additional rare disorders of childhood gastritis are autoimmune gastritis, often associated with pernicious anemia, and varioliform or lymphocytic gastritis, sometimes referred to as erosive gastritis. The association of autoimmune gastritis with intrinsic factor antibodies, manifestations of cobalamin malabsorption (pernicious anemia), and achlorhydria are rare in children but have been described in adults.[103, 104] Autoimmune gastritis, the presence of systemic autoantibodies against antral gastrin-producing cells or parietal cells, is rarely associated with mucosal ulceration and more frequently with atrophic gastritis. In addition, a decreased gastric acidity state in autoimmune gastritis is thought to be caused in part by antibodies directed against the proton pump of the parietal cell apical membrane.[105, 106] It is still controversial as to whether there is an increased prevalence of *H. pylori* in patients with atrophic gastritis. A study in Japan demonstrated that although the association with atrophic gastritis is high, the association of *H. pylori* with atrophic gastritis and pernicious anemia is quite low.[107] A similar finding of decreased *H. pylori* infection prevalence in adults having varioliform gastritis has also been reported.[108] Lymphocytic gastritis or varioliform gastritis is extremely rare in childhood, more common in adult males, and associated with a diffuse infiltration of the gastric epithelium by small lymphocytes.[109–111]

### Stress-Related Gastritis and Ulcers

The overall prevalence of stress-related gastritis and ulcers in children is not known. However, stress-related gastric mucosal inflammation and ulceration is one of the more commonly reported sequelae among critically ill hospitalized patients.[11, 112, 113] In adults it is associated with significant morbidity and mortality.[114] In infants, shock resulting from prenatal asphyxia, traumatic delivery, or overwhelming sepsis causes stress-related gastric and/or duodenal ulcers. In older children, motor vehicle trauma or other related traumatic injuries and shock are associated with stress-related ulcers. Gastroduodenal inflammation, as determined by histology, accompanied by multiple erosions of the gastric and duodenal mucosa seen at endoscopy, is common in the patient with stress-related peptic ulceration.[115] Major surgical procedures, severe head and body trauma, burns, and overwhelming sepsis are often implicated as causes of gastroduodenal ulceration.[112, 116] Most patients with severe burns or multiple-organ injuries from trauma-related incidents have acute mucosal inflammation in the stomach and duodenum and, depending on the severity of the injury or burn, frank ulcers in multiple areas of the upper gastrointestinal tract.[11, 117, 118]

In adults, gastric erosions or ulcers are observed in most patients with severe systemic stress, but up to 75% of these patients are asymptomatic. In one large study of critically ill adult patients, only mechanical ventilation and pre-existing coagulopathy were clearly demonstrated to be independent risk factors for overt bleeding from the gastrointestinal tract and subsequent hemodynamic compromise.[112] Pediatric studies performed to date have been limited.[119–122]

Animal studies have suggested that epithelial damage to the gastroduodenal mucosa, in association with microcirculatory changes and nitric oxide–induced injury as well as vagal hyperactivity causing excessive gastric acid production, results in stress-related ulcers due to systemic stress.[123, 124] Further studies have described peptides produced in the central nervous system as the result of gastric hyperacidity caused by increased stomach parietal cell acid secretion and pepsin secretion from body cells.

Prophylaxis with some form of acid-blocking agent is of value in the patient at risk for stress-induced gastroduodenal inflammation and ulceration.[113, 116, 125] A cytoprotective, acid-buffering agent such as sucralfate was better than placebo in decreasing the incidence of gastric erosions in critically ill patients.[126] The administration of an $H_2$ receptor antagonist (e.g., ranitidine) or proton-pump inhibitor (e.g., omeprazole) has also been suggested for critically ill patients who are at risk for stress ulcers.[115, 127]

## DRUG-RELATED GASTRITIS AND ULCERS

Numerous pharmacologic agents are noxious to the gastroduodenal mucosa and cause mucosal inflammation and ulceration. Infants with meconium aspiration syndrome who develop persistent fetal circulation or persistent pulmonary hypertension are often given medications that decrease pulmonary vascular resistance (e.g., tolazoline [Priscoline]).[128, 129] These infants have been shown to be at increased risk for the development of duodenal ulcers, in part because of increased gastrin and pepsin release as a result of mast cell degranulation and histamine stimulation. These infants are critically ill, usually are receiving ventilatory assistance, and frequently have coagulopathies, all risk factors for significant gastric or duodenal ulceration in adult studies.[112]

### Nonsteroidal Anti-inflammatory Agents and Aspirin

There is still a relative paucity of information on gastroduodenal injury induced by nonsteroidal anti-inflammatory agents (NSAIDs) in children, and even less on aspirin-induced injury. However, both NSAIDs and aspirin result in significant gastroduodenal injury, patient morbidity, and health care cost.[130, 131] Aspirin, even at low doses (75–325 mg/day) used for antiplatelet therapy in cardiovascular disorders, has been shown to induce either bleeding ulcers or gastric erosions.[132] Many studies have shown that in adult patients taking 1 g or more of aspirin per day the risk for gastric ulcer is 10 to 20 times higher than in controls.[133, 134]

One analysis demonstrated that NSAIDs are associated with a strong dose-response effect on the gastroduodenal mucosa with resultant injury, inflammation, and often erosions and ulceration.[135] The same study demonstrated that corticosteroid administration alone produced a risk for ulcer development and that corticosteroids were synergistic in the mucosal injury observed when given concurrently with NSAIDs.[135] Although there was an early suggestion that tolerance to NSAIDs might develop,[136–138] there are probably no "safe" NSAIDs.

There is some controversy about the extent of NSAID-induced gastroduodenal injury in children. One study demonstrated that only 5 of 702 pediatric patients had documented gastropathy determined by symptoms, barium swallow, or endoscopy. However, because of the criteria used to determine adverse effects of NSAIDs, this study may have underestimated the extent of the problem; many NSAID-induced gastroduodenal ulcers are silent,[139] and only a fraction of the patient cohort had endoscopy. In contrast, another study[140] showed that abdominal pain was reported in 27.9% of 344 pediatric arthritic patients taking some form of NSAIDs. A relative risk for gastroduodenal injury of 4.8 for patients who were taking NSAIDs, compared with those who were not, was seen. Based on adult studies,[141] there is concern that as pediatric use of NSAIDs as antipyretics and for other indications (e.g., athletic injury) increases, the prevalence of gastric and duodenal mucosal injury will also increase.

NSAIDs and aspirin mediate injury to the gastric and duodenal mucosa via a number of pathophysiologic mechanisms. Both compounds produce local injury directly. Aspirin decreases gastric epithelial cell apical surface pH and impairs vital cell functions.[142–143] Aspirin also decreases bicarbonate secretion. NSAIDs induce gastroduodenal injury by several mechanisms, including increased platelet-activating factor, platelet dysfunction, inhibition of prostaglandin synthesis, increased oxygen free radicals, enhanced mast cell histamine release, and increased mucosal capillary damage. Both drugs cause microvascular damage and delayed epithelial healing. In one large, multicenter, adult study, NSAID intake and aspirin use were two of the most commonly identified risk factors for ulcer bleeding.[144]

The distinction between NSAID injury and other causes of inflammation may be difficult.[145, 146] Foveolar hyperplasia, although considered a characteristic of NSAID injury, may still be absent more than 50% of the time.[145]

Misoprostol and its analogues may have benefit in the control of NSAID-induced gastropathy.[147–149] Diarrhea has been a complication of this therapy. One pediatric study from Canada showed, in a small cohort of arthritic children, that misoprostol (9.8 ± 2.5 μg/kg/day) given during NSAID therapy reduced symptoms in 82% of the patients with gastrointestinal complaints, whereas 18% had recurrence of symptoms after initial improvement.[150] However, this study was limited in that there were no controls and it was retrospective and based on symptomatology only.

## *HELICOBACTER PYLORI*

### Epidemiology

The epidemiology of *H. pylori* infection in humans is interesting, particularly in regard to gastroduodenal disease associated with gastric colonization by the organism.[32, 151] However, despite many studies of the prevalence of *H. pylori* infection, our understanding of the incidence of this infection is lacking.[1, 37] Most epidemiologic studies of *H. pylori* infection have been performed in adults, who probably were infected for decades before diagnosis.[152] Acute *H. pylori* infection is not known to be present with specific diagnostic symptoms.

Data on the incidence of *H. pylori* infection in children are limited.[153–155] The incidence of *H. pylori* infection in industrialized countries has been estimated to be about 0.5%

of the susceptible population per year. This incidence is thought to be decreasing, so that infected adults are more likely to have been infected in childhood.[156, 157] The incidence of *H. pylori* infection continues to be high in developing countries, with estimates of 3% and 10% per year. Throughout the world, the incidence of *H. pylori* infection appears to be higher in children than in adults.[37]

The route of transmission of *H. pylori* is postulated to be fecal-oral or oral-oral.[158, 159] In several studies, *H. pylori* DNA was identified in the dental plaque and saliva of adults and children by polymerase chain reaction (PCR) techniques.[160–162] The mouth may be a reservoir for this infection, or it may be an initial site of colonization before seeding of the stomach and colonization of the gastric epithelia. The fecal-oral route of transmission has been definitively characterized in ferrets.[163] Gastric colonization of ferret stomachs by *Helicobacter mustelae* results in similar pathology as in human infection with *H. pylori.*[164] Ferrets get chronic gastritis, duodenal and gastric ulcers, and gastric carcinoma as the end result of long-term *H. mustelae* infection.[165–167]

Humans appear to be the primary natural reservoir of *H. pylori* infection, though others exist, including water[168] and domestic cats.[169, 170] Water, as an environmental source of *H. pylori* infection, was first described in a study of Peruvian infants; $^{13}$C-labeled breath testing was used as the measure of infection, and an epidemiologic association was made between contaminated water and the high prevalence of this infection. The specific viability of this organism in water has not been definitively described, but the methodologies used to identify organisms in water (immunomagnetic beads, fluorescent microscopy, PCR) and the techniques of epidemiologic association have been well done.[171] Domestic cats have been shown to harbor *H. pylori,*[167, 170] although the organism was not found in stray cats.[172] Finally, investigations from two different groups have led to contradicting theories regarding the housefly as a potential vector for *H. pylori* transmission.[173, 174]

*H. pylori* primarily infects children, and the risk factors that have been described include familial overcrowding, endemic country of origin, poor socioeconomic circumstances, and certain ethnicities. In particular, in the United States, the prevalence rates among African-Americans and Hispanics are similar to those of people residing in developing countries.[153] Little is known, however, about the phenotype and genotype of *H. pylori* strains infecting children and, in particular, the epidemiology of infecting pediatric *H. pylori* strains.

In addition to chronic superficial gastritis, *H. pylori* has been associated with chronic active gastritis and with primary duodenal ulcers in more than 90% of infected adults and children.[30, 32, 175–177] It is estimated that the lifetime risk for development of peptic ulcer disease among *H. pylori*-infected persons is higher than 10%.[37] The recurrence rate of duodenal ulcers is markedly reduced after successful treatment of *H. pylori* infection.[178, 179] *H. pylori* infection is less commonly associated with gastric ulcers, and its associations with Barrett's esophagus and with nonulcer dyspepsia are still controversial.[180–182] Of particular interest is the association of *H. pylori* infection, particularly if acquired in early childhood, with gastric cancer.[40] Multiple studies have demonstrated that concurrent or previous *H. pylori* infection is associated with a 2.7- to 12-fold increased risk for development of gastric cancer.[177, 183] In regions of the world with high rates of gastric cancer, the prevalence of *H. pylori* infection is also high, and infection tends to be acquired early in life. In addition to the link between *H. pylori* infection and gastric cancer, this organism is also thought to play a role in the development of low-grade B cell lymphomas of the gastric mucosa-associated lymphoid tissue type (MALT)[184] (see Chapter 45).

## Pathogenesis

A proposed schematic of the natural history of *H. pylori* infection is depicted in Figure 18–1. However, the interaction between bacterial virulence properties and the host immune response that results in mucosal disease is still not clearly characterized. Many bacterial virulence factors have been described for *H. pylori.*[185] Specifically, urease (*ure*A, *ure*B, and *ure*C genes) is produced in large quantities by all *H. pylori* isolates and also by the other gastric *Helicobacter* species identified.[186] This organism is highly motile and uses its flagella (*fla*A, *fla*B genes) to navigate through the thick, viscous gastric mucus to reach the apical surface of the gastric epithelial cells, where it adheres, replicates, and occupies its biologic niche.[187] More recently, attention has been given to the vacuolating cytotoxin produced by at least half of *H. pylori* strains isolated. This cytotoxin, first described in the late 1980s, produces vacuoles in the cytoplasm of eukaryotic cells in vitro.[188, 189] The gene (*vac*A) for this vacuolating cytotoxin, an 87-kd protein, has at least two alleles and is variably expressed among *H. pylori* isolates.[190] In addition to cytotoxin activity, *H. pylori* strains also differ in regard to a high-molecular-weight protein, designated CagA, which ranges from 105 to 140 kd.[191] About 60% of *H. pylori* isolates produce this protein, and its presence is thought to correlate strongly with expression of the vacuolating cytotoxin. The *cag*A gene is absent from those strains lacking the CagA protein product. The presence or absence of the cytotoxin has prompted some researchers to classify *H. pylori* strains into type I (cytotoxin-positive) and type II (cytotoxin-negative) strains.[192] Type I strains have been shown to be associated with more severe gastric or duodenal disease than type II strains. A major part of the *H. pylori* genome has been found to confer pathogenicity to the organism; this *pathogenicity island,* as it is now called, may contain a number of genes that confer virulence to the particular organism in a susceptible host.[193–195]

A vigorous local and systemic host immune response is observed after gastric colonization by *H. pylori.*[196] A monocyte and macrophage response can be seen in infected gastric mucosa, with both polymorphonuclear cells and plasma cells also present in the inflammatory infiltrate.[197, 198] It is still not clear whether T cells play a major role in the inflammation associated with *H. pylori* infection, but increased levels of interleukin-1 (IL-1), IL-2, IL-6, IL-8, and tumor necrosis factor-α, are detectable in the gastric epithelium of infected persons.[199] Circulating immunoglobulin G (IgG) antibodies are easily detectable in *H. pylori*-infected individuals, and they form the basis of many of the diagnostic assays that are used.[200]

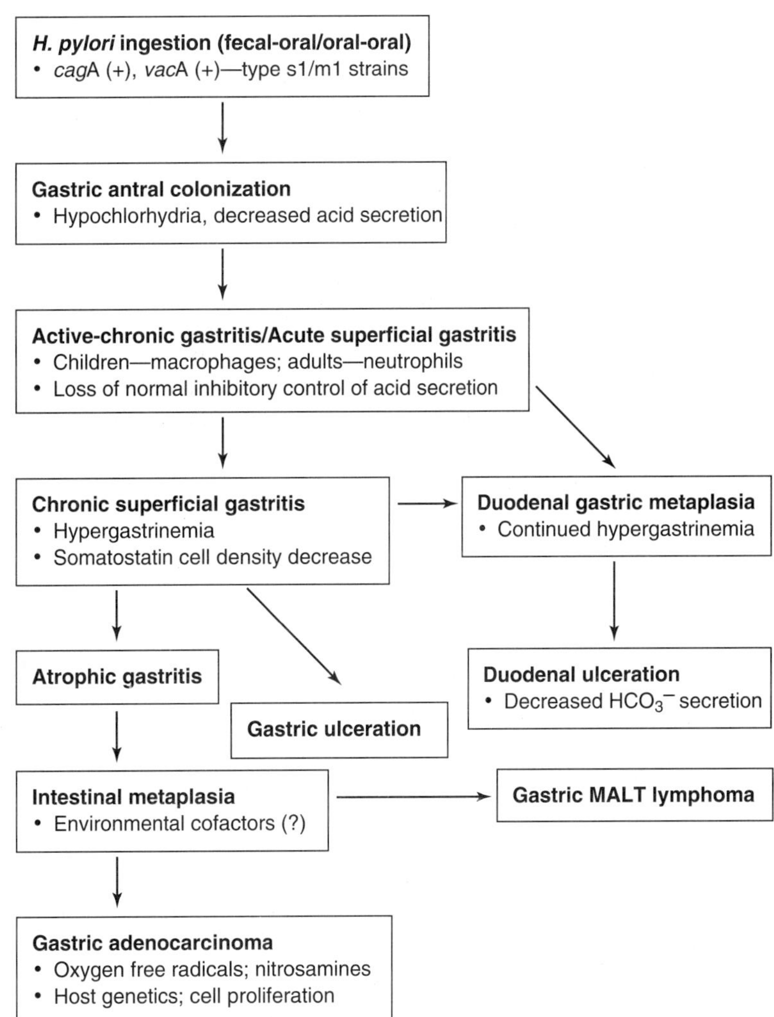


**FIGURE 18–1.** Proposed schematic of *H. pylori* infection and resultant gastroduodenal disease.

## Microbiology

Bacteria have been described as using one or more of three basic mechanisms,[105] called virulence determinants, to cause host disease.[201] These mechanisms are adhesion, invasion, and toxin elaboration. *H. pylori* is a gram-negative organism that resides under microaerobic conditions (approximately 80% $N_2$, 10% $CO_2$, 5% $H_2$, and 5% $O_2$), in a neutral microenvironment away from the acidic gastric milieu, in the overlying mucus and adherent to the gastric epithelial cells primarily in the gastric antrum.[202, 203] Two primary morphologic shapes, bacillary and coccoid, have been described for this organism.[204] The biologic relevance of each form is not clearly understood, although it is believed that the bacillary form is the more virulent.

This organism is highly motile, with multiple unipolar flagella, and the genetic basis for this virulence determinant has been well characterized.[205] Biochemically, *H. pylori* produces catalase, oxidase, and urease enzymes. The urease enzyme allows the bacterium to metabolize the urea that is present in the gastric mucus to create the neutral microenvironment in which it lives and replicates. It is the urease that biochemically separates *H. pylori* from the intestinal campylobacters.[206, 207] The urease enzyme has received much attention and provides a useful, rapid diagnostic tool both in the endoscopy suite and for noninvasive $^{13}C$- or $^{14}C$-labeled breath testing.[208, 209] The urease enzyme is the specific virulence determinant on which most of the attention has been focused in the development of vaccine constructs against *H. pylori* infection.[210]

At least 11 other species of *Helicobacter* have been identified.[211] *Helicobacter fennellieae* and *Helicobacter cinaedi* are both human pathogens that reside in the lower gastrointestinal tract and cause diarrheal disease in immunocompromised patients. Most of the other *Helicobacter* species are animal pathogens. Much attention has been given to *Helicobacter felis,* an organism that infects domestic and wild cats and causes chronic gastritis in the feline stomach.[212] Researchers have been using *H. felis* in a mouse model of chronic and acute gastritis in the development of vaccine against gastric *Helicobacter* infection.[213] Another helicobacter of great interest is *Helicobacter hepaticus,* which infects certain strains of mice and has satisfied Koch's postulates as a causative agent of hepatocellular carcinoma in these murine strains.[214] *Gastrospirillum hominis,* or *H. helmannii,* has been observed by histologic staining of gastric biopsies obtained at upper endoscopy on patients with chronic-active gastritis.[211] However, primary culture of these organisms has not been successfully performed, and the clinical relevance of these gastric spirochetes remains unclear.

## Methods for Detection

The gold standard for the diagnosis of active *H. pylori* infection is esophagogastroduodenoscopy with gastric biopsies. However, there are numerous, fairly accurate detection assays that have become commercialized and available for clinical use. Invasive techniques are based on endoscopy and multiple biopsies for the detection of *H. pylori.* Histologic demonstration of *H. pylori* or its identification by microbiologic means (i.e., culture) constitutes direct evidence of the presence of this microorganism. Most noninvasive techniques rely on detection of a characteristic of *H. pylori* (e.g., the ability to hydrolyze urea) or the response of the immune system to its presence (i.e., specific antibodies).

### *Invasive Techniques*

**HISTOLOGIC IDENTIFICATION.** The characteristic histologic appearance of *H. pylori* is a $3.0 \times 0.5$ μm spiral rod located adjacent to the gastric epithelium. Although the Steiner stain or a modified silver stain (Warthin-Starry) is considered the best method for the identification of *H. pylori* organisms (Fig. 18–2), a trained pathologist can readily see the curved, spiral organisms on a Giemsa stain of the gastric biopsy sections (Fig. 18–3).

In addition to the stain used, a second factor that influences the histologic detection of *H. pylori* is the uneven distribution of the organism throughout the gastric mucosa. A considerable variation in the numbers of bacteria can be observed in biopsy specimens from a single source, and in 10% of all positive cases there are sections completely free of organisms.[215, 216] Two biopsies taken from within 2 to 5 cm of the pylorus are generally considered to be sufficient for diagnosis.[217]

Because histologic gastritis may be present in the absence of macroscopic mucosal abnormalities, this examination permits a better correlation between the presence of *H. pylori* and its pathologic result.[218, 219] The observation of histologic chronic (active) gastritis without evidence of *H. pylori* should prompt a careful re-examination of the sections to exclude the bacterium. Histologic examination of gastric biopsies can provide important information about the presence of *H. pylori* and the condition of the mucosa.

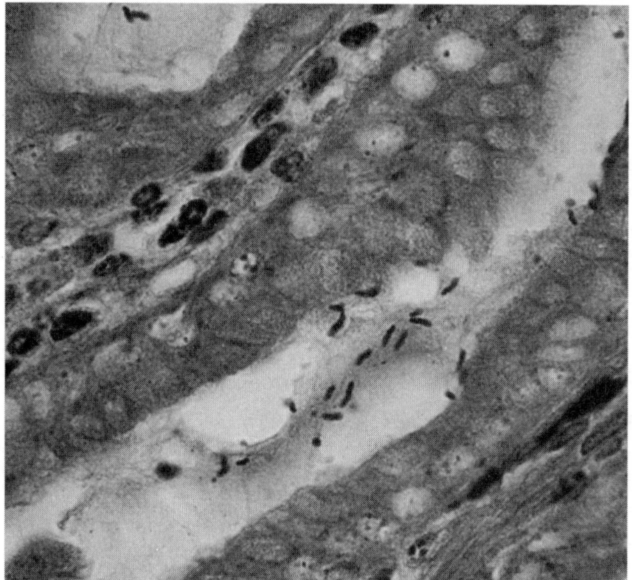

**FIGURE 18–2.** Warthin-Starry stain of *H. pylori.* Organisms can be seen both in the mucous layer overlying the gastric epithelium and adherent to the apical epithelial cell surface.

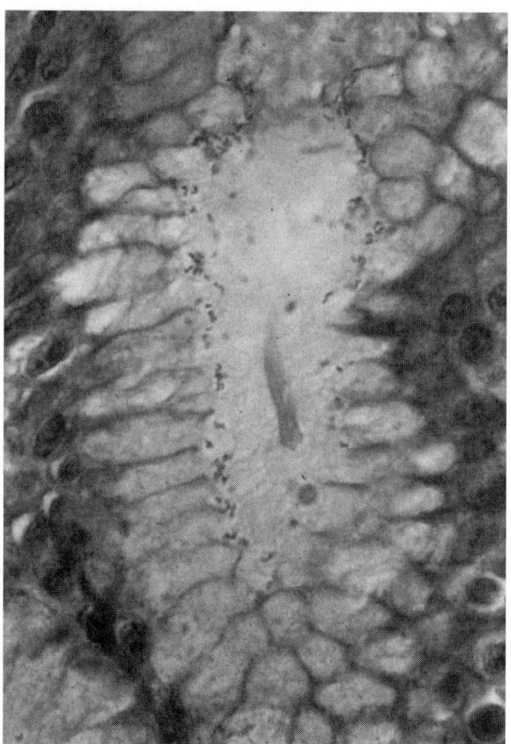

**FIGURE 18–3.** Giemsa stain of *H. pylori.*

**CULTURE.** *H. pylori* is obligately microaerophilic. The problem of uneven distribution of the organism may contribute to falsely negative cultures. However, this seems not to be an important problem, since even a single bacterium can give rise to a positive culture. Other factors that have been implicated in unsuccessful culturing of *H. pylori* include recent antibiotic use, ingestion of topical anesthetic or simethicone during endoscopy, and contamination of the biopsy forceps with other organisms or glutaraldehyde. An important application for culture is the determination of the antibiotic susceptibility profile of treatment-resistant organisms.[220]

An important characteristic of *H. pylori* that forms the basis of several diagnostic tests is the ability of the organism to produce urease in a 1,000-fold higher concentration than any other known bacterium that may inhabit the human stomach.[221, 222] Urease catalyzes the degradation of urea to ammonia and bicarbonate (Fig. 18–4). This reaction causes an increase in the pH of the surrounding medium, which can be detected with a pH indicator as a color change.[223] A number of tests have been developed, ranging from simple solutions of urea, water, and phenol to the various commercially produced tests, of which the CLO test (Delta West Ltd., Bentley, Western Australia) is the most frequently used. Positive results are obtained with good sensitivity and specificity within a few hours after addition of the biopsy specimen to the medium. Urease tests are also dependent on the

$$\begin{matrix} NH_2 \\ \diagdown \\ {}^{*}C = O + 2\,H_2O + H^+ \xrightarrow{\text{urease}} 2\,NH_3 + 2\,{}^{*}CO_2 \uparrow + 2\,H_2O \\ \diagup \\ NH_2 \end{matrix}$$

**FIGURE 18–4.** Principle of the urea breath test. The patient ingests a certain quantity of labeled urea. Urease produced by *H. pylori* transforms urea into ammonia and labeled* $CO_2$. The $CO_2$ is transported to the lungs and exhaled.

density of the bacteria and therefore are most sensitive when performed on antral tissue.

### Noninvasive Techniques

The most promising noninvasive method is based on urease enzyme production by *H. pylori* organisms and involves the administration of a $^{13}C$- or $^{14}C$-labeled urea meal, followed by testing of expired breath samples over a 2-hour period. In *H. pylori*-colonized patients, the urea is metabolized to ammonia and labeled bicarbonate, and the latter is carried to the lungs and excreted in the expired breath as labeled carbon dioxide (see Fig. 18–4). The labeled carbon excreted can then be quantified. This test is semiquantitative in that it measures the approximate bacterial load in the entire stomach, and of all the noninvasive tests it may be the best predictor of treatment success. The amount of labeled carbon dioxide in single, pooled, or serial breath samples is directly related to the extent of urea hydrolysis and the presence or absence of *H. pylori.* The original description of this technique in humans used the stable, naturally occurring isotope, $^{13}C$.[209] Although $^{13}C$ has the advantage of being nonradioactive, its measurement requires an expensive and complicated gas isotope ratio mass spectrometer. Because this equipment is not widely available, an adaptation of this method, using $^{14}C$, has been devised.[224–226] $^{14}C$ can easily be quantified with the use of a scintillation counter. It has been estimated that a single upper gastrointestinal series produces more bone marrow exposure than a hundred $^{14}C$-urea breath tests.[227] Although this noninvasive technique has the disadvantage of not allowing actual culture of the organism, the urea breath test detects *H. pylori* over a much greater surface area of the stomach.

**SEROLOGY.** Soon after the isolation of *H. pylori,* it became clear that virtually all infected subjects develop a local and a systemic immune response against this organism.[228, 229] Several serologic techniques have been used to determine the antibody response to *H. pylori,* including hemagglutination, bacterial agglutination, complement fixation, indirect immunofluorescence, immunoblotting, and enzyme-linked immunosorbent assays (ELISA).[200] In general, ELISA has been found to be more sensitive in detecting *H. pylori* antibodies than bacterial agglutination or complement fixation.[230] Commercially available serologic assays, primarily based on IgG antibody levels against *H. pylori* antigens, have reasonable accuracy in detecting the presence of *H. pylori* infection.[200] However, caution must be used when relying on the results of these assays for patient management, particularly when deciding on therapy. The assays may be limited in their accuracy if they are used in populations different from those in which they were developed (e.g., in a developing country instead of the United States). In addition, most commercially available assays have been standardized and validated (against esophagogastroduodenoscopy with biopsy) in adult populations, and their cutoff values may be different from what might be appropriate for use in children. It has been demonstrated that results obtained from serologic tests for the detection of *H. pylori* in adults cannot necessarily be extrapolated to the pediatric age group.[231, 232] Although the reason for this discrepancy is not yet fully understood, it has been suggested that a difference in *H. pylori* antigen recognition may be responsible for the decreased sensitivity and specificity in children. Conversely, because of the variable immune response in children, a significant difference in cutoff values between the adult and pediatric populations may be the causative factor.[233, 234] Finally, the IgG response to *H. pylori* infection persists for at least 3 months and even longer than 1 year in the face of successful antimicrobial treatment of the infection; therefore, the use of serology for post-treatment monitoring may be limited.

**POLYMERASE CHAIN REACTION.** PCR techniques in capable hands are exquisitely sensitive but can be fraught with false-positives, such as from contaminated forceps or endoscopy equipment. This technique has been able to detect *H. pylori* in biopsy specimens,[235, 236] gastric juice and saliva,[237] dental plaque,[235, 238] and feces.[239] However, because of the relatively high cost and time consumption of PCR as a diagnostic tool for the detection of *H. pylori,* this technique does not yet belong among the routine diagnostic possibilities in clinical practice.

## *H. PYLORI*-ASSOCIATED GASTRODUODENAL DISEASE IN CHILDREN

Soon after Warren and Marshall[240] reported an association between the presence of *H. pylori* in the gastric mucosa and antral gastritis in adults, this association was also noted in children.[26] Studies in adults established the presence of the organism in almost all cases of chronic gastritis.[241] However, because gastritis is a common finding in adults, it was originally suggested that *H. pylori* was colonizing inflamed tissue rather than causing the inflammation.[242] The significantly less frequent finding of gastritis in children allowed for investigation of whether *H. pylori* was a cause for gastritis or an opportunistic colonizer of inflamed tissue.[26] Although the bacteria are not commonly found on the gastric mucosa of children with secondary causes of gastritis (e.g., eosinophilic gastroenteritis, Crohn's disease),[28] *H. pylori* was present in most children with gastritis.[26] This observation was a strong factor in the implication of *H. pylori* as a cause of chronic antral gastritis.

In 1986, Hill and associates[243] reported that four children with chronic gastritis were infected with *H. pylori.* Later that year, Cadranel and colleagues[244] found the organism to be present in a group of eight patients with chronic gastritis. Shortly thereafter, Drumm and coworkers[26] observed the bacteria in 70% of their 67 pediatric patients with chronic active gastritis. Similar observations were made by Mahony and colleagues[245] in 38 pediatric patients and by Czinn and coworkers[31] in 25 children. Numerous additional studies confirmed that *H. pylori* colonization of the gastric mucosa is virtually always associated with chronic gastritis in children.[28, 246, 247] Despite the well-known predominance of gastrointestinal pathology in males, *H. pylori*-associated gastritis has been shown to be equally as common in boys as in girls.[248] Finally, eradication of *H. pylori* from the gastric mucosa is associated with healing of the antral gastritis, another finding in favor of *H. pylori* as the cause of primary gastritis in children.[247]

*H. pylori*-associated gastritis in children is often not apparent at endoscopy.[26, 233] In a prospective study, the endoscopic findings were normal in 8 of 10 children who had histologic antral gastritis. A nodularity of the antral mucosa has also been described to occur in association with *H. pylori* gastritis in children (Figs. 18–5 and 18–6).[249] This finding has rarely been observed in adults.[222, 250]

## Peptic Ulcer Disease in Children

The prevalence of peptic ulcer disease in childhood is extremely low. Large pediatric endoscopy centers report an incidence of 5 to 7 children with peptic ulcer disease per year.[4] Almost all peptic ulcers in children are located in the duodenum; gastric ulcers are extremely rare in children.[230] A strong correlation has been demonstrated between duodenal ulceration and *H. pylori* gastritis in children.[28] In fact, *H. pylori* gastritis has been found in 90% to 100% of pediatric patients with duodenal ulcer disease.[246] As in adults,[183] duodenal ulcerations in the absence of *H. pylori* are extremely rare in childhood, and duodenal ulcer disease in children does not relapse if *H. pylori* is cleared from the gastric mucosa.[247, 251] Yeung and colleagues[247] treated 23 children with *H. pylori* gastritis associated with duodenal ulcer disease, using either cimetidine alone or a combination of cimetidine and amoxicillin. Although only a small portion of the children in this study remained uninfected, when the gastric mucosa did remain clear of *H. pylori* (combination therapy) no recurrence of duodenal ulcer disease was detected 6 months after the end of treatment. In contrast, 50% of patients whose ulcers were originally healed but who remained colonized with *H. pylori* (cimetidine-only therapy) had a recurrence of their ulcers by 6 months.

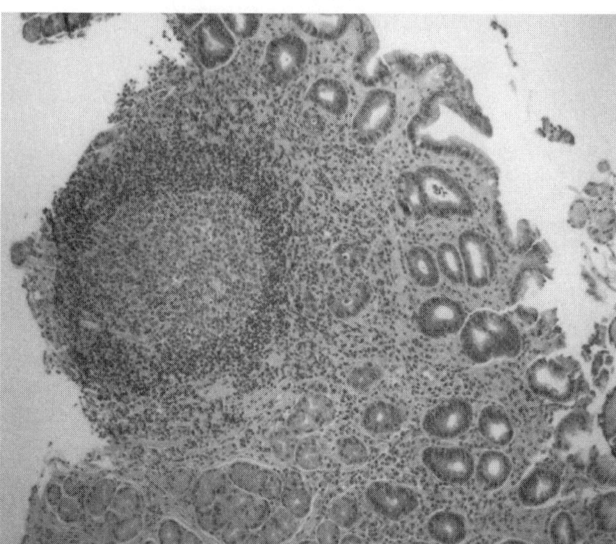

**FIGURE 18–6.** Gastric antral biopsy obtained from a 13-year-old girl with endoscopic pyloric channel ulcers, demonstrating large lymphoid follicle with lamina propria inflammation, predominant lymphocytes, macrophages, plasma cells, few to no polymorphonuclear cells, and denudement of the superficial epithelium (hematoxylin and eosin stain; original magnification ×60).

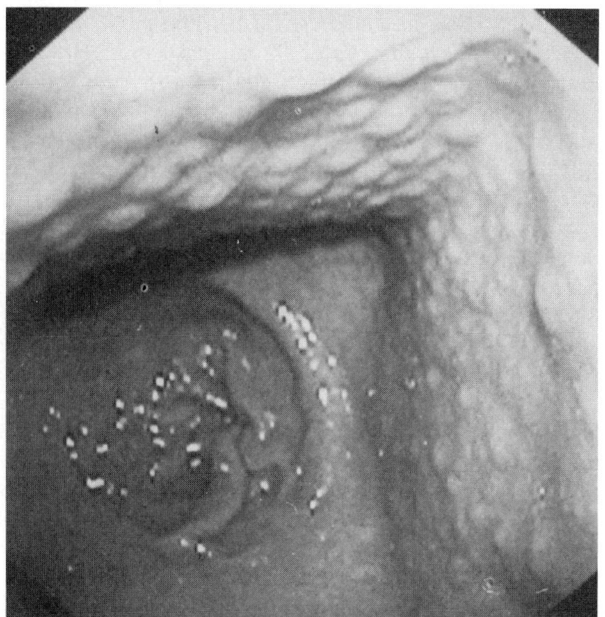

**FIGURE 18–5.** *H. pylori*–associated nodular gastritis observed at the time of endoscopy. Note the large, readily apparent lymphoid nodules.

## Gastric Cancer

Support for the role of *H. pylori* in gastric cancer comes from three sources: studies paralleling the epidemiologic features of cancer with those of *H. pylori* infection,[252, 253] cross-sectional studies of *H. pylori* infection in patients with cancer,[254] and prospective studies of *H. pylori* infections.[40, 255] Gastric cancer appears to be more common in areas of poverty, afflicting people in developing nations and those in the lower socioeconomic classes of the industrialized world.[256] In many countries of Latin America and Asia, gastric cancer remains the most common malignancy among men and the second most common among women.[257, 258] Incidence rates are as high as 80 per 100,000 population in regions of Colombia and Japan. By contrast, gastric cancer afflicts fewer than 10 per 100,000 people per year in the United States and western Europe.[259] Within low-risk countries, there are ethnic groups with increased risk. In the United States, for example, the prevalence of gastric cancer among blacks, Asians, and Hispanics is almost double that among whites.[259]

Clues to the decline in gastric cancer incidence derive from studies of people who moved from regions of high gastric cancer risk to regions of low risk. People who moved from Japan, a high-risk country, to regions of lower risk in the United States only moderately decreased their cancer risk, even if they immigrated at a young age.[260] Second-generation immigrants, however, adopted a gastric cancer risk much closer to that of their new country. Similar results have been found among European immigrants to Australia,[261] and Puerto Rican migrants to New York.[262] From these studies it was concluded that environmental factors initiate malignant transformation in the stomach.

*H. pylori* infection is a marker of increased risk of gastric adenocarcinoma. Definite proof of cause, however, can be accomplished only when controlled trials demonstrate that elimination or prevention of infection prevents malignancy. Short-term studies documenting reversal of *preneoplastic* conditions with anti-*H. pylori* therapy lend support to the association of *H. pylori* and cancer. It is generally believed that intestinal metaplasia, and in particular dysplasia, are by nature irreversible.[263, 264]

## Gastric Lymphomas

Unlike the intestine, the stomach is not functionally a lymphoid organ.[265] In infancy and early childhood, the stomach lacks a significant number of immunocompetent lymphocytes and plasma cells. With age, however, chronic inflammation can develop, leading lymphocytes to accumulate in the submucosa and gradually to increase their depth of penetration. *H. pylori* infection causes almost all cases of chronic gastritis.[266] With the eradication of this microorganism, chronic inflammation decreases and the density of submucosal lymphocytes dramatically declines.[267] Because most gastric lymphomas arise in areas of chronic inflammation,[268] it seems likely that prior *H. pylori* infection and gastric lymphomas are linked.

Primary non-Hodgkin's lymphoma of the stomach is an uncommon cancer, accounting for only 10% of lymphomas and 3% of gastric neoplasms.[269] However, gastric non-Hodgkin's lymphoma is the most common extranodal form of this lymphoma, accounting for 20% of primary extranodal disease.[270] Immunologic studies have shown these tumors to be of B cell lineage.[271] Evidence suggests that infection with *H. pylori* may increase the risk of gastric non-Hodgkin's lymphoma.[254, 268, 272–276]

Low-grade B cell lymphomas that arise in the stomach, lung, salivary gland, and thyroid recapitulate the structural features of MALT, as typified in Peyer's patches.[277] These lymphomas, together with the high-grade lesions that may evolve from them,[278] are collectively known as MALT lymphomas.[277] MALT lymphomas were first described in the early 1980s, when Isaacson and Wright[279] noted that the histology of certain low-grade B cell gastrointestinal lymphomas was unlike that of comparable low-grade nodal lymphomas but was similar to that of MALT. However, MALT is not present in the normal stomach, nor in other sites in which MALT lymphomas arise.

In the stomach, lymphoid tissue is acquired as a result of colonization of the gastric mucosa by *H. pylori*.[280] Wotherspoon and colleagues[276] demonstrated that this *H. pylori*-associated lymphoid tissue is of MALT type. They subsequently suggested that MALT acquired in response to *H. pylori* infection provides the background on which other, unidentified factors act, and that this leads to the development of lymphoma in a small proportion of cases. Hussell and colleagues[281] demonstrated that cellular proliferation of low-grade B cell gastric MALT lymphomas in reaction to *H. pylori* is dependent on *H. pylori*-specific T cells and their products, rather than the bacteria themselves.

The specific colonization of lymphoid follicle centers by neoplastic cells[282] and the binding of specific antibodies[283] suggest that MALT tumors are immunologically responsive. Given the close association between gastric MALT lymphoma and *H. pylori,* it is possible that this organism evokes the immunologic response and that eradication of *H. pylori* might inhibit the tumor. Several studies have suggested that anti-*H. pylori* therapy may eradicate MALT lymphoma in some cases.[284, 285]

Our group recently described the case of a 14-year-old girl presenting with severe cachexia, abdominal pain, and nausea who was diagnosed with *H. pylori* chronic-active gastritis and associated gastric lymphoproliferative disease of the low-grade MALT type (Fig. 18–7).[286] Eradication of the infection was followed by complete resolution of her lymphoproliferative disorder without the use of any adjuvant chemotherapy or surgery, and with no relapse after a 7-year follow-up.

## Treatment of *H. pylori* Infection and Vaccine Development

The recurrence of duodenal ulcers can be dramatically reduced and prevented by a single course of antimicrobial therapy directed at the eradication of *H. pylori* organisms infecting the gastric mucosa. Because of the economic impact of peptic ulcer disease (i.e., treatment costs, morbidity and mortality) as well as the prevalence of *H. pylori* worldwide, a Consensus Development Conference of the National Institutes of Health (NIH) recommended that all patients with ulcers who are also infected by *H. pylori* receive antimicrobial therapy. There is a notable lack of consensus on

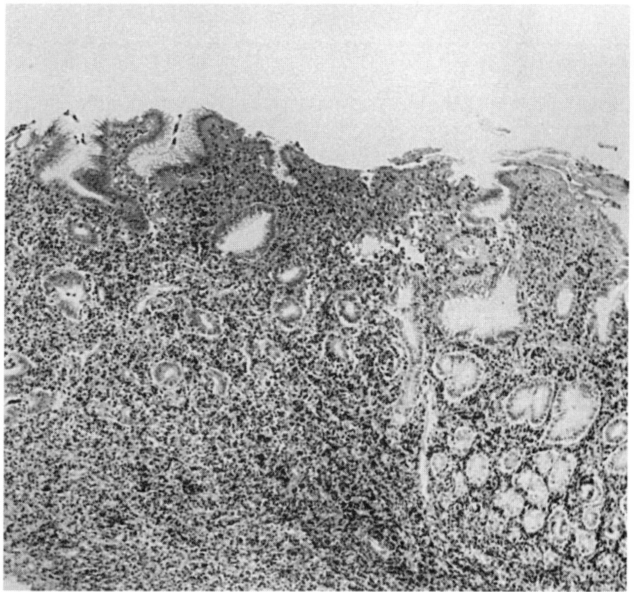

**FIGURE 18–7.** MALToma in a *H. pylori*-infected child. Antral biopsy specimen showing the infiltrate of monotonous-appearing, small lymphoid cells with lymphoepithelial lesions and gland destruction (hematoxylin and eosin stain; original magnification ×20).

which patients who are infected by *H. pylori* and manifesting other gastroduodenal disease (e.g., gastritis) should receive therapy. Reports of reinfection rates vary in the literature, but cross-infection may occur and can be quite high in families with small children.[287]

*H. pylori* is a difficult organism to treat, and success of therapy requires the concurrent administration of two or more antimicrobial drugs. In treatment trials, the success of therapy usually has been arbitrarily defined as the absence of detectable organisms on tissue sampling or carbon-labeled urea breath tests 1 month or longer after treatment is discontinued. Most treatment trials have been performed in adults, and there is a notable lack of available information on treatment of *H. pylori*-infected children. None of the drug regimens currently used to treat *H. pylori* eradicates the organism successfully 100% of the time, and some regimens are associated with a relatively high frequency of side effects. In addition, *H. pylori* is resistant to only a few antimicrobial agents (vancomycin, nalidixic acid), but it can readily become resistant to metronidazole and, to a lesser extent, clarithromycin. Therefore, the success of the therapeutic regimen depends highly on the patient's compliance, the resistance that may develop in *H. pylori* strains colonizing the infected patient, and any adverse reactions.

Many therapeutic regimens have been suggested (Table 18–3). The recommended duration is 2 weeks, although some treat for longer periods.

The most promising treatment and possible prevention of *H. pylori* infection and its significant gastroduodenal disease sequelae lies in the development of an efficacious vaccine. Given the long-term risk of gastric cancer associated with *H. pylori* infection and the varied rates of eradication with antimicrobial regimens, a vaccination approach to prevent the late and life-threatening manifestations of *H. pylori* infection should be considered. Extensive efforts in many laboratories are underway worldwide. Prophylaxis by vaccination seems essential because host natural immunity is inadequate to clear this infection, despite a seemingly vigorous local and systemic immune response.[288]

### Indications for Treatment of *H. pylori*-Infected Children

It is recommended that a child with refractory abdominal symptoms and documented *H. pylori* infection with histopathologic findings (i.e., chronic-active gastritis) should be treated with antimicrobial agents. Patients who have failed empiric acid-blockade therapy (i.e., $H_2$ receptor antagonists), should be evaluated for *H. pylori* infection before initiation of antimicrobial therapy. Evaluation should be performed by upper endoscopy and biopsies with, at minimum, histologic evaluation and appropriate staining (i.e., Giemsa, Warthin-Starry). Urea breath testing should be used as a screen until appropriate controlled trials in children are performed. If serology is used as a screening method, a careful understanding of the assay chosen and the study population used for validation (age, diagnosis, geographic location) should be undertaken before the patient is subjected to the test and charge. Patients who are undergoing maintenance antisecretory therapy and are subsequently diagnosed with *H. pylori*-associated peptic ulcer disease should be treated for the infection, regardless of whether they are in the initial disease stages or are experiencing a recurrence. Controlled prospective studies are needed to assess the benefits of treating children with nonulcer dyspeptic conditions and *H. pylori* infection.[289]

## CLINICAL FINDINGS

The clinical findings of primary and secondary gastritis and primary and secondary peptic ulcer disease are summarized in Table 18–4.

**TABLE 18–3. Triple-Therapy Combinations**

| COMBINATION THERAPY | INVESTIGATORS | NO. OF PATIENTS | DAYS | ERADICATION RATE (%) |
|---|---|---|---|---|
| Tetracycline-bismuth-metronidazole | Labenz et al | 19 | 14 | 84.2 |
| | Cutler et al | 118 | 28 | 96.6 |
| | Graham et al | 93 | 14 | 87.0 |
| | Wilhelmsen et al | 152 | 14 | 89–98 |
| | Hosking et al | 76 | 7 | 94.0 |
| | Iser et al | 101 | 14 | 90.0 |
| | Thijs et al | 100 | 15 | 93.0,* 98.4,† 50.0‡ |
| | Bell et al | 43 | 14 | 90.9,† 33.3‡ |
| Amoxicillin-bismuth-metronidazole | Burette et al | 36 | 14 | 95.0,† 63.0‡ |
| | Seppala et al | 93 | 14 | 84.0 |
| | Rautelin et al | 86 | 14 | 91.0 |
| Amoxicillin-bismuth-tinidazole | Bianchi Porro et al | 17 | 14 | 83.0 |
| | Di Napoli et al | 50 | 10 | 69.0 |
| Omeprazole-tetracycline-metronidazole | McCarthy et al | 43 | 7 | 58.0 |
| Omeprazole-amoxicillin-metronidazole | Bell et al | 127 | 14 | 96.4,† 75.0‡ |
| Omeprazole-clarithromycin-tinidazole | Bazzoli et al | 65 | 7 | 95.0 |
| Omeprazole-clarithromycin-metronidazole | Labenz et al | 80 | 7 | 95.0 |
| Tetracycline-bismuth-amoxicillin | Graham et al | 16 | 14 | 43.0 |
| Amoxicillin-furazolidone-metronidazole | Coelho et al | 47 | 5 | 75.0 |
| Omeprazole-clarithromycin-amoxicillin | Lind et al | 787 | 7 | 96.0 |

*Overall eradication.
†Metronidazole-sensitive strains.
‡Metronidazole-resistant strains.
Adapted from Blecker U, Gold BD: Treatment of *Helicobacter pylori* infection: a review. Pediatr Infect Dis J 1997;16:391–399, with permission.

**TABLE 18–4. Clinical Findings in Primary and Secondary Gastritis and Peptic Ulcer Disease**

| DISEASE ENTITY | SIGNS AND SYMPTOMS |
|---|---|
| Primary gastritis | Asymptomatic (most common)<br>Recurrent abdominal pain (any location)<br>Epigastric pain<br>Water brash, heartburn (gastroesophageal reflux disease symptoms)<br>Vomiting, nausea, anorexia<br>Iron deficiency anemia<br>Short stature, growth failure (?) |
| Secondary gastritis | Abdominal pain<br>Upper gastrointestinal blood loss—hematemesis, melena<br>Epigastric pain localization ("crampy")<br>Irritability, change in feeding patterns<br>Fatigue<br>Iron deficiency anemia |
| Primary peptic ulcer disease | Chronic, recurrent abdominal pain<br>Episodic epigastric pain<br>Vomiting, particularly recurrent<br>Nocturnal wakening<br>Anemia |
| Secondary peptic ulcer disease | Life-threatening gastrointestinal bleeding<br>Gastric or duodenal perforation<br>Shock<br>Abdominal pain (rare) |

## Primary Gastritis and Peptic Ulcer Disease

Nonulcer dyspepsia and its association with *H. pylori* is controversial in both the adult and pediatric populations.[290, 291] Studies that have attempted to determine cost-effective methods to diagnose and treat nonulcer dyspepsia associated with *H. pylori* have been inconclusive.[292] A decision analysis was performed by Silverstein and coworkers,[292] in which empiric therapy for the initial management of dyspepsia was compared with initial endoscopy with or without testing for *H. pylori*; the choice for management conclusions by these authors was a "toss-up." The analysis demonstrated that there were only marginal savings resulting from empiric therapy for adult patients with dyspepsia. As with adults, the majority of children with *H. pylori*-associated gastritis are asymptomatic.[293–295] Although studies of *H. pylori*-associated duodenal ulcer disease in children have provided more conclusive evidence that symptoms may be present, there can be "silent" duodenal ulcers. One study performed by Lai and colleagues[296] evaluated 348 patients with nonulcer dyspepsia in relation to *H. pylori* infection and topographic pathology using the revised Sydney classification for gastritis.[215] In this study, age was observed to be the most important determinant of dyspeptic symptoms, in that ulcer-like pain was negatively related to age. The older the patient, the less likely it was that there would be pain symptoms on initial presentation with dyspeptic symptoms.[296]

Many clinicians use the criteria of "recurrent, persistent abdominal pain" to determine both the institution of diagnostic assays and treatment for *H. pylori* infection. However, recurrent abdominal pain does not appear to be a symptom complex that is associated with increased prevalence of *H. pylori*.[230, 297] Children with *H. pylori*-associated primary gastritis also do not appear to have specific symptomatology that would differentiate them from those with abdominal pain significant enough to warrant upper endoscopy who have "normal" gastric mucosal histology.[298] In addition, there is a lack of consensus among gastroenterologists regarding objective symptom scoring methods, which makes studies that evaluate the association of symptoms with *H. pylori* difficult to interpret.[299] For reasons not completely understood, the placebo effect appears to be significant in children, although no prospective placebo-controlled, randomized trials in this population have been performed.[291, 300]

Treatment studies in children with duodenal ulcers and *H. pylori* infection provide circumstantial evidence that the symptoms of primary ulcers are more specific and different from the symptoms of *H. pylori*-associated primary gastritis.[291] Children with duodenal ulcers frequently have recurring symptoms such as epigastric pain, nausea, and vomiting.[24, 291, 301] As indicated in Table 18–4, nocturnal awakening is a consistent feature of children with duodenal ulcer disease. Children undergoing diagnostic upper endoscopy who have demonstrable ulcer on histology and macroscopic analysis have more than a 90% prevalence of abdominal pain symptoms.[4] The association with meals is also controversial in children compared with adults, and studies are limited owing to the varying diagnostic criteria used to characterize ulcers (i.e., endoscopy, symptomatology).[291, 302]

## Secondary Gastritis and Peptic Ulcer Disease

Symptoms that occur in secondary gastritides and secondary ulcers can be variable. For example, the symptoms associated with an ulcer resulting from NSAID use and one caused by CMV-associated hypertrophic gastropathy can be quite different. These symptoms can range from abdominal pain localized to the epigastric area or bright-red hematemesis in NSAID-induced gastric ulcers to pedal and presacral edema and watery vomiting in the protein-losing enteropathy and gastric dysmotility of CMV-associated Ménétrier's disease.[303, 304] In many children, secondary gastritis results in a microcytic, hypochromic anemia that can be associated with decreased energy at school and daily activities or frank fatigue and excessive sleeping.

Symptoms that result from secondary ulcers are also dependent on the underlying cause and can range from minimal to acute, life-threatening emergencies such as gastrointestinal hemorrhage or perforation.[4] Secondary ulcers manifesting acutely in children are often associated with excessive morbidity and usually do not develop a chronic component, because they resolve once the underlying disease is treated.[120, 305]

# DIAGNOSIS OF GASTRITIS

Standard practice among gastroenterologists should be the use of upper endoscopy as the method of choice for the diagnosis of gastritis and peptic ulcer disease in children.[306] Radiologic studies such as a single-contrast barium swallow can be useful to evaluate the anatomy of the esophagus, stomach, and upper small intestine (usually to the ligament of Treitz), the rapidity of clearance of the esophagus and stomach, and the more obvious mucosal abnormalities. Double-contrast studies can increase the sensitivity of this diagnostic method, but only to a certain degree.[307] The upper gastrointestinal series is only moderately sensitive in defining ulcers. In one study, only 14% of duodenal ulcers detected at endoscopy were found on radiography.[4] Ulcers in children can be subtle and are often "disguised" in the anterior wall of the duodenum.[302] As observed through the video endoscope, both secondary and particularly primary ulcers in children appear more like the aphthous ulcers seen in the mouth with active herpes viral infections or in the colon with active Crohn's disease. False-positive test results are common with contrast radiography.[308] Although useful in the initial evaluation of the child with significant abdominal symptoms, contrast radiography is not as sensitive nor as specific as endoscopy in the diagnosis of gastroduodenal inflammation.

## Classification

Many of the key classifications of gastritis were devised before the epidemiology of *H. pylori* and its association with antral gastritis, duodenal ulcer, and possibly gastric carcinoma were recognized. Originally, chronic gastritis was characterized as *superficial, atrophic,* or *hypertrophic.*[309, 310] Strickland and Mackay[311] considered atrophic gastritis and introduced the important topographic division between type A (involving atrophy of the corpus and associated with pernicious anemia) and type B (antral atrophy). Correa introduced an epidemiologic aspect, linking the terms *hypersecretory gastritis* to an association with duodenal ulcer disease (type B) and *autoimmune gastritis* with pernicious anemia (type A) to a high-cancer-risk group.[312] These terms were further modified to *diffuse antral gastritis, diffuse corporal gastritis,* and *multifocal atrophic gastritis.*[313] Type *A* (autoimmune), *B* (bacterial), and *C* (chemical damage) were advocated by Wyatt and Dixon later that same year.[314]

Because of the multiplicity of classifications with consequent confusion and attendant difficulties in comparing data between various centers, and because of the pivotal role that infection with *H. pylori* is now known to play in the pathogenesis of gastritis, the classification of gastritis and the responses of the gastric mucosa to injury were reconsidered in 1990 by the Sydney Working Party on Gastritis. It was decided to name the new classification "The Sydney System for the Classification of Gastritis." The Sydney system consists of two main divisions: *histologic* and *endoscopic.* The histologic classification of the Sydney system draws on the key elements from the classifications outlined previously, perhaps most from that of Whitehead and associates.[310] The system's backbone is the recognition of the topographic distribution of abnormalities to the gastric antrum alone, to the gastric corpus alone, or to both (pangastritis). The previous categories of gastritis (e.g., types A, B, and C) are no longer used.

Because most clinicians first encounter gastritis as viewed through the endoscope, a system for classifying endoscopic gastritis has been developed in parallel with the histologic system, recognizing that the correlation between the two is less than perfect. The aim of producing an endoscopic system of classification was to encourage and facilitate the reporting of endoscopic appearances in a standard way.

### Histologic Classification of the Sydney System

The Sydney system recognizes only three basic morphologies: *acute gastritis, chronic gastritis,* and *special forms.* Chronic gastritis is the most common form. Acute gastritis is transient and seldom biopsied, and special forms are uncommon. The variables in the morphologic descriptions pertinent to chronic gastritis are as follows.

**Normal mucosa:** Contains scattered mononuclear cells, lymphocytes, and plasma cells. In the corpus, small lymphocyte aggregates are occasionally present at the base of the glands. Granulocytes are absent.

**Acute versus chronic:** If neutrophils are the dominant inflammatory cell, the gastritis is acute. If there is a concomitant increase in chronic inflammatory cells, the gastritis is classified as chronic.

**Inflammation:** Refers to the presence of chronic inflammatory cells in the lamina propria. Their distribution (superficial or deep) in the mucosa is disregarded in the Sydney classification.

**Atrophy:** Refers to the loss of gastric glands.

**Activity:** Refers to the presence of neutrophil granulocytes in the lamina propria, in intraepithelial sites, or both.

**Intestinal metaplasia:** The individual patterns of intestinal metaplasia may be commented on but are not graded.

***H. pylori:*** A simple stain (e.g., Giemsa, not necessarily a silver stain) is recommended for its detection. The stain used is that best suited to the particular laboratory's practice.

The main morphologic changes of inflammation, atrophy, activity (density of neutrophil polymorphs), metaplasia, and density of *H. pylori* are classified according to a standard classification into four grades: (1) none, (2) mild, (3) moderate, and (4) severe. Other variables, such as cell mucin content, epithelial degeneration, foveolar hyperplasia, edema, erosions, fibrosis, or vascularity, are documented but not graded. Specific variables that would determine the final classification are documented as one of the special types of gastritis. Examples of such specific variables are granulomas, eosinophils, *Gastrospirillum,* CMV, and radiation damage.

The **topography** aspect of the Sydney system summarizes the morphology and describes the topographic distribution of the gastritis. The system is finally completed by the addition, when possible, of an **etiology.** The term "idiopathic" is used when the cause is unknown. Common examples are (1) *H. pylori*-associated chronic gastritis of the antrum; (2) autoimmune-associated chronic pangastritis, corpus predominant with severe atrophy; (3) drug-associated acute gastritis of the antrum; and (4) idiopathic chronic pangastritis. Finally, biopsies from patients in whom *H. pylori* was previously documented but is no longer seen are increasingly common. This should be recognized by the prefix term "*H. pylori*-free," implying the previous presence of the organism.

### Endoscopic Classification of the Sydney System

Virtually all gastric biopsies are obtained under endoscopic control, and the endoscopist must formulate a description of endoscopic appearances for diagnostic or research purposes. The term *endoscopic gastritis* is adopted for the description of all macroscopic abnormalities of the gastric lining that do not fall into the category of specific entities such as gastric ulcer, carcinoma, or polyps. It is recognized that at present the correlations between the macroscopically abnormal appearance of the gastric lining (endoscopic gastritis) and the histologic classification (or the symptoms) are rather imperfect.

Parallel with the histologic division, the severity of the various features of endoscopic gastritis should be graded as *absent, mild, moderate,* or *severe.* They should also be described topographically as affecting the antrum, the corpus, or the whole stomach (pangastritis). Pangastritis can also be described as corpus or antrum predominant.

**Edema:** Readily diagnosed when severe, with opalescent tinge of the mucosa and an accentuated areae gastricae pattern. Rarely the most conspicuous abnormality.

**Erythema:** Patchy erythema is easily discernible. It consists of minute (1–3 mm diameter), red patches that can be focal, segmental, or widespread. Occasionally it can take the form of reddish streaks.

**Friability:** Present when there is punctate hemorrhage due to minimal trauma and the mucosa appears dull.

**Exudate:** May be punctate (especially with *H. pylori* infection) or patchy, resistant to vigorous rinsing. Exudate must be distinguished from food residues.

**Flat erosion:** A break in the mucosal continuity. Corresponds to solitary or few (mild), multiple (moderate), or innumerable (severe) foci of necrosis, which vary in size from pinpoint to 1 cm in diameter. They may have a red halo. Distinction between a large erosion and an ulcer is arbitrary; ulcers must have a depth of at least 1 mm. Flat erosions are found mainly in the antrum or on prepyloric folds.

**Raised erosion:** These may be in the antrum, but usually they are corpus predominant. They appear as elevated mounds of mucosa, capped by a central defect. When severe, they may mimic gastric polyposis. They are graded as described for flat erosions.

**Rugal hyperplasia (hyperrugosity):** Exists when rugal folds do not flatten on insufflation, but estimation of size can be difficult. Folds approximately 5 mm in diameter are classified as mild hyperrugosity; those 5 to 10 mm in diameter are moderate; and folds more than 10 mm thick represent severe hyperrugosity. These folds are the dominant abnormality in the rugal hyperplastic gastropathies.

**Rugal atrophy (hyporugosity):** The opposite of hyperrugosity. It is mainly corpus predominant and should be graded as mild, moderate, or severe (complete absence of rugae).

**Visibility of vascular pattern:** Vessels are visible even in the slightly distended stomach.

**Intramural bleeding spots:** They stem from the loss of vascular integrity and appear as dark, irregular spots, streaks, or flecks that are often multiple and may extravasate into the lumen. They are mild when only a few are present, moderate if more than 10 are visible, and severe when they involve extensive areas of mucosa.

**Nodularity:** May be fine (mild) or coarse (severe). Antral nodularity is a common finding in *H. pylori* gastritis in children.[249, 315, 316] It is generally associated histologically with lymphoid hyperplasia. Studies have demonstrated that antral nodularity, although rare, can be observed in adults.[250] However, lymphoid hyperplasia is not a striking feature of *H. pylori* gastritis in adults.

**Erythematous/exudative endoscopic gastritis:** The most common form encountered in clinical practice. It consists of patchy erythema, fine granularity, loss of luster, and punctate exudates. Occasionally, mild friability may be present. This type of endoscopic gastritis usually is antral predominant but may be pangastritic in distribution. It is graded as mild, moderate, or severe.

**Endoscopic flat erosive gastritis:** Flat erosions predominate. They may be antral predominant or pangastritic. A layer of exudate may cover the lesions. Occasionally there is a linear alignment of the erosions along the mucosal folds and focal erythema. It is graded as mild, moderate, or severe.

**Endoscopic raised erosive gastritis:** Raised erosions predominate. Grading (mild, moderate, or severe) is based on the number of lesions.

**Endoscopic gastritis with atrophy:** The vascular pattern is visible in the slightly distended stomach, which has absent or flattened folds. Intestinal metaplasia may be visible as grayish patches with a villous appearance on close inspection. This lesion is graded as mild, moderate, or severe, according to the visibility of the vascular pattern.

**Endoscopic hemorrhagic gastritis:** Characterized by punctate ecchymoses or frank bleeding into the lumen. The number of bleeding spots determine the grade (mild, moderate, or severe).

**Endoscopic enterogastric reflux gastritis:** Exhibits erythema, edema of the rugae, and refluxed bile in the lumen. There may be intense, beefy-red discoloration, and the gastric folds near the stoma may be erythematous to the point of appearing polypoid. It is graded into the usual categories.

**Endoscopic rugal hyperplastic gastritis:** Diagnosed in the presence of striking hyperrugosity that cannot be obliterated by inflation of the stomach. In Ménétrier's disease there is copious mucus, and in gastrinoma there may be conspicuous accentuation of areae gastricae, with abundant, clear secretion in the lumen. In hyperplastic hypersecretory gastritis, there is irregular discoloration of the thickened folds, loss of luster, and flecks of exudate.

## Histopathology of *H. pylori*-Associated Gastritis

*H. pylori*-infected gastric mucosa almost always shows a combination of inflammation and epithelial changes. The classic feature caused by this organism is chronic-active gastritis. The inflammatory infiltrate generally consists of monocytes and neutrophils. *H. pylori*-associated gastritis is also characterized by the presence of acute or chronic inflammation, with immature surface epithelial cells. Syncytia and mucus loss are often present as a result of overactive cell renewal. According to the Sydney system for the gradation of gastritis, this type of gastritis is termed "*H. pylori*-associated chronic gastritis with polymorphonuclear cell activity."[317] The degree of inflammation varies in severity from a minimal inflammatory infiltrate in the lamina propria, with preserved architecture, to severe gastritis with dense inflammation. In very severe cases, intra-epithelial neutrophils can be detected both in the surface epithelium and in the gastric pits as microabscesses.[266] However, a neutrophilic infiltrate is almost invariably seen only in adults infected by *H. pylori* or, at times, in children living in developing countries where infection rates are high and infection occurs at very young ages.[197, 318]

Usually in *H. pylori* gastritis, the fundic inflammation is less important than that of the antral mucosa.[319–321] In addition, in the rare cases in which *H. pylori* was found in normal mucosa, its localization was almost always in the fundus. This difference between the two zones, fundus and antrum, has practical implications for the detection of *H. pylori* by means of biopsy. In many persons, the fundic gland mucosa extends well into the anatomic antrum.[322] Therefore, at least two biopsies should be taken within 2 to 5 cm of the pylorus to be sure to obtain a sample from the antral mucosa.

## TREATMENT

A complete review of the treatment of *H. pylori* infection in children has already been given. There are a number of other agents that can be tried empirically in the treatment of gastric inflammation.

### Mucosal Cytoprotection

As mentioned in the discussion of the treatment of NSAID-induced injury, prostaglandins, and in particular prostaglandin E, are believed to be cytoprotective to the gastric mucosa, and their coadministration can be helpful to reduce gastroduodenal injury in chronic NSAID users.[148, 323, 324] The synthetic analogues, misoprostol and enprostil, have been shown to be useful in mucosal healing even in the absence of changes in gastric secretion. Prostaglandins are believed to stimulate mucus and bicarbonate secretion, enhance mucosal blood flow, stimulate surface-active phospholipids, and inhibit acid output.[149, 325] Although there have not been many reports describing the tolerability of prostaglandins, side effects in adults have been minimal to moderate (i.e., diarrhea, abdominal cramping).

### Enhancement of Mucosal Barrier Function

The gastric mucosal barrier can be both enhanced and allowed to repair itself by administration of the sulfated sucrose aluminum salt, sucralfate. This compound forms a "proteinaceous" paste at the ulcer surface and has been reported to increase mucosal blood flow, gastric mucus production, and bicarbonate secretion.[326, 327] This drug is tolerated well with minimal to no reported side effects, and it has been effective in promoting ulcer healing when used alone.[328] In a small case series of pediatric ulcer patients, Chiang and colleagues reported that there was a 92% rate of healing with 1 g of sucralfate administered four times per day.[329] Only 2 of the 16 patients who were kept on maintenance therapy relapsed. However, *H. pylori* status was not determined, and this may have been a significant confounding variable in the patients who relapsed. In one study evaluating the use of stress ulcer prophylaxis in ventilated trauma patients, it was observed that use of sucralfate alone resulted in no difference in the incidence of nosocomial infections and actually produced a trend of decreasing pneumonia after study day 4, compared with $H_2$ receptor antagonists.[330]

### Acid Secretion Inhibition and Acid Neutralization

Compounds that promote healing of ulcers and gastroduodenal mucosal inflammation can be divided into two categories: those that neutralize acid and those that inhibit acid secretion.[141] Over-the-counter antacids can be beneficial both in resolving pain and in promoting some mucosal healing.[331, 332] It is postulated that use of antacids promotes mucosal microcirculation and mucosal prostaglandin release. Antacids are often ineffective against more severe ulcers and in particular have no mechanism of action against *H. pylori* in vitro or in vivo. Side effects include constipation with aluminum hydroxide compounds and diarrhea with magnesium hydroxide compounds.

Inhibition of acid secretion can be achieved by two classes of compounds. The first group works by antagonism of the histamine $H_2$ receptors on the parietal cells. Compounds that perform this function include cimetidine, ranitidine, famotidine, and nizatidine. These agents are useful in the prophylaxis of gastrointestinal bleeding in critically ill patients.[333] More recently, a series of compounds have been tried that are directed at antagonism of the $H^+K^+$-ATPase proton pump in the apical portion of the parietal cell membrane. One additional class of compound that is rarely used in children because of the high incidence of side effects is the anticholinergics, such as pirenzepine.[334, 335] Anticholinergics are potent acid inhibitory agents but have side effects such as dizziness, constipation, dry mouth, urinary retention, and blurred vision; they are poorly tolerated and have had limited study in children.

Proton-pump inhibitors are extremely effective in the inhibition of parietal cell acid secretion. Omeprazole, the most commonly used proton-pump inhibitor in children, has been shown to be highly effective in children for the treatment of disorders with acid hypersecretion, such as G-cell hyperplasia.[336] Omeprazole alone is more effective in the treatment of peptic ulcers in adults than $H_2$ receptor antagonists.[337, 338] Concern has been raised about the tumorigenic potential of the proton-pump inhibitors as a result of studies performed in rodents using supraphysiologic doses for prolonged durations.[339, 340] However, there have been no reports in humans to associate long-term use of omeprazole or other proton-pump inhibitors and neoplasia of gastrin-producing cells.[341] Kato and coworkers demonstrated the efficacy of omeprazole administered once daily in the endoscopically confirmed healing of esophagitis, gastric, and duodenal ulcers.[342] They demonstrated a cumulative healing of 46%, 85%, 92%, and 92%, at 2, 4, 6, and 8 weeks of therapy, respectively, with no adverse side effects or gastrin cell hyperplasia at follow-up endoscopy. Finally, one long-term study of omeprazole use for a mean of 48 months (range, 6–84 months) in the treatment of ranitidine-resistant ulcers demonstrated moderate hypergastrinemia and a significant argyrophil cell hyperplasia that correlated with the grade of corpus gastritis.[343] Because hypergastrinemia and gastritis are closely related, the authors were unable to conclude the role of each in the findings at the end of omeprazole therapy. Therefore, more data are necessary, particularly from pediatric studies, to determine the overall safety of omeprazole and its potential long-term side effects.

Finally, omeprazole has a biochemical structure similar to that of the macrolide antibiotics (a substituted benzimidazole) and has demonstrated a mean inhibitory concentration against *H. pylori* in vitro. The sole administration of omeprazole for *H. pylori* infection has demonstrated short-term clearance of the organism but ineffective long-term eradication.[344] In another study of omeprazole monotherapy in six children and one adult infected by *H. pylori*, none of the seven patients had clearance of their infection at the conclusion of 8 weeks of therapy.[345] Moreover, DNA fingerprinting of the infecting *H. pylori* isolates showed that the inability to clear the infection did not appear to be related to acquired antibiotic resistance to the drug or to reinfection of the stomach with a different *H. pylori* strain.[345] However, in dual therapy with omeprazole and one antibiotic—and, more importantly, in triple therapeutic regimens with omeprazole and two antibiotics—eradication rates of *H. pylori* infection increased dramatically.[346, 347] Finally, in a small cohort study evaluating 2-week triple therapy of *H. pylori*-infected children with omeprazole, metronidazole, and clarithromycin, successful eradication was demonstrated in 93% of the 15 patients with no adverse effects.[348] These studies clearly demonstrate the importance of omeprazole in the regimens that result in successful eradication of *H. pylori* in both adults and children.

## REFERENCES


1. Sonnenberg A, Everhart JE: The prevalence of self reported peptic ulcer in the United States. Am J Pub Health 1996;86:200–205.
2. Sonnenberg A: Temporal trends and geographical variations of peptic ulcer disease. Aliment Pharmacol Ther 1995;2:3–12.
3. Sonnenberg A: Factors which influence the incidence and the course of peptic ulcer. Scand J Gastroenterol 1988;23:119–140.
4. Drumm BD, Rhoades JM, Stringer DA, et al: Peptic ulcer disease in children: etiology, clinical findings, and clinical course. Pediatrics 1988;82:410–414.
5. Loof L, Adami HO, Agenas I, et al: The Diagnosis and Therapy Survey, October 1978–March 1983: health care and consumption and current drug therapy in Sweden with respect to the clinical diagnosis with gastritis. Scand J Gastroenterol Suppl 1985;109:35–39.
6. Kurata JH, Haile BM: Epidemiology of peptic ulcer disease. Clin Gastroenterol 1984;13:289–307.
7. Eastham EJ: Peptic ulcer. In Walker WA, Durie PR, Hamilton JR, et al (eds): Pediatric Gastrointestinal Disease: Pathophysiology, Diagnosis and Management, vol 1. Toronto, BC Decker, 1991, pp 438–451.
8. Macarthur C, Saunders N, Feldman W: *Helicobacter pylori,* gastroduodenal disease, and recurrent abdominal pain in children. JAMA 1995;273:729–734.
9. Gold BD: *Helicobacter pylori* infection and peptic ulcer disease. Semin Pediatr Infect Dis 1996;7:265–271.
10. Drumm B, Gormally S, Sherman PM: Gastritis and peptic ulcer disease. In Walker AW, Durie PR, Hamilton JR, Walker-Smith J (eds): Pediatric Gastrointestinal Disease: Pathophysiology, Diagnosis and Management, vol. 1. St. Louis, BC Decker, 1996, pp 506–518.
11. Silen W: The clinical problem of stress ulcers. Clin Invest Med 1987;10:270–274.
12. Kurata JH, Nogawa AN: Meta-analysis of risk factors for peptic ulcer disease: nonsteroidal antiinflammatory drugs, *Helicobacter pylori*, and smoking. J Clin Gastroenterol 1997;24:2–17.
13. Hirschowitz BI: Zollinger-Ellison syndrome: pathogenesis, diagnosis and management. Am J Gastroenterol 1996;92(suppl 4):445–485.
14. Moonka D, Lichtenstein GR, Levine MS, et al: Giant gastric ulcers: an unusual manifestation of Crohn's disease. Am J Gastroenterol 1993;88:297–299.
15. Ruuska T, Vaajalahti P, Arajarvi P, Maki M: Prospective evaluation of upper gastrointestinal mucosal lesions in children with ulcerative colitis and Crohn's disease. J Pediatr Gastroenterol Nutr 1994;19:181–186.
16. Serjeant GR, May H, Patrick A, Slifer E: Duodenal ulceration in sickle cell anemia. Trans R Soc Trop Med Hyg 1973;67:59–63.
17. Rao S, Royal LE, Conrad HA, et al: Duodenal ulcer in sickle cell disease. J Pediatr Gastroenterol Nutr 1990;10:117–120.
18. Oppenheimer EH, Esterly JR: Pathology of cystic fibrosis: review of the literature and comparison of 146 autopsied cases. Perspect Pediatr Pathol 1975;2:241–278.
19. Rosenstein B, Perman JA, Kramer SS: Peptic ulcer disease in cystic fibrosis: an unusual occurrence in black adolescents. Am J Dis Child 1986;140:66–69.
20. Bourke B, Jones N, Sherman P: *Helicobacter pylori* infection and peptic ulcer disease in children. Pediatr Infect Dis J 1996;15:1–13.
21. Sherman PM: Peptic ulcer disease in children. Gastroenterol Clin North Am 1994;23:707–725.
22. Mitchell HM, Bohane TD, Tobias V, et al: *Helicobacter pylori* infection in children: potential clues to pathogenesis. J Pediatr Gastroenterol Nutr 1993;16:120–125.
23. Habbick BF, Melrose AG, Grant JC: Duodenal ulcer in childhood. Arch Dis Child 1968;43:23–28.
24. Murphy MS, Eastham EJ, Jimenez M, et al: Duodenal ulceration: a review of 110 cases. Arch Dis Child 1987;62:544–548.
25. Jackson RH: Genetic studies of peptic ulcers disease in children. Paediatr Scand 1972;61:493–494.
26. Drumm B, Sherman P, Cutz E, Karmali M: Association of *Campylobacter pylori* on the gastric mucosa with antral gastritis in children. N Engl J Med 1987;316:1557–1561.
27. Goodwin CS, Armstrong JA, Chilvers T, Peters M: Transfer of *Campylobacter pylori* and *Campylobacter mustelae* to *Helicobacter* gen. nov. as *Helicobacter pylori* comb. nov. and *Helicobacter mustelae* comb. nov., respectively. Int J Syst Bacteriol 1989;39:397–405.
28. Drumm B, Perez-Perez GI, Blaser MJ, Sherman PM: Intrafamilial clustering of *Helicobacter pylori* infection. N Engl J Med 1990;322:359–363.
29. Wang JT, Shen JC, Lin JT, et al: Direct DNA amplification and restriction pattern analysis of *Helicobacter pylori* in patients with duodenal ulcers and their families. J Infect Dis 1993;169:1544–1548.
30. Drumm B: *Helicobacter pylori* in the pediatric patient. Gastroenterol Clin North Am 1993;22:169–182.
31. Czinn S, Dahms B, Jacobs G, et al: Campylobacter-like organisms in association with symptomatic gastritis in children. J Pediatr 1986;109:80–83.
32. Blaser MJ: *Helicobacter pylori*: its role in gastroduodenal disease. Clin Infect 1992;15:386–393.
33. Akamatsu T, Ota H, Shimizu T, et al: Histochemical study of *Helicobacter pylori* and surface mucous gel layer in various gastric lesions. Acta Histochem Cytochem 1995;28:181–185.
34. Marshall BJ, Armstrong JA, McGechie DB, Glancy RJ: Attempts to fulfill Koch's postulates for pyloric *Campylobacter.* Med J Aust 1985;142:436–439.
35. Prieto G, Polanco I, Larrauri J, et al: *Helicobacter pylori* infection in children: clinical, endoscopic, and histologic correlations. J Pediatr Gastroenterol Nutr 1992;14:420–425.
36. Yeung CK, Fu KH, Yuen KY, et al: *Helicobacter pylori* and associated duodenal ulcer. Arch Dis Child 1990;65:1212–1216.
37. Parsonnet J: The incidence of *Helicobacter pylori* infection. Aliment Pharmacol Ther 1995;9:45–51.

38. Veldhuyzen van Zanten SJO, Pollack PT, Best LM, et al: Increasing prevalence of *Helicobacter pylori* infection with age: continuous risk of infection in adults rather than cohort effect. J Infect Dis 1994;169:434–437.
39. Mitchell HM, Li YY, Hu PJ, et al: Epidemiology of *Helicobacter pylori* in southern China: identification of early childhood as the critical period for acquisition. J Infect Dis 1992;166:149–153.
40. Forman D, Newell DG, Fullerton F, et al: Association between infection with *Helicobacter pylori* and risk of gastric cancer: evidence from a prospective investigation. Br Med J 1991;302:1302–1305.
41. Correa P: *Helicobacter pylori* and gastric carcinogenesis. Am J Surg Pathol 1995;19:S37–S43.
42. Warren JR, Marshall BJ: Unidentified curved bacilli on gastric epithelium in active chronic gastritis. Lancet 1983;1:1273–1275.
43. Marshall BJ, Warren JR: Unidentified curved bacilli in the stomach of patients with gastritis and peptic ulceration. Lancet 1984;1:1311–1315.
44. Kobel FB, Barbero GJ: Gastric secretion in infancy and childhood. Gastroenterology 1967;52:1101–1112.
45. Harad T, Hyman PE, Everett S, et al: Meal-stimulated gastric acid secretion in premature infants. J Pediatr 1984;104:534–538.
46. Seabrook M, Amarnath RP, Amarnath M, et al: Twenty four hour intragastric profiles in fed and fasted premature infants. Gastroenterology 1991;100:A546.
47. Lambert J, Mobassaleh M, Grand RI: Efficacy of cimetidine for gastric acid suppression in pediatric patients. J Pediatr 1992;120:478–488.
48. Baron JH: Studies of basal and peak acid output with an augmented histamine test. Gut 1963;4:136–144.
49. Christie DL, Ament ME: Gastric acid hypersecretion in children with duodenal ulcer. Gastroenterology 1976;71:242–244.
50. Mohammed R, Hearns JB, Cream GP: Gastric acid secretion in children with duodenal ulceration. Scand J Gastroenterol 1982;17:289–292.
51. Gear MWL, Truelove SC, Whitehead R: Gastric ulcer and gastritis. Gut 1971;12:639–645.
52. Tatsuta M, Ishi H, Okuda S: Location of peptic ulcers in relation to antral and fundic gastritis by chromoendoscopic follow up examinations. Dig Dis Sci 1986;31:7–11.
53. Carrick J, Lee A, Hazell S, et al: *Campylobacter pylori*, duodenal ulcer, and gastric metaplasia: possible role of functional heterotopic tissue in ulcerogenesis. Gut 1989;30:790–797.
54. Hyman PE, Hassall E: Marked basal gastric acid hyper-secretion and peptic ulcer disease: medical management with a combination of H2 receptor antagonist and anti-cholinergic. J Pediatr Gastroenterol Nutr 1988;7:57–63.
55. Ghai OP, Singh M, Walia BNS, Gadekar NG: An assessment of gastric secretory response with "maximal" augmented histamine stimulation in children with peptic ulcer. Arch Dis Child 1965;40:77–79.
56. Robb JDA, Thomas PS, Orszulok J, Odling-Smee GW: Duodenal ulcer in childhood. Arch Dis Child 1972;47:688–696.
57. Euler AR, Byrne WJ, Campbell MF: Basal and pentagastrin-stimulated gastric acid secretory rates in normal children and in those with peptic ulcer disease. J Pediatr 1982;103:766–768.
58. Nagita A, Amemoto K, Yoden A, et al: Diurnal variation in intragastric pH in children with and without peptic ulcers. Pediatr Res 1996;40:528–532.
59. Yamashiro Y, Shioya T, Ohtsuka Y, et al: Patterns of 24 h intragastric acidity in duodenal ulcers in children: the importance of monitoring and inhibiting nocturnal activity. Acta Paediatr Jpn 1995;37:557–561.
60. Mcqueen S, Hutton DA, Allen A, Garner A: Gastric and duodenal surface mucus gel thickness in the rat: effect of prostaglandins and damaging agents. Am J Physiol 1983;8:388–394.
61. Isenberg JI, Selling JA, Hogan DL, Koss MA: Impaired proximal duodenal mucosal bicarbonate secretion in patients with duodenal ulcer. N Engl J Med 1987;316:374–379.
62. Mertz-Nielsen AJH, Frokiare H, Bukhave K, Rask-Madsen J: Gastric bicarbonate secretion and release of prostaglandin E2 are increased in duodenal ulcer patients but not in *Helicobacter pylori* positive healthy subjects. Scand J Gastrenterol 1996;31:38–43.
63. Gold BD, Islur P, Policova Z, et al: Surface properties of *Helicobacter mustelae* and ferret gastrointestinal mucosa. Clin Invest Med 1996;19:92–100.
64. Lichtenberger LM, Romero JJ: Effect of ammonium ion on the hydrophobic and barrier properties of the gastric mucus gel layer: implications on the role of ammonium in *H. pylori* induced gastritis. J Gastroenterol Hepatol 1994;9(suppl 1):513–519.
65. Go MF, Lew GM, Lichtenberger LM, et al: Gastric mucosal hydrophobicity and *Helicobacter pylori*: response to antimicrobial therapy. Am J Gastroenterol 1993;88:1362–1365.
66. Younan R, Pearson J, Allen A, Venables C: Changes in the structure of the mucus gel on the mucosal surface of the stomach in association with peptic ulcer disease. Gastroenterology 1982;82:827–831.
67. Taylor IL: Gastrointestinal hormones in the pathogenesis of peptic ulcer disease. Clin Gastroenterol 1984;13:355–382.
68. Defize J, Meuwissen SGM: Pepsinogens: an update of biochemical, physiological, and clinical aspects. J Pediatr Gastroenterol Nutr 1987;6:493–508.
69. Rotter JI, Sones JQ, Samloff IM, et al: Duodenal ulcer disease associated with elevated serum pepsinogen I: an autosomal inherited disorder. N Engl J Med 1979;300:63–66.
70. Oderda G, Vaira D, Dell'Olio D, et al: Serum pepsinogen I and gastrin concentrations in children positive for *Helicobacter pylori*. J Clin Pathol 1990;43:762–765.
71. Dolwaczny D, Noehl N, Tschop K, et al: Goblet cell antibodies in patients with inflammatory bowel disease and their first degree relatives. Gastroenterology 1997;113:101–107.
72. Polito JM, Childs B, Mellits ED, et al: Crohn's disease: concordance for site and clinical type in affected family members—potential hereditary influences. Gastroenterology 1996;111:573–580.
73. Buchta RM, Kaplan JM: Zollinger Ellison syndrome in a 9 year old child: case report and review of this entity in childhood. Pediatrics 1971;47:594–598.
74. Zollinger RM, Ellison EH: Primary peptic ulcerations of the jejunum associated with islet cell tumours of the pancreas. Ann Surg 1955;142:709–713.
75. Meko JB, Norton JA: Management of patients with Zollinger-Ellison. Ann Rev Med 1995;46:395–411.
76. Maton PN: Zollinger-Ellison syndrome: recognition. Drugs 1996;52:33–44.
77. Wilson SD: The role of surgery in children with Zollinger Ellison syndrome. Surgery 1982;92:682–692.
78. Jaros W, Biller J, Flores A, et al: Significance of antral G cell hyperplasia in young patients. Gastroenterology 1985;88:A1432.
79. Friesen ST, Tomita T: Hypergastrinemia, hyperchlorhydria without tumour. Ann Surg 1981;194:481–493.
80. Zaatar R, Younoszai MK, Mitros F: Pseudo-Zollinger Ellison syndrome in a child presenting with anemia. Gastroenterology 1987;92:508–512.
81. Snyder M, Scurry M, Hughes W: Hypergastrinemia in familial endocrine adenomatosis. Ann Intern Med 1974;80:321–325.
82. Gustavsson S, Kelly RA, Melton LJ, Zinsmeister AR: Trends in peptic ulcer surgery: a population based study in Rochester, Minnesota, 1956–1985. Gastroenterology 1988;94:688–694.
83. Kettelhut BV, Metcalfe DD: Pediatric mastocytosis (review). Ann Allergy 1994;73:197–202.
84. Miner PB: The role of the mast cell in clinical gastrointestinal disease with special reference to systemic mastocytosis. J Invest Dermatol 1991;96:S40–S44.
85. Cherner JA, Jensen RT, Dubois A, et al: Gastrointestinal dysfunction in systemic mastocytosis. Gastroenterology 1988;95:657–667.
86. Ueyama T, Ureshino J, Motooka M, Masuda K: Isolated Crohn's disease of the gastroduodenum: a case. Radiat Med 1993;11:167–169.
87. Yardley JH, Hendrix TR: Histological findings in gastroduodenal mucosa in patients with gastroduodenal Crohn's disease: the focus. Pol J Pathol 1996;47:115–118.
88. Griffiths AM, Alemayehu E, Sherman PM: Clinical features of gastroduodenal Crohn's disease in adolescents. J Pediatr Gastroenterol Nutr 1989;8:166–171.
89. Lanaerts C, Roy CC, Vaillancourt M, et al: High incidence of upper gastrointestinal tract involvement in children with Crohn's disease. Pediatrics 1989;83:777–781.
90. Korelitz BI, Waye JD, Kreuning J, et al: Crohn's disease in endoscopic biopsies of the gastric antrum and duodenum. Am J Gastroenterol 1981;76:103–109.
91. Cameron DJS: Upper and lower gastrointestinal endoscopy in children and adolescents with Crohn's disease: a prospective study. J Gastroenterol Hepatol 1991;6:355–358.
92. Snyder JD, Rosenblum N, Wershil B, et al: Pyloric stenosis and eosinophilic gastroenteritis. J Pediatr Gastroenterol Nutr 1987;6:543–547.
93. Whitington PF, Whitington GL: Eosinophilic gastroenteropathy in childhood. J Pediatr Gastroenterol Nutr 1988;7:379–385.

94. Steffen RM, Wyllie R, Petras RE, et al: The spectrum of eosinophilic gastroenteritis. Clin Pediatr 1991;30:404–411.
95. Beneck D: Hypertrophic gastropathy in a newborn: a case report and review of the literature. Pediatr Pathol 1994;14:213–221.
96. Faure C, Besnard M, Hirsch A, et al: Chronic hypertrophic gastropathy in a child resembling adult Menetrier's disease. J Pediatr Gastroenterol Nutr 1996;23:419–421.
97. Hochman JA, Witte DP, Cohen MB: Diagnosis of cytomegalovirus infection in pediatric Menetrier's disease by in situ hydridization. J Clin Microbiol 1996;34:2588–2589.
98. Occena RO, Taylor SE, Robinson CC, Sokol RJ: Association of cytomegalovirus with Menetrier's disease in childhood: report of two new cases with a review of the literature. J Pediatr Gastroenterol Nutr 1993;17:217–224.
99. Cieslak TJ, Mullett CT, Puntel RA, Latimer IS: Menetrier's disease associated with cytomegalovirus infection in children: report of two cases and review of the literature. Pediatr Infect Dis J 1993;12:340–343.
100. Drut RM, Gomez MA, Lojo MM, Drut R: Cytomegalovirus-associated Menetrier's disease in adults: demonstration by polymerase chain reaction (PCR). Medicina 1995;55:659–664.
101. Bayerdörffer E, Ritter MM, Hatz R, et al: Healing of protein losing hypertrophic gastropathy by eradication of *Helicobacter pylori*: is *Helicobacter pylori* a factor in Menetrier's disease? Gut 1994;35:701–704.
102. Wolfsen HC, Carpenter HA, Talley NJ: Menetrier's disease: a form of hypertrophic gastropathy. Gastroenterology 1993;104:1310–1319.
103. De Aizpurua HJ, Cosgrove LJ, Unger B, Toh BH: Autoantibodies cytotoxic to gastric parietal cells in serum of patients with pernicious anemia. N Engl J Med 1983;309:625–629.
104. Vandelli C, Bottazzo GF, Daniach O, Frangeschi F: Autoantibodies to gastrin-producing cells in antral (type B) chronic gastritis. N Engl J Med 1979;300:1406–1410.
105. Karlsson FA, Burman P, Loof L, Marsh S: Major parietal cell antigen in autoimmune gastritis with pernicious anemia is the acid producing $H^+$, $K^+$-adenosine triphosphate of the stomach. J Clin Invest 1988;81:475–479.
106. Miyazaki Y, Shinomura Y, Murayam Y, et al: Marked increase in fundic mucosal histidine decarboxylase activity in a patient with $H^+$,$K^+$-ATPase antibody positive autoimmune gastritis. Int Med 1993;32:602–606.
107. Haruma K, Komoto K, Kawaguchi H, et al: Pernicious anemia and *Helicobacter pylori*. Am J Gastroenterol 1995;90:1107–1110.
108. Dixon MF, Brown LJ, Burke DA, Rathbone BJ: Lymphocytic gastritis: relationship to *Campylobacter pylori* infection. J Pathol 1988;154: 125–132.
109. Couper R, Lashi B, Drumm B, et al: Chronic varioliform gastritis in childhood. J Pediatr 1989;115:441–444.
110. Caporali R, Luciano S: Diffuse varioliform gastritis. Arch Dis Child 1986;61:405–407.
111. Farahat K, Hainaut P, Jamar F, et al: Lymphocytic gastritis: an unusual cause of hypoproteinemia. J Intern Med 1993;234:95–100.
112. Cook DJ, Fuller HD, Guyatt GH, et al: Risk factors for gastrointestinal bleeding in critically ill patients. N Engl J Med 1994;330:377–381.
113. Eddleston JM, Pearson RC, Holland J, et al: Prospective endoscopic study of stress erosions and ulcers in critically ill adult patients treated with either sucralfate or placebo. Crit Care Med 1994;22:1949–1954.
114. Hsu HY, Chang MH, Wang TH, et al: Acute duodenal ulcer. Arch Dis Child 1989;64:774–779.
115. Miller TA: Stress erosive gastritis: what is optimal therapy and who should undergo it. Gastroenterology 1995;109:626–628.
116. Carroll TA, Morris K, Rawluk D: Gastroprotection in neurosurgery: the practice in Great Britain. Br J Neurosurg 1997;11:39–42.
117. O'Keefe G, Maier RV: Current management of patients with stress ulceration. Adv Surg 1996;30:155–177.
118. Lucas CE: Natural history and surgical dilemma of "stress" gastric bleeding. Arch Surg 1971;102:266–273.
119. Morden RS, Mollitt DL, Santulli TV: Operative management of stress ulcers in children. Ann Surg 1982;172:523–531.
120. Dunn S, Weber TR, Grosfeld JL, et al: Acute peptic ulcer in childhood: emergency surgical therapy in 39 cases. Arch Surg 1983;196:18–20.
121. Krasna IH, Schneider KM, Becker JM: Surgical management of stress ulcerations in childhood: report of 5 cases. J Pediatr Surg 1971;6:301–306.
122. Bell MJ, Keating JP, Ternberg JL, et al: Perforated stress ulcer in infants. J Pediatr Surg 1987;16:998–1002.
123. Hisanaga Y, Goto H, Tachi K, et al: Implication of nitric oxide synthase activity in the genesis of water. Aliment Pharmacol Ther 1996;10:933–940.
124. Cho CH, Qui BS, Bruce IC: Vagal hyperactivity in stress induced gastric ulceration in rats. J Gastroenterol Hepatol 1996;11:125–128.
125. Vorder Bruegge WF, Peura DA: Stress-related mucosal damage: review of drug therapy. J Clin Gastroenterol 1990;12:S35–S40.
126. Navab F, Steingrub J: Stress ulcer: is routine prophylaxis necessary? Am J Gastroenterol 1995;90:708–712.
127. Balaban DH, Duckworth CW, Peura DA: Nasogastric omeprazole: effects on gastric pH in critically ill patients. Am J Gastroenterol 1997;92:79–83.
128. Butt W, Auldist A, McDougal P, Duncan A: Duodenal ulceration: a complication of tolazoline therapy. Aust Paediatr J 1986;22:221–223.
129. Adams J, Hyde W, Procianoy R, Rudolph AJ: Hypochloremic metabolic alkalosis following tolazoline-induced gastric hypersecretion. Pediatrics 1980;65:298–300.
130. Dajani EZ, Agrawal NM: Prevention and treatment of ulcers induced by non-steroidal anti-inflammatory drugs: an update. J Physiol Pharmacol 1995;46:3–16.
131. Smalley WE, Griffin MR, Fought RL, Ray WA: Excess costs from gastrointestinal disease associated with nonsteroidal antiinflammatory drugs. J Gen Intern Med 1996;11:461–469.
132. Guslandi M: Gastric toxicity of antiplatelet therapy with low-dose aspirin. Drugs 1997;53:1–5.
133. Piper DW, McIntosh JH, Ariotti DF, et al: Analgesic ingestion and chronic peptic ulcer. Gastroenterology 1981;80:427–432.
134. McIntosh HH, Byth K, Piper DW: Environmental factors in aetiology of chronic gastric ulcer: a case control study of exposure variables before first symptoms. Gut 1985;26:789–798.
135. Griffin MR, Smalley WE: Drugs and ulcers: clues about mucosal protection from epidemiologic studies. J Clin Gastroenterol 1995;21:S113–S119.
136. Graham DY, Smith JL: Aspirin and the stomach. Ann Intern Med 1986;104:390–398.
137. Graham DY: Prevention of gastroduodenal injury induced by chronic non-steroidal antiinflammatory injury. Gastroenterology 1989;96:675–681.
138. Langman MJS: Epidemiologic evidence on the association between peptic ulceration and antiinflammatory drug use. Gastroenterology 1989;96:640–646.
139. Pearson SP, Kelberman I: Gastrointestinal effects of NSAIDs: difficulties in management and detection. Postgrad Med 1996;100:131–132, 135–136, 141–143.
140. Dowd JE, Cimaz R, Fink CW: Nonsteroidal antiinflammatory drug-induced gastroduodenal injury in children. Arthritis Rheum 1995;38:1225–1231.
141. Soll AH: Consensus conference: medical treatment of peptic ulcer disease. Practice guidelines. Practice Parameters Committee of the American College of Gastroenterology. JAMA 1996;275:622–629.
142. Rowe PHMJS, Kason I, Marrone G, Silen W: Effect of stimulated systemic administration of aspirin, salicylate, and indomethacin on amphibian gastric mucosa. Gastroenterology 1986;90:559–569.
143. Meyer RA, McGinley D, Posalaky Z: Effects of aspirin on tight junction structure on the canine gastric mucosa. Gastroenterology 1986;91:1390–1395.
144. Imhof MCO, Hartwig A, Thon KP, et al: Which peptic ulcers bleed? Results of a case-control study, DUSUK study group. Scand J Gastroenterol 1997;32:131–138.
145. El-Zimaity HMT, Genta RM, Graham DY: Histologic features do not define NSAID-induced gastritis. Hum Pathol 1996;27:1348–1354.
146. Caelli M, LaCorte R, DeCarlo L, et al: Histopathology of patients treated with non-steroidal anti-inflammatory drugs. J Clin Pathol 1995;48:553–555.
147. Graham DY, White RH, Moreland LW, et al: Duodenal and gastric ulcer prevention with misoprostol in arthritis patients taking NSAIDs: misoprostol study group. Ann Intern Med 1993;119:257–262.
148. Silverstein FE, Graham DY, Senior JR, et al: Misoprostol reduces serious gastrointestinal complications in patients with rheumatoid arthritis receiving non-steroidal anti-inflammatory drugs: a randomized, double-blind, placebo-controlled trial. Ann Intern Med 1995;123:241–249.
149. Sontag SJ, Schnell TG, Budiman-Mak E, et al: Healing of NSAID-induced gastric ulcers with a synthetic prostaglandin analog (Enprostil). Am J Gastroenterol 1994;89:1014–1020.

150. Gazarian M, Berkovitch M, Koren G, et al: Experience with misoprostol therapy for NSAID gastropathy in children. Ann Rheum Dis 1995;54:277–280.
151. Blaser MJ: Not all *Helicobacter pylori* strains are created equal: should all be eliminated? Lancet 1997;349:1020–1022.
152. Webb PM, Night T, Greaves S, et al: Relationship between infection with *Helicobacter pylori* and living conditions in childhood: evidence for person to person transmission in early life. Br Med J 1994;308:750–753.
153. Staat MA, Kruszon-Moran D, McQuillan GM, Kaslow RA: A population-based serologic survey of *Helicobacter.* J Infect Dis 1996;174:1120–1123.
154. Ashorn M, Miettinen A, Ruuska T, et al: Seroepidemiological study of *Helicobacter pylori* infection in infancy. Arch Dis Child Fetal Neonatal Ed 1996;74:F141–F142.
155. Malaty HM, Graham DY: Importance of childhood socioeconomic status on the current prevalence of *Helicobacter pylori* infection. Gut 1994;35:742–745.
156. Malaty HM, Kim JG, Kim SD, Graham DY: Prevalence of *Helicobacter pylori* infection in Korean children: inverse relation to socioeconomic status despite a uniformly high prevalence in adults. Am J Epidemiol 1996;143:257–262.
157. Van Zanten SJOV, Pollack PT, Best LM, et al: Increasing prevalence of *Helicobacter pylori* infection with age: continuous risk of infection in adults rather than cohort effect. J Infect Dis 1994;169:434–437.
158. Megraud F: Transmission of *Helicobacter pylori*: faecal-oral versus oral-oral. Aliment Pharmacol Ther 1995;9:85–91.
159. Goodman KJ, Correa P: The transmission of *Helicobacter pylori*: a critical review of the evidence. Int J Epidemiol 1995;24:875–887.
160. Chow TKF, Lambert JR, Wahlqvist ML, Hsu-Hage BHH: *Helicobacter pylori* in Melbourne Chinese immigrants: evidence for oral-oral transmission via chopsticks. J Gastroenterol Hepatol 1995;10:562–569.
161. Luzza F, Maletta M, Imeneo M, et al: Evidence against an increased risk of *Helicobacter pylori* infection in dentists: a serological and salivary study. Eur J Gastroenterol Hepatol 1995;7:773–776.
162. Banatvala NYA, Clements L, Herbert A, et al: *Helicobacter pylori* infection in dentists: a case-control study. Scand J Infect Dis 1995;27:149–151.
163. Fox JG, Blanco MC, Yan L, et al: Role of gastric pH in isolation of *Helicobacter mustelae* from the feces of ferrets. Gastroenterology 1993;104:86–92.
164. Fox JG, Correa P, Taylor NS, et al: *Helicobacter mustelae*-associated gastritis in ferrets: an animal model of *Helicobacter pylori* gastritis in humans. Gastroenterology 1990;99:352–362.
165. Lee A: *Helicobacter* infections in laboratory animals: a model for gastric neoplasia. Ann Med 1995;27:575–582.
166. Perkins SE, Fox JG, Walsh JH: *Helicobacter mustelae*-associated hypergastrinemia in ferrets *(Mustelae putorius furo).* Am J Vet Res 1996;57:147–150.
167. Yu J, Russell M, Salomen RN, et al: Effect of *Helicobacter mustelae* infection on ferret gastric epithelial cell proliferation. Carcinogenesis 1995;16:1927–1931.
168. Klein PD, Graham DY, Opekun AR, O'Brian-Smith E: Water as a risk factor for *Helicobacter pylori* infection in Peruvian children. Lancet 1991;337:1503–1506.
169. Handt LK, Fox JG, Dewhirst FE, et al: *Helicobacter pylori* isolated from the domestic cat: public health implications. Infect Immun 1994;62:2367–2374.
170. Handt LK, Fox JG, Stalis IH, et al: Characterization of feline *Helicobacter pylori* strains and associated gastritis in a colony of domestic cats. J Clin Microbiol 1995;33:2280–2289.
171. Enroth H, Engstrand L: Immunomagnetic separation and PCR for detection of *Helicobacter pylori* in water and stool specimens. J Clin Microbiol 1995;33:2162–2165.
172. El-Zaatari FA, Woo JS, Badr A, et al: Failure to isolate *Helicobacter pylori* from stray cats indicates that *H. pylori* in cats may be an anthroponosis: an animal infection with a human pathogen. J Med Microbiol 1997;46:372–376.
173. Osato MS, Le HH, Ayoub C, Graham DY: Houseflies as a reservoir for *Helicobacter pylori.* Gastroenterology 1997;112:A247.
174. Grubel P, Hoffman JS, Chong FK, et al: Vector potential of houseflies *(Musca domestica)* for *Helicobacter pylori.* J Clin Microbiol 1997;35:1300–1303.
175. Parsonnet J: Bacterial infection as a cause of cancer. Environ Health Perspect 1995;103:263–268.
176. Parsonnet J: *Helicobacter pylori* in the stomach: a paradox unmasked. N Engl J Med 1996;335:278–280.
177. Blaser MJ, Parsonnet J: Parasitism by the "slow" bacterium *Helicobacter pylori* leads to altered gastric homeostasis and neoplasia. J Clin Invest 1994;94:4–8.
178. Bell GD: Conference report: duodenal ulcer trials reported at the European *Helicobacter pylori* study group workshops, Edinburgh, 1995. Aliment Pharmacol Ther 1996;10:49–54.
179. Miehlke S, Bayerdorffer E, Lehn N, et al: Recurrence of duodenal ulcer during five years of follow up after cure of *Helicobacter pylori* infection. Eur J Gastroenterol Hepatol 1995;7:975–978.
180. Seppala K, Pikkarained P, Sipponen P, et al: Cure of peptic gastric ulcer associated with eradication of *Helicobacter pylori.* Gut 1995;36:834–837.
181. Tucci A, Corinaldesi R, Stanghellini V, et al: *Helicobacter pylori* infection and gastric function in patients with chronic idiopathic dyspepsia. Gastroenterology 1992;103:768–774.
182. Newton M, Bryan R, Burnham WR, Kamm MA: Evaluation of *Helicobacter pylori* in reflux esophagitis and Barrett's esophagus. Gut 1997;40:9–13.
183. Blaser MJ, Chyou PH, Normura A: Age at establishment of *Helicobacter pylori* infection and gastric carcinoma, gastric ulcer and duodenal ulcer risk. Cancer Res 1995;55:562–565.
184. Crabtree JE, Spencer J: Immunologic aspects of *Helicobacter pylori* infection and malignant transformation of B cells. Semin Gastroinest Dis 1996;7:30–40.
185. Figura N, Tabaqchali S: Bacterial pathogenic factors. Curr Opin Gastroenterol 1996;12:11–15.
186. Mobley HLT, Island MD, Hausinger RP: Molecular biology of microbial ureases. Microbiol Rev 1995;59:451–480.
187. O'Toole PW, Kostrzynska M, Trust TJ: Non-motile mutants of *Helicobacter pylori* and *Helicobacter mustelae* defective in hook production. Mol Microbiol 1994;14:691–703.
188. Figura N, Guglielmetti P, Rossolini A, et al: Cytotoxin production by *Campylobacter pylori* strains isolated from patients with peptic ulcers and from patients with chronic gastritis only. J Clin Microbiol 1989;27:225–226.
189. Leunk RD, Johnson PT, David BC, et al: Cytotoxic activity in broth culture filtrates of *Campylobacter pylori.* J Med Microbiol 1988;26:93–99.
190. Atherton JC, Cao P, Peek J, et al: Mosaicism in vacuolating cytotoxin alleles of *Helicobacter pylori*: Association of vacA types with cytotoxin production and peptic ulceration. J Biol Chem 1995;270:17771–17777.
191. Tummuru MKR, Cover TL, Blaser MI: Cloning and expression of a high molecular weight major antigen of *Helicobacter pylori*: evidence of linkage to cytotoxin production. Infect Immun 1993;61:1799–1809.
192. Xiang Z, Censini S, Bayelli PF, et al: Analysis of expression of CagA and VacA virulence factors in 43 strains of *Helicobacter pylori* reveals that the clinical isolates can be divided into two major types and that CagA is not necessary for expression of the vacuolating cytotoxin. Infect Immun 1995;63:94–98.
193. Censini S, Lange C, Xiang ZY, et al: *cag*, a pathogenicity island of *Helicobacter pylori*, encodes type I-specific and disease-associated virulence factors. Proc Nat Acad Sci U S A 1996;93:14648–14653.
194. Atherton JC, Peek RM Jr, Tham KT, et al: Clinical and pathological importance of heterogeneity in *vac*A, the vacuolating cytotoxin gene of *Helicobacter pylori.* Gastroenterology 1997;112:92–99.
195. Blaser MJ: Intrastrain differences in *Helicobacter pylori*: a key question in mucosal damage? Ann Med 1995;27:559–563.
196. Wyatt JI: Histopathology of gastroduodenal inflammation: the impact of *Helicobacter pylori.* Histopathology 1995;26:1–15.
197. Ashorn M: What are the specific features of *Helicobacter pylori* gastritis in children. Ann Med 1995;27:617–620.
198. Whitney AEW, Emory TS, Marty AM, et al: Macrophage infiltration of the gastric mucosa in children with and without *Helicobacter pylori* infection. J Pediatr Gastroenterol Nutr 1996;23:348.
199. Anderson LP, Crabtree JI: Immunological aspects of *Helicobacter pylori.* Curr Opin Gastroenterol 1994;10:26–29.
200. Cutler AF, Havstad S, Ma CK, et al: Accuracy of invasive and noninvasive tests to diagnose *Helicobacter pylori* infection. Gastroenterology 1995;109:136–141.
201. Gotschlich EC: Thoughts on the evolution of strategies used by bacteria for evasion of host defenses. Rev Infect Dis 1983;5:S778–S783.

202. McGowan FD, Cover TL, Blaser MJ: *Helicobacter pylori* and gastric acid: biological and therapeutic implications. Gastroenterology 1996;110:926–938.
203. Dekigai H, Murakami M, Kita T: Mechanism of *Helicobacter pylori* associated gastric mucosa injury. Dig Dis Sci 1995;40:1332–1339.
204. Chan WY, Hui PK, Leung KM, et al: Coccoid forms of *Helicobacter pylori* in the human stomach. Clin Microbiol Infect Dis 1994;102:503–507.
205. Schmitz A, Josenhans C, Suerbaum S: The *H. pylori* flagellar biosynthesis regulatory protein FlbA affects the expression of flagellar components on the transciptional level and is probably a membrane protein. Gut 1995;37:A245.
206. Owen RJ, Bickley J, Hurtado A, et al: Comparison of PCR-based restriction length polymorphism analysis of urease genes with rRNA gene profiling for monitoring *Helicobacter pylori* infections in patients on triple therapy. J Clin Microbiol 1994;32:1203–1210.
207. Karita M, Tsuda M, Nakazawa T: Essential role of urease in vitro and in vivo *Helicobacter pylori* colonisation study using a wild-type and isogenic mutant strain. J Clin Gastroenterol 1995;21:S160–S163.
208. Steen T, Berstad K, Meling T, Berstad A: Reproducibility of the $^{14}$C urea breath test repeated after 1 week. Am J Gastroenterol 1995;90:2103–2105.
209. Graham DY, Klein PD, Evans DJ Jr, et al: *Campylobacter pylori* detected noninvasively by the $^{13}$C-urea breath test. Lancet 1987;1:1174–1177.
210. Corthesy-Theulaz I, Ferrero RL: Vaccines. Clin Opin Gastroenterol 1996;12:41–44.
211. Fox JG: Non-human reservoirs of *Helicobacter pylori*. Aliment Pharmacol Ther 1995;9:93–103.
212. Lee A, Hazell SL, O'Rourke J, Kouprach S: Isolation of a spiral-shaped bacterium from the cat stomach. Infect Immun 1988;56:2843–2850.
213. Czinn S, Ja JGN: Oral immunization against *Helicobacter pylori*. Infect Immun 1991;59:2359–2363.
214. Fox JG, Li X, Yan L, et al: Chronic proliferative hepatitis in A/JCr mice associated with persistent *Helicobacter* hepaticus infection: a model of *Helicobacter*-induced carcinogenesis. Infect Immun 1996;64:1548–1558.
215. Dixon MF, Genta RM, Yardley JH, Correa P, and the participants of the International Workshop on the Histopathology of Gastritis, Houston, 1994: Classification and grading of gastritis: the updated Sydney system. Am J Surg Pathol 1996;20:1161–1181.
216. Wyatt JI, Primrose J, Dixon MF: Distribution of *Campylobacter pylori* in gastric biopsies. J Pathol 1988;155:350.
217. El-Zimaity HMT, Al-Assi MR, Genta RM, Graham DY: Confirmation of successful therapy of *Helicobacter pylori* infection: number and site of biopsies or a rapid urease test. Am J Gastroenterol 1995;90:1962–1964.
218. Elta GH, Appelman HD, Behler EM, et al: A study of the correlation between endoscopic and histological diagnoses in gastroduodenitis. Am J Gastroenterol 1987;82:749–753.
219. Sauerbruch T, Schreiber MA, Schüssler P, Permanetter W: Endoscopy in the diagnosis of gastritis: diagnostic value of endoscopic criteria in relation to histologic diagnosis. Endoscopy 1984;16:101–104.
220. McNulty CA, Dent JC: Susceptibility of clinical isolates of *Campylobacter pylori* to twenty-one antimicrobial agents. Eur J Clin Microbiol 1988;7:566–569.
221. Hazell SL, Lee A: *Campylobacter pylori*, urease, hydrogen ion back diffusion, and gastric ulcers. Lancet 1986;2:15–17.
222. Marshall BJ, Langton SR: Urea hydrolysis in patients with *Campylobacter pylori* infection. Lancet 1986;2:965–966.
223. Abdalla S, Marco F, Perez RM, et al: Rapid detection of gastric *Campylobacter pylori* colonization by a simple biochemical test. J Clin Microbiol 1989;27:2604–2605.
224. Debognie JC, Pauwels S, Raat A, et al: Quantification of *Helicobacter pylori* infection in gastritis and ulcer disease using a simple and rapid carbon-14 urea breath test. J Nucl Med 1991;32:1192–1198.
225. Henze E, Malfertheiner P, Clausen M, et al: Validation of a simplified carbon-14-urea breath test for routine use for detecting *Helicobacter pylori* noninvasively. J Nucl Med 1990;31:1940–1944.
226. Marshall BJ, Surveyor I: Carbon-14 urea breath tests for the diagnosis of *Campylobacter pylori*-associated gastritis. J Nucl Med 1988;29:11–16.
227. Marshall BJ, Plankey MW, Hoffman SR, et al: A 20-minute breath test for *Helicobacter pylori*. Am J Gastroenterol 1991;86:438–445.
228. Newell DG, Rathbone BJ: The serodiagnosis of *Campylobacter pylori* infection. Serodiagn Immunother Infect Dis 1989;3:1–6.
229. Newell DG, Stacey AR: The serology of *Helicobacter pylori* infection, in Rathbone BJ (ed): *Helicobacter pylori* and gastroduodenal disease, vol 1. London: Blackwell Scientific Publications, 1992:64–73.
230. Chong SK, Lou Q, Asnicar MA, et al: *Helicobacter pylori* infection in recurrent abdominal pain in childhood: comparison of diagnostic tests and therapy. Pediatrics 1995;96:211–215.
231. Westblom TU, Madan E, Gudipati S, et al: Diagnosis of *Helicobacter pylori* infection in adult and pediatric patients by using Pyloriset, a rapid latex agglutination test. J Clin Microbiol 1992;30:96–98.
232. Megraud F: Epidemiology of *Helicobacter pylori* infection. Gastroenterol Clin North Am 1993;22:73–88.
233. Czinn SJ, Carr HS: Rapid diagnosis of *Campylobacter pyloridis* associated gastritis. J Pediatr 1987;110:569–570.
234. Khanna B, Cutler A, Perry M, et al: Sensitivity of commercially available serology tests to detect *Helicobacter pylori* infection in children. Gastroenterology 1997;112:A172.
235. Bickley J, Owen RJ, Fraser AG, Pounder RE: Evaluation of the polymerase chain reaction for detecting the urease C gene of *Helicobacter pylori* in gastric biopsy samples and dental plaque. J Med Microbiol 1993;39:338–344.
236. Kooistra-Smid AM, Schirm J, Snijder JA: Sensitivity of culture compared with that of polymerase chain reaction for detection of *Helicobacter pylori* from antral biopsy samples. J Clin Microbiol 1993;31:1918–1920.
237. Westblom TU, Phadnis S, Yang P, Czinn SJ: Diagnosis of *Helicobacter pylori* infection by means of a polymerase chain reaction assay for gastric juice aspirates. Clin Infect Dis 1993;16:367–371.
238. Nguyen AM, Engstrand L, Genta RM, Graham DY, et al: Detection of *Helicobacter pylori* in dental plaque by reverse transcription polymerase chain reaction. J Clin Microbiol 1993;31:783–787.
239. Mapstone NP, Lynch DA, Lewis FA, et al: PCR identification of *Helicobacter pylori* in faeces from gastritis patients. Lancet 1993;341:447.
240. Warren JR, Marshall BJ: Unidentified curved bacilli on gastric epithelium in active chronic gastritis. Lancet 1983;1:1273–1275.
241. Cheng EH, Bermanski P, Silversmith M, et al: Prevalence of *Campylobacter pylori* in esophagitis, gastritis, and duodenal disease. Arch Intern Med 1990;150:1132–1134.
242. Peterson WL: *Helicobacter pylori* and peptic ulcer disease. N Engl J Med 1991;324:1043–1048.
243. Hill R, Pearman J, Worthy P, et al: *Campylobacter pyloridis* and gastritis in children. Lancet 1986;1:387.
244. Cadranel S, Goossens H, DeBoeck M, et al: *Campylobacter pyloridis* in children. Lancet 1986;1:735–736.
245. Mahony MJ, Wyatt JI, Littlewood JM: *Campylobacter pylori* gastritis. Arch Dis Child 1988;63:654–655.
246. Kilbridge PM, Dahms BB, Czinn SJ: *Campylobacter pylori* associated gastritis and peptic ulcer disease in children. Am J Dis Child 1988;142:1149–1152.
247. Yeung CK, Fu KH, Yuen KY, et al: *Helicobacter pylori* and associated duodenal ulcer. Arch Dis Child 1990;65:1212–1216.
248. Blecker U, Mehta DI, Vandenplas Y: Sex-ratio of *Helicobacter pylori* infection in childhood. Am J Gastroenterol 1994;89:243.
249. Bujanover Y, Konikoff F, Baratz M: Nodular gastritis and *Helicobacter pylori*. J Pediatr Gastroenterol Nutr 1990;11:41–44.
250. Sbeih F, Abdullah A, Sullivan S, Merenkov Z: Antral nodularity, gastric lymphoid hyperplasia, and *Helicobacter pylori* in adults. J Clin Gastroenterol 1996;22:227–230.
251. Dooley CP, Cohen H: The clinical significance of *Campylobacter pylori*. Ann Intern Med 1988;108:70–79.
252. Recavarren-Arce S, Leon-Barua R, Cok J, et al: *Helicobacter pylori* and progressive gastric pathology that predisposes to gastric cancer. Scand J Gastroenterol 1991;18:51–57.
253. Correa P, Fox J, Fontham E, et al: *Helicobacter pylori* and gastric carcinoma: serum antibody prevalence in populations with contrasting cancer risks. Cancer 1990;66:2569–2574.
254. Parsonnet J, Vandersteen D, Goates J, et al: *Helicobacter pylori* infection in intestinal and diffuse type gastric adenocarcinoma. J Natl Cancer Inst 1991;83:640–643.
255. Parsonnet J, Friedman GD, Vandersteen DP, et al: *Helicobacter pylori* infection and the risk of gastric carcinoma. N Engl J Med 1991;325:1127–1131.
256. Fox JG, Correa P, Taylor NS, et al: *Campylobacter pylori*-associated

gastritis and immune response in a population at increased risk of gastric carcinoma. Am J Gastroenterol 1989;84:775–781.

257. Joly DJ: Resources for the control of cancer in Latin America: preliminary survey. Bol Sanit Panam 1977;83:330–345.
258. Parkin DM: Cancer occurrence in developing countries. Lyon: IARC Scientific Publications, 1986;75:1–39.
259. Young JJ, Percy CL, Asire AJ, et al: Cancer incidence and mortality in the United States, 1973–1977. NCI Monogr 1981;57:1–187.
260. Haenszel W, Kurihara M, Segi M, et al: Stomach cancer among Japanese in Hawaii. J Natl Cancer Inst 1972;49:969–988.
261. McMichael AJ, McCall MG, Hartshorne JM, et al: Patterns of gastrointestinal cancer in European migrants to Australia: the role of dietary change. Int J Cancer 1980;25:431–437.
262. Rosenwaike I: Cancer mortality among Puerto Rican-born residents in New York City. Am J Epidemiol 1984;119:177–185.
263. Correa P, Haenszel W, Cuello C, et al: Gastric precancerous process in a high risk population: cohort follow-up. Cancer Res 1990;50:4737–4740.
264. Lansdown M, Quirke P, Dixon M, et al: High grade dysplasia of the gastric mucosa: a marker for gastric carcinoma. Gut 1990;31:977–983.
265. Ming SC: Adenocarcinoma and other malignant epithelial tumors of the stomach. In Ming SC, Goldman H (eds): Pathology of the Gastrointestinal Tract, vol 1. Philadelphia: WB Saunders, 1992, pp 584–618.
266. Robert ME, Weinstein WM: *Helicobacter pylori*-associated gastric pathology. Gastroenterol Clin North Am 1993;22:59–72.
267. Kosunen TU, Seppälä K, Sarna S, et al: Diagnostic value of decreasing IgG, IgA, and IgM antibody titres after eradication of *Helicobacter pylori*. Lancet 1992;339:893–895.
268. Brooks JJ, Enterline HT: Primary gastric lymphomas: a clinicopathologic study of 58 cases with long-term follow-up and literature review. Cancer 1983;51:701–711.
269. Spiro HM: Gastric lymphomas. In Spiro HM (ed): Clinical Gastroenterology. New York: Macmillan, 1983, pp 292–297.
270. Rubin E, Farber JL: The gastrointestinal tract. In Rubin E, Farber, JL (eds): Essential pathology, vol 1. Philadelphia: JB Lippincott, 1990, pp 352–392.
271. Villar HV, Wong R, Paz B, et al: Immuno-phenotyping in the management of gastric lymphoma. Am J Surg 1991;161:171–175.
272. Doglioni C, Wotherspoon AC, Moschini A, et al: High incidence of primary gastric lymphoma in Northeastern Italy. Lancet 1992;339:834–835.
273. Forman D, Sitas F, Newell DG, et al: Geographic association of *Helicobacter pylori* antibody prevalence and gastric cancer mortality. Int J Cancer 1990;46:608–611.
274. Parsonnet J, Hansen S, Rodriguez L, et al: *Helicobacter pylori* infection and gastric lymphoma. N Engl J Med 1994;330:1267–1271.
275. Talley NJ, Zinsmeister AR, Weaver A, et al: Gastric adenocarcinoma and *Helicobacter pylori* infection. J Natl Cancer Inst 1991;83:1734–1739.
276. Wotherspoon AC, Ortiz-Hidalgo C, Falzon MR, et al: *Helicobacter pylori*-associated gastritis and primary B-cell gastric lymphoma. Lancet 1991;338:1175–1176.
277. Isaacson PG, Spencer J: Malignant lymphoma of mucosa-associated lymphoid tissue. Histopathology 1987;11:445–462.
278. Chan JKC, Ng CS, Isaacson PG: Relationship between high-grade lymphoma and low-grade B-cell mucosa associated lymphoid tissue lymphoma (MALToma) of the stomach. Am J Pathol 1990;136:1153–1164.
279. Isaacson PG, Wright DH: Malignant lymphoma of mucosa-associated lymphoid tissue: a distinctive type of B-cell lymphoma. Cancer 1983;52:1410–1416.
280. Stolte M, Eidt S: Lymphoid follicles in the antral mucosa: immune response to *Campylobacter pylori*. J Clin Pathol 1989;42:1269–1271.
281. Hussell T, Isaacson PG, Crabtree JE, et al: The response of cells from low-grade B-cell gastric lymphomas of mucosa-associated lymphoid tissue to *Helicobacter pylori*. Lancet 1993;342:571–574.
282. Isaacson PG, Wotherspoon AC, Diss TC, et al: Follicular colonization in B-cell lymphoma of mucosa-associated lymphoid tissue. Am J Surg Pathol 1991;15:819–828.
283. Greiner A, Marx A, Schausser B, Muller-Hermelink HK: The pivotal role of the immunoglobulin receptor of tumor cells from B-cell lymphomas of mucosa associated lymphoid tissue (MALT). Adv Exp Med Biol 1994;355:189–193.
284. Wotherspoon AC, Doglioni C, Diss TC, et al: Regression of primary low-grade B-cell gastric lymphoma of mucosa-associated lymphoid tissue type after eradication of *Helicobacter pylori*. Lancet 1993;342:575–577.
285. Bayerdörffer E, Neubauer A, Eidt S, et al: Double-blind treatment of early gastric malt-lymphoma patients by *H. pylori* eradication (abstract). Gastroenterology 1994;106:370.
286. Blecker U, McKeithan TW, Hart J, Kirschner BS: Resolution of *Helicobacter pylori* associated gastric lymphoproliferative disease in a child. Gastroenterology 1995;109:973–977.
287. Rowland M, Kuman D, O'Connor P, et al: Reinfection with *Helicobacter pylori* in children. Gastroenterology 1997;112:A273.
288. Wyatt JI, Rathbone BJ: Immune response of the gastric mucosa to *Campylobacter pylori*. Scand J Gastroenterol 1988;23:44–49.
289. Anonymous. NIH Consensus Conference: *Helicobacter pylori* in peptic ulcer disease. JAMA 1994;272:65–69.
290. Gormally S, Drumm B: *Helicobacter pylori* and gastrointestinal symptoms. Arch Dis Child 1994;70:165–166.
291. Gormally SM, Prakash N, Durnin MT, et al: Symptoms in children before and after treatment of *Helicobacter pylori* infection. J Pediatr 1995;126:753–756.
292. Silverstein MD, Peterson T, Talley NJ: Initial endoscopy or empirical therapy with or without testing for *Helicobacter pylori* for dyspepsia: a decision analysis. Gastroenterology 1996;110:72–83.
293. Reifen R, Rasooly I, Drumm B, et al: *Helicobacter pylori* infection in children: Is there specific symptomatology? Dig Dis Sci 1994;39:1488–1492.
294. Blecker U, Hauser B, Lanciers S, et al: Symptomatology of *Helicobacter pylori*. Acta Paediatr 1996;85:1156–1158.
295. Blecker U, Hauser B, Lanciers S, et al: The prevalence of *Helicobacter pylori*-positive serology in asymptomatic children. J Pediatr Gastroenterol Nutr 1993;16:252–256.
296. Lai ST, Fung KP, Ng FH, Lee KC: A quantitative analysis of non-ulcer dypepsia as related to age, pathology and *Helicobacter pylori* infection. Scand J Gastroenterol 1996;31:1078–1082.
297. Fiedorek SC, Malaty HM, Evans DL, et al: Factors influencing the epidemiology of *Helicobacter pylori* infection in children. Pediatrics 1991;88:578–582.
298. Mahoney MJ, Wyatt JI: Management and response to treatment of *Helicobacter pylori* gastritis. Arch Dis Child 1992;67:940–943.
299. van Zanten S, Sherman P: A systematic overview of *Helicobacter pylori* infection as the cause of gastritis, duodenal ulcer, gastric cancer and non-ulcer dyspepsia: applying eight diagnostic criteria in establishing causation. Can Med Assoc J 1994;150:177–185.
300. Talley NJ: A critique of therapeutic trials in *Helicobacter pylori*-positive functional dyspepsia. Gastroenterology 1994;106:1174–1183.
301. Puri P: Duodenal ulcer in childhood: a continuing disease in adult life. J Pediatr Surg 1978;13:525–526.
302. Deckelbaum RJ, Roy CC, Lussier-Lazaroff J: Peptic ulcer disease: a clinical study of 73 children. Can Med Assoc J 1974;111:225–228.
303. Levy M, Miller DR, Kaufman DW, et al: Major upper gastrointestinal tract bleeding: relation to the use of aspirin and other non-narcotic analgesics. Arch Intern Med 1988;148:281–285.
304. Stillman AE, Mantheir U, Pinnas J: Transient protein-losing enteropathy and enlarged gastric rugae. Am J Dis Child 1981;135:29–33.
305. Adeyemi SD, Ein SH, Simpson JS: Perforated stress ulcer in infants. Ann Surg 1979;190:706–708.
306. Hargrove CB, Ulshen MH, Shub MD: Upper gastrointestinal endoscopy in infants: diagnostic usefulness and safety. Pediatrics 1984;74:828–831.
307. Dooley CP: Double contrast barium meal and upper gastrointestinal endoscopy. Ann Intern Med 1984;101:538–545.
308. Miller V, Doig CM: Upper gastrointestinal tract endoscopy. Arch Dis Child 1984;59:1100–1102.
309. Roca MSCT, Whitehead R: The histological state of the gastric and duodenal mucosa in healthy volunteers. Gut 1975;16:404–410.
310. Whitehead R, Truelove SC, Gear MW: The histological diagnosis of chronic gastritis in fibreoptic gastroscope biopsy specimens. J Clin Pathol 1972;25:1–11.
311. Strickland RG, Mackay IR: A reappraisal of the nature and significance of chronic atrophic gastritis. Dig Dis Sci 1973;18:426–440.
312. Correa P: The epidemiology and pathogenesis of chronic gastritis: three etiologic entities. Front Gastrointest Res 1980;6:98–108.
313. Correa P: Chronic gastritis: a clinico-pathological classification. Am J Gastroenterol 1988;83:504–509.
314. Wyatt J, Dixon MF: Chronic gastritis: a pathogenetic approach. J Pathol 1988;154:113–124.

315. Hassall E, Israel DJ: Unique features of *Helicobacter pylori* disease in children. Dig Dis Sci 1991;36:417–423.
316. Rosh JR, Kurfist LA, Benkov KJ, et al: *Helicobacter pylori* and gastric lymphonodular hyperplasia in children. Am J Gastroenterol 1992;87:135–139.
317. Price A: The Sydney System: histological division. J Gastroenterol Hepatol 1991;6:209–222.
318. Quieroz DMM, Rocha GA, Mendes EN, et al: Differences in the distribution and severity of *Helicobacter pylori* gastritis in children and adults with duodenal ulcer disease. J Pediatr Gastroenterol Nutr 1991;12:178–181.
319. Collins JS, Sloan JM, Hamilton PW, et al: Investigation of the relationship between gastric antral inflammation and *Campylobacter pylori* using graphic tablet planimetry. J Pathol 1989;159:281–285.
320. Loffeld RJLF, Potters HV, Arends JW, et al: *Campylobacter pylori* associated gastritis in patients with non-ulcer dyspepsia. J Pathol 1988;41:85–88.
321. Siurala M, Sipponen P, Kekki M: *Campylobacter pylori* in a sample of Finnish population: relations to morphology and functions of the gastric mucosa. Gut 1988;29:909–915.
322. Tominag K: Distribution of parietal cells in the antral mucosa of human stomachs. Gastroenterology 1975;69:1201–1207.
323. Robert A: Cytoprotection by prostaglandins. Gastroenterology 1979;77:761–767.
324. Konturek SJ, Brzozowski T, Drozdow D, et al: Healing of chronic gastroduodenal ulcerations by antacids, role of prostaglandins and epidermal growth factor. Dig Dis Sci 1990;35:1121–1129.
325. Sontag SJ: Prostaglandins in peptic ulcer disease: an overview of current status and future directions. Drugs 1986;32:445–457.
326. Szabo S: The mode of action of sucralfate: the $1 \times 1 \times 1$ mechanism of action. Scand J Gastroenterol 1991;185:7–12.
327. Szabo S, Hollander D: Pathways of gastrointestinal protection and repair: mechanism of action of sucralfate. Am J Med 1989;83:91–94.
328. McCarthy DM: Sucralfate. N Engl J Med 1991;325:1017–1025.
329. Chiang BL, Chiang MH, Lin MI, et al: Chronic duodenal ulcer in children: clinical observation and response to treatment. J Pediatr Gastroenterol Nutr 1989;8:161–165.
330. Thomason MH, Payseur ES, Hakeneworth AM, et al: Nosocomial pneumonia in ventilated trauma patients during stress ulcer prophylaxis with sucralfate, antacid, and ranitidine. J Trauma 1996;41:503–508.
331. Peterson WL: Healing of duodenal ulcer with antacids. N Engl J Med 1977;297:341–345.
332. Weberg R, Aubert E, Dahlberg O, et al: Low-dose antacids or cimetidine for duodenal ulcer? Gastroenterology 1988;95:1465–1469.
333. Cook DJ, Reeve BK, Guyatt GH, et al: Stress ulcer prophylaxis in critically ill patients: resolving discordant meta-analysis. J Am Med Assoc 1996;275:308–314.
334. Feldman M: Inhibition of gastric acid secretion by selective and non-selective anticholinergics. Gastroenterology 1984;86:361–366.
335. Texter ED, Reilly PA: The efficacy and selectivity of pirenzepine: review and commentary. Scand J Gastroenterol 1982;72:237–246.
336. DeGiacomo C, Fiocca R, Villani L, et al: Omeprazole treatment of severe peptic disease associated with antral G cell hyperfunction and hyperpepsinogenemia I in an infant. J Pediatr 1990;117:989–993.
337. Sanders SW: Pathogenesis and treatment of acid peptic disorders: comparison of proton pump inhibitors with other antiulcer agents. Clin Ther 1996;18:2–34.
338. Maton PN: Omeprazole. N Engl J Med 1991;324:965–975.
339. Ekman L, Hansson E, Havu N, et al: Toxicologic studies on omeprazole. Scand J Gastroenterol 1985;108:53–69.
340. Walan A: Clinical utility and safety of omeprazole: the first proton pump inhibitor. Med Res Rev 1990;10:1–54.
341. Freston JW: Long-term acid control and proton pump inhibitors: interactions and safety issues in perspective. Am J Gastroenterol 1997;92:51S–55S.
342. Kato S, Ebina K, Fujii K, et al: Effect of omeprazole in the treatment of refractory acid-related diseases in childhood: endoscopic healing and twenty-four hour intragastric acidity. J Pediatr 1996;128:415–421.
343. Lamberts R, Creutzfeldt W, Struber HG, et al: Long-term omeprazole therapy in peptic ulcer disease: gastrin, endocrine cell growth, and gastritis. Gastroenterology 1993;104:1356–1370.
344. Solcia E, Villani L, Fiocca R, et al: Effects of eradication of *Helicobacter pylori* on gastritis in duodenal ulcer patients. Scand J Gastroenterol 1994;201:28–34.
345. Sherman P, Shames B, Loo V, et al: Omeprazole therapy for *Helicobacter pylori* infection. Scand J Gastroenterol 1992;27:1018–1022.
346. Logan RP, Gummett PA, Schaufelberger HD, et al: Eradication of *Helicobacter pylori* with clarithromycin and omeprazole. Gut 1994;35:323–326.
347. Lind T, van Zanten SV, Unge P, et al: Eradication of *Helicobacter pylori* using one-week triple therapies combining omeprazole with two antimicrobials: the MACH I study. Helicobacter 1996;1:138–144.
348. Dohil R, Israel DM, Hassall E: Effective 2-week therapy for *Helicobacter pylori* disease in children. Am J Gastroenterol 1997;92:244–247.

# Chapter 19

# Gastropathies: Pathophysiology and Clinical Features

*Nicola L. Jones and Philip M. Sherman*

Since the advent of fiberoptic endoscopy and mucosal biopsy, identification and investigation of disorders affecting the gastric mucosa have increased greatly. Gastritis and peptic ulcer disease were previously classified as being of either primary (idiopathic) or secondary origin.[1] Most cases of "primary" gastritis are caused by previously unrecognized *Helicobacter pylori* infection. Secondary gastritis and associated ulceration are caused by specific diseases (e.g., Crohn's disease, eosinophilic gastroenteritis, infections) or the use of exogenous agents such as nonsteroidal anti-inflammatory drugs (NSAIDs).

The precise pathogenic mechanisms resulting in gastritis and subsequent peptic ulceration are not clearly understood. It has long been suggested that an imbalance between aggressive factors that damage the mucosal integrity and protective mucosal defenses (cytoprotection) play a role in the development of gastric inflammation.[2, 3] The host and bacterial factors related to disease pathogenesis after *H. pylori* infection are current areas of intense investigation.[4] *H. pylori* infection and disease pathogenesis are discussed in detail in Chapter 18 and therefore are only briefly covered in this chapter.

## ETIOLOGY

### Infections

The infectious causes of gastritis are summarized in Table 19–1.

#### *Helicobacter pylori*

*H. pylori* infection fulfills each of Koch's postulates as a cause of chronic active gastritis in humans.[5] Although this is not true for *H. pylori* as a cause of peptic ulcer disease,[6] the evidencc is compelling. Eradication of infection decreases the recurrence rate of duodenal ulcer from approximately 80% to 3% at 1 year of follow-up.[7] Therefore, eradication of *H. pylori* alters the natural history of peptic ulcer disease. In addition, *H. pylori* infection is epidemiologically associated with the subsequent development of gastric cancers, including adenocarcinoma, lymphoma, and mucosa-associated lymphoid tissue (MALT) lymphoma.[7]

#### *Helicobacter heilmannii*

Previously known as *Gastrosporillum hominis*,[8] *Helicobacter heilmannii* is genetically closely related to the cat and dog helicobacter, *Helicobacter felis*.[9] The organism is larger and more elongated than *H. pylori*.[9] In the largest published series, *H. heilmannii* was identified in 39 of 15,180 gastric biopsy specimens.[10] In children, a prevalence of infection of 0.3% was reported by Oliva and colleagues.[11] The majority of infected patients have evidence of mild chronic gastritis. A comparative analysis of 202 matched patients identified a milder severity of gastritis in patients with *H. heilmannii* infection compared with those infected with *H. pylori*.[12] The presence of peptic ulceration in association with this infection has been reported on rare occasions both in adults and children.[13, 14] In addition, cases of gastric cancer and MALT

**TABLE 19–1. Infectious Causes of Gastritis**

| | |
|---|---|
| Bacteria | *Helicobacter pylori*<br>*Helicobacter heilmannii*<br>*Mycobacterium avium–intracellulare*<br>*Mycobacterium tuberculosis*<br>*Treponema pallidum* |
| Virus | Cytomegalovirus<br>Herpes simplex virus<br>Varicella-zoster virus |
| Fungal | *Pneumocystis carinii*<br>*Rhizopus oryzae* (Zygomycetes) |
| Parasitic | *Anisakis simplex* |
| Protozoa | *Cryptosporidium parvum* |

lymphoma in association with *H. heilmannii* infection have been described.[12, 15, 16]

To date, it has not been possible to culture this fastidious organism by standard microbiologic techniques. Therefore, the potential virulence factors of *H. heilmannii* have not been formally evaluated. However, the colonization of a specific-pathogen-free murine model has allowed molecular characterization of certain features of the organism, such as the presence of the urease enzyme.[9, 17]

### Other Bacteria

Compared with infection with helicobacters, gastritis caused by infection with other bacterial, viral, or parasitic pathogens occurs only rarely. However, in immunocompromised children the frequency of infections increases substantially.[18, 19] Other rare gastric infections in immunodeficient patients include *Mycobacterium avium-intracellulare,* which causes refractory gastric ulceration.[20]

### Viruses

Isolated reports have identified herpes simplex virus as a cause of gastritis in patients with primary or secondary immunodeficiencies.[21] Both gastritis and esophagitis with histopathologic evidence of eosinophilic nuclear inclusion bodies typical for herpes simplex virus were described in a patient receiving immunosuppressive agents. Rare cases of gastric involvement during disseminated varicella-zoster virus (VSV) infection in immunocompromised patients were also reported.[22] A bone marrow transplant recipient with disseminated VSV underwent endoscopic evaluation for severe abdominal pain and vomiting. Histopathologic assessment of gastric biopsies showed nonspecific gastritis with the presence of herpes viral particles detected by electron microscopy and VSV-specific DNA detected with the use of the polymerase chain reaction. For cytomegalovirus (CMV), see the discussion of Ménétrier's disease in a later section.

### Parasites

Acute gastric anisakiasis has been reported in immunocompetent adults after consumption of raw fish, particularly in the form of sushi or sashimi.[23] Symptoms consisting of epigastric pain, nausea, vomiting, and urticaria typically occur within 1 to 12 hours after the ingestion of raw fish. Endoscopic findings include severe erosive gastritis, edema, and the presence of single or multiple worms. So far, no cases of gastric anisakiasis have been reported in children.

### Fungi

Gastric fungal infection is an infrequent occurrence in immunocompetent patients. In contrast, the risk of infection is increased in persons with primary or secondary immunodeficiencies. For example, *Pneumocystis carinii* infection of the stomach is described in patients with the acquired immunodeficiency syndrome.[24, 25] Among 37 patients with extrapulmonary infection with *P. carinii* identified at autopsy, 22% had evidence of gastrointestinal involvement.[25] Isolated cases of zygomycosis, also known as mucormycosis,[26, 27] caused by infection with the Zygomycetes class of fungi have also been reported. These ubiquitous organisms are not pathogenic in the normal host but can produce serious infections in immunocompromised individuals. *Rhizopus oryzae* infection resulting in gastric perforation in a neonate was believed to be contracted from elastic bandages.[26] Both gastric and small bowel perforations were reported in a neonate with zygomycosis.[27]

### Protozoa

*Cryptosporidium parvum* infection typically causes an enteritis.[28] However, cases of partial gastric outlet obstruction caused by cryptosporidium occur in immunocompromised patients.[29] A patient with the acquired immunodeficiency syndrome and diarrhea due to cryptosporidiosis developed symptoms suggestive of gastric outlet obstruction. Endoscopic findings included evidence of inflammation and partial obstruction of the pyloric channel with cryptosporidial organisms identified in the gastric biopsy specimen.

## Ménétrier's Disease

Ménétrier's disease in childhood and infancy is a relatively uncommon disorder characterized by hypertrophy of gastric rugae in the body of the stomach and a protein-losing gastropathy. It has several features that distinguish it from the adult form of the disease. Symptoms in children often begin abruptly and resolve spontaneously, with a mean duration of symptoms of approximately 6 weeks.[30, 31] In contrast, adults develop a more severe and chronic condition.[32] The average age at presentation in children is 5 years, and there is a slight predilection for males.[30]

Edema and vomiting are the most frequent presenting symptoms. Radiographically, the characteristic hypertrophied gastric rugae are identified by upper gastrointestinal series predominantly in the fundic region (Fig. 19–1).[33] The demonstration of a thickened gastric lining by additional diagnostic imaging modalities, including ultrasound and computed axial tomography, have also been reported.[34, 35] Endoscopically, most patients have swollen gastric rugae with large quantities of adherent gelatinous material.[30] Microscopic findings include hypertrophic and dilated gastric glands filled with mucus and occasionally exhibiting a sawtooth appearance, referred to as hypertrophic gastropathy. An inflammatory infiltrate consisting of neutrophils, eosinophils, and lymphocytes is present within the lamina propria.

Ménétrier's disease in childhood has been identified as having an infectious origin, and CMV appears to be the causal agent.[31, 36] Although CMV can infect any part of the gastrointestinal tract, gastric involvement in immunocompetent children frequently is associated with Ménétrier's disease. The presence of CMV infection can be identified in approximately 30% of children with Ménétrier's disease, either by culture of the virus from gastric tissue[30] or by serologic techniques.[30, 36] In immunodeficient patients, thickened folds, erosions, and ulcerations may be seen endoscopically. Gastric infection is frequently found in association with other organ involvement in patients who have undergone organ transplantation.[37, 38] CMV infection is diagnosed by endoscopy and biopsy. CMV-infected cells appear enlarged, with intranuclear acidophilic and cytoplasmic baso-

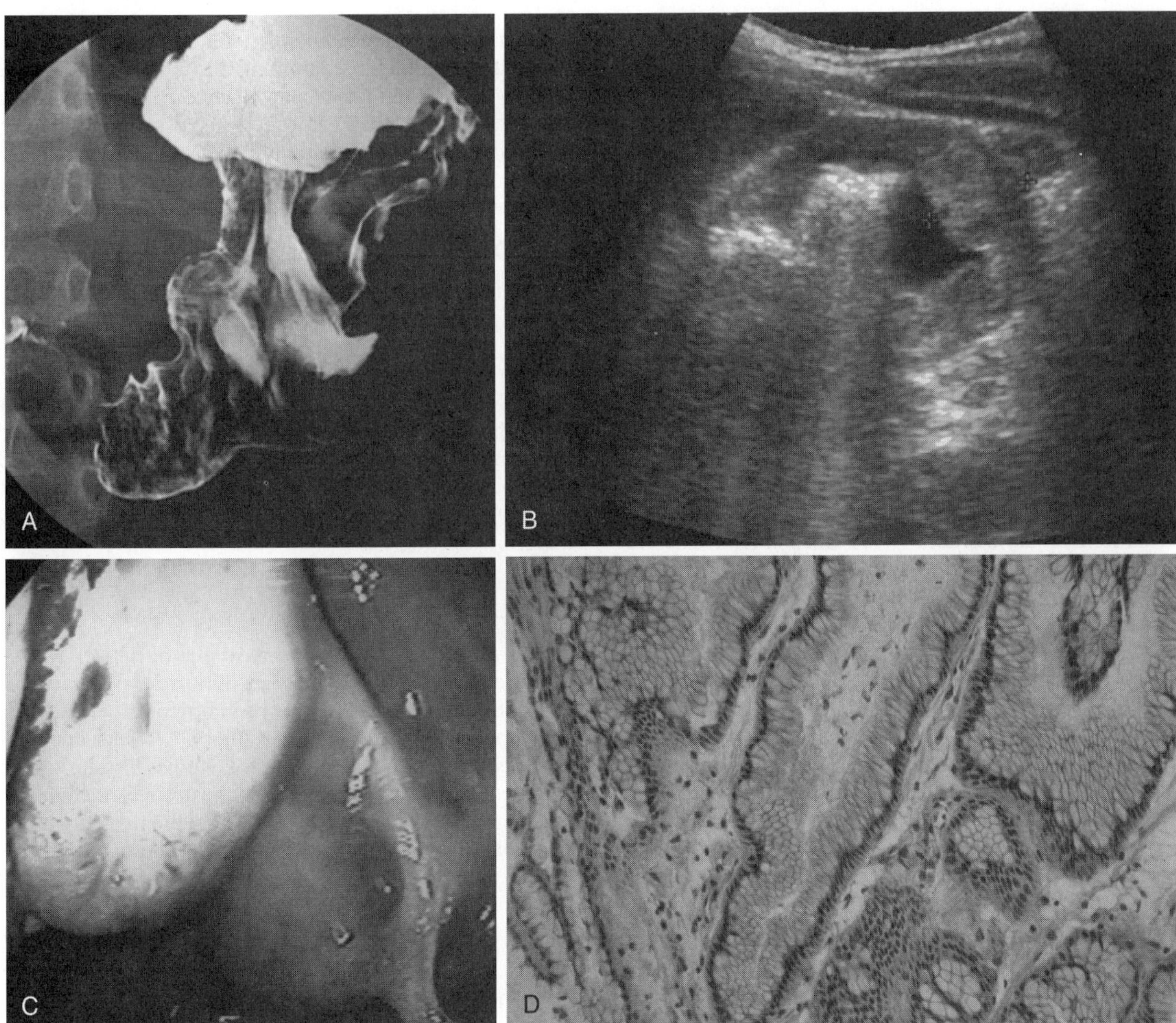


**FIGURE 19–1.** Diagnostic studies of a 5-year-old boy who presented with vomiting and hypoproteinemia. *A,* Upper gastrointestinal study demonstrating thickened folds in the body of the stomach. *B,* Abdominal sonogram of the stomach demonstrating thickening of the mucosal folds as outlined by cursors. *C,* Endoscopic findings of prominent gastric rugae with adherent gelatinous material. *D,* Histolopathologic findings of biopsy from the gastric body. Hypertrophic gastric glands are filled with mucus and exhibit a sawtooth appearance characteristic of Ménétrier's disease. (*A* and *B*, Courtesy of Dr. B. Shuckett, The Hospital for Sick Children, Toronto.)

philic inclusion bodies.[39] If findings on hematoxylin and eosin staining are equivocal, special techniques such as immunohistochemistry, in situ hybridization, and polymerase chain reaction can be used to confirm CMV infection.[40, 41]

The presence of intranuclear inclusion bodies in gastric biopsy specimens obtained from children with Ménétrier's disease is indirect evidence suggestive of a role for CMV in this disease. In one case report, the presence of acute infection with CMV in a child was associated with Ménétrier's disease.[42] The child presented with a 12-day history of vomiting, epigastric pain, weight loss, and hypoalbuminemia. Radiographic and pathologic findings were consistent with Ménétrier's disease. At presentation, an increase in CMV-specific immunoglobulin M (IgM) in serum and detection of early antigen of CMV in the gastric biopsy specimen was followed by conversion to CMV-specific IgG antibodies at follow-up. Thus, virologic studies confirmed acute infection with CMV.

Infection with *H. pylori* and a protein-losing hypertrophic gastropathy also has been reported both in adults and children.[43–45] However, the classic histologic features of Ménétrier's disease are not present. Moreover, a low frequency of *H. pylori* infection was identified in adult patients with Ménétrier's disease.[32] These data indicate that *H. pylori* infection is probably not an important factor in disease pathogenesis.

A potential role for transforming growth factor-α (TGF-α) in disease pathogenesis is provided by studies of transgenic mice.[46] Transgenic mice with inducible overexpression of TGF-α exhibit clinical and histologic features resembling those of Ménétrier's disease in humans.[47] On induction of TGF-α overexpression, the mice develop an enlarged stomach with nodular mucosal lesions. A phenotype of foveolar hyperplasia similar to that found in Ménétrier's disease is observed histologically in association with an increase in TGF-α in both glandular and surface epithelia. In pediatric and adult patients with Ménétrier's disease, increased levels of TGF-α messenger RNA and translated protein are detectable in the gastric mucosa.[31, 46] These studies provide evidence for a role of elevated TGF-α in disease pathogenesis, possibly as a result of infection with CMV.

## Drugs/Toxins

### Nonsteroidal Anti-inflammatory Agents

NSAID use is associated with hemorrhagic gastric erosions most often in the fundus and with gastric ulcerations in the antrum of the stomach[48] (see Chapter 18). The frequency of such complications even in adult patients is low but rises with advancing age.[49] Prospective studies to examine the frequency of upper gastrointestinal disease related to NSAID use among children are lacking. Retrospective studies among children with juvenile rheumatoid arthritis receiving a variety of NSAIDs indicate that the incidence of significant gastrointestinal side effects is low.[50, 51] However, severe complications of mucosal erosions and ulceration, including gastrointestinal bleeding, have been described in association with high-dose aspirin therapy used in the treatment of Kawasaki's disease[52] and when oral sulindac was used for treatment of a patent ductus arteriosus.[53]

Histopathologic features characteristic of NSAID-induced gastropathy include foveolar hyperplasia, vasodilation, edema, a notable lack of inflammatory cells, and the presence of muscle fibers in the lamina propria.[54] These features are not consistently present nor specific to NSAID-induced gastritis and therefore cannot be relied on to establish a conclusive diagnosis of chemical gastritis.[55]

Several mechanisms could explain the increased risk of gastric mucosal damage with NSAID use, including suppression of prostaglandin synthesis, increased neutrophil adherence, decreased mucosal blood flow, and alterations in the mucus gel layer.[56] Current evidence does not provide support for an interaction with *H. pylori* infection in the pathogenesis of NSAID-related gastric disease.[57] NSAIDs reduce prostaglandin synthesis by inhibiting cyclo-oxygenase. Two forms of cyclo-oxygenase exist—COX-1, which is constitutively active, and COX-2, which is inducible during inflammation.[58] Evidence suggests that the inhibition of COX-1 activity produces the adverse effects of NSAIDs.[58] The side effect profiles of various NSAIDs are closely related to the level of inhibition of COX-1.[56, 58] However, the report of a transgenic COX-1 knockout mouse that does not develop spontaneous gastric injury but still develops gastric erosions in response to oral NSAID administration has raised some questions regarding the biologic plausibility of this theory.[59]

Misoprostol, a prostaglandin analogue, is beneficial in preventing NSAID-related gastropathy. [60] In a retrospective chart review of children attending a rheumatology clinic over a 3-year period, 22 children were prescribed misoprostol for gastrointestinal symptoms considered to be related to NSAID use.[61] In 82%, symptoms resolved completely in association with an increase in mean hemoglobin concentration. To date, no controlled studies examining the effect of misoprostol therapy in children have been reported. However, concerns raised about both the cost-effectiveness of prophylaxis with misoprostol[62, 63] and the side effects associated with its use[64] do not support widespread prophylactic therapy at this time.

The efficacy of prophylaxis with acid-suppression therapy for NSAID-induced gastric damage also remains controversial.[60, 65–67] Acid suppression with histamine $H_2$ receptor antagonists or proton-pump inhibitors during NSAID use may reduce gastric ulcer formation.[65, 66] However, evidence in an animal model suggests that antisecretory agents also reduce the therapeutic activity of NSAIDs.[67] A recent meta-analysis showed that treatment with $H_2$ blockers was without benefit in the prevention of NSAID-induced gastric ulcers.[60] Additional novel approaches under evaluation include NSAIDs in association with other compounds such as nitric oxide[68] or zwitterionic phospholipids,[69] and highly selective COX-2 inhibitors.[70]

### Corticosteroids

The ability of steroids to cause gastric mucosal damage had been controversial since an initial meta-analysis failed to identify an association between corticosteroid use and the development of gastric mucosal injury.[71] A subsequent meta-analysis pooled the data from 71 studies in adult patients and identified an increased risk for gastrointestinal ulceration and hemorrhage among patients who were treated with corticosteroids that was proportional to the dosage employed.[72] Similar studies have not been performed in children. The mechanism for induction of gastric mucosal damage is not known but could relate to effects on prostanoid synthesis.[73]

### Ethanol

Ethanol ingestion in humans causes petechiae, mucosal erosions, and hemorrhage from the stomach.[74, 75] A single dose of 40% alcohol causes mucosal congestion and hemorrhage within minutes of intake.[74] Superficial gastric mucosal hemorrhages were observed in 20 of 125 adults who regularly consumed alcohol and underwent diagnostic upper endoscopy.[75]

### Gastrostomy Tubes

The use of gastrostomy tubes for supplemental enteral nutrition in a variety of chronic conditions (e.g., cystic fibrosis, cerebral palsy, Crohn's disease) is increasing.[76] There have been case reports describing injury to the lining of the stomach after placement of gastrostomy feeding tubes.[77] Whether the mucosal injury is directly associated with symptomatology other than focal hemorrhage remains unclear.

### Other Agents

Gastric ulceration has been reported in association with stimulant abuse, including abuse of cocaine and methamphetamines.[78] Additional exogenous agents reported to cause gastritis include antibiotics (e.g., penicillin, ampicillin, chloramphenicol, tetracycline, cephalosporins), the anticonvulsant valproic acid,[79, 80] and 5-amino-salicylic acid (ASA) compounds.

## Stress

Several clinical conditions are associated with stress-induced gastric ulceration, including sepsis, brain injuries,[81] and burns.[82] The results of several large prospective studies in both adult and pediatric patients suggest that the incidence of clinically significant gastrointestinal bleeding in critically ill patients is low.[83] For example, a prospective study found that only 4 of 984 children admitted to a pediatric intensive care unit had significant gastrointestinal bleeding—defined as bleeding requiring transfusion, causing hypotension, or resulting in death.[84] Risk factors for gastrointestinal bleeding that were identified in these children included coagulopathy and prolonged mechanical ventilation.

## Crohn's Disease

Crohn's disease is covered in detail in Chapter 32 and therefore is covered only briefly in this section. Studies in pediatric populations have identified gastroduodenal inflammation in a significant proportion of patients with Crohn's disease.[85, 86] Children with gastroduodenal involvement are more likely to have extensive disease involving both the small bowel and the large intestine.[87] A review of 25 patients with Crohn's disease undergoing upper gastrointestinal endoscopy and biopsy identified acute and chronic gastritis in 10 subjects, with granulomas present in the mucosa of 3 of the 10 cases.[88] The presence of coexisting infection with *H. pylori* in pediatric studies has not been determined. However, in two studies of adult patients with Crohn's disease, evidence of gastritis was present in 34% and 76% of patients after exclusion of *H. pylori* infection.[89, 90]

## Eosinophilic Gastritis

Eosinophilic gastritis is a condition of unknown cause identified by the histopathologic finding of extensive eosinophilic infiltration of gastric tissue.[91] Frequently, a peripheral eosinophilia and an increased level of serum IgE coexist.[92] More diffuse mucosal involvement, extending beyond the stomach to include other areas of the gastrointestinal tract, is referred to as eosinophilic gastroenteritis.[92, 93] Additional details regarding this entity are described in Chapter 27.

## Lymphocytic Gastritis in Celiac Disease

Lymphocytic gastritis is characterized by an intense lymphocytic infiltration of the pit and surface gastric epithelium.[94] Lymphocytic gastritis is associated with the endoscopic appearance of varioliform gastritis in adults.[95, 96] A similar association has not been identified in children.[97]

Although the cause of lymphocytic gastritis remains unclear, an association between untreated celiac disease and lymphocytic gastritis has been identified in both adult and pediatric populations.[98, 99] In a study of 60 children with chronic gastritis, lymphocytic gastritis was identified in 9 of the 15 children with gluten-sensitive enteropathy but in none of the 45 children without celiac disease.[100]

In contrast to adults with lymphocytic gastritis who are asymptomatic,[101] children with celiac disease and associated lymphocytic gastritis more often have symptoms of upper gastrointestinal tract disease, including recurrent vomiting.[100] In addition, resolution of the lymphocytic infiltrate was documented[100] after treatment with a gluten-free diet in all children who underwent an endoscopic re-evaluation. Studies using sucrose as a marker of permeability of the gastric mucosa identified an increase in gastric permeability in adults with untreated celiac disease,[101, 102] suggesting that celiac disease is not limited to the small bowel.

## Autoimmune Gastritis

Chronic atrophic gastritis associated with pernicious anemia is characterized by circulating parietal cell autoantibodies directed against the gastric $H^+,K^+$-ATPase and mucosal mononuclear cell infiltrates with associated loss of both parietal cells and chief cells.[103, 104] Animal models of autoimmune gastritis suggest a potential role for CD4-positive T cell cytotoxicity in disease pathogenesis.[105] Studies also implicate Fas-mediated induction of target cell apoptosis in murine autoimmune gastritis.[106] There is no unifying hypothesis that accounts for the development of autoimmune gastritis. In children, autoimmune gastritis is a rare entity, but it has been reported in association with other autoimmune disorders such as thyroiditis.[107]

## Bile Reflux Gastritis

Reflux of duodenal fluid into the stomach has been implicated in the pathogenesis of gastritis that occurs after partial gastric resection. Histologic changes ascribed to bile reflux include foveolar hyperplasia, mucosal edema, and vasodilation but with a paucity of inflammatory cells in the mucosa.[108]

Both animal and human studies have demonstrated that bile acids can induce alterations in the gastric mucosa.[109] Patients who have undergone partial gastrectomy have an elevation in gastric bile acid concentration in association with gastritis.[110] In addition, these patients have both a higher mast cell density and a higher gastric mucosal histamine content than normal controls. Mast cell–derived mediators such as histamine are also implicated in duodenal reflux related gastric injury. Bile acids can directly stimulate histamine release from mast cells.[111]

Controversy exists regarding the etiopathogenic significance of bile reflux in patients who have not undergone gastric resection or drainage procedures.[112, 113] Among 316 adult patients with dyspepsia undergoing endoscopy, 15% had histologic findings characteristic of bile reflux gastritis.[113] There was no correlation between the presence of gastritis and elevations in gastric bile acid concentration indicative of duodenal reflux.

## Portal Hypertensive Gastropathy

Portal hypertensive gastropathy is frequently identified in children with portal hypertension.[114, 115] Endoscopic findings, usually localized to the fundus and corpus of the stomach, include a mosaic appearance resembling snake skin, a diffuse scarlatiniform erythema, and petechial hemorrhages. The more severe manifestations include a gastric "cherry-red" spot pattern and diffuse mucosal hemorrhage.[116] Histologically, there is extensive edema with capillary and venous dilatation without significant mucosal inflammation.[116] Studies in children indicate that portal hypertensive gastropathy is a rare cause of upper gastrointestinal bleeding and that most children are asymptomatic.[114]

It has been postulated that esophageal variceal sclerotherapy can increase the likelihood of the development of gastropathy by increasing hyperdynamic congestion[115] (see Chapter 51).

## Chronic Granulomatous Disease

The term *chronic granulomatous disease* refers to a group of inherited disorders characterized by impairment of intracellular killing of catalase-positive organisms that results in recurrent infections of the skin, lungs, and reticuloendothelial organs.[117] Owing to a deficient nicotinamide adenine dinucleotide phosphate (NADPH) oxidase activity, phagocytes are unable to produce superoxide and other reactive oxygen species.[117] Several different mutations are associated with chronic granulomatous disease, with both autosomal recessive and X-linked inheritances.[118, 119]

Gastrointestinal involvement in chronic granulomatous disease includes gastric outlet obstruction caused by antral narrowing. Vomiting, postprandial epigastric pain, and weight loss are associated symptoms.[120–124] Radiologic examination demonstrates concentric, smooth narrowing of the antrum with varying degrees of pyloric obstruction.

Histologic assessment of the gastric mucosa characteristically demonstrates the presence of granulomas with histiocytes containing granules that stain positively with the periodic acid–Schiff reaction.[125] Therapy for gastric involvement includes antimicrobial agents and anti-inflammatory drugs such as sulfasalazine and corticosteroids.[120–123, 125]

## Graft-Versus-Host Disease

Acute graft-versus-host disease affecting the upper gastrointestinal tract occurs in up to 44% of allogenic bone marrow transplant recipients.[126] Symptoms of gastric graft-versus-host disease include anorexia, nausea, and vomiting with or without concomitant diarrhea and signs of involvement of other organs such as skin and liver.

The diagnosis is based on histologic findings of gastric epithelial cell apoptosis with a predominantly lymphocytic infiltrate in the lamina propria (Fig. 19–2). Graft-versus-host disease affecting the upper gastrointestinal tract can occur in the absence of both histologic abnormalities in the intestinal mucosa and symptoms of lower gastrointestinal graft-versus-host disease (e.g., diarrhea).[127] Upper endoscopy and biopsy of the fundus and antrum is warranted for accurate diagnosis.

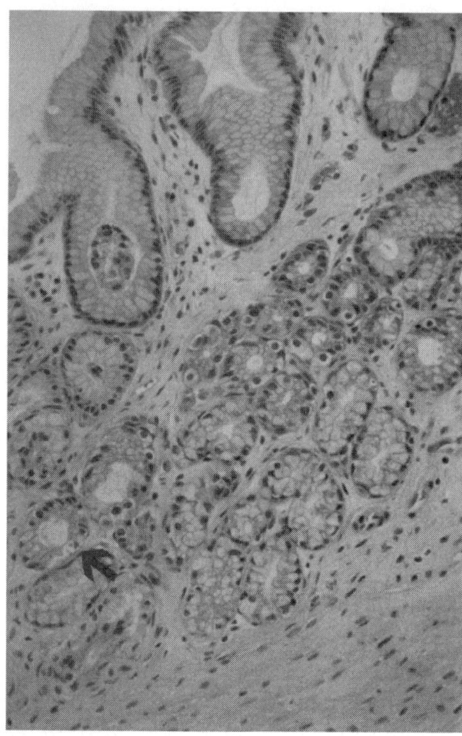

**FIGURE 19–2.** Gastric antral biopsy from an 8-year-old boy after bone marrow transplantation, exhibiting clinical features consistent with graft-versus-host disease. Apoptotic crypt epithelial cells are evident *(arrow)*.

## Pseudo–Zollinger-Ellison Syndrome

Pseudo–Zollinger-Ellison syndrome (pseudo-ZES)—also referred to as antral G-cell hyperplasia syndrome[128]—is characterized by an exaggerated serum gastrin release in response to feeding, and unchanged or decreased gastrin levels in response to stimulation with secretin. Antral G-cell hyperfunction can also occur in the absence of detectable G-cell hyperplasia.[129] This syndrome is distinct from ZES, in which hypergastrinemia is caused by the presence of a gastrinoma.[130, 131] ZES can be distinguished by a marked elevation in gastrin in response to provocative testing with secretin and the lack of an increase in response to a test meal.[132, 133] In addition, the presence of a gastrinoma can be identified in most cases preoperatively by imaging procedures[134–136] or intraoperatively.

Clinical manifestations of this syndrome mimic those of ZES and are related to the presence of multiple gastric or duodenal ulcers.[137] Signs and symptoms include isolated anemia, abdominal pain, vomiting, weight loss, and gastrointestinal bleeding.[138] Diarrhea is an additional presenting symptom in some patients.[128] Endoscopic findings include gastric antral or duodenal ulceration. Histologically, acute or chronic inflammation in the antrum is present. Elevated numbers of G cells in the antrum are detected histologically.[139]

# CLINICAL PRESENTATION

The differential diagnosis of gastritis is presented in Table 19–2.

**TABLE 19–2. Differential Diagnosis of Gastritis**

| | |
|---|---|
| **Associated with Epigastric Pain** | |
| | Pancreatitis<br>Disorders of the biliary tract<br>Nonulcer dyspepsia<br>Urinary tract infection, urolithiasis<br>Functional |
| **Associated with Gastrointestinal (GI) Bleeding** | |
| GI cause | Esophagitis<br>Mallory-Weiss tear<br>Varices<br>Erosions/ulcerations<br>Polyp<br>Ectopic pancreas, pancreatitis<br>Duodenitis<br>Duplication cyst<br>Hematobilia |
| Vascular cause | Hemangioma (Klippel-Trénaunay-Weber syndrome, blue rubber bleb nevus syndrome)<br>Arteriovenous malformation<br>Connective tissue disorders (Ehlers-Danlos syndrome, pseudoxanthoma elasticum)<br>Telangiectasia (CREST syndrome, hereditary hemorrhagic telangiectasia)<br>Bleeding diathesis |
| Non-GI cause | Nasopharynx<br>Maternal blood<br>Munchausen's syndrome by proxy |

CREST, calcinosis cutis, Raynaud's phenomenon, esophageal dysfunction, sclerodactyly, and telangiectasia.

### *Helicobacter pylori*

*H. pylori*–induced gastritis is asymptomatic in the majority of infected persons, including children.[6] In addition, it is not possible to distinguish clinically the small subset of patients who are likely to develop the specific complications of peptic ulcers and gastric cancers. The clinical outcome of *H. pylori* infection is probably determined by both host and bacterial factors. Several bacterial virulence factors have been implicated in specific disease pathogenesis.[140–144]

The role of *H. pylori* infection in the clinical setting of recurrent abdominal pain of childhood has received much attention.[145, 146] Overall, the evidence does not support an increased prevalence of *H. pylori* infection in children with recurrent abdominal pain. A meta-analysis of 45 pediatric studies by Macarthur and associates[145] found no association between *H. pylori* infection and recurrent abdominal pain of childhood. Therefore, the chronic-active gastritis induced by helicobacter infection does not equate with the development of clinical symptomatology.

The presenting symptoms of secondary gastritis are not specific, particularly in young children. Epigastric pain, vomiting, and signs of upper gastrointestinal blood loss can occur.[50, 85, 92, 100, 114, 125, 126] Symptoms related to gastrointestinal blood loss include fatigue, hematemesis or melena, and hematochezia with vigorous hemorrhage.

### Associated Peptic Ulcer Disease

Peptic ulcer disease is rare in children.[147–149] Children with *H. pylori*–related peptic ulcer disease have chronic recurrent symptoms. Epigastric and abdominal pain and vomiting are frequent presenting symptoms. An important feature which distinguishes *H. pylori*–infected children with ulcer from those with gastritis alone is the presence of nocturnal awakening.[150] Hematemesis may also occur.[147] Secondary peptic ulcer disease may manifest with symptoms that are indistinguishable from those of *H. pylori*–related ulceration, and it is important to inquire about other potential known causes of gastritis in all patients with symptoms suggestive of ulcer disease.

## DIAGNOSIS

### Diagnostic Imaging

Studies document the lack of sensitivity of both single- and double-contrast barium studies in the diagnosis of gastritis and peptic ulceration in children.[151, 152] In addition, radiographic studies carry a high false-positive rate of diagnosis.[151, 153] False-positive results are related primarily to the region of the first and second parts of the duodenum, owing to the motility of this area.

Barium contrast studies of the upper gastrointestinal tract detect abnormalities in at most 50% of patients with gastric Crohn's disease (Fig. 19–3).[85] This is not unexpected, because the mucosa also appears to be endoscopically normal in many patients.[85, 90]

An upper gastrointestinal series identified the characteristic hypertrophied gastric rugae of Ménétrier's disease in most reports.[31–33] Ultrasound or computed tomographic scanning may also be used to demonstrate the thickened gastric folds.[34]

### Endoscopy

Upper endoscopy is a safe procedure in children, including newborns and small infants,[154] and is considered the diagnos-

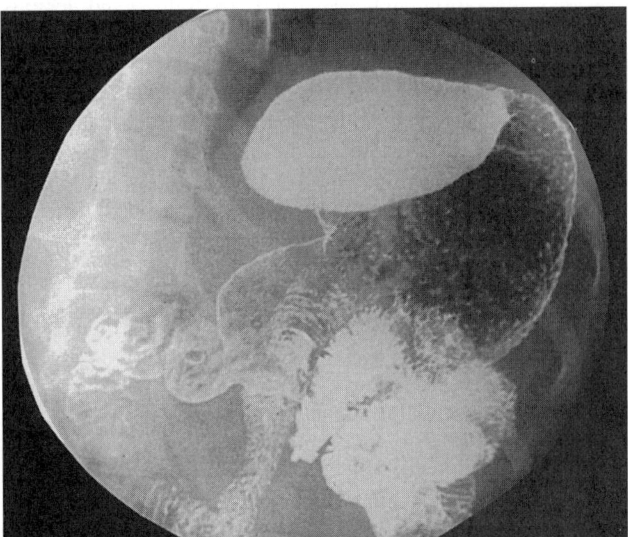

**FIGURE 19–3.** Multiple aphthous ulcers in a 15-year-old adolescent girl with Crohn's disease.

tic modality of choice for gastric diseases.[151, 152, 155–158] Endoscopically, active peptic ulceration usually appears as a white-based oval or round region with surrounding hyperemia. A diagnosis of gastritis can be considered based on the particular endoscopic findings (e.g., erythema, loss of vascular pattern) but must be confirmed by histopathology.

Antral nodularity noted at endoscopy has been considered a unique feature of *H. pylori*–related disease, particularly in children.[149] Several studies have documented the presence of nodularity of the antrum in association with *H. pylori* infection in children.[148, 149, 159–161] However, *H. pylori*–infected gastric mucosa can also appear unremarkable on endoscopy.[160, 162] Histologic assessment of biopsies taken at the time of upper endoscopy is required to confirm gastritis and the infection.[6]

### Histopathology

Because the correlation between endoscopic and histologic findings is low,[163] a diagnosis of gastritis should always be confirmed by histopathologic examination of gastric biopsies. Current recommendations for the accurate histologic diagnosis of *H. pylori* infection in adults suggest the biopsies should be obtained from both the antrum and the body.[164] Most published studies in children diagnose *H. pylori* infection based on biopsies obtained from the antrum alone.[147, 150] In one study of *H. pylori*–infected children, the diagnosis of infection in biopsies obtained from the body correlated with those obtained from the antrum in all cases.[148]

Ménétrier's disease most frequently involves the body of the stomach in children.[30, 33] Therefore, biopsies of this region should be taken if the diagnosis is being considered.

## TREATMENT

### Prevention

The use of prophylactic therapy (e.g., cytoprotection, reduction or neutralization of gastric acid) for the prevention of stress ulceration and associated gastroduodenal lesions remains controversial.[165] In a double-blind, controlled study of patients in a pediatric intensive care unit, prophylaxis with cimetidine increased gastric pH but was unable to prevent upper gastrointestinal bleeding.[84] Results of a meta-analysis including 56 adult studies identified a decrease in clinically significant bleeding with prophylaxis with histamine $H_2$-receptor antagonists.[165] However, a concurrent reduction in mortality rate was not detected.

### Management of Acute Hemorrhage

Treatment for acute massive hemorrhage caused by secondary gastritis includes adequate resuscitation and supportive care in the intensive care unit (see Chapter 6). There is no evidence to support the use of gastric saline lavage to stop bleeding or to prevent recurrent bleeding.[166] Similarly, agents that reduce splanchnic blood flow (e.g., octreotide, somatostatin, vasopressin) are not effective in the setting of acute nonvariceal upper gastrointestinal bleeding.[166, 167] In a double-blind, placebo-controlled trial of oral omeprazole in patients with recent bleeding, both further bleeding and the need for surgery were reduced.[168] Whether these findings are applicable to pediatric patients, however, remains to be established.

Therapeutic endoscopy is widely employed in adult patients with acute upper gastrointestinal bleeding. In a meta-analysis of 30 randomized controlled trials, patients with active bleeding who received hemostatic endoscopic treatment had less continued bleeding, a reduced need for surgery, and lowered mortality.[169] When analyzed separately, thermal contact devices (including monopolar and bipolar electrocoagulation and heater probe), laser treatment, and injection therapy all reduced further bleeding and surgery, but only laser therapy was associated with a reduction in mortality.

Therapeutic endoscopy by an experienced endoscopist could also prove efficacious in the care of highly selected pediatric patients.[170] Studies to address this issue formally are needed, because most upper gastrointestinal bleeds, even if massive, subside within 24 hours with supportive care alone.[171]

### Specific Therapy

Treatment of *H. pylori*–associated duodenal or gastric ulceration is aimed at eradication of the organism.[7] Treatment options are considered in detail in Chapter 18.

Eosinophilic gastritis is traditionally treated with corticosteroids.[92] Ketotifen therapy may be a useful alternative for some patients.[93] Conservative management is sufficient for children with Ménétrier's disease, because the disease is self-limited.[30]

Optimal therapy for Crohn's gastritis is not known. However, a response to therapy with corticosteroids and $H_2$ receptor antagonists has been reported.[87] Therapy with a proton-pump inhibitor appears to provide a promising therapeutic advantage for patients with symptomatic gastroduodenal Crohn's disease.[172]

Gastrectomy was initially the treatment of choice for patients with the pseudo–ZES or ZES.[128] However, the successful treatment of a child with pseudo-ZES with a proton-pump inhibitor suggests that medical treatment alone may be beneficial.[137] Further trials are needed to determine the long-term efficacy and safety of such medical therapy.

Treatment for peptic ulcer disease is discussed in detail in Chapter 18.

## REFERENCES


1. Drumm B, Rhoads JM, Stringer DA, et al: Peptic ulcer disease in children: etiology, clinical findings, and clinical course. Pediatrics 1988;82:410–414.
2. Scheiman JM: NSAIDs, gastrointestinal injury and cytoprotection. Gastroenterol Clin North Am 1996;25:279–298.
3. Hills BA: Gastric surfactant and the hydrophobic mucosal barrier. Gut 1996;39:621–624.
4. Hunt RH, Tytgat GNJ: *Helicobacter pylori:* Basic Mechanisms to Clinical Cure. Norwell, MA, Kluwer Academic Publishers, 1996.
5. Veldhuyzen van Zanten SJO, Sherman PM: *Helicobacter pylori* infection as a cause of gastritis, duodenal ulcer, gastric cancer and nonulcer

dyspepsia: a systematic overview. Can Med Assoc J 1994;150:177–185.

6. Bourke B, Jones N, Sherman P: *Helicobacter pylori* infection and peptic ulcer disease in children. Pediatr Infect Dis J 1996;15:1–13.
7. Veldhuyzen van Zanten SJO, Sherman PM, Hunt RH: *Helicobacter pylori:* new developments and treatments. Can Med Assoc J 1997;156:1565–1574.
8. McNulty CAM, Dent JC, Curry A, et al: New spiral bacterium in gastric mucosa. J Clin Pathol 1989;42:585–591.
9. Solnick JV, O'Rourke J, Lee A, et al: An uncultured gastric spiral organism is a newly identified helicobacter in humans. J Infect Dis 1993;168:379–385.
10. Heilmann KL, Borchard F: Gastritis due to spiral shaped bacteria other than *Helicobacter pylori*: clinical, histologic, and ultrastructural findings. Gut 1991;32:137–140.
11. Oliva MM, Lazenby AJ, Perman JA: Gastritis associated with *Gastrosporillum hominis* in children: comparison with *Helicobacter pylori* and review of the literature. Mod Pathol 1993;6:513–515.
12. Stolte M, Kroher G, Meining A, et al: A comparison of *Helicobacter pylori* and *Helicobacter heilmannii* gastritis: a matched control study involving 404 patients. Scand J Gastroenterol 1997;32:28–33.
13. Chone L, Flejou JF, Gringnon Y, et al: *Helicobacter heilmannii*: new spiral shaped bacterium responsible for acute gastric ulcerations. Gastroenterol Clin Biol 1995;19:447–448.
14. Akin OY, Tsou VM, Werner AL: *Gastrosporillum hominis*-associated chronic active gastritis. Pediatr Pathol Lab Med 1995;15:429–435.
15. Yang H, Li X, Xu Z, et al: *Helicobacter heilmannii* infection in a patient with gastric cancer. Dig Dis Sci 1995;40:1013–1014.
16. Morgner A, Bayerdorffer E, Meining A, et al: *Helicobacter heilmannii* and gastric cancer. Lancet 1995;346:511–512.
17. Solnick JV, O' Rourke J, Lee A, et al: Molecular analysis of urease genes from a newly identified uncultured species of *Helicobacter.* Infect Immun 1994;62:1631–1638.
18. Rotterdam H, Tsang P: Gastrointestinal disease in the immunocompromised patient. Hum Pathol 1994;25:1123–1140.
19. Jones B, Wall SD: Gastrointestinal disease in the immunocompromised host. Radiol Clin North Am 1992;30:555–577.
20. Cappell MS, Taunk JL: A chronic gastric ulcer refractory to conventional antiulcer therapy associated with localized gastric *Mycobacterium avium intracellulare* infection in a homosexual man with acquired immunodeficiency syndrome. Am J Gastroenterol 1991;86:654–657.
21. Howiler W, Goldberg HI: Gastroesophageal involvement in herpes simplex. Gastroenterology 1976;70:775–778.
22. McCluggage WG, Fox JD, Baillie KEM, et al: Varicella zoster gastritis in a bone marrow transplant recipient. J Clin Pathol 1994;47:1054–1056.
23. Muraoka A, Suehiro I, Fujii M, et al: Acute gastric anisakiasis: 28 cases during the last 10 years. Dig Dis Sci 1996;41:2362–2365.
24. Dieterich DT, Lew EA, Bacon DJ, et al: Gastrointestinal pneumocystosis in HIV-infected patients on aerosolized pentamidine: report of five cases and literature review. Am J Gastroenterol 1992;87:1763–1770.
25. Cohen OJ, Stoeckle MY: Extrapulmonary *Pneumocystis carinii* infections in the acquired immunodeficiency syndrome. Arch Intern Med 1991;151:1205–1214.
26. Dennis JE, Rhodes KH, Cooney DR, et al: Nosocomial *Rhizopus* infection (zygomycosis) in children. J Pediatr 1980;96:824–828.
27. Vadeboncoeur C, Walton JM, Raisen J, et al: Gastrointestinal mucormycosis causing an acute abdomen in the immunocompromised pediatric patient: three cases. J Pediatr Surg 1994;29:1248–1249.
28. Sharpstone D, Gazzard B: Gastrointestinal manifestations of HIV infection. Lancet 1996;348:379–383.
29. Garone MA, Winston BJ, Lewis JH: Cryptosporidiosis of the stomach. Am J Gastroenterol 1986;81:465–470.
30. Occena RO, Taylor SF, Robinson CC, et al: Association of cytomegalovirus with Ménétrier's disease in childhood: report of two new cases with a review of literature. J Pediatr Gastroenterol Nutr 1993;17:217–224.
31. Sferra TJ, Pawel BR, Qualman SJ, et al: Ménétrier disease of childhood: role of cytomegalovirus and transforming growth factor alpha. J Pediatr 1996;128:213–219.
32. Wolfsen HC, Carpenter HA, Talley NJ: Ménétrier's disease: a form of hypertrophic gastropathy or gastritis? Gastroenterology 1993;104:1310–1319.
33. Kovacs AAS, Churchill MA, Wood D, et al: Molecular and epidemiologic evaluations of a cluster of cases of Ménétrier's disease associated with cytomegalovirus. Pediatr Infect Dis J 1993;12:1011–1014.
34. Takaya J, Kawamura Y, Kino M, et al: Ménétrier's disease evaluated serially by abdominal ultrasonography. Pediatr Radiol 1997;27:178–180.
35. Palmer WE, Bloch SM, Chew FS: Ménétrier disease. AJR Am J Roentgenol 1992;158:62.
36. Cieslak TJ, Mullett CT, Puntel RA, et al: Ménétrier's disease associated with cytomegalovirus infection in children: report of two cases and review of the literature. Pediatr Infect Dis J 1993;12:340–343.
37. Arabia FA, Rosado LJ, Huston CL, et al: Incidence and recurrence of gastrointestinal cytomegalovirus infection in heart transplantation. Ann Thorac Surg 1993;55:8–11.
38. Sakr M, Hassanein T, Gavaler J, et al: Cytomegalovirus infection of the upper gastrointestinal tract following liver transplantation: incidence, location, and severity in cyclosporine- and FK506-treated patients. Transplantation 1992;53:786–791.
39. Rosen P, Armstrong D, Rice N: Gastrointestinal cytomegalovirus infection. Arch Intern Med 1973;132:274–281.
40. Strickler JG, Manivel JC, Copenhaver CM, et al: Comparison of in-situ hybridization and immunohistochemistry for detection of cytomegalovirus and herpes simplex virus. Hum Pathol 1990;21:443–448.
41. Wu GD, Shintaku P, Chien K, et al: A comparison of routine light microscopy, immunohistochemistry, and in-situ hybridization for the detection of cytomegalovirus in gastrointestinal biopsies. Am J Gastroenterol 1989;84:1517–1520.
42. Eisenstat DDR, Griffiths AM, Cutz E, et al: Acute cytomegalovirus infection in a child with Ménétrier's disease. Gastroenterology 1995;109:592–595.
43. Bayerdorffer E, Ritter MM, Hatz R, et al: Healing of protein losing hypertrophic gastropathy by eradication of *Helicobacter pylori:* Is *Helicobacter pylori* a pathogenic factor in Ménétrier's disease? Gut 1994;35:701–704.
44. Milov DE, Bailey DJ: Infantile *Helicobacter pylori* associated with thickened gastric folds. J Pediatr Gastroenterol Nutr 1995;21:107–109.
45. Hill ID, Sinclair-Smith C, Lastovica AJ, et al: Transient protein losing enteropathy associated with acute gastritis and *Campylobacter pylori.* Arch Dis Child 1987;62:1215–1219.
46. Takagi H, Jhappan C, Sharp R, et al: Hypertrophic gastropathy resembling Ménétrier's disease in transgenic mice overexpressing transforming growth factor alpha in the stomach. J Clin Invest 1992;90:1161–1167.
47. Dempsey PJ, Goldenring JR, Soroka CJ, et al: Possible role of transforming growth factor alpha in the pathogenesis of Ménétrier's disease: supportive evidence from humans and transgenic mice. Gastroenterology 1992;103:1950–1963.
48. Soll AH, Weinstein WM, Kurata J, et al: Nonsteroidal anti-inflammatory drugs and peptic ulcer disease. Ann Intern Med 1991;114:307–319.
49. Silverstein FE, Graham DY, Senior JR, et al: Misoprostol reduces serious gastrointestinal complications in patients with rheumatoid arthritis receiving nonsteroidal anti-inflammatory drugs. Ann Intern Med 1995;123:241–249.
50. Keenan GF, Giannini EH, Athreya BH: Clinically significant gastropathy associated with nonsteroidal anti-inflammatory drug use in children with juvenile rheumatoid arthritis. J Rheumatol 1995;22:1149–1151.
51. Dowd JE, Cimaz R, Fink CW: Nonsteroidal anti-inflammatory drug–induced gastroduodenal injury in children. Arthritis Rheum 1995;38:1225–1231.
52. Matsubara T, Mason W, Kashani IA, et al: Gastrointestinal hemorrhage complicating aspirin therapy in acute Kawasaki disease. J Pediatr 1996;128:701–703.
53. Ng PC, So KW, To KF, et al: Fatal hemorrhagic gastritis associated with oral sulindac treatment for patent ductus arteriosus. Acta Paediatr 1996;85:884–886.
54. Taha AS, Nakshabendi I, Lee FD, et al: Chemical gastritis and *Helicobacter pylori*-related gastritis in patients receiving non-steroidal anti-inflammatory drugs: comparison and correlation with peptic ulceration. J Clin Pathol 1992;45:135–139.
55. El-Zimaity HM, Genta RM, Graham DY: Histological features do not define NSAID-induced gastritis. Human Pathol 1996;27:1348–1354.
56. Wallace JL: Nonsteroidal anti-inflammatory drugs and gastroenteropathy: the second hundred years. Gastroenterology 1997;112:1000–1016.

57. Jones, NL, Sherman P, Wang B, et al: *Helicobacter pylori* and nonsteroidal anti–inflammatory drugs: partners in crime? Bull Rheum Dis 1997;46(8):6–7.
58. Hayllar J, Bjarnason I: NSAIDs, COX-2 inhibitors, and the gut. Lancet 1995;346:521–522.
59. Langenbach R, Morham SG, Tiano HF, et al: Prostaglandin synthesis 1 gene disruption in mice reduces arachidonic acid-induced inflammation and indomethacin-induced gastric ulceration. Cell 1995;83:483–492.
60. Koch M, Dezi A, Ferrario F, et al: Prevention of nonsteroidal anti-inflammatory drug-induced gastrointestinal mucosal injury. Arch Intern Med 1996;156:2321–2332.
61. Gazarian M, Berkovitch, Koren G, et al: Experience with misoprostol therapy for NSAID gastropathy in children. Ann Rheum Dis 1995;54:277–280.
62. Stucki G, Johannesson M, Liang MH: Is misoprostol cost-effective in the prevention of nonsteroidal anti-inflammatory drug-induced gastropathy in patients with chronic arthritis? A review of conflicting economic evaluations. Arch Intern Med 1994;154:2020–2025.
63. Edelson JT, Tosteson ANA, Sax P: Cost-effectiveness of misoprostol for prophylaxis against nonsteroidal anti-inflammatory drug-induced gastrointestinal tract bleeding. JAMA 1990;264:41–47.
64. Herting RL, Clay GA: Overview of clinical safety with misoprostol. Dig Dis 1985;30(suppl):185S–193S.
65. Taha AS, Hudson N, Hawkey CJ, et al: Famotidine for the prevention of gastric and duodenal ulcers caused by nonsteroidal anti-inflammatory drugs. N Engl J Med 1996;334:1435–1439.
66. Cullen D, Bardhan KD, Eisner M, et al: Primary gastroduodenal prophylaxis with omeprazole for NSAID users. Gastroenterology 1996;110:A86.
67. Lichtenberger LM, Ulloa C, Romero JJ, et al: Omeprazole reduces both the GI toxicity and therapeutic activity of NSAIDs in rats. Gastroenterology 1996;110:A176.
68. Davies NM, Roseth AG, Appleyard CB, et al: NO-naproxen vs. naproxen: ulcerogenic, analgesic and anti-inflammatory effects. Aliment Pharm Ther 1997;11:69–79.
69. Lichtenberger LM, Ulloa C, Vanous AL, et al: Zwitterionic phospholipids enhance aspirin's therapeutic activity, as demonstrated in rodent model systems. J Pharmacol Exp Ther 1996;277:1221–1227.
70. Chan CC, Boyce S, Brideau C, et al: Pharmacology of a selective cyclooxygenase-2 inhibitor, L-745,337: a novel nonsteroidal anti-inflammatory agent with an ulcerogenic sparing effect in rat and nonhuman primate stomach. J Pharmacol Exp Ther 1995;274:1531–1537.
71. Conn HO, Blitzer BL: Nonassociation of adrenocorticosteroid therapy and peptic ulcer. N Engl J Med 1976;294:473–479.
72. Messer J, Reitman D, Sacks HS, et al: Association of adrenocorticosteroid therapy and peptic-ulcer disease. N Engl J Med 1983;309:21–24.
73. Ligumsky M, Karmeli F, Sharon P, et al: Enhanced thromboxane $A_2$ and prostacyclin production by cultured rectal mucosa in ulcerative colitis and its inhibition by steroids and sulfasalazine. Gastroenterology 1981;81:444–449.
74. Tarnawski A, Hollander D, Stachura J, et al: Alcohol injury to the normal human gastric mucosa: endoscopic, histologic and functional assessment. Clin Invest Med 1987;10:259–263.
75. Laine L, Weinstein WM: Histology of alcoholic hemorrhagic "gastritis": a prospective evaluation. Gastroenterology 1988;94:1254–1262.
76. Chait PG, Weinberg J, Connolly BL, et al: Retrograde percutaneous gastrostomy and gastrojejunostomy in 505 children: a 4½-year experience. Radiology 1996;201:691–695.
77. Kazi S, Gunasekaran TS, Berman JH, et al: Gastric mucosal injuries in children from inflatable low-profile gastrostomy tubes. J Pediatr Gastroenterol Nutr 1997;24:75–78.
78. Pecha RE, Prindiville T, Pecha BS, et al: Association of cocaine and methamphetamine use with giant gastroduodenal ulcers. Am J Gastroenterol 1996;91:2523–2527.
79. Marks WA, Morris MP, Bodensteiner JB, et al: Gastritis with valproate therapy. Arch Neurol 1988;45:903–905.
80. Cheili R, Perasso A, Giacosa A: Gastritis: A Critical Review. Berlin, Springer-Verlag, 1987.
81. Cushing H: Peptic ulcers and the interbrain. Surg Gynecol Obstet 1932;55:1–34.
82. Czaja C, Mcalhany JC, Pruitt BA: Acute gastroduodenal disease after thermal injury. N Engl J Med 1974;291:925–929.
83. Cook DJ, Fuller HD, Guyatt G, et al: Risk factors for gastrointestinal bleeding in critically ill patients. N Engl J Med 1994;330:377–381.
84. Lacroix J, Nadeau D, Laberge S, et al: Frequency of upper gastrointestinal bleeding in a pediatric intensive care unit. Crit Care Med 1992;20:35–42.
85. Ruuska T, Vaajalahti P, Arajarvi P, et al: Prospective evaluation of upper gastrointestinal mucosal lesions in children with ulcerative colitis and Crohn's disease. J Pediatr Gastroenterol Nutr 1994;19:181–186.
86. Cameron DJS: Upper and lower gastrointestinal endoscopy in children and adolescents with Crohn's disease: a prospective study. J Gastroenterol Hepatol 1991;6:355–358.
87. Lenaerts C, Roy CC, Vaillancourt M, et al: High incidence of upper gastrointestinal tract involvement in children with Crohn disease. Pediatrics 1989;83:777–781.
88. Griffiths AM, Alemayehu E, Sherman P: Clinical features of gastroduodenal Crohn's disease in adolescents. J Pediatr Gastroenterol Nutr 1989;8:166–171.
89. Halme L, Rautelin H, Leidenius M, et al: Inverse correlation between *Helicobacter pylori* infection and inflammatory bowel disease. J Clin Pathol 1996;49:65–67.
90. Oberhuber G, Puspok A, Oesterreicher C, et al: Focally enhanced gastritis: a frequent type of gastritis in patients with Crohn's disease. Gastroenterology 1997;112:698–706.
91. Wehut WD, Olmsted WW, Neiman HL, et al: Eosinophilic gastritis: radiologic-pathologic correlation (RPC) from the Armed Forces Institute of Pathology (AFIP). Radiology 1976;120:85–89.
92. Whitington PF, Whitington GL: Eosinophilic gastroenteropathy in childhood. J Pediatr Gastroenterol Nutr 1988;7:379–385.
93. Melamed I, Feanny SJ, Sherman PM, et al: Benefit of ketotifen in patients with eosinophilic gastroenteritis. Am J Med 1991;90:310–314.
94. Haot J, Jouret A, Willette M, et al: Lymphocytic gastritis: prospective study of its relationship with varioliform gastritis. Gut 1990;31:282–285.
95. Haot J, Hamichi L, Wallez L, et al: Lymphocytic gastritis: a newly described entity. A retrospective endoscopic and histologic study. Gut 1988;29:1258–1264.
96. Haot J, Berger F, Andre C, et al: Lymphocytic gastritis versus varioliform gastritis: a historical series revisited. J Pathol 1989;158:19–22.
97. Couper R, Laski B, Drumm B, et al: Chronic varioliform gastritis in childhood. J Pediatr 1989;115:441–444.
98. Wolber R, Owen D, Del Buono L, et al: Lymphocytic gastritis in patients with celiac sprue or spruelike intestinal disease. Gastroenterology 1990;98:310–315.
99. Lynch DAF, Sobala GM, Dixon MF, et al: Lymphocytic gastritis and associated small bowel disease: a diffuse lymphocytic gastroenteropathy? J Clin Pathol 1995;48:939–945.
100. De Giacomo C, Gianatti A, Negrini R, et al: Lymphocytic gastritis: a positive relationship with celiac disease. J Pediatr 1994;124:57–62.
101. Vogelsang H, Oberhuber G, Wyatt J: Lymphocytic gastritis and gastric permeability in patients with celiac disease. Gastroenterology 1996;111:73–77.
102. Meddings J: Sucrose: how sweet it is? J Pediatr Gastroenterol Nutr 1997;24:621–622.
103. Wang XH, Miyazaki Y, Shinomura Y, et al: Characterization of human autoantibodies reactive to gastric parietal cells. Biochem Biophys Res Commun 1993;190:207–214.
104. Kaye M: Immunologic aspects of gastritis and pernicious anemia. Baillieres Clin Gastroenterol 1987;1:487–506.
105. Martinelli TM, van Drile IR, Alderuccio F, et al: Analysis of mononuclear cell infiltrate and cytokine production in murine autoimmune gastritis. Gastroenterology 1996;110:1791–1802.
106. Nishio A, Katakai T, Oshima C, et al: A possible involvement of Fas-Fas ligand signaling in the pathogenesis of murine autoimmune gastritis. Gastroenterology 1996;111:959–967.
107. Kuitunen P, Maenpaa J, Krohn K, et al: Gastrointestinal findings in autoimmune thyroiditis and non-goitrous juvenile hypothyroidism in children. Scand J Gastroenterol 1971;6:336–341.
108. Sobala GM, King RF, O'Connor HJ, et al: Bile reflux and intestinal metaplasia in gastric mucosa. J Clin Pathol 1993;46:235–240.
109. Stern AI, Hogan DL, Isenberg JI: Effect of sodium taurocholate on the human gastric mucosa at acid and neutral pH's. Gastroenterology 1984;87:1272–1276.
110. Bechi P, Amorosi A, Mazzanti R, et al: Reflux-related gastric mucosal injury is associated with increased mucosal histamine content in humans. Gastroenterology 1993;104:1057–1063.
111. Quist RG, Ton-Nu H, Lillienau J, et al: Activation of mast cells by bile acids. Gastroenterology 1991;101:446–456.

112. Hughes K, Robertson DA, James WB: Duodeno-gastric reflux in normal and dyspeptic subjects. Clin Radiol 1982;33:461–466.
113. Sobala GM, King RFG, Axon ATR, et al: Reflux gastritis in the intact stomach. J Clin Pathol 1990;43:303–306.
114. Hyams JS, Treem WR: Portal hypertensive gastropathy in children. J Pediatr Gastroenterol Nutr 1993;17:13–18.
115. Yachha SK, Ghoshal UC, Gupta R, et al: Portal hypertensive gastropathy in children with extrahepatic portal venous obstruction: role of variceal obliteration by endoscopic sclerotherapy and *Helicobacter pylori* infection. J Pediatr Gastroenterol Nutr 1996;23:20–23.
116. Payen JL, Cales P, Voigt JJ, et al: Severe portal hypertensive gastropathy and antral vascular ectasia are distinct entities in patients with cirrhosis. Gastroenterology 1995;108:138–144.
117. Leusen JHW, de Klein A, Hilarius PM, et al: Disturbed interaction of p21-*rac* with a mutated p67-*phox* causes chronic granulomatous disease. J Exp Med 1996;184:1243–1249.
118. Royer-Pokora B, Kunkel LM, Monaco AP, et al: Cloning the gene for an inherited human disorder—chronic granulomatous disease—on the basis of its chromosomal location. Nature 1986;322:32–38.
119. Dinauer MC, Pierce EA, Bruns GA, et al: Human neutrophil cytochrome $b_{558}$ light chain (p22-*phox*): Gene structure, chromosomal location, and mutations in cytochrome-negative autosomal recessive chronic granulomatous disease. J Clin Invest 1990;86:1729–1737.
120. Chin TW, Steihm ER, Falloon J, et al: Corticosteroids in treatment of obstructive lesions of chronic granulomatous disease. J Pediatr 1987;111:349–352.
121. Griscom NT, Kirkpatrick JA, Girdany BR, et al: Gastric antral narrowing in chronic granulomatous disease of childhood. Pediatrics 1974;54:456–460.
122. Stopyrowa J, Fyderek K, Sikorska B, et al: Chronic granulomatous disease of childhood: disease manifestation and response to salazosulfapyridine therapy. Pediatrics 1989;149:28–30.
123. Mulholland MW, Delaney JP, Simmons RL: Gastrointestinal complications of chronic granulomatous disease: surgical implications. Surgery 1983;94:569–574.
124. Hirsch BZ, Whitington PF, Kirschner BS, et al: Isolated granulomatous gastritis in an adolescent. Dig Dis Sci 1989;34:292–296.
125. Rosh JR, Tang HB, Mayer L, et al: Treatment of intractable gastrointestinal manifestations of chronic granulomatous disease with cyclosporine. J Pediatr 1995;126:143–145.
126. Weisdorf DJ, Snover DC, Haake R, et al: Acute upper gastrointestinal graft-versus-host disease: clinical significance and response to immunosuppressive therapy. Blood 1990;76:624–629.
127. Roy J, Snover D, Weisdorf S, et al: Simultaneous upper and lower endoscopic biopsy in the diagnosis of intestinal graft-versus-host disease. Transplantation 1991;51:642–646.
128. Freisen SR, Tomito T: Pseudo-Zollinger-Ellison syndrome: Hypergastrinemia, hyperchlorrhydria without tumor. Ann Surg 1981;194:481–493.
129. Annibale B, Bonamico M, Rindi G, et al: Antral gastric cell hyperfunction in children: a functional and immunocytochemical report. Gastroenterology 1991;101:1547–1551.
130. Ellison EH, Wilson SD: The Zollinger-Ellison syndrome: re-appraisal and evaluation of 260 registered cases. Ann Surg 1964;160:512–530.
131. Buchta RM, Kaplan JM: Zollinger-Ellison syndrome in a nine-year-old child: a case report and review of this entity in childhood. Pediatrics 1971;47:594–598.
132. Wolfe MM, Jain DK, Edgerton JR: Zollinger-Ellison syndrome associated with persistently normal fasting serum gastrin concentrations. Ann Intern Med 1985;103:215–217.
133. Frucht H, Howard JM, Slaff JI, et al: Secretin and calcium provocative tests in the Zollinger-Ellison syndrome: a prospective study. Ann Intern Med 1989;111:713–722.
134. Zimmer T, Ziegler K, Bader M, et al: Localisation of neuroendocrine tumors of the upper gastrointestinal tract. Gut 1994;35:471–475.
135. Rosch T, Lightdale CJ, Botet JF, et al: Localization of pancreatic endocrine tumors by endoscopic ultrasonography. N Engl J Med 1992;326:1721–1726.
136. Lamberts SWJ, Bakker WH, Reubi JC, et al: Somatostatin-receptor imaging in the localization of endocrine tumors. N Engl J Med 1990;323:1246–1249.
137. Zaatar R, Younoszai MK, Mitros F: Pseudo-Zollinger-Ellison syndrome in a child presenting with anemia. Gastroenterology 1987;92:508–512.
138. De Giacomo C, Fiocca R, Villani L, et al: Omeprazole treatment of severe peptic disease associated with antral G cell hyperfunction and hyperpepsinogenemia I in an infant. J Pediatr 1990;117:989–993.
139. Rindi G, Annibale B, Bonamico M, et al: *Helicobacter pylori* infection in children with antral gastrin cell hyperfunction. J Pediatr Gastroenterol Nutr 1994;18:152–158.
140. Blaser MJ: Not all *Helicobacter pylori* strains are created equal: should all be eliminated? Lancet 1997;349:1020–1022.
141. Atherton JC, Cao P, Peek RM, et al: Mosaicism in vacuolating cytotoxin alleles of *Helicobacter pylori*. J Biol Chem 1995;270:17771–17777.
142. Atherton JC, Peek RM Jr, Tham KT, et al: Clinical and pathologic importance of heterogeneity in *vacA*, the vacuolating cytotoxin gene of *Helicobacter pylori*. Gastroenterology 1997;112:92–99.
143. Censini S, Lange C, Xiang Z, et al: *cag*, a pathogenicity island of *Helicobacter pylori*, encodes type I-specific and disease-associated virulence factors. Proc Natl Acad Sci U S A 1996;93:14648-14653.
144. Tummuru MKR, Sharma SA, Blaser MJ: *Helicobacter pylori picB*, a homologue of the *Bordetella pertussis* toxin secretion protein, is required for the induction of IL-8 in gastric epithelial cells. Mol Microbiol 1995;18:867–876.
145. Macarthur C, Saunders N, Feldman W: *Helicobacter pylori*, gastroduodenal disease, and recurrent abdominal pain in children. JAMA 1995;273:729–734.
146. Kugathasan S, Czinn SJ: Gastroduodenal inflammation and related disorders in children. Curr Opin Gastroenterol 1996;12:537–543.
147. Drumm B, Sherman P, Cutz E, et al: Association of *Campylobacter pylori* on the gastric mucosa with antral gastritis in children. N Engl J Med 1987;316:1557–1561.
148. Mitchell HM, Bohane TD, Tobias V, et al: *Helicobacter pylori* infection in children: potential clues to pathogenesis. J Pediatr Gastroenterol Nutr 1993;16:120–125.
149. Hassall E, Dimmick JE: Unique features of *Helicobacter pylori* disease in children. Dig Dis Sci 1991;36:417–423.
150. Gormally SM, Prakash N, Durnin MT, et al: Association of symptoms with *Helicobacter pylori* infection in children. J Pediatr 1995;126:753–756.
151. Gyepes MT, Smith LE, Ament ME: Fiberoptic endoscopy and upper gastrointestinal series: comparative analysis in infants and children. AJR Am J Roentgenol 1977;128:53–56.
152. Cox K, Ament ME: Upper gastrointestinal bleeding in children and adolescents. Pediatrics 1979;63:408–413.
153. Miller V, Doig CM: Upper gastrointestinal tract endoscopy. Arch Dis Child 1984;59:1100–1102.
154. Ruuska T, Fell JME, Bisset WM, et al: Neonatal and infantile upper gastrointestinal endoscopy using a new small diameter fiberoptic gastroscope. J Pediatr Gastroenterol Nutr 1996;23:604–608.
155. Sukhabote J, Freeman HJ: Granulomatous (Crohn's) disease of the upper gastrointestinal tract: a study of 22 patients with mucosal granulomas. Can J Gastroenterol 1993;7:605–609.
156. Tam PKH, Saing H: Pediatric upper gastrointestinal endoscopy: a 13 year experience. J Pediatr Surg 1989;24:443–447.
157. Ashorn M, Maki M, Ruuska T, et al: Upper gastrointestinal endoscopy in recurrent abdominal pain of childhood. J Pediatr Gastroenterol Nutr 1993;16:273–277.
158. Miller TL, McQuinn LB, Orav EJ: Endoscopy of the upper gastrointestinal tract as a diagnostic tool for children with human immunodeficiency virus infection. J Pediatr 1997;130:766–773.
159. Czinn SJ, Dahms BB, Jacobs GH, et al: Campylobacter-like organisms in association with symptomatic gastritis in children. J Pediatr 1986;109:80–83.
160. Prieto G, Polanco I, Larrauri J et al: *Helicobacter pylori* infection in children: clinical, endoscopic, and histologic correlations. J Pediatr Gastroenterol Nutr 1992;14:420–425.
161. Bujanover Y, Konikoff F, Baratz M: Nodular gastritis and *Helicobacter pylori*. J Pediatr Gastroenterol Nutr 1990;11:41–44.
162. Queiroz DMM, Rocha GA, Mendes EN, et al: Differences in distribution and severity of *Helicobacter pylori* gastritis in children and adults with duodenal ulcer disease. J Pediatr Gastroenterol Nutr 1991;12:178–181.
163. Black DB, Haggitt RC, Whitington PF: Gastroduodenal endoscopic-histologic correlation in pediatric patients. J Pediatr Gastroenterol Nutr 1988;7:353–358.
164. Goodwin CS, Mendall MM, Northfield TC: *Helicobacter pylori* infection. Lancet 1997;349:265–269.
165. Cook DJ, Reeve BK, Guyatt GH, et al: Stress ulcer prophylaxis

in critically ill patients: resolving discordant meta-analyses. JAMA 1996;275:308–314.
166. Laine L, Peterson WL: Bleeding peptic ulcer. N Engl J Med 1994;331:717–727.
167. Thomson ABR: Therapeutic options for patients with bleeding with peptic ulcers. Can J Gastroenterol 1994;8:269–274.
168. Khuroo MS, Yattoo GN, Javid G, et al: A comparison of omeprazole and placebo for bleeding peptic ulcer. N Engl J Med 1997;336:1054–1058.
169. Cook DJ, Guyatt GH, Salena BJ, et al: Endoscopic therapy for acute nonvariceal upper gastrointestinal hemorrhage: a meta-analysis. Gastroenterology 1992;102:139–148.
170. Wyllie R, Kay MH: Therapeutic intervention for nonvariceal gastrointestinal hemorrhage. J Pediatr Gastroenterol Nutr 1996;22:123–133.
171. Sherman PM: Peptic ulcer disease in children: diagnosis, treatment, and the implication of *Helicobacter pylori*. Gastroenterol Clin North Am 1994;23:707–725.
172. Woolfson K, Greenberg GR: Symptomatic improvement of gastroduodenal Crohn's disease with omeprazole. Can J Gastroenterol 1992;6:21–24.

# Chapter 20

# Gastric Motility Disorders

*Aliye Uc and Paul E. Hyman*

## GASTRIC MOTILITY

The healthy stomach expands to receive a meal, mixes and grinds the food into small particles, and discriminates between solids and liquids and between digestible and indigestible particles. Through connections with the enteric nervous system, gastric emptying mechanisms adapt to the diet, regulating the delivery of nutrients to the small bowel for digestion and absorption. If a toxic or irritant compound is ingested, the stomach participates in the vomiting reflex, to expel the noxious gastric contents.

Gastric fundic, antral, and pyloric smooth muscles act in concert with duodenal sensory and motor functions to regulate gastric emptying according to food composition and physiologic and emotional states. These gastric motor functions are regulated by intrinsic and extrinsic nerves and by hormones.

### Gastric Motor Physiology and Gastric Emptying

Anatomically, the stomach is divided into three portions: fundus, body (corpus), and antrum. Functionally, there are two regions: proximal and distal stomach. The proximal stomach consists of the gastric fundus and the oral third of the corpus; the distal stomach consists of the aboral two thirds of the corpus, the antrum, and the pylorus. The proximal stomach functions as an alternately expanding and contracting reservoir. It relaxes to accommodate the meal and contracts to squeeze its contents toward the antrum. Antral peristalsis functions to grind and triturate solids.[1–3]

#### *Proximal Stomach*

With each swallow the proximal stomach relaxes to allow food to enter without increasing intragastric pressure. This phenomenon, called *receptive relaxation*, is regulated by inhibitory vagal nerves.[4, 5] Eventually fundic wall tension increases in a slow, sustained contraction that moves gastric contents toward the antrum. A pressure gradient between stomach and duodenum is necessary for the emptying of liquids. If intragastric pressures do not exceed those in the duodenum, liquids will not transit through the pylorus.

#### *Distal Stomach*

The distal stomach grinds solid food and pumps it into the duodenum. The electrical activity of the distal stomach is characterized by a cycle of depolarizations and repolarizations that gives rise to slow waves about three times each minute. The slow wave pattern is generated from the pacemaker region, located in the midcorpus along the greater curvature. Slow waves propagate distally from the pacemaker region to the pylorus. Slow waves consist of an initial upstroke potential and a plateau potential.[4, 5] Contractions are generated only when the plateau potential exceeds a certain threshold, creating an action potential. The amplitude and duration of each contraction is related to the time the plateau potential remains above this threshold. Acetylcholine acts on the smooth muscle to increase the plateau phase of the slow wave, leading to more forceful contractions.[4, 5] Sympathetic nerve stimulation, such as occurs with stress or fright, causes release of norepinephrine, which reduces the plateau potential and decreases the amplitude of antral contractions. Therefore, gastric emptying slows down during stressful situations.

During fasting the distal esophagus, stomach, small bowel, and gallbladder participate in a cycle of alternating periods of motor quiescence and activity. This cycle, known as the *migrating motor complex* (MMC), moves down the bowel in intervals ranging from less than 1 hour to 5 or 6 hours. Because the MMC was first described in the small bowel, the nomenclature applies best to the small bowel. The MMC consists of three sequential phases: a quiescent phase (phase 1); followed by a period of irregular contractions of variable amplitude, some of which are propagating (phase 2); and finally a short period of intense activity (phase 3) with regular, strong, propagating contractions occurring at a maximum rate for the organ, 3 per minute for the antrum and 11 to 13 per minute for the duodenum (Fig. 20–1). During phase 3, there is strong propulsion through a wide-open pylorus. This is the period when undigested food residues or foreign bodies leave the stomach. Feeding interrupts the MMC, replacing the cycle with a postprandial pattern, including phasic antral contractions that mix and grind the food.

Peristaltic contractions push food particles from the antrum to the pylorus. When the antral contraction approaches the pylorus, the pylorus closes. The antral contraction against

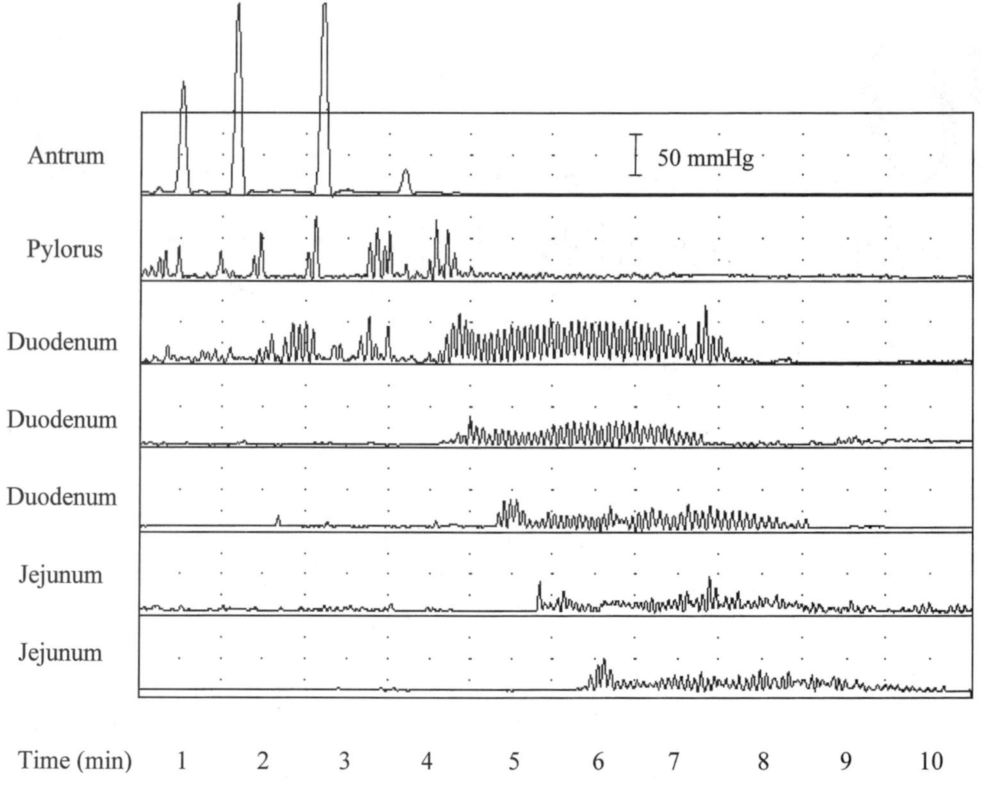


**FIGURE 20–1.** Phase 3 of the migrating motor complex is a marker for neuromuscular integrity. (Courtesy of S. N. Reddy, D.Eng.)

a closed pylorus creates a forceful retropulsion of the gastric contents. This to and fro movement creates shearing forces and breaks food particles into smaller pieces (1–2 mm) that can be expelled through the pylorus. This phenomenon is known as grinding or *trituration* of the solids by the distal stomach. During trituration, solids do not empty, so there is a delay, or *lag phase*, in gastric emptying. The duration of the lag phase is related to the size and consistency of the solid component of the meal. After a typical adult's meal of both solids and liquids, the lag phase lasts about 1 hour. Once the particles are liquefied, emptying proceeds. Solids that cannot be broken down to small particles are retained in the stomach until the next phase 3.

## Regulation of Gastric Emptying

Several factors affect the gastric emptying rate (Table 20–1). The fraction of a liquid meal that empties per unit time remains constant.[6] Gastric emptying of neutral, iso-osmolar, and calorically inert solutions (e.g., normal saline) is rapid, in the range of 10% to 20% per minute, reaching a simple exponential rate.[7] Solutions that are hypertonic or contain acid, fat, or certain amino acids delay gastric emptying by acting on duodenal receptors. There are five types of small bowel receptors regulating gastric emptying: lipid receptors, osmoreceptors, amino acid receptors, glucoreceptors, and pH receptors. The regulation of gastric emptying by these small bowel chemoreceptors is known as small intestinal feedback inhibition. Acidic solutions empty slowly from the stomach, with higher acid concentrations causing more profound inhibition.[8] Fatty acids, monoglycerides, and diglycerides all delay gastric emptying. The fatty acid chain length determines the degree of inhibition, with 10- to 14-carbon chains causing the greatest delay.[9] The emptying of amino acids is determined by the osmolality of the solution, except that L-tryptophan delays gastric emptying.[10] Lipid infused into the ileum delays gastric emptying possibly by raising the plasma peptide YY level, a phenomenon known as the *ileal brake*.[11]

The gastric emptying rate is influenced by nutritive density, or the kilocalories per unit volume. Isocaloric concentrations of fats, carbohydrates, and proteins—4, 9, and 9 g per 100 mL, respectively—leave the stomach at similar rates.[12]

The stomach discriminates among different meal components. For example, if a liquid, a digestible solid, and an indigestible solid are ingested simultaneously, the pattern of emptying for each is different. In experiments by Hinder

**TABLE 20–1. Factors That Modulate the Rate of Gastric Emptying in Health**

| FACTOR | EFFECT |
|---|---|
| **Meal Factors** | |
| Volume | Rate proportional to volume |
| Acidity | Slows |
| Osmolarity | Hypertonic meals empty more slowly |
| Nutrient density | Rate inversely proportional to nutrient density |
| Fat | Slows |
| L-Tryptophan | Slows |
| **Other Factors** | |
| Ileal fat | Slows (ileal brake) |
| Rectal/colonic distention | Slows |
| Pregnancy | Slows |

From Quigley EMM: Gastric and small intestinal motility in health and disease. Gastroenterol Clin North Am 1996;25:119, with permission.

and Kelly,[13] dogs were given a meal of 1% dextrose, cubed liver, and plastic spheres. The liquid emptied rapidly, with only 10% of the initial volume remaining in the stomach at 1 hour. The digestible solids emptied more slowly: almost 4 hours was required for 90% of the liver to pass out of the stomach. The indigestible solids, plastic spheres awaiting phase 3 to be propelled from the stomach, did not empty during the study period.

### Development of Gastric Motility

Gastric motility is immature in premature infants and limits feeding readiness. The inability to provide enteral nutrition in preterm infants—owing to poor suck and swallow, decreased lower esophageal sphincter tone, and delayed gastric emptying—obliges clinicians to use parenteral nutrition.[14]

**GASTRIC EMPTYING.** The human fetus empties swallowed amniotic fluid from the stomach at 30 weeks' gestation.[15] Small intestinal feedback inhibition exists in full-term infants and in preterm infants 32 weeks' gestational age and older. Stimulation of duodenal receptors by fat, carbohydrate, acid, tryptophan, or increasing osmolality slows gastric emptying. Glucose solutions empty slower than plain water.[16] Starches empty at the same rate as water, perhaps because of failed hydrolysis of the starch in the proximal small bowel of the full-term infant.[17]

**GASTRIC MOTILITY.** Between 25 and 30 weeks' postconceptual age, the antrum but not the duodenum displays phasic contractions. The MMC appears between 32 and 35 weeks after conception.[18] The motilin receptor agonist erythromycin stimulates antral contractions at all ages tested but induces phase 3 only in newborns with at least 32 weeks' gestation, suggesting that functioning motilin receptors appear before mature antroduodenal coordination.[19] In infants tested before 32 weeks' gestational age, gastric and duodenal contractions consist of nonpropagating clusters alternating with quiescence. With increasing postnatal age the frequency of clusters decreases and cluster duration increases.[20] The amplitude of antral contractions increases with gestational age, from 10 mm Hg at 28 weeks to 40 mm Hg at 38 weeks.[21] The propagation velocity of phase 3 increases with postnatal age.[22] A volume as small as 4 mL/kg stimulated a fed response in neonates. However, motor activity did not change in response to feeding formula diluted from 0.67 to 0.22 Kcal/mL, suggesting that dilute formula does not stimulate a fed response.[23]

Decreased gastric emptying rates in infants may reflect immature gastric and duodenal motor function and an absence of coordination between antrum and duodenum. Results from antroduodenal manometry in preterm and full-term infants suggest that gastrointestinal motility at birth is a work in progress and that neuromuscular maturation is completed after birth.

## ASSESSMENT OF GASTRIC MOTOR AND SENSORY FUNCTIONS

### Tests of Gastric Emptying

#### *Barium Contrast Studies*

Barium contrast studies detect retained food particles or bezoars and mechanical obstruction. Barium may delay gastric emptying and should not be used to assess gastric function.[24]

#### *Gastric Emptying Scintigraphy*

Scintigraphy is available at most medical centers for quantification of gastric emptying. Rapid access to results and a high rate of patient acceptability are features that make scintigraphy the favored method of screening for gastric emptying disorders.

In older children and adults, emptying of solids is a more sensitive and earlier predictor of impaired stomach function.[25] Infants are tested with the formula they normally drink, mixed with 1 mCi technetium 99m–sulphur colloid. The type and volume of formula varies from infant to infant. After a fast of 2 to 4 hours, some centers give the formula in a bottle, and others use gavage feeding. The advantage to bottle feeding is that it approximates the child's routine; the disadvantages are that the child may not voluntarily drink enough to stimulate a postprandial motility response, and the radionuclide (if given at the beginning of the session) may not mix completely with the meal. The advantage to gavage feeding is that a specific volume is ingested in a fixed time; the disadvantage is that natural conditions are not reproduced, including the physiologic responses to eating. The child is placed supine under a gamma camera, and images are acquired each minute for 1 hour. The supine posture is excellent for provoking gastroesophageal reflux but may retard gastric emptying.[26] Delayed gastric emptying during a study with the infant supine may be an artifact that corrects when the child is placed in the right lateral decubitus position or held upright[27] (Fig. 20–2).

In most cases, test data fit a simple exponential curve: $f = ae^{-kt}$. In this equation, $f$ is the fraction of the meal in the stomach at time $t$, $a$ is the fraction present at $t = 0$, $e$ is the natural logarithmic constant 2.718, and $k$ is the rate of gastric emptying. Commonly, results are reported as the percentage of emptying at a specific time (e.g., 30 minutes, 1 hour, 2 hours) or the time required to empty 50% of radioactive material from the stomach ($t_{1/2}$). In adults, a $t_{1/2}$ longer than 120 minutes for emptying of two eggs was considered abnormal.[28]

#### *Indicator Dilution Tests*

Indicator dilution methods assess the gastric secretion and emptying of liquids by repeated sampling of gastric contents after the addition of a small amount of a nonabsorbable dye such as phenol red (for clear liquids) or a marker such as polyethylene glycol (for opaque liquids).[29] The advantages of a marker dilution method are that it provides simultaneous measurements of total gastric volume and secretion as well as emptying. The disadvantages include the requirement for gastric intubation and the operator time commitment, not only at the bedside but also in the laboratory and at the computer. Many research studies employ a marker dilution technique, but this method is impractical for clinical practice.

#### *Ultrasound Imaging*

Real-time ultrasonography has been used in the evaluation of gastric emptying to make serial measurements of antral

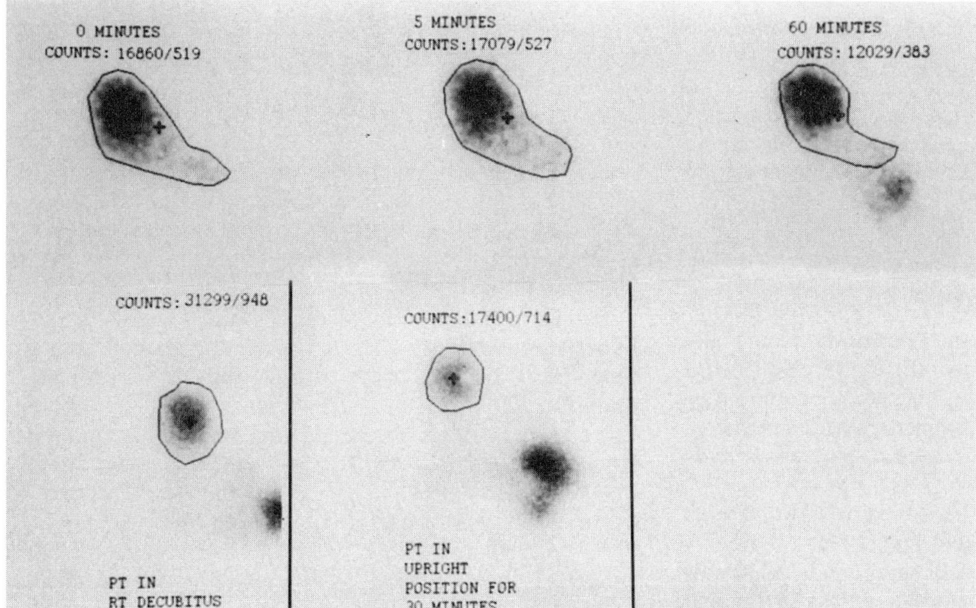


**FIGURE 20–2.** Radionuclide scintiscan of gastric emptying in a 3-week-old girl with vomiting. *Top row:* Three posterior views show activity in the stomach at times 0, 5, and 60 minutes. The percentage of the marker emptied at 60 minutes is 29% (normal, >40%). *Second row:* The percentage emptying after 30 minutes in the right lateral decubitus position is 63%, and after 30 minutes in the upright position it is 80%. In this study, the infant has positionally delayed gastric emptying. (Courtesy of Javier Villaneuva-Meyer, MD.)

cross-sectional area before and after a meal (Fig. 20–3). In contrast to gastric scintigraphy, which measures emptying of the radioactive meal only, ultrasound estimates both the meal and gastric secretions. It is noninvasive, reproducible, and can be performed easily even in young infants,[30, 31] but it is operator dependent, and specials skills are required to perform and interpret the study. Ultrasound is more accurate for gastric emptying of liquids than of solids.

## Tests of Gastric Myoelectric Activity

### *Electrogastrography*

Gastric myoelectric activity, first recorded in infants from serosal electrodes,[32] is now measured from pairs of Ag/AgCl electrodes on the skin surface overlying the stomach. Electrogastrography (EGG) is the measurement of the amplitude and frequency of gastric slow waves. Certain steps ensure signal fidelity: (1) accurate placement is facilitated with ultrasound or comparable guidance to locate the stomach; (2) the skin must be slightly abraded with sandpaper before the electrodes are placed; and (3) the raw signal is amplified and filtered to exclude cardiac and small intestinal electrical activity, as well as respiratory and movement artifacts.

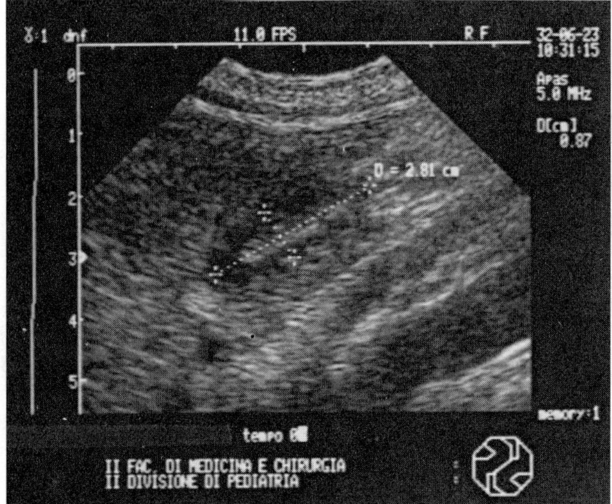


**FIGURE 20–3.** Ultrasonic view of the gastric antrum. The antrum is visible as the dark area between the markers in the anteroposterior and longitudinal diameters. (Courtesy of Salvatore Cucchiara, MD.)

EGG measures the basal electrical rhythm of the stomach or the frequency of the gastric slow waves. Normal frequencies are between 2.5 and 3.5 per minute. Dysrhythmias detected by EGG include tachygastria (5–9 waves per minute for at least 1 minute), bradygastria (fewer than 2 per minute for at least 1 minute), a mixed pattern (bradytachyarrhythmia), or absent electrical activity (flat line) (Fig. 20–4). Variation in the signal amplitude is measured as *power*: the amplitude squared divided by time. EGG power is a function of both the amplitude and the regularity of the slow waves. Typically, power increases after meals.

EGG is an attractive test because of its noninvasive character.[33] Measurements are influenced by electrode placement, subcutaneous fat tissue (less reliability in obese patients), and movements of the stomach within the abdomen. Children are prone to move without regard to the examiner's instructions, creating motion artifacts. Special expertise is required for the computer analysis and data interpretation. EGG has been used to evaluate children with enteric neuromuscular disorders. In neuropathic pseudo-obstruction, there is persistent tachygastria; if there is no dominant frequency, the disorder is usually myopathic.[34] Abnormal rhythms occur in children with functional dyspepsia.[35]

# DISORDERS OF GASTRIC EMPTYING

## Gastroparesis

Gastroparesis is defined as delayed gastric emptying in the absence of a demonstrable mechanical or mucosal lesion

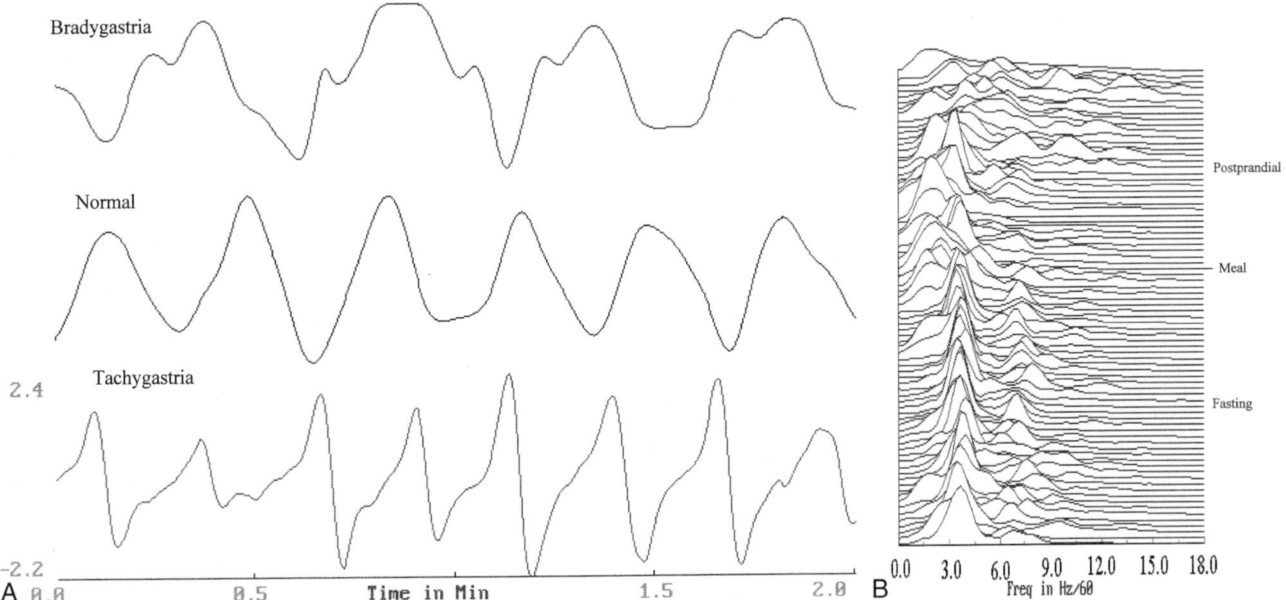


**FIGURE 20–4.** *A,* Typical EGG waveforms in bradygastria, normal rhythm, and tachygastria. *B,* A three-dimensional diagram of EGG results after fast Fourier transform analysis. Each horizontal line represents 1 minute of recording. Note that the dominant frequency is normal before the meal but becomes disorganized in a mixed arrhythmia after the meal in a patient with postprandial antral hypomotility. (Courtesy of S. N. Reddy, D.Eng.)

by radiologic or endoscopic studies. Signs and symptoms of gastroparesis include nausea, vomiting, abdominal distention, and epigastric pain in older children, and regurgitation, irritability, food refusal, and failure to thrive in infants and toddlers. Vomiting many hours after eating suggests a diagnosis of gastroparesis, especially if the vomitus contains recognizable food.[36] Delayed gastric emptying is commonly associated with gastroesophageal reflux disease in infants.[37] The physiology responsible for gastroparesis may include reduced contractions in the stomach; failed relaxation of the duodenum; impaired coordination among stomach, pylorus, and duodenum; or some combination of these factors.

## *Gastroparesis of Prematurity*

Gastroparesis commonly complicates the feeding of premature infants. Retained gastric contents may be regurgitated, causing obstructive apnea or aspiration pneumonia. Gastroparesis of prematurity is transient, disappearing with advancing age.

Berseth and Nordyke characterized the preterm infant postprandial responses (i.e., motor activity) as increased (mature fed response), unchanged (indeterminate fed response), or decreased (immature fed response). These postprandial motor responses change with gestational age.[38] Approximately two thirds of infants with less than 36 weeks' gestation display an immature response, 10% have an indeterminate response, and 25% have a mature response. Only 15% of full-term infants display an immature response. The immature response, postprandial duodenal hypomotility, is associated with delayed gastric emptying.[39] In preterm infants, gastric emptying slowed and there were fewer duodenal contractions as the size of the meal increased. In contrast, healthy adults increased the number of duodenal contractions as the size of the meal increased, and the rate of gastric emptying stayed constant.

The decreased motility and slowed gastric emptying with increasing meal size may represent a "duodenal brake" protecting the immature intestine from exposure to excessive amounts of substrate. Therefore, gastroparesis may be a normal developmental finding, and not a disease state, in the preterm infant. Remnants of the duodenal brake persisting into infancy may provide a physiologic explanation for why overfeeding associated with postprandial emesis or why cisapride, which increases the number and strength of duodenal contractions,[40] is a useful drug for many infants with gastroesophageal reflux.

## *Drug-Associated Gastroparesis*

Drugs such as morphine and other narcotic agonists, cholinergic antagonists, β-adrenergic agonists, and tricyclic antidepressants delay gastric emptying.[41]

## *Postviral Gastroparesis*

Isolated gastroparesis occurs as an acute complication of local inflammation, as in rotavirus gastroparesis.[42] Chronic gastroparesis acquired after infection by rotaviruses or other organisms is rare. Infectious agents such as herpes zoster,[43] Epstein-Barr virus,[44] and cytomegalovirus[45] can cause severe generalized disturbances in gastrointestinal motor function, especially in the immunocompromised patient or after organ transplantation. In otherwise healthy children, viral gastroparesis is usually transient, lasting months rather than years, and spontaneous recovery is seen in most cases.[46] Small bowel manometry shows postprandial antral hypomotility. It is not clear whether postviral gastroparesis is related to prolonged infection of the myenteric plexus, to an autoimmune inflammatory response to antigens common to myenteric neurons and the virus, or to some other cause.

### Gastroparesis Associated with Systemic Disease

Abnormal gastric emptying occurs as part of a diffuse disorder of gastrointestinal motor function, such as chronic intestinal pseudo-obstruction,[47] progressive systemic sclerosis,[48] dermatomyositis,[49] or Duchenne's muscular dystrophy.[50] The delayed gastric emptying observed in many patients with anorexia nervosa may reflect a hypersensitivity of the small intestinal chemoreceptor feedback mechanism after prolonged nutrient deprivation.[51]

Chronic gastroparesis due to autonomic neuropathy is an unusual complication in children and young adults with insulin-dependent diabetes mellitus, with onset occasionally as early as 1 to 7 years after diagnosis.[52] Hyperglycemia slows gastric emptying. Poorly controlled diabetes mellitus results in gastroparesis that further complicates postprandial glucose control. The best screening test for diabetic gastroparesis is scintigraphy to measure gastric emptying of a solid meal at a time when the patient is euglycemic. The most common manometric finding in diabetic gastroparesis is postprandial antral hypomotility. Acute gastroparesis may develop secondary to metabolic disorders such as hypokalemia, hyperglycemia, or hypothyroidism.

### Treatment of Gastroparesis

Diet changes reduce symptoms and gastric retention in some patients with gastroparesis. Patients may benefit from low-fat, low-fiber, high-protein, high-caloric-density liquid meals; smaller and more frequent feedings; or the substitution of pureed foods for solids. In severe cases, it is possible to bypass the gastroparetic stomach by placing a feeding tube into the small bowel, thus avoiding parenteral nutrition. Nasojejunal tube feedings may be especially helpful when respiratory distress accompanies gastroparesis, as in the acute to subacute phases of diaphragmatic hernia. For chronic gastroparesis, gastrojejunal or jejunostomy tubes are a management option.

Cisapride binds to serotonin receptors on myenteric plexus motor neurons, enhancing the release of acetylcholine.[53] It accelerates gastric emptying in preterm infants and children.[54–57] Cisapride is commonly used in the long-term treatment of patients with diabetic gastroparesis.[52] The dosage of cisapride in children is 0.15 to 0.3 mg/kg three to four times daily; in adults, it is 10 to 20 mg four times daily. Common adverse effects at therapeutic doses are transient diarrhea and abdominal cramps. Serious adverse effects are uncommon. Life-threatening cardiac arrhythmias were associated with excessive cisapride serum concentrations caused by overdose or by concomitant use of antifungals (ketoconazole, fluconazole, itraconazole, miconazole) or macrolides (erythromycin, clarithromycin, troleandomycin).[58, 59] These medications compete for a cytochrome P-450 isozyme. Oral dosing may be problematic in patients with gastroparesis, but the absorption of cisapride in the small bowel is excellent, so the drug may be given by jejunal tube.

Metoclopramide is a dopamine antagonist with gastrointestinal prokinetic and central nervous system antiemetic properties. Intravenous metoclopramide, 1 mg/kg, improved liquid gastric emptying in children with gastroesophageal reflux and postsurgical gastroparesis but not in those with gastroparesis of prematurity.[60] Drug tolerance to metoclopramide developed after several months of use, a factor that limited its usefulness for persistent symptoms.[61] Central nervous system side effects may develop in 20% to 30% of children treated with effective doses of metoclopramide. Irritability, sedation, and extrapyramidal side effects such as torticollis are transient or reversible with diphenhydramine in almost all cases, although irreversible changes have occurred.[62] The effective oral dosage of metoclopramide in children is 0.25 to 0.3 mg/kg four times daily,[63] although at least one expert recommended doses no higher than 0.1 mg/kg four times daily, a dose that is likely to be safe but ineffective.[64] Subcutaneous administration of metoclopramide gave serum concentrations equal to 80% of those obtained with intravenous administration and three times higher than with oral dosing.[65] The benefit of subcutaneous administration is that it avoids the variable absorption of oral drug in a patient with gastroparesis but does not require intravenous access.

Bethanechol is a muscarinic cholinergic agonist that enhances gastric motor activity. Because it is not selective for the gastrointestinal smooth muscle, it has a low therapeutic index. Subcutaneous administration of bethanechol improved gastric emptying in patients with diabetic gastroparesis.[24] Bethanechol is rarely used because of its cholinergic side effects at effective doses and the development of alternative agents with more favorable side effect profiles.

Erythromycin binds to motilin receptors, stimulating gastric antral contractions. Erythromycin accelerated gastric emptying in patients with diabetic gastroparesis.[66] The long-term efficacy of erythromycin is limited by the development of drug tolerance. Erythromycin given intravenously, 1 to 3 mg/kg over 30 to 60 minutes, stimulated clusters of gastric antral contractions in children with chronic functional gastrointestinal symptoms.[67]

Drug combinations using several prokinetics simultaneously, each with a different mechanism of action, have not been studied systematically. Anecdotal evidence suggests that in some patients the response to cisapride plus a cholinesterase inhibitor is better than the response to cisapride alone. Similarly, in patients with nausea as a prominent component of their gastroparesis, it may be beneficial to begin with metoclopramide, to reduce the nausea, before adding cisapride to stimulate contractions.

Gastroparesis is usually transient, resolving in weeks or months. Surgery has little role in the management of children with gastroparesis except in a few special circumstances. Rare patients with persistent, isolated gastroparesis may benefit from gastric drainage procedures such as subtotal distal gastrectomy with gastrojejunostomy, extensive gastric resection with Roux-en-Y drainage, and pyloroplasty. Pyloroplasty accompanying fundoplication failed to change the incidence of postoperative complications.[68] Gastric antroplasty, using a 2.5- to 3.5-cm incision through the antral muscularis down to the duodenum without mucosal incision, decreased the incidence of postoperative dumping syndrome, compared with pyloroplasty, in children with gastroesophageal reflux and delayed gastric emptying.[69] Gastric drainage procedures are not helpful in children with motility disorders involving the small bowel. Antroduodenal and colonic manometry are helpful in the assessment of bowel physiology before gastric drainage surgery; children with small bowel or colonic motility disorders do not benefit from gastric surgery. Electrical stimulation, or gastric pacing, is a research procedure that holds promise for those with chronic gastroparesis.[70]

## Accelerated Gastric Emptying

Accelerated gastric emptying is a complication of gastric surgery. Proximal gastric vagotomy impairs gastric receptive relaxation and accommodation and consequently speeds the emptying of liquids, with variable effects on the emptying of solids. Truncal vagotomy combines these effects with the denervation of the distal stomach and slows the emptying of solids. Liquids empty quickly, especially in the upright position. Pyloroplasty has little effect on the functions of the proximal stomach (i.e., emptying of liquids). However, the disruption of the pylorus by pyloroplasty results in impaired trituration, rapid gastric emptying of solids, and increased duodenogastric reflux.

*Dumping syndrome* is a cluster of symptoms resulting from rapid gastric emptying of carbohydrate-rich meals. In older children, symptoms include abdominal discomfort, palpitations, sweating, faintness, and diarrhea. Symptoms in younger children include irritability, sweating, emesis, and diarrhea. Early symptoms (epigastric pain and fullness, nausea, vomiting, diarrhea, weakness) occur 10 to 30 minutes after meals. Late symptoms (palpitations, sweating, weakness) occur 1 to 3 hours after meals as the result of hypoglycemia. In children, the diagnosis is easily overlooked because of the nonspecific nature of the symptoms. The most common cause of dumping syndrome in pediatric patients is the unintentional migration of the feeding end of a gastrostomy tube through the pylorus and into the duodenum. Dumping syndrome in children has been described rarely and almost exclusively after Nissen fundoplication.[71,72] The symptoms emerge shortly after surgery and often are transient. The diagnosis is based on a typical history, provocation of symptoms and hyperglycemia and/or hypoglycemia by a glucose meal, and the results of gastric emptying scintigraphy. The treatment for dumping syndrome is diet modification: small, frequent meals; increased fat intake; thickened feedings; continuous nasogastric or gastrostomy feeding; restricted fluid intake during meals; increased viscosity of meals (with the use of guar gum or pectin); or addition of complex carbohydrates such as uncooked starches.[73–75] Long-acting somatostatin analogues (e.g., octreotide) improve symptoms in some patients, perhaps by slowing gastric emptying and transit of the small intestine.[76]

### REFERENCES


1. Quigley EMM: Gastric and small intestinal motility in health and disease. Gastroenterol Clin North Am 1996;25:113–145.
2. Cannon WB, Lieb CM: The receptive relaxation of the stomach. Am J Physiol 1911;29:267–273.
3. Kelly KA: Gastric emptying of liquids and solids: roles of proximal and distal stomach. Am J Physiol 1980;239:71–76.
4. Sanders KM, Publicover NG: Electrophysiology of the gastric musculature. In Handbook of Physiology: The Gastrointestinal System. Motility and Circulation. Sect 6, vol I, chapt 23. Bethesda, American Physiology Society, 1989, pp 187–216.
5. Szurszewski JH: Electrophysiologic basis of gastrointestinal motility. In Johnson LR (ed): Physiology of the Gastrointestinal Tract, 2nd ed. New York, Raven Press, 1987, pp 383–422.
6. Hunt JN, Spurrell WR: The pattern of emptying of the human stomach. J Physiol 1951;113:157–168.
7. Hunt JN: Some properties of an alimentary osmoreceptor mechanism. J Physiol 1956;132:267–288.
8. Hunt JN, Knox MT: The slowing of gastric emptying by four strong acids and three weak acids. J Physiol 1972;222:187–208.
9. Hunt JN, Knox MT: A relationship between the length of the fatty acids and the slowing of gastric emptying. J Physiol 1968;194:327–336.
10. Stephens JR, Woolson RF, Cooke AR: Effects of essential and nonessential amino acids on gastric emptying in the dog. Gastroenterology 1975;69:920–927.
11. Spiller RC, Adrian TE, Trotman IF, et al: Further characterization of the "ileal brake" in man: effect of ileal infusion of partial digests of fat, protein and starch on jejunal motility and release of neurotensin, enteroglucagon and peptide YY. Gut 1988;29:1042–1051.
12. Hunt JN, Stubbs DF: The volume and energy content of meals as determinants of gastric emptying. J Physiol 1975;245:209–225.
13. Hinder RA, Kelly KA: Canine gastric emptying of solids and liquids. Am J Physiol 1977;233:E335–E340.
14. Berseth CL: Gastrointestinal motility in the neonate. Clin Perinatol 1996;23:179–190.
15. McLain C: Amniography studies of the gastrointestinal motility of the human fetus. Am J Obstet Gynecol 1963;86:1079–1087.
16. Cavell B: Gastric emptying in preterm infants. Acta Paediatr Scand 1979;68:725–730.
17. Husband J, Husband P, Mallinson C: Gastric emptying of starch meals in the newborn. Lancet 1970;2:290–292.
18. Ittmann PI, Amarnath R, Berseth CL: Maturation of antroduodenal motor activity in preterm and term infants. Dig Dis Sci 1992;37:14–19.
19. Tomomasa T, Miyazaki M, Koizumi T, et al: Erythromycin increases gastric antral motility in human premature infants. Biol Neonate 1993;63:349–352.
20. Amarnath RP, Berseth CL, Malagelada J-R, et al: Postnatal maturation of the small intestinal motility in preterm infants. J Gastrointest Motility 1989;1:138–143.
21. Tomomasa T, Itoh Z, Koizumi T, et al: Nonmigrating rhythmic activity in the stomach and the duodenum of neonates. Biol Neonate 1985;48:1–9.
22. Uc A, Hoon A, Di Lorenzo C, Hyman PE: Antroduodenal manometry in children with no upper gastrointestinal symptoms. Scand J Gastroenterol 1997;32:681–685.
23. Koenig WJ, Amarnath R, Hench V, et al: Manometrics for preterm and term infants: a new tool for old questions. J Pediatr 1995;95:203–206.
24. Malagelada J-R, Rees WDW, Mazzotta LJ, Go VLW: Gastric motor abnormalities in diabetics and postvagotomy gastroparesis. Gastroenterology 1980;78:286–293.
25. Chaudhuri TK, Fink S: Gastric emptying in human disease states. Am J Gastroenterol 1991;86:533–538.
26. Moore JG, Datz FL, Greenberg CE, et al: Effect of body posture on radionuclide measurements of gastric emptying. Dig Dis Sci 1988;33:1592–1595.
27. Villaneuva-Meyer J, Swischuk LE, Cesani F, et al: Pediatric gastric emptying: value of right lateral and upright positioning. J Nucl Med 1996;8:1356–1358.
28. Parkman HP, Harris AD, Krevsky B, et al: Gastroduodenal motility and dysmotility: an update on techniques available for evaluation. Am J Gastroenterol 1995;90:869–892.
29. Dubois A, Mizrahi M: New PC-based program to calculate gastric secretion and emptying using a marker dilution technique. Dig Dis Sci 1992;37:1302–1304.
30. Newel SJ, Chapman S, Booth IW: Ultrasonic assessment of gastric emptying in the preterm infant. Arch Dis Child 1993;69:32–36.
31. Carlos MA, Babyn PS, Marcon MAA, Moore AM: Changes in gastric emptying in early postnatal life. J Pediatr 1997;130:931–937.
32. Telander RL, Morgan KG, Kroelen DL, et al: Human gastric atony with tachygastria and gastric retention. Gastroenterology 1978;75:497–501.
33. Chen JDZ, McCallum RW: Clinical applications of electrogastrography. Am J Gastroenterol 1993;88:1324–1336.

34. Devane SP, Ravelli AM, Bisset WM, et al: Gastric antral dysrhythmias in children with chronic intestinal pseudo-obstruction. Gut 1992;33:1477–1481.
35. Cucchiara S, Riezzo G, Minella R, et al: Electrogastrography in nonulcer dyspepsia. Arch Dis Child 1992;67:613–617.
36. Horowitz M, Dent J: Disordered gastric emptying: mechanical basis, assessment and treatment. Baillieres Clin Gastroenterol 1991;5:371–407.
37. Cucchiara S, Salvia G, Borrelli O, et al: Gastric electrical dysrhythmias and delayed gastric emptying in gastroesophageal reflux disease. Am J Gastroenterol 1997;92:1103–1108.
38. Berseth CL, Nordyke CK: Manometry can predict feeding readiness in preterm infants. Gastroenterology 1992;103:1523–1528.
39. Knapp E, Berseth CL: Immature duodenal motor responses to bolus feedings are associated with delayed gastric emptying in preterm infant. Pediatr Res 1996;39:313A.
40. DiLorenzo C, Reddy SN, Villaneuva-Meyer J, et al: Cisapride in children with chronic intestinal pseudo-obstruction: an acute, double-blind crossover, placebo controlled trial. Gastroenterology 1991;101:1564–1570.
41. Nimmo WS: Drugs, diseases and altered gastric emptying. Clin Pharmacokinet 1976;1:189–203.
42. Bardhan PK, Salam MA, Molla AM: Gastric emptying of liquid in children suffering from acute rotaviral gastroenteritis. Gut 1992;33(1):26–29.
43. Kebede D, Barthel JS, Singh A: Transient gastroparesis associated with cutaneous herpes zoster. Dig Dis Sci 1987;32:318–322.
44. Yahr MD, Frontera AT: Acute autonomic neuropathy: its occurrence in infectious mononucleosis. Arch Neurol 1975;32:132–133.
45. Press MF, Riddell RH, Ringus J: Cytomegalovirus inclusion disease: its occurrence in the myenteric plexus of a renal transplant patient. Arch Pathol Lab Med 1980;104:580–583.
46. Sigurdsson L, Flores AF, Putnam PE, et al: Postviral gastroparesis: presentation, treatment, outcome. J Pediatr 1997;131:751–754.
47. Hyman PE: Chronic intestinal pseudo-obstruction in childhood: progress in diagnosis and management. Scand J Gastroenterol 1995;213:39–46.
48. Greydanus MP, Camilleri M: Abnormal postcibal antral and small bowel motility due to neuropathy or myopathy in systemic sclerosis. Gastroenterology 1989;96:110–115.
49. Kelckner FS: Dermatomyositis and its manifestations in the gastrointestinal tract. Am J Gastroenterol 1970;53:141–146.
50. Staiano A, Corraziari E, Andreotti MR, et al: Upper gastrointestinal tract motility in children with progressive muscular dystrophy. J Pediatr 1992;121:720–724.
51. Rigaud D, Bedig G, Merrouche M, et al: Delayed gastric emptying in anorexia nervosa is improved by completion of a renutrition program. Dig Dis Sci 1988;33:919–925.
52. Reid B, Di Lorenzo C, Travis L, et al: Diabetic gastroparesis due to postprandial antral hypomotility in childhood. Pediatrics 1992;90:43–46.
53. Cucchiara S: Cisapride therapy for gastrointestinal disease. J Pediatr Gastroenterol Nutr 1996;22:259–269.
54. Janssens G, Melis K, Vaerenberg M: Long-term use of cisapride in premature infants of <34 weeks gestational age. J Pediatr Gastroenterol Nutr 1990;11:420–422.
55. Cucchiara S, Bortolotti M, Minella R, et al: Children with functional gastrointestinal symptoms: effect of cisapride on fasting antroduodenal motility, gastric emptying of liquids, and symptoms. Eur J Gastroenterol Hepatol 1992;4:627–633.
56. Carroccio A, Ianoco G, Li Voti G, et al: Gastric emptying in infants with gastroesophageal reflux: ultrasound evaluation before and after cisapride administration. Scand J Gastroenterol 1992;27:799–804.
57. Riezzo G, Cucchiara S, Chiloiro M, et al: Gastric emptying and myoelectrical activity in children with non-ulcer dyspepsia: effect of cisapride treatment. Dig Dis Sci 1995;40:1428–1434.
58. Pettignano R, Chambliss CR, Darsey E, et al: Cisapride-induced dysrhythmia in a pediatric patient receiving extracorporeal life support. Crit Care Med 1996;24:1268–1271.
59. Lewin MB, Bryant RM, Fenrich AL, et al: Cisapride-induced long QT interval. J Pediatr 1996;128:279–281.
60. Hyman PE, Abrams CE, Dubois A: Gastric emptying in infants: response to metoclopramide depends on the underlying condition. J Pediatr Gastroenterol Nutr 1988;7:181–184.
61. Schade RR, Dugas MC, Lhotsky DM, et al: Effect of metoclopramide on gastric liquid emptying in patients with diabetic gastroparesis. Dig Dis Sci 1985;30:10–15.
62. Putnam PE, Orenstein SR, Wessel HB, Stowe RM: Tardive dyskinesia associated with metoclopramide use in a child. J Pediatr 1992;121:983–985.
63. Hyams JS, Leichtner AM, Zamett LO, Walters JK: Effects of metoclopramide on prolonged intraesophageal pH testing in infants with gastroesophageal reflux. J Pediatr Gastroenterol Nutr 1986;5:716–720.
64. Orenstein SR: Gastroesophageal reflux. In Hyman PE (ed): Pediatric Gastrointestinal Motility Disorders. New York, Academy Professional Information Services, 1994, p 76.
65. McCallum RW, Valenzuela G, Polepalle SC, et al: Subcutaneous metoclopramide in the treatment of symptomatic gastroparesis: clinical efficacy and pharmacokinetics. J Pharmacol Exp Ther 1991;258:136–142.
66. Janssens J, Peeters T, Vantrappen G, et al: Improvement of gastric emptying in diabetic gastroparesis by erythromycin. N Engl J Med 1990;322:1028–1031.
67. Di Lorenzo C, Flores AF, Tomomasa T, Hyman PE: Effect of erythromycin on antroduodenal motility in children with chronic functional gastrointestinal symptoms. Dig Dis Sci 1994;39:1399–1404.
68. Maxson RT, Harp S, Jackson RJ, et al: Delayed gastric emptying in neurologically impaired children with gastroesophageal reflux: the role of pyloroplasty. J Pediatr Surg 1994;29:726–729.
69. Fonkalsrud EW, Ament ME, Vargas J: Gastric antroplasty for the treatment of delayed gastric emptying and gastroesophageal reflux in children. Am J Surg 1992;164:327–331.
70. Hocking MP, Vogel SB, Sninsky CA: Human gastric myoelectric activity and gastric emptying following gastric surgery and with pacing. Gastroenterology 1992;103:1811–1816.
71. Meyer S, Deckelbaum RJ, Lax E, Schiller M: Infant dumping syndrome after esophageal reflux surgery. J Pediatr 1981;99:235–237.
72. Caulfield ME, Wyllie R, Firor HV, Michener W: Dumping syndrome in children. J Pediatr 1987;110:212–215.
73. Leeds AR, Ralphs DNL, Ebied F, et al: Pectin in the dumping syndrome: reduction of volumes and plasma volume changes. Lancet 1981;1:1075–1078.
74. Harju E, Larmi TKI: Efficacy of guar gum in preventing the dumping syndrome. J Parenter Enterol Nutr 1983;7:470–472.
75. Gitzelmann R, Hirsig J: Infant dumping syndrome: reversal of symptoms by feeding uncooked starch. Eur J Pediatr 1986;145:504–506.
76. Primrose JN, Johnston D: Somatostatin analogue SMS201–995 (octreotide) as a possible solution to the dumping syndrome after gastrectomy or vagotomy. Br J Surg 1989;76:140–144.

# Chapter 21

# Bezoars

Daniel L. Preud'Homme and Adam G. Mezoff

Bezoars are aggregates of undigested material such as plant fibers, hair, medication, or other inedible material found in the esophagus, stomach, small intestine, or colon. The term *bezoar* comes from the Arabic *badzehr* or the Persian *panzehr,* which refer to masses of fibers or foreign material found in sacrificed animals such as goats.[1, 1a] In ancient times, these animal bezoars were considered to have magical or medicinal qualities and were used as antidotes to poisons from snake bites, diverse diseases, and aging. Charak, an Indian physician, reported the presence of bezoars in his work in the 2nd and 3rd centuries B.C.[2] In the western world, Baudamant first described this finding in an autopsy performed in 1779.[3] The first extensive review was done in 1915 by Matas, followed by the landmark review by DeBakey and Oschner in 1938.[1, 1a] Surgical removal of bezoars was first described in the 19th century by Schonbon.[2]

## PATHOGENESIS

The formation of bezoars depends on both the specific character of the indigestible material that is ingested and clinical characteristics of the patient that affect digestion and gastric emptying (Table 21–1). Phytobezoars result from rapid accumulation of vegetable matter in the stomach. They occur primarily in patients with poor mastication or altered gastric anatomy or physiology. Delayed gastric emptying secondary to disease states (diabetes mellitus, scleroderma, muscular dystrophy), surgical intervention in the upper intestinal tract (Billroth I and II), vagotomy, or the use of medications that decrease gastric acidity (antacids, histamine $H_2$ receptor antagonists, proton-pump inhibitors) may all contribute to formation of a bezoar.[4] In the specific instance of persimmon bezoars, the action of gastric acidity on fiber such as tannin or cellulose forms an insoluble coagulum, which grows with the continued ingestion of the fruit.[5]

Trichobezoars occur primarily in children with behavioral disorders. The ingestion of hair usually starts in childhood, when formation of the hairball occurs in the stomach, and continues for years. The bezoar slowly grows and eventually occupies the whole stomach cavity. These masses are then referred to as hair casts. Extension of these casts may occur upward to the esophagus or downward to the small intestine. There usually are no underlying anatomic or physiologic defects in these patients, such as those found in patients with phytobezoars.

## CLASSIFICATION

### Phytobezoars

Phytobezoars are the most frequently observed type and account for approximately 40% of the total number of reported bezoars. They are composed of indigestible vegetable fibers, most commonly from pulpy fruits, orange pits, seeds, roots, or leaves. A case of a "cotton" bezoar was reported in a heroin addict who swallowed the cotton ball used to filter a water-methadone pill preparation for intravenous infusion.[6] These bezoars are usually found in the stomach (78%), although up to 17% may occur in the small intestine.[4] Sunflower seed concretions have been described in the colons of children.[7]

### Diospyrobezoar (Persimmon Bezoar)

Although made of vegetable matter, persimmon bezoars represent a class by themselves and account for up to 29% of all bezoars.[1] Persimmon bezoars are named for a native American tree that also is present in Iran and the Middle East, *Diospyros virginiana.* Its fruit, a berry, contains a material called shiboul or phobatanin. This substance is present in the unripened fruit and under the skin of the ripe fruit.[8]

**TABLE 21–1. Factors Predisposing to the Formation of Phytobezoars**

| FACTOR | PREVALENCE IN PATIENTS (%) |
|---|---|
| Poor mastication | 80 |
| Gastric surgery with vagotomy | 56 |
| Gastroparesis | 20 |
| Histamine $H_2$ receptor antagonists | 12 |
| Diabetes mellitus | 6 |
| Excessive intake of fibers | 44 |

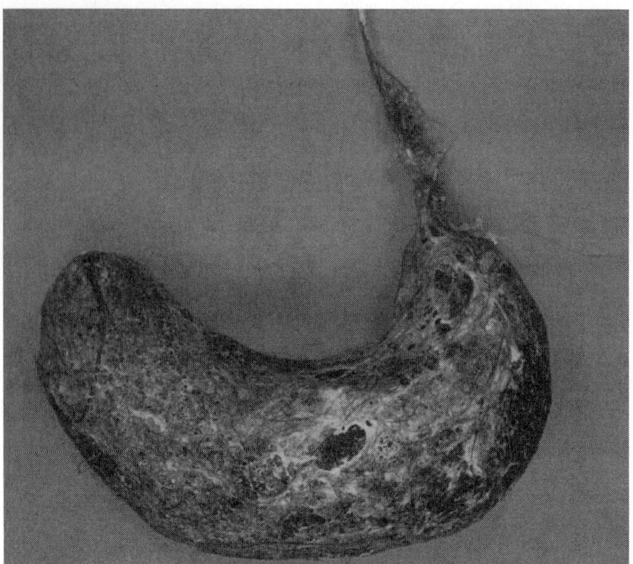

**FIGURE 21–1.** Hair cast of the stomach. (Courtesy of D. Mirkin, MD, Children's Medical Center, Dayton, OH.)

## Trichobezoar

Trichobezoars occur predominantly (up to 90%) in females under the age of 20, often in children.[1] They have been described in children as young as 1 year old. They consist of an aggregation of hair and foodstuff and are black regardless of the patient's hair color, because of the chemical reaction of hair with gastric acidity (Fig. 21–1). The hair in the trichobezoar is usually from the patient, although hair from animals, carpet, or toys is occasionally recovered.[9] Trichobezoars are usually the site for intense food putrefaction and can generate a very foul-smelling odor and halitosis. The act of hair swallowing is thought to be akin to pica or nail-biting. Only about 9% of patients with trichobezoars have proven psychiatric problems.[10] Trichobezoars usually are present in the stomach but may have very long tails. These tails can invade the esophagus proximally and expand to the colon distally. The extension of a trichobezoar from the stomach to the entire length of the small intestine is referred to as Rapunzel syndrome.[2] Trichobezoars may weight up to 6.5 pounds.

## Lactobezoar

Lactobezoars are gastric masses made of milk protein. They occur primarily in premature, low-birth-weight infants. Although the exact cause remains unclear, it is thought to be related to formula composition, protein flocculation, thickening agents, immature gastric motility, and rapidity of feeding.[11] Most reported cases have occurred in infants fed high-calorie formula for premature babies.[12] However, human milk bezoars have also been described.[13] The formation of lactobezoars may be precipitated by the addition of thickening agents, such as gel of pectin, to the infant's formula.[14] Lactobezoars have also been reported in adults fed Osmolite (Ross Nutritionals, Columbus, OH).[15]

## Paper Bezoar

At least two case reports of paper bezoars, one in a child and one in an adult, have been described. The undigested material was toilet paper, ingested over several days.[16]

## Medication Bezoar

A large number of case reports have documented the formation of concretions from various medications, leading to gastric bezoars. The medications implicated were nifedipine XL,[17] sucralfate,[18] bromide,[19] enteric-coated aspirin,[20] calcium or sodium polystyrene sulfonate (Kayexalate),[21] iron,[22] meprobamate,[23] slow-release theophylline,[24] and antacid.[25] Along with the typical obstructive symptoms of bezoars, these foreign bodies may also induce symptoms based on their intrinsic pharmacologic effects. Bezoar formation is probably related to the composition of the inert compound in the medication (e.g., cellulose). This has been a particular problem with medications packaged in insoluble material for long, continuous delivery of the active drug.[17]

## Cement Bezoars

Cement contains oxide of silica, aluminum, iron, and calcium; sulphuric anhydroxide; magnesium hydroxide; and calcium carbonate. It is easily accessible to children. Several cases of cement bezoars have been reported in young children, with the formation of solidified concretions. Different types of cement require various lengths of time to "set." After this time has elapsed, attempts at gastric lavage are futile and surgery is required.[26]

## Yeast Bezoars

Yeast bezoars have been reported primarily in patients undergoing gastric surgery, particularly vagotomy, although one was described in a newborn and was composed of *Candida albicans* and polystyrene resin.[27] Of the 43 patients with yeast bezoars reported in a Finnish study in 1974, 48% had undergone a Billroth I procedure and vagotomy. The most common species of fungus noted were *C. albicans* and *Torulopsis glabrata*.[28] Yeast bezoars are usually asymptomatic and are discovered incidentally. They have a tendency to recur.

## Shellac Bezoars

Although glue bezoars have been described in experimenting adolescents, most shellac bezoars occur in adult alcoholics who drink shellac to intensify the effect of their alcohol. Shellac can be found in furniture polish and is readily available to children.[1]

## Polybezoars

The term *polybezoars* refers to bezoars composed of multiple objects (metallic, plastic, or even wood) encased in

**TABLE 21–2. Clinical Manifestation of Bezoars**

| CHARACTERISTIC | INCIDENCE IN PATIENTS (%) |
|---|---|
| Halitosis | 20–40 |
| Abdominal/epigastric pain | 40–70 |
| Fullness after meal | 20–60 |
| Nausea/vomiting | 10–50 |
| Abdominal mass | 10–88 |
| Perforation/pneumatosis/acute abdomen | 7–10 |
| Dysphagia | 5 |
| Intestinal obstruction, partial or complete | up to 75 |
| Weakness/weight loss | 6–30 |
| Peptic ulcer disease | 10–24 |
| Hematemesis | up to 71 |

trichobezoars. These usually are found in children or in neurologically impaired adults. Polybezoars often contain a large number of metal pins or clips.[29]

## CLINICAL PRESENTATION

A summary of the clinical manifestations of bezoars is shown in Table 21–2.[1, 29a, 30–33] The initial presentation of many bezoars depends on their type. In premature infants and newborns, the most common bezoar is the lactobezoar. The most common symptom is feeding intolerance.[11] With time, symptoms may include abdominal distention, irritability, and vomiting. Physical examination often discloses a palpable mid-abdominal mass.

Trichobezoars and phytobezoars are more common in older children and adults. Trichobezoars form over long periods (several years), and early in their course their signs and symptoms can be subtle (early satiety or nausea).[1] These bezoars can grow to a substantial size and mass, causing pressure necrosis of the gastric mucosa, ulceration, gastrointestinal bleeding, and even gastric perforation.[32] Most trichobezoars have "tails," either up the esophagus (leading to dysphagia) or down the small intestine (leading to partial or complete obstruction). Trichobezoars can often be identified by abdominal palpation. Crepitus, caused by putrefaction and bacterial growth, may be elicited. Phytobezoars are formed much more rapidly than trichobezoars. Symptoms include nausea, vomiting, and signs of gastric outlet obstruction, which may persist even after the bezoar has been removed. Serious complications such as gastric perforation are rare but have been the subject of case reports in both adult and pediatric patients.[32] Pharmacobezoars not only may induce symptoms as a result of their gastric mass, but they also carry the potential for drug intoxication.[17–24] Concretion of foreign objects in the duodenum and in the biliary tract can cause pancreatitis (toxic "sock" syndrome).[34] Symptoms such as malabsorption and protein-losing enteropathy can also arise from bezoars in these locations.[1]

## DIAGNOSIS

The diagnosis of bezoars in adult patients can often be made by history and physical examination. Knowledge of predisposing factors may heighten clinical suspicion. Laboratory studies are of limited value, although, occasionally, a mild microcytic anemia or leukocytosis may develop. Imaging studies such as plain abdominal radiographs are the initial diagnostic modality identifying most bezoars. Barium studies may be useful to identify the bezoar and to determine the extent of the mass (Fig. 21–2). However, upper gastrointestinal series may fail to diagnose bezoars in 36% to 50% of patients.[25, 34] Moreover, in a reported case of enteric-coated aspirin bezoar, the use of barium changed the acid environment of the bezoar, leading to its disruption and subsequent increase in the salicylate level.[20] Other methods, such as ultrasound or computed tomography, have also been used to document gastric bezoars.[35, 36] These studies do not add to the diagnostic accuracy. Endoscopy remains the diagnostic modality of choice for identifying the type of gastric bezoar. Endoscopy also allows further therapeutic interventions.[25]

## TREATMENT

Gastric lavage with or without endoscopy has been used in an attempt to dissolve the bezoar mass. Instillation of various pharmacologic agents has also been attempted in an effort to increase the chance of chemical dissolution. These agents used include the following.

1. Acetylcysteine. One case reported by Schlang describes lavage with 15 mL acetylcysteine diluted in 50 mL of 0.9% NaCl per nasogastric tube. This treatment was repeated 8 hours later, and the bezoar was successfully dissolved.[37]

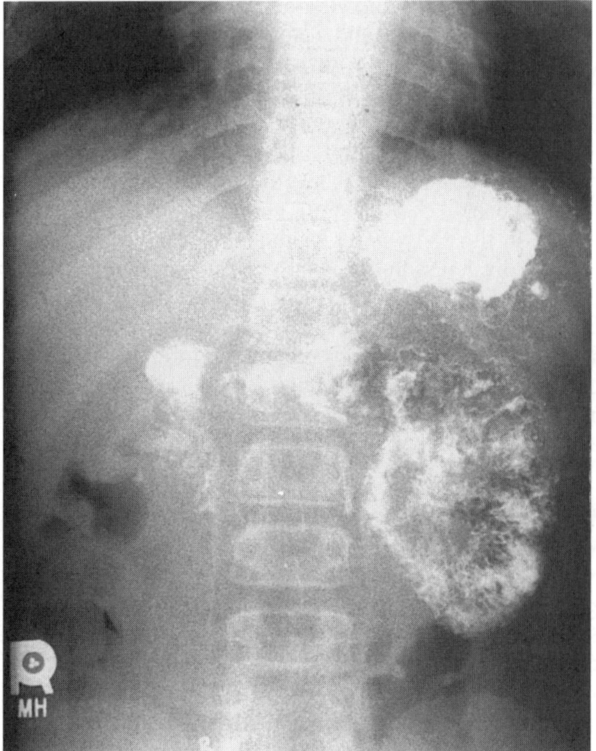


**FIGURE 21–2.** Barium swallow showing a mass effect in the body of the stomach. This mass was a trichobezoar that had to be removed by surgical intervention. (Courtesy of F. Unger, MD, Children's Medical Center, Dayton, OH.)

2. Papain. This enzyme is no longer available in tablet form in the United States. However, papain is present in high concentration in commercial meat tenderizer, along with a high concentration of sodium (1,880 mg/5 mL).[38] It has been used successfully to enzymatically break protein bonds in a phytobezoar. It can be administered as a lavage or in a diluted beverage. In small series of selected cases (15 patients), it has proved to be quite useful.[39] Complications such as hypernatremia or perforation of the esophagus or stomach have been reported.[40, 41]

3. Cellulase. It is believed that this enzyme cleaves the bond between leucoanthocyanidine-hemicellulose-cellulose.[42] A collection of 19 reported cases revealed a 100% success rate with the use of 3 to 5 g of cellulase diluted with 300 to 500 mL of water administered orally for 2 to 5 days.[39, 42]

4. Metoclopramide. Delayed gastric emptying is a major predisposing factor in the formation of gastric bezoars. Metoclopramide has been used acutely and in long-term maintenance to help clear and prevent the recurrence of phytobezoars.[43]

Endoscopy has been used to physically disrupt the bezoar. This can be done with a high-pressure water system (waterpick), a snare, or forceps.[25] The bezoar fragments are then withdrawn through the suction channel of the instrument. Other techniques using extracorporeal shock-wave lithotripsy, endoscopic drill, or a neodymium:yttrium-aluminum-garnet laser have also been reported.[25]

Gastric lavage and antimycotics usually are successful in breaking down yeast bezoars. Pharmacobezoars are a serious challenge in view of the potential toxicity of the medications involved. Endoscopy and vigorous lavage have been successful in the dissolution and detoxification of the pill mass. Conservative treatment with bowel rest and slow refeeding is the only treatment for lactobezoars in infants.[10, 11, 13]

The success rates of the different therapies are difficult to compare. Significant complications arising from the use of various dissolution agents have been reported. Surgery was the treatment of choice before endoscopic techniques came into use in the early 1970s. Although conservative management, medical dissolution, and endoscopic removal are the best options in the treatment of most bezoars, surgery remains the therapy of choice for the more significant complications (gastrointestinal obstruction, perforation) and for bezoars made of unusual foreign substances (e.g., cement, shellac). On occasion, trichobezoars can be milked down the cecum and allowed to pass.[31]

## PREVENTION

Gastric motility disorders, previous gastric surgery, poor mastication, and hypochlorhydria are major risk factors for the development and recurrence of many forms of gastric phytobezoars. Dietary counseling to avoid pulpy and fiber-rich foods should be provided to patients with these problems. Prokinetic agents such as metoclopramide or cisapride may be useful in preventing recurrences in certain patient populations. Identification of pica-like behavior in children should initiate counseling to prevent the ingestion of foreign substances. A history of significant trichotillomania may prompt psychological evaluation.

## REFERENCES


1. DeBakey M, Ochsner A: Bezoars and concretions. Surgery 1938;4:934–963.

1a. DeBakey M, Ochsner A: Bezoars and corrections. Part 2. Surgery 1939;5:132–160.

2. Deslypere JP, Praet M, Verdonk G: An unusual case of trichobezoar: the Rapunzel syndrome. Am J Gastroenterol 1982;7:467–470.

3. Baudamant WW: Memoire sur des cheveux trouves dans l'estomac et dans les intestins greles. J Med Chir Pharm 1779;52:507–514.

4. Tebar TC, Robles Campos R, Parilla Paricio P, et al: Gastric surgery and bezoars. Dig Dis Sci 1992;11:1694–1696.

5. Hayes PG, Rotstein OD: Gastrointestinal phytobezoars: presentation and management. Can J Surg 1986;6:419–420.

6. Kaden W: Phytobezoar in an addict: the cottonpicking stomach syndrome. JAMA 1969;209:1367.

7. Tsou VM, Bishop PR, Nowicki MJ: Colonic sunflower seed bezoars. Pediatrics 1997;6:896–897.

8. Izumi S, Isida K, Iwamoto M: Mechanism of formation of phytobezoar with special reference to a persimmon ball. Jpn J Med Sc Tr, II Biochemistry 1933;2:21.

9. Sidhu BS, Singh G, Khanna S: Trichobezoar. J Indian Med Assoc 1993;4:100–101.

10. Bhatnagar V, Mitra DK: Childhood trichobezoar. Indian J Pediatr 1984;51:489–492.

11. Schreiner RL, Brady MS, Franken EA, et al: Increased incidence of lactobezoars in low birth weight infant. Am J Dis Child 1979;133:936–939.

12. Schreiner RL, Brady MS, Ernst JA, et al: Lack of lactobezoars in infants given predominantly whey containing formula. Am J Dis Child 1982;136:437–439.

13. Yoss B: Human milk bezoars. J Pediatr 1984;5:819–822.

14. Faverge B, Gratecos LA: Lactobezoar gastrique du nourrisson induit par Gelopectose. Pediatrie 1987;42:685–686.

15. Chintapalli KN: Gastric bezoar causing intramural pneumatosis. J Clin Gastroenterol 1994;3:264–266.

16. Majeski JA: Paper bezoars in the stomach. South Med J 1985;12:1520.

17. Stack PE, Patel NR, Young MF, et al: Pharmacobezoars: the irony of the antidote. First case report of nifedipine XL bezoars. J Clin Gastroenterol 1994;3:264–265.

18. Strozik KS, Walele AH, Hoffman H: Bezoar in a preterm baby associated with sucralfate. Clin Pediatr 1996;8:423–424.

19. Iberti TJ, Patterson BK, Fisher CJ: Prolonged bromide intoxication resulting from a gastric bezoar. Arch Intern Med 1984;144:402–403.

20. Boghacz K, Caldron P: Enteric coated aspirin: elevation of the serum salicylate level by barium study. Case report and review of the medical management. Am J Med 1987;83:783–787.

21. Towsend C, Remmers A, Sarles II, et al: Intestinal obstruction from medication bezoar in patients with renal failure. N Engl J Med 1973;288:1058–1059.

22. Landsman I, Bricker JT, Reid BS, et al: Emergency gastrectomy: treatment of choice for iron bezoar. J Pediatr Surg 1987;22:184–185.

23. Schwartz HS: Acute meprobamate poisoning with gastrostomy and removal of a drug containing mass. N Engl J Med 1976;295:1177–1178.

24. Cereda JM, Scott J, Quigley EM: Endoscopic removal of a pharmacobezoar of slow release theophylline. BMJ 1986;293:1143–1144.

25. Lee J: Bezoars and foreign bodies of the stomach. Gastrointest Endosc Clin North Am 1996;6:605–619.

26. Visvanathan R: Cement bezoar of the stomach. Br J Surg 1986;73:381–382.

27. Metlay L, Klionsky B: An unusual gastric bezoar in a newborn: polystyrene resin and *Candida albicans*. J Pediatr 1983;1:121–123.

28. Perttala Y, Peltokallio P, Leiviska T, et al: Yeast bezoar formation following gastric surgery. Am J Roentgenol Radium Ther Nucl Med 1975;2:365–373.

29. Bitar D: Polybezoar and gastrointestinal foreign bodies in the mentally retarded. Am Surg 1975;41:497–499.

29a. Raffin SB: Bezoars. In Sleisenger MH, Fortran JS (eds): Gastrointestinal Disease: Pathophysiology, Diagnosis, Management, 4th ed. Philadelphia, WB Saunders, 1989, pp 741–745.

30. Zarling EJ, Thompson L: Nonpersimmon gastric phytobezoar, a benign recurrent condition. Arch Intern Med 1994;144:959–961.

31. Robles R, Parrilla P, Escamilla C, et al: Gastrointestinal bezoars. Br J Surg 1994;81:1000–1001.

32. Lagios MD: Emphysematous gastritis with perforation complicating a phytobezoar. Am J Dis Child 1968;116:202–204.
33. Brady PG: Gastric phytobezoar consequent to delayed gastric emptying. Gastrointest Endosc 1978;24:159–161.
34. Adler AI, Olscamp A: Toxic "sock" syndrome: bezoar formation and pancreatitis associated with iron deficiency and pica. West J Med 1995;163:480–481.
35. Naik DR, Bolia A, Boon AW: Demonstration of a lactobezoar by ultrasound. Br J Radiol 1987;60:506–508.
36. Tamminen J, Rosenfeld D: CT diagnosis of a gastric trichobezoar. Comput Med Imaging Graph 1988;6:339–341.
37. Schlang HA: Acetylcysteine in the removal of a bezoar. JAMA 1970;214:1329.
38. Zarling EJ, Moeller DD: Bezoar therapy: complication using Adolph meat tenderizer and alternatives from literature review. Arch Intern Med 1981;141:1669–1670.
39. Walker-Renard P: Update on the medical management of phytobezoar. Am J Gastroenterol 1993;10:1663–1666.
40. Dugan FA, Lilly JO, McCaffey TD: Dissolution of a phytobezoar with short term medical management. South Med J 1972;65:313–316.
41. Holsinger JW, Fuson RL, Sealy WC: Esophageal perforation following meat impaction and papain ingestion. JAMA 1968;204:188–189.
42. Lee P, Holloway WD, Nicholson GI: The medicinal dissolution of phytobezoar using cellulase. Br J Surg 1977;64:403–405.
43. Delpre G, Kadish U, Glanz I: Metoclopramide in the treatment of gastric bezoar. Am J Gastroenterol 1984;79:739–740.

SECTION FOUR

# THE SMALL AND LARGE INTESTINE

# Chapter 22

# Maldigestion and Malabsorption

*Elizabeth E. Mannick and John N. Udall, Jr.*

The gastrointestinal tract receives ingested nutrients, digests them, and absorbs the simple constituents. Normal intestinal digestion and absorption can be divided into sequential stages: (1) luminal hydrolysis and solubilization, (2) hydrolysis at the enterocyte membrane, (3) absorption across the enterocyte membrane and cellular processing, and (4) uptake from the enterocyte into blood and lymph. In the luminal stage, proteins, carbohydrates, and lipids are hydrolyzed by enzymes released from salivary glands, the stomach, and the pancreas. Bile from the liver participates in this process by creating a solubilizing organic environment in which lipids can be digested. Digestion continues at the level of intestinal cell membrane, where hydrolysis of peptides and disaccharides by brush border enzymes takes place. This is followed by the cellular absorption of amino acids, small peptides, monosaccharides, monoglycerides, and fatty acids. Once inside the enterocyte, nutrients are processed. (Water and small molecules may also be absorbed by a paracellular route.) Absorbed nutrients are then transported into blood and lymph and carried into distant organs for storage or metabolism. Diseases that interrupt any of these stages may lead to maldigestion and malabsorption. Generally speaking, malabsorption can be defined as "subnormal intestinal absorption of dietary constituents, and thus excessive loss of nutrients in the stool; it may be due to a digestive defect, a mucosal abnormality, or lymphatic obstruction."[1]

## PATHOPHYSIOLOGIC MECHANISMS

A list of maldigestive and malabsorptive disorders is shown in Table 22–1. They are reviewed in this chapter, and an approach to diagnosis and management of these disorders is presented.

### Digestion in the Lumen

#### *Mouth*

Although there are obvious differences between the mouth and the rest of the gastrointestinal tract, there are similarities in terms of exocrine secretion.[2] Saliva, the exocrine secretion present in the mouth, is important for normal digestion. Three pairs of salivary glands help in elaborating the fluid: the parotid, submandibular, and sublingual glands. These three glands contribute 20%, 60%, and 20%, respectively, to the total amount of saliva.[3] Numerous smaller glands are located in the lips, palate, tongue, and cheeks; these glands also contribute to the exocrine fluid. Saliva contains amylase and lipase; both hydrolytic enzymes are important to digestion. The amylase is almost entirely derived from the parotid glands. Lingual lipase is secreted by the serous glands (Ebner's glands) under the circumvallate papillae of the tongue. Also present in the saliva is a carrier protein for vitamin $B_{12}$. This carrier protein, or haptocorrin, is known as R binder protein.[4] Knowledge of the mechanisms of transfer of vitamin $B_{12}$ from one carrier to another in the intestinal tract is incomplete.[5]

One disease that may have an unexpected effect on digestion in the mouth is cystic fibrosis (CF). CF is now recognized as a generalized abnormality of the exocrine glands of the body secondary to a dysfunctional cystic fibrosis transmembrane conductance regulator protein.[6] In CF, the submandibular glands may enlarge, with an associated reduction in salivary fluid volume. Parotid glands and amylase production seem less affected.[2] Studies of lingual lipase suggest that salivary lipase activity is higher in CF patients than in controls. This results in increased intragastric lipolysis of a triglyceride test meal.[7]

In Sjögren's syndrome, there is little or no saliva, yet maldigestion does not seem to be a feature of this disease.[8]

#### *Stomach*

The stomach is essential for normal digestion. Gastric acid, pepsinogen, lipase, and intrinsic factor produced by the gastric mucosa all participate in the intraluminal stage of digestion. The production of hydrochloric acid by parietal cells is important, because a low pH facilitates the conversion of pepsinogen to pepsin.[3] Gastric lipase, produced by chief cells of the fundus, is necessary for complete digestion of the fat present in human milk.[9, 10] In addition, intrinsic factor, a protein elaborated by the gastric mucosa, binds

**TABLE 22–1. Gastrointestinal Diseases Associated with Maldigestion and Malabsorption**

| DISEASE/CONDITION | PATHOPHYSIOLOGY |
|---|---|
| | **Intraluminal Digestion** |
| Stomach | |
| Protein-calorie malnutrition[13, 14] | Decreased acid production, hypochlorhydria |
| Zollinger-Ellison syndrome[20] | Inactivation of pancreatic enzymes at a low duodenal pH, and decreased ionization of conjugated bile salts |
| Pernicious anemia[23–25] | Decreased intrinsic factor secretion, vitamin $B_{12}$ malabsorption |
| Dumping syndrome[26–28] | Rapid emptying of stomach contents into the small intestine, dilution of enzymes |
| Pancreas[50] | |
| Cystic fibrosis | Impaired secretion of enzymes and bicarbonate |
| Shwachman-Diamond syndrome | Impaired secretion of enzymes |
| Acute/chronic pancreatitis | Impaired secretion of enzymes and bicarbonate |
| Protein-caloric malnutrition[134] | Impaired secretion of enzymes |
| Trypsinogen deficiency[30–32] | Impaired secretion of enzymes |
| Lipase deficiency[34] | Impaired secretion of enzymes |
| Amylase deficiency[35, 36] | Impaired secretion of enzymes |
| Liver | |
| Cholestasis syndromes | Impaired secretion of bile salts with deficient micelle formation |
| Ileal disease or surgery | Intestinal malabsorption of bile salts, deficient bile salt pool |
| Intestine | |
| Enterokinase deficiency[38–40] | Impaired activation of luminal pancreatic enzymes |
| Protein-caloric malnutrition[41–44] | Bacterial overgrowth with consumption of nutrients, toxin production, and deconjugation of bile acids |
| Anatomic duplication | Bacterial overgrowth with consumption of nutrients |
| Blind loop syndrome[45] | Bacterial overgrowth with consumption of nutrients |
| Short bowel syndrome[46, 47] | Bacterial overgrowth with consumption of nutrients |
| Pseudo-obstruction[48, 49] | Bacterial overgrowth with consumption of nutrients |
| | **Digestion at the Enterocyte Membrane** |
| Congenital disaccharidase deficiency | Impaired digestion of a specific disaccharide leading to bacterial fermentation in the colon |
| Lactase[57–61] | |
| Sucrase-isomaltase[63–67] | |
| Trehalase[73] | |
| Acquired/late-onset disaccharidase deficiency | Loss of enzyme activity due to mucosal injury or loss of activity with age |
| Lactase[62] | |
| Sucrase-isomaltase[69] | |
| Glucoamylase[70, 71] | |
| | **Enterocyte Absorption** |
| Protein-calorie malnutrition[134] | "Damage" vs. "adaptive regulation," altered mucosal architecture |
| Hartnup's disease[74–76] | Transport defect of neutral amino acids |
| Lysinuric protein intolerance[74, 82, 83] | Transport defect of dibasic amino acids in intestine and kidney |
| Blue diaper syndrome[74, 85] | Transport defect of tryptophan |
| Oasthouse syndrome[86, 87] | Transport defect of methionine in intestine and kidney |
| Lowe's syndrome[88, 89] | X-linked trait with defect in transport of lysine and arginine |
| Glucose-galactose malabsorption[90–97] | Selective defect in glucose and galactose sodium cotransport system |
| Congenital chloride diarrhea[165–167] | Selective defect in chloride transport by the intestine |
| Abetalipoproteinemia[100, 102] | Absent production of apolipoprotein B, lipoproteins, and chylomicrons |
| Hypobetalipoproteinemia[74, 102] | Impaired production of apolipoprotein B |
| Celiac disease | Damage to absorptive/digestive surface |
| Short bowel syndrome | Loss of absorptive/digestive surface, abnormal transit |
| Mucosal injury syndromes | Damage to digestive/absorptive surface |
| Milk/soy protein intolerance | |
| Postenteritis syndrome | |
| Tropical sprue | Damage to digestive/absorptive surface |
| Whipple's disease | Lymphatic obstruction, impaired lipid transport (?), patchy enteropathy |
| Bacterial infection/inflammation | |
| *Shigella* | Damage to digestive/absorptive surface, abnormal motility |
| *Salmonella* | Damage to digestive/absorptive surface, abnormal motility |
| *Campylobacter* | Damage to digestive/absorptive surface, abnormal motility |
| Cholera | Secretory water and electrolyte loss |
| Giardiasis | Disruption of epithelial function secondary to adhesion or toxin(?) |
| Crohn's disease | Damage to digestive/absorptive surface, chronic gastrointestinal blood loss |
| Viral infection | |
| Rotavirus | Damage to digestive/absorptive area |
| Human immunodeficiency virus[168–170] | Damage to digestive/absorptive area, bacterial overgrowth, exocrine pancreatic and hepatic insufficiency |
| Acrodermatitis enteropathica | Impaired absorption of zinc |
| | **Uptake into Blood and Lymph** |
| Congestive heart failure[103] | Venous distention, bowel wall edema |
| Intestinal lymphangiectasia[101, 104–107] | Obstructed lymphatic transport of lipid and fat-soluble vitamins, intestinal protein loss |
| Intestinal lymphoma | Obstructed lymphatic transport of lipid and fat-soluble vitamins |
| Carcinoid syndrome | Obstructed lymphatic transport of lipid and fat-soluble vitamins |
| | **Miscellaneous Disorders** |
| Immune deficiency syndromes | Altered bacterial flora |
| Allergic gastroenteropathy | Unknown immune mechanism |
| Eosinophilic gastroenteropathy | Unknown immune mechanism |
| Drugs | |
| Methotrexate | Damage to mucosal surface by interference with enterocyte replication |
| Cholestyramine | Blocked reabsorption of bile salts in the ileum by drug; malabsorption of calcium, fat, bile acids, and fat-soluble vitamins |
| Phenytoin | Calcium, folic acid malabsorption |
| Sulfasalazine | Folic acid malabsorption |
| Histamine $H_2$ receptor antagonists | Impaired acid/proteolytic liberation of vitamin $B_{12}$ |

vitamin $B_{12}$ in the duodenum after it is released from an R binder. Vitamin $B_{12}$ bound to intrinsic factor is protected from luminal hydrolysis.[4, 11, 12]

When acid production of the stomach is decreased due to malnutrition,[13, 14] disease,[15] or medication,[16] the conversion of pepsinogen to pepsin is retarded. With decreased levels of pepsin, protein digestion may be compromised. When acid production of the stomach is suppressed by proton-pump inhibitors, bacterial overgrowth may also occur.[17, 18] This contributes to malabsorption and has been reported to decrease absorption of vitamin $B_{12}$.[19] The production of excessive quantities of acid, as in Zollinger-Ellison syndrome, depresses the luminal pH in the duodenum and thereby inactivates hydrolytic enzymes of the pancreas that are important for normal digestion.[20]

Pernicious anemia is a chronic disease characterized by the absence of intrinsic factor. Normally, vitamin $B_{12}$ binds stoichiometrically with intrinsic factor. The intrinsic factor–$B_{12}$ complex is resistant to digestion in the small intestine, and the vitamin is then absorbed by receptor-mediated endocytosis in the ileum.[21, 22] This sequence does not occur when there is no intrinsic factor. Pernicious anemia is not common in infancy and childhood but can occur in this age group.[23–25]

Hemigastrectomy for peptic ulcer disease decreases gastric mass and may result in the dumping syndrome. Other surgical procedures more common in childhood, such as the Nissen fundoplication, may also result in the dumping syndrome.[26–29] The syndrome is the result of pyloric sphincter malfunction and altered digestion and motility, which lead to the rapid emptying of a meal into the duodenum. This produces hyperglycemia, which triggers insulin release. Later, hypoglycemia, pallor, diaphoresis, and diarrhea can develop.

## *Pancreas*

The pancreas is both an exocrine and an endocrine organ and is essential for normal digestion. Pancreatic juice has two functionally important constituents: bicarbonate ions and digestive enzymes. The digestive enzymes play a major role in the digestion of ingested nutrients: proteins (Fig. 22–1), carbohydrates (Fig. 22–2), and lipids (Fig. 22–3). Hydrolysis of proteins and carbohydrates requires only the enzymes of the pancreas and the gastrointestinal tract. However, complete digestion and solubilization of dietary triglycerides requires not only pancreatic lipase, colipase, and intestinal lipase but also bile acids to provide the appropriate milieu.[9, 10]

Diseases of the pancreas, such as CF, Shwachman-Diamond syndrome, and acute and chronic pancreatitis, may be associated with a decrease in hydrolytic enzyme secretion. A deficiency of pancreatic enzymes also occurs in severe protein-calorie malnutrition. In addition, pancreatic proteases are important for vitamin $B_{12}$ absorption. These enzymes help release vitamin $B_{12}$ from R binder proteins, allowing the vitamin to bind intrinsic factor.[4, 21, 22] Although there may be a failure to degrade R proteins and free vitamin $B_{12}$ for binding to intrinsic factor in diseases of the pancreas, vitamin

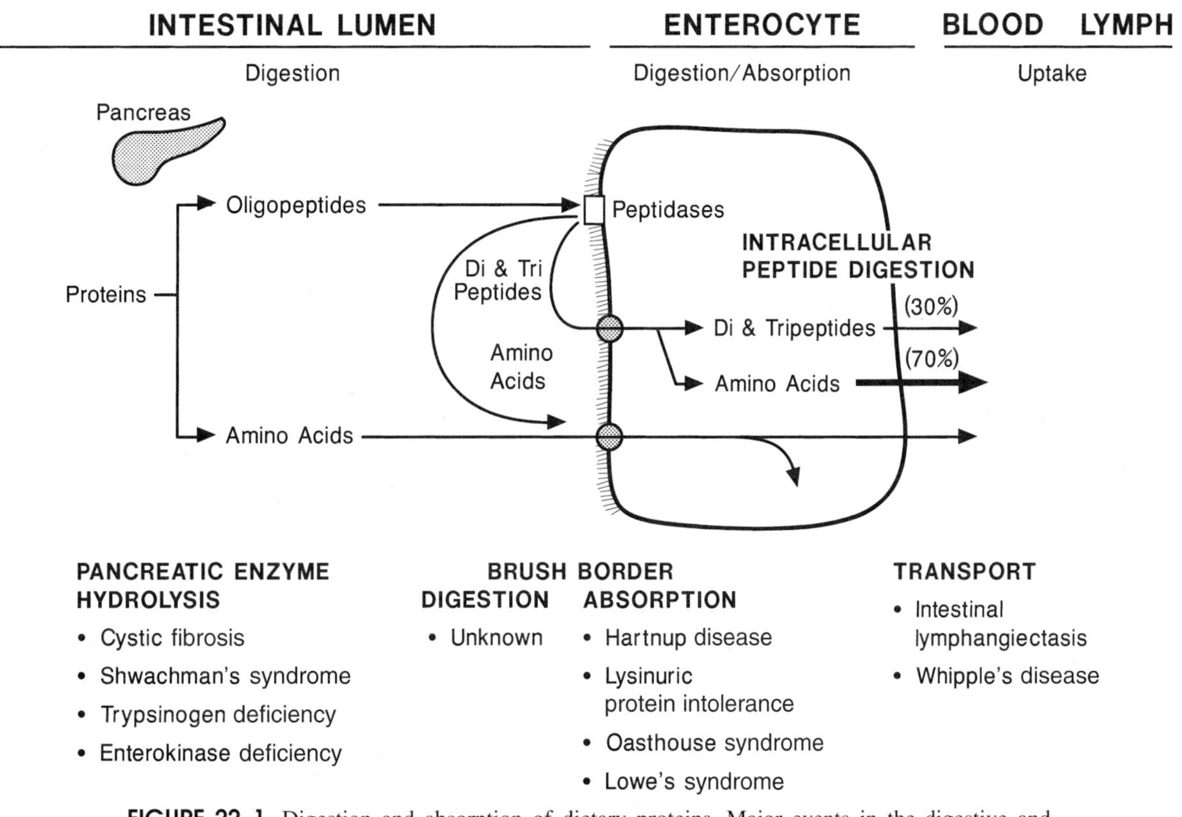


**FIGURE 22–1.** Digestion and absorption of dietary proteins. Major events in the digestive and absorptive process are shown with some of the associated disease states that result in the maldigestion and malabsorption of proteins. (Modified from Silverman A, Roy CC: Pediatric Clinical Gastroenterology, 3rd ed. St. Louis, CV Mosby, 1983, with permission.)

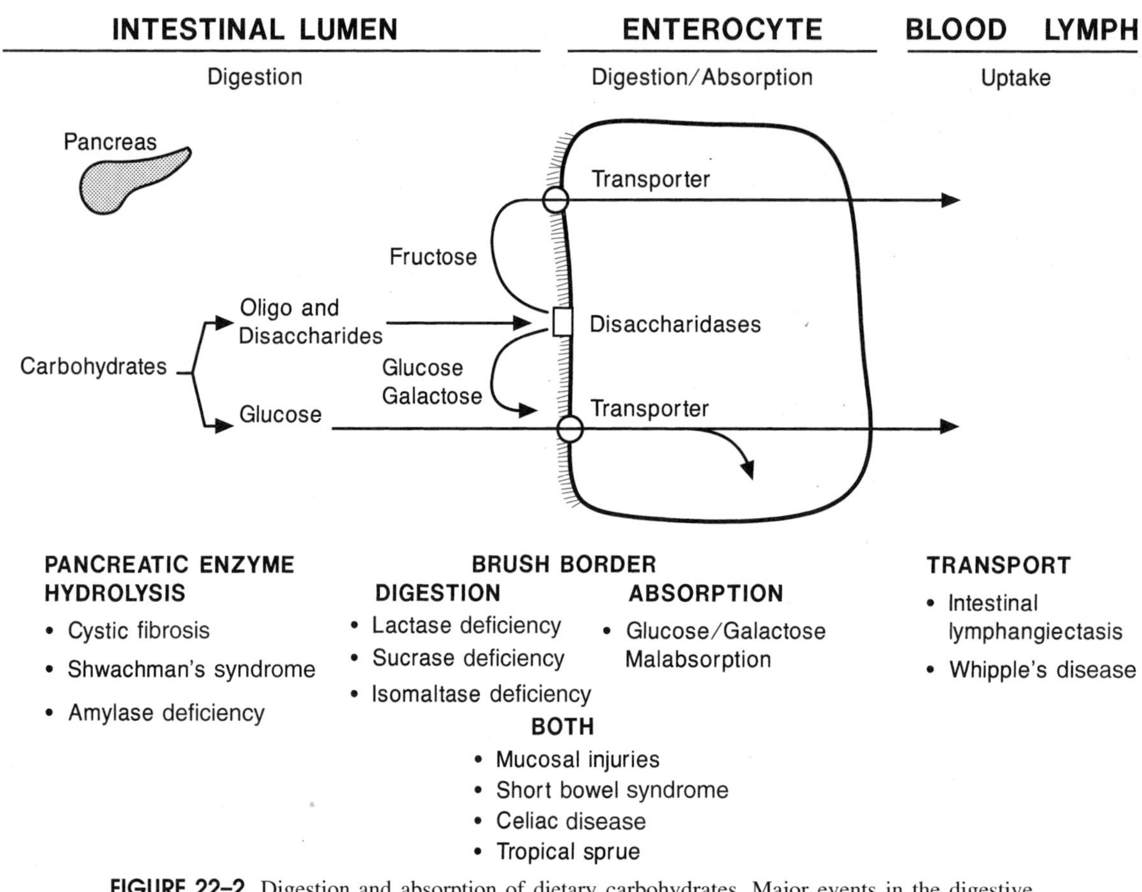


**FIGURE 22–2.** Digestion and absorption of dietary carbohydrates. Major events in the digestive and absorptive process are shown with some of the associated disease states that result in the maldigestion and malabsorption of carbohydrates. (Modified from Silverman A, Roy CC: Pediatric Clinical Gastroenterology, 3rd ed. St. Louis, CV Mosby, 1983, with permission.)

$B_{12}$ deficiency is very rare in exocrine pancreatic dysfunction.[4]

Deficiencies of pancreatic trypsinogen, lipase, and amylase have been described. In 1965, Townes described a 6-week-old white male infant with chronic diarrhea, failure to gain weight, hypoproteinemia, and edema.[30] The infant was unable to hydrolyze dietary protein owing to a singular deficiency of pancreatic trypsinogen. Morris and Fisher reported a second child with trypsinogen deficiency disease.[31] Since then, an additional patient has been reported.[32] The diagnosis of trypsinogen deficiency in these three patients was made on the basis of undetectable tryptic activity in duodenal juice. It has been suggested that these three children may have had low trypsin activity, on the basis of enteropeptidase (enterokinase) deficiency, and not trypsinogen deficiency.[33] Sheldon described five children with congenital pancreatic lipase deficiency.[34] All five had decreased lipase in duodenal fluid aspirates. Sheldon suggested that the deficiency was attributable to an autosomal recessive gene. Pancreatic amylase deficiency has also been described. Lowe and May reported a 13-year-old boy whose duodenal juice showed a persistent absence of amylase with a decreased level of trypsin but a normal amount of lipase.[35] Another case of amylase deficiency was reported by Lilibridge and Townes.[36] They described a 2-year-old child who showed poor weight gain on a diet containing starch, despite a more than adequate caloric intake. Weight gain and growth improved when starch was eliminated from the diet and replaced by disaccharides.

## Liver

The products of triglyceride hydrolysis, fatty acids and monoglycerides, are solubilized by bile salts to form micelles.[37] The fatty acids and monoglycerides are then absorbed in the small intestine. Disorders that interrupt the delivery of bile salts to the small intestine or interrupt the enterohepatic circulation of bile salts result in impaired micelle formation and fat maldigestion. These diseases are also usually associated with malabsorption of fat-soluble vitamins (vitamins A, D, E, and K), which can lead to clinical manifestations of vitamin deficiencies. Tables 22–2 and 22–3 list the numerous diseases that can impair hepatic function and result in maldigestion and malabsorption of nutrients.

## Small Intestine

Biochemical and anatomic abnormalities of the small intestine may contribute to maldigestion. Congenital enterokinase deficiency is a condition that is associated with decreased amounts of enterokinase in the brush border. The enzyme is necessary for the activation of trypsinogen and other luminal proteases. Deficiency of the enzyme was first reported by Hadorn and associates, and its occurrence in

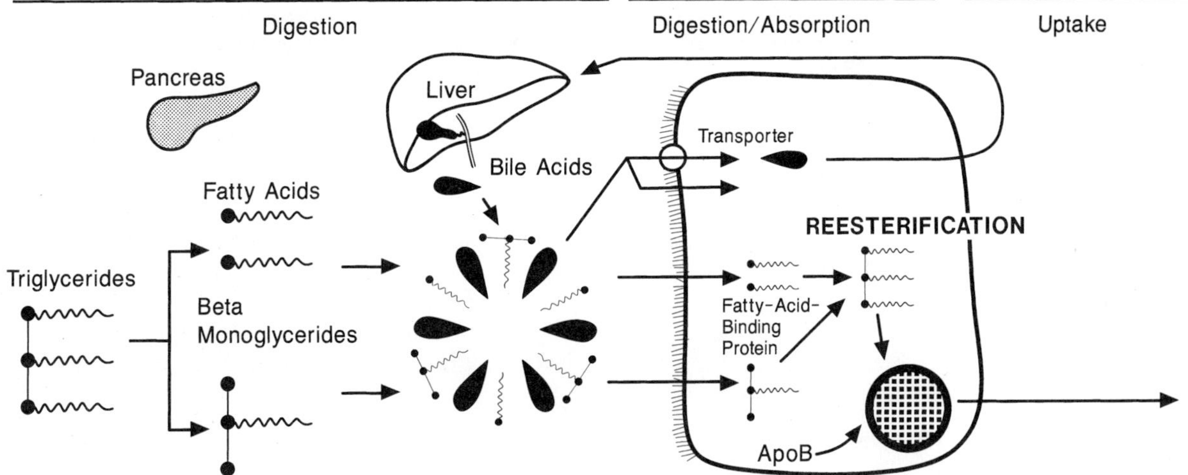


**PANCREATIC ENZYME LIPOLYSIS**
- Cystic fibrosis
- Shwachman's syndrome
- Enterokinase deficiency
- Pancreatitis

**BILE ACID MICELLAR SOLUBILIZATION**
- Cholestatic liver disease
- Bile Acid Pool Depletion

**BRUSH BORDER ABSORPTION**
- Ileal resection
- Celiac disease
- Short bowel syndrome

**CHYLOMICRON FORMATION**
- Abeta-lipoproteinemia
- Hypobeta-lipoproteinemia

**TRANSPORT**
- Intestinal lymph-angiectasis
- Whipple's disease

**FIGURE 22–3.** Digestion and absorption of dietary triglycerides. Major events in the digestive and absorptive process are shown with some of the associated disease states that result in the maldigestion and malabsorption of triglycerides. (Modified from Silverman A, Roy CC: Pediatric Clinical Gastroenterology, 3rd ed. St. Louis, CV Mosby, 1983, with permission.)

**TABLE 22–2. Neonatal Cholestatic Disorders Associated with Malabsorption**

**Anatomic**
Extrahepatic disorders[141, 142]
- Biliary atresia
- Biliary hypoplasia or stenosis
- Sclerosing cholangitis[136]

Mixed extrahepatic/intrahepatic disorders[141, 142]
- Congenital hepatic fibrosis/infantile polycystic disease
- Caroli's disease

**Idiopathic**
"Idiopathic" neonatal hepatitis
Arteriohepatic dysplasia—Alagille's syndrome
Nonsyndromic paucity of intrahepatic bile ducts
Byler's disease
Familial benign recurrent cholestasis
Hereditary cholestasis with lymphedema

**Metabolic Diseases Affecting the Hepatocyte**
Tyrosinemia
Wolman's disease
Niemann-Pick disease
Gaucher's disease
Galactosemia
Fructosemia
Glycogen storage disease type III or IV
Alpha$_1$-antitrypsin deficiency
Cystic fibrosis
Neonatal iron storage disease
Multiple acyl–coenzyme A dehydrogenation deficiency

**Inflammatory/Hepatitis**
Viral infections
- Cytomegalovirus
- Hepatitis B virus
- Hepatitis C virus—suspected[137–139]
- Varicella
- Rubella
- Herpesvirus

Bacterial and parasitic infections
- Tuberculosis
- Listeriosis
- Syphilis
- Toxoplasmosis

Toxin-induced
- Total parenteral nutrition–associated cholestasis
- Sepsis with an infection at a distant site; endotoxin mediated (?)
- Drugs
- Breast milk-secreted drugs[140]

**Miscellaneous**
Histiocytosis syndromes
Neonatal lupus

Modified from Balistreri WF: Neonatal cholestasis. J Pediatr 1985;106: 171–189, with permission.

**TABLE 22–3. Cholestatic Disorders in Children and Young Adults That May Be Associated with Malabsorption**

**Anatomic**
Extrahepatic disorders
  Choledochal cyst
  Bile duct stenosis
  Biliary tract neoplasms[143]
  Cholelithiasis with obstruction[144]
  Primary sclerosing cholangitis[145, 146]
Mixed extrahepatic/intrahepatic disorders
  Congenital hepatic fibrosis
  Infantile polycystic disease of liver and/or kidney
  Caroli's disease

**Idiopathic**
Hepatic tumor[147]
Familial benign recurrent cholestasis—Summerskill's syndrome
Hereditary cholestasis with lymphedema—Aagenaes' syndrome
Arteriohepatic dysplasia—Alagille's syndrome
Nonsyndromatic paucity of intrahepatic bile ducts
Indian childhood cirrhosis[148]

**Metabolic Diseases Affecting the Hepatocyte**
Gaucher's disease
$Alpha_1$-antitrypsin deficiency
Cystic fibrosis
Hepatolenticular degeneration—Wilson's disease[149]
Porphyria[150]

**Infectious/Drug Induced**
Viral infections
  Cytomegalovirus
  Hepatitis B virus
  Chronic active hepatitis
  Hepatitis C virus[151]
  Herpesvirus
  Varicella virus
Bacterial and parasitic infections
  Tuberculosis
  Syphilis
  Leptospirosis
  Malaria[152]
Toxin/drug-induced
  Parenteral nutrition–associated
  Sepsis with an infection at a distant site—endotoxin mediated (?)
  Pregnancy, estrogen, progesterone[153–161]
  Drug

**Miscellaneous**
Inflammatory bowel disease[162]
Histiocytoses syndromes
Autoimmune liver disease[163]
Graft-versus-host liver disease[164]

Data from Balistreri WF: Neonatal cholestasis: lessons from the past, issues for the future (foreword). Semin Liver Dis 1987;7:1–7, Thieme Medical Publishers, Inc.; and Alagille D, Odievre M: Liver and Biliary Tract Disease in Children. New York, John Wiley & Sons, 1979, pp 163–252.

siblings supports an autosomal recessive mode of inheritance.[38] Individuals with the disease present with diarrhea, edema, severe growth retardation, and hypoproteinemia. The initial report noted that, with enterokinase deficiency, the lipase concentration in unstimulated duodenal fluid was normal but fat was still malabsorbed; this may have been related to failure of activation of procolipase to colipase by enterokinase. The specific diagnosis of enterokinase deficiency rests on the generation of normal tryptic activity when exogenous enterokinase is added to duodenal juice. Pancreatic enzyme supplementation in children with this deficiency generates normal proteolytic activity in the duodenum, and clinical problems appear to resolve.[39] It has been suggested that a form of acquired enterokinase deficiency may occur in certain acquired diseases of the small intestine.[40]

Availability of ingested nutrients for absorption may also be compromised by overgrowth of the bowel with bacteria, as occurs in malnutrition,[41–44] the blind loop syndrome,[45] short bowel syndrome,[46, 47] and pseudo-obstruction.[48, 49] In addition, the pH in the proximal small intestine reflects the net effect of gastric acid secretion, pancreatic bicarbonate production, and the buffering action of food. One study has provided evidence for the hypothesis that the postprandial duodenal pH is excessively acid in patients with CF and that this may be an important element in continuing fat malabsorption in patients in this disease.[50] This malabsorption may limit the efficacy of the newer high-lipase pancreatic enzyme supplements and lead to delayed enzyme release, a possible factor in the reports of proximal colonic strictures.[50] Finally, substances present in the diet in high concentrations may bind and inhibit the efficient absorption of certain nutrients, such as the binding of oxalates or fatty acids to calcium and the binding of phytates to iron and zinc.

## Digestion at the Enterocyte Membrane

A continuous sheet of epithelial cells (enterocytes) covers the surface of the villi and crypts. Other cells are interspersed in this epithelial carpet, including goblet cells, endocrine cells, intraepithelial lymphocytes, Paneth cells, caveolated cells, and mucous cells.[3] Some of the cell types are common to both villous and crypt epithelium, and others are found exclusively in only one of these regions. Disruption or damage of the epithelium can occur in celiac disease, in Crohn's disease, or secondary to pathogens and may result in malabsorption.

Colonization of the small intestine with the actinomyces, *Tropheryma whippelii*, is the proposed cause of Whipple's disease, and this infection can also lead to malabsorption.[51–53] The disorder most commonly affects middle-aged men but has been described in a child.[54] The major clinical features are diarrhea, weight loss, and arthropathy. The diagnosis is established by duodenal biopsy, which shows the pathognomonic periodic acid–Schiff (PAS)–positive infiltrates in the lamina propria. Reverse-transcriptase–polymerase chain reaction of tissue can be used to verify the presence of *T. whippelii*.[51] In most cases, patients can be treated successfully with the prolonged administration of antimicrobials such as trimethoprim-sulfamethoxazole.

At the surface of the epithelium, aminopeptidases present in the brush border hydrolyze most, but not all, of the remaining oligopeptides and dipeptides produced by luminal digestion of proteins (see Fig. 22–1). In addition, there are specific hydrolysis-transport proteins for dipeptides, which simultaneously hydrolyze dipeptides and transport them into the enterocyte.

Carbohydrates are also hydrolyzed by membrane-associated enzymes (see Fig. 22–2). The pattern of carbohydrate ingestion changes with age.[55] During infancy the disaccharide lactose accounts for most of the dietary carbohydrate. However, in older children and adults, starch makes up about 60% of ingested carbohydrate, with sucrose and lactose constituting 30% and 10%, respectively.[55, 56] The complex carbohydrates present in the diet of the older child and adult are hydrolyzed to disaccharides and monosaccharides. The disaccharides are hydrolyzed to monosaccharides by specific disaccharidases located in the brush border membrane of intestinal epithelial cells. Monosaccharides are then transported across the enterocyte membrane. When there is a deficiency of a brush border disaccharidase, the maldigested disaccharide moves with luminal contents into the colon, where it is metabolized by colonic bacteria. Carbon dioxide, hydrogen, other gases, and organic acids are produced, with consequent abdominal distention, flatulence, and diarrhea. Although a number of disaccharidase deficiencies have been described, the most common is lactase deficiency.

There are several types of lactase deficiency. Congenital lactase deficiency is rare and is associated with symptoms occurring a short time after birth, when lactose is present in the diet.[57–61] The largest group of patients with this disorder is from Finland, where 16 cases have been described.[61] No more than 40 cases have been reported altogether. Adult-onset lactase deficiency, or primary adult-type hypolactasia, is caused by the physiologic decline in lactase that occurs with age in mammals. The persistence of the enzyme in some Caucasian groups should be considered the exception. Some ethnic groups with adult-onset lactase deficiency begin losing the enzyme in very early childhood; in others the loss of lactase occurs later.[56, 62] A third type of lactase deficiency may occur when there is loss or destruction of small intestinal epithelial cells as the result of intestinal disease or inflammation.

Congenital sucrase-isomaltase deficiency is a less common form of disaccharidase deficiency. It was first described in 1961 by Weijers and coworkers.[63] Although it is generally considered to be a rare condition, the heterozygote frequency in white American subjects is 2%,[64] and the homozygote frequency in Eskimos is as high as 10%.[65–67] The entity also appears to be common in Greenland.[56] Recently, a point mutation in the sucrase-isomaltase gene was identified that leads to a transport block of sucrase-isomaltase in a pre-Golgi compartment.[68] Symptoms of congenital sucrase-isomaltase deficiency vary from severe diarrhea in infancy to intermittent, bothersome symptoms in the older child. The correct diagnosis may be missed for several months or years, with symptoms being attributed to "toddler diarrhea" or "maternal anxiety." The diagnosis is established by the demonstration of deficient sucrase and isomaltase activities in a morphologically normal jejunal biopsy. Maltase activity is also reduced, since sucrase accounts for a large proportion of the total maltase activity. One report described 22 cases of sucrase-isomaltase deficiency occurring over a period of 20 years.[69] The authors noted a change in the presentation of this condition over time and related this to the delay in introduction of sucrose to the diets of infants. They also found that the hydrogen breath test failed to detect all subjects with the disease and concluded that disaccharidase determination remains the key to diagnosis.[69] As with many other congenital disorders of digestion, dietary withdrawal of sucrose results in prompt symptomatic improvement.

Glucoamylase or maltase is a brush border enzyme important in hydrolyzing linear alpha-1-4 glucose polymers. Glucose is produced in this process. All the alpha-glucosidases except trehalase can hydrolyze maltose to yield glucose and are therefore called maltases. A deficiency of maltase activity has been described in patients with severe mucosal injury.[70] Theoretically, it may lead to carbohydrate maldigestion, although its clinical significance appears to be minimal. To determine the prevalence of small intestinal glucoamylase deficiency in children with chronic diarrhea, Lebenthal and associates studied small bowel biopsy specimens from 511 children (aged 1 month to 9 years) with chronic diarrhea evaluated at 54 medical centers.[71] Fifteen of these children had glucoamylase deficiency. Six had significant small intestinal mucosal injury and disaccharidase deficiencies and were defined as having secondary glucoamylase deficiency; the other nine patients had normal mucosal morphologic features and were defined as having primary glucoamylase deficiency.[71] A congenital gamma-glucoamylase deficiency has been described in CBA/Ca mice.[72]

Trehalose (alpha-D-glucopyranoside) is a nonreducing disaccharide that occurs in plants such as mushrooms, in some microorganisms, and in many insects. Trehalase deficiency has been documented in a family who developed symptoms following the ingestion of mushrooms.[73] An autosomal dominant type of inheritance has been suggested. Trehalose maldigestion is not rare in Greenland.[56]

## Absorption into the Enterocyte

### *Amino Acids*

Amino acids are rapidly absorbed by a group of sodium-coupled cotransport systems, similar to those present in the proximal tubular cells of the kidney (see Fig. 22–1). Absorption of some dipeptides is more rapid than absorption of the constituent amino acids. Amino acids, once absorbed, pass through the enterocyte rapidly, with only a small fraction being used for protein synthesis within the enterocyte. The small fraction of dipeptides and tripeptides that enter the enterocyte is mostly hydrolyzed within the enterocyte. Carrier proteins for amino acid exit from the enterocyte are probably located on basolateral membranes, but they have not been well characterized.

Defective protein absorption because of impaired dipeptide or amino acid transport by the enterocyte is extremely rare, perhaps because of the redundancy of substrate specificity. A generalized defect in protein absorption would be fatal. However, there are several diseases of amino acid transport worth mentioning.

*Hartnup's disease* is a condition that results from a defect in the transport of free neutral amino acids in the small intestine and the proximal renal tubule.[74] The discovery that Hartnup's disease is an inherited disorder is told best by Dr. Harvey Levy.[75] In 1951, a 12-year-old boy, E. Hartnup (E.H.), was admitted to the Middlesex Hospital, London, England, with mild cerebellar ataxia and a red, scaly rash on the exposed areas of his body. His mother believed that he had pellagra, for her eldest daughter (P.H.) had identical symptoms and had been treated at the hospital in 1937 for that disease. Although the rash in E.H. was quite consistent with pellagra, other findings were not. Apart from variable cerebellar signs and retarded mental development of E.H., the only abnormality detected at that time was in the urinary excretion of free amino acids. Paper chromatography of the urine disclosed an excretion pattern of amino acids quite unlike that seen in any other disease. At the same time, P.H., then age 19, had a recurrence of ataxia (without a rash), similar to that which she had in childhood when the pellagra-like rash was most severe. The excretion pattern of amino acids in her urine was identical to that of her brother E.H., and it was then clear that these two siblings were affected by the same disorder. An inherited condition seemed probable when it was learned that the parents were first cousins.[75] The disease was not fully described in the medical literature, however, until 1956.[76]

The onset of Hartnup's disease usually occurs in early childhood with attacks of cerebellar ataxia and a pellagra-like rash appearing after exposure to sunlight. However, some reports suggest that the disease may also manifest in adulthood.[77, 78] In one case, a young woman was diagnosed with pellagra. Her symptoms were precipitated by prolonged lactation and increased activity.[78] Her dietary niacin intake was within recommended guidelines. Chromatography of urinary amino acids was diagnostic of Hartnup's disease. Her symptoms resolved with oral nicotinamide. In most cases of Hartnup's disease, mental retardation and/or a dementing psychiatric disturbance similar to that seen in pellagra can occur. These clinical manifestations are, however, intermittent and variable, and skin rash is the primary cause of most referrals. The pellagra results from the abnormally small proportion of dietary tryptophan available for the nutritionally important kynurenine-nicotinamide pathway. Unabsorbed free tryptophan is metabolized by intestinal bacteria to produce metabolites such as indoles, some of which may be potent inhibitors of the kynurenine-nicotinamide pathway and may, therefore, further decrease the already diminished production of nicotinamide. Since tryptophan can be absorbed in the form of dipeptides and tripeptides, it is perhaps surprising that clinical symptoms occur at all. However, all clinical attacks are associated with an inadequate or irregular diet, and this may well result in insufficient absorption of peptide-bound tryptophan. The metabolism of the other neutral amino acids in this disorder does not seem to present the same difficulties. There is no specific treatment for the condition other than supplements of nicotinamide. It has been suggested that the cause of Hartnup's disease is multifactorial.[79] This may explain why some patients do not respond to tryptophan and/or nicotinamide but do have a reversal of symptoms with trihexyphenidyl.[80] Other patients have responded to a lipid-soluble tryptophan derivative.[81] The ultimate prognosis is good, with some amelioration of the condition in later life.[74, 75]

*Lysinuric protein intolerance* causes severe symptoms including marked failure to thrive, diarrhea, vomiting, protein intolerance, hepatosplenomegaly, and often mental retardation.[82, 83] The defect is in the transport of dibasic amino acids and is inherited as an autosomal recessive trait. The transport defect has been demonstrated in the small intestine, the liver, and the proximal renal tubules.[74, 81, 82] Onset is in infancy, commencing at the time of weaning from the breast to a cow's milk formula. Generally, after the first year of life, protein aversion is common, and symptoms ameliorate with a decreased protein intake. If a high protein intake is maintained, hyperammonemia, hepatosplenomegaly, and sometimes coma develop. The disease has been diagnosed in a 35-year-old woman with a history of almost two decades of relapsing coma with hyperammonemia.[84] The cornerstone of treatment is a low-protein diet. in the range of 1.5 g per kilogram of body weight per day or less. Early attempts at preventing hyperammonemia with arginine or ornithine supplements were not entirely successful, presumably because of poor intestinal absorption. Diarrhea occurs if more than 22 g of arginine is ingested. However, the use of this urea-cycle intermediate may allow the use of a low-protein diet and result in catch-up growth.[74, 82] Rajantie and colleagues[82, 83] showed that another urea-cycle intermediate, citrulline, is absorbed normally and is capable of preventing the ornithinopenic hyperammonemia in lysinuric protein intolerance. This may allow a higher intake of dietary protein.

*Blue diaper syndrome* results from the isolated malabsorption of tryptophan. The disease is also associated with an increased absorption of calcium.[74] Thier and Alpers[85] suggested that a specific tryptophan transport system is defective in blue diaper syndrome, rather than a group-specific transport system, as in Hartnup's disease. The disease is inherited as an autosomal recessive trait and manifests in the neonatal period with failure to thrive, recurrent pyrexia, irritability, constipation, and a blue discoloration of diapers.[74] The stools contain large quantities of indoles, tryptophan, tryptamine, and indolic acid. The blue discoloration results from the presence of indigotin (indigo blue), an oxidation product of urinary indicans.

*Oasthouse syndrome* (methionine malabsorption) is a very rare condition. It was first described by Smith and Strang.[86] They described a neonate who was developmentally retarded, had recurrent episodes of edema, and had excessive urinary excretion of alpha-hydroxybutyric acid (a bacterial breakdown product of methionine), which gave the infant an unusual odor similar to that of an oasthouse (the British word for a kiln for drying hops or malt). Later, Hooft and associates[87] described a similar child who malabsorbed methionine and excreted large amounts of alpha-hydroxybutyric acid in the urine, which gave the child an oasthouse odor. The infant they described presented with convulsions, diarrhea, and severe mental retardation. On treating the patient with a methionine-free diet, the symptoms improved.

*Lowe's syndrome,* unlike the conditions already mentioned, is inherited as a sex-linked trait and is characterized by mental retardation, cataracts, and renal tubular acidosis with aminoaciduria. Defective absorption of lysine and arginine has been demonstrated,[88, 89] but the pathologic significance of this finding is not clear.

## Monosaccharides

Monosaccharides produced by the action of brush border oligosaccharidases are small hydrophilic molecules that do not penetrate cell membranes rapidly (see Fig. 22–2). Simple diffusion of these compounds across membranes is slow, but diffusion is an important means of uptake when monosaccharides are at high luminal concentrations. For the most part, however, specific sodium-coupled transport systems mediate efficient transport or absorption of monosaccharides, including glucose. These transport systems are presumably integral membrane proteins and use energy to transport glucose and other monosaccharides. The monosaccharides glucose, galactose, xylose, and fructose may also enter enterocytes by means of a third mechanism, facilitated diffusion. In this type of transport, a molecule to be transported (e.g., fructose) couples with its carrier on the external side of the membrane, and the complex either diffuses or rotates within the membrane. At the inner side of the membrane, the transported molecule dissociates from its carrier. An important difference exists between simple diffusion and facilitated diffusion. Facilitated diffusion depends on a fixed number of carrier protein sites; therefore, this process is saturable, unlike simple diffusion.[3]

Glucose-galactose malabsorption was first described in 1962 by Lindquist and Meeuwisse.[90] In vivo[91, 92] and in vitro[93, 94] studies have shown markedly impaired or absent sodium-coupled mucosal uptake of glucose. In many patients, clinical intolerance to the offending carbohydrates improves with age, despite the fact that the enzyme deficiency and transport defect persist. Wozniak and coworkers[95] showed that there are at least two molecular variants of the transport defect. One results from deletion of the transport site and does not change with age. In the other there is a reduced number of normally functioning transport sites, but they appear to increase in number with age. Absorption of fructose, xylose, leucine, and alanine is intact. Defects in $Na^+$/glucose cotransporter trafficking and function have been noted in this condition, and gene mutations have been linked to phenotype.[96]

An infant who suffered from not only malabsorption of glucose-galactose but also fructose has been reported.[97] This is the first report of congenital malabsorption of the three main monosaccharides that constitute a normal diet—glucose, galactose, and fructose (see Fig. 22–1). Malabsorption of fructose has been postulated to be one of the causes of "toddler's diarrhea."[98] Malabsorbed carbohydrates are fermented by anaerobic bacteria of the colon to short-chain fatty acids.[99] The production of short-chain fatty acids from dietary carbohydrates that are malabsorbed is a mechanism whereby considerable amounts of calories can be salvaged.

### *Fatty Acids and Monoglycerides*

The products of lipid digestion, including fatty acids, monoglycerides, cholesterol, sterol vitamins, and other lipids, pass from the intestinal lumen through the intestinal water into the enterocyte cytoplasm (see Fig. 22–3). Lipolysis products move through the intestinal aqueous milieu and across the peripheral unstirred water layer and mucous gel by diffusion of large liposomes and mixed micelles or diffusion of lipid monomers in free solution.[3] Medium-chained triglycerides, 6 to 12 carbon units in length, are rapidly and completely hydrolyzed by pancreatic lipase to fatty acids and glycerol, both of which are rapidly taken up by enterocytes.

Abetalipoproteinemia is a rare disorder of lipid processing within the enterocyte. Lipids, once absorbed as monoglycerides and fatty acids into the enterocyte, are reassembled as triglycerides and incorporated into chylomicrons, which are then transported into the blood. In abetalipoproteinemia there is inefficient or defective chylomicron formation. The triglyceride in the affected cells does not appear to receive the normal apoprotein coating. The defect is presumed to involve the synthesis of apo B or intracellular assembling of apo B with lipid.[100] In order to explain all the manifestations of the disease, which affects a number of organ systems, a hypothesis of some generalized defect in cell membranes has been put forward. The disease is characterized by malformed erythrocytes (acanthocytes), retinal atrophy and clumping of retinal pigment (retinitis pigmentosa), and a form of Friedreich's ataxia. Biochemically there is profound hypocholesterolemia and a total absence of low-density lipoproteins in the plasma. The mode of inheritance is autosomal dominant, and the condition appears more predominantly in males (70%). Treatment consists of dietary restriction of triglycerides. Medium-chain triglycerides should be substituted for long-chain triglycerides, and adequate fat-soluble vitamins and linoleic acid should be provided.[101]

Familial hypobetalipoproteinemia is similar to abetalipoproteinemia. In the heterozygote state of this condition, the intestinal mucosa and fat absorption are probably normal.[74, 102] In homozygotes, the intestinal tract findings mimic those of abetalipoproteinemia, including fat malabsorption and extensive neutral fat accumulation in enterocytes. Various forms of hypobetalipoproteinemia have been described, indicating that the intestinal transport of triglyceride to the plasma is under complex genetic control.

### Uptake into Blood and Lymph

Cardiac failure can cause bowel edema and lead to malabsorption.[103] Another disease that results in malabsorption at the level of uptake into blood and lymph is intestinal lymphangiectasia.[104–107] This is a condition in which the subepithelial lymph ducts are dilated and functionally obstructed. Consequently, removal of chylomicrons in the lymph is abnormally slow. A small bowel biopsy may not help in the diagnosis of this disease process.[107] Treatment is with a low-fat diet in which predominantly medium-chain triglycerides are ingested. Infiltrative diseases of the small intestine (e.g., tuberculous enteritis, intestinal lymphoma, Whipple's disease) may compress lymphatic vessels in the small intestinal wall and retard chylomicron removal. In addition, enlargement of regional lymph nodes, such as occurs in tuberculosis, lymphoma, metastatic carcinoma, and metastatic carcinoid disease, may produce obstruction and fat malabsorption.

## DIAGNOSIS

A good history, a physical examination, and judicious use of laboratory studies usually provide the information necessary to diagnose a maldigestion or malabsorption disorder.

### History

The symptoms of diarrhea, weight loss, and poor growth are not unique to malabsorption. Many nongastrointestinal disorders, such as urinary tract infections or central nervous system disorders, produce similar symptoms. However, with other clues from a complete and accurate clinical history, a cause can often be postulated. Important aspects of the history include the following.

1. A chronologic description of all symptoms (e.g., fever, diarrhea, abdominal pain), the relation of symptoms to changes in lifestyle or stress, and information concerning the introduction of antibiotics or other medications should be obtained. Exacerbation of chronic medical problems should also be considered.
2. Assessment of appetite, activity, and sleeping habits before the onset of the symptoms is important.
3. A dietary history is necessary to assess intake in terms of nutritional type and quantity. Note should be made of the dietary manipulations employed in an attempt to resolve symptoms. The physician should ascertain whether there has been prolonged dietary restriction initiated to control diarrhea. Dietary restrictions can result in malnutrition.
4. A perinatal history should be obtained. Signs and symptoms present from birth suggest a congenital disorder but do not rule out acquired causes of malabsorption. A history of prior abdominal surgery can suggest an anatomic cause for malabsorption, such as an intestinal stricture or partial small bowel obstruction.
5. A history of serial infections can implicate CF or an immune deficiency syndrome as a possible cause of maldigestion or malabsorption.
6. Inquire about recent travel on the part of the patient or immediate family members to tropical or underdeveloped areas. If a child is cared for in a daycare nursery, infections such as giardiasis may be implicated as a cause of malabsorption.
7. Many maldigestive and malabsorptive disorders affect organ systems other than the intestinal tract. Systemic complaints not directly related to the digestive tract (e.g., malaise, edema, fever, delayed onset of menses, secondary amenorrhea, weight loss) may suggest inflammatory bowel disease or early liver disease. Evidence of bleeding, bruising, or rashes may be secondary to a deficiency state that accompanies malabsorption.
8. A family history should be obtained, because other family members may have similar signs and symptoms. This can suggest a genetically determined or infectious disorder.

## Physical Examination

The number and prominence of physical findings may parallel the severity and chronicity of the malabsorptive disorder. The physical examination may be unremarkable or show subtle abnormalities known to be associated with mild malabsorption. During the examination it may be noticed that the child is depressed and passive in response. This is common in moderate to severe malnutrition. Many chronically malnourished children also show evidence of developmental delay. Accurate measurement of height, weight, and head circumference; calculation of weight for length; and construction of a growth curve are fundamental parts of the physical examination. The plotted growth curves for weight and length can provide valuable information in the assessment of growth problems secondary to the nutritional inadequacies of chronic maldigestive and malabsorptive disorders.[108] Examination of the head, face, and neck may reveal evidence of fat-soluble or water-soluble vitamin deficiencies (e.g., xerophthalmia in vitamin A deficiency, cheilitis and smooth tongue in vitamin B complex deficiencies). Examination of the trunk, buttocks, and extremities can give a subjective impression of muscle wasting or decreased fat stores. A more accurate measurement of muscle mass and fat stores can be provided by skinfold thickness measurements.

The cardiac examination may reveal a rapid heart rate from anemia, or bradycardia secondary to protein-calorie malnutrition. Abdominal distention may be detected, reflecting fatty infiltration of the liver, laxity of abdominal musculature, or both. This can be associated with protein-calorie malnutrition. Tenderness of the liver may be present secondary to fatty infiltration or congestive heart failure. A prominent abdominal venous pattern, a palpable spleen, or a noticeable fluid wave on abdominal examination may herald chronic liver disease with portal hypertension and ascites. A delay in the appearance of secondary sex characteristics is common with chronic malabsorption in older children. Nail bed pallor from decreased blood hemoglobin and clubbing of the nail beds can occur in both celiac disease[109] and inflammatory bowel disease.[110, 111] Joint pain, swelling, and erythema can be extraintestinal manifestations of inflammatory bowel disease. Abnormalities of color and texture of the skin and hair can be seen in fat-soluble vitamin and trace element deficiency states. The neurologic examination may reveal the abnormal reflexes of Chvostek's or Trousseau's sign from hypocalcemia. There may also be abnormal cerebellar signs from a vitamin E or vitamin B-complex deficiency.

## Laboratory Testing

Laboratory studies can help confirm the presence of maldigestion and malabsorption and, more importantly, help identify the cause. They can elucidate specific vitamin or trace element deficiency states as well as document adequate serum levels during supplemental vitamin therapy. Studies can be divided into three categories based on availability, expense, and invasiveness (Table 22–4).

### *Initial Screening Tests*

**STOOL EXAMINATION.** The identification of occult blood and fecal leukocytes in a stool specimen suggests an inflammatory condition of the lower colon. Decreased stool pH may reflect carbohydrate maldigestion and malabsorption in the small intestine and subsequent fermentation by colonic bacteria. Overt carbohydrate malabsorption is associated with reducing substances in stool samples. A test for qualitative fecal fat excretion or stain for fat globules can be a quick and simple way to screen for fat malabsorption.[112] If there is suspicion of a gastrointestinal pathogen, stool samples should be obtained for bacterial culture and examination for ova and parasites.

For some enteric pathogens, the diagnostic value of fecal testing is lost if the stool is not taken to the laboratory quickly and tested immediately. Collection of a stool sample can be a challenge for the mother of a child with liquid stools. Rectal aspiration using an 8F to 10F feeding tube

**TABLE 22–4. Diagnostic Studies in the Evaluation of Maldigestion and Malabsorption**

**Initial Studies**

Stool examination for blood, leukocytes, reducing substances, and *Clostridium difficile* toxin; stool examination for ova and parasites and cultures for infectious bacterial pathogens
Complete blood count
Serum electrolytes, blood urea nitrogen, creatinine, calcium, phosphorus, albumin, total protein
Urinalysis and culture

**Second-Phase Studies**

Sweat chloride test
Breath analysis
D-Xylose test
Serum carotene, folate, $B_{12}$, and iron levels
Fecal alpha$_1$-antitrypsin level
Fecal fat studies or coefficient of fat absorption studies
Fatty test meal,[117] Lundh test meal[116]

**Third-Phase Studies**

Fat-soluble vitamin levels: A, 25-hydroxy D, and E
Contrast radiographic studies: upper gastrointestinal series or barium enema
Small intestinal biopsy for histology and mucosal enzyme determination
Bentiromide excretion test

**Specialized Studies**

Schilling test
Serum/urine bile acid determination
Endoscopic retrograde pancreatography
Provocative pancreatic secretion testing

and a 20-mL syringe may be tried.[112] Other techniques include lining a disposable diaper with plastic wrap to prevent absorption and using a urine collection bag that has been placed over the anus. Stool samples that cannot be processed immediately and examined for bacterial pathogens, ova, and parasites can be placed in an appropriate preservative or transport medium for later analysis.

**COMPLETE BLOOD COUNT.** Anemia is common in malabsorption syndromes, including celiac disease, CF, and inflammatory bowel disease. The microcytic, hypochromic anemia of iron deficiency is prevalent and may be caused either by chronic blood loss through the gastrointestinal tract or by iron malabsorption. Less commonly, megaloblastic anemia can occur. In untreated celiac disease, this can result from reduced serum and red blood cell folate levels.[113] The chronic malabsorption of folate and vitamin $B_{12}$ may also produce megaloblastic anemia.[114] In CF, iron deficiency anemia with low serum ferritin is seen frequently, even in stable patients.[115] In CF patients with advanced pulmonary disease, polycythemia is seen less frequently than with other pulmonary disorders of comparable severity. The anemia associated with inflammatory bowel disease can present as an iron deficiency anemia, megaloblastic anemia, or the anemia of chronic disease.

**ADDITIONAL BLOOD TESTS.** In patients with malabsorption, the chronic loss of electrolytes and base can be reflected by low serum levels of sodium, potassium, chloride, and bicarbonate. Depending on the degree of malnutrition, total serum proteins, including albumin, can be depressed. Because of its relatively long half-life, serum albumin may not reflect current nutritional status. Serum proteins with a relatively shorter half-life may be used as nutritional markers. These include prealbumin (transthyretin), somatomedin C, retinol-binding protein, and transferrin.

## *Second-Phase Testing*

Serum concentrations of carotene, folate, and vitamins $B_{12}$, A, and E have also been used to assess maldigestive and malabsorptive states. Monitoring of absorbed lipids after a standardized meal may be helpful in assessing maldigestion and malabsorption.[116, 117]

In mild to moderate malabsorption, quantitative fat excretion measured in a 72-hour stool collection provides the most accurate estimation of fat malabsorption. This information, along with a 72-hour dietary history, can be used to calculate a coefficient of fat absorption. A fecal fat excretion study does not identify the pathophysiologic cause of malabsorption; it documents only the presence of fat maldigestion and/or malabsorption. A 72-hour stool collection is difficult to obtain from a small child. For these reasons, quantitative fecal fat excretion studies are not commonly used.

The steatocrit is a newer measurement to assess fat malabsorption.[118] It is based on the principle that when a stool sample is homogenized and centrifuged at 15,000 rpm for 15 minutes, the lipid portion rises to the top and the solid aqueous portion gravitates to the bottom. If this is done in a hematocrit tube, the amount of fat in a given stool sample can be estimated. This provides a crude estimate of fat malabsorption.[118] However, its value in assessing fat malabsorption has been challenged.[119]

**BREATH TEST.** Breath hydrogen testing is performed principally for the investigation of lactose malabsorption or bacterial overgrowth of the small intestine, although other applications show promise. Similarly, malabsorption of sucrose, fructose, and other sugars can be diagnosed by breath hydrogen testing.

**D-XYLOSE TEST.** The absorption of D-xylose is thought to be a passive process that reflects the functional surface area of the proximal small intestine. The test is not dependent on bile salts, pancreatic exocrine secretion, or intestinal brush border enzymes. A standard dose is given by mouth. It is based on body surface area (14.5 g/m$^2$ up to a maximum dose of 25 g as a 10% aqueous solution). Approximately 50% of the absorbed dose is metabolized in the liver, and the remainder is excreted in the urine. The serum D-xylose concentration at 1 hour can be used to assess D-xylose absorption after the standard dose. The serum level should exceed 25 mg/dL. A timed urine collection after the standard oral dose can also be used to approximate D-xylose absorption. The sensitivity and specificity of this test is somewhat controversial.[120–125] However, it does remain a relatively noninvasive screen for adequate proximal small intestinal surface area.

## *Third-Phase Testing*

**INTESTINAL BIOPSY.** The diagnostic value of small intestinal biopsy varies with the disease process. Capsule biopsy specimens are obtained from the area of the duodenojejunal junction, and endoscopic biopsies are usually obtained from the proximal to middle duodenum. Serial biopsy specimens from other areas of the proximal small bowel can be considered when intermittent or patchy disease distribution is suspected. The careful mounting of the biopsy sample before fixation allows for proper orientation.

**PANCREATIC TESTING.** Finally, a variety of specific tests exist for assessment of pancreatic secretory function. These include provocative pancreatic secretion testing, the bentiromide excretion test, and, most recently, a noninvasive stable-isotope method to assess pancreatic exocrine function.[126]

## Management

Only selected management principles are outlined here, because treatment principles have been noted elsewhere in the chapter and text.

Therapy for malabsorptive disorders is based on first identifying the disease process and then applying specific treatment principles for the disease. Second, if protein-calorie malnutrition and/or any vitamin or trace mineral deficiency is present, it should be vigorously treated enterally, parenterally, or both. The goal of nutritional support in pediatric practice is to provide adequate protein, calories, lipids, vitamins, and trace minerals for catch-up growth and maintenance of normal growth.

### *Maldigestion*

For altered luminal digestion, specific therapies can be initiated, depending on the cause. Supplemental enzymes may be provided to augment depressed enzyme secretion by the pancreas, as in CF and Shwachman-Diamond syndrome. The enzymes can be given along with a histamine $H_2$ receptor antagonist to help minimize acid-mediated degradation in the stomach. However, with the high-potency pancreatic enzyme supplements used today, colonic strictures (fibrosing colonopathy) have been described, and there are now specific recommendations for the use of these replacement enzymes.[127, 128] Fat-soluble vitamin supplements can be provided in an attempt to overcome disorders of absorption. New pharmacologic strategies have been developed to enhance thc absorption of vitamin E with the use of polyethylene glycol.[129, 130] Dietary medium-chain triglycerides can improve fat absorption in patients with impaired triglyceride digestion and absorption. Liver disease and cholestasis can occur with CF. Some disorders of cholestasis can be improved by the use of ursodeoxycholic acid, which stimulates bile flow, resulting in improvement in fat digestion. Cotting and colleagues demonstrated improved liver function and nutritional status in eight CF patients treated with ursodeoxycholic acid.[131]

As noted previously, the dumping syndrome has been shown to be a complication of the Nissen fundoplication. Symptoms associated with dumping syndrome can be alleviated with the use of uncooked starch.[132]

### *Malabsorption*

In patients with mild to moderate malabsorption, a slow continuous infusion of nutrients by way of a nasogastric tube or through a gastrostomy may increase absorption. The slow rate increases the contact time between nutrients and the absorptive surface. This form of therapy is ideal for nocturnal feedings, but an enteral infusion pump is necessary. Other methods, such as the use of taurine, may improve fat absorption in patients with CF.[133]

Patients with severe malabsorption that has resulted in significant protein-calorie malnutrition may require parenteral nutritional support, which can provide the necessary nutrients, including minerals, vitamins, and iron.

In the future, new drugs as well as designer formulas and nutrients may allow health care professionals to optimize intestinal digestion and absorption in patients with diseases of the intestinal tract.

## REFERENCES


1. O'Toole M (ed): Miller-Keane Encyclopedia and Dictionary of Medicine, Nursing, & Allied Health, 6th ed. Philadelphia, WB Saunders, 1997, p 955.
2. Basu MK, Chisholm DM: Oral manifestation of gastrointestinal disease. In Bouchier IAD, Allan RN, Hodgson HJF, et al (eds): Textbook of Gastroenterology. London, Bailliere Tindall, 1984, pp 1–10.
3. Granger DN, Barrowman JA, Kvietys PR: Eating: salivation, mastication, and deglutition. In Clinical Gastrointestinal Physiology: A Saunders Monograph in Physiology. Philadelphia, WB Saunders, 1985, pp 31–51.
4. Gueant JL, Champigneulle B, Gaucher P, et al: Malabsorption of vitamin $B_{12}$ in pancreatic insufficiency of the adult and of the child. Pancreas 1990;5:559–567.
5. Fedosov SN, Petersen TE, Nexo E: Binding of cobalamin and cobinamide to transcobalamin from bovine milk. Biochemistry 1995;34:16082–16087.
6. Cheng SH, Gregory RJ, Marshall J: Defective intracellular transport and processing of CFTR is the molecular basis of most cystic fibrosis. Cell 1990;63:827–834.
7. Fredrikzon B, Blackberg L: Lingual lipase: An important lipase in the digestion of dietary lipids in cystic fibrosis? Pediatr Res 1980;14:1387–1390.
8. Talal N: Sjögren's syndrome. In Samter M (ed): Immunological Diseases, 4th ed. Boston, Little, Brown, 1988, pp 1501–1507.
9. Moreau H, Bernadac A, Gargouri Y, et al: Immunocytolocalization of human gastric lipase in chief cells of the fundic mucosa. Histochemistry 1989;91:419–423.
10. Bernback S, Blackberg L, Hernell O: The complete digestion of human milk triacylglycerol in vitro requires gastric lipase, pancreatic colipase-dependent lipase, and bile-salt stimulated lipase. J Clin Invest 1990;85:1221–1226.
11. Allen RH, Seetharam B, Podell E, et al: Effect of proteolytic enzymes on the binding of cobalamin to R protein and intrinsic factor. J Clin Invest 1978:61:47–54.
12. Allen RH, Seethadam B, Allen NC, et al: Correction of cobalamin malabsorption in pancreatic insufficiency with a cobalamin analogue that binds with high affinity to R protein but not to intrinsic factor. J Clin Invest 1978;61:1628–1634.
13. Adesola AO: The influence of severe protein deficiency (kwashiorkor) on gastric acid secretion in Nigerian children. Br J Surg 1968;55:866.
14. Gracey M, Cullity GJ, Suharjono, et al: The stomach in malnutrition. Arch Dis Child 1977;52:325–327.
15. Verner JV, Morrison AB: Endocrine pancreatic islet disease with diarrhea: Report of a case due to diffuse hyperplasia of non-beta islet tissue with a review of 54 additional cases. Arch Intern Med 1974;133:492–500.
16. Koop H, Kuly S, Flug M, et al: Intragastric pH and serum gastrin during administration of different doses of pantoprazole in healthy subjects. Eur J Gastroenterol Hepatol 1996;8:915–918.
17. Thorens J, Froechlich F, Schwizer W, et al: Bacterial overgrowth during treatment with omeprazole compared with cimetidine: a prospective randomised double blind study. Gut 1996;39:54–59.
18. Lewis SJ, Franco S, Young G, et al: Altered bowel function and duodenal bacterial overgrowth in patients treated with omeprazole. Aliment Pharmacol Ther 1996;10:557–561.
19. Saltzman JR, Kemp JA, Golner BB, et al: Effect of hypochlorhydria due to omeprazole treatment or atrophic gastritis on protein-bound vitamin $B_{12}$ absorption. J Am Coll Nutr 1994;13:584–591.

20. Isenberg JI, Walsh JH, Grossman MI: Zollinger-Ellison syndrome. Gastroenterology 1973;65:140–165.
21. Robertson JA, Gallagher ND: In vivo evidence that cobalamin is absorbed by receptor-mediated endocytosis in the mouse. Gastroenterology 1985;88:908–912.
22. Gueant JL, Gerard A, Monin B, et al: Radioautographic localization of iodinated human intrinsic factor in the guinea pig ileum using electron microscopy. Gut 1988;29:1370–1378.
23. Fakatselli NM, Delta BG, Hudaverdi EY, et al: Pernicious anemia in childhood. Am J Med Sci 1978;276:144–151.
24. Heisel MA, Siegel SE, Falk RE, et al: Congenital pernicious anemia: report of seven patients, with studies of the extended family. J Pediatr 1984;105:564–568.
25. Levine JS, Allen RH: Intrinsic factor within parietal cells of patients with juvenile pernicious anemia: a retrospective immunohistochemical study. Gastroenterology 1985;88:1132–1136.
26. Meyer S, Deckelbaum RJ, Lax E, et al: Infant dumping syndrome after gastroesophageal reflux surgery. J Pediatr 1981;99:235–237.
27. Caulfield ME, Wyllie R, Firor HV, et al: Dumping syndrome in children. J Pediatr 1987;110:212–215.
28. Rivkees SA, Crawford JD: Hypoglycemia pathogenesis in children with dumping syndrome. Pediatrics 1987;80:937–942.
29. Samuk I, Afriat R, Horne T, et al: Dumping syndrome following Nissen fundoplication, diagnosis, and treatment. J Pediatr Gastroenterol Nutr 1996;23:235–240.
30. Townes PL: Trypsinogen deficiency disease. J Pediatr 1965;66:275–285.
31. Morris MD, Fisher DA: Trypsinogen deficiency disease. Am J Dis Child 1967;114:203–208.
32. Townes PL, Bryson MF, Miller G: Further observations on trypsinogen deficiency disease: report of a second case. J Pediatr 1967;71:220–224.
33. Green JR, Bender SW, Posselt HG, et al: Case report: primary intestinal enteropeptidase deficiency. J Pediatr Gastroenterol Nutr 1984;3:630–633.
34. Sheldon W: Congenital pancreatic lipase deficiency. Arch Dis Child 1964;39:268–271.
35. Lowe CV, May DC: Selective pancreatic deficiency: absent amylase, diminished trypsin, and normal lipase. Am J Dis Child 1951;82:459–464.
36. Lilibridge CB, Townes PL: Physiologic deficiency of pancreatic amylase in infancy: a factor in iatrogenic diarrhea. J Pediatr 1973;82:279–282.
37. Krag E, Thaysen EH: Bile acids in health and disease. Scand J Gastroenterol 1996;31:73–81.
38. Hadorn B, Tarlow MJ, Lloyd JK, et al: Intestinal enterokinase deficiency. Lancet 1969;1:812–813.
39. Ghishan FK, Lee PC, Lebenthal E, et al: Isolated congenital enterokinase deficiency: recent findings and review of the literature. Gastroenterology 1983;85:727–731.
40. Mann NS, Mann SK: Enterokinase. Proc Soc Exp Biol Med 1994;206:114–118.
41. Mata LJ, Jimenez F, Cordon M, et al: Gastrointestinal flora of children with protein-calorie malnutrition. Am J Clin Nutr 1972;25:1118–1126.
42. Heyworth B, Brown J: Jejunal microflora in malnourished Gambian children. Arch Dis Child 1975;50:27–33.
43. Gracey M, Suharjono, Sunoto, et al: Microbial contamination of the gut: another feature of malnutrition. Am J Clin Nutr 1973;26:1170–1174.
44. Gilman RH, Partanen R, Brown KH, et al: Decreased gastric acid secretion and bacterial colonization of the stomach in severely malnourished Bangladesh children. Gastroenterology 1988;94:1308–1314.
45. Toskes PP, Donaldson RM: The blind loop syndrome. In Sleisenger MH, Fordtran JS (eds): Gastrointestinal Disease: Pathophysiology, Diagnosis, Management, 4th ed. Philadelphia, WB Saunders, 1989, pp 1289–1297.
46. Thompson JS: Management of the short bowel syndrome. Gastroenterol Clin North Am 1994;23:403–420.
47. Vanderhoof JA: Short bowel syndrome in children and small intestinal transplantation. Pediatr Clin North Am 1996;43:533–550.
48. Husebye E, Skar V, Hoverstad T: Abnormal intestinal motor patterns explain enteric colonization with gram-negative bacilli in late radiation enteropathy. Gastroenterology 1995;109:1078–1089.
49. Basilisco G: Hereditary megaduodenum. Am J Gastroenterol 1997;92:150–153.
50. Barraclough M, Taylor CJ: Twenty-four hour ambulatory gastric and duodenal pH profiles in cystic fibrosis: effect of duodenal hyperacidity on pancreatic enzyme function and fat absorption. J Pediatr Gastroenterol Nutr 1996;23:45–50.
51. Marth T, Strober W: Whipple's disease. Semin Gastrointest Dis 1996;7:41–48.
52. Von Herbay A, Maiwald M, Ditton HJ, et al: Histology of intestinal Whipple's disease revisited: a study of 48 patients. Virchows Arch 1996;429:335–343.
53. Schnider PJ, Reisinger EC, Gerschlager W, et al: Long-term follow-up in cerebral Whipple's disease. Eur J Gastroenterol Hepatol 1996;8:899–903.
54. Duprez TP, Grandin CB, Bonnier C, et al: Whipple disease confined to the central nervous system in childhood. AJNR Am J Neuroradiol 1996;17:1589–1591.
55. Burke V: Mechanisms of intestinal digestion and absorption. In Anderson CM, Burke V, Gracey M (eds): Paediatric Gastroenterology, 2d ed. Melbourne, Blackwell Scientific Publications, 1987, pp 137–184.
56. Gudmand-Hoyer E, Skovbjerg H: Disaccharide digestion and maldigestion. Scand J Gastroenterol 1996;31(suppl 216):111–21.
57. Holzel A, Schwarz V, Sutcliffe KW: Defective lactose absorption causing malnutrition in infancy. Lancet 1959;1:1126–1128.
58. Lifshitz F: Congenital lactase deficiency. J Pediatr 1966;66:229–237.
59. Launiala K, Kuitunen P, Visakorpi JK: Disaccharidases and histology of duodenal mucosa in congenital lactose malabsorption. Acta Paediatr Scand 1966;55:257–263.
60. Levin B, Abraham JM, Burgess EA, et al: Congenital lactose malabsorption. Arch Dis Child 1970;45:173–177.
61. Savilahti E, Launiala K, Kuitunen P: Congenital lactase deficiency: a clinical study on 16 patients. Arch Dis Child 1983;58:246–252.
62. Koldovsky O: Digestion and absorption of carbohydrates, protein and fat in infants and children. In Walker WA, Watkins JB (eds): Nutrition in Pediatrics: Basic Science and Clinical Application. Boston, Little, Brown, 1985, pp 253–277.
63. Weijers HA, Van de Kamer JH, Dicke WK, et al: Diarrhoea caused by deficiency of sugar splitting enzymes I. Acta Paediatr Scand 1961;50:55–71.
64. Welsh JD, Poley JR, Bhatia M, et al: Intestinal disaccharidase activities in relation to age, race, and mucosal damage. Gastroenterology 1978;75:847–855.
65. Ellestad-Sayed JJ, Haworth JC: Disaccharide consumption and malabsorption in Canadian Indians. Am J Clin Nutr 1977;30:698–703.
66. Ellestad-Sayed JJ, Haworth JC, Hildes JA: Disaccharide malabsorption and dietary patterns in two Canadian Eskimo communities. Am J Clin Nutr 1978;31:1473–1478.
67. Gudmand-Hoyer E: Sucrose malabsorption in children: a report of thirty-one Greenlanders. J Pediatr Gastroenterol Nutr 1985;4:873–877.
68. Ouwendijk J, Moolenaar CEC, Peters WJ, et al: Congenital sucrase-isomaltase deficiency. J Clin Invest 1996;97:633–641.
69. Baudon JJ, Veinberg F, Thioulouse E, et al: Sucrase-isomaltase deficiency: changing pattern over two decades. J Pediatr Gastroenterol Nutr 1996;22:284–288.
70. Lebenthal E, Lee PC: Glucoamylase and disaccharidase activities in normal subjects and in patients with mucosal injury of the small intestine. J Pediatr 1980;97:389–393.
71. Lebenthal E, Khin-Maung-U, Zheng BY, et al: Small intestinal glucoamylase deficiency and starch malabsorption: a newly recognized alpha-glucosidase deficiency in children. J Pediatr 1994;124:541–546.
72. Quezada-Calvillo R, Senchyna M, Underdown BJ: Characterization of intestinal gamma-glucoamylase deficiency in CBA/Ca mice. Am J Physiol 1993;265:G1150–G1157.
73. Madzarovova-Nohejlova J: Trehalase deficiency in a family. Gastroenterology 1973;65:130–133.
74. Muller DPR, Milla PJ: Selective inborn errors of absorption. In Milla PJU, Muller DPR (eds): Harries' Paediatric Gastroenterology. Edinburgh, Churchill Livingstone, 1988, pp 211–238.
75. Levy HL: Hartnup disorder. In Scriver CR, Beaudet AL, Sly WS, et al (eds): The Metabolic Basis of Inherited Disease. New York, McGraw-Hill, 1989, pp 2515–2527.
76. Baron DN, Dent CE, Harris H, et al: Hereditary pellagra-like skin rash with temporary cerebellar ataxia: constant renal aminoaciduria and other bizarre biochemical features. Lancet 1956;2:421–428.
77. Mori E, Yamadori A, Tsutsumi A, et al: Adult-onset Hartnup disease presenting with neuropsychiatric symptoms but without skin lesions. Rinsho Shinkeigaku 1989;29:687–692.
78. Oakley A, Wallace J: Hartnup disease presenting in an adult. Clin Exp Dermatol 1994;19:407–408.

79. Scriver CR, Mahon B, Levy HL, et al: The Hartnup phenotype: mendelian transport disorder, multifactorial disease. Am J Hum Genet 1987;40:401–412.
80. Darras BT, Ampola MG, Dietz WH, et al: Intermittent dystonia in Hartnup disease. Pediatr Neurol 1989;5:118–120.
81. Jonas AJ, Butler IJ: Circumvention of defective neutral amino acid transport in Hartnup disease using tryptophan ethyl ester. J Clin Invest 1989;84:200–204.
82. Rajantie J, Simell O, Perheentupa J: Lysinuric protein intolerance: basolateral transport defect in renal tubuli. J Clin Invest 1981;67:1078–1082.
83. Rajantie J, Simell O, Perheentupa J: Intestinal absorption in lysinuric protein intolerance: impaired for diamino acids, normal for citrulline. Gut 1980;21:519–524.
84. Ono N, Kishida K, Tokumoto K: Lysinuric protein intolerance presenting deficiency of argininosuccinate synthetase. Intern Med 1992;31:55–59.
85. Thier SO, Alpers DH: Disorders of intestinal transport of amino acids. Am J Dis Child 1969;117:13–23.
86. Smith AJ, Strang LB: An inborn error of metabolism with the urinary excretion of alpha-hydroxy-butyric acid and phenylpyruvic acid. Arch Dis Child 1958:33:109–113.
87. Hooft C, Timmermans J, Snoeck J, et al: Methionine malabsorption in a mentally defective child. Lancet 1964;2:20.
88. Bartsocas CS, Levy HL, Crawford JD, et al: A defect in intestinal amino acid transport in Lowe's syndrome. Am J Dis Child 1969;117:93–95.
89. Hayashi Y, Hanioka K, Kanomata N: Clinicopathologic and molecular-pathologic approaches to Lowe's syndrome. Pediatr Pathol Lab Med 1995;15:389–402.
90. Lindquist B, Meeuwisse GW: Chronic diarrhea caused by monosaccharide malabsorption. Acta Paediatr 1962;51:674–685.
91. Hughes WS, Senior JR: The glucose-galactose malabsorption syndrome in a 23-year-old woman. Gastroenterology 1975;68:142–145.
92. Fairclough PD, Clark ML, Dawson AM, et al: Absorption of glucose and maltose in congenital glucose-galactose malabsorption. Pediatr Res 1978;12:1112–1114.
93. Stirling CE, Schneider AJ, Wong MD, et al: Quantitative radioautography of sugar transport in intestinal biopsies from normal humans and a patient with glucose-galactose malabsorption. J Clin Invest 1972;51:438–451.
94. Booth IW, Patel PB, Sule D, et al: Demonstration of defective jejunal brush border $NA^+$-coupled glucose transport in congenital glucose-galactose malabsorption (abstract). Pediatr Res 1987;22:98.
95. Wozniak E, Fenton TR, Walker-Smith JA, et al: Glucose absorption in congenital glucose-galactose malabsorption: a kinetic basis for clinical remission (abstract). Pediatr Res 1984;18:1063.
96. Martin MG, Turk E, Lostao MP, et al: Defects in $Na^+$/glucose cotransporter (SGLT1) trafficking and function cause glucose-galactose malabsorption. Nat Genet 1996;12:216–20.
97. Iacono G, Carroccio A, Cavataio F, et al: Congenital fructose-glucose-galactose malabsorption. J Pediatr Gastroenterol Nutr 1995;21:95–99.
98. Hoekstra JH: Fructose breath hydrogen tests in infants with chronic non-specific diarrhoea. Eur J Pediatr 1995;154:362–64.
99. Mortensen PB, Clausen MR: Short-chain fatty acids in the human colon: relation to gastrointestinal health and disease. Scand J Gastroenterol 1996;31(suppl 216):132–148.
100. Havel RJ, Kane JP: Structure and metabolism of plasma lipoproteins. In Scriver CR, Beaudet AL, Sly WS, et al (eds): The Metabolic Basis of Inherited Disease. New York, McGraw-Hill, 1989, pp 1129–1164.
101. Pomerantz M, Waldman TA: Systemic lymphatic abnormalities associated with gastrointestinal protein loss secondary to intestinal lymphangiectasia. Gastroenterology 1963;45:703–711.
102. Schonfeld G: The hypobetalipoproteinemias. Annu Rev Nutr 1995;15:23–34.
103. Davidson JD, Waldmann TA, Goodman DS, et al: Protein-losing gastroenteropathy in congestive heart-failure. Lancet 1961;1:899–902.
104. Mistilis SP, Skyring AP, Stephen DD: Intestinal lymphangiectasia: mechanism of enteric loss of plasma-protein and fat. Lancet 1965;1:77–80.
105. Vardy PA, Lebenthal E, Schwachmann H: Intestinal lymphangiectasia: a reappraisal. Pediatrics 1975;55:842–851.
106. Bolton RP,Cotter KL, Losowsky MS: Impaired neutrophil function in intestinal lymphangiectasia. J Clin Pathol 1986;39:876–880.
107. Hart MH, Vanderhoof JA, Antonson DL: Failure of blind small bowel biopsy in the diagnosis of intestinal lymphangiectasia. J Pediatr Gastroenterol Nutr 1987;6:803–805.
108. Silverman A, Roy CC: Physical signs. In Pediatric Clinical Gastroenterology, 3d ed. St. Louis, CV Mosby, 1983, pp 38–43.
109. Benson GD, Kowlessar OD, Sleisenger MH: Adult celiac disease with emphasis upon response to the gluten-free diet. Medicine (Baltimore) 1964;43:1–40.
110. Fielding JF, Cooke WT: Finger clubbing and regional enteritis. Gut 1971;12:442–444.
111. Hamilton JR, Bruce GA, Abdourhaman M, et al: Inflammatory bowel disease in children and adolescents. Adv Pediatr 1979;26:311–341.
112. Sondheimer JM: Office stool examination: a practical guide. Contemporary Pediatrics 1990;7:63–82.
113. Dormandy KM, Waters AH, Molin DL: Folic acid deficiency in celiac disease. Lancet 1963;1:632–635.
114. Hoffbrand AV, Douglas AP, Fry T, et al: Malabsorption of dietary folate (pteroylglutamates) in adult coeliac disease and dermatitis herpetiformis. Br Med J 1970;4:85–89.
115. Ater JL, Herbst JJ, Landaw SA, et al: Relative anemia and iron deficiency in cystic fibrosis. Pediatrics 1983;71:810–814.
116. Lundh G: Pancreatic exocrine function in neoplastic and inflammatory disease: a simple and reliable new test. Gastroenterology 1962;42:275–280.
117. Goldstein R, Blodheim O, Levy E, et al: The fatty meal test: an alternative to stool fat analysis. Am J Clin Nutr 1983;38:763–768.
118. Columbo C, Maiavacca R, Ronchi M, et al: The steatocrit: a simple method for monitoring fat malabsorption in patients with cystic fibrosis. J Pediatr Gastroenterol Nutr 1987;6:926–930.
119. Addison GM: Acid steatocrit. J Pediatr Gastroenterol Nutr 1996;22:227.
120. Rolles CJ, Nutter S, Kendal MJ, et al: One-hour blood-xylose screening-test for coeliac disease in infants and young children. Lancet 1973;2:1043–1045.
121. Christie DL: Use of the one-hour blood xylose test as an indicator of small bowel mucosal disease. J Pediatr 1978;92:725–728.
122. Buts JP, Morin CL, Roy CC, et al: One-hour blood xylose test: a reliable index of small bowel function. J Pediatr 1978;90:729–733.
123. Levine JJ, Seidman E, Walker WA: Screening tests for enteropathy in children. Am J Dis Child 1987;141:435–438.
124. Urban E: The A, B, C, of D-xylose absorption. Gastroenterology 1989;97:512–513.
125. Lifschitz CH, Polanco I: The D-xylose test in pediatrics: Is it useful? Gastroenterology 1989;97:246–247.
126. Deutsch JC, Santhosh-Kumar CR, Kolli VR: A noninvasive stable-isotope method to simultaneously assess pancreatic exocrine function and small bowel absorption. Am J Gastroenterol 1995;90:2182–2185.
127. Borowitz DS, Grand RJ, Durie PR, et al: Use of pancreatic enzyme supplements for patients with cystic fibrosis in the context of fibrosing colonopathy. J Pediatr 1995;127:681–684.
128. Littlewood JM: Management of malabsorption in cystic fibrosis: influence of recent developments on clinical practice. Postgrad Med J 1996;72(suppl 2):S56–S62.
129. Sokol RJ, Henbi JE, Butler-Simon N: Treatment of vitamin E deficiency during chronic childhood cholestasis with oral D-alpha-tocopheryl polyethylene glycol-1000 succinate. Gastroenterology 1987;93:975–985.
130. Sokol RJ: Vitamin E and neurologic deficits. Adv Pediatr 1990;37:119–148.
131. Cotting J, Lentze MJ, Reichen J: Effects of ursodeoxycholic acid treatment on nutrition and liver function in patients with cystic fibrosis and longstanding cholestasis. Gut 1990;31:918–921.
132. Girtzelmann R, Hirsig J: Infant dumping syndrome: reversal of symptoms by feeding uncooked starch. Eur J Pediatr 1986;145:504–506.
133. Belli DC, Levy E, Darling P, et al: Taurine improves the absorption of a fat meal in patients with cystic fibrosis. Pediatrics 1987;80:517–523.
134. Solomons NW, Molina S, Bulux J: Effect of protein-energy malnutrition on digestive and absorptive capacities of infants and children. In Lebenthal E (ed): Textbook of Gastroenterology and Nutrition in Infancy, 2d ed. New York, Raven Press, 1989, pp 517–533.
135. Balistreri WF: Neonatal cholestasis. J Pediatr 1985;106:171–189.
136. Amedee-Manesme O, Bernard O, Brunelle F, et al: Sclerosing cholangitis with neonatal onset. J Pediatr 1987;111:225–229.
137. Tong MJ, Thursby M, Rakela J, et al: Studies on the maternal-infant transmission of the viruses which cause acute hepatitis. Gastroenterology 1981;80:999–1004.

138. Giovannini M, Tagger A, Ribero ML, et al: Maternal-infant transmission of hepatitis C virus and HIV infections: a possible interaction (letter). Lancet 1990;335:1166.
139. Wejstal R, Hermodsson S, Iwarson S, et al: Mother to infant transmission of hepatitis C virus infection. J Med Virol 1990;30:178–180.
140. Frey B, Schubiger G, Musy JP: Transient cholestatic hepatitis in a neonate associated with carbamazepine exposure during pregnancy and breast-feeding. Eur J Pediatr 1990;150:136–138.
141. Balistreri WF: Foreword: Neonatal cholestasis: lessons from the past, issues for the future. Semin Liver Dis 1987;7:1–7.
142. Alagille D, Odievre M: Liver and Biliary Tract Disease in Children. New York, John Wiley & Sons, 1979, pp 163–252.
143. Akers DR, Needham ME: Sarcoma botryoides (rhabdomyosarcoma) of the bile ducts with survival. J Pediatr Surg 1971;6:474–479.
144. Shaffer EA: Gallbladder disease. In Walker WA, Duric PR, Hamilton JR, et al (eds): Pediatric Gastrointestinal Disease. Philadelphia, BC Decker, 1991, pp 1152–1170.
145. Classen M, Gotze H, Richter HJ, et al: Primary sclerosing cholangitis in children. J Pediatr Gastroenterol Nutr 1987;6:197–202.
146. Spivak W, Grand RJ, Eraklis A: A case of primary sclerosing cholangitis in childhood. Gastroenterology 1982;82:129–132.
147. Horowitz ME, Etcubanas E, Webber BL, et al: Hepatic undifferentiated (embryonal) sarcoma and rhabdomyosarcoma in children. Cancer 1987;59:396–402.
148. Bhave SA, Pandit AN, Pradhan AM, et al: Liver disease in India. Arch Dis Child 1982;57:922–928
149. Perman JA, Welin SL, Grand RJ, et al: Laboratory measures of copper metabolism in the differentiation of chronic active hepatitis and Wilson disease in children. J Pediatr 1979;94:564–568.
150. Meyer UA: Hepatic porphyrias: New findings on the nature of metabolic defects. In Popper H, Schaffner F (eds): Progressive Liver Diseases. New York, Grune & Stratton, 1976, pp 280–293.
151. Sherlock S: Hepatitis C viral infection: an update (supplement). In Sherlock S: Diseases of the Liver and Biliary System, 8th ed. Oxford, Blackwell, 1989, pp 1–9.
152. Davenport M. Neonatal malaria and obstructive jaundice. Arch Dis Child 1986;61:515–517.
153. Orellana-Alcalde JM, Dominguez JP: Jaundice and oral contraceptive drugs. Lancet 1966;2:1278–1280.
154. Stoll BA, Andrews JT, Motteram R: Preliminary communications: liver damage from oral contraceptives. Br Med J 1966;1:960–961.
155. Ockner RK, Davidson CS: Hepatic effects of oral contraceptives. N Engl J Med 1967;276:331–334.
156. Davis RA, Kern F Jr, Showalter R, et al: Alterations of hepatic $Na^+,K^+$-ATPase and bile flow by estrogen: effects on liver surface membrane lipid structure and function. Proc Natl Acad Sci U S A 1978;75:4130–4134.
157. Kern F Jr, Everson GT, DeMark B, et al: Biliary lipids, bile acids, and gallbladder function in the human female: effects of contraceptive steroids. J Lab Clin Med 1982;99:798–805.
158. Royal College of General Practitioners Oral Contraception Study: Oral contraceptives and gallbladder disease. Lancet 1982;2:957–959.
159. Lieberman DA, Keeffe EB, Stenzel P: Severe and prolonged oral contraceptive jaundice. J Clin Gastroenterol 1984;6:145–148.
160. Frezza M, Pozzato G, Chiesa L, et al: Reversal of intrahepatic cholestasis of pregnancy in women after high dose *S*-adenosyl-L-methionine administration. Hepatology 1984;4:274–278.
161. Vose M: Estrogen cholestasis: Membranes, metabolites or receptors? Gastroenterology 1987;93:643–649.
162. Schrumpf E, Fausa O, Kolmannskog F, et al: Sclerosing cholangitis in ulcerative colitis: a follow-up study. Scand J Gastroenterol 1982;17:33–39.
163. Mieli-Vergani G, Mowat AP: The immunology of autoimmune chronic active hepatitis. In Branski D, Dinari G, Rosen P, et al (eds): Paediatric Gastroenterology: Aspects of Immunology and Infections. Basel, Karger, 1986, pp 256–265.
164. Ferrara JLM, Deeg HJ: Graft-versus-host disease. N Engl J Med 1991;324:667–674.
165. Gamble JL, Fahey KR, Appleton J, et al: Congenital alkalosis with diarrhea. J Pediatr 1945;26:509–518.
166. Darrow DC: Congenital alkalosis with diarrhea. J Pediatr 1945;26:149–152.
167. Holmberg C: Electrolyte economy and its normal regulation in congenital chloride diarrhea. Pediatr Res 1978;12:82–86.
168. McLoughlin LC, Nord KS, Joshi VV, et al: Severe gastrointestinal involvement in children with acquired immunodeficiency syndrome. J Pediatr Gastroenterol Nutr 1987;6:517–524.
169. Castaldo A, Tarallo L, Palomba E, et al: Iron deficiency and intestinal malabsorption in HIV disease. J Pediatr Gastroenterol Nutr 1996;22:359–363.
170. Steuerwald M, Bucher HC, Müller-Brand J, et al: HIV-enteropathy and bile acid malabsorption: response to cholestyramine. Am J Gastroenterol 1995;90:2051–2053.

# Chapter 23

# Protracted Diarrhea

*Roy Proujansky*

The syndrome of protracted diarrhea, also known as intractable diarrhea of infancy, was originally defined in 1968 by Avery and colleagues as diarrhea of longer than 2 weeks' duration occurring in a child younger than 3 months of age.[1] Associated features were a negative evaluation for infectious agents, requirement for intravenous hydration, persistence of severe symptoms in the hospital, and a high mortality rate. Since this original description, numerous subsequent reports have resulted in modification of this definition and have helped to characterize the heterogeneous nature of the diagnostic entities that result in this clinical syndrome.[2–6] Protracted diarrhea of infancy is now more commonly defined as severe diarrhea, usually occurring in a child younger than 1 year of age, which is prolonged and often associated with poor nutrition requiring aggressive enteral or parenteral nutrition support.[6] Some authors have chosen to further narrow this definition by excluding common infectious causes, celiac disease, and protein-sensitive enteropathies.

Since these original descriptions great progress has been made toward identifying the unique pathophysiology of some of the individual diagnostic entities that present as protracted diarrhea. For instance, congenital microvillus atrophy and autoimmune enteropathy are now both known to make up significant percentages of those cases with a more severe and protracted course associated with higher morbidity and mortality. For the purposes of this discussion, these disorders can be classified into conditions that are (1) caused by primary defects of the structure or function of the intestinal epithelium or (2) secondary to infectious, inflammatory, or immunologic mechanisms (Table 23–1). However, there continue to be a number of patients whose disease remains "idiopathic" after extensive evaluation, for whom prognosis is variable, and for whom therapeutic interventions are supportive (parenteral nutrition) or nonspecific (antibiotics, corticosteroids). This chapter describes the clinical presentation of the typical patient with protracted diarrhea and highlights specific disorders that may manifest in this manner. Key features necessary in the diagnostic evaluation and management of such patients are also reviewed.

## IDIOPATHIC PROTRACTED DIARRHEA

Patients with protracted diarrhea usually come to medical attention in the first several months of life with persistent diarrhea that is severe, is associated with poor weight gain or weight loss, and does not respond to dietary manipulation.[2–4] Persistent symptoms despite outpatient evaluation for common infectious agents usually result in hospitalization for more aggressive diagnostic evaluation and nutritional support. At the time of hospitalization, these infants are often severely wasted and malnourished and showing signs of both acute and subacute dehydration. They are often quite irritable and may have some degree of anorexia or vomiting. Diarrhea may cease when the patient is fasted, suggesting a predominantly malabsorptive cause, or it may continue despite fasting if a secretory component is contributing to the diarrhea. For many infants, an underlying inflammatory process may also affect the colon, resulting in stools which are described as containing mucus and blood.[6]

For these often quite ill infants, diagnostic and therapeutic interventions must proceed simultaneously. Establishment of sustainable venous access and subsequent fluid and electrolyte balance are essential as the initial diagnostic evaluation is proceeding. In addition, cautious introduction of enteral or

**TABLE 23–1. Etiology of Protracted Diarrhea**

**Idiopathic**

**Disorders of Intestinal Epithelial Structure or Function**
- Congenital microvillus atrophy
- Tufting enteropathy
- Congenital transport defects
  - Congenital glucose-galactose malabsorption
  - Congenital chloride diarrhea
  - Congenital sodium diarrhea
  - Primary bile salt malabsorption
- Hormonally-mediated secretory diarrhea
- Mitochondrial disease

**Infectious, Inflammatory, and Immunologically-based Disorders**
- Infection
- Cow's milk– and soy protein–sensitive enteropathy
- Celiac disease
- Immunodeficiency
  - X-linked agammaglobulinemia
  - T cell and combined immunodeficiencies
  - Human immunodeficiency virus infection
  - Miscellaneous immunodeficiencies associated with protracted diarrhea
- Autoimmune enteropathy

**Miscellaneous Disorders**
- Hirschsprung's disease

parenteral nutrition, or both, should be initiated. Appropriate testing for infectious causes should be done, and, after the patient is in stable condition, more aggressive diagnostic studies such as biopsy of the small intestinal mucosa and endoscopic and histologic evaluation of the colonic mucosa should be performed (see later discussions). These studies are directed toward documentation of (1) the presence of an intestinal and/or colonic mucosal lesion that is responsible for the patient's symptoms or (2) identification of one of the specific diagnostic entities noted in Table 23–1. Infants with idiopathic protracted diarrhea often are found to have some degree of partial or total villous atrophy or blunting associated with varying degrees of mucosal inflammation, with a cellular infiltrate including neutrophils, eosinophils, and plasma cells.[2–6] The severity of the mucosal lesion, however, does not appear to correlate with the response to therapeutic intervention or the duration of hospitalization or aggressive nutritional support.[7, 8]

Several common mechanisms are often invoked to explain the possible etiology for those patients whose protracted diarrhea is idiopathic. For some, diagnostic challenge with the suspected dietary antigen ultimately establishes a diagnosis of protein-sensitive enteropathy.[6–8] Protein-sensitive enteropathy may also occur during or after the course of an intercurrent infectious process, exacerbating mucosal inflammation and malnutrition associated with the initial intestinal injury.[9] The ongoing identification of new infectious agents causing diarrhea suggests that some cases of protracted diarrhea result from as yet unidentified infectious agents. In addition, opportunistic pathogens may potentially prolong diarrhea in patients with an established insult from another process.

The prognosis for these children has improved significantly since the original descriptions of the protracted diarrhea syndrome. Initial reports identified mortality rates as high as 45%, but in more recent studies mortality is in the range of 5% to 7%. This improvement is the result of several factors. More recent studies concerning idiopathic protracted diarrhea no longer include specific entities such as congenital microvillus atrophy and autoimmune enteropathy, which are associated with a more severe clinical course. Similarly, cases of protracted diarrhea resulting from protein-sensitive enteropathies (reactions to cow's milk or soy) are often considered "idiopathic" until a later date, when the patient is cautiously challenged with the offending antigen and the diagnosis is proven. These patients tend to have a good prognosis and are often included in reported series of patients with protracted diarrhea.[7, 8] In addition, significant improvements in enteral and parenteral nutrition support techniques since the 1970s have greatly improved patient outcomes for this disorder.

In one series,[4] a familial nature to the protracted diarrhea syndrome was associated with an especially poor prognosis; however, the patients in this series were ultimately shown to have congenital microvillus atrophy. Other studies have documented a familial nature to idiopathic protracted diarrhea not associated with any alteration in morbidity or mortality.[10]

## DEFECTS OF EPITHELIAL STRUCTURE OR FUNCTION

For a number of the causes of the protracted diarrhea syndrome, the primary pathophysiologic process relates to an abnormality or severe alteration in normal epithelial absorptive mechanisms, secretory processes, or both. This may be associated with structural abnormalities of the enterocyte brush border, defects in individual transport proteins, or abnormal stimulation of normally functioning secretory processes as a result of excessive endogenous secretagogues.

### Congenital Microvillus Atrophy

Congenital microvillus atrophy, microvillus inclusion disease, and familial microvillus atrophy are all pseudonyms for a rare disorder in which infants present with intractable diarrhea associated with characteristic abnormalities of the intestinal epithelial surface. In an initial study by Davidson and associates,[11] three of five infants with intractable diarrhea beginning at birth had ultrastructural abnormalities of the microvillus surface, and one had intracellular inclusions. Several subsequent studies have characterized a fairly typical pattern of clinical presentation and associated histologic and ultrastructural findings.[12–14]

Diarrhea characteristically begins in the first few days of life. Most infants have had an uneventful antenatal course, and there is no history of polyhydramnios, distinguishing this disorder from some of the congenital secretory diarrheas. In a number of reported cases, a sibling or other relative was previously affected and consanguinity was identified, suggesting an autosomal recessive pattern of inheritance.[11, 13–15] The diarrhea is described as watery, nonbloody, and voluminous. Stool volumes ranging from 100 to 500 mL/kg per day in fed infants; they diminish but remain excessive, at 50 to 300 mL/kg per day, in fasted infants.[14] Stool pH is usually neutral, and stool sodium concentration is usually elevated (54–120 mmol/L).

The findings on mucosal biopsy of the small intestine that are characteristic of congenital microvillus atrophy include diffuse and severe villous atrophy, crypt hypoplasia, and normal (or decreased) numbers of inflammatory cells in the lamina propria (Fig. 23–1). In addition, periodic acid–Schiff (PAS) staining frequently reveals the presence of PAS-positive material within the apical cytoplasm of epithelial cells. Ultrastructural changes detected by electron microscopy include absence or shortening of microvilli, abnormally shaped or disordered microvilli, and microvilli lining membrane-bound vacuoles within the apical cytoplasm of enterocytes.[13, 14] PAS-positive staining and electron microscopic abnormalities can also be detected in rectal biopsy specimens.[13, 14] The rectal biopsy findings in one case enabled specific diagnosis several months before the demonstration of the histologic findings in a jejunal biopsy.[13]

Mucosal biopsies from patients with congenital microvillus atrophy have been documented to have reduced levels of lactase and sucrase in most cases.[13, 14] Ussing's chamber studies of a jejunal segment from one affected patient demonstrated unidirectional ion fluxes that were 30% of normal and a net secretory state with respect to sodium and chloride.[16]

Weight loss and ongoing malabsorption are uniform in this disorder, and all affected infants have required total parenteral nutrition to maintain adequate fluid and nutritional status. Limited improvement in stool volume has been achieved with loperamide and somatostatin for a small number of patients. Elemental and modified diets have been

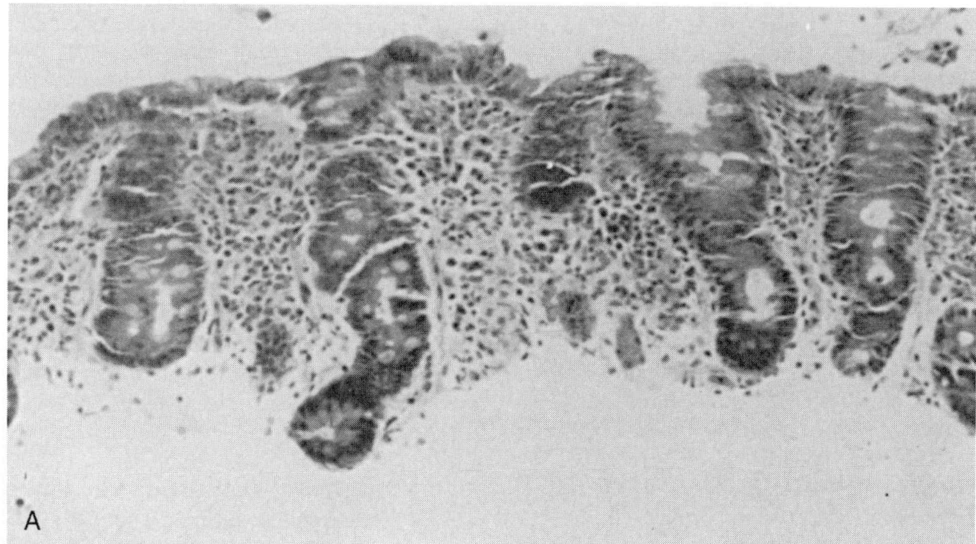


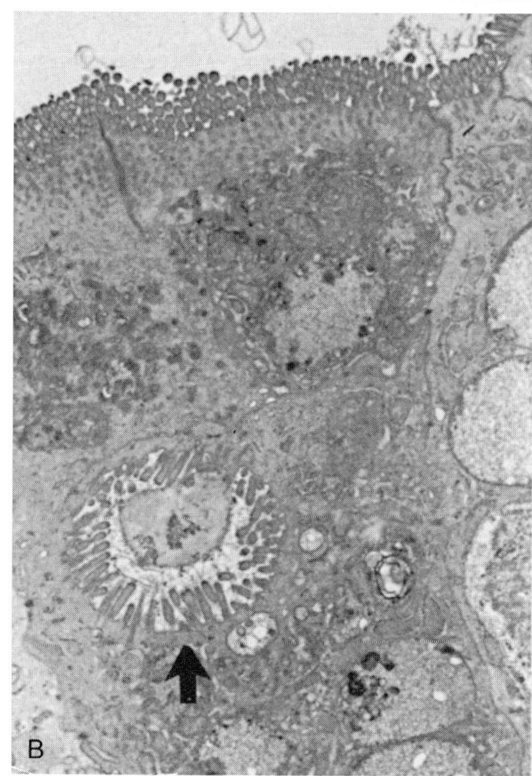


**FIGURE 23–1.** *A,* Jejunal biopsy specimen from an infant with congenital microvillus atrophy. Total villus atrophy and mild nonspecific increase in cellularity are seen (light micrograph; original magnification, ×100). *B,* Electron micrograph showing intact brush border and well-formed microvillus inclusion present within the enterocyte cell cytoplasm (*arrow*). Atypical cytoplasmic vesicular bodies are seen. (From Rhoads JM, Vogler RC, Lacey SE, et al: Microvillus inclusion disease: *in vitro* jejunal electrolyte transport. Gastroenterology 1991;100:811–817, with permission.)

tried without success, and more novel treatments such as corticosteroids, exogenous epidermal growth factor, and colostrum have likewise been ineffective. Most patients have died from complications of their disease or of long-term parenteral nutrition. Successful outcomes from transplantation of the small intestine or combined bowel-liver transplantation have been described.[17, 18]

Although the characteristic form of congenital microvillus atrophy manifests in the first few days of life and is quite severe, several authors have documented the occurrence of less severe disorders with similar features which may be variants of this disorder. Phillips and coworkers[14] described a later onset of symptoms, between the sixth and ninth weeks of life, in four infants. Three of these infants were among the small number of survivors in their survey of patients with congenital microvillus atrophy. Raafat and associates described three infants from two families with protracted diarrhea beginning after the first week of life associated with abnormal PAS staining of mucosal biopsies and disordered microvilli seen by electron microscopy. No intracytoplasmic microvillus inclusions were identified. Two of the three infants died. The authors referred to these findings as "intestinal microvillous dystrophy" and suggested that there may be a varied spectrum of the severity of the mucosal abnormality.[19]

## Tufting Enteropathy

Tufting enteropathy is a more recently described cause of protracted diarrhea that is also associated with abnormalities of the epithelial surface but with clinical and histologic features that suggest it is a distinct clinical disorder.[20] The three infants described all experienced during the first 4 weeks of life the onset of severe, watery diarrhea that was not responsive to dietary manipulation or immunosuppressive therapy. Discontinuation of enteral feedings was associated with drastic reduction in stool volume. Two of the three patients survived but were dependent on total parenteral nutrition. Extensive investigations disclosed only the unique histopathologic findings of this disorder. Jejunal mucosal biopsy revealed partial villous atrophy with crypt hyperplasia and normal numbers of mononuclear inflammatory cells. On the surface epithelium, focal "tufts" of densely packed enterocytes projecting off of the epithelial surface were seen. Ultrastructural studies revealed relatively normal-appearing microvilli that were slightly reduced in length. None of the intracellular inclusions typically seen in congenital microvillus atrophy were identified.

A subsequent report by Goulet and colleagues identified six children with similar histologic findings.[21] These authors emphasized the secretory nature of the diarrheal process and the frequent association of a family history of consanguinity or previously affected siblings. In addition to the unique histologic features, immunostaining revealed significant alterations in the distribution of laminin and heparan sulfate proteoglycan in the basement membrane. Multiple nutritional, antibiotic, and immunosuppressive treatment regimens were unsuccessful, and all of the patients remained dependent on total parenteral nutrition.

## Disorders of Epithelial Transport

There are several disorders that manifest clinically as protracted diarrhea of infancy and are caused by abnormalities of specific intestinal transport processes. Progress in the biochemistry and molecular biology of the affected transport proteins has greatly enhanced the understanding of these conditions.

*Congenital glucose-galactose malabsorption* is a rare, autosomal recessive disorder caused by defects in the intestinal Na+/glucose transporter, known as SGLT1. This illness is characterized by the onset in the first few days of life of severe, watery diarrhea associated with acidic stools which contain sugar.[22–24] The inability to transport glucose or galactose across the intestinal epithelial surface results in severe osmotic diarrhea after exposure to milk or formula containing glucose, galactose, or lactose. This usually leads to severe dehydration and metabolic acidosis, often associated with hypernatremia. Some patients also exhibit glycosuria. The diagnosis is suggested by the striking improvement observed after removal of glucose and galactose from the diet and by the successful feeding of a fructose-based milk formula. Breath hydrogen testing can be used to confirm malabsorption of glucose or galactose. Confirmation of the diagnosis has been done in the past by in vitro measurement of abnormal glucose transport in a jejunal mucosal biopsy specimen. However, since the cloning of the SGLT1 gene (SLC5A1), documentation of genetic mutations has become possible, enabling molecular diagnosis and genetic counseling.[25, 26]

*Congenital chloride diarrhea* is another uncommon autosomal recessive disorder characterized by severe, watery diarrhea beginning at birth.[26–29] Most of these infants are born prematurely, and polyhydramnios is uniformly present. Profuse, watery diarrhea beginning on the first day of life may be thought to be urine initially. Abdominal distention is present initially or develops rapidly. Urinary chloride concentrations are in the range of 100 to 150 mmol/L and are associated with a stool pH of 4 to 6. Serum sodium and chloride concentrations usually are both low, serum pH is alkalotic, and patients are often quite dehydrated at presentation. This fairly characteristic presentation is diagnostic of this disorder. The primary defect is a disturbance in normal chloride-bicarbonate exchange in the distal ileum and right colon. Mapping of a gene locus for congenital chloride diarrhea has led to the discovery of mutations in the *DRA* (*d*own-*r*egulated in *a*denoma) gene, which segregates with the clinical phenotype in many patients.[30] This finding is likely to lead in the future to molecular diagnosis and to further characterization of the nature of the chloride secretory defect. Current treatment requires lifelong supplementation with sodium chloride and potassium chloride to maintain normal serum sodium, potassium, and chloride concentrations and to correct alkalosis. With appropriate supplementation, the prognosis is good, and normal growth, development, and intelligence can be expected.

*Congenital sodium diarrhea* has been described for a small number of patients.[31, 32] These infants clinically are quite similar to those with congenital chloride diarrhea, with prematurity, polyhydramnios and neonatal onset of watery diarrhea and abdominal distention. Fecal electrolytes are most notable for the high sodium concentration (100 to 145 mEq/L). Fecal chloride concentration may be increased but is much lower than that seen in congenital chloride diarrhea, and the stool pH is normal or slightly alkalotic. The primary defect in transport affects the brush border sodium-hydrogen ion exchanger. These patients have been treated with a sodium-potassium-citrate solution, which has normalized electrolytes and serum pH despite persistence of the diarrhea.

*Primary bile acid malabsorption* has been characterized as a rare cause for protracted diarrhea in infancy.[33, 34] Patients were described as having the onset of diarrhea in the first week of life, with persistent symptoms unresponsive to dietary change. Carbohydrate and fat malabsorption were present. Radiolabeled bile acid absorptive studies showed excessive fecal losses of bile salts and decreased ileal bile salt absorption. Parenteral alimentation was required for survival during infancy.

## Disorders of Epithelial Energy Metabolism

Disorders of mitochondrial energy metabolism have been identified as an important cause of a variety of previously poorly understood neuromuscular disorders affecting children and adults. These unique disorders of oxidative phosphorylation have also been shown to be responsible for disease in other organ systems, including bone marrow, liver, and kidney. Cormier-Daire and coworkers described two children with severe diarrhea and villous atrophy who ultimately were shown to have rearrangements in their mitochondrial DNA.[35] Initial, recurrent episodes of lactic acidosis suggested a mitochondrial disorder, although neurologic symptoms compatible with mitochondrial disease did not occur until later. Mitochondrial DNA alterations detected in muscle were retrospectively shown to have been present in biopsy specimens of the colon and rectum. The authors suggested that mitochondrial disease be considered in patients with chronic diarrhea associated with elevation of serum lactic acid or other nonintestinal symptoms or signs compatible with this group of disorders.

### Hormonally-Mediated Secretory Diarrhea

Secretory diarrhea resulting from excessive endogenous release of a hormonal stimulus is a relatively uncommon cause of diarrhea in childhood. However, secretory diarrhea caused by excessive secretion of vasoactive intestinal peptide (VIP) from neural crest tumors is an important diagnostic entity because of its implications for appropriate diagnosis and management. Secretory diarrhea caused by VIP-secreting tumors has been seen in both infants and older children in association with ganglioneuroblastomas and neuroblastomas.[36–39] In addition to persistent diarrhea, patients may also experience flushing episodes and may be found to be hypokalemic. Pseudo-obstructive symptoms have also been described as part of this clinical syndrome.[40] Fecal electrolytes may reveal marked elevations in sodium and potassium concentration, although this may fluctuate. This disorder should be suspected in cases of protracted diarrhea in which the diarrhea is secretory in nature and associated with normal intestinal mucosal histology. Elevated VIP levels in this setting should lead to an aggressive search for an underlying neural crest tumor.

## INFECTIOUS, INFLAMMATORY, AND IMMUNOLOGICALLY-BASED DISORDERS

### Infection

Most cases of diarrhea caused by an infectious agent in childhood are self-limited, and such agents are unlikely to cause protracted diarrhea in an infant. Nevertheless, pathogens that are more commonly associated with acute, self-limited illness, such as *Campylobacter, Yersinia enterocolitica,* and enteroadherent *Escherichia coli,* can be associated with more prolonged illness.[41–43] Similarly, several parasitic infections, such as giardiasis and cryptosporidiosis, may cause protracted symptoms, although prolonged, severe disease is relatively uncommon.[44, 45]

### Protein-Sensitive Enteropathy and Celiac Disease

Protein-sensitive enteropathies and celiac disease are both reviewed more extensively elsewhere in this text; however, a few issues are worth noting here. Cow's milk– and soy protein–sensitive enteropathies have both been associated with protracted diarrhea in infancy, of varying severity.[46, 47] In addition to severe enteritis, many patients also have significant colitis with grossly bloody stools.[48] As noted previously, protein-sensitive enteropathy may also be an important cause of prolonged diarrhea after an infectious process.[9] Protracted diarrhea in infancy is an uncommon presentation for celiac disease, because patients often are not exposed to gluten-containing foods at an early age, and the symptoms usually respond relatively promptly to gluten withdrawal.

### Immunodeficiency

Gastrointestinal symptoms, and diarrhea in particular, are well recognized manifestations of congenital and acquired immunodeficiencies. These disorders may manifest with recurrent or atypical infections that provide a clue to the underlying immunodeficiency, or they may initially manifest with predominantly gastrointestinal symptoms before the development of other infectious complications suggesting an underlying immunodeficiency disorder. The impact of immunodeficiency on gastrointestinal function is discussed elsewhere in this text. This section focuses on immunodeficiencies that may be associated with protracted diarrhea.

In general, pure antibody deficiency syndromes are an uncommon cause of protracted diarrhea in infancy. For the first 6 months of life, protective maternal antibodies often delay the onset of infectious symptoms from disorders such as *X-linked agammaglobulinemia.* Patients with this disorder may have severe and persistent diarrhea secondary to infections such as giardiasis or chronic rotavirus infection.[49, 50] However, other systemic infectious complications are more common than diarrheal disease for these patients. *Transient hypogammaglobulinemia of infancy* has also been associated with chronic diarrhea that is usually less severe, and associated with less significant malabsorption, than that seen in protracted diarrhea of infancy.[51, 52] Some patients with *common variable immunodeficiency* with evidence of predominantly B cell dysfunction have persistent *Giardia* infection or diarrhea associated with variable degrees of villous atrophy.[49]

More significant gastrointestinal disease can be seen in a number of immunodeficiency disorders with T cell dysfunction or combined B cell and T cell dysfunction. *Severe combined immunodeficiency* is often associated with very severe diarrhea and failure to thrive, along with severe systemic infections with a variety of common and opportunistic agents.[53] The diarrhea in this disorder is caused both by infectious agents and by other, poorly understood mechanisms related to the impact of severe immunodeficiency on normal intestinal function. Patients with the *Wiskott-Aldrich syndrome* may have severe diarrhea, usually infectious in origin, that occurs before or is unassociated with the other classic features of this (i.e., thrombocytopenia, eczema).[54] Recurrent or protracted diarrhea has been identified as a common manifestation of other, poorly characterized, T cell immunodeficiencies.[55] Severe and persistent diarrhea is a common occurrence during the course of symptomatic *human immunodeficiency virus* infection.[56]

Several clinical syndromes associated with both protracted diarrhea and variable degrees of immunodeficiency have been characterized to occur during infancy. The association of erythroderma, failure to thrive, protracted diarrhea, and immunodeficiency has been described by a number of authors.[57–59] Previously referred to as Leiner's disease, this condition is associated with severe erythema and scaling of the skin as a prominent clinical feature. The onset of erythroderma and diarrhea is during the first several weeks of life. Immunologic features are quite variable and may include low immunoglobulins, decreased neutrophil chemotaxis, and alterations in T cell number and function. Diarrhea has eventually resolved in most described patients.

Protracted diarrhea associated with dysmorphic features, hypertelorism, woolly hair, and immunodeficiency has been described in eight patients and in other reports.[60, 61] The facial features and hair abnormality, including easy loss of hair and its brittle nature, were similar in all patients. Defects in both humoral and cell-mediated immunity were noted. Most patients had severe diarrhea, which continued when they were not being fed, and required parenteral nutrition to thrive. Death from infection or complications of long-term parenteral nutrition was common.

## Autoimmune Enteropathy

Several authors have described a subset of patients with protracted diarrhea in infancy whose clinical presentation is associated with the presence of circulating autoantibodies directed against intestinal epithelial cells.[62–65] These patients initially come to medical attention during the first year of life, usually between 3 and 6 months of age, or occasionally earlier. Diarrhea and failure to thrive are the usual presenting symptoms. The diarrhea often has both malabsorptive and secretory components, and the secretory nature of the diarrhea may be quite severe. Diarrheal stools may also be grossly bloody when there is an associated colitis. There may be a family history of other affected siblings or relatives. Other autoimmune or atopic disease may be seen at presentation or during the subsequent clinical course; reported cases have included alopecia, atopic dermatitis, asthma, formula protein intolerance, diabetes, hypothyroidism, autoimmune hepatitis, autoimmune thrombocytopenia, hemolytic anemia, neutropenia, interstitial nephropathy, glomerulonephritis, and systemic vasculitis.[66]

Mucosal biopsy of the small intestine usually reveals severe villous atrophy associated with a prominent increase in the cellularity of the lamina propria (Fig. 23–2). The crypts are usually hyperplastic, but crypt hypoplasia has also been described. Associated inflammatory cell infiltrates may be identified frequently in the colon and have also been found to affect the gastric mucosa and the pancreas.

The presence of autoantibodies to intestinal epithelial cells has usually been documented by indirect immunofluorescence using normal human duodenum or jejunum as the tissue substrate. Immunofluorescent staining tends to be more prominent along the villi, with prominent staining of the epithelial brush border having been noted frequently. A similar pattern of epithelial immunofluorescence has also been seen in the proximal tubules of the kidney in a patient with associated glomerulonephritis. Autoantibodies are usually immunoglobulin G (IgG), but IgM and IgA autoantibodies may also be seen. In addition, a variety of other autoantibodies have been detected in individual patient sera, including antinuclear antibody, islet cell antibody, thyroglobulin antibody, parietal cell antibody, and smooth muscle antibody. Variants of this disorder associated with the presence of autoantibodies to goblet cells and antibullous pemphigoid antigens have also been reported.[67, 68] Intestinal epithelial autoantibodies have been characterized as either complement-fixing autoantibodies, which bind to the apical portion of the intestinal epithelial cell, or autoantibodies that show a cytoplasmic staining pattern and do not fix complement.[69] The detection of such antibodies in patients without gastrointestinal disease and lack of correlation of the autoantibody titer with clinical disease severity in some patients has put in question the pathogenic role of antibodies directed against intestinal epithelial cells. Despite the prominent autoimmune features that are present in these patients, extensive immunologic investigations of T cell, B cell, com-

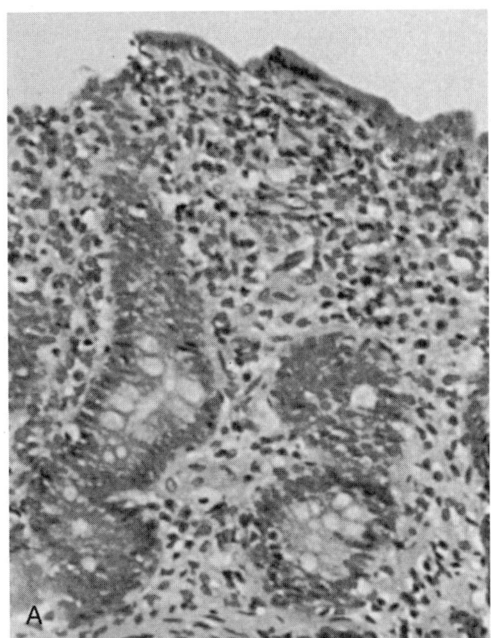


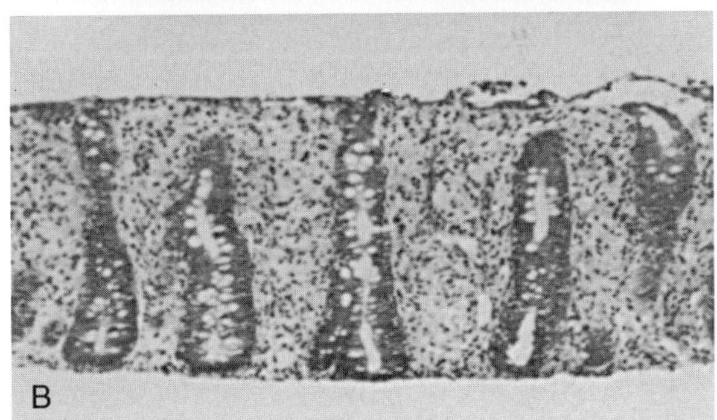


**FIGURE 23–2.** *A,* Jejunal biopsy specimen from an infant with autoimmune enteropathy. Severe villus atrophy and crypt hyperplasia are present (original magnification, ×250). *B,* Histologic appearance of typical autoimmune colitis. Note preservation of crypt architecture, irregularity of surface epithelium, and increased cellularity of the lamina propria (original magnification ×250). (*A,* From Colletti RB, Guillot AP, Rosen S, et al: Autoimmune enteropathy and nephropathy with circulating autoantibodies. J Pediatr 1991;118:853–864, with permission. *B,* From Hill SM, Milla PJ, Bottazzo GF, et al: Autoimmune enteropathy and colitis: is there a generalized autoimmune gut disorder? Gut 1991;32:36–42, with permission.)

plement, and neutrophil function usually have been unrevealing, although a few cases have been associated with selective IgA deficiency.[62, 69]

The treatment options for patients with autoimmune enteropathy usually have included supportive nutritional management combined with varying levels of immunosuppression. Patients with severe disease often require total parenteral nutrition for support until their disease improves or is under better control with immunosuppressive therapy. Prednisone, prednisone plus azathioprine, cyclophosphamide, and cyclosporin have all been used with success. Some patients appear to be resistant to all forms of immunosuppression.[65, 67]

## DIAGNOSTIC EVALUATION

The initial evaluation of the patient with protracted diarrhea should include a detailed assessment of the critical historical features and physical findings that might suggest one of the specific diagnoses outlined in the previous discussion. A history of the presence or absence of polyhydramnios, consanguinity, or previously affected siblings in association with diarrhea beginning at birth or in the first week of life is suggestive of a congenital transport defect or congenital microvillus atrophy. A careful dietary history should be obtained, including variations in the diarrhea that occurred with particular formulas or feedings. The physical examination should include a careful assessment for dysmorphic features, abdominal distention, and abdominal masses. Gentle digital rectal examination should be performed, and the stool should be tested for occult blood. The presence of grossly bloody stool or occult blood should suggest an inflammatory process as the basis for the patient's diarrheal disorder.

The character of the diarrhea and some simple biochemical analyses are extremely useful in classifying the predominantly malabsorptive, secretory, or mixed nature of the diarrhea. Cessation of the diarrhea within 24 to 48 hours after discontinuation of all oral intake indicates a predominantly malabsorptive process. Continuation of diarrhea after institution of bowel rest should suggest a significant secretory component and should guide the subsequent evaluation in this direction. For some patients, diarrhea decreases but still continues when feeding is stopped, suggesting both malabsorptive and secretory components. Inflammatory processes in particular are often associated with both malabsorptive and secretory contributions to the diarrheal process.

If the diarrheal process appears to be malabsorptive in nature, it is valuable to attempt to determine whether there is generalized malabsorption or an osmotic diarrhea caused by malabsorption of a specific carbohydrate. Protracted diarrhea can occur as the result of malabsorption of specific carbohydrates, as in *congenital glucose-galactose malabsorption* or *isolated congenital lactase deficiency*.[70] These possibilities can be tested by trying formulas of different carbohydrate content and determining whether the diarrhea persists and whether malabsorbed carbohydrate can be detected in stools (i.e., by testing for the presence of reducing substances). An alternative approach involves the use of specialized carbohydrate-free formulas, with a specific carbohydrate added to evaluate malabsorption of that particular sugar. Diarrhea that persists despite attempts at feeding with multiple different carbohydrates suggests a generalized malabsorptive disorder, which can be evaluated further with tests such as the oral D-xylose test. The stool "osmotic gap" can be measured to document the osmotic nature of diarrhea caused by malabsorbed carbohydrate. This is done by checking the osmolality of a fresh stool specimen (approximately 290 mOsm/kg) and comparing it with a number equal to twice the sum of the fecal concentrations of sodium and potassium in milliequivalents per liter:

$$\text{Osmotic gap} = \text{stool osmolality} - 2(\text{stool sodium} + \text{stool potassium})$$

An osmotic gap is indicated when the difference is greater than 50 mOsm. The presence of a persistent osmotic gap in the absence of demonstrable carbohydrate malabsorption should raise concern about the possible surreptitious administration of a laxative as a form of *Munchausen's syndrome by proxy*.[71]

Measurement of fecal electrolyte concentrations is also a useful adjunct to the evaluation of secretory processes and may point to specific diagnoses such as *congenital chloride diarrhea* or *congenital sodium diarrhea*. Stool sodium concentrations are usually greater than 90 mEq/L in secretory diarrheas, and the stool osmotic gap is usually less than 50 mOsm and may even be negative.

Included in the initial evaluation of the stools in patients with protracted diarrhea should be testing for infectious agents, including routine bacterial pathogens, *Clostridium difficile* toxin, and ova and parasites. For patients with negative evaluations for infectious agents who are subsequently shown to have an underlying immunodeficiency, more aggressive evaluation for infectious causes, including electron microscopy of small intestinal mucosal biopsies, is indicated.

Extensive immunologic testing for immunodeficiency, analysis of serum specimens for anti-intestinal epithelial antibodies, or measurements of circulating VIP levels should probably be reserved until evaluation of a small intestinal mucosal biopsy has occurred. Small intestinal mucosal biopsy should be included in the diagnostic evaluation of all patients with protracted diarrhea and is usually the key diagnostic test for distinguishing between specific causes. The primary role of intestinal mucosal biopsy is to establish whether the villous structure and epithelial morphology are normal or abnormal and whether changes are associated with mucosal inflammation. In the setting of normal mucosal histology and the absence of inflammation, consideration should be given to primary transport defects, hormonally-mediated secretory processes, or the possibility of disease restricted to the colon as the cause for the protracted diarrhea. Significant mucosal inflammation should suggest protein-sensitive enteropathies, infections, immunodeficiency, or the possibility of autoimmune enteropathy. Abnormal villous morphology with little or no mucosal inflammation should lead to consideration of congenital microvillus atrophy or one of its variants.

In addition to routine hematoxylin and eosin staining of mucosal biopsies, additional studies may be useful for the evaluation of specific diagnostic entities. Abnormalities discovered by PAS staining and electron microscopy facilitate the diagnosis of congenital microvillus atrophy and tufting disease. Electron microscopy can also be useful for documenting the presence of intracellular pathogens such as *Microsporidia* in patients with underlying immunodeficiencies such as *human immunodeficiency virus infection*. Mucosal biopsy samples can also be assayed for disaccharidase levels when specific disaccharidase deficiencies are being considered as primary causes of diarrhea. At the time of small intestinal biopsy, collection of intestinal fluid may be useful for additional studies for infectious agents.

Colonoscopy and biopsy may also be a useful adjunct to small intestinal mucosal biopsy in selected patients. Epithelial abnormalities have been detected in the colon of patients with congenital microvillus atrophy before their detection in intestinal mucosal biopsies, as noted previously.[13] In addition, disparities that sometimes occur when patients with severe diarrhea have relatively mild inflammation on intestinal mucosal biopsy may at times be resolved by the demonstration of a more severe inflammatory process in the colon.

## TREATMENT

Treatment modalities for protracted diarrhea can be classified as general measures used to ensure appropriate nutritional status and to pharmacologically treat diarrheal processes and more specific therapies directed at specific causes identified after diagnostic evaluation (Table 23–2). In addition, there are several treatment approaches that may be applied to complicating pathophysiologic processes such as secondary bile salt malabsorption or bacterial overgrowth of the small intestine.

### Nutritional Therapy

The primary goal for the delivery of appropriate nutrition for patients with protracted diarrhea is to provide adequate calories and nutrients for normal growth and weight gain and to preferentially deliver these by the enteral route. The specific approach applied must be tailored to the individual clinical diagnosis. For transport defects such as congenital chloride diarrhea and hormone-secreting tumors, intestinal absorption should be intact and delivery of adequate nutrients should not be problematic. Glucose-galactose malabsorption can be treated with a glucose- and galactose-free diet, substituting fructose as the major carbohydrate, and similar approaches can be used as treatment for other primary and secondary disorders of carbohydrate malabsorption. Severe formula protein sensitivity usually requires the delivery of a formula with hydrolyzed protein or free amino acids.

**TABLE 23–2. Therapeutic Options for Protracted Diarrhea**

| |
|---|
| **Nutritional Therapy** |
| Carbohydrate-specific formulas and diets |
| Elemental formulas |
| Total parenteral nutrition |
| **Antibiotic Therapy** |
| Broad-spectrum oral antibiotics (neomycin, colistin) |
| Bowel cocktail (metronidazole, gentamycin, cholestyramine) |
| **Anti-inflammatory Therapy** |
| Corticosteroids |
| Antimetabolites (6-mercaptopurine, azathioprine) |
| Immunosuppressives (cyclosporin, FK506) |
| **Immunotherapy** |
| Intravenous immunoglobulin |
| Oral immunoglobulin |
| **Antidiarrheal Agents** |
| Cholestyramine |
| Bismuth subsalicylate |
| Loperamide |
| Octreotide |

For more severe enteropathies with generalized malabsorption, enteral formulations that are elemental in nature are often the preferred source of nutrients. In addition to containing protein hydrolysates or free amino acids, these formulas usually contain glucose polymers as the primary carbohydrate source. This allows minimization of the impact of osmotic diarrhea from carbohydrate malabsorption as a contributor to ongoing diarrhea and dehydration. These formulas can be delivered orally with formula advancement titrated based on the presence of diarrhea or chemical demonstration of ongoing carbohydrate malabsorption. Enteral formula also can be delivered as a continuous infusion via a nasogastric feeding tube, or via a nasojejunal feeding tube in the patient with recurrent vomiting, and may be better tolerated than oral, bolus-type feedings.[72] This approach has been shown to be very effective when compared with parenteral nutrition and is associated with faster resolution of diarrhea and reduced length of hospitalization for patients with protracted diarrhea.[8] A variation of this approach, using a semi-elemental formula with a higher percentage of total calories delivered as fat in the form of medium-chain triglycerides, has also been shown to be effective and to produce more rapid weight gain.[73]

For patients with significant fluid and electrolyte imbalance due to ongoing stool losses from a secretory process or severe malabsorption unresponsive to enteral therapy, total parenteral nutrition is the treatment of choice. When there is clearcut evidence of a severe secretory process or severe malabsorption early in the evaluation of a patient with protracted diarrhea, central venous access should be obtained and parenteral nutrition instituted early to begin nutritional restitution while attempts at introducing and advancing enteral feedings are progressing. Delay in institution of parenteral nutrition can be associated with life-threatening metabolic and infectious complications owing to the severity of ongoing malnutrition.

Careful monitoring of serum electrolytes, phosphorus, and magnesium should occur in the early stages of nutritional therapy to detect early evidence of *refeeding syndrome,* which can occur in severely malnourished patients with overzealous nutritional therapy.[74] When refeeding syndrome occurs, it may associated with arrhythmias and even sudden death. Patients at risk for refeeding syndrome can usually be identified by the presence of low serum levels of phosphorus, potassium, and/or magnesium before institution of nutritional therapy. It can be prevented by advancing total calorie administration slowly until electrolyte abnormalities have corrected.

### Treatment of Infection, Inflammation, and Immunodeficiency

Appropriate antibiotic therapy should be an obvious addition to the treatment regimen for patients with protracted diarrhea when a specific infectious pathogen has been diagnosed by routine microbiologic methods. In addition, antibiotic therapy aimed at the possible presence of significant pathogens that remain undiagnosed or at *bacterial overgrowth* of the small intestine has been used as adjunctive treatment. Bacterial overgrowth has been identified as a potentially important contributor to ongoing malabsorption in the malnourished patient with protracted diarrhea.[75, 76] Because of this phenomenon, as well as the possible contribution of undiagnosed pathogens to ongoing protracted diarrhea, the use of nonabsorbable, broad-spectrum antibiotics has received some attention as an adjunct to treatment in this setting. This has led some investigators to use a "bowel cocktail" of oral gentamycin, metronidazole, and cholestyramine.[77, 78] The cholestyramine is added to bind bile salts that may be malabsorbed as a result of either the primary enteropathic process or bacterial overgrowth. This approach has been shown to significantly reduce diarrhea and to lead to more rapid nutritional restitution associated with improved nitrogen balance and fat absorption.

Aggressive anti-inflammatory therapy has generally been reserved for patients with autoimmune enteropathy who have been treated with corticosteroids, antimetabolites, and more potent immunosuppressives. Isolated reports identify the attempted use of corticosteroids in patients with idiopathic protracted diarrhea with significant inflammation present on intestinal mucosal biopsy. However, there are no controlled studies demonstrating the value of this approach as a standard treatment.

Treatment for protracted diarrhea associated with underlying immunodeficiency is based on appropriate therapy for the immunodeficient state. Occasionally, a specific diagnosis for the underlying immunodeficiency is difficult to ascertain or is confused owing to the contribution of intestinal protein loss to low serum immunoglobulin levels and to anergy associated with malnutrition. Novel attempts for additional immunotherapy in these situations have been described. Repeated infusions of fresh-frozen plasma to reverse enterocolitis associated with immunodeficiency was described for two patients initially believed to have a primary underlying immunodeficiency disorder.[79] Oral immunoglobulin therapy has also been shown to reduce diarrhea and to improve serum immunoglobulin levels in children with immunodeficiency and diarrhea.[80]

## Pharmacologic Therapy for Diarrhea

The primary treatment for the infant with protracted diarrhea is based on minimizing stool losses caused by malabsorption through alteration of carbohydrate and other nutrient intake as noted previously. However, a number of patients have a significant secretory component contributing to their diarrhea that prevents discontinuation of parenteral fluid therapy or is associated with significant irritability and perianal irritant dermatitis. In these situations, the addition of an antidiarrheal agent such as loperamide or a bile-salt binding agent such as cholestyramine may be useful. For patients with significant ongoing fluid secretion, the use of octreotide, a synthetic analogue of somatostatin, may be warranted. Octreotide has been used effectively to treat secretory diarrhea caused by VIP-secreting tumors and has been evaluated in a limited series for patients with protracted diarrhea of infancy.[81] In that study, octreotide was of limited value for reducing diarrhea for patients with congenital microvillus atrophy and autoimmune enteropathy but was effective for one patient with idiopathic protracted diarrhea. Nevertheless, anecdotal reports of good or partial success with this agent in patients with protracted diarrhea suggest that additional studies of its potential efficacy are warranted.

## REFERENCES


1. Avery GB, Villavicencio O, Lilly JR, Randolph JG: Intractable diarrhea in early infancy. Pediatrics 1968;41:712.
2. Larcher VF, Shepherd R, Francis DEM, Harries JT: Protracted diarrhoea in infancy: analysis of 82 cases with particular reference to diagnosis and management. Arch Dis Child 1977;52:597.
3. Rossi TM, Lebenthal E, Nord KS, Fazili RR: Extent and duration of small intestinal mucosal injury in intractable diarrhea of infancy. Pediatrics 1980;66:730.
4. Candy DCA, Larcher VF, Cameron DJS, et al: Lethal familial protracted diarrhoea. Arch Dis Child 1981;56:15.
5. Cuenod B, Brousse N, Goulet O, et al: Classification of intractable diarrhea in infancy using clinical and immunohistological criteria. Gastroenterology 1990;99:1037.
6. Walker-Smith JA: Intractable diarrhoea in infancy: a continuing challenge for the pediatric gastroenterologist. Acta Pediatr Suppl 1994;395:6.
7. Goldgar CM, Vanderhoof JA: Lack of correlation of small bowel biopsy and clinical course of patients with intractable diarrhea of infancy. Gastroenterology 1986;90:527.
8. Orenstein SR: Enteral versus parenteral therapy for intractable diarrhea of infancy: a prospective, randomized trial. J Pediatr 1986;109:277.
9. Iyngkaran N, Robinson MJ, Sumithran E, et al: Cow's milk protein-sensitive enteropathy: an important factor in prolonging diarrhoea of acute infective enteritis in early infancy. Arch Dis Child 1978;53:150.
10. Vanderhoof JA, Murray ND, Antonson DL, Kaufman SS: Familial occurrence of protracted diarrhea of infancy. J Pediatr 1986;109:845.
11. Davidson GP, Cutz E, Hamilton JR, Gall DG: Familial enteropathy: a syndrome of protracted diarrhea from birth, failure to thrive, and hypoplastic villus atrophy. Gastroenterology 1978;75:783.
12. Phillips AD, Jenkins P, Raafat F, Walker-Smith JA: Congenital microvillous atrophy: specific diagnostic features. Arch Dis Child 1985;60:135.
13. Cutz E, Rhoads JM, Drumm B, et al: Microvillus inclusion disease: an inherited defect of brush-border assembly and differentiation. N Engl J Med 1989;320:646.
14. Phillips AD, Schmitz J: Familial microvillous atrophy: a clinicopathological survey of 23 cases. J Pediatr Gastroenterol Nutr 1992;14:380.
15. Nathavitharana KA, Green NJ, Raafat F, Booth IW: Siblings with microvillous inclusion disease. Arch Dis Child 1994;71:71.
16. Rhoads JM, Vogler RC, Lacey SR, et al: Microvillus inclusion disease: in vitro jejunal electrolyte transport. Gastroenterology 1991;100:811.
17. Oliva MM, Perman JA, Saavedra JM, et al: Successful intestinal transplantation for microvillus inclusion disease. Gastroenterology 1994;106:771.
18. Herzog D, Atkinson P, Grant D, et al: Combined bowel-liver transplantation in an infant with microvillous inclusion disease. J Pediatr Gastroenterol Nutr 1996;22:405.
19. Raafat F, Green NJ, Nathavitharana KA, Booth IW: Intestinal microvillous dystrophy: a variant of microvillous inclusion disease or a new entity? Hum Pathol 1994;25:1243.
20. Reifen RM, Cutz E, Griffiths A-M, et al: Tufting enteropathy: a newly recognized clinicopathological entity associated with refractory diarrhea in infants. J Pediatr Gastroenterol Nutr 1994;18:379.
21. Goulet O, Kedinger M, Brousse N, et al: Intractable diarrhea of infancy with epithelial basement membrane abnormalities. J Pediatr 1995;127:212.
22. Lindquist B, Meeuwisse GW: Chronic diarrhoea caused by monosaccharide malabsorption. Acta Paediatr 1962;51:674.
23. Evans L, Grasset E, Heyman M, et al: Congenital selective malabsorption of glucose and galactose. J Pediatr Gastroenterol Nutr 1985;4:878.

24. Turk E, Zabel B, Mundlos S, et al: Glucose/galactose malabsorption caused by a defect in Na+/glucose cotransporter. Nature 1991;350:354.
25. Martin MG, Turk E, Lostao MP, et al: Defects in Na+/glucose cotransporter (SGLT1) trafficking and function cause glucose-galactose malabsorption. Nat Genet 1996;12:216.
26. Holmberg C, Perheentupa J, Launiala K, Hallman N: Congenital chloride diarrhoea: clinical analysis of 21 Finnish patients. Arch Dis Child 1977;52:255.
27. Norio R, Perheentupa J, Launiala K, Hallman N: Congenital chloride diarrhea, an autosomal recessive disease: genetic study of 14 Finnish and 12 other families. Clin Genet 1971;2:182.
28. Holmberg C, Perheentupa J, Launiala K: Colonic electrolyte transport in health and in congenital chloride diarrhea. J Clin Invest 1975;56:302.
29. Holmberg C: Electrolyte economy and its hormonal regulation in congenital chloride diarrhea. Pediatr Res 1978;12:82.
30. Hoglund P, Haila S, Socha J, et al: Mutations of the down-regulated in adenoma (DRA) gene cause congenital chloride diarrhoea. Nat Genet 1996;14:316.
31. Holmberg C, Perheentupa J: Congenital Na+ diarrhea: a new type of secretory diarrhea. J Pediatr 1985;106:56.
32. Booth IW, Murer H, Stange G, et al: Defective jejunal brush-border Na+/H+ exchange: a cause of congenital secretory diarrhoea. Lancet 1985;1:1066.
33. Heubi JE, Balistreri WF, Partin JC, et al: Refractory infantile diarrhea due to primary bile acid malabsorption. J Pediatr 1979;94:546.
34. Heubi JE, Balistreri WF, Fondacaro JD, et al: Primary bile acid malabsorption: defective in vitro ileal active bile acid transport. Gastroenterology 1982;83:804.
35. Cormier-Daire V, Bonnefont J-P, Rustin P, et al: Mitochondrial DNA rearrangements with onset as chronic diarrhea with villous atrophy. J Pediatr 1994;124:63.
36. Mitchell CH, Sinatra FR, Crast FW, et al: Intractable watery diarrhea, ganglioneuroblastoma, and vasoactive intestinal peptide. J Pediatr 1976;89:593.
37. Hansen LP, Lund HT, Fahrenkrug J, Sogaard H: Vasoactive intestinal polypeptide (VIP)–producing ganglioneuroma in a child with chronic diarrhea. Acta Paediatr Scand 1980;69:419.
38. Scheibel E, Rechnitzer C, Fahrenkrug J, Hertz H: Vasoactive intestinal poypeptide (VIP) in children with neural crest tumors. Acta Paediatr Scand 1982;71:721.
39. Socha J, Dobrzanska A, Rowecka K, et al: Chronic diarrhea due to VIPoma in two children. J Pediatr Gastroenterol Nutr 1984;3:143.
40. Malik M, Connors R, Schwarz KB, O'Dorisio TM: Hormone-producing ganglioneuroblastoma simulating intestinal pseudoobstruction. J Pediatr 1990;116:406.
41. Blaser MJ, Reller LB: *Campylobacter* enteritis. N Engl J Med 1981;305:1444.
42. Marks MI, Pai CH, Lafleur L, et al: *Yersinia enterocolitica* gastroenteritis: a prospective study of clinical, bacteriologic, and epidemiologic features. J Pediatr 1980;96:26.
43. Cantey JR: *Escherichia coli* diarrhea. Gastroenterol Clin North Am 1993;22:609.
44. DuPont HL, Sullivan PS: Giardiasis: the clinical spectrum, diagnosis and therapy. Pediatr Infect Dis 1986;5:S131.
45. Macfarlane DE, Horner-Bryce J: Cryptosporidiosis in well-nourished and malnourished children. Acta Paediatr Scand 1987;76:474.
46. Halpin TC, Byrne WJ, Ament ME: Colitis, persistent diarrhea, and soy protein intolerance. J Pediatr 1977;91:404.
47. Powell GK: Milk- and soy-induced enterocolitis of infancy. J Pediatr 1978;93:553.
48. Odze RD, Wershil BK, Leichtner AM, Antonioli DA: Allergic colitis in infants. J Pediatr 1995;126:163.
49. Ament ME, Ochs HD, Davis SD: Structure and function of the gastrointestinal tract in primary immunodeficiency syndromes: a study of 39 patients. Medicine (Baltimore) 1973;52:227.
50. Saulsbury FT, Winkelstein JA, Yolken RH: Chronic rotavirus infection in immunodeficiency. J Pediatr 1980;97:61.
51. Perlmutter DH, Leichtner AM, Goldman H, Winter HS: Chronic diarrhea associated with hypogammaglobulinemia and enteropathy in infants and children. Dig Dis Sci 1985;30:1149.
52. Glassman M, Grill B, Gryboski J, Dwyer J: High incidence of hypogammaglobulinemia in infants with diarrhea. J Pediatr Gastroenterol Nutr 1983;2:465.
53. Stephan JL, Vlekova V, LeDeist F, et al: Severe combined immunodeficiency: a retrospective single-center study of clinical presentation and outcome in 117 patients. J Pediatr 1993;123:564.
54. Sullivan KE, Mullen CA, Blaese RM, Winkelstein JA: A multiinstitutional survey of the Wiskott-Aldrich syndrome. J Pediatr 1994;125:876.
55. Berthet F, LeDeist F, Duliege AM, et al: Clinical consequences and treatment of primary immunodeficiency syndromes characterized by functional T and B lymphocyte anomalies (combined immune deficiency). Pediatrics 1994;93:265.
56. Falloon J, Eddy J, Wiener L, Pizzo PA: Human immunodeficiency virus infection in children. J Pediatr 1989;114:1.
57. Glover MT, Atherton DJ, Levinsky RJ: Syndrome of erythroderma, failure to thrive, and diarrhea in infancy: a manifestation of immunodeficiency. Pediatrics 1988;81:66.
58. Jacobs JC, Miller ME: Fatal familial Leiner's disease: a deficiency of the opsonic activity of serum. Pediatrics 1972;49:255.
59. Leiner C: Erythroderma desquamativa (universal dermatitis of children at the breast). Br J Dis Child 1908;5:244.
60. Girault D, Goulet O, LeDeist F, et al: Intractable infant diarrhea associated with phenotypic abnormalities and immunodeficiency. J Pediatr 1994;125:36.
61. Stankler L, Lloyd D, Pollitt RJ, et al: Unexplained diarrhoea and failure to thrive in 2 siblings with unusual facies and abnormal scalp hair shafts: a new syndrome. Arch Dis Child 1982;57:212.
62. McCarthy DM, Katz SI, Gazze L, et al: Selective IgA deficiency associated with total villous atrophy of the small intestine and an organ-specific anti-epithelial cell antibody. J Immunol 1978;120:932.
63. Mirakian R, Richardson A, Milla PJ, et al: Protracted diarrhoea of infancy: evidence in support of an autoimmune variant. Br Med J 1986;293:1132.
64. Seidman EG, Lacaille F, Russo P, et al: Successful treatment of autoimmune enteropathy with cyclosporine. J Pediatr 1990;117:929.
65. Colletti RB, Guillot AP, Rosen S, et al: Autoimmune enteropathy and nephropathy with circulating anti-epithelial cell antibodies. J Pediatr 1991;118:858.
66. Jenkins HR, Jewkes F, Vujanic GM: Systemic vasculitis complicating infantile autoimmune enteropathy. Arch Dis Child 1994;71:534.
67. Moore L, Xu Xiaoning, Davidson G, et al: Autoimmune enteropathy with anti-goblet cell antibodies. Hum Pathol 1995;26:1162.
68. Lachaux A, Bouvier R, Cozzani E, et al: Familial autoimmune enteropathy with circulating anti-bullous pemphigoid antibodies and chronic autoimmune hepatitis. J Pediatr 1994;125:858.
69. Martin-Villa JM, Regueiro JR, de Juan D, et al: T-lymphocyte dysfunctions occurring together with apical gut epithelial cell autoantibodies. Gastroenterology 1991;101:390.
70. Savilahti E, Launiala K, Kuitunen P: Congenital lactase deficiency: a clinical study on 16 patients. Arch Dis Child 1983;58:246.
71. Fleisher D, Ament ME: Diarrhea, red diapers, and child abuse. Clin Pediatr 1977;17:820.
72. Parker P, Stroop S, Greene H: A controlled comparison of continuous versus intermittent feeding in the treatment of infants with intestinal disease. J Pediatr 1981;99:360.
73. Jirapinyo P, Young C, Nualanong S, et al: High-fat semielemental diet in the treatment of protracted diarrhea of infancy. Pediatrics 1990;86:902.
74. Solomon SM, Kirby DF: The refeeding syndrome: a review. JPEN J Parenter Enteral Nutr 1990;14:90.
75. Challacombe DN, Richardson JM, Rowe B, Anderson CM: Bacterial microflora of the upper gastrointestinal tract in infants with protracted diarrhoea. Arch Dis Child 1974;49:270.
76. deBoissieu D, Chaussain M, Badoual J, et al: Small-bowel bacterial overgrowth in children with chronic diarrhea, abdominal pain, or both. J Pediatr 1996;128:203.
77. Bowie MD, Mann MD, Hill ID: The bowel cocktail. Pediatrics 1981;67:920.
78. Hill ID, Mann MD, Househam KC, Bowie MD: Use of oral gentamicin, metronidazole, and cholestyramine in the treatment of severe persistent diarrhea in infants. Pediatrics 1986;77:477.
79. Cannon RA, Blum PM, Ament ME, et al: Reversal of enterocolitis-associated combined immunodeficiency by plasma therapy. J Pediatr 1982;101:711.
80. Melamed I, Griffiths AM, Roifman CM: Benefit of oral immune globulin therapy in patients with immunodeficiency and chronic diarrhea. J Pediatr 1991;119:486.
81. Bisset WM, Jenkins H, Booth I, et al: The effect of somatostatin on small intestinal transport in intractable diarrhoea of infancy. J Pediatr Gastroenterol Nutr 1993;17:169.

# Chapter 24

# Protein-Losing Enteropathy

Wallace A. Gleason, Jr.

"Idiopathic catabolic hypoproteinemia" was described by Gordon in 1959.[1] He found that loss of serum proteins into the intestine caused by a process that he called "exudative enteropathy" was responsible. Although this term implies an active, exudative process localized to the small and large intestine, more recent reports have described enteric protein loss into the esophagus, as a result of reflux esophagitis, and into the stomach, as a result of hypertrophic gastropathy, as well as transudative loss of proteins into the gastrointestinal system. A broader term proposed by Waldmann,[2, 3] *gastrointestinal protein loss*, seems more precise, reflecting a wider distribution of lesions and the transudative character of the protein loss in many of the processes described. Nonetheless, the term most commonly used to describe this situation is *protein-losing enteropathy.*

## PATHOPHYSIOLOGY

The gastrointestinal tract may be responsible for as much as 10% of total body protein catabolism. Normally, less than 2% of circulating albumin is lost per day. Gastrointestinal protein catabolism, in which circulating proteins are imported into enterocytes and degraded within lysosomes, is distinct from protein-losing enteropathy, in which proteins are spilled into the gastrointestinal lumen. Under normal circumstances, the cell membranes of enterocytes, joined at apical tight junctions, form a highly impermeable barrier. Compromise of this barrier, allowing serum proteins to enter the gastrointestinal lumen, results from mucosal erosion or ulceration; increased pressure in the lymphatic vessels draining the intestine that is transmitted distally to the lacteals, the thin-walled lymphatic channels within the core of the intestinal villi, resulting in rupture and loss of the constituents of lymph (fluid, proteins, lymphocytes); or surface cell loss or damage with disruption of the mucosal barrier.[4]

Virtually any serum protein may be lost during this process, but because albumin is responsible for most of the oncotic pressure holding fluid within the vascular space, consequences of its loss are more dramatic. Edema, resulting from decreased plasma oncotic pressure and subsequent leakage of fluid out of capillaries, is usually the most prominent sign of protein-losing enteropathy. Loss of immunoglobulins and lymphocytes may result in recurrent infections.

The degree of hypoalbuminemia depends on at least three variable processes: (1) the rate of albumin loss, (2) the increase in the rate of synthesis of albumin in the liver, and (3) the decrease in the nonenteric catabolism of albumin in response to lower serum levels.

## DIAGNOSIS

Protein-losing enteropathy is not a specific disease but a pathophysiologic process.[5] Successful treatment requires precise diagnosis of the underlying disease with its extensive differential diagnosis.[6] This discussion is limited to those disorders that have been associated with protein-losing enteropathy in children.

Symptoms of the underlying illness may include diarrhea, abdominal pain, and allergic phenomena and may be elicited in the medical history. Edema, usually positional, is a frequent complaint and finding. In infants, edema frequently manifests itself as facial and periorbital swelling. Older children, because they spend more time erect, are more likely to develop ankle and leg edema. Asymmetric lymphedema of a limb may be a clue to underlying lymphatic dysplasia associated with primary intestinal lymphangiectasia.

The goal of initial laboratory investigations is to ascertain and explain hypoalbuminemia, taking into account the lower normal values for serum albumin in infants and children (Table 24–1) and other possible causes, such as renal or hepatic disease or malnutrition.

Anthropometric data, including weight for age, height (length in infants) for age, and weight for height, are readily determined and can be compared with normative data on National Center for Health Statistics growth charts. These are reliable data that can exclude malnutrition of a degree required to produce hypoalbuminemia. Routine findings on urinalysis rule out proteinuria, and normal levels of transaminases exclude liver dysfunction. A convenient and reliable estimate of hepatic synthetic function can be obtained with measurement of the prothrombin time. In the setting of possible intestinal disease, vitamin K deficiency due to intes-

**TABLE 24–1. Normal Values for Serum Proteins by Age**

| AGE | TOTAL PROTEIN (g/dL) | ALBUMIN (g/dL) |
|---|---|---|
| Cord | 4.8–8.0 | 2.2–4.0 |
| Newborn | 4.4–7.6 | 3.2–4.8 |
| 1 day–1 mo | 4.4–7.6 | 2.5–5.5 |
| 1–3 mo | 3.6–7.4 | 2.1–4.8 |
| 4–6 mo | 4.2–7.4 | 2.8–5.0 |
| 7–12 mo | 5.1–7.5 | 3.2–5.7 |
| 13–24 mo | 3.7–7.5 | 1.9–5.0 |
| 25–36 mo | 5.3–8.1 | 3.3–5.8 |
| 3–5 yr | 4.9–8.1 | 2.9–5.8 |
| 6–8 yr | 6.0–7.9 | 3.3–5.0 |
| 9–11 yr | 6.0–7.9 | 3.2–5.0 |
| 12–16 yr | 6.0–7.9 | 3.2–5.1 |
| Adult | 6.0–8.0 | 3.1–5.4 |

From Barone MA, ed: The Harriet Lane Handbook: A Manual for Pediatric House Officers, 14th ed. St. Louis, Mosby-Year Book, 1996, p 122.

tinal malabsorption could prolong the prothrombin time, but it should correct promptly with a dose of parenteral vitamin K.

## DEMONSTRATION OF PROTEIN-LOSING ENTEROPATHY

Demonstration of protein-losing enteropathy requires the detection in stool of a circulating macromolecule that is not absorbed, secreted, or degraded in the gastrointestinal tract. The easier it is to measure the marker, the more useful the test will be. Most such techniques involve identification of markers that have been injected or secreted into the blood compartment.

The original demonstration of exudative enteropathy used iodine 131–labeled polyvinyl pyrrolidone.[1] Because the rate of protein loss may be affected by the size, shape, and charge of the labeled macromolecule, $^{131}$I-albumin was substituted as a more physiologic marker. Although the technique for iodination of albumin was straightforward and iodinated albumin was easy to detect, thyroid uptake of the radioactive iodine and luminal digestion of the radiolabeled albumin with subsequent absorption of the iodine confounded interpretation.[7] Most of these problems were solved with the introduction of chromium 51–labeled albumin,[2] which became the most widely used radiolabeled macromolecule for the study of protein-losing enteropathy.[3]

Radiolabeled macromolecules impose hazards and inconveniences, limiting their attractiveness for use in children. Exposure to ionizing radiation prohibits their use in pediatric clinical research. Six to 10 days of hospitalization are required, as is a 48- to 72-hour stool collection with meticulous avoidance of urine contamination—a difficult task in infants and children. These inconveniences, and the emergence of better techniques, have made interest in radiolabeled macromolecules largely historical.

Extensive clinical experience using sodium pertechnetate technetium 99m–labled human serum albumin for scintigraphy has revealed that less than 0.5% of an intravenous dose normally appears in stool or urine within 24 hours.[8] Based on this observation, scintigraphic imaging has been used to demonstrate gastrointestinal protein loss.[9–11] Unlike other techniques, scintigraphic imaging localizes the site of gastrointestinal protein loss, but it is not yet clear how that information is useful. Exposure to radiation limits its utility in pediatric medicine. Although this technique may be helpful in documenting protein-losing enteropathy, experience is too limited to allow such a judgment at present.

## FECAL EXCRETION OF ALPHA$_1$-ANTITRYPSIN

In 1977, Crossley and Elliot showed that children with gastrointestinal protein loss documented by $^{51}$Cr-labeled albumin had levels of fecal alpha$_1$-antitrypsin (FA1-AT), measured by radial immunodiffusion, that were 10-fold higher than levels from adults or from children with no evidence of protein-losing enteropathy.[12] FA1-AT was independent of the serum concentration of alpha$_1$-antitrypsin (A1-AT) and of fecal water content. Random samples varied no more than twofold, validating the use of random samples as a screening test for protein-losing enteropathy.

FA1-AT fulfills the criteria as a marker for protein-losing enteropathy and has the following advantages:

1. It is a serum protein.
2. It is not present in the diet; therefore fecal levels reflect only protein entering the intestine from the intravascular space.
3. Its molecular weight of 50,000 is similar to that of albumin.
4. As a protease inhibitor, it resists intraluminal proteolysis and is excreted without degradation in the stool.
5. Urine contamination of the stool specimen does not invalidate the result—a feature particularly helpful in pediatric patients.

The original description of this technique emphasized its simplicity.[12] Further studies in which FA1-AT clearance (FA1-AT times the weight of the stool excreted in 24 hours, divided by A1-AT) was determined provided no convincing evidence that the increase in precision to be gained by that method justifies the inconvenience of prolonged stool collection. However, these studies provided further validation of the use of random samples. For example, there is a linear correlation between the clearances of radiolabeled serum albumin and FA1-AT,[13–15] and there is little day-to-day variation in the excretion of FA1-AT during several consecutive days of stool collection.[14, 16, 17] FA1-AT is excreted as two forms: alone and complexed with enzyme.[18] As a result, radial immunodiffusion slightly underestimates the total amount of FA1-AT present and may account for the slight differences noted between the clearances of FA1-AT and radiolabeled serum albumin.[4, 13]

Levels of FA1-AT in stool are stable. Ninety-three percent of the FA1-AT remained after 72 hours of incubation at 37°C, allowing transport of specimens before assay. A1-AT is undetectable in gastric secretions, and exogenous A1-AT is destroyed in vitro after 1 hour of incubation at 37°C in gastric juice but not in duodenal juice. The reliability of FA1-AT in detecting esophageal or gastric protein loss is therefore questionable. Because meconium contains higher levels of A1-AT than stool,[19] this technique is not recommended in neonates younger than 1 week of age. Premature

**TABLE 24–2. Protein-Losing Enteropathy in Infants and Children**

**Low Serum Albumin**

- ***Infectious Causes***
  - *Giardia lamblia*
  - Hypertrophic gastropathy
  - Cytomegalovirus
  - *Helicobacter pylori*
  - *Strongyloides stercoralis*
- ***Noninfectious Causes***
  - Enterocyte heparan suphate deficiency
  - Crohn's disease
  - Graft-versus-host disease
  - Henoch-Schönlein purpura
  - Intestinal lymphangiectasia
    - Primary
    - Secondary
      - Multifocal lymphatic dysplasia
      - Heart disease
      - Noonan syndrome
      - Nephrotic syndrome
      - Arsenic poisoning
  - Juvenile rheumatoid arthritis
  - Multiple polyposis
  - Peptic (reflux) esophagitis
  - Systemic lupus erythematosus
  - Systemic phenobarbital hypersensitivity

**Normal Serum Albumin**

- ***Infectious Causes***
  - *Clostridium dificile*
  - *Clostridium perfringens*
  - Measles
  - Rotavirus
  - Salmonellosis
  - Neonatal necrotizing enterocolitis
- ***Noninfectious Causes***
  - Allergic gastroenteropathy
  - Cow's milk feeding (? enteropathy)
  - Gluten-sensitive enteropathy
  - Colonic malakoplakia
  - Malnutrition

infants, however, have normal levels of FA1-AT.[20] Although it might be expected that patients with low levels of circulating A1-AT would have falsely low levels of FA1-AT, increased levels of FA1-AT have been reported in patients with homozygous $P_iZZ$ A1-AT deficiency, the most common phenotype in children with A1-AT deficiency. Although the mechanism of excretion of A1-AT in this condition is unclear and is not related to the presence of liver disease, it is not thought to contribute to the low circulating levels of A1-AT.[21]

With the wide use of this simple, accurate test, subclinical protein-losing enteropathy has been found in many disorders in which it was unexpected (Table 24–2). This discovery has broadened the scope and expanded the differential diagnosis of protein-losing enteropathy to include disorders other than those causing hypoalbuminemia, in which levels of FA1-AT are no more than two to four times normal. In one series, 24% of the children had normal serum albumin values.[22] Although this may reflect the insensitivity of serum albumin as a test for protein-losing enteropathy, it also questions the clinical importance of gastrointestinal protein loss of this extent, particularly in view of the demonstration that A1-AT is synthesized by Paneth cells and a line of colonic epithelial cells, so that low levels of FA1-AT may result from shedding of enteric epithelial cells rather than from protein-losing enteropathy.[23]

In view of the distinction between small increases in FA1-AT associated with normal levels of serum albumin and more substantial increases associated with hypoalbuminemia, the differential diagnosis of protein-losing enteropathy is presented according to its association with hypoalbuminemia in Table 24–2, and pathophysiologically in Table 24–3 and in the following discussion.

## SPECIFIC ENTITIES

### Infections

Protein-losing enteropathy is seen in a number of gastrointestinal infections characterized by mucosal erosion or ulceration (see Table 24–3). Forty percent of children with acute diarrheal illnesses have increased levels of FA1-AT, up to

**TABLE 24–3. Pathophysiologic Classification of Protein-Losing Enteropathy in Infants and Children**

**Mucosal Erosion or Ulceration**

- ***Infectious Causes***
  - *Clostridium dificile*
  - *Clostridium perfringens*
  - Colonic malakoplakia
  - Cytomegalovirus
  - *Giardia lamblia*
  - *Helicobacter pylori*
  - Hypertrophic gastropathy (Ménétrier's disease)
  - Measles
  - Rotavirus
  - Salmonellosis
  - Strongyloides stercoralis
- ***Noninfectious Causes***
  - Allergic gastroenteropathy
  - Anastomotic ulceration/ischemia
  - Atopic dermatitis
  - Burns
  - Cow's milk feeding (?enteropathy)
  - Gluten-sensitive enteropathy
  - Graft-versus-host disease
  - Henoch-Schönlein purpura
  - Inflammatory bowel disease
  - Juvenile rheumatoid arthritis
  - Malnutrition
  - Multiple polyposis
  - Neonatal necrotizing enterocolitis
  - Peptic (reflux) esophagitis
  - Systemic lupus erythematosus
  - Systemic phenobarbital hypersensitivity

**Lymphatic Obstruction**

- Intestinal lymphangiectasia
  - Primary
  - Secondary
    - Arsenic poisoning
    - Familial
    - Heart disease
    - Inflammatory
    - Nephrotic syndrome
    - Noonan syndrome

four times the upper limit of normal, and increases commonly accompany inflammatory conditions such as salmonellosis and parasitic infections.[24–27] Increased FA1-AT occurs in enterocolitis caused by *Clostridium dificile*[28] or *Clostridium perfringens*[29] and serves to differentiate active enterocolitis from asymptomatic colonization with *C. dificile*.[30] FA1-AT is transiently increased in rotavirus diarrhea,[24–27] although studies on this point are not unanimous.[26] Increased FA1-AT excretion rarely persists beyond 5 days in these infections, an important point in the commonly encountered clinical problem of distinguishing between an acute, self-limited infection and a chronic enteric disorder.[27] These diagnoses are best approached by microbiologic studies identifying these agents or their enterotoxins in stool specimens. Cytomegalovirus and *Helicobacter pylori* have both been implicated in the pathogenesis of hypertrophic gastropathy (see later discussion).

The observation that measles commonly precipitates kwashiorkor in children in developing nations led to studies in the mid-1970s demonstrating protein-losing enteropathy in malnourished African children with measles infection.[31, 32] Protein-losing enteropathy is more likely to complicate enteric infection in children within 2 weeks of measles infection than in those with a remote history or no history of measles.[33] A more recent study found that malnourished Transkeian children in South Africa with marasmus had increased excretion of FA1-AT, but those with kwashiorkor did not.[34]

The clinical importance of the relatively small gastrointestinal loss of protein in these children is uncertain. Gastrointestinal protein loss in enteric infections may be important in the development of malnutrition in children with diarrhea,[24–27] but children with marasmus or marasmic kwashiorkor without enteric infection[35, 36] also have increased gastrointestinal protein loss, suggesting a self-perpetuating abnormality of intestinal function resulting from mucosal edema regardless of the inciting factor.

In distinction to the conditions just described, giardiasis[37–39] and strongyloidiasis[40] can cause gastrointestinal protein loss in sufficient quantity to result in hypoalbuminemia and edema. Both conditions are diagnosed by identifying the parasites or their cysts or ova in stool or, more dependably, by duodenal intubation or a string test, such as the Enterotest (see Chapter 29).

## Noninfectious Inflammatory Disorders

In 1967, Waldmann and colleagues described six children presenting with edema, growth retardation, extreme hypoalbuminemia (1.5–2.4 g/dL), hypogammaglobulinemia, anemia, eosinophilia, and other manifestations of allergy, such as asthma, eczema, and allergic rhinitis.[41] Although most of these patients were infants, one was 14 years old. Normal absorption of D-xylose and the absence of steatorrhea excluded gluten-sensitive enteropathy, cystic fibrosis, and intestinal lymphangiectasia. All had protein-losing enteropathy that responded to an elimination diet or corticosteroids. These patients were found to be allergic to cow's milk, based on the reversal of gastrointestinal protein loss when cow's milk was excluded from the diet and the development of vomiting, diarrhea, and exacerbation of gastrointestinal protein loss when it was reintroduced, leading to the designation "allergic gastroenteropathy." Similar, steroid-responsive protein-losing enteropathy has been encountered in patients with Henoch-Schönlein purpura.[42]

Although protein-losing enteropathy was indirectly implicated as the mechanism of hypoalbuminemia in a child with atopic dermatitis,[43] a more formal assessment found no greater increase in the incidence of gastrointestinal protein loss in children with atopic dermatitis than in normal children.[44] Anastomotic ulceration after distal small bowel resection can result in protein-losing enteropathy with or without hypoalbuminemia.[45, 46] A similar picture can be seen as a repercussion of intestinal ischemia.[47] In both of these entities, recurrent iron deficiency anemia due to chronic gastrointestinal bleeding, visible or occult, is more prominent than protein-losing enteropathy.

Twenty-five percent of patients undergoing bone marrow transplantation develop graft-versus-host disease involving the intestine, a disorder causing hypoproteinemia that results, in part, from protein-losing enteropathy.[48] This disorder is more common in children older than 13 years of age, and it is heralded by the development of diarrhea more than 20 days after transplantation.[49] Important in the differential diagnosis for patients with abdominal symptoms and hypoproteinemia after bone marrow transplantation are typhlitis (neutropenic colitis, see Chapter 46) and veno-occlusive disease of the liver (see Chapter 52), which may contribute to the symptoms of diarrhea and ascites, respectively. A similar clinical syndrome of protein-losing enteropathy with fever, rash, alopecia, icterus, myositis, and nephritis has been ascribed to phenobarbital hypersensitivity.[50]

Inflammatory bowel disease is an important cause of protein-losing enteropathy. In general, the degree of hypoalbuminemia and protein loss is greater in patients with Crohn's disease than in those with ulcerative colitis, and greater in those with diffuse small bowel disease than in those with limited small bowel disease or colonic disease.[22, 50, 51] Classically, 50% to 60% of children with Crohn's disease have at least mild hypoalbuminemia.[52–54] An even greater proportion, 70% to 80%, have protein-losing enteropathy demonstrable with radiolabeled albumin even though serum albumin levels are normal. In these children with normal serum albumin, there is little correlation between measures of severity or extent of disease and the amount of gastrointestinal protein loss.[55]

In young women, systemic lupus erythematosus can manifest with hypoalbuminemia and edema caused by gastrointestinal protein loss,[56] and this presentation has also been recorded in children.[57, 58]

A curious syndrome of gastroesophageal reflux, protein-losing enteropathy, and finger clubbing has been reported in three patients. The mechanism of protein loss was presumably exudation from the inflamed esophageal mucosa, since it was accompanied by bleeding and completely resolved after successful surgical treatment by fundoplication.[59]

Children with untreated celiac disease have FA1-AT levels that are roughly three times normal at the time of diagnosis. Levels progressively decrease with the duration of dietary gluten elimination.[16, 60] Increased levels of FA1-AT are also seen in neonatal necrotizing enterocolitis.[61] Although correlation between hemoglobin in the stools and levels of FA1-AT might intuitively be expected in inflammatory intestinal disorders such as these, none has been found in several studies,[22, 54, 62, 63] probably because the mass ratio of hemoglobin to A1-AT in plasma is roughly 160:1 at normal levels of both proteins.[18]

Infants fed cow's milk–based formulas have higher levels of FA1-AT than do exclusively breast-fed infants or infants fed breast milk supplemented with cow's milk–based formulas.[62] This finding adds to other evidence (see Chapter 27) that a subtle enteropathy is caused by cow's milk in some infants. As with the other inflammatory disorders discussed, there is no correlation between levels of A1-AT and hemoglobin in the stool in cow's milk–fed infants.

Three infants have been reported in whom severe protein-losing enteropathy was associated with complete absence of heparan sulfate in enterocytes, as determined by histochemistry.[64] These infants, who presented with massive enteric protein loss and secretory diarrhea in the first weeks of life and required total parenteral nutrition and repeated albumin infusions, had intestinal biopsies that were repeatedly normal. The distribution of the vascular and lamina propria glycosaminoglycans was normal. This report suggests another mechanism of intestinal protein loss. Retention of proteins in vascular or tissue compartments is dependent on molecular size and charge. The loss or reduction of endothelial anions greatly increases albumin and water leakage from biologic membranes by negating the effect of charge. This mechanism has been implicated in urinary protein loss in congenital and minimal-change nephrotic syndromes,[65] and loss of sulfated glycosaminoglycans from the epithelium and basement membrane of inflamed intestine has been demonstrated and suggested as the mechanism of intestinal protein loss in inflammatory enteropathy.[66, 67]

Juvenile colonic polyps are usually solitary, histologically benign lesions with no premalignant potential that cause painless hematochezia or, less commonly, intussusception. A syndrome of multiple juvenile polyps with chronic gastrointestinal bleeding and protein-losing enteropathy can lead to inanition. Unlike solitary juvenile colonic polyps, which are seen most commonly in preschool-age children, these lesions appear in infancy.[68–70] Macrocephaly, in one case caused by intracranial cysts, has been reported in several cases.[71, 72] The mechanism of gastrointestinal protein loss is unknown, but inflammation has been incriminated in the pathogenesis of both solitary and juvenile polyps. The prognosis is poor because of the hundreds of polyps throughout the stomach, small bowel, and colon. Malakoplakia of the colon, typically associated with abdominal tuberculosis, produces a similar clinical picture, with chronic gastrointestinal bleeding and gastrointestinal protein loss as a result of polypoid lesions throughout the colon. These lesions have characteristic histiocytic infiltration and Michaelis-Gutmann bodies, intracellular and extracellular inclusion bodies, when examined histologically.[73]

FA1-AT levels are increased in burned children. Claimed to be caused by an alteration in intestinal mucosal permeability demonstrable in burned patients, FA1-AT correlates with the surface area of the burn.[74] The levels in even the most severely burned children are only slightly increased, and the clinical significance of this degree of protein loss is limited.

Because fecal excretion of A1-AT tends to decrease as inflammatory gastrointestinal disorders resolve, FA1-AT may be a convenient, noninvasive way to monitor the activity of these disorders in infants and children.

## Lymphatic Obstruction

The term *intestinal lymphangiectasia* describes a group of disorders in which dilatation of the lacteals—the fine, thin-walled lymphatic channels extending up into the small bowel villi—results from obstruction of the flow of lymph through the thoracic duct and into the superior vena cava.[75] Fat intake, digestion, and absorption lead to further engorgement and rupture of lacteals, resulting in steatorrhea and drainage of lymph into the intestinal lumen. The resulting losses of proteins, lymphocytes, and immunoglobulins ultimately results in hypoalbuminemia, lymphopenia, and hypogammaglobulinemia, respectively. These findings can represent important clues to the diagnosis, and the presence of all three is virtually pathognomonic.

Intestinal lymphangiectasia may occur as a primary disorder or secondary to other causes of lymphatic obstruction. Familial forms with various patterns of inheritance have been described,[76, 77] including the Hennekam syndrome, an autosomal recessive syndrome of gastrointestinal protein loss with facial anomalies and mild mental retardation.[78, 79] Fleisher and associates described a patient with intestinal lymphangiectasia thought to be caused by an inflammatory disorder because of its response to corticosteroid therapy.[80] Lymphatic obstruction may be limited to the intestine, or it may coexist with multifocal lymphatic dysplasia, as in Noonan's syndrome.[81, 82] Intestinal lymphangiectasia has been described as a manifestation of arsenic poisoning.[83]

Cardiac disorders and surgical procedures resulting in transmission of elevated pressure from the right atrium into the superior vena cava and thoracic duct, including clinically silent constrictive pericarditis,[84] have been complicated by the development of intestinal lymphangiectasia.[85–89] Several reports describe successful treatment of this problem by percutaneous fenestration of the conduit,[90–92] heart transplantation,[93] or redesign of the operation.[94] Resolution of protein-losing enteropathy has also been reported with corticosteroid therapy.[95, 96] The response of these patients, some of whom were gravely ill with severe diarrhea, anasarca, and inanition, only after 15 days of intravenous corticosteroids attests that patience and persistence are important in managing this difficult clinical situation. The corticosteroid responsiveness of some forms of secondary intestinal lymphangiectasia may result from influences other than the anti-inflammatory effects of these agents. Postulated mechanisms include stabilization of lymphatic and capillary membranes and a decrease in the volume of lymphoid tissue. A serendipitous observation made by a parent of an adolescent with protein-losing enteropathy complicating the Fontan operation and cerebral venous thrombosis led to a promising new therapy and, perhaps, the beginning of a better understanding of this problem. Donnelly and coworkers interpreted the parent's observation that whenever heparin was substituted for warfarin, the patient's diarrhea and peripheral edema improved.[97] Further refinement of this observation led to early clinical experience with three patients, which showed that low-dose heparin therapy, in the range of 5,000 U/$m^2$/day and well below the anticoagulant dose of heparin, decreases intestinal protein loss and normalizes serum albumin. These authors speculated that exogenous heparin, a lipophilic proteoglycan with strong ionic charge known to be internalized by endothelial cells, makes up for a deficiency in endogenous proteoglycans, similar to the mechanism highlighted by the cases of enterocyte heparan sulfate deficiency discussed previously.

Gastrointestinal protein loss occurs in the acute phase of idiopathic nephrotic syndrome. Its cause is unknown, but histologic features of intestinal lymphangiectasia have been found in intestinal biopsies of some children with nephrotic syndrome.[98] Perhaps the known variability of the extent and severity of the intestinal lesion in patients with intestinal lymphangiectasia explains why it can be demonstrated only in some nephrotic patients.[99]

## Hypertrophic Gastropathy (Ménétrier's Disease)

A syndrome of gastrointestinal protein loss and giant hypertrophy of the gastric rugae has been recognized to have radiologic, endoscopic, and histologic features suggestive of what is called Ménétrier's disease in adults.[100, 101] Because there are distinctions between the adult disease and its pediatric imitator, notably its transience and benign prognosis, hypertrophic gastropathy is probably a better term.[102, 103] These children present with abdominal pain and vomiting and with the gradual development of edema and ascites. The cause is unknown, but an allergic cause has been proposed because of its occurrence in several children with a history of atopy.[104] Several cases have been associated with cytomegalovirus infection,[105, 106] and the finding of localization of cytomegalovirus and transforming growth factor-alpha in four children similar to that seen in adults with Ménétrier's disease seems to support a role for this agent.[107] Increased width of tight junctions between gastric epithelial cells has been proposed as being responsible for gastrointestinal protein loss.[108] Recovery of *H. pylori* from children with hypertrophic gastropathy[109, 110] and the observation of severe gastrointestinal protein loss in children with *H. pylori* gastritis[111] have engendered the speculation that this organism may also be responsible for transient hypertrophic gastropathy in children. All reports emphasize that transient hypertrophic gastropathy is benign and self-limited, requiring no specific therapy. These distinctions between the pediatric syndrome and true Ménétrier's disease, as it is encountered in adults, together with the association of hypertrophic gastropathy with infectious agents, serves as the rationale for its classification in the category of infections in Table 24–2.

## TREATMENT

Two reports, each of single adult patients, indicate that octreotide, a synthetic analogue of somatostatin, is effective in treating protein-losing enteropathy caused, in one case, by intestinal lymphangiectasia[112] and in the other by Ménétrier's disease.[113] In general, however, the treatment of protein-losing enteropathy is the treatment of the underlying disease. The reader is therefore referred to the sections of this text in which the specific diagnostic entities are discussed.

## REFERENCES


1. Gordon RS: Exudative enteropathy: abnormal permeability of the gastrointestinal tract demonstrable with labeled polyvinyl pyrrolidone. Lancet 1959;1:325–332.
2. Waldmann TA: Gastrointestinal protein loss demonstrated by $^{51}$Cr-labeled albumin. Lancet 1961;2:121–123.
3. Waldmann TA: Gastrointestinal protein loss in pediatrics. In James AE, Wagner HN, Cooke RE (eds): Pediatric Nuclear Medicine. Philadelphia, WB Saunders, 1974, pp 442–445.
4. Perrault J, Markowitz H: Protein-losing gastroenteropathy and the intestinal clearance of serum alpha$_1$-antitrypsin. Mayo Clin Proc 1984;59:278–279.
5. Parfitt AM: Familial neonatal hypoproteinemia with exudative enteropathy and intestinal lymphangiectasis. Arch Dis Child 1966;41:54–62.
6. Colon AR, Sandberg DH: Protein-losing enteropathy in children. South Med J 1973;66:641–644.
7. Freeman T, Gordon AH: Measurement of albumin leak into the gastrointestinal tract using $^{131}$I-albumin and ion exchange resins by mouth. Gut 1964;5:155–157.
8. McAfee JG, Stern GF, Fueger MS, et al: $^{99m}$Tc-labeled serum albumin for scintillation scanning of the placenta. J Nucl Med 1964;5:936–946.
9. Digvi CR, Lisann NM, Yeh SDJ, et al: $^{99m}$Technetium-albumin scintigraphy in the diagnosis of protein-losing enteropathy. J Nucl Med 1986;27:1710–1712.
10. Lan JA, Chervu LR, Marans Z, et al: Protein-losing enteropathy detected by $^{99m}$Tc-labeled human serum albumin abdominal scintigraphy. J Pediatr Gastroenterol Nutr 1988;7:872–876.
11. Kashiwagi T, Fukui H, Jyoku T, et al: Imaging diagnosis of protein-losing enteropathy by $^{99m}$Tc-labeled serum albumin. Kaku Igaku 1990;27:1361–1368.
12. Crossley JR, Elliot RB: Simple method for diagnosing protein-losing enteropathies. Lancet 1977;1:428–429.
13. Florent C, L'Hirondel C, Desmazures C, et al: Intestinal clearance of alpha-antitrypsin: a sensitive method for the detection of protein-losing enteropathy. Gastroenterology 1981;81:777–780.
14. Hill RE, Hercz A, Corey ML, et al: Fecal clearance of alpha$_1$-antitrypsin: a reliable measure of enteric protein loss in children. J Pediatr 1981;99:416–418.
15. Karbach U, Ewe K, Bodenstein H: Alpha$_1$-antitrypsin, a reliable endogenous marker for intestinal protein loss and its application in patients with Crohn's disease. Gut 1983;24:718–723.
16. Dinari G, Rosenbach Y, Zahavi I, et al: Random fecal alpha$_1$-antitrypsin excretion in children with intestinal disorders. Am J Dis Child 1984;138:971–973.
17. Maggazzu G, Jacono G, DiPasquale G, et al: Reliability and usefulness of random fecal alpha$_1$-antitrypsin concentration: further simplification of the method. J Pediatr Gastroenterol Nutr 1985;4:402–407.
18. Buffone GJ, Shulman RJ: Characterization and evaluation of immunochemical methods for the measurement of fecal alpha$_1$-antitrypsin. Am J Clin Pathol 1985;83:326–330.
19. Ryley HC, Lynne N, Brogan TD, et al: Plasma proteins in meconium from normal infants and from babies with cystic fibrosis. Arch Dis Child 1974;49:901–904.
20. Sivan Y, Dinari G, Weilunsky E, et al: Protein conservation by the immature intestine. Biol Neonate 1985;47:32–35.
21. Grill BB, Tinghitella T, Hillemeier AC, et al: Increased intestinal clearance of alpha$_1$-antitrypsin in patients with alpha$_1$-antitrypsin deficiency. J Pediatr Gastroenterol Nutr 1983;2:95–98.
22. Thomas DW, Sinatra FR, Merritt RJ: Random fecal alpha$_1$-antitrypsin concentration in children with gastrointestinal disease. Gastroenterology 1981;80:776–782.
23. Molmenti EP, Perlmutter DH, Rubin DC: Cell-specific expression of alpha 1-antitrypsin in human intestinal epithelium. J Clin Invest 1993;92:2022–2034.
24. Maki M, Harmionen A, Vesikari T, et al: Fecal alpha$_1$-antitrypsin excretion in acute diarrhea. Arch Dis Child 1982;57:154–156.
25. Fontana M, Zuin G, Galli L, et al: Fecal alpha$_1$-antitrypsin excretion in acute diarrhea: relationship with causative pathogens. Helv Pediatr Acta 1988;43:211–218.
26. Hoffman HD, Hanekom C: Random fecal alpha$_1$-antitrypsin in children with acute diarrhea. J Trop Pediatr 1987;33:299–301.
27. Zuin G, Fontana M, Nicoli S, et al: Persistence of protein loss in

acute diarrhea: a follow-up study by fecal alpha$_1$-antitrypsin measurement. Acta Pediatr Scand 1991;80:961–993.
28. Rybolt AH, Bennett RG, Laughon BE, et al: Protein-losing enteropathy with *Clostridium dificile* infection. Lancet 1989;1:1353–1355.
29. Ehringhaus C, Dominick H-C, Schuller M: Protein-losing enteropathy associated with *Clostridium perfringens*. Lancet 1989;2:268–269.
30. Dansinger ML, Johnson S, Jansen PC, et al: Protein-losing enteropathy is associated with *Clostridium dificile* diarrhea but not with asymptomatic colonization: a prospective case-control study. Clin Infect Dis 1996;22:932–937.
31. Dossetor JFB, Whittle HC: Protein-losing enteropathy and malabsorption in acute measles enteritis. Br Med J 1975;2:592–593.
32. Axton JHM: Measles: a protein-losing enteropathy. Br Med J 1975;2:79–80.
33. Sarker SA, Wahed MA, Rahaman MM, et al: Persistent protein-losing enteropathy in post measles diarrhea. Arch Dis Child 1986;61:739–743.
34. Iputo JE: Protein-losing enteropathy in Transkeian children with morbid protein-energy malnutrition. South Afr Med J 1993;83:588–589.
35. Madina EH, Soliman AT, Morsi MR: Protein-losing enteropathy in the different forms of protein-energy malnutrition. J Trop Pediatr 1987;33:254–256.
36. Lunn PG, Whitehead RG, Coward WA: Two pathways to kwashiorkor? Trans R Soc Trop Med Hyg 1979;73:438–444.
37. Sherman P, Leibman WM: Apparent protein-losing enteropathy associated with giardiasis. Am J Dis Child 1980;134:893–894.
38. Sutton DL, Kamath KR: Giardiasis with protein-losing enteropathy. J Pediatr Gastroenterol Nutr 1985;4:56–59.
39. Korman SH, Bar-Oz B, Mandelberg A, et al: Giardiasis with protein-losing enteropathy: diagnosis by fecal alpha$_1$-antitrypsin determination. J Pediatr Gastroenterol Nutr 1990;10:249–252.
40. Sullivan PB, Lunn PG, Northrup-Clewes CA, et al: Parasitic infection of the gut and protein-losing enteropathy. J Pediatr Gastroenterol Nutr 1992;15:404–407.
41. Waldmann TA, Wochner RD, Laster L, et al: Allergic gastroenteropathy: a cause of excessive protein loss. N Engl J Med 1967;276:761–769.
42. Reif S, Jain A, Santiago J, et al: Protein-losing enteropathy as a manifestation of Henoch-Schonlein purpura. Acta Pediatr Scand 1991;80:482–485.
43. Jenkins HR, Walker-Smith JA, Atherton DJ: Protein-losing enteropathy in atopic dermatitis. Pediatr Dermatol 1986;3:125–129.
44. Pike MG, Riches P, Atherton DJ: Fecal alpha$_1$-antitrypsin and gastrointestinal permeability to oligosaccharides in atopic dermatitis. Pediatr Dermatol 1989;6:10–12.
45. Parashar K, Kyawhla S, Booth IW, et al: Ileocolonic ulceration: a long-term complication following ileocolic anastomosis. J Pediatr Surg 1988;23:226–228.
46. Couper RTL, Durie PR, Stafford SE, et al: Late gastrointestinal bleeding and protein loss after distal small bowel resection in infancy. J Pedaitr Gastroenterol Nutr 1989;9:454–460.
47. Thompson JF, Levy J, Stolar CJH, et al: Protein-losing enteropathy in prolonged post-ischemic ileitis. J Pediatr Gastroenterol Nutr 1986;5:504–507.
48. Weisdorf SA, Salati LM, Longsdorf JA, et al: Graft-versus-host disease of the intestine: a protein-losing enteropathy characterized by fecal alpha$_1$-antitrypsin. Gastroenterology 1983;85:1076–1081.
49. Papadopoulou A, Lloyd DR, Williams MD, et al: Gastrointestinal and nutritional sequelae of bone marrow transplantation. Arch Dis Child 1996;75:208–1357.
50. Knutsen AP, Shah M, Schwarz, KB, et al: Graft versus host-like illness in a child with phenobarbital hypersensitivity. Pediatrics 1986;78:581–584.
51. Grill BB, Hillemeier AC, Gryboski JD: Fecal alpha$_1$-antitrypsin clearance in patients with inflammatory bowel disease. J Pediatr Gastroenterol Nutr 1984;3:56–61.
52. Thomas DW, Sinatra FR, Merritt RJ: Fecal alpha$_1$-antitrypsin excretion in young people with Crohn's disease. J Pediatr Gastroenterol Nutr 1983;2:491–496.
53. Roy CC, Silverman A, Alagille D: Pediatric Clinical Gastroenterology, 4th ed. St. Louis, CV Mosby, 1995, p 474.
54. Beeken WL, Busch HJ, Sylvester DL: Intestinal protein loss in Crohn's disease. Gastroenterology 1972;62:207–215.
55. Herzog D, DeLvin E, Seidman E: Fecal alpha$_1$-antitrypsin: a marker of intestinal versus systemic inflammation in pediatric Crohn's disease. Inflammatory Bowel Dis 1996;2:236–243.
56. Perednia DA, Curosh NA: Lupus-associated protein-losing enteropathy. Arch Intern Med 1990;150:1806–1810.
57. Tsukahara M, Matsuo K, Kojima H: Protein-losing enteropathy in a boy with systemic lupus erythematosus. J Pediatr 1980;97:778–779.
58. Molina JF, Brown RF, Gedalia A, et al: 1996. Protein-losing enteropathy as the initial manifestation of childhood systemic lupus erythematosus. J Rheumatol 23:1269–1271.
59. Herbst JJ, Johnson DG, Oliveros MA: Gastroesophageal reflux and protein-losing enteropathy and finger clubbing. Am J Dis Child 1976;130:1256–1258.
60. Catassi C, Cardinali E, D'Angelo G, et al: Reliability of random fecal alpha-antitrypsin determination on nondried stools. J Pediatr 1986;109:500–502.
61. Shulman RJ, Buffone G, Wise L: Enteric protein loss in necrotizing enterocolitis as measured by fecal alpha$_1$-antitrypsin excretion. J Pediatr 1985;107:287–289.
62. Woodruff C, Fabacher D, Latham C: Fecal alpha$_1$-antitrypsin and infant feeding. J Pediatr 1985;106:228–232.
63. Morrow RJ, Lawson N, Hussaini SH, et al: The usefulness of fecal hemoglobin, albumin and alpha$_1$-antitrypsin in the detection of gastrointestinal bleeding. Ann Clin Biochem 1990;27:208–212.
64. Murch SH, Winyard PJ, Koletzko S, et al: Congenital enterocyte heparan sulphate deficiency with massive albumin loss, secretory diarrhea, and malnutrition. Lancet 1996;347:1299–1301.
65. Vernier RL, Klein DJ, Sisson SP, et al: Heparan sulphate–rich anionic sites in the human glomerular basement membrane: decreased concentration in congenital nephrotic syndrome. N Engl J Med 1983;309:1001–1009.
66. Murch SH, MacDonald TT, Walker-Smith JA, et al: Disruption of sulphated glycosaminoglycans in intestinal inflammation. Lancet 1993:341:711–14.
67. Murch SH: Sulphation of proteoglycans and intestinal function. J Gastroenterol Hepatol 1995;10:210–212.
68. Arbeter AM, Courtney RA, Gaynor MF: Diffuse gastrointestinal polyposis associated with chronic blood loss, hypoproteinemia and anasarca in an infant. J Pediatr 1970;76:609–611.
69. Soper RT, Kent TH: Fatal juvenile polyposis in infancy. Surgery 1971;69:692–698.
70. Gourley GR, Odell GB, Selkurt J, et al: Juvenile polyps associated with protein-losing enteropathy. Dig Dis Sci 1982;27:941–945.
71. Schwartz AM, McCauley RKG: Juvenile gastrointestinal polyposis. Radiology 1976;121:441–444.
72. Scharf GM, Becker JHR, Laage NJ: Juvenile gastrointestinal polyposis or the infantile Cronkite-Canada syndrome. J Pediatr Surg 1986;21:953–954.
73. Satti MB, Abu-Mehla A, Taha OMA, et al: Colonic malakoplakia and abdominal tuberculosis in a child: report of a case with review of the literature. Dis Colon Rectum 1985;28:353–357.
74. Matoth I, Granot E, Gorenstein A, et al: Gastrointestinal protein loss in children recovering from burns. J Pediatr Surg 1991;26:1175–1178.
75. Waldmann TA, Steinfeld JL, Dutcher TF, et al: The role of the gastrointestinal system in idiopathic hypoproteinemia. Gastroenterology 1961;41:197–207.
76. Bronspiegel N, Zelnick N, Rabinowitz H, et al: Aplasia cutis congenita and intestinal lymphangiectasia: an unusual association. Am J Dis Child 1985;139:509–513.
77. Mucke J, Hoepffner W, Scheerschmidt G, et al: Early onset lymphedema, recessive form: a new form of genetic lymphedema syndrome. Eur J Pediatr 1986;145:195–198.
78. Hennekam RCM, Geerdink RA, Hamel BCJ, et al: Autosomal recessive intestinal lymphangiectasia and lymphedema with facial anomalies and mental retardation. Am J Med Genet 1989;34:593–600.
79. Yasunaga M, Yamanaka C, Mayumi M, et al: Protein-losing gastroenteropathy with facial anomaly and growth retardation: a mild case of Hennekam syndrome. Am J Med Genet 1993;45:477–480.
80. Fleisher TA, Strober W, Muchmore AV, et al: Corticosteroid responsive intestinal lymphangiectasia secondary to an inflammatory process. N Engl J Med 1979;300:605–606.
81. Vallet HL, Holtzapple PG, Eberlein WR, et al: Noonan syndrome with intestinal lymphangiectasis: a metabolic and anatomic study. J Pediatr 1972;80:269–274.
82. Herzog DB, Logan R, Kooistra JB: The Noonan syndrome with intestinal lymphangiectasia. J Pediatr 1976;88:270–272.
83. Kobayashi A, Ohbe Y: Protein-losing enteropathy associated with arsenic poisoning. Am J Dis Child 1972;121:515–517.

84. Vesin P, Cattan D: Constrictive pericarditis with protein-losing enteropathy: role of the lymphatic system. In Dirke G, Norberg R, Plantin L (eds): Physiology and Pathophysiology of Plasma Protein Metabolism. London, Pergamon Press, 1968, pp 115–162.
85. Sondheimer JM, Hamilton JR: Intestinal function in infants with severe congenital heart disease. J Pediatr 1978;92:572–578.
86. Gleason WA, Roodman ST, Laks H: Protein-losing enteropathy and intestinal lymphangiectasia after superior vena cava-right pulmonary artery (Glenn) shunt. J Thorac Cardiovasc Surg 1979;77:606–609.
87. Hess J, Kruizinga K, Bijleveld CMA, et al: Protein-losing enteropathy after Fontan operation. J Thorac Cardiovasc Surg 1984;88:606–609.
88. Kirk CR, Gibbs JL, Wilkinson JL, et al: Protein-losing enteropathy caused by baffle obstruction after Mustard's operation. Br Heart J 1988;59:69–72.
89. Feldt RH, Driscoll DJ, Offord KP, et al: Protein-losing enteropathy after the Fontan operation. J Thorac Cardiovasc Surg 1996;112:672–680.
90. Warnes CA, Feldt RH, Hagler DJ: Protein-losing enteropathy after the Fontan operation: successful treatment by percutaneous fenestration of the atrial septum. Mayo Clin Proc 1996;71:378–379.
91. Jacobs ML, Rychick J, Bynum CJ, et al: Protein-losing enteropathy after Fontan operation: resolution after baffle fenestration. Ann Thorac Surg 1996;61:206–208.
92. Mertens L, Dumoulin M, Gewillig M: Effect of percutaneous fenestration of the atrial septum on protein-losing enteropathy after the Fontan operation. Br Heart J 1994;72:591–592.
93. Sierra C, Calleja F, Picazo B, et al: Protein-losing enteropathy secondary to Fontan procedure resolved after cardiac transplantation. J Pediatr Gastroenterol Nutr 1997;24:229–230.
94. Kreutzer J, Keane JF, Lock JE, et al: Conversion of modified Fontan procedure to lateral atrial tunnel cavopulmonary anastomosis. J Thorac Cardiovasc Surg 1996;111:1169–1188.
95. Rothman A, Snyder J: Protein-losing enteropathy following the Fontan operation: resolution with prednisone therapy. Am Heart J 1991;121:618–619.
96. Rychik J, Piccoli DA, Barber G: Usefulness of corticosteroid therapy for protein-losing enteropathy after the Fontan procedure. Am J Cardiol 1991;68:819–821.
97. Donnelly JP, Rosenthal A, Castle VP, et al: Reversal of protein-losing enteropathy with heparin therapy in three patients with univentricular hearts and Fontan palliation. J Pediatr 1997;130:474–478.
98. Salasar de Sousa J, Guerreiro O, Cunha A, et al: Association of nephrotic syndrome with intestinal lymphangiectasia. Arch Dis Child 1968;43:245–248.
99. Vardy PA, Lebenthal E, Schwachman H: Intestinal lymphangiectasia: a reappraisal. Pediatrics 1975;55:842–851.
100. Sandberg DH: Hypertrophic gastropathy (Ménétrier's disease) in childhood. J Pediatr 1971;78:866–868.
101. Tokatli A, Ozsoylu S: Ménétrier disease in a child. J Pediatr Gastroenterol Nutr 1991;12;404–406.
102. Lachman RS, Martin DJ, Vawter GF: Thick gastric folds in childhood. Am J Radiol 1971;112:83–92.
103. Pesce F, Barbino A, Dufour C, et al: Hypertrophic gastropathy with transient sessile polyps. J Pediatr Gastroenterol Nutr 1992;14:323–326.
104. Marks MP, Lanza MV, Kahlstrom EJ, et al: Pediatric hypertrophic gastropathy. Am Radiol 1986;147:1031–1034.
105. Stillman AE, Sieber O, Manthei U, et al: Transient protein-losing enteropathy and enlarged gastric rugae in childhood. Am J Dis Child 1981;135:29–33.
106. Leonidas JC, Beatty EC, Wenner HA: Ménétrier's disease and cytomegalovirus in childhood. Am J Dis Child 1973;126:806–808.
107. Sferra TJ, Pawel BR, Qualman SJ, et al: Ménétrier's disease of childhood: role of cytomegalovirus and transforming growth factor alpha. J Pediatr 1996;128:213–219.
108. Oderda G, Cinti S, Cangiotti AM, et al: Increased tight junction width in two children with Ménétrier's disease. J Pediatr Gastroenterol Nutr 1990;11:123–127.
109. Hill ID, Sinclair-Smith C, Lastovica AJ, et al: Transient protein-losing enteropathy associated with acute gastritis and *Campylobacter pylori*. Arch Dis Child 1987;62:1215–1219.
110. *Campylobacter pylori* and protein-losing enteropathy in children (editorial). Lancet 1988;1:865–866.
111. Cohen HA, Shapiro RP, Frydman M, et al: Childhood protein-losing enteropathy associated with *Helicobacter pylori* infection. J Pediatr Gastroenterol Nutr 1991;13:201–203.
112. Bac DJ, Van Hagen PM, Postema PTE, et al: Octreotide for protein-losing enteropathy with intestinal lymphangiectasia. Lancet 1995;345:1639.
113. Yeaton P, Frierson HF Jr: Octreotide reduces enteral protein losses in Ménétrier's disease. Am J Gastroenterol 1993;88:95–98.

# Chapter 25

# Celiac Disease

*Riccardo Troncone and Salvatore Auricchio*

## DEFINITION

Celiac disease (CD), also called *gluten-sensitive enteropathy,* is a permanent intestinal intolerance to dietary wheat gliadin and related proteins that produces mucosal lesions in genetically susceptible individuals.

## HISTORICAL BACKGROUND

CD was first accurately described by Samuel Gee in 1888, but it was not until the early 1950s that Dicke in Holland established the role of wheat and rye flour in the pathogenesis of the disease and identified the protein known as *gluten* as the harmful factor in those cereals.[1] A major contribution to the understanding of the disease came from the development of methods for peroral biopsy of the small intestinal mucosa, which allowed definition of the mucosal lesion,[2] and from the definition of diagnostic criteria published in 1969 by the European Society of Paediatric Gastroenterology and Nutrition (ESPGAN)[3] (see section on diagnosis).

## CEREAL PROTEINS AND OTHER ENVIRONMENTAL FACTORS

### Cereal Proteins

The cereals that are toxic for patients with CD are wheat, rye, and barley; rice and maize are nontoxic and are usually used as wheat substitutes in the diet of patients with CD. The toxicity of oats is still controversial. It has recently been shown that the use of oats as part of a gluten-free diet had no unfavorable effects on adult patients in remission and did not prevent mucosal healing in patients with newly diagnosed disease.[4, 5] Nevertheless, the finding that avenin seems to be able to activate mucosal cell–mediated immunity in in vitro cultured celiac biopsies and in in vivo challenged rectal mucosa (see section on pathogenesis)[6, 7], and the fear that small amounts of gliadin could contaminate oats, suggests caution before the inclusion of oats is advocated in the diet of celiac patients. Cereal grains belong to the grass family (Gramineae). Grains considered toxic for celiac patients (rye, barley, and to a lesser extent, oats) bear a close taxonomic relationship to wheat, whereas nontoxic grains (rice and maize) are taxonomically dissimilar[8] (Fig. 25–1). Wheat seed endosperm contains heterogeneous protein classes differentiated according to their extractability and solubility in different solvents into albumins, globulins, gliadins, and glutenins. The wheat toxicity results from the gliadin protein fraction,[9] and the toxicity of cereals other than wheat is most likely associated with prolamin fractions equivalent to gliadins in the grain of these other species.[10] Gliadins are single polypeptide chains ranging in molecular weight from 30,000 to 75,000 daltons. They have a low charge and a remarkably high glutamine and proline content. They have been classified according to their electrophoretic mobilities into groups designated α, β, γ, and ω. More recently they have been classified on the basis of their N terminal amino acid sequences into α, γ, and ω types. A-gliadin is one of the major α-gliadin components that is known to activate CD; its primary amino acid sequence has been determined.[11] The amino acid sequence(s) responsible for the disease have not been fully elucidated. From in vitro organ culture systems 31–43 and 44–45 sequences of the A-gliadin molecule seem to be immunogenic.[12] Even if useful, there is no doubt that in vitro methodology must be paralleled by in vivo challenge studies. In fact, histologic changes have been shown to occur in the celiac intestinal mucosa after challenge with 200 mg of a synthetic peptide encompassing the 31–49 sequence of A-gliadin[13]; subsequently, the sequences 31–43 and 44–55 have also been found to induce changes when instilled in the jejunum in vivo.[14] Studies are in progress in several laboratories investigating the binding of peptides to the CD-associated HLA-DQ 2 molecule.[15]

### Other Environmental Factors

The relevance of environmental factors other than gluten in CD is suggested by the significant changes in the incidence of the disease by time, and place, and by the reported discordance of about 30% of monozygotic twins. Feeding practices seem to be relevant; the protective effect of breast feeding has been well documented in case-control studies.[16] More recently, Scandinavian studies[17] have pointed out that the type and the amount of cereals introduced in infants' diets have profound effects on the clinical features and the actual incidence of the disease.

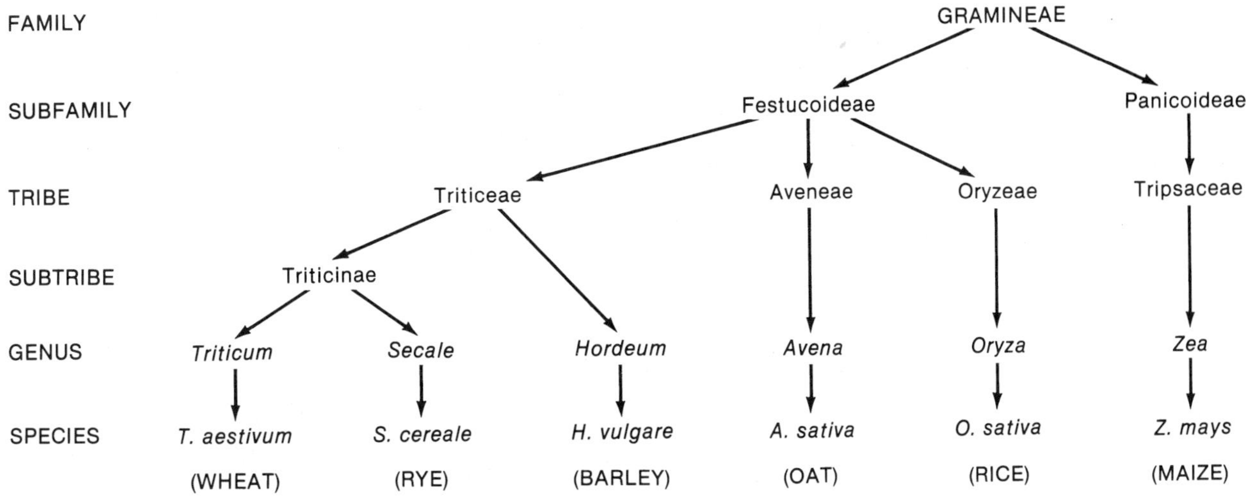


**FIGURE 25–1.** Taxonomic relationships of major cereal grains. (From Kasarda DD, Qualset CO, Mecham DK, et al: A test of toxicity of bread made from wheat lacking alpha-gliadins coded for by the 6A chromosome. In McNicholl B, McCarthy CF, Fottrell PF [eds]: Perspectives in Celiac Disease. Lancaster, UK, MTP Press, 1978, p 55, with permission.)

Among environmental factors that could play a possible role in CD, infective factors must also be considered. Adenovirus serotype 12 is of particular interest because one of its proteins (E1b) shows significant amino acid sequence homology with an antigenically active gluten peptide.[18] Viral infection and subsequent exposure to gliadin could trigger the development of the enteropathy as result of immunologic cross-reactivity, but experimental evidence is far from conclusive.

## GENETICS OF CELIAC DISEASE

### Family Studies

Susceptibility to CD is determined to a significant extent by genetic factors. That is suggested by the occurrence of multiple cases in families, the prevalence of CD found among first-degree relatives being approximately 10%.[19] Moreover, as many as 75% of monozygotic twins have been found to be concordant with the disease.[20] The concordance rate among HLA-identical siblings is about 30%, indicating that a great part of the genetic susceptibility maps to the HLA region on chromosome 6.

### Genetic Markers

The strongest association of CD is with the HLA class II D region markers, class I and class III region gene associations being secondary to linkage disequilibrium. More recently, convergent evidence from different populations has suggested that the primary association of CD is with the DQ α/β heterodimer encoded by the *DQA1*0501* and the *DQB1*0201* genes, located either in *cis* (in DR3 DQ2-positive subjects) or in *trans* (in DR5 DQ7/DR7 DQ2-heterozygous individuals)[21] (Fig. 25–2). Such a DQ molecule has been found to be present in 95% or more of celiac patients compared with 20% to 30% of controls. The data available on DQ2-negative celiac patients indicate that they almost invariably express the HLA alleles DR4 DQw8.[22] A gene dosage effect has been suggested, because subjects carrying a double dose of *DQB1*0201* have been found to have a greater risk of developing CD.[23] The most likely mechanism to explain the association with HLA class II genes is that the DQ molecule binds a peptide fragment of an antigen involved in the pathogenesis of CD to present it to T cells.

Other non-HLA genes could confer susceptibility to CD. Considering the relevance of the immune response in the pathogenesis of the disease, candidate genes are those influencing the T cell response. Among those, there are T cell receptor (TCR) genes, genes involved in processing or transport of peptides within the cell, and genes controlling the synthesis of cytokines or cytokine receptor. In this regard, a rarer allele of tumor necrosis factor (TNF)-α (promoter region polymorphism) is associated with CD.[24] More data on the identification of CD-associated genes are expected to come from the whole genome screening currently being performed in several laboratories analyzing affected sibling pairs.

## EPIDEMIOLOGY

The reported prevalence of symptomatic CD is 1 in 1000 live births, with a range from 1 in 250 (observed in Sweden) to 1 in 4000 (observed in Denmark).[25] The prevalence in women appears to be greater than in men. The reported incidence of CD is higher in Europe than in the United States, even in populations with similar genetic background. Asymptomatic or silent cases of CD have been identified by screening programs in at-risk groups (e.g., first-degree relatives or patients affected by diseases known to be associated with CD) or even in healthy people. Among blood donors, the prevalence of asymptomatic CD has been found to be as high as 1 in 266.[26] Catassi and associates[27] determined the prevalence of subclinical or silent CD among

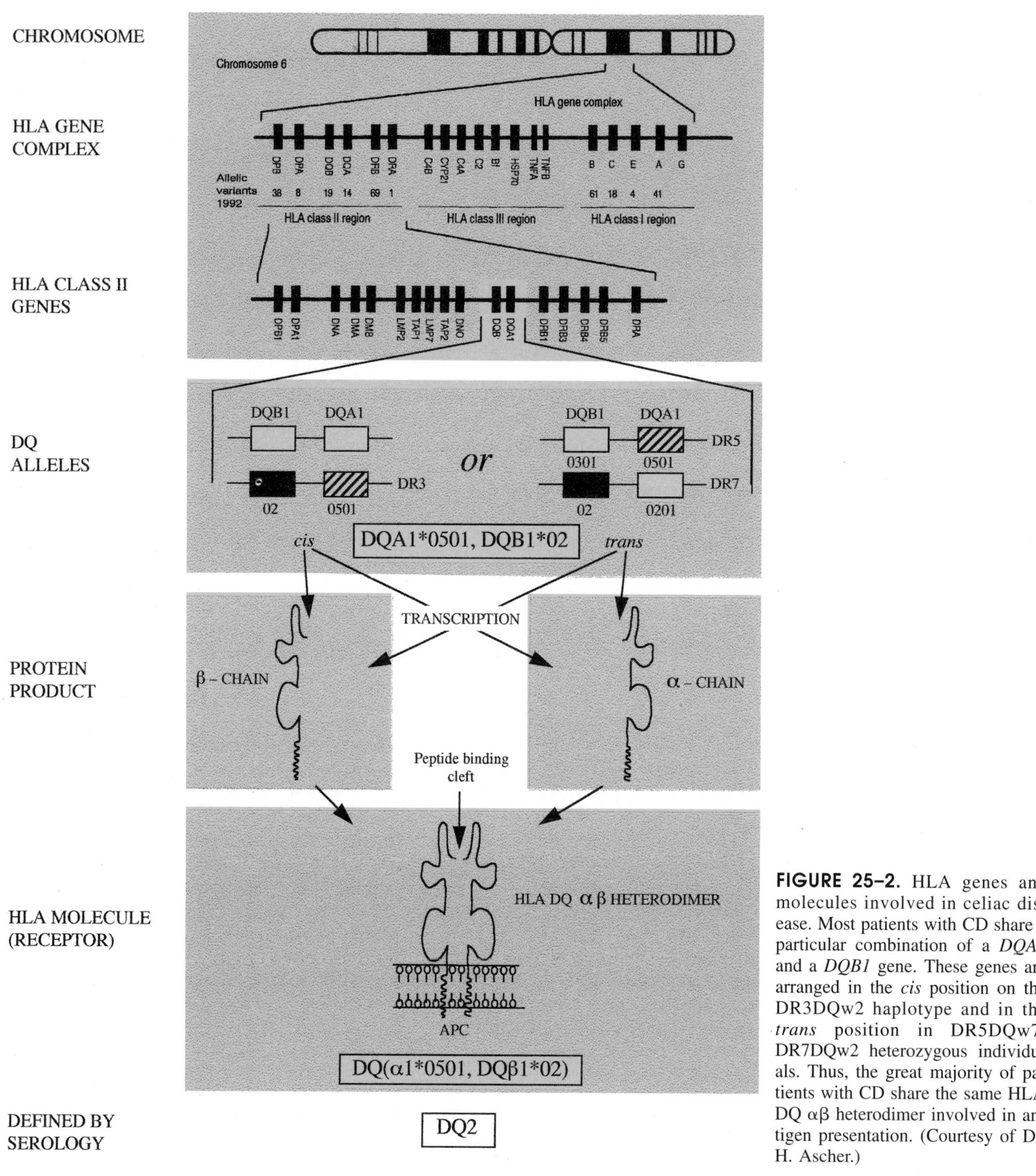


**FIGURE 25–2.** HLA genes and molecules involved in celiac disease. Most patients with CD share a particular combination of a *DQA1* and a *DQB1* gene. These genes are arranged in the *cis* position on the DR3DQw2 haplotype and in the *trans* position in DR5DQw7/DR7DQw2 heterozygous individuals. Thus, the great majority of patients with CD share the same HLA DQ αβ heterodimer involved in antigen presentation. (Courtesy of Dr. H. Ascher.)

asymptomatic school students in Italy and found it to be 3.28 in 1000. Not and colleagues[28] reported positive antiendomysial antibodies in 8 of 2000 healthy blood donors in the United States. If the presumed diagnosis of CD in these subjects is confirmed, then the prevalence of CD in the United States is comparable to that in Europe.[28]

Significant changes in prevalence have been noted not only by place but also by time. Some of these variations may be consequence of environmental factors other than dietary gluten. Changes in infant feeding practices, such as prolonged breast feeding, lower antigenicity of the formulas used, and later introduction of gluten into the diet all have been considered to explain the reported decline in the incidence of CD. Nevertheless, it is now becoming clear that in the countries where a decreasing incidence of CD has been noted, the disease is not really disappearing but only changing in clinical presentation. In Finland, CD is rarely diagnosed in children younger than the age of 5 years, presenting in the majority of cases in school-age children and adolescents.[29]

## PATHOGENESIS

It is now generally accepted that CD is an immunologically mediated small intestinal enteropathy. The mucosal lesion shows features suggesting both humoral- and cell-mediated immunologic overstimulation. Analogies with in vivo and in vitro models in which delayed-type hypersensitivity has been induced support the hypothesis that a key role in the induction of the mucosal damage is played by cell-mediated mechanisms. Flattening of the small intestinal mucosa occurs in vivo during the evolution of intestinal graft-versus-host disease or the rejection of small bowel transplants.[30] The parallelism between such models and the celiac mucosa where a similar sequence of events triggered by gliadin ultimately leads to mucosal atrophy suggests a common immunopathogenic mechanism. Most favor the hypothesis that the activation of lamina propria T cells by class II HLA-restricted antigen-presenting cells is one of the first events driven by gliadin.[31] Antigen recognition leads to up-regulation of interleukin-2 (IL-2) receptor expression and production of cytokines. In the untreated celiac mucosa a significant increase in the percentage of mononuclear cells expressing the IL-2 receptor (CD25+ cells) has been noted.[32]

Intercellular adhesion molecule type 1 (ICAM-1), which is necessary for T cell adherence at sites of inflammation, is also up-regulated.[33] Data have been recently obtained from gliadin-reactive CD4+, CD25+ T cell clones from celiac biopsies in vitro challenged with gliadin, which were found to secrete interferon-$\gamma$ at very high levels, and often TNF-$\alpha$, as well.[34] Some T cell clones also secreted IL-4, IL-5, and IL-6, suggesting that more studies are needed to map the role of different cytokines in the pathogenesis of mucosal damage.

The other important feature of celiac mucosa is the infiltration of the epithelium by lymphocytes. More than 90% of intraepithelial lymphocytes (IELs) express CD8 and less than 10% express CD4. The normal mucosal T IELs may express either the $\alpha/\beta$ (90% of cells) or the $\gamma/\delta$ form (10% of cells) of the TCR. In the celiac mucosa the percentage of TCR $\gamma/\delta$+ IELs is increased both in treated and untreated patients,[35] but their role remains elusive.

Untreated CD also presents a condition of enhanced humoral immunity. In the untreated celiac mucosa, there is a significant increase in the number of IgA-secreting plasma cells, with high frequency of J chain expression.[36] This observation agrees with the increased generation of secretory IgA observed in organ cultures of untreated celiac mucosa.[37] Altogether, these findings, along with the marked increase of mucosal IgM production and the cytokine-induced epithelial secretory component overexpression, reflect a condition of enhanced secretory immunity. Particularly intriguing is the gliadin-triggered production of autoantibodies directed to noncollagenous proteins of the extracellular matrix (antireticulin or antiendomysial antibodies).[38] The autoantigen(s) remain to be identified, but transglutaminase is one of the putative candidates.[39] It is still unclear if these autoantibodies, whose diagnostic relevance is discussed later in this chapter, have a role in the pathogenesis of mucosal damage and/or in the clinical expression of gluten sensitivity. Some of the extraintestinal manifestations of the disease could be explained by the development of organ-specific autoantibodies.

The in vivo immune activation of mucosal cell–mediated immunity can be reproduced in vitro using the organ culture of treated celiac mucosa. In such a system a gliadin digest is able to induce early overexpression of HLA-DR molecules by the epithelial cells and subsequently full activation of T cells. CD4+ lymphocytes showing signs of activation migrate in the higher lamina propria compartments, whereas CD8+ lymphocytes infiltrate the epithelium.[40] Similar phenomena (T cell activation, infiltration of epithelium by lymphocytes) also occur in the rectal mucosa of celiac patients in vitro cultured with gliadin (Troncone and coworkers, unpublished observations). Such models may prove useful to clarify the distinctive pathogenic mechanisms leading to disease and may help in defining novel therapeutic approaches.[41]

In conclusion, all the evidence available suggests a gluten-dependent activation of mucosal immunity in CD. Nevertheless, there is not only a cell-mediated abnormal immune response in the celiac mucosa but also a mucosal immunoglobulin hyperproduction and immunohistochemical evidence of subepithelial complement activation that could contribute to the pathogenesis of the mucosal lesion. On the other hand, not all the features of the celiac lesion can be reproduced in such systems; the enterocyte damage present in the celiac mucosa is absent in animal models of mucosal-delayed hypersensitivity. Finally, models of in vitro and in vivo challenges represent, from an immunologic point of view, a "recall" response. It remains to be understood which is the primary event leading to sensitization to gluten and the consequent deranged mucosal immune response.

## PATHOLOGY

CD manifests itself pathologically as a disease of the small intestine. A distinct pattern of abnormalities has been observed; the features include (1) partial to total villous atrophy; (2) elongated crypts; (3) increased mitotic index in the crypts; (4) increased IELs; (5) infiltrations of plasma cells and lymphocytes as well as mast cells, eosinophils, and basophils in the lamina propria; and (6) absence of identifiable brush border and abnormalities in the epithelial cells, which become flattened, cuboidal, and pseudostratified. However, these changes are not pathognomic of CD, and most of them may be seen in other entities, such as cow's milk or soy protein hypersensitivity, intractable diarrhea of infancy, heavy infestation with *Giardia lamblia,* primary immunodeficiencies, tropical sprue, bacterial overgrowth, and intestinal lymphoma. Hence, it is crucial to establish the gluten dependence of the jejunal lesion.

In recent years it has been recognized that the evolution of the mucosal lesion in CD requires transition from an earlier phase characterized by an infiltrative pattern (epithelium filled with numerous small nonmitotic lymphocytes), through a hyperplastic lesion (crypt hyperplasia without villous atrophy), to the destructive picture of the flat mucosa.[31] Moreover, it has now been accepted that the gluten-dependent enteropathy is not restricted to patients with flat mucosa on a gluten-containing diet; there are patients who have a high count of IELs in an otherwise normal jejunal mucosa while taking a normal diet, this count falling on gluten-free diet and rising again on gluten reintroduction. Furthermore, not only subtle pathologic abnormalities but also immunologic tests have been proposed to identify subjects with "gluten sensitivity" but without "overt" CD. The abnormalities detected by such tests include the presence of serum endomysial antibodies, and/or an increased number of γδ+ IELs, and/or positive response to rectal gluten challenge. To this regard, first-degree relatives of celiac patients are a special population where sensitivity to gluten is likely to be more prevalent. Forty one percent of healthy relatives have an increased density of γδ+ IELs[42] and the presence of inflammatory changes detectable by immunohistochemistry.[43] In our experience approximately the same percentage have been shown to mount an inflammatory rectal response to the rectal gluten challenge, a dynamic test that more specifically may indicate gluten sensitivity.[44] From a clinical point of view, most "gluten-sensitive" subjects have no symptoms; others present mild symptoms of enteropathy.[45] The evolution toward more severe forms of enteropathy probably depends on the genetic make-up of the subject and on environmental factors such as the amount of dietary gluten and/or intercurrent infections. For these subjects the term *potential CD* has been suggested. It is also possible that during life the severity of the gluten-dependent enteropathy may change. Patients have been reported who have a normal mucosa on a normal diet and, at some other time before or since, have had a flat jejunal mucosa that recovers on a gluten-free diet. For such patients the term *latent CD* has been proposed.[46]

## CLINICAL PRESENTATION

Clinical features of CD differ considerably, most depending on the age at presentation. Intestinal symptoms are common in children diagnosed within the first 2 years of life. Failure to thrive, chronic diarrhea, abdominal distention, muscle wasting, anorexia, and irritability are often present. Vomiting may occur in a third of such early-presenting patients. The clinical history reveals that growth has been normal in the first months of life, but within weeks or months after the introduction of wheat into the diet, stools become foul, greasy, and bulky and the abdomen becomes distended. The gain in weight stops, the appetite wanes, and the child becomes miserable and depressed. A small number of patients may present as very ill, with profuse diarrhea leading to dehydration and shock (celiac crisis).

CD presentating later in childhood are characterized by the prevalence of extraintestinal symptoms, this pattern being close to the adult type of the disease. In the Tampere region in Finland, CD is rarely diagnosed in children younger than 5 years of age, manifesting mostly with minor abdominal symptoms, short stature, delayed puberty, anemia, and joint complaints.[47] Among extraintestinal symptoms, short stature has been recognized as one of the commoner presenting symptoms of CD; approximately 10% of patients with isolated short stature undergoing jejunal biopsy have been found to have total villous atrophy.[48] More recent is the recognition of arthritis[49, 50] and chronic "cryptogenetic" hepatitis[51] as presenting symptoms of CD; in both cases symptoms resolved on a gluten-free diet. CD without any symptoms or signs of malabsorption can be found among patients suffering from neurologic dysfunctions of otherwise unknown causes, mainly ataxia and peripheral neuropathy.[52] The combination of CD (mainly silent), epilepsy, and bilateral occipital calcifications has recently been reported.[53] Finally, it has become evident, mostly from family studies, that CD may be completely silent clinically.[19]

## ASSOCIATED DISEASES

### Dermatitis Herpetiformis

Dermatitis herpetiformis (DH) is characterized by a symmetric pruritic skin rash with subepidermal blisters and granular subepidermal deposits of IgA in remote uninvolved skin. Most patients with DH have abnormal small intestinal biopsy pathology, histologically indistinguishable from that of CD, although usually less severe. Approximately 60% of children with DH have been reported to have subtotal villous atrophy, and 30% have partial villous atrophy on jejunal biopsy.[54] The histologic changes return to normal after dietary exclusion of gluten. Therapy with dapsone usually leads to prompt clinical improvement; a strict gluten-free diet permits a reduction or discontinuation of dapsone over a period of months. Improvement of skin lesions on a gluten-free diet seems to occur also in patients with no evident mucosal abnormality; in the same patients the rash recurs with a gluten rechallenged.

### Autoimmunity and Celiac Disease

Some diseases, many with an autoimmune pathogenesis, are found with a higher than normal frequency in celiac patients; among these are thyroid diseases,[55] Addison's disease,[56] pernicious anemia,[57] autoimmune thrombocytopenia,[58] sarcoidosis,[59] insulin-dependent diabetes mellitus,[60] and alopecia.[61] Such associations have been interpreted as a consequence of the sharing of identical HLA haplotypes (e.g., B8, DR3). Nevertheless, the relation between CD and autoimmunity is more complex. In CD patients there is evidence that the risk of developing autoimmune diseases is directly correlated to the duration of gluten exposure. Furthermore, CD patients have in their serum not only autoantibodies directed to noncollagenous matrix proteins (e.g., endomysial antibodies) but also a series of organ-specific autoantibodies (Ventura and associates, personal communication), their titer declining on a gluten-free diet. All this evidence favors the hypothesis that CD is an autoimmune disease triggered in genetically susceptible individuals by the ingestion of gluten.

### Other Diseases

An increased incidence of Down syndrome has been found in CD patients compared with the general population.[62] Selective IgA deficiency is also a condition associated with celiac disease.[63] Screening test alternatives to those based on the measurement of IgA isotype antibodies must be adopted in such patients. Finally, there are reports of associations between CD and other diseases of the gastrointestinal tract, such as cystic fibrosis[64] and cow's milk protein intolerance.[65]

## LABORATORY FINDINGS

### Tests for Malabsorption

Tests for malabsorption may be of help in approaching the diagnosis of CD. Determination of hemoglobin, serum iron, calcium, phosphorus, alkaline phosphatase, magnesium, and protein levels may be indicative of malabsorption. In particular, red blood cell folate levels have been found to be a sensitive index.[19] Prothrombin levels should be checked in any case before intestinal biopsy is performed.

Fat balance studies remain the most satisfactory method of demonstrating malabsorption of fat, but among absorption tests the 1-hour blood xylose test has been the most used.[66] An oral dose of 5 g for children below 30 kg in weight, followed by a 60-minute blood level determination, leads to good separation between untreated patients and controls; nevertheless, the rate of false-positive and false-negative results is high.

### Permeability Test

Over the last few years, tests based on intestinal permeability to sugars have been found of value as a noninvasive screening tool. Most of them are based on the differential intestinal absorption of two nonmetabolized sugars. In untreated CD the absorption of the smaller probe (mannitol, rhamnose) is reduced owing to the loss of intestinal surface area, and that of the larger one (lactulose, cellobiose) is reported as increased, because paracellular pathways are "leakier" and/or increased in number. Expression of the results as a ratio of disaccharide: monosaccharide recovery gives clear separation between normal cases and patients with CD.[67, 68] Although this test has a sufficient sensitivity for abnormalities of jejunal mucosa, it is also characterized by a low specificity for CD and false-positive results occurring mainly in patients with mucosal abnormalities due to other causes (e.g., Crohn's disease, atopic eczema, food allergy, and damage induced by nonsteroidal anti-inflammatory agents).

### Serologic Tests

Among noninvasive screening tests the measurement of serum antigliadin antibodies (AGAs) has found great application over the last few years.[69] The sensitivity of the tests has proved to be high, although it does not reach 100%. When IgG and IgA isotypes are considered separately, IgG AGAs show a higher sensitivity than IgA, but at the cost of many false-positive results. Postinfection malabsorption, Crohn's disease, and cow's milk protein intolerance are common gastrointestines disorders with IgG AGA. Atopic eczema, pemphigus, and pemphigoid among are the commonest nongastrointestinal disease in the false-positive subjects. A practical problem to be borne in mind in relation to the use of IgA AGA in diagnosis is the high prevalence of IgA deficiency (about 1 in 50) in CD.

AGAs are not the only antibodies present in elevated titers in the serum of celiac patients. Among nondietary antibodies of special interest are reticulin antibodies. They were first reported in celiac patients in the early 1970s. Antibodies belonging to the IgG class are of limited diagnostic value in CD, whereas IgA antibodies show high sensitivity and specificity for the diagnosis.[70] Celiac patients' sera react not only with rat and other rodent tissue but also with primate tissue. Chorzelski and colleagues[71] first described the endomysium antibodies directed against reticulin-like connective tissue around smooth muscle fibers in the monkey esophagus. The test gives an almost 100% sensitivity and specificity for CD.[71–78] Burgin-Wolff and coworkers reported only 90% sensitivity; many of the false-negative results occurred in children younger than 2 years of age.[73] More recently, a new substrate for such antibodies has been found in the umbilical cord,[79] an easily and commonly available, inexpensive human tissue.[80]

Serologic screening tests have been used to assess the prevalence of CD in at-risk groups and the general population. The meaning of "false positivity" (presence of such antibodies in subjects with apparently normal mucosa) remains to be established. In a family study, positivity of gliadin antibodies in first-degree relatives without gross histologic lesions but with minor morphometric abnormalities of the jejunal mucosa has been interpreted as latent CD. Similarly, patients with positive reticulin antibodies and normal small bowel mucosal architecture rebiopsied after 1 to 7 years were found to have villous atrophy.[81] Similar results were obtained in a cohort of diabetic children.[82] Therefore, these studies imply that the patients with so-called false-positive IgA AGA or reticulin (endomysium) antibody test should be carefully followed up, because "latent" CD is suspected.

No test has so far shown sensitivity and specificity sufficient to replace the small bowel biopsy. Normal results of any such tests should not dissuade a suspicious clinician from performing a biopsy in a patient whose clinical history and physical findings suggest CD. Nevertheless, some of them (particularly endomysial antibodies) remain useful tools for screening subjects belonging to at-risk groups (e.g., first-degree relatives of celiac patients). These tests may also be of value in assessing compliance with the gluten-free diet, although they are not sensitive enough to detect slight transgressions; they are also useful during challenge, as an early predictor of relapse with the aim of obtaining the definitive diagnosis in the shortest time and with minimum side effects.

## DIAGNOSIS

In 1969, ESPGAN recommended three intestinal biopsies for the diagnosis of CD in childhood: one performed at the time of presentation, another after the patient has been on a gluten-free diet when the mucosa is expected to have returned to normal, and the final biopsy after the patient has been rechallenged with gluten, when villous atrophy is expected to have recurred.[3]

Twenty years later a working group from the ESPGAN

reconsidered such diagnostic criteria.[83] The two requirements mandatory for the diagnosis of CD remain: (1) the finding of villous atrophy with hyperplasia of the crypts and abnormal surface epithelium, while the patient is eating adequate amounts of gluten; and (2) a full clinical remission after withdrawal of gluten from the diet. The finding of circulating IgA antibodies to gliadin, reticulin, and endomysium at the time of diagnosis, and their disappearance on a gluten-free diet, adds weight to the diagnosis. A control biopsy to verify the consequences on the mucosal architecture of the gluten-free diet is considered mandatory only in patients with equivocal clinical response to the diet and in patients asymptomatic at first presentation (as is often the case in patients diagnosed during screening programs, e.g., first-degree relatives of celiac patients).

Gluten challenge is not considered mandatory, except under unusual circumstances. These include situations where there is doubt about the initial diagnosis, for example when no initial biopsy was done, or when the biopsy specimen was inadequate or not typical of CD. Again, the diagnostic challenge may be necessary to exclude other causes (e.g., cows' milk–sensitive enteropathy, postenteritis syndrome, and giardiasis) that could be responsible for the flat mucosa. As most of these disorders occur in the first 2 years of life, gluten challenge is recommended more often in patients diagnosed when they are younger than 2 years of age.

With regard to the age when the challenge should be performed, it is not advisable to challenge children too soon after the first biopsy. It has been noted that children challenged before the age of 3 years showed enamel defects in the permanent central incisors. Furthermore, growth is affected by gluten challenge. When children are older and usually better able to cooperate while having a procedure, it is technically easier to obtain a specimen of small bowel for histologic examination. Gluten challenge should be discouraged before the age of 7 years and during the pubertal growth spurt.

Once decided, gluten challenge should always been performed under strict medical supervision. It should be preceded by an assessment of mucosal histology and performed with a standard dose of at least 10 g of gluten per day without disrupting established dietary habits. A further biopsy is taken when there is a noticeable clinical relapse or, in any event, after 3 to 6 months. Laboratory tests (IgA gliadin, reticulin and endomysium antibodies, absorptive and permeability tests), more than clinical symptoms, can be of help in assessing the timing of the biopsy to shorten the duration of the challenge.[84] If no or only minimal changes of mucosal architecture become evident, patients should be strictly followed up and a further biopsy obtained, in the absence of symptoms or altered laboratory tests, at 2 years. If the histologic picture is still unchanged, long-term follow-up into adult life is vital, with further biopsies taken if symptoms recur or if an antibody test result becomes abnormal.

## THERAPY

### Gluten-Free Diet

Since the identification of gluten as etiologic factor in CD, a strict gluten-free diet has become the cornerstone of the management of such patients. Their diet should exclude wheat, rye, and barley; oats should be excluded as well, because the toxicity has not been definitively disproved and because of the fear that small amounts of gliadin could contaminate oats; rice and maize are nontoxic and are usually used as wheat substitutes.

The clinical response to withdrawal of gluten is often dramatic, but it must be stressed that the gluten-free diet is recommended for both symptomatic and asymptomatic patients with CD. Normalization of the jejunal histology occurs after about 6 months. The most likely cause of lack of response is failure to adhere strictly to the diet, but the possibility of sensitivity to other dietary proteins, lymphoma, and immunodeficiency should also be considered.

All the present evidence strongly supports the view that restriction of gliadin and related prolamines should be complete and for life for all patients. In fact, it has now been demonstrated that the risk of developing small intestinal lymphoma later is increased only in patients taking a reduced-gluten or a normal diet, whereas for patients who have taken a gluten-free diet for 5 years or more the risk of developing malignancies over all sites (increased morbidity for cancer of the mouth, pharynx, and esaphagus has also been noted in celiac patients) is not increased when compared with the general population.[85] Further confirming the protective role of a gluten-free diet against malignancies is the finding that in the series from Scotland the mortality rate in patients with CD diagnosed in childhood was similar to that of the general population, no deaths from malignancies having been registered among such patients.[86] Malignancies are not the only risk that celiac patients not compliant with gluten-free diet are exposed to; nutritional deficiencies,[87] and more recent evidence that the risk of developing autoimmune diseases is related to the duration of exposure to gluten are additional concerns.[88]

### Other Therapeutic Measures

Specific vitamin, mineral, and trace element deficiencies should be corrected. Replacement therapy can generally be discontinued after clinical and histologic recovery on gluten-free diet has been documented.

Other dietary measures are rarely needed. The disaccharidase activity is greatly depressed in atrophic celiac mucosa, but it is advisable to remove milk and lactose-containing products only if intolerance is clinically manifest. Secondary lactase deficiency resolves rapidly after institution of a gluten-free diet, and milk can usually be tolerated after 2 to 4 weeks of the diet.

When patients present in celiac crisis, rapid correction of volume depletion and fluid and electrolyte abnormalities is crucial; steroid therapy is helpful. Short-term administration of steroids (2 mg/kg per 24 hours of prednisone for 1–2 weeks) may also be used in severely ill infants in whom anorexia and malabsorption do not rapidly respond to the gluten-free diet.

## REFERENCES

1. Dicke WM, Weijers HA, Van de Kamer JK: The presence in wheat of a factor having a deleterious effect in cases of coeliac disease. Acta Pediatr 1953;42:34–42.

2. Shiner M, Doniach I: Histopathologic studies in steatorrhoea. Gastroenterology 1960;38:419–440.
3. Meeuwisse G: Diagnostic criteria in coeliac disease. Acta Pediatr Scand 1970;59:461–463.
4. Janatuinen EK, Pikkarainem PH, Kemppainen TA, et al: A comparison of diets with and without oats in adults with celiac disease. N Engl J Med 1995;333:1033–1037.
5. Srinivasan U, Leonard N, Jones E, et al: Absence of oats toxicity in adult coeliac disease. BMJ 1996;313:1330–1331.
6. Troncone R, Maiuri L, Leone A, et al: Oat prolamines activate mucosal immune response in the in vitro–cultured treated coeliac mucosa. J Pediatr Gastroenterol Nutr 1996;22:414.
7. Mayer M, Troncone R, Mazzarella G, et al: Oats prolamines induce lymphocytic infiltration when instillated in the coeliac rectal mucosa. J Pediatr Gastroenterol Nutr 1997;24:453.
8. Kasarda DD, Qualset CO, Mecham DK, et al: A test of toxicity of bread made from wheat lacking alpha-gliadins coded for by the 6A chromosome. In McNicholl B, McCarthy CF, Fottrell PF (eds): Perspectives in Coeliac Disease. Lancaster, UK, MTP Press, 1978;55–61.
9. Van de Kamer JH, Weijers HA, Dicke WK: An investigation into the injurious constituents of wheat in connection with their action on patients with coeliac disease. Acta Pediatr 1953;42:223–231.
10. Auricchio S, Cardelli M, de Ritis G, et al: An in vitro animal model for the study of cereal components toxic in coeliac disease. Pediatr Res 1984;18:1372–1378.
11. Kasarda DD, Okita TW, Bernardin JE, et al: Nucleic acid (cDNA) and amino acid sequences of alpha-type gliadins from wheat (*Triticum aestivum L.*). Proc Natl Acad Sci USA 1984;81:4712–4716.
12. Maiuri L, Troncone R, Mayer M, et al: In vitro activities of A-gliadin–related synthetic peptides: damaging effect on the atrophic coeliac mucosa and activation of mucosal immune response in the treated coeliac mucosa. Scand J Gastroenterol 1996;31:247–253.
13. Sturgess R, Day P, Ellis HJ, et al: Wheat peptide challenge in coeliac disease. Lancet 1994;343:758–761.
14. Marsh MN, Morgan S, Ensari A, et al: In vivo activity of peptides 31–43, 44–55, 55–68 of A-gliadin in gluten-sensitive enteropathy (GSE). Gastroenterology 1995;108:A871.
15. Johansen BH, Vartdal F, Eriksen JA, et al: Identification of a putative motif for binding of peptides to HLA-DQ2. Int Immunol 1996;8:177–182.
16. Auricchio S, Follo D, de Ritis G, et al: Working hypothesis: does breast feeding protect against the development of clinical symptoms of coeliac disease in children? J Pediatr Gastroenterol Nutr 1983;2:428–433.
17. Ascher H, Krantz I, Kristiansson B: Increasing incidence of coeliac disease in Sweden. Arch Dis Child 1991;66:608–611.
18. Kagnoff MF, Austin RK, Hubert JJ, Kasarda DD: Possible role for a human adenovirus in the pathogenesis of celiac disease. Exp Med 1984;160:1544–1557.
19. Auricchio S, Mazzacca G, Tosi R, et al: Coeliac disease as a familial condition: identification of asymtomatic coeliac patients within family groups. Gastroenterol Int 1988;1:25–31.
20. Polanco I, Biemond I, van Leeuwen A, et al: Gluten-sensitive enteropathy in Spain: genetic and environmental factors. In McConnell RB (ed): Genetics of Coeliac Disease. Lancaster, UK, MTP Press, 1981, pp 211–231.
21. Sollid ML, Markussen G, Ek J, et al: Evidence for a primary association of celiac disease to a particular HLA-DQ alpha/beta heterodimer. J Exp Med 1989;169:345–350.
22. Mantovani V, Corazza GR, Bragliani M, et al: Asp57-negative HLA-DQβ chain and *DQA1*0501* allele are essential for the onset of DQw2-positive and DQw2-negative coeliac disease. Clin Exp Immunol 1993;91:153–156.
23. Ploski R, Ek J, Thorsby E, Sollid LM: On the HLA-DQ (alpha 1*0501, beta 1*0201)-associated susceptibility in celiac disease: a possible gene dosage effect of *DQB1*0201*. Tissue Antigens 1993;41:173–177.
24. McManus R, Wilson AG, Mansfield J, et al: TNF-2, a polymorphism of the tumour necrosis-α gene promoter, is a component of the celiac disease major histocompatibility complex haplotype. Eur J Immunol 1996;26:2113–2118.
25. Greco L, Maki M, Di Donato F, Visakorpi JK: Epidemiology of coeliac disease in Europe and the Mediterranean area: a summary report on multicentre study by the European Society of Paediatric Gastroenterology and Nutrition. In Auricchio S, Visakorpi JK (eds): Common Food Intolerances. Vol 1: Epidemiology of Coeliac Disease. Basel, Karger, 1992, pp 25–44.
26. Hed J, Lieden G, Ottosson E, et al: IgA antigliadin antibodies and jejunal mucosal lesions in healthy blood donors. Lancet 1986;2:215.
27. Catassi C, Ratsch I-M, Fabiani E, et al: Coeliac disease in the year 2000: exploring the iceberg. Lancet 1994;343:200–203.
28. Not T, Horvath K, Mill I, et al: Coeliac disease risk in USA: high prevalence of antigliadin and entiendomisyum antibodies in healthy blood donors in the USA. Seventh International Symposium on Coeliac Disease, Tampere, Finland, 1996.
29. Maki M, Holm K: Incidence and prevalence of coeliac disease in Tampere: coeliac disease is not disappearing. Acta Pediatr Scand 1990;79:380–382.
30. Ferguson A: Models of immunologically driven small intestinal damage. In Marsh MN (ed): The Immunopathology of the Small Intestine. New York, Wiley, 1987, pp 225–252.
31. Marsh MN: Gluten, major histocompatibility complex, and the small intestine: a molecular and immunobiologic approach to the spectrum of gluten sensitivity ("celiac sprue"). Gastroenterology 1992;102:330–354.
32. Halstensen TS, Brandtzaeg P: Activated T lymphocytes in the celiac lesion: nonproliferative activation (CD25) of CD4+ αβ cells in the lamina propria but proliferation (Ki-67) of αβ and γδ cells in the epithelium. Eur J Immunol 1993;23:505–551.
33. Sturgess R, Kontakou M, Spencer J, et al: Effects of interferon-γ and tumour necrosis factor-α on ICAM-1 expression on jejunal mucosal biopsies cultured in vitro. Gut 1993;34:S31.
34. Nilsen EM, Lundin KEA, Krajci P, et al: Cytokine profiles of gluten-responsive intestinal T cell clones from coeliac disease patients. Gut 1995;35:766–776.
35. Halstensen TS, Scott H, Brandtzaeg P: Intraepithelial T cells of the TCR γδ CD8− and Vδ1/Jδ1 + phenotypes are increased in coeliac disease. Scand J Immunol 1989;30:665–672.
36. Kett K, Scott H, Fausa O, et al: Secretory immunity in celiac disease: cellular expression of immunoglobulin A subclass and joining chain. Gastroenterology 1990;99:386.
37. Wood GM, Howdle PD, Trejdosiewicz LK, et al: Jejunal plasma cells and in vitro immunoglobulin production in adult coeliac disease. Clin Exp Immunol 1987;69:123.
38. Picarelli A, Maiuri L, Frate A, et al: Production of antiendomysial antibodies after in vitro gliadin challenge of small intestinal biopsy samples from patients with coeliac disease. Lancet 1996;348:1065–1067.
39. Dieterich W, Volta U, Donner P, et al: Identification of the autoantigen in coeliac disease. Presented at the American Gastroenterological Association Meeting, Washington, DC, May 10–13, 1997.
40. Maiuri L, Picarelli A, Boirivant M, et al: Definition of the initial immunologic modifications upon in vitro gliadin challenge in the small intestine of celiac patients. Gastroenterology 1996;110:1368–1378.
41. Maiuri L, Picarelli A, Coletta S, et al: CTLA4 inhibits T cell–mediated gliadin-induced immune response in treated coeliac intestinal explants. J Paediatr Gastroenterol Nutr 1996;22:428.
42. Holm K, Maki M, Savilahti E, et al: Intraepithelial γδ T cell receptor lymphocytes and genetic susceptibility to coeliac disease. Lancet 1992;339:1500.
43. Holm K, Savilahti E, Koskimies S, et al: Immunohistochemical changes in the jejunum in first-degree relatives of patients with coeliac disease and the coeliac disease marker DQ genes: HLA class II antigen expression, interleukin-2 receptor–positive cells, and dividing crypt cells. Gut 1994;35:55.
44. Troncone R, Greco L, Mayer M, et al: Rectal gluten challenge reveals gluten sensitization not restricted to celiac HLA in siblings of children with celiac disease. Gastroenterology 1996;111:318–324.
45. Picarelli A, Maiuri L, Mazzilli MG, et al: Gluten-sensitive disease with mild enteropathy. Gastroenterology 1996;111:608–616.
46. Troncone R: Latent coeliac disease in Italy and the SIGEP Working Group on Latent Coeliac Disease. Acta Paediatr 1995;84:1252–1257.
47. Maki M, Kallonen K, Lahdeaho ML, Visakorpi JK: Changing pattern of childhood coeliac disease in Finland. Acta Pediatr Scand 1988;77:408–412.
48. Cacciari E, Salardi S, Lazzari R, et al: Short stature and coeliac disease: a relationship to consider even in patients with no gastrointestinal tract symptoms. J Pediatr 1983;103:708–711.
49. Pinals RS: Arthritis associated with gluten-sensitive enteropathy. J Rheumatol 1986;13:201–204.
50. Bourne JT, Kumar P, Huskisson EC, et al: Arthritis and coeliac disease. Ann Rheumatic Dis 1985;44:592–598.

51. Vajro P, Fontanella A, Mayer M, et al: Elevated serum aminotransferase activity as an early manifestation of gluten-sensitive enteropathy. J Pediatr 1993;122:416–419.
52. Hadjivassiliou M, Gibson A, Davies Jones GA, et al: Does cryptic gluten sensitivity play a part in neurological illness? Lancet 1996;347:369–371.
53. Gobbi G, Bouquet F, Greco L, et al: Coeliac disease, epilepsy, and cerebral calcifications. Lancet 1992;340:439–443.
54. Reunala T, Kosnai T, Karpati S, et al: Dermatitis herpetiformis: jejunal findings and skin response to gluten-free diet. Arch Dis Child 1984;59:517–522.
55. Mulder CJJ, Tytgat GNJ, Groenland F, Pena AS: Combined coeliac disease and thyroid disease: a study of 17 cases. J Clin Nutr Gastroenterol 1988;3:89–92.
56. Reunala T, Salmi J, Karvonen J: Dermatitis herpetiformis and coeliac disease associated with Addison's disease. Arch Dermatol 1987;123:930–932.
57. Stene-Larsen G, Mosvold J, Ly B: Selective vitamin $B_{12}$ malabsorption in adult coeliac disease: report on three cases with associated autoimmune diseases. Scand J Gastroenterol 1988;23:1105–1108.
58. Stenhammar L, Ljunggren CG: Thrombocytopenic purpura and coeliac disease. Acta Paediatr Scand 1988;77:764–766.
59. Douglas JD, Gillon J, Logan RFA, et al: Sarcoidosis and coeliac disease: an association. Lancet 1984;2:13–14.
60. Savilahti E, Simell O, Koskimes S, et al: Coeliac disease in insulin-dependent diabetes mellitus. J Pediatr 1986;108:690–693.
61. Corazza GR, Andreani ML, Venturo N, et al: Coeliac disease and alopecia areata: report of a new association. Gastroenterology 1995;109:1333–1337.
62. Amil Dias J, Walker-Smith J: Down's syndrome and coeliac disease. J Pediatr Gastroenterol Nutr 1990;10:41–43.
63. Savilahti E, Pelkonen P, Visakorpi JK: IgA deficiency in children: a clinical study with special reference to intestinal findings. Arch Dis Child 1971;46:665–670.
64. Goodchild MC, Nelson R, Anderson CM: Cystic fibrosis and coeliac disease: co-existence in two children. Arch Dis Child 1973;48:684–691.
65. Watt J, Pincott JR, Harries JT: Combined cow's milk protein and gluten-induced enteropathy: common or rare? Gut 1983;24:165–170.
66. Rolles CJ, Kendall MJ, Nutter S, Anderson CM: one-hour blood xylose screening test for coeliac disease in infants and young children. Lancet 1973;2:1043–1045.
67. Juby LD, Rothwell J, Axon ATR: Lactulose/mannitol test: an ideal screen for coeliac disease. Gastroenterology 1989;96:79–85.
68. Juby LD, Rothwell J, Axon ATR: Cellobiose/mannitol sugar test—a sensitive tubeless test for coeliac disease: results on 1010 unselected patients. Gut 1989;30:476–480.
69. Troncone R, Ferguson A: Antigliadin antibodies. J Pediatr Gastroenterol Nutr 1991;12:150–158.
70. Maki M, Hallstrom O, Vesikari T, Visakorpi JK: Evaluation of serum IgA-class reticulin antibody test for the detection of childhood celiac disease. J Pediatr 1984;105:901–905.
71. Chorzelski TP, Beutner EH, Suley J, et al: IgA anti-endomysium antibody: a new immunological marker of dermatitis herpetiformis and coeliac disease. Br J Dermatol 1984;111:395–402.
72. Karpati S, Bukgin-Wolff A, Krieg T, et al: Binding to human jejunum of serum IgA antibody from children with coeliac disease. Lancet 1990;336:1335.
73. Burgin-Wolff A, Gaze H, Hadziselimovic F, et al: Antigliadin and antiendomysium antibody determination for coeliac disease. Arch Dis Child 1991;66:941.
74. Hallstrom O: Comparison of IgA-class reticulin and endomysium antibodies in coeliac disease and dermatitis herpetiformis. Gut 1989;30:1255.
75. McMillian SA, Haughton DJ, Biggart JD, et al: Predictive value for coeliac disease of antibodies to gliadin, endomysium, and jejunum in patients attending for jejunal biopsy. BMJ 1991;303:1163–1165.
76. Ferreira M, Lloyd Davies S, Butler M, et al: Endomysial antibody: is it the best screening test for coeliac disease? Gut 1992;33:1633.
77. Chan KN, Phillips AD, Mirakian R, et al: Endomysial antibody screening in children. J Pediatr Gastroenterol Nutr 1994;18:316.
78. Volta U, Molinaro N, Fusconi M, et al: IgA antiendomysial antibody test: a step forward in coeliac disease screening. Dig Dis Sci 1991;36:752.
79. Landinser B, Rossipal E, Pittschieler K: Endomysium antibodies in coeliac disease: an improved method. Gut 1994;35:776.
80. Karpati S, Burgin-Wolff A, Krieg T, et al: Binding to human jejunum of serum IgA antibody from children with coeliac disease. Lancet 1990;336:1335.
81. Collin P, Helin H, Maki M, et al: Follow-up of patients positive in reticulin and gliadin antibody tests with normal small bowel biopsy findings. Scand J Gastroenterol 1993;28:595.
82. Maki M, Huupponen T, Holm K, et al: Seroconversion of reticulin autoantibodies predicts coeliac disease in insulin-dependent diabetes mellitus. Gut 1995;36:239.
83. Walker-Smith JA, Guandalini S, Schmitz J, et al: Revised criteria for the diagnosis of coeliac disease. Arch Dis Child 1990;65:909–911.
84. Mayer M, Greco L, Troncone R, et al: Early prediction of relapse during gluten challenge in childhood coeliac disease. J Pediatr Gastroenterol Nutr 1989;8:474–479.
85. Holmes GKT, Prior P, Lane MR, et al: Malignancy in coeliac disease: effect of a gluten-free diet. Gut 1989;30:333–338.
86. Logan RFA, Rifkind EA, Turner ID, Ferguson A: Mortality in celiac disease. Gastroenterology 1989;97:265–271.
87. Holmes GKT: Long-term health risks for unrecognized coeliac patients. In Auricchio S, Visakorpi JK (eds): Common Food Intolerances: Vol 1. Epidemiology of Coeliac Disease. Basel, Karger, 1992, 105–118.
88. Ventura A, Magazzu G, Greco L, et al: Autoimmune disorders in coeliac disease: relationship with duration of exposure to gluten. J Pediatr Gastroenterol Nutr 1997;24:463.

# Chapter 26

# Short Bowel Syndrome

*William R. Treem*

Management of the child with short bowel syndrome (SBS) is one of the greatest challenges facing those caring for infants and children. Providing adequate nutrition and avoiding complications are critical, since children have a remarkable capacity to achieve normal enteral feeding. Two major developments have altered the prognosis for even the most severely affected infants and children. More than 30 years ago, the first patient given total parenteral nutrition (TPN) was an infant with SBS.[1] Since then, parenteral nutrition has become an indispensable part of the acute and chronic management of SBS. More recently, success with small bowel transplantation has offered hope to those without sufficient intestinal adaptation to support enteral feedings.[2]

## DEFINITION

SBS is defined as malabsorption, fluid and electrolyte loss, and malnutrition following massive small bowel resection. As much as half of the small intestine may be lost without significant long-term problems in sustaining normal nutrition, provided the duodenum, distal ileum, and ileocecal valve (ICV) are spared. In contrast, distal ileal resections that include the ICV may induce severe diarrhea even though only 25% of the small bowel has been resected. Resection of more than 75% of the small intestine with preservation of the ICV invariably produces initial intractable malabsorption and diarrhea. Wilmore[3] reviewed the case histories of 50 infants younger than 2 months of age and defined SBS as less than 75 cm of residual small intestine. Since the length of the small intestine is estimated to be 200 to 300 cm at birth in a full-term neonate,[4] these infants underwent a greater than 50% resection. This definition may not be applicable in preterm infants because the total intestinal length normally doubles from the 26th to the 38th week of gestation.[5] Thereafter the length of the small intestine increases to 600 to 800 cm in the adult; intestinal diameter also changes from 1.5 cm to 3 to 4 cm.[6] These changes and the development of the plicae circulares, villi, and microvilli combine to enlarge the absorptive surface area from approximately 950 cm$^2$ at birth to 7,500 cm$^2$ in the adult.[7] The infant does not tolerate massive small bowel resection initially as well as the adult because of a lack of intestinal reserve. Conversely, the infant has a more favorable long-term prognosis because of a greater residual capacity for growth and development.[8]

## ETIOLOGY

Table 26–1 summarizes the causes of SBS in infants collated from several published series.[3, 9–14] The most common causes include necrotizing enterocolitis, volvulus, jejunoileal atresia(s), and gastroschisis. Midgut volvulus and diffuse small bowel Crohn's disease predominate in the older child.[15] Less frequent etiologies of SBS include trauma to the gastrointestinal tract[16] and total colonic aganglionosis with proximal extension into the small bowel.[12]

## PATHOPHYSIOLOGY

The basic defect of SBS is a markedly decreased intestinal surface area for absorption of fluid, electrolytes, and nutrients coupled with a rapid and often disordered transit of intestinal contents, which compromises intraluminal digestion. The effect of the intestinal resection depends on six main factors: (1) the amount of remaining small intestine, (2) whether it is proximal (jejunal) or distal (ileal), (3) whether the ICV has been resected, (4) whether the colon has been resected as well, (5) the degree of intestinal adaptation over time, and (6) the presence of residual bowel disease or surgical complications. These factors influence the fluid, electrolyte, and nutrient requirements for each individual patient and determine the time required until full intestinal adaptation.

## SITE-SPECIFIC PATHOPHYSIOLOGY

It is rare that the duodenum must be resected with other segments of the small bowel. Duodenal resection or bypass results in malabsorption of iron, folate, and calcium and puts the patient at risk for anemia and osteopenia. A lack of coordinated mixing of bile and pancreatic secretions with duodenal contents may also affect intraluminal digestion and absorption of fat- and lipid-soluble vitamins.

Selective proximal jejunal resections generally result in

**TABLE 26–1. Summary of Series on the Etiology of Short Bowel Syndrome in Infants**

| | NO. OF SUBJECTS | | | | | | |
|---|---|---|---|---|---|---|---|
| ETIOLOGIC DISORDER | Wilmore[3] (1972) | Bohane et al[9] (1979) | Cooper et al[10] (1984) | Dorney et al[11] (1985) | Grosfeld et al[12] (1986) | Caniano et al[13] (1989) | Goulet et al[14] (1991) |
| Volvulus | 30 | 2 | 6 | 6 | 5 | 1 | 22 |
| Atresia(s) | 14 | 6 | 3 | 3 | 13 | 5 | 36 |
| Gastroschisis | 5 | 3 | 2 | 1 | 5 | 5 | 10 |
| Necrotizing enterocolitis | 0 | 4 | 5 | 2 | 24 | 2 | 11 |
| Other* | 1 | 0 | 0 | 1 | 7 | 1 | 8 |
| Total | 50 | 15 | 16 | 13 | 54 | 14 | 87 |

*Meconium peritonitis, extensive intestinal angioma, complicated intussusception, congenital short bowel syndrome.

little chronic diarrhea because the intact ileum and colon adapt to reabsorb nutrients and excess fluid and electrolytes.[17] However, duodenal and jejunal mucosa is also the site of secretin and cholecystokinin synthesis and, theoretically, extensive loss of jejunum should result in decreased hormonal stimulation of pancreatic and biliary secretion. This hypothesis is open to question, since studies in animals have shown that pancreatic enzyme synthesis and secretion are well maintained after major small bowel resection.[18] Extensive jejunal resection may lead to a reduction in intestinal lactase (or other disaccharidase) activity. Undigested lactose undergoes bacterial fermentation, with production of lactate and other volatile short-chain fatty acids (SCFAs), and contributes to an osmotic diarrhea. Nonhydrolyzed and nonabsorbed sugars also provide a fertile milieu for bacterial overgrowth and the production of potentially toxic metabolic by-products of bacterial metabolism such as D-lactate. Measurements of carbohydrate excretion in children with large resections of both jejunum and ileum show fecal loss of up to 65% of dietary carbohydrate and a direct correlation between stool weight and fecal carbohydrate excretion.[19]

In the jejunum, there is back-diffusion of fluid and electrolytes into the lumen due to leaky epithelial junctions, and the luminal contents remain isotonic even as the bulk of nutrients is being absorbed. Conversely, in the ileum, the tight junctions are less permeable; there is less back-diffusion and an increased concentration of the luminal contents. Thus, resection of the ileum has more profound effects on the volume and tonicity of intestinal contents reaching the colon.

Moderate loss of the terminal ileum and right colon may also contribute to diarrhea because of a reduced capacity to absorb sodium chloride. Only the ileum and colon can absorb sodium chloride against a steep concentration gradient.[20] Sodium chloride absorption against electrochemical gradients is a prerequisite to continued fluid absorption in this area, since most sodium chloride has been absorbed proximally, and poorly absorbed solutes (such as potassium, divalent cations, and carbohydrates) become concentrated in luminal fluid within the lower ileum and colon.

Resection of the ileum also causes diarrhea and steatorrhea secondary to the malabsorption of bile salts. After entry into the intestinal tract, the large majority (95–98%) of conjugated bile salts are absorbed either passively in the proximal small intestine or actively in the distal ileum.[21] The bulk of intestinal reabsorption takes place in the terminal ileum via an active carrier-mediated system that is sodium dependent. Active ileal absorption is necessary to maintain the bile salt pool, and resection of the ileum can lead to loss of bile salts at a rate that cannot be compensated by increased liver synthesis.

Figure 26–1 summarizes the consequences of the malabsorption of bile salts in SBS. In an adult, if less than 100 cm of distal ileum is resected, watery diarrhea (termed *cholerrheic diarrhea*) will result without significant steatorrhea. Increased amounts of bile salts reach the colon and are lost in the feces, but the liver compensates by increasing bile acid synthesis up to 20-fold.[22] Intraluminal concentrations of bile salts are maintained, and there is normal fat digestion and absorption in the proximal small bowel. In the colon, the high concentration of secondary bile acids produced by bacterial deconjugation and dehydroxylation induces reversible secretion of sodium and water via mechanisms of increased mucosal cyclic adenosine monophosphate levels and direct damage by bile salts to the colonic epithelium.[23, 24] The bile acid concentration in the fecal aqueous phase may exceed the concentration of 3 mmol/L sufficient to produce water and electrolyte secretion from the colon.[25]

If more than 100 cm of ileum has been resected, massive bile salt loss, which overwhelms the liver's ability to compensate, will result in steatorrhea. The resultant drop below the critical micellar concentration of intraluminal bile acids necessary for absorption of dietary fat and fat-soluble vitamins leads to an increase in fatty acids entering the colon. Fatty acids, like bile acids, impair colonic water and ion absorption, stimulate colonic fluid secretion (especially when they are hydroxylated by colonic bacteria), and lower stool pH. Following ileal resection, children also have interruption of the enterohepatic circulation of bile acids, increased fecal bile acid excretion, accelerated disappearance of isotopically labeled bile acids from the duodenal bile, reduced pool sizes after an overnight fast, and a reduced magnitude of rise in postprandial serum bile acid concentrations.[26]

Resection of the ICV is associated with increased severity of disease and prolonged reliance on nutritional supplementation. An intact ICV prevents reflux of colonic bacteria and bacterial overgrowth. Without the ICV, bacterial colonization of the ileum will not only impair bile salt reabsorption but also aggravate the malabsorption of vitamin $B_{12}$.

Patients who have undergone a partial or total colectomy in addition to extensive small bowel resection (particularly ileal) are more prone to develop severe dehydration, hypovolemia, hypokalemia, hypomagnesemia, and hyponatremia, or the "end-jejunostomy syndrome."[27] The large potential reserve capacity of the intact healthy adult human colon has been demonstrated by the absorption of 6 L of water and

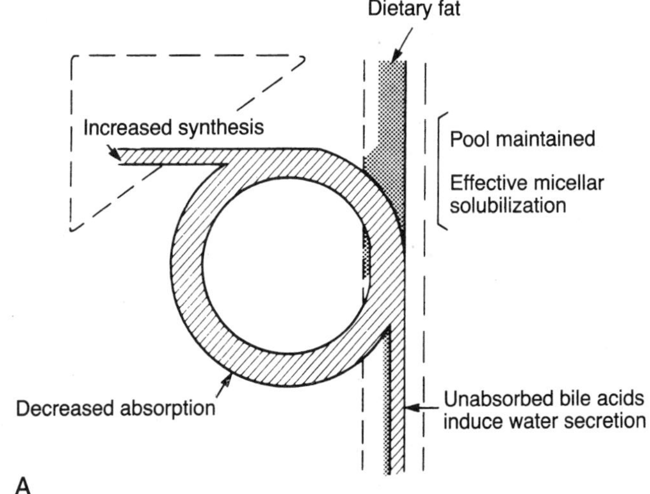


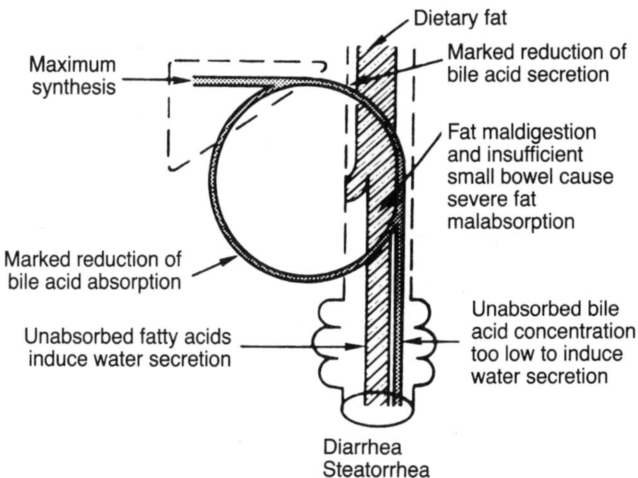


**FIGURE 26–1.** Mechanisms of diarrhea in patients with ileal resections. In ileal resections less than 100 cm *(A)*, malabsorbed bile acids are entirely replaced by increased liver synthesis of bile acids, and proximal small bowel fat absorption is preserved. Unabsorbed bile acids induce water secretion in the colon (cholerrheic diarrhea). In larger resections, greater than 100 cm *(B)*, liver synthesis cannot compensate for fecal bile salt loss, and the total bile acid pool and proximal luminal bile salt concentration are reduced, leading to fat malabsorption. Malabsorbed fatty acids induce water secretion in the colon (steatorrhea). (Adapted from Hofman AF, Poley JR: Role of bile acid malabsorption in pathogenesis of diarrhea and steatorrhea in patients with ileal resection: I. Response to cholestyramine or replacement of dietary long-chain triglyceride by medium-chain triglyceride. Gastroenterology 1972;62:931; with permission.)

800 mEq of sodium slowly perfused into the cecum.[28] The colon also salvages malabsorbed carbohydrate by bacterial fermentation to SCFA, which are absorbed and utilized as fuel by colonic epithelial cells. In patients with combined ileal and colonic resections, the severity of diarrhea and fecal electrolyte composition is more closely related to the amount of residual colon than to the degree of ileal resection.[29] Adult patients with a jejunostomy and less than 100 cm of jejunum usually need long-term parenteral support, whereas 50 cm or more of jejunum usually suffices for adequate oral nutrition if the colon is preserved.[30]

## MOTILITY DISTURBANCES

Intestinal resection can have profound effects on small bowel motility, disrupting the normal patterns necessary for effective intraluminal contact of nutrients with enzymes or absorptive surfaces. Motility disturbances depend once again on the site and extent of resection. The consequence of proximal small bowel resection is primarily a decrease in the inhibition of gastric emptying by intestinal chyme.[27] The faster emptying rate appears to correlate directly with the remaining jejunal length, suggesting a loss of a small intestinal brake on gastric emptying.[31] Despite an increase in the rate of gastric emptying in patients with proximal small bowel resections, small bowel transit remains normal because of slow transit through the intact ileum.

When the distal bowel is resected, the slowing effect of the ileum is lost. Total intestinal transit is also correlated with the length of remaining colon in patients with colonic resection.[32]

## MALABSORPTION OF SPECIFIC ELECTROLYTES, VITAMINS, AND TRACE ELEMENTS

Deficiencies of divalent cations are not uncommon after intestinal resection, leading to symptoms of tetany, osteopenia, osteomalacia, and spontaneous fracture. Even though the rate of absorption of iron, calcium, and magnesium is maximal in the duodenum, these cations are absorbed throughout the small bowel. Luminal availability of calcium may be decreased by sequestration as insoluble calcium soaps in patients with steatorrhea. Calcium absorption may be further compromised by fat-soluble vitamin D malabsorption, since intestinal calcium transport is dependent on adequate levels of active vitamin D.[33] Magnesium and zinc can also form complexes with unabsorbed fatty acids, preventing normal transport.[34] Hypomagnesemia may further aggravate calcium homeostasis because of the role of magnesium as a cofactor for parathormone, which stimulates bone resorption and renal hydroxylation of vitamin D to its active form. Zinc deficiency also develops in the setting of fat malabsorption. In addition to the clinical consequences, zinc deficiency may have a detrimental effect on small bowel adaptation after bowel resection.

Malabsorption of the fat-soluble vitamins increases with increasing steatorrhea, and deficiencies of vitamins A, D, E, and K all have been described in patients with SBS. Iron deficiency also occurs owing to a loss of the proximal small bowel absorptive surface area. Some patients also develop small intestinal mucosal blood loss from chronic stasis, mucosal injury, and even mucosal ulceration, especially at the site of a previous anastomosis.[35] A syndrome of noninfectious colitis and hematochezia has been described in infants with SBS, which may contribute to iron deficiency.[36]

Vitamin $B_{12}$ malabsorption is almost invariably present when more than 100 cm of terminal ileum has been resected. Because $B_{12}$ receptors are restricted to the ileum, there is no adaptation of vitamin $B_{12}$ absorption after a large ileal resection. Less extensive resection does result in decreased absorption, provided there is no residual ileal disease and no bacterial overgrowth. In the setting of bacterial overgrowth, there is competitive uptake of intrinsic factor–bound vitamin $B_{12}$ by anaerobic bacteria[37] and/or conversion of some of the ingested vitamin $B_{12}$ by bacterial flora to vitamin $B_{12}$ analogues, making less active vitamin available to the host.[38] Vitamin $B_{12}$ deficiency may also affect small bowel adaptation, since it alters both small bowel mucosal cell morphology and transport functions.[39, 40] Deficiencies of other water-soluble vitamins are uncommon in all except those patients with minimal remaining small bowel. Folate is normally absorbed in the proximal small intestine after deconjugation of dietary folates by the mucosa to pteroylmonoglutamates. Conservation of body folate stores is enhanced by a significant enterohepatic recirculation.[41] In the setting of proximal small bowel bacterial overgrowth and extensive duodenojejunal resection, absorption and the enterohepatic circulation may be sufficiently impaired to result in significant folate malabsorption.

## SPECIFIC CLINICAL CONSEQUENCES OF BOWEL RESECTION

Although the primary causes of deficient absorption in SBS are a loss of absorptive surface and disruption of normal motility patterns, there are also major secondary effects of small bowel resection that exacerbate the malabsorption, may delay small bowel adaptation, and complicate the management of patients with SBS.

### Gastric Acid Hypersecretion

Gastric acid hypersecretion occurs after massive small bowel resection in both experimental animals[42] and approximately 50% of adult patients.[43] It is a transient phenomenon, returning to normal in most patients within 1 year of the resection.[44] Gastric acid hypersecretion may interfere with intraluminal digestion by lowering the pH of the duodenum, inactivating pancreatic enzymes, and impairing micelle formation and lipolysis.[45] The increased secretion of acid can also cause direct mucosal damage, including peptic ulcer disease in the proximal small bowel. The high-solute load of excessive gastric secretions may add to the diarrhea by presenting the small intestinal remnant with an increased fluid and electrolyte load and by stimulating peristalsis.[46]

Gastric hypersecretion after massive resection has been attributed to hypergastrinemia and an increase in parietal cell mass due to either a loss of small bowel tissue responsible for gastrin degradation[47] or a decrease in levels of an intestinal gastrin inhibitory factor.[48] Hypergastrinemia may persist months or years after small bowel resection.[44] In both adult and pediatric studies, the presence and magnitude of gastric acid hypersecretion appear to be proportional to the length of intestine resected.[48]

### Bacterial Overgrowth

Chronic bacterial overgrowth is a frequent complication of SBS and may play a large role in perpetuating malabsorption. Factors that promote bacterial overgrowth include (1) absence of the ICV; (2) presence of a partial small bowel obstruction from a tight anastomosis, an ischemic stricture, or an adhesion; (3) presence of a dilated, hypotonic bowel segment with disordered motility; (4) presence of an enteroenteral fistula secondary to an underlying inflammatory disease such as Crohn's disease or a surgical complication; and (5) relative achlorhydria secondary to the prolonged use of acid blockers to prevent gastric acid hypersecretion.

Patients with bacterial overgrowth may have depressed levels of maltase, sucrase, lactase, and enterokinase in jejunal biopsies.[49] Depressed serum protein levels are also seen. In addition to the effect on brush border peptidases, there is evidence to suggest that small bowel bacteria deaminate dietary protein moieties,[50] interrupting normal uptake of peptides and amino acids. Protein-losing enteropathy and even a flat villous lesion resembling celiac sprue have been documented in occasional patients with bacterial overgrowth.

### D-Lactic Acidosis

D-Lactic acidosis is a rare complication of SBS and intestinal bypass surgery.[51, 52] Patients present with symptoms of confusion, slurred speech, unsteady gait, stupor, and even coma and physical findings of dysarthria, nystagmus, and Kussmaul breathing. In some cases, milder episodes of behavioral changes, dizziness, and incoordination may precede the more serious episode. The patients have a metabolic acidosis with an increased anion gap, elevated plasma levels of D-lactate, and normal levels of L-lactate. Prerequisites for this syndrome are small bowel bacterial overgrowth and exposure of these bacteria to fermentable carbohydrate. In several children, D-lactic acidosis has followed liberalization of their diet to take in more carbohydrate, including lactose.[51, 53] Malabsorption leads to bacterial generation of progressively larger amounts of lactic acid. Accumulation of lactic acid in the lumen results in a drop in luminal pH, which favors the growth of acid-producing and acid-tolerant bacteria, such as *Lactobacillus,* at the expense of the normally predominant gut bacteria.

Effective treatment consists of correction of the acidosis with bicarbonate infusion, cessation of enteral carbohydrate, and reduction of the colonic flora with antibiotics such as oral vancomycin, neomycin, or metronidazole.

### Renal Stones and Gallstones

Dietary oxalate reacts with calcium within the lumen to form highly insoluble complexes of calcium oxalate that are not absorbed. In patients with fat malabsorption, dietary calcium binds with unabsorbed fatty acids, is unavailable to complex with dietary oxalate, and frees oxalate to be absorbed primarily in the colon and eventually excreted in the urine.[54] Patients with SBS, large ileal resections, and an intact colon are at risk of hyperoxaluria.[55]

The incidence of gallstones in adult patients who have undergone ileal resection may be as much as threefold greater than in the normal population.[56] This is presumably secondary to depletion of the bile salt pool, giving rise to lithogenic bile.[57]

Biliary stasis and obstruction have also been associated with the formation of biliary sludge and pigment stones in the gallbladder and common duct.[58, 59] Analysis of biliary sludge has shown predominantly calcium bilirubinate granules, few cholesterol crystals, and a high proportion of unconjugated bilirubinate.[60] Gallstones in patients treated with prolonged TPN are pigment stones and have a very high calcium bilirubinate content, suggesting that stasis is a factor in their formation.[61] Fasting, lack of hormonal stimuli that regulate gallbladder emptying, and prolonged sequestration of gallbladder bile appear to be important factors leading to the formation of sludge and pigment gallstones in children with SBS maintained on TPN.

In four reviews of SBS in infancy and childhood, 20 (12%) of 174 patients developed cholelithiasis and 16 of the 20 required cholecystectomy for acute cholecystitis, biliary colic, or both.[11–14] Because of the high incidence of this complication in children with significant ileal resections, and the ever greater occurrence in adult patients (up to 40%), some centers perform cholecystectomy routinely during the initial bowel resection or at the time of re-establishment of intestinal continuity.[14]

## SMALL BOWEL ADAPTATION

Modern techniques of parenteral nutrition have allowed time for adaptation to take place, improving the prospects for survival with normal growth and eventual enteral feedings in children with as little as 11 cm of small bowel and an intact ICV or 25 cm of small bowel without an ICV.[11, 62, 63] Many factors stimulate the intestinal epithelium to become hyperplastic and increase its absorptive capacity. A proposed scheme of interwoven stimuli is outlined in Figure 26–2. A discussion of mechanisms of bowel adaptation can be divided into the roles of (1) luminal nutrients, (2) endogenous fuels for the gut, (3) pancreatic secretions, (4) circulating hormones, (5) growth factors, and (6) intracellular modulators.

### General Evidence for Intestinal Adaptation

Resection of the small bowel in animals results in mucosal hyperplasia of the remaining small intestine, provided the animal is fed orally.[64] The major morphologic changes are increased height of the villi and elongation of the crypts (Fig. 26–3), resulting from increased numbers of cells but not increased size of individual cells.[65, 66] The morphologic changes are accompanied by functional increases in the absorption of most nutrients. An increase in nutrient absorption per centimeter of remaining bowel has been shown for fat, protein, glucose, galactose, sucrose, maltose, sodium, water, bile acids, vitamin $B_{12}$, calcium, and zinc.[67]

There are few studies that document similar morphologic changes of adaptation in the human small intestine. Studies of patients with jejunoileal bypass surgery have shown that the jejunoileum left in continuity becomes elongated and the villi increase in height both in the jejunum (24–40%) and in the ileum (38–70%).[68, 69] These data confirm the animal work cited earlier, showing greater adaptation in the distal bowel.

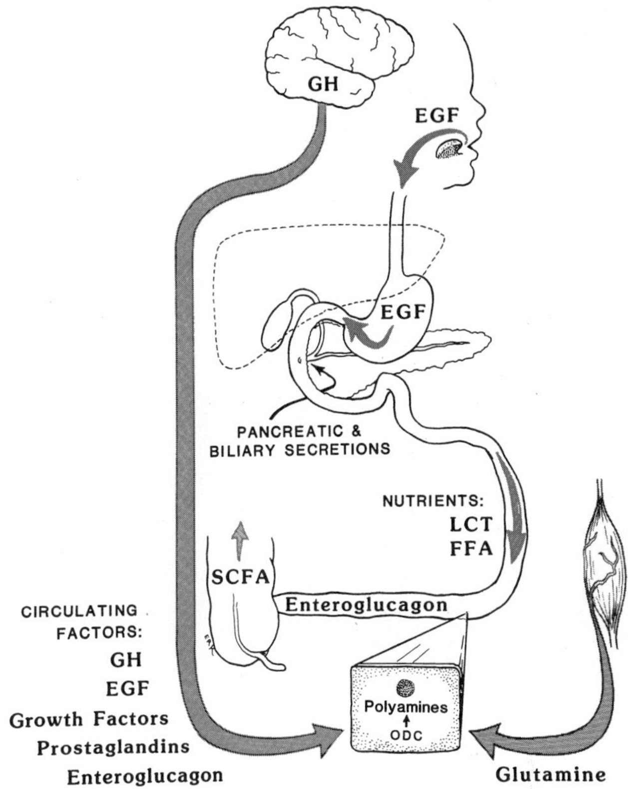


**FIGURE 26–2.** Multifactorial schematic of influences on small bowel adaption, including (1) luminal nutrients, (2) gastrointestinal and systemic hormones, (3) growth factors, (4) pancreatic and biliary secretions, (5) substrates for enterocyte metabolism, and (6) intracellular mediators of DNA and protein synthesis. GH, growth hormone; EGF, epidermal growth factor; LCT, long-chain triglycerides; FFA, free fatty acids; SCFA, short-chain fatty acids; ODC, ornithine decarboxylase.

### The Importance of Luminal Nutrients

Nutrients in the lumen of the small intestine are essential for the maintenance of mucosal mass. Not only starvation, but even the provision of adequate protein and calories exclusively via TPN, results in mucosal hypoplasia.

Nutrients may stimulate mucosal adaptation by several interrelated mechanisms, including (1) direct contact with and uptake by the mucosal surface, (2) stimulus of local gut and extraintestinal hormones, and (3) release of pancreatic secretions and other potential growth factors. The direct stimulatory effect of nutrients on growth of the absorptive mucosa is thought to be responsible for the normal proximal-to-distal absorptive gradient; proximal jejunal villi are taller and have greater absorptive capacity because of abundant exposure to nutrients, most of which are depleted by the time intestinal chyme reaches the distal small bowel. Jejunectomy results in increased exposure of the ileum to nutrients and marked hyperplasia. Similarly, when a segment of ileum is transplanted proximally and exposed to the jejunal nutrient environment, that segment becomes hyperplastic and takes on the morphologic and functional absorptive characteristics of proximal intestine.[70] Conversely, a jejunal segment transposed to the ileal environment undergoes opposite changes and decreases its mucosal mass.[71] Thus, the proximal intes-

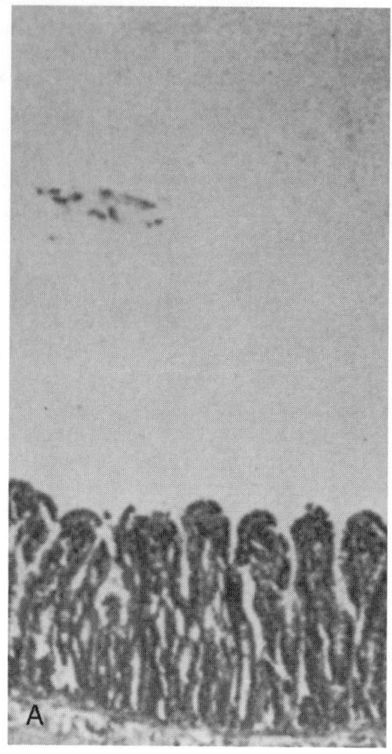


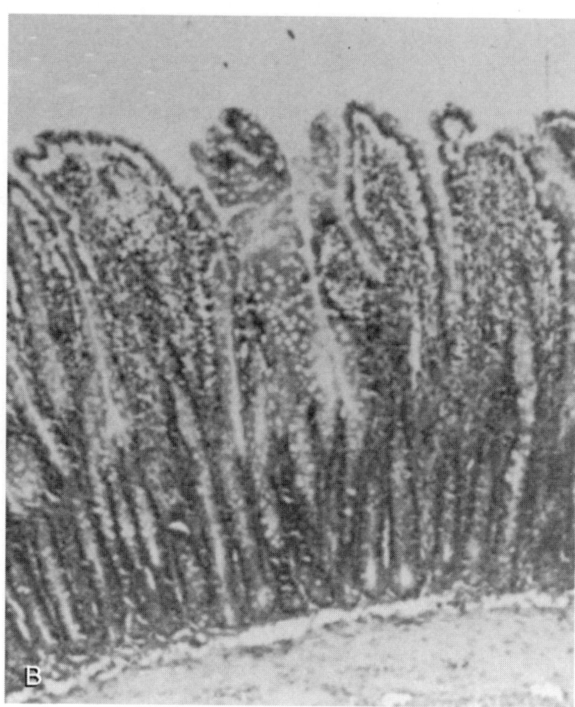


**FIGURE 26–3.** Ileal hyperplasia 1 month after jejunal resection in a rat maintained on a chow diet. *A,* Normal ileum. *B,* Ileum after jejunal resection. Hematoxylin and eosin, ×1,400. (From Weser E: Nutritional aspects of malabsorption: Short gut adaptation. Am J Med 1979;67:116; with permission.)

tine may normally function at a level close to the limit of its capacity to differentiate and adapt. The distal intestine, as a result of proximal absorption, may receive fewer nutrients ordinarily and function at less than full potential. Numerous studies have demonstrated that even in the presence of small bowel resection (the most potent trigger of small intestinal mucosal hyperplasia), no adaptation takes place unless luminal nutrients are provided. After intestinal resection, parenteral nutrition should be supplemented with enteral nutrients as soon as possible to stimulate adaptation.

An attempt has been made to determine the specific nutrients responsible for stimulating the adaptive response by infusing single nutrients into the gastrointestinal tract while the experimental animal is otherwise nourished with TPN. Among the micronutrients, long-chain triglycerides (LCT) given intragastrically after resection promote intestinal adaptation to a greater extent than proteins and polysaccharides.[72] The same effect is not seen with medium-chain triglycerides (MCT),[73] which are often used to provide a major source of fat calories to patients with SBS because they do not require digestion by pancreatic enzymes and colipase and are not as dependent on bile acids for micellar solubilization and absorption.

The effects of individual infusions of sugars on small bowel adaptation have also been studied. When infusions of 5% sucrose, maltose, and lactose are given, significantly greater mucosal growth is seen throughout the small bowel than with equal concentrations of glucose, fructose, and galactose.[74] These studies have given rise to the concept that the functional work of hydrolysis of disaccharides, which is necessary for their absorption, is more important to small bowel adaptation than simply luminal contact of the substrate with the enterocyte or even mucosal metabolism by the enterocyte of the resulting monosaccharides.[75]

Proteins also contribute to adaptive changes in the small intestine after resection. Some studies suggest that whole proteins such as casein are more potent than hydrolysates in inducing mucosal hyperplasia in rats undergoing small bowel resection.[76] However, even amino acids infused into the ileum have been shown to produce significant hyperplasia in rats maintained on TPN and to prevent hypoplasia of the jejunum when infused into the proximal small bowel.[77]

## The Role of Metabolic "Fuels" for the Enterocyte

### *Glutamine*

Glutamine is the preferred substrate for small bowel oxidative metabolism. When rats are fed with a standard formula lacking in glutamine, mucosal atrophy takes place.[78–80] Some animal studies have suggested a therapeutic effect of oral diets supplemented with glutamine fed to rats undergoing massive small bowel resections.[78–80] The provision of glutamine-enriched parenteral solutions as the sole source of nutrition is associated with relative preservation of small bowel mucosa in rats.[81] In these formulations, glutamine is substituted for other nonessential amino acids, and a direct correlation is found between glutamine intake and intestinal DNA content, mucosal wet weight, sucrase, maltase, and villous height.

Glutamine is absent from all but a few currently available elemental diets. No amino acid preparation for use in TPN contains glutamine because of poor stability and spontaneous degradation to pytoglutamic acid and ammonia. To overcome these problems, peptide analogues of glutamine have been developed.[82, 83]

### *Short-Chain Fatty Acids*

SCFAs, including primarily acetate, propionate, and butyrate, are produced by bacterial fermentation of dietary carbohydrates and fiber in the colon.[84] They are avidly absorbed by the colonic mucosa and, at the same time, stimulate colonic sodium and water absorption.[85, 86] SCFAs, especially butyrate, have been shown to be the preferred substrate for energy metabolism in isolated colonocytes.[87] Depending on the quantity of fiber and complex polysaccharides in the diet, colonic absorption of SCFA may normally supply 5 to 10% of the daily energy requirements.[88] The small intestine also has the capacity to absorb SCFA. Although normal SCFA concentrations within the small bowel are low, small intestinal mucosal absorption is as efficient as colonic absorption when SCFAs are available.[89]

Numerous animal studies have documented that removal of fiber from the diet results in reversible ileal and colonic mucosal atrophy.[90, 91] The adaptive effect of a fiber-supplemented diet is inhibited by antibiotics, suggesting that it is due to bacterial fermentation of available fiber and the production of SCFA.[92]

Preliminary investigations of the effect of SCFA or fermentable fiber supplementation in animal models of SBS have been published. Pectin is completely fermented by colonic bacteria to SCFA. In rats undergoing an 80% small bowel resection, pectin supplementation of an elemental diet resulted in increases in mucosal weight, DNA, RNA, and protein in the colon and small bowel compared with resected rats fed an elemental diet alone. Villus height, crypt depth, and mucosal thickness in the ileum were all significantly greater in the pectin-supplemented rats.[93] The addition of SCFA to TPN following massive small bowel resection in the adult rat prevented the usual small intestinal mucosal atrophy seen in rats maintained on SCFA-free TPN.[94]

## Trophic Effects of Enteric Hormones

The stimulus of mucosal adaptation in the proximal small bowel after infusion of nutrients into the distal segments, or the amelioration of mucosal atrophy in segments not in continuity with the nutrient stream, suggests that circulating gut hormones released by nutrient exposure play an important role.[95]

### *Enteroglucagon*

Interest in the hormone enteroglucagon was stimulated by the observation that a patient with an enteroglucagon-producing tumor of the kidney had intestinal mucosal hyperplasia that disappeared when the tumor was resected.[96] In animal models of bowel resection, plasma enteroglucagon levels are increased and correlate with the degree of resection and the crypt cell production rate in the remaining segment.[97, 98] Proglucagon-derived peptides may be responsible for some of the previously observed enteroglucagon effects.[99, 100]

### *Cholecystokinin, Secretin, and Pancreaticobiliary Secretions*

Diversion of pancreaticobiliary secretions into the ileum stimulates ileal mucosal growth, suggesting a role in small bowel adaptation.[101, 102] Complex diets are more effective than elemental diets, and TPN is less effective in stimulating endogenous pancreatic secretions. Studies in rats and dogs have shown that parenteral injections of cholecystokinin combined with secretin can prevent hypoplasia of intestinal mucosa associated with TPN.[103, 104] Experimental evidence suggests that the trophic effects of cholecystokinin seen in animal TPN models are secondary to hormonal stimulation of pancreaticobiliary secretions.[105]

### *Prostaglandins*

Prostaglandin $E_2$ ($PGE_2$) induces a proliferative response in the duodenum and proximal jejunum, particularly in suckling rats.[106] Studies of small intestinal adaptation suggest that prostaglandins stimulate mucosal hyperplasia by prolonging mucosal cell survival.[107, 108]

### *Growth Factors*

Epidermal growth factor (EGF) is a polypeptide hormone that is secreted directly into the small intestine by Brunner's glands and produces stimulation of DNA synthesis throughout the gastrointestinal tract.[109] When administered parenterally, EGF causes precocious development of the small intestine in suckling rats.[110] Parenteral administration of EGF significantly reduces the hypoplasia produced throughout the gastrointestinal tract by 10 days of TPN in adult rats and stimulates crypt cell production rates.[111] Saliva, duodenal secretions, and bile are rich sources of EGF, and this hormone may be an important factor in the maintenance of mucosal mass in the proximal small bowel and the mucosal proliferation in the ileum exposed to proximal intestinal contents after jejunectomy.[112] Growth hormone has also been implicated in the response to small bowel resection because hypophysectomized animals do not undergo mucosal hyperplasia following enterectomy in spite of the provision of sufficient enteral calories.[113] However, studies have not shown that growth hormone induces intestinal adaptation in rats after small bowel resection.[114] IgGl, a growth factor stimulated by growth hormone, does appear capable of inducing intestinal adaptation in this model.[115]

The role of other growth factors such as transforming growth factor-α is currently under investigation.[116]

## Polyamines in Intestinal Adaptation

Rapid tissue and cell growth is associated with the rapid accumulation of tissue polyamines. Ornithine is the starting substrate for the biosynthesis of the polyamines: putrescine, spermidine, and spermine. Decarboxylation of ornithine to form putrescine is the rate-limiting step in polyamine biosynthesis catalyzed by ornithine dicarboxylase (ODC). An increase in ODC activity is one of the earliest events that occurs during the transition of cells from dormancy to active proliferation.[117] Polyamines have been shown in vitro to facilitate nearly all aspects of DNA, RNA, and protein synthesis.

The question of the benefit of exogenously administered polyamines is raised by studies showing that spermine and spermidine given orally to neonatal rats induce precocious mucosal structural and biochemical changes characteristic of postweaning maturation.[118] One study in patients with SBS correlated postprandial jejunostomy fluid polyamine levels with intestinal remnant length and carbohydrate absorption,[119] suggesting that polyamine content might serve as an indicator of mucosal hyperplasia and prove useful in assessing the response to specific diets.

## MANAGEMENT OF THE PATIENT WITH SHORT BOWEL SYNDROME

The management of infants and children with massive intestinal resections can be divided into acute and chronic phases. The acute phase encompasses the stabilization of fluid and electrolyte needs, the early provision of parenteral nutrition to reverse catabolism, the judicious use of pharmacologic agents to combat gastric acid hypersecretion and loss of luminal fluid and electrolytes, and the limited provision of enteral glucose and electrolyte solutions and elemental diets to stimulate small bowel adaptation. The chronic phase includes the gradual transition from parenteral to enteral nutrition; determination of supplemental enteral fluid, electrolyte, divalent cation, trace element, and vitamin needs; and specific treatment of complications of SBS. Long-term management involves careful monitoring of growth and nutritional parameters and close surveillance for the potential complications of parenteral nutrition, including catheter-related sepsis, cholestatic liver disease, and gallstones. Loss of oral motor skills and aversion to oral feeding are particular problems in infants with SBS that must be addressed early, long before any substantial intake of nutrients by the oral route.

### Total Parenteral Nutrition and Fluid and Electrolyte Therapy

Infants and children undergoing massive intestinal resection require the immediate placement of a nutritional central venous catheter to allow for the management of their fluid, electrolyte, and nutritional needs in the postoperative period. In patients with less extensive resections, usually those with a remaining long jejunal segment, an intact ICV, and a colon in continuity, enteral feedings may be well tolerated after the initial brief postoperative ileus and period of anastomotic and wound healing. The purposes of the initial phase of therapy are to assess fluid and electrolyte losses and replace them in the parenteral fluid, and to provide adequate amino acids to maintain the synthesis of essential proteins and avoid excessive muscle catabolism.

Table 26–2 provides the approximate fluid and electrolyte composition of intestinal luminal contents at various segments. A key tenet of managing patients with SBS is to individualize their care by assessing and anticipating their specific needs. Excessive fluid losses via gastrostomy, jejunostomy, ileostomy, enterocutaneous fistula, or feces should be quantified by measuring the volume and electrolyte composition at each site. A comparable mixture of fluid and electrolytes can then be replaced prophylactically on a volume-per-volume basis. In the initial phases of acute management, when stool and ostomy output may be rapidly changing, the use of a second pump may be necessary, with a reassessment of the composition of the infused solution more than once a day. Later, when losses are more predictable, appropriate electrolytes can be added to the TPN solution to account fully for the proper balance. In addition to extra sodium and potassium, acetate (over and above the acetate salts of amino acids contained in many TPN solutions) will often be included to compensate for excessive losses of bicarbonate. Ostomy losses may change with time and must be periodically reviewed. An infant with a newly created ileostomy absorbs approximately 80% of the small bowel fluid load,[120] whereas a child with an established ileostomy absorbs more than 90% of the same volume.[121] This may be secondary to recruitment of an ileal amiloride-inhibitable sodium channel, which is normally present only in the distal colon and is stimulated by increased intestinal fluid losses and resulting mineralocorticoid excess.[122]

Patients with large volume and electrolyte losses benefit from early reanastomosis of the small intestine to the colon. In some patients with all or part of the colon bypassed, colonic infusion of fluid and electrolytes via a mucous fistula may be useful in maintaining plasma volume and positive fluid and electrolyte balance.[123] Reinfusion of secretions from the proximal stoma into the mucous fistula may allow reabsorption of up to 70% of the reinfused secretions and also prevent hypoplasia of the unused distal segment, thereby facilitating the eventual reanastomosis.[124, 125]

Standard quantities of vitamins and trace minerals are added to the parenteral nutrition solution and usually are sufficient. In patients with high-output proximal fistulas,

**TABLE 26–2. Fluid and Electrolyte Composition of Intestinal Luminal Contents of Infants**

| TYPE OF FLUID | AMOUNT (mL/kg/24 hr) | ION CONCENTRATION (mEq/L) | | |
|---|---|---|---|---|
| | | $Na^+$ | $K^+$ | $Cl^-$ |
| Dietary | 100 | 30 | 20 | 30 |
| Saliva | 70 | 3 | 25 | 20 |
| Gastric juice | 50 | 50 | 7.5 | 140 |
| Pancreaticobiliary secretions | 45 | 100 | 3 | 30 |
| Duodenum | 285 | — | — | — |
| Distal ileum* | 60 (new) | — | — | — |
| | 25 (established) | 100 | 26 | — |
| Rectum | 5–10 | 22 | 54 | 21 |

*Data from new ileostomies and established ileostomies.

Adapted from Rhodes JM, Powell DW: Diarrhea. In Walker WA, Durie PR, Hamilton JR, et al (eds): Pediatric Gastrointestinal Disease: Pathophysiology, Diagnosis, Management. Philadelphia, BC Decker, 1991, p. 63, with permission.

and in premature infants, additional zinc may be required. Deficiencies of zinc, copper, chromium, carnitine, manganese, selenium, and molybdenum all have been described in patients receiving prolonged TPN.[126] Prevention of the cardiomyopathy, macrocytosis, and depigmentation of skin and hair associated with selenium deficiency[127, 128] requires the addition of 20 μg/L of selenium to the TPN solution.[129] Monitoring blood levels of the above trace elements, as well as iron, biotin, vitamin $B_{12}$, folate, carnitine, and fat-soluble vitamins, every 3 to 6 months is mandatory in patients dependent on TPN.[130]

## ENTERAL FEEDINGS

Enteral feedings are of primary importance in stimulating the adaptive response to bowel resection. There has been a trend away from a prolonged period of "bowel rest" and toward earlier introduction of luminal nutrients in patients with SBS. In preparation for early feeding, a gastrostomy tube is often surgically placed at the time of the original intestinal resection. This facilitates enteral feeding in patients who may be too sick or unwilling to take appropriate formulas by mouth. The placement of a long-term nasogastric feeding tube may exacerbate upper respiratory problems or lead to the development of aversive feeding behavior and is a less attractive alternative. Regardless of the technique used to deliver nutrients, sucking behavior in infants should be encouraged to ease the eventual transition to oral feeding and contribute to more complete digestion of formula by stimulating the elaboration of lingual lipase and salivary amylase.[131] In general, continuous infusion is preferred over bolus administration of nutrients because of documentation of improved fat, nitrogen, calcium, zinc, and copper absorption in infants with SBS.[132] A significant increase in body weight during continuous feeding as compared with intermittent feeding has also been demonstrated in patients with SBS, chronic diarrhea, and congenital heart disease.[132, 133]

Glucose-containing fluid and electrolyte solutions are often the earliest enteral feedings employed. This first step in enteral feedings permits an assessment of the possible response to a more complex meal. A high-sodium–containing solution (approximately 85 mEq/L) used in conjunction with glucose or glucose polymers is well absorbed.[27, 134–136]

The optimal nutrient composition of enteral feedings in short bowel patients is controversial. Some studies have challenged previously held views that low-fat, elemental diets are best tolerated. Increased knowledge of small bowel adaptation has prompted investigation of new formulations designed to enhance mucosal hyperplasia and nutrient absorption.[137] In an effort to supply the gut with some luminal nutrients, the initial feeding is most often an elemental formula supplying less than 10% of the total daily caloric intake via constant intragastric feedings. Stool volume, pH, and reducing substances are closely monitored for signs of severe malabsorption, which would compromise fluid and electrolyte balance and mitigate against continued increases in enteral feeding. Advances must be slow, and parenteral nutrition must be reduced concurrently without compromising total protein and caloric intake. There is no evidence that diluting an enteral formula helps, and this practice only substitutes hypocaloric fluid for an equivalent volume of more complete parenteral nutrition. If marked carbohydrate intolerance is documented, a carbohydrate-free elemental formula can be used to supply some stimulus for mucosal adaptation. Glucose polymers or fructose may be added in graded concentrations as tolerated.

Previous studies in patients with SBS documented the efficacy of elemental diets with protein hydrolysates or amino acids, glucose polymers, and MCTs in the early adaptive stages of SBS.[138–140] These formulas were thought to be more easily absorbed and to stimulate less endogenous gastrointestinal secretions. However, more recent studies have shown that elemental diets are no better absorbed than polymeric ones even in the early phases of enteral feeding.[137, 141] In patients with jejunostomies, there is no difference in caloric absorption, stomal output, and electrolyte losses between an elemental and polymeric diet. Potential disadvantages of an elemental diet are the high cost, the high osmolality, and the lack of stimulation of colonic mucosal proliferation.[142]

Protein hydrolysates are typically used for the protein source. There is no clear indication that hydrolysates are better at inducing small bowel adaptation than intact proteins, but the former are more rapidly absorbed[143] and result in improved nitrogen balance in patients with end jejunostomies.[144] Since protein absorption occurs predominantly by intact dipeptide and tripeptide absorption, free amino acids are not necessary. In the presence of normal renal function, blood urea nitrogen (BUN) can be used as a rough guide to the adequacy of protein intake, both enteral and parenteral. A BUN level less than 4 mg/dL likely reflects too low a nitrogen intake, whereas a BUN greater than 20 mg/dL probably indicates an excessive nitrogen intake.

Carbohydrate is generally provided in the form of glucose polymers or sucrose. Lactose is poorly tolerated in most patients in the early phase after significant small bowel resection and should be avoided until adequate documentation of lactose tolerance. With increasing time for mucosal adaptation, carbohydrate absorption increases, improving to approximately 70% of the total carbohydrate ingested.[145, 146] Increased absorption is found in patients with a colon incontinuity, in whom salvage of carbohydrate by bacterial fermentation appears to be important in overall gut conservation of carbohydrate-derived energy.[147] In these patients, restriction of dietary lactose and sucrose and provision of some carbohydrate as complex polysaccharide (starch) or in the form of nonstarch fermentable fiber may improve overall energy utilization from carbohydrate, reduce colonic luminal osmolality, and facilitate colonic reabsorption of water. The addition of the fermentable fiber pectin to a diarrhea-inducing polymeric formula that was tube-fed to normal subjects reversed diarrhea and normalized low levels of fecal SCFAs.[148]

Documentation of the contribution of carbohydrate malabsorption to diarrhea has led to a re-evaluation of earlier observations that a high-carbohydrate, low-fat diet of predominantly MCTs was better for patients with SBS.[149, 150] Low-fat diets theoretically decrease the possibility that malabsorption of long-chain fatty acids will cause colonic water secretion and contribute to poor absorption of divalent cations. Some studies have contradicted these assumptions. In patients with jejunostomies, a high-fat diet induced a linear increase in the fat absorbed, an increased caloric intake, no increase in ostomy fluid output, but an increased loss of divalent cations.[151, 152] In a controlled crossover study of a high-fat versus a high-carbohydrate diet in adults with greater than 50% small bowel resection, there were no differences in the calcium, magnesium, and zinc absorbed, the volume of stool or ostomy output, urine volume, or electrolyte excretion between the dietary periods regardless of whether the patient had a jejunostomy, ileostomy, or enterocolonic anastomosis. Although the fecal fat excretion was three times higher on the high-fat than on the high-carbohydrate diet, the proportion of ingested fat absorbed was unchanged, and the mean percentage of total calories absorbed averaged 65% of intake on both diets.[153] A study of six infants with intractable diarrhea, including four with SBS, also demonstrated satisfactory weight gain and no differences in stool weight, electrolyte losses, and the enteral absorption of fat in infants fed a lower-carbohydrate, higher-fat formula.[154] The preponderance of fecal energy loss was from carbohydrate-derived energy irrespective of formula consumed. These studies, and the increased palatability of higher-fat diets, suggest that many patients with SBS need not be relegated to low-fat diets for a prolonged period.

The transition to oral bolus feedings from parenteral nutrition and constant enteral tube feedings is often very gradual and may take months or even years. The rapidity of this transition depends not only on the length and health of the remaining intestine but also on the avoidance of medical and surgical complications. With the advent of home parenteral nutrition, it is routine for the patient to be sent home on some combination of cycled parenteral and enteral nasogastric or gastrostomy feedings even while the transition to oral formula and solid foods is being made. Several studies have assessed the absorptive capacity of stable short-bowel patients in an attempt to define their nutritional needs and predict the eventual transition to a full oral diet.[145, 146] Stable adults with SBS ingesting an ad libitum oral diet absorb approximately two thirds of total ingested calories and up to three fourths of dietary protein. These studies dictate that for eventual autonomy from parenteral nutrition, the patient must have the capacity to ingest at least 150% of expected kilocalories per kilogram and 130% of expected grams per kilogram protein for ideal body weight to counteract the increased losses of nutrients. Adaptive hyperphagia has been observed in several studies of ambulatory patients allowed ad libitum oral intake.[155, 156] Compensatory hyperphagia would be expected to develop only in infants and children with no active bowel disease, no stricture or severe motility disturbance, and no aversion to oral feedings.

Poor absorption of fat-soluble vitamins, calcium, magnesium, and zinc is common in children with SBS. Without supplementation, complications of rickets or tetany may accompany calcium, magnesium, and vitamin D malabsorption, especially in infants and children with less than 50 cm of remaining small intestine at the time of the original surgery.[157] Oral administration of most minerals and vitamins is usually sufficient to maintain serum levels, although intermittent parenteral administration of vitamins K and D may occasionally be necessary. Availability of newer preparations of vitamins E and D complexed with polyethylene-glycol succinate enhance absorption even in a bile salt—deficient luminal environment.[158] In patients with ileal resections greater than 100 cm, vitamin $B_{12}$ malabsorption is invariably present. Periodic screening of blood cell counts, blood smears, and serum $B_{12}$ levels is important, and, if necessary, a Schilling's test can be performed. Replacement of calcium is often mandatory, especially in patients consuming a lactose-free diet. Parenteral injections of magnesium sulfate or citrate may be necessary because oral magnesium supplements often lead to increased diarrhea.

Oxalate excretion should be monitored in those with steatorrhea and an intact colon. If hyperoxaluria is demonstrated (urinary oxalate excretion $>$ 50 mg/day), a low-oxalate diet is instituted eliminating chocolate, tea, cola, and vegetables such as spinach, celery, and carrots. The addition of oral calcium supplements may also help decrease oxalate absorption and excretion in the urine, decreasing the risk of oxalate renal stones. Inability to achieve therapeutic blood levels with oral antibiotics may also be a problem in children with SBS. Absorption appears to be proportional to the length of the remaining bowel, and significant malabsorption is common in infants who have undergone greater than a 50% small bowel resection.[159] In these patients, parenteral antibiotics are necessary for even routine infections such as otitis media.

## PHARMACOLOGIC THERAPY

The goals of drug therapy in patients with SBS are to reduce incapacitating diarrhea, help control fluid and electrolyte loss, and treat intervening complications. Pharmacologic manipulations cannot compensate for lack of absorption and may be detrimental if used indiscriminately, but judicious use of drugs may permit the patient to control symptoms sufficiently to leave the hospital. Both cimetidine and ranitidine effectively suppress gastric acid hypersecretion and reduce gastric secretory volume after massive small bowel resection.[160, 161] Cimetidine and, more recently, omeprazole also decrease jejunostomy fluid volume and excretion of sodium and potassium in adults with severe SBS.[162] Cimetidine prevents marked drops in jejunal pH and enhances fatty acid absorption in adults with massive small bowel resection and a jejunocolostomy.[45] Intravenous administration of an $H_2$ receptor antagonist should start immediately after the bowel resection. Oral treatment is rarely necessary for longer than 1 year post resection.

Several antidiarrheal drugs including codeine, diphenoxylate, and anticholinergic agents have been used in patients with SBS. In children, the only drug of this kind that has gained widespread acceptance is loperamide because of its lack of extraintestinal opiate effects at therapeutic doses. Loperamide decreases ileal output in patients with ileostomies.[163] Other factors such as the known antisecretory activity or effects on colonic motility may play a role in the drug's antidiarrheal activity.[164] Doses from 0.1 to 1.0 mg/kg per day have been used in children with SBS. Some caution must be exercised in those patients with risk factors for bacterial overgrowth, since delay in intestinal transit would be expected to promote proliferation of small bowel flora.

Cholestyramine, an ion-exchange resin that binds intraluminal dihydroxy bile acids, is often given to reduce the effects of malabsorbed bile salts on the colon.[165] In children, an appropriate dose is 100 to 250 mg/kg per day in three divided doses. Cholestyramine also binds dietary oxalate and prevents its absorption. Disadvantages of cholestyramine therapy include further depletion of an already shrunken bile salt pool in those patients with steatorrhea. In these cases, the drug may actually worsen the diarrhea and steatorrhea. With this concern in mind, some clinicians will use cholestyramine only in conjunction with high MCT formulas or a low-fat diet.[14, 22] A therapeutic trial may be necessary to determine the drug's potential benefit in the individual patient. Cholestyramine also binds vitamin D and may exacerbate malabsorption of other fat-soluble vitamins as well as folate.[166] In large doses, cholestyramine can cause a hyperchloremic metabolic acidosis. Aluminum hydroxide antacids also bind bile salts but are associated with depletion of phosphorus and calcium and resultant osteomalacia.[167, 168]

Octreotide is an octapeptide somatostatin analogue that has been used successfully to partially control diarrhea associated with vasoactive intestinal polypeptide–secreting tumors and carcinoid syndrome in adults[169–171] and with idiopathic secretory diarrhea and congenital microvillous atrophy in children.[172, 173] Somatostatin is known to inhibit exocrine secretions from the stomach, pancreas, and small intestine and to reduce splanchnic blood flow and slow gastrointestinal motility.[174, 175] Octreotide can be administered subcutaneously. The clinical effect peaks 2 hours after injection and lasts for up to 12 hours. The use of intravenous and subcutaneous octreotide has been investigated in patients with SBS.[176] In a 5-year-old patient, octreotide reduced massive ileostomy fluid losses by two thirds and prolonged transit time from mouth to ileostomy from 20 to 360 minutes.[177]

In the few long-term studies of octreotide in the management of patients with SBS, drug tolerance has been good, with no significant changes in glucose homeostasis, thyroid function, or fat malabsorption. Data on growth hormone secretion and growth velocity in children treated with long-term octreotide are not available. At present, it appears that octreotide may reduce stomal or fecal water and sodium loss and decrease reliance on parenteral supplementation or oral rehydration solutions. However, tachyphylaxis to octreotide may occur. The drug may also increase the risk of cholelithiasis, and by its inhibition of pancreatic and biliary secretions, could inhibit small intestinal adaptation.[178, 179]

Treatment of chronic bacterial overgrowth may result in profound improvement of diarrhea. The diagnosis should be suspected in the child with SBS whose intolerance to enteral feedings is out of proportion to the residual length of small intestine or whose diarrhea significantly worsens, with excessive bloating, eructation, and flatulence. Megaloblastic anemia is typically present. Folate levels are usually normal or even high, since intestinal bacteria produce folic acid, but serum vitamin $B_{12}$ levels are low, and vitamin $B_{12}$ absorption with or without added intrinsic factor is abnormal. Less commonly, iron deficiency anemia or a mixed picture results from mucosal damage and chronic blood loss secondary to bacterial overgrowth. Some patients with bacterial overgrowth develop colitis or ileitis with large ulcerations that appear similar to Crohn's disease. This form of colitis occasionally responds to antimicrobial therapy, although sulfasalazine and occasionally a short course of corticosteroids are necessary. Deficiencies in fat-soluble vitamins may appear with the patient presenting with purpura, osteomalacia, or night blindness. Hypoproteinemia is common and may reflect a protein-losing enteropathy. Small bowel barium roentgenograms should be performed in any patient with these findings to show the site and extent of any structural lesion. Enteroclysis can better delineate a discrete stricture or mucosal disease.

The gold standard for the diagnosis of bacterial overgrowth has been proximal small bowel intubation and the demonstration of the presence of a complex flora of strict anaerobes and coliforms in numbers greater than $10^6$ organisms per ml.[180] Because of the difficulty performing this test on infants and small children, the possible contamination with mouth and upper respiratory flora, and the requirement for strict anaerobic culture techniques, other less invasive tests have been developed. A single elevated fasting breath hydrogen sample[181] or a combination of a high fasting breath hydrogen and a rise in breath hydrogen 2 hours after a 50-g oral glucose challenge has been advocated as an indicator of bacterial overgrowth.[182] Many of these breath tests suffer from difficulty in separating patients with massive small bowel resection (whose rapid transit and subsequent colonic bacterial action on the fermentable or labeled substrate would be expected to yield an early peak) from those with true proximal small bowel bacterial overgrowth. In this respect, the $^{14}C$ D-xylose breath test may have an advantage, since a small dose should be totally absorbed even in a short proximal bowel, provided the mucosa is intact.[183]

The choice of antimicrobial therapy has largely been empiric. Tetracycline enjoys popularity in adult patients because of its effectiveness against *Bacteroides* species. In pediatric patients, combinations of metronidazole and trimethoprim-sulfamethoxazole or oral vancomycin and gentamicin have been used with success. Cyclic treatment of 1 week every 1 to 2 months may be necessary. Surgical procedures to resect a stricture or taper a dilated hypotonic segment have been reported to be effective in small numbers of cases (see later). Prokinetic agents such as metaclopromide and cisapride may be useful in patients with dilated proximal segments, bile reflux, pseudo-obstruction, and bacterial overgrowth.[184] In some patients, the judicious use of balanced polyethylene glycol–electrolyte solutions to promote defecation and reduce stasis and bacterial proliferation has been advocated.

One study reported the beneficial effects of combination therapy with growth hormone, oral and/or parenteral glutamine supplementation, and a diet high in complex carbohydrates (60% of total calories) in adult patients with SBS, many of whom were able to wean from or reduce their parenteral nutrition requirement substantially with this treatment.[185] Balance studies were performed that showed that patients receiving the special diet and both glutamine and growth hormone experienced a reduction in stool weight and an increase in protein absorption, whereas no such effects were seen in the groups receiving the diet alone or the diet supplemented with either glutamine or growth hormone.

## LONG-TERM PARENTERAL NUTRITION THERAPY

The development of TPN is the most important technical advance in improving growth, development, and survival in infants and children with SBS. The advent of home parenteral nutrition has revolutionized long-term care and allowed children and families to enjoy a more normal life in spite of severe gastrointestinal pathology. Often, the parenteral nutrition infusion can be limited to the night-time hours, allowing routine daily activities and school attendance. Several studies have demonstrated that children with SBS receiving home TPN therapy can achieve normal growth rates, anthropometric measurements, and visceral protein levels.[186, 187] However, with prolonged use of TPN has come the recognition of major complications. Morbidity and mortality are most commonly related to central venous catheter infections and progressive liver disease, which accounted for 11 deaths in 102 patients over a 10-year period in one review.[188]

## Catheter-Related Infections

In 104 cases of infants and children collated from three series of neonatal SBS patients who were receiving TPN at home, the rate of catheter-related sepsis approximated 2.0 episodes per 1,000 days.[11, 13, 14] Gram-positive cocci dominate the list of organisms responsible for Broviac catheter sepsis, accounting for approximately 60 to 75% of all isolates.[189] Coagulase-negative *Staphylococcus* is the most common isolate in our experience. *Staphylococcus aureus* and streptococcal species are also important pathogens, and gram-negative rods including *Pseudomonas* species account for about 25% of blood isolates. Fungal infections are uncommon but result in a high degree of mortality. We currently prescribe oral antifungal prophylaxis to all patients with SBS maintained on home TPN. Antibiotic prophylaxis should also be considered prior to dental work, gastrointestinal endoscopies or cystoscopies, incision and drainage of abscesses, and after any episode of catheter breakage and repair.

Every patient with SBS and a fever, no obvious focal infection, and a central venous catheter should be treated for potential catheter-related sepsis. A high white blood cell count is suggestive but is not always present. New onset of glucose intolerance and glycosuria may be helpful clues. In many cases, eradication of the organism causing sepsis can be accomplished without removal of the catheter.[190, 191] A response to therapy with resolution of fever is usually seen within a 5-day period, and lack of response has been associated with the presence of an abscess, endocarditis, septic venous thrombosis, pulmonary embolism, immunocompromised status, and the organisms *Pseudomonas aeruginosa* and *Candida albicans*.[192, 193] Infections with these organisms are absolute indications to remove the catheter. If blood cultures remain positive for 48 hours after isolation of an organism and treatment with appropriate antibiotics, strong consideration should be given to removing the catheter. Because of the high incidence of infections with non-*aureus* staphylococcal species, treatment should be initiated with vancomycin plus an antibiotic to cover aerobic gram-negative enteric organisms.

## TPN-Associated Liver Disease

The etiology of progressive cholestatic liver disease associated with prolonged TPN is not fully elucidated.[194] Retrospective studies of premature neonates receiving TPN have found that intestinal resection for necrotizing enterocolitis and other congenital abnormalities is a strong risk factor for the development of cholestasis.[195–197] Intestinal bacterial proliferation, particularly of anaerobic organisms, may be involved in the pathogenesis of cholestatic liver injury in patients with SBS.[198]

Mechanisms postulated to link hepatic disease with intestinal bacterial proliferation include bacterial deconjugation of bile salts and production of hepatotoxic bile acids,[199] release of bacterial endotoxin,[200] or release of bacterial cell wall components such as peptidoglycan-polysaccharide polymers directly into the portal circulation.[201]

Death from severe progressive liver disease was documented in 10 out of 190 pediatric patients with SBS on long-term TPN.[10–14] Early institution of enteral feedings to promote intestinal motility, avoidance of iron overload,[198] and attention to the treatment of bacterial overgrowth with antibiotics, prokinetic agents, and surgical procedures may significantly reduce the morbidity and mortality associated with this complication.

# SURGICAL THERAPY

Surgical therapy should be reserved for patients with specific complications such as strictures or partial obstruction with resulting dilatation, stasis, and bacterial overgrowth; or for those whose anatomy precludes sufficient adaptation to allow autonomy from parenteral nutrition.[202, 203] The risk of making the patient worse by further resection or creation of new adhesions or strictures must be balanced against the risk of recurrent catheter-related sepsis, progressive liver disease, or loss of available sites for nutritional catheters. Though some of the procedures described in the following sections have shown remarkable anecdotal success, controlled, prospective long-term studies are lacking, and firm conclusions about their merits are difficult to reach.

## Intestinal Interpositions

Based on studies in animals, reversal of short segments of small intestine (3–15 cm) or interposition of isoperistaltic or antiperistaltic segments of colon has been advocated to delay gastric emptying, slow intestinal transit, and increase absorption.[204–207] Warden and Wesley[208] reversed 3-cm segments of distal ileum in five infants with greater than 25 cm of residual small bowel at the time of the reversal. All patients had at least initial improvements, with two showing an increase in mouth-to-anus transit time; however, diarrhea recurred in one, and another died of overwhelming pneumonia soon after surgery.[208] Other reports also describe initial improvement followed by a return to the preoperative status.[203]

Glick and coworkers[209] reported the interposition of 8 to 14 cm of isoperistaltic colon, just distal to the ligament of Treitz, in six infants with SBS. It was not clear why only three of the infants responded and were able to discontinue parenteral nutrition. The major disadvantage of interposition of both small intestinal and colonic reversed segments is that they cause an element of functional obstruction that may favor stasis and an increased tendency for bacterial overgrowth.

### Intestinal Lengthening and Tapering Procedures

In 1980, Bianchi[210] devised a method in pigs that had undergone massive small bowel resection for doubling the length of the dilated remaining small bowel based on the arrangement of the blood vessels of the mesentery. These vessels divide into anterior and posterior branches, permitting longitudinal splitting of the gut between them, reconstruction of the split gut into narrower tubes, and reanastomosis of these tubes in continuity. Four children underwent the tube intestinal lengthening procedure, increasing their small bowel length from 30 to 54 cm to 42 to 101 cm. All were able to wean from TPN to full enteral feedings. However, one required a second laparotomy for intestinal obstruction, and in three of the children, the operation was performed before full intestinal adaptation had taken place.[211] Tapering the dilated segment of small bowel is as important as, if not more important than, lengthening it to restore coaptation of the walls and more normal peristalsis in patients with stasis and bacterial overgrowth.[212] Tapering enteroplasty is effective at the time of an original operation for intestinal atresia as well.[213] Other strategies to preserve intestinal length include stricturoplasty and serosal patching,[214] particularly in those with Crohn's disease in whom discrete strictures or perforations may develop, otherwise necessitating multiple small bowel resections.

### Artificial Enteric Sphincters

The importance of a functioning ICV to prolong small bowel transit and prevent bacterial overgrowth has prompted efforts to construct an artificial ICV. Studies have shown benefits of surgically constructed valves in experimental animals[215, 216]; however, attempts in humans have yielded inconclusive results and, in certain cases, have led to obstruction.[217, 218] Most artificial valves are created by deliberately fashioning a short jejunocolic or colojejunal intussusception or fashioning a small bowel–to–colon anastomosis via a submucosal tunnel in the receiving colon.

## SMALL BOWEL TRANSPLANTATION

Although technically easier to perform than liver transplantation, small bowel and multivisceral tranplantation has lagged behind in development because of the complexity of immunosuppression required to prevent both rejection and graft-versus-host disease (GVHD) after the procedure. With the discovery and use of tacrolimus (FK506), successes with both small bowel and combined small bowel and liver transplantation have increased, and these procedures have become accepted modalities of therapy for patients who fail to undergo adequate bowel adaptation and remain wedded to parenteral nutrition to survive.

Table 26–3 summarizes the disorders resulting in intestinal transplantation in children at the University of Pittsburgh between 1990 and 1993. These include many of the most prominent causes of SBS in children but also encompass other causes of gut failure, including microvillus inclusion disease, intestinal pseudo-obstruction, and polyposis syndromes.[219] Other series in children include patients with congenital defects in intestinal electrolyte transport and autoimmune enteritis.[220, 221] In adults, diseases that are more likely to lead to small bowel transplantation include Crohn's disease, mesenteric ischemia and infarction, and inoperable intestinal tumors. Dependency on TPN must not be the sole criterion for transplantation, because many children on TPN can expect a year of survival with an excellent quality of life. Factors that raise consideration of small intestinal or liver–small bowel transplant include the development of end-stage liver disease; impending loss of venous access and catheter sites for the administration of TPN; recurrent episodes of potentially fatal complications (such as catheter-related sepsis, esophageal and small bowel variceal bleeding, pulmonary embolism); and reasonable certainty that intestinal dysfunction is permanent. That certainty exists for children with microvillus inclusion disease, generalized polyposis syndromes, congenital transport defects, or bowel resections leaving less than 15 cm of remaining jejunum (especially without an ICV). Children left with more than 15 cm of jejunum in infancy should not be subjected to small intestinal transplantation unless adaptation fails to occur within 2 or 3 years or prolonged TPN is impossible or unsafe.

**TABLE 26–3. Disorders Resulting in Intestinal Transplant at the University of Pittsburgh, 1990–1993**

| DIAGNOSIS | NO. OF PATIENTS |
|---|---|
| Midgut volvulus | 8 |
| Gastroschisis | 8 |
| Necrotizing enterocolitis | 6 |
| Microvillus inclusion disease | 2 |
| Small bowel atresia | 3 |
| Neuropathic pseudo-obstruction | 2 |
| Hollow viscus myopathy | 1 |
| Hirschsprung's disease | 1 |
| Multiple juvenile polyposis | 1 |

Adapted from Kocoshis SA: Small bowel transplantation in infants and children. Gastroenterol Clin North Am 1994;23:727–742, with permission.

Since 1985, more than 180 small bowel transplantations have been done, involving the isolated small bowel with or without the colon (38%), the liver and small bowel (46%), or several organs, including at times the stomach and pancreas (16%).[222, 223] Two thirds of the recipients were younger than 20 years of age with 46% younger than 5 years of age and 18% 5 to 20 years of age. Fifty-one percent of patients have survived for more than 2 years after the graft (Table 26–4). Death was caused mainly by infections (42%), multiorgan failure (30%), or lymphoma (post-transplant lymphoproliferative disease) (11%). Eighty percent of the survivors had a functional intestinal graft and were no longer receiving parenteral nutrition. As Table 26–4 shows, the patient and graft survival depended on the type of primary immunosuppression used, with a distinct advantage seen in patients treated with tacrolimus versus cyclosporine. Subsequent results in children whose transplants took place at mature small bowel transplant centers reflect improved outcomes gained by experience. Four-year survival rates at Pittsburgh Children's Hospital in 37 children are 40% in those undergoing combined liver–small bowel transplants and 60% in

**TABLE 26–4. Graft and Patient Survival 1 and 3 Years After Transplantation: International Intestinal Transplant Registry (1985–1995)**

| TYPE OF TRANSPLANTATION | IMMUNOSUPPRESSIVE TREATMENT | NUMBER OF GRAFTS | % GRAFT SURVIVAL/ % PATIENT SURVIVAL AT 1 YEAR | % GRAFT SURVIVAL/ % PATIENT SURVIVAL AT 3 YEARS |
|---|---|---|---|---|
| Small bowel | Tacrolimus | 48 | 65/83 | 29/47 |
| Small bowel | Cyclosporine | 21 | 17/57 | 11/50 |
| Small bowel + liver | Tacrolimus | 64 | 64/66 | 38/40 |
| Small bowel + liver | Cyclosporine | 19 | 44/44 | 28/28 |
| Multivisceral | Tacrolimus | 17 | 51/59 | 37/43 |
| Multivisceral | Cyclosporine | 11 | 41/41 | 41/41 |

Adapted from Goulet O: Intestinal transplantation. J Pediatr Gastroenterol Nutr 1997;25:1–11, with permission.

those with isolated small intestinal transplantation. Twenty-six pediatric transplantations, 17 combined and 8 intestine alone, have been performed at the University of Nebraska with 1-year patient survival rates of 73% and 100%, respectively. In six combined small bowel–liver transplants performed in Paris since late 1994, five patients are alive and free from parenteral nutrition with a follow-up of 8 to 26 months.

All patients undergoing intestinal transplantation experience at least one episode of intestinal rejection, and most programs create an ileostomy at the time of insertion of the graft to facilitate frequent protocol-driven endoscopic and histologic monitoring. Tacrolimus and corticosteroids are administered immediately to prevent rejection. In addition, other drugs including $PGE_1$, broad-spectrum antibiotic and antifungal drugs, gancyclovir or acyclovir, and intravenous immunoglobulin are variously used to prevent infection and bowel ischemia. Clinical observations, endoscopic examination, and bowel histologic findings are used to monitor for intestinal rejection. Clinical features that correlate well with histologic rejection are sudden onset of fever, abdominal distention, ileus, increased ileostomy output, hematemesis, stomal bleeding, and discoloration of the stoma. Septicemia due to enteric organisms also correlates strongly with intestinal rejection. The earliest endoscopic signs of rejection are edema, erythema, and aperistalsis. More advanced rejection is characterized by aphthous ulcers advancing to broad-based ulcers, or even completely denuded mucosa at times covered by a pseudomembrane. Acute cellular rejection is marked by the presence of activated lymphocytes attacking crypt epithelium and apoptosis of crypt cells.[224] Because cytomegalovirus (CMV) infections are a major risk to intestinal transplant recipients and because the signs and histologic features of CMV enteritis can mimic graft rejection, it is essential to rule out CMV in all intestinal biopsies using immune histochemistry or in situ hybridization techniques. Changes of rejection may involve the entire bowel or they may be patchy. Usually the ileum is more severely involved than the jejunum but not always. Hepatic and intestinal rejection may occur simultaneously, and often upper and lower (ileoscopy) endoscopy and biopsy as well as liver biopsy must be performed to make a diagnosis.

In addition to rejection and infection, post-transplant lymphoproliferative disease (PTLD) caused by infection with Epstein-Barr virus (EBV) remains a difficult complication of small bowel transplantation. Patients who develop PTLD have generally received substantially more immunosuppression prior to the onset of their tumors than those children without PTLD. These patients are treated with a reduction or cessation of their immunosuppression, intravenous immunoglobulin, acyclovir, and α-interferon. Unfortunately, in spite of EBV-induced suppression of helper T cells, intestinal transplant patients often experience rejection soon after their immunosuppressive regimen is curtailed.

As soon as the postoperative ileus resolves, most children undergoing intestinal transplantation are fed continuously with elemental formulas composed of amino acids or hydrolyzed proteins and relatively low in fat or high in MCTs. These are given to compensate for the postoperative dysfunction of mesenteric lymphatics. Although lymphatics generally recanalize, this process usually takes several weeks, after which a more complex formula containing LCT can be introduced. Chylous ascites has been recognized during this phase in several patients. Most of these patients are susceptible to osmotic diarrhea, and secretory diarrhea frequently develops in the presence of intercurrent infections or mild rejection. Stool losses are often high in fluid and sodium content and mandate prompt intervention with careful replacement of ongoing fluid losses intravenously. Rotaviral infection can be fatal in these patients. Patients and parents must be trained in techniques to recognize signs of dehydration, to measure ostomy and stool losses, and to replace those losses immediately with supplemental oral rehydration solutions even before the start of intravenous therapy.

## PROGNOSIS OF INFANTS AND CHILDREN WITH SHORT BOWEL SYNDROME

The prognosis of SBS has dramatically improved since the advent of TPN. With the advent of small bowel transplantation as a viable therapeutic option, even those infants with intestinal loss so massive as to make the possibility of enteral nutrition unlikely may be candidates for support with TPN.[315] Decisions about rational treatment must be made on an individual basis. Most infants are currently treated with lifesaving surgery and prolonged nutritional support to buy time for further development and refinement of clinical small bowel transplantation.

Table 26–5 summarizes the most recent collected series of infants with SBS. Prior to the routine use of long-term TPN, Wilmore and Dudrick collected much of the published pediatric experience through 1972.[1] The survival rate was

**TABLE 26–5. Prognosis of Short Bowel Syndrome in Infants**

| | WILMORE[3] | BOHAN[9] | COOPER[10] | DORNEY[11] | GROSFELD[12] | CANIANO[13] | GOULET[14] | |
|---|---|---|---|---|---|---|---|---|
| Total no. of patients | 50 | 15 | 16 | 13 | 54 | 14 | 87 | |
| Residual length of jejunoileum (cm) | 0–75 | 25–150 | 15–105 | 0–30 | 13–120 | 15–53 | <40 | 40–80 |
| No. (%) of patients who survived | 26 (52) | 13 (86) | 13 (81) | 9 (69) | 45 (83) | 12 (86) | 24 (67) | 47 (92) |
| No. reaching full adaptation* | 26 (52%) | 12/13 | 13/13 | 5/9 | ? | 8/12 | 18/24 | 44/47 |
| Time (mean or range) to full adaptation (mo) | ? | 2–10 | 14 | 4–32 | 13/14 | 18 | 27 | 14 |
| No. (%) of deaths | 24 (48) | 2 (14) | 3 (19) | 4 (31) | 9 (17) | 2 (14) | 16 (18) | |
| Causes of death | | | | | | | | |
| Sepsis | ? | 2/2 | 0/3 | 2/4 | 3/9 | 0/2 | 12/16 | |
| Hepatic failure | ? | 0/2 | 3/3 | 2/4 | 5/9 | 2/2 | 0/16 | |
| Gallstones and cholangitis | ? | ? | ? | 6/13 | 2/54 | 3/14 | 9/87 | |

*Full adaptation is defined as complete autonomy from parenteral nutrition and full enteral feedings.

95% in 20 infants with a jejunoileal length of 38 to 75 cm, both with and without an ICV. Infants with 15 to 38 cm of jejunoileum survived 50% of the time, provided the ICV was intact; those without an ICV all died. All infants with less than 15 cm of small intestine with or without an ICV died. Overall survival was 52%.

Since that time, survival has improved, and the length of viable residual jejunoileum deemed necessary for survival and eventual small bowel adaptation has decreased. Most series have documented greater than 80% overall survival.[10–14] In infants with only 0 to 30 cm of residual jejunoileum, the survival rate was still 69%.[11] Goulet and colleagues documented a 94% survival rate in infants with less than 40 cm of small bowel born after 1980 (when home parenteral nutrition was introduced) compared with a 65% survival rate for those treated prior to 1980.[14] Survival continues to be correlated with the length of remaining jejunoileum: 92% of infants with 40 to 80 cm of residual small intestine survived versus 66% of those with less than 40 cm.[14]

## REFERENCES

1. Wilmore DW, Dudrick SJ: Growth and development of an infant receiving all nutrients exclusively by vein. JAMA 1968; 203:860–864.
2. Schroeder P, Goulet O, Lear PA: Small bowel transplantation: European experience. Lancet 1990; 336:110–111.
3. Wilmore DW: Factors correlating with a successful outcome following extensive intestinal resection in newborn infants. J Pediatr 1972; 80:88–95.
4. Siebert JR: Small intestine length in infants and children. Am J Dis Child 1980; 134:593–595.
5. Touloukian RJ, Walker Smith GJ: Normal intestinal length in preterm infants. J Pediatr Surg 1983; 18:720–723.
6. Trier JS, Winter HS: Anatomy, embryology, and developmental abnormalities of the small intestine and colon. *In* Sleisenger MH, Fordtran JS, eds: Gastrointestinal Disease: Pathophysiology, Diagnosis, and Management. Philadelphia, WB Saunders, 1989, pp 991–1021.
7. Klish WJ, Putnam TC: The short gut. Am J Dis Child 1981; 135:1056–1061.
8. Ziegler MM: Short bowel syndrome in infancy: Etiology and management. Clin Perinatol 1986; 13:163–173.
9. Bohane TD, Haka-Ikse K, Biggar WD, et al: A clinical study of young infants after small intestinal resection. J Pediatr 1979; 94:552–558.
10. Cooper A, Floyd TF, Ross AJ, et al: Morbidity and mortality of short-bowel syndrome acquired in infancy: An update. J Pediatr Surg 1984; 19:711–717.
11. Dorney SFA, Ament ME, Berquist WE, et al: Improved survival in very short small bowel of infancy with use of long-term parenteral nutrition. J Pediatr 1985; 107:521–525.
12. Grosfeld JL, Rescorla FJ, West JW: Short bowel syndrome in infancy and childhood. Am J Surg 1986; 151:41–46.
13. Caniano DA, Starr J, Ginn-Pease ME: Extensive short bowel syndrome in neonates: Outcome in the 1980s. Surgery 1989; 105:119–124.
14. Goulet OJ, Revillon Y, Jan D, et al: Neonatal short bowel syndrome. J Pediatr 1991; 119:18–23.
15. Ricour C, Duhamel JF, Arnaud-Battandier F, et al: Enteral and parenteral nutrition in the short-bowel syndrome in children. World J Surg 1985; 9:310–315.
16. Grosfeld JL, Rescorla FJ, West KW: Gastrointestinal injuries in childhood: Analysis of 53 patients. J Pediatr Surg 1989; 24:580–583.
17. Appleton GVN, Bristol JB, Williamson RCH: Proximal enterectomy provides a stronger systemic stimulus to intestinal adaption than distal enterectomy. Gut 1987; 28(S1):165–168.
18. Gelinas MD, Morin CL, Morrisset J: Exocrine pancreatic function following proximal small bowel resection in rats. J Physiol 1982; 322:71–82.
19. Ameen VZ, Powell GK, Jones LA: Quantitation of fecal carbohydrate excretion in patients with short bowel syndrome. Gastroenterology 1987; 92:493–500.
20. Fordtran JS, Rectror FC, Carter NW: The mechanisms of sodium absorption in the human intestine. J Clin Invest 1968; 47:884–900.
21. Schiff ER, Small NC, Dietschy JM: Characterization of the kinetics of the passive and active transport mechanisms of bile acid absorption in the small intestine and colon of the rat. J Clin Invest 1972; 51:1351–1362.
22. Hofmann AF, Poley JR: Role of bile acid malabsorption in pathogenesis of diarrhea and steatorrhea in patients with ileal resection: I. Response to cholestyramine or replacement of dietary long-chain triglyceride by medium-chain triglyceride. Gastroenterology 1972; 62:918–934.
23. Chadwick VS, Gaginella TS, Carlson GL, et al: Effect of molecular structure on bile acid–induced alterations in absorptive function, permeability, and morphology in the perfused rabbit colon. J Lab Clin Med 1979; 94:661–674.
24. Saunders DR, Hedges JR, Sillery J, et al: Morphological and functional effects of bile salts on rat colon. Gastroenterology 1975; 68:1236–1245.
25. Mekhjian HS, Phillips SF, Hofmann AF: Colonic secretion of water and electrolytes induced by bile acids: Perfusion studies in man. J Clin Invest 1971; 50:1569–1577.
26. Heubi JE, Ballstren WF, Partin JC, et al: Enterohepatic circulation of bile acids in infants and children with ileal resection. J Lab Clin Med 1980; 95:231–240.
27. Allard JP, Jeejeebhoy KN: Nutritional support and therapy in the short bowel syndrome. Gastroenterol Clin 1989;18:589–601.
28. Debongnie JC, Phillips SF: Capacity of the human colon to absorb fluid. Gastroenterology 1978; 74:698–703.
29. Mitchel JE, Breuer RI, Zuckerman L, et al: The colon influences ileal resection diarrhea. Dig Dis Sci 1980; 25:33–41.

30. Nightingale JM, Lennard-Jones JE: The short bowel syndrome: What's new and old. Dig Dis 1993; 11:12–31.
31. Nightingale JMD, van der Sijp JRM, Kamm MA: Disturbed gastric emptying in short bowel syndrome: Correlation with jejunal length and evidence for a "colonic brake" (abstract). Gastroenterology 1991; 100:A235.
32. Cummings JH, James WPT, Wiggins HS: Role of the colon in ileal-resection diarrhea. Lancet 1973; 1:344–347.
33. Weser E, Fletcher JT, Urban E: Short bowel syndrome. Gastroenterology 1979; 77:572–579.
34. Ladefoged K, Nicolaidou P, Jarnum S: Calcium, phosphorus, magnesium, zinc, and nitrogen balance in patients with severe short bowel syndrome. Am J Clin Nutr 1980; 33:2137–2144.
35. Couper RTL, Durie PR, Stafford SE, et al: Late gastrointestinal bleeding and protein loss after distal small bowel resection in infancy. J Pediatr Gastroenterol Nutr 1989; 9:454–460.
36. Taylor SF, Sondheimer JM, Sokol RJ, et al: Noninfectious colitis associated with short gut syndrome in infants. J Pediatr 1991; 119:24–28.
37. Welkos SL, Toskes PP, Baer H: Importance of anaerobic bacteria in the cobalamin malabsorption of the experimental rat blind loop syndrome. Gastroenterology 1981; 80:313–320.
38. Schjonsky H: Vitamin $B_{12}$ absorption and malabsorption. Gut 1989; 30:1686–1691.
39. Arvanitakis C: Functional and morphologic abnormalities of the small intestinal mucosa in pernicious anemia. Acta Hepatogastroenterol 1978; 25:313–318.
40. Joshi M, Hyams JS, Treem WR: Cytoplasmic vacuolization of enterocytes: An unusual histopathologic finding in juvenile nutritional megaloblastic anemia. Mod Pathol 1991; 4:62–65.
41. Steinberg SE, Campbell CL, Hellman RS: Kinetics of the normal folate enterohepatic cycle. J Clin Invest 1979; 64:83–88.
42. Landor JH, Baker WK: Gastric hypersecretion produced by massive small bowel resection in dogs. J Surg Res 1964; 4:518–522.
43. Straus E, Gerson GD, Yalow RS: Hypersecretion of gastrin associated with short bowel syndrome. Gastroenterology 1974; 66:175–180.
44. Williams NS, Evans P, King RFGJ: Gastric acid secretion and gastrin production in the short bowel syndrome. Gut 1985; 26:914–919.
45. Cortot A, Fleming CR, Malagelada JR: Improved nutrient absorption after cimetidine in short-bowel syndrome with gastric hypersecretion. N Engl J Med 1979; 300:79–81.
46. Dubois A, van Eerdewegh P, Gardner JD: Gastric emptying and secretion in Zollinger-Ellison syndrome. J Clin Invest 1977; 59:255–263.
47. Becker HD, Reeder DD, Thompson JC: Extraction of circulating endogenous gastrin by the small bowel. Gastroenterology 1973; 65:903–906.
48. Hyman PE, Everett SL, Harada T: Gastric acid hypersecretion in short bowel syndrome in infants: Association with extent of resection and enteral feeding. J Pediatr Gastroenterol Nutr 1986; 5:191–197.
49. King CE, Toskes PP: Small intestine bacterial overgrowth. Gastroenterology 1979; 76:1035–1055.
50. Curtis KJ: Protein digestion and absorption in the blind-loop syndrome. Dig Dis Sci 1979; 24:923–929.
51. Perlmutter DH, Boyle JT, Campos JM, et al: D-Lactic acidosis in children: An unusual metabolic complication of small bowel resection. J Pediatr 1983; 102:234–238.
52. Carr DB, Shih VE, Richter JM, et al: D-Lactic acidosis simulating a hypothalamic syndrome after bowel bypass. Ann Neurol 1982; 11:195–197.
53. Rosenthal P, Pesce M: Long-term monitoring of D-lactic acidosis in a child. J Pediatr Gastroenterol Nutr 1985; 4:674–676.
54. Chadwick VS, Modha K, Dowling RH: Mechanism for hyperoxaluria in patients with ileal dysfunction. N Engl J Med 1973; 289:172–176.
55. Dobbins JW, Binder HJ: Importance of the colon in enteric hyperoxaluria. N Engl J Med 1977; 296:298–300.
56. Heaton KW, Read AF: Gallstones in patients with disorders of the terminal ileum and disturbed bile salt metabolism. Br Med J 1969; 3:494–496.
57. Hill GL, Mair WSJ, Golligher JC: Gallstones after ileostomy and ileal resection. Gut 1975; 16:932–936.
58. Bernhoft RA, Pellegrini CA, Broderick WC, et al: Pigment sludge and stone formation in the acutely ligated dog gallbladder. Gastroenterology 1983; 85:1166–1171.
59. Boonyapisit ST, Trotman BW, Ostrow DW: Unconjugated bilirubin and the hydrolysis of conjugated bilirubin in gallbladder bile of patients with cholelithiasis. Gastroeterology 1978; 24:70–74.
60. Allen B, Bernhoft R, Blanckaert N, et al: Sludge is calcium bilirubinate associated with bile stasis. Am J Surg 1981; 141:51–56.
61. O'Brien CB, Berman JM, Fleming CR, et al: Total parenteral nutrition gallstones contain more calcium bilirubinate than sickle cell gallstones (abstract). Gastroenterology 1986; 90:1752.
62. Postuma R, Moroz S, Friesen F: Extreme short bowel syndrome in an infant. J Pediatr Surg 1983; 18:264–268.
63. Kurz R, Sauer H: Treatment and metabolic findings in extreme short bowel syndrome with 11-cm jejunal remnant. J Pediatr Surg 1983; 18:257–263.
64. Weser E, Hernandez MH: Studies of small bowel adaptation after intestinal resection in the rat. Gastroenterology 1971; 60:69–75.
65. Weser E: Nutritional aspects of malabsorption: Short gut adaptation. Am J Med 1979; 67:1014–1020.
66. Williamson RCN: Intestinal adaptation: Structural, function, and cytokinetic changes. N Engl J Med 1978; 298:1393–1402.
67. Weser E: Nutritional aspects of malabsorption: Short-gut adaptation. Clin Gastroenterol 1983; 12:443–461.
68. Iverson BM, Schjonsby H, Skagen DW, et al: Intestinal adaptation after jejunoileal bypass operation for massive obesity. Eur J Clin Intest 1976; 6:355–360.
69. Dudrick SJ, Daly JM, Castro G, et al: Gastrointestinal adaptation following small bowel bypass for obesity. Ann Surg 1977; 185:642–648.
70. Mienge H, Robinson JWL: Functional and structural characteristics of the rat intestinal mucosa following ileojejunal transposition. Acta Hepatogastroenterol 1978; 25:150–154.
71. Gronqvist B, Engstrom B, Grimelius L: Morphologic studies of the rat small intestine after jejunoileal transposition. Acta Chiurgica Scand 1975; 141:208–217.
72. Lentze MJ: Intestinal adaptation in short-bowel syndrome. Eur J Pediatr 1989; 148:294–299.
73. Vanderhoof JA, Grandjean CJ, Kaufman SS, et al: Effect of high-percentage medium-chain triglyceride diet on mucosal adaptation following massive bowel resection in rats. J. Parenter Enter Nutr 1984; 8:685–698.
74. Weser E, Babbitt J, Hoban M: Intestinal adaptation: Different growth responses to disaccharides compared with monosaccharides in rat small bowel. Gastroenterology 1986; 91:1521–1527.
75. Clark RM: "Luminal nutrition" versus "functional work load" as controllers of mucosal morphology and epithelial replacement in rat small intestine. Digestion 1977; 15:411–424.
76. Vanderhoof JA, Grandjean CJ, Burkley KT, et al: Effect of casein versus casein hydrolysate on mucosal adaptation following massive bowel resection in infant rats. J Pediatr Gastroenterol Nutr 1984; 3:262–267.
77. Spector MH, Levine GM, Deren JJ: Direct and indirect effects of dextrose and amino acids on gut mass. Gastroenterology 1977; 72:706–710.
78. Booth IW: Enteral nutrition os primary therapy in short bowel syndrome. Gut 1994; (1 Suppl): S69–S72.
79. Vanderhoof JA, Blackwood DA, Mohammadpour H, et al: Effects of oral supplementation of glutamine on small intestinal mucosal mass following resection. J Am Coll Nutr 1992; 11:223–227.
80. Michail S, Mohammadpour H, Park JHY, et al: Effect of glutamine-supplemented elemental diet on mucosal adaptation following bowel resection in rats. J Pediatr Gastroenterol Nutr 1995; 21:394–398.
81. Hwang TL, O'Dwyer ST, Smith RJ, et al: Preservation of small bowel mucosa using glutamine-enriched parenteral nutrition. Surg Forum 1986; 37:56–58.
82. Magnusson I, Kihlberg R, Alvestrand A. et al: Utilization of intravenously administered *N*-acetyl-L-glutamine in humans. Metabolism 1989; 38:82–88.
83. Tamada H, Nezu R, Imamura I, et al: The dipeptide alanyl-glutamine prevents intestinal mucosal atrophy in parenterally fed rats. JPEN J Parenter Enteral Nutr 1992; 16:110–116.
84. Roediger WEW: Role of anaerobic bacteria in the metabolic welfare of the colonic mucosa in man. Gut 1980; 21:793–798.
85. Ruppin H, Bar-Meir S, Soergel KH, et al: Absorption of short-chain fatty acids by the colon. Gastroenterology 1980; 78:1500–1507.
86. Binder HJ, Mehta P: Short-chain fatty acids stimulate active sodium and chloride absorption in vitro in the rat distal colon. Gastroenterology 1989; 96:989–996.

87. Roediger WEW: Utilization of nutrients by isolated epithelial cells of the rat colon. Gastroenterology 1982; 83:424–429.
88. Cummings JH, Branch WJ: The importance of short-chain fatty acids in man. Scand J Gastroenterol 1984; 20:88–99.
89. O'Dwyer ST, Smith RJ, Kripke SA, et al: New fuels for the gut. *In* Rombeau JL, Caldwell MD, eds: Clinical Nutrition: Enteral and Tube Feeding. 2d ed. Philadelphia, WB Saunders, 1990, pp 540–555.
90. Ecknauer R, Sircar B, Johnson LR: Effect of dietary bulk on small bowel intestinal morphology and cell renewal in the rat. Gastroenterology 1981; 81:781–786.
91. Jacobs LR, Lupton JR: Effect of dietary fibers on rat large bowel mucosal growth and cell proliferation. Am J Physiol 1984; 246:G378–G385.
92. Kelberman I, Cheetham B, Rosenthal J, et al: Short-chain fatty acids overcome antibiotic inhibition of colonic adaptation (abstract). Gastroenterology 1991: 100:A527.
93. Koruda MU, Rolandelli RH, Settle RG: The effect of a pectin-supplemented elemental diet on intestinal adaptation to massive small bowel resection. J Parenter Enter Nutr 1986; 10:343–350.
94. Koruda MJ, Rolandelli RH, Settle RG, et al: Effect of parenteral nutrition supplemented with short-chain fatty acids on intestinal adaptation to massive small bowel resection. J Parenter Enter Nutr 1986; 10:343–350.
95. Dworkin LD, Levine GM, Farber NJ, et al: Small intestinal mass of the rat is partially determined by indirect effects of intraluminal nutrition. Gastroenterology 1976; 71:626–630.
96. Gleeson MH, Bloom SR, Polak JM, et al: An endocrine tumor in kidney affecting small bowel structure, motility, and absorptive function. Gut 1971; 12:733–742.
97. Jacobs LR, Polak JM, Bloom SR, et al: Intestinal mucosal and fasting plasma levels of immunoreactive enteroglucagon in three animal models of intestinal adaptation: Resection, hypothermic hyperphagia, and lactation in the rat. *In* Robinson JWL, Dowling RH, Riecken EO, eds: Mechanisms of Intestinal Adaptation. Lancaster, England, MTP Press, 1982, pp 231–240.
98. Bloom SR: Gut hormones in adaptation. Gut 1987; 28(S1):31–35.
99. Fuller PJ, Beveridge DJ, Taylor RG: Ileal proglucagon gene expression in the rat: Characterization in intestinal adoptation using in situ hybridization. Gastroenterology 1993; 104:459–466.
100. Drucker DJ, Ehrlich P, Asa SL, et al: Induction of intestinal epithelial proliferation by glucagon-like peptide 2. Proc Natl Acad Sci USA 1996; 93:7911–7916.
101. Weser E, Drummond A, Tawil T: Effect of diverting bile and pancreatic secretions into the ileum on small bowel mucosa in rats fed a liquid formula diet. J Parenter Enter Nutr 1982; 6:39–42.
102. Aiman GC: Influence of bile and pancreatic secretions on the size of the intestinal villi in the rat. Am J Anat 1971; 132:167–178.
103. Hughes CA, Bates T, Dowling RH: Cholecystokinin and secretin prevent the intestinal mucosal hypoplasia of total parenteral nutrition in the dog. Gastroenterology 1987; 75:34–41.
104. Weser E, Bell D, Tawil T: Effects of octapeptide cholecystokinin, secretin, and glucagon on intestinal mucosal growth in parenterally nourished rats. Dig Dis Sci 1981; 26:409–416.
105. Fine H, Levine GM, Shiau YF: Effects of cholecystokinin and secretin on intestinal structure and function. Am J Physiol 1983; 245:G358–G363.
106. Koetz HR, Lentz MJ, Muller OM, et al: Effect of 16,16-dimethyl prostaglandin $E_2$ on small intestinal mucosa in suckling rats. Eur J Clin Invest 1987; 17:293–300.
107. Vanderhoof JA, Grandjean CJ, Baylor JM, et al: Morphological and functional effects of 16,16 dimethyl prostaglandin-$E_2$ on mucosal adaptation after massive distal small bowel resection in the rat. Gut 1988; 29:802–808.
108. Hollworth ME, Granger DN, Ulrich-Baker MG, et al: Pharmacologic enhancement of adaptive growth after extensive small bowel resection. Pediatr Surg Int 1988; 3:55–61.
109. Marti U, Burwen SJ, Jones AL: Biological effects of epidermal growth factor with emphasis on the gastrointestinal tract and liver: An update. Hepatology 1989; 9:126–138.
110. Malo C, Menard D: Influence of epidermal growth factor on the development of suckling mouse intestinal mucosa. Gastroenterology 1982; 83:28–35.
111. Goodlad RA, Wilson TJG, Lenton W, et al: Proliferative effects of urogastrone-EGF on the intestinal epithelium. Gut 1987; 28(S1):37–43.
112. Ulshen MH, Lynn-Cook LE, Raasch RH: Effects of intraluminal epidermal growth factor on mucosal proliferation in the small intestine of adult rats. Gastroenterology 1986; 91:1134–1140.
113. Taylor B, Murphy GM, Dowling RH: Effect of food intake and the pituitary on intestinal structure and function after resection (abstract). Gut 1975; 16:397–398.
114. Park JHY, Vanderhoof JA: Growth hormone did not enhance mucosal hyperplasia after small bowel resection. Scand J Gastroenterol 1996; 31:349–354.
115. Vanderhoof JA, McCusker RH, Clark R, et al: Truncated and native insulin-like growth factor I enhance mucosal adaptation after jejunoileal resection. Gastroenterology 1992; 102:1949–1956.
116. Selub SE, Roundtree DB, Ulshen MH, et al: Transforming growth factor mRNA abundance in massive small bowel resection (abstract). Gastroenterology 1991; 100:A547.
117. Luk GD, Yang P. Polyamines in intestinal and pancreatic adaptation. Gut 1987; 28(S1):95–101.
118. Dufour C, Dandrifosse G, Forget P, et al: Spermine and spermidine induce intestinal maturation in the rat. Gastroenterology 1988; 95:112–116.
119. Thompson JS, Laughlin BS: Relationship of jejunostomy and urine polyamine content to refeeding and intestinal structure and function. J Parenter Enter Nutr 1989; 13:13–17.
120. Ho TF, Yip WCL, Tay JSH, et al: Rice water and milk: Effect on ileal fluid osmolality and volume. Lancet 1982; 1:169.
121. Schwartz KB, Ternberg JL, Bell MJ, et al: Sodium needs of infants and children with ileostomy. J Pediatr 1983; 102:509–513.
122. Will PC, Cortright RN, Grosedose RG, et al: Amiloride-sensitive salt and fluid absorption in small intestine of sodium-depleted rats. Am J Physiol 1985; 248:G133–G141.
123. Rodgers JB, Bernard HR, Balint JA: Colonic infusion in the management of the short bowel syndrome. Gastroenterology 1976; 70:186–189.
124. Puppala BL, Mangurtan HH, Kraut JR, et al: Distal ileostomy drip feedings in neonates with short bowel syndrome. J Pediatr Gastroenterol Nutr 1985; 4:489–494.
125. Levy E, Frileux P, Sandrucci S, et al: Continuous enteral nutrition during the early adaptive stage of the short bowel syndrome. Br J Surg 1988; 75:549–553.
126. Purdum PP, Kirky DF: Short-bowel syndrome: A review of the role of nutrition support. J Parenter Enter Nutr 1991; 15:93–101.
127. Van Rij AM, Thomson CD, McKenzie JM: Selenium deficiency in total parenteral nutrition. Am J Clin Nutr 1970; 32:2076–2085.
128. Reeves WC, Marcuard SP, Willis SE, et al: Reversible cardiomyopathy due to selenium deficiency. J Parenter Enter Nutr 1989; 13:663–665.
129. Dahlstrom KA, Ament ME, Medhin MG, et al: Serum trace elements in children receiving long-term parenteral nutrition. J Pediatr 1986; 109:625–630.
130. Mock DM, Baswell DL, Baker H, et al: Biotin deficiency complicating parenteral alimentation: Diagnosis, metabolic repercussions, and treatment. J Pediatr 1985; 106:762–769.
131. Hamosh M, Scanlon JW, Ganot D, et al: Fat digestion in the newborn: Characterization of lipase in gastric aspirates of premature and term infants. J Clin Invest 1981; 67:838–846.
132. Parker P, Stroop S, Greene H: A controlled comparison of continuous versus intermittent feeding in the treatment of infants with intestinal disease. J Pediatr 1981; 99:360–364.
133. Schwartz SM, Gewitz MH, Sec CC, et al: Enteral nutrition in infants with congenital heart disease and growth failure. Pediatrics 1990; 86:368–373.
134. Griffin GE, Fagan EF, Hodgson HJ, et al: Enteral therapy in the management of massive gut resection complicated by chronic fluid and electrolyte depletion. Dig Dis Sci 1982; 27:902–908.
135. MacMahon RA: The use of the World Health Organization oral rehydration solution in patients on home parenteral nutrition. J Parenter Enter Nutr 1984; 8:720–723.
136. Beaugerie L, Cosnes J, Verwaerde F, et al: Isotonic high-sodium oral rehydration solution (ORS) for increasing sodium reabsorption in short bowel syndrome (abstract). Gastroenterology 1990; 98:A158.
137. Young EA, Cioletti LA, Winborn WB, et al: Comparative study of nutritional adaptation to defined formula diet in rats. Am J Clin Nutr 1980; 33:2106–2110.
138. Voitk AJ, Echave V, Brown RA, et al: Use of elemental diet during the adaptive stage of short gut syndrome. Gastroenterology 1973; 65:419–426.

139. Simko V, Linscheer WG: Absorption of different elemental diets in short bowel syndrome lasting 15 years. Dig Dis Sci 1976; 21:419–425.
140. Christie DS, Ament ME: Dilute elemental diet and continuous-infusion technique for management of short bowel syndrome. J Pediatr 1975; 87:705–708.
141. McIntyre PB: The short bowel. Br J Surg 1985; 72:592–593.
142. Janne P, Carpentier Y, Williems G, et al: Colonic mucosal atrophy induced by a liquid elemental diet in rats. Am J Dig Dis 1977; 22:808–812.
143. Vanderhoof JA, Grandjean CJ, Burkley KT, et al: Effect of casein versus casein hydrolysate on mucosal adaptation following massive bowel resection in growing rats. J Pediatr Gastroenterol Nutr 1984; 3:262–267.
144. Cosnes J, Evard D, Beaugerie JG, et al: Prospective, randomized trial comparing small peptides versus whole proteins in patients with a high jejunostomy (abstract). Gastroenterology 1990; 98:A165.
145. Messing B, Pigot F, Rongier M, et al: Intestinal absorption of free oral hyperalimentation in the very short bowel syndrome. Gastroenterology 1991; 100:1502–1508.
146. Woolf GM, Miller C, Kurian R, et al: Nutritional absorption in short bowel syndrome: Evaluation of fluid, calorie, and divalent cation requirements. Dig Dis Sci 1987; 32:8–15.
147. Bond JH, Currier BE, Buchwald H, et al: Colonic conservation of malabsorbed carbohydrate. Gastroenterology 1980; 78:444–447.
148. Zimmaro DM, Rolandelli RH, Koruda MJ, et al: Isotonic tube feeding formula induces liquid stool in normal subjects: Reversal by pectin. J Parenter Enter Nutr 1989; 13:117–123.
149. Bochenek W, Rodgers JB, Balint JA: Effects of changes in dietary lipids on intestinal fluid loss in the short bowel syndrome. Ann Intern Med 1970; 72:205–213.
150. Andersson H, Isaksson B, Sjogren B: Fat-reduced diet in the symptomatic treatment of small bowel disease. Gut 1974; 15:351–359.
151. Simko V, McCarroll AM, Goodman S, et al: High-fat diet in the short-bowel syndrome: Intestinal absorption and gastroenteropancreatic hormone responses. Dig Dis Sci 1980; 25:333–339.
152. Oveson L, Chu R, Howard L: The influence of dietary fat on jejunostomy output in patients with severe short bowel syndrome. Am J Clin Nutr 1983; 38:270–277.
153. Woolf GM, Miller C, Kurian R, et al: Diet for patients with a short bowel: High fat or high carbohydrate. Gastroenterology 1983; 84:823–828.
154. Galeano NF, Leroy C, Belli D, et al: Comparison of two special infant formulas designed for the treatment of protracted diarrhea. J Pediatr Gastroenterol Nutr 1988; 7:76–83.
155. DeCecco S, Nelson J, Burnes J, et al: Nutritional intake of gut failure patients on home parenteral nutrition. J Parenter Enter Nutr 1987; 11:529–532.
156. Cosnes J, Lamy PH, Beaugerie L, et al: Adaptive hyperphagia in patients with postsurgical malabsorption. Gastroenterology 1990; 99:1814–1819.
157. Ohkobchi N, Igarashi Y, Tazawa Y, et al: Evaluation of the nutritional condition and absorptive capacity of nine infants with short bowel syndrome. J Pediatr Gastroenterol Nutr 1986; 5:198–206.
158. Sokol RJ, Heubi JE, Butler-Simon N, et al: Treatment of vitamin E deficiency during chronic childhood cholestasis with oral d-d tocopheryl polyethylene glycol-1000 succinate. Gastroenterology 1987; 93:975–985.
159. Menardi G, Guggenbichler JP: Bioavailability of oral antibiotics in children with short-bowel syndrome. J Pediatr Surg 1984; 19:84–86.
160. Murphy JP, King DR, Dubois A: Treatment of gastric hypersecretion with cimetidine in the short bowel syndrome. N Engl J Med 1979; 300:80–81.
161. Hyman PE, Garvey TQ, Harada T: Effect of ranitidine on gastric acid hypersecretion in an infant with short bowel syndrome. J Pediatr Gastroenterol Nutr 1985; 4:316–319.
162. Nightingale JMD, Walker ER, Burnham WR, et al: Omeprazole reduces secretory diarrhea in some patients with the short bowel syndrome (SBS) (abstract). Gut. 1989; 30:A179.
163. Tytgat GN, Hiubregtsc K, Dagevor J, et al: Effect of loperamide on fecal output and composition in well-established ileostomy and ileorectal anastomosis. Am J Dig Dis 1977; 22:669–676.
164. Sandhu BK, Tripp JH, Candy DCA, et al: Loperamide studies on its mechanism of action. Gut 1981; 22:658–662.
165. Hofmann AF, Poley JR: Cholestyramine treatment of diarrhea associated with ileal resection. N Engl J Med 1969; 281:397–402.
166. West RJ, Lloyd JK: The effect of cholestyramine on intestinal absorption. Gut 1975; 16:93–98.
167. Sali A, Murray WR, Mackay C: Aluminium hydroxide in bile salt diarrhea. Lancet 1977; 2:1051–1053.
168. Spencer H, Kramer L: Antacid-induced calcium loss. Arch Intern Med 1983; 143:657–659.
169. Matron PN, O'Dorisio TM, Howe BA: Effect of a long-acting somatostatin analogue (SMS 201–995) in a patient with pancreatic cholera. N Engl J Med 1985; 312:17–21.
170. Kvols LK, Moertel CG, O'Connell MJ, et al: Treatment of the malignant carcinoid syndrome: Evaluations of a long-acting somatostatin analogue. N Engl J Med 1986; 315:663–666.
171. Vinik AI, Tasi ST, Moattari AR: Somatostatin analogue (SMS 201–995) in the management of gastroenteropancreatic tumors and diarrhea syndromes. Am J Med 1986; 81(Suppl 6B):23–40.
172. Jaros W, Biller J, Green S, et al: Successful treatment of idiopathic secretory diarrhea of infancy with the somatostatin analogue SMS 201–995. Gastroenterology 1988; 94:189–193.
173. Couper RTL, Berzen A, Berall G, et al: Clinical response to the long-acting somatostatin analogue SMS 201–995 in a child with congenital microvillus atrophy. Gut 1989; 30:1020–1024.
174. Krejs GJ: Physiological role of somatostatin in the digestive tract: Gastric acid secretion, intestinal absorption, and motility. Scand J Gastroenterol 1986; 21(Suppl 119):47–53.
175. Reichlin S: Somatostatin. N Engl J Med 1983; 309:1495–1501, 1556–1563.
176. Williams NS, Cooper JC, Axon AT, et al: Use of a long-acting somatostatin analogue in controlling lifethreatening ileostomy diarrhea. Br Med J 1984; 289:1027–1028.
177. Ohlbaum PH, Galperine RI, Demarquez JL, et al: Use of a long-acting somatostatin analogue (SMS 201–995) in controlling a significant ileal output in a five-year-old child. J Pediatr Gastroenterol Nutr 1987; 6:466–470.
178. Rosen GH: Somatostatin and its analogs in the short bowel syndrome. J Parenter Enter Nutr 1992; 7:81–87.
179. Burroughs AK, Malagelada R: Potential indications for octrectide in gastroenterology: Summary of workshop. Digestion 1993; 54(suppl 1):59–66.
180. Corazza GR, Menozzi MG, Strocchi A, et al: The diagnosis of small bowel bacterial overgrowth: Reliability of jejunal culture and inadequacy of breath hydrogen testing. Gastroenterology 1990; 98:302–309.
181. Perman JA, Modler S, Barr RG, et al: Fasting breath hydrogen concentration: Normal values and clinical application. Gastroenterology 1984; 87:1358–1363.
182. Kerlin P, Wong L: Breath hydrogen testing in bacterial overgrowth of the small intestine. Gastroenterology 1988; 95:982–988.
183. Craig RM, Atkinson AJ: D-Xylose testing: A review. Gastroenterology 1988; 95:223–231.
184. Puntis JWL, Booth IW, Buick R: Cisapride in neonatal short gut. Lancet 1986; 2:108–109.
185. Byrne TA, Persinger RL, Young LS, et al: A new treatment for patients with short-bowel syndrome. Growth hormone, glutamine and a modified diet. Ann Surg 1995; 222:243–254.
186. Dahlstrom KA, Strandvik B, Kopple J, et al: Nutritional status in children receiving home parenteral nutrition. J Pediatr 1985; 107:219–224.
187. Lin CH, Rossi TM, Heitlinger LA, et al: Nutritional assessment of children with short bowel syndrome receiving home parenteral nutrition. Am J Dis Child 1987; 141:1093–1098.
188. Vargas JH, Ament ME, Berquist WE, et al: Long-term home parenteral nutrition in pediatrics: Ten years' experience in 102 patients. J Pediatr Gastroenterol Nutr 1987; 6:24–32.
189. Decker MD, Edwards KM: Central venous catheter infections. Pediatr Clin North Am 1988; 35:579–612.
190. Wang EEL, Prober CG, Ford-Jones L: The management of central intravenous catheter infections. Pediatr Infect Dis 1984; 3:110–113.
191. Prince A, Heller B, Levy J, et al: Management of fever in patients with central venous catheters. Pediatr Infect Dis 1986; 5:20–24.
192. Pollard AJ, Sreeram N, Wright JG, et al: ECG and echocardiographic diagnosis of pulmonary thromboembolism associated with central venous lines. Arch Dis Child. 1995; 73:147–150.
193. Nahata MC, King DR, Powell DA, et al: Management of catheter-related infections in pediatric patients. J Parenter Enter Nutr 1988; 12:58–59.
194. Merritt RJ: Cholestasis associated with total parenteral nutrition. J Pediatr Gastroenterol Nutr 1986; 5:9–22.

195. Pereira GR, Sherman MS, DiGiacomo J, et al: Hyperalimentation-induced cholestasis: Increased incidence and severity in premature infants. Am J Dis Child 1981; 135:842–845.
196. Dahms BB, Halpin TC: Serial liver biopsies in parenteral nutrition–associated cholestasis of early infancy. Gastroenterology 1981; 81:136–144.
197. Postuma R, Trevenen CL: Liver disease in infants receiving total parenteral nutrition. Pediatrics 1979; 63:110–115.
198. Colomb V, Goulet O, Rambaud C, et al: Long-term parenteral nutrition in children: Liver and gallbladder disease. Transplant Proc 1992; 24:1054–1055.
199. Palmer RH: Bile acids, liver injury, and liver disease. Arch Intern Med 1972; 130:606–617.
200. Nolan JP: Endotoxin, reticuloendothelial function, and liver injury. Hepatology 1981; 5:458–465.
201. Lichtman SN, Sartor RB, Keku J, et al: Hepatic inflammation in rats with experimental small intestinal overgrowth. Gastroenterology 1990; 98:414–423.
202. Thompson JS, Rikkers LF: Surgical alternatives for the short bowel syndrome. Am J Gastroenterol 1987; 82:97–106.
203. Devine RM, Kelly KA: Surgical therapy of the short bowel syndrome. Gastroenterol Clin North Am 1989; 18:603–618.
204. Barros D'Sa AB: An experimental evaluation of segmental reversal after massive small bowel resection. Br J Surg 1979; 66:493–500.
205. Tanner WA: The effect of reversed jejunal segments on the myoelectrical activity of the small bowel. Br J Surg 1978; 65:567–571.
206. Hutzer NE, Salzberg AM: Preileal transposition of colon to prevent the development of short bowel syndrome in puppies with 90% small intestinal resection. Surgery 1971; 70:189–197.
207. Sidhu GS, Narasimharao KL, Rani VU, et al: Absorptive studies after massive small bowel resection and antiperistaltic colon interposition in rhesus monkey. Dig Dis Sci 1985; 30:483–488.
208. Warden MJ, Wesley JR: Small bowel reversal procedure for treatment of the "short gut" body. J Pediatr Surg 1978; 13:321–323.
209. Glick PL, deLorimier AA, Adzick NS, et al: Colon interposition: An adjuvant operation for short gut syndrome. J Pediatr Surg 1984; 19:719–725.
210. Bianchi A: Intestinal loop lengthening: A technique for increasing small intestinal length. J Pediatr Surg 1980; 15:145–151.
211. Bianchi A: Intestinal lengthening: An experimental and clinical review. J R Soc Med 1984; 77:35–41.
212. Thompson JS, Vanderhoof JA, Antonson DL: Intestinal tapering and lengthening for short bowel syndrome. J Pediatr Gastroenterol Nutr 1985; 4:495–497.
213. Weber TR, Vane DW, Grosfeld JL: Tapering enteroplasty in infants with bowel atresia and short gut. Arch Surg 1982; 117:684–688.
214. Thompson JS: Strategies for preserving intestinal length in the short bowel syndrome. Dis Col Rec 1986; 30:208–213.
215. Vinograd I, Merguerian P, Udassin R, et al: An experimental model of a submucosally tunneled valve for the replacement of the ileocecal valve. J Pediatr Surg 1984; 19:726–731.
216. Lopez-Perez GA, Martinez AJ, Machuca J, et al: Experimental antireflux intestinal valve. Am J Surg 1981; 141:597–600.
217. Waddell WR, Kern F, Halgrimson CG, et al: A simple jejunocolic valve for relief of rapid transit and the short bowel syndrome. Arch Surg 1970; 100:438–444.
218. Ricotta J, Zuidema GD, Gadacz TR, et al: Construction of an ileocecal valve and its role in massive resection of the small intestine. Surg Gynecol Obstet 1981; 151:310–314.
219. Kocoshes SA: Small bowel transplantation in infants and children. Gastroenterol Clin North Am 1994; 23:727–742.
220. Langnas AN, Shaw BW, Antonson DL, et al: Preliminary experience with intestinal transplantation in infants and children. Pediatrics 1996; 97:443–448.
221. Asfar S, Atkison P, Ghent C, et al: Small bowel transplantation: A life-saving option for selected patients with intestinal failure. Dig Dis and Sci 1996; 41:875–883.
222. Grant D: Intestinal Transplantation registry on behalf of the current results of intestinal transplantation. Lancet 1996; 347:1801–1803.
223. Goulet O, Jan D, Brousse N, et al: Intestinal transplantation. J Pediatr Gastroenterol Nutr 1997; 25:1–11.
224. Abu-Elmagd KM, Tzukis AG, Todo S, et al: Monitoring and treatment of intestinal allograft rejection in humans. Transplant Proc 1993; 25:1202–1207.

Chapter 27

# Allergic Bowel Disease and Eosinophilic Gastroenteritis

Christopher Justinich

Despite many advances in the area of mucosal immunology of the gastrointestinal (GI) tract and increased understanding of the pathophysiology of inflammatory bowel disease, the patient with presumed food hypersensitivity continues to present a challenge for the clinician.[1] In certain instances, it is clear that food protein antigens induce objective signs and symptoms and that these can be reproduced by reexposure to the offending antigen. Examples include immunoglobulin E (IgE)–mediated anaphylactic reactions and infantile cow's milk protein–induced colitis. However, GI disorders characterized by predominantly eosinophilic inflammation in tissue may not be associated with known sensitization to specific, identifiable food antigens. Are these "idiopathic" eosinophilic gastroenteropathies (EGEs) similar to allergic disease, or do different insults to the intestinal tract lead to similar signs, symptoms, and pathologic findings? There is considerable overlap in what is observed in food allergy and in idiopathic EGE, with eosinophilic inflammation of tissue occurring in either condition.

The goal of this chapter is to provide an overview of food hypersensitivity and EGE. It also provides a brief review of intestinal immunology and pathophysiology, specifically as they pertain to allergy and eosinophilic inflammation in the gut. The clinical spectrum of presentation of allergic disease of the intestinal tract is outlined, with special reference to IgE-mediated anaphylaxis and evidence for allergic disease caused by different mechanisms (e.g., cell-mediated immune reactions). Cow's milk allergy is used as a model for the effects of food allergens on the GI tract. Gluten-induced enteropathy is discussed in Chapter 25. The role of ancillary testing is discussed, including the IgE-radioallergosorbent test (IgE-RAST), skin prick tests, food challenge tests, and more specialized tests that may have clinical relevance. Finally, the clinical, pathologic, and radiographic features of idiopathic EGE are outlined, with a discussion of the differential diagnosis, investigations, treatment, and outcome.

## DEFINITIONS

Any adverse reaction to the ingestion of food can be termed *intolerance* or *sensitivity*.[2–10] This definition does not imply any specific underlying mechanism, but by definition it excludes true allergic reactions and therefore encompasses symptoms caused by nonimmunologic mechanisms. For example, chemicals in food such as caffeine or selective malabsorption of lactose may cause GI symptoms. Reactions to the ingestion of these foods are reproducible but are not mediated by immunologic mechanisms.

On the other hand, true *food allergy* or *food hypersensitivity* is defined as a reproducible adverse reaction to a food protein antigen that is immune mediated. This implies that elimination of the offending protein will lead to resolution of the symptoms, with return of symptoms on reintroduction. The classic example is an IgE-mediated anaphylactic reaction to food, although other immune mechanisms are possible.

The term *eosinophilic gastroenteropathy* is defined as GI disease characterized by abnormal numbers of eosinophils in tissue but with no proven relation to demonstrable food protein allergy. This definition attempts to distinguish for the clinician idiopathic EGE from proven allergy, which is likely to have a different pathophysiology, treatment, and natural history. This distinction is somewhat arbitrary, because both entities may be characterized by tissue eosinophilia, and a reaction that is considered idiopathic may respond to the elimination of food protein antigens even though a defined immune mechanism cannot be documented.

## PATHOPHYSIOLOGY OF FOOD ALLERGY

Type I (immediate hypersensitivity) reactions represent the classic immune response, in which antigens form cross-links with specific IgE-bound mucosal mast cells, causing degranulation.[11] The roles of type II (cytotoxicity) and type III (immune complex disease) reactions have not been established. The sera of normal and atopic individuals contain small quantities of food antigens and IgG antibodies against food proteins.[12, 13] This phenomenon is enhanced by conditions predisposing to increased intestinal permeability, such as prematurity[14, 15] and IgA deficiency.[16] There is evidence to support the presence of type IV (delayed hypersensitivity) reactions, which cause immune-mediated damage to the GI tract without the involvement of IgE.[17] It is likely that, in some patients, more than one mechanism can be implicated.

The following is a brief overview of mucosal immunology as it pertains to food allergy; more comprehensive reviews are available elsewhere.[11, 18–21] In order to develop specific reactivity to foods, the immune system must be sensitized to food proteins that cross the epithelial barrier of the gut (Fig. 27–1).[22] Under normal circumstances, this is accomplished by means of specialized M cells, which transport antigen into the areas overlying Peyer's patches, where mucosal macrophages and dendritic cells process the antigen in order to present it to lymphocytes in association with human leukocyte antigen (HLA) class II antigens.[23] There is evidence that small bowel epithelium, which also can express class II antigens, may also participate in antigen presentation.[23, 24] Lymphocytes that have been exposed to antigens circulate through lymphatics and the blood stream, then selectively repopulate the GI mucosa—a process determined by cell surface adhesion markers.[22]

B lymphocytes differentiate into polymeric immunoglobulin-producing plasma cells, from which IgA and IgM antibodies are transported with secretory component to the surface, where they play an important role in immunity by providing a barrier to absorption of macromolecules.[22, 25] Immune dysregulation in atopic persons may allow B cells to differentiate preferentially into IgE-producing plasma cells. T lymphocytes differentiate into specialized subpopulations of cells. Intraepithelial lymphocytes often express CD8 surface markers (suppressor cells), and lamina propria T cells more often express CD4 surface markers. These are increased in patients with food-sensitive enteropathy.[26] CD8-positive cells may play a role in the development of tolerance to proteins, by suppressing the immune response to presented antigens. T lymphocytes can also be grouped by the array of cytokines they produce. In allergic disease, antigen-specific clones ($T_{H2}$ cells) producing eosinophil chemoattractants such as interleukin-5 may predominate, perpetuating the allergic response.[27, 28] The same has been shown in EGE.[29, 30] However, elaboration of $T_{H1}$ cytokines has been shown in milk-allergic infants,[31] making the distinction between $T_{H1}$ and $T_{H2}$ somewhat arbitrary.[32]

Eosinophils are increased at sites of allergic inflammation, and they contribute to symptoms on activation by releasing a variety of inflammatory mediators.[33, 34] Because eosinophils also produce cytokines that perpetuate allergic inflammation, it is conceivable that eosinophils play a causal role in the pathogenesis of EGE,[35] since this disorder is not simply a response to food antigens.[36]

Mucosal mast cells play multiple roles in allergic inflammation.[19, 33, 37–39] The cross-linking of antigen to IgE-bound mast cells results in degranulation and release of a myriad of inflammatory mediators, including histamine, lysosomal enzymes, leukotrienes, and proinflammatory cytokines, leading to increased vascular permeability, edema, and inflam-

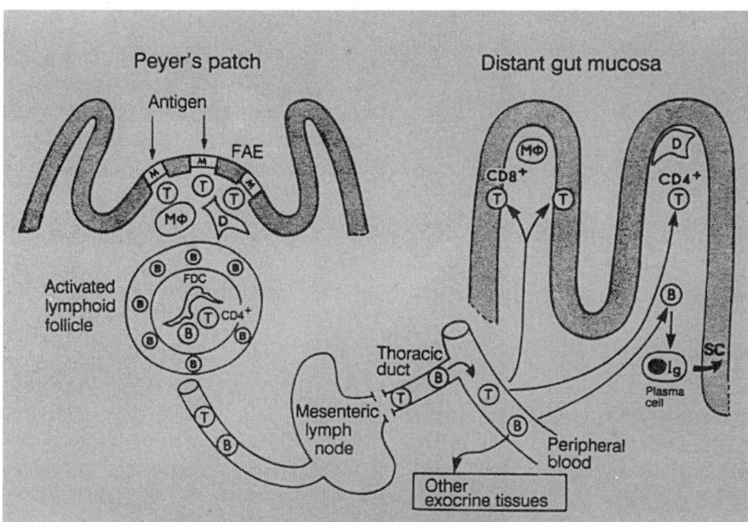


**FIGURE 27–1.** Schematic representation of initiation of mucosal immune responses and cell traffic in the mucosal immune system. Luminal antigen is transported mainly into Peyer's patch through M cells (M) of follicle-associated epithelium (FAE) and presented to T cells (T) by HLA class II-positive dendritic cell (D) or macrophage (Mϕ) after being processed. Antigen is presented to B cells by follicular dendritic cell (FDC) under the influence of CD4-positive regulatory T cells. Stimulated T and B memory cells migrate through lymph to the peripheral blood circulation and extravasate mainly in the gut lamina propria but also to some extent in other endocrine tissues, including the upper digestive tracts. Intestinal B cells that remain in the lamina propria differentiate under the influence of D, Mϕ, and CD4-positive T cells to plasma cells producing polymeric Ig, which is transported to the lumen by epithelial secretory component (SC). Most CD8-positive T cells migrate into the villous epithelium, perhaps to mediate oral tolerance to food antigens. (From Brandtzaeg P, Nilssen DE, Rognum TO, et al: Ontogeny of the mucosal immune system and IgA deficiency. In Macdermott RP, Elson CO (eds): Mucosal Immunology I: Basic Principles. Gastroenterol Clin North Am 1991;20:401, with permission.)

mation. Mast cells are capable of degranulating via mechanisms independent of IgE, which may help to explain the variability of clinical expression of allergic reactions.[40]

## PREVALENCE

Food allergy is perceived as being common, especially in children.[41] Difficulties encountered when studying this problem include differences in the definition of food allergy versus nonimmunologic intolerance, difficulty defining and performing objective tests that confirm the diagnosis, and the fact that many young children "outgrow" their allergies with time. Studies vary widely in reported incidence of food allergy in general and cow's milk allergy in particular. One adult population study[42] demonstrated that almost 20% of a large cohort of patients perceived intolerance to eight common foods, but after double-blind, placebo-controlled food challenges, only 19.4% of those who reported intolerance were confirmed by a positive test. The overall prevalence of allergy was 1.4%. Among patients with GI problems seen in an outpatient setting, food allergy was confirmed in 3.2%.[43]

In the pediatric literature, a prospective study by Bock examined 480 infants from birth to age 3 years and investigated those thought to have adverse reactions to food by open food challenges and by blinded food challenges in equivocal cases.[44] Initial complaints of food-induced reactions were greatest in the first year of life (80%), decreasing thereafter. Of the 480 infants, 133 (28%) had symptoms suspected as being related to specific foods; however, this was confirmed by open or blinded challenges in only 37 (8%). Two thirds of these adverse reactions were attributable to cow's milk. This study excluded reactions caused by fruit and fruit juices, which yielded positive open challenges in 56 patients (12%), because of the difficulty in attributing diarrhea to an immunologic reaction as opposed to osmotic diarrhea in this age group. However, data from Israel indicate that allergy to fruits may be more common than previously thought, especially in older children.[45]

Two large, prospective studies of cow's milk allergy in infants have been published. In Sweden,[46] cow's milk allergy, defined by improvement after elimination of cow's milk formula with recurrence of symptoms on challenge, occurred in 20 (1.9%) of 1,079 infants. However, more than one third of the patients in one group were lost to follow-up. In the most closely followed group, 328 of 332 patients completed the study, and 12 infants (3.7%) were diagnosed with cow's milk allergy. In the second study, from Canada,[47] cow's milk protein allergy was similarly diagnosed by elimination and rechallenge. Allergy was found in 59 (7.5%) of 787 infants. Both studies included infants who were breast-fed and exposed to cow's milk protein from the maternal diet transmitted through breast milk. The incidence figures are in keeping with Bock's results,[44] in which cow's milk allergy was responsible for 25 adverse reactions (5.2%) among 480 children younger than 3 years old.

## IMMEDIATE HYPERSENSITIVITY REACTIONS TO FOOD

Type I (IgE-mediated) immediate hypersensitivity reactions to foods are most common in young children, with 50% of these reactions occurring in the first year of life. The majority are reactions to cow's milk or to soy protein from infant formulas.[1] Twenty percent of these reactions occur in the second year of life, and 10% thereafter. Other food allergies begin to predominate in older children, including egg, fish, peanut, and wheat. Together with milk and soy, these account for more than 90% of food allergy in children.[48] It is commonly thought that these patients are allergic to multiple foods. However, double-blind food challenges demonstrate that more than 80% of these children respond to only one or two foods.[48, 49]

The importance of a thorough history cannot be overemphasized, because patients may have hypersensitivity to bizarre and unexpected proteins. For example, sensitivities to lactase enzyme added to milk[50] and to maple syrup sap in a tree pollen–sensitive child[51] have been described. Immediate hypersensitivity reactions including anaphylactic reactions to breast milk,[52] protein hydrolysate formulas,[53, 54] and rice cereal[55] in infants have been reported, even though these foods are generally considered to be well tolerated. In addition, milk protein may be present in foods thought to be "dairy free."[56] Similar "occult" exposures may occur to various proteins as a result of improper labeling, changes in product composition with time, or contamination of foods by improper preparation techniques.[57]

Blinded food challenges have shown that symptoms referable to the GI tract in IgE-mediated allergy typically begin within minutes of the ingestion, although occasionally may be delayed for up to 2 hours. They tend to be short-lived, lasting 1 to 2 hours.[49, 58] Symptoms include nausea, vomiting, abdominal pain, and diarrhea; they may also include oral symptoms, skin manifestations, wheezing, or airway edema (Table 27–1).

The rapid onset of these symptoms after food ingestion correlates highly with positive IgE-RAST or skin prick tests to the offending antigen, making confirmation of the clinical suspicion of immediate hypersensitivity straightforward. Caution must be used, however, because positive responses on these tests do not always predict clinically relevant reactions in blinded food challenges.[59] If the clinical history is equivocal, then double-blind food challenges in a controlled environment are needed to prove or disprove a reaction.

### Anaphylactic Reactions

Anaphylactic reactions to food ingestion are life-threatening. For the purpose of this discussion, and the recommenda-

**TABLE 27–1. Manifestations of Immediate (IgE-Mediated) Food Allergy**

| | |
|---|---|
| Generalized | Gastrointestinal |
| Anaphylaxis | Vomiting |
| Cutaneous | Diarrhea |
| Urticaria | Malabsorption/protein-losing enteropathy |
| Angioedema | Bleeding/anemia |
| Atopic dermatitis | Infantile colic |
| Respiratory | |
| Rhinoconjunctivitis | |
| Asthma | |

Adapted from Sampson HA: Differential diagnosis in adverse reactions to foods. J Allergy Clin Immunol 1986;78:212–219, with permission.

tions given, the term anaphylaxis is limited to those IgE-mediated reactions causing upper airway obstruction, hypotension, and circulatory collapse. Although any protein may be implicated, certain foods have a propensity to cause severe reactions in susceptible persons: cow's milk, egg, peanut, and shellfish. The altering of food protein antigens through cooking or prior hydrolysis does not preclude a type I allergic reaction, because some proteins are relatively resistant to denaturation.

Experience with fatal and near-fatal anaphylactic reactions to foods in 13 children and adolescents has been reported.[60] All of the patients had a history of asthma. The most common foods implicated were nuts (including peanut), egg, and milk. Although the children had a history of serious reactions to the same foods and were educated in their avoidance, they or their families were unaware of the offending antigen disguised in food. The majority of ingestions did not occur at home. Comparison of the six fatal reactions with the seven near-fatal cases indicated that early administration of epinephrine after symptom onset was associated with survival. The reactions were either rapidly progressive or followed a biphasic pattern, with a symptom-free interval of up to 2½ hours before the return of severe symptoms. Families, caregivers, and patients with a history of anaphylaxis to food, especially those with a history of asthma, require education on avoidance of offending foods and the use of epinephrine (see later discussion) and need several hours of observation in a hospital setting after a significant reaction.

Exercise-induced anaphylaxis to specific foods has been reported in children[61, 62] and underscores the importance of good history taking, blinded food challenges, and, when necessary, recreation of the conditions that caused the anaphylactic reaction.[63] These patients often have a history of atopy and may have mild asthma. Double-blind food challenges demonstrate that ingestion of the food in question does not induce symptoms; however, the combination of ingestion followed by exercise minutes to hours after ingestion leads to anaphylaxis. The mechanism underlying exercise-induced anaphylaxis is not completely understood, but similar recommendations for education, prevention, and treatment of anaphylactic reactions should be given. Patients should avoid offending foods for 12 hours before exercise, and they should exercise in the presence of a companion who is prepared to administer epinephrine if necessary.[61]

## Other Type I Reactions

*Oral allergy syndrome (OAS)* is a clinical syndrome in which fresh foods, often fruits and vegetables, provoke local symptoms of itching of the mouth and pharynx. It is thought to result from a cross-reactivity between tree pollens and food antigens. OAS may be limited to local reactions in the mouth, although some series describe a progression of OAS to true systemic anaphylactic reactions, especially if the antigen is ingested.[64, 65] These patients are typically atopic and exhibit positive IgE-RAST and skin prick tests to the antigens in question.[66]

It has been reported that *chronic urticaria* can be caused by adverse reactions to foods, especially with acute urticarial reactions. However, in one large series, only 1.4% of 554 adults with urticaria had positive RAST or skin prick tests to food.[67] Similarly, 2% of 94 children reported an association with food.[68] Open challenges can be used to verify the presence of food allergy in these patients.

*Atopic dermatitis (AD)* is a chronic pruritic skin condition found in atopic persons, with a characteristic distribution varying with age. Patients with this condition often have a history of adverse reactions to food, but this is a poor predictor of documented food hypersensitivity.[69] In a study of 113 children with AD,[70] double-blind food challenges were used to determine the prevalence of food allergy. Sixty-three children (56%) had a total of 101 positive challenges; of these, 84% involved cutaneous symptoms and 52% involved GI symptoms, although frequently these patients denied GI symptoms by history. Ninety percent were sensitive to one or two foods. After 1 to 2 years, 40% of these patients outgrew their food sensitivities. Repeated rechallenge over time is indicated, because skin prick tests may remain positive after clinical tolerance is attained.

## Investigation and Management

An approach to the evaluation of IgE-mediated hypersensitivity to food is the subject of more comprehensive reviews.[49, 71] Briefly, patients with a history of a significant reaction to one or more foods should be tested by skin prick against those foods and against a limited battery of common food allergens (milk, soy, egg, peanut, fish, wheat). It may be necessary to skin test with natural foods if skin tests are negative to commercially prepared extracts.[72] Skin testing has a sensitivity of 90% to 100% depending on the antigen, so patients with negative skin testing are very unlikely to have IgE-mediated disease and should be challenged openly with the food in question. Non-IgE-mediated hypersensitivity may still cause symptoms on challenge, but these may be delayed for hours or days. IgE-RAST testing for specific foods does not have greater positive or negative predictive value than skin prick testing, and combining the two does not improve the diagnostic yield.[59] If IgE-RAST or skin prick tests are positive, the food is avoided for 3 weeks; if symptoms improve, the elimination diet is continued. If there is no improvement, then open or single-blind challenges with the food are given to try to elicit a response. These challenges should be performed in a setting in which access to emergency treatment of allergic reactions is available.

Positive challenges should lead to consultation with a dietitian to educate the patient and family concerning avoidance of the food and to ensure that adequate nutrition is maintained. Groups such as The Food Allergy Network provide support and educational materials for families. Patients with a history of serious reactions to foods should be provided with an epinephrine kit for home use, proper instruction on how the device is used, and a MedicAlert bracelet. Two different kits with preloaded syringes are available for self-administration. The Ana-Kit (Bayer Corporation, West Haven, CT) can deliver two 0.3-mL doses of epinephrine (1:1000) for intramuscular or subcutaneous injection. It has a graduated syringe that can deliver smaller doses for younger children. Recommended dosing is as follows: infants to 2 years, 0.05 to 0.1 mL; 2 to 6 years, 0.15 mL; 6 to 12 years, 0.2 mL; and older than 12 years, 0.3 mL.

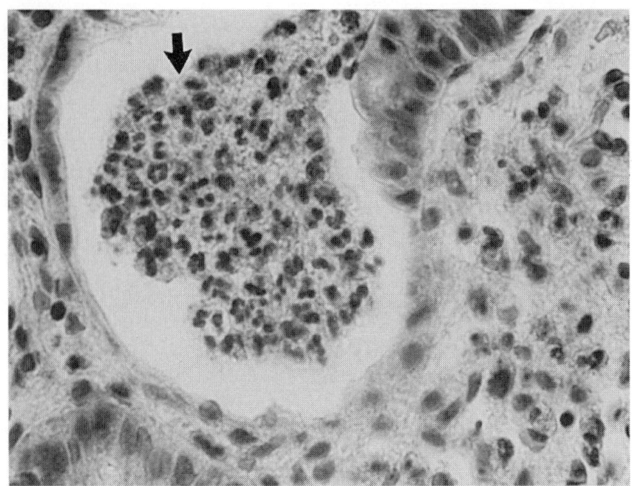

**FIGURE 27–2.** Marked eosinophilic colitis with eosinophilic crypt abscess *(arrow)*. Hematoxylin-eosin stain, ×40. (Courtesy of David Mack, MD.)

The second device is the EpiPen (Center Laboratories, Port Washington, NY) for intramuscular use, which delivers 0.3 mL of epinephrine 1:1000 for older children; the EpiPen Jr delivers 0.15 mL. If a kit is used, the patient should go to a hospital emergency room and stay for 3 to 4 hours, regardless of whether additional treatment is required. It is imperative for any health care provider presented with a patient at risk for anaphylactic reaction to foods to ensure that the patient obtain a kit for administration of epinephrine and be properly trained in its use.

## NON-IgE-MEDIATED FOOD ALLERGY

Milk protein allergy can be used as a model for non-IgE-mediated food allergy, although theoretically the same discussion could be applied to any number of food allergies. Much of the study in this area involves infants with milk protein intolerance, both because it is common and because young infants frequently have only milk protein in the diet.[73] The clinical spectrum of cow's milk protein allergy is varied, and the presenting features often parallel the site of involvement, similar to idiopathic EGE (Table 27–2). Avoidance of cow's milk resolves the symptoms and histologic findings; rechallenge reproduces the injury.

**TABLE 27–2. Clinical Presentation of Cow's Milk Protein Allergy**

| | |
|---|---|
| Vomiting | Iron deficiency anemia |
| Diarrhea | Eosinophilic colitis |
| Failure to thrive | Atopic dermatitis |
| Protein-losing enteropathy, edema | Infantile colic |

### Clinical Presentation

*Eosinophilic colitis* in young infants is probably the most common manifestation of cow's milk protein allergy and has been the subject of several reviews.[74–76] It is characterized by diarrhea with blood and mucous, typically in otherwise healthy, predominantly male infants. It has been described in exclusively breast-fed infants, presumably as a result of transmission of maternal dietary antigens through breast milk.[77, 78] Symptoms can occur soon after birth, suggesting that sensitization may occur in utero.[79, 80] In the absence of infection, sigmoidoscopy is helpful to exclude other causes of bleeding and to document eosinophilic colitis by mucosal biopsy. The gross features of erythema, edema, lymphoid hyperplasia, and occasionally erosions are nonspecific, so mucosal biopsies are required to make the diagnosis. These biopsies show inflammation predominated by eosinophils. Studies vary in the extent of eosinophilia needed to confirm the diagnosis: more than 60 per six high-power fields (hpf),[81] more than 20/hpf in the maximally involved area,[76] or more than 25% of the inflammatory infiltrate.[82] The epithelial layer of the colon is generally normal, and in most cases intraepithelial eosinophils are present, which is thought to indicate disease activity.[75] In severe cases, eosinophilic crypt abscesses can be seen (Fig. 27–2). The eosinophils may be clustered in foci within the same area, and the intensity may vary considerably between sites. The rectosigmoid is usually representative, so multiple biopsies should be taken from this region. Removal of milk protein from the infant or breast-feeding mother usually leads to prompt resolution in symptoms, although microscopic or gross blood can persist

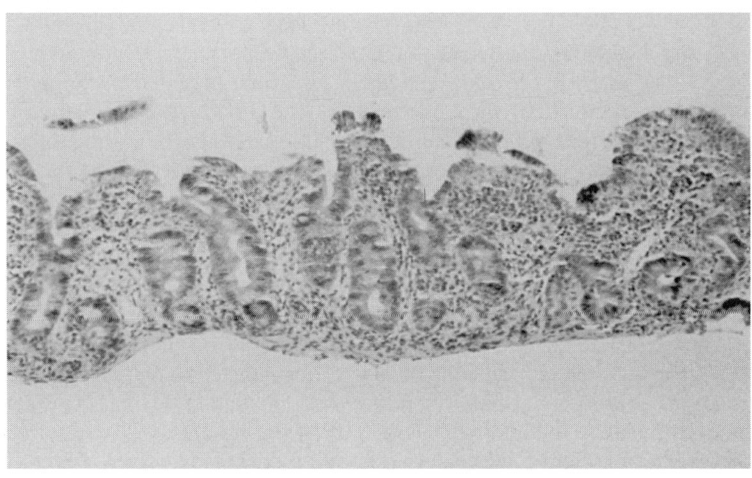

**FIGURE 27–3.** Histologic features of cow's milk protein–induced enteropathy. Duodenal biopsy from a 6-month-old with cow's milk protein–induced duodenitis with partial villous atrophy and diffuse chronic inflammatory infiltrate. Symptoms of diarrhea and failure to thrive resolved on a cow's milk protein-free diet. Hematoxylin-eosin stain, ×40.

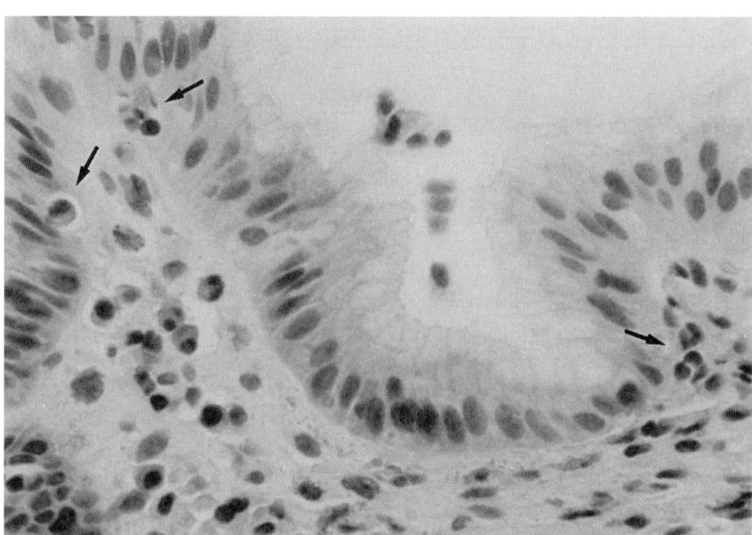

**FIGURE 27–4.** Gastric biopsy from a teenage girl with abdominal pain and vomiting. Note intraepithelial eosinophils *(arrows)*. Hematoxylin-eosin stain, ×40.

for several weeks. Evidence suggests that immunoglobulin and other immune deficiencies may predispose infants to allergic colitis.[83]

Cow's milk allergy can also cause a *small bowel enteropathy* leading to chronic inflammation with villous atrophy[84–89] (Fig. 27–3); the same type of enteropathy can be seen with soy and other proteins.[90, 91] Most patients present with diarrhea and failure to thrive, often characterized by peripheral blood eosinophilia, iron deficiency anemia, and hypoalbuminemia from protein-losing enteropathy. At times, patients may present without overt GI symptoms but with profound anemia or hypoalbuminemia. Careful morphometric studies have shown that the villous atrophy in this disorder is associated not only with increased numbers of eosinophils but also with increased intraepithelial lymphocytes and IgE-containing cells in the lamina propria.[89] Treatment with a milk-free diet leads to rapid resolution of symptoms and the return of normal villi. Rechallenge with milk protein reproduces symptoms, and villous atrophy can be reestablished even within 24 to 48 hours of rechallenge.[87]

*Allergic gastritis* is a common feature of both cow's milk protein allergy and idiopathic EGE. Symptoms include pain and vomiting, especially if the gastric outlet is narrowed by mucosal or muscle wall involvement. Mucosal biopsies demonstrate eosinophilia with intraepithelial eosinophils (Fig. 27–4). This condition may mimic hypertrophic pyloric stenosis in infants but responds to removal of cow's milk protein from the diet. Clues to the diagnosis include an atypical age for hypertrophic pyloric stenosis, peripheral blood eosinophilia, and eosinophilia in mucosal biopsies.[92]

*Allergic esophagitis* is characterized by dysphagia, pain, and symptoms mimicking gastroesophageal reflux; pH probe studies showing no acid reflux; and intense eosinophilia on esophageal biopsy[93] (Fig. 27–5). Infants may also present with feeding aversion in the absence of other symptoms. This has been seen in association with cow's milk allergy in infants. Treatment with elemental formula leads to resolution of symptoms and histologic findings. We have found increased mucosal mast cells in allergic esophagitis, distinguishing these patients from those with inflammation caused by gastroesophageal reflux.[94] Allergy should be considered in patients with gastroesophageal reflux symptoms who are unresponsive to reflux therapy, especially if eosinophilic inflammation of the esophagus is marked.

Milk allergy can cause *irritability and infantile colic*-like symptoms in some infants. By definition, colic is an idiopathic condition with increased crying behavior in infants, and therefore it is not an allergic disease. However, because allergy can potentially lead to inflammation and pain, cow's milk protein allergy is often considered in infants with colic.[95] Studies evaluating treatment of colic with protein hydrolysate formulas have been inconclusive. In one study, Taubman demonstrated that parental counseling was more effective than protein hydrolysate formulas in decreasing colic, and when infants went back to cow's milk or soy formulas after 18 days no infant had increased crying with this "challenge."[96] On the other hand, a second study dem-

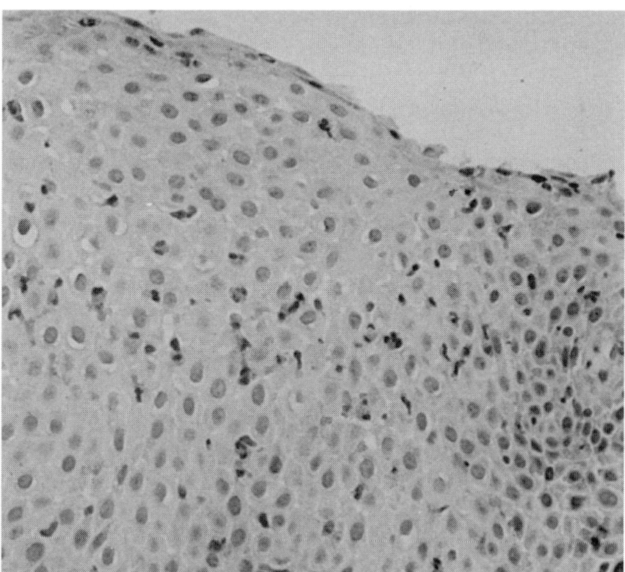

**FIGURE 27–5.** Distal esophageal biopsy from a teenage girl with dysphagia, unresponsive to antacid therapy. A pH probe did not demonstrate acid reflux. The biopsy revealed marked eosinophilic inflammation. Symptoms resolved with corticosteroid therapy. Hematoxylin-eosin stain, ×40.

onstrated decreased crying with the use of protein hydrolysate in the majority of colicky infants, with crying time increasing significantly after a placebo-controlled, double-blind whey challenge.[97] A third study, also randomized and double-blinded, showed increased crying behavior in infants receiving cow's milk formula compared with those receiving semielemental formula.[98] These studies support the idea that cow's milk protein allergy may play a role in some infants with colic. A limited trial of protein hydrolysate formula and early rechallenge to confirm the findings may be indicated.[99]

There are poorly controlled studies describing a variety of other problems potentially caused by food protein allergy, including joint disease, migraine, and behavior problems. Causal relations between food allergy and these entities are unproved, and their discussion is beyond the scope of this chapter.

### Investigation and Management

Classic tests of allergy (IgE-RAST and skin prick tests) will be negative unless the patient has both IgE- and non-IgE-mediated disease. Therefore investigators have looked for tests of cell-mediated immunity, such as lymphocyte proliferation assays (LPA). Peripheral blood mononuclear cells are collected from patients and incubated in the presence of food antigens.[100] The proliferative response of these cells to specific antigens is measured. These are labor-intensive investigations, and proponents of LPA try to extrapolate findings from clones of isolated peripheral blood mononuclear cells, which may not be representative of the situation in vivo.[101, 102] Patients who are allergic to foods, with or without AD, have increased reactivity to food antigens,[101, 103–106] and this responsiveness seems to diminish if these proteins are eliminated from the diet.[103] An earlier study reported increased response by LPA to milk and soy proteins in infants with allergic enterocolitis,[107] but this was not confirmed by a more recent report.[108] Differences in technique, including the nature and source of the antigens used, and heterogeneity of patient populations may account for these differences, and until more data are available it is difficult to define a clinical role for these tests.

Patch testing of the skin with food antigens to demonstrate delayed (type IV) hypersensitivity after 48 to 72 hours is another modality that deserves further study.[109] However, local skin reactions may not be representative of reactions in the GI tract.

If commonly available ancillary testing is not helpful, then the diagnosis rests on the resolution of symptoms in response to an elimination diet, with return of symptoms on rechallenge.[110] In difficult cases it may be necessary to perform double-blind food challenges. Unlike the rapid response that is characteristic of IgE-mediated disease, a prolonged challenge may identify delayed reactions with predominantly GI symptoms up to 6 days after exposure.[111–113] In infants, avoidance of food protein antigens with the use of hypoallergenic casein or whey hydrolysate formulas is safe and effective in the majority of infants.[114–117] Soy formulas may be tolerated by infants who are allergic to cow's milk.[118] Bock found that only 7% of milk-allergic infants and children were allergic to soy by double-blind challenge. However, the highest reported incidence of soy allergy in cow's milk–sensitive infants is 35%.[46] The difference may be a reflection of differences in milk-soy cross-reactivity between IgE and non-IgE-mediated disease.

Amino acid–based products are now available for infants and older children who are highly sensitized to food antigens.[119, 120] Elemental diet can be used as a treatment or as a diagnostic tool to assess complex food allergies, by eliminating dietary protein antigens completely and then systematically rechallenging the patient with offending foods.[121–123] Avoidance of specific allergens remains the mainstay of therapy.[124, 125]

Although antihistamines and corticosteroids are used to treat acute allergic reactions, pharmacologic therapy has not been effective in preventing manifestations of food allergy.[126] Randomized trials of mast cell stabilizers such as oral cromolyn and ketotifen have not demonstrated efficacy in children with AD and food hypersensitivity,[127–129] although trials in non-IgE-mediated allergy are lacking. One report suggests that the immune response to antigens can be altered by altering gut flora.[130] In infants with AD and cow's milk allergy, *Lactobacillus GG* with protein hydrolysate formula caused significant improvement in AD compared with formula hydrolysate alone.

## NATURAL HISTORY OF FOOD ALLERGY

The natural history of both IgE and non-IgE-mediated food allergies in young children suggests that tolerance develops with time. In a cohort of 100 children observed prospectively for immediate and delayed sensitivity to foods, 28% developed clinical tolerance by 2 years, 56% by 4 years, and 78% by 6 years.[131] However, sensitivity in children with IgE-mediated disease persisted longer than in those with delayed reactions (22% versus 59% at 2 years). In addition, the group with persistent cow's milk allergy tended to have higher IgE levels, milk-specific IgE, and sensitization to other foods, suggesting a more pronounced immune dysregulation.[132, 133] Similarly, infants with milk-induced enteropathy and colitis tend to outgrow the problem by 1 to 2 years of age. It is recommended that the initial reexposure to the offending antigen be done in a stepwise fashion[111, 113] in a setting in which acute allergic reactions can be treated. Food-specific quantitative IgE-RAST tests are now available that help predict when patients with previous anaphylactic reactions have outgrown their allergy.[133a]

Bock reported follow-up of nine children who had a history of severe reactions to foods, most commonly milk protein, most of whom were younger than 1 year of age at time of first reaction.[134] Three of these children could eventually tolerate the offending food, four could tolerate small quantities without a life-threatening reaction, and two continued to have significant reactions. Some patients retained positive skin prick tests even though the challenges were negative, a previously described phenomenon. Anaphylactic reactions to certain foods such as peanut or shellfish tend to persist.

## PREVENTION OF FOOD ALLERGY

Children with allergy to milk have greater numbers of hospitalizations, more episodes of anaphylaxis, and an increased incidence of AD,[135] so prevention in high-risk infants becomes an important issue.[136] Studies have compared exclusive breast-feeding, with mothers on regular or "hypoallergenic" diets, with standard and hydrolysate formulas for prevention or postponement of atopy in infants at risk (i.e., those with a strong family history of atopy and or high cord blood IgE levels). A 15-year prospective, uncontrolled study compared breast-feeding with cow's milk and soy formula; the incidence of atopy was twice as high in the formula-fed groups.[137] Similar studies with a follow-up of 1 to 2 years showed a lower incidence of atopic disorders, but it was unclear whether the effect would be long-lasting.[138]

Three randomized, controlled trials have described dietary interventions to prevent atopy in infants considered to be at high risk, with long-term follow-up. One study showed no benefit after 7 years of follow-up in infants randomly assigned to receive breast-feeding supplemented by cow's milk formula versus breast-feeding with mothers avoiding cow's milk, egg, and peanut during the last trimester of pregnancy and lactation, supplementing with a casein hydrolysate formula.[139] However, only 57% of the patients were available for follow-up at 7 years. A second study compared casein hydrolysate formula with cow's milk formula alone or as a supplement to breast milk.[140] At 4 years, the hydrolysate group had a significantly lower incidence of eczema, but not of asthma or milk allergy. The third study examined 216 high-risk infants, comparing breast milk with cow's milk, soy, and a partial whey hydrolysate formula.[141] In a 5-year follow-up with a low dropout rate, the breast-fed and partial whey hydrolysate groups had significantly less atopy, including asthma and eczema, and a lower rate of positive double-blind food challenges.

In summary, for high-risk infants, breast-feeding, or alternatively, formula-feeding with hydrolysate formulas, seems to be beneficial for long-term prevention of some manifestations of atopy.

## IDIOPATHIC EOSINOPHILIC GASTROENTEROPATHY (EGE)

Idiopathic EGE is an inflammatory condition of the GI tract characterized by eosinophilic inflammation in tissue. Frequently it is accompanied by peripheral blood eosinophilia. It should be a "diagnosis of exclusion" and therefore requires the clinician to eliminate known causes of peripheral blood and tissue eosinophilia. As described by Katz and colleagues,[92] the clinical presentation and pathologic features of this disease closely resemble the enteropathy caused by hypersensitivity to milk protein antigens. Every effort should be made to exclude known allergies, by appropriate IgE-RAST and skin prick tests. Cow's milk protein remains the most common food allergen, and standard ancillary testing may not identify sensitivity to foods. Care must be taken to totally exclude a protein that has been implicated, because continued inadvertent ingestion of offending antigens may perpetuate the disease.

### Differential Diagnosis

As shown in Table 27–3, the differential diagnosis of eosinophilia of the GI tract includes simple food allergy, parasitic infection (e.g., dog hookworm),[142] connective tissue diseases including vasculitis,[143, 144] Ménétrier's disease,[145] and congenital intestinal obstruction.[146] Eosinophilia of the antral mucosa can be associated with *Helicobacter pylori* infection,[147] so appropriate studies for *H. pylori* should be performed. Increased numbers and activation of eosinophils have been described in both ulcerative colitis and Crohn's disease,[148] and early inflammatory bowel disease may mimic EGE. In these instances, a prolonged follow-up interval may be needed before a definitive diagnosis is made. Hypersensitivity to medications should always be considered if appropriate; tissue eosinophilia secondary to medication, including anticonvulsants[149] and gold therapy,[150] has been described. Hypereosinophilic syndrome may affect the GI tract; extreme eosinophilia with involvement of multiple organ systems points to this diagnosis as opposed to isolated EGE.[151] When the muscular form of EGE affects the gastric outlet, it may resemble hypertrophic pyloric stenosis[152] or outlet obstruction from chronic granulomatous disease.[153] Upper GI involvement with muscle layer thickening can be difficult to distinguish from Crohn's disease[154] or small bowel malignancy.

**TABLE 27–3. Differential Diagnosis of Eosinophilic Gastroenteropathy**

| | |
|---|---|
| Mucosal disease | Muscle disease |
| Inflammatory bowel disease | Hypertrophic pyloric stenosis (infancy) |
| Connective tissue disease | Chronic granulomatous disease |
| Food allergy | Crohn's disease |
| Drug allergy | Lymphoma, other malignancy |
| Hypereosinophilic syndrome | Serosal disease (ascites) |
| Gluten-sensitive enteropathy | Malignancy |
| Autoimmune enteropathy | Liver disease |

### Clinical Presentation

The presenting symptoms and signs of EGE depend on the distribution of the involved areas of the GI tract and the extent to which the depth of the bowel wall is affected. Klein and associates[155] described a classification for this disease, distinguishing mucosal, muscle layer, and serosal disease, and the clinical presentation in children has been reported in other studies (Table 27–4).[82, 92, 156, 157] Each of these three forms of the disease is associated with peripheral blood eosinophilia or increased eosinophil precursors in bone marrow, but it is uncertain why only some areas of the bowel are affected. There is no consistent response to elimination diets,[36] so by definition EGE is not a food hypersensitivity.

*Mucosal disease* is the most common form of EGE. Patients typically present with abdominal pain, vomiting and/or diarrhea, and rectal bleeding.[82, 92, 157–160] The diarrhea may arise from mucosal disease leading to malabsorption and growth delay, or it may arise from colonic disease with blood and net fluid secretion. Protein-losing enteropathy with hypoalbuminemia is a common finding. Peripheral blood eosinophilia (absolute count >660/mm$^3$) is common but may not be found at presentation, and some authors have advocated examination of bone marrow to demonstrate increased eosinophil precursors. Diagnosis is best made by endoscopic

**TABLE 27–4. Clinical Presentation of Eosinophilic Gastroenteropathy**

| | NO. WITH SYMPTOM/TOTAL | PERCENTAGE |
|---|---|---|
| **Common Symptoms** | | |
| Vomiting | 40/80 | 50 |
| Diarrhea | 39/79 | 49 |
| Growth delay | 36/78 | 46 |
| Abdominal pain | 26/79 | 33 |
| Rectal bleeding | 14/73 | 19 |
| **Uncommon Symptoms** | | |
| Anemia | | |
| Edema/protein-losing enteropathy | | |
| Pyloric obstruction | | |
| Small bowel obstruction | | |
| Perforation | | |
| Ascites | | |
| Pancreatitis | | |
| Cholecystitis | | |
| **Laboratory Features** | | |
| Peripheral blood eosinophilia | 62/80 | 78 |
| Hypoalbuminemia | 15/23 | 65 |
| Increased serum IgE | 42/61 | 69 |
| Positive IgE-RAST to foods | 16/35 | 46 |
| Positive skin prick to foods | 9/26 | 35 |

Data from Katz et al,[92] Justinich et al,[157] Talley et al,[158] and Moon and Kleinman.[159]

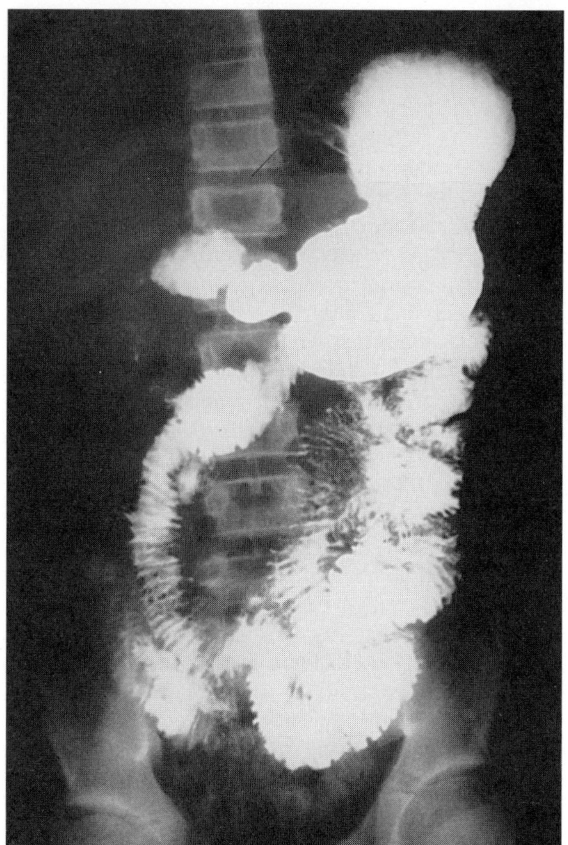

FIGURE 27–6. Diffuse thickening of small bowel folds in mucosal eosinophilic gastroenteropathy.

biopsies at multiple sites, because the characteristic mucosal eosinophilia may be patchy. The disease may affect the GI tract diffusely, with obvious thickening of intestinal mucosa (Fig. 27–6), or it may affect only specific sites. Eosinophilic colitis may mimic the signs, symptoms, and early pathologic findings of inflammatory bowel disease.[154, 160] Eosinophilic esophagitis manifests with dysphagia, pain, and even stricture formation.[161, 162] Rare manifestations include obstruction,[163] perforation,[164–166] hepatobiliary disease,[163, 167] and pancreatitis.[168]

*Muscle layer disease* causes obstruction and can affect any area of the bowel.[158] However, the classic site of involvement in childhood is at the gastric outlet (Fig. 27–7).[152, 169] The condition may mimic hypertrophic pyloric stenosis or other causes of gastric outlet obstruction, inflammatory bowel disease, or malignancy of the GI tract.

*Serosal eosinophilic gastroenteropathy* is rare and typically causes abdominal pain and ascites.[170] Underlying liver disease, renal disease, or malignancy must be ruled out. A diagnostic paracentesis shows marked eosinophilia.

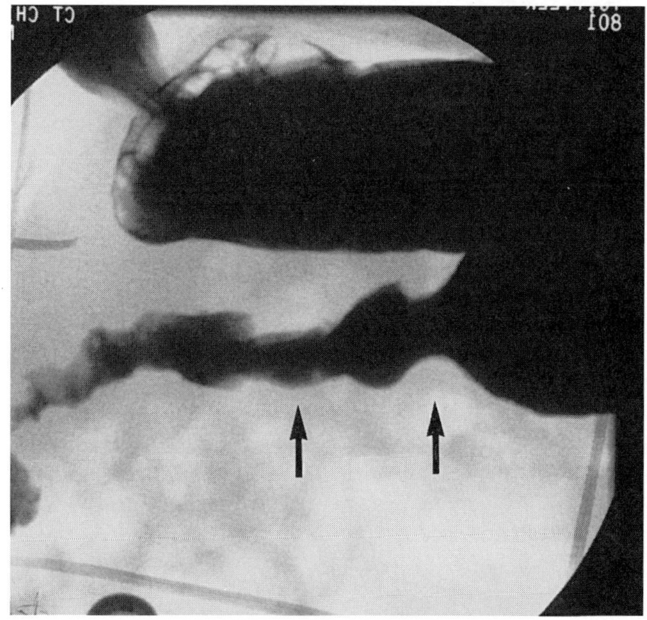


FIGURE 27–7. Pyloric narrowing *(arrows)* caused by eosinophilic thickening in the muscular form of eosinophilic gastroenteropathy. (Courtesy of C. Foley, MD.)

## Pathologic Findings

EGE is characterized by increased eosinophils in tissue, although there are no widely accepted criteria for the pathologic diagnosis. For mucosal biopsies, emphasis is placed on a minimum number of eosinophils (e.g., >20/hpf[156, 158] or >25% of the inflammatory infiltrate[82]). Some authors attach greater significance to the finding of intraepithelial eosinophils and degranulating eosinophils, as indicators of activity of disease.[157] A review of 180 biopsies from the upper GI tract in children undergoing endoscopy for a variety of reasons did not reveal more than 10 eosinophils per high-power field,[171] and similar studies of rectosigmoid biopsies considered normal showed fewer than 60 eosinophils per 6 high-power fields.[81] A pediatric autopsy series from Texas[172] called into question what is considered "normal" for eosinophils in the GI tract, unless geographical differences are present. The authors found that 52% of cases had at least one site with more than 20 eosinophils per high-power field; mean mucosal eosinophil counts ranged from 35/hpf in the cecum to 15/hpf in the duodenum and 5/hpf in the antrum. It is important to consider other causes of increased eosinophils in tissue and to correlate the findings with the clinical presentation.

## Radiographic Findings

The radiographic findings of EGE are nonspecific. The abnormalities seen relate to the site of involvement and also to the predominant layer of bowel involved with the disease (Table 27–5).[173, 174] These studies may be useful in the evaluation of site and extent of involvement, especially when they are considered in the context of a patient with a history of atopy, peripheral blood eosinophilia, and hypoalbuminemia. The most characteristic signs in young children are antral and pyloric abnormalities, including thickening of the muscular layer causing obstruction similar to hypertrophic pyloric stenosis (see Fig. 27–7)[169] and a "lacy" pattern and nodularity of the antrum. The small bowel mucosa may similarly show nodularity, thickening of folds (see Fig. 27–6), and signs of malabsorption with increased small bowel fluid. Eosinophilic esophagitis may cause diffuse stricturing of the esophagus, often more proximal to that expected from peptic disease.[161, 162] Serosal disease characteristically manifests with eosinophilic ascites.[170] More rare findings include ulcers with or without perforation,[164–166] bowel obstruction,[163] and evidence of cholecystitis and pancreatitis.[168]

## Management

Despite the fact that "idiopathic" EGE responds poorly to dietary therapy, an attempt should be made to identify potential food allergens and eliminate these proteins first. If allergy is suspected or if biopsies reveal evidence of eosinophilia, our practice is to perform a complete blood count and differential, serum albumin, serum IgA, and serum IgE determinations as a general indication of atopy. Specific IgE-RASTs for milk, soy, egg, and peanut are performed along with tests for any specific food that may be implicated in the development of symptoms, as determined by a careful history. If duodenal villous atrophy is profound, antigliadin and antiendomysial antibodies for celiac disease are included. We also enlist the help of a clinical allergist to perform skin tests as indicated, in an attempt to document specific food allergens.

If these tests are unrevealing, or if the patient has not responded to elimination of suspected foods, then a milk-protein-free diet is tried for 2 to 3 weeks to see whether symptoms improve, even in the absence of objective evidence of milk sensitivity. It is essential to enlist the help of a qualified dietitian who can educate families properly to avoid unintentional ingestions by reading food labels and to ensure that nutritional requirements are being met. We have also used elimination diets to try to improve symptoms and investigate which foods may be implicated. Ultimately, complete exclusion of intact food protein (exclusive elemental diet) can be used to determine whether food antigens are implicated in disease.[122, 123] One report has described reversal of symptoms, growth delay, laboratory abnormalities, and long-term dependence on corticosteroids in response to an exclusive elemental diet, although it is uncertain whether the improvement was caused by removal of food antigens or some other mechanism.[175]

Corticosteroids are the mainstay of pharmacologic therapy for idiopathic EGE. We start with prednisone or equivalent at 2 mg/kg per day (maximum 40 mg), with tapering to low-dose alternate-day therapy within 6 to 8 weeks. Eosinophilic inflammation typically responds to treatment with corticosteroids, and symptoms resolve quickly. A subgroup of patients relapse when tapered and may do well with a low-dose alternate-day regimen.

Agents that stabilize mast cells have been used to treat this disorder even though it is not established that mast cells are implicated in the pathophysiology of the disease. Sodium cromoglycate has been used, although this medication is thought to be degraded in the stomach when taken orally. Anecdotal evidence from case reports argues both for and against its efficacy.[167, 175–179] Ketotifen is a mast cell–stabilizing agent that has effects on eosinophil migration and activation. It can be efficacious to treat EGE, has minimal side effects, and has been reported to enable chronic corticosteroid-dependent patients to discontinue corticosteroids.[180] Budesonide, a topically active corticosteroid, was used successfully to treat one case of ileocolonic disease.[179]

These is no established usefulness for antihistamines, although there is one case report of decreased symptoms from food allergy with the use of cetirizine, a histamine $H_1$ receptor antagonist.[181]

**TABLE 27–5. Radiographic Features of Eosinophilic Gastroenteropathy**

| Predominant Mucosal Disease | Predominant Serosal Disease |
|---|---|
| Thickened folds | Ascites |
| Polyps | Pleural effusion |
| Gastric or duodenal ulcers | Adherent loops of bowel |
| Spasm | Omental/mesenteric thickening |
| Hypersecretion | Eosinophilic lymphadenopathy |
| Areae gastricae (antral abnormality) | |
| **Predominant Muscularis Disease** | |
| Stenosis including pyloric stenosis | |
| Rigidity | |
| Dysmotility | |

Adapted from Vilettas KM, Bennett WF, Bova JG, et al: Radiographic manifestations of eosinophilic gastroenteritis. Abdom Imaging 1995;20:406–413; and Littlewood Teele RL, Katz AJ, Goldman H, Kettell RM: Radiographic features of eosinophilic gastroenteritis (allergic gastroenteropathy) of childhood. AJR Am J Roentgenol 1979;132:575–580, with permission.


**REFERENCES**

1. Esteban MM: Adverse food reactions in childhood: concept, importance and present problems. J Pediatr Gastroenterol Nutr 1992;121:S1–S3.

2. Sampson HA: Differential diagnosis in adverse reactions to foods. J Allergy Clin Immunol 1986;78:212–219.
3. Ferguson A: Definitions and diagnosis of food allergy: consensus and controversy. J Pediatr 1992;121:S7–S11.
4. The European Society for Pediatric Gastroenterology and Nutrition Working Group for the Diagnostic Criteria for Food Allergy: Diagnostic criteria for food allergy with predominantly intestinal symptoms. J Pediatr Gastroenterol Nutr 1992;14:108–112.
5. Walker-Smith JA: Diagnostic criteria for gastrointestinal food allergy in childhood. Clin Exp Allergy 1995;25(suppl 1):20–22.
6. Ferguson A: Scope and diagnostic criteria of food hypersensitivity. Clin Exp Allergy 1995;25:111–113.
7. May CD: Are confusion and controversy about food hypersensitivity really necessary? J Allergy Clin Immunol 1985;75:329–333.
8. Hide DW: Food allergy in children. Clin Exp Allergy 1994;24:1–2.
9. Warner JO: Food and behaviour. Clin Exp Allergy 1995;25(suppl 1):23–26.
10. Roesler TA, Barry PC, Bock A: Factitious food allergy and failure to thrive. Arch Pediatr Adolesc Med 1994;148:1150–1155.
11. Lee TGD, Swieter M, Befus D: Mast cells, eosinophils, and gastrointestinal hypersensitivity. Immunol Allergy Clin North Am 1988;8: 469–483.
12. Kletter B, Gery I, Freier S, et al: Immune responses of normal infants to cow milk: antibody type and kinetics of production. Int Arch Allergy Immunol 1971;40:656–666.
13. Udall JN: Serum antibodies to endogenous proteins: the significance? J Pediatr Gastroenterol Nutr 1989;8:145–147.
14. Muller G, Bernsau I, Muller W, et al: Cow milk protein antigens and antibodies in serum of premature infants during the first 10 days of life. J Pediatr 1986;109:869–873.
15. Axelsson I, Jakobsson I, Lindberg T, et al: Macromolecular absorption in preterm and term infants. Acta Paediatr Scand 1989;78:532–537.
16. Cunningham-Rundles C, Brandeis WE, Good RA, et al: Milk precipitins, circulating immune complexes, and IgA deficiency. Immunology 1978;75:3378–3389.
17. Macdonald TT: Evidence for cell-mediated hypersensitivity as an important pathogenic mechanism in food intolerance. Clin Exp Allergy 1995;25(suppl 1):10–13.
18. Metcalfe DD, Sampson HA, Simon RA (eds): Food Allergy: Adverse Reactions to Foods and Food Additives, 2nd ed. Cambridge, MA, Blackwell Science, 1997.
19. Crowe SE, Perdue MH: Gastrointestinal food hypersensitivity: basic mechanisms of pathophysiology. Gastroenterology 1992;103:1075–1095.
20. Macdermott RP, Elson CO (eds): Mucosal Immunology I: Basic Principles. Gastroenterol Clin North Am 1991;20(3).
21. Metcalfe DD: Food hypersensitivity. J Allergy Clin Immunol 1984;73:749–762.
22. Brandtzaeg P, Nilssen DE, Rognum TO, et al: Ontogeny of the mucosal immune system and IgA deficiency. In Macdermott RP, Elson CO (eds): Mucosal Immunology I: Basic Principles. Gastroenterol Clin North Am 1991;20:397–440.
23. Bland PW, Kambarage DM: Antigen handling by the epithelium and lamina propria macrophages. In Macdermott RP, Elson CO (eds): Mucosal Immunology I: Basic Principles. Gastroenterol Clin North Am 1991;20:577–596.
24. Russell GJ, Bhan AK, Winter HS: The distribution of T and B lymphocyte populations and MHC class II expression in human fetal and postnatal intestine. Pediatr Res 1990;27:239–244.
25. Davin J-C, Senterre J, Mahieu PR: The high lectin-binding capacity of human secretory IgA protects nonspecifically mucosae against environmental antigens. Biol Neonate 1991;59:121–125.
26. Nagata S, Yamashiro Y, Ohtsuka Y, et al: Quantitative analysis and immunohistochemical studies on small intestinal mucosa of food sensitive enteropathy. J Pediatr Gastroenterol Nutr 1995;20:44–48.
27. de Jong EC, Spanhaak S, Martens BPM, et al: Food allergen (peanut)-specific TH2 clones generated from the peripheral blood of a patient with food allergy. J Allergy Clin Immunol 1996;98:73–81.
28. Andre F, Pene J, Andre C: Interleukin-4 and interferon-gamma production by peripheral blood mononuclear cells from food-allergic patients. Allergy 1996;51:350–355.
29. Desreumaux P, Bloget F, Seguy D, et al: Interleukin 3, granulocyte-macrophage colony-stimulating factor, and interleukin 5 in eosinophilic gastroenteritis. Gastroenterology 1996;110:768–774.
30. Jaffe JS, James SP, Mullins GE, et al: Evidence for an abnormal profile of interleukin-4 (IL-4), IL-5, and interferon-gamma (γ-INF) in peripheral blood T cells from patients with allergic eosinophilic gastroenteritis. J Clin Immunol 1994:14:299–309.
31. Heyman M, Darmon N, Dupont C, et al: Mononuclear cells from infants allergic to cow's milk secrete tumor necrosis factor α, altering intestinal function. Gastroenterology 1994;106:1514–1523.
32. Borish L, Rosenwasser L: $T_{H1}/T_{H2}$ lymphocytes: Doubt some more. J Allergy Clin Immunol 1997;99:161–164.
33. Bischoff SC: Mucosal allergy: role of mast cells and eosinophil granulocytes in the gut. Baillieres Clin Gastroenterol 1996;10:443–459.
34. Weller PF: The immunobiology of eosinophils. N Engl J Med 1991;324:1110–1118.
35. Levy AM, Kita K: The eosinophil in gut inflammation: effector or director? Gastroenterology 1996;110:952–954.
36. Leinbach GE, Rubin CE: Eosinophilic gastroenteritis: a simple reaction to food allergens? Gastroenterology 1970;59:874–889.
37. Church MK, Levi-Schaffer F: The human mast cell. J Allergy Clin Immunol 1997;99:155–160.
38. Saavedra-Delgado AM, Metcalfe DD: The gastrointestinal mast cell in food allergy. Ann Allergy 1983;51:185–189.
39. Moller A, Grabbe J, Czarnetzki BM: Mast cells and their mediators in immediate and delayed immune reactions. Skin Pharmacol 1991;4(suppl 1):56–63.
40. Knutson TW, Bengtsson U, Dannaeus A, et al: Intestinal reactivity in allergic and non-allergic patients: an approach to determine the complexity of the mucosal reaction. J Allergy Clin Immunol 1993;91:553–559.
41. Altman DR, Chiaramonte LT: Public perception of food allergy. J Allergy Clin Immunol 1996;97:1247–1251.
42. Young E, Stoneham MD, Petruchevitch A, et al: A population study of food intolerance. Lancet 1994;343:1127–1130.
43. Bischoff SC, Herrmann A, Manns MP: Prevalence of adverse reactions to food in patients with gastrointestinal disease. Allergy 1996;51:811–818.
44. Bock SA: Prospective appraisal of complaints of adverse reactions to foods in children during the first 3 years of life. Pediatrics 1987;79:683–688.
45. Kivity S, Dunner K, Marian Y: The pattern of food hypersensitivity in patients with onset after 10 years of age. Clin Exp Allergy 1994;24:19–22.
46. Jakobsson I, Lindberg T: A prospective study of cow's milk protein intolerance in Swedish infants. Acta Paediatr Scand 1979;68:853–859.
47. Gerrard JW, MacKenzie JWA, Goluboff N, et al: Cow's milk allergy: prevalence and manifestations in an unselected series of newborns. Acta Paediatr Scand 1973;234 (suppl):1–21.
48. Bock SA, Atkins FM: Patterns of food hypersensitivity during sixteen years of double-blind, placebo-controlled food challenges. J Pediatr 1990;117:561–567.
49. Sampson HA: IgE-mediated food intolerance. J Allergy Clin Immunol 1988;81:495–504.
50. Binkley KE: Allergy to supplemental lactase enzyme. J Allergy Clin Immunol 1996;97:1414–1416.
51. Binkley KE: Making maple syrup: hazardous vocational ingestion of raw sap in a patient with nut and tree pollen sensitivity. J Allergy Clin Immunol 1994;94:267–268.
52. Lifschitz CH, Hawkins HK, Guerra C, et al: Anaphylactic shock due to cow's milk protein hypersensitivity in a breast-fed infant. J Pediatr Gastroenterol Nutr 1988;7:141–144.
53. Saylor JD, Bahna SL: Anaphylaxis to casein hydrolysate formula. J Pediatr 1991;118:71–73.
54. Ellis MH, Short JA, Heiner DC: Anaphylaxis after ingestion of a recently introduced hydrolyzed whey protein formula. J Pediatr 1991;118:74–77.
55. Cavataio F, Carroccio A, Montalto G, et al: Isolated rice intolerance: clinical and immunologic characteristics in four infants. J Pediatr 1996;128:558–560.
56. Gern JE, Yang E, Evrard HM, et al: Allergic reactions to milk-contaminated "non-dairy" products. N Engl J Med 1991;324:976–979.
57. Steinman HA: "Hidden" allergens in foods. J Allergy Clin Immunol 1996;98:241–250.
58. Atkins FM, Steinberg SS, Metcalfe DD: Evaluation of immediate adverse reactions to foods in adult patients: II. A detailed analysis of reaction patterns during oral food challenge. J Allergy Clin Immunol 1985;75:356–363.

59. Sampson HA, Albergo R: Comparison of results of skin tests, RAST, and double-blind food challenges in children with atopic dermatitis. J Allergy Clin Immunol 1984;74:26–33.
60. Sampson HA, Mendelson L, Rosen JP: Fatal and near fatal anaphylactic reactions to food in children and adolescents. N Engl J Med 1992;327:380–384.
61. Tilles S, Schocket A, Milgrom H: Exercise-induced anaphylaxis related to specific foods. J Pediatr 1995;127:587–589.
62. Caffarelli C, Terzi V, Perrone F, et al: Food related, exercise induced anaphylaxis. Arch Dis Child 1996;75:141–144.
63. Kaplan MS: The importance of appropriate challenges in diagnosing food sensitivity. Clin Exp Allergy 1994;24:291–293.
64. Amlot PL, Kemeny DM, Zachary C, et al: Oral allergy syndrome (OAS): symptoms of IgE-mediated hypersensitivity to foods. Clin Exp Allergy 1987;17:33–42.
65. Ortolani C, Ispano M, Pastorello E, et al: The oral allergy syndrome. Ann Allergy 1988;61:47–52.
66. Ortolani C, Ispano M, Pastorello EA, et al: Comparison of results of skin prick tests (with fresh foods and commercial food extracts) and RAST in 100 patients with oral allergy syndrome. J Allergy Clin Immunol 1989;83:683–690.
67. Champion RH, Roberts SOB, Carpenter RG, et al: Urticaria and angioedema: a review of 554 patients. Br J Dermatol 1969;81:588–597.
68. Harris A, Twarog FJ, Geha RF: Chronic urticaria childhood: natural course and etiology. Ann Allergy 1983;51:161–165.
69. Burks AW, Mallory SB, Williams LW, et al: Atopic dermatitis: clinical relevance of food hypersensitivity reactions. J Pediatr 1988;113:447–451.
70. Sampson HA, McCaskill CC: Food hypersensitivity and atopic dermatitis: evaluation of 113 patients. J Pediatr 1985;107:669–675.
71. Patel L, Radivan FS, David TJ: Management of anaphylactic reactions to food. Arch Dis Child 1994;71:370–375.
72. Rosen JP, Selcow JE, Mendelson LM, et al: Skin testing with natural foods in patients suspected of having food allergies: Is it a necessity? J Allergy Clin Immunol 1994;93:1068–1070.
73. Businco L, Benincori N, Cantani A: Epidemiology, incidence and clinical aspects of food allergy. Ann Allergy 1984;53:615–622.
74. Odze RD, Wershil BK, Leichtner AM, et al: Allergic colitis in infants. J Pediatr 1995;126:163–170.
75. Odze RD, Bines J, Leichtner AM, et al: Allergic proctocolitis in infants. Hum Pathol 1993;24:668–674.
76. Machida HM, Catto Smith AG, Gall DG, et al: Allergic colitis in infancy: clinical and pathologic aspects. J Pediatr Gastroenterol Nutr 1994;19:22–26.
77. Lake AM, Whitington PF, Hamilton SR: Dietary protein-induced colitis in breast-fed infants. J Pediatr 1982;101:906–910.
78. Pittscheiler K: Cow's milk protein-induced colitis in the breast-fed infant. J Pediatr Gastroenterol Nutr 1990;10:548–549.
79. Piastra M, Stabile A, Fioravanti G, et al: Cord blood mononuclear cell responsiveness to beta-lactoglobulin: T-cell activity in "atopy-prone" and "non-atopy-prone" newborns. Int Arch Allergy Immunol 1994;104:358–365.
80. Szepfalusi Z, Nentwich I, Gerstmayr M, et al: Prenatal allergen contact with milk proteins. Clin Exp Allergy 1997;27:28–35.
81. Winter HS, Antonioli DA, Fukagawa N, et al: Allergy-related proctocolitis in infants: diagnostic usefulness of rectal biopsy. Mod Pathol 1990;3:5–10.
82. Goldman H, Proujansky R: Allergic proctitis and gastroenteritis in children: clinical and mucosal biopsy features in 53 cases. Am J Surg Pathol 1986;10:75–86.
83. Ojuawo A, St Louis D, Lindley KJ, et al: Non-infective colitis in infancy: evidence in favour of minor immunodeficiency in its pathogenesis. Arch Dis Child 1997;76:345–348.
84. Kuitunen P, Visakorpi JK, Savilahti E, et al: Malabsorption syndrome with cow's milk intolerance: clinical findings and course in 54 cases. Arch Dis Child 1975;50:351–356.
85. Manuel PD, Walker-Smith JA, France NE: Patchy enteropathy in childhood. Gut 1979;20:211–215.
86. Walker-Smith JA: Cow milk-sensitive enteropathy: predisposing factors and treatment. J Pediatr 1992;121:S111–S115.
87. Iyngkaran N, Yadav M, Boey CG, et al: Severity and extent of upper small bowel mucosal damage in cow's milk protein-sensitive enteropathy. J Pediatr Gastroenterol Nutr 1988;7:667–674.
88. Challacomb DN, Wheeler EE, Campbell PE: Morphometric studies and eosinophil counts in the duodenal mucosa of children with chronic nonspecific diarrhea and cow's milk allergy. J Pediatr Gastroenterol Nutr 1986;5:887–891.
89. Rosekrans PCM, Meijer CJLM, Cornelisse CJ, et al: Use of morphometry and immunohistochemistry of small intestinal biopsy specimens in the diagnosis of food allergy. J Clin Pathol 1980;33:125–130.
90. Ament ME, Rubin CE: Soy protein: another cause of the flat intestinal lesion. Gastroenterology 1972;62:227–229.
91. Vitoria JC, Camarero C, Sojo A, et al: Enteropathy related to fish, rice and chicken. Arch Dis Child 1982;57:44–48.
92. Katz AJ, Twarog FJ, Zeiger RS, et al: Milk-sensitive and eosinophilic gastroenteropathy: similar clinical features with contrasting mechanisms and clinical course. J Allergy Clin Immunol 1984;74:72–78.
93. Kelly KJ, Lazenby AJ, Rowe PC, et al: Eosinophilic esophagitis attributed to gastroesophageal reflux: improvement with an amino acid-based formula. Gastroenterology 1995;109:1503–1512.
94. Kalafus D, Ricci A, Hyams J, et al: Demonstration of increased mucosal mast cells in esophagitis in children. Gastroenterology 1996:110:A148.
95. Sampson HA: Infantile colic and food allergy: fact or fiction? J Pediatr 1989;115:583–584.
96. Taubman B: Parental counseling compared with elimination of cow's milk or soy protein for the treatment of infant colic syndrome: a randomized trial. Pediatrics 1988;83:756–761.
97. Lothe L, Lindberg T: Cow's milk whey protein elicits symptoms of infantile colic in colicky formula-fed infants. Pediatrics 1989;83:262–266.
98. Forsyth BWC: Colic and the effect of changing formulas: a double-blind multiple crossover study. J Pediatr 1989;115:521–526.
99. Kahn A, Mozin MJ, Rebuffat E, et al: Milk intolerance in children with persistent sleeplessness: a prospective double-blind crossover evaluation. Pediatrics 1989;84:595–603.
100. Kondo N, Fukutomi O, Agata H, et al: The role of T lymphocytes in patients with food-sensitive atopic dermatitis. J Allergy Clin Immunol 1993;91:658–668.
101. Sampson HA: Food antigen-induced lymphocyte proliferation in children with atopic dermatitis and food hypersensitivity. J Allergy Clin Immunol 1993;91:549–551.
102. Frew AJ: How useful are T cell clones in investigating allergy? Clin Exp Allergy 1995;25:1143–1144.
103. Iida S, Kondo N, Agata H, et al: Differences in lymphocyte proliferative responses to food antigens and specific IgE antibodies to foods with age among food sensitive patients with atopic dermatitis. Ann Allergy Asthma Immunol 1995;74:334–340.
104. Fukutomi O, Kondo N, Agata H, et al: Timing of onset of allergic symptoms as a response to a double-blind, placebo-controlled food challenge in patients with food allergy combined with a radioallergosorbent test and the evaluation of proliferative lymphocyte responses. Int Arch Allergy Immunol 1994;104:352–357.
105. Werfel T, Ahlers G, Schmidt P, et al: Detection of a κ-casein-specific lymphocyte response in milk-responsive atopic dermatitis. Clin Exp Allergy 1996;26:1380–1386.
106. Reekers R, Beyer K, Niggemann B, et al: The role of circulating food antigen-specific lymphocytes in food allergic children with atopic dermatitis. Br J Dermatol 1996;135:935–941.
107. Van Sickle GJ, Keating Powell G, McDonald PJ, et al: Milk and soy protein-induced enterocolitis: evidence for lymphocyte sensitization to specific food proteins. Gastroenterology 1985;88:1915–1921.
108. Eigenmann PA, Belli DC, Ludi F, et al: In vitro lymphocyte proliferation with milk and casein-whey protein hydrolyzed formula in children with cow's milk allergy. J Allergy Clin Immunol 1995;96:549–557.
109. Breneman JC, Sweeney M, Robert A, et al: Patch tests demonstrating immune reaction to foods. Ann Allergy 1989;62:461–469.
110. Burks AW, Sampson HA: Diagnostic approaches to the patient with suspected food allergy. J Pediatr 1992;121:S64–S71.
111. Baehler P, Chad Z, Gurbindo C, et al: Distinct patterns of cow's milk allergy in infancy defined by prolonged, two-stage double-blind, placebo-controlled food challenges. Clin Exp Allergy 1996;26:254–261.
112. Bengtsson U, Nilsson-Balknas U, Hanson LA, et al: Double blind, placebo controlled food reactions do not correlate to IgE allergy in the diagnosis of staple food related gastrointestinal symptoms. Gut 1996;39:130–135.
113. Hill DJ, Firer MA, Shelton MJ, et al: Manifestations of milk allergy in infancy: clinical and immunologic findings. J Pediatr 1986;109:270–276.

114. Kleinman RE: Cow milk allergy in infancy and hypoallergenic formulas. J Pediatr 1992;121:S116–S121.
115. Sampson HA, Bernhisel-Broadbent J, Yang E, et al: Safety of casein hydrolysate formula in children with cow milk allergy. J Pediatr 1991;118:520–525.
116. Wahn U, Wahl R, Rugo E: Comparison of the residual allergenic activity of six different hydrolyzed protein formulas. J Pediatr 1992;121:S80–S84.
117. Hide DW, Gant C: Hypoallergenic formulae: have they a therapeutic role? Clin Exp Allergy 1994;24:3–5.
118. Businco L, Bruno G, Gianni Giampietro P, et al: Allergenicity and nutritional adequacy of soy protein formulas. J Pediatr 1992;121:S21–S28.
119. McLeish CM, Macdonald A, Booth IW: Comparison of an elemental with a hydrolysed whey formula in intolerance to cow's milk. Arch Dis Child 1995;73:211–215.
120. Sampson HA, James JM, Bernhisel-Broadbent J: Safety of an amino-acid derived infant formula in children allergic to cow milk. Pediatrics 1992;90:463–464.
121. Hill DJ, Cameron DJS, Francis DEM: Challenge confirmation of late-onset reactions to extensively hydrolyzed formulas in infants with multiple food protein intolerance. J Allergy Clin Immunol 1995;96:386–394.
122. Dockhorn RJ, Smith TC: Use of a chemically defined hypoallergenic diet (Vivonex®) in the management of suspected food allergy. Ann Allergy 1981;47:264–266.
123. Justinich CJ, Seidman E, Roy CC: Elemental diet in food hypersensitivity. In Bounos G (ed): Elemental Diets. Boca Raton, FL, CRC Press, 1993, pp 281–296.
124. Zanussi C, Pastorello E: Dietary treatment of food allergy. In Brostoff J, Challacombe SJ (eds): Food Allergy and Intolerance. London, Bailliere Tindall, 1987, pp 971–976.
125. Smith LJ, Munoz-Furlong A: The management of food allergy. In Metcalfe DD, Sampson HA, Simon RA (eds): Food Allergy: Adverse Reactions to Foods and Food Additives, 2nd ed. Cambridge, MA, Blackwell Science, 1997, pp 431–444.
126. Sogn D: Medications and their use in the treatment of adverse reactions to foods. J Allergy Clin Immunol 1986;78:238–243.
127. Burks AW, Sampson HA: Double-blind placebo-controlled trial of oral cromolyn in children with atopic dermatitis and documented food hypersensitivity. J Allergy Clin Immunol 1988;81:417–423.
128. Businco L, Benincori N, Nini G, et al: Double-blind crossover trial with oral sodium cromoglycate in children with atopic dermatitis due to food allergy. Ann Allergy 1986;57:433–438.
129. Osvath P, Kelenhegyi K, Micskey E: Comparison of ketotifen and DSCG in treatment of food allergy in children. Allergol Immunopathol (Madr) 1986;14:515–518.
130. Majamaa H, Isolauri E: Probiotics: a novel approach in the management of food allergy. J Allergy Clin Immunol 1997;99:179–185.
131. Bishop JM, Hill DJ, Hosking CS: Natural history of cow's milk allergy: clinical outcome. J Pediatr 1990;116:862–867.
132. Hill DJ, Firer MA, Ball G, Hosking CS: Natural history of cow's milk allergy in children: immunological outcome over 2 years. Clin Exp Allergy 1993;23:124–131.
133. James JM, Sampson HA: Immunologic changes associated with the development of tolerance in children with cow milk allergy. J Pediatr 1992;121:371–377.
133a. Sampson HA, Ho DG: Relationship between food-specific IgE concentrations and the risk of positive food challenges in children and adolescents. J Allergy Clin Immunol 1997;100:444–451.
134. Bock SA: Natural history of severe reactions to foods in young children. J Pediatr 1985;107:676–680.
135. Kaplan MS: Complications in children with severe allergy to cow milk. Ann Allergy 1993;71:529–532.
136. Kerner JA: Use of infant formulas in preventing or postponing atopic manifestations. J Pediatr Gastroenterol Nutr 1997;24:442–446.
137. Gruskay FL: Comparison of breast, cow, and soy feedings in the prevention of onset of allergic disease: a 15-year prospective study. Clin Pediatr 1982;21:486–491.
138. Zeiger RS: Prevention of food allergy in infancy. Ann Allergy 1990;65:430–441.
139. Zeiger RS, Heller S: The development and prediction of atopy in high risk children: follow-up at age seven years in a prospective randomized study of combined maternal and infant food allergen avoidance. J Allergy Clin Immunol 1995;95:1179–1190.
140. Mallet E, Henocq A: Long-term prevention of allergic diseases by using protein hydrolysate formula in at risk infants. J Pediatr 1992;121:S95–S100.
141. Chandra RK: Five-year follow-up of high risk infants with family history of allergy who were exclusively breast-fed or fed partial whey hydrolysate, soy, and conventional cow's milk formulas. J Pediatr Gastroenterol Nutr 1997;24:380–388.
142. Khoshoo V, Schantz P, Craver R, et al: Dog hookworm: a cause of eosinophilic enterocolitis in humans. J Pediatr Gastroenterol Nutr 1994;19:448–452.
143. DeSchryver-Kecskemeti N, Clouse RF: A previously unrecognized subgroup of "eosinophilic gastroenteritis": association with connective tissue diseases. Am J Surg Pathol 1984;8:171–180.
144. Buchman AL, Wolf D, Gramlich T: Eosinophilic gastrojejunitis associated with connective tissue disease. South Med J 1996;89:327–330.
145. Fishbein M, Kirschner BS, Gonzales-Vallina R, et al: Ménétrier's disease associated with formula protein allergy and small intestinal injury in an infant. Gastroenterology 1992;103:1664–1668.
146. Olson AD, Fukui-Miner K: Eosinophilic mucosal infiltrate in infants with congenital gastrointestinal obstruction. Am J Gastroenterol 1994;89:934–936.
147. McGovern TW, Talley NJ, Kephart GM, et al: Eosinophil infiltration and degranulation in *Helicobacter pylori*-associated chronic gastritis. Dig Dis Sci 1991;36:435–440.
148. Walsh RE, Gaginella TS: The eosinophil in inflammatory bowel disease. Scand J Gastroenterol 1991;26:1217–1224.
149. Anttilla VJ, Valtonen M: Carbamazepine-induced eosinophilic colitis. Epilepsia 1992;33:119–121.
150. Martin DM, Goldman JA, Gilliam J, et al: Gold-induced eosinophilic enterocolitis: response to oral cromolyn sodium. Gastroenterology 1981;80:1567–1570.
151. Falade AG, Darbyshire PJ, Raafat F, et al: Hypereosinophilic syndrome in childhood appearing as inflammatory bowel disease. J Pediatr Gastroenterol Nutr 1991;12:276–279.
152. Snyder JD, Rosenblum N, Weshil B, et al: Pyloric stenosis and eosinophilic gastroenteritis in infants. J Pediatr Gastroenterol Nutr 1987;6:543–547.
153. Griscom NT, Kirkpatrick JA, Girdany BR, et al: Gastric antral narrowing in chronic granulomatous disease of childhood. Pediatrics 1974;54:456–460.
154. Haberkern CM, Christie DL, Haas JE: Eosinophilic gastroenteritis presenting as ileocolitis. Gastroenterology 1978;74:896–899.
155. Klein NC, Hargrove RL, Sleisenger MH, et al: Eosinophilic gastroenteritis. Gastroenterology 1970;49:299–319.
156. Whitington PF, Whitington GL: Eosinophilic gastroenteropathy in childhood. J Pediatr Gastroenterol Nutr 1988;7:379–385.
157. Justinich C, Matte C, Russo P, et al: Eosinophilic gastroenteropathy in childhood. Gastroenterology 1991;100:A219.
158. Talley NJ, Shorter RG, Phillips SF, et al: Eosinophilic gastroenteritis: a clinicopathological study of patients with disease of the mucosa, muscle layer, and subserosal tissues. Gut 1990;31:54–58.
159. Moon A, Kleinman RE: Allergic gastroenteropathy in children. Ann Allergy Asthma Immunol 1995;74:5–12.
160. Moore D, Lichtman S, Lentz J, et al: Eosinophilic gastroenteritis presenting in an adolescent with isolated colon involvement. Gut 1986;29:1219–1222.
161. Attwood SEA, Smyrk TC, Demeester TR, et al: Esophageal eosinophilia with dysphagia: a distinct clinicopathologic syndrome. Dig Dis Sci 1993;38:109–116.
162. Van Rosendaal GMA, Anderson MA, Diamant NE: Eosinophilic esophagitis: case report and clinical perspective. Am J Gastroenterol 1997;92:1054–1056.
163. Rumans MC, Lieberman DA: Eosinophilic gastroenteritis presenting with biliary and duodenal obstruction. Am J Gastroenterol 1987;82:775–778.
164. Felt-Bersma RJF, Meuwissen SGM, van Velzen D: Perforation of the small intestine due to eosinophilic gastroenteritis. Am J Gastroenterol 1984;79:442–445.
165. Walia HS, Abraham TK, Walia HK: Eosinophilic enteritis with perforation. Can J Surg 1988;31:268–269.
166. Deslandres C, Russo P, Gould P, et al: Perforated duodenal ulcer in a pediatric patient with eosinophilic enteritis. Can J Gastroenterol 1997:11:208–212.
167. Steffen RM, Wyllie R, Petras RE, et al: The spectrum of eosinophilic gastroenteritis. Clin Pediatr 1991;30:404–411.

168. Flejou JF, Potet F, Bernades P: La pancreatite a eosinophils: une manifestation rare de l'allergie digestive? Gastroenterol Clin Biol 1989;13:731–733.
169. Blankenberg FG, Parker BR, Sibley E, et al: Evolving asymmetric hypertrophic pyloric stenosis associated with histologic evidence of eosinophilic gastroenteritis. Pediatr Radiol 1995;25:310–311.
170. Hyams JS, Treem WR, Schwartz AN: Recurrent abdominal pain and ascites in an adolescent. J Pediatr 1988;113:569–574.
171. Black DD, Haggitt RC, Whitington PF: Gastroduodenal endoscopic-histologic correlation in pediatric patients. J Pediatr Gastroenterol Nutr 1988;7:361–366.
172. Lowichik A, Weinburg AG: A quantitative evaluation of mucosal eosinophils in the pediatric gastrointestinal tract. Mod Pathol 1996;9:110–114.
173. Vitellas KM, Bennett WF, Bova JG, et al: Radiographic manifestations of eosinophilic gastroenteritis. Abdom Imaging 1995;20:406–413.
174. Littlewood Teele R, Katz AJ, Goldman H, et al: Radiographic features of eosinophilic gastroenteritis (allergic gastroenteropathy) of childhood. AJR Am J Roentgenol 1979;132:575–580.
175. Justinich C, Katz A, Gurbindo C, et al: Elemental diet improves steroid dependent eosinophilic gastroenteropathy and reverses growth failure. J Pediatr Gastroenterol Nutr 1996;23:81–85.
176. Moots RJ, Prouse P, Gumpel JM: Near fatal eosinophilic gastroenteritis responding to oral sodium cromoglycate. Gut 1988;29:1282–1285.
177. Heatley RV, Harris A, Atkinson M: Treatment of a patient with clinical features of both eosinophilic gastroenteritis and polyarteritis nodosa with oral sodium cromoglycate. Dig Dis Sci 1980;25:470–473.
178. Kravis LP, South MA, Rosenlund ML: Eosinophilic gastroenteritis in the pediatric patient. Clin Pediatr 1982;21:713–717.
179. Russel MGVM, Zeijen RNM, Brummer R-JM, et al: Eosinophilic enterocolitis diagnosed by means of technetium-99m albumin scintigraphy and treated with budesonide. Gut 1994;35:1490–1492.
180. Melamed I, Feanny SJ, Sherman PM, et al: Benefit of ketotifen in patients with eosinophilic gastroenteritis. Am J Med 1991;90:310–314.
181. Shaikh WA: Cetirizine: effective treatment for food (egg) allergy. Allergy 1996;51:275–276.

# Chapter 28

# Infectious Diarrhea

*Mitchell B. Cohen and D. Wayne Laney, Jr.*

In the United States, an estimated 21 to 37 million episodes of diarrhea occur annually in children younger than 5 years of age.[1] Ten percent of these children are seen by a physician, more than 200,000 are hospitalized, and between 300 and 400 die from the illness. Worldwide, the number of childhood deaths from diarrhea is higher than 4 million per year.

Knowledge of diarrheal disease has increased remarkably during the past few decades.[2, 3] Numerous bacterial pathogens and an increasing number of viral pathogens have been demonstrated to cause diarrhea. This increased understanding of pathogenic mechanisms has led to improvements in therapy. This chapter discusses the major viral and bacterial agents of infectious diarrhea, including their epidemiology, pathogenesis, clinical manifestations, diagnosis, and therapy.

## VIRAL GASTROENTERITIS

Diarrheal disease caused by viral agents occurs far more frequently than does similar disease of bacterial origin. In fact, viral gastroenteritis is the second most common illness in the United States, after the common cold.[4] Despite the frequent occurrence of viral enteritides, the identification of a specific virus as causative agent is a relatively recent development.[5] Rotavirus and a number of other small round structured viruses have been identified as a major cause of nonbacterial gastroenteritis in children and adults. This discussion focuses on these established pathogens, then continues with a brief summary of several newer viral enteropathogens and the current status of several candidate pathogens.

### Rotavirus

Rotavirus was first identified as a specific viral pathogen in duodenal cells of children with diarrhea by Bishop and associates in 1973.[6] Subsequent studies indicated that rotavirus is responsible not only for more cases of diarrheal disease in infants and children than any other single cause but also for a significant portion of deaths caused by diarrhea in both developed and developing countries throughout the world.[7] Rotavirus is responsible for 20% to 70% of hospitalizations for diarrhea among children worldwide.[8]

#### *Virology*

The genus Rotavirus is classified as a member of the family Reoviridae of the RNA viruses. Rotaviruses are round particles 68 nm in diameter and are composed of two separate shells (capsids). The capsids surround a 38-nm icosahedral core structure, which in turn encloses the 11 double strands of RNA in the core. This structure gives the virus its characteristic appearance of a wide-rimmed wheel with spokes radiating from the hub, from which its name was derived (*rota* is Latin for "wheel") (Fig. 28–1).[9]

Rotaviruses are classified based on antigenic properties of various proteins found in the capsid stricture. The VP6 protein on the inner capsid of the virus determines the rotavirus group.[5] Most viruses infecting humans are classified as group A, although rotaviruses from groups B and C have occasionally been associated with human diarrheal disease as well. The next level of classification is the subgroup, which is determined by other antigenic differences among the VP6 proteins. At least two subgroups are known to exist.[5] Subgroup typing has proved important in the study of patients who experience more than one episode of rotaviral infection. In these patients, recurrent infections usually but not necessarily involve agents of different subgroups, which suggests that subgroup antigens are not sufficient for inducing the production of protective antibodies.[10] Finally, the rotaviruses are classified into a variety of serotypes based on the antigenic differences of VP7 glycoprotein or the VP4 protease-sensitive hemagglutinin proteins that are found in the outer capsid.[3] VP7-based serotypes are now referred to as G types (for glycoprotein in VP7); G types 1 through 4 are responsible for most infections in children. VP4 serotypes are called P types (representing protease sensitivity of VP4). Reassortments of VP7 and VP4 have been used in candidate rotavirus vaccines.

#### *Epidemiology*

Rotavirus infection appears to occur throughout the world. In temperate climates, a sharp increase in incidence of cases occurs during the winter months.[7] In the United States, the peak rotavirus season begins in November in the Southwest and ends in the Northeast in April.[7] In the tropics, year-round transmission occurs, with seasonal variation in some areas.[11] Transmission is primarily from person to person,

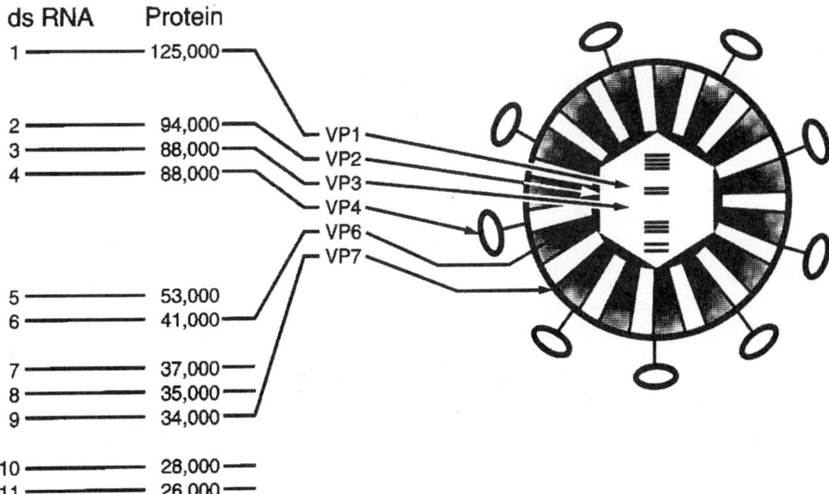


**FIGURE 28–1.** Rotavirus gene products. Schematic representation of rotavirus particle and viral proteins (VP). (From Kapikian AZ, Hoshino Y, Chanock RM, Perez-Schael, I: Efficacy of a quadrivalent rhesus rotavirus–based human rotavirus vaccine aimed at preventing severe rotavirus diarrhea in infants and young children. J Infect Dis 1996; 174[suppl 1]:S65–S72, with permission.)

through contact with feces or contaminated fomites. Spread by water is likely. Respiratory transmission has been suggested but not proved.[12]

Although the virus may affect all age groups, it most commonly produces disease in children between 6 and 24 months of age. A study in Washington, DC, found that most children have developed rotavirus antibodies by the age of 2 years, which helps to explain the observed decreased incidence of rotaviral infection in later childhood.[13] The disease does occur in the adult population, however, and has even been known to produce epidemics.[14, 15] A prospective study by Wenman and coworkers[16] found that rotavirus infection occurs in adult populations with approximately half the frequency seen in children. Those adults whose children had rotavirus were more likely to be infected than were adults without infected children. Most adults found to have rotavirus infection were asymptomatic; if symptoms were present, they were generally mild. This would seem to indicate that the antibody acquired earlier in life provides protective benefit.

The other age group that appears to have protection from rotavirus infection is the neonate. The virus can be found in stool samples from asymptomatic neonates. Neonatal epidemics of rotavirus excretion have been described in which approximately half of the nursery patients examined were found to have rotavirus. Many of these infants were asymptomatic, and those with disease had only mild symptoms.[17, 18] Breast-fed infants are less likely to be infected, and, when infected, these infants are apparently less likely than their bottle-fed counterparts to suffer symptoms of disease. This may reflect the protective effect of maternal antibodies in colostrum and breast milk.[19] Nosocomial spread of rotaviral illness among hospitalized infants has also been documented.[20]

## Clinical Manifestations

Once a susceptible patient has come in contact with rotavirus, a 48- to 72-hour incubation period occurs before the onset of symptoms.[12] Illness typically begins with the sudden onset of diarrhea and vomiting. The diarrhea usually is watery and rarely may be associated with gross or occult blood in the stool.[21] The fluid loss from diarrhea and vomiting is often severe enough to cause dehydration. Fever is present in most patients.[12] A comparison of the characteristics of rotaviral infections with those of other enteric viruses is presented in Table 28–1.

Diarrhea caused by rotavirus usually lasts from 2 to 8 days.[22] Shedding of virus into the intestinal lumen begins about 3 days after infection and may persist for as long as 3 weeks.[23, 24]

In addition to gastrointestinal symptoms, patients with rotavirus often have respiratory tract symptoms.[12] Of 150 patients hospitalized with acute gastroenteritis, 26% had rhinitis, 8% had abnormal breath sounds, 49% had pharyngeal erythema, and 18% had palpable cervical adenopathy.[25] In addition, 19% had signs of otitis media. Unlike the fever and vomiting, none of these manifestations associated with rotavirus infection seemed helpful in the recognition of rotaviral disease, because the group infected with nonrotavirus organisms had similar signs and symptoms. The clinical symptoms of rotavirus infection are more severe in patients with underlying malnutrition. In the malnourished murine rotavirus model, a smaller inoculum is required for infection,

**TABLE 28–1. Viral Enteric Pathogens**

| VIRUS | PREDOMINANT AGE GROUP AFFECTED | SEASONALITY | DURATION OF SYMPTOMS |
|---|---|---|---|
| Rotavirus | 6–24 mo | ↑ in winter months | 2–8 days |
| Norwalk virus/calciviruses | Older children, adults, ? infants | Winter and summer | 12–48 hr |
| Enteric adenovirus | <2 yr | ↑ in summer months | up to 14 days |
| Astrovirus | 1–3 yr | Unknown | 1–4 days |

less time is required for incubation, and the symptoms are more severe.[26] In addition, rotavirus replication can occur in the liver and kidney, at least in immunocompromised hosts.[27]

### Pathophysiology

Rotavirus invades the villus intestinal epithelial cells and replicates, causing cell death and sloughing. Histologically, this is manifested as blunting of the intestinal villi.[28] In response to the loss of villus cells, there is crypt hypertrophy. The lytic infection of highly differentiated absorptive enterocytes and the sparing of undifferentiated crypt cells results in both a loss of absorptive capacity with "unopposed" crypt cell secretion (i.e., secretory diarrhea) and loss of brush border hydrolase activity (i.e., osmotic diarrhea).

Another possible mechanism for rotaviral diarrhea also has been demonstrated. The rotavirus nonstructural glycoprotein NSP4 has been shown to mediate age-dependent intestinal secretion in mice.[29] The relevance of this novel viral enterotoxin to human rotaviral infection is uncertain. Other models, including vasoactive inflammatory agents, have also been proposed; consistent with this, in rotavirus infection there may be an increase in the number of inflammatory cells in the lamina propria. Disease effects are apparently limited to the duodenum and the proximal jejunum,[12] since studies in patients with known rotavirus disease have yielded normal gastric and rectal biopsies.[30]

### Diagnosis

Rotavirus was initially linked to acute gastroenteritis through electron microscopic evidence of viral particles in biopsy specimens of affected patients.[6] This technique continues to be useful in rotavirus detection, especially in conjunction with monoclonal or polyclonal antibodies (immunoelectron microscopy).[22] The obvious drawback of this approach is the need for specialized personnel and equipment. Consequently, a variety of immunoassays have been developed for detecting group A rotavirus antigen in stools[30, 31]; most immunoassays have sensitivities and specificities in the range of 90%.

### Treatment and Prevention

Currently, supportive care with oral or intravenous rehydration is the mainstay of therapy.[32, 33] No antiviral agents effective against rotavirus have yet been developed. However, probiotic therapy has been shown to be effective in preventing and treating rotaviral infection. Treatment with *Lactobacillus GG* has been shown to shorten the course of rotaviral diarrhea from 2.5 to 1.1 days in a study performed in Finland.[34, 35] In addition, other probiotic agents (*Bifidobacterium bifidum* and *Streptococcus thermophilus*) have been shown to prevent diarrheal disease and shedding of rotavirus in a chronic hospital setting when given to formula-fed infants.[36] Oral administration of immunoglobulin has been shown to promote faster recovery from rotaviral infection[37]; this therapy may be reserved for severely affected hospitalized infants.

In infants, natural rotavirus infection confers protection against subsequent infection. This protection increases with each new infection and reduces the severity of diarrhea.[38] The strategy for developing effective oral rotavirus vaccine involves the use of live, attenuated strains that should protect an infant by the same mechanism as natural infection. The most extensively studied strategy for rotavirus vaccination has been the Jennerian approach, which uses an antigenically related rotavirus strain from an animal host as the immunogen to induce protection. Attenuated bovine strains were initially tried[39]; these were protective in some populations but not others. This variability was in part attributed to the antigenic differences in circulating strains and the failure of animal strains to elicit heterotypic protection in some studies. To increase the efficacy of the Jennerian approach, second-generation polyvalent reassortment vaccines have been developed. These contain neutralization antigens that can provide homotypic (serotype-specific) immunity against the four epidemiologically important group A rotavirus VP7 serotypes. These vaccines, which are based on attenuated human and rhesus strains, are not highly effective at preventing infection but do have an efficacy of more than 80% in preventing dehydration associated with severe diarrhea.[40–42] A rotavirus vaccine (Rotashield J, Wyeth-Ayerst, St. David's, PA) has been approved for use in the United States. It is likely that more of these vaccines will be licensed in the near future.[43]

## Small Round Structured Viruses

### Caliciviruses

"Winter vomiting disease" was thought to be caused by nonbacterial gastroenteritis for decades before an etiologic agent was identified from an outbreak, in 1968, in Norwalk, Ohio.[44] In this outbreak, only some of the patients had diarrhea; the predominant clinical manifestation was vomiting and nausea.[44] Virus particles were visualized by immune electron microscopy on fecal material derived from the Norwalk outbreak.[5] This represented the first definitive association between a specific virus (Norwalk virus) and acute gastroenteritis. Subsequently a number of similar etiologic agents were identified; before the cloning of the prototype Norwalk virus genome,[45, 46] these viruses, which were a group of morphologically diverse, positive-stranded RNA viruses that caused acute gastroenteritis, were identified as Norwalk-like agents. These organisms were also named for the communities in which they were first isolated (e.g., Montgomery County, Hawaii, Snow Mountain, Taunton, Otofuke, and Sapporo viruses). Based on reverse transcription–polymerase chain reaction (PCR), the sequence structure of these viruses has enabled their classification as human caliciviruses (HuCV).

With the use of molecular tools, HuCV have now been preliminarily classified into four genotypes, represented by Norwalk virus, Snow Mountain agent, Sapporo virus, and hepatitis E virus.[47–49] This classification system may allow the development of assays based on recombinant HuCV antigens or PCR products rather than the current cumbersome classification schemes that rely on human reagents (convalescent outbreak sera) of varying sensitivity and specificity. Molecular tools have already allowed the identification of HuCV as agents of both pediatric and adult viral gastroenteritis in foodborne outbreaks as well as outbreaks in nursing homes, hospitals, and a university setting. Despite the potential for future understanding of the contribution of individual

HuCV to outbreaks of nonbacterial gastroenteritis, Norwalk virus still remains the prototypic agent of HuCV, and it is described in greater detail in the following section.

### *Norwalk Virus*

**EPIDEMIOLOGY.** Although the Norwalk virus has been most extensively studied in the United States, it is apparently worldwide in distribution.[50] Of patients exposed to the Norwalk virus either naturally or experimentally, 50% develop clinical symptoms.[51] Studies evaluating the prevalence of anti-Norwalk antibody among populations of various age groups initially demonstrated the group from 3 months to 12 years of age had only a 5% antibody-positive rate. More recent epidemiologic studies, using bacculovirus-expressed recombinant Norwalk virus antigen in an enzyme-linked immunosorbent assay (ELISA), have demonstrated a serologic response in 49% of Finnish infants between 3 and 24 months of age.[52] These data contradict previous beliefs that Norwalk virus most often caused disease in older children and adults.

Transmission of the Norwalk virus is most often fecal-oral. Unlike rotavirus, this usually involves the spread of infection to a large population through a common source rather than from direct, person-to-person contact.[53] In one outbreak, an infected bakery employee transmitted the virus through food products to approximately 3,000 people.[54] Outbreaks have also been related to ingestion of raw oysters and clams[55] and to contaminated water supplies. Nosocomial spread of this disease has been documented. In addition to its fecal-oral spread, there is some evidence that the Norwalk virus is transmitted through a respiratory route in the form of aerosolized particles from vomitus.[56] Although previously referred to as "winter vomiting disease"[44] the Norwalk agent produces outbreaks of disease that can occur throughout the year.

**PATHOPHYSIOLOGY.** The histologic changes induced by the Norwalk virus in an infected host have been studied in small bowel biopsies from infected volunteers.[57] Those volunteers who remained free of clinical symptoms had normal biopsy specimens, whereas those with symptoms exhibited marked, but not specific, changes, including focal areas of villous flattening and disorganization of epithelial cells. On electron microscopy, microvilli were shortened, and there was dilatation of the endoplasmic reticulum. These volunteers had repeat biopsies 2 weeks after the illness, and normal histology was again present. Other investigators have demonstrated the presence of normal gastric and rectal histology in patients affected by the Norwalk agent, as is typical of viral gastroenteritis.[50]

**CLINICAL MANIFESTATIONS.** The clinical manifestations of disease produced by the Norwalk virus include nausea, vomiting, and cramping abdominal pain (see Table 28–1). Diarrhea is said to be a less consistent feature of this illness. In the original outbreak, only 44% of patients experienced diarrhea, whereas 84% had vomiting.[44] Other studies, however, have found that diarrhea occurs in most children and experimentally infected adult volunteers who become ill from this virus.[51, 58, 59] Fever occurs in approximately one third of affected patients, but respiratory symptoms are not typically a part of this illness. An incubation period of approximately 24 to 48 hours has been noted before the onset of symptoms,[44, 51] and symptoms persist for 12 to 48 hours.

**DIAGNOSIS AND TREATMENT.** Development of techniques for diagnosis of the Norwalk virus has been difficult owing to the lack of methods for culturing the virus in vitro and the lack of an appropriate animal model. The use of molecular-based diagnostic assays is likely to improve our ability to recognize these infections and better understand their importance.[47–49, 51, 52, 60]

The treatment for Norwalk illness is supportive; oral rehydration solutions are used if necessary. Significant dehydration is uncommon, and the need for hospitalization is rare.

### *Enteric Adenovirus*

The enteric adenoviruses are among the more recently recognized viral pathogens that cause acute gastroenteritis. Adenoviruses are a large group of viruses long recognized for their role in the pathogenesis of respiratory infections and keratoconjunctivitis. Most of the 47 serotypes are known to be shed in the feces of infected patients. In patients with predominantly gastrointestinal symptoms, the organisms are detectable by electron microscopy of stool samples; however, they fail to grow in standard tissue culture conditions.[23] Their unique cell culture requirements allow for the differentiation of nonenteric adenoviruses from the enteric serotypes (Ad40 and Ad41), which are recognized to be among the common causes of viral childhood gastroenteritis.[61, 62]

Infection with enteric adenoviruses apparently occurs throughout the year, with only slight seasonal variation.[63, 64] This disease tends to affect predominantly younger children, with most patients being younger than 2 years of age.[64, 65] Enteric adenovirus is spread by the fecal-oral route. Transmission of the disease to family contacts is unusual.

Diarrhea is the most commonly reported symptom of enteric adenoviral infection. In contrast with diarrhea from other viral enteritides, diarrhea from enteric adenovirus typically persists for a prolonged period, sometimes as long as 14 days. Viruses may be excreted in the feces of infected patients for 1 to 2 weeks.[63] Vomiting frequently occurs but is usually mild and of a much shorter duration than is the diarrhea. Dehydration has been seen in approximately half of affected patients, and hospitalization is sometimes necessary. The frequency of association of respiratory symptoms with enteric adenovirus infection is unclear.[65]

The diagnosis of enteric adenovirus is best made by electron microscopy or immunoelectron microscopy of stool samples or from intestinal biopsy specimens. ELISA[66] and PCR[67] techniques have also been used successfully in enteric adenovirus diagnosis. Treatment is mainly supportive, and oral rehydration solutions are useful in cases of dehydration.

### *Astrovirus*

Astrovirus, similar to HuCV, is a single-stranded RNA virus grouped with the small round structured viruses. However, the recently derived sequence of the astrovirus RNA genome reveals that this agent is sufficiently different to be classified in its own family as Astroviridae.[68] Astrovirus is worldwide in distribution and tends to infect mainly children in the 1- to 3-year age group. In controlled studies in Thailand, astrovirus infection was the second most common cause of enteritis, after rotavirus infection, in symptomatic children.[69] Astrovirus infection occurred in 9% of children with diarrhea, compared with 2% of controls. Comparable findings have been reported in daycare centers in North America and Japan.[70, 71] Most children infected with astrovirus develop symptoms. Vomiting, diarrhea, abdominal pain, and fever all are commonly seen with infection by this agent, and symptoms typically last 1 to 4 days. Spread of the virus may occur via the fecal-oral route from person-to-person contact or through contaminated food or water. Asymptomatic shedding of astrovirus has also been reported.[72]

### *Other Viruses*

A variety of other viruses are being studied to determine what role, if any, they may play in the pathogenesis of human enteric infections. With the exception of those viruses previously discussed in detail, insufficient data are available to ascertain clinical and epidemiologic differences, if any, among the various small round viruses.

Pestivirus, a single-stranded RNA virus of the togavirus family, has been found in the feces of 24% of children living on an American Indian reservation who had diarrhea attributable to no other infectious agent.[73] These children experienced only mild diarrhea but had more severe respiratory complaints.

Coronavirus is known to cause an upper respiratory illness in humans and has been shown to cause diarrhea in some animals.[74] The role of this agent in human diarrheal disease is unclear, and at least one study found coronavirus more commonly in children without diarrhea than in those who were ill.[75] Coronavirus was implicated in an outbreak of necrotizing enterocolitis.[76]

Toroviruses are pleomorphic viruses recognized to cause enteric illness in a variety of animals.[77] Members of this group, originally described in Berne, Switzerland, and Breda, Iowa, and named for those cities, have been seen in the feces of humans with diarrheal disease.[78] Because of the pleomorphic structure of toroviruses, electron microscopy was inadequate to prove an etiopathogenic role of these viruses in diarrheal disease. The more recent findings of torovirus-like particles by immunoassay, using validated anti–Breda virus antiserum, lends additional weight to the hypothesis that these are agents of human gastroenteritis.[79] Their causative role in human disease, however, remains unproved. Similarly, picobirnavirus is known to cause disease in animals and has been isolated from stools of humans with diarrheal illness.[80]

Cytomegalovirus has been associated with enteritis and colitis. Except for Ménétrier's disease, caused by gastric cytomegalovirus infection, enteritis and colitis seem to occur almost exclusively among immunocompromised patients. In this population, cytomegalovirus causes viremia and is carried by the blood stream to a variety of sites, including organs of the gastrointestinal tract. Diagnosis may be made by virus detection in feces, by demonstration of typical cytomegalic inclusion cells, or by in situ hybridization.[81]

## BACTERIAL GASTROENTERITIS

### Host-Defense Factors

For an infecting bacterial agent to cause diarrhea, it must first overcome the following gastrointestinal tract defenses: (1) gastric acidity, (2) intestinal motility, (3) mucus secretion, (4) normal intestinal microflora, and (5) specific mucosal and systemic immune mechanisms. Gastric acidity is the first barrier encountered by infecting organisms.[82] Many studies have demonstrated the bactericidal properties of gastric juice at pH less than 4.[83] In patients with achlorhydria or decreased gastric acid secretion, the gastric pH is higher, and this bactericidal effect is diminished. Gastric acidity serves to decrease the number of viable bacteria that proceed to the small intestine.

Organisms surviving the gastric acidity barrier are trapped within the mucus layer of the small intestine, facilitating their movement through the intestine by peristalsis. If motility in the intestine is abnormal or absent, organisms are more readily able to initiate the infectious process. Some organisms can elaborate toxic substances that impair intestinal motility. Increased intestinal peristalsis, which occurs during some enteric infections, may be an attempt by the host to rid itself of infective organisms.

In addition to its role in conjunction with intestinal motility, mucus also serves to provide a nonspecific barrier to bacterial proliferation and mucosal colonization. This barrier has been shown to be effective in preventing toxins from exerting their effects. Exfoliated mucosal cells trapped in the mucous layer may trap invading microorganisms. Mucus also contains carbohydrate analogues of surface receptors, which may prevent invading organisms from binding to actual receptors.

The normal endogenous microflora of the gut serves as its next line of defense. Anaerobes, which are a large component of the normal flora, elaborate short-chain fatty acids and lactic acid, which are toxic to many potential pathogens. In breast-fed infants, this line of defense is enhanced by the presence of anaerobic lactobacilli, which produce fermentative products that act as toxins to foreign bacteria. Further evidence in support of the importance of endogenous microflora is the increase in susceptibility to infection after one's normal flora has been reduced by antibiotic administration, as is seen with *Clostridium difficile* infection.

The most complex element in the host-defense armamentarium involves the mucosal and systemic immune systems. Both serum and secretory antibodies may exert their protective effects at the intestinal level, even though the serum components are produced outside the gut. An immune response may be *specific* to a particular infective agent or *generalized* to a common group of bacterial antigens.

### Mechanisms of Bacterial Disease Production

Bacteria have developed a variety of virulence factors (Table 28–2) to overcome host defense mechanisms: (1) *invasion* of the mucosa, followed by intraepithelial cell multiplication or invasion of the lamina propria; (2) production of *cytotoxins*, which disrupt cell function via direct alteration of the mucosal surface; (3) production of *enterotoxins*, polypeptides that alter cellular salt and water balance yet leave cell morphology undisturbed; and (4) *adherence* to the mucosal surface with resultant flattening of the microvilli and disruption of normal cell functioning. Each of the bacterial virulence mechanisms acts on specific regions of the intestine. Enterotoxins are primarily effective in the small bowel

**TABLE 28–2. Bacterial Pathogens Grouped by Pathogenic Mechanism**

| INVASIVE | CYTOTOXIC | TOXIGENIC | ADHERENT |
|---|---|---|---|
| *Shigella* | *Shigella* | *Shigella* | Enteropathogenic *E. coli* |
| *Salmonella* | Enteropathogenic *Escherichia coli* | Enterotoxigenic *E. coli* | Enterohemorrhagic *E. coli* |
| *Yersinia enterocolitica* | Enterohemorrhagic *E. coli* | *Yersinia enterocolitica* | Enteroaggregative *E. coli* |
| *Campylobacter jejuni* | *Clostridium difficile* | *Aeromonas* | Diffuse-adherent *E. coli* |
| *Vibrio parahaemolyticus* | | *V. cholerae* and non-01 vibrios | |

Modified from Cohen MB: Etiology and mechanisms of acute infectious diarrhea in infants in the United States. J Pediatr 1991;118:S34–S43, with permission.

but can affect the colon; the effects of cytotoxins and direct epithelial cell invasion occur predominantly in the colon. Enteroadhesive mechanisms appear to function in both the small intestine and colon.

## *Salmonella*

Members of the species *Salmonella* are currently recognized as the most common cause of bacterial diarrhea among children in the United States. Surveillance data from the Centers for Disease Control and Prevention indicate that the incidence of disease caused by this bacteria is increasing.[84] Infection caused by *Salmonella* may result in several different clinical syndromes, including (1) acute gastroenteritis; (2) focal, nonintestinal infections; (3) bacteremia; (4) asymptomatic carrier state; and (5) enteric fever (including typhoid fever). Each of these entities may be caused by any of the commonly recognized species of *Salmonella*.

### Microbiology

*Salmonella* is a motile, gram-negative bacillus of the family Enterobacteriaceae. It can be identified on selective media because it does not ferment lactose. Three distinct species of *Salmonella* are recognized: *Salmonella enteritidis, Salmonella choleraesuis,* and *Salmonella typhi. S. enteritidis* is further subdivided into approximately 1,700 serotypes. Each serotype is referred to by its genus and serotype names (e.g., *Salmonella typhimurium*) rather than the formally correct *S. enteritidis*, serotype *typhimurium. S. choleraesuis* and *S. typhi* are known to have only one serotype each.

### Epidemiology

*Salmonella* is estimated to cause 1 to 2 million gastrointestinal infections each year in the United States.[84] At Children's Hospital Medical Center, Cincinnati, salmonellae are the most commonly isolated bacterial enteropathogens (Fig. 28–2). The highest attack rate for salmonellosis is in infancy, with a lower incidence of symptomatic infection in patients older than 6 years of age.[84, 85] Nontyphoidal *Salmonella* is usually spread via contaminated water supplies or foods, with meat, fresh produce, fowl, eggs, and raw milk frequently implicated.

A large outbreak involved contaminated alfalfa sprouts which were shipped worldwide.[86] Most of the egg-associated outbreaks have involved products such as mayonnaise, ice cream,[87] and cold desserts, in which salmonella can multiply profusely and which are eaten without cooking after the addition of, or contamination by, raw egg. Although "shell" eggs are frequently contaminated, the number of bacteria in infected eggs is often near or below the human infective dose.[88] In contrast, with a generation time of 80 minutes at 20°C, one bacterium can become a billion in 40 hours, and with a generation time of 40 minutes at 25°C, it can do so in 20 hours.

Although any of these food sources may become contaminated through contact with an infected food handler, the farm animals themselves are often infected. Pets, notably cats, turtles, lizards, snakes, and chicks, may also harbor *Salmonella*. Person-to-person spread of infection also occurs and is especially common in cases involving infants.[89]

### Pathogenesis

Inocula of fewer than $10^3$ salmonellae are probably sufficient to cause disease.[89] Patients in whom host defenses are diminished are more likely to develop clinical manifestations of the disease. This has been demonstrated in patients who have reduced levels of gastric acid.[82] Patients with lymphoproliferative diseases and hemolytic diseases, especially sickle cell anemia, are more likely to experience severe disease and develop complications from *Salmonella* infection. The mechanisms for this increased susceptibility may involve altered macrophage function, defective complement activation, or damage to the bones from thromboses.

Having overcome host defenses, *Salmonella* produces disease through a process that begins with colonization of the ileum and the colon. The organisms next invade enterocytes and colonocytes and proliferate within epithelial cells and in

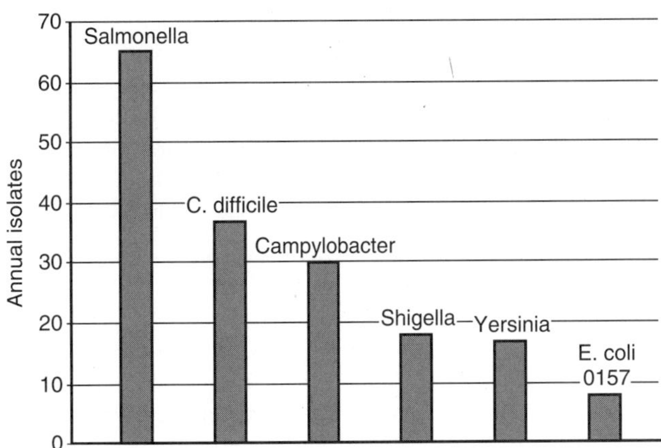


**FIGURE 28–2.** Bacterial enteropathogens isolated at Children's Hospital Medical Center, 1994. (Data from the Infection Control Office, Children's Hospital Medical Center, Cincinnati, OH.)

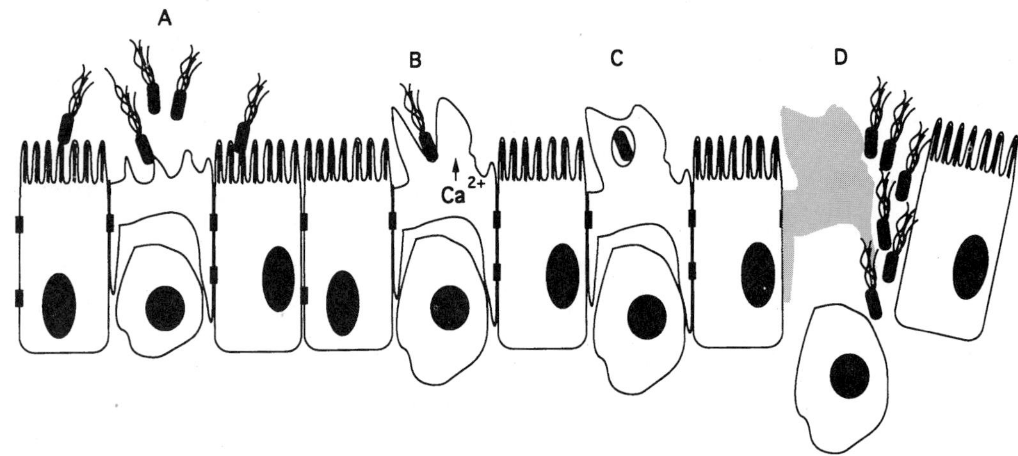


**FIGURE 28–3.** Interaction of enteropathogenic *Salmonella* species with the intestinal epithelium. Diagrammed are the interaction and invasion of salmonellae with an M cell and an absorptive epithelial cell overlying the Peyer's patch follicle. *Salmonella* invasion is shown for an M cell. Adherence of salmonellae to an M cell (A) is followed by *Salmonella* invasion-induced membrane ruffle (B). C, Bacterium localized within an intracellular vacuole. D, Destruction of the invaded M cell followed by an influx of bacteria into the epithelial cell breach and entry into Peyer's patch. (From Hromockyj A, Falkow S: Interactions of bacteria with the gut epithelium. In Blaser MJ, Smith PD, Ravdin JI, et al [eds]: Infections of the Gastrointestinal Tract. New York, Raven Press, 1995. Courtesy of Brad Jones, Ph.D.)

the lamina propria (Fig. 28–3).[90] From the lamina propria, *Salmonella* may then move to the mesenteric lymph nodes and eventually to the systemic circulation, causing bacteremia. Because these organisms invade enterocytes and colonocytes, both enteritis, with watery diarrhea, and colitis, with bloody diarrhea, may result.

### Clinical Manifestations

After an incubation period of 12 to 72 hours, *Salmonella* usually produces a mild, self-limited illness characterized by fever and watery diarrhea. Blood, mucus, or both are commonly present in the stool. Bacteremia occurs in approximately 6% of *Salmonella* infections in children but much less frequently in adults.[91] Patients may develop sequelae after *Salmonella* infection, including pneumonia, meningitis, and osteomyelitis.

Even in those patients in whom no sequelae occur, excretion of the organisms may persist for several weeks. In patients younger than 5 years of age, the median time of excretion has been shown to be 7 weeks, with 2.6% of patients continuing to shed organisms for 1 year or longer.[92] Studies have also shown a higher incidence of the carrier state among children with salmonellosis than is seen in adults.[92] Localization of *Salmonella* organisms in chronic carriers is often in the biliary tract and is frequently associated with cholelithiasis.

### Diagnosis and Treatment

Diagnosis of *Salmonella* infection can be made through stool or blood culture. Use of enriched media and culture of material from freshly passed stools, rather than from rectal swab, increase the likelihood of recovering the organism.[92] Owing to the increased risk of developing the carrier state, antimicrobial treatment of uncomplicated cases of *Salmonella* gastroenteritis is not recommended.[93] Treatment is recommended in patients at high risk for the development of disseminated disease, including those who are immunocompromised, those with hematologic disease, patients with artificial implants, those with severe colitis, and pregnant women. Treatment is also recommended for patients at any age who appear toxic.

Treatment of children younger than 1 year of age with salmonellosis remains controversial because of the risk of bacteremia and secondary infections. Antimicrobial therapy is recommended for infants with *Salmonella* bacteremia. Parenteral antibiotics are recommended for any infant (younger than 3 months of age) with a stool culture that is positive for *Salmonella*.[94]

Most *Salmonella* are sensitive to a wide variety of antibiotics, including ampicillin (35 mg/kg [maximum 1 g] per dose, given every 4 hours, intravenously, for 14 days), chloramphenicol (20 mg/kg [maximum 1 g] per dose, given every 6 hours, intravenously or orally, for 14 days), trimethoprim-sulfamethoxazole (trimethoprim, 5 mg/kg [maximum 160 mg], plus sulfamethoxazole, 25 mg/kg [maximum 800 mg] per dose, given every 12 hours, orally, for 14 days), and the third-generation cephalosporins.[95] Resistance to ampicillin is increasing.[96] Ceftriaxone, cefotaxime, or a fluoroquinolone (not approved for use in children younger than 18 years of age) are often effective when resistance to other agents is demonstrated.

A follow-up stool culture usually is not warranted unless the patient is employed in the preparation of food. If evidence of a "cure" is necessary, two to three consecutive negative stool cultures, obtained 1 to 3 days apart, are sufficient.

## Typhoid Fever

Although uncommon in the United States, typhoid fever, caused by *S. typhi*, commonly affects children in developing countries. *S. typhi* differs from other salmonellae in that it requires a human host. The disease it causes also differs in severity from the typically mild gastroenteritis caused by other members of the genus; *S. typhi* infection also has a higher case-fatality rate.

Typhoid fever typically begins with a period of fever lasting approximately 1 week. Patients then complain of headache and abdominal pain. Diarrhea is not usually a manifestation of typhoid fever, and many patients experience constipation. Hepatomegaly and splenomegaly have also been frequently noted.[97] The characteristic "rose spots" (palpable, erythematous lesions), typical in adult cases of typhoid fever, occur with far less frequency in pediatric patients.[97] Patients may become chronic carriers.

Diagnosis of typhoid fever is made on the basis of positive blood cultures. *S. typhi* is usually sensitive to several antimicrobial agents, including ampicillin, chloramphenicol, trimethoprim-sulfamethoxazole, cefotaxime, and ceftriaxone. Drug choice is based on site of infection and susceptibility of the organism.

A live oral vaccine from an attenuated strain of *S. typhi* (Ty21a) has been available in the United States since 1989; one recommended dosing schedule is four doses given every other day.[98] Current efforts are directed toward development of other attenuated strains, which may provide successful immunization in single-dose therapy.[98] Vaccine based on the Vi antigen from the *S. typhi* polysaccharide capsule produces seroconversion in 90% of subjects, lasting 3 years.[99]

## Shigella

Bacillary dysentery, an illness caused by *Shigella*, was described in ancient Greece. Osler,[100] in 1892, referred to the disease as "one of the four great epidemic diseases of the world." He further stated: "In the tropics it destroys more lives than cholera, and it has been more fatal to armies than powder and shot." Despite our increased knowledge of the pathogenesis and treatment of shigellosis, this organism continues to be a significant cause of diarrheal disease.

### Microbiology

*Shigella* is a gram-negative, nonmotile, non-lactose-fermenting aerobic bacillus, closely related to members of the genus *Escherichia*. The organisms are classified into four species or groups known as *Shigella dysenteriae, Shigella flexneri, Shigella boydii,* and *Shigella sonnei* (groups A, B, C and D, respectively). Members of groups A, B, and C exist in numerous serotypes, but only one serotype of group D is known.[101] *S. sonnei* is the most commonly recovered *Shigella* species in the developed world, accounting for 70% of isolates in the United States. *S. dysenteriae* and *S. flexneri* are the most commonly recovered species of *Shigella* in the developing world.[101]

### Epidemiology

*Shigella* is worldwide in its distribution, and the incidence and severity of shigellosis span an equally broad range. In Highland Mayan Indian children, the incidence of shigellosis is 1,900 cases per 1,000 children per year in the third year of life.[102] In the developed world, *Shigella* occurs much less frequently. However, in some studies *Shigella* is the second most common pathogen identified in cases of bacterial diarrhea in children aged 6 months to 10 years.[103] It may also be the most common bacterial cause of outbreaks of diarrhea in daycare settings. Outbreaks of shigellosis have also been described in residential institutions and on cruise ships. This disease is endemic on American Indian reservations in the Southwest.

*Shigella* is predominantly spread via the fecal-oral route, with person-to-person contact the most likely method. Secondary spread to household contacts may occur. The infection may be spread through contamination of food and water, as often occurs in areas of poor sanitation and inadequate personal hygiene. Spread of *Shigella* has also been documented to occur venereally among homosexual men.

### Clinical Manifestations

Patients infected with *Shigella* may experience a mild, self-limited, watery diarrhea that is clinically indistinguishable from gastroenteritis caused by a variety of other agents. The more classic form of shigellosis, however, is bacillary dysentery. This illness usually begins with fever and malaise, followed by watery diarrhea and cramping abdominal pain. By the second day of illness, blood and mucus are usually present in the stools, and tenesmus has become a prominent symptom. At this point, in approximately 50% of affected patients, the stool volume decreases, with only scant amounts of blood and mucus being passed.[101] This pattern of bloody, mucus-containing stools is referred to as *dysentery.* Bacteremia is an uncommon feature of this illness, but several other complications have been reported, including seizures (in children), arthritis, purulent keratitis, and the hemolytic-uremic syndrome (HUS). Nonsupperative arthritis is the most commonly occurring extraintestinal complication of shigellosis. Patients who carry the histocompability locus antigen HLA-B27 may be predisposed to the development of this complication as well as to the development of Reiter's syndrome.[104] The association of seizures with shigellosis was earlier attributed to the neurotoxic effect of the *Shigella* toxin (Shiga toxin). It now seems likely, however, that the seizures may simply represent a subgroup of common febrile seizures and have no direct relation to the effects of Shiga toxin.

### Pathogenesis

*Shigella* has been found to cause disease only in humans and in the higher apes.[101] The organisms are potent, with as few as 10 organisms being able to cause disease in a healthy adult.[101] Patients infected with *Shigella* may excrete $10^5$ to $10^8$ organisms per gram of feces. This high rate of excretion and the relatively low number of organisms required to produce disease make possible the widespread distribution of disease.

For *Shigella* to exert its pathologic effect on a host, the bacteria must first come into contact with the surface of an intestinal epithelial cell and induce cytoskeletal rearrangements resulting in phagocytosis.[90, 105, 106] The bacteria then secrete enzymes that degrade the phagosomal membrane, releasing the bacteria into the host cytoplasm. Intracytoplasmic bacteria move rapidly, in association with a comet tail made up of host cell actin filaments. When moving

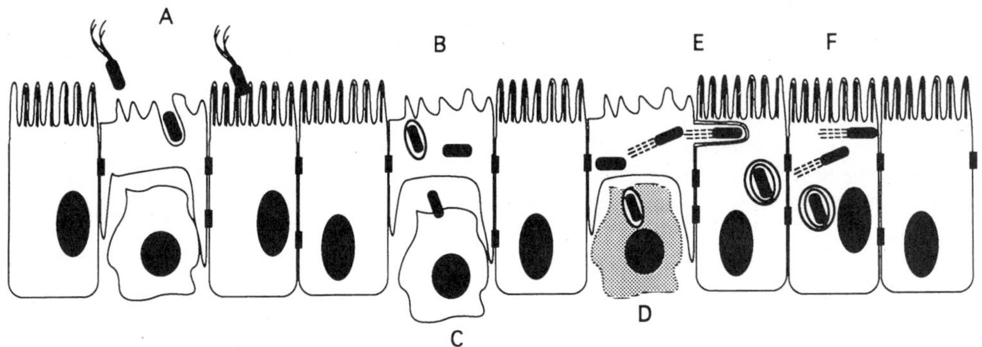


**FIGURE 28–4.** Interaction of *Shigella* species with the gut epithelium. Diagrammed is the putative interaction of shigellae with M cells overlying Peyer's patch follicles as well as absorptive epithelial cells. Invasion is diagrammed for an M cell. A and B, Adherence to and intimate association of shigellae with an M cell followed by localization of the invading organism with an intracellular cytoplasmic vacuole. C, D, and E, Bacteria, having transcytosed the M cell, may interact with Peyer's patch macrophages and induce macrophage apoptosis. Bacteria free within the target cell cytoplasm also move within the host cell via an actin-associated tail. F, Shigella intercellular invasion through a host cell membrane protrusion, followed by residence of the invading organism wihin a double-membraned intracellular cytoplasmic vacuole and escape from that vacuole. (From Hromockyj A, Falkow S: Interactions of bacteria with the gut epithelium. In Blaser MJ, Smith PD, Ravdin JI, et al [eds]: Infections of the Gastrointestinal Tract. New York, Raven Press, 1995, with permission.)

bacteria reach the cell margin, they push out long protrusions with the bacteria at the tips that are then taken up by neighboring cells, allowing the infection to spread from cell to cell (Fig. 28–4).[90]

Shiga toxin is elaborated by all species, although in greater amounts by *S. dysenteriae* than by other species,[101] and may play a role in the pathogenesis of *Shigella* infection. The toxin has neurotoxic, enterotoxic, and cytotoxic effects.[101] Structurally, it is composed of an active, or A, subunit (molecular weight 32 kd) surrounded by five binding, or B, subunits (77 kd).[101] The B subunits bind to cell-specific receptors and are taken up by endocytosis. Within the cells, the B subunits are cleaved away, and the remaining A subunit is shortened by proteolysis. This molecule is thought then to bind to the 60S ribosome and inhibit protein synthesis, leading to cell death and sloughing.[107] This is the presumed mechanism for the cytotoxic effect. An enterotoxic effect of Shiga toxin in the ileum may account for the early watery diarrhea.

### Diagnosis and Treatment

In patients with signs and symptoms of colitis, the diagnosis of shigellosis should be considered. Stool culture provides the only definitive means to differentiate this organism from other invasive pathogens. *Shigella* may be cultured from stool specimens or rectal swabs, especially if mucopus is present, but there may be a delay of several days from the onset of symptoms to the recovery of organisms. Sigmoidoscopy or colonoscopy typically reveals a friable mucosa, possibly with discrete ulcers. Rectal biopsy may be useful to differentiate shigellosis from ulcerative colitis.[108]

In addition to rehydration, antimicrobial therapy has been recommended for *Shigella* (1) to shorten the course of the disease, (2) to decrease the period of excretion of the organisms,[109] and (3) to decrease the secondary attack rate, since humans provide the only reservoir for the organism. However, handwashing, rather than use of antimicrobials, is the most effective method to prevent person-to-person spread. Those clinicians who advise against the routine treatment of shigellosis with antibiotics argue that (1) the disease is most often self-limited and (2) the use of antibiotics may facilitate the development of resistant strains[110] and may increase the likelihood developing HUS as a sequela.[102] We recommend antibiotic therapy only for patients who are severely ill at the time of diagnosis or who remain ill at the time of identification of *Shigella* in a stool culture.

A wide range of antibiotics has been used to treat *Shigella,* necessitated by the development of resistant strains. Currently, the agent of choice is trimethoprim-sulfamethoxazole (trimethoprim, 5 mg/kg [maximum 160 mg], plus sulfamethoxazole, 25 mg/kg [maximum 800 mg] per dose, given every 12 hours, orally or intravenously, for 5 days). Ampicillin (25 mg/kg [maximum 500 mg] per dose, given every 6 hours, orally or intravenously, for 5 days) may be used if local strains are typically susceptible.[95] Amoxicillin is ineffective against *Shigella.*[111] Nalidixic acid (55 mg/kg per day given every 6 hours for 5 days) has also proved effective. Cefixime and ceftriaxone are alternative agents for resistant organisms.[101] Tetracycline, ciprofloxacin, and norfloxacin have been used successfully for the treatment of *Shigella*, but these agents are approved for use only in adult patients. Multidrug-resistant strains have occurred in Latin America, Central Africa, and Southeast Asia.[112]

Development of a vaccine for shigellosis is currently being pursued. These efforts include vaccines using a modified *Escherichia coli* strain; one using a mutant strain of *S. flexneri*, which lacks the ability to proliferate intracellularly; and one based on a strain with mutations in its virulence genes.[101]

## Campylobacter

*Campylobacter* is a gram-negative, motile, curved or spiral-shaped rod, exhibiting a "seagull" appearance when identified in stained stool smears.[113] Multiple species of *Campylobacter* have been recognized, including *Campylobacter jejuni, Campylobacter fetus, Campylobacter coli,* and *Campylobacter laridis,* with *C. jejuni* being the one most commonly associated with disease in humans.[114] *Campylobacter upsaliensis* has been reported as another member of this group that causes diarrhea,[115] and it seems probable that still others may be identified.

### Epidemiology

*Campylobacter* is recognized to be worldwide in distribution. In developing countries, *Campylobacter* is a significant bacterial cause of diarrhea in children younger than 2 years of age, yet it rarely occurs in developing nations in older children and adults. When infection does occur in the population older than 2 years of age it tends to be asymptomatic.[116] It is likely that patients in these countries are infected with *Campylobacter* early in life and then develop immunity, thus making asymptomatic infection more typical in older children and adults.

In the industrialized world, most patients infected with *Campylobacter* develop symptoms.[116] The number of *Campylobacter* infections in these countries is now recognized to be quite high, with some studies finding this organism to be the most common cause of bacterial diarrhea. *Campylobacter* tends to infect people in two distinct age groups: children in the first year of life and young adults.[117]

*Campylobacter* may be spread by direct contact or through contaminated sources of food and water. Milk, meat, and eggs, especially if undercooked, have been implicated in outbreaks. These sources may be contaminated from human fecal shedding, or the organisms may be harbored in the asymptomatic farm animals. *Campylobacter* is commonly spread among populations of children in daycare centers.

### Pathogenesis

The mechanisms through which *Campylobacter* produces disease are not fully understood. Walker and coworkers[114] identified three potential mechanisms: (1) adherence to the intestinal mucosa followed by the elaboration of toxin; (2) invasion of the mucosa in the terminal ileum and colon; and (3) "translocation," in which the organisms penetrate the mucosa and replicate in the lamina propria and mesenteric lymph nodes. The variety of pathogenic mechanisms may account for the spectrum of disease caused by *Campylobacter.* It is also conceivable that different strains or serotypes of *Campylobacter* may demonstrate different pathogenic mechanisms, as is seen with *E. coli*.

### Clinical Manifestations

*Campylobacter* may cause disease ranging from mild diarrhea to frank dysentery. Typically, patients experience fever and malaise followed by diarrhea, nausea, and abdominal pain that may mimic appendicitis[85] or inflammatory bowel disease. The symptoms usually resolve in less than 1 week.[118] Bacteremia may rarely occur, with some species implicated more often than are others.[119] *Campylobacter* is also known to cause meningitis, abscesses, septic abortions, pancreatitis, and pneumonia. Guillain-Barré syndrome and Reiter's syndrome are documented to occur as sequelae of *Campylobacter* infection. Increasing evidence has implicated *C. jejuni* as the most common antecedent of Guillain-Barré syndrome and the variant form, Miller-Fisher syndrome, a neuropathy associated with ataxia, areflexia, and ophthalmoplegia.[120, 121] Although evidence for molecular mimicry is still preliminary, it is likely that peripheral nerves share epitopes with *C. jejuni*; therefore, the immune response initially mounted to attack *C. jejuni* is misdirected to peripheral nerves.[121]

After the resolution of symptoms, patients may continue to shed organisms for as long as 7 weeks.[122]

### Diagnosis and Treatment

Culture of the organisms, the gold standard for diagnosis, is routinely accomplished in most laboratories if selective media are used and cultures are incubated at 42°C. Because disease caused by *Campylobacter* is usually mild and self-limited, supportive treatment alone should suffice. In cases of severe disease, erythromycin (10 mg/kg [maximum 500 mg] per dose, given every 6 hours for 5 to 7 days) has been recommended.[95] The need for antibiotic therapy has been questioned, based in part on several studies demonstrating a decrease in the duration of excretion of *Campylobacter* after antibiotic treatment but no decrease in the duration of symptoms. In general, in these studies, antimicrobial therapy was begun late in the course of the illness. In a placebo-controlled, double-blind trial, Salazar-Lindo and colleagues[123] demonstrated a shortened duration of illness, from 4.2 to 2.5 days, in patients who received erythromycin by day 4 of their illness. For cases of *Campylobacter* septicemia, gentamicin (1.5 to 2.5 mg/kg per dose, intramuscularly or intravenously, given every 8 hours) is recommended, with chloramphenicol and erythromycin acceptable as alternatives. Tetracycline (250 to 500 mg per dose, intravenously, given every 6 to 12 hours) may be used in patients older than 8 years of age.[95] Ciprofloxacin is an effective alternative agent but is not approved for use in children younger than 18 years of age. Antibiotic treatment is recommended for outbreaks of *Campylobacter* in daycare settings, because treatment has been shown to eliminate fecal shedding of organisms within 48 hours.[114]

## Yersinia

### Microbiology

The genus *Yersinia* includes the species *Yersinia pestis*, which causes plague; *Yersinia pseudotuberculosis*, known to cause pseudoappendicitis, mesenteric adenitis, and gastroenteritis; and *Yersinia enterocolitica*, recognized with increasing frequency as a cause of bacterial diarrhea. *Yersinia* is a gram-negative, coccoid bacillus that is facultatively anaerobic. It is non-lactose-fermenting and is observed to be motile at temperatures of 25°C but nonmotile at 37°C.

### Epidemiology

*Yersinia* was initially thought to occur with greater frequency in countries with cooler climates but is now recognized to be worldwide in distribution. Although the true incidence and prevalence of this organism are not known, in some areas yersiniosis occurs more frequently than does shigellosis.[124] Outbreaks due to *Yersinia* have been associated with spread through contaminated water and foods, including bean sprouts, tofu, and chocolate milk.[124, 125] Pork has also been implicated as a source, as in the Fulton County, Georgia, outbreak in 1990, in which chitterlings were found to be the vehicle of infection.[126, 127] The organism tends to cause disease more frequently in young children, with 24 months the median age in one study.[128] *Yersinia* may also be spread among household contacts. In addition, there may be an increased incidence in the summer months.[124, 128]

### Pathogenesis

*Y. enterocolitica* constitutes a heterogeneous group of serotypes with many identified virulence factors.[129] *Y. enterocolitica* produces disease in the intestine through an invasive route. After penetrating the mucosal epithelium, primarily in the ileum, organisms replicate in Peyer's patches and accumulate in the mesenteric lymph nodes.[124] Most serotypes produce an enterotoxin similar to the *E. coli* heat-stable toxin but only at temperatures lower than 30°C; therefore, this toxin may *not* have an important role in disease production by *Yersinia* in the human intestine. There is speculation on the role of preformed toxin in causing disease, because toxin may be produced when the organisms are present in refrigerated foods.[124]

The virulence of *Y. enterocolitica* has been shown to be plasmid related. Different serotypes exhibit different degrees of virulence. Serotypes O:3, and O:9 are the ones most frequently associated with diarrheal disease in Europe and Japan, whereas a larger number of serotypes are seen in North America.[129]

### Clinical Manifestations

The most frequent clinical syndrome caused by *Y. enterocolitica* is gastroenteritis, which typically affects young children. After an incubation period of 1 to 11 days, patients develop diarrhea, fever, and abdominal pain.[124] A marked increase in the leukocyte count is common. The symptoms usually resolve in 5 to 14 days but have been known to persist for several months. Excretion of organisms occurs for about 6 weeks.[128] Several complications, including appendicitis, have been documented after *Y. enterocolitica* infection.

In older children and young adults, *Yersinia* is more likely to produce the pseudoappendicular syndrome, in which the signs and symptoms mimic appendicitis.[124] In this same age group, there has also been an association of *Y. enterocolitica* with nonspecific abdominal pain.[130] Radiographic changes in the terminal ileum more often associated with Crohn's disease, namely mucosal thickening and aphthous ulcers, have been seen with yersiniosis in young adults.[85]

*Yersinia* bacteremia occurs and, despite therapy with appropriate antibiotics, has a case-fatality rate of 34% to 50%. The finding of *Yersinia* in blood from asymptomatic donors, however, makes the possibility of transient bacteremia seem likely as well.[124]

Sequelae of *Yersinia* infection include erythema nodosum and reactive arthropathy; however, these are more commonly seen in adults.[129] This arthropathy tends to involve the weight-bearing joints of the lower extremities and has been noted to occur most often in *Yersinia* patients who carry the histocompatibility antigen HLA-B27.[131]

### Diagnosis and Treatment

*Yersinia* may be cultured with the use of selective media, preferably with "cold enrichment." Despite the best of methods, culture of *Yersinia* may require as long as 4 weeks. In addition to diagnosis by culture, *Yersinia* may also be detected serologically, through the use of agglutinin titers. These measurements appear to be useful only in conjunction with cultures, because agglutinin titers may be affected by a number of factors, including the patient's age, the underlying disease, and previous use of antibiotics and immunosuppressive agents.[132] These titers may also be more useful in Europe and Japan, where infection is caused by a restricted number of serotypes.

Antibiotics have not been proved effective in alleviating symptoms of *Yersinia* or in shortening the period of its excretion.[124] Pai and associates[133] compared the efficacy of trimethoprim-sulfamethoxazole versus placebo in the treatment of *Yersinia* gastroenteritis and found no significant difference. It should be noted, however, that therapy was not begun until near the end of the course of the illness.[133] In cases of severe disease and in patients with underlying illness, treatment is recommended. Trimethoprim-sulfamethoxazole, aminoglycosides, chloramphenicol, and third-generation cephalosporins are generally recommended. Tetracycline and quinolones are alternative choices for adult patients.[95] Gentamicin or chloramphenicol is recommended for treatment of septicemia. Because septicemia may be associated with an iron overload state,[134, 135] cessation of iron therapy is also recommended during infection.

## Cholera

Although cholera is a disease rarely encountered in developed countries, it remains an important entity. Investigation of the pathogenesis of cholera led to the recognition and understanding of the mechanism of action of cholera toxin, which remains the prototype for bacterial enterotoxins. Cholera is also important, from a therapeutic perspective, in that initial efforts in the use of oral rehydration solutions were carried out in patients with cholera. However, most importantly, on a worldwide basis, cholera continues to be a major public health problem in almost all developing countries.[136, 137] Cholera afflicts both children and adults, and cholera exists as an endemic disease in more than 100 countries of the world. The death rate is highly dependent on the treatment facilities; the highest mortality rates are in Africa, where case-fatality rates have approximated 10%, especially during epidemic attacks. It is likely that cholera as an endemic infection causes 100,000 to 150,000 deaths annually.

### Microbiology

*Vibrio cholerae* is a gram-negative, motile, curved bacillus that is free-living in bodies of salt water.[138] *V. cholerae* is classified on the basis of lipopolysaccharide antigens. Until recently, all epidemic strains of *V. cholerae* were of the O1 serotype. Group O1 is further subdivided into two biotypes: classic and El Tor. Other serotypes were thought to cause sporadic cases of diarrhea but not epidemic disease. This dictum was discarded by the development of an ongoing epidemic in Asia and South America caused by a new serotype, O139, synonym Bengal.[139, 140] Although the pathogenesis and clinical features of O139 cholera are identical to those of O1 cholera, persons having immunity to serotype O1 are not immune to the Bengal serotype. This lack of immunity is primarily a result of the unique O139 cell surface antigen.

## Epidemiology

*V. cholerae* is spread via contamination of food and water supplies. There is no evidence of an animal reservoir, but humans may serve as transient carriers.[141] On rare occasions, humans may chronically carry the organism.[142] Owing to the nature of its spread, persons living in areas with adequate sanitation are at minimal, if any, risk for encountering cholera. Cholera does occur in the United States, but usually as a result of imported food brought back by returning international travelers. Travelers from the United States to endemic areas are at low risk (about 1 per 30,000 travelers).[144] Cholera has also been isolated from oysters in the Gulf Coast.[143] However, owing to the frequency of international travel, it is important for the clinician who encounters a patient with severe cholera symptoms (dehydration and rice-water stools) to suspect this infection even in nonendemic areas.

## Pathogenesis

*V. cholerae* enters its potential host through the oral route, usually in contaminated food or water. Volunteer studies have shown that a relatively large number of organisms (approximately $10^{11}$) must be ingested to produce symptoms.[145] Similar to other ingested organisms, *V. cholerae* must survive the acidic gastric environment. The importance of gastric acidity as a host-protective factor is borne out by the increased occurrence of cholera in patients with absent or reduced gastric acidity.[82, 145]

The organisms travel to the small intestine, where they adhere to the epithelium. This process may be aided by production of mucinase.[145] The intestinal epithelium remains intact with normal morphology.[146] *Vibrio* species produce a toxin that is composed of a central subunit (A) surrounded by five B subunits; the latter bind to a ganglioside, $GM_1$, which serves as the toxin receptor. This binding facilitates the transfer of the A subunit across the cell membrane, where it is cleaved into two components, denoted $A_1$ and $A_2$. The disulfide linkage between $A_1$ and $A_2$ is reduced to liberate an active $A_1$ peptide, which acts as a catalyst to facilitate the transfer of adenosine diphosphate-ribose from nicotinamide adenine dinucleotide to a guanyl nucleotide-binding regulatory protein ($G_s$). $G_s$ then stimulates adenylate cyclase, located on the basolateral membrane, thereby increasing cyclic adenosine monophosphate. This result in turn leads to chloride secretion and a net flux of fluid into the intestinal lumen.[147]

Although this mechanism of toxin action adequately explains the clinical symptoms of cholera, similar symptoms have been noted in patients infected with strains that do *not* produce the classic cholera toxin. This has led to the recognition that *V. cholerae* harbors additional virulence factors in the bacterial genome that may contribute to diarrheal disease and must be considered in the design of a nonreactigenic vaccine. Newly recognized toxins produced by *V. cholerae* include zonula occludens toxin and the accessory cholera toxin.[148, 149]

## Clinical Manifestations

After an incubation period, commonly 1 to 3 days, the symptoms of cholera usually begin abruptly with vomiting and profuse, watery diarrhea. The stool soon becomes clear, with bits of mucus giving it the so-called rice-water appearance. Patients do not experience tenesmus but rather a sense of relief with defecation.[138] Typically there is no fever. The rate of fluid loss with cholera can be remarkable in severe disease, with purging rates in excess of 1 L/hour reported in adult patients.[146] Despite the dramatic presentation and health risk of "cholera gravis," most patients with cholera infection are asymptomatic or experience mild symptoms. In addition to people with reduced gastric acidity, people with blood group O are at increased risk for more severe disease. Other host factors that predispose to increased purging are less clear.

## Diagnosis and Treatment

*V. cholerae* is identified by colonial morphology and pigmentation on selective agar (e.g., thiosulfate citrate bile salt–sucrose agar). Further identification depends on biochemical markers (e.g., positive oxidase reaction) and motility of the organism. Specific serotyping is used to confirm the identification

The mainstay of cholera treatment is rehydration. In cases in which the disease is less severe and is recognized early, oral rehydration solutions are appropriate and effective. When purging is excessive (more than 10 mL/kg per hour), intravenous rehydration is required.

Antibiotics have been shown to cause a decrease in duration of the diarrhea, total amount of fluid lost, and length of time organisms are excreted.[138] Tetracycline (250 to 500 mg per dose, given every 6 hours for 3 to 5 days) has been recommended as an appropriate antibiotic for adults,[146] and furazolidone (1.25 mg/kg [maximum 100 mg] per dose, given every 6 hours for 10 days) has been suggested for children and pregnant patients. Ampicillin, chloramphenicol, trimethoprim-sulfamethoxazole, and doxycycline may also be used. Single-dose ciprofloxacin has also been shown to be effective in the treatment of *V. cholerae* O1 or O139,[150] although this drug is not approved for use in children.

Despite much progress, an ideal cholera vaccine is not yet available. An ideal vaccine would provide a high level of long-term protection even to those at high risk for severe illness (e.g., people with blood group type O), and this protection would commence shortly after administration of a single oral dose.[151] New oral vaccines have been developed for cholera, including both killed vaccines and live attenuated strains.[152, 153] Although some of these vaccines are now in field trial and one effective vaccine (CVD103-HgR) has

**TABLE 28–3. Diarrheogenic *Escherichia coli***

| NAME | ABBREVIATION | PATHOGENIC MECHANISMS | ILLNESS |
|---|---|---|---|
| Enteropathogenic *E. coli* | EPEC | Adherence to enterocytes | Infantile diarrhea in developing countries |
| Enterotoxigenic *E. coli* | ETEC | Enterotoxin elaboration | Infantile diarrhea in developing countries; traveler's diarrhea |
| Enteroinvasive *E. coli* | EIEC | Invasion of epithelial cells; toxin elaboration | Watery diarrhea/dysentery |
| Enterohemorrhagic *E. coli* | EHEC | Cytotoxin elaboration<br>Adherence | Hemorrhagic colitis; hemolytic-uremic syndrome |
| Diffuse-adherent *E. coli* | DAEC | ?Adherence | ?Diarrhea |
| Enteroaggregative *E. coli* | EAEC | ?Adherence<br>Enterotoxin elaboration | Persistent diarrhea in developing countries |

been licensed on three continents, there remains a need to continue development of nonreactigenic O1 vaccines and vaccines against the new O139 epidemic strain. Neither the killed nor the live O1 vaccines protect against the new serotype O139, since most of the protection is lipopolysaccharide-mediated and the new serotype has a unique lipopolysaccharide. Therefore, the appearance of the new serotype reinforces the need for testing additional vaccine candidates.

## Other Vibrios

The noncholera vibrios, *V. parahaemolyticus, V. pluvialis, V. mimicus, V. hollisae, V. furnissii,* and *V. vulnificans*, have been shown to cause gastrointestinal illness, wound infections, and septicemia.[154] Although each organism has its own characteristics, most noncholera vibrios produce a protein toxin identical to the classic cholera toxin.[138] Some species also produce a heat-stable toxin similar to *E. coli* heat-stable toxin.[155] Although these organisms produce a cholera-like illness, the stool may sometimes contain blood and leukocytes, and sepsis can occur. This has led to speculation that some members of this group, namely *V. parahaemolyticus*, may be capable of invasiveness as well as toxin production.[154] In the United States, gastroenteritis caused by these vibrios is most often associated with the ingestion of raw oysters.[156]

Gastroenteritis caused by non-O1 vibrios tends to be far milder than that caused by *V. cholerae*. In severe cases of diarrhea or septicemia, antibiotics may be helpful, with the agents used for *V. cholerae* recommended.

## *Escherichia coli*

*E. coli* constitutes a diverse group of organisms, including nonpathogenic strains, which are among the most common bacteria in the normal flora of the human intestine, and pathogenic strains. Pathogenic *E. coli* strains that cause diarrheal illness have been recognized since the 1940s.[157, 158]

These diarrheogenic *E. coli* have been studied extensively and are currently classified, on the basis of serogrouping or pathogenic mechanisms, into five major groups: (1) enteropathogenic *E. coli* (EPEC), an important cause of diarrhea in infants in developing countries; (2) enterotoxigenic *E. coli* (ETEC), a cause of diarrhea in infants in developing areas of the world and a cause of traveler's diarrhea in adults; (3) enteroinvasive *E. coli* (EIEC), which cause either a watery ETEC-like illness or, less commonly, a dysentery-like illness; (4) enterohemorrhagic *E. coli* (EHEC), which cause hemorrhagic colitis and HUS; and (5) enteroaggregative *E. coli* (EAEC) and diffuse-adherent *E. coli* (DAEC), which along with EPEC have been implicated as causes of persistent diarrhea. Each of these groups of *E. coli* has unique properties (Table 28–3).

### *Enteropathogenic* Escherichia coli

EPEC is a major cause of diarrhea in developing countries. As much as 30% to 40% of infant diarrhea, particularly in the 0- to 6-month age group, may be caused by EPEC, and in some studies EPEC infection exceeds that of rotavirus.[159–162] In North America and the United Kingdom, EPEC infections were common during the 1940s through the 1960s; now they are most commonly associated with sporadic cases and nosocomial or daycare outbreaks.[163, 164] However, because of the general unavailability of serotyping, the true incidence of EPEC-associated diarrhea may be underestimated. A 1997 study in Seattle children with diarrhea, in which DNA probes were used to screen *E. coli* present in stool, found a high incidence of EPEC-like organisms in this population.[165]

The hallmark of EPEC infection is the "attaching and effacing" lesion seen in the intestine.[164, 166] This lesion is characterized by destruction of microvilli and intimate adherence between the bacterium and the epithelial cell membrane. Directly beneath the surface of the adherent organism, there are marked cytoskeletal changes in the enterocyte, including accumulation of actin polymers. Often, the bacteria are raised on a pedestal-like structure as a result of this actin accumulation. A number of steps are probably responsible for the development of this attaching and effacing lesion. As proposed by Donnenberg and Kaper,[167] EPEC pathogenesis consists of three phases: (1) localized adherence, which brings the bacteria in close contact with the enterocyte (e.g., docking); (2) signal transduction, including increases in intracellular calcium and protein phosphorylation; and (3) intimate adherence, a multigene process encoded in the bacterium by a locus of enterocyte effacement.[168, 169] The dramatic loss of absorptive microvilli in the intestine presumably leads to diarrhea via malabsorption. Although this is probably the predominant mechanism, some evidence suggests that a separate secretory mechanism is also involved.

Patients with symptomatic EPEC infection typically experience diarrhea, vomiting, malaise, and fever. The stool may contain mucus but does not usually contain blood. Symptoms with EPEC infection are more severe than with some other enteric infections and may persist for 2 weeks or longer.[157] In some patients, EPEC has caused protracted diarrhea with dehydration, malnutrition, and zinc deficiency as complications; treatment with parenteral hyperalimentation has been required.[164] EPEC can be detected by serotyping of isolated *E. coli*,[163, 170] by demonstration of the presence of the enterocyte adherence factor or other virulence genes using molecular probes,[171] or by identification of the attaching and effacing phenotype using tissue culture cells.[172] These assays are not commonly used in the clinical microbiology laboratory. Diagnosis of EPEC may be made by demonstrating the presence of adherent organisms on small intestinal or rectal biopsy.[163, 164, 170]

Although controlled studies of antibiotic therapy for EPEC have been few, the significant morbidity associated with this agent argues for treatment with antibiotics in most cases. Trimethoprim-sulfamethoxazole (trimethoprim, 5 mg/kg [maximum 160 mg], plus sulfamethoxazole, 25 mg/kg [maximum 800 mg] per dose, given every 12 hours) has been used with some success, as have oral neomycin and gentamicin.

## *Enterotoxigenic* Escherichia coli

ETEC are recognized as an important cause of diarrhea in infants in developing areas of the world. In endemic areas, children in the first few years of life may be infected several times each year.[173] In the United States, cases of ETEC among children are uncommon.[174] ETEC is also a major cause of traveler's diarrhea in adults. Fecal-oral transmission and consumption of heavily contaminated food or water are the most common vehicles for ETEC infection.

The production of disease by ETEC begins with colonization of the small intestine. There the bacteria depend on fimbriae (also called *pili*) to facilitate attachment to the mucosal surface and overcome the forward motion of peristalsis. This attachment process causes no detectable structural changes in the architecture of the brush border membrane but does allow the bacteria to release their enterotoxins, heat-labile toxin (LT) and heat-stable toxin (ST), in close proximity to the enterocyte brush border membrane where toxin receptors are present.[175] These toxins in turn stimulate adenylate cyclase (in the case of LT) or guanylate cyclase (in the case of ST), and both ultimately result in a net fluid secretion from the intestine (see the reviews by Cohen and Giannella[176] and by Sears and Kaper[177]). Two endogenous ligands for the ST receptor, guanylin and uroguanylin, have been identified.[178, 179] This discovery is consistent with the hypothesis that ST is a superagonist and exerts its diarrheal action by means of usurping a normal secretory mechanisms in the intestine (e.g., by molecular mimicry of these less potent endogenous ligands).

Clinically, ETEC infection causes nausea, abdominal pain, and watery diarrhea. Stools typically contain neither mucus nor leukocytes. ETEC can be diagnosed with the use of bioassays such as the suckling mouse assay,[180] immunoassays, or gene probes specific for either ST[181] or LT.[182] PCR assays are also available. However, none of these assays is commonly used in the clinical microbiology laboratory. Supportive measures are sufficient therapy for most cases of ETEC diarrhea, with oral rehydration a mainstay of therapy. Antibiotics, including trimethoprim-sulfamethoxazole, have been shown to decrease the duration of fecal excretion of the organisms.[183] Quinolone antibiotics may be more effective,[184] but they are not recommended for use in children.

## *Enteroinvasive* Escherichia coli

EIEC share many common features, including virulence mechanisms, with shigella. These organisms preferentially colonize the colon and invade and replicate within epithelial cells, where they cause cell death.[157] In addition, both organisms elaborate one or more secretory enterotoxins. Clinically, both shigella and EIEC infections are characterized by a period of watery diarrhea that precedes the onset of dysentery (scanty stools containing mucus, pus, and blood). More commonly, in contrast to shigella, only this first phase of watery diarrhea is seen in EIEC infection.[185] This illness is clinically indistinguishable from other causes of bacterial diarrhea (e.g., ETEC) or nonbacterial infectious diarrhea. In a minority of patients with EIEC infections, the dysentery syndrome of characteristic stools, tenesmus, and fever is also seen. Bacteremia is not reported.

Infection due to EIEC is uncommon, but foodborne outbreaks of disease have occurred in the United States and aboard cruise ships. Diagnosis is dependent on bioassay (the Sereny test), serotyping, ELISA, or DNA probe techniques. None of these tests is commonly available in the clinical laboratory. Treatment is currently limited to supportive measures, although ampicillin given intramuscularly has been associated with bacteriologic cure and clinical improvement.[185]

## *Enterohemorrhagic* Escherichia coli

EHEC are a distinct class of organisms that have been identified since 1983 as the cause of two recognizable syndromes: hemorrhagic colitis and HUS.[186, 187] Hemorrhagic colitis is an illness characterized by crampy abdominal pain, initial watery diarrhea, and subsequent development of grossly bloody diarrhea with little or no fever. Although there may be more than 100 serotypes in this class of diarrheogenic *E. coli*, in North America the *E. coli* serotype O157:H7 is the prototypic member of this family of organisms. *E. coli* O157:H7 is the most common cause of infectious bloody diarrhea in the United States.[188] Similarly, HUS, which is defined as the triad of acute renal failure, thrombocytopenia, and microangiopathic hemolytic anemia, is also highly associated with antecedent *E. coli* O157:H7 infection.

EHEC infections may occur in sporadic cases, but they have also been associated with outbreaks of disease in nursing homes, daycare centers, and other institutions; several reviews have been published.[189–192] It is estimated that *E. coli* O157:H7 causes approximately 10,000 to 20,000 infections per year in the United States alone and may be responsible for 250 deaths annually.[193] Inadequately cooked hamburgers were most likely the source of the first outbreak[186] and remain the most common vehicle of transmission. In 1993 there was a large epidemic in the western United States; inadequately cooked hamburgers were again implicated as the cause. Other, small epidemics have been attributed to apple juice or cider, and large-scale outbreaks in Japan have been associated with bean sprouts. Contaminated water has also been a source of infection.[194, 195] Common to all of these outbreaks is a reservoir of EHEC in the intestines of cattle and other animals who are asymptomatic. Infection is spread either by direct contact with intestinal contents or through droppings or water runoff from contaminated pastures. A low infectious dose for EHEC and the resistance of these organisms to gastric acid and to the food preserving process (high salt and drying) contribute to the high attack rate. The low infectious dose also contributes to frequent person-to-person transmission.[189–192]

Genetic evidence and experimental observations regarding common pathogenic mechanisms (attaching and effacing lesions) suggest that *E. coli* O157:H7 and this class of organisms represent a new pathogen that has evolved from EPEC.[196, 197] Although the term EHEC, initially proposed by Levine,[157] is descriptive of the most common illness caused by these organisms, it is not the only term associated with these pathogens. Toxins produced by these organisms are important in the pathogenesis of disease; these toxins are similar to Shiga toxin, a cytotoxin produced by *S. dysenteriae* type 1, and are cytotoxic for Vero cells. Therefore, these toxins have also been referred to as Shiga-like toxins or verotoxins, and the organisms that produce these toxins have been called Shiga-like toxin–producing *E. coli* (SLTEC) or verotoxic *E. coli* (VTEC). More recently, these toxins have been collectively referred to as a family of *Stx,* or Shiga toxins. However, toxin production in the absence of other virulence factors (e.g., adherence) may not be sufficient to cause disease. This has important implications for diagnostic tests that simply identify the presence of one or more cytotoxins.

Both the very old and the very young appear to be at increased risk for EHEC infection and its complications.[189–192] Clinical features and complications of *E. coli* O157:H7 infection include bloody diarrhea, nonbloody diarrhea, HUS, thrombotic thrombocytopenic purpura, and, uncommonly, asymptomatic infection.[189] Symptoms may persist for several days or, less commonly, for several weeks. Early reports suggested that carriage of the organism was brief and that prompt culture was necessary to recover these organisms.[198, 199] More recently, prolonged shedding has been observed.[200, 201] This has led to the recommendation that two negative stool cultures be obtained before a child is allowed to return to daycare.[200]

The identification of EHEC is made difficult because it is not possible to differentiate disease-producing *E. coli* from normal enteric flora on the basis of standard microbiologic techniques. There are currently six techniques for identification of EHEC: biochemical markers with serotyping (most commonly used), serum antibody tests, cytotoxin bioassays, DNA hybridization, PCR-based tests, and cytotoxin detection (including ELISAs). Some of these methods (e.g., toxin-based assays) detect the presence of cytotoxin-producing organisms, including non-O157 serotypes.

Prevention of disease transmission is made difficult by the fact that these organisms colonize the intestine of healthy cattle and other food animals, including beef, pork, lamb, and poultry. Therefore, they can survive and multiply in the food chain. Proper cooking destroys these organisms; in hamburgers, an internal cooking temperature of 70°C (157°F) renders the meat safe. Practically, safe cooking most commonly results in a gray hamburger (not pink), with clear juices. Risk can be lowered by educating consumers about cross-contamination, use of warning labels now affixed to meat in the United States, and improvements in meat processing and microbial contamination detection.

At present there is no effective therapy to treat *Stx*-producing *E. coli* disease, so prevention is the most important strategy. Hemorrhagic colitis has been confused with a number of other conditions, including ischemic colitis, appendicitis, Crohn's disease, ulcerative colitis, cecal polyp, pseudomembranous colitis, and an acute abdomen (ileitis). Therefore, an important aspect of treatment of EHEC-associated hemorrhagic colitis is making the correct diagnosis and avoiding unnecessary diagnostic studies such as angiography and laparotomy. The mainstay of therapy for hemorrhagic colitis is the management of dehydration, electrolyte abnormalities, and gastrointestinal blood loss. Antimicrobial agents may help by killing the bacterial pathogens, but they may also cause harm by increasing the release and subsequent absorption of Shiga-like toxin.[202] Trials of antibiotic treatment of EHEC infection are inconclusive. Although these organisms are uniformly sensitive to antimicrobials in vitro, at present there is no evidence that antimicrobial therapy is helpful in diminishing the severity of illness, shortening the duration of fecal excretion, or preventing HUS.[203, 204] A double-blind, placebo-controlled study has begun to evaluate a novel treatment strategy for preventing HUS.[205] This strategy is based on the use of a chemically synthesized Shiga-like toxin receptor attached to an inert, sandlike material (Synsorb-Pk from Synsorb Biotech, Calgary, Alberta). Trials are under way to test the hypothesis that exogenous, free luminal receptor can adsorb unbound toxin and prevent intestinal uptake and subsequent toxin-mediated systemic complications.

### *Enteroaggregative and Diffuse-Adherent* Escherichia coli

The initial observation of adherence by EPEC served as the foundation for the identification of two other classes of diarrheogenic *E. coli.* Although EPEC demonstrates localized adherence to human laryngeal tumor (HEp-2) cells in tissue culture, EAEC demonstrates a pattern of aggregative or stacked-brick adherence, and DAEC demonstrates a pattern of diffuse adherence.[206] The relation of these adherence patterns to the pathogenic mechanisms of these organisms, which are poorly described, is not certain. EAEC characteristically enhances intestinal mucus secretion[207] and may possess both cytotoxins and enterotoxins.[208] Less is known about the mechanisms of DAEC, which has been shown to produce fingerlike projections in intestinal cell lines in tissue culture, embedding the bacteria in these projections.[159] The clinical features of EAEC infection include a watery, mucoid, secretory diarrheal illness with low-grade fever and little or no vomiting.[209, 210] EAEC has been associated with sporadic cases and outbreaks[211]; moreover, there is a strong association between EAEC and persistent diarrhea.[212] For example, Cravioto and colleagues identified EAEC in 51% of Mexican children with persistent diarrhea but in only 5% of asymptomatic age-matched infants.[159] DAEC has been isolated in

France from a large proportion of hospitalized patients with diarrhea who had no other identified enteropathogen.[213] Both the HEp-2 cell assay and DNA probes have been used to identify EAEC and DAEC; however, these are not routinely available in the clinical microbiology laboratory.

## *Clostridium difficile*

*C. difficile* is a gram-positive anaerobic bacillus. Disease caused by this organism can manifest in a variety of ways, ranging from asymptomatic carriage to potentially life-threatening pseudomembranous colitis. This organism has been primarily, but not exclusively, associated with illness occurring after disruption of the normal intestinal flora by antibiotics.

### Epidemiology

Of great interest in the study of *C. difficile* is the difference in the incidence of isolation of the organism and its toxin in various age groups. *C. difficile* toxin has been found in the feces of 10% of normal-term neonates and 55% of those in a neonatal intensive care unit.[214] Most infants found to have toxin in their stools are asymptomatic. A small group of toxin-positive infants have signs and symptoms of necrotizing enterocolitis, but no clear relation to *C. difficile* or its toxin has been demonstrated. The presence of *C. difficile* toxin in these asymptomatic infants may indicate the coexistence of some protective antitoxic substance[215] or may reflect a lack of appropriate toxin receptors in patients in this age group.[216]

The incidence of *C. difficile* toxin positivity decreases beyond the neonatal period. The incidence of asymptomatic carriage in children older than 2 years of age approaches that in healthy adults (about 3%). Furthermore, not all of these organisms are toxin producers. Adults who develop disease from *C. difficile* infection are also more likely than children to experience severe colitis symptoms.

### Pathogenesis

*C. difficile* elaborates two important toxins. Toxin A probably mediates human disease; it is called an enterotoxin despite the fact that it causes cytotoxicity with hemorrhage and mucosal destruction in addition to having enterotoxic effects. Toxin A is a large protein (308 kd) that binds to an enterocyte surface receptor and activates an intracellular G protein–dependent signal transduction mechanism.[217] Bound toxin results in altered permeability, inhibition of protein synthesis, and direct cytotoxicity. Toxin B is thought not to be an important mediator of human disease. However, this "cytotoxin" is almost always found with toxin A, and toxin B is the basis for the "gold standard" cytotoxic tissue culture assay.

### Clinical Manifestations

*C. difficile*–related diarrhea almost always occurs in the setting of antimicrobial administration. Less commonly, the syndrome of pseudomembranous enterocolitis is seen after surgery (without antimicrobial agents) and after antineoplastic therapy. Any mucosal disease, including inflammatory bowel disease, is thought to be a risk factor, but only 1.7% of pediatric patients with inflammatory bowel disease were found to have *C. difficile* toxin in stool while in good control.[218] Hospitalization is a major risk factor for the acquisition of infection. Most patients experience mild, watery diarrhea that lasts only a few days and spontaneously resolves. In some patients, symptoms persist for weeks to months. Pseudomembranous colitis develops in a subset of patients. Patients with this disease are often extremely ill, with high fever, leukocytosis, and hypoalbuminemia.

### Diagnosis and Treatment

*C. difficile* should be suspected in cases of colitis or mild diarrhea in which blood and leukocytes are noted in the stools. Concurrent or recent exposure (within several weeks) to antibiotics should increase the suspicion of *C. difficile* as the causative agent. The use of virtually any antibiotic may predispose to *C. difficile* disease.

Diagnosis of *C. difficile* can be made by culture of the organism or by examination for the presence of toxin in feces. The "gold standard" for laboratory detection of *C. difficile* toxin requires the use of a tissue culture system, with demonstration of a cytopathic effect that can be neutralized by specific antitoxin. Other assays, including a rapid toxin ELISA assay, have sensitivities and specificities approaching those of the tissue culture system and can be interpreted within hours. Sigmoidoscopy in cases of pseudomembranous colitis typically reveals friable white exudate overlying multiple ulcerated areas.[219] The histologic findings of such lesions are depicted in Figure 28–5. Less commonly, pseudomembranes may not be present in the rectosigmoid but may be present in the more proximal colon.

In cases of mild diarrheal illness caused by *C. difficile*, discontinuation of any antibiotics the patient is receiving may be sufficient therapy. In cases of severe illness and especially in cases of pseudomembranous colitis, treatment should also include oral vancomycin (5–10 mg/kg [maximum 500 mg] per dose, given every 6 hours for 7 days) or metronidazole (5–10 mg/kg [maximum 500 mg] per dose, given every 8 hours for 7 days).[220] Compared with vancomycin, metronidazole is much less expensive and has similar efficacy.

There is a fairly high rate of relapse of illness, generally 15% to 20%, after treatment of *C. difficile*. These relapses usually occur within 1 month of completion of therapy and have been thought to result from the activation of *C. difficile* spores remaining from the primary infection.[221] Most of these cases of relapse are responsive to a second course of vancomycin or metronidazole or to repeated short courses of these drugs. There are reports of multiple relapses in which cholestyramine, given as a slurry (120 mg/kg per dose every 8 hours) for 4 weeks and tapered over the following 3 weeks, was effective in eradication of the organism.[221] Intravenously administered gamma globulin is an alternative therapy for chronic *C. difficile* enterocolitis.[222] *Lactobacillus GG* has also been used successfully in a few pediatric patients with recurrent or persistent infection.[223]

## *Aeromonas* and *Plesiomonas*

Within the past decade, several organisms not previously recognized as enteric pathogens have been linked to diarrheal

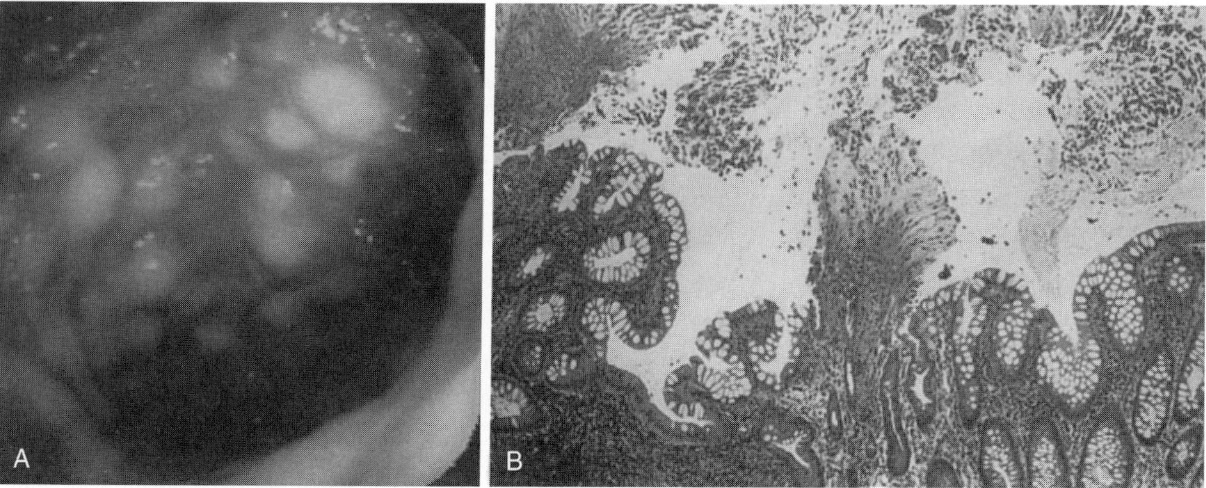


**FIGURE 28–5.** *A,* The endoscopic appearance of the sigmoid colon with multiple densely adherent plaques (pseudomembranes). *B,* Mucosal biopsy shows a focus of necrotizing enterocolitis with a typical volcano lesion (accumulated fibropurulent exudate intermixed with mucus). (From Bates M, Bove K, Cohen MB: Pseudomembranous colitis caused by *C. difficile*. J Pediatr 1997;130:146, with permission.)

disease. This includes organisms of the genus *Aeromonas* and the closely related bacterium *Plesiomonas shigelloides* (previously classified as *Aeromonas shigelloides*). These organisms are gram-negative, facultatively anaerobic bacilli classified in the family Vibrionaceae. They are oxidase-positive, differentiating them from members of the Enterobacteriaceae.[224]

## Aeromonas

Several members of the genus *Aeromonas*, including *Aeromonas hydrophila,* are common inhabitants of fresh and brackish water in the United States. These organisms were initially recognized as opportunistic pathogens in immunocompromised hosts, especially those with malignant hematologic diseases. The organisms also have been known to cause disease in patients with underlying hepatobiliary disease.[224] *Aeromonas* has been isolated from healthy persons as well and has therefore been thought to be part of the normal flora. Despite initial studies that yielded conflicting results,[225] it is now generally accepted that *A. hydrophila* is an enteric pathogen.

Studies in Australian children with diarrhea have found *Aeromonas* species present in 10% of patients.[226] Infection appears to occur most frequently in children younger than 2 years of age.[227] Of patients with *Aeromonas* isolated from stool cultures at Children's Hospital Medical Center, Cincinnati, approximately 50% were younger than 3 months. *Aeromonas* infection is also seasonal, occurring more often in the summer months.[224]

Not all *Aeromonas* species are pathogenic. The method of pathogenesis remains unclear. Both cytotoxic[227] and enterotoxic[224] properties have been observed, but neither these nor other pathogenic mechanisms are found consistently in strains isolated from patients with *Aeromonas*-associated disease.[225] *Aeromonas caviae*, a commonly isolated species, demonstrates both adherence and cytotoxin production.[228]

Clinical symptoms attributed to *Aeromonas* can be grouped into three categories: (1) acute watery diarrhea, the most common syndrome; (2) dysentery, which usually is self-limited; and (3) persistent watery diarrhea. Cramping abdominal pain and vomiting may also occur.[227] Symptoms may occasionally be severe and, especially when dysentery is present, have been incorrectly diagnosed as ulcerative colitis.[226]

In mild cases of *Aeromonas* infection, supportive treatment should suffice. In patients who are immunocompromised, are otherwise acutely ill, or have persistent illness, treatment with antibiotics is recommended. Trimethoprim-sulfamethoxazole is usually effective (trimethoprim, 5 mg/kg [maximum 160 mg], plus sulfamethoxazole, 25 mg/kg [maximum 800 mg] per dose, given every 12 hours for 14 days), as are tetracycline, chloramphenicol, and the aminoglycosides.[224] Most strains of *Aeromonas* are resistant to the penicillins, including ampicillin.[224]

## Plesiomonas

*P. shigelloides*, like *Aeromonas*, is commonly found in the environment,[229] especially in bodies of water, including water from a home aquarium.[230] Unlike *Aeromonas*, however, *Plesiomonas* has been reported to occur in epidemics, with contaminated water often found to be the cause.[229] *Plesiomonas* is also known to be spread through improperly cooked seafood.[231]

The pathogenesis of disease caused by *P. shigelloides* is not well understood. A cytotoxin has been found in some strains[229] but not in others. An invasive mechanism is also suspected, because of the colitis symptoms.[231] In addition to small-volume stools with leukocytes and possible blood, patients may also experience severe abdominal pain. Fever has been seen in approximately one third of patients.[231] In one group of adult patients, symptoms persisted longer than 2 weeks in 75% and longer than 4 weeks in 32%.[231]

Diagnosis of *P. shigelloides* is made by stool culture. Although this illness is usually self-limited, treatment with antimicrobial agents has been shown to decrease the duration of symptoms,[231] with trimethoprim-sulfamethoxazole or aminoglycosides suggested as appropriate choices. There are no controlled trials of antimicrobial treatment of gastroenteritis caused by this organism.

### *Mycobacterium avium-intracellulare*

*Mycobacterium avium* and *Mycobacterium intracellulare*, known collectively as *Mycobacterium avium-intracellulare* or *Mycobacterium avium* complex (MAC), are acid-fast bacilli that have been recognized primarily for their role in cases of atypical tuberculosis. These organisms are now recognized as causative agents of diarrheal symptoms as well. In a review of pediatric cases of atypical mycobacterial infections, Lincoln and Gilbert[232] described two immunocompetent patients whose clinical findings included diarrhea and colonic ulceration.

Of even greater significance than these sporadic cases of MAC infection in immunocompetent hosts is its occurrence among immunocompromised patients. In patients with the acquired immunodeficiency syndrome, MAC is among the most commonly isolated agents causing systemic bacterial infections.[233] These patients may also have chronic diarrhea and abdominal pain.[234, 235] MAC has also been noted to cause diarrhea in patients undergoing bone marrow transplantation[236] and in a patient with cystic fibrosis.[237]

The MAC organisms may be cultured from gastric and duodenal aspirates obtained endoscopically and from the stool, the bone marrow, and the blood.[233] Endoscopic examination in patients with MAC may reveal findings similar to those seen in Whipple's disease, with minute superficial ulcerations in the small bowel.[235] Treatment of MAC infections with conventional antituberculosis agents usually is unsuccessful in eradicating the organisms or alleviating symptoms.[233]

## POTENTIAL DIARRHEOGENIC ORGANISMS

### Enterotoxigenic *Bacteroides fragilis*

*Bacteroides fragilis* is an anaerobic organism that is commonly isolated from normal stool flora. However, some investigators have identified a toxin-producing variant that is enteropathogenic.[238] Enterotoxigenic organisms have been isolated from both healthy persons and those with diarrhea.[239] Epidemiologic associations with diarrhea have been shown for enterotoxigenic *B. fragilis* in several studies[240–243] but not others.[244] Additional investigation is required to fulfill Koch's postulates for this organism.

### *Brachyspira aalborgi*

Intestinal spirochetosis, or the colonization of the large bowel by *Brachyspira aalborgi* and related spirochetes, has recently been implicated as a cause of diarrhea.[245] Some studies have shown an association between this organism and bloody diarrhea,[246] although asymptomatic colonization has also been reported.[247] The potential of this organism to cause diarrhea requires further evaluation.

### *Hafnia alvei*

This organism has been associated with diarrhea in sporadic cases and in at least one hospital outbreak. Although a causal relation between *Hafnia alvei* and diarrhea has not been clearly established, a subset of this organism may be enteropathogenic. Organisms isolated from patients with diarrhea typically demonstrate the attaching and effacing lesion seen with EPEC, whereas nonpathogenic isolates do not show this characteristic.[248]

### *Listeria monocytogenes*

Invasive illness caused by *Listeria* is well known. An outbreak of *Listeria* gastroenteritis and fever without invasive disease was reported in persons who had consumed contaminated chocolate milk.[249] The importance of *L. monocytogenes* in outbreaks of gastroenteritis caused by contaminated food has yet to be adequately determined.

## CONCLUSION

Despite this chapter's catalog of both bacterial and viral infectious agents, from 40% to 60% of cases of diarrhea are currently not attributable to any known cause. Undoubtedly, as techniques for identification and culture become more sophisticated, other causative agents will be identified and the percentage of diarrheal illnesses described as idiopathic or nonspecific will continue to decline. Advances in the widespread use of improved oral rehydration solutions have led to a decline in the morbidity and mortality associated with diarrhea. Future advances in preventive measures, including vaccines, may lead to a reduction of the incidence of diarrheal disease.

## REFERENCES


1. Glass RI, Lew JF, Gangarosa RE, et al: Estimates of morbidity and mortality rates for diarrheal diseases in American children. J Pediatr 1991;118:527–533.
2. Guerrant RL, Bobak DA: Bacterial and protozoal gastroenteritis. N Engl J Med 1991;325:327–340.
3. Blacklow NR, Cukor G: Viral gastroenteritis. N Engl J Med 1991;325:252–264.
4. Blacklow NR, Cukor G: Viral gastroenteritis N Engl J Med 1981;304:397–406.
5. Kapikian AZ, Wyatt RG, Dolin R, et al: Visualization by immune electron microscopy of a 27 nm particle associated with acute infectious nonbacterial gastroenteritis. J Virol 1972;10:1075–1081.
6. Bishop RF, Davidson GP, Holmes IH, et al: Virus particles in epithelial cells of duodenal mucosa from children with acute non-bacterial gastroenteritis. Lancet 1973;2:1281–1283.
7. Ho MS, Glass RI, Pinsky PF, et al: Rotavirus as a cause of diarrheal morbidity and mortality in the United States. J Infect Dis 1988;158:1112–1116.
8. Kapikian AZ, Chanock RM: Rotaviruses. In Fields BN, Knipe DM, Howley PM, et al (eds): Fields Virology, 3rd ed, vol 2. Philadelphia, Lippincott-Raven Press, 1996, pp 1657–1708.

9. Kapikian AZ, Hoshino Y, Chanock RM, Perez-Schael I: Efficacy of a quadrivalent Rhesus rotavirus-based human rotavirus vaccine aimed at preventing severe rotavirus diarrhea in infants and young children. J Infect Dis 1996;174:S65–S72.
10. Simhon A, Crystie IL, Totterdell BM, et al: Sequential rotavirus diarrhea caused by virus of same subgroup. Lancet 1981;1:1174.
11. Steinhoff MC: Rotavirus: the first five years. J Pediatr 1980;96:611–622.
12. Santosham M, Yolken RH, Wyatt RG, et al: Epidemiology of rotavirus diarrhea in a prospectively monitored American Indian population. J Infect Dis 1985;152:778–783.
13. Yolken RH, Wyatt RG, Zissis G, et al: Epidemiology of human rotavirus types 1 and 2 and as studied by enzyme-linked immunosorbent assay. N Engl J Med 1978;299:1156–1161.
14. Lycke E, Blomberg J, Berg G, et al: Epidemic acute diarrhea in adults associated with infantile gastroenteritis virus. Lancet 1978;2:1056–1057.
15. Meurman OH, Laine MJ: Rotavirus epidemic in adults. N Engl J Med 1977;296:1298–1299.
16. Wenman WM, Hinde D, Feltham S, et al: Rotavirus infection in adults: results of a prospective family study. N Engl J Med 1979;301:303–306.
17. Totterdell BM, Chrystie IL, Banatvala JE: Rotavirus infections in a maternity unit. Arch Dis Child 1976;51:924–928.
18. Bishop RF, Hewstone AZ, Davidson GP, et al: An epidemic of diarrhea in human neonates involving a reovirus-like agent and "enteropathogenic" serotypes of *E. coli*. J Clin Pathol 1976;29:46–49.
19. Crystie IL, Totterdell BM, Banatvala JE: Asymptomatic endemic rotavirus infections in the newborn. Lancet 1978;1:1176–1178.
20. Ryder RW, McGowan JE, Hatch MH, et al: Reovirus-like agent as a cause of nosocomial diarrhea in infants. J Pediatr 1977;90:698–702.
21. Delage G, McLaughlin B, Berthiaume L: A clinical study of rotavirus gastroenteritis. J Pediatr 1978;93:455–457.
22. Bartlett AS III, Bednarz-Prashad AJ, DuPont HL, et al: Rotavirus gastroenteritis. Annu Rev Med 1987;38:399–415.
23. Flewett TH, Bryden AS, Davies H, et al: Epidemic viral enteritis in a long-stay children's ward. Lancet 1975;1:4–5.
24. Wilde J, Yolken R, Willoughby R, et al: Improved detection of rotavirus shedding by polymerase chain reaction. Lancet 1991;337:323–326.
25. Rodriguez WJ, Kim HW, Arrobio JO, et al: Clinical features of acute gastroenteritis associated with human reovirus-like agent in infants and young children. J Pediatr 1977;91:188–193.
26. Riepenhoff-Talty M, Offor E, Klossner K, et al: Effect of age and malnutrition on rotavirus infection in mice. Pediatr Res 1985;19:1250–1253.
27. Gilger MA, Matson DO, Conner ME, et al: Extraintestinal rotavirus infections in children with immunodeficiency. J Pediatr 1992;120:912–917.
28. Davidson GP, Barnes GL: Structural and functional abnormalities of the small intestine in infants and young children with rotavirus enteritis. Acta Paediatr Scand 1979;68:181–186.
29. Ball JH, Peng T, Zeng C Q-Y, et al: Age-dependent diarrhea induced by a rotaviral nonstructural glycoprotein. Science 1996;272:101–104.
30. Christy C, Vosefski D, Madore HP: Comparison of three enzyme immunoassays to tissue culture for the diagnosis of rotavirus gastroenteritis in infants and young children. J Clin Microbiol 1990;28:1428–1430.
31. Yolken RH, Leggiadro RJ: Immunoassays for the diagnosis of viral enteric pathogens. Diagn Microbiol Infect Dis 1986;4:S61–S69.
32. Nazarian LF, Berman JH, Brown G, et al: Practice parameter: the management of acute gastroenteritis in young children. Pediatrics 1996;97:424–435.
33. Duggan C, Santosham M, Glass RI: The management of acute diarrhea in children: oral rehydration, maintenance, and nutritional therapy. MMWR Morb Mortal Wkly Rep 1992;41(RR-16):1–20.
34. Isolauri E, Juntunen M, Rautanen T, et al: A human *Lactobacillus* strain (*Lactobacillus casei*, sp strain GG) promotes recovery from acute diarrhea in children. Pediatrics 1991;88:90–97.
35. Kaila M, Isolauri E, Soppi E, et al: Enhancement of the circulating antibody secreting cell response in human diarrhea by a human *Lactobacillus* strain. Pediatr Res 1992;32:141–144.
36. Saavedra JM, Bauman NA, Orung I, et al: Feeding *Bifidobacterium bifidum* and *Streptococcus thermophilus* to infants in hospital for prevention of diarrhoea and shedding of rotavirus. Lancet 1994;334:1046–1049.
37. Guarino A, Canani RB, Russo S, et al: Oral immunoglobulins for treatment of acute rotaviral gastroenteritis. Pediatrics 1994;93:12–16.
38. Velazquez FR, Matson DO, Calva JJ, et al: Rotavirus infection in infants as protection against subsequent infections. N Engl J Med 1996:335:1022–1028.
39. Clark HF, Offit PA, Ellis RW, et al: The development of multivalent bovine rotavirus (strain WC3) reassortment vaccine for infants. J Infect Dis 1996;174:S73–S80.
40. Treanor JJ, Clark HF, Pichichero M, et al: Evaluation of the protective efficacy of a serotype 1 bovine-human rotavirus reassortment vaccine in infants. Pediatr Infect Dis J 1995;14:301–307.
41. Rennels MB, Glass RI, Dennehy PH, et al: Safety and efficacy of high-dose rhesus-human reassortant rotavirus vaccines: report of the National Multicenter Trial. United States Rotavirus Vaccine Efficacy Group. Pediatrics 1996;97:7–13.
42. Bernstein DI, Glass RI, Rodgers G, et al: Evaluation of rhesus rotavirus monovalent and tetravalent reassortant vaccines in US children. United States Rotavirus Vaccine Efficacy Group. JAMA 1995;273:1191–1196.
43. Glass RI, Compans R, Lang D (eds): Fifth Rotavirus Vaccine Workshop: Current Issues and Future Developments, Atlanta, GA, October 1995. J Infectious Dis 1996;174:S1–S126.
44. Adler JL, Zickl R: Winter vomiting disease. J Infect Dis 1969;119:668–673.
45. Jiang X, Wang M, Graham DY, Estes MK: Norwalk virus genome cloning and characterization. Science 1990;250:1580–1583.
46. Jiang X, Wang M, Wang K, Estes MK: Sequence and genomic organization of Norwalk virus. Virology 1993;195:51–61.
47. Jiang X, Wang J, Estes MK: Characterization of SRSVs using RT-PCR and new antigen ELISA. Arch Virol 1995;140:363–374.
48. Matson DO, Zhong WM, Nakata S, et al: Molecular characterization of a human calicivirus with closer genetic relationships to feline calicivirus than other human caliciviruses. J Med Virol 1995;45:215–222.
49. Wang JX, Jiang X, Madore P, et al: Sequence diversity of SRSVs in the Norwalk virus group. J Virol 1994;68:5982–5990.
50. Cukor G, Blacklow NR: Human viral gastroenteritis. Microbiol Rev 1984;48:157–179.
51. Graham DY, Jiang X, Tanaka T, et al: Norwalk virus infection of volunteers: new insights based on improved assays. J Infect Dis 1994;170:34–43.
52. Lew JF, Valdesuso J, Vesikari T, et al: Detection of Norwalk virus or Norwalk-like infections in Finnish infants and young children. J Infect Dis 1994;169:1364–1367.
53. Jenkins S, Horman JR, Israel E, et al: An outbreak of Norwalk-related gastroenteritis at a boy's camp. Am J Dis Child 1985;139:787–789.
54. Kuritsky JN, Osterholm MT, Greenberg HB, et al: Norwalk gastroenteritis: a community outbreak associated with bakery product consumption. Ann Intern Med 1984;100:519–521.
55. Morse DL, Guzewich JJ, Hanrahan JP, et al: Widespread outbreaks of clam- and oyster-associated gastroenteritis: role of Norwalk virus. N Engl J Med 1986;314:678–681.
56. Greenberg HB, Wyatt RG, Kapikian AZ: Norwalk virus in vomitus. Lancet 1979;1:55.
57. Agus SG, Dolin R, Wyatt RG, et al: Acute infectious nonbacterial gastroenteritis: intestinal histopathology. Ann Intern Med 1973;79:18–25.
58. Storr J, Rice S, Phillips AD, et al: Clinical associations of Norwalk-like virus in the stools of children. J Pediatr Gastroenterol Nutr 1986;5:576–580.
59. Kjeldsberg E, Anestad G, Greenberg H, et al: Norwalk virus in Norway: an outbreak of gastroenteritis studied by electron microscopy and radioimmunoassay. Scand J Infect Dis 1989;21:521–526.
60. Matsui SM, Kim JP, Greenberg HB, et al: The isolation and characterization of a Norwalk virus-specific cDNA. J Clin Invest 1991;87:1456–1461.
61. Wadeli G, Allard A, Johansson M, et al: Enteric adenoviruses. In Bock G, Whelan J (eds): Novel Diarrhoea Viruses: CIBA Foundation Symposium 128. Chichester, England, John Wiley, 1987, pp 63–91.
62. Kotloff KL, Losonsky GA, Morris JG Jr, et al: Enteric adenovirus infection and childhood diarrhea: an epidemiologic study in three clinical settings. Pediatrics 1989;84:219–225.
63. Uhnoo I, Wadell G, Svensson L, et al: Importance of enteric adenoviruses 40 and 41 in acute gastroenteritis in infants and young children. J Clin Microbiol 1984;20:365–372.

64. Grimwood K, Carzino R, Barnes GL, Bishop RF: Patients with adenovirus gastroenteritis admitted to an Australian pediatric teaching hospital from 1981–1992. J Clin Microbiol 1995;33:131–136.
65. Wood DJ: Adenovirus gastroenteritis. Br Med J 1988;296:229–230.
66. Martin AL, Kudesia G: Enzyme linked immunosorbent assay for detecting adenoviruses in stool specimens: comparison with electron microscopy and isolation. J Clin Pathol 1990;43:514–515.
67. Allard A, Girones R, Juto P, et al: Polymerase chain reaction for detection of adenoviruses in stool samples. J Clin Microbiol 1990:28;2659–2667.
68. Jiang B, Monroe SS, Koonin EV, et al: RNA sequence of astrovirus: distinctive genetic organization and a putative retrovirus-like ribosomal frameshifting signal that directs the viral replicase synthesis. Proc Natl Acad Sci U S A 1993;90:10539–10543.
69. Herrmann J, Taylor D, Echeverria P, et al: Astroviruses as a cause of gastroenteritis in children. N Engl J Med 1991;324;1757–1760.
70. Lew JF, Moe CL, Monroe SS, et al: Astrovirus and adenovirus associated with diarrhea in children in day care settings. J Infect Dis 1991;164:673–678.
71. Utagawa ET, Nishizawa S, Sekine S, et al: Astrovirus as a cause of gastroenteritis in Japan. J Clin Microbiol 1994;32:1841–1845.
72. Ashley CR, Caul EO, Paver WK: Astrovirus-associated gastroenteritis in children. J Clin Pathol 1978;31:939–943.
73. Yolken R, Dubovi E, Leister F, et al: Infantile gastroenteritis associated with excretion of pestivirus antigens. Lancet 1989;1:517–520.
74. Centers for Disease Control and Prevention: Viral agents of gastroenteritis: public health importance and outbreak management. MMWR Morb Mortal Wkly Rep 1990;39(RR-5):1–23.
75. Flewett TH, Beards GM, Brown DWG, et al: The diagnostic gap in diarrheal aetiology. In Bock G, Whelan J (eds): Novel Diarrhoea Viruses: CIBA Foundation Symposium 128. Chichester, England, John Wiley, 1987, pp 238–249.
76. Resta S, Luby JP, Rosenfled CR, Siegel JD: Isolation and propagation of a human enteric coronavirus. Science 1985;229:978–981.
77. Woode GN: Breda and Breda-like viruses: diagnosis, pathology and epidemiology. In Bock G, Whelan J (eds): Novel Diarrhoea Viruses: CIBA Foundation Symposium 128. Chichester, England, John Wiley, 1987, pp 175–191.
78. Horzinek MC, Weiss M, Ederveen J: Toroviridae: a proposed new family of enveloped RNA viruses. In Bock G, Whelan J (eds): Novel Diarrhoea Viruses: CIBA Foundation Symposium 128. Chichester, England, John Wiley, 1987, pp 162–174.
79. Koopmans M, Petric M, Glass RI, et al: Enzyme-linked immunosorbent assay reactivity of torovirus-like particles in fecal specimens for humans with diarrhea. J Clin Microbiol 1993;31:2738–2744.
80. Pereira HG, Fialho AM, Flewett TH, et al: Novel viruses in human faeces. Lancet 1988;2:103–104.
81. Hochman JA, Witte DP, Cohen MB: Diagnosis of cytomegalovirus in pediatric Ménétrier's disease with *in situ* hybridization. J Clin Microbiol 1996;34:2588–2589.
82. Giannella RA, Broitman SA, Zamcheck N: Influence of gastric acidity on bacterial and parasitic enteric infections. Ann Intern Med 1973;78:271–276.
83. Giannella RA, Broitman SA, Zamcheck N: Gastric acid barrier to ingested microorganisms in man: studies in vivo and in vitro. Gut 1972;13:251–256.
84. Hargrett-Bean NT, Pavia AT, Tauxe RT: *Salmonella* isolates from humans in the United States, 1984–1986. MMWR Morb Mortal Wkly Rep 1988;3(SS 2):25–31.
85. Bishop WP, Ulshen MH: Bacterial gastroenteritis. Pediatr Clin North Am 1988;35:69–87.
86. Mahon BE, Ponka A, Hall WN, et al: An international outbreak of salmonella infections caused by alfalfa sprouts grown from contaminated seeds. J Infect Dis 1997;175:876–882.
87. Hennessy TW, Hedberg CW, Slutsker L, et al: A national outbreak of *Salmonella enteritidis* infections from ice cream. N Engl J Med 1994;334:1281–1286.
88. Duguid JP, North RAE: Eggs and salmonella food-poisoning: an evaluation. J Med Microbiol 1991;34:65–72.
89. Blaser MJ, Newman LS: A review of human salmonellosis: I. Infective dose. Rev Infect Dis 1982;4:1096–1106.
90. Hromockyj AE, Falkow S: Interactions of bacteria with the gut epithelium. In Blaser MJ, Smith PD, Ravdin JI, et al (eds): Infections of the Gastrointestinal Tract. New York, Raven Press, 1995, pp 603–616.
91. Torrey S, Fleisher G, Jaffe D: Incidence of *Salmonella* bacteremia in infants with *Salmonella* gastroenteritis. J Pediatr 1986;108:718–721.
92. Buchwald DS, Blaser MJ: A review of human salmonellosis: II. Duration of excretion following infection with nontyphi *Salmonella*. Rev Infect Dis 1984;6:345–356.
93. Aserkoff B, Bennett JV: Effect of antibiotic therapy in acute salmonellosis on the fecal excretion of salmonellae. N Engl J Med 1969;281:636–640.
94. St. Geme HW III, Hodes HL, March SM, et al: Consensus: management of the *Salmonella* infection in the first year of life. Pediatr Infect Dis J 1988;7:615–521.
95. Pickering LK: Therapy for acute infectious diarrhea in children. J Pediatr 1991;118:S118–S128.
96. Lee LA, Puhr ND, Maloney EK, et al: Increase in antimicrobial resistant *Salmonella* infections in the United States, 1989–1990. J Infect Dis 1994;170:128–134.
97. Colon AR, Gross DR, Tamer MA: Typhoid fever in children. Pediatrics 1975;56:606–609.
98. Levine MM, Hone D, Stocker BAD, et al: Vaccines to prevent typhoid. In Woodrow G, Levine MM (eds): New-Generation Vaccines. New York, Marcel Dekker, 1990, pp 269–287.
99. Plotkin SA, Bouveret-Le Cam N: A new typhoid vaccine composed of the Vi capsular polysaccharide. Arch Intern Med 1995;155:2293–2299.
100. Osler W: The Principles and Practice of Medicine. New York, D Appleton & Company, 1892.
101. Acheson DWK, Keusch GT: *Shigella* and enteroinvasive *Escherichia coli*. In Blaser MJ, Smith PD, Ravdin JI, et al (eds): Infections of the Gastrointestinal Tract. New York, Raven Press, 1995, pp 763–784.
102. Mata LJ: The children of Santa Maria Caugué: a prospective field study of health and growth. Cambridge, MA, MIT Press, 1978.
103. Cohen MB: Etiology and mechanisms of acute infectious diarrhea in infants in the United States. J Pediatr 1991;4:S34–S39.
104. Calin A, Fries JF: An "experimental" epidemic of Reiter's syndrome revisited: follow-up evidence on genetic and environmental factors. Ann Intern Med 1976;84:564–566.
105. Theriot JA: The cell biology of infection by intracellular bacterial pathogens. Ann Rev Cell Dev Biol 1995;11:213–239.
106. Hale TL: Genetic basis of virulence in *Shigella* species. Microbiol Rev 1991;55:206–224.
107. O'Brien AD, Holmes RK: Shiga and shiga-like toxins. Microbiol Rev 1987;51:206–220.
108. Surawicz CM, Belic L: Rectal biopsy helps to distinguish acute self-limited colitis from idiopathic inflammatory bowel disease. Gastroenterology 1984;86:104–113.
109. Tong MJ, Martin DG, Cunningham JJ, Gunning J: Clinical and bacteriological evaluation of antibiotic treatment in shigellosis. JAMA 1970;214:1841–1844.
110. Ross S, Controni G, Khan W: Resistance of shigellae to ampicillin and other antibiotics. JAMA 1972;221:45–47.
111. Nelson JD, Haltalin KC: Amoxicillin less effective than ampicillin against *Shigella* in vitro and in vivo: relationship of efficacy to activity in serum. J Infect Dis 1974;129:S222–S227.
112. Shears P: *Shigella* infections. Ann Trop Med Parasitol 1996;90:104–114.
113. Williams EK, Lohr JA, Guerrant RL: Acute infectious diarrhea: II. Diagnosis, treatment and prevention. Pediatr Infect Dis J 1986;5:458–465.
114. Walker RI, Caldwell MB, Lee EC, et al: Pathophysiology of *Campylobacter* enteritis. Microbiol Rev 1986;50:81–94.
115. Goosens H, Vlaes L, DeBoeck M, et al: Is *Campylobacter upsaliensis* an unrecognised cause of human diarrhoea? Lancet 1990;335:584–586.
116. Sjögren E, Ruiz-Palacios G, Kaijser B: *Campylobacter jejuni* isolations from Mexican and Swedish patients, with repeated symptomatic and/or asymptomatic diarrhoea episodes. Epidemiol Infect 1989;102:47–57.
117. Tauxe RT, Hargrett-Bean, Patton CM, et al: *Campylobacter* isolates in the United States, 1982–1986. MMWR Morb Mortal Wkly Rep 1988;37(SS-2):1–13.
118. Blaser MJ, Reller LB: *Campylobacter* enteritis. N Engl J Med 1981;305:1444–1452.
119. Spelman DW, Davidson N, Buckmaster ND, et al: *Campylobacter* bacteraemia: a report of 10 cases. Med J Aust 1986;145:503–505.
120. Rees JH, Soudain SE, Gregson NA, Hughes RAC: *Campylobacter jejuni* infection and Guillain-Barré syndrome. N Engl J Med 1995;333:1374–1379.

121. Salloway S, Mermel LA, Seamans M, et al: Miller-Fisher syndrome associated with *Campylobacter jejuni* bearing lipopolysaccharide molecules that mimic human ganglioside $GB_3$. Infect Immun 1996;64:2945–2949.
122. Karmali MA, Fleming PC: *Campylobacter* enteritis in children. J Pediatr 1979;94:527–533.
123. Salazar-Lindo E, Sack RB, Chea-Woo E, et al: Early treatment with erythromycin of *Campylobacter jejuni* associated dysentery in children. J Pediatr 1986;109:355–360.
124. Cover TL, Aber RC: *Yersinia enterocolitica*. N Engl J Med 1989;321:16–24.
125. Black RE, Jackson RJ, Tsai T, et al: Epidemic *Yersinia enterocolitica* infection due to contaminated chocolate milk. N Engl J Med 1978;298:76–79.
126. Lee LA, Gerber AR, Lonsway DR, et al: *Yersinia enterocolitica* O:3 infections in infants and children, associated with the house-hold preparation of chitterlings. N Engl J Med 1990;322:984–987.
127. Lee LA, Taylor J, Carter GP, et al: *Yersinia enterocolitica* O:3: an emerging cause of pediatric gastroenteritis in the United States. J Infect Dis 1991;163:660–663.
128. Marks MI, Pai CH, Lafleur L, et al: *Yersinia enterocolitica* gastroenteritis: a prospective study of clinical, bacteriological, and epidemiologic features. J Pediatr 1980;96:26–31.
129. Cover TL. *Yersinia enterocolitica* and *Yersinia pseudotuberculosis*. In Blaser MJ, Smith PD, Ravdin JI, et al (eds): Infections of the Gastrointestinal Tract. New York, Raven Press, 1995, pp 811–823.
130. Attwood SEA, Mealy K, Cafferkey MI, et al: *Yersinia* infection and acute abdominal pain. Lancet 1987;1:529–533.
131. Dequeker J, Jamar R, Walravens M: HLA-B27, arthritis and *Yersinia enterocolitica* infection. J Rheumatol 1980;7:706–710.
132. Bottone EJ, Sheehan DJ: *Yersinia enterocolitica*: guidelines for serologic diagnosis of human infections. Rev Infect Dis 1983;5:898–906.
133. Pai CH, Gillis F, Tuomanes E, et al: Placebo-controlled double-blind evaluation of trimethoprim-sulfamethoxazole treatment of *Yersinia* enterocolitica gastroenteritis. J Pediatr 1984;104:308–311.
134. Gayraud M, Scavizzi MR, Mollaret HH, et al: Antibiotic treatment of *Yersinia enterocolitica* septicemia: a retrospective review of 43 cases. Clin Infect Dis 1993;17:405–410.
135. Mofenson HC, Caraccio TR, Sharieff N: Iron sepsis: *Yersinia enterocolitica* septicemia possibly caused by an overdose of iron. N Engl J Med 1987;316:1092–1093.
136. Kaper JB, Morris JG Jr, Levine MM: Cholera. Clin Microbiol Rev 1995;8:48–86.
137. Blake PA: Epidemiology of cholera in the Americas. Gastroenterol Clin North Am 1993;3:639–660.
138. Morris JG Jr, Black RE: Cholera and other vibrioses in the United States. N Engl J Med 1985;312:343–350.
139. Ramamurthy T, Garg S, Sharma R, et al: Emergence of novel strain of *Vibrio cholerae* with epidemic potential in southern and eastern India. Lancet 1993;341:703–704.
140. Albert MJ, Siddique AK, Islam MS, et al: Large outbreak of clinical cholera due to *Vibrio cholerae* non-O1 in Bangladesh. Lancet 1993;341:704.
141. Finkelstein RA: Cholera. Crit Rev Micriobiol 1973;2:553–623.
142. Azurin JC, Kobari K, Barua D, et al: A long-term carrier of cholera: Cholera dolores. Bull World Health Organ 1967;37:745–749.
143. DePaola A, Capers GM, Mote ML, et al: Isolation of Latin American epidemic strain of *Vibrio cholerae* O1 from US Gulf coast. Lancet 1992;339:624.
144. Weber JT, Levine WC, Hopkins DP, Tauxe RV: Cholera in the United States, 1965–1991: risks at home and abroad. Arch Intern Med 1994;154:551–556.
145. Carpenter CCJ: Clinical and pathophysiologic features of diarrhea caused by *Vibrio cholerae* and *Escherichia coli*. In Field M, Fordtran JS, Schutz SG (eds): Secretory Diarrhea. Bethesda MD, American Physiological Society, 1980, pp 66–73.
146. Carpenter CCJ: Cholera and other enterotoxin-related diarrheal diseases. J Infect Dis 1972;126:551–564.
147. Moss J, Burns DL, Hsia JA, et al: Cyclic nucleotides: mediators of bacterial toxin action in disease. Ann Intern Med 1984;101:653–666.
148. Fasano A, Baudry B, Pumplin DW, et al: *Vibrio cholerae* produces a second enterotoxin which affects intestinal tight junctions. Proc Natl Acad Sci U S A 1991;88:5242–5246.
149. Trucksis M, Galen JE, Michalski J, et al: Accessory cholera enterotoxin (Ace), the third toxin of a *Vibrio cholerae* virulence cassette. Proc Natl Acad Sci U S A 1993;90:5267–5271.
150. Khan WA, Bennish ML, Seas C, et al: Randomized controlled comparison of single dose ciprofloxacin and doxycycline for cholera caused by *Vibrio cholerae* O1 or O139. Lancet 1996;348:296–300.
151. Levine MM: Development of bacterial vaccines. In Blaser MJ, Smith PD, Ravdin JI, et al (eds): Infections of the Gastrointestinal Tract. New York, Raven Press, 1995, pp 1441–1470.
152. Levine MM, Kaper JB: Live oral vaccines against cholera: an update. Vaccine 1993;11:207–212.
153. Trach DD, Clemens JD, Ke NT, et al: Field trial of a locally produced, killed, oral cholera vaccine in Vietnam. Lancet 1997;349:231–235.
154. Morris JG Jr: Noncholera vibrio species. In Blaser MJ, Smith PD, Ravdin JI, et al (eds): Infections of the Gastrointestinal Tract. New York, Raven Press, 1995, pp 671–685.
155. Honda T, Arita M, Takeda T, et al: Non-O1 *Vibrio cholerae* produces two newly identified toxins related to *Vibrio* parahaemolyticus hemolysin and *Escherichia coli* heat-stable enterotoxin. Lancet 1985;2:163–164.
156. Wilson R, Lieb S, Roberts A, et al: Non-O group 1 *Vibrio cholerae* gastroenteritis associated with eating raw oysters. Am J Epidemiol 1981;114:293–298.
157. Levine MM: *Escherichia coli* that cause diarrhea: enterotoxigenic, enteropathogenic, enteroinvasive, enterohemorrhagic and enteroadherent. J Infect Dis 1987;155:377–389.
158. Levine MM: *Escherichia coli* infections. N Engl J Med 1985;313:445–447.
159. Cravioto A, Reyes RE, Ortega R: Prospective study of diarrhoeal disease in a cohort of rural Mexican children: incidence and isolated pathogens during the first two years of life. Epidemiol Rev 1988;101:123.
160. Gomes TAT, Blake PA, Trabulsi LR: Prevalence of *Escherichia coli* strains with localized, diffuse and aggregative adherence to HeLa cells in infants with diarrhea and matched controls. J Clin Microbiol 1989;27:266–269.
161. Gomes TAT, Rassi V, MacDonald KL, et al: Enteropathogens associated with acute diarrheal disease in urban infants in Sao Paulo, Brazil. J Infect Dis 1991;164:331–337.
162. Robbins-Browne R, Still CS, Miliotis MD, et al: Summer diarrhea in African infants and children. Arch Dis Child 1980;55:923–928.
163. Sherman P, Drumm B, Karmali M, Cutz E: Adherence of bacteria to the intestine in sporadic cases of enteropathogenic *Escherichia coli*-associated diarrhea in infants and young children: a prospective study. Gastroenterology 1989;96:86–94.
164. Rothbaum R, McAdams AJ, Giannella R, et al: A clinicopathologic study of enterocyte-adherent *Escherichia coli*: a cause of protracted diarrhea in infants. Gastroenterology 1982;83:441–454.
165. Bokete TN, Whittam TS, Wilson RA, et al: Genetic and phenotypic analysis of *Escherichia coli* with enteropathogenic characteristics isolated from Seattle children. J Infect Dis 1997;175:1382–1389.
166. Moon HW, Whipp SC, Argenzio RA, et al: Attaching and effacing activities of rabbit and human enteropathogenic *Escherichia coli* in pig and rabbit intestines. Infect Immun 1983;41:1340–1351.
167. Donnenberg MS, Kaper JB: Enteropathogenic *Escherichia coli*. Infect Immun 1992;60:3953–3961.
168. McDaniel TK, Jarvis KG, Donnenberg MS, Kaper JB: A genetic locus of enterocyte effacement conserved among diverse enterobacterial pathogens. Proc Nat Acad Sci U S A 1995;92:1664–1668.
169. McDaniel TK, Kaper JB: A cloned pathogenicity island from enteropathogenic *Escherichia coli* confers the attaching and effacing phenotype on *E. coli* K-12. Mol Microbiol 1997;23:399–407.
170. Bhan MK, Raj P, Levine MM, et al: Enteroaggregative *Escherichia coli* associated with persistent diarrhea in a cohort of rural children in India. J Infect Dis 1989;159:1061–1064.
171. Gicquelais KG, Baldini MM, Martinez J, et al: Practical and economical method for using biotinylated DNA probes with bacterial colony blots to identify diarrhea-causing *Escherichia coli*. J Clin Microbiol 1990;28:2485–2490.
172. Knutton S, Baldwin T, Williams PH, McNeish AS: Actin accumulation at sites of bacterial adhesion to tissue culture cells: basis of a new diagnostic test for enteropathogenic and enterohemorrhagic *Escherichia coli*. Infect Immun 1989;57:1290–1298.
173. Black RE, Brown KH, Becker S, et al: Longitudinal studies of infectious diseases and physical growth of children in rural Bangladesh: II. Incidence of diarrhea and association with known pathogens. Am J Epidemiol 1982;115:315–324.
174. Gorbach SL, Kean BH, Evans DG, et al: Traveler's diarrhea and toxigenic *Escherichia coli*. N Engl J Med 1975;292:933–936.

175. Cohen MB, Guarino A, Shukla R, et al: Age-related differences in receptors for *Escherichia coli* heat-stable enterotoxin in the small and large intestine of children. Gastroenterology 1988;94:367–373.
176. Cohen MB, Giannella RA: Enterotoxigenic *E. coli.* In Blaser MJ, Smith PD, Ravdin JI, et al (eds): Infections of the Gastrointestinal Tract. New York, Raven Press, 1995, pp 691–708.
177. Sears CL, Kaper JB: Enteric bacterial toxins: mechanisms of action and linkage to intestinal secretion. Microbiol Rev 1996;60:167–215.
178. Currie MG, Gok KF, Kato J, et al: Guanylin: an endogenous activator of intestinal guanylate cyclase. Proc Natl Acad Sci U S A 1992;89:947–951.
179. Kita T, Smith CE, Fok KF, et al: Characterization of human uroguanylin: a member of the guanylin peptide family. Am J Physiol 1994;266:F342–F348.
180. Giannella RA: The suckling mouse model for the detection of heat-stable *Escherichia coli* enterotoxin: characteristics of the model. Infect Immun 1976;14:95–99.
181. Moseley SL, Hardy JW, Huq MI, et al: Isolation and nucleotide sequence determination of a gene encoding a heat-stable enterotoxin of *Escherichia coli*. Infect Immun 1983;39:1167–1174.
182. Moseley SL, Escheverria P, Seriwatana J, et al: Identification of enterotoxigenic *Escherichia coli* using three enterotoxin gene probes. J Infect Dis 1982;145:863–869.
183. Black RE, Levine MM, Clements ML, et al: Treatment of experimentally induced enterotoxigenic *Escherichia coli* diarrhea with trimethoprim, trimethoprim-sulfamethoxazole, or a placebo. Rev Infect Dis 1982;4:540–545.
184. Heck JE, Staneck JL, Cohen MB, et al: Prevention of traveler's diarrhea: ciprofloxacin vs. trimethoprim-sulfamethoxazole in adult volunteers working in Latin America and the Caribbean. J Travel Med 1992;1:136–142.
185. DuPont HL, Formal SB, Hornick RB, et al: Pathogenesis of *Escherichia coli* diarrhea. N Engl J Med 1971;285:1–9.
186. Riley LW, Remis RS, Helgerson SD et al. Hemorrhagic colitis associated with a rare *Escherichia coli* serotype. N Engl J Med 1983;308:681–685.
187. Karmali MA, Steele BT, Petric M, Lim C: Sporadic cases of hemolytic uremic syndrome associated with fecal cytotoxin and cytotoxin-producing *Escherichia coli* in stools. Lancet 1983;1:619–620.
188. Slutsker LA, Ries AA, Greene KD, et al: *Escherichia coli* O157:H7 diarrhea in the United States: clinical and epidemiologic features. Ann Intern Med 1997;126:505–513.
189. Cohen MB. *E. coli* O157:H7 infections: a frequent cause of bloody diarrhea and the hemolytic uremic syndrome. Adv Pediatr 1996;43:171–207.
190. Cohen MB, Giannella RA: Hemorrhagic colitis associated with *E. coli* O157:H7. Adv Intern Med 1991;37:173–195.
191. Griffin PM, Olmstead LC, Petras RE: *Escherichia coli* O157:H7-associated colitis. Gastroenterology 1990;99:142–149.
192. Tarr PI: *E. coli* O157:H7: clinical, diagnostic, and epidemiological aspects of human infection. Clin Infect Dis 1995;20:1–10.
193. Boyce TG, Swerdlow DL, Griffin PM: *E. coli* O157:H7 and the hemolytic uremic syndrome. N Engl J Med 1995;333:364–368.
194. Swerdlow DL, Woodruff BA, Brady RC, et al: A waterborne outbreak in Missouri of *E. coli* O157:H7 associated with bloody diarrhea and death. Ann Intern Med 1992;117:812–819.
195. Keene WF, McAnulty JM, Hoesly FC et al: A swimming-associated outbreak of hemorrhagic colitis caused by *E. coli* O157:H7 and *Shigella sonnei*. N Engl J Med 1994;331:579–584.
196. Whittam TS, Wachsmuth IK, Wilson RA: Genetic evidence of clonal descent of *Escherichia coli* O157:H7 associated with hemorrhagic colitis and hemolytic uremic syndrome. J Infect Dis 1988;157:1124–1133.
197. Whittam TS, Wolfe ML, Wachsmuth IK, et al: Clonal relationships among *E. coli* strains that cause hemorrhagic colitis and infantile diarrhea. Infect Immun 1993;61:1619–1629.
198. Milford DV, Taylor CM, Guttridge B, et al: Hemolytic uraemic syndromes in the British Isles 1985–1988: association with verocytotoxin producing *E. coli.* I: Clinical and epidemiological aspects. Arch Dis Child 1990:65:716–722.
199. Bitzan M, Ludwig K, Klemt M, et al: The role of *E. coli* O157 infections in the classical (enteropathic) haemolytic uraemic syndrome: results of a Central European, multicentre study. Epidemiol Infect 1993;110:183–196.
200. Belongia EA, Osterholm MT, Soler JT, et al: Transmission of *E. coli* O157:H7 infection in Minnesota child day-care facilities. JAMA 1993;269:883–888.
201. Karch H, Russmann H, Schmidt H, et al: Long-term shedding and clonal turnover of enterohemorrhagic *E. coli* O157 in diarrheal diseases. J Clin Microbiol 1995:33:1602–1605.
202. Walterspiel JN, Ashkenazi S, Morrow AL, et al: Effect of subinhibitory concentrations of antibiotics on extracellular Shiga-like toxin: I. Infection 1992;20:25–29.
203. Griffin PM: *E. coli* O157:H7 and other enterohemorrhagic *E. coli.* In Blaser MJ, Smith PD, Ravdin JI, et al (eds): Infections of the Gastrointestinal Tract. New York, Raven Press, 1995, pp 739–761.
204. Proulx F, Turgeio JP, Delage G, et al: Randomized, controlled trial of antibiotic therapy for *E. coli* O157:H7 enteritis. J Pediatr 1992;121:299–303.
205. Armstrong GD, Rowe PC, Goodyer P, et al: A phase I study of chemically synthesized verotoxin (Shiga-like toxin) Pk-trisaccharide receptors attached to chromosorb for preventing hemolytic uremic syndrome. J Infect Dis 1995;171:1042–1045.
206. Nataro JP, Kaper JB, Robins Browne R, et al: Patterns of adherence of diarrheagenic *Escherichia coli* to Hep-2 cells. Pediatr Infect Dis J 1987;6:829–831.
207. Tzipori S, Montanaro J, Robins Browne RM, et al: Enteropathogenic *Escherichia coli* enteritis: evaluation of the gnotobiotic piglet model of human infection. Gut 1985;26:570–578.
208. Savarino SJ, Fasano A, Robertson DC, Levine MM: Enteroaggregative *Escherichia coli* elaborate a heat-stable enterotoxin demonstrable in an in vitro rabbit intestinal model. J Clin Invest 1991;87:1450–1455.
209. Bhan MK, Raj P, Levine MM, et al: Enteroaggregative *Escherichia coli* associated with persistent diarrhea in a cohort of rural children in India. J Infect Dis 1989;1061–1064.
210. Paul M, Tsukamato T, Ghosh AR, et al: The significance of enteroaggregative *Escherichia coli* in the etiology of hospitalized diarrhoea in Calcutta, India and the demonstration of a new honey-combed pattern of aggregative adherence. FEMS Microbiol Lett 1994;117:319–326.
211. Smith HR, Scotland SM, Willshaw GA, et al: Isolates of *Escherichia coli* O44:H18 of diverse origin are enteroaggregative. J Infect Dis 1994;170:1610–1613.
212. Fang GD, Lima AAM, Martin CV, et al: Etiology and epidemiology of persistent diarrhea in Northeastern Brazil: a hospital based prospective, case-controlled study. J Pediatr Gastroenterol Nutr 1995;21:137–144.
213. Jallat C, Livrelli V, Darfeuille-Michaud A, et al: *Escherichia coli* strains involved in diarrhea in France: high prevalence and heterogeneity of diffusely adhering strains. J Clin Microbiol 31:2031–2037.
214. Donta ST, Myers MG: *Clostidium difficile* toxin in asymptomatic neonates. J Pediatr 1982;100:431–434.
215. Rolfe RD: Binding kinetics of *Clostridium difficile* toxins A and B to intestinal brush border membranes from infant and adult hamsters. Infect Immun 1991;59:1223–1230.
216. Eglow R, Pothoulakis C, Itzkowitz S, et al: Diminished *Clostridium difficile* toxin A (TxA) receptors in newborn rabbit ileum is associated with decreased toxin A receptor. J Clin Invest 1992;90:82–829.
217. Pothoulakis C, LaMont JT, Eglow R, et al: Characterization of rabbit ileal receptors for *Clostridium difficile* toxin A: evidence for a receptor coupled G protein. J Clin Invest 1991;88:119–125.
218. Hyams J, McLaughlin JC: Lack of relationship between *C. difficile* toxin and inflammatory bowel disease in children. J Clin Gastroenterol 1985;7:387–390.
219. Bates M, Bove K, Cohen MB: Pseudomembranous colitis caused by *C. difficile*. J Pediatr 1997;130:146.
220. Teasley DG, Gerding DN, Olson GM: Prospective randomized trial of metronidazole versus vancomycin for *Clostridium difficile*-associated diarrhoea and colitis. Lancet 1983;2:1043–1046.
221. Fekety R, Shah AB: Diagnosis and treatment of *Clostridium difficile* colitis. JAMA 1993;269:71–75.
222. Leung DYM, Kelly CP, Boguniewicz M, et al: Treatment with intravenously administered gamma globulin of chronic relapsing colitis induced by *Clostridium difficile* toxin. J Pediatr 1991;118:633–637.
223. Biller JA, Katz AJ, Flores AF, et al: Treatment of recurrent *Clostridium difficile* colitis with Lactobacillus GG. J Pediatr Gastroenterol Nutr 1995;21:224–226.
224. Holmberg SD, Farmer JJ III: *Aeromonas hydrophila* and *Plesiomonas shigelloides* as causes of intestinal infections. Rev Infect Dis 1984;6:663–669.
225. Challapalli M, Tess BR, Cunningham DG, et al: *Aeromonas*-associated diarrhea in children. Pediatr Infect Dis J 1988;7:693–698.

226. Gracey M, Burke V, Robinson J. *Aeromonas*-associated gastroenteritis. Lancet 1982;2:1304–1306.
227. Agger WA, McCormick JD, Gurwith MJ: Clinical and microbiological features of *Aeromonas hydrophila*-associated diarrhea. J Clin Microbiol 1985;21:909–913.
228. Namdari H, Bottone EJ: Microbiologic and clinical evidence supporting the role of *Aeromonas caviae* as a pediatric enteric pathogen. J Clin Microbiol 1990;28:837–840.
229. Olsvik O, Wachsmuth K, Kay B, et al: Laboratory observations on *Plesiomonas shigelloides* strains isolated from children with diarrhea in Peru. J Clin Microbiol 1990;28:886–889.
230. Centers for Disease Control and Prevention. Aquarium-associated *Plesiomonas shigelloides* infection—Missouri. MMWR Morb Mortal Wkly Rep 1989;38:617–619.
231. Kain KC, Kelly MT: Clinical features, epidemiology, and treatment of *Plesiomonas shigelloides* diarrhea. J Clin Microbiol 1989;27:998–1001.
232. Lincoln EM, Gilbert LA: Disease in children due to mycobacteria other than *Mycobacterium tuberculosis*. Am Rev Respir Dis 1972;105:683–714.
233. Young LS: *Mycobacterium avium* complex infections. J Infect Dis 1988;157:863–867.
234. Hawkins CC, Gold JWM, Whimbey EW, et al: *Mycobacterium avium* complex infections in patients with the acquired immunodeficiency syndrome. Ann Intern Med 1986;105:184–188.
235. Gillin JS, Urmacher C, West R, et al: Disseminated *Mycobacterium avium-intracellulare* infection in acquired immunodeficiency syndrome mimicking Whipple's disease. Gastroenterology 1983;85:1187–1191.
236. Ozkaynak MF, Lenarsky C, Kohn D, et al: *Mycobacterium avium-intracellulare* infections after allogeneic bone marrow transplantation in children. Am J Pediatr Hematol Oncol 1990;12:220–224.
237. Kinney JS, Little BJ, Yolken RH, et al: *Mycobacterium avium* complex in a patient with cystic fibrosis: disease vs. colonization. Pediatr Infect Dis J 1989;8:393–396.
238. Weikel CS, Grieco FD, Reuben J, et al: Human colonic epithelial cells, HT29/C1, treated with crude *Bacteroides fragilis* enterotoxin dramatically alter their morphology. Infect Immun 1992;60:321–327.
239. Myers LL, Shooop DS, Stackhouse LL, et al: Isolation of enterotoxigenic *Bacteroides fragilis* from humans with diarrhea. J Clin Microbiol 1987;25:2330–2333.
240. Sack RB, Myers LL, Almeido-Hill J, et al: Enterotoxigenic *Bacteroides fragilis*: epidemiologic studies of its role as a human diarrheal pathogen. J Diarrheoeal Dis Res 1992;10:4–9.
241. Sack RB, Albert MJ, Alam K, et al: Isolation of enterotoxigenic *Bacteroides fragilis* from Bangladeshi children with diarrhea: a controlled study. J Clin Microbiol 1994;32:960–963.
242. Sears CL, Myers LL, Lazemby A, Van Tassell RL: Enterotoxigenic *Bacteroides fragilis*. Clin Infect Dis 1995;20:S142–S148.
243. San Joaquin VH, Gaffis JC, Lee C, Sears CL: Association of *Bacteroides fragilis* with childhood diarrhea. Scand J Infect Dis 1995;61:3202–3207.
244. Pantosti A, Menozzi MG, Frate A, et al: Detection of enterotoxigenic *Bacteroides fragilis* and its toxin in stool samples from adults and children in Italy. Clin Infect Dis 1997;24:12–16.
245. Lee JI, Hampson DJ: Genetic characterization of intestinal spirochaetes and their association with disease. J Med Microbiol 1994;40:365–371.
246. daCunha Ferreira RM, Phillips AD, Stevens CR, et al: Intestinal spirochaetosis in children. J Pediatr Gastroenterol Nutr 1993:17:333–336.
247. Surawicz CM, Roberts PL, Rompalo A, et al: Intestinal spirochetosis in homosexual men. Am J Med 1987;82:587–592.
248. Ismaili A, Bourke B, DeAzavedo JCS, et al: Heterogeneity in phenotypic and genotypic characteristics among strains of *Hafnia alvei*. J Clin Microbiol 1996;34:2973–2979.
249. Balton CB, Austin CC, Sobel J, et al: An outbreak of gastroenteritis and fever due to *Listeria monocytogenes* in milk. N Engl J Med 1997;336:100–105.

# Chapter 29

# Enteric Parasites

Dorsey M. Bass

Enteric parasites are important agents of disease throughout the world. Although the frequency and severity of parasitic diseases are most extreme in the developing world, changes in worldwide travel, immigration, commerce, and daycare for young children and increasing numbers of patients with immune compromise have led to increased incidences of parasitic diseases in the developed world. Parasitic disease may mimic other gastrointestinal disorders, such as inflammatory bowel disease, hepatitis, sclerosing cholangitis, peptic ulcer disease, and celiac disease. Parasitic infection can also trigger overt manifestations of quiescent chronic intestinal disorders.

## EPIDEMIOLOGY

A variety of epidemiologic factors predispose patients to parasitic infestation worldwide, but the single most important factor is socioeconomic status. It has been shown repeatedly, in both the developed and developing world, that children of lower socioeconomic status have higher parasite loads and a greater prevalence of multiple infestations.[1, 2] Travel to developing countries can expose an individual to parasites that may not cause symptoms until weeks, months, or years later. Immigrants from developing countries often harbor pathogens that are unfamiliar to physicians in their new homelands and may pass them on to their new countrymen. Less obvious sources of parasites include foodstuffs increasingly imported from all areas of the world. The United States has experienced outbreaks of intestinal cyclosporiasis from imported raspberries.[3]

Protozoan infections endemic to the developed world, such as giardiasis, are transmitted with great efficiency in daycare centers, where fecal-oral contamination is quite common. Institutions for the mentally retarded are also common reservoirs for *Giardia, Entamoeba histolytica,* and other protozoans. Pets and livestock are potential sources of *Cryptosporidium, Giardia,* and *Toxocara* species, canine hookworm, *Balantidium coli,* and other organisms.

Dietary habits can also be risk factors. Consumption of raw or undercooked fish can lead to *Diphyllobothrium latum, Capillaria philippinensis,* or *Anisakis* infection. Inadequate cooking of pork predisposes to *Taenia solium* and *Trichenella* infections. Beefsteak tartare and other raw or rare bovine delicacies can harbor *Taenia saginata.* Furthermore a variety of protozoan organisms can be transmitted via produce that has been exposed to human or animal waste. Unpasteurized apple juice has been reported as a cause of *Cryptosporidium* outbreaks.[4]

## HOST FACTORS

Children, particularly toddlers, are more susceptible to these infestations, owing to their habits of "mouthing" all sorts of environmental objects, their propensity to go barefoot, and their immunologic "naiveté." Patients with compromised immune systems, whether due to congenital defects, infections such as human immunodeficiency virus (HIV), or medical ministrations (transplant and oncology patients) may have severe, protracted, or unusual manifestations of parasitic disease. Patients with hypogammaglobulinemia and immunoglobulin A (IgA) deficiency may suffer severe protozoan infections such as giardiasis. Patients with acquired immunodeficiency syndrome (AIDS) infected with *Cryptosporidium* organisms may have severe, prolonged diarrhea as well as unusual manifestations in the biliary tree and lungs, despite high levels of luminal IgA antibody directed against *Cryptosporidium.*[4a] Sexual practices, particularly those that involve anal penetration, are also associated with parasitic diseases.[5, 6]

## CLINICAL PRESENTATIONS

Enteric parasites most often produce gastrointestinal symptoms—abdominal pain, diarrhea, flatulence, and distention.[7] In a children's hospital laboratory survey of stool ova and parasite tests, it was found that stools sent from the gastroenterology clinic were most likely to be positive, as compared with stools submitted from other outpatient clinics, the emergency room, or inpatient settings.[7a] Heavy infestations of large worms such as *Ascaris* can lead to intestinal obstruction or, if they wander into the biliary system, biliary obstruction with cholangitis or pancreatitis. *Amoeba* and *Trichuris* organisms can cause enterocolitis with tenesmus and mucoid, bloody stool.

Liver disease from enteric parasites can be due to bile duct obstruction by organisms such as *Ascaris* worms or liver flukes or from portal hypertension due to inflammatory reactions to ova, as in schistosomiasis. Some protozoans such as *Cryptosporidium* can infect biliary epithelium and produce syndromes such as cholangitis and cholecystitis. Other protozoans such as *E. histolytica* can cause hepatic parenchymal necrosis resulting in liver abscesses.

Systemic manifestations of parasitic infestation are also common. Intestinal luminal blood and protein loss can lead to anemia and edema. Fever is often the most prominent feature of amebic liver abscess. Malabsorption is common in giardiasis and cryptosporidiosis and can lead to wasting, fat soluble–vitamin deficiency, and failure to thrive.

## DIAGNOSIS

**STOOL EXAMINATION.** The mainstay of diagnosing enteric parasites is a skilled microscopist in the parasitology laboratory. At least 35 species of enteric parasites may be identified by stool examination.[8] Furthermore, the observation of fecal leukocytes, eosinophils, and macrophages in preserved specimens may provide clues to nonparasitic gastrointestinal diseases. Because microscopists' skills vary, clinicians are advised to select reference laboratories with care. Careful attention to the appropriate collection, preservation, and examination of samples is critical to successful diagnosis of enteric parasites.

Appropriate sample collection begins with ascertaining that no interfering substances are present in the stool that will invalidate the results. Common interfering substances include barium (from contrast radiography), bismuth preparations, antacids, and mineral oil. Antibiotics can also make detection of protozoans difficult. It is preferable to wait 2 weeks after the ingestion of any of these substances before obtaining a specimen. Clinicians evaluating gastrointestinal symptoms should obtain stool specimens before initiating gastrointestinal radiology studies and certain forms of empiric therapy. Water and urine contamination of stool lead to rapid lysis of trophozoites and should be avoided.

Although examination of a fresh stool specimen is useful for identification of motile trophozoites, it is rarely performed in laboratories in the United States. Most stools are collected in preservatives, which allows for convenience in both collection and examination. The commonly used preservatives, such as formalin and polyvinyl alcohol, are quite toxic if ingested.

The appropriate number and frequency of stool examinations are matters of some controversy. It is clear that repeated samples obtained on separate days enhance sensitivity at least 20%, owing to variable shedding of eggs, cysts, and trophozoites.[8a] For patients with very low clinical-epidemiologic risk factors, one sample may be adequate, but for those with a high index of suspicion, more than three samples may be needed, particularly for *E. histolytica* and *Dientamoeba fragilis.*

Some enteric parasites, most notably *Cryptosporidium* and *Cyclospora* species, are not detected on routine ova and parasite examinations. These organisms require either acid-fast staining or special immunofluorescence techniques.

**IMMUNOASSAY.** Enzyme-linked immunoassay (ELISA) tests for antigen in stool samples are widely available for *Giardia* and *Cryptosporidium* species. These sensitive and specific assays can be useful adjuncts to standard stool examinations. Because several common organisms can cause the clinical picture of giardiasis, ELISA is not recommended as the sole means of evaluating patients, except in the context of a known outbreak.

**MACROSCOPIC EXAMINATION.** *Ascaris lumbricoides* worms can be passed intact in the stool or vomited, particularly during febrile illness. They are easily recognized because of their size (15 to 40 cm) and resemblance to earthworms. Cestodes, or more commonly, segments of cestodes, can also be passed per rectum. Species identification is possible by microscopic examination. *Enterobius* organisms venture nocturnally onto the perianal area to lay eggs. The small threadlike worms may be visualized or the "Scotch tape" test may be employed to identify the eggs of this common parasite.

**SEROLOGY.** Serologic detection of antibodies to *E. histolytica* is possible in 85% of dysentery and 95% of liver abscess patients. Specific IgM serology for *Giardia* may be useful in obscure cases.

**INTESTINAL FLUID AND BIOPSY.** Duodenal fluid may be useful in diagnosis of giardiasis or strongyloidiasis when stool specimens are negative. Fluid may be obtained by duodenal intubation or during endoscopy. It should be examined immediately. The Entero-Test is a gelatin capsule that contains a string that adsorbs duodenal fluid. It is swallowed and then retrieved by a string taped to the patient's cheek. The author has found this technique difficult to perform in young children, and not particularly sensitive.

In selected patients, duodenal biopsy may reveal *Giardia, Cryptosporidium,* Microsporidia, or *Strongyloides* organisms. Biopsy of the edges of colon ulcers may reveal trophozoites of *E. histolytica.* The sensitivity of intestinal biopsy for diagnosis of parasitic disease depends to a large degree on the interest and experience of the pathologist.

## PATHOGENIC ORGANISMS

### Protozoa

#### *Giardia lamblia*

Giardiasis is the most common pathogenic intestinal protozoan infection in the world. It has been estimated that some 2% to 5% of the population of the industrialized world and 20% of those in the developing world are infected at any time.[9–12] The majority of these infections are asymptomatic. *Giardia* were also the first described human protozoan agents of intestinal disease. Von Leeuwenhoek observed them in 1681 in his own diarrheal stool and described them as "animalcules." *Giardia* are also of interest because of their relationship to archeobacteria by comparison of ribosomal RNA sequence.[13] This relationship suggests that organisms such as *Giardia* may have been among the first eukaryotic life forms.

*G. lamblia* exists in two forms, the encysted, environmentally stable form that is responsible for transmission, and the small intestine–dwelling trophozoite, which is the motile form observed by von Leeuwenhoek. In the small intestine the trophozoites adhere to enterocytes by a ventral disc, causing local effacement of the microvilli. A variety of mammals, including dogs, cats, gerbils, beaver, raccoons, and sheep, can harbor the organism and participate in disease transmission.[14–16]

The pathophysiology of giardiasis is unclear. Pathologic changes in the small intestine are quite variable. Although most symptomatic patients have normal or nearly normal villi,[17] 5% to 10% or more have subtotal villus atrophy. Patients with immunoglobulin deficiency are particularly prone to histologic abnormality.[18] Most symptomatic patients have lactose intolerance, both clinically and as measured by the hydrogen breath test.

Symptoms of giardiasis can include diarrhea, flatulence, malabsorption with weight loss, constipation, and abdominal pain. Symptoms can be intermittent or continuous. Stools may be watery, malabsorptive, or formed, but are not bloody and do not contain leukocytes.

Laboratory findings are generally nonspecific. Fat may be found in the stool. Rarely, serum albumin is decreased and fecal $\alpha_1$-antitrypsin is increased. Eosinophilia does not occur. Radiologic findings are generally nonspecific. Giardiasis localized to the terminal ileum may radiologically mimic Crohn's disease.[19]

Diagnosis is based on demonstration of *Giardia* trophozoites, cysts, or antigen in stool, duodenal fluid, or intestinal biopsy specimens. Microscopic examination of a single stool specimen is approximately 70% sensitive for detection. Sensitivity increases to approximately 85% with three samples. Examination of duodenal fluid has been reported to be 40% to 90% sensitive. Antigen detection assays offer 85% to 95% sensitivity on a single specimen but do not identify other protozoans that can cause similar symptoms.

Treatment options for giardiasis include metronidazole (and its derivatives), quinacrine, and furazolidone (Table 29–1). Immunocompromised patients may require prolonged therapy to clear the organism. Some apparent clinical treatment failures are due to lactose intolerance, which can persist for weeks after successful treatment.

## *Entamoeba histolytica*

Although a variety of species of amebae inhabit the human intestine, only *E. histolytica* is clearly pathogenic. In addition, only certain strains of *E. histolytica* are capable of invading the mucosa and causing disease. Biochemical, immunologic, and more recently DNA analyses have shown that markers exist that distinguish between pathogenic and nonpathogenic strains.[20–22] It has been proposed that nonpathogenic strains be designated *Entamoeba dispar.* Clinical assays distinguishing between virulent and nonvirulent strains or species of *Entamoeba* are not yet routinely available.

The life cycle of these protozoans is quite similar to that of *Giardia.* Ingested cysts are stimulated by gastric acid to excystate in the small intestine. The resulting trophozoites colonize the large intestine, where they multiply, invade the mucosa, or encystate, depending on local conditions and the nature of the particular strain. Invading trophozoites destroy epithelial target cells by releasing substances such as hemolysins, which disrupt cell membranes, as well as a variety of proteases that disrupt the extracellular matrix. Injury to epithelial cells triggers release of cytokines leading to chemotaxis of leukocytes, which also contribute to the local inflammatory response. Eventually, ulceration of the mucosa occurs and invading amebae may enter the portal circulation, and eventually the liver. Unlike intestinal lesions, hepatic abscesses contain almost no inflammatory cells, consisting almost entirely of necrotic liver cells. In patients treated with large doses of steroids, amebae may spread to a variety of organs, including lungs, brain, and eyes. For reasons unknown, such systemic dissemination is not common in AIDS patients, who are often infected with *Entamoeba* species.[23]

Risk factors for amebiasis include poverty, crowding, poor hygiene, travel in endemic areas, and male homosexual promiscuity. Risk factors for severe disease include age (particularly infants), malnutrition, and corticosteroid use. Although physicians in the United States think of amebic disease as exotic, prevalence of infection here has been estimated as high as 5% among the general population and 30% among homosexual men.[6] Most of these infections are clinically silent and are due to noninvasive strains (*E. dispar*).[23]

Symptoms of intestinal amebiasis vary with the location and extent of the infection. *E. histolytica* may invade any portion of the colon but prefer the cecum and ascending colon. Patients often complain of abdominal pain, anorexia, malaise, and intermittent diarrhea. Patients with rectosigmoid involvement suffer from tenesmus and more frequent diarrhea. Patients with extensive involvement have symptoms similar to those of ulcerative colitis, with frequent mucous, bloody stools. In nonfulminant cases, fever is uncommon, but with fulminant colitis or hepatic abscess, fever can be prominent. Toxic megacolon or perforation can occur, and they are leading causes of mortality in untreated patients. In some cases a localized granulomatous reaction to *E. histolytica* known as *ameboma* occurs. Amebomas are difficult to distinguish from colon carcinoma. Amebic dysentery may mimic inflammatory bowel disease leading to institution of high-dose steroid therapy, which can be lethal in persons with amebiasis.

Amebic liver abscess is manifested by right upper quadrant pain, leukocytosis, fever, and hepatomegaly. *Liver abscess usually occurs in the absence of current or recent overt intestinal disease.* Liver function tests, including bilirubin and transaminases, are often normal. Ultrasonography shows one or more cystic masses in the hepatic parenchyma. Complications of abscesses include rupture, with possible pericardial or pleural spread.

Diagnosis of colonic amebiasis is best made by microscopic examination of fresh stool. Three to six samples should be adequate to identify 90% of cases. Biopsies taken from the edge of colon ulcers may also be useful in identifying trophozoites, particularly with periodic acid–Schiff (PAS) stain. ELISA and polymerase chain reaction (PCR) assays may soon offer increased sensitivity as well as the potential to discriminate between *E. histolytica* and *E. dispar.*

Serologic testing is particularly useful for suspected amebic liver abscess. Most patients have neither overt intestinal symptoms nor detectable cysts or trophozoites in their stool. Approximately 90% of patients with amebic liver abscess have high titers on a variety of assays and after 2 weeks are universally positive. In nonendemic areas, suspected liver abscesses may require aspiration to exclude bacterial causes.

Treatment of amebiasis is highly effective. The drug of choice for invasive colon or liver disease is metronidazole (or the related drugs, tinidazole and ornidazole). The recommended dosage (10 to 15 mg/kg tid to a maximum of 750

**TABLE 29–1. Treatment of Enteric Parasites**

| DISEASE | DRUG | DOSAGE | COMMENTS |
|---|---|---|---|
| Amebiasis (*E. histolytica*) | | | |
| Asymptomatic | Iodoquinol or | 30–40 mg/kg/day in 3 doses × 20 days (max. 2 g/day) | Currently suggested that asymptomatic cyst passers in nonedemic areas be treated |
| | Paromomycin | 25–35 mg/kg/day in 3 doses × 7 days | |
| Colitis, liver abscess | Metronidazole or | 35–50 mg/kg/day in 3 doses (max. 2.25 g/day) × 10 days | Metronidazole absorbed very well orally |
| | Tinidazole | 50 mg/kg/day in 3 doses (max. 2 g/day) × 3 days | |
| *Ancylostoma caninum* (dog hookworm, eosinophilic enterocolitis) | Mebendazole or | 100 mg bid × 3 days | Serologic/clinical diagnosis; no ova or parasites are found in stool |
| | Pyrantel pamoate or | 11 mg/kg (max. 1 g)/day × 3 days | |
| | Albendazole | 400 mg once | |
| Anisakiasis (fish worm) | Surgical or endoscopic removal | | |
| Ascariasis | Mebendazole or | 100 mg bid × 3 days | For symptoms of obstruction, pyrantel pamoate is drug of choice |
| | Pyrantel pamoate or | 11 mg/kg (max. 1 g)/day × 3 days | |
| | Albendazole | 400 mg once | |
| *Balantidium coli* | Tetracycline or | 40 mg/kg/day in 4 doses × 10 days (max. 2 g/day) | |
| | Iodoquinol or | 40 mg/kg/day in 3 doses × 20 days (max. 2 g/day) | |
| | Metronidazole | 35–50 mg/kg/day in 3 doses × 5 days (max. 2.25 g/day) | |
| *Blastocystis hominis* | Metronidazole or | 35–50 mg/kg/day in 3 doses × 5 days (max. 2.25 g/day) | Clinical importance of infection is debatable |
| | Iodoquinol | 40 mg/kg/day in 3 doses × 20 days (max. 2 g/day) | |
| *Capillaria philippinensis* | Mebendazole or | 200 mg bid × 20 days | Noncompliance with prolonged course leads to frequent relapse |
| | Albendazole or | 200 mg bid × 10 days | |
| | Thiabendazole | 25 mg/kg/day in 2 doses × 30 days | |
| Cryptosporidiosis | Azithromycin (?) or | 25 mg/kg/day bid × 14 days | Partial clinical response has been reported. Improved immune function is best prognosis. |
| | Paromomycin | 40–50 mg/kg/day in 4 doses | |
| *Cyclospora* | Trimethoprim-sulfamethoxazole (TMP-SMZ) | TMP 5 mg/kg/day, SMZ 25 mg/kg/day bid × 7 days | |
| *Dientamoeba fragilis* | Tetracycline or | 40 mg/kg/day in 4 doses × 10 days (max. 2 g/day) | |
| | Iodoquinol or | 40 mg/kg/day in 3 doses × 20 days (max. 2g/day) | |
| | Metronidazole or | 35–50 mg/kg/day in 3 doses × 10 days (max. 2.25 g/day) | |
| | Paromomycin | 25–30 mg/kg/day in 3 doses × 7 days | |
| *Enterobius vermicularis* (pinworm) | Mebendazole or | 100 mg once; repeat in 2 wk | Treatment of household contacts is often advised |
| | Pyrantel pamoate or | 11 mg/kg (max. 1 g) once; repeat in 2 weeks | |
| | Albendazole | 400 mg × once; repeat in 2 weeks | |
| Giardiasis | Metronidazole or | 15 mg/kg/day in 3 doses × 5 days (max. 750 mg/day) | |
| | Tinidazole or | 50 mg/kg once (max. 2 g) | |
| | Furazolidone or | 6 mg/kg/day in 4 doses × 10 days (max. 400 mg/day) | |
| | Paromomycin | 25–35 mg/kg/day in 3 doses × 7 days | |
| Hookworm | Mebendazole or | 100 mg bid × 3 days | |
| | Pyrantel pamoate or | 11 mg/kg (max. 1 g)/day × 3 days | |
| | Albendazole | 400 mg once | |
| *Isospora belli* | TMP-SMZ | TMP 5 mg/kg/day, SMZ 25 mg/kg/day tid × 10 days, then bid × 3 wk | |
| Microsporidiosis *Enterocytozoon bieneusi* *Septata intestinalis* | Albendazole | 400 mg bid | *S. intestinalis* responds much better to treatment. |
| Schistosomiasis | Praziquantel | | Treatment does not reverse established portal hypertension. |
| *S. japonicum* | | 60 mg/kg in 3 doses once | |
| *S. mansoni* | | 40 mg/kg in 2 doses once | |
| *S. haematobium* | | 40 mg/kg in 2 doses once | |
| *S. mekongi* | | 40 mg/kg in 2 doses once | |
| Strongyloidiasis | Thiabendazole or | 25–50 mg/kg/day in 2 doses × 2 days (max. 3 g/day) | Discontinuing large doses of steroids is important in fulminant, disseminated disease. |
| | Ivernectin | 200 μg/kg/day × 1–2 days | |
| Tapeworm (adult worm) *D. latum, T. solium, T. saginata* | Praziquantel | 5–10 mg/kg once | |
| Tapeworm *Hymenolepis nana* | Praziquantel | 25 mg/kg once | |
| *Trichuris trichiura* | Mebendazole or | 100 mg bid × 3 days | |
| | Albendazole | 400 mg × 1–3 days | |

Data from Drugs for parasitic infections. Med Lett 1995;37:99–108; and Morrow JD, Neuzil KM: Pharmacology of antimicrobial agents in the therapy of gastrointestinal infections. In Blaser MJ, et al (eds): Infections of the Gastrointestinal Tract. New York, Raven Press, 1995, pp 967–983.

mg per day) is three times that employed for giardiasis. The drug is absorbed extremely well from the gut, and oral therapy is usually quite effective. Drainage of liver abscesses is indicated for diagnosis, imminent rupture (cavity greater than 10 cm in adults), or failure to respond to 72 hours of metronidazole. All symptomatic patients as well as asymptomatic cyst passers require a luminal agent to prevent disease spread. Iodoquinol or paromomycin is administered for this purpose (see Table 29–1).

## *Dientamoeba fragilis*

*D. fragilis* is a binucleate flagellate, 5 to 12 μm in diameter, that inhabits the large intestine. It has worldwide distribution, and infection is found most often in children, daycare center attendees, and persons with poor hygiene.[24] Seroprevalence studies suggest that 90% of children have experienced infection by age 5 years.[25] The vast majority of infections are asymptomatic. There is an association with pinworm infestation: patients with *D. fragilis* are eight to 20 times more likely than uninfected persons to have pinworms.[26] Experimental ingestion of pinworm ova has led to *D. fragilis* infection. *D. fragilis* alone has not been shown to infect volunteers, and the organism is unstable in water and gastric juice.

Symptoms of *D. fragilis* infestation include diarrhea (predominantly during the first week or two), abdominal pain, flatulence, and weight loss.[27] Occasionally mild colitis has been described. Unlike most protozoan infections, eosinophilia is reported to be associated with *D. fragilis,* although this may be due to associated pinworm infestation. Diagnosis is made by stool examination. Invasive organisms have not been reported in biopsy specimens. A Scotch tape test for pinworm should be performed to look for concurrent *Enterobius* infestation. Treatment is usually metronidazole, although iodoquinol, tetracycline, and paromomycin have also been effective.

## *Blastocystis hominis*

*B. hominis* is a strict anaerobic protozoan that is a common inhabitant of the human cecum and colon. Its pathogenic role is controversial, as some studies have failed to note different prevalences of infection in symptomatic and asymptomatic persons.[28, 29] At least one study has shown such a difference in children in Malaysia.[30] Some studies suggest that the number of organisms observed in fecal smears correlates with symptoms. Symptoms are similar to those with *D. fragilis* and may be chronic.[31] Diagnosis is by stool examination. Treatment is usually metronidazole; furazolidine, emetine, cotrimazole, and iodoquinol are alternatives.

## *Balantidium coli*

*B. coli* is a very large (50 to 200 μm) ciliate protozoan that may invade the colonic mucosa to induce abdominal pain, diarrhea, and frank dysentery. Distribution is worldwide, although most infections occur in the tropics, in association with poor hygiene and intimate contact with livestock. Swine are a major reservoir of *B. coli,* and farmers and abattoir workers are at increased risk. Diagnosis is made by finding the characteristic large trophozoites in fresh stool. Tetracycline, metronidazole, paromomycin, and iodoquinol are used to treat this infection.

## *Cryptosporidium*

*Cryptosporidium* organisms were described early in this century as a veterinary pathogen, but it was not until 1976 that human disease began to be recognized.[32] These small protozoans are classified in the order Eucoccidiida, along with *Plasmodium* (malaria), *Isospora,* and *Toxoplasma gondii.* Cryptosporidia infect a wide variety of mammals and may complete their complex life cycle, which involves both asexual and sexual multipication, in the intestinal epithelia of one host. They are intracellular but do not enter the cytoplasm of host cells. The final product of the life cycle is the oocyst, which measures 4 to 6 μm in diameter and contains four infectious sporozoites.

With the advent of improved diagnostic testing and increased physician awareness, a great deal has been learned about the epidemiology of *Cryptosporidium* infection. *Cryptosporidium parvum* is quite prevalent among livestock such as cattle and sheep and domestic pets such as kittens and puppies. *Cryptosporidium* is a relatively common cause of human diarrhea, accounting for as many as 6% of cases in the developing world and 1.5% in the developed world. Furthermore, because the oocyts are chlorine resistant and small enough to pass through conventional water purification filtration devices, huge waterborne outbreaks affecting hundreds of thousands of people are possible.[33] Aside from contact with animals, other known risk factors include daycare center attendance, employment in hospitals, travel, and immunosuppression.

Parasite replication occurs mainly in the apical border of jejunal, ileal, and colonic enterocytes. Pathologic examination shows variable villus atrophy with crypt hyperplasia, usually with a mild mixed inflammatory infiltrate.

The associated clinical illness begins after approximately a week's incubation and consists of voluminous watery stools, flatulence, malaise, and abdominal pain lasting from 3 to 30 days in a normal host. Fever is not a major feature. Considerable weight loss can occur, and the disease can be devastating to previously malnourished hosts. In immunocompromised hosts such as patients with AIDS the diarrhea can be severe and "cholera-like." Immunocompromised patients may develop symptomatic *Cryptosporidium* infection of pancreatic ducts, the biliary tree and gallbladder, lungs, and sinuses.[34]

Diagnosis usually requires using special stains of stool samples. Acid-fast and immunofluorescence techniques can reliably identify infection. In many laboratories these special stains must be specifically requested. Commercial ELISA kits with good sensitivity and specificity are also available. Cryptosporidia can also be found in bronchial wash material and in biopsies of affected organs.

Treatment remains problematic. Normal hosts recover spontaneously in 1 to 3 weeks, but the immunocompromised host may suffer unremitting severe disease. Such patients may require meticulous supportive care, including intravenous fluids and nutritional support. A variety of drugs have been used with limited efficacy for *Cryptosporidium* infections in patients with AIDS, including metronidazole, sulfonamides, and spiromycin. The luminal amebicide paromomycin has been helpful in reducing oocyst shedding and improving symptoms in some patients, but it does not clear the organism from extraluminal sites such as the biliary system. Azithromycin has shown promise in recent studies but has not yet been formally evaluated with placebo controls.[35] Enteric immunoglobulins from either human serum or bovine colostrum have also been administered, with varying results.[36, 37] Reversal of immunosuppression by effective antiretroviral therapy usually leads to improvement in diarrhea.

## Other Coccidia

*Sarcocystis, Cyclospora,* and *Isospora belli* are obligate intracellular protozoans that less often produce intestinal coccidian infestations. *Sarcocystis* organisms produce a zoonosis in carnivores and can also cause human disease after consumption of undercooked beef or pork.[38] It seems to be most prevalent in Southeast Asia. Infection of intestine and skeletal muscle can occur in humans. Intestinal symptoms range from mild abdominal pain to acute obstruction requiring resection of heavily infested small bowel. Other than surgical resection, optimal therapy is not known.

*Cyclospora species* are Coccidia that produce a spectrum of infection quite similar to that of *Cryptosporidium.*[39] Oocysts of *Cyclospora* are larger than those of *Cryptosporidium,* measuring 8 to 10 μm in diameter, and are best seen with acid-fast stains. Prolonged illness has been reported in patients with AIDS. Most reported cases to date have originated in developing countries. Recently in the United States a multistate outbreak was traced to raspberries imported from Guatemala.[3] Treatment is trimethoprim-sulfamethoxazole.

*I. belli* is a cause of traveler's diarrhea in normal hosts and of protracted diarrhea in immunocompromised hosts.[40] Although infection is much more common in the tropics, daycare outbreaks have been reported in the United States. Unlike *cryptosporidia,* scant numbers of the large 30-μm oocysts are excreted in the stool, making diagnosis difficult. Small intestine biopsy may be helpful in establishing the diagnosis. Accurate diagnosis is important because the organism is sensitive to trimethoprim-sulfamethoxazole. Maintenance therapy may be necessary for immunocompromised patients, to prevent relapses.

*Microsporidia. Enterocytozoon bieneusi* and *Septata intestinalis* are intracellular parasites that have been reported principally in patients with AIDS.[41–43] The illness is similar to that found with *Cryptosporidium* infection: prolonged watery diarrhea with weight loss. Microsporidia can also cause cholangiopathy, keratoconjunctivitis, and sinusitis in patients with AIDS.[34, 44–46] Although special techniques for visualizing spores are reported, diagnosis often requires intestinal biopsy, preferably jejunal. The more common *E. bieneusi* is difficult to recognize in standard paraffin hematoxylin and eosin sections and may require embedding in plastic resin, special stains, or electron microscopy. *S. intestinalis* is larger and more easily seen on routine sections. Albendazole has been reported helpful for these infections, particularly for *S. intestinalis.*

## Nematodes (Roundworms)

### *Ascaris lumbricoides*

*A. lumbricoides* is the largest and most common helminthic infection worldwide.[47] Adult worms live in the jejunum, where the 20- to 49-cm long females may produce 200,000 eggs per day. The fertilized eggs are excreted in the feces and must mature in the soil for 10 to 14 days before the first-stage larvae, which are infectious, develop. When such embryonated eggs are ingested and reach the intestine, second-stage larvae develop that penetrate the intestinal mucosa to migrate via the liver to the lungs. The tiny larvae then pass through the alveolar wall, to the respiratory tract, and back to the gut after being swallowed. Then mature worms develop that may live 12 to 18 months. The respiratory phase may induce an eosinophilic pneumonitis, Loeffler's syndrome, which may clinically resemble seasonal asthma.

Under normal circumstances the intestinal phase of infection is asymptomatic. Serious complications arise either during heavy infestations, which may produce intestinal obstruction, or during migration of worms, which is frequently precipitated by an unrelated febrile illness. Infected patients may vomit or cough up the large earthwormlike ascarids during such illnesses (Fig. 29–1). Alternatively, the worms can obstruct the biliary or pancreatic ducts, producing cholangitis or pancreatitis.[48–50] *Ascaris* obstruction of the bowel lumen may lead to volvulus or perforation.[51]

The role of *Ascaris* worms in chronic malnutrition of children in the tropics is unclear. Heavy infestation is probably one of many factors affecting such children. Some studies have shown improvement in nutritional status after ascaris eradication.[52]

Diagnosis of ascariasis can be made by finding the eggs in stools. Adult worms may be expelled from the mouth or anus, observed during endoscopy, or outlined by barium during radiologic studies. Eosinophilia is prominent only during larval migrations through tissues.

Treatments include pyrantel pamoate, which paralyzes *Ascaris worms* and can be given by nasogastric tube for cases of intestinal obstruction. Mebendazole and albendazole are also effective in uncomplicated cases. Endoscopic or surgical therapy is necessary for some complications. Mass treatment

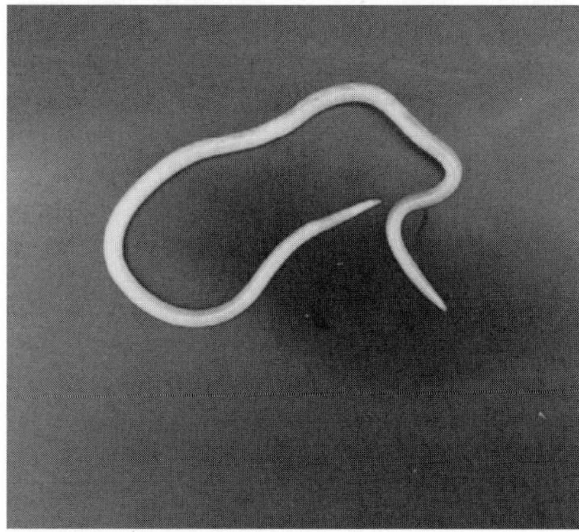

**FIGURE 29–1.** *Ascaris* worm vomited by a Cambodian child with cerebral malaria.

programs are useful in communities with high prevalences of infection.

### *Trichuris trichiura*

*T. trichiura* (whipworm) is named for the morphology of adult worms. *Trichuris* worms differ from other human nematodes in two ways. First, there is no tissue migration during its life cycle. Second, adult *Trichuris* worms reside in the colon rather than the small intestine. Like *Ascaris* eggs, those of *Trichuris* must mature in the soil before being ingested, making direct person-to-person transmission impossible. The larvae hatch and mature in the distal small bowel before migrating to the cecum, where they attach to the bowel wall via their narrow anterior ("whip") end. They may reside in the colon for as long as 8 years.

*Trichuris* has a worldwide distribution similar to that of *Ascaris.* The infection is most common in the tropics, especially Asia, but an estimated 2 million people are infected in the United States. Toddlers and young children tend to have the heaviest worm burdens.

Most light infections are asymptomatic. Moderate infections produce a picture of chronic colitis with diarrhea, abdominal pain, and weight loss. Heavy infections can produce a dysentery-like picture that may feature rectal prolapse.[53] Chronic infections in children are associated with stunted growth, anemia, and delayed cognitive development.

### *Necator americanus* and *Ancylostoma duodenale* (Hookworms)

Hookworm infestation affects approximately 1 billion people.[53, 54] There are two species of human hookworms, *N. americanus* and *A. duodenale.* Transmission of hookworm requires contamination of soil with human fecal material and an unshod population (usually young children). Filiform infective larvae in the contaminated soil invade the host via the skin (usually the bare foot) and are carried by the circulation to the lungs, where they penetrate the alveoli. They then proceed up the airway until they are swallowed into the gut. Hookworms reside in the small intestine, where they attach to the mucosa with their specialized mouth parts. Each worm is capable of ingesting up to 250 μL of blood per day. Symptoms of hookworm are the sequelae of this blood loss—mainly anemia and hypoproteinemia.[55] Patients may also report intense pruritic rashes on the feet during the initial larval penetration. Some patients with heavy worm burdens also report epigastric distress. Diagnosis of significant hookworm infection is made by finding the characteristic ova in fresh or preserved stool specimens. Treatment of choice is mebendazole or albendazole (see Table 29–1).

### *Strongyloides stercoralis*

*Strongyloides* is a small (1- to 10-mm long) nematode that is capable of replicating completely within the host.[56] Because of this capability, patients with suppressed immune systems can acquire an enormous worm burden, with potentially fatal dissemination. Infection begins when filiform larvae in contaminated soil penetrate the skin. The larvae then migrate via blood or lymph to the lungs, where they penetrate the alveoli and proceed up the airway to the pharynx and are swallowed. The larvae mature in the proximal small intestine, and females burrow into the lamina propria to lay eggs. The eggs hatch locally and the resulting rhabditiform larvae migrate into the intestinal lumen. Most of the rhabditiform larvae are passed with stool into the environment, where they mature into infectious filiform larvae. A variable number are able to differentiate into filiform larvae in the host colon. These infectious progeny are capable of reinfecting the host and maintaining a state of chronic infection.

In most hosts an equilibrium state seems to be reached in which a small number of adult worms are maintained. In severely malnourished or steroid-treated hosts the equilibrium becomes impaired and huge worm burdens can develop. In such circumstances larvae may disseminate to all organs, carrying with them associated enteric bacteria. This syndrome, known as *disseminated strongyloidiasis,* is usually fatal.[57] *Strongyloides* organisms are present in virtually all tropical and subtropical regions. They are also found in the southern United States and in small pockets of industrialized nations. Institutionalized patients are often infected.

Whereas most normal patients with chronic low-grade infections are asymptomatic, *Strongyloides* can cause significant gastrointestinal illness. Most common is a syndrome similar to giardiasis, with bloating, heartburn, and malabsorptive stools. Intractable diarrhea has been described in infants. Rarely, an ulcerative colitis–like picture may be seen with prominent pseudopolyp formation.[58]

The disseminated strongyloidiasis syndrome most often follows high-dose corticosteroid therapy.[59] Interestingly, the hyperinfection syndrome does not appear to be very common in patients with AIDS, even in tropical areas.[60] The hyperinfection syndrome usually results in a severe mucoid, bloody diarrhea, as a result of millions of adult worms and larvae migrating through the mucosa of the intestine. Prostration, shock, perforation, and associated gram-negative sepsis are common. Larvae can carry gram-negative organisms to every organ including those of the central nervous system.

Diagnosis of *S. stercoralis* infection is principally by identification of larvae in the stool. Eggs and adult worms are seldom identified. Duodenal fluid or biopsy may also be helpful in the diagnosis. Eosinophilia is common but often not impressive and is not a feature of the disseminated disease. Serologic assays are becoming available that will be helpful in selected cases.[61]

Treatment of choice is thiabendazole 25 mg/kg per day, which may require multiple courses for complete eradication. Larger doses, up to 50 mg/kg per day, are suggested for disseminated disease. Albendazole and mebendazole have some efficacy as well. Ivermectin, which is used for onchocerciasis, has shown promise in treatment of strongyloidiasis.[62]

### *Capillaria philippinensis*

*C. philippinensis* normally parasitizes fresh-water fish and birds, but it can be acquired by humans who consume raw or undercooked fish. Like *S. stercoralis,* a complete cycle of reproduction can occur within the human host, allowing for great amplification of the worm burden. The worms primarily colonize the upper small intestine. The human disease has been mainly reported in Southeast Asia, Thailand, and the Philippines. Symptoms are chronic abdominal pain, diarrhea, severe wasting, and edema.[63] The disease is often fatal when untreated. Eggs, larvae, and adult worms may be found in the stool or in duodenal aspirates. Treatment is a prolonged (30-day) course of mebendazole or albendazole.

### *Enterobius vermicularis* (Pinworm)

These small nematodes, a common infection of children throughout the world, cause anal pruritus when the females emerge from the rectum to lay eggs in the perianal skin. The migrating females can also cause urinary tract infections, vaginitis, and salpingitis in girls. The eggs are best found by placing a piece of clear adhesive tape sticky side down over the perianal area and then examining it under the microscope. Treatment is with mebendazole. Because of frequent environmental contamination, most clinicians treat the household.

## Cestodes (Tapeworms)

The most important tapeworms of humans are *D. latum, T. saginata, T. solium,* and *Hymenolepis nana.* The first three are spread by the ingestion of undercooked fish or meat, whereas *H. nana* has a classic fecal-oral route of contagion. All of the adult worms consist of a scolex, or head, which attaches to the host intestine, and numerous proglottids, the egg-producing segments.

*D. latum* is a fish tapeworm that can measure 3 to 10 m in length. Most infections are asymptomatic, although vitamin $B_{12}$ deficiency may occur due to competition with the host. Diagnosis is made by finding eggs or proglottids in the stool. Treatment is praziquantel.

### *Taenia solium*

*T. solium* is the pork tapeworm. Humans acquire the intestinal infection by eating undercooked pork containing the infectious cysticerci. Intestinal infection is largely asymptomatic, but a potentially serious condition can be transmitted by eggs passed in the stools of humans infected with the pork tapeworm. Cysticercosis results from ingestion of eggs from *T. solium*–infected humans. The ingested eggs hatch into onchospheres, which penetrate the mucosa and are carried by the blood to a variety of tissues, including muscle and brain. Seizures and other neurologic problems may follow.

### *Taenia saginata*

*T. saginata,* the beef tapeworm, is acquired by eating undercooked beef. This largest human parasite may be 25 m long. Nevertheless, infection is usually asymptomatic except for the passage of proglottids in the feces or the occasional crawling out of the anus of active proglottids. The eggs of *T. saginata* are not infectious in humans so there is no equivalent of cysticercosis from the beef tapeworm.

### *Hymenolepis nana*

*H. nana* does not require an intermediate host and spreads easily via the fecal-oral route. Furthermore autoinfection may allow the worm burden to increase without additional exposure. Symptoms of heavy worm burden may include diarrhea, cramping, and anorexia. The diagnosis is made by finding ova in the stool. Niclosamide and praziquantel are the drugs of choice.

## Flukes

### *Schistosomiasis*

*Schistosoma mansoni, S. japonicum,* and *S. haematobium* are trematodes whose complex life cycles require an intermediate snail host.[64–66] *S. mansoni* is found in the Caribbean, South America, the Middle East, and Africa. *S. japonicum* is found in the Far East: Japan, China, and the Philippines. *S. haematobium* is mainly in the Nile valley and elsewhere in Africa. Humans are infected when skin is exposed to contaminated water containing cercariae, which penetrate the skin and are carried to the lungs. They eventually reach the systemic circulation and the intrahepatic portal circulation, where they mature into adult forms. As the male and female worms couple, they migrate upstream to the terminal mesenteric venules, where the female lays 300 to 3000 eggs per day for several years. Some eggs erode into the gut lumen and are excreted with feces, to continue their life cycle in snails; other eggs remain trapped in tissues or are swept upstream into the liver. As the eggs erode into the bowel lumen they evoke an inflammatory response which may produce a dysentery-like picture with bleeding, ulceration, and pseudopolyp formation. With severe chronic infection, eggs that have been carried to the liver cause fibrosis and severe portal hypertension. Diagnosis can be made by stool examination in the more acute phases. Rectal biopsy and liver biopsy can also be diagnostic. Serologic testing is also available (but not helpful) for persons in endemic regions, where light exposure is common. Treatment with praziquantel is effective but does not reverse the severe chronic portal hypertension seen in longstanding cases.

## Zoonotic Infections

For most of the parasitic infections described above, humans are primary, or at least intermediate, hosts (i.e., the infecting parasites· can complete or partially complete their reproductive cycle humans). Infection with parasites from other native hosts can lead to unusual manifestations, as these "strangers in a strange land" often migrate aimlessly away from the intestine.

### Cutaneous Larva Migrans

Nematode larvae from a variety of species can wander in the skin producing severe pruritus. "Swimmer's itch" is usually due to cercariae from bird schistosomes, whereas "ground itch" syndromes may be due to a variety of nematodes.

### Anisakiasis

*Anisakis* larvae (from raw or undercooked fish) can produce intense abdominal distress as they flee the gastric or intestinal lumen across the epithelium.[67] These parasites are quite common in a variety of popular food fish, such as salmon, mackerel, rockfish, and cod.[67] Symptoms usually begin within 12 hours of eating the fish. The worms have a propensity for the greater curve of the stomach and can produce an impressive local inflammatory response as well as systemic leukocytosis.[68] Some data suggest that symptoms result from hypersensitivity to the worms. Diagnosis is based on history, radiology, and endoscopy. Treatment consists of physically removing the worms by endoscopy or surgery.

### *Ancylostoma caninum*

Canine hookworms can cause eosinophilic ileocolitis during their abortive infection of humans.[67, 69] Although most cases have been reported from western Australia, at least one case has been described in the southern United States.[70] *A. caninum* is common in dogs worldwide, and further reports are anticipated. Because the canine hookworm does not produce eggs in human hosts, diagnosis has depended on finding the usually solitary worm during colonoscopy or by serology. Mebendazole and albendazole are said to be helpful.

### Visceral Larva Migrans

The larvae of ascarids of cats and dogs (*Toxocara cati* and *T. canis*) disseminate in the viscera and eyes of the child host who ingests the ova, which are common in sandboxes and playground soil.[71, 72] Typical clinical manifestations include fever, hepatomegaly, lymphadenopathy, cough, and wheezing. Serious sequelae, including blindness, can result from ocular involvement. Diagnosis is based on the clinical picture and serology. Although most cases resolve spontaneously, severe pulmonary disease responds to steroids. Larvicidal drugs such as diethylcarbamazine and albendazole are also used.

## REFERENCES


1. Holland CV, Taren DL, Cropton DW: Intestinal helminthiasis in relation to socioeconomic environment of Panamanian children. Soc Sci Med 1988;26:209–213.
2. Guerrant RL, Bobak D: Bacterial and parasitic gastroenteritis. N Engl J Med 1991;325:327–333.
3. Herwaldt BL, Ackers M-L: An outbreak in 1996 of cyclosporiasis associated with imported raspberries. N Engl J Med 1997;336:1548–1556.
4. Millard PS, Gensheimer KF, Addiss DG, et al: An outbreak of cryptosporidiosis from fresh-pressed apple cider [published erratum appears in JAMA 1995 Mar 8;273(10):776]. JAMA 1994;272:1592–1596.

4a. Benhamou Y, Kapel N, Hoang K, et al: Inefficacy of intestinal secretory immune response to *Cryptosporidium* in acquired immunodeficiency syndrome. Gastroenterology 1995;108:627–635.

5. Esfandiari A, Jordan WC, Brown CP: Prevalence of enteric parasitic infection among HIV-infected attendees of an inner city AIDS clinic. Cell Mol Biol 1995;41:S19–23.
6. Allason-Jones E, Mindel A, Sargeaunt P, Williams P: *Entamoeba histolytica* as a commensal intestinal parasite in homosexual men. N Engl J Med 1986;315:353–356.
7. Genta RM: Diarrhea in helminthic infections. Clin Infect Dis 1993;16:S122–S129.

7a. Kabani A, Cadrain G, Trevenen C, et al: Practice guidelines for ordering stool ova and parasite testing in a pediatric population. The Alberta Children's Hospital. Am J Clin Pathol 1995;104:272–278.

8. Desowitz RS: 1989. Fecal, blood, and urine examinations in parisitology. In Goldsmith R, Heyneman D (eds): Tropical Medicine and Parisitology. Norwalk, CT, Appleton & Lange, 1989, pp 866–875.

8a. Hiatt RA, Markell EK, Ng E: How many stool examinations are necessary to detect pathogenic intestinal protozoa? Am J Trop Med Hyg 1995;53:36–39.

9. Grimmond TR, Radford AJ, Brownridge T, et al: *Giardia* carriage in aboriginal and non-aboriginal children attending urban day-care centers in South Australia. Aust Paediatr J 1988;24:304–305.
10. Pickering LK, Engelkirk PG: *Giardia lamblia.* Pediatr Clin North Am 1988;35:565–577.
11. Mason PR, Patterson BA: Epidemiology of *Giardia lamblia* infection in children: cross-sectional and longitudinal studies in urban and rural communities in Zimbabwe. Am J Trop Med Hyg 1987;37:277–282.
12. Woo PT, Paterson WB: *Giardia lamblia* in children in day-care centres in southern Ontario, Canada, and susceptibility of animals to *G. lamblia.* Trans R Soc Trop Med Hyg 1986;80:56–59.
13. Kabnick K, Peattie DA: Giardia: a missing link between prokaryotes and eukaryotes. Am Scientist 1991;79:34–43.
14. Collins GH, Pope SE, Griffin DL. et al: Diagnosis and prevalence of *Giardia* spp in dogs and cats. Aust Vet J 1987;64:89–90.
15. Kiorpes AL, Kirkpatrick CE, Bowman DD: Isolation of *Giardia* from a llama and from sheep. Can J Vet Res 1987;51:277–280.
16. Pacha RE, Clark GW, Williams EA, et al: Small rodents and other mammals associated with mountain meadows as reservoirs of *Giardia* spp. and *Campylobacter* spp. Appl Environ Microbiol 1987;53:1574–1579.
17. Oberhuber G, Kastner N, Stolte M: Giardiasis: a histologic analysis of 567 cases. Scand J Gastroenterol 1997;32:48–51.
18. Washington K, Stenzel TT, Buckley RH, Gottfried MR: Gastrointestinal pathology in patients with common variable immunodeficiency and X-linked agammaglobulinemia. Am J Surg Pathol 1996;20:1240–1252.
19. Gunasekaran TS, Hassall E: Giardiasis mimicking inflammatory bowel disease. J Pediatr 1992;120:424–426.
20. Cevallos MA, Porta H, Alagon AC, Lizardi PM: Sequence of the 5.8S ribosomal gene of pathogenic and non-pathogenic isolates of *Entamoeba histolytica.* Nucleic Acids Res 1993;21:355.
21. Chapman A, Vallejo V, Mossie KG, et al: Isolation and characterization of species-specific DNA probes from *Taenia solium* and *Taenia saginata* and their use in an egg detection assay. J Clin Microbiol 1995;33:1283–1288.
22. Carrero JC, Laclette JP: Molecular biology of *Entamoeba histolytica:* a review. Arch Med Res 1996;27:403–412.
23. Allason-Jones E, Mindel A, Sargeaunt P, Katz D: Outcome of untreated infection with *Entamoeba histolytica* in homosexual men with and without HIV antibody. Br Med J 1988;297:654–657.
24. Butler WP: *Dientamoeba fragilis.* An unusual intestinal pathogen. Dig Dis Sci 1996;41:1811–1813.
25. Chan F, Stewart N, Guan M, et al: Prevalence of *Dientamoeba fragilis* antibodies in children and recognition of a 39 kDa immunodominant protein antigen of the organism. Eur J Clin Microbiol Infect Dis 1996;15:950–954.
26. Chang SL: Parisitization of the parasite. JAMA 1973;223:1510–1513.
27. Grendon JH, DiGiacomo RF, Frost FJ: Descriptive features of *Dientamoeba fragilis* infections. J Trop Med Hyg 1995;98:309–315.
28. Shlim DR, Hoge CW, Rajah R, et al: Is *Blastocystis hominis* a cause of diarrhea in travelers? A prospective controlled study in Nepal [see Comments]. Clin Infect Dis 1995;21:97–101.
29. Markell EK: Is there any reason to continue treating *Blastocystis infections?* (Editorial; Comment). Clin Infect Dis 1995;21:104–105.
30. Sinniah B, Rajeswari B: *Blastocystis hominis* infection, a cause of human diarrhea. Southeast Asian J Trop Med Public Health 1994;25:490–493.
31. O'Gorman MA, Orenstein SR, Proujansky R, et al: Prevalence and characteristics of *Blastocystis hominis* infection in children. Clin Pediatr 1993;32:91–96.
32. Nine FA, Burek JD, Page DL, et al: Acute enterocolitis in a human being infected with the protozoan *Cryptosporidium.* Gastroenterology 1976;70:592–598.
33. MacKenzie WR: A massive outbreak in Milwaukee of *Cryptosporidium* infection transmitted through the public water supply. N Engl J Med 1994;331:161–168.
34. Bouche H, Housset C, Dumont JL, et al: AIDS-related cholangitis: diagnostic features and course in 15 patients. J Hepatol 1993;17:34–39.
35. Hicks P, Zwiener RJ, Squires J, Savell V: Azithromycin therapy for

*Cryptosporidium parvum* infection in four children infected with human immunodeficiency virus. J Pediatr 1996;129:297–300.
36. Greenberg PD, Cello JP: Treatment of severe diarrhea caused by *Cryptosporidium parvum* with oral bovine immunoglobulin concentrate in patients with AIDS. J Acquir Immune Defic Syndr Hum Retrovirol 1996;13:348–354.
37. Kuhls TL, Orlicek SL, Mosier DA, et al: Enteral human serum immunoglobulin treatment of cryptosporidiosis in mice with severe combined immunodeficiency. Infect Immun 1995;63:3582–3586.
38. Ackers JP: Gut coccidia—*Isospora, Cryptosporidium, Cyclospora* and *Sarcocystis.* Semin Gastrointest Dis 1997;8:33–44.
39. Brennan MK, MacPherson DW, Palmer J, Keystone JS: Cyclosporiasis: a new cause of diarrhea. Can Med Assoc J 1996;155:1293–1296.
40. Marshall MM, Naumovitz D, Ortega Y, Sterling CR: Waterborne protozoan pathogens. Clin Microbiol Rev 1997;10:67–85.
41. Schwartz DA, Sobottka I, Leitch GJ, et al: Pathology of microsporidiosis: emerging parasitic infections in patients with acquired immunodeficiency syndrome. Arch Pathol Lab Med 1996;120:173–188.
42. Croft SL, Williams J, McGowan I: Intestinal microsporidiosis. Semin Gastrointest Dis 1997;8:45–55.
43. Asmuth DM, DeGirolami PC, Federman M, et al: Clinical features of microsporidiosis in patients with AIDS. Clin Infect Dis 1994;18:819–825.
44. Didier ES, Rogers LB, Brush AD, et al: Diagnosis of disseminated microsporidian *Encephalitozoon hellem* infection by PCR-Southern analysis and successful treatment with albendazole and fumagillin. J Clin Microbiol 1996;34:947–952.
45. Garvey MJ, Ambrose PG, Ulmer JL: Topical fumagillin in the treatment of microsporidial keratoconjunctivitis in AIDS. Ann Pharmacother 1995;29:872–874.
46. Rossi RM, Wanke C, Federman M: Microsporidian sinusitis in patients with the acquired immunodeficiency syndrome. Laryngoscope 1996;106:966–971.
47. Khuroo MS: Ascariasis. Gastroenterol Clin North Am 1996;25:553–577.
48. Asrat T, Rogers N: Acute pancreatitis caused by biliary ascaris in pregnancy. J Perinatol 1995;15:330–332.
49. Kuzu MA, Ozturk Y, Ozbek H, Soran A: Acalculous cholecystitis: ascariasis as an unusual cause. J Gastroenterol 1996;31:747–749.
50. Parenti DM, Steinberg W, Kang P: Infectious causes of acute pancreatitis. Pancreas 1996;13:356–371.
51. Holcombe C: Surgical emergencies in tropical gastroenterology. Gut 1995;36:9–11.
52. Hlaing T: Ascariasis and childhood malnutrition. Parasitology 1993;107:S125–S136.
53. Grencis RK, Cooper ES: *Enterobius, Trichuris, Capillaria,* and hookworm including *Ancylostoma caninum.* Gastroenterol Clin North Am 1996;25:579–597.
54. Hotez PJ, Pritchard DI: Hookworm infection. Sci Am 1995;272:68–74.
55. Yu SH, Jiang ZX, Xu LQ: Infantile hookworm disease in China. A review. Acta Trop Med 1995;59:265–270.
56. Grove DI: Human strongyloidiasis. Adv Parasitol 1996;38:251–309.
57. Haque AK, Schnadig V, Rubin SA, Smith JH: Pathogenesis of human strongyloidiasis: autopsy and quantitative parasitological analysis. Mod Pathol 1994;7:276–288.
58. Choudhry U, Choudhry R, Romeo DP, et al: Strongyloidiasis: new endoscopic findings. Gastrointest Endosc 1995;42:170–173.
59. Hagelskjaer LH: A fatal case of systemic strongyloidiasis and review of the literature. Eur J Clin Microbiol Infect Dis 1994;13:1069–1074.
60. Celedon JC, Mathur-Wagh U, Fox J, et al: Systemic strongyloidiasis in patients infected with the human immunodeficiency virus. A report of 3 cases and review of the literature. Medicine 1994;73:256–263.
61. Sato Y, Kobayashi J, Shiroma Y: Serodiagnosis of strongyloidiasis. The application and significance. Rev Inst Med Trop Sao Paulo 1995;37:35–41.
62. Ottesen EA, Campbell WC: Ivermectin in human medicine. J Antimicrob Chemother 1994;34:195–203.
63. Lee SH, Hong ST, Chai JY, et al: A case of intestinal capillariasis in the Republic of Korea. Am J Trop Med Hyg 1993;48:542–546.
64. Lucey DR, Maguire JH: Schistosomiasis. Infect Dis Clin North Am 1993;7:635–653.
65. Strickland GT: Gastrointestinal manifestations of schistosomiasis. Gut 1994;35:1334–1337.
66. Elliott DE: Schistosomiasis. Pathophysiology, diagnosis, and treatment. Gastroenterol Clin North Am 1996;25:599–625.
67. Muraoka A, Suehiro I, Fujii M, et al: Acute gastric anisakiasis: 28 cases during the last 10 years. Dig Dis Sci 1996;41:2362–2365.
68. Kakizoe S, Kakizoe H, Kakizoe K, et al: Endoscopic findings and clinical manifestation of gastric anisakiasis. Am J Gastroenterol 1995;90:761–763.
69. Croese J, Fairley S, Loukas A, et al: A distinctive aphthous ileitis linked to *Ancylostoma caninum.* J Gastroenterol Hepatol 1996;11:524–531.
70. Khoshoo V, Schantz P, Craver R, et al: Dog hookworm: a cause of eosinophilic enterocolitis in humans. J Pediatr Gastroenterol Nutr 1994;19:448–452.
71. Glickman LT, Magnaval JF: Zoonotic roundworm infections. Infect Dis Clin North Am 1993;7:717–732.
72. Hotez PJ: Visceral and ocular larva migrans. Semin Neurol 1993;13:175–179.
73. Drugs for parasitic infections. Med Lett 1995;37:99–108.
74. Morrow JD, Neuzil KM: Pharmacology of antimicrobial agents used in the therapy of gastrointestinal infections. In Blaser MJ, et al (eds): Infections of the Gastrointestinal Tract. New York, Raven Press, 1995, pp 967–983.

# Chapter 30

# Gastrointestinal Manifestations of Primary Immunodeficiencies

*Athos Bousvaros*

In 1995, an expert panel of the World Health Organization identified more than 80 primary and secondary immunodeficiency syndromes.[1] If selective immunoglobulin A (IgA) deficiency is excluded, approximately 400 children with primary immunodeficiency syndromes are born in the United States each year,[2] whereas human immunodeficiency virus infects 1,000 to 2,000 American children born each year.[3] This chapter reviews the gastrointestinal manifestations and complications of the more common immunodeficiency syndromes (Table 30–1). A more detailed discussion of the systemic complications of each syndrome can be found elsewhere.[4]

## COMPONENTS OF THE IMMUNE RESPONSE

The immune response is a complex process involving epithelial cells, monocytes, T and B lymphocytes, and effector cells (neutrophils, eosinophils, and mast cells). To trigger the cascade of immunologic events summarized in Table 30–2, an exogenous antigen must penetrate the physical barriers at epithelial surfaces. The gastrointestinal tract has multiple host defenses, including gastric acid, digestive enzymes, intestinal mucin, and normal bacterial flora, that reduce the amount of antigen that reaches the epithelium. The human gut epithelial cells are joined by tight junctions that limit macromolecular permeability.[5, 6] However, in certain specialized regions of gut epithelium, termed *follicle-associated epithelium (dome epithelium),* modified epithelial cells (M cells) preferentially bind bacteria and viruses. These M cells are located over lymphoid nodules and Peyer's patches in the gut. They provide a portal of entry that directly exposes potential pathogens to the systemic and mucosal immune systems.[5, 7]

On exposure to cells of the immune system, antigen is endocytosed and processed by antigen-presenting cells (APCs). Although many different types of cells can present antigen to T cells, two principle APCs in the body are monocyte/macrophages and dendritic cells. APCs are characterized by their ability to phagocytose proteins or peptides, degrade them intracellularly, complex these peptides with proteins of the major histocompatibility complex (MHC), and transport the peptide-MHC protein to the APC cell surface.[8] *Antigen presentation* to a CD4 (helper) T lymphocyte occurs when a peptide complexed to an MHC class II protein on the surface of an APC comes in contact with the T cell receptor complex on the surface of the lymphocyte. Stimulation of the T cell receptor alone is not sufficient to promote T lymphocyte activation, and a second signal (either through another cell surface molecule such as CD28, through surface cell adhesion molecules such as LFA-1, or through cytokine signaling) is necessary to activate a T cell.[9, 10] After a T cell is stimulated by primary and secondary signals, two primary intracellular signal transduction pathways (one involving protein-kinase C and diacylglycerol, and the other involving inositol triphosphate and calcineurins) are thought to result in *T lymphocyte activation*[11, 12] (Fig. 30–1).

Helper (CD4) T lymphocytes have been categorized into two broad types. $T_{H1}$ helper T cells promote cellular immune responses and delayed-type hypersensitivity by secreting interleukin-2 (IL-2), interferon-γ (IFN-γ), and tumor-necrosis factor-β (TNF-β). $T_{H2}$ cells promote humoral responses by secreting IL-4, IL-5, and IL-6,[13] which in turn promote B lymphocyte differentiation into plasma cells and antibody synthesis.

Humoral immunity is generated by B lymphocytes, which, on exposure to antigen, proliferate and differentiate into plasma cells.[14] The mechanisms of B cell activation have been reviewed elsewhere.[15, 16] Immunodeficiencies that inhibit T cell differentiation and proliferation commonly impair B cell function and humoral immunity.

The activated monocytes, T lymphocytes, and B lymphocytes produce a wide array of cytokines (interleukins). More than 20 such cytokines have now been isolated. Their effects include promotion of lymphocyte growth and differentiation, MHC up-regulation, stimulation of cytotoxic (CD8) T cell proliferation, recruitment and activation of neutrophils (IL-

**TABLE 30–1. Classification and Etiology of Primary Immunodeficiency Diseases with Prominent Gastrointestinal Manifestations**

| DISEASE | PROPOSED CAUSE |
|---|---|
| Predominantly antibody deficiencies | |
| X-linked agammaglobulinemia | Absence of BtK gene in B cells |
| Hyper-IgM syndrome | Absence of gp39 (CD40 ligand) on T cells |
| Selective IgA deficiency | Impaired IgA synthesis; molecular defect unknown |
| Transient hypogammaglobulinemia of infancy | Unknown |
| Combined cellular/humoral defects | |
| Common variable immunodeficiency | Impaired B cell differentiation; molecular defect unknown |
| Severe combined immunodeficiency | Multiple causes, including adenosine deaminase deficiency, purine nucleotidyl phosphorylase deficiency, absence of IL-2 receptor gamma chain (in X-linked SCID), T cell maturation defects (e.g., ZAP-70 kinase mutation) |
| Bare lymphocyte syndrome | MHC class I and/or class II deficiency |
| Immunodeficiency with other systemic disease | |
| Ataxia-telangiectasia | Phosphatidylinositol 3-kinase defect |
| Wiskott-Aldrich syndrome | Altered WAS gene/protein |
| DiGeorge syndrome | Thymic hypoplasia |
| Other primary immunodeficiency diseases | |
| Defects of phagocytic function | |
| Chronic granulomatous disease | |
| Leukocyte-adhesion deficiency | |
| Schwachman's syndrome | |
| Complement deficiencies | |
| Immunodeficiency associated with other diseases (e.g., Down syndrome, Fanconi's anemia, xeroderma) | |
| Glycogen storage disease 1B | |
| Dubowitz' syndrome | |
| Intestinal lymphangiectasia | |
| Chronic mucocutaneous candidiasis | |
| Malnutrition | |
| Malignancy | |
| Drug-induced | |
| Acquired immunodeficiency syndrome | |

Adapted from Rosen F, Wedgwood R, Eibl M, et al: Primary immunodeficiency disease: report of a WHO scientific group. Clin Exp Immunol 1995;1(suppl 99):1–24.

8), and promotion of eosinophil differentiation.[17] The end result of the immune response is the recruitment of activated effector cells (cytotoxic lymphocytes, macrophages, neutrophils, eosinophils, and mast cells) to an infected or inflamed tissue. In bacterial infections, neutrophils can phagocytose and degrade microorganisms; this process is facilitated by opsonization of bacteria by immunoglobulin and complement.[18] In viral infections, infected cells are typically lysed by CD8 (cytotoxic) T cells containing cytolytic proteins (e.g., perforin, granzymes).[19]

Derangements at any point in this complex pathway result in three principal types of disorders in immunodeficient patients. First, an individual's susceptibility to *infection* may be increased. Second, *autoimmune disease* (including enteropathy, colitis, and hepatitis) may occur because dysfunctional mononuclear cells may be unable to properly suppress unwanted immune responses. (Colitis occurs in animals missing a wide variety of immune response genes, suggesting that bowel inflammation is a nonspecific response that may occur in a wide variety of immunoregulatory defects.[20–23]) Finally, many individuals with immunodeficiency are at increased risk for *malignancies*.

**TABLE 30–2. Components of the Immune Response**

| |
|---|
| Antigen uptake |
| Antigen processing |
| Antigen presentation to T cells |
| T lymphocyte activation |
| B cell activation, switching, and immunoglobulin production |
| Leukocyte homing and adhesion to tissues |
| Effector cell recruitment |
| Release of inflammatory mediators (e.g., prostaglandin, leukotriene, complement) |

From Bousvaros A: Immunosuppressive therapies in pediatric gastroenterology. In Walker WA, Durie P, Hamilton JR, et al (eds): Pediatric Gastrointestinal Disease, 2nd ed. St. Louis, CV Mosby, 1995, with permission.

## GASTROINTESTINAL MANIFESTATIONS OF PRIMARY IMMUNODEFICIENCIES

### Humoral Immunodeficiencies

#### *Selective Immunoglobulin A Deficiency*

Selective IgA deficiency is the most common primary immunodeficiency, with a prevalence of approximately 1 in 500.[24] The decreased IgA production probably results from a wide variety of potential immunologic derangements.[14, 25–27] Individuals with this disorder have extremely low levels (less than 5 mg/dL) of serum and mucosal IgA; in addition, 15% to 20% of patients with selective IgA deficiency also

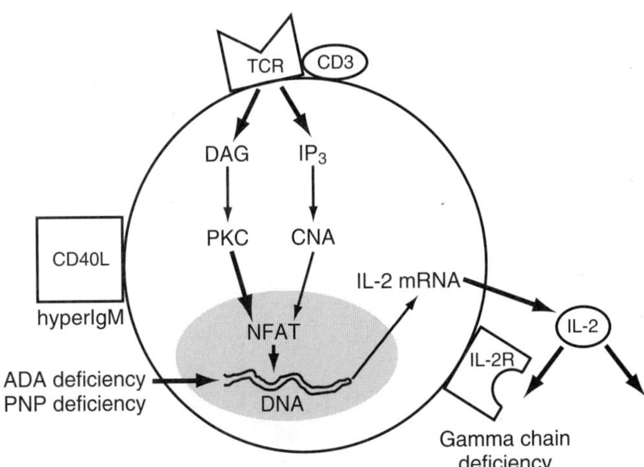


**FIGURE 30–1.** Signaling effects in T lymphocyte activation and sites of effects of immunodeficiency syndromes. Binding of antigen (in association with MHC proteins) to the T cell receptor (TCR)–CD3 complex activates two intracellular pathways of signaling. The first pathway involves diacylglycerol (DAG) and protein kinase C (PKC); the second involves inositol triphosphate ($IP_3$) and calcineurin A (CNA). The end result of this intracellular signaling is increased DNA synthesis by T cells and increased synthesis of cytokine (e.g., IL-2) mRNA as mediated by the nuclear factor of activated T cells (NFAT). The activated T cell expresses CD40 ligand (CD40L). Patients with adenosine deaminase (ADA) deficiency and purine nucleotidyl phosphorylase (PNP) deficiency have impaired synthesis of DNA; patients with X-linked severe combined immunodeficiency have defective IL-2 receptor gamma chain expression. Patients with hyper-IgM syndrome have defective expression of CD40 ligand (CD40L). (Adapted from Bousvaros A: Immunosuppressive therapies in pediatric gastroenterology. In Walker WA, Durie P, Hamilton JR, et al (eds): Pediatric Gastrointestinal Disease, 2nd ed. St. Louis, CV Mosby, 1995, p 2029, with permission.)

have low levels of IgG subclasses IgG2 and IgG4. A compensatory increase in biologically active secretory IgM frequently protects against infection.[28, 29]

Most persons with selective IgA deficiency are asymptomatic. However, they are at increased risk for infections and autoimmune disease[30] (Table 30–3). Recurrent giardiasis refractory to antibiotic therapy may result in partial villus atrophy and secondary malabsorption.[24] Chronic *Strongyloides* infection poorly responsive to anthelminthic therapy has also been reported.[31]

The most common noninfectious complication of selective IgA deficiency is celiac disease. Antigliadin IgA and antiendomysial IgA antibodies commonly yield false-negative results and are unreliable screening tools in this population.[32] In one prospective study in which jejunal biopsy was performed in 65 consecutive children with selective IgA deficiency, 7.7% showed diagnostic features of celiac disease.[33] In addition, there are increased incidences of nodular lymphoid hyperplasia, food allergy, pernicious anemia, and idiopathic villus atrophy in IgA-deficient patients.[24] There is one reported case of a patient with selective IgA deficiency, celiac disease, and ulcerative colitis.[34]

Antibiotic therapy with metronidazole, furazolidone, or quinacrine should be administered to the patient with selective IgA deficiency and giardiasis.[35] If diarrhea persists and biopsy demonstrates villus atrophy, a gluten-free diet may be therapeutic. Intravenous immunoglobulin (IVIG) should be avoided in patients with selective IgA deficiency, because it does not cross mucosal surfaces and may result in systemic anaphylaxis.[36] Finally, a small number of patients with selective IgA deficiency may develop common variable immunodeficiency (CVI), which has a much higher prevalence of gastrointestinal complications[37] (see later discussion).

## X-Linked Agammaglobulinemia

X-linked (Bruton's) agammaglobulinemia (XLA) manifests with recurrent infections after 9 months of age. Affected boys have a paucity of peripheral lymphoid tissue and low serum levels of all classes of immunoglobulins. Humoral responses to specific antigens are markedly depressed or absent. The gene for XLA has been localized to chromosome Xq22. B cells from affected persons have a defect in a B cell–specific tyrosine kinase gene (*BtK*).[38, 39]

Recurrent sinusitis, otitis media, pneumonia, and bronchitis are the most common reported illnesses in persons with XLA. Autoimmune disease (including arthritis and dermatomyosis) may also develop.[40] Patients with XLA are at risk for disseminated echovirus infection with central nervous system involvement. Chronic enteritis develops in 10%; identifiable causes of the enteritis include *Giardia, Salmonella, Campylobacter, Cryptosporidium,* rotavirus, coxsackievirus, and poliovirus. Associations with sclerosing cholangitis and a sprue-like illness have also been noted.[41–44] Patients with XLA, small bowel strictures, and transmural intestinal fissures resembling Crohn's disease have been seen. In contrast to Crohn's disease, however, no granulomas or plasma cells are identified when strictures are resected.[40, 45] Patients with XLA may also be at increased risk for small and large bowel cancers.[42, 46]

## Hyper-IgM Syndrome

X-linked immunodeficiency with hyper-IgM syndrome (hyper-IgM) is a rare disorder characterized by impaired humoral immunity; low serum levels of IgG, IgA, and IgE;

**TABLE 30–3. Disorders Associated with Selective Immunoglobulin A (IgA) Deficiency**

| |
|---|
| Upper respiratory infections |
| Otitis media |
| Sinusitis |
| Bronchiectasis |
| Allergic disorders (including food allergies) |
| Anaphylaxis to intravenous immunoglobulin |
| Giardiasis |
| Strongyloidiasis |
| Nodular lymphoid hyperplasia |
| Celiac disease (with false-negative antiendomysial antibody) |
| Achlorhydria |
| Henoch-Schönlein purpura |
| Inflammatory bowel disease |
| Gastrointestinal lymphoma |
| Primary biliary cirrhosis |
| Cholelithiasis |
| Hepatitis C |

Data from Cunningham-Rundles,[24] Leung et al,[31] and Meini et al.[33]

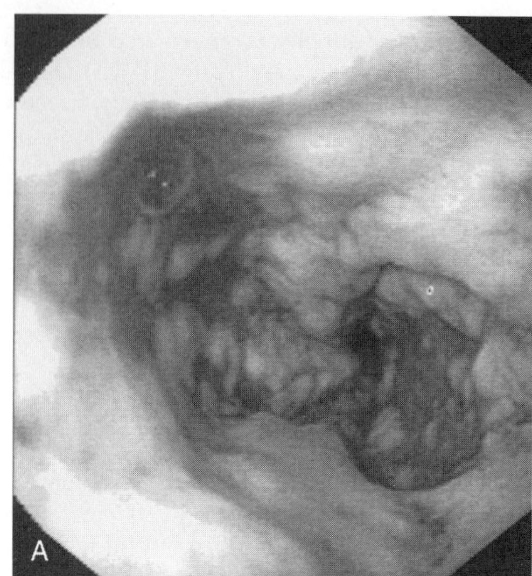


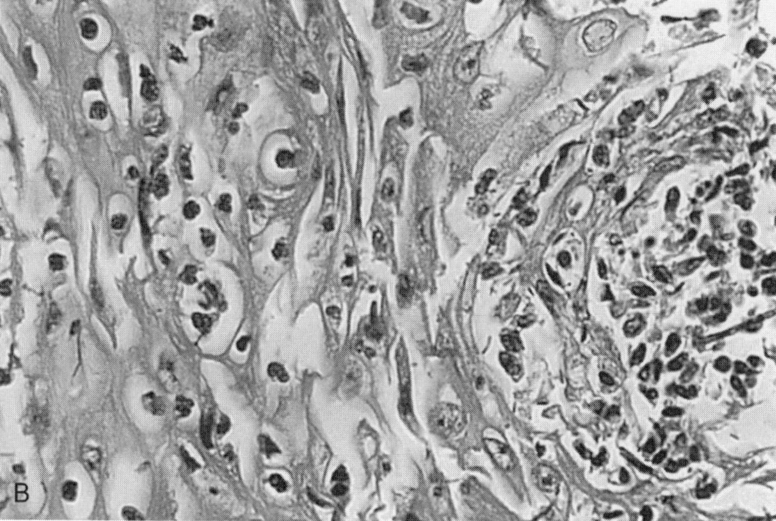


**FIGURE 30–2.** Esophageal candidiasis in a patient with the hyper-IgM syndrome. *A,* Endoscopic view of the esophagus demonstrates near-complete coating of the esophageal mucosa with a creamy white exudate. *B,* Esophageal histology demonstrates inflammatory cells and pseudohyphae. (*A,* Courtesy of Drs. Carine Lenders and Samuel Nurko; *B,* courtesy of Dr. Kameran Badizadegan, Children's Hospital, Boston.)

and normal or increased IgM levels. The molecular cause of hyper-IgM is impaired production of the gp39 molecule by activated T cells, which results in impairment of functional antibody production.[38, 47, 48]

Boys with hyper-IgM present between 1 month and 10 years of life with opportunistic infections. Chronic encephalitis and idiopathic neurologic deterioration may occur.[49] Gastrointestinal complications reported include histoplasmosis of the esophagus, cryptosporidiosis, giardiasis, hepatosplenomegaly, and intestinal lymphoid hyperplasia[44, 49, 50] (Figs. 30–2 and 30–3). Patients with hyper-IgM are also at increased risk for intestinal lymphoma.

Abnormal transaminase and alkaline phosphatase levels are seen in 50% of patients. Two separate series suggest that sclerosing cholangitis and cirrhosis occur in up to 35% of patients older than 10 years of age.[49, 51] Pancreatic and hepatobiliary malignancies have been reported in patients as young as 7 years of age.[51]

### Transient Hypogammaglobulinemia of Infancy

Transient hypogammaglobulinemia of infancy is a poorly defined condition characterized by low serum immunoglobulin levels in infancy, with attainment of normal levels at a later time. Serum IgG is typically low, without any subclass specificity; IgA or IgM levels may also be decreased. The prevalence of this condition in infants with recurrent infections ranges from 0.1% to 5% in different studies.[52, 53] Children with transient hypogammaglobulinemia of infancy typically present with recurrent respiratory infections at 6 to 12 months of age. Although the immunoglobulin deficiency usually resolves in later childhood, a subset of children have persistent hypogammaglobulinemia, which may evolve into common variable immunodeficiency.[54]

Chronic diarrhea is the second most common complication in these patients after respiratory illness. Lactose intolerance, *Giardia lamblia* infestation, or *Clostridium difficile* infection were found in one third of 55 children with low serum immunoglobulins and chronic diarrhea. Small bowel histology demonstrated enteritis or villus atrophy in up to 50% of these patients. It is unclear whether these patients had transient hypogammaglobulinemia of infancy or enteric protein loss from the intestinal illness.[55] In children with recurrent *C. difficile* infection unresponsive to antibiotics and low antibody titers to *C. difficile,* IVIG has resulted in clearance of the infection.[56]

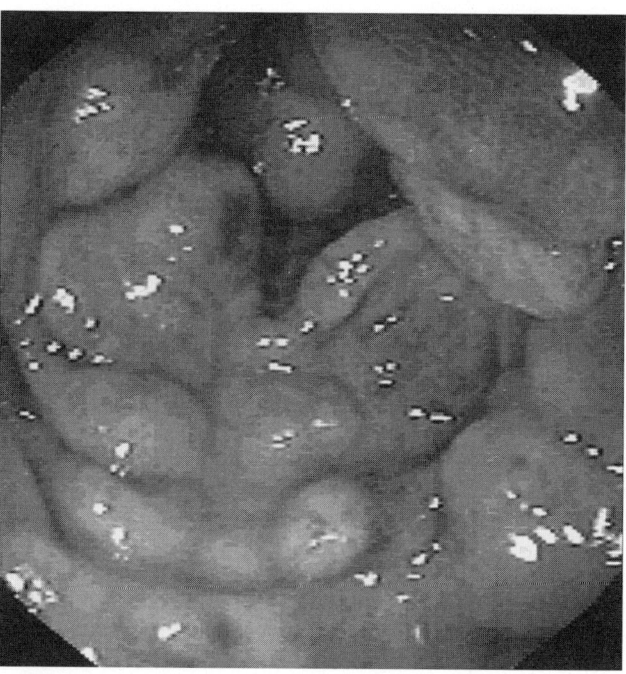

**FIGURE 30–3.** Massive lymphoid nodular hyperplasia seen in the colon of a patient with hyper-IgM syndrome. (Courtesy of Dr. Victor Fox, Children's Hospital, Boston.)

## Combined Cellular/Humoral Immunodeficiencies

### Common Variable Immunodeficiency

CVI is a rare syndrome, affecting between 1 in 50,000 and 1 in 200,000 persons; it is characterized by hypogammaglobulinemia, recurrent infections, enteropathy, autoimmune disease, and malignancy. Up to 45% of cases are diagnosed in childhood.[57] The cause of CVI is unknown, but B lymphocyte differentiation into plasma cells is impaired.[58–61]

Patients typically present in late childhood and young adulthood with recurrent sinusitis, bronchitis, and pneumonia. Common causes of the respiratory illness include *Streptococcus pneumoniae, Haemophilus influenzae,* and *Mycoplasma pneumoniae*; mycobacteria, *Pneumocystis,* and fungi are less frequent pathogens. Diagnosis of CVI is established by demonstration of persistently low antibody levels over time and impaired responses to standard pediatric immunizations; in a male, XLA must be excluded.[58, 62]

Gastrointestinal disease occurs in up to 70% of patients and accounts for much of the morbidity (Table 30–4). Infectious diarrhea caused by a wide variety of pathogens may occur. Nodular lymphoid hyperplasia is detected radiographically or endoscopically in up to 20% of patients and may predispose to either malabsorption or gastrointestinal bleeding.[64, 65]

Between 10% and 20% of patients with CVI have an enteropathy characterized by weight loss, abdominal pain, and severe diarrhea in the absence of enteric infection. Small bowel biopsy in these patients demonstrates partial or subtotal villus atrophy, hyperplastic crypts, and apoptotic bodies.[45, 66] Gluten-free or lactose-free diets may help a subset of patients, but most improve when treated with an elemental diet, although parenteral nutrition may also be required.[63, 66–68] The severe malabsorption may result in vitamin $B_{12}$ deficiency and/or zinc deficiency.[63, 69]

An inflammatory bowel disease–like syndrome, characterized by small intestinal strictures and microscopic colitis, may occur.[40, 66] Unlike Crohn's disease, there is generally no granulomatous inflammation in this enteropathy. A necrotizing variant of this enteropathy requiring colectomy at 10 months of age was reported in an infant with CVI.[70] Another condition that may be confused with inflammatory bowel disease is a noninfectious granulomatous illness, resembling sarcoidosis, which also involves the skin and lung.[71, 72]

Patients with CVI are at a 30-fold increased risk for the development of gastric carcinoma or malignant lymphoma. The small bowel lymphomas reported may manifest with intestinal malabsorption.[45, 58] In addition, a cecal carcinoma of neuroendocrine origin was reported in a 16-year-old with CVI.[73]

Twenty percent of CVI patients have a persistent mild elevation in transaminases. The cause is unknown, with liver biopsies demonstrating mild periportal changes or granulomas.[40] Hepatitis C is now reported as a complication of IVIG infusion in CVI patients,[74, 75] and it may progress rapidly to cirrhosis.[76, 77]

Therapy for CVI consists of monthly IVIG infusions and symptomatic treatment of infections and malabsorption.[78] Epstein-Barr virus infections in CVI patients may respond to IFN-α.[79]

**TABLE 30–4. Gastrointestinal Complications of Common Variable Immunodeficiency**

| |
|---|
| Enteric infections (including *Shigella, Salmonella,* and dysgonic fermenter 3) |
| Giardiasis |
| Cryptosporidiosis |
| Nodular lymphoid hyperplasia |
| Enterocolitis |
| Enteropathy/malabsorption/wasting syndrome |
| Perirectal abscess |
| Short stature |
| Zinc deficiency |
| Inflammatory bowel disease |
| Ménétrier's disease |
| Atrophic gastritis/pernicious anemia |
| Gastric adenocarcinoma |
| Intestinal lymphoma |
| Cecal carcinoma (undifferentiated) |
| Hepatitis C with cirrhosis |

Data from Sneller et al,[58] Cunningham-Rundles,[62] Sperber and Mayer,[63] deBruin et al,[73] Quinti et al,[74] and Eisenstein and Sneller.[78]

### Severe Combined Immunodeficiency

The term *severe combined immunodeficiency* (SCID) refers to a group of diseases characterized by molecular defects interfering with T and/or B cell differentiation and resulting in an infant with failure to thrive and extreme susceptibility to infections.[80] Several molecular causes of SCID have been identified[38, 81, 82] (see Table 30–1). Presenting features include growth impairment, chronic diarrhea, persistent thrush or candidiasis, or overwhelming sepsis. Graft-versus-host disease from transfusions of nonirradiated blood or disseminated illness from live vaccines may occur if the diagnosis is delayed. Diagnosis is established by the demonstration of low or absent T lymphocyte numbers in peripheral blood; B cell and neutrophil counts may also be depressed, depending on the variant of SCID.[80]

Gastrointestinal illness occurs in up to 90% of patients. Organisms frequently associated with illness include rotavirus, *Candida*, cytomegalovirus, Epstein-Barr virus, and *Escherichia coli*. Although candidiasis rarely involves the intestine, candidal esophagitis should be suspected in infants with SCID and decreased oral intake.[44, 83] Chronic viral infection is the most frequent cause of enteritis and may be responsible for death in 80% of cases.[84] Other less common causes of enteropathy include *Salmonella*, *Shigella*, and *Cryptosporidium* infections.[41, 44]

Autoimmune enteropathy has been described in at least one patient with defective T lymphocyte function[85]; in addition, patients with SCID are prone to various autoimmune complications (including hemolytic anemia and glomerulonephritis).[83]

Hepatic abnormalities are also common in SCID patients and include graft-versus-host disease of the liver, adenovirus and cytomegalovirus hepatitis, rotavirus hepatitis, parenteral nutrition–associated liver disease, and lymphoproliferative disorder.[86, 87] Pancreatic infection by viruses has also been described.[88]

One variant of SCID that seems to render a patient particularly prone to gastrointestinal complications is *bare lympho-*

*cyte syndrome.* Gastrointestinal candidiasis is common in addition to giardiasis, cryptosporidiosis, and other bacterial enteritides. A high incidence of hepatobiliary abnormalities is noted, including sclerosing cholangitis associated with biliary cryptosporidiosis. Bacterial cholangitis secondary to *Pseudomonas, Enterococcus,* and *Streptococcus* infections has been described.[89]

The principal therapy for patients with SCID is bone marrow transplantation, ideally from a matched sibling. In SCID patients with adenosine deaminase deficiency, infusions of a long-acting form of adenosine deaminase correct metabolic abnormalities and provide some restoration of immune function.[90] In addition, gene replacement therapy has also been used in these patients with some success.[91]

## Other Primary Immunodeficiencies

*Wiskott-Aldrich syndrome* is an X-linked immunodeficiency characterized by the classic triad of severe eczema, thrombocytopenia, and recurrent infections. The gene for this syndrome has been described.[92] Children are usually diagnosed before 2 years of age, after presenting with epistaxis, purpura, recurrent otitis, sinusitis, pneumonia, opportunistic infections, or diarrhea.[93]

Gastrointestinal complications occur in 10% to 30% of patients. Gastrointestinal bleeding from thrombocytopenia can antedate the diagnosis. Infectious diarrhea occurs in up to 25% of cases, though opportunistic pathogens are unusual. Henoch-Schönlein purpura may occur in up to 5% of patients, and necrotizing enterocolitis has been reported in one patient.[93] A steroid-responsive inflammatory bowel disease characterized by bloody diarrhea and colonic pseudopolyps has been seen.[94] Finally, patients with Wiskott-Aldrich syndrome are at a 100-fold increased risk of developing lymphoma, which may originate in the gut.[93]

*Chronic granulomatous disease (CGD)* refers to a group of immunodeficiencies characterized by the inability of an affected patient's neutrophils to generate superoxide and hydrogen peroxide, leaving the patient susceptible to infections with catalase-positive organisms.[95] The disease has an estimated incidence of 1 in 250,000 persons, with an X-linked inheritance pattern seen in two thirds of patients and autosomal recessive inheritance in the remainder.[96, 97] The most common presenting features involve suppurative infections by catalase-positive organisms, such as *Staphylococcus aureus, Serratia, Aspergillus, Candida,* and *Nocardia.*[98, 99]

Gastrointestinal involvement is often pronounced. Many patients with CGD present with gastric outlet obstruction secondary to pronounced antral narrowing[98, 100] (Fig. 30–4). The antral narrowing is usually caused by a combination of infection and granulomatous inflammation. It may resolve with a combination of antibiotics and corticosteroid therapy but may also require surgical intervention.[100, 101] Similar obstructive lesions of the esophagus occur less frequently.[98] Small bowel involvement may mimic Crohn's disease, with multifocal abscesses, fistulas, and granulomatous colitis. The presence of lipid-containing histiocytes in the mucosa and submucosa of colonic biopsies strongly suggests CGD colitis.[102, 103] Such colitis may respond to therapy with corticosteroids, IFN-γ, or cyclosporine, but surgical resection may be necessary for intractable colitis or acute obstruction.[102–104]

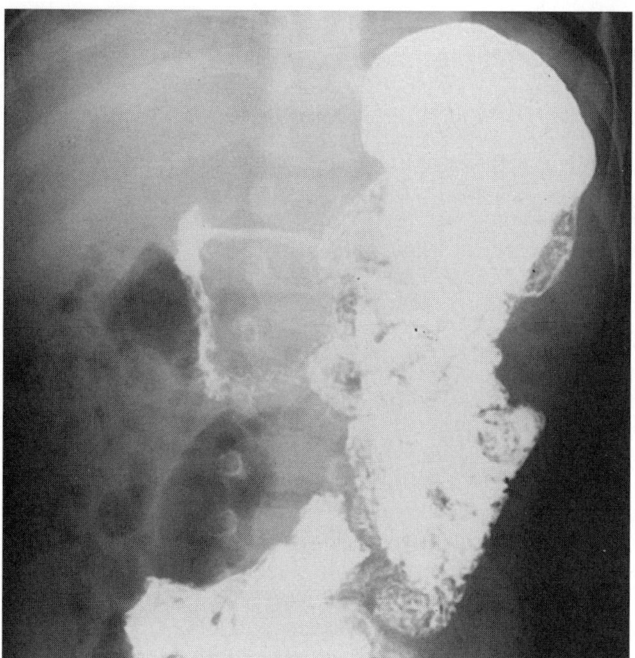

**FIGURE 30–4.** Gastric outlet obstruction secondary to antral narrowing in a patient with chronic granulomatous disease. The patient underwent partial gastrectomy, with inflammatory cells and granulomas identified in the hypertrophied antral tissue. (Courtesy of Dr. Thorne Griscom and Children's Hospital, Boston, Radiology Teaching File.)

Pyogenic or fungal liver abscess is also a common complication of CGD; it is treated with appropriate antimicrobial agents, surgical drainage, and possibly IFN-γ.[105] Prophylactic IFN-γ may reduce the frequency of opportunistic infections.[99, 106]

*Chronic mucocutaneous candidiasis* is characterized by a diminished T cell response to candidal antigens. Infants with this disorder present with persistent thrush or candidal dermatitis, failure to thrive, and dystrophic nails. Candidal esophagitis may result in refusal of foods. A polyglandular endocrinopathy syndrome characterized by hypoparathyroidism, hypothyroidism, adrenal insufficiency, and pernicious anemia develops in up to 70% of older children. Malabsorption secondary to pancreatic insufficiency contributes to the poor weight gain in 10% of patients. Therapy includes eradication of candida with topical antibiotics plus ketoconazole or fluconazole, as well as hormone or pancreatic enzyme replacement when appropriate.[107, 108]

*Leukocyte-adhesion deficiency* is characterized by impaired phagocytic function secondary to deficiencies of adhesion molecules (CD18/Mac-1) necessary for cell migration and interactions. Necrotic infections of the skin (including pyoderma gangrenosum) and mucous membranes, otitis media, and episodes of microbial sepsis are the principal features.[109, 110] Gastrointestinal complications include intraoral infections and periodontitis, candidal esophagitis, gastritis, appendicitis, necrotizing enterocolitis, and perirectal abscess.[109, 111, 112] Fatal enterocolitis similar to that of necrotizing enterocolitis or Hirschsprung's disease has been described in an infant with leukocyte-adhesion deficiency.[113, 114]

Patients with *glycogen storage disease type 1B (GSD 1B)* present with severe hypoglycemia, failure to thrive, and hepatomegaly. In contrast to von Gierke's disease (GSD 1A), these patients have severe neutropenia and phagocytic dysfunction.[115] GSD 1B is characterized by absence of the hepatic glucose 6-phosphate transport protein.[116]

Patients with GSD 1B may develop an idiopathic colitis clinically similar to Crohn's disease.[117, 118] Granulocyte-macrophage colony stimulating factor was used in the treatment of two patients with GSD 1B, and increased neutrophil counts with concurrent improvement in the bowel inflammation were noted.[119]

*Ataxia-telangiectasia* (AT) is a recessive disorder characterized by progressive neurologic degeneration, ocular and skin telangiectasias, and immunodeficiency predisposing to infections and malignancies.[120] Chronic diarrhea and gastrointestinal cancers have both been reported as complications of AT.[121, 122]

*Shwachman's syndrome,* characterized by pancreatic insufficiency, neutropenia, and metaphyseal dysostosis, is reviewed in Chapter 54.

## REFERENCES


1. Rosen F, Wedgwood R, Eibl M, et al: Primary immunodeficiency diseases: report of a WHO scientific group. Clin Exp Immunol 1995;1(suppl 99):1–24.
2. Conley M, Stiehm E: Immunodeficiency disorders: general considerations. In Stiehm E (ed): Immunologic Disorders in Infants and Children. Philadelphia, WB Saunders, 1996, pp 201–252.
3. Centers for Disease Control and Prevention: AIDS among children—United States, 1996. MMWR Morb Mortal Wkly Rep 1996;45:1005–1010.
4. Stiehm E: Immunologic Disorders in Infants and Children. Philadelphia, WB Saunders, 1996.
5. Sanderson I, Walker W: Uptake and transport of macromolecules by the intestine: possible role in clinical disorders. Gastroenterology 1993;104:622–639.
6. Udall J, Walker W: The physiologic and pathologic basis for the transport of macromolecules across the intestinal tract. J Pediatr Gastroenterol Nutr 1982;1:295–301.
7. Pabst E: The anatomical basis for the immune function of the gut. Anat Embryol (Berl) 1987;176:135–143.
8. Grey H, Sette A, Buus S: How T cells see antigen. Sci Am 1989;261:56–64.
9. Abbas A, Lichtman A, Pober J: Molecular basis of T cell recognition and activation. In Cellular and Molecular Immunology. Philadelphia, WB Saunders, 1994, pp 136–167.
10. Shimizu Y, Van Seventer GA, Ennis E, et al: Crosslinking of the T cell specific molecules CD7 and CD28 modulates T cell adhesion. J Exp Med 1992;17:S77–S82.
11. Masuda E, et al: Expression of lymphokine genes in T cells. Immunologist 1993;1:198–203.
12. Sigal N, Dumont F: Cyclosporin A, FK-506, and rapamycin: pharmacologic probes of lymphocyte signal transduction. Annu Rev Immunol 1992;10:519–560.
13. Mosmann T, Coffman R: TH1 and TH2 cells: different patterns of lymphokine secretion lead to different functional properties. Annu Rev Immunol 1989;7:145–173.
14. Strober W, Harriman G: The regulation of IgA B cell differentiation. Gastroenterol Clin North Am 1991;20:473–494.
15. Parker D: T cell dependent B cell activation. Annu Rev Immunol 1993;11:331–360.
16. Marshall L, Aruffo A, Ledbetter J, Noelle R: The molecular basis for T cell help in humoral immunity: CD40 and its ligand, gp39. J Clin Immunol 1993;13:165–174.
17. Plaeger S: Principal human cytokines. In Stiehm E (ed): Immunologic Disorders in Infants and Children. Philadelphia, WB Saunders, 1996, pp 1063–1065.
18. Abramson J, Wheeler J, Quie P: The polymorphonuclear leukocyte system. In Stiehm E (ed): Immunologic Disorders in Infants and Children. Philadelphia, WB Saunders, 1996, pp 94–112.
19. Kupfer A, Singer S: Cell biology of cytotoxic and T helper functions. Annu Rev Immunol 1989;7:309–337.
20. Kuhn R, Lohler J, Rennick D, et al: Interleukin-10 deficient mice develop chronic enterocolitis. Cell 1993;75:263–274.
21. Hammer R, Maika S, Richardson J, et al: Spontaneous inflammatory disease in transgenic rats expressing HLA-B27 and human beta-2 microglobulin: an animal model of HLA-B27 associated human disorders. Cell 1990;63:1099–1112.
22. Mombaerts P, Mizoguchi E, Grusby M, et al: Spontaneous development of inflammatory bowel disease in T cell receptor mutant mice. Cell 1993;75:275–282.
23. Sadlack B, Merz H, Schorle H, et al: Ulcerative colitis like disease in mice with a disrupted interleukin-2 gene. Cell 1993;75:253–261.
24. Cunningham-Rundles C: Selective IgA deficiency and the gastrointestinal tract. Immunol Allergy Clin North Am 1988;8:435–449.
25. Strober W, Krakauer R, Klaeveman H, et al: Secretory component deficiency: a disorder of the IgA immune system. N Engl J Med 1976;294:351–356.
26. Conley M, Cooper M: Immature IgA B cells in IgA deficient patients. N Engl J Med 1981;305:475–479.
27. Briere F, Bridon J, Chevet D, et al: Interleukin 10 induces B lymphocytes from IgA deficient patients to secrete IgA. J Clin Invest 1994;94:97–104.
28. Morgan G, Levinsky R: Clinical significance of IgA deficiency. Arch Dis Child 1988;63:579–581.
29. Oxelius V, Laurell A, Lindquist B, et al: IgG subclasses in selective IgA deficiency: common occurrence of IgG2-IgA deficiency. N Engl J Med 1981;304:1476–1477.
30. Zinneman H, Kaplan A: The association of giardiasis with reduced secretory immunoglobulin A. Am J Dig Dis 1972;17:793–797.
31. Leung V, Liew C, Sung J: Strongyloidiasis in a patient with IgA deficiency. Trop Gastroenterol 1995;16:27–30.
32. Rittmeyer C, Rhoads J: IgA deficiency causes false-negative endomysial antibody results in celiac disease. J Pediatr Gastroenterol Nutr 1996;23:504–506.
33. Meini A, Pillan N, Villanacci V, et al: Prevalence and diagnosis of celiac disease in IgA deficient children. Ann Allergy Asthma Immunol 1996;77:333–336.
34. Falchuk K, Falchuk Z: Selective immunoglobulin A deficiency, ulcerative colitis, and gluten-sensitive enteropathy: a unique association. Gastroenterology 1975;69:503–506.
35. Shepherd R, Boreham P: Recent advances in the diagnosis and management of giardiasis. Scand J Gastroenterol 1989;24(suppl 169):60–64.
36. Burks A, Sampson H, Buckley R: Anaphylactic reactions following gammaglobulin administration in patients with hypogammaglobulinemia: detection of IgE antibodies to IgA. N Engl J Med 1986;314:560–564.
37. Espanol T, Catala M, Hernendez M, et al: Development of a common variable immunodeficiency in IgA deficient patients. Clin Immunol Immunopathol 1996;80:333–335.
38. Ochs H, Aruffo A: Advances in X-linked immunodeficiency diseases. Curr Opin Pediatr 1993;5:684–691.
39. Tsukada S, Saffran D, Rawlings D, et al: Deficient expression of a B cell cytoplasmic tyrosine kinase in human X-linked agammaglobulinemia. Cell 1993;72:279–290.
40. Hermaszewski R, Webster A: Primary hypogammaglobulinemia: a survey of clinical manifestations and complications. QJM 1993;86:31–42.
41. Arbo A, Santos J: Diarrheal diseases in the immunocompromised host. Pediatr Infect Dis 1987;6:894–906.
42. Lederman H, Winkelstein J: X-linked agammaglobulinemia: an analysis of 96 patients. Medicine (Baltimore) 1985;64:145–156.
43. Sisto A, Feldman P, Garel L, et al: Primary sclerosing cholangitis in children: study of 5 cases and review of the literature. Pediatrics 1987;80:918–923.
44. Stiehm E, Chin T, Haas A, Peerless A: Infectious complications of the primary immunodeficiencies. Clin Immunol Immunopathol 1986;40:69–86.
45. Washington K: Gastrointestinal pathology in patients with common variable immunodeficiency and X-linked agammaglobulinemia. Am J Surg Pathol 1996;20:1240–1252.
46. vanderMeer J, Weening R, Schellekens P, et al: Colorectal cancer in patients with X-linked agammaglobulinemia. Lancet 1993;341:1439–1440.

47. Fuleihan R, Ramesh N, Loh R, et al: Defective expression of the CD40 ligand in X chromosome linked immunoglobulin deficiency with normal or elevated IgM. Proc Natl Acad Sci U S A 1993;90:2170–2173.
48. Allen R, Armitage R, Conley M, et al: CD40 ligand defects responsible for X-linked hyper-IgM syndrome. Science 1993;259:990–993.
49. Banatvala N, Davies J, Kanariou M, et al: Hypogammaglobulinemia associated with normal or increased IgM (the hyper IgM syndrome): a case series review. Arch Dis Child 1994;71:150–152.
50. Hostohoffer R, Berger M, Clark H, Schreiber J: Disseminated *Histoplasma capsulatum* infection in a patient with hyper IgM immunodeficiency. Pediatrics 1994;94:234–236.
51. Hayward A, Levy J, Facchetti F, et al: Cholangiopathy and tumors of the pancreas, liver and biliary tree in boys with X-linked immunodeficiency and hyper-IgM. J Immunol 1997;158:977–983.
52. Cano F, Mayo D, Ballow M: Absent viral antibodies in patients with transient hypogammaglobulinemia of infancy. J Allergy Clin Immunol 1990;85:510–513.
53. Dressler F, Peter H, Muller W, Rieger C: Transient hypogammaglobulinemia of infancy: five new cases, review of the literature, and redefinition. Acta Paediatr Scand 1989;78:767–774.
54. McGeady S: Transient hypogammaglobulinemia of infancy: need to reconsider name and definition. J Pediatr 1987;110:47–50.
55. Perlmutter D, Leichtner A, Goldman H, Winter H: Chronic diarrhea associated with hypogammaglobulinemia and enteropathy in infants and children. Dig Dis Sci 1985;30:1149–1155.
56. Leung D, Kelly C, Boguniewicz M, et al: Treatment with intravenously administered gamma globulin of chronic relapsing colitis induced by *Clostridium difficile* toxin. J Pediatr 1991;118:633–637.
57. Cunningham-Rundles C: Clinical and immunologic studies of common variable immunodeficiency. Curr Opin Pediatr 1994;6:676–681.
58. Sneller M, Strober W, Eisenstein E, et al: New insights into common variable immunodeficiency. Ann Intern Med 1993;118:720–730.
59. Farrington M, Grosmaire L, Nonoyama S, et al: CD40 ligand expression is defective in a subset of patients with common variable immunodeficiency. Proc Natl Acad Sci U S A 1994;91:1099–1103.
60. Nonoyama S, Farrington M, Ishida H, et al: Activated B cells from patients with common variable immunodeficiency proliferate and synthesize immunoglobulin. J Clin Invest 1993;92:1282–1287.
61. Punnonen J, Kainulainen L, Ruuskanen O, et al: IL-4 synergizes with IL-10 and anti-CD40 MoAbs to induce B-cell differentiation in patients with common variable immunodeficiency. Scand J Immunol 1997;45:203–212.
62. Cunningham-Rundles C: Clinical and immunologic analyses of 103 patients with common variable immunodeficiency. J Clin Immunol 1989;9:22–33.
63. Sperber K, Mayer L: Gastrointestinal manifestations of common variable immunodeficiency. Immunol Allergy Clin North Am 1988;8:423–434.
64. Bastlein C, Burlefinger R, Holzberg E: Common variable immunodeficiency syndrome and nodular lymphoid hyperplasia in the small intestine. Endoscopy 1988;20:272–275.
65. Bennett W, Watson R, Heard J, et al: Home hyperalimentation for common variable hypogammaglobulinemia with malabsorption secondary to intestinal nodular lymphoid hyperplasia. Am J Gastroenterol 1987;82:1019–1095.
66. Teahon K, Webster A, Price A, et al: Studies on the enteropathy associated with primary hypogammaglobulinemia. Gut 1994;35:1244–1249.
67. Conley M, Park C, Douglas S: Childhood common variable immunodeficiency with autoimmune disease. J Pediatr 1986;108:915–922.
68. Catassi C, Mirakian R, Natalini G, et al: Unresponsive enteropathy associated with circulating antienterocyte antibodies in a boy with common variable hypogammaglobulinemia and type I diabetes. J Pediatr Gastroenterol Nutr 1988;7:608–613.
69. Litzman J, Dastych M, Hegar P: Analysis of zinc, iron, and copper serum levels in patients with common variable immunodeficiency. Allergol Immunopathol (Madr) 1995;23:117–120.
70. John H, Sullivan K, Smith C, Mulberg A: Enterocolitis in common variable immunodeficiency. Dig Dis Sci 1996;41:621–623.
71. Pierson J, Camisa C, Lawlor K, Elston D: Cutaneous and visceral granulomas in common variable immunodeficiency. Cutis 1993;52:221–222.
72. Spickett G, Zhang J, Green T, Shriminkar J: Granulomatous disease in common variable immunodeficiency: effect on immunoglobulin replacement therapy and response to steroids and splenectomy. J Clin Pathol 1996;49:431–434.
73. deBruin N, deGroot R, denHollander J, et al: Small cell undifferentiated (neuroendocrine) carcinoma of the cecum in a child with common variable immunodeficiency. American Journal of Pediatric Hematology/Oncology 1993;15:258–261.
74. Quinti I, Pandolti F, Paganelli R, et al: HCV infection in patients with primary defects of Ig production. Clin Exp Immunol 1995;102:11–16.
75. Webster A, Brown D, Franz A, Dusheiko G: Prevalence of hepatitis C in patients with primary antibody deficiency. Clin Exp Immunol 1996;103:5–7.
76. Smith M, Webster D, Dhillon A, et al: Orthotopic liver transplantation for chronic hepatitis in two patients with common variable immunodeficiency. Gastroenterology 1995;108:879–884.
77. Sumazaki R, Matsubara T, Moki T, et al: Rapidly progressive hepatitis C in a patient with common variable immunodeficiency. Eur J Pediatr 1996;155:532–534.
78. Eisenstein E, Sneller M: Common variable immunodeficiency: diagnosis and management. Ann Allergy 1994;73:285–294.
79. Toraldo R, D'Avanzo M, Tolone C, et al: Effect of interferon-gamma in a patient with common variable immunodeficiency and chronic Epstein-Barr virus infection. Pediatr Hematol Oncol 1995;12:489–493.
80. Stephan J, Vlekova V, LeDiest F, et al: Severe combined immunodeficiency: a retrospective single-center study of clinical presentation and outcome in 117 patients. J Pediatr 1993;123:564–572.
81. Leonard W: The molecular basis of X-linked severe combined immunodeficiency: the role of the interleukin-2 receptor gamma chain as a common gamma chain. Immunol Rev 1994;138:61–86.
82. Leonard W: The molecular basis of X-linked severe combined immunodeficiency: defective cytokine receptor signaling. Annu Rev Med 1996;47:229–239.
83. Berthet F, LeDiest F, Dulliege A, et al: Clinical consequences and treatment of primary immunodeficiency syndromes characterized by functional T and B lymphocytes anomalies (combined immune deficiency). Pediatrics 1994;93:265–270.
84. Jarvis W, Middleton P, Gelfand E: Significance of viral infections in severe combined immunodeficiency disease. Pediatr Infect Dis 1983;2:187–192.
85. Murch S, Meadows N, Morgan G, et al: Severe enteropathy and immunodeficiency in interleukin-2 deficiency (abstract). J Pediatr Gastroenterol Nutr 1994;19:A335.
86. Washington K, Gossage D, Gottfried M: Pathology of the liver in severe combined immunodeficiency and DiGeorge syndrome. Pediatr Pathol 1993;13:485–504.
87. Gilger M, Matson D, Conner M, et al: Extraintestinal rotavirus infections in children with immunodeficiency. J Pediatr 1992;120:912–917.
88. Washington K, Gossage D, Gottfried M: Pathology of the pancreas in severe combined immunodeficiency and DiGeorge syndrome. Hum Pathol 1994;25:908–914.
89. Klein C, Lisowska-Grospierre B, LeDiest F, et al: Major histocompatibility complex class II deficiency: clinical manifestations, immunologic features, and outcome. J Pediatr 1993;123:921–928.
90. Hershfield M: PEG-ADA: an alternative to haploidentical bone marrow transplantation and an adjunct to gene therapy for adenosine deaminase deficiency. Hum Mutat 1995;5:107–112.
91. Blaese R, Culver K, Miller A, et al: T lymphocyte directed gene therapy for ADA-SCID: initial trial results after 4 years. Science 1995;270:475–480.
92. Kirchhausen T, Rosen F: Disease mechanism: unraveling Wiskott-Aldrich syndrome. Curr Biol 1996;6:676–678.
93. Sullivan K, Mullen C, Blaese R, Winkelstein J: A multiinstitutional survey of the Wiskott-Aldrich syndrome. J Pediatr 1994;125:876–885.
94. Hsieh K, Chang M, Lee C, Wang C: Wiskott-Aldrich syndrome and inflammatory bowel disease. Ann Allergy 1988;60:429–431.
95. Roos D, deBoer M, Kuribayashi F, et al: Mutations in the X-linked and autosomal recessive forms of chronic granulomatous disease. Blood 1996;87:1663–1681.
96. Liese J, Jendrossek V, Jansson A, et al: Chronic granulomatous disease in adults. Lancet 1995;346:220–223.
97. Hadzic N, Heaton N, Baker A, et al: Successful orthotopic liver transplantation for fulminant liver failure in a child with autosomal recessive chronic granulomatous disease. Transplantation 1995;60:1185–1186.
98. Eckert J, Abramson S, Starke J, Brandt M: The surgical implications of chronic granulomatous disease. Am J Surg 1995;169:320–323.

99. Fischer A, Segal A, Seger R, Weening R: The management of chronic granulomatous disease. Eur J Pediatr 1993;152:896–899.
100. Griscom N, Kirkpatrick J, Girdany B, et al: Gastric antral narrowing in chronic granulomatous disease of childhood. Pediatrics 1974;54:456–460.
101. Danziger R, Goren A, Becker J, et al: Outpatient management with oral corticosteroid therapy for obstructive conditions in chronic granulomatous disease. J Pediatr 1993;122:303–305.
102. Werlin S, Chusid M, Caya J, Oechler H: Colitis in chronic granulomatous disease. Gastroenterology 1982;82:328–331.
103. Sloan J, Cameron C, Maxwell R, et al: Colitis complicating chronic granulomatous disease: a clinicopathological case report. Gut 1996;38:619–622.
104. Rosh J, Tang H, Mayer L, et al: Treatment of intractable gastrointestinal manifestations of chronic granulomatous disease with cyclosporine. J Pediatr 1995;126:143–145.
105. Hague R, Eastham E, Lee R, Cant A: Resolution of hepatic abscess after interferon gamma in chronic granulomatous disease. Arch Dis Child 1993;69:443–445.
106. International Chronic Granulomatous Disease Study Group: A controlled trial of interferon gamma to prevent infection in chronic granulomatous disease. N Engl J Med 1991;324:509–516.
107. Herrod H: Chronic mucocutaneous candidiasis in childhood and complications of non-*Candida* infection. J Pediatr 1990;116:377–382.
108. Kirkpatrick C: Chronic mucocutaneous candidiasis. Eur J Clin Microbiol Infect Dis 1989;8:448–456.
109. Anderson D, Springer T: Leukocyte-adhesion deficiency: an inherited defect in the Mac-1, LFA-1, and p150,95 glycoproteins. Annu Rev Med 1987;38:175–194.
110. Voss L, Rhodes K: Leukocyte adhesion deficiency presenting with recurrent otitis media and persistent leukocytosis. Clin Pediatr 1992;31:442–445.
111. Todd R, Freyer D: The CD11/CD18 leukocyte glycoprotein deficiency. Hematol Oncol Clin North Am 1988;2:13–31.
112. Roberts M, Atkinson J: Oral manifestations associated with leukocyte adhesion deficiency: a five year case study. Pediatr Dent 1990;12:107–111.
113. Hawkins H, Heffelfinger S, Anderson D: Leukocyte adhesion deficiency: clinical and postmortem observations. Pediatr Pathol 1992;12:119–130.
114. Rivera-Matos I, Rakita R, Marisalco M, et al: Leukocyte-adhesion deficiency mimicking Hirschsprung disease. J Pediatr 1995;127:755–757.
115. Gitzelmann R, Bosshard N: Defective neutrophil and monocyte functions in glycogen storage disease Ib: a literature review. Eur J Pediatr 1993;152(suppl 1):S33–S38.
116. Nordlie R, Sukalskie K: Human microsomal glucose-6 phosphatase system. Eur J Pediatr 1993;152:S2–S6.
117. Couper R, Kapelushnik J, Griffiths A: Neutrophil dysfunction in glycogen storage disease Ib: association with Crohn's like colitis. Gastroenterology 1991;100:549–554.
118. Roe T, Thomas D, Gilsanz V, et al: Inflammatory bowel disease in glycogen storage disease Ib. J Pediatr 1986;109:55–59.
119. Roe T, Coates T, Thomas D, et al: Treatment of chronic inflammatory bowel disease in glycogen storage disease Ib with colony stimulating factors. N Engl J Med 1992;326:1666–1669.
120. Lavin M, Shiloh Y: Ataxia telangiectasia: a multifaceted genetic disorder associated with defective signal transduction. Curr Opin Immunol 1996;8:459–464.
121. Abdullah A: Aetiology of chronic diarrhoea in children: experience at King Khalid University Hospital, Riyadh, Saudi Arabia. Ann Trop Pediatr 1994;14:111–117.
122. Ceroni M, Karau J, Pergami P, et al: High incidence of gastrointestinal cancer in a family with ataxia telangiectasia. Acta Neurologica 1994;16:33–37.

Chapter 31

# Gastrointestinal Complications of Secondary Immunodeficiency Syndromes

*Tracie L. Miller*

The first cases of the acquired immunodeficiency syndrome (AIDS) were described in the early 1980s. Later, in 1984,[1] the human immunodeficiency virus (HIV) was determined to be the pathogen, and HIV infection was recognized as a spectrum of disease, ranging from asymptomatic infection to full-blown AIDS. Since the initial description of HIV, the Centers for Disease Control and Prevention has reported a total of 566,002 cases of AIDS in the United States; 7,472 of affected persons are children under the age of 13 years.[2] An additional 1,000 to 2,000 children per year acquire HIV "vertically,"[3] most from their mother, and more than 8.8 million women of childbearing age are infected with HIV.

HIV is an RNA virus that belongs to the lentivirus family. It has a particular tropism for the CD4 surface antigen of cells, and the binding of HIV to the CD4 receptor initiates the viral cycle. The virus may subsequently replicate within the host cell, or, alternatively, the proviral DNA within the host cells may remain latent until cellular activation occurs. Human T lymphocytes and monocytes-macrophages are the primary cells that are infected with HIV, although other cell lines can be infected as well. The net effect is suppression of the immune system and a progressive decline in CD4-positive T lymphocytes, which leaves patients susceptible to opportunistic and recurrent bacterial infections.

## CELLULAR COMPONENTS OF GASTROINTESTINAL TRACT

A dysfunctional gastrointestinal (GI) tract can produce significant clinical symptoms that contribute to both morbidity and mortality in children with HIV infection. These symptoms include weight loss, diarrhea, and malabsorption. In addition, the GI tract is a potential route of viral entry, although this is less relevant in the pediatric population.

It is reasonable to expect the GI tract to be a major target for HIV, because it houses 60% of all the lymphocytes in the body.[4] The presence of HIV proteins and nucleic acids has been demonstrated in the mucosa of small intestine and colon biopsy specimens from adult patients with HIV infection, as demonstrated by in situ hybridization. There is controversy, however, about the target cells of the virus. Nelson and coworkers[5] showed the presence of HIV RNA in the enterochromaffin cells of rectal crypts. Other studies failed to confirm these findings but identified viral nucleic acid and proteins in cells in the lamina propria.[6] It has also been reported that colon carcinoma cells in vitro can be infected with HIV,[7] although those cells expressed CD4 receptors, which usually are not found on intestinal epithelial cells.

The cellular profile of the lamina propria is altered with HIV infection. Normal human lamina propria T cells have a CD4-CD8 ratio similar to that of circulating peripheral T cells, whereas intraepithelial T cells are predominantly CD8. One study of HIV-infected patients[8] detected an early, preferential loss of duodenal CD4 T lymphocyte cells in the lamina propria, as well as intraepithelial lymphocytes. These abnormalities were found well before there was a significant drop in peripheral CD4 T lymphocyte counts. The results showed that the proportion of CD4-positive T cells was five times lower in the duodenal mucosa than in the peripheral blood. A 200- to 1,000-fold higher HIV P24 content per wet weight on intestinal biopsy specimens, as compared with serum, has been reported.[9] Replication of HIV may be promoted by intestinal T cells, which are usually more activated than peripheral blood T cells. Other studies have shown that plasma cell immunoglobulins A and M (IgA, IgM) are decreased in AIDS patients, suggesting less cytoplasmic immunoglobulin per cell.[10]

## ABNORMALITIES IN STRUCTURE AND FUNCTION OF THE GASTROINTESTINAL TRACT

Distinctive changes in the cellular components of the GI tract are associated with HIV infection. Previous studies have shown that activated mucosal T cells play a role in the pathogenesis of enteropathy in the human small intestine[11] and can affect the morphology of the villi and crypts in a manner similar to what is seen in patients with HIV infection. A distinct enteropathy with HIV was first described by Kotler and coworkers[12] when they studied 12 homosexual men with HIV, as well as controls. Seven of the patients had diarrhea, weight loss, an abnormally low *d*-xylose absorption, as well as steatorrhea, without evidence of intestinal infection. Jejunal and rectal biopsy specimens were obtained from all patients with diarrhea, and jejunal biopsy showed partial villus atrophy with crypt hyperplasia and increased numbers of intraepithelial lymphocytes. This was the first histologic description of a specific pathologic process that occurs in the lamina propria of the small intestine in some patients with HIV. Additionally, Ullrich and associates[13] described the small intestine's structure in adult patients with HIV. Histologically, they found low-grade small bowel atrophy and maturational defects of enterocytes in HIV-infected patients.

Recently, histologic findings in 43 children with HIV infection were reported.[14] The majority of patients had normal villus architecture, and many of the children with villus blunting had an associated intercurrent enteric infection. Distinctive features of hyperplasia of the lamina propria and increased intraepithelial lymphocytes were not apparent.

To link the altered morphology with abnormal intestinal function, Bjarnason and colleagues[15] studied intestinal inflammation and ileal structure and function in patients whose HIV infections were at various stages of progression. HIV-infected patients who were relatively asymptomatic had normal intestinal absorption and permeability, yet both functions became impaired as the disease progressed to AIDS. Patients with AIDS and diarrhea had significant malabsorption of bile acids and vitamin $B_{12}$, which was more severe than that of Crohn's ileitis. Morphometric analysis of ileal biopsies was unremarkable in patients with AIDS. These findings suggest that patients with AIDS have a low-grade enteropathy with relatively minor ileal morphologic changes and suffer severe ileal malabsorption. Malabsorption of bile acids may play a pathogenic role in these patients. The absorptive defect of AIDS enteropathy was studied using a *d*-xylose kinetic model of proximal absorption[16] and correlated with the results of a Schilling's test for cobalamin absorption, which measures distal intestinal function. There were minimal histologic abnormalities in both the proximal and distal biopsy sites in patients with diarrhea and no enteric infection. Histologically, the proximal and distal biopsy sites were similar. Absorption of *d*-xylose was low, and the absorptive defect was more severe and greater than would have been expected from histologic abnormalities found. Little information was obtained by more distal biopsy samplings. Thus, these findings support other studies that showed little association between histologic characteristics of the small bowel and its absorptive function in patients with HIV infection.

Other investigators have found some correlation between histologic abnormalities and altered GI function, yet most studies do not support a direct role for GI malabsorption in growth failure or weight loss. Ullrich and coworkers[13] described GI malabsorption in HIV-infected patients: there were low levels of lactase enzyme in the brush border, crypt death, decreased villus surface area, and fewer mitotic figures per crypt as compared with control patients. In addition, Keating and associates[17] described absorptive capacity and intestinal permeability in HIV-infected patients. Malabsorption was prevalent in all groups of patients with AIDS but was not as common in asymptomatic, "well" HIV-infected patients. Malabsorption correlated significantly with the degree of immune suppression and with body mass index. There were mild decreases in the jejunal villus height–crypt depth ratio, yet not as severe as the subtotal villus atrophy found in celiac disease. Lim and colleagues[18] found disaccharidase activity to decrease in direct proportion to increasing severity of HIV disease, although there was no association between disaccharidase levels and weight loss. In addition, Mosavi and coworkers[19] found no correlation between diarrhea and weight loss in HIV-positive patients.

Formal studies of GI absorption in children with HIV are more limited. GI malabsorption occurs frequently in HIV-infected children and may progress with the disease. In one study, 40% of children had nonphysiologic lactose malabsorption and 61% had generalized carbohydrate malabsorption that was not associated with GI symptoms or nutritional status.[20] These findings have been confirmed by others.[21] Another study in children revealed an association between diarrhea and nutrition.[22] Abnormal *d*-xylose absorption has also been associated with enteric infections in children.[20] Fat and protein loss or malabsorption have been described in children as well.

The cause of GI malabsorption in HIV infection is unclear and may be multifactorial. The cellular milieu of the lamina propria is altered significantly by HIV infection.[8] This would imply that abnormal cytokine concentrations, as well as activated cells, are present and might alter intestinal function. The depletion of the CD4-positive T lymphocytes in the intestinal tract may suggest changes in the cytokine environment. It also appears that viral load may be considerably higher in the GI tract than that measured peripherally, and this can also affect mucosal GI structure and function. Studies that suggest these hypotheses include ones by Kotler and coworkers,[23] who studied intestinal mucosal inflammation of 74 HIV-infected persons. They observed an abnormal histopathologic picture in 69% of the patients, and this finding was associated with altered bowel habits. They found high tissue P24 antigen levels, and these were correlated with more advanced HIV disease. Tissue P24 detection was associated with both altered bowel habits and histologic mucosal abnormalities. The tissue content of cytokines such as tumor necrosis factor, interferon alfa, and interleukin 1β were higher in HIV-infected individuals than in controls, and the elevations were independent of intestinal infection. They concluded that in the absence of other enteric pathogens,

HIV reactivation in the intestinal mucosa may be associated with an inflammatory bowel syndrome.

Other potential causes of GI dysfunction include the child's susceptibility to small bowel bacterial overgrowth, which can result in malabsorption. Bacterial overgrowth may be due to AIDS gastropathy,[24, 25] a condition in which the stomach produces only small amounts of hydrogen chloride, allowing bacterial pathogens to escape the acid barrier of the stomach and colonize the duodenum. Additionally, iatrogenic hypochlorhydria may be due to the administration of acid-blocking agents as treatment for ongoing peptic disease.

## INFECTIONS OF THE GASTROINTESTINAL TRACT

The GI tract is a major target for opportunistic infections in HIV-infected children. As children with HIV infection survive longer, new pathogens and previously non-pathogenic organisms are becoming increasingly problematic. Such infections include cytomegalovirus (CMV), herpes simplex virus (HSV), *Cryptosporidium*, and *Microsporidia*. The assumption that much of the diarrhea of children with HIV infection is not associated with enteric pathogens has been recently challenged. Unusual viral infections, as well as parasites, are being diagnosed with increasing frequency owing to better diagnostic techniques.

### Viral Infections

The most common GI viral pathogen in HIV-infected children is CMV. Other pathogens, such as HSV, adenovirus, Epstein-Barr virus, and a variety of other newly discovered ones can also contribute to intestinal dysfunction and diarrhea.

#### *Herpes Simplex Virus*

HSV infection in an immunocompromised child is thought to represent reactivation of a latent virus acquired earlier in life. GI infection with HSV most often involves the esophagus and is characterized by multiple, small, discrete ulcers along the esophagus. HSV can also involve other areas of the intestinal tract, including the colon and small bowel, although less frequently than the esophagus. The diagnosis of HSV relies on recognition of the multinucleate, intranuclear inclusion bodies (Cowdry type A), ground-glass appearance, and molding of the nuclei. The squamous epithelium is usually infected, although there may be involvement of intestinal glandular epithelium in the mesenchymal cells as well. HSV monoclonal antibody staining confirms the diagnosis of herpes. With extensive involvement there may be transmural necrosis and development of tracheoesophageal fistulas. Treatment of HSV is outlined in Table 31–1.

**TABLE 31–1. Primary Sites of Gastrointestinal Involvement and Treatment for Common Enteric Pathogens of HIV-Positive Children**

| PATHOGEN | DRUG |
|---|---|
| **Bacteria** | |
| *Salmonella* (SI, C) | Ampicillin, TMP-SMZ |
| *Shigella* (SI, C) | Ampicillin, TMP-SMZ |
| *Campylobacter* (SI) | Erythromycin |
| *Yersina* (SI, C) | TMP-SMZ; tetracycline |
| *Aeromonas* (SI) | |
| *C. difficile* (C) | Metronidazole, vancomycin, bacitracin |
| **Mycobacteria** | |
| *M. tuberculosis* (SI) | Isoniazid, rifampin, pyrazinamide, ethambutol, aminoglycoside |
| MAC (SI) | Clarithromycin, azithromycin, ethambutol, rifabutin, rifampin, clofazimine, amikacin, fluoroquinolones |
| **Viruses** | |
| CMV (SI, C) | Ganciclovir, foscarnet, CMV-IVIG |
| HSV (OP, E) | Acyclovir, foscarnet |
| **Fungi** | |
| *Candida albicans* (OP, E) | Fluconazole, itraconazole, ketoconazole, amphotericin B |
| *Histoplasma* (SI) | Amphotericin B, fluconazole, itraconazole |
| *Cryptococcus* (SI) | Amphotericin B, fluconazole, itraconazole |
| *P. carinii* (SI) | TMP-SMZ; pentamidine; atovaquone |
| **Parasites** | |
| *Cryptosporidium* (SI) | Azithromycin, paromomycin, octreotide, bovine hyperimmune colostrum |
| Microsporidia (SI) | Albendazole, metronidazole |
| *I. belli* (SI) | TMP-SMZ; pyrimethamine |
| *G. lamblia* (SI) | Metronidazole, furazolidone |

C, colon; CMV-IVIG, cytomegalovirus intravenous immunoglobulin; E, esophagus; OP, oropharynx; S, stomach; SI, small intestine; TMP-SMZ, trimethoprim-sulfamethoxazole.

#### *Cytomegalovirus*

CMV in an immunocompromised child is similar to HSV and represents reactivation of a latent virus acquired earlier in life. Reported incidences of GI involvement vary from a low of 4.4% up to 52% of patients studied, and this may be due to the variability in diagnosing CMV from endoscopic biopsy specimens.[26] CMV may involve any part of the GI tract but more often affects the esophagus or colon. Typically, CMV infection is represented by one or two discrete, single, large ulcers of the esophagus and colon. Lesions may lead to severe GI bleeding. CMV inclusion bodies can be discovered incidentally in an asymptomatic patient, and this does not necessarily reflect disease.

Patients with upper gastrointestinal CMV disease typically complain of dysphagia and upper abdominal symptoms, whereas colitis is more likely to present with diarrhea, which may be watery or bloody. The colitis from CMV infection is typically patchy and can be associated with severe necrotizing colitis and hemorrhage. CMV usually affects the cecum and the right colon. Diagnosis is confirmed by endoscopy and biopsy. The histologic appearance of CMV-infected cells is quite unique (Fig. 31–1). The cells are enlarged and contain intranuclear and cytoplasmic inclusion bodies. The nuclear inclusion bodies are acidophilic and are often surrounded by a halo. Cytoplasm inclusion bodies are multiple,

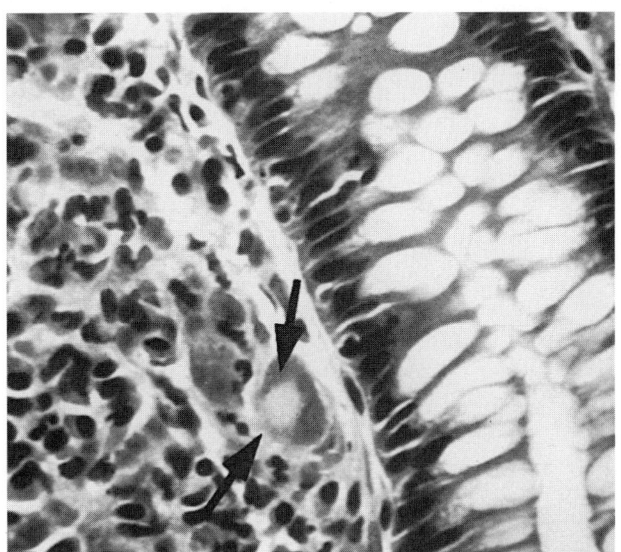

**FIGURE 31–1.** Small bowel biopsy of a child with HIV infection showing cytomegalovirus inclusion *(arrows)* within the lamina propria.

granular, and often basophilic. Cells that are dying may appear smaller and smudged and will have ill-defined inclusion bodies. Staining for CMV antigen shows that many of the infected cells are endothelial cells, many others being perivascular mesenchymal cells. CMV can cause vasculitis because of its target cell population. Thus, the spread of CMV occurs with circulating infected endothelial cells. Treatment options are outlined in Table 31–1.

### *Other Viral Infections*

Infection with unusual viral pathogens has been described. These include the human papillomavirus and Epstein-Barr virus, which have been identified in esophageal ulcers of patients with HIV. Adenovirus infections of the stomach and colon has both been reported. There are novel enteric viruses that have been associated with diarrhea in HIV-infected children.[27] These viruses, among others, include astrovirus and picornavirus. Cegielski and coworkers,[28] studying 59 children with HIV infection in Tanzania, found small round-structured viruses (SRSV) to be more common in HIV-infected than in uninfected children with chronic diarrhea. Rotavirus and coronavirus-like particles were not associated with HIV infection. The investigators felt that these SRSV may be associated with HIV infection and could lead to chronic diarrhea in Tanzanian children.

## Bacterial Infections

Bacterial infections that involve the GI tract of children with HIV infection can be divided into three groups: bacterial overgrowth of normal gut flora; pathogens that can affect immunocompromised children as well as immunocompetent ones (*Salmonella, Shigella, Campylobacter, Clostridium difficile*, and *Aeromonas*); and bacterial infections that are more common in immunocompromised children (*Mycobacterium avium intracellulare* complex [MAC]).

Very few studies have evaluated bacterial overgrowth in HIV-infected children, although there has been an association of gastric hypoacidity with opportunistic enteric infections and bacterial overgrowth in adult patients with HIV.[29] Lactose hydrogen breath testing has shown high baseline readings in children, which can suggest bacterial overgrowth in the small intestine.[20] Bacterial overgrowth in the small bowel is usually detected by quantitative duodenal aspirate for bacterial culture; therapy is directed at the organism, which is often anaerobic.

Common bacterial pathogens include *Salmonella, Shigella, Campylobacter, C. difficile*, and *Aeromonas.* These infections occur more frequently in immunocompromised patients such as children with HIV than in immunocompetent patients. HIV-infected patients with *Campylobacter* infection have also been shown to have higher rates of bacteremia than the general population. *C. difficile* colitis is more common in the immunosuppressed population. Treatment options are outlined in Table 31–1.

Intestinal infections with *Mycobacterium* include *Mycobacterium tuberculosis,* MAC, and other atypical mycobacteria. In some adult studies, MAC is the second most common pathogen recognized in biopsy specimens from the intestinal tract, occurring in 10% of patients.[30] Infection with MAC typically occurs in the very late stages of AIDS in children, typically when CD4 counts are lower than 200 cells per cubic millimeter. The most common clinical manifestation of GI infections with MAC are fever, weight loss, malabsorption, and diarrhea. Intestinal obstruction resulting from lymph node involvement and intussusception, terminal ileitis, which resembles Crohn's disease, and refractory gastric ulcers are often found. Endoscopically, fine, white nodules may be seen in the duodenum or the duodenal mucosa may look velvety and grayish. Segments of the GI tract can become infected with MAC. Histologically, there is a diffuse histiocytic infiltrate in the lamina propria with blunting of the small intestinal villi. These histiocytic infiltrates can be recognized with hematoxylin and eosin and acid-fast stains (Fig. 31–2). Appropriate therapies are outlined in Table 31–1, yet MAC infection is often frustrating to treat.

Other entities such as bacterial enteritis have been de-

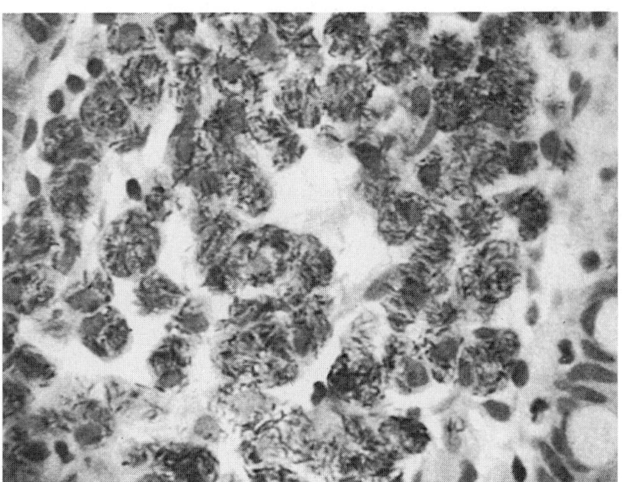

**FIGURE 31–2.** Small bowel biopsy of a child with HIV infection showing histiocytes infiltrated with *Mycobacterium avium intracellulare* within the lamina propria.

scribed in adults with HIV. A study by Orenstein and Kotler evaluated ileal and colonic biopsy specimens in AIDS patients with diarrhea[31] and found bacteria similar to adherent *Escherichia coli* along the intestinal epithelial border. Similar studies documented by Kotler's group[32] showed adherent bacteria in 17% of all adult patients with AIDS. The infection was localized principally to the cecum and right colon, and three distinct histopathologic patterns of adherence were observed: attachment on effacing lesions; bacteria intercalated between microvilli; and aggregates of bacteria attached more loosely to the damaged epithelium. The bacterial cultures of frozen rectal biopsies yielded *E. coli* in 12 of the 18 cases. These findings suggest that chronic infection with adherent bacteria can also produce the syndrome of AIDS-associated diarrhea.

## Parasitic Infections

### *Cryptosporidium parvum*

Gastrointestinal infection with *C. parvum* can occur in as many as 20% of symptomatic adult patients with HIV infection.[33] Although *Cryptosporidium* was initially isolated in animals, it was first noted to cause enterocolitis in both immunocompromised and immunocompetent humans in 1976.[34, 35] *Cryptosporidium* infection usually affects the GI tract, although it has been known to affect other organs, including the biliary tree, pancreas, gallbladder, and respiratory tract. In immunocompetent persons the diarrhea is self-limited, but in immunocompromised patients it can be protracted and associated with significant malabsorption and nutritional compromise. The small intestine is the primary target, although infection can involve any part of the intestinal tract. Esophageal cryptosporidiosis has been described in one child[36] and in adult patients. Clayton and associates[37] described two patterns of enteric cryptosporidiosis. One was associated with severe clinical disease with significant malabsorption, and the majority of the organisms were found in the proximal small bowel. Clinical disease was less severe in patients with colon disease or with infection noted only in the stool. Patients with proximal small bowel infection with *Cryptosporidium* showed crypt hyperplasia, villus atrophy, lamina propria inflammatory infiltrates, abnormal *d*-xylose absorption, more weight loss, and shorter survival, with greater need for intravenous hydration and hyperalimentation than patients with colon disease. In other studies, absorption of nutrients correlates inversely with active infection,[38] as shown by altered vitamin $B_{12}$ and *d*-xylose absorption and lactulose and mannitol urinary excretion ratios. Intestinal function improved in patients whose oocyte counts were reduced by treatment with paromomycin

In a pediatric study,[39] symptomatic cryptosporidiosis was documented in 6.4% of immunocompetent children and 22% of immunodeficient children, whereas in an asymptomatic population *Cryptosporidium* organisms were found in 4.4% of immunocompetent and 4.8% of immunodeficient children. Children were treated with spiramycin for 14 days, and the authors found a significant reduction in the shedding of infectious oocysts and reported that children treated for asymptomatic infection with *Cryptosporidium* developed no GI symptoms, whereas children who were not treated developed GI symptoms.

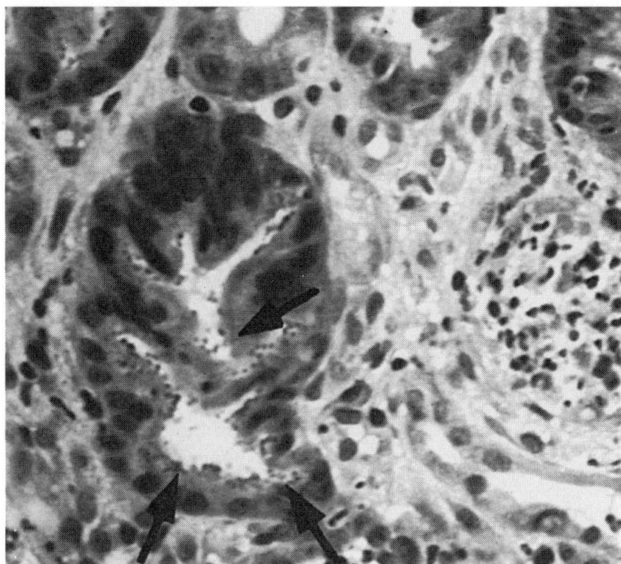

**FIGURE 31–3.** Small bowel biopsy of a child with HIV infection showing *Cryptosporidium* attached to the villus *(arrows).*

The diagnosis of cryptosporidiosis can be made by identifying the organisms in a duodenal aspirate, stool, or tissue biopsy samples. On hematoxylin and eosin–stained sections, these organisms can be found as rows or clusters of basophilic spherical structures 2 to 4 μm in diameter attached to the microvillus border of the epithelial cells (Fig. 31–3). The tips in the lateral aspect of the villi show the greatest number of organisms in the small intestine. In the colonic epithelium, crypt and surface epithelial involvement appear equal. Cryptosporidia also stain with Giemsa but not with mucous stains. The acid-fast stain on a stool sample is one of the most widely used methods for determining whether a patient has cryptosporidiosis. More recent sensitive and specific methods for diagnosing cryptosporidiosis include fluorescein-labeled IgG monoclonal antibodies.[40, 41]

Treating children with HIV infection for cryptosporidiosis can often be difficult. The disease can be chronic and protracted, with diffuse, watery diarrhea and dehydration. Several different agents have been used to eradicate the organism, with varying success. The most effective treatment is to improve immune function and nutritional status. The former may be difficult in children with HIV, although with the advent of protease inhibitor therapy it may be possible. Octreotide therapy of acute and chronic diarrhea and the resulting improvement in nutritional status eradicated cryptosporidia from one patient.[41, 42] Other investigators have used bovine hyperimmune colostrum with benefit.[43, 44] Recently, the macrolides, such as azithromycin, have shown some promise in the treatment of *Cryptosporidium* infection.[45]

### *Microsporidia*

Microsporidians are obligate intracellular protozoal parasites that infect a variety of cell types in many different animal species. The organisms were first described in 1857, when they were recognized as a cause of disease in nonhuman hosts.[46] The first description of a microsporidian, *En-*

*terocytozoon bieneusi,* as a human pathogen was in 1985, and it has since been described as a more common human pathogen.[47] This organism typically infects patients with severely depressed CD4 T lymphocyte counts. One of the largest case studies of intestinal microsporidiosis in patients with HIV infection was described by Orenstein and coworkers[48] in 67 adult patients with AIDS and AIDS-related complex and chronic, nonpathogenic diarrhea. *E. bieneusi* was diagnosed by electron microscopy in 20 of the patients; more jejunal biopsy specimens than duodenal ones were positive. The parasites and spores were clearly visible by light microscopy in 17 of the 21 specimens. Infection was confined to enterocytes located at the tip of the intestinal villus, and the histologic findings included villus atrophy, cell degeneration, necrosis, and sloughing. Other investigators[49–51] have found microsporidians in as many as 50% of HIV-infected patients with chronic and unexplained diarrhea. Other species of Microsporidia, including *Encephalitozoon (septata) intestinalis,* can cause significant enteric disease with diarrhea, malabsorption, and wasting. *E. septata intestinalis* differs from *E. bieneusi* in its tendency to disseminate and can infect enterocytes as well as macrophages, fibroblasts, and endothelial cells.

Albendazole therapy reportedly relieved clinical symptoms and eliminated microsporidian spores in the feces. Autopsy-proven clearance of microsporidians also occurred in a single patient after albendazole therapy. Other therapies show atovaquone to be an effective treatment as well.[52]

### *Isospora belli*

*I. belli* has been recognized as an opportunistic small bowel pathogen in patients with HIV infection. This organism is most common in tropical and subtropical climates. Isosporiasis can be diagnosed by identifying the oocyte in the stool or by biopsy. The diagnosis is critical, since, unlike cryptosporidiosis or microsporidiosis, therapy is very effective. *I. belli* is found within enterocytes and within the cytoplasm. The organism stains poorly, although the central nucleus, large nucleolus, and perinuclear halo give it a characteristic appearance. The infection produces mucosal atrophy and tissue eosinophilia. A 10-day course of trimethoprim-sulfamethoxazole (TMP-SMX) is effective therapy, and recurrence can be prevented by ongoing prophylaxis with the same drug. Other therapies for *Isospora* infection include pyrimethamine, especially for patients with sulfa allergy.[53]

### Other Parasites

Infection by *Blastocystis hominis,* which is usually considered a nonpathogenic parasite, has been described in patients with chronic diarrhea and HIV. This organism is more pathogenic for immunocompromised patients and can cause mild, prolonged diarrhea or recurrent diarrhea. Effective therapy include diiodohydroxyquin, 650 mg orally tid for 21 days in adults and children older than 12 years. Other protozoans that can infect HIV-infected patients include *Entamoeba histolytica, Entamoeba coli, Entamoeba hartmanni, Endolimax nana, Giardia lamblia* (and others in 4% of the cases).

## Fungal Infections

### *Candida albicans*

Candidiasis of the GI tract is the most common fungal infection in HIV-infected children. In children with HIV, the esophagus is the principal target of *Candida* organisms, and the majority of patients develop esophageal candidiasis during the course of their illness. It is also an AIDS-defining disease, second only in prevalence to *Pneumocystis carinii* pneumonia. Patients with *Candida* esophagitis complain of odynophagia or dysphagia and often have vomiting and recurrent abdominal pain. Children often have oral thrush intercurrent with more disseminated and invasive *Candida* esophagitis, although the absence of oral thrush does not preclude the diagnosis of *Candida* esophagitis in children.[14] Histopathologically, invasive disease is documented by yeast forms within intact mucosa, compared with colonization, where the yeast is found on intact mucosal surfaces or necrotic tissue. These organisms are best seen by Gomori's methenamine silver or periodic acid–Schiff (PAS) stain. Upper GI studies can suggest *Candida* esophagitis when diffuse mucosal irregularities are seen on radiographs (Fig. 31–4). The most sensitive test for invasive candidiasis of the esophagus includes upper gastrointestinal endoscopy and biopsy with appropriate staining. Candidiasis can affect the stomach and the small bowel if the acid barrier has been suppressed, either through decreased gastric acid production or iatrogenically with potent acid blockers. Numerous effective therapies have been described to treat *Candida* infection of the upper

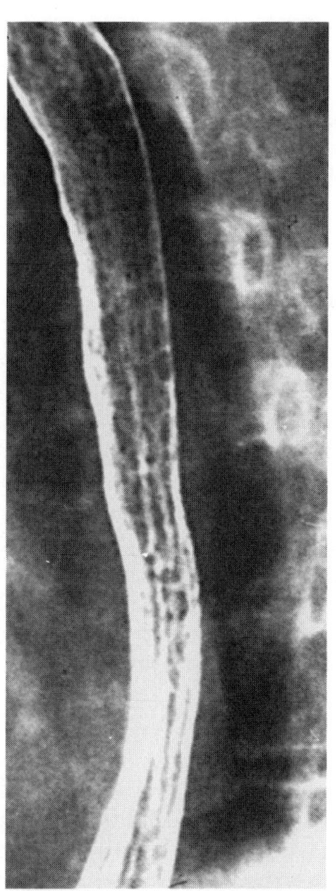

**FIGURE 31–4.** Radiographic contrast study showing mucosal irregularities seen with *Candida* esophagitis.

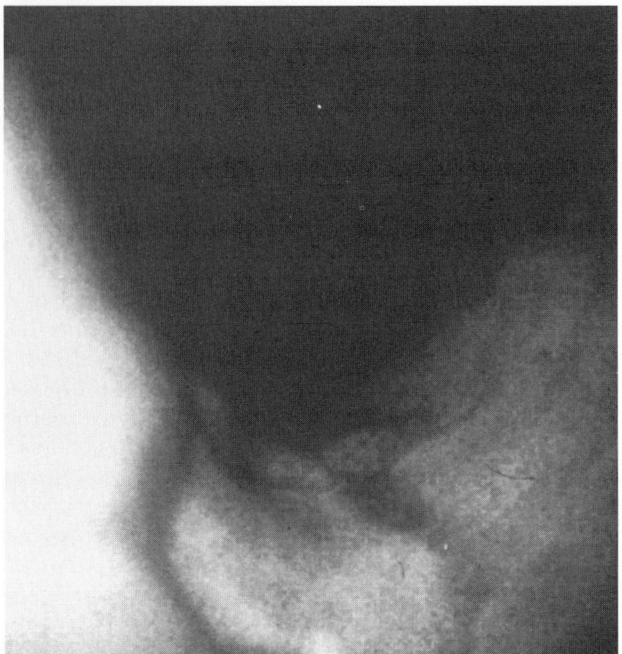

**FIGURE 31–5.** Endoscopic view of the esophagus in an HIV-infected child with a large, idiopathic esophageal ulcer.

gastrointestinal tract, including fluconazole and ketoconazole. Ketoconazole has more hepatic side effects than fluconazole. Finally, for very severe and invasive disease, either topical or intravenous amphotericin can be used. Agents such as oral miconazole or nystatin are not indicated for invasive *Candida.*

### *Other Fungal Infections*

Some 5% of adult patients with AIDS in the American Midwest develop disseminated histoplasmosis. There is enterocolitis associated with infection, and at colonoscopy plaques, ulcers, pseudopolyps, and skip areas are frequently seen. Cryptococcal GI disease has been identified in patients with disseminated *Cryptococcus* infection. The esophagus and colon are involved most frequently. *P. carinii* infection involving the GI tract has been described as well.[54] GI pneumocystosis develops after hematogenous or lymphatic dissemination from the lungs or reactivation of latent GI infection. The administration of aerosolized pentamidine has increased the risk of extrapulmonary spread of *P. carinii. P. carinii* infection can occur throughout the GI tract. In the lamina propria are foamy exudates that contain *P. carinii* organisms. Although more rarely, infection of the colon can cause diarrhea.

## NONINFECTIOUS CHRONIC DIARRHEA

In as many as 15% to 25% of HIV-infected children, the cause of their diarrhea is indeterminate. It is possible that these children have infectious diarrhea from a pathogen that escapes detection. Rarer viruses have been described that could cause chronic diarrhea. Autonomic dysfunction is another potential mechanism of noninfectious diarrhea not previously described. Clinically, children with autonomic neuropathy have sweating, urinary retention, and abnormal cardiovascular hemodynamics. It is possible that this autonomic denervation contributes to the diarrhea in patients with HIV infection, as Griffin and coworkers have suggested,[55] who applied neuron-specific polyclonal antibodies to jejunal specimens. There was a significant reduction in axonal density in both villi and pericryptal lamina propria in patients with HIV infection as compared with controls, and the reduction was greater in patients with diarrhea.

## IDIOPATHIC ESOPHAGEAL ULCERATION

Esophageal ulceration in children with HIV is typically a result of an intercurrent opportunistic infection. Idiopathic oral and esophageal ulcers have been described in both children and adults with HIV. These ulcers are characteristically large and may be single or multiple (Fig. 31–5). They are located in the middle to distal esophagus. Whether HIV itself is involved in the pathogenesis of these ulcers is a matter of controversy.[56] Treatment options for these ulcers are limited but include steroid therapy (which has produced encouraging results[57]) and thalidomide.[58] A significant portion of children receiving thalidomide develop a rash that precludes therapeutic use of the drug.

## CLINICAL MANAGEMENT OF GASTROINTESTINAL DISORDERS

The diagnostic approach to the child with GI symptoms is outlined in Table 31–2. A comprehensive clinical and nutritional history should be taken. Growth history should be reviewed. The physical examination should focus on an assessment of nutritional status and the possibility of intestinal or hepatobiliary disease. Every HIV-infected child with diarrheal symptoms should have a complete evaluation for bowel pathogens before any other diagnostic studies, as

**TABLE 31–2. Approach to Diagnosis of Gastrointestinal Tract Disease in HIV-Infected Children**

**Preliminary Evaluation**

1. Complete history and physical examination
   - Calorie intake, anthropometrics, GI symptoms
   - Oropharyngx, abdominal and rectal examinations
2. Evaluation for enteric pathogens
   - Bacterial, viral, parasite cultures, stool examination

**Secondary Evaluation**

1. Malabsorption studies
   - Hydrogen breath test analysis
   - Fecal fat determination
   - *d*-Xylose absorption
   - Stool alpha$_1$-antitrypsin
2. Radiographic studies (contrast, ultrasound)

**Tertiary Evaluation**

1. Upper gastrointestinal tract endoscopy
   - Biopsy specimens for H&E staining
   - Brushings for cytology
   - Duodenal aspirate (for quantitative bacterial culture, ova and parasite)
   - Electron microscopy

treatment of the pathogen may resolve the symptoms. Evaluations for enteric infections should include studies for the organisms outlined in the preceding section on infectious diarrhea. The clinician should keep in mind that children with active enteric infections can also have secondary problems with malabsorption. If the clinical history and physical examination are suspicious for GI malabsorption without enteric infection, the next step should be a lactose breath hydrogen test, which measures hydrogen production as a response to an oral lactose load. Elevated baseline breath hydrogen value or early peak of hydrogen production suggests bacterial overgrowth. Testing *d*-xylose absorption also helps to determine the absorptive capacity of the GI tract. Fat malabsorption is determined by a 72-hour fecal fat collection.

If noninvasive studies such as those described above are not helpful in documenting and determining the cause of the malabsorption disorder, endoscopy with biopsy and a quantitative bacterial culture of the duodenal fluid may be useful. We have found that a histologic abnormality is confirmed in 72% of children who undergo endoscopy, and clinical management is changed in 70% of them because of the endoscopic evaluation.[14] A high diagnostic yield has been supported by other investigators as well.[59] Specific gastrointestinal symptoms have not been predictive of abnormal endoscopic findings; rather, advanced-stage HIV disease and increased numbers of symptoms seem to be more predictive.[14] Histologic studies of the small bowel may help to determine the degree of villus blunting, and electron microscopy and special staining for opportunistic pathogens can be performed. Samples for quantitative bacterial cultures and parasite evaluation of the duodenal fluid should be obtained when endoscopy is performed. Characteristically, the detection of more than $10^5$ organisms per milliliter of duodenal fluid confirms bacterial overgrowth. It is important to obtain both anaerobic and quantitative cultures.

Treatment of intestinal infections has been outlined in Table 31–1 and in previous sections. When symptomatic lactose malabsorption is found, a lactose-free diet is initiated. Children can limit lactose in their diet by taking exogenous lactase or lactase-treated milk. For malabsorption of protein and fat, a protein hydrolysate diet should be tried. Many of these supplements are tolerated poorly because they are unpalatable. In many circumstances, special supplements may need to be administered through a feeding tube.[60, 61]

## OTHER SECONDARY IMMUNODEFICIENCIES

A variety of other disorders (Table 31–3) can cause secondary immunodeficiency with effects on the gastrointestinal tract. Overall, these disorders are more prevalent than either primary or HIV-associated immunodeficiencies. Premature infants, children with cancer and associated exposure to immunosuppressant and cytotoxic medications (including graft-versus-host disease), and children with protein-losing enteropathy and associated loss of immunoglobulins from the gastrointestinal tract can all be immunodeficient because of the underlying disorder. In general, children with these immunodeficiencies are at risk for many of the same complications experienced by children with HIV infection.

**TABLE 31–3. Secondary Causes of Immunodeficiencies Known to Affect the Gastrointestinal Tract**

| |
|---|
| Prematurity |
| Malnutrition, micronutrient deficiency |
| Immunosuppression |
| Graft-versus-host disease |
| Protein-losing enteropathy |
| Inflammatory bowel disease |
| Malignancy |

### Malnutrition and Micronutrient Deficiencies

Malnutrition is the most common cause of immunodeficiency worldwide. Before HIV was described, *P. carinii* pneumonia and Kaposi's sarcoma, known opportunistic diseases, were first described in otherwise healthy but malnourished children and adults in developing nations.[62, 63] This association led investigators to conclude that nutrition alone can affect the human immune response. Malnourished children exhibit profound involution of lymphoid tissues, including thymic atrophy and diminished paracortical regions of lymph nodes.[64] In young infants and children, protein-calorie malnutrition increases the risk of death severalfold by increasing susceptibility to infection.[65] In many countries, mortality rates increase from 0.5% in children whose weight-for-height percentage of standard is greater than 80%, to a mortality rate of 18% in children whose weight-for-height percentage of standard is less than 60%.[66] In other diseases such as cystic fibrosis and cancer, nutritional status has been linked closely to survival rates and morbidity. In leukemia and lymphoma patients, the incidence of infection with *P. carinii* is higher in those with protein-calorie malnutrition.[62]

Biochemically, protein-calorie malnutrition leads to changes in several aspects of the immune system. Cell-mediated immunity, microbial function of phagocytes, complement systems, secretory antibodies, and antibody affinity are consistently impaired in patients with significant malnutrition. Additionally, deficiencies of micronutrients, especially zinc and iron, as well as many others, may also have deleterious effects on the immune system. Other immune alterations secondary to protein-calorie malnutrition include impaired chemotaxis of neutrophils, decreased lysozyme levels in serum and secretions, and interferon production in antibody response to T cell–dependent antigens. A child with protein-calorie malnutrition may also have impaired mucosal immunity with lower concentrations of secretory IgA in saliva, nasopharynx, tears, and GI tract, as compared with well-nourished control children.

As in children and adults with HIV infection, T cell function is depressed not only in the peripheral circulation but in the intestinal tract as well. Subsequently, plasma cell function and macrophage activity may be impaired, leading to more frequent intestinal infections in children with severe protein-calorie malnutrition. Not only does nutrition improve the immune function of the intestinal tract, but nutrients themselves are trophic and essential for the maintenance of the absorptive capacity of the intestines. In some studies, weight loss of more than 30%, due to other disorders, was associated with a reduction in pancreatic enzyme secretion of over 80%, villus atrophy, and impaired carbohydrate and fat absorption.[67] These disorders are promptly reversed with appropriate nutritional rehabilitation. In addition, with villus blunting, increased antigen uptake can also occur, leaving the child at higher risk for enteric infections. The pathogenesis of villus blunting is currently unclear, but it may be due to crypt hyperplasia as the primary event with premature sloughing at the villus tip[68]; alternatively, there may be loss of enterocytes at the villus tip with resultant proliferation at the crypts.[69]

## Immunosuppressive Therapy

Immunosuppressant medications are the mainstay of therapy for many children with autoimmune disorders, inflammatory bowel disease, chronic pulmonary disease, cancer, and organ transplantation. The best-known immunosuppressants are corticosteroids, azathioprine, cyclosporin, tacrolimus, and antithymocyte globulin. Unfortunately, these medications' effects are not targeted to specific organs; rather, they suppress immune function indiscriminately throughout the child. Thus, several immune malfunctions, including decreased monocyte adherence, neutrophil chemotaxis, and overall suppression of the inflammatory response are found. Children are at risk for enteric infections similar to those described in children with HIV infection.

### REFERENCES


1. Gallo RC, Salahuddin SZ, Popovic M, et al: Frequent detection and isolation of cytopathic retroviruses (HTLV-III) from patients with AIDS and at risk for AIDS. Science 1984; 224:500–503.
2. Centers for Disease Control and Prevention: AIDS among children—United States, 1996. MMWR 1996; 45:1005–1010.
3. Davis SF, Byers RH Jr, Lindegren ML, et al: Prevalence and incidence of vertically transmitted acquired human immunodeficiency virus infection in the United States. JAMA 1995; 274:952–955.
4. Fauci AS: Multifactorial nature of human immunodeficiency virus disease: implications for therapy. Science 1993; 262:1011.
5. Nelson JA, Wiley CA, Reynolds-Kohler C, et al: Human immunodeficiency virus detected in bowel epithelium from patients with gastrointestinal symptoms. Lancet 1988; 1:259–262.
6. Fox C, Kotler D, Tierney A, et al: Detection of HIV-1 RNA in the lamina propria of patients with AIDS and gastrointestinal disease. J Infect Dis 1989; 159:467–471.
7. Adachi A, Koenig S, Gendelman HE, et al: Productive, persistent infection of human colorectal cell lines with HIV. J Virol 1987; 61:209–211.
8. Schneider T, Jahn HU, Schmidt W, et al: Loss of CD4 T lymphocytes in patients infected with human immunodeficiency virus type 1 is more pronounced in the duodenal mucosa than in the peripheral blood. Gut 1995; 37:524–529.
9. Kotler DP, Reka S, Borcich A, Cronin WJ: Detection, localization, and quantitation of HIV-associated antigens in the intestinal biopsies from patients with human immunodeficiency virus. Am J Pathol 1991; 139:823–830.
10. Kotler DP, Scholes JV, Tierney AR: Intestinal plasma cell alterations in the acquired immunodeficiency syndrome. Dig Dis Sci 1987; 32:129–138.
11. MacDonald T, Spencer J: Evidence that activated mucosal T-cells play a role in the pathogenesis of enteropathy in human small intestine. J Exp Med 1988; 167:1341–1349.
12. Kotler DP, Gaetz HP, Lange M, et al: Enteropathy associated with the acquired immunodeficiency syndrome. Ann Intern Med 1984; 104:421–428.
13. Ullrich R, Zeitz M, Heise W, et al: Small intestinal structure and function in patients infected with human immunodeficiency virus (HIV): evidence for HIV-induced enteropathy. Ann Intern Med 1989; 111:15–21.
14. Miller TL, McQuinn LB, Orav ZEJ: Endoscopy of the upper gastrointestinal tract as a diagnostic tool for children with human immunodeficiency infection. J Pediatr 1997; 130:766–773.
15. Bjarnason I, Sharpstone DR, Frances DR, et al: Intestinal inflammation, ileal structure and function in HIV. AIDS 1996; 10:1385–1391.
16. Carlson S, Yokoo H, Craig RM: Small intestinal human immunodeficiency virus–associated enteropathy: evidence for panintestinal enterocyte dysfunction. Lab Clin Med 1994; 124:652–659.
17. Keating J, Bjarnason I, Somasundaram S, et al: Intestinal absorptive capacity, intestinal permeability and jejunal histology in human immunodeficiency virus and their relation to diarrhea. Gut 1995; 37:623–629.
18. Lim SG, Menzles IS, Nukajam WS, et al: Intestinal disaccharidase activity in human immunodeficiency virus disease. Scand J Gastroenterol 1995; 30:235–241.
19. Mosavi AJ, Hussain MF, DuPont HL, et al: Lack of correlation between diarrhea and weight loss in HIV-positive outpatients in Houston, Texas. J Clin Gastroenterol 1995; 21:61–64.
20. Miller TL, Orav EJ, Martin SR, et al: Malnutrition and carbohydrate malabsorption in children with vertically-transmitted human immunodeficiency virus-1 infection. Gastroenterology 1991; 100:1296–1302.
21. The Italian Pediatric Intestinal HIV Study Group: Intestinal malabsorption of HIV-infected children: relationship to diarrhoea, failure to thrive, enteric micro-organisms and immune impairment. AIDS 1993; 7:1435–1440.
22. Yolken RH, Hart W, Oung I, et al: Gastrointestinal dysfunction and disaccharide intolerance in children infected with human immunodeficiency virus. J Pediatr 1991; 118:359–363.
23. Kotler DP, Reka S, Clayton F: Intestinal mucosal inflammation associated with human immunodeficiency virus infection. Dig Dis Sci 1993; 38:1119–1127.
24. Lake-Bakaar G, Quadros E, Beidas S, et al: Gastric secretory failure in patients with the acquired immunodeficiency syndrome (AIDS). Ann Intern Med 1988; 109:502–504.
25. Lake-Bakaar G, Tom W, Lake-Bakaar D, et al: Gastropathy and ketoconazole malabsorption in the acquired immunodeficiency syndrome (AIDS). Ann Intern Med 1988; 109:471–473.
26. Smith PD, Lane HC, Gill VJ, et al: Intestinal infections in patients with the acquired immunodeficiency syndrome (AIDS): etiology and response to therapy. Ann Intern Med 1988; 108:328–333.
27. Grohmann GS, Glass RI, Pereira HG, et al: Enteric viruses and diarrhea in HIV-infected patients. N Engl J Med 1993; 329:14–20.
28. Cegielski JP, Msengi AE: Enteric viruses associated with HIV infection in Tanzanian children with chronic diarrhea. Pediatric AIDS and Infectious Disease: Fetus to Adolescent 1994; 5:296–299.
29. Belitsos PC, Greenson JK, Yardley JH, et al: Association of gastric hypoacidity with opportunistic enteric infections in 12 patients with AIDS. J Infect Dis 1992; 166:277–284.
30. Vazquez M, Rotterdam H, Vamvakas E: Diagnostic yields of surgical specimens from patients with AIDS or at risk for AIDS. Prog AIDS Pathol 1990; 2:187–194.
31. Orenstein JM, Kotler DP: Diarrheogenic bacterial enteritis in acquired immunodeficiency syndrome: a light and electron microscopy study of 52 cases. Hum Pathol 1995; 26:481–492.
32. Kotler DP, Giang TT, Thiim M, et al: Chronic bacterial enteropathy in patients with AIDS. J Infect Dis 1995; 171:552–558.
33. Rene E, Marche C, Regnier B, et al: Intestinal infections in patients with AIDS. A prospective study in 132 patients. Dig Dis Sci, 1989; 34:774–780.
34. Nime FA, Burek JD, Page DL, et al: Acute enterocolitis in a human being infected with the protozoon *Cryptosporidium.* Gastroenterology 1976; 70:592–598.
35. Meisel JL, Perera DR, Meligro C, Rubin CE: Overwhelming watery diarrhea associated with a *Cryptosporidium* in an immune compromised patient. Gastroenterology 1976; 70:1156–1160.
36. Kazlow PG, Shah K, Benkov KJ, et al: Oesophageal cryptosporidiosis in a child with acquired immunodeficiency syndrome. Gastroenterology 1986; 91:1301–1303.
37. Clayton F, Heller T, Kotler DP: Variation in the enteric distribution of *cryptosporidia* in acquired immunodeficiency syndrome. Am J Clin Pathol 1994; 102:420–425.
38. Goodgame RW, Kimball K, Ou CN, et al: Intestinal function and injury

in acquired immunodeficiency-related cryptosporidiosis. Gastroenterology 1995; 108:1075–1082.

39. Pettoello-Mantovani M, DiMartino L, Dettori G, et al: Asymptomatic carriage of intestinal *Cryptosporidia* in immunocompetent and immunodeficent children. A prospective study. Pediatr Infect Dis J 1995; 14:1042–1047.
40. Soave R, Johnson WD Jr: *Cryptosporidium* and *Isospora belli* infections. J Infect Dis 1988; 157:225–229.
41. Kreinik G, Burstein O, Landor M, et al: Successful management of intractable cryptosporidial disease with intravenous octreotide, a somatostatin analogue. AIDS 1991; 5:765–767.
42. Simon D, Weiss L, Tanowitz HB, Wittner M: Resolution of *Cryptosporidium* infection in an AIDS patient after improvement of nutritional and immune status with octreotide. Am J Gastroenterol 1991; 86:615–618.
43. Nord J, Ma P, DiJohn D, et al: Treatment with bovine hyperimmune colostrum of cryptosporidial diarrhea in AIDS patients. AIDS 1990; 4:581–584.
44. Ungar BL, Ward DJ, Fayer R, Quinn CA: Cessation of *Cryptosporidium*-associated diarrhea in an acquired immunodeficiency patient after treatment with hyperimmune bovine colostrum. Gastroenterology 1990; 98:486–489.
45. Hicks P, Zwiener RJ, Squires J, Savell V: Azithromycin therapy for *Cryptosporidium parvum* infection in 4 children infected with HIV. J Pediatr 1996; 129:297–300.
46. Bryan RT, Cali A: *Microsporidia:* opportunistic pathogens in patients with AIDS. In Sun T (ed): Progress in Clinical Parasitology. New York, Field and Wood, 1990, pp 1–26.
47. Desportes I, LeCharpentier Y, Galian A, et al: Occurrence of a new microsporidian: *Enterocytozoon bieneusi* ng. n. sp., in the enterocytes of a human patient with AIDS. J Protozool 1985; 32:250–254.
48. Orenstein JM, Chiang J, Steinberg W, et al: Intestinal microsporidiosis as a cause of diarrhea in human immunodeficiency virus infected patients: a report of 20 cases. Hum Pathol 1990; 21:475–481.
49. Molina JM, Sarfati C, Beauvais B, et al: Intestinal microsporidiosis in HIV-infected patients with chronic unexplained diarrhea: prevalence and clinical biological features. J Infect Dis 1993; 167:217–221.
50. Coyle CM, Wittner M, Kotler DP, et al: Prevalence of microsporidiosis due to *Enterocytozoon bieneusi* and *Enterocytozoon (septata) intestinalis* among patients with AIDS-related diarrhea: determination of polymerase chain reaction to the microsporidian small-subunit rRNA gene. Clin Infect Dis 1996; 23:1002–1006.
51. Kotler DP, Orenstein JM: Prevalence of intestinal microsporidiosis in HIV-infected individual referred for gastroenterological evaluation. Am J Gastroenterol 1994; 89:1998–2002.
52. Anwar-Bruni DM, Hogan SE, Schwartz DA, et al: Atovaquone is effective treatment for the symptoms of gastrointestinal microsporidiosis in human immundeficiency virus-1 infected patients. AIDS 1996; 10:619–623.
53. Weiss LM, Perlman DC, Sherman J, et al: *Isospora belli* infection: treatment with pyrimethamine. Ann Intern Med 1988; 109:474–475.
54. Ramos-Soriano AG, Saavedra JM, Wu TC, et al: Enteric pathogens associated with gastrointestinal dysfunction in children with HIV infection. Mol Cell Probes 1996; 10:67–73.
55. Griffin GE, Miller A, Batman P, et al: Damage to jejunal intrinsic autonomic nerves in HIV infection. AIDS 1988; 2:379–382.
56. Wilcox CM, Schwartz DA, Clark WS: Esophageal ulceration in human immunodeficiency virus infection. Ann Intern Med 1995; 123:143–149.
57. Kotler DP, Reka S, Orenstein JM, Fox CH: Chronic idiopathic esophageal ulceration in the acquired immunodeficiency syndrome. Characterization and treatment with corticosteroids. J Clin Gastroenterol 1992; 15:284–290.
58. Naum SM, Molloy PJ, Kania RJ, et al: Use of thalidomide in treatment and maintenance of idiopathic esophageal ulcers in HIV+ individuals. Dig Dis Sci 1995; 40:1147–1148.
59. Bashir RM, Wilcox CM: Symptom-specific use of upper gastrointestinal endoscopy in human immunodeficiency virus–infected patients yields high dividends. J Clin Gastroenterol 1996; 23:292–298.
60. Miller TL, Awnetwant EL, Evans S, et al: Gastrostomy tube supplementation for HIV-infected children. Pediatrics 1995; 96:696–702.
61. Henderson RA, Saavedra JM, Perman JA, et al: Effect of enteral tube feeding on growth of children with symptomatic human immunodeficiency virus infection. J Pediatr Gastroenterol Nutr 1994; 18:429–434.
62. Chandra RK (ed): Immunocompetence of Nutritional Disorders. London, Arnold, 1980.
63. Centers for Disease Control: Task Force on Kaposi's Sarcoma and Opportunistic Infections: epidemiologic aspects of the current outbreak of Kaposi's sarcoma and opportunistic infection. N Engl J Med 1982; 306:248–252.
64. Chandra RK, Newbuerne PM: Nutrition, Immunity and Infection: Mechanisms of Interactions. New York, Plenum, 1977.
65. Scrimshaw NS, Taylor CE, Gordon JE.: Interactions of nutrition and infection. WHO Monogr Ser 1968; 57.
66. Hughes WT, Price RA, Sisko F, et al: Protein-calorie malnutrition: a host determinant for *Pneumocystis carinii* infection. Am J Dis Child 1974; 128:44–52.
67. O'Keefe SJ: Nutrition and gastrointestinal disease. Scand J Gastroenterol 1996; 220S:52–59.
68. MacDonald TT: Pathogenesis of intestinal inflammation. In Pediatric Gastrointestinal Disease: Pathophysiology, Diagnosis, and Management. Philadelphia, BC Decker, 1991.
69. Booth CC: The enterocyte in celiac disease. Br Med J 1970; 3:725–731.

# Chapter 32

# Crohn's Disease

*Jeffrey S. Hyams*

Despite more than 60 years of observation and research since its classic description in 1932 by Crohn, Ginzburg, and Oppenheimer,[1] the cause of Crohn's disease remains unknown. This chapter provides an overview of the current understanding of possible pathogenetic mechanisms involved in Crohn's disease, describes its pathologic and clinical expression, and provides a detailed guideline to its management.

## EPIDEMIOLOGY

Insidious onset of disease, lack of universal diagnostic criteria, and occasional misclassification of patients has made the study of the epidemiology of inflammatory bowel disease (IBD) difficult.[2] Reports of adults have indicated greatly disparate trends in the incidence of this disorder.[3–5] A threefold increase (to 3.11 cases per 100,000 population per year) in the incidence of Crohn's disease in children has been noted in Wales, while the incidence of ulcerative colitis remained constant (0.71/100,000 per year).[6] In France, four new cases of Crohn's disease have been noted for each new case of ulcerative colitis.[7] The prevalence of IBD in children younger than 15 years of age in Wales was 20 per 100,000 population; the comparable rates for Crohn's disease and ulcerative colitis were 16.6 and 3.4, respectively.

Crohn's disease affects males and females equally; it is more common in whites than in nonwhites, in northern than in southern areas, and in urban than in rural areas.[8] It is more common in Jews than in non-Jews, and in the Jewish population the disease is more common in families of middle European origin compared with those of Polish or Russian origin.[9] Crohn's disease occurs with a higher frequency in patients with Turner's syndrome, Hermansky-Pudlak syndrome, and glycogen storage disease type 1B.

Passive smoking exposure and maternal smoking at birth increased the likelihood of developing IBD (particularly Crohn's disease) in one study,[10] but another study showed no such relation.[11] Breast feeding has been noted to be negatively associated with the development of Crohn's disease,[11] although this observation remains controversial. Viral infections in early life have been noted to be associated with the future development of IBD,[12] although conditions of improved domestic hygiene in infancy have been associated with a higher likelihood of disease.[13] Finally, a Swedish study suggested that the consumption of "fast foods" at least twice a week, daily ingestion of soft drinks, or increased consumption of sucrose were each associated with an increased risk of developing Crohn's disease.[14]

## ETIOLOGY

### Genetic Observations

The single greatest known risk factor for the development of IBD is having a first-degree relative with Crohn's disease or ulcerative colitis. For a first-degree relative of a proband with Crohn's disease, the age-adjusted risk of developing Crohn's disease during a lifetime is about 4%, with a slightly greater risk for females than for males.[15] Daughters of a person with Crohn's disease have a 12.6% lifetime risk of developing IBD, compared with a 7.9% risk for male offspring.[15] At the time of diagnosis of Crohn's disease, the likelihood of finding IBD in a first-degree relative of the proband is 10% to 25%.[15, 16] Concordance in monozygotic twins is greater for Crohn's disease than for insulin-dependent diabetes, asthma, or schizophrenia.[17] Studies of families with multiple affected members[18–21] have suggested genetic anticipation (earlier onset of disease, increased severity, or both, in succeeding generations of affected families).[20, 21] Clustering of disease among siblings noted in one study was suggested to imply an infectious cause.[18]

Crohn's disease is not inherited in a simple Mendelian manner or in a polygenic fashion (multiple genes, each with a small effect).[22] An oligogenic model (limited number of genes acting together) has been proposed, as has a genetic-heterogeneity model.[23] Human leukocyte antigen studies have revealed evidence for genetic heterogeneity in IBD.[24, 25] The alleles DRB1*01 and DRB1*07 were associated with increased "susceptibility" to Crohn's disease, whereas DRB1*03 had a strong negative association with this disorder.[25] It has been suggested that susceptibility loci for Crohn's disease may exist on chromosomes 6[26] and 16.[27] Within close distance to the chromosome 16 locus are genes involved in complement receptors, mycobacterial cell adhesion, B lymphocyte function, leukocyte adhesion, and the interleukin-4 (IL-4) receptor.[24]

## Infection

Conflicting data continue to arise concerning a potential role for *Mycobacterium paratuberculosis.* DNA from the organism has been found in Crohn's disease tissue in some studies[28] but not in others.[29] Immunocytochemistry has demonstrated the presence of *Listeria, Escherichia coli,* and *Streptococcus* in Crohn's disease tissue, but it is unclear whether these organisms were part of the primary disease process or secondary invaders of damaged tissue.[30]

Other studies have focused on a potential relation between measles virus infection resulting in microvascular injury and the pathogenesis of Crohn's disease.[31–33] It has been proposed that measles infection early in life, in genetically susceptible individuals, causes a granulomatous vasculitis of the mesenteric vessels, leading to microvascular thrombosis, multifocal gastrointestinal infarction, and, eventually, gross pathologic sequelae such as inflammation, fistulas, fibrosis, and strictures.[31] IBD occurs less frequently than expected in persons with hemophilia or von Willebrand's disease, inherited disorders of coagulation that might be expected to protect against microvascular thrombosis.[34]

## Immunologic Mechanisms

As depicted in Figure 32–1, an antigenic presence, of either dietary or infectious origin, stimulates the normally rich immune system of the intestinal mucosa. Mucosal inflammation occurs in a controlled and protective fashion ("physiologic inflammation"), and in a normal host the inflammation is self-limited. It has been proposed that in certain genetically susceptible hosts, or in someone with previous mucosal injury, the inflammatory cascade is not self-limited, and the continued production of inflammatory mediators by activated immune cells leads to tissue injury and fibrosis characteristic of IBD.[35] Increased intestinal permeability has been suggested as a factor that may allow increased antigenic stimulation of the gut.[36]

Activated immune cells present in the intestinal mucosa secrete a number of soluble mediators of inflammation, including cytokines, arachidonic acid metabolites, reactive oxygen intermediates, and growth factors.[37, 38] Increased mucosal levels of proinflammatory cytokines have been found in mucosa from patients with Crohn's disease,[39] as have decreased levels of the inhibitory IL-4.[40] A diminished ratio of

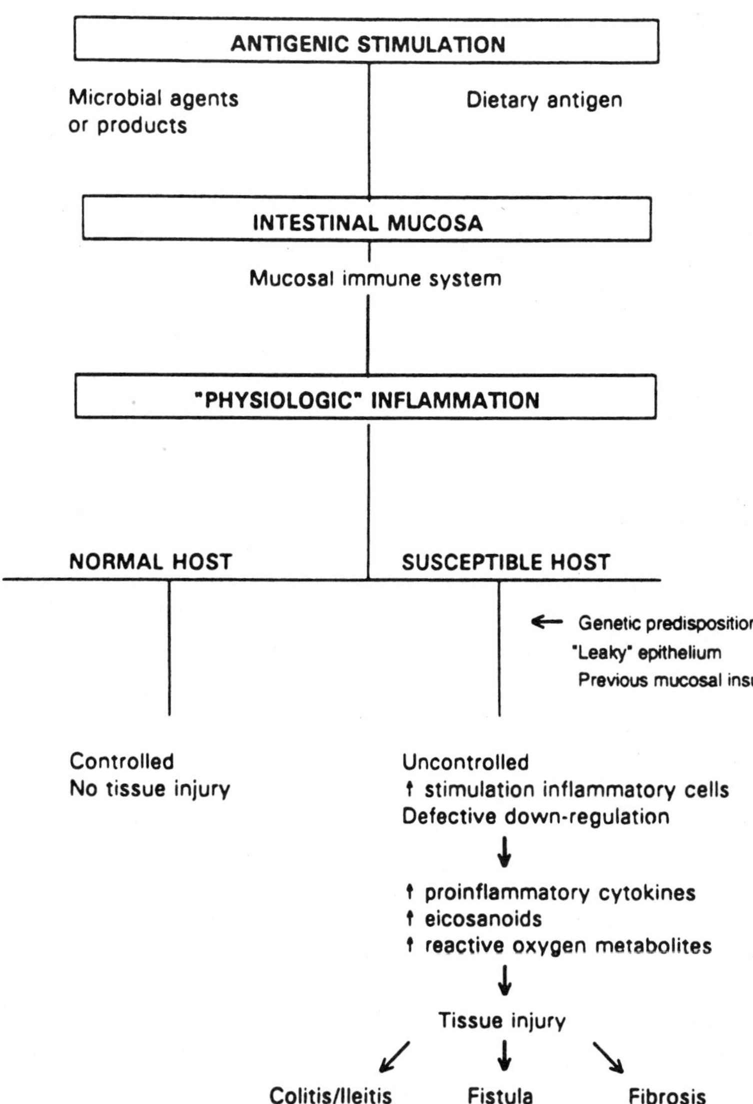


**FIGURE 32–1.** Proposed schema for the pathogenesis of Crohn's disease. (Adapted from Hyams JS: Crohn's disease. Pediatr Clin North Am 1996;43:257, with permission.)

IL-1 receptor antagonist to IL-1β in inflamed tissue has been reported.[41] Effects of proinflammatory cytokines (IL-1, IL-6, IL-8, tumor necrosis factor-α) include recruitment of inflammatory cells through increased expression of vascular adhesion cell molecules,[42] increased neutrophil eicosanoid production,[43] eosinophil degranulation,[44] induction of nitric oxide synthase in macrophages and neutrophils,[45] and increased collagen production.[46] Reactive oxygen metabolites produced by neutrophils are potent cytotoxins and cause cell injury or death.[45] Products of inflammatory cells such as histamine, prostaglandins, and leukotrienes cause chloride secretion by epithelial cells, contributing to diarrhea.[47]

T cell populations extracted from Crohn's disease tissue overproduce interferon-γ and underproduce IL-4 when stimulated in vitro.[48] This has prompted labeling of Crohn's disease as a disorder characterized by an abnormal $T_{H1}$ (T helper 1) response.[48, 49] A dysregulated $T_{H1}$ response to common luminal bacterial antigens may be crucial to the conversion of physiologic to pathologic inflammation. In a germ-free rat model of colitis, *Bacteroides* species were most responsible for inducing a chronic inflammatory response.[50]

## Neuroendocrine Mechanisms

The neuroendocrine system starts with the hypothalamic-pituitary axis and ends with the enteric nervous system and intestinal immune cells. The production of neuropeptides, including substance P, vasoactive intestinal peptide, and somatostatin, is affected by cytokines, and these products in turn may alter cytokine production.[51] These neuropeptides affect intestinal motility, increase water and electrolyte secretion, and activate mast cells. The potential relation between stress or emotional state and disease activity in IBD may have its foundation in the neuroendocrine modulation of intestinal inflammation.[52]

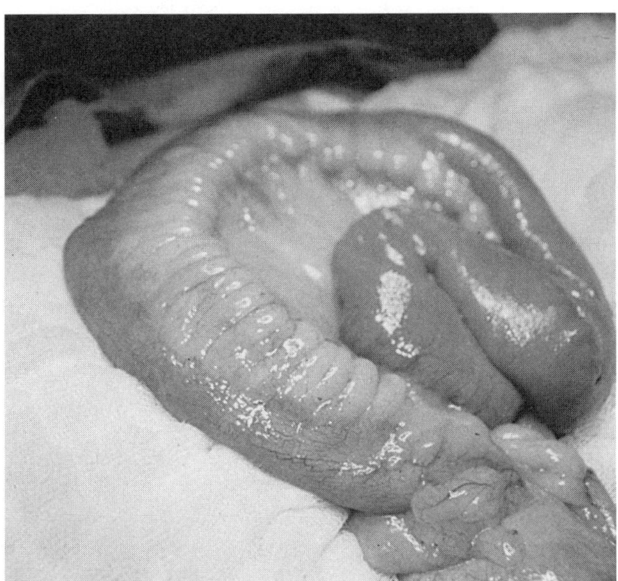

**FIGURE 32–2.** Mesenteric fat creeping over inflamed bowel.

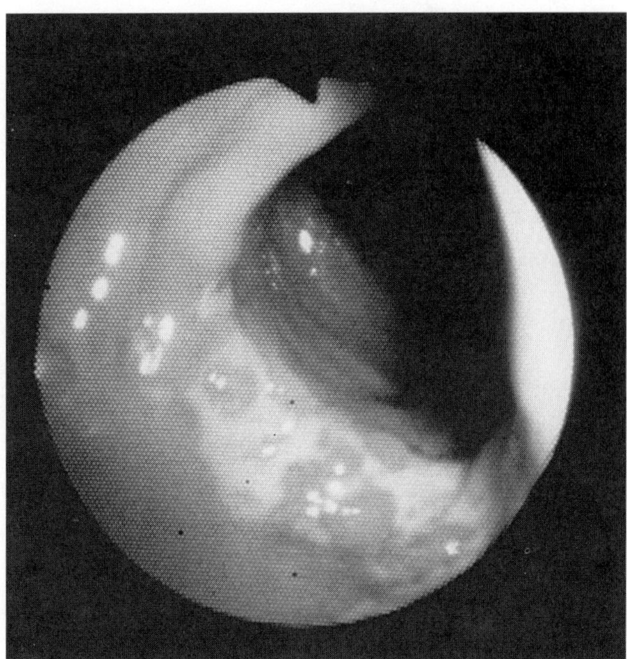

**FIGURE 32–3.** Deep irregular ulcer in Crohn's disease of the large bowel.

# PATHOLOGY

## Macroscopic Pathology

Gross inspection of the bowel in well-established Crohn's disease reveals marked wall thickening caused by transmural edema and chronic inflammation. Mural thickening is accompanied by narrowing of the bowel lumen, which may be severe enough to cause clinical obstruction. The mesentery is thickened with edematous, indurated fat that migrates over the serosal surface of the bowel (Fig. 32–2). Mesenteric lymph nodes are frequently enlarged. The bowel mucosa may reveal small aphthous lesions that may coalesce into larger, irregular and deeper ulcers (Fig. 32–3). Bowel inflammation and ulceration may be confluent; however, more characteristically it is punctuated by "skip areas" of grossly and even microscopically normal mucosa. Cobblestoning of the surface lining may occur as a result of extensive linear and serpiginous mucosal ulceration with associated regeneration and hyperplasia, in addition to marked submucosal thickening (Fig. 32–4). Stricture formation may occur in the setting of chronic inflammation as a result of fibrous tissue proliferation involving first the submucosa and then the deeper layers of the bowel wall. Cytokine production in inflamed tissue may act as a stimulus to the local production of excessive amounts of collagen.[46]

Loops of adjacent bowel may become matted together because of serosal and mesenteric inflammation. Fistulas are thought to arise when transmural bowel inflammation extends through the serosa into adjacent structures, such as bowel, abdominal wall, bladder, vagina, or perineum. Frequently, a fistulous tract ends blindly in an inflammatory mass (phlegmon) adjacent to the bowel and involves the bowel itself as well as the mesentery, lymph nodes, and occasionally a chronic active abscess cavity.

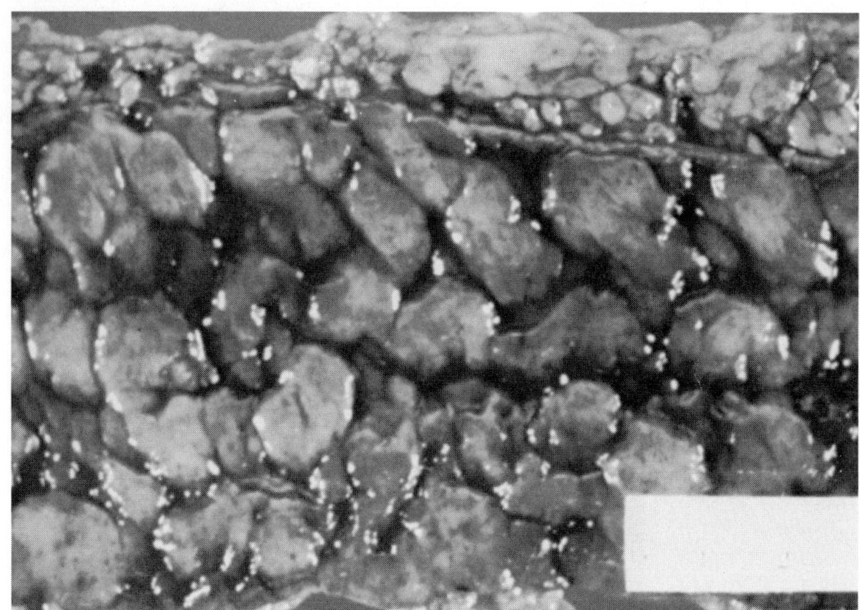

**FIGURE 32–4.** Resection specimen from patient with Crohn's disease of the large intestine revealing marked bowel wall thickening with cobblestoning.

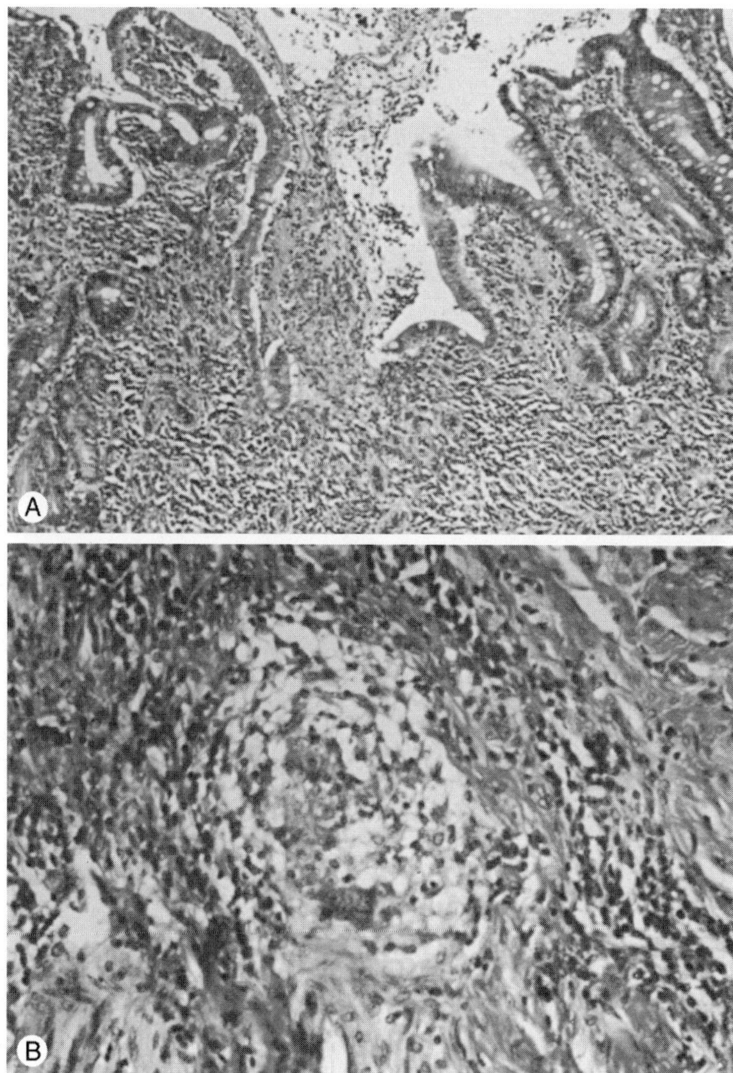


**FIGURE 32–5.** *A,* Solitary aphthoid ulcer overlying a lymphoid nodule in early Crohn's disease. *B,* Well-formed submucosal epithelial granuloma. (Courtesy of Andrew Ricci, Jr., MD.)

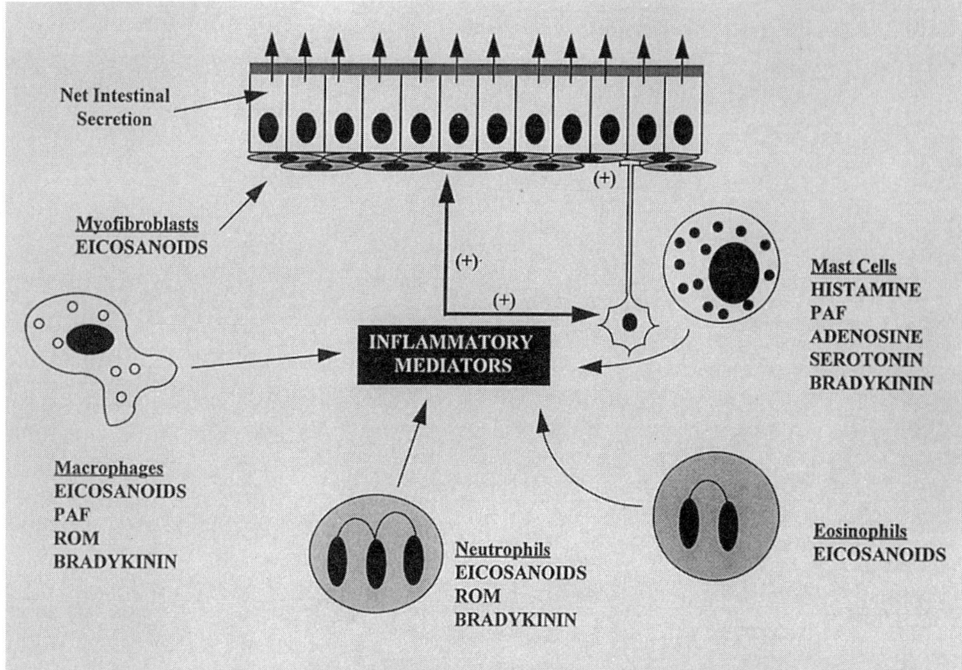


**FIGURE 32–6.** Inflammatory mediators in inflammatory bowel disease cause direct and indirect stimulation of intestinal secretion. (Adapted from Musch MW, Chang EB: Diarrhea in inflammatory bowel disease. In Targan SR, Shanahan F [eds]: Inflammatory Bowel Disease: From Bench to Bedside. Baltimore, Williams & Wilkins, 1994, p 242, with permission.)

## Microscopic Appearance

The findings on histologic examination of the bowel in Crohn's disease are highly dependent on the duration of disease involvement.[53, 54] Early disease may manifest as superficial aphthoid lesions of the mucosa, usually overlying a lymphoid follicle (Fig. 32–5*A*). Mucosal ulcers may become confluent, producing broad, depressed ulcer beds. There is sequential progression from mucosal disease to profound transmural infiltration of the bowel with lymphocytes, histiocytes, and plasma cells. The inflammation is typically extensive in the submucosa and is characterized by edema, lymphatic dilatation, and collagen deposition. The latter is responsible for obliteration of the submucosa, which results in stricture, obstruction, or both. Deep fissuring ulceration into the muscularis propria frequently occurs; when prominent, it is highly characteristic of Crohn's disease even in the absence of granulomas. Crypt abscesses and goblet cell depletion are common but may not be as marked as in ulcerative colitis. Mucosa that is thought to be normal grossly often reveals abnormalities such as edema and an increase in mononuclear cell density in the lamina propria.[55]

Granulomas are not always found in pathologic specimens from patients with Crohn's disease, being absent in up to 40% of surgically resected specimens and 60% to 80% of mucosal biopsies.[56–58] Granulomas may be found in any layer of the bowel wall, although they are most commonly located in the superficial submucosa (Fig. 32–5*B*). They may also be present in extraintestinal structures such as lymph nodes, mesentery, and peritoneum. It has been suggested that granulomas may be a secondary phenomenon caused by breaks in mucosal integrity and subsequent host inflammatory response to bacterial antigens.[59]

## PATHOPHYSIOLOGY OF GASTROINTESTINAL SYMPTOMS

The presence of inflammation in the small and large intestine, bowel wall thickening, or both, leads to a number of derangements that culminate in diarrhea, gastrointestinal bleeding, and abdominal pain. Extensive jejunal and ileal disease may lead to malabsorption. Malabsorbed fatty acids entering the colon impair electrolyte and water absorption.[60] Abnormal terminal ileal function may result in bile acid loss, with an eventual decrease in luminal bile acid concentration worsening steatorrhea.[61] Bile salts may significantly impair colonic absorption of electrolytes.[62] Bacterial overgrowth in the small intestine, associated with obstruction, stasis, or enteroenteric fistula, may lead to mucosal damage and bile salt deconjugation, further worsening symptoms. Inflammatory mediators released by activated immune cells lead to increased mucosal electrolyte secretion[47] (Fig. 32–6).

Diffuse mucosal disease leads to exudation of serum proteins and bleeding. Cramping abdominal pain may result from gut distention, usually in association with obstruction or abnormalities in intestinal motility.[63] The pain of Crohn's disease may also result from inflammation-mediated recruitment of silent nociceptors in the ileocecal region.[64]

## CLASSIFICATION OF SUBGROUPS IN CROHN'S DISEASE

Subgroups of persons with Crohn's disease have been observed based on anatomic distribution, extent of disease, biologic behavior, and laboratory findings (Table 32–1).

**TABLE 32–1. Subgroups of Patients with Crohn's Disease**

| CHARACTERISTIC | PERCENTAGE OF PATIENTS |
|---|---|
| **Anatomic Location** | |
| Gastroduodenal | 30–40 |
| Jejunoileal | 15–20 |
| Ileal | 30–35 |
| Ileocolonic | 50–60 |
| Colonic | 15–20 |
| Perirectal | 20–30 |
| **Biologic Behavior** | |
| Fibrostenosing (nonperforating) | |
| Fistulizing (perforating) | |
| Inflammatory | |
| **Laboratory Markers** | |
| ANCA-positive | |
| ANCA-negative | |

## Anatomic Location and Extent of Disease

Anatomic classification systems, primarily based on radiographic appearance of the gut, may still have value although endoscopy has now clearly shown that even parts of the bowel thought to be normal radiographically and visually may contain microscopic inflammation.[65, 66] The common anatomic subgroups and their relative frequencies are shown in Table 32–1. Involvement of the esophagus, stomach, or duodenum is found to affect 30% to 40% of children when careful endoscopy and biopsy techniques are applied.[67, 68]

## Biologic Behavior

Fistulizing, fibrostenosing, and inflammatory types of Crohn's disease have been described.[69–71] The fistulizing subgroup includes any patient with internal or external fistulas, except minor anal fissure. The fibrostenosing category includes patients with persistent abdominal pain and radiologic documentation of marked stenosis of a segment of the small or large intestine. The inflammatory group includes patients not readily classified into one of the other categories. There may be overlap between subgroups. The fibrostenosing and fistulizing subgroups tend to have a more aggressive course with a greater need for surgery.[71] A very high degree of concordance for anatomic site and biologic type of Crohn's disease has been noted in families with more than one affected member.[72]

## Laboratory Markers

Although serum perinuclear antineutrophil cytoplasmic antibodies (pANCA) are usually associated with ulcerative colitis (see Chapter 33), there exists a subgroup of patients with Crohn's disease who also express this autoantibody.[73] The presence of pANCA in patients with Crohn's disease may define a clinical subgroup including those with endoscopically or histopathologically documented left-sided colitis, an absence of disease confined to the small bowel, and symptoms of left-sided colonic inflammation (bleeding, urgency).[74] Recent studies have suggested that antibodies to oligomannosidic epitopes of the yeast *Saccharomyces cervisiae* may be a marker of Crohn's disease, especially when the small bowel is involved.[74a, 74b]

# CLINICAL FEATURES

The presenting clinical features of Crohn's disease are depicted in Table 32–2.[75–79] Terminal ileal and cecal disease is associated with right lower quadrant discomfort, and examination often reveals tenderness on palpation and a fullness or distinct mass in this area. Periumbilical pain is common with colonic disease or more diffuse small bowel disease. Epigastric pain is seen in children with gastroduodenal involvement,[80] whereas odynophagia and dysphagia are observed in most patients with Crohn's disease of the esophagus.[81] The abdominal pain associated with Crohn's disease tends to be persistent and severe and frequently awakens the child from sleep. At times, the acute development of right lower quadrant pain without a well-established previous history of illness suggests a diagnosis of appendicitis, but at laparotomy findings consistent with Crohn's disease are discovered.

Diarrhea is seen in two thirds of affected children and may be severe and nocturnal. Gross blood in the stools is unusual with isolated small bowel disease and more common when the colon is involved. However, severe hemorrhage may be seen in the setting of small bowel disease when bowel ulceration extends deeply into the bowel wall and involves a larger blood vessel.

Fever (approximately 50% of patients) may be low grade or spiking and may persist for extended periods before a diagnosis is made. Nausea and vomiting are frequent and may be seen with involvement of any part of the bowel. Fatigue is also a common complaint. Anorexia, weight loss, and diminution in growth velocity may be seen in 20% to 60% of children (see later discussion).

Perirectal inflammation with fissures, fistulas, or tags develops in approximately 25% to 30% of affected children and may be misdiagnosed as hemorrhoids or perianal condyloma.[82–84] The perirectal disease may prompt suspicion of abuse.[85] Drainage from these fistulas may be impressive, but perirectal pain is unusual unless there is actual abscess formation.

**TABLE 32–2. Presenting Clinical Features of Children with Crohn's Disease**

| FEATURE | PERCENTAGE AFFECTED |
|---|---|
| Abdominal pain | 75 |
| Diarrhea | 65 |
| Weight loss | 65 |
| Growth retardation | 25 |
| Nausea/vomiting | 25 |
| Perirectal disease | 25 |
| Rectal bleeding | 25 |
| Extraintestinal manifestations | 25 |

Data compiled from Gryboski and Spiro[75]; Burbige, Huang, and Bayless[76]; Posthuma and Moroz[77]; Raine[78]; and Barton and Ferguson.[79]

## Gastrointestinal Complications

**HEMORRHAGE.** Massive acute gastrointestinal hemorrhage is seen in fewer than 1% of patients with Crohn's disease,[86] but it can be so severe as to cause exsanguination. Mesenteric angiography is used to guide surgical resection.

**OBSTRUCTION.** Intestinal obstruction may occur secondary to severe bowel wall inflammation with or without localized phlegmon or abscess formation, stricture formation associated with chronic inflammation, undigested food occluding the lumen of a strictured bowel, carcinoma, or adhesions associated with previous surgery.[87] Chronic low-grade obstruction may lead to proximal small bowel bacterial overgrowth.

**PERFORATION.** Free perforation (i.e., that not accompanying an abscess or chronic fistula) is unusual in Crohn's disease. It is most common in the ileum. Rarely it may be the initial presentation of the disease. No relation to perforation has been established for corticosteroid therapy, duration of disease, toxic dilatation, or obstruction.[88] Classic signs of peritonitis may be masked in the presence of high doses of corticosteroids.

**ABSCESS.** Transmural bowel inflammation with fistulization and perforation may lead to the formation of abscesses. Fever and abdominal pain are invariably present, although it may be difficult to differentiate clinically between an abscess and an exacerbation of the underlying disease with phlegmon formation.[89] Fecal flora is found when these abscesses are cultured. Hip pain may indicate the presence of an iliopsoas abscess.

**FISTULA FORMATION.** Although perianal and perirectal fistulization are most common, enteroenteric, enterovesical, enterovaginal, and enterocutaneous fistulas also occur. A small percentage of children have highly destructive perianal disease, which often does not respond well to medical therapy.[84] The most common enteroenteric fistula is between the ileum and the sigmoid colon. Enterocolic fistulas may lead to bacterial overgrowth of the proximal bowel.

**TOXIC MEGACOLON.** Toxic megacolon is very rare in Crohn's disease.[90]

**CARCINOMA.** Persons with Crohn's colitis may be at similar risk to develop carcinoma of the colon as those with ulcerative colitis. The absolute cumulative frequency of risk for development of colorectal cancer in extensive Crohn's colitis was reported to be 8% after two decades of disease, compared with 7% for a group of subjects with ulcerative colitis.[91] Colorectal carcinoma has been reported in a 21-year-old who was diagnosed with Crohn's disease at the age of 8 years.[91a] Because many patients with Crohn's disease undergo resection of diseased colon within one to two decades, the absolute number of those developing carcinoma is small. Carcinoma may also arise in the small bowel.[92]

## Extraintestinal Manifestations

Extraintestinal manifestations are seen in 25% to 35% of patients with IBD and can be classified into four groups: (1) those directly related to intestinal disease activity, which usually respond to therapy directed against bowel disease; (2) those whose course appears to be unrelated to bowel disease activity; (3) those that are a direct result of the presence of diseased bowel, such as ureteral obstruction or nephrolithiasis; and (4) complications arising from therapy.[93, 94]

**JOINTS.** A peripheral form (colitic arthritis or enteropathic synovitis) and an axial form (including ankylosing spondylitis or sacroiliitis[95, 96]) have been described. Peripheral arthritis (10% of patients) may involve any joint, most commonly, in decreasing order of frequency, the knees, ankles, hips, wrists, and elbows. It is more commonly observed when the colon is involved, and joint activity often corresponds to clinical bowel activity. Involvement of the points of attachment of tendons and ligaments to bone (enthesopathy) is frequent.[97] Data have been published demonstrating a relation between gut inflammation resembling early Crohn's disease and seronegative spondyloarthropathy.[98] Clubbing, a form of hypertrophic osteoarthropathy, is common in children with Crohn's disease, particularly when the small bowel is affected.[75]

**MUSCULOSKELETAL.** Muscle diseases described include vasculitic myositis,[99] granulomatous myositis,[100] pyomyositis,[101] and dermatomyositis.[102] Proximal muscle weakness is rarely associated with high-dose daily corticosteroid therapy.[103]

**SKIN.** Erythema nodosum, pyoderma gangrenosum, epidermolysis bullosa acquisita, polyarteritis nodosa, and "metastatic" Crohn's disease have been described.[104–106] Acne can be exacerbated by corticosteroid therapy. Trace metal deficiency (zinc) and vitamin deficiency (pyridoxine) may be complicated by rashes.[107, 108]

**ORAL.** Canker sores are noted by many patients and range in severity from painless to severe. They may occasionally contain granuloma if biopsied.[109] Care must be taken to distinguish true Crohn's disease lesions from irritation or ulceration associated with dental braces. Granulomatous tonsillitis has been described.[110]

**OCULAR.** Ocular problems such as uveitis, episcleritis, and iritis are often seen in the setting of other extraintestinal manifestations such as arthritis and erythema nodosum.[111] Slit-lamp examination reveals uveitis in about 6% of children with Crohn's disease, and most are asymptomatic.[112] Increased intraocular pressure[113] and posterior subcapsular cataracts[114] may be seen with prolonged corticosteroid therapy.

**VASCULAR.** Hypercoagulability from thrombocytosis, hyperfibrinogenemia, elevated factor V and factor VIII, and depression of antithrombin III is seen in some patients with IBD.[115, 116] Vascular complications have included deep vein thrombosis, pulmonary emboli, and neurovascular disease.[117, 118]

**RENAL.** Urinary tract abnormalities may include ureteral obstruction and hydronephrosis secondary to an ileocecal phlegmon encasing the right ureter,[119] enterovesical fistula, perinephric abscess, and nephrolithiasis.[120, 121] Oxalate, urate, and phosphate stones may be found.[121] Amyloidosis is a rare complication of Crohn's disease and has been reported in children.[122] The development of proteinuria or elevated creatinine in a patient with long-standing Crohn's disease should suggest this entity.

**HEPATOBILIARY.** Abnormal serum aminotransferases are seen during the course of disease in approximately 14% of children with IBD.[123] When enzyme elevation is prolonged (longer than 6 months) the patient usually has either sclerosing cholangitis or chronic hepatitis.[123] Further discussion of sclerosing cholangitis can be found in Chapter 33. Brief elevation of serum aminotransferase can be associated with increased bowel disease activity, medications (e.g., 6-mercaptopurine), parenteral nutrition, and massive weight gain. Other disorders described have included hepatic granuloma,[124] hepatic abscess,[125] cholelithiasis,[126] and acalculous cholecystitis.[127] Terminal ileal resection or significant disease is associated with increased enteric bile acid loss and an interruption of the enterohepatic circulation of bile acids.[128] Bile may then become supersaturated with cholesterol, leading to gallstone formation.

**PANCREAS.** Pancreatitis may develop as a reaction to drug therapy (6-mercaptopurine, sulfasalazine), as a result of duodenal disease, in association with sclerosing cholangitis, or in an idiopathic form.[94, 129, 130]

**BONE.** Osteopenia may result from malnutrition, inadequate calcium intake or malabsorption, vitamin D deficiency, excessive proinflammatory cytokine production by diseased bowel, prolonged inactivity, and corticosteroid therapy.[94] Decreased bone density has been found at diagnosis[131] as well as during the course of disease.[132] It has been proposed that bone formation may be inhibited in the presence of bowel inflammation.[133] Both cortical and trabecular bone loss may occur, with resultant fractures, loss of height, severe pain, and disability. Aseptic necrosis (osteonecrosis) is very rare in the pediatric population with IBD.

**HEMATOLOGIC.** Anemia may occur secondary to iron deficiency, folic acid deficiency, vitamin $B_{12}$ deficiency, hemolysis (drug-induced or autoimmune), and bone marrow suppression (6-mercaptopurine). Immune activation with the elaboration of proinflammatory cytokines may suppress erythrocyte production.[134] It may also be the operative mechanism for the thrombocytosis seen in many patients.[135] Neutropenia is a rare accompanying condition.[136]

## Malnutrition

Weight loss is seen in more than 50% of children with Crohn's disease at the time of presentation. Causes of malnutrition in these patients include suboptimal dietary intake, increased gastrointestinal losses, malabsorption, and possibly increased requirements associated with marked inflammatory activity (Fig. 32–7). Anorexia may be severe enough to mimic anorexia nervosa. Children who fear exacerbation of gastrointestinal symptoms from eating decrease their intake. Delayed gastric emptying noted in some children may be associated with early satiety.[137] Marked mucosal inflammation leads to the loss of cellular constituents and hematochezia, with the development of protein-losing enteropathy and iron-deficiency anemia. Fecal calcium and magnesium losses may be increased.[138] Deficiency states for iron, folic acid, vitamin $B_{12}$, nicotinic acid, vitamin D, vitamin K, calcium, magnesium, and zinc have been noted.[139]

Studies in adults have suggested that total energy expenditure—which is a function of resting metabolic expenditure, diet-induced thermogenesis, and activity energy expenditure—is not raised and that approximately 35 Kcal/kg per day is sufficient to achieve energy balance.[140, 141] A study of growing adolescents with inactive Crohn's disease demonstrated resting expenditure at 15% greater than predicted.[142] Weight loss usually is caused more by a decrease in fat than by loss of protein stores.[143]

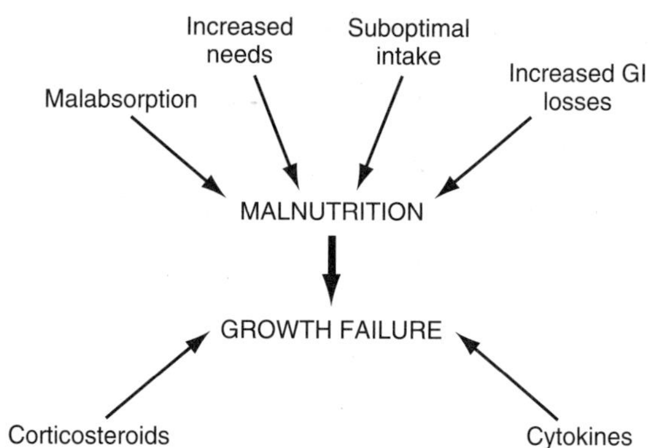


**FIGURE 32–7.** Contributing factors to the development of malnutrition and growth failure in children and adolescents with Crohn's disease.

## Growth Failure

A decrease in growth velocity may precede overt gastrointestinal symptoms in up to 20% of children with Crohn's disease,[144] and absolute height deficiency at the time of diagnosis may be present in 30%.[144–148] Permanent growth failure has been reported.[147]

There are probably several pathogenetic mechanisms that lead to growth failure (see Fig. 32–7), including chronic undernutrition.[149–151] In the presence of malnutrition and poor growth, serum levels of insulin-like growth factor I (IGF-I) are low and increase with nutritional restitution.[152] Levels of IGF-I–binding protein are similar in both normally grown and growth-retarded children with Crohn's disease.[152] Growth hormone levels have generally been shown to be normal in children with Crohn's disease.[149]

Chronic administration of high-dose daily corticosteroid therapy may be an iatrogenic cause of growth failure. Daily corticosteroid therapy for a period as short as 7 to 14 days is associated with decreased type I collagen production, a prerequisite for linear growth.[153] Alternate-day therapy appears to have little impact on growth velocity[153] or on type I or III collagen production.[154] It is often difficult to separate the growth-retarding effects of increased disease severity from those of the concomitant use of high doses of corticosteroids. It has been suggested that disease activity may have a more deleterious impact on growth than does corticosteroid therapy.[145, 146]

## Psychological Disturbances

Depression and anxiety may be present at diagnosis or during the course of the disease.[155–157] Neither disease activity nor the use of corticosteroids has been correlated with the development of depression.[155, 156]

## DIAGNOSIS

The diagnosis of Crohn's disease is suspected in the presence of a combination of clinical and laboratory observations

**TABLE 32–3. Clinical and Laboratory Findings Used to Establish a Diagnosis of Crohn's Disease**

| | |
|---|---|
| **History** | **Laboratory Tests** |
| Abdominal pain | Anemia |
| Diarrhea | Elevated ESR |
| Rectal bleeding | Hypoalbuminemia |
| Fever | Thrombocytosis |
| Arthritis | Positive guaiac |
| Rash | **Radiography** |
| Family history of IBD | Nodularity |
| **Physical Examination** | Skip areas |
| Abdominal tenderness | String sign |
| Mass | Fistula |
| Perirectal disease | Ulceration |
| Clubbing | **Endoscopy** |
| Stomatitis | Ulcers |
| Erythema nodosum | Cobblestoning |
| Pyoderma gangrenosum | Rectal sparing |
| **Growth Data** | |
| Height and weight velocity decreases for age | |

IBD, inflammatory bowel disease; ESR, erythrocyte sedimentation rate.

and then confirmed with radiologic, endoscopic, and histologic findings (Table 32–3). Because the clinical findings can involve systems outside of the gastrointestinal tract, the diagnosis may be delayed for months or years before the appropriate diagnostic studies are performed.

## History and Physical Examination

A complete clinical history is mandatory to elicit both gastrointestinal and extraintestinal manifestations. Physical examination should include careful abdominal palpation with particular attention to tenderness, fullness, or mass. Careful inspection of the perirectal area and perineum is mandatory. A rectal examination and stool guaiac test should be part of the routine physical examination. The presence of stomatitis, clubbing, arthritis, erythema nodosum, or pyoderma gangrenosum is suggestive of IBD. Height and weight should be measured and compared with previous values to calculate the rate of change.

## Laboratory Evaluation

Appropriate stool cultures and examination should be made to exclude enteric bacterial pathogens and parasites such as *Salmonella, Shigella, Campylobacter, E. coli* 0157:H7, *Yersinia, Aeromonas, Clostridium difficile, Cryptosporidium,* and *Giardia.* Acute onset of bloody diarrhea with fever and vomiting is more suggestive of a bacterial pathogen than of Crohn's disease.

Laboratory abnormalities frequently found include anemia (70% of cases), elevated erythrocyte sedimentation rate (80%), hypoalbuminemia (60%), and guaiac-positive stools (35%).[158] Although thrombocytosis is common (60%), the total leukocyte count is commonly normal. There may be a left shift with an increased percentage of band forms. In the nutritionally depleted patient, serum zinc, magnesium, calcium, and phosphorus levels may be low. Serum aminotransferases are elevated at the time of diagnosis in approximately 10% of patients.[123]

Breath hydrogen testing for lactose malabsorption may be helpful in subsequent dietary management. Urinalysis should be performed to exclude pyuria or infection associated with enterovesical fistula.

## Radiographic Evaluation

An upper gastrointestinal series with small-bowel follow-through is required in all patients with Crohn's disease. It can be performed with oral ingestion of contrast medium or by enteroclysis. Careful fluoroscopy with abdominal palpation is used to identify irregular, nodular (cobblestoned), and thickened bowel loops as well as stenotic areas (string sign), ulcers, and fistulas (Fig. 32–8). Pathologic terminal ileal nodularity, which is common in Crohn's disease, must be distinguished from nonpathologic nodular lymphoid hyperplasia; in the latter condition, the nodules are usually 3 mm or less in diameter. Antegrade filling of the colon can help identify areas of gross colonic involvement (Fig. 32–9).

The presence of a tender mass in the right lower quadrant in a patient with Crohn's disease suggests the presence of an inflammatory phlegmon or abscess. Ultrasound examination may reveal bowel wall thickening and extraluminal fluid, suggesting abscess. Computed tomography may be useful to delineate extramural extension of inflammation by fistulization to adjacent structures and in the diagnosis of

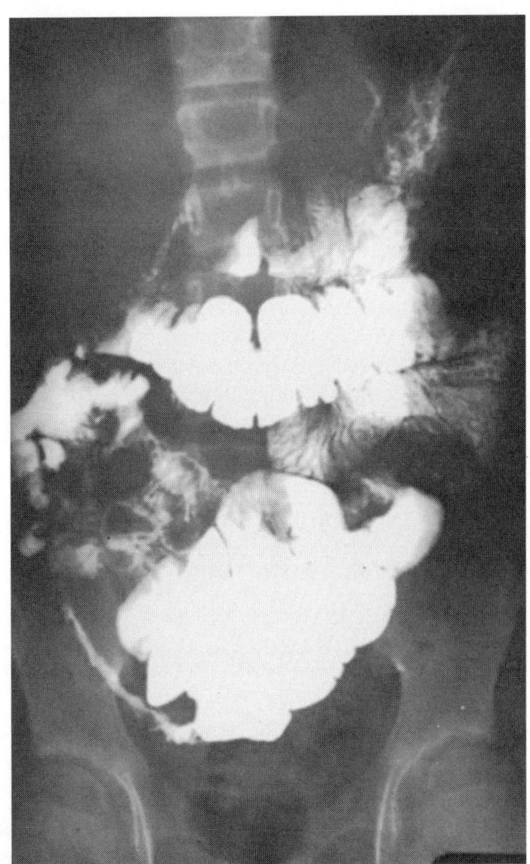

**FIGURE 32–8.** Crohn's disease of the terminal ileum with narrowing, irregularity, and mass effect.

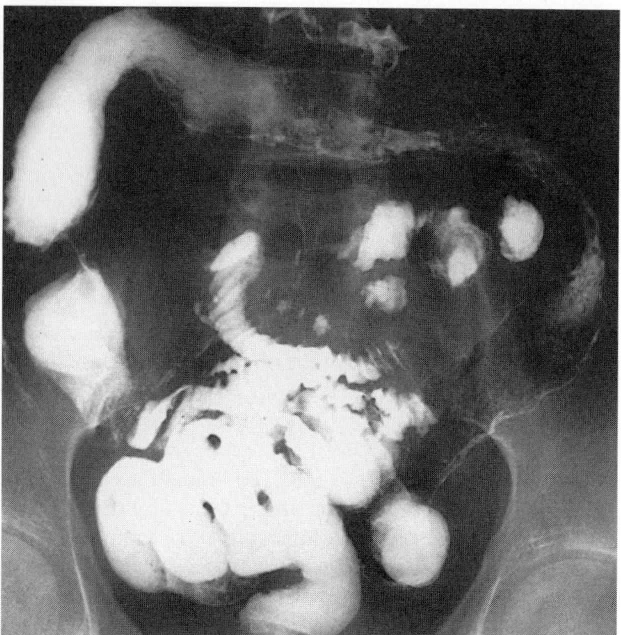

**FIGURE 32–9.** Crohn's disease of the colon with foreshortening, stricture formation, and marked mucosal irregularity.

abscesses. Radioisotope studies (usually indium 111) are limited by the relatively long half-life and radiation dose of the isotope.

### Endoscopic and Histologic Evaluation

Examination of the colon is often performed early in the evaluation of a child with chronic bloody diarrhea with the aim of distinguishing ulcerative colitis from Crohn's disease. The finding of aphthous lesions (small ulcers on an erythematous base) in the midst of an otherwise normal-looking colon is highly suggestive of Crohn's disease. Rectal sparing is unusual in ulcerative colitis and common in Crohn's disease. Patchiness of inflammation, with abnormal areas interspersed with grossly normal-appearing areas, is characteristic of Crohn's disease. Deep fissuring ulcers and heaped-up edematous mucosa (pseudopolyps) may be present. The ileocecal valve may appear granular, friable, and edematous. Intubation of the terminal ileum may reveal marked nodularity, inflammation, and ulceration.

Mucosal biopsies should be taken from normal- and abnormal-appearing areas. Biopsies of normal-appearing areas may reveal inflammation and, rarely, granuloma, which is diagnostic of Crohn's disease.[159]

## DIFFERENTIAL DIAGNOSIS

The protean manifestations of Crohn's disease lead to a long differential diagnosis (Table 32–4). Right lower quadrant pain may suggest appendicitis, infection, neoplasm (especially lymphoma), ovarian pathology, intussusception, mesenteric adenitis, or Meckel's diverticulum (torsion, diverticulitis). If bloody diarrhea is part of the presentation, then infection with a bacterial pathogen or invasive parasite is considered. Hemolytic-uremic syndrome may closely mimic IBD,[160, 161] as may Henoch-Schönlein purpura.[162] Perirectal inflammation or fissures or tags may be confused with perianal streptococcal infection, hemorrhoids, and condyloma. Short stature and delayed pubertal development may be considered to represent an endocrinopathy before Crohn's disease is diagnosed. Anorexia and weight loss may be confused with anorexia nervosa. Persistent joint symptoms, and particularly frank arthritis, are often considered to represent juvenile rheumatoid arthritis if gastrointestinal symptoms are not present.

## THERAPY

Currently available medical, surgical, and nutritional interventions are directed toward decreasing inflammation with the hope of controlling symptoms, addressing complications, and preventing recurrent or worsening disease. Treatment should be directed primarily by the symptoms and not by abnormal laboratory tests, biopsies, or radiographs. There may be a considerable dissociation between abnormal tests and clinical activity,[163, 164] especially when obstruction is secondary to bowel stenosis. Assessment of disease activity must include not only the usual signs and symptoms of Crohn's disease, but growth activity and quality of life. A pediatric Crohn's disease activity index has been published to standardize assessment of disease activity.[165]

**TABLE 32–4. Differential Diagnosis of Presenting Symptoms of Crohn's Disease**

| PRIMARY PRESENTING SYMPTOM | DIAGNOSTIC CONSIDERATIONS |
|---|---|
| Right lower quadrant abdominal pain, with or without mass | Appendicitis, infection (e.g., *Campylobacter, Yersinia*), lymphoma, intussusception, mesenteric adenitis, Meckel's diverticulum, ovarian cyst |
| Chronic periumbilical or epigastric abdominal pain | Irritable bowel, constipation, lactose intolerance, peptic disease |
| Rectal bleeding, no diarrhea | Fissure, polyp, Meckel's diverticulum, rectal ulcer syndrome |
| Bloody diarrhea | Infection, hemolytic-uremic syndrome, Henoch-Schönlein purpura, ischemic bowel, radiation colitis |
| Watery diarrhea | Irritable bowel, lactose intolerance, giardiasis, cryptosporidium, sorbitol, laxatives |
| Perirectal disease | Fissure, hemorrhoid (rare), streptococcal infection, condyloma (rare) |
| Growth delay | Endocrinopathy |
| Anorexia, weight loss | Anorexia nervosa |
| Arthritis | Collagen vascular disease, infection |
| Liver abnormalities | Chronic hepatitis |

**TABLE 32–5. Pharmacotherapy of Crohn's Disease**

| CATGORY | DAILY DOSAGE Usual (mg/kg) | Maximum |
|---|---|---|
| ***Aminosalicylates*** | | |
| Sulfasalazine | 30–50 | 3 g |
| Mesalamine | 40–60 | 4.8 g |
| Asacol | | |
| Pentasa | | |
| ***Corticosteroids*** | | |
| Prednisone | 1–2 | 40–80 mg |
| Budesonide | — | 9–15 mg |
| ***Immunomodulators*** | | |
| 6-Mercaptopurine | 1–1.5 | 100 mg |
| Azathioprine | 2–2.5 | 150 mg |
| Methotrexate* | | |
| Cyclosporine* | | |
| ***Antibiotics*** | | |
| Metronidazole | 10–20 | 1 g |
| Ciprofloxacin | — | 1 g |

*Specific pediatric dosing guidelines not available.

## Pharmacologic Therapy

Medications used to treat Crohn's disease can be divided into the following categories: aminosalicylates, corticosteroids, immunomodulators, and antibiotics[166] (Table 32–5). Each medication may be used to treat active disease or to maintain remission.

**AMINOSALICYLATES.** Further discussion of the pharmacology of these agents can be found in Chapter 33. The two generic preparations are sulfasalazine (Azulfidine) and mesalamine (Asacol, Pentasa, Claversal, Salofalk).[167] Asacol (Eudragit-S coating) is active in the terminal ileum and colon, whereas Pentasa (ethylcellulose microgranules) has activity from the proximal jejunum to the colon. All controlled studies with these medications have been performed in adults.

***Active Disease***. Sulfasalazine is usually effective for mild to moderate Crohn's colitis but has no documented efficacy in small bowel disease.[168] The efficacy of mesalamine in the treatment of active Crohn's disease of the distal small bowel or large bowel is largely dose related. In adults, 3.2 g/day of Asacol[169] or 4 g/day Pentasa[170] was shown to be more effective than placebo in inducing remission. In children, mesalamine doses administered are usually approximately 50 mg/kg/day.[171] Mesalamine enemas may be used for distal colonic disease.

***Maintenance Therapy.*** Pentasa (4 g/day in adults) has been shown to facilitate steroid withdrawal after a steroid-induced remission and may reduce the relapse rate after discontinuation of the steroids.[172] Two meta-analyses have suggested that aminosalicylate preparations decrease the risk of relapse in patients in remission,[173, 174] especially in those with ileal disease rather than ileocolitis or colitis. The postoperative administration of mesalamine decreases the likelihood of recurrent disease after resection of the terminal ileum or ileocecal region.[175, 176]

***Toxicity.*** Mesalamine is usually well tolerated. Side effects reported include worsening of diarrhea and rectal bleeding, nephritis, pancreatitis, hair loss, hepatitis, and pericarditis.[166, 177] Sulfasalazine may be associated with a higher frequency of side effects, particularly nausea, abdominal pain, headache, and rash.

**CORTICOSTEROIDS.** The potential mechanisms of action have been reviewed previously[178] and are thought to be largely secondary to an inhibition of expression or production of polypeptides involved in the inflammatory response (e.g., adhesion molecules, cytokines, leukotrienes).

***Active Disease.*** The efficacy of systemic corticosteroids in the treatment of active disease in virtually all distributions of Crohn's disease has been demonstrated.[168, 179] Oral therapy is usually initiated with prednisone at a dose of 1 to 2 mg/kg/day, with a maximum of 40 to 60 mg/day. Intravenous therapy is occasionally used for particularly severe disease. The dose is tapered over several weeks to months to an alternate-day schedule and then discontinued depending on the patient's response. Budesonide, a synthetic steroid with high affinity for the glucocorticoid receptor, potent anti-inflammatory activity, and low systemic bioavailability, is now being used in the treatment of Crohn's disease.[180–182] At a dose of 9 to 15 mg/day, approximately 50% of adult patients achieved remission compared with 20% of those receiving placebo.[180] Budesonide (9 mg/day) had slightly less efficacy than prednisolone (40 mg/day) in decreasing Crohn's disease activity in adults but had less of an inhibitory effect on the pituitary-adrenal axis.[181] Budesonide (9 mg/day) was more effective than mesalamine (4 g/day) in the treatment of active Crohn's disease.[181a] Corticosteroid enemas may be used for relief of symptoms caused by inflammation of the sigmoid and rectum.

***Maintenance Therapy.*** Most evidence suggests that prednisone has little efficacy in preventing recurrence of symptoms in those in remission.[168, 179] In a study of adults, 6 mg/day of budesonide was more efficacious than placebo in decreasing the likelihood of recurrent symptoms after remission and in prolonging time to recurrent symptoms in those that did relapse.[182] Although alternate-day prednisone therapy is often used in a maintenance regimen in both children and adults, there are no data supporting its efficacy.

***Toxicity.*** The toxicity of corticosteroid therapy largely relates to the dose administered and the duration of therapy.[183] The major side effects relevant to its use in children are listed in Table 32–6.[184] Growth inhibition is a major problem with daily therapy, but normal growth rates may

**TABLE 32–6. Side Effects of Corticosteroid Therapy**

| | |
|---|---|
| **Cosmetic** | **Musculoskeletal** |
| Moon facies | Osteopenia |
| Acne | Aseptic necrosis of bone |
| Hirsutism | Vertebral collapse |
| Striae | Myopathy |
| Central obesity | **Psychological** |
| **Metabolic** | Mood swings |
| Hypokalemia | Psychosis |
| Hyperglycemia | **Other** |
| Hyperlipidemia | Hypertension |
| **Endocrinologic** | Intraocular hypertension |
| Growth suppression | Cataracts |
| Delayed puberty | Immunosuppression |
| Adrenal suppression | Pseudotumor cerebri |

be preserved with alternate-day therapy.[185] Compliance with therapy may be problematic in children and adolescents who have mood swings and cosmetic problems associated with corticosteroid therapy. Adequate calcium intake and maintenance of physical activity are important to prevent corticosteroid-induced bone disease.

**IMMUNOMODULATORS.** Immunomodulator therapy is commonly used in the treatment of Crohn's disease that is refractory to corticosteroids and for patients who cannot be weaned from corticosteroids.[186] The potential mechanisms of action[166, 183] and pharmacology[186] of these medications have been reviewed previously.

***Active Disease.*** 6-Mercaptopurine (1–1.5 mg/kg/day) and azathioprine (2–2.5 mg/kg/day) are effective in patients with active disease when added to corticosteroid therapy. They facilitate the development of remission and promote tapering of the corticosteroid dosage.[187–190] Either medication usually requires 3 to 6 months to show efficacy, and neither is effective as primary therapy (single agent). It has been suggested that a large intravenous loading dose of azathioprine given at the initiation of therapy might decrease the response time to less than 1 month.[191] Those patients in whom leukopenia develops during therapy appear to have a greater likelihood of achieving improvement of symptoms.[192] Recent data suggest that 6-mercaptopurine started in the first month of therapy for children with moderate to severe disease may decrease the total amount of prednisone used in the first year of treatment.[192a]

Methotrexate (25 mg, intramuscularly, once weekly) was more effective than placebo for facilitating remission in adult patients receiving prednisone for chronically active disease.[193] In a placebo-controlled blinded study, oral cyclosporine facilitated remission in patients with active disease that was resistant to corticosteroids,[194] but recurrence of symptoms was frequent as the medication was discontinued.[195] Another study of adults found no benefit of oral cyclosporine.[196] Oral cyclosporine was not as effective as prednisolone in newly diagnosed children with Crohn's disease.[197] Intravenous cyclosporine was helpful in improving symptoms in a small group of children with active, refractory colitis[198] and in closing severe fistula in adults.[199] It has been suggested that malabsorption of oral cyclosporine is common in Crohn's disease and that intravenous therapy may be preferable at initiation of therapy. Studies have suggested a role for biologic agents in the treatment of Crohn's disease. A chimeric human-mouse IgG1 monoclonal antibody to tumor necrosis factor-α resulted in clinical improvement in more than 60% of patients compared with 17% for the control population.[200] Similar results were obtained with a non-chimeric anti-TNF-α antibody.[200a] This type of antibody has shown efficacy in treating perirectal disease.[200b] Interleukin-10, a cytokine that has anti-inflammatory activity, showed some clinical promise in one limited study.[200b]

***Maintenance Therapy.*** 6-Mercaptopurine and azathioprine have been shown to significantly decrease the likelihood of recurrent disease in those patients in remission.[201, 202] Once remission has been maintained for 4 years without steroids, the risk of relapse is the same whether either medication is stopped or continued.[203] A small, uncontrolled study of children suggested that azathioprine or 6-mercaptopurine could maintain a cyclosporine-induced remission.[204] Neither methotrexate nor cyclosporine has been shown to maintain remission. A small pilot study suggested 6-mercaptopurine may decrease the likelihood of postoperative recurrence.[204a]

***Toxicity.*** All immunomodulators predispose patients to an increased risk of infection. Myelosuppression is a potentially serious side effect of azathioprine or 6-mercaptopurine and may be more likely in individuals who lack the enzyme thiopurine methyltransferase.[166] Bone marrow toxicity may be seen shortly after therapy is begun or many years into therapy, and regular blood testing is mandatory.[205] Other side effects associated with azathioprine or 6-mercaptopurine include pancreatitis, hepatitis, fever, rash, and arthralgias.[166, 186, 206] A theoretic risk for the development of malignancy has been suggested with long-term therapy, but the risk is thought to be quite low.[186] Methotrexate therapy has been associated with hepatitis, nausea, and rash.[186] The risk of hepatic fibrosis is thought to be low in patients with IBD treated with methotrexate. Renal disease (azotemia, hypertension), hypertrichosis, gingival hyperplasia, and tremor are the more common side effects of cyclosporine,[186] although opportunistic infection and a potentially increased risk of malignancy are a concern.

**ANTIBIOTICS.** These medications have long been used both for primary treatment and to address complications of Crohn's disease. Their precise mechanisms of action in this disorder are not clear.

***Active Disease.*** Metronidazole has efficacy similar to that of sulfasalazine in the treatment of Crohn's disease of the colon.[207] It has been used as the drug of choice for perirectal fistula, although the problem usually flares on discontinuation of therapy.[208] Metronidazole plus ciprofloxacin had similar efficacy to methylprednisolone in a small group of adults with active disease.[209] Ciprofloxacin is commonly used to treat perirectal disease, but controlled data are lacking.

***Maintenance Therapy.*** Metronidazole (20 mg/kg/day) decreases the likelihood of endoscopic recurrence at 3 months and clinical recurrence at 1 year after ileal resection.[210]

***Toxicity.*** Peripheral neuropathy is the most serious side effect of metronidazole therapy.[211] Rarely, paresthesias may persist despite discontinuation of the medication. Nausea and a metallic taste are common. The author has seen *Candida* esophagitis in adolescents treated with broad-spectrum antibiotics who are also receiving immunosuppressive therapy.

**ADJUNCTIVE THERAPY.** An enteric-coated fish oil preparation has been used to maintain remission.[211a] Loperamide may help control diarrhea. Anticholinergics such as dicyclomine and low-dose tricyclic antidepressant medications (e.g., amitriptyline) may be helpful in subjects with Crohn's disease who also have symptoms of irritable bowel syndrome. Cholestyramine, a bile acid–binding resin, may decrease diarrhea in those patients who have had terminal ileal resection or extensive ileal disease with attendant loss of bile acids into the colon, stimulating colonic secretion. Persons with extensive resection of the terminal ileum are at risk for development of vitamin $B_{12}$ deficiency and should receive parenteral supplementation. Calcium supplementation should be provided to at least meet the recommended daily allowance (RDA), if it is not met by dietary intake. There is theoretic evidence to suggest that nonsteroidal anti-inflammatory agents exacerbate Crohn's disease, and they should be avoided if possible.[212]

## Nutritional Therapy

Nutritional therapy can be used as primary therapy without accompanying pharmacologic intervention or as adjunctive therapy with medications. It has been postulated that bowel rest decreases luminal antigenic stimulation, resulting in a decrease in bowel inflammation.

### Active Disease

Total parenteral nutrition and bowel rest may be effective in inducing remission in as many as 60% to 80% of subjects.[213, 214] A large meta-analysis of exclusive enteral nutritional therapy, with either elemental or polymeric diets, showed a large range (20–80%) in remission of subjects.[215] In general, enteral therapy was less effective than corticosteroids in effecting remission in those studies in which a comparison was made.[215] No differences have been demonstrated between elemental and nonelemental diets.[216] The relapse rate after enteral nutrition–induced remission is greater than after remission achieved with prednisolone.[217] In selected children with growth failure, enteral nutritional therapy may be preferable to corticosteroids as initial therapy.

### Maintenance Therapy

Data are limited. One study showed that after successful treatment of active Crohn's disease in children and adolescents by exclusive enteral nutritional therapy, supplementary enteral nutrition prolonged remission and was associated with improved growth.[218] Gastrostomy placement is safe and well tolerated for those children being treated with long-term enteral therapy who do not want to use a nasogastric tube.[219]

### Other Indications

Intensive nutritional support, primarily through enteral supplementation via tube feedings, has been shown to be effective in reversing growth retardation in most patients.[148, 150, 151] It is imperative that nutritional support be started well before physiologic bone maturation and fusion of epiphyses if catch-up growth is to be expected.

## Surgery

Surgery is required in 50% to 70% of affected children or adults within the first 10 to 15 years after diagnosis.[220, 221] Intractable symptoms despite medical therapy, obstruction, abdominal abscess, fistulas, and severe perirectal disease are the most common reasons for surgery.[222] Long-standing ileal disease is associated with a higher likelihood of obstruction requiring surgery than is colonic disease.[75]

Resectional therapy is not curative. Endoscopic evidence of recurrent disease is present at the neoterminal ileum in more than 70% of adults at 1 year after terminal ileal resection, although only 35% are symptomatic.[223] Approximately 80% of children with terminal ileal or ileocecal resection are clinically well 4 years after surgery.[220] Segmental colonic resection is followed by relapse within 5 years in 70% of cases.[220] The recurrence rate at the neoterminal ileum 5 to 10 years after panproctocolectomy and ileostomy is 70% if ileal disease was present at the time of surgery but only 10% if disease was limited to the colon.[224] Children undergoing intestinal resection within 1 year of onset of symptoms have a delayed recurrence of active disease, compared with patients whose preoperative duration of symptomatic disease was longer.[225]

Strictureplasty is a well accepted method in the surgical management of adult and pediatric patients with Crohn's disease.[226, 227] In this procedure, a longitudinal incision is made through the stenotic bowel, and the opening is then closed transversely. The risk of reoperation after strictureplasty is not greater than after resection.[226] Strictureplasty is generally performed on small intestinal strictures or at an ileocolonic anastomosis in the presence of mostly fibrotic disease. Mild inflammation does not preclude performance of strictureplasty.

A variety of surgical techniques have been developed to help address severe perirectal disease.[228, 229] Skin tags should virtually never be excised. Abscess formation requires drainage. Superficial fistulas can be treated successfully with fistulotomy (lay-open technique). Complex fistulas may require long-term drainage and partial fistulotomy. Control of symptoms—not cure—is the realistic goal of such therapy. Proctectomy and diversion of the fecal stream may be required for particularly severe perirectal disease.[229] Marked rectal disease, with or without complex fistula formation, may eventually lead to rectal stenosis. Frequently, this can be managed with dilatation.

Despite intensive medical and nutritional therapy, growth failure still persists in some children with Crohn's disease. Surgery may significantly improve growth in most of these children, provided they are prepubertal or in early puberty, good nutrition can be maintained, and corticosteroid therapy can be discontinued or weaned to an alternate-day schedule.[220, 230, 231]

## Psychological Therapy

Many fears can be diminished with a thorough explanation of the course of the disease, discussion of the rationale for the use of certain medications and surgery, and an understanding of the difficulty of the child and family in coping with a chronic illness. Counseling and interaction with age- and sex-matched peer groups may be helpful.

## NATURAL HISTORY

Crohn's disease is marked by periods of exacerbation and remission. Only 1% of patients with well-documented Crohn's disease do not have at least one relapse after diagnosis and initial therapy.[232] Data suggest that markers of inflammation such as C-reactive protein, orosomucoid, and erythrocyte sedimentation rate identify patients at higher risk for recurrence.[233, 234] Patients with ileocolitis usually have a poorer response to medications and a greater need for surgery than those with small bowel disease alone.[75] Younger age (less than 25 years) appears to be associated with a greater risk of relapse.[233] A history of multiple previous relapses is probably the greatest predictor of subsequent relapses.

Death from Crohn's disease in the pediatric population is extremely rare. Adults with Crohn's disease appear to have an increased mortality risk compared with age-matched controls (standardized mortality ratio 1.51).[235]

*Acknowledgment*

The author is indebted to Andrew Ricci, Jr., MD, for his contribution to the pathology section of this chapter.

## REFERENCES

1. Crohn BB, Ginzburg L, Oppenheimer GD: Regional ileitis: a pathologic and clinical entity. JAMA 1932;99:1323–1329.
2. Eisen GM, Sandler RS: Update on the epidemiology of IBD. Progress in Inflammatory Bowel Disease (Crohn's & Colitis Foundation of America) 1994;15:1–7.
3. Lindberg E, Jarnerot G: The incidence of Crohn's disease is not decreasing in Sweden. Scand J Gastroenterol 1991;26:495–500.
4. Sandler RS, Golden AL: Epidemiology of Crohn's disease. J Clin Gastroenterol 1986;8:160–165.
5. Munkholm P, Langholz E, Nielson OH, et al: Incidence and prevalence of Crohn's disease in the county of Copenhagen, 1962–1987: a sixfold increase in incidence. Scand J Gastroenterol 1992;27:609–614.
6. Cosgrove M, Al-Atia RF, Jenkins HR: The epidemiology of paediatric inflammatory bowel disease. Arch Dis Child 1996;74:460–461.
7. Gottrand F, Colombel JF, Moreno L, et al: Incidence of inflammatory bowel diseases in children in the Nord-Pas-de-Calais region. Arch Fr Pediatr 1991;48:25–28.
8. Shivananda S, Lennard-Jones J, Logan R, et al: Incidence of inflammatory bowel disease across Europe: is there a difference between north and south? Results of the European collaborative study on inflammatory bowel disease. Gut 1996;39:690–697.
9. Roth MP, Peterson GM, McElree C, et al: Geographic origins of Jewish patients with inflammatory bowel disease. Gastroenterology 1989;97:900–904.
10. Lashner BA, Shaheen NJ, Hanauer SB, Kirschner BS: Passive smoking is associated with an increased risk of developing inflammatory bowel disease in children. Am J Gastroenterol 1993;88:356–359.
11. Rigas A, Rigas B, Glassman M, et al: Breast feeding and maternal smoking in the etiology of Crohn's disease and ulcerative colitis in childhood. Ann Epidemiol 1993;3:387 392.
12. Ekbom A, Adami HO, Helmick CG, et al: Perinatal risk factors for inflammatory bowel disease: a case-control study. Am J Epidemiol 1990;132:1111–1119.
13. Gent AE, Hellier MD, Grace RH, et al: Inflammatory bowel disease and domestic hygiene in infancy. Lancet 1994;343:766–767.
14. Persson PG, Ahlbom A, Hellers G: Diet and inflammatory bowel disease: a case-control study. Epidemiology 1992;3:47–52.
15. Peeters M, Nevens H, Baert F, et al: Familial aggregation in Crohn's disease: increased age-adjusted risk and concordance in clinical characteristics. Gastroenterology 1996;111:597–603.
16. Meucci G, Vecchi M, Torgano G, et al: Familial aggregation of inflammatory bowel disease in Northern Italy: a multicenter study. Gastroenterology 1992;103:514–519.
17. Tysk C, Lindberg E, Jarnerot G, Floderus-Myrhed B: Ulcerative colitis and Crohn's disease in an unselected population of monozygotic and dizygotic twins: a study of heritability and the influence of smoking. Gut 1988;29:990–996.
18. Van Kruiningen HJ, Colombel JF, Cartun RW, et al: An in-depth study of Crohn's disease in two French families. Gastroenterology 1993;104:351–360.
19. Lee JCW, Lennard-Jones JE: Inflammatory bowel disease in 67 families each with three or more affected first degree relatives. Gastroenterology 1996;111:587–596.
20. Colombel JF, Grandbastien B, Gower-Rousseau C, et al: Clinical characteristics of Crohn's disease in 72 families. Gastroenterology 1996;111:604–607.
21. Polito JM II, Rees RC, Childs B, et al: Preliminary evidence for genetic anticipation in Crohn's disease. Lancet 1996;347:798–800.
22. Duerr RH: Genetics of inflammatory bowel disease. Inflamm Bowel Dis 1996;2:48–60.
23. Yang H, Rotter JI: Genetics of inflammatory bowel disease. In Targan SR, Shanahan F (eds): Inflammatory bowel disease: from bench to bedside. Baltimore, Williams & Wilkins, 1994, pp 32–64.
24. Satsangi J, Welsh KI, Bunce M, et al: Contribution of genes of the major histocompatibility complex to susceptibility and disease phenotype in inflammatory bowel disease. Lancet 1996;347:1212–1217.
25. Danze PM, Colombel JF, Jacquot S, et al: Association of HLA class II genes with susceptibility to Crohn's disease. Gut 1996;39:69–72.
26. Plevy SE, Targan SR, Yang H, et al: Tumor necrosis factor microsatellites define a Crohn's disease associated haplotype on chromosome 6. Gastroenterology 1996;110:1053–1060.
27. Hugot JP, Laurent-Puig P, Gower-Rousseau C, et al: Mapping of a susceptibility locus for Crohn's disease on chromosome 16. Nature 1996;379:821–823.
28. Lisby G, Andersen J, Engbaek K, Binder V: *Mycobacterium paratuberculosis* in intestinal tissue from patients with Crohn's disease demonstrated by a nested primer polymerase chain reaction. Scand J Gastroenterol 1994;29:923–929.
29. Rowbotham DS, Mapstone NP, Trejdosiewicz LK, et al: *Mycobacterium paratuberculosis* DNA not detected in Crohn's disease tissue by fluorescent polymerase chain reaction. Gut 1995;37:660–667.
30. Liu Y, Van Kruiningen HJ, West AB, et al: Immunocytochemical evidence of *Listeria, Escherichia coli,* and *Streptococcus* antigens in Crohn's disease. Gastroenterology 1995;108:1396–1404.
31. Wakefield AJ, Ekbom A, Dhillon AP, et al: Crohn's disease: pathogenesis and persistent measles virus infection. Gastroenterology 1995;108:911–916.
32. Wakefield AJ, Pittilo RM, Sim R, et al: Evidence of persistent measles virus infection in Crohn's disease. J Med Virol 1993;39:345–353.
33. Thompson NP, Montgomery SM, Pounder RE, Wakefield AJ: Is measles vaccination a risk factor for inflammatory bowel disease? Lancet 1995;345:1071–1074.
34. Thompson NP, Wakefield AJ, Pounder RE: Inherited disorders of coagulation appear to protect against inflammatory bowel disease. Gastroenterology 1995;108:1011–1015.
35. James SP, Klapproth JM: Major pathways of mucosal immunity and inflammation: cell activation, cytokine production and the role of bacterial factors. Aliment Pharmacol Ther 1996;10(suppl 2):1–9.
36. May GR, Sutherland LR, Meddings JB: Is small intestinal permeability really increased in relatives of patients with Crohn's disease? Gastroenterology 1993;104:1627–1632.
37. Sartor RB: Cytokines in intestinal inflammation: pathophysiological and clinical considerations. Gastroenterology 1994;106:533–539.
38. Isaacs KL, Sartor RB, Haskill JS: Cytokine mRNA profiles in inflammatory bowel disease mucosa detected by PCR amplification. Gastroenterology 1992;103:1587–1595.
39. Reimund JM, Wittersheim C, Dumont S, et al: Increased production of tumour necrosis factor-α, interleukin-1β, and interleukin-6 by morphologically normal intestinal biopsies from patients with Crohn's disease. Gut 1996;39:684–689.
40. Nielsen OH, Koppen T, Rudiger N, et al: Involvement of interleukin-4 and -10 in inflammatory bowel disease. Dig Dis Sci 1996;41:1786–1793.
41. Hyams JS, Fitzgeral JE, Wyzga N, et al: Relationship of interleukin-1 receptor antagonist to mucosal inflammation in inflammatory bowel disease. J Pediatr Gastroenterol 1995;21:419–425.
42. Pedersen G, Brynskov J, Nielsen OH, Bendtzen K: Adhesion molecules in inflammatory and neoplastic intestinal diseases. Dig Dis 1995;13:322–336.
43. Eberhart CE, Dubois RN: Eicosanoids and the gastrointestinal tract. Gastroenterology 1995;109:285–301.
44. Eliakim R, Rachmilewitz D: Inflammatory bowel disease: the asthma of the intestine? Inflamm Bowel Dis 1996;2:122–132.
45. Conner EM, Brand SJ, Davis JM, et al: Role of reactive metabolites of oxygen and nitrogen in inflammatory bowel disease: toxins, mediators, and modulators of gene expression. Inflamm Bowel Dis 1996;2:133–147.
46. Graham MF: Pathogenesis of intestinal strictures in Crohn's disease: An update. Inflamm Bowel Dis 1995;1:220–227.
47. Musch MW, Chang EB: Diarrhea in inflammatory bowel disease. In

Targan SR, Shanahan F (eds): Inflammatory bowel disease: from bench to bedside. Baltimore, Williams & Wilkins, 1994, pp 239–254.

48. Fuss IJ, Neurath M, Boirivant M, et al: Disparate CD4+ lamina propria (LP) lymphokine secretion profiles in inflammatory bowel disease: Crohn's disease LP cells manifest increased secretion of IFN-γ, whereas ulcerative colitis LP cells manifest increased secretion of IL-5. J Immunol 1996;157:1261–1270.
49. Desreumaux P, Brandt E, Gambiez L, et al: Distinct cytokine patterns in early and chronic ileal lesions of Crohn's disease. Gastroenterology 1997;113:118–126.
50. Rath HC, Herfarth HH, Ikeda JS, et al: Normal luminal bacteria, especially *Bacteroides* species mediate chronic colitis and arthritis in HLA-B27/human β2 microglobulin transgenic rats. J Clin Invest 1996;98:945–953.
51. Ottaway CA: Role of the neuroendocrine system in cytokine pathways in inflammatory bowel disease. Aliment Pharmacol Ther 1996;10(suppl 2):10–15.
52. Mayer EA: Breaking down the functional and organic paradigm. Curr Opin Gastroenterol 1996;12:3–7.
53. Morson BC, Dawson IMP: Inflammatory disorders. In Gastrointestinal Pathology, 2nd ed. London, Blackwell Scientific, 1979, pp 272–336.
54. Rickert RR, Carter HW: The "early" ulcerative lesion of Crohn's disease: correlative light and scanning electron microscopic studies. J Clin Gastroenterol 1980;2:11–19.
55. Goodman MJ, Skinner JM, Truelove SC: Abnormalities in apparently normal bowel mucosa in Crohn's disease. Lancet 1976;1:275–278.
56. Riddell RH: Pathology of idiopathic inflammatory bowel disease. In Kirsner JB, Shorter RG (eds): Inflammatory Bowel Disease, 4th ed. Philadelphia, Lea & Febiger, 1995, pp 517–552.
57. Chong SKF, Blackshaw AJ, Boyle S, et al: Histologic diagnosis of chronic inflammatory bowel disease in childhood. Gut 1985;26:55–59.
58. Surawicz CM, Meisel JL, Ylvisaker T, et al: Rectal biopsy in the diagnosis of Crohn's disease: value of multiple biopsies and serial sectioning. Gastroenterology 1981;81:66–71.
59. Cartun RW, Van Kruiningen HJ, Berman MM: An immunohistochemical search for infectious agents in Crohn's disease. Mod Pathol 1993;6:212–219.
60. Riedel BD, Ghishan FK: Acute diarrhea. In Walker WA, Durie PR, Hamilton JR, et al (eds): Pediatric Gastrointestinal Disease: Pathophysiology, Diagnosis, Management, 2nd ed. Philadelphia, Mosby, 1996, pp 251–262.
61. Hofman AF: Bile acid malabsorption caused by ileal resection. Arch Intern Med 1972;130:597–605.
62. Phillips SF, Gaginella TS: Intestinal secretion as a mechanism in diarrheal disease. In Jerzy Glass GB (ed): Progress in Gastroenterology, vol 3. New York, Grune & Stratton, 1977, pp 481–504.
63. Collins SM: The immunomodulation of enteric neuromuscular function: implications for motility and inflammatory disorders. Gastroenterology 1996;111:1683–1699.
64. Mayer EA: Pain. In Targan SR, Shanahan F (eds): Inflammatory Bowel Disease: From Bench to Bedside. Baltimore, Williams & Wilkins, 1994, pp 255–269.
65. Elliott PR, Lennard-Jones JE, Bartram GE, et al: Colonoscopic diagnosis of minimal change colitis in patients with a normal sigmoidoscopy and normal air-contrast barium enema. Lancet 1982;1:650–651.
66. Heyman MB, Perman JA, Ferrell LD, Thaler MM: Chronic nonspecific inflammatory bowel disease of the cecum and proximal colon in children with grossly normal-appearing colonic mucosa: diagnosis by colonscopic biopsies. Pediatrics 1987;80:255–261.
67. Lenaerts C, Roy CC, Vaillancourt M, et al: High incidence of upper gastrointestinal tract involvement in children with Crohn's disease. Pediatrics 1989;83:777–781.
68. Mashako MNL, Cezard JP, Navarro J, et al: Crohn's disease lesions in the upper gastrointestinal tract: correlation between clinical, radiological, endoscopic, and histological features in adolescents and children. J Pediatr Gastroenterol Nutr 1989;8:442–446.
69. Greenstein AJ, Lachman P, Sachar DB, et al: Perforating and nonperforating indications for repeated operations in Crohn's disease: evidence for two clinical forms. Gut 1988;29:588–592.
70. Sachar DB, Andrews HA, Farmer RG, et al: Proposed classification of patient subgroups in Crohn's disease. Gastroent Intern 1992;5:141–154.
71. Perri F, Annese V, Napolitano G, et al: Sub-groups of patients with Crohn's disease have different clinical outcomes. Inflamm Bowel Dis 1996;2:1–5.
72. Bayless TM, Tokayer AZ, Polito JM II, et al: Crohn's disease: concordance for site and clinical type in affected members. Potential hereditary influences. Gastroenterology 1996;111:573–579.
73. Proujansky R, Fawcett PT, Gibney KM, et al: Examination of antineutrophil cytoplasmic antibodies in childhood inflammatory bowel disease. J Pediatr Gastroenterol Nutr 1993;17:193–197.
74. Vasilauskas EA, Plevy SE, Landers CJ, et al: Perinuclear antineutrophil cytoplasmic antibodies in patients with Crohn's disease define a clinical subgroup. Gastroenterology 1996;110:1810–1819.
74a. Ruemmele FM, Targan SR, Levy G, et al: Diagnostic accuracy of serological assays in pediatric inflammatory bowel disease. Gastroenterology 1998;115:822–829.
74b. Quinton JF, Sendid B, Reumaux D, et al: Anti-saccharomyces cerevisiae mannan antibodies combined with antineutrophil cytoplasmic autoantibodies in inflammatory bowel disease: prevalence and diagnostic role. Gut 1998;42:788–791.
75. Gryboski JD, Spiro HM: Prognosis in children with Crohn's disease. Gastroenterology 1978;74:807–817.
76. Burbige EJ, Huang SS, Bayless TM: Clinical manifestations of Crohn's disease in children and adolescents. Pediatrics 1975;55:866–871.
77. Posthuma R, Moroz SP: Pediatric Crohn's disease. J Pediatr Surg 1985;20:478–482.
78. Raine PAM: BAPS collective review: Chronic inflammatory bowel disease. J Pediatr Surg 1984;19:18–23.
79. Barton JR, Ferguson AA: Clinical features, morbidity and mortality in Scottish children with inflammatory bowel disease. QJM 1990;75:423–439.
80. Griffiths AM, Alemayehu E, Sherman P: Clinical features of gastroduodenal disease in adolescents. J Pediatr Gastroenterol Nutr 1989;8:166–171.
81. D'Haens G, Rutgeerts P, Geboes K, Vantrappen G: The natural history of esophageal Crohn's disease: three patterns of evolution. Gastrointest Endosc 1994;40:296–300.
82. Tolia V: Perianal Crohn's disease in children and adolescents. Am J Gastroenterol 1996;91:922–926.
83. Stratakis CA, Graham W, DiPalma J, Leibowitz I: Misdiagnosis of perianal manifestations of Crohn's disease: two cases and review of the literature. Clin Pediatr 1994;33:631–633.
84. Markowitz J, Grancher K, Rosa J, et al: Highly destructive perianal disease in children with Crohn's disease. J Pediatr Gastroenterol Nutr 1995;21:149–153.
85. Sellman SPB, Hupertz VF: Crohn's disease presenting as suspected abuse. Pediatrics 1996;272–274.
86. Cirocco WC, Reilly JC, Rusin LC: Life-threatening hemorrhage and exsanguination from Crohn's disease: report of four cases. Dis Colon Rectum 1995;38:85–95.
87. Kirchmann HMA, Bender SW: Intestinal obstruction in Crohn's disease in childhood. J Pediatr Gastroenterol Nutr 1987;6:79–83.
88. Katz S, Schulman N, Levin L: Free perforation in Crohn's disease: a report of 33 cases and review of the literature. Am J Gastroenterol 1986;81:38–43.
89. Biller JA, Grand RJ, Harris BH: Abdominal abscesses in adolescents with Crohn's disease. J Pediatr Surg 1987;22:873–876.
90. Grieco MD, Bordan DL, Geiss AC, Beil AR Jr: Toxic megacolon complicating Crohn's colitis. Ann Surg 1980;191:75–80.
91. Gillen CD, Walmsley RS, Prior P, et al: Ulcerative colitis and Crohn's disease: a comparison of the colorectal cancer risk in extensive colitis. Gut 1994;35:1590–1592.
91a. Ribeiro MB, Greenstein AJ, Sachar DS, et al: Colorectal adenocarcinoma in Crohn's disease. Ann Surg 1996;223:186–193.
92. Bernstein D, Rogers A: Malignancy in Crohn's disease. Am J Gastroenterol 1996;91:434–440.
93. Mayer L, Janowitz H: Extraintestinal manifestations of inflammatory bowel disease. In Kirsner JB, Shorter RG (eds): Inflammatory Bowel Disease. Philadelphia, Lea & Febiger, 1988, pp 299–317.
94. Hyams JS: Extraintestinal manifestations of inflammatory bowel disease in children. J Pediatr Gastroenterol Nutr 1994;19:7–21.
95. Passo MH, Fitzgerald JF, Brandt KD: Arthritis associated with inflammatory bowel disease in children: relationship of joint disease to activity and severity of bowel lesion. Dig Dis Sci 1986;31:492–497.
96. Weiner SR, Clarked J, Taggart NA, Utsinger PD: Rheumatic manifestations of inflammatory bowel disease. Semin Arthritis Rheum 1991;20:353–366.
97. Leirisalo-Repo M, Repo H: Gut and spondyloarthropathies. Rheum Dis Clin North Am 1992;18:23–35.

98. De Vos M, Mielants H, Cuvelier C, et al: Long-term evolution of gut inflammation in patients with spondyloarthropathy. Gastroenterology 1996;110:1696–1703.
99. Gilliam JH III, Challa VR, Agudelo CA, et al: Vasculitis involving muscle associated with Crohn's colitis. Gastroenterology 1981;81:787–790.
100. Menard DB, Haddad H, Blain JG, et al: Granulomatous myositis and myopathy associated with Crohn's colitis. N Engl J Med 1976;295:818–819.
101. Lao J, Bostwick HE, Berezin S, et al: Pyomyositis in a patient with Crohn's disease. J Pediatr Gastroenterol Nutr 1995;20:347–350.
102. Leibowitz G, Eliakim R, Amir G, Rachmilewitz D: Dermatomyositis associated with Crohn's disease. J Clin Gastroenterol 1994;18:48–52.
103. Kirsner JB: The local and systemic complications of inflammatory bowel disease. JAMA 1979;242:1177–1183.
104. Apgar JT: Newer aspects of inflammatory bowel disease and its cutaneous manifestations: a selective review. Semin Dermatol 1991;10:138–147.
105. Levitt MD, Ritchie JK, Lennard-Jones JE, Phillips RKS: Pyoderma gangrenosum in inflammatory bowel disease. Br J Surg 1991;78:676–678.
106. Peltz S, Vestey JP, Ferguson A, et al: Disseminated metastatic cutaneous Crohn's disease. Clin Exp Dermatol 1993;18:55–59.
107. Heimburger CD, Tamura T, Marks RD: Rapid improvement in dermatitis after zinc supplementation in a patient with Crohn's disease. Am J Med 1990;88:71–73.
108. Paller AS: Cutaneous changes associated with inflammatory bowel disease. Pediatr Dermatol 1986;3:439–445.
109. Plauth M, Jenss H, Meyle J: Oral manifestations of Crohn's disease: an analysis of 79 cases. J Clin Gastroenterol 1991;13:29–37.
110. Bozkurt T, Langer M, Fendel K, et al: Granulomatous tonsillitis: a rare extraintestinal manifestation of Crohn's disease. Dig Dis Sci 1992;37:1127–1130.
111. Petrelli EA, McKinley M, Troncale FJ: Ocular manifestations of inflammatory bowel disease. Ann Ophthalmol 1982;14:356–360.
112. Hofley P, Roarty J, McGinnity G, et al: Asymptomatic uveitis in children with chronic inflammatory bowel disease. J Pediatr Gastroenterol Nutr 1993;17:397–400.
113. Tripathi RC, Kirschner BS, Kipp M, et al: Corticosteroid treatment for inflamatory bowel disease in pediatric patients increases intraocular pressure. Gastroenterology 1992;102:1957–1961.
114. Urban RC, Cotlier E: Corticosteroid-induced cataracts. Surv Ophthalmol 1986;31:102–110.
115. Lake AM, Stauffer JQ, Marie Stuart MJ: Hemostatic alterations in inflammatory bowel disease. Dig Dis Sci 1978;23:897–902.
116. Webberley MJ, Hart MT, Melikian V: Thromboembolism in inflammatory bowel disease: role of platelets. Gut 1993;34:247–251.
117. Talbot RW, Heppell J, Dozois RR, Beart RW Jr: Vascular complications of inflammatory bowel disease. Mayo Clin Proc 1986;61:140–145.
118. Gormally SM, Bourke W, Kierse B, et al: Isolated cerebral thromboembolism and Crohn disease. Eur J Pediatr 1995;154:815–818.
119. Kent GG, McGowan GE, Hyams JS, Leichtner AM: Hypertension associated with unilateral hydronephrosis as a complication of Crohn's disease. J Pediatr Surg 1987;22:1049–1050.
120. Shield DE, Lytton B, Weiss RM, Schiff M Jr: Urologic complications of inflammatory bowel disease. J Urol 1976;115:701–706.
121. Clark JH, Fitzgerald JF, Bergstein JM: Nephrolithiasis in childhood inflammatory bowel disease. J Pediatr Gastroenterol Nutr 1985;4:829–834.
122. Kahn E, Markowitz J, Simpser E, et al: Amyloidosis in children with inflammatory bowel disease. J Pediatr Gastroenterol Nutr 1989:8:447–453.
123. Hyams J, Markowitz J, Treem W, et al: Characterization of hepatic abnormalities in children with inflammatory bowel disease. Inflamm Bowel Dis 1995;1:27–33.
124. Danzi JT: Extraintestinal manifestations of idiopathic inflammatory bowel disease. Arch Intern Med 1988;148:297–302.
125. Mir-Madjlessi SH, McHenry MC, Farmer RG: Liver abscess in Crohn's disease: report of four cases and review of the literature. Gastroenterology 1986;91:987–993.
126. Lorusso D, Leo S, Mossa A, et al: Cholelithiasis in inflammatory bowel disease: a case-control study. Dis Colon Rectum 1990;33:791–794.
127. Hyams JS, Baker E, Schwartz AN, et al: Acalculous cholecystitis in Crohn's disease. J Adolesc Health Care 1988;10:151–154.
128. Rutgeerts P, Ghoos Y, Vantrappen G, Fevery J: Biliary lipid composition in patients with nonoperated Crohn's disease. Dig Dis Sci 1986;31:27–32.
129. Keljo DJ, Sugerman KS: Pancreatitis in patients with inflammatory bowel disease. J Pediatr Gastroenterol Nutr 1997;25:108–112.
130. Evans JS, George DE, Barwick KW, Lafer DJ: Crohn's disease presenting as chronic pancreatitis with biliary tract obstruction. J Pediatr Gastroenterol Nutr 1996;22:384–388.
131. Ghosh S, Cowen S, Hannan WJ, Ferguson A: Low bone mineral density in Crohn's disease, but not in ulcerative colitis at diagnosis. Gastroenterology 1994;107:1031–1039.
132. Abitbol V, Roux C, Chaussade S, et al: Metabolic bone assessment in patients with inflammatory bowel disease. Gastroenterology 1995;108:417–422.
133. Hyams JS, Wyzga N, Kreutzer DL, et al: Inhibition of bone formation in children with Crohn's disease: an in vitro study. J Pediatr Gastroenterol Nutr 1997;24:289–295.
134. Means RT Jr, Krantz SB: Progress in understanding the pathogenesis of the anemia of chronic disease. Blood 1992;80:1639–1647.
135. Hyams JS, Fitzgerald JE, Treem WR, et al: Relationship of functional and antigenic interleukin-6 to disease activity in inflammatory bowel disease. Gastroenterology 1993;104:1285–1292.
136. Stevens C, Peppercorn MA, Grand RJ: Crohn's disease associated with autoimmune neutropenia. J Clin Gastroenterol 1991;13:328–330.
137. Grill BB, Lange R, Markowitz R, et al: Delayed gastric emptying in children with Crohn's disease. J Clin Gastroenterol 1985;7:216–226.
138. Motil KJ, Altschuler SI, Grand RJ: Mineral balance during nutritional supplementation in adolescents with Crohn disease and growth failure. J Pediatr 1985;107:473–479.
139. Motil KJ, Grand RJ: Nutritional management of inflammatory bowel disease. Pediatr Clin North Am 1985;32:447–469.
140. Stokes MA, Hill GL: Total energy expenditure in patients with Crohn's disease: measurement by the combined body scan technique. J Parenter Enterol Nutr 1993;17:3–7.
141. Kushner RF, Schoeller DA: Resting and total energy expenditure in patients with inflammatory bowel disease. Am J Clin Nutr 1991;53:161–165.
142. Zoli G, Katelaris PH, Garrow J, et al: Increased energy expenditure in growing adolescents with Crohn's disease. Dig Dis Sci 1996;41:1754–1759.
143. Royall D, Greenberg GR, Allard JP, et al: Total enteral nutrition support improves body composition of patients with active Crohn's disease. J Parenter Enterol Nutr 1995;19:95–99.
144. Kanof ME, Lake AM, Bayless TM: Decreased height velocity in children and adolescents before the diagnosis of Crohn's disease. Gastroenterology 1988;95:1523–1527.
145. Motil KJ, Grand RJ, Davis-Kraft L, et al: Growth failure in children with inflammatory bowel disease: a prospective study. Gastroenterology 1993;105:681–691.
146. Walker-Smith JA: Management of growth failure in Crohn's disease. Arch Dis Child 1996;75:351–354.
147. Markowitz J, Grancher K, Rosa J, et al: Growth failure in pediatric inflammatory bowel disease. J Pediatr Gastroenterol Nutr 1993;16:373–380.
148. Ferry GD, Buller HA: Mechanisms of growth retardation, drug therapy, and nutritional support in pediatric inflammatory bowel disease. Inflamm Bowel Dis 1995;1:313–330.
149. Kelts DG, Grand RJ, Shen G, et al: Nutritional basis of growth failure in children and adolescents with Crohn's disease. Gastroenterology 1979;76:720–727.
150. Belli DC, Seidman E, Bouthillier L, et al: Chronic intermittent elemental diet improves growth failure in children with Crohn's disease. Gastroenterology 1988;94:603–610.
151. Polk DB, Hattner JT, Kerner JA Jr: Improved growth and disease activity after intermittent administration of defined formula diet in children with Crohn's disease. J Parenter Enterol Nutr 1992;16:499–504.
152. Thomas AG, Holly JMP, Taylor F, Miller V: Insulin like growth factor-I, insulin like growth factor binding protein-I, and insulin in childhood Crohn's disease. Gut 1993;34:944–947.
153. Hyams JS, Moore RE, Leichtner AM, et al: Relationship of type I procollagen to corticosteroid therapy in children with inflammatory bowel disease. J Pediatr 1988;112:893–898.
154. Hyams JS, Treem WE, Carey DE, et al: Comparison of collagen propeptides as growth markers in children with inflammatory bowel disease. Gastroenterology 1991;100:971–975.

155. Wood B, Watkins JB, Boyle JT, et al: Psychological functioning in children with Crohn's disease and ulcerative colitis: implications for models of psychobiological interaction. J Am Acad Child Adolesc Psychiatry 1987;26:774–781.
156. Burke P, Kocoshis SA, Chandra R, et al: Determinants of depression in recent onset pediatric inflammatory bowel disease. J Am Acad Child Adolesc Psychiatry 1990;29:608–610.
157. Szanjberg N, Krall V, Davis P, et al: Psychopathology and relationship measures in children with inflammatory bowel disease and their parents. Child Psychiatry Hum Dev 1993;23:215–232.
158. Thomas DW, Sinatra FR: Screening laboratory tests for Crohn's disease. West J Med 1989;150:163–164.
159. Hyams JS, Goldman H, Katz A: Differentiating small bowel Crohn's disease from lymphoma: role of rectal biopsy. Gastroenterology 1980;79:340–343.
160. Whitington PF, Friedman AL, Chesney RW: Gastrointestinal disease in the hemolytic uremic syndrome. Gastroenterology 1979;76:728–733.
161. Loirat C, Sonsino E, Moreno AV, et al: Hemolytic-uremic syndrome: an analysis of the natural history and prognostic features. Acta Paediatr Scand 1984;73:505–541.
162. Allen DM, Diamond LK, Howell DA: Anaphylactoid purpura in children (Schönlein-Henoch syndrome): review with a follow-up of the renal complications. Am J Dis Child 1960;99:833–854.
163. Modigliani R, Mary JY, Simon JF, et al: Clinical, biological, and endoscopic picture of attacks of Crohn's disease: evolution on prednisolone. Gastroenterology 1990;98:811–818.
164. Hyams JS, Mandel F, Ferry GD, et al: Relationship of common laboratory parameters to the activity of Crohn's disease in children. J Pediatr Gastroenterol Nutr 1992;14:216–222.
165. Hyams JS, Ferry GD, Mandel FS, et al: Development and validation of a pediatric Crohn's disease activity index. J Pediatr Gastroenterol Nutr 1991;10:439–447.
166. Elton E, Hanauer SB: Review article: the medical management of Crohn's disease. Aliment Pharmacol Ther 1996;10:1–22.
167. Leichtner AM: Aminosalicylates for the treatment of inflammatory bowel disease. J Pediatr Gastroenterol Nutr 1995;21:245–252.
168. Malchow H, Ewe K, Brandes JW, et al: European Cooperative Crohn's Disease Study (ECCDS): results of drug treatment. Gastroenterology 1984;86:249–266.
169. Tremaine WJ, Schroeder KW, Harrison JM, Zinsmeister AR: A randomized, double-blind, placebo-controlled trial of oral mesalamine (5-ASA) preparation, Asacol, in the treatment of symptomatic Crohn's colitis or ileocolitis. J Clin Gastroenterol 1994;19:278–282.
170. Singleton JW, Hanauer SB, Gitnick GL, et al: Mesalamine capsules for the treatment of active Crohn's disease: results of a 16-week trial. Gastroenterology 1993;104:1293–1301.
171. Griffiths A, Koletzko S, Sylvester F, et al: Slow-release 5-aminosalicylic acid therapy in children with small intestinal Crohn's disease. J Pediatr Gastroenterol Nutr 1993;17:186–192.
172. Modigliani R, Colombel JF, Dupas JL, et al: Mesalamine in Crohn's disease with steroid-induced remission: effect on steroid withdrawal and remission maintenance. Gastroenterology 1996;110:688–693.
173. Messori A, Brignola C, Trallori G, et al: Effectiveness of 5-aminosalicylic acid for maintaining remission in patients with Crohn's disease: a meta-analysis. Am J Gastroenterol 1994;89:692–698.
174. Steinhart HA, Hemphill D, Greenberg R: Sulfasalazine and mesalazine for maintenance therapy of Crohn's disease: a meta-analysis. Am J Gastroenterol 1994;89:216–224.
175. Sutherland LR, Martin F, Bailey RJ, et al: A randomized, placebo-controlled, double-blind trial of mesalamine in the maintenance of remission of Crohn's disease. Gastroenterology 1997;112:1069–1077.
176. Brignola C, Cottone M, Pera A, et al: Mesalamine in the prevention of endoscopic recurrence after intestinal resection for Crohn's disease. Gastroenterology 1995;108:345–349.
177. Marteau P, Nelet F, LeLu M, et al: Adverse events in patients treated with 5-aminosalicylic acid: 1993–1994 Pharmacovigilance report for Pentasa in France. Aliment Pharmacol Ther 1996;10:949–956.
178. Thiesen A, Thomson ABR: Older systemic and newer topical glucocorticosteroids and the gastrointestinal tract. Aliment Pharmacol Ther 1996;10:487–496.
179. Summers RW, Switz DM, Sessions JT Jr, et al: National Cooperative Crohn's Disease Study: results of drug treatment. Gastroenterology 1979;77:847–869.
180. Greenberg GR, Feagan BG, Martin F, et al: Oral budesonide for active Crohn's disease. N Engl J Med 1994;331:836–841.
181. Rutgeerts P, Lofberg R, Malchow H, et al: A comparison of budesonide with prednisolone for active Crohn's disease. N Engl J Med 1994;331:842–845.
181a. Thomsen OO, Cortot A, Jewell D, et al: A comparison of budesonide and mesalamine for active Crohn's disease. N Engl J Med 1998; 339:370–374.
182. Lofberg R, Rutgeerts P, Malchow H, et al: Budesonide prolongs time to relapse in ileal and ileocaecal Crohn's disease: a placebo controlled one year study. Gut 1996;39:82–86.
183. Hanauer SB: Inflammatory bowel disease. N Engl J Med 1996;334: 841–848.
184. Spahn JD, Kamada AK: Special considerations in the use of glucocorticoids in children. Pediatr Rev 1995;16:266–272.
185. Hyams JS, Moore RE, Leichtner AM, et al: Relationship of type I procollagen to corticosteroid therapy in children with inflammatory bowel disease. J Pediatr 1988;112:893–898.
186. Sandborn WJ: A review of immune modifier therapy for inflammatory bowel disease: azathioprine, 6-mercaptopurine, cyclosporine, and methotrexate. Am J Gastroenterol 1996;91:423–433.
187. Present DH, Korelitz BI, Wisch N, et al: Treatment of Crohn's disease with 6-mercaptopurine: a long term randomized double blind study. N Engl J Med 1980;302:981–987.
188. Ewe K, Press AG, Singer CC, et al: Azathioprine combined with prednisolone or monotherapy with prednisolone in active Crohn's disease. Gastroenterology 1993;105:367–372.
189. Verhave M, Winter HS, Grand RJ: Azathioprine in the treatment of children with inflammatory bowel disease. J Pediatr 1990;117:809–814.
190. Markowitz J, Rosa J, Grancher K, et al: Long-term 6 mercaptopurine treatment in adolescents with Crohn's disease. Gastroenterology 1990;99:1347–1351.
191. Sandborn WJ, Van Os EC, Zins BJ, et al: An intravenous loading dose of azathioprine decreases the time to response in patients with Crohn's disease. Gastroenterology 1995;109:1808–1817.
192. Colonna T, Korelitz BI: The role of leukopenia in the 6-mercaptopurine-induced remission of refractory Crohn's disease. Am J Gastroenterol 1994;89:362–366.
192a. Markowitz J, Grancher K, Mandel F, et al: 6-Mercaptopurine (6MP) + prednisone therapy for newly diagnosed pediatric Crohn's disease (CD): a prospective, multicenter, placebo-controlled clinical trial (abstract). Gastroenterology 1998;114:1032A.
193. Feagan BG, Rochon J, Fedorak RN, et al: Methotrexate for the treament of Crohn's disease. N Engl J Med 1995;332:292–297.
194. Brynskov J, Freund L, Rasmussen SN, et al: A placebo-controlled, double-blind, randomized trial of cyclosporine therapy in active chronic Crohn's disease. N Engl J Med 1989;321:845–850.
195. Brynskov J, Freund L, Rasmussen SN, et al: Final report of a placebo-controlled, double-blind, randomized, multicentre trial of cyclosporin treatment in active chronic Crohn's disease. Scand J Gastroenterol 1991;26:689–695.
196. Jewell DP, Lennard-Jones JE: Oral cyclosporine for chronic active Crohn's disease: a multicentre controlled trial. The cyclosporin study group of Great Britain and Ireland. Eur J Gastroenterol Hepatol 1994;6:499–505.
197. Nicholls S, Domizio P, Williams CB, et al: Cyclosporin as initial treatment for Crohn's disease. Arch Dis Child 1994;71:243–247.
198. Mahdi G, Israel DM, Hassall E: Cyclosporine and 6-mercaptopurine for active, refractory Crohn's colitis in children. Am J Gastroenterol 1996;91:1355–1359.
199. Present DH, Lichtiger S: Efficacy of cyclosporine in treatment of fistula of Crohn's disease. Dig Dis Sci 1994;39:374–380.
200. Targan SR, Hanauer SB, Van Deventer SJH, et al: Short-term study of chimeric monoclonal antibody cA2 to tumor necrosis factor alpha for Crohn's disease. N Engl J Med 1997;337:1029–1035.
200a. Stack WE, Mann SD, Roy AJ, et al: Randomized controlled trial of CDP571 antibody to tumour necrosis factor alpha in Crohn's disease. Lancet 1997;349:521–524.
200b. van Deventer SJH, Elson CO, Fedorak RN: Multiple doses of intravenous interleukin 10 in steroid refractory Crohn's disease. Gastroenterology 1997;113:383–389.
201. O'Donoghue DP, Dawson AM, Powell-Tuck J, et al: Double-blind withdrawal trial of azathioprine as maintenance treatment for Crohn's disease. Lancet 1978;2:955–957.
202. Candy S, Wright J, Gerber M, et al: A controlled double blind study of azathioprine in the management of Crohn's disease. Gut 1995;37:674–678.

203. Bouhnik Y, Lemann M, Mary JY, et al: Long-term follow-up of patients with Crohn's disease treated with azathioprine or 6-mercaptopurine. Lancet 1996;347:215–219.
204. Ramakrishna J, Langhans N, Calenda K, et al: Combined use of cyclosporine and azathioprine or 6-mercaptopurine in pediatric inflammatory bowel disease. J Pediatr Gastroenterol Nutr 1996;22:296–302.
204a. Kader HA, Raynor SC, Young R, et al. Introduction of 6-mercaptopurine in Crohn's disease patients during the perioperative period: a preliminary evaluation of recurrence of disease. J Pediatr Gastroenterol Nutr 1997;25:93–97.
205. Connell WR, Kamm MA, Ritchie JK, Lennard-Jones JE: Bone marrow toxicity caused by azathioprine in inflammatory bowel disease: 27 years of experience. Gut 1993;34:1081–1085.
206. Cuffari C, Theoret Y, Latour S, et al: 6-Mercaptopurine metabolism in Crohn's disease: correlation with efficacy and toxicity. Gut 1996;39:401–406.
207. Sutherland L, Singleton J, Sessions J, et al: Double blind, placebo-controlled trial of metronidazole in Crohn's disease. Gut 1991;32:1071–1075.
208. Brandt LJ, Bernstein LH, Boley SJ, et al: Metronidazole therapy for perineal Crohn's disease: a follow-up study. Gastroenterology 1994;107:1856–1860.
209. Prantera C, Zannoni F, Scribano ML, et al: An antibiotic regimen for the treatment of active Crohn's disease: a randomized, controlled clinical trial of metronidazole plus ciprofloxacin. Am J Gastroenterol 1996;91:328–332.
210. Rutgeerts P, Hiele M, Geboes K, et al: Controlled trial of metronidazole treatment for prevention of Crohn's recurrence after ileal resection. Gastroenterology 1995;108:1617–1621.
211. Duffy LF, Daum F, Fisher SE, et al: Peripheral neuropathy in Crohn's disease patients treated with metronidazole. Gastroenterology 1985;88:681–684.
211a. Belluzzi A, Brignola C, Campieri M, et al: Effect of an enteric-coated fish-oil preparation on relapses in Crohn's disease. N Engl J Med 1996;334:1557–1560.
212. Bjarnason I, Hayllar J, MacPherson A, et al: Side effects of nonsteroidal anti-inflammatory drugs on the small and large intestine in humans. Gastroenterology 1993;104:1832–1847.
213. Ostro MJ, Greenberg GR, Jeejeebhoy KN: Total parenteral nutrition and complete bowel rest in the management of Crohn's disease. J Parenter Enteral Nutr 1985;9:280–287.
214. Jeejeebhoy KN: Nutritional aspects of inflammatory bowel disease. In Kirsner JB, Shorter RG (eds): Inflammatory Bowel Disease, 4th ed. Baltimore, Williams & Wilkins, 1995, pp 734–749.
215. Griffiths AM, Ohlsson A, Sherman PM, et al: Meta-analysis of enteral nutrition as a primary treatment of active Crohn's disease. Gastroenterology 1995;108:1056–1067.
216. Bernstein CN, Shanahan F: Critical appraisal of enteral nutrition as primary therapy in adults with Crohn's disease. Am J Gastroenterol 1996;91:2075–2079.
217. Gorard DA, Hunt JB, Payne-James JJ, et al: Initial response and subsequent course of Crohn's disease treated with elemental diet or prednisolone. Gut 1993;34:1198–1202.
218. Wilschanski M, Sherman P, Pencharz P, et al: Supplementary enteral nutrition maintains remission in paediatric Crohn's disease. Gut 1996;38:543–548.
219. Israel DM, Hassall E: Prolonged use of gastrostomy for enteral hyperalimentation in children with Crohn's disease. Am J Gastroenterol 1995;90:1084–1088.
220. Davies G, Evans CM, Whand WS, et al: Surgery for Crohn's disease in childhood: influence of site of disease and operative procedure on outcome. Br J Surg 1990;77:891–894.
221. Farmer RG, Michener WM: Prognosis of Crohn's disease with onset in childhood or adolescence. Dig Dis Sci 1979;24:752–757.
222. Telander RL, Schmeling DJ: Current surgical management of Crohn's disease in childhood. Semin Pediatr Surg 1994;3:19–27.
223. Rutgeerts P, Gebhoes K, Vantrappen G, et al: Predictability of the postoperative course of Crohn's disease. Gastroenterology 1990;99:956–963.
224. Hyams JS, Grand RJ, Colodny AH, et al: Course and prognosis after colectomy and ileostomy for inflammatory bowel disease in childhood and adolescence. J Pediatr Surg 1982;17:400–405.
225. Griffiths AM, Wesson DE, Shandling B, et al: Factors influencing postoperative recurrence of Crohn's disease in childhood. Gut 1991;32:491–495.
226. Ozuner G, Fazio VW, Lavery IC, et al: Reoperative rates for Crohn's disease following strictureplasty: long-term analysis. Dis Colon Rectum 1996;39:1199–1203.
227. Oliva L, Wyllie R, Alexander F, et al: The results of strictureplasty in pediatric patients with multifocal Crohn's disease. J Pediatr Gastroenterol Nutr 1994;18:306–310.
228. Schutz DJ Jr: Management of anal fistulas in Crohn's disease: a surgical perspective. Inflamm Bowel Dis 1996;2:61–63.
229. Pescatori M, Interisano A, Basso L, et al: Management of perianal Crohn's disease: results of a multicenter study in Italy. Dis Colon Rectum 1995;38:121–124.
230. Hyams JS, Moore RE, Leichtner AM, et al: Longitudinal assessment of type I procollagen in children with inflammatory bowel disease subjected to surgery. J Pediatr Gastroenterol Nutr 1989;8:68–74.
231. McClain BI, Davidson PM, Stokes KB, Beasley SW: Growth after gut resection for Crohn's disease. Arch Dis Child 1990;65:760–762.
232. Binder V, Hendriksen C, Kreiner S: Prognosis in Crohn's disease based on results from a regional patient group from the county of Copenhagen. Gut 1985;26:146–150.
233. Sahmoud T, Hoctin-Boes G, Modigliani R, et al: Identifying patients with a high risk of relapse in quiescent Crohn's disease. Gut 1995;37:811–818.
234. Prantera C, Pallone F, Brunetti G, et al: Oral 5-aminosalicylic acid (Asacol) in the maintenance of Crohn's disease: The Italian IBD study group. Gastroenterology 1992;103:363–368.
235. Persson PG, Bernell O, Leijonmarck CE, et al: Survival and cause-specific mortality in inflammatory bowel disease: a population-based cohort study. Gastroenterology 1996;110:1339–1345.

# Chapter 33

# Ulcerative Colitis

James F. Markowitz

Ulcerative colitis (UC) is an important pediatric gastrointestinal disease given its potential for significant morbidity and even mortality during childhood, its chronicity, and its premalignant nature. Although significant advances in the understanding of its immunologic basis have led to novel therapeutic approaches, UC remains medically incurable. Nevertheless, current medical and surgical therapeutic options have improved the overall outlook for children with this condition.

## EPIDEMIOLOGY

As opposed to the documented rise in incidence of pediatric Crohn's disease over the last 30 years, incidence of UC in children appears to have remained fairly stable or to have decreased slightly. Various studies report the incidence in children to be 1.5 to 10 cases per 100,000 population.[1–5] The prevalence appears to be 18 to 30 per 100,000.[1–5] Males and females are equally affected. Although most pediatric UC patients present as adolescents (87% of subjects in a recent review from the Cleveland Clinic[6]), it is not unusual to see young children with UC.[7] A review of the combined experience from two tertiary care pediatric centers in the northeast United States reported that 38% of children with UC present by the age of 10 years.[8] UC may develop before 1 year of age.[9]

Risk factors associated with the development of UC during childhood include ethnic background (Ashkenazic Jews are affected more often than other whites, and whites more often than blacks) and a positive family history for inflammatory bowel disease (IBD). Overall, 10% to 15% of children with UC have first-degree relatives with IBD.[8, 10] However, 22.6% of Jewish children with UC have affected relatives, compared with only 13.7% of non-Jewish children.[10] Children with UC are more likely than their unaffected siblings to have had diarrhea during infancy.[11] Children who received formula feedings as infants appear to be at no greater risk for development of UC than those who received breast milk.[12] Although cigarette smoking apparently protects against the development of UC in adult populations, the data in childhood are less clear-cut. Epidemiologic studies have documented that passive smoking during childhood protects against development of UC in adulthood.[13] Although passive smoking may increase the risk of developing Crohn's disease as a child, a protective effect against UC in childhood has not been clearly demonstrated.[11, 14]

## GENETICS

UC can increasingly be differentiated from Crohn's disease genetically. Although both illnesses are often familial, studies consistently demonstrate a lower rate of IBD among relatives of probands with UC versus Crohn's disease, in both Jewish and non-Jewish families.[10, 15, 16] Similarly, the rate of concordant disease is much less for monozygotic twin pairs with UC than with Crohn's disease.[17]

Although they are less important in UC than in Crohn's disease, genetic factors clearly affect the development of UC. The human leukocyte antigen allele HLA-DR2 was found in 40% of a U.S. population with UC, confirming previous studies in which 70% of a Japanese UC population was found to have the same association.[18–20] Similar HLA class II allele associations have not been seen in Crohn's disease. The putative Crohn's disease susceptibility gene (*IBD1*), localized on chromosome 16, does not appear to be important in UC.[21, 22]

Other subclinical markers of disease have been used to further clarify the genetic basis of UC. The best defined is pANCA, a distinct subset of perinuclear antineutrophil cytoplasmic antibodies that is highly specific for UC and may well represent a marker of a genetically controlled immunoregulatory disturbance. pANCA is present in about 70% of UC patients but in only 6% of those with Crohn's disease and 3% of healthy controls.[23] The presence or absence of pANCA is concordant within families[24] and also tends to correlate with the presence of HLA-DR2.[19] The fact that not all UC patients manifest these markers strongly suggests that UC is a genetically heterogeneous disorder.

## ETIOLOGY

Despite significant advances in unraveling the pathophysiology of UC, its cause remains unknown. Numerous theories have been proposed over the years; they are described in the following sections.

## Infectious Agents

Although there is great clinical similarity between UC and infectious colitides, no solid evidence supports the theory that an infectious agent is the primary cause of colonic inflammation in UC.

## Food Allergy

Allergic reactions, especially to dietary antigens such as milk, have been extensively investigated, but data supporting an allergic origin for UC are lacking. High titers of antibodies to dietary antigens such as milk are not specific to UC.[25, 26] Patients with UC at times respond to elemental or elimination diets, but when the particular food that appeared to induce symptoms is reintroduced symptoms are only rarely reproduced consistently.[27]

## Psychological Factors

In the past, UC was considered to be a psychosomatic disorder. However, although children with UC often demonstrate psychological profiles that distinguish them from healthy children and control subjects with other chronic diseases,[28–32] these traits do not appear to be the cause of the illness. An analysis of the literature on the psychosomatic origin of UC demonstrates many methodologic deficiencies, including lack of controls, lack of diagnostic criteria, and nonblinded collection of data.[33] None of the well-designed studies in the literature shows an association between UC and psychiatric disturbance.

## Metabolic Deficiencies

Short-chain fatty acids extracted from the luminal contents are a major source of energy for the colonocyte. The observation that fecal butyrate is increased in UC suggests the possibility that UC may represent a form of colonic mucosal "malnutrition."[34, 35] Further testing of this hypothesis should help unravel whether this apparent inability to utilize short-chain fatty acids in UC is important etiologically.

## Immunity

Current opinion appears to favor an autoimmune origin for UC. The immunologic profile of patients with UC is characterized by a predominantly humoral response.[36] This profile is distinctly different from the predominantly cell-mediated response seen in Crohn's disease. In UC, there is marked overproduction of immunoglobulin G1 (IgG1) by both intestinal lymphocytes and those in the peripheral circulation.[37] Autoantibodies have been identified that are directed against colonic epithelial proteins such as the cytoskeletal protein tropomyosin.[38] In addition, these autoantibodies cross-react with antigens in tissues commonly affected by the extraintestinal manifestations of UC, including biliary epithelium, skin, chondrocyte, and eye ciliary body.[39] The factor or factors that initiate this autoimmune process remain to be elucidated.

# PATHOLOGY

## Anatomic Distribution

Before the mid-1970s, extent of disease in UC was determined largely by barium enema and sigmoidoscopy. With these techniques, 60% of 388 children were found to have pancolitis, 22% left-sided colitis, and 17% proctitis or proctosigmoiditis.[40, 41] With colonoscopy 41% of 180 children were found to have pancolitis, 34% left-sided disease, and 26% proctitis or proctosigmoiditis.[8] These latter data are comparable to those from a Danish study, in which only 30% of 77 children diagnosed before the age of 15 years were found to have pancolitis.[42] In that study only 13% of children diagnosed before 10 years of age had pancolitis, but a U.S. report noted that 71% of such children had pancolitis at diagnosis.[7] The more recent data may reflect an increased awareness of the disease in children, leading to earlier recognition of milder cases of disease. Support for this concept can be found in the more recent studies on the evolution of proctosigmoiditis in children, in which proximal extension of disease is estimated to be 25% within 3 years of initial diagnosis and 29% to 70% over the course of follow-up.[42–44]

## Macroscopic Findings

The inflammatory changes characteristic of UC are confined to the mucosa. The external surface of the colon appears normal. Classically, mucosal abnormalities begin at the anal verge and extend proximally to a variable extent. In the untreated patient, rectal sparing should suggest Crohn's disease, although a few children with well documented UC have been described to have rectal sparing at initial presentation.[45] Because treatment (both systemic and rectal) can significantly change the appearance of the mucosa, particular care must be taken in interpreting the finding of rectal sparing in a child undergoing endoscopy after therapy has been initiated.

The gross appearance of the mucosa in UC depends on the severity of inflammation. Mild disease is characterized by diffuse erythema and loss of the normal mucosal vasculature pattern. A fine granularity can also be present. Moderate inflammation results in numerous small surface ulcerations, scattered flecks of exudate, and spontaneous or contact bleeding from the mucosal surface. With more active disease, larger, deep ulcerations covered with shaggy exudate become widespread. As these ulcers surround less involved areas of mucosa, single or multiple pseudopolyps form (Fig. 33–1). Although all of these changes are present diffusely in involved areas of the large bowel, the severity of the inflammatory process can vary from location to location.

## Microscopic Findings

Neutrophilic infiltration of crypts (cryptitis) is often accompanied by crypt abscesses, depletion of goblet cell mu-

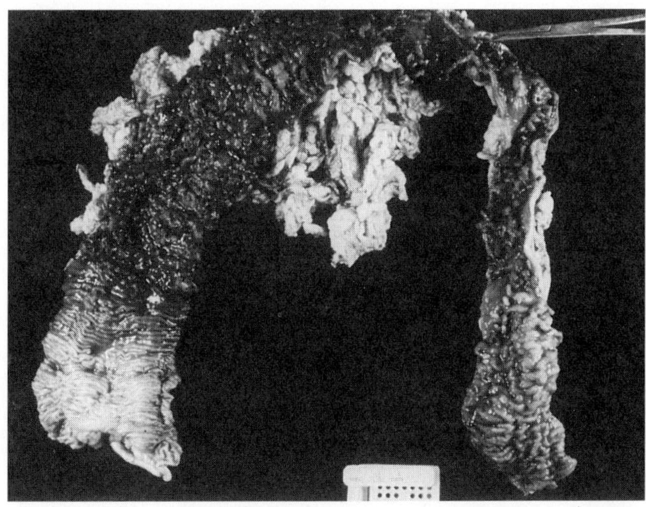

**FIGURE 33–1.** Macroscopic appearance of the colon of a 16-year-old with ulcerative colitis at the time of subtotal colectomy. Note mucosa characterized by diffuse ulceration and multiple pseudopolyps. (Courtesy of Ellen Kahn, MD.)

cin, and chronic inflammatory cells in the lamina propria, and these constitute the primary histologic findings in UC (Fig. 33–2). In addition, signs of chronicity include evidence of crypt damage, such as crypt distortion, a papillary configuration to the surface epithelium, and Paneth cell metaplasia. None of these findings is pathognomonic for UC, because similar changes can be seen in severe Crohn's colitis. Infectious colitis may also have a similar appearance, although histologic differentiation of UC from acute, self-limited colitis usually is possible.[46] In surgical specimens obtained from patients with severe or fulminant disease, ulceration can extend into the submucosa or, rarely, into the deeper layers of the bowel wall.[47]

## CLINICAL FEATURES

Children with UC most commonly present with diarrhea, rectal bleeding, and abdominal pain (Table 33–1). Frequent watery stools can contain either streaks of blood or clots and are most common on arising in the morning, after eating, and during the night. Children often describe both tenesmus and urgency, although the former symptom is at times misinterpreted as constipation by the child or parent. Although acute weight loss is common, abnormalities of linear growth are unusual (see later discussion).

The severity of symptoms at presentation is variable. Forty percent to 50% of children and adolescents present with mild symptoms, characterized by fewer than four stools per day, only intermittent hematochezia, and minimal (if any) systemic symptoms or weight loss.[8, 48] These children generally have normal physical examinations or only minimal tenderness on palpation of the lower abdomen. Stools can have streaks of blood, or they may only be guaiac-positive. Laboratory studies can reveal mild anemia and elevated acute phase reactants (e.g., erythrocyte sedimentation rate). However, some children have entirely normal laboratory studies.

Another third of children with UC are moderately ill, often displaying weight loss, more frequent diarrhea, and systemic symptoms. Physical examination demonstrates abdominal tenderness, and laboratory studies often are characterized by moderate leukocytosis, mild anemia, and elevated acute phase reactants.

The final 10% to 15% of the pediatric UC population have acute, fulminant disease presentation. These patients appear moderately to severely toxic and have severe crampy abdominal pain, fever, more than six diarrheal stools per day, and, at times, copious rectal bleeding. They frequently manifest tachycardia, orthostatic hypotension, diffuse abdominal tenderness without peritoneal signs, and abdominal distention. Laboratory studies reveal leukocytosis, often with numerous band forms, anemia, thrombocytosis, and hypoproteinemia. Toxic megacolon represents the most dangerous extreme of acute, fulminant colitis; it is rare in the pediatric age group.

## EXTRAINTESTINAL MANIFESTATIONS

Extraintestinal manifestations are common in children with UC and can affect almost every organ system of the body. The more common sites of involvement are the skin, eyes, biliary tree, and joints. Although the cause of these extraintestinal manifestations remains unknown, an anti-colonocyte antibody detectable in the sera of patients with UC has been shown to cross-react with antigens present in the skin, ciliary body of the eye, bile duct and joints.[38, 39, 49] Many of the extraintestinal manifestations tend to occur at times of increased colitis activity. It is therefore tempting to speculate that extraintestinal symptoms result when autoantibodies capable of recognizing these nonintestinal tissues develop as part of the humoral response characteristic of UC. (See Chapter 32 for further details of extraintestinal manifestations of IBD.)

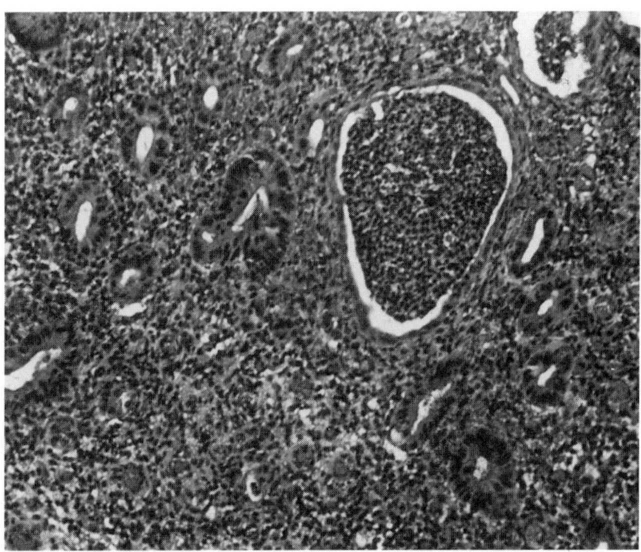

**FIGURE 33–2.** Colonic biopsy. Active ulcerative colitis, characterized by neutrophilic infiltration of the crypts, crypt abscesses, and crypt distortion. Hematoxylin-eosin stain, × 125.

**TABLE 33–1. Symptoms at Diagnosis of Ulcerative Colitis**

| SYMPTOMS AND SIGNS | PATIENTS DIAGNOSED 1970–1978 (N = 87)* | | PATIENTS DIAGNOSED BEFORE 1967 (N = 125)† | |
|---|---|---|---|---|
| | No. of Patients | % of Population | No. of Patients | % of Population |
| Hematochezia | 84 | 96 | 107 | 86 |
| Diarrhea | 82 | 94 | 116 | 93 |
| Abdominal pain | 77 | 88 | 107 | 86 |
| Anorexia | 44 | 50 | — | — |
| Nocturnal diarrhea | 43 | 49 | — | — |
| Weight loss | 37 | 42 | 64 | 51 |
| Fever | 12 | 13 | 46 | 37 |
| Vomiting | 10 | 11 | 53 | 42 |

*Hamilton JR, Bruce GA, Abdourhaman M, Gall DG: Inflammatory bowel disease in children and adolescents. (Barness LA, ed). Adv Pediatr 1979;26:311–341.

†Michener WM: Ulcerative colitis in children: problems in management. Pediatr Clin North Am 1967;14:159–163.

## Hepatobiliary Disorders

The most serious hepatobiliary diseases associated with UC are primary sclerosing cholangitis (PSC) and autoimmune hepatitis. The presentation and severity of these manifestations are generally independent of the activity of colitis and often do not appear to be affected by medical management of UC or by colectomy. PSC occurs in 3.5% of children and adolescents with UC.[50] It may be present before or at the time of the initial diagnosis of UC, or it can develop during the course of the illness. Although most children described in the literature appear to have mild liver disease, patients occasionally have been described as progressing to end-stage liver disease requiring transplantation or death from cholangiocarcinoma.[50–52] Patients with UC and PSC do not appear to have a more severe or benign course of colitis than those without the hepatobiliary disease, but the presence of PSC in UC has been shown to enhance the risk of colorectal aneuploidy, dysplasia, and cancer.[53] Absolute cumulative risk for colorectal cancer in UC patients with PSC after 10, 20, and 25 years of disease is 9%, 31%, and 50%, respectively, compared with 2%, 5%, and 10%, respectively, in UC patients without PSC.[54] In addition, those with PSC and UC complicated by colorectal cancer are at increased risk of cholangiocarcinoma, compared with patients with PSC and UC but no colorectal malignancy.[54]

Autoimmune hepatitis is unusual in children with UC, having been identified in only 1 (0.4%) of 237 children and adolescents with UC in the series previously described.[50] In addition, serum aminotransferase abnormalities can be seen in a variety of other clinical circumstances: during periods of increased colitis activity; in association with specific therapies used for colitis, including corticosteroids, sulfasalazine, parenteral hyperalimentation, azathioprine, and 6-mercaptopurine; or with the fatty changes associated with massive acute weight gain.[50]

## Joint Disorders

Arthralgias have been described in up to 32% of children with UC at some time during their course.[55] Arthritis, either a peripheral migratory type affecting the large joints or a monoarticular, nondeforming arthritis primarily affecting the knees or ankles, is reported in 10% to 20% of children.[55, 56] The presence and activity of arthritis and arthralgias usually (but not invariably) correlate with the activity of the bowel disease. Ankylosing spondylitis occurs in up to 6% of adults with UC[57] but is rare during childhood.

## Skin Disorders

Cutaneous manifestations occur during periods of enhanced colitis activity, with erythema nodosum occurring more commonly than pyoderma gangrenosum.[58, 59] Erythema nodosum lesions appear as raised, erythematous, painful, circular nodules that usually occur over the tibia but may also be present on the lower leg, ankle, or extensor surface of the arm. Lesions persist from several days to a few weeks and usually remit in association with treatments directed at the enhanced colitis activity.[58, 59] Pyoderma gangrenosum usually appears as small, painful, sterile pustules that coalesce into a larger sterile abscess (Fig. 33–3). This ultimately drains, forming a deep, necrotic ulcer. Lesions usually occur on the lower extremities, although the upper extremities, trunk, and head are not spared. A variety of possibly beneficial therapies have been reported, but at present systemic or local cyclosporine appears to be the treatment of choice.[60, 61]

## Thromboembolic Disorders

Case reports document the occurrence of thromboembolic complications in children with UC. Sites of venous or arterial thrombosis include the extremities, portal or hepatic vein, lung, and central nervous system.[62, 63]

## Ocular Disorders

Eye involvement in UC is rare in children, although episcleritis and asymptomatic uveitis have been described.[64, 65] Other ocular disorders, such as posterior subcapsular cataracts or increased ocular pressure, may result from corticosteroid therapy.[66, 67]

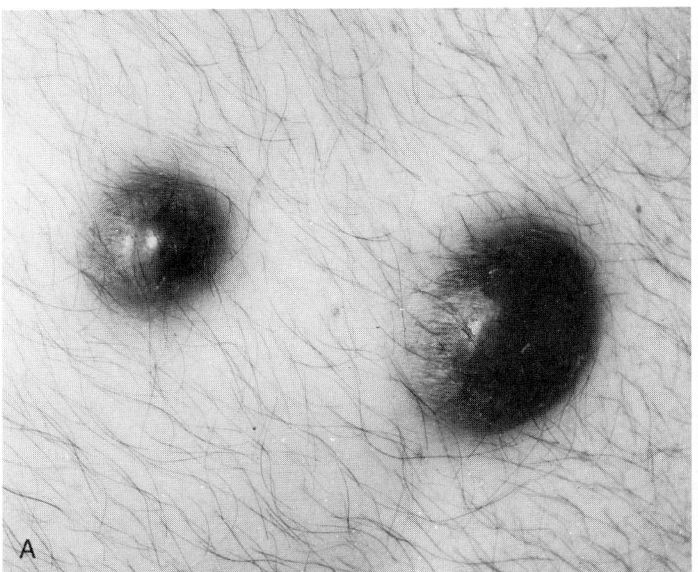


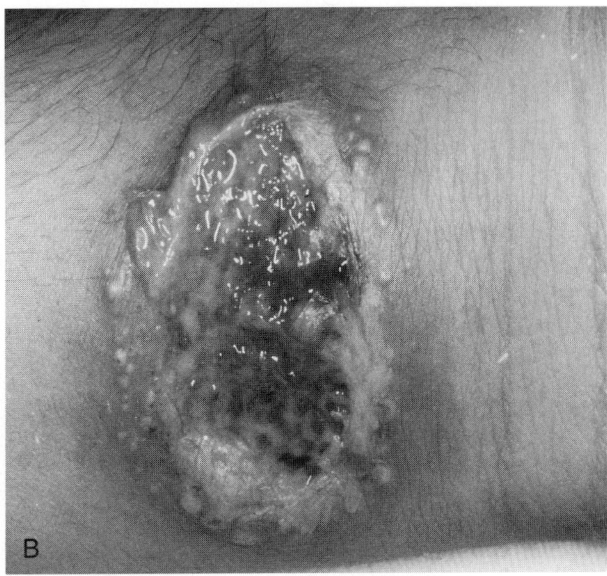


**FIGURE 33–3.** *A,* Pustular phase of pyoderma gangrenosum in a 15-year-old boy with ulcerative colitis. Cutaneous lesions began 2 weeks after initial gastrointestinal symptoms. *B,* Typical chronic ulcer of pyoderma gangrenosum from the same patient, located on the dorsal surface of the forearm.

## COMPLICATIONS

### Bleeding

Hematochezia is almost universal in UC, but severe hemorrhage requiring urgent or multiple transfusions occurs in fewer than 5% of cases. When present, severe hemorrhage is usually the result of diffuse, active mucosal ulceration. Children who continue to require blood transfusions after 14 days of intensive medical therapy have been shown to be at risk for significant complications and colectomy,[68] although more recent data suggest that such children may be successfully managed with intensive medical therapy for longer periods without significant morbidity or need for eventual colectomy.[69]

### Perforation

Free perforation of the colon is a rare emergency complication of UC. Circumstances that predispose to perforation include acute fulminant colitis, toxic megacolon, and diagnostic interventions such as barium enema or colonoscopy. In these settings, gaseous distention or direct pressure from an endoscope can generate sufficient force to perforate the inflamed colon. Peritonitis and septic shock can result. Fluid resuscitation, broad-spectrum antibiotics, and emergency surgery are required. Plain radiographs of the abdomen may be used to identify a possible free perforation in children with UC who have worsening symptoms or shoulder pain, since concomitant corticosteroid therapy may mask physical findings such as board-like rigidity or diffuse rebound tenderness.

### Toxic Megacolon

This complication has been described in up to 5% of children and adolescents with UC, and it represents a medical and potentially surgical emergency.[40, 68] Improper diagnosis or treatment can lead to a rapidly progressive deterioration complicated by severe electrolyte disturbances, hypoalbuminemia, hemorrhage, perforation, sepsis, and/or shock. Precipitating factors include the use of antidiarrheal agents such as anticholinergics or opiates and excessive colonic distention during barium enema or colonoscopy. Possibly because of recognition and minimization of these factors, the frequency of toxic megacolon in the pediatric population appears to be decreasing. In a review of the clinical outcome of children with UC treated at two tertiary centers between 1975 and 1994, only 1 case of toxic megacolon was seen in 171 children monitored for a total of 823 patient-years.[8]

### Carcinoma

The colorectal tumors that develop in the setting of chronic UC are adenocarcinomas. In contrast to sporadic adenocarcinomas, those that arise in UC do not begin as adenomatous polyps but rather as flat lesions characterized by the presence of dysplasia.[70] The genetic alterations that precede the development of dysplasia occur multifocally in the colon, so that the resulting adenocarcinomas are evenly distributed about the colon.[71] Multifocal or synchronous tumors are present in 10% to 20% of patients.[72]

Patients who are diagnosed with colitis during childhood are at particularly high lifetime risk of colorectal cancer, because duration (longer than 10 years) and extent of colitis (pancolitis, left-sided colitis, and proctitis, in order of greater to lesser risk) are the two most critical risk factors for cancer in these conditions.[73–75] Other, less well characterized risk factors include concomitant PSC[53, 54]; an excluded, defunctionalized, or bypassed segment[76]; and depressed red blood cell folate levels.[77] Patients as young as 16 years of age have been demonstrated to have colonic aneuploidy, dysplasia, or cancer; however, as in adults, the risk for these changes does not appear to be significant in the first decade of illness.[40, 73, 78]

Population-based studies support the observation that children with UC have an increased lifetime risk of colorectal cancer.[79–82] A large Swedish study examined the standardized incidence ratio (the ratio of observed to expected cases) of colorectal cancer in relation to age. Children with onset of UC before 15 years of age had a ratio of 118 (162 for those with pancolitis), compared with 2.2 to 16.5 for patients older than 15 years at diagnosis.[79] These figures translate to cumulative colorectal cancer incidence rates of 5% at 20 years and 40% at 35 years for patients with colitis onset before the age of 15 years, and 5% and 30%, respectively, for those whose colitis began between ages 15 and 39 years.[79] These values are strikingly similar to those originally reported by Devroede and colleagues from the Mayo Clinic in children with onset of colitis before 14 years of age (3% in the first 10 years, 43% at 35 years).[73] In addition, 52% to 68% of colitis-associated cancers detected because of symptoms have regional node involvement or distant metastasis, resulting in overall 5-year survival rates of 31% to 55%.[83–85] Therefore, it is estimated that there is an 8% risk of dying from colon cancer 10 to 25 years after diagnosis of UC if colectomy is not performed for control of disease symptoms.[86]

Given the high risks of colorectal cancer, surveillance colonoscopy has been advocated (often uncritically) as an approach that may lessen the need for prophylactic proctocolectomy. Surveillance programs, as currently practiced, suffer from a lack of objective premalignant markers and the problems associated with invasive testing. A standardized definition of dysplasia (negative, indefinite, low-grade, or high-grade[70]) is in widespread use, but interobserver variability using these definitions results in major discrepancy rates of 4% to 7.5% between expert pathologists reviewing the same slides.[87, 88] In addition, evaluations must be made, but have not always been reported, based on an "intent to treat" model, because noncompliance with the surveillance protocol (refusal to enroll or maintain the regular examination schedule) and inability to adequately evaluate the entire colon owing to stricture, poor bowel preparation, or active disease constitute realities of surveillance that bear directly on the efficacy of the surveillance strategy.

The literature generally reflects the practice of performing colectomy only after high-grade dysplasia or cancer has been detected. A review of prospective cohort studies revealed that, with this approach, surveillance detects cancer at an early and potentially curable stage 65% of the time, thereby reducing the frequency of detection of advanced lesions from 60% to 35%.[86] However, the data suggest that 33 patients would have to be under regular surveillance for 15 years to prevent 1 incurable cancer. With biannual examinations resulting in 7 to 8 colonoscopies per patient, a total of about 250 procedures would be performed to prevent 1 incurable cancer.[86] Analyses such as these have led to a vigorous discussion regarding the cost-effectiveness of surveillance as it is currently practiced.[89, 90]

Better markers are being sought to enhance the predictive accuracy of surveillance. Expanding indications for surgery to include the identification of low-grade dysplasia might enhance the effectiveness of surveillance, because low-grade dysplasia has been shown to advance to high-grade dysplasia or cancer in 54% of cases within 5 years.[91] Other markers, including aneuploidy,[78, 92–94] loss of tumor suppressor gene (e.g., *p53*[95]) function, expression of proto-oncogenes (e.g., K-*ras*[96]), and expression of abnormal mucin-associated antigens (e.g., sialosyl-Tn[97]), have also been investigated as adjuncts to surveillance for dysplasia.

No prospective studies have assessed the optimal schedule of surveillance, although a cost-benefit analysis suggested colonoscopies every 3 years for the first 10 years of surveillance, with more frequent investigations as the duration of colitis increases.[98] Current practice usually mandates biyearly colonoscopies beginning at 7 to 10 years after diagnosis. Although many advocate initiating surveillance only after 15 to 20 years of disease in adults with left-sided colitis or proctosigmoiditis, the frequent proximal extension of these disease distributions in patients with onset during childhood suggests that all patients with childhood-onset UC of any extent should be enrolled in a surveillance program within 10 years of initial diagnosis. Procedures require panendoscopy to the cecum, with two to four biopsies every 10 cm from the cecum to the sigmoid, and every 5 cm in the sigmoid and rectum. Additional biopsies must be performed if a mass or other suspicious lesion is identified. Current recommendations for colectomy include any identification of dysplasia (low-grade or high-grade) confirmed by two independent, experienced pathologists. Repeat colonoscopy for confirmation of dysplasia on new biopsies is not recommended, because there is no way to guarantee that the identical site can be biopsied on a subsequent procedure. If indefinite dysplasia is identified, aggressive medical management to reduce active inflammation, followed by repeat surveillance colonoscopy within 3 to 6 months, is indicated.

### Growth and Development

About 10% of children with ulcerative colitis demonstrate significantly impaired linear growth,[3, 99] and, for many patients, periods of poor caloric intake associated with episodes of active disease can result in acute weight loss. Why linear growth impairment is so unusual in UC compared with Crohn's disease remains to be explained, although the different cytokine profiles seen in the two diseases may be important. In one study, serum from children with Crohn's disease caused marked impairment in bone growth in an animal model, but serum from children with UC was no different than that from healthy controls.[100] Further study is necessary before it can be determined whether this effect is mediated by circulating proinflammatory cytokines or by some other serum factor.

## DIAGNOSIS

### History

Many children present with obvious symptoms of diarrhea and rectal bleeding. In others, symptoms are less obvious and more difficult to elicit, especially in children or adolescents who are unwilling or too embarrassed to discuss the frequency and consistency of their bowel movements. Awakening with pain or the need to defecate is an especially important symptom to elicit, because it often helps differentiate the child with organic illness from one with a functional condition. The history should seek to identify evidence of recent weight loss, poor growth, arrested sexual development, or, in the postmenarchal adolescent, secondary amenorrhea. When family history reveals other relatives with IBD, the possibility that UC is present is increased.

## Physical Examination

Children with active colitis often have mild to moderate abdominal tenderness, especially in the left lower quadrant or in the midepigastric area. Tender bowel loops may be palpable, but inflammatory masses are lacking. With fulminant disease, marked tenderness can be present. Perianal inspection is generally normal, and the presence of perianal tags or fistulas suggests Crohn's disease. The presence of arthritis or of skin lesions such as erythema nodosum, pyoderma gangrenosum, or cutaneous vasculitis is an important clue to the autoimmune nature of the child's illness.

## Laboratory Studies

Once UC is suspected, the laboratory studies outlined in Table 33–2 help exclude other illnesses and provide evidence to support proceeding to more invasive radiologic and endoscopic diagnostic procedures. Microcytic anemia, mild to moderate thrombocytosis, elevated erythrocyte sedimentation rate, and hypoalbuminemia are present in 40% to 80% of cases. The total leukocyte count is normal to only mildly elevated, unless the illness is complicated by acute fulminant colitis. Elevated serum aminotransferase levels are present in 3% of children at the time of initial diagnosis and reflect signs of potentially serious concomitant liver disease (chronic active hepatitis or PSC) in about half of them.[50] In a number of children, however, all laboratory studies are normal.

Enteric pathogens must be excluded in all patients. Particular attention must be given to the possibility of *Clostridium difficile*–mediated colitis, given the frequency with which many children are exposed to antibiotics. If a pathogen is identified, it must be treated and the patient must be monitored, because it is not unusual for children with UC to present initially with superimposed infection. If symptoms persist despite eradication of the identified pathogen, workup should continue.

**TABLE 33–2. Laboratory Studies in Suspected Ulcerative Colitis**

| |
|---|
| Complete blood count, differential, reticulocyte count |
| Erythrocyte sedimentation rate, C-reactive protein |
| Electrolytes, serum chemistries (including total protein, albumin, liver functions) |
| Serum iron, total iron-binding capacity, ferritin |
| Stools for enteric pathogens (including *Salmonella, Shigella, Campylobacter, Yersinia, Aeromonas, Escherichia coli*) |
| Stool for *Clostridium difficile* toxin |
| Direct microscopic examination of the stool for ova and parasites, Charcot-Leyden crystals, leukocytes |
| Perinuclear antineutrophil cytoplasmic antibody (pANCA) |

More specific diagnostic laboratory studies are moving from the research bench to clinical practice. In particular, serologic tests for the detection of circulating pANCA can be useful in differentiating UC from other colitides, including Crohn's disease.[23] pANCA can be detected in about 70% of adults with UC but in only 6% of Crohn's patients and 3% of controls. One pediatric study demonstrated that a detection system for pANCA had a 67% sensitivity, 97% specificity, 67% negative predictive value, and 97% positive predictive value for identifying UC in children.[101]

## Radiography

Traditionally, when UC was suspected, a barium enema was performed to identify radiographic signs of inflammation. Although the barium enema can, at times, differentiate between Crohn's and UC, the classic radiographic findings attributed to one form of colitis can be mimicked by the other. It is now increasingly common to eliminate the study in favor of colonoscopy. In most circumstances, however, the child with suspected UC should still undergo an upper gastrointestinal series with small bowel follow-through to help exclude the possibility of Crohn's disease.

Abdominal ultrasound, computed tomography, and various scintigraphic techniques, including technetium 99m–hexamethylpropyleneamineoxime ($^{99m}$Tc-HMPAO)–labeled leukocyte scan,[102, 103] can be used to assess the presence and extent of intestinal inflammation, although these studies are not widely used to establish the initial diagnosis. Overall, these modalities are more useful in identifying complications associated with Crohn's disease than UC.

## Endoscopy

Colonoscopy allows accurate determination of the extent and distribution of colitis through direct visualization and biopsy of the affected segments. UC is characterized by diffuse inflammation that begins at the anal verge and progresses proximally to a variable degree. Although rectal sparing is generally associated with Crohn's disease, untreated children can have rectal sparing at initial colonoscopy yet subsequently have typical UC.[45] In mild UC, the rectal and colonic mucosa appears erythematous, the normal vascular markings are lost, and there is increased friability evidenced by petechiae or contact hemorrhage. With more active disease, exudate, ulcerations, and marked hemorrhage are evident. Skip lesions, aphthous ulcerations, and significant ileal inflammation are indicative of Crohn's disease. All children who undergo endoscopy should be biopsied, because the histologic appearance can often help differentiate between acute, self-limited colitis, Crohn's disease, and UC.[46]

# DIFFERENTIAL DIAGNOSIS

The differential diagnosis is summarized in Table 33–3. Most of these conditions can easily be excluded by history, physical examination, laboratory evaluation, or endoscopy and biopsy. In contrast to the situation in adults, neoplastic

**TABLE 33–3. Differential Diagnosis of Ulcerative Colitis**

Crohn's disease
Enteric infection
- *Salmonella*
- *Shigella*
- *Campylobacter*
- *Aeromonas*
- *Yersinia*
- Enterohemorrhagic *Escherichia coli*
- *Entamoeba histolytica*

Pseudomembranous (post-antibiotic) enterocolitis
- *Clostridium difficile*

Carbohydrate intolerance
- Lactose
- Sucrose
- Sorbitol, xylitol

Vasculitis
- Henoch-Schönlein purpura
- Hemolytic-uremic syndrome

Allergic enterocolitis/eosinophilic gastroenteritis
Laxative abuse
Neoplasms
- Adenocarcinoma
- Intestinal polyposis

disease, ischemia, and radiation-induced injury are rarely significant diagnostic concerns in children and adolescents.

## MEDICAL THERAPIES

Because curative medical therapy does not exist, current treatment is symptomatic and supportive. Treatment aims include the suppression of symptoms and the control of unavoidable complications. In many cases, UC and Crohn's disease respond to the same therapeutic modalities, and the reader may want to review Chapter 32 for additional details of the various pharmacologic agents discussed here. Therapeutic options are listed in Table 33–4. Much of the data supporting the use of these medications have been extrapolated from adult studies. The following discussion focuses on those aspects of treatment that have been shown to be particularly effective in the pediatric population.

**TABLE 33–4. Medical Therapeutic Options in Ulcerative Colitis**

**Nutritional Therapy**
- Appropriate dietary intake (with or without food supplements)
- Short-chain fatty acids
- n-3 Fatty acids (fish oils)

**Anti-inflammatory Agents**
- Corticosteroids
  - Prednisone, prednisolone, hydrocortisone
  - Budesonide*
  - Fluticasone propionate*
- 5-Aminosalicylates
  - Sulfasalazine
  - Olsalazine
  - Mesalamine
  - Balsalazide*

**Immunomodulators**
- 6-Mercaptopurine
- Azathioprine
- Cyclosporine
- Tacrolimus
- Methotrexate

*Not commercially available in the United States.

### Nutritional Therapy

Nutritional therapies such as elemental diets have a role as primary treatment in Crohn's disease, but UC is less amenable to such interventions.[104] Although "bowel rest" can ameliorate symptoms in Crohn's disease of the small bowel, it is often ineffective in UC, possibly because the colonocyte derives energy from the fecal stream in the form of short-chain fatty acids. Nutritional interventions in UC are generally adjunctive to other treatments. In UC, assurance of an adequate dietary intake promotes normal growth and prevents catabolism, thereby enhancing the effect of other treatment modalities.[105] Nutritional support can be accomplished successfully by a number of approaches, including dietary supplementation and enteral or parenteral nutrition.

The therapeutic use of short chain fatty acids is one area in which a nutritional intervention can offer benefit as primary therapy in UC. Adults with UC have been shown to have impaired colonic butyrate metabolism.[106] Similarly, fecal concentrations of *n*-butyrate are elevated in children with inactive or mild UC, suggesting impaired utilization of this metabolic fuel.[35] Three placebo-controlled trials of short-chain fatty acid or butyrate enemas demonstrated limited improvement in symptom score and endoscopic appearance in actively treated adult subjects, although statistical significance was reached in only one study.[107–109] An additional study in adults reported decreased mucosal hyperproliferation after short-chain fatty acid or butyrate enemas, suggesting that such treatment may have a role in decreasing the colon cancer risk in UC.[110] No pediatric trials have been reported.

Initial studies of n-3 fatty acids derived from fish oil suggested that early relapse of UC in remission could be delayed by supplementing the diet with 5.1 g/day of n-3 fatty acids, although relapses rates after 3 months were comparable to those seen in placebo-treated controls.[111] Similarly, n-3 fatty acids provided no[112] or only modest[113] steroid-sparing effect compared with placebo in the treatment of acute UC. However, a novel, enteric-coated fish oil preparation delivering 2.7 g/day of n-3 fatty acids demonstrated steroid-sparing effects in an open-label trial in a group of adults with chronic, steroid-dependent UC.[114]

### Corticosteroids

Corticosteroids appear to down-regulate multiple steps in the inflammatory cascade that results in UC.[115, 116] The initial use of corticosteroids as treatment for children with UC was largely based on extrapolation from studies in adults.[117] Pediatric treatment regimens have evolved through empiric use and clinical experience rather than controlled clinical trial. Prednisone, methylprednisolone, and hydrocortisone are the agents most frequently used. Commonly prescribed dosages are comparable to those prescribed for children with Crohn's disease, as summarized in Chapter 32. Oral corticosteroids are well absorbed,[118] although occasionally a child with poor absorption or corticosteroid resistance may benefit from intravenous bolus or continuous infusion dosing. Rectal corticosteroids are particularly beneficial in children with severe tenesmus and urgency, but many children have difficulty retaining enema formulations, so foam-based treatments or suppositories may be preferable in selected patients. One adult study demonstrated better efficacy for systemically administered corticotropin (ACTH), compared with intravenous hydrocortisone, although pediatric experience with this therapy is lacking.[119]

The decision to use corticosteroids must be balanced by their potential adverse effects. A wide spectrum of complications can occasionally occur (see Table 32–6). Systemically active corticosteroids can interfere with linear bone growth even in the face of adequate dietary intake.[120] Alternate-day dosing minimizes these effects while maintaining reduced disease activity[121–123] and appears to have no deleterious effect on bone mineralization in children.[124] However, in patients who have not completed their linear growth and whose disease activity cannot be controlled by alternate-day dosing regimens, the anti-inflammatory effects of daily corticosteroids must be weighed against the coincident suppression of linear growth.

Newer topically active corticosteroids (budesonide, fluticasone propionate) have the potential to provide anti-inflammatory activity to the gut without systemic toxicity because of their high first-pass metabolism.[125] These agents may offer particular advantages for the treatment of children if they prove to be minimally growth suppressive, but pediatric studies have yet to be reported. The enema formulation of budesonide is as effective as rectal mesalazine[126] and rectal prednisolone or hydrocortisone[127, 128] in the treatment of left-sided and distal colitis. In adults, budesonide enemas (2 mg) cause fewer abnormal ACTH stimulation tests than rectal hydrocortisone (100 mg).[128] Multiple courses of rectal budesonide are safe and effective for recurrent flares of UC.[129] Data on the effect of oral budesonide in UC are limited. A single study in adults with active extensive and distal UC demonstrated that oral budesonide (10 mg) delivered as a controlled-release preparation is as effective as oral prednisolone (40 mg) but does not suppress plasma cortisol levels.[130] Additional studies are required to determine whether the current oral formulation, which is designed to deliver active budesonide to the ileum and right colon, is an effective therapy in children with UC.

## 5-Aminosalicylates

It is postulated that the 5-aminosalicylate (5-ASA) drugs (sulfasalazine, mesalamine, olsalazine, balsalazide) exert local anti-inflammatory effects through a number of different mechanisms. These include inhibition of 5-lipoxygenase with resulting decreased production of leukotriene B4, scavenging of reactive oxygen metabolites, prevention of the upregulation of leukocyte adhesion molecules, and inhibition of interleukin-1 (IL-1) synthesis.[116, 131] 5-ASA is rapidly absorbed from the upper intestinal tract on oral ingestion, and various delivery systems have been employed to prevent absorption until the active drug can be delivered to the distal small bowel and colon. Sulfasalazine (Azulfidine) links 5-ASA via an azo bond to sulfapyridine. Bacterial enzymes in the colon break the azo linkage, releasing 5-ASA to exert its anti-inflammatory effect in the colon. Because the sulfapyridine moiety causes most of the untoward reactions to sulfasalazine and is thought to have no therapeutic activity, newer agents have been designed to deliver 5-ASA without sulfapyridine. Olsalazine (Dipentum) links two molecules of 5-ASA via an azo bond, whereas balsalazide (Colazide) links 5-ASA via an azo bond to an inert, nonabsorbed carrier. A number of other delayed release preparations (Asacol, Claversal, Mesasal, Salofalk) prevent rapid absorption of 5-ASA (generically called mesalamine) by coating it with Eudragit, a pH-sensitive acrylic resin. Another preparation (Pentasa) coats micrograules of mesalamine with ethylcellulose, releasing it in a time-dependent fashion. Uncoated mesalamine is also available as a rectal suppository or enema formulation (Rowasa).

Overall, the 5-ASA drugs have been shown to be effective in controlling mild to moderate UC in adults in 50% to 90% of cases, and they are effective in maintaining remission in 70% to 90% of cases.[132] Despite extensive studies in adults, few pediatric studies exist. Clinical experience with sulfasalazine in children with UC has generally mirrored the adult experience.[133] One pediatric study directly compared the efficacy of sulfasalazine and olsalazine.[134] In this study, 79% of children with mildly to moderately active UC treated with sulfasalazine (60 mg/kg/day) clinically improved, compared with only 39% of those treated with olsalazine (30 mg/kg per day). Several smaller, open-label or double-blind pediatric trials and one larger retrospective analysis of 10 years' clinical experience with Eudragit-coated 5-ASA preparations in children reported therapeutic benefits in active UC as well as in active Crohn's colitis and active small bowel Crohn's disease.[135–138] Adverse reactions to all of the 5-ASA preparations have been described and have required discontinuation of treatment in 5% to 15% of cases. The more serious complications reported in children have included pancreatitis,[139–141] nephritis,[142] exacerbation of disease,[135] and sulfa- or salicylate-induced allergic reactions.

## Antibiotics

There is little role for antibiotics in the primary therapy of active UC.[143, 144] Based on experience in adults, metronidazole is occasionally used for the treatment of mild to moderate UC or for maintenance of remission in the 5-ASA–intolerant or allergic patient.[145] A controlled trial of ciprofloxacin as an adjunct to corticosteroids in adults with active UC demonstrated no benefit compared with placebo.[146]

## Immunomodulators

### *6-Mercaptopurine and Azathioprine*

Despite the surgically curable nature of UC (see later discussion), many parents and physicians are reluctant to perform colectomy in children with even severely active UC. As a consequence, immunomodulators are increasingly being used therapeutically. The most commonly prescribed agents are 6-mercaptopurine and azathioprine.[147] These purine analogues inhibit RNA and DNA synthesis, thereby down-regulating cytotoxic T cell activity and delayed hypersensitivity reactions.[148]

Clinical experience in children with UC has mirrored adult studies demonstrating that 6-mercaptopurine and azathioprine can act as steroid-sparing agents and can induce and maintain remission in 60% to 75% of patients.[147, 149] Onset of action is delayed, with a mean time to response of 4.5 ± 3.0 months.[147] At 6-mercaptopurine doses of 1.0 to 1.5 mg/kg/day, adverse reactions requiring discontinuation of treatment (e.g., allergic reactions, pancreatitis, severe leukopenia) occur in fewer than 5% of pediatric patients.[147] Sixty-five percent of adults with UC who achieve complete remission with 6-mercaptopurine maintain continuous remission for 5 years if they remain on the medication, compared with only 13% of those who electively discontinue 6-mercaptopurine after induction of remission.[150] These data are comparable to those from an earlier study using azathioprine, in which 64% of adults maintained on azathioprine after induction of remission remained well at 1 year, compared with only 41% of those switched to placebo after remission induction.[151] No comparable pediatric data have been published. Finally, studies have shown that azathioprine and 6-mercaptopurine are effective agents for maintaining long-term remission induced by intravenous cyclosporine in both children and adults with severe UC.[152, 153]

### *Cyclosporine and Tacrolimus*

Cyclosporine and tacrolimus (FK506) are potent inhibitors of cell-mediated immunity. Both agents bind to their respective intracellular receptors (immunophilins). The resulting drug-immunophilin complex inhibits the action of another intracellular mediator, calcineurin, which in turn inactivates the genes responsible for the production of IL-2 and IL-4.[154] As a consequence, T cell and, to a lesser extent, B cell function is impaired.

The use of cyclosporine for the treatment of severe UC in children has had mixed results. The initial rate of response, defined as avoidance of imminent surgery and discharge from the hospital, has been reported to be 20% to 80% with either oral or intravenous routes of administration.[155, 156] Responses usually occur within 7 to 14 days after the initiation of treatment, but relapses necessitating colectomy occur within 1 year in 70% to 100% of initial responders during or after discontinuation of cyclosporine.[155, 156] However, it has been shown in both children and adults that, if 6-mercaptopurine or azathioprine is added to the regimen once cyclosporine has induced remission, 60% to 90% of treated patients maintain long-term remission.[153, 157] Tremors, hirsutism, and systemic hypertension are the most common toxic effects of cyclosporine that have been described in children with IBD. However, isolated reports of *Pneumocystis carinii* pneumonia, lymphoproliferative disease, and serious bacterial and fungal infections in cyclosporine-treated patients merit careful monitoring of all children treated with cyclosporine, especially those treated in combination with corticosteroids and 6-mercaptopurine or azathioprine.

One preliminary experience with oral tacrolimus (FK506) as treatment for fulminant colitis in children has been reported in abstract form.[158] After treatment with 0.1 mg/kg per dose every 12 hours with whole blood trough levels adjusted to 10 to 15 ng/mL, five of six children improved and avoided surgery. By 14 days, stool frequency significantly decreased and rectal bleeding subsided. Ultimately, three of the five responding patients were successfully weaned off tacrolimus to 6-mercaptopurine. Further experience with this agent is required before its efficacy and safety profile can be compared with those of cyclosporine.

### *Methotrexate*

Methotrexate has been used with beneficial effects in a few children with severe Crohn's disease, but pediatric experience in UC is lacking. Preliminary studies in adult patients suggest that methotrexate may provide beneficial effects in the induction and maintenance of remission.[159] However, a double-blind trial demonstrated no benefit compared with placebo for either indication.[160]

## Other Medical Therapies

Other new and potentially revolutionary therapies for the treatment of IBD are evolving.[161] These "biologic" therapies offer the potential to interfere selectively at various points in the immune-mediated inflammatory process that characterizes UC. Work progresses on agents such as anti–tumor necrosis factor antibodies,[162, 163] anti-inflammatory cytokines such as IL-10 and IL-11,[164] and antisense oligonucleotides designed to inhibit expression of genes central to the inflammatory process (e.g., NFκB[165]) or central to the expression of cell adhesion molecules (e.g., intercellular adhesion molecule-1).[166]

## SURGERY

UC is a surgically curable condition, and within 5 years of diagnosis intractable or fulminant symptoms necessitate colectomy in 19% of affected children and adolescents (see Course and Prognosis).[8] Indications for surgery in UC are summarized in Table 33–5. Curative surgery requires total mucosal proctocolectomy. Although proctocolectomy and ileostomy result in a healthy patient with no risk of future recurrence, few children or parents readily accept the option of a permanent ileostomy. Most instead opt for restorative surgery that allows the child to continue to defecate by the normal route.

Because it is often difficult to definitively distinguish between fulminant UC and Crohn's colitis preoperatively,

**TABLE 33–5. Indications for Surgery in Ulcerative Colitis**

| |
|---|
| Failure of medical therapy |
| Intractable symptoms |
| Drug toxicity |
| Persistent hemorrhage requiring transfusion |
| Perforation |
| Toxic megacolon |
| Low- or high-grade dysplasia |
| Carcinoma |

many centers perform a staged procedure in the child with active colitis who requires surgery. Initially subtotal colectomy and ileostomy are performed, followed at a later date by restorative surgery if the colectomy specimen confirms a diagnosis of UC. The most commonly performed surgery is the ileal pouch anal anastomosis (IPAA). The continent ileostomy (Kock's pouch) is rarely, if ever, performed in children given the success of the IPAA. Summaries of pediatric surgical experience document that IPAA using an ileal J-pouch (or, less commonly, a W- or S-pouch) results in fewer daytime and nocturnal bowel movements and less fecal soiling than an ileoanal anastomosis without a pouch.[167, 168] Anorectal function is well preserved in children, and postoperative fecal soiling is unusual.[169] When growth retardation is evident preoperatively, significant increases in height velocity can be expected postoperatively.[170]

Small bowel obstruction is the most common early postoperative complication of IPAA surgery.[171] Pouchitis is the most common late complication described; it occurs in 19% of operated children and adolescents. It generally responds to treatment with metronidazole, ciprofloxacin, 5-ASA, or corticosteroids.[167, 168, 171]

## COURSE AND PROGNOSIS

The course and prognosis of UC in children based on clinical experience derived after 1975 has been reported.[8] Seventy percent of children can be expected to enter remission within 3 months of initial diagnosis, regardless of the character of their initial attack (mild, moderate, or severe), and 45% to 58% remain inactive over the first year after diagnosis.[8] However, 10% of those whose symptoms are characterized as moderate to severe can be expected to remain continuously symptomatic. Over ensuing 7- to 10-year intervals, approximately 55% of all patients have inactive disease, 40% have chronic intermittent symptoms, and 5% to 10% have continuous symptoms. These data are similar to those reported in adult populations.[172, 173] Colectomy is required in 5% of all children with UC within the first year after diagnosis, and in 19% to 23% by 5 years after diagnosis.[8, 42] These rates rise to 9% and 26%, respectively, in the subgroup of children initially presenting with moderate to severe symptoms.[8] Overall, these rates appear comparable to those reported in a Swedish pediatric population treated between 1961 and 1990[173] and lower than those from older U.S. data that revealed colectomy rates of almost 50% by 5 years after diagnosis in children presenting between 1955 and 1964, and 26% in those presenting between 1965 and 1974.[40]

Children with proctitis or proctosigmoiditis appear to follow a somewhat more benign course. More than 90% are asymptomatic within 6 months of diagnosis. In any given year of follow-up, 55% remain asymptomatic and fewer than 5% have continuously active disease.[43] In contrast to adults, proximal extension of disease occurs frequently, so that within 3 years of initial diagnosis as many as 25% of children may demonstrate signs of proximal extension. This rate may increase up to 70% over the course of follow-up.[42–44] Colectomy may eventually be required in 5% of patients.

## REFERENCES


1. Olafsdottir EJ, Fluge G, Haug K: Chronic inflammatory bowel disease in children in western Norway. J Pediatr Gastroenterol Nutr 1989;8:454–458.
2. Binder V, Both H, Hansen PK, et al: Incidence and prevalence of UC and CD in the County of Copenhagen 1962–1978. Gastroenterology 1982;83:563–568.
3. Hildebrand H, Fredrikzon B, Holmquist L, et al: Chronic inflammatory bowel disease in children and adolescents in Sweden. J Pediatr Gastroenterol Nutr 1991;13:293–297.
4. Barton JR, Gillon S, Ferguson A: Incidence of inflammatory bowel disease in Scottish children between 1968 and 1983: marginal fall in ulcerative colitis, three-fold rise in Crohn's disease. Gut 1989;30:618–622.
5. Cosgrove M, Al-Atia RF, Jenkins HR: The epidemiology of pediatric inflammatory bowel disease. Arch Dis Child 1996;74:460–461.
6. Michener WM, Caulfield ME, Wyllie RW, Farmer RG: Management of inflammatory bowel disease: 30 years of observation. Cleve Clin J Med 1990;58:685–691.
7. Gryboski JD: Ulcerative colitis in children 10 years old or younger. J Pediatr Gastroenterol Nutr 1993;17:24–31.
8. Hyams JS, Davis P, Grancher K, et al: Clinical outcome of ulcerative colitis in children. J Pediatr 1996;129:81–88.
9. Dady IM, Thomas AG, Miller V, Kelsen AJ: Inflammatory bowel disease in infancy: an increasing problem? J Pediatr Gastroenterol Nutr 1996;23:569–576.
10. Griffiths A, Harris K, Smith C, et al: Prevalence of inflammatory bowel disease in first-degree relatives of children with IBD (abstract). Gastroenterology 1997;112:A985.
11. Gilat T, Hacohen D, Lilos P, Langman MJS: Childhood factors in ulcerative colitis and Crohn's disease: an international cooperative study. Scand J Gastroenterol 1987;22:1009–1024.
12. Koletzko S, Griffiths A, Corey M, et al: Infant feeding practices and ulcerative colitis in children. Br Med J 1991;302:1580–1581.
13. Sandler RS, Sandler DP, McDonnell CW, Wurzelman JI: Childhood exposure to environmental tobacco smoke and the risk of ulcerative colitis. Am J Epidemiol 1992;135:603–608.
14. Lashner BA, Shaheen NJ, Hanauer SB, Kirschner BS: Passive smoking is associated with an increased risk of developing inflammatory bowel disease in children. Am J Gastroenterol 1993;88:356–359.
15. Roth M-R, Petersen GM, McElree C, et al: Familial empiric risk estimates of inflammatory bowel disease in Ashkenazi Jews. Gastroenterology 1989;96:1016–1020.
16. Yang H, McElree C, Roth M-P, et al: Familial empiric risks for inflammatory bowel disease: differences between Jews and non-Jews. Gut 1993;34:517–524.
17. Tysk C, Lindberg E, Jarenot G, Floderus-Myrhed B: Ulcerative colitis and Crohn's disease in an unselected population of monozygotic and dizygotic twins: a study of heredibility and the influence of smoking. Gut 1988;29:990–996.
18. Toyoda H, Wang SJ, Yang HY, et al: Distinct associations of HLA class II genes with IBD. Gastroenterology 1993;104:741–748.
19. Yang H, Rotter JI, Toyoda H, et al: Ulcerative colitis: a genetically heterogeneous disorder defined by genetic (HLA class II) and subclinical (antineutrophil cytoplasmic antibodies) markers. J Clin Invest 1993;92:1080–1084.
20. Asakura H, Tsuchiya M, Aiso S, et al: Association of human lymphocyte-DR2 antigen with Japanese ulcerative colitis. Gastroenterology 1982;82:413–418.
21. Ohmen JD, Yang HY, Yamamoto KK, et al: Susceptibility locus for inflammatory bowel disease on chromosome 16 has a role in Crohn's disease, but not ulcerative colitis. Hum Mol Genet 1996;5:1679–1683.
22. Cho JH, Fu Y, Kirschner BS, Hanauer SB: Confirmation of a susceptibility locus (IBD1) for Crohn's disease on chromosome 16 (abstract). Gastroenterology 1997;112:A948.
23. Duerr RH, Targan SR, Landers CJ, et al: Anti-neutrophil cytoplasmic antibodies in ulcerative colitis: comparison with other colitides/diarrheal illnesses. Gastroenterology 1991;100:1590–1596.
24. Shanahan F, Duerr RH, Rotter JI, et al: Neutrophil autoantibodies in ulcerative colitis: familial aggregation and genetic heterogeneity. Gastroenterology 1992;103:456–461.
25. Jewell DP, Truelove SC: Circulating antibodies to cow's milk proteins in ulcerative colitis. Gut 1972;13:796–801.

26. Taylor KB, Truelove SC: Circulating antibodies to cow's milk proteins in ulcerative colitis. Br Med J 1961;2:924.
27. Candy S, Borok G, Wright JP, et al: The value of an elimination diet in the management of patients with ulcerative colitis. S Afr Med J 1995;85:1176–1179.
28. Bruce T: Emotional sequelae of chronic inflammatory bowel disease in children and adolescents. Clin Gastroenterol 1986;15:89–104.
29. Burke P, Meyer V, Kocoshis S, et al: Depression and anxiety in pediatric inflammatory bowel disease and cystic fibrosis. J Am Acad Child Adolesc Psychiatry 1989;28:948–951.
30. Wood B, Watkins JB, Boyle JT, et al: Psychological functioning in children with Crohn's disease and ulcerative colitis: implications for models of psychobiological interaction. J Am Acad Child Adolesc Psychiatry 1987;26:774–781.
31. Burke P, Meyer V, Kocoshis S, et al: Obsessive-compulsive symptoms in childhood inflammatory bowel disease and cystic fibrosis. J Am Acad Child Adolesc Psychiatry 1989;28:525–527.
32. Krall V, Szajnberg NM, Hyams JS, et al: Projective personality tests of children with inflammatory bowel disease. Percept Mot Skills 1995;80:1341–1342.
33. North CS, Clouse RE, Spitznagel EL, Alpers DH: The relation of ulcerative colitis to psychiatric factors: a review of findings and methods. Am J Psychiatry 1990;147:974–981.
34. Roediger WE: The colonic epithelium in ulcerative colitis: an energy-deficiency disease? Lancet 1980;2:712–715.
35. Treem WR, Ahsan N, Shoup M, Hyams JS: Fecal short-chain fatty acids in children with inflammatory bowel disease. J Pediatr Gastroenterol Nutr 1994;18:159–164.
36. Sartor RB: Cytokines in intestinal inflammation: pathophysiological and clinical considerations. Gastroenterology 1994;106:533–539.
37. MacDermott RP, Nash GS, Auer IO, et al: Alterations in serum immunoglobulin G subclasses in patients with ulcerative colitis and Crohn's disease. Gastroenterology 1989;96:764–768.
38. Das KM, Dasgupta A, Mandal A, Geng X: Autoimmunity to cytoskeletal protein tropomyosin(s): a clue to the pathogenetic mechanism for ulcerative colitis. J Immunol 1993;150:2487–2493.
39. Bhagat S, Das KM: A shared unique peptide in human colon, eye, and joint detected by a novel monoclonal antibody. Gastroenterology 1994;107:103–108.
40. Michener WM, Farmer RG, Mortimer EA: Long-term prognosis of ulcerative colitis with onset in childhood or adolescence. J Clin Gastroenterol 1979;1:301–305.
41. Hamilton JR, Bruce GA, Abdourhaman M, Gall DG: Inflammatory bowel disease in children and adolescents. (Barness LA, ed.) Adv Pediatr 1979:26:311–341.
42. Langholz E, Munkholm P, Krasilnikoff PA, Binder V: Inflammatory bowel diseases with onset in childhood: clinical features, morbidity, and mortality in a regional cohort. Scand J Gastroenterol 1997;32:139–147.
43. Hyams J, Lerer T, Colletti R, et al: Clinical outcome of ulcerative proctitis in children. J Pediatr Gastroenterol Nutr 1997;25:149–152.
44. Mir-Madjlessi SH, Michener WM, Farmer RG: Course and prognosis of idiopathic ulcerative proctosigmoiditis in young patients. J Pediatr Gastroenterol Nutr 1986;5:571–575.
45. Markowitz J, Kahn E, Grancher K, et al: Atypical rectosigmoid histology in children with newly diagnosed ulcerative colitis. Am J Gastroenterol 1993;88:2034–2037.
46. Surawicz CM, Haggitt RC, Husseman M, McFarland LV: Mucosal biopsy diagnosis of colitis: acute self-limited colitis and inflammatory bowel disease. Gastroenterology 1994;107:755–763.
47. Riddell RH: Pathology of idiopathic inflammatory bowel disease. In Kirsner JB (ed): Inflammatory Bowel Disease. Philadelphia, Lea & Febiger, 1988, pp 329–350.
48. Michener WM: Ulcerative colitis in children: problems in management. Pediatr Clin North Am 1967;14:159–163.
49. Das KM, Squillante L, Chitayet D, Kalousek DK: Simultaneous appearance of a unique common epitope in fetal colon, skin and biliary epithelial cells: a possible link for extracolonic manifestations in ulcerative colitis. J Clin Gastroenterol 1992;15:311–316.
50. Hyams J, Markowitz J, Treem W, et al: Characterization of hepatic abnormalities in children with inflammatory bowel disease. Inflamm Bowel Dis 1995;1:27–33.
51. Quigley EMM, LaRusso NF, Ludwig J, et al: Familial occurrence of primary sclerosing cholangitis and ulcerative colitis. Gastroenterology 1983;85:1160–1165.
52. Wilschanski M, Chait P, Wade JA, et al: Primary sclerosing cholangitis in 32 children: clinical, laboratory, and radiographic features, with survival analysis. Hepatology 1995;22:1415–1422.
53. Broome U, Lindberg B, Lofberg R: Primary sclerosing cholangitis in ulcerative colitis: a risk factor for the development of dysplasia and DNA aneuploidy? Gastroenterology 1992;102:1877–1880.
54. Broome U, Lofberg R, Veress B, Eriksson LS: Primary sclerosing cholangitis and ulcerative colitis: evidence for increased neoplastic potential. Hepatology 1995;22:1404–1408.
55. Passo MH, Fitzgerald JF, Brandt KD: Arthritis associated with inflammatory bowel disease in children: relationship of joint disease to activity and severity of bowel lesion. Dig Dis Sci 1986;31:492–497.
56. Lindsey CB, Schaller JG: Arthritis associated with inflammatory bowel disease in children. J Pediatr 1974;84:16–20.
57. Greenstein AJ, Janowitz HD, Sachar DB: The extra-intestinal complications of Crohn's disease and ulcerative colitis: a study of 700 patients. Medicine (Baltimore) 1976;55:401–412.
58. Mir-Madjlessi SH, Taylor JS, Farmer RG: Clinical course and evolution of erythema nodosum and pyoderma gangrenosum in chronic ulcerative colitis: a study of 42 patients. Am J Gastroenterol 1985;80:615–620.
59. Levitt MD, Ritchie JK, Lennard-Jones JE, Phillips RKS: Pyoderma gangrenosum in inflammatory bowel disease. Br J Surg 1991;78:676–678.
60. Matis, WL, Ellis CN, Griffiths CEM, Lazarus GS: Treatment of pyoderma gangrenosum with cyclosporine. Arch Dermatol 1992;128:1060–1064.
61. Friedman S, Marion JF, Scherl E, et al: The treatment of choice for pyoderma gangrenosum complicating IBD: intravenous cyclosporine (abstract). Gastroenterology 1997;112:A975.
62. Paradis K, Bernstein ML, Adelson JW: Thrombosis as a complication of inflammatory bowel disease in children: a report of 4 cases. J Pediatr Gastroenterol Nutr 1985;4:659–662.
63. Markowitz RL, Ment LR, Gryboski JD: Cerebral thromboembolic disease in pediatric and adult inflammatory bowel disease: case report and review of the literature. J Pediatr Gastroenterol Nutr 1989;8:413–420.
64. Daum F, Gould HB, Gold D, et al: Asymptomatic uveitis in children with inflammatory bowel disease. Am J Dis Child 1979;133:170–171.
65. Hofley P, Roarty J, McGinnity G, et al: Asymptomatic uveitis in children with chronic inflammatory bowel diseases. J Pediatr Gastroenterol Nutr 1993;17:397–400.
66. Tripathi RC, Kipp MA, Tripathi BJ, et al: Ocular toxicity of prednisone in pediatric patients with inflammatory bowel disease. Lens Eye Toxic Res 1992;9:469–482.
67. Tripathi RC, Kirschner BS, Kipp M, et al: Corticosteroid treatment for inflammatory bowel disease in pediatric patients increases intraocular pressure. Gastroenterology 1992;102:1957–1961.
68. Werlin SL, Grand RJ: Severe colitis in children and adolescents: diagnosis, course, and treatment. Gastroenterology 1977;73:828–832.
69. Gold DM, Levine JL, Weinstein TA, et al: Prolonged medical therapy for severe pediatric ulcerative colitis. Am J Gastroenterol 1995;90:732–735.
70. Riddell RH, Goldman H, Ransohoff DF, et al: Dysplasia in inflammatory bowel disease: standardized classification with provisional clinical applications. Hum Pathol 1983;14:931–968.
71. Itzkowitz S: Colorectal cancer in inflammatory bowel disease. Prog Inflamm Bowel Dis 1993;14:1–5.
72. Ransohoff DF: Colon cancer in ulcerative colitis. Gastroenterology 1988;94:1089–1091.
73. Devroede GJ, Taylor WF, Sauer WG, et al: Cancer risk and life expectancy of children with ulcerative colitis. N Engl J Med 1971;285:17–21.
74. Sugita A, Sachar DB, Bodian C, et al: Colorectal cancer in ulcerative colitis: influence of anatomical extent and age at onset on colitis-cancer interval. Gut 1991;32:167–169.
75. Gillen CD, Walmsley RS, Prior P, et al: Ulcerative colitis and Crohn's disease: a comparison of the colorectal cancer risk in extensive colitis. Gut 1994;35:1590–1592.
76. Lavery IC, Jagelman DG: Cancer in the excluded rectum following surgery for inflammatory bowel disease. Dis Colon Rectum 1982;25:522–524.
77. Lashner BA: Red blood cell folate is associated with the development of dysplasia and cancer in ulcerative colitis. J Cancer Res Clin Oncol 1993;119:549–554.

78. Markowitz J, McKinley M, Kahn E, et al: Endoscopic screening for dysplasia and mucosal aneuploidy in adolescents and young adults with childhood onset colitis. Am J Gastroenterol 1997;92:2001–2006.
79. Ekbom A, Helmick C, Zack M, Adami H-O: Ulcerative colitis and colorectal cancer: a population-based study. N Engl J Med 1990;323:1228–1233.
80. Ekbom A, Helmick C, Zack M, Adami H-O: Increased risk of large-bowel cancer in Crohn's disease with colonic involvement. Lancet 1990;336:357–359.
81. Brostrom O, Lofberg R, Nordenvall B, et al: The risk of colorectal cancer in ulcerative colitis: an epidemiologic study. Scand J Gastroenterol 1987;22:1193–1199.
82. Langholz E, Munkholm P, Davidsen M, Binder V: Colorectal cancer risk and mortality in patients with ulcerative colitis. Gastroenterology 1992;103:1444–1451.
83. Lavery IC, Chiulli RA, Jagelman DG, et al: Survival with carcinoma arising in mucosal ulcerative colitis. Ann Surg 1982;195:508–512.
84. Gyde SN, Prior P, Thompson H, et al: Survival of patients with colorectal cancer complicating ulcerative colitis. Gut 1984;25:228–231.
85. Choi PM, Nugent FW, Schoetz DJ Jr, et al: Colonoscopic surveillance reduces mortality from colorectal cancer in ulcerative colitis. Gastroenterology 1993;105:418–424.
86. Griffiths AM, Sherman PM: Colonoscopic surveillance for cancer in ulcerative colitis: a critical review. J Pediatr Gastroenterol Nutr 1997;24:202–210.
87. Dixon MF, Brown LJ, Gilmour HM, et al: Observer variation in the assessment of dysplasia in ulcerative colitis. Histopathology 1988;13:385–397.
88. Melville DM, Jass JR, Shepherd NA, et al: Dysplasia and deoxyribonucleic acid aneuploidy in the assessment of precancerous changes in chronic ulcerative colitis: observer variation and correlations. Gastroenterology 1988;95:668–675.
89. Jonsson B, Ahsgren L, Andersson LO, et al: Colorectal cancer surveillance in patients with ulcerative colitis. Br J Surg 1994;81:689–691.
90. Axon AT: Colonic cancer surveillance in ulcerative colitis is not essential for every patient. Eur J Cancer 1995;31A:1183–1186.
91. Lennard-Jones JE, Melville DM, Morson BC, et al: Precancer and cancer in extensive ulcerative colitis: findings among 401 patients over 22 years. Gut 1990;31:800–806.
92. Lofberg R, Brostrom O, Karlen P, et al: DNA aneuploidy in ulcerative colitis: reproducibility, topographic distribution and relation to dysplasia. Gastroenterology 1992;102:1149–1154.
93. Rubin CE, Haggitt RC, Burmer GC, et al: DNA aneuploidy in colonic biopsies predicts future development of dysplasia in ulcerative colitis. Gastroenterology 1992;103:1611–1620.
94. Befrits R, Hammarberg C, Rubio C, et al: DNA aneuploidy and histologic dysplasia in long-standing ulcerative colitis: a 10-year follow-up study. Dis Colon Rectum 1994;37:313–319.
95. Yin J, Harpaz N, Tong Y, et al: p53 point mutations in dysplastic and cancerous ulcerative colitis lesions. Gastroenterology 1993;104:1633–1639.
96. Burmer GC, Levine DS, Kulander BG, et al: C-Ki-*ras* mutations in ulcerative colitis and sporadic colon carcinoma. Gastroenterology 1990;99:416–420.
97. Itzkowitz SH, Young E, Dubois D, et al: Sialosyl-Tn antigen is prevalent and precedes dysplasia in ulcerative colitis: a retrospective case-control study. Gastroenterology 1996;110:694–704.
98. Lashner BA: Recommendations for colorectal cancer screening in ulcerative colitis: a review of research from a single university-based surveillance program. Am J Gastroenterol 1992;87:168–175.
99. Markowitz J, Grancher K, Rosa J, et al: Growth failure in pediatric inflammatory bowel disease. J Pediatr Gastroenterol Nutr 1993;16:373–380.
100. Hyams JS, Wyzga N, Kreutzer DL, et al: Alterations in bone metabolism in children with inflammatory bowel disease: an in vitro study. J Pediatr Gastroenterol Nutr 1997;24:289–295.
101. Seidman EG, Ruemmele FM, Landers C, et al: Disease specific diagnostic accuracy of new serological tests in pediatric IBD (abstract). Gastroenterology 1997;112:A1087.
102. Charron M, Orenstein SR, Bhargava S: Detection of inflammatory bowel disease in pediatric patients with technetium-99m-HMPAO-labelled leukocytes. J Nucl Med 1994;35:451–455.
103. Jobling JC, Lindley KJ, Yousef Y, et al: Investigating inflammatory bowel disease: white cell scanning, radiology, and colonoscopy. Arch Dis Child 1996;74:22–26.
104. Seidman E, LeLeiko N, Ament M, et al: Nutritional issues in pediatric inflammatory bowel disease. J Pediatr Gastroenterol Nutr 1991;12:424–438.
105. Kleinman RE, Balistreri WF, Heyman MD, et al: Nutritional support for pediatric patients with inflammatory bowel disease. J Pediatr Gastroenterol Nutr 1989;8:8–12.
106. Den Hond E, Hiele M, Ghoos Y, Rutgeerts P: In vivo colonic butyrate metabolism in extensive ulcerative colitis (abstract). Gastroenterology 1996;110:A893.
107. Vernia P, Marcheggiano A, Caprilli R, et al: Short-chain fatty acid topical treatment in distal ulcerative colitis (abstract). Aliment Pharmacol Ther 1995;9:309–313.
108. Breuer RI, Soergel KH, Lashner BA, et al: Short chain fatty acid rectal irrigation for left-sided ulcerative colitis: a randomized, placebo-controlled trial (abstract). Gastroenterology 1996;110:A873.
109. Scheppach W and the German-Austrian SCFA Study Group: Treatment of distal ulcerative colitis with short-chain fatty acid enemas: a placebo-controlled trial. Dig Dis Sci 1996;41:2254–2259.
110. Scheppach W, Muller JG, Boxberger F, et al: Histological changes in the colonic mucosa following irrigation with short-chain fatty acids. Eur J Gastroenterol Hepatol 1997;9:163–168.
111. Loeschke K, Ueberschaer B, Pietsch A, et al: n-3 Fatty acids only delay early relapse of ulcerative colitis in remission. Dig Dis Sci 1996;41:2087–2094.
112. Stack WA, Cole AT, Makhdoom Z, et al: A randomized controlled trial of essential fatty acids in acute ulcerative colitis (abstract). Gastroenterology 1997;112:A1095.
113. Hawthorne AB, Daneshmend TK, Hawkey CJ, et al: Treatment of ulcerative colitis with fish oil supplementation: a prospective 12 month randomised controlled trial. Gut 1992;33:922–928.
114. Belluzzi A, Brignola C, Boschi S, et al: A novel enteric coated preparation of Ω-3 fatty acids in a group of steroid-dependent ulcerative colitis: an open study (abstract). Gastroenterology 1997;112:A930.
115. Thiesen A, Thomson ABR: Older systemic and newer topical glucocorticosteroids and the gastrointestinal tract. Aliment Pharmacol Ther 1996;10:487–496.
116. Zimmerman MJ, Jewell DP: Cytokines and mechanisms of action of glucocorticoids and aminosalicylates in the treatment of ulcerative colitis and Crohn's disease. Aliment Pharmacol Ther 1996;10(suppl 2):93–98.
117. Truelove SC, Witts LJ: Cortisone in ulcerative colitis: final report on a therapeutic trial. Br Med J 1955;2:1041.
118. Milsap RL, George DE, Szefler SJ, et al: Effect of inflammatory bowel disease on absorption and disposition of prednisolone. Dig Dis Sci 1983;28:161–168.
119. Meyers S, Sachar DB, Goldberg JD, Janowitz HD: Corticotropin versus hydrocortisone in the intravenous treatment of ulcerative colitis: a prospective, randomized, double-blind clinical trial. Gastroenterology 1983;85:351–357.
120. Hyams JS, Moore RE, Leichtner AM, et al: Relationship of type I procollagen to corticosteroid therapy in children with inflammatory bowel disease. J Pediatr 1988;112:893–898.
121. Hyams JS, Carey DE, Leichtner AM, Goldberg BD: Type I procollagen as a biochemical marker of growth in children with inflammatory bowel disease. J Pediatr 1986;109:619–624.
122. Hyams JS, Treem WR, Carey DE, et al: Comparison of collagen propeptides as growth markers in children with inflammatory bowel disease. Gastroenterology 1991;100:971–975.
123. Whittington PF, Barnes V, Bayless TM: Medical management of Crohn's disease in adolescence. Gastroenterology 1977;72:1338–1344.
124. Issenman RM, Atkinson SA, Radoja C, Fraher L: Longitudinal assessment of growth, mineral metabolism and bone mass in pediatric Crohn's disease. J Pediatr Gastroenterol Nutr 1993;17:401–406.
125. Lofberg R: New steroids for inflammatory bowel disease. Inflamm Bowel Dis 1995;1:135–141.
126. Lemann M, Galian A, Rutgeerts P, et al: Comparison of budesonide and 5-aminosalicylic acid enemas in active distal ulcerative colitis. Aliment Pharmacol Ther 1995;9:557–562.
127. Lofberg R, Ostergaard Thomsen O, Langholz E, et al: Budesonide versus prednisolone retention enemas in active distal ulcerative colitis. Aliment Pharmacol Ther 1994;8:623–629.
128. Bayless T, Sninsky C, for the U.S. Budesonide Enema Study Group: Budesonide enema is an effective alternative to hydrocortisone enema in active distal ulcerative colitis (abstract). Gastroenterology 1995;108:A778.

129. Pruitt R, Kayz S, Bayless T, Levine J, for the U.S. Budesonide Enema Study Group: Repeated use of budesonide enema is safe and effective for the treatment of acute flares of distal ulcerative colitis (abstract). Gastroenterology 1996;110:A995.
130. Lofberg R, Danielsson A, Suhr O, et al: Oral budesonide versus prednisolone in patients with active extensive and left-sided ulcerative colitis. Gastroenterology 1996;110:1713–1718.
131. Greenfield SM, Punchard NA, Teare JP, Thompson RPH: Review article: the mode of action of the aminosalicylates in inflammatory bowel disease. Aliment Pharmacol Ther 1993;7:369–383.
132. Hanauer SB: Aminosalicylates: old and new. Mt Sinai J Med 1990;57:283–287.
133. Leichtner AM: Aminosalicylates for the treatment of inflammatory bowel disease. J Pediatr Gastroenterol Nutr 1995;21:245–252.
134. Ferry GD, Kirschner BS, Grand RJ, et al: Olsalazine versus sulfasalazine in mild to moderate childhood ulcerative colitis: results of the Pediatric Gastroenterology Collaborative Research Group Clinical Trial. J Pediatr Gastroenterol Nutr 1993;17:32–38.
135. Tolia V, Massoud N, Klotz U: Oral 5-aminosalicylic acid in children with colonic inflammatory bowel disease: clinical and pharmacokinetic experience. J Pediatr Gastroenterol Nutr 1989;8:333–338.
136. Barden L, Lipson A, Pert P, Walker-Smith JA: Mesalazine in childhood inflammatory bowel disease. Aliment Pharmacol Ther 1989;3:597–603.
137. Griffiths A, Koletzko S, Sylvester F, et al: Slow-release 5-aminosalicylic acid therapy in children with small intestinal Crohn's disease. J Pediatr Gastroenterol Nutr 1993;17:186–192.
138. D'Agata ID, Vanounou T, Seidman E: Mesalamine in pediatric inflammatory bowel disease: a 10 year experience. Inflamm Bowel Dis 1996;2:229–235.
139. Garau P, Orenstein SR, Neigut DA, Kocoshis SA: Pancreatitis associated with olsalazine and sulfasalazine in children with ulcerative colitis. J Pediatr Gastroenterol Nutr 1994;18:481–485.
140. Radke M, Bartolomaeus G, Muller M, Richter I: Acute pancreatitis in Crohn's disease due to 5-ASA therapy. J Pediatr Gastroenterol Nutr 1993;16:337–339.
141. Abdullah AM, Scott RB, Martin SR: Acute pancreatitis secondary to 5-aminosalicylic acid in a child with ulcerative colitis. J Pediatr Gastroenterol Nutr 1993;17:441–444.
142. Behrens R, Ruder H: Chronisch-entzundliche darmerkrankung und nephritis. Klin Padiatr 1992;204:61–64.
143. Chapman RW, Selby WS, Jewell DP: Controlled trial of intravenous metronidazole as an adjunct to corticosteroids in severe ulcerative colitis. Gut 1986;27:1210–1212.
144. Davies PS, Rhodes J, Heatley RV, Owen E: Metronidazole in the treatment of chronic proctitis: a controlled trial. Gut 1977;18:680–681.
145. Gilat T, Leichtman G, Delpre G, et al: A comparison of metronidazole and sulfasalazine in the maintenance of remission in patients with ulcerative colitis. J Clin Gastroenterol 1989;11:392–395.
146. Mantzaris GJ, Archavlis E, Christoforidis P, et al: A prospective randomized controlled trial of oral ciprofloxacin in acute ulcerative colitis. Am J Gastroenterol 1997;92:454–456.
147. Markowitz J, Grancher K, Mandel F, Daum F: Immunosuppressive therapy in pediatric inflammatory bowel disease: results of a survey of the North American Society for Gastroenterology and Nutrition. Am J Gastroenterol 1993;88:44–48.
148. Sandborn WJ: A review of immune modifier therapy for inflammatory bowel disease: azathioprine, 6-mercaptopurine, cyclosporine, and methotrexate. Am J Gastroenterol 1996;91:423–433.
149. Verhave M, Winter HS, Grand RJ: Azathioprine in the treatment of children with inflammatory bowel disease. J Pediatr 1990;117:809–814.
150. George J, Present DH, Pou R, et al: The long-term outcome of ulcerative colitis treated with 6-mercaptopurine. Am J Gastroenterol 1996;91:1711–1714.
151. Hawthorne AB, Logan RFA, Hawkey CJ, et al: Randomised controlled trial of azathioprine withdrawal in ulcerative colitis. Br Med J 1992;305:20–22.
152. Fernandez-Banares F, Bertran X, Esteve-Comas M, et al: Azathioprine is useful in maintaining long-term remission induced by intravenous cyclosporine in steroid-refractory severe ulcerative colitis. Am J Gastroenterol 1996;91:2498–2499.
153. Ramakrishna J, Langhans N, Calenda K, et al: Combined use of cyclosporine and azathioprine or 6-mercaptopurine in pediatric inflammatory bowel disease. J Pediatr Gastroenterol Nutr 1996;32:296–302.
154. Ho S, Clipstone N, Timmermann L, et al: The mechanism of action of cyclosporin A and FK506. Clin Immunol Immunopathol 1996;80:S40–S45.
155. Benkov KJ, Rosh JR, Schwerenz AH, et al: Cyclosporine as an alternative to surgery in children with inflammatory bowel disease. J Pediatr Gastroenterol Nutr 1994;19:290–294.
156. Treem WR, Cohen J, Davis P, et al: Cyclosporine for the treatment of fulminant ulcerative colitis in children. Dis Colon Rectum 1995;38:474–479.
157. Bousvaros A, Kirschner B, Werlin S, et al: Oral tacrolimus treatment of severe colitis in children (abstract). Gastroenterology 1997;112:A941.
158. Egan LJ, Sandborn WJ: Methotrexate for inflammatory bowel disease: pharmacology and preliminary results. Mayo Clin Proc 1996;71:69–80.
159. Oren R, Arber N, Odes S, et al: Methotrexate in chronic active ulcerative colitis: a double-blind, randomized, Israeli multicenter trial. Gastroenterology 1996;110:1416–1421.
160. Sands B: Biologic therapy for inflammatory bowel disease. Inflamm Bowel Dis 1997;3:95–113.
161. Evans RC, Clark L, Heath P, Rhodes JM: Treatment of ulcerative colitis with an engineered human anti-TNF$\alpha$ antibody CDP571 (abstract). Gastroenterology 1996;110:A905.
162. Sands BE, Podolsky DK, Tremaine WJ, et al: Chimeric monoclonal anti–tumor necrosis factor antibody (cA2) in the treatment of severe, steroid-refractory ulcerative colitis (UC) (abstract). Gastroenterology 1996;110:A1008.
163. Kucharzik T, Lugering N, Domschke W, Stoll R: Synergistic effect of immunoregulatory cytokines on peripheral blood monocytes: potential therapeutic approach in IBD? Gastroenterology 1996;110:A943.
164. Neurath MF, Petterson S, zum Buschenfelde K-H M, Strober W: Local administration of antisense phosphorothioate oligonucleotides to the p65 subunit of NF-$\kappa$B abrogates established experimental colitis in mice. Nat Med 1996;2:998–1004.
165. Yacyshyn B, Woloschuk B, Yacyshyn MB, et al: Efficacy and safety of ISIS 2302 (ICAM-1 antisense oligonucleotide) treatment of steroid-dependent Crohn's disease (abstract). Gastroenterology 1997;112:A1123.
166. Rintala RJ, Lindahl H: Restorative proctocolectomy for ulcerative colitis in children: is the J-pouch better than the straight pull-through? J Pediatr Surg 1996;31:530–533.
167. Fonkalsrud EW: Long-term results after colectomy and ileoanal pull-through procedure in children. Arch Surg 1996;131:881–885.
168. Shamberger RC, Lillehei CW, Nurko S, Winter HS: Anorectal function in children after ileoanal pull-through. J Pediatr Surg 1994;29:329–332.
169. Nicholls S, Vieira MC, Majrowski WH, et al: Linear growth after colectomy for ulcerative colitis in childhood. J Pediatr Gastroenterol Nutr 1995;21:82–86.
170. Sarigol S, Caulfield M, Wyllie R, et al: Ileal pouch-anal anastomosis in children with ulcerative colitis. Inflamm Bowel Dis 1996;2:82–87.
171. Langholz E, Munkholm P, Davidsen M, Binder V: Course of ulcerative colitis: analysis of changes in disease activity over years. Gastroenterology 1994;107:3–11.
172. Hendriksen C, Kreiner S, Binder V: Long term prognosis in ulcerative colitis—based on results from a regional patient group from the county of Copenhagen. Gut 1985;26:158–163.
173. Ahsgren L, Jonsson B, Stenling R, Rutegard J: Prognosis after early onset of ulcerative colitis: a study from an unselected patient population. Hepatogastroenterology 1993;40:467–470.

Chapter 34

# Chronic Intestinal Pseudo-obstruction

*Paul E. Hyman*

A group of experts met recently to clarify the definition of chronic intestinal pseudo-obstruction in the pediatric population. The rationale for this heuristic endeavor was concern that overuse of the term was resulting in unnecessary and inappropriate treatments, including parenteral nutrition, in children who had been misdiagnosed. They wrote, "Chronic intestinal pseudo-obstruction is a rare, severe, disabling disorder characterized by repetitive episodes or continuous symptoms and signs of bowel obstruction, including radiographic documentation of dilated bowel with air-fluid levels, in the absence of a fixed, lumen-occluding lesion."[1] Chronic intestinal pseudo-obstruction is a clinical diagnosis based on phenotype, not pathology or manometry. The most common signs are abdominal distention and failure to thrive. The most common symptoms are abdominal pain, vomiting, and constipation or diarrhea. Chronic intestinal pseudo-obstruction represents a number of different conditions that vary in cause, severity, course, and response to therapy (Table 34–1). Examples of genetic heterogeneity in pseudo-obstruction include, but are not limited to, a wide spectrum of abnormal gastric, small intestinal, and colonic myoelectrical activity and contractions as well as histologic abnormalities in nerve and muscle. Although these diseases have distinctive pathophysiologic characteristics, they are considered together because of their clinical and therapeutic similarities.

## ETIOLOGY

Pseudo-obstruction may occur as a primary disease or as a secondary manifestation of a large number of other conditions that transiently (e.g., hypothyroidism, phenothiazine overdose) or permanently (e.g., scleroderma, amyloidosis) alter bowel motility (Table 34–2).

Most congenital forms of neuropathic and myopathic pseudo-obstruction are both rare and sporadic, possibly representing new mutations. That is, there is no family history of pseudo-obstruction, no associated syndrome, and no evidence of other predisposing factors such as toxins, infections, ischemia, or autoimmune disease. In some cases, chronic intestinal pseudo-obstruction results from a familial inherited disease. There are reports of autosomal-dominant[2, 3] and -recessive[4–6] neuropathic, and dominant[7–9] and recessive[10, 11] myopathic, patterns of inheritance. In the autosomal-dominant diseases, expressivity and penetrance are variable; some of those affected die in childhood, but those less handicapped are able to reproduce. An X-linked recessive form of neuropathic pseudo-obstruction has been mapped to its locus, Xq28.[12] When counseling families, a thorough family history

**TABLE 34–1. Features of Chronic Intestinal Pseudo-obstruction in Pediatric Patients**

| |
|---|
| **Onset** |
| Congenital |
| Acquired |
| Acute |
| Gradual |
| **Presentation** |
| Megacystis—microcolon intestinal hypoperistalsis syndrome |
| Acute neonatal bowel obstruction, with or without megacystitis |
| Chronic vomiting and failure to thrive |
| Chronic abdominal distention and failure to thrive |
| **Cause** |
| Sporadic |
| Familial |
| Toxic |
| Ischemic |
| Viral |
| Inflammatory |
| Autoimmune |
| **Area of Involvement** |
| Entire gastrointestinal tract |
| Segment of gastrointestinal tract |
| Megaduodenum |
| Small bowel |
| Colon |
| **Pathology** |
| Myopathy |
| Neuropathy |
| Absent neurons |
| Immature neurons |
| Degenerating neurons |
| Intestinal neuronal dysplasia |
| No microscopic abnormality |

**TABLE 34–2. Causes of Chronic Pseudo-obstruction in Children**

**Primary Pseudo-obstruction**

- Visceral myopathy: sporadic or familial
- Visceral neuropathy: sporadic or familial

**Secondary Pseudo-obstruction: Related or Associated Recognized Causes**

- Muscular dystrophies
- Scleroderma and other connective tissue diseases
- Postischemic neuropathy
- Postviral neuropathy
- Generalized dysautonomia
- Hypothyroidism
- Diabetic autonomic neuropathy
- Drugs: anticholinergics, opiates, calcium channel blockers, many others
- Severe inflammatory bowel disease
- Organ transplantation
- Amyloidosis
- Chagas' disease
- Fetal alcohol syndrome
- Chromosome abnormalities
- Multiple endocrine neoplasia IIB
- Radiation enteritis

is essential, and screening tests of relatives should be considered to seek milder phenotypic expression.

Pseudo-obstruction may result from exposure to toxins during critical developmental periods in utero. A few children with fetal alcohol syndrome[13] and a few exposed to narcotics in utero have neuropathic forms of pseudo-obstruction. Presumably, any substance that alters neuronal migration or maturation might affect the development of the myenteric plexus and cause pseudo-obstruction.

Children with chromosomal abnormalities or syndromes may suffer from pseudo-obstruction. Children with Down syndrome have a higher incidence of Hirschsprung's disease than the general population and may have abnormal esophageal motility[14] and neuronal dysplasia in the myenteric plexus. Rare children with Down syndrome have a myenteric plexus neuropathy so generalized and so severe that they present with pseudo-obstruction. Children with neurofibromatosis, multiple endocrine neoplasia type IIB (MEN IIB), and other chromosome aberrations and autonomic neuropathies may suffer from neuropathic constipation. Children with Duchenne's muscular dystrophy sometimes develop pseudo-obstruction, especially in the terminal stages of life. Esophageal manometry and gastric emptying are abnormal in Duchenne's dystrophy, suggesting that the myopathy includes gastrointestinal smooth muscle even in asymptomatic children.[15]

Acquired pseudo-obstruction may be a rare complication of infection from cytomegalovirus[16] or Epstein-Barr virus.[17] Immunocompromised children and immunosuppressed transplant recipients seem at higher risk than the general population. Many of the acquired cases of pseudo-obstruction might be a result of myenteric plexus neuritis from persistent viral infection or an autoimmune inflammatory response. Mucosal inflammation causes abnormal motility. With celiac disease,[18] Crohn's disease, and the chronic enterocolitis associated with Hirschsprung's disease some patients develop dilated bowel and symptoms due, not to anatomic obstruction, but to a neuromuscular disorder presumably related to the effects of inflammatory mediators on mucosal afferent sensory nerves or motor nerves in the enteric plexuses. Other rare causes of pseudo-obstruction associated with inflammation include myenteric neuritis associated with antineuronal antibodies[19] and intestinal myositis.[20]

## PATHOLOGY

There may be histologic abnormalities in the muscle or nerve or, rarely, both.[21] Histology is normal in about 10% of cases that are studied appropriately. In such cases there may be an abnormality in some biochemical aspect of stimulus-contraction coupling.

When laparotomy is imminent for a child with pseudo-obstruction, there must be timely communication between the surgeon and the pathologist. A laparotomy is not indicated for biopsy alone,[22] perhaps because a pathologic diagnosis usually does not alter the clinical management or the clinical course. When surgery is indicated (e.g., for colectomy, cholecystectomy or creation of an ileostomy) a plan should be made to obtain a full-thickness bowel biopsy specimen at least 2 cm in diameter. The tissues should be processed for studies: histology, histochemistry for selected peptides and enzymes, electron microscopy, and silver stains.

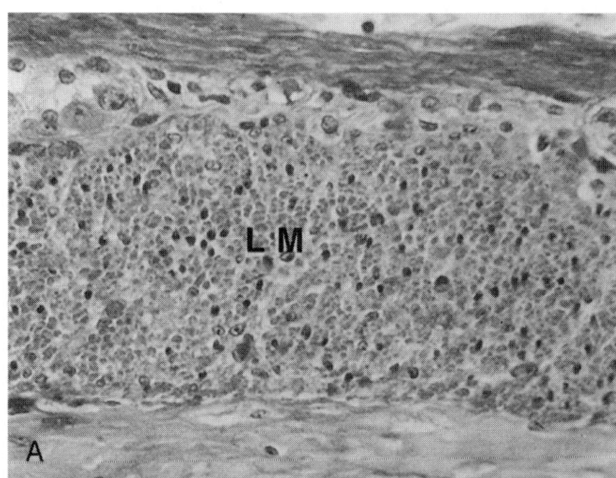


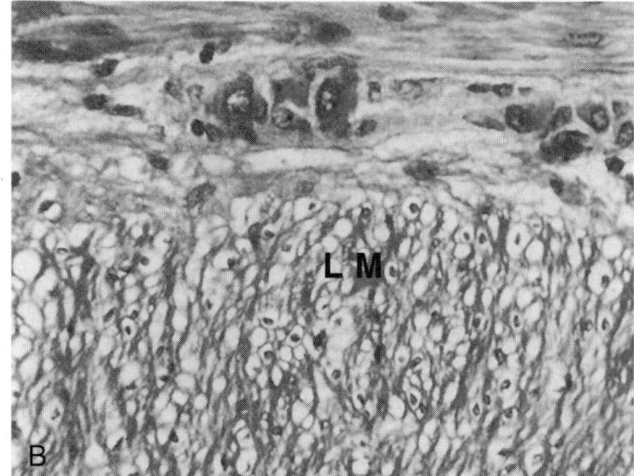


**FIGURE 34–1.** Visceral myopathy. *A*, Longitudinal muscle cut in cross section from the small intestine of a control infant. *B*, Longitudinal muscle from an infant with visceral myopathy shows classic vacuolar degeneration. Note the normal neurons in the myenteric plexus above the longitudinal muscle. × 136. (Courtesy of Dr. Michael D. Schuffler.)

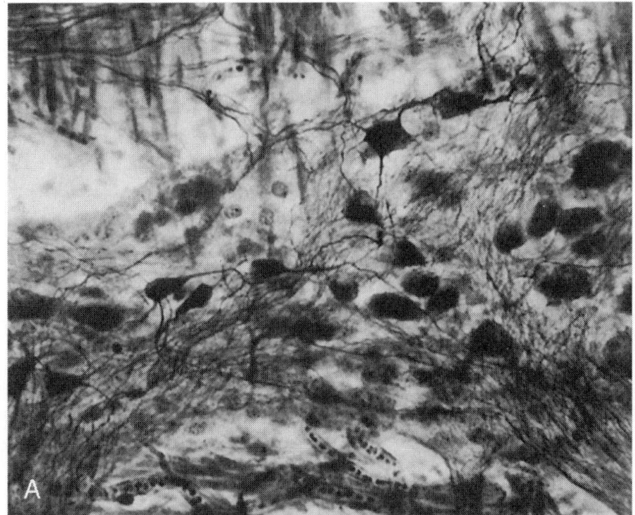


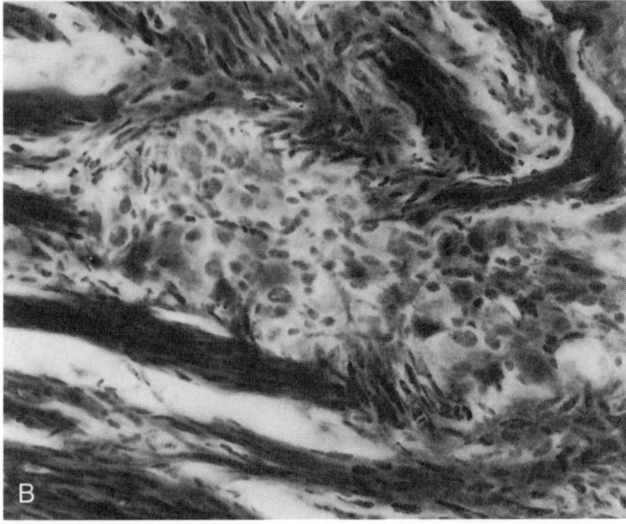


**FIGURE 34–2.** Maturational arrest of myenteric plexus. *A*, Ganglionic area of myenteric plexus from the small intestine of a control infant. Note the numerous argyrophilic neurons and axons. *B*, Ganglionic area of myenteric plexus from the small intestine of an infant with chronic intestinal pseudo-obstruction caused by maturational arrest. Note the absence of argyrophilic neurons and axons. The ganglion is filled with numerous cells, which are probably glial cells and immature neurons. × 544. (Courtesy of Dr. Michael D. Schuffler.)

Muscle disease may be inflammatory but more often is not. In light microscopy of both familial and sporadic forms of hollow visceral myopathy, the muscularis appears thin. The external longitudinal muscle layer is more involved than the internal circular muscle, and there may be extensive fibrosis in the muscle tissue. By electron microscopy there are vacuolar degeneration and disordered myofilaments (Fig. 34–1).

Neuropathic disease is best examined with silver stains of the myenteric plexus[23, 24] and routine histologic techniques. The presence of neurons in the submucous plexus of a suction biopsy specimen eliminates Hirschsprung's disease as a diagnostic possibility but is inadequate for the evaluation of other neuropathies. There may be maturational arrest of the myenteric plexus (Fig. 34–2). This hypoganglionosis is characterized by fewer neurons, which may be smaller than normal. Maturational arrest can be a primary congenital disorder or can occur secondary to ischemia or infection. Changes can be patchy or generalized.

Intestinal neuronal dysplasia,[25] or hyperganglionosis, is a histologic diagnosis defined by these findings: (1) hyperplasia of the parasympathetic neurons and fibers of the myenteric (and sometimes submucous) plexus, characterized by increases in the number and size of ganglia, thickened nerves, and increases in neuron cell bodies; (2) increased acetyl cholinesterase–positive nerve fibers in the lamina propria; (3) increased acetylcholine esterase–positive nerve fibers around submucosal blood vessels; (4) heterotopic neuron cell bodies in the lamina propria, muscle, and serosal layers. The first two criteria are obligatory.

Children with intestinal neuronal dysplasia are a heterogeneous group. Children with primary pseudo-obstruction due to neuronal dysplasia may have disease that is limited to the colon or disseminated. Other children may have neuronal dysplasia associated with prematurity, protein allergy, chromosome abnormalities, MEN IIB, and neurofibromatosis; however, intestinal neuronal dysplasia is an occasional incidental finding in bowel specimens examined for reasons unrelated to motility. Intestinal neuronal dysplasia correlates poorly with motility-related symptoms.[26] Thus, a pathologic diagnosis of intestinal neuronal dysplasia neither predicts clinical outcome nor influences management.

## CLINICAL FEATURES

### Presentation

More than half the affected children develop symptoms at or shortly after birth. A few cases are diagnosed in utero, by ultrasound findings of polyhydramnios and megacystis and marked abdominal distention (Fig. 34–3). Intestinal malrotation is found in both neuropathic and myopathic congenital forms of pseudo-obstruction. Of children who present at birth, about 40% have an intestinal malrotation. In the most severely affected infants symptoms of acute bowel obstruction appear within the first hours of life. Less severely affected infants present months later with symptoms of vomiting, diarrhea, and failure to thrive. A few patients have megacystis at birth and insidious onset of gastrointestinal symptoms over the first few years. More than three quarters of the children develop symptoms by the end of the first year of life, and the remainder present sporadically through the first two decades.

Although there is individual variation in the number and intensity of signs and symptoms, it may be useful to note the relative frequencies in this population. Abdominal distention and vomiting are the most common features, complaints of about three quarters of the patients. Constipation, episodic or intermittent abdominal pain, and poor weight gain are features in about 60% of cases. Diarrhea is a complaint in one third. Urinary tract smooth muscle is affected in those with both hollow visceral neuropathy and hollow visceral myopathy, about one fifth of all pseudo-obstruction patients. Often these children are severely affected at birth and are described by the phenotype *megacystis-microcolon intestinal hypoperistalsis syndrome*.[27]

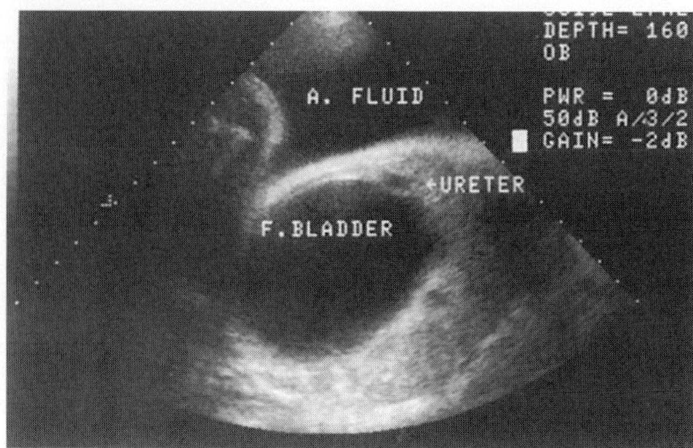


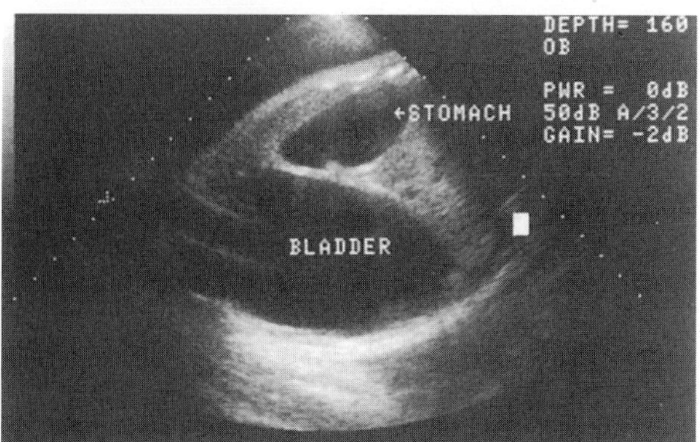


**FIGURE 34–3.** Ultrasound of infant with pseudo-obstruction diagnosed in utero. There is polyhydramnios as well as distention of the stomach and urinary bladder. (Courtesy of Radha Cherukuri, MD.)

The majority of children's clinical course is characterized by relative remissions and exacerbations. Many are able to identify factors that precipitate deteriorations, including intercurrent infections, general anesthesia, psychological stress, and poor nutritional status.

The radiographic signs are those of intestinal obstruction, with air-fluid levels (Fig. 34–4), dilated stomach, small intestine, and colon, or microcolon in those studied because of obstruction at birth.[28] There may be prolonged stasis of contrast material placed into the affected bowel, so it is prudent to plan how to evacuate the contrast fluid or to use a nontoxic, isotonic, water-soluble medium to prevent barium from solidifying into a true anatomic obstruction. Children who feel well can still show radiographic evidence of bowel obstruction. The greater problem arises when children develop an acute deterioration. Radiographs demonstrate the same patterns of bowel obstruction that are seen when the child feels well. In children who previously had surgery, it can be difficult to discriminate between physical obstruction related to adhesions and an episodic increase in the symptoms of pseudo-obstruction.

**FIGURE 34–4.** Upright abdominal radiograph in a 4-year-old boy with hollow visceral myopathy. Note massive bowel dilatation and air-fluid levels, central venous catheter in the inferior vena cava, and antroduodenal manometry catheter in the stomach and duodenum.

## Diagnosis

An incorrect diagnosis of pseudo-obstruction can result from misdiagnosis of infant and toddler victims of Münchausen's syndrome by proxy.[29] Well-meaning clinicians inadvertently co-create disease as they respond to a parent's symptom fabrications by performing tests and procedures, including parenteral nutrition support, repeated surgery, and even small bowel transplantation.[30] Adolescents with disabling abdominal pain arising from psychiatric diseases such as visceral pain disorder, post-traumatic stress disorder, and Asperger's syndrome may also confuse gastroenterologists.[31, 32]

Diagnostic testing provides information about the nature and severity of the pathophysiology. Manometric studies are more sensitive than radiographic tests to evaluate the strength and coordination of contraction and relaxation in the esophagus, gastric antrum, small intestine, colon, and anorectal area.

In affected children scintigraphy demonstrates delayed gastric emptying of solids or liquids and reflux of intestinal contents back into the stomach. Dilated loops of bowel predispose to bacterial overgrowth, so breath hydrogen testing may reveal elevations in fasting breath hydrogen and a rapid increase in breath hydrogen with a carbohydrate meal.

Esophageal manometry is abnormal in about half those affected by pseudo-obstruction. In children with myopathy, contractions are low amplitude but coordinated in the distal two thirds of the esophagus. Lower esophageal sphincter pressure is low, and sphincter relaxation is complete. When the esophagus is affected by neuropathy, contraction amplitude in the esophageal body may be high, normal, low, or absent. There may be simultaneous, spontaneous, or repetitive contractions. Relaxation of the lower esophageal sphincter may be incomplete or absent.

Antroduodenal manometry findings are always abnormal with intestinal pseudo-obstruction involving the upper gastrointestinal tract; however, manometry is often abnormal in partial or complete small bowel obstruction. Although the manometric patterns of true obstruction differ from those of pseudo-obstruction in adults,[33, 34] such a distinction was not possible in children we have studied. Antroduodenal manometry should not be used as a test to differentiate true bowel obstruction from pseudo-obstruction. Manometry should be done after a diagnosis of pseudo-obstruction is established, to determine the physiologic correlates for the symptoms, to assess drug responses, and for prognosis.[35–37] Contrast radiography and, as a last resort, exploratory laparotomy are best for differentiating true obstruction from pseudo-obstruction.

As in the esophagus, intestinal myopathy causes low-amplitude coordinated contractions, and neuropathy causes uncoordinated contractions. Interpretation of antroduodenal manometry requires recognition of normal and abnormal features (Table 34–3). The abnormalities in pseudo-obstruction are commonly discrete and easily interpreted by eye (Fig. 34–5). They contrast markedly with normal features of antroduodenal manometry (Fig. 34–6).

In most cases the manometric abnormality correlates with clinical severity of the disease. For example, children with total aganglionosis have contractions of normal amplitude that are never organized into migrating motor complexes (MMCs), fed patterns, or even bursts or clusters of contractions but are simply a monotonous pattern of random events. Children with such a pattern are dependent on total parenteral nutrition (TPN). More than 80% of children with MMCs are nourished enterally, but more than 80% of children without MMCs require partial or total parenteral nutrition. Discrete abnormalities in the organization of intestinal contractions are listed in Table 48–3.

**TABLE 34–3. Antroduodenal Manometric Features from Studies of 300 Children***

| |
|---|
| **Normal Features** |
| Migrating motor complex (MMC) (fasting) |
| Postprandial (phase 2–like) pattern |
| **Abnormal Features in Duodenum** |
| Absent MMC phase 3 |
| Sustained tonic contractions |
| Retrograde propagation of phase 3 |
| Giant single-propagating contractions |
| Absent phase 2 with increased phase 3 frequency |
| Persistently low-amplitude or absent contractions |
| Prolonged nonpropagating clusters |
| **Postprandial Abnormalities** |
| Antral hypomotility after a solid nutrient meal |
| Absent or decreased motility |
| Failure to induce a fed pattern (MMC persists) |

*Each of these features is easily recognized by visual inspection of the recording.

From Tomomasa T, DiLorenzo C, Morikawa A, et al: Analysis of fasting antroduodenal manometry in children. Dig Dis Sci 1996;41:195–203.

Normal antroduodenal manometry and absence of dilated bowel in a patient with symptoms of chronic intestinal pseudo-obstruction shifts the emphasis from medical to psychological illness. It is often difficult for families to consider and engage in psychological intervention, especially when the decision is based on a "lack of medical findings." Thus it is important to interpret the antroduodenal manometry as a positive diagnostic indicator, *especially* when the results are normal.

Colonic manometry is abnormal in colonic pseudo-obstruction.[38] The normal features of colon manometry in children include (1) high-amplitude propagating contractions (phasic contractions stronger than 60 mm Hg amplitude propagating over at least 30 cm; Fig. 34–7); (2) a gastrocolic response (the increase in motility that follows a meal); and (3) an absence of discrete abnormalities. With neuropathic disease contractions are normal or reduced in amplitude, but there are no high-amplitude propagating contractions or gastrocolic response. With myopathy there are usually no colonic contractions.

There are several pitfalls with intestinal and colonic manometry. In dilated bowel no contractions are recorded and manometry is not diagnostic. Recordings filled with respiratory and movement artifacts from an agitated, angry, crying patient are uninterpretable. Acute pseudo-obstruction is usually associated with ileus, so that an absence of contractions may not reflect the underlying abnormality. Manometry is most likely to be helpful when performed in a cooperative patient at a time when the patient is feeling well.

Anorectal manometry is usually normal in chronic intestinal pseudo-obstruction. There is an absence of the rectoinhibitory reflex only in Hirschsprung's disease and in some patients with intestinal neuronal dysplasia.

In a few specialized centers, electrogastrography is a noninvasive screening test for evaluation of children thought to have pseudo-obstruction.[39] Skin electrodes are placed over the stomach, just as surface electrodes are placed over the heart to perform electrocardiography. The electrical slow-wave rhythms of the gastric body and antrum are recorded. Gastric slow waves normally occur at a rate of 3 per minute. Gastric neuropathies are characterized by decreases (bradygastria) or increases (tachygastria) in slow-wave frequency.

## TREATMENT

### Nutrition Support

The goal of nutrition support is to achieve normal growth and development with the fewest possible complications and the greatest patient comfort. In children with pseudo-obstruction, motility improves as nutritional deficiencies resolve and worsens as malnutrition recurs.

Roughly a third of affected children require partial or total parenteral nutrition. One third require total or partial tube feedings, and the rest eat by mouth. TPN is the least desirable means of achieving nutritional sufficiency because of the high rate of complications. In the absence of enteral nutrients, the gastrointestinal tract does not grow or mature normally. In the absence of the postprandial rise in trophic

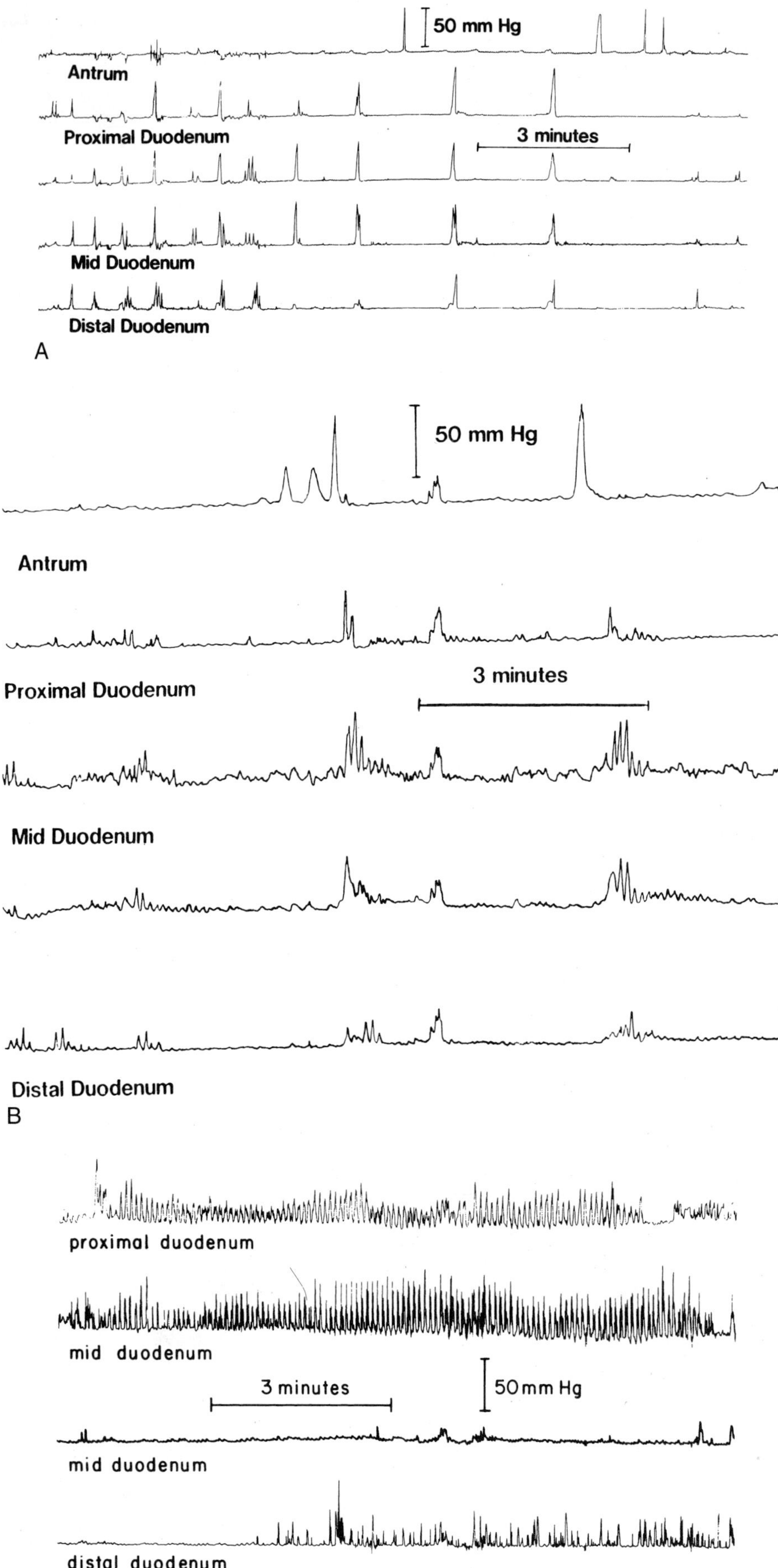


**FIGURE 34–5.** Discrete abnormalities in antroduodenal manometry. *A*, Single propagating high-amplitude duodenal contractions. These "single ring" contractions are associated with irritable bowel disorders when the migrating motor complex is present. *B*, Nonpropagating, simultaneous, short clusters in monotonous pattern continuing uninterrupted for a 6-hour study. *C*, Long burst of nonpropagating duodenal contractions.

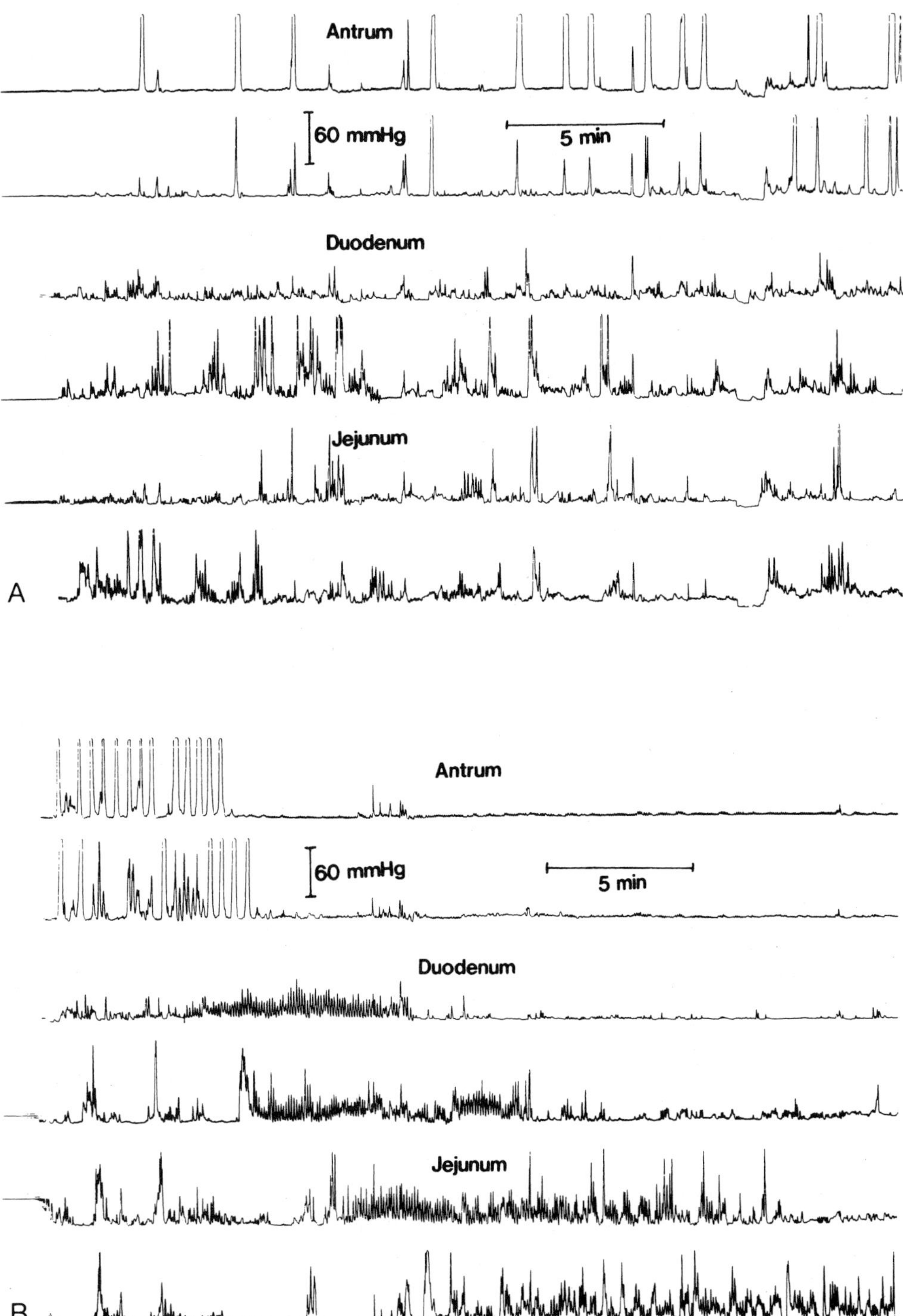


**FIGURE 34–6.** *A*, Phase 2–like activity, consisting of random, intermittent, variable-amplitude contractions in the gastric antrum and the duodenum. This is also the postprandial pattern that interrupts the migrating motor complex (MMC). *B*, Phase 3 of the MMC.

and stimulant gastrointestinal hormones, bile stasis and liver disease develop.[40] TPN-associated cholelithiasis[41] and progressive liver disease are important causes of morbidity and mortality in children with pseudo-obstruction. The minimal volume, composition, and route of enteral support required to reverse or prevent the progression of gastrointestinal complications have not been determined. It seems likely that a complex liquid formula containing protein and fat, given by mouth or gastrostomy tube, and contributing 10% to 25% of the child's total calorie requirement would be sufficient to stimulate postprandial increases in splanchnic blood flow and plasma concentrations of gastrin and other trophic factors. Every effort should be extended to maximize enteral nutritional support in parenteral nutrition–dependent children.

Continuous feeding via gastrostomy or jejunostomy may be effective when bolus feedings fail. Most children with visceral myopathy and a few with neuropathy have an atonic stomach and almost no gastric emptying. In these children, a feeding jejunostomy may be helpful for the administration of medications and for drip feedings.[42] Care must be taken to place a jejunostomy into an undistended bowel loop.

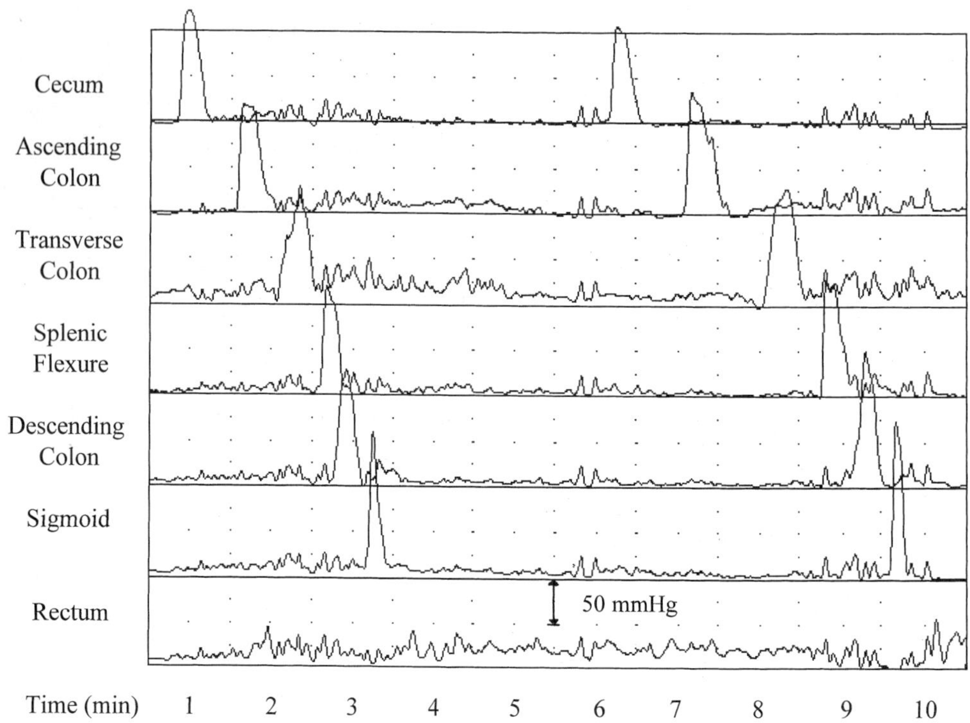


**FIGURE 34–7.** High-amplitude propagating contractions are a marker of colonic neuromuscular integrity in children.

## Drugs

Drugs to stimulate intestinal contractions are helpful in a minority of children with pseudo-obstruction. Bethanechol, neostigmine, metoclopramide, and domperidone have not been useful. Cisapride has been helpful in a minority of children. Cisapride's mechanism of action is to bind to serotonin receptors on the motor nerves of the myenteric plexus, facilitating release of acetylcholine and stimulating gastrointestinal smooth muscle contraction. Cisapride is most likely to work in children with MMC and without dilated bowel.[36] Cisapride increases the number and strength of contractions in the duodenum of children with pseudo-obstruction but does not initiate the MMC in patients without it or inhibit discrete abnormalities.[43]

A trial of cisapride is appropriate for every child with pseudo-obstruction. For children on TPN the trial should be initiated when there is no acute illness and no malnutrition, coincident with initiation of enteral feedings. Liquid suspension, 1 mg per mL, or tablet, 5 or 10 mg, is administered at 0.1 to 0.3 mg/kg per dose three or four times daily. Side effects—gastrointestinal complaints and irritability—are observed in about 5% of children. Cisapride overdose, or intercurrent dosing with macrolide antibiotics or antifungal agents is associated with a rare but serious risk of cardiac ventricular arrhythmias. The addition of an anticholinesterase inhibitor such as neostygmine or physostygmine may improve the response to cisapride in some patients.

Erythromycin, a motilin receptor agonist, appears to facilitate gastric emptying in those with neuropathic gastroparesis by stimulating high-amplitude 3-minute antral contractions, relaxing the pylorus, and inducing antral phase 3 episodes in doses of 1 to 3 mg/kg intravenously[44] or 3 to 5 mg orally. Erythromycin does not appear to be effective for more generalized motility disorders.

Antibiotics are used for bacterial overgrowth. Bacterial overgrowth is associated with steatorrhea, fat-soluble vitamin malabsorption, and malabsorption of the intrinsic factor–vitamin $B_{12}$ complex. It is possible that bacterial overgrowth contributes to bacteremia and frequent episodes of central venous catheter-related sepsis and to TPN-associated liver disease. Further, bacterial overgrowth, mucosal injury, malabsorption, fluid secretion, and gas production may contribute to chronic intestinal dilatation. Chronic antibiotic use may result in the emergence of resistant strains of bacteria or overgrowth with fungi. Thus, treating bacterial overgrowth must be considered on an individual basis.

Excessive gastrostomy drainage may result from retrograde flow of intestinal contents into the stomach or from gastric acid hypersecretion. Gastric secretory function or gastric pH should be tested before beginning antisecretory drugs. Histamine $H_2$-receptor antagonists may be used to suppress gastric acid hypersecretion. Tolerance develops after a few months of intravenous use,[45] so the drug should be given orally when possible. When a drug is added to TPN, gastric pH should be assessed at regular intervals to monitor drug efficacy. Induction of achlorhydria is inadvisable because it promotes bacterial overgrowth in the stomach.

Constipation is treated with mineral oil, suppositories, or enemas. Oral enteral lavage solutions usually cause acute abdominal distention in children with pseudo-obstruction. Acute pain due to episodes of pseudo-obstruction is best treated by decompressing distended bowel. It is appropriate to consider nonsteroidal anti-inflammatory agents (e.g., ketorolac) and epidural anesthetics as alternatives to, or in combination with, systemic narcotics.

Chronic pain is rarely a problem in children with congenital pseudo-obstruction but is more common in adolescents who have autoimmune or inflammatory disease and progressive loss of intestinal function. Pain consists of a nociceptive component and an affective component. Patients with chronic pain benefit from a multidisciplinary approach including not only attention to gastrointestinal disease but also mental health assessment and treatment for the affective component. Collaboration with pain management specialists is beneficial for optimizing the care of pseudo-obstruction patients who complain of chronic pain. Multiple modalities for pain relief are useful: massage, relaxation, hypnosis, psychotherapy, and drugs all have shown positive effects. Drugs that reduce afferent signaling, improving chronic visceral pain, include the tricyclic antidepressants, clonidine, and gabapentin.[46] Long-term narcotic therapy is inadvisable, because narcotics cause disorganization of intestinal motility, tolerance to narcotics develops rapidly, and narcotic withdrawal can simulate the visceral pain of acute pseudo-obstruction.

## Surgery

One of the management challenges in pseudo-obstruction is the evaluation and re-evaluation of newborns and children with episodic acute obstructive symptoms. Although most acute episodes represent pseudo-obstruction, it is important to intervene with surgery when the episode is a true bowel obstruction, appendicitis, or another surgical condition. Many children with episodes of acute pseudo-obstruction undergo repeated exploratory laparotomies. It is especially important to avoid unnecessary abdominal surgery in children with pseudo-obstruction for several reasons: (1) They often suffer from prolonged postoperative ileus: (2) Adhesions create a diagnostic problem each time there is a new obstructive episode: (3) Adhesions following laparotomy may distort normal tissue planes and make future surgery riskier in terms of bleeding and organ perforation. After several laparotomies turn up no evidence of mechanical obstruction, the surgeon may choose a more conservative management plan for subsequent episodes, including pain management, nutritional support, and abdominal decompression.

Gastrostomy was the only procedure that reduced the number of hospitalizations in adults with pseudo-obstruction,[47] and the experience with children seems to be similar. Gastrostomy provides a quick and comfortable means of evacuating gastric contents and relieves pain and nausea related to gastric and bowel distention. Continued "venting" may decompress more distal regions of small bowel, obviating nasogastric intubation and pain medication. Gastrostomy is used for enteral feeding and enteral administration of medication. Gastrostomy placement should be considered for those receiving parenteral nutrition and for children who will need tube feedings longer than 2 months. In many patients, endoscopic gastrostomy placement is ideal. In those with contraindications to endoscopic placement, surgical placement is appropriate. Care must be taken to place the ostomy in a suitable position, above the gastric antrum in the midbody.

Fundoplication is rarely indicated for pseudo-obstruction. After fundoplication, symptoms can change from vomiting to repeated retching.[48] In children with pseudo-obstruction, vomiting is reduced by venting the gastrostomy. Acid reflux is controlled with antisecretory medication.

Results of pyloroplasty or Roux-en-Y gastrojejunostomy to improve gastric emptying in pseudo-obstruction have been poor; gastric emptying remains delayed. Altering the anatomy rarely improves the function of the dilated fundus and body. Small bowel resections or tapering operations may provide relief for months or even years; however, when the lesion is present in other areas of bowel those areas gradually dilate and symptoms recur.

Ileostomy can decompress dilated distal small bowel and provide further benefit by removing the high-pressure zone at the end of the bowel, the anal sphincter. Transit of luminal contents is always from a high-pressure zone to a lower-pressure one. In pseudo-obstruction patients with gastric antral contractions but no effective small bowel contractions, bowel transit improves with the creation of an ileostomy because of the absence of resistance to flow at the ostomy site.

Colectomy is sometimes necessary in congenital forms of generalized pseudo-obstruction to decompress an abdomen so distended that respiration is impaired. In general, colon diversions are inadvisable because of a high incidence of diversion colitis.[49] Diversion colitis can cause abdominal pain, tenesmus, and hematochezia.

Subtotal colectomy with ileoproctostomy cures rare children with neuropathic pseudo-obstruction confined to the colon. Typically these children are able to eat normally and grow, but they are unable to defecate spontaneously. They differ from children with functional fecal retention in that their stools are never huge or hard, there is no retentive posturing, the history of constipation begins at birth, and there are often extrarectal fecal masses. Colon pathology may show neuronal dysplasia, maturational arrest, or no diagnostic abnormality, but colon manometry is always abnormal, without high-amplitude propagating contractions or a postprandial rise in motility index. Before colectomy for constipation, antroduodenal manometry is necessary to determine whether the upper gastrointestinal tract is involved. Abnormal antroduodenal manometry is a relative contraindication to colectomy because upper gastrointestinal symptoms appear after colon resection. Before surgery, a psychological evaluation may help to assess the possibility of psychiatric disease and somatization masquerading as colon disease and to prepare the patient for the procedures.

A cecostomy using a small "button" ostomy appliance for regular infusion of colonic lavage solution has not been effective for colonic pseudo-obstruction. The abdomen distends, but the colon does not empty.

Failure of medical management may signal a need for total bowel resection. Rarely, a mucosal secretory disorder complicates the management of pseudo-obstruction. Several liters of intestinal secretions drain from enteric orifices each day. When secretions cannot be controlled with opiates, anticholinergics, antibiotics, steroids, or somatostatin analogue, it may be necessary to resect the entire bowel to avoid life-threatening electrolyte abnormalities and nutritional disturbances caused by the large volume losses. Total bowel resection may reduce episodes of bacterial transmigration across dilated bowel, causing repeated life-threatening central venous catheter infections. Total bowel resection should be considered alone or in combination with small bowel transplantation. Small bowel or combined liver-bowel transplants have the potential to cure children with pseudo-obstruction. Intestinal transplantation offers great promise for the future.[50]

## REFERENCES


1. Rudolph CD, Hyman PE, Altschuler SM, et al: Diagnosis and treatment of chronic intestinal pseudo-obstruction in children: report of consensus workshop. J Pediatr Gastroenterol Nutr 1997;24:102–112.
2. Roy AD, Bharucha H, Nevin NC, et al: Idiopathic intestinal pseudo-obstruction: a familial visceral neuropathy. Clin Genet 1980;18:291–297.
3. Mayer EA, Schuffler MD, Rotter JI, et al: Familial visceral neuropathy with autosomal dominant transmission. Gastroenterology 1986;91:1528–1535.
4. Schuffler MD, Bird TD, Sumi SM, et al: A familial neuronal disease presenting as intestinal pseudo-obstruction. Gastroenterology 1978;75:889–898.
5. Haltia M, Somer H, Palo J, et al: Neuronal intranuclear inclusion disease in identical twins. Ann Neurol 1984;15:316–321.
6. Patel H, Norman MG, Perry TL, et al: Multiple system atrophy with neuronal intranuclear hyaline inclusions. Report of a case and review of the literature. J Neurol Sci 1985;67:57–65.
7. Faulk DL, Anuras S, Gardner D: A familial visceral myopathy. Ann Intern Med 1987;89:600–606.
8. Schuffler MD, Pope CE: Studies of idiopathic intestinal pseudo-obstruction. II. Hereditary hollow visceral myopathy: family studies. Gastroenterology 1977;73:339–344.
9. Schuffler MD, Lowe MC, Bill AH: Studies of idiopathic intestinal pseudo-obstruction: I. Hereditary hollow visceral myopathy: clinical and pathological studies. Gastroenterology 1977;73:327–328.
10. Anuras S, Mitros FA, Nowak TV, et al: A familial visceral myopathy with external ophthalmoplegia and autosomal recessive transmission. Gastroenterology 1983;84:346–353.
11. Ionasescu V, Thompson SH, Ionasescu R, et al: Inherited ophthalmoplegia with intestinal pseudo-obstruction. J Neurol Sci 1983;59:215–228.
12. Auricchio A, Brancolini V, Casari G, et al: The locus for a novel syndromatic form of neuronal intestinal pseudo-obstruction maps to Xq28. Am J Hum Genet 1996;58:743–748.
13. Uc A, Vasiliauskas E, Piccoli D, et al: Chronic intestinal pseudo-obstruction associated with fetal alcohol syndrome. Dig Dis Sci 1997;42:1163–1167.
14. Hillemeier C, Buchin PJ, Gryboski J: Esophageal dysfunction in Down syndrome. J Pediatr Gastroenterol Nutr 1982;1:101–104.
15. Staiano A, Corraziari E, Andriotti MR, et al: Upper gastrointestinal tract motility in children with progressive muscular dystrophy. J Pediatr 1992;121:720–724.
16. Sonsino E, Movy R, Foucaud P, et al: Intestinal pseudo-obstruction related to cytomegalovirus infection of the myenteric plexus. N Engl J Med 1984;311:196–197.
17. Vassallo M, Camilleri M, Caron BL, et al: Intestinal pseudo-obstruction from selective cholinergic dysautonomia due to infectious mononucleosis. Gastroenterology 1990;98:A400.
18. Cucchiara S, Bassotti G, Castellucci G, et al: Upper gastrointestinal motor abnormalities in children with celiac disease. J Pediatr Gastroenterol Nutr 1995;21:435–442.
19. Smith VV, Gregson N, Foggensteinor L, et al: Acquired intestinal aganglionosis and circulating autoantibodies without neoplastic or other neuronal involvement. Gastroenterology 1997;112:1366–1371.
20. Ginies JL, Francois H, Joseph MG, et al: A curable cause of chronic idiopathic intestinal pseudo-obstruction in children: idiopathic myositis of the small intestine. J Pediatr Gastroenterol Nutr 1996;23:426–429.
21. Krishnamurthy S, Schuffler MD: Pathology of neuromuscular disorders of the small intestine and colon. Gastroenterology 1987;93:610–639.
22. Schuffler MD: Chronic intestinal pseudo-obstruction: progress and problems. J Pediatr Gastroenterol Nutr 1990;10:157–163.
23. Smith B: The Neuropathology of the Alimentary Tract. London, Edward Arnold, 1972.
24. Schuffler MD, Jonak Z: Chronic idiopathic intestinal pseudo-obstruction caused by a degenerative disorder of the myenteric plexus: the use of Smith's method to define the neuropathology. Gastroenterology 1982;82:476–486.
25. Schofield ED, Yunis EJ: Intestinal neuronal dysplasia. J Pediatr Gastroenterol Nutr 1991;12:182–189.
26. Cord-Udy CL, Smith VV, Ahmed S, et al: An evaluation of the role of suction rectal biopsy in the diagnosis of intestinal neuronal dysplasia. J Pediatr Gastroenterol Nutr 1997;24:1–6.
27. Granata C, Puri P: Megacystis-microcolon-hypoperistalsis syndrome. J Pediatr Gastroenterol Nutr 1997;25:12–19.
28. Vargas JH, Sachs P, Ament ME: Chronic intestinal pseudo-obstruction syndrome in pediatrics: results of a national survey by members of the North American Society of Pediatric Gastroenterology and Nutrition. J Pediatr Gastroenterol Nutr 1988;7:323–332.
29. Baron HI, Beck DC, Vargas JH, et al: Overinterpretation of gastroduodenal motility studies: two cases involving Munchausen syndrome by proxy. J Pediatr 1995;126:397–400.
30. Kosmach B, Tarbell S, Reyes J, et al: "Munchausen by proxy" syndrome in a small bowel transplant recipient. Transplant Proc 1996;28:2790–2791.
31. Zeltzer LK, Hyman PE, Heyman MB, et al: Persistent visceral pain in adolescents. J Pediatr Gastroenterol Nutr 1995;22:92–98.
32. Stam R, Akkermans LMA, Weigant VM: Trauma and the gut: interactions between stressful experience and intestinal function. Gut 1997;40:704–709.
33. Summers RW, Anuras S, Green J: Jejunal manometry patterns in health, partial intestinal obstruction, and pseudo-obstruction. Gastroenterology 1983;85:1301–1306.
34. Camilleri M: Jejunal manometry in distal subacute mechanical obstruction: significance of prolonged simultaneous contractions. Gut 1989;30:468–475.
35. Tomomasa T, DiLorenzo C, Morikawa A, et al: Analysis of fasting antroduodenal manometry in children. Dig Dis Sci 1996;41:195–203.
36. Hyman PE, DiLorenzo C, McAdams L, et al: Predicting the clinical response to cisapride in children with chronic intestinal pseudo-obstruction. Am J Gastroenterol 1993;88:832–836.
37. Fell JME, Smith VV, Milla PJ: Infantile chronic idiopathic intestinal pseudo-obstruction: the role of small intestinal manometry as a diagnostic tool and prognostic indicator. Gut 1996;39:306–311.
38. DiLorenzo C, Flores AF, Reddy SN, et al: Colonic manometry in children with chronic intestinal pseudo-obstruction. Gut 1993;34:803–807.
39. Devane SP, Ravelli AM, Bisset WM, et al: Gastric antral dysrhythmias in children with chronic idiopathic intestinal pseudo-obstruction. Gut 1992;33:1477–1481.
40. Dahms BB, Halpin TC Jr: Serial liver biopsies in parenteral nutrition–associated cholestasis of early infancy. Gastroenterology 1981;81:136–144.
41. Roslyn JJ, Berquist WE, Pitt HA, et al: Increased risk of gallstones in children receiving total parenteral nutrition. Pediatrics 1983;71:784–789.
42. Di Lorenzo C, Flores A, Hyman PE: Intestinal motility and jejunal feeding in children with chronic intestinal pseudo-obstruction. Gastroenterology 1995;108:1379–1385.
43. DiLorenzo C, Reddy SN, Villanueva-Meyer J, et al: Cisapride in children with chronic intestinal pseudo-obstruction: an acute, double-blind crossover placebo controlled trial. Gastroenterology 1991;101:1564–1570.
44. DiLorenzo C, Flores AF, Tomomasa T, et al: Effect of erythromycin on antroduodenal motility in children with chronic functional gastrointestinal symptoms. Dig Dis Sci 1994;39:1399–1404.
45. Hyman PE, Garvey TQ, Abrams CE: Tolerance to intravenous ranitidine. J Pediatr 1987;110:794–796.
46. Rosner H, Rubin L, Kestenbaum A: Gabapentin adjunctive therapy in neuropathic pain states. Clin J Pain 1996;12:56–58.
47. Pitt HA, Mann LL, Berquist WE, et al: Chronic intestinal pseudo-obstruction: management with total parenteral nutrition and a venting enterostomy. Arch Surg 1985;120:614–618.
48. DiLorenzo C, Flores A, Hyman PE: Intestinal motility in symptomatic children with fundoplication. J Pediatr Gastroenterol Nutr 1991;12:169–173.
49. Ordein J, DiLorenzo C, Flores A, Hyman PE: Diversion colitis in children with pseudo-obstruction. Am J Gastroenterol 1992;87:88–90.
50. Goulet O, Jan D, Brousse N, et al: Intestinal transplantation. J Pediatr Gastroenterol Nutr 1997;25:1–11.

Chapter 35

# Polyps and Polyposis Syndromes

*Regino P. González-Peralta and Joel M. Andres*

Intestinal polyps are tumors that protrude into the lumen of the bowel. They are characterized by their gross appearance, location, number per unit area of intestinal surface, presence or absence of a stalk (pedunculated versus sessile), association with extraintestinal lesions, and histologic features that determine the relative risk of malignant transformation.

In adults, most intestinal polyps are either true neoplastic polyps, that is, adenomatous lesions, or benign hyperplastic polyps. These polyps occur infrequently in children and are mainly discussed with the inherited polyposis syndromes—familial polyposis coli, Gardner's syndrome, and Peutz-Jeghers syndrome.

Juvenile polyps are the most common type of intestinal tumor in children and are a common cause of rectal bleeding. Generally, polyps are asymptomatic; the greatest concern is the propensity of certain polyps to become malignant. Juvenile polyps may be classified as hamartomatous, but some authors refer to them as inflammatory or retention polyps. Most of the inherited polyposis syndromes are autosomal dominant, except for Turcot's syndrome, which is probably autosomal recessive. These inherited conditions are either hamartomatous or adenomatous polyposis syndromes (Table 35–1). Carcinomas generally do not evolve from the hamartomatous syndromes, whereas malignant change is a major concern in the adenomatous syndromes. Mixed juvenile-adenomatous polyps have been reported. The noninherited polyposes include nodular lymphoid hyperplasia, inflammatory polyps, and the rare syndromes described by Cronkhite-Canada and Ruvalcaba-Myhre-Smith.

**TABLE 35–1. Classification of Polyps and Polyposis Syndromes**

| |
|---|
| **Juvenile Polyp(s)** |
| **Inherited Hamartomatous Polyposis Syndromes** |
| Juvenile polyposis |
| Peutz-Jeghers syndrome |
| Cowden's syndrome |
| **Inherited Adenomatous Polyposis Syndromes** |
| Familial polyposis coli |
| Gardner's syndrome |
| Turcot's syndrome |
| **Noninherited Polyposis** |
| Lymphoid polyposis |
| Inflammatory polyposis |
| Cronkhite-Canada syndrome |
| Ruvalcaba-Myhre-Smith syndrome |

## JUVENILE POLYPS

### Clinical Characteristics

The origin of and the genetic predisposition for juvenile polyps are unknown; they are believed to have either a hamartomatous or an inflammatory cause. Juvenile polyps, also referred to as retention polyps, are the most common polypoid lesion of the colon in children, accounting for nearly 90% of colorectal polyps. These polyps are rarely discovered in children younger than 1 year of age and are usually diagnosed between age 2 and 10 years. Early (precolonoscopy) reports indicated that juvenile polyps were usually solitary and invariably were located in the rectosigmoid colon. In more recent studies, the incidence of multiple polyps has substantially increased. Further, more juvenile polyps were noted to occur in the right colon. None were described proximal to the descending colon in the period from 1974 to 1975, whereas the incidence was 44% in the period from 1982 to 1984.[1] Similar results were reported by other investigators,[2] who noted that 58% of patients had more than one polyp and that 26% of the polyps were located proximal to the transverse colon. The differences in these findings probably represent more extensive use of colonoscopy in the evaluation of rectal bleeding in children.

Children with juvenile polyps characteristically present with asymptomatic hematochezia, usually mild, although the associated rectal bleeding can be profuse. As many as one third of affected children can experience microcytic, hypochromic anemia related to chronic blood loss.[2] Diarrhea and tenesmus can occur, especially when the polyps are located in the distal colon. Similarly, rectal prolapse or prolapse of a rectal polyp is occasionally seen. Colocolonic intussusception associated with pedunculated polyps is rare. Juvenile polyps have been noted at ureterosigmoidostomy anastomosis sites.[3]

## Pathology

Grossly (Fig. 35–1*A*), juvenile polyps are large (0.5 to 3 cm) and usually erythematous, which contrasts with the normal pink colonic mucosa. The polyp surface glistens, and large fluid-filled cystic areas are typically noted on cut-section examination. They are often friable and bleed easily when manipulated by the colonoscope. Most juvenile polyps are pedunculated; sessile polyps are rare. Histologically (Fig. 35–1*B*), they are mucosal lesions that consist of dilated, mucus-filled, tortuous cystic glands and inflammatory cells in a prominent lamina propria. The glands are composed of well-formed mucus-secreting cells. Occasionally, dilated glands rupture into the stroma, eliciting a foreign giant cell reaction.[4]

### *Juvenile Polyps, Adenoma, and Cancer*

Numerous reports have documented adenomatous changes in juvenile polyps.[2, 3, 5–13] Juvenile polyps are not neoplastic per se, but focal adenomatous areas[2, 5–9] and epithelial dysplasia[14] in these polyps may confer a risk of carcinoma, even in children.[6–9] Most if not all colorectal carcinomas arise from pre-existing adenomas of the colon.[11] In one study, a significant increase in ornithine decarboxylase and tyrosine kinase enzyme activity (markers for rapid cell proliferation) was noted in juvenile polyps, suggesting a higher level of cellular proliferation, but there was a normal DNA aneuploidy score and no expression of p53 gene (indicative of late malignant changes).[15] Relatives of patients with juvenile polyposis syndrome are at risk of developing cancer.[6, 10] In addition, in patients with juvenile polyposis, adenomatous epithelium can be found within the juvenile polyps or arising separately from nonpolypoid mucosa.[16] Patients with juvenile polyposis syndromes carry a more significant risk of colon carcinoma than is generally appreciated.[17] Because of these facts, it has been suggested that juvenile polyposis (in contradistinction to isolated juvenile polyps) should be considered as seriously as the familial adenomatous polyposis syndromes, except that regular colonoscopic surveillance may obviate prophylactic colectomy.[13, 14] Even though the degree of association between juvenile polyps and gastrointestinal carcinoma is probably low, this pathogenetic sequence needs to be studied more carefully. A large family was reported who had a tendency to develop colonic polyps of three mixed histologic types—juvenile, adenomatous, and hyperplastic.[18] The characteristic lesion, however, was the atypical juvenile polyp with mixed juvenile and adenomatous histopathology. Some affected persons developed polyps of more than one type. Typically, fewer than 15 polyps were found at colonoscopy, and no extracolonic disease was associated with the development of polyps. Analysis of the family pedigree supported autosomal dominant inheritance, and genetic linkage studies did not reveal candidate gene loci (e.g., adenomatous polyposis coli [APC]) important in colorectal tumorigenesis. Despite lack of a gene locus, adenocarcinoma occurred at a young age in members of this family, indicating a predisposition to malignancy. The authors proposed a new polyposis disorder they have named *hereditary mixed polyposis syndrome* (HMPS). Because histopathologic classification is not perfect, others have suggested that HMPS could be a variant of juvenile polyposis syndrome.[19]

## Diagnosis and Management

Specific guidelines for the management of children with juvenile polyps are difficult to establish, because the natural

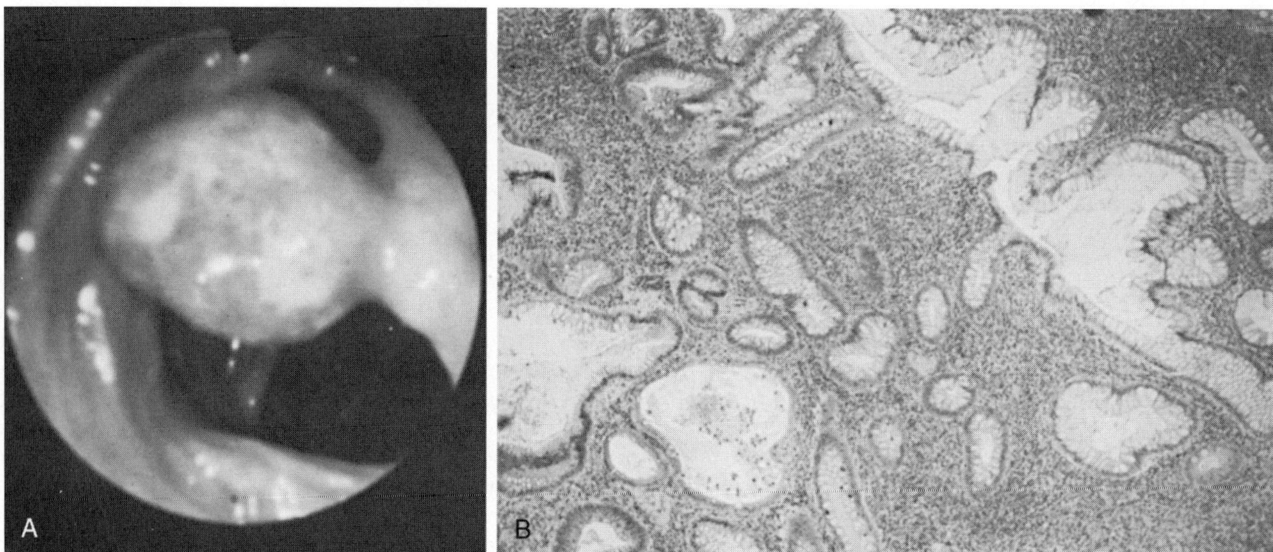


**FIGURE 35–1.** Juvenile polyp. *A,* Large pedunculated polyp in distal colon as seen through the colonoscope. (Courtesy of William R. Treem, MD.) *B,* This low-power (× 63) photomicrograph of a juvenile polyp demonstrates the typical cystic, mucus-filled glands and prominent lamina propria with inflammatory cells.

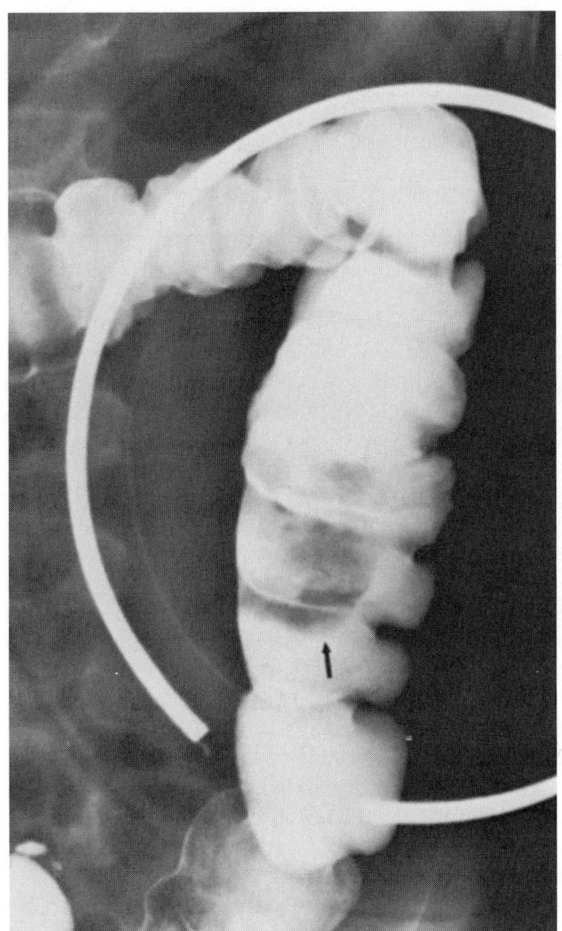

**FIGURE 35–2.** This barium enema spot film of the distal colon demonstrates a large juvenile polyp *(arrow)*.

history of this common problem is not clearly understood. Unfortunately, there is a paucity of literature to support the general belief that most juvenile polyps outgrow their vascular supply, become necrotic, and subsequently autoamputate. However, because of significant anemia and the possibility that adenomatous polyps may be more common in children than was previously believed, the diagnosis by colonoscopy and removal of all juvenile polyps may be warranted. After conscious sedation, colonoscopy and polypectomy can be safely accomplished with snare electrocauterization[2]; general anesthesia is rarely required. After the removal of mixed juvenile adenomatous polyps, children should be carefully monitored. Although the appropriate frequency of endoscopic evaluation is not known in such instances, surveillance colonoscopy is suggested at least every 2 years, or earlier if rectal bleeding recurs. For the newly referred child, a colonoscopy to the cecum is prudent when polyps are noted by barium contrast study (Fig. 35–2) or suspected because of prolapse of a rectal mass, and in the presence of unexplained rectal bleeding.[2] After removal of an isolated juvenile polyp, a child does not require any further evaluation unless there is a recurrence of rectal bleeding. Compared with an age- and sex-matched group of the general population, patients with a solitary juvenile polyp are not at increased risk of developing colon cancer.[20]

## INHERITED HAMARTOMATOUS POLYPOSIS SYNDROMES

There are familial syndromes that are characterized by hamartomatous polyps of the gastrointestinal tract. These include juvenile polyposis, Peutz-Jeghers syndrome, and Cowden's syndrome (Table 35–2).

### Juvenile Polyposes

This group of rare familial syndromes includes juvenile polyposis, juvenile polyposis of infancy, and generalized gastrointestinal polyposis.[21, 22]

The commonest of these polyposis syndromes is juvenile polyposis, which is usually diagnosed in the first decade of life in children with multiple colonic polyps.[21, 22] An autosomal-dominant gene is suspected but not proved, as approximately 50% of affected persons have a positive family history. The diagnosis of juvenile polyposis is likely when five or more juvenile polyps are discovered in the colorectum or throughout the gastrointestinal tract, *or* with the presence of any number of juvenile polyps plus a family history of juvenile polyposis.[14, 23] Associated anomalies include hypertelorism, intestinal malrotation, hydrocephalus, undescended testis, and Meckel's diverticulum.[21] Similar findings characterize juvenile polyposis of infancy, in addition to involvement of the stomach and the small intestine. Bloody or mucoid diarrhea usually occurs in the first few weeks of life. Rectal prolapse and intussusception may develop, the latter leading to death in a few instances.[24] In these children, diarrhea and intestinal protein losses lead to severe malnutrition and failure to thrive. There is some evidence that this form of juvenile polyposis represents autosomal-recessive inheritance.[25] In generalized juvenile polyposis, there are multiple polyps throughout the gastrointestinal tract,[26] but sometimes they are confined exclusively to the stomach.[27]

### Peutz-Jeghers Syndrome

#### *Clinical Characteristics*

Peutz[28] first noted the association of mucocutaneous pigmentation with intestinal polyposis in three generations of a Dutch family. Twenty-eight years later, Jeghers and associates[29] reported 10 similar cases, and Peutz-Jeghers syndrome became widely recognized. By 1969, it was described in 321 patients of wide ethnic and geographic distribution.[30] A mendelian dominant mode of inheritance was first suggested by Jeghers and associates.[29] In one study of five generations of a family, only three persons were free of abnormal pigmentation or polyps.[31] However, only 50% of people with Peutz-Jeghers syndrome report a family history. This probably represents an incomplete diagnosis of the disorder in relatives. Moreover, it is estimated that fewer than 5% of people with polyposis do not have hyperpigmentation, and fewer than 5% have hyperpigmentation without gastrointestinal polyps.[23] These variations suggest an autosomal-dominant gene with high penetrance and variable expression.[30]

The abnormal pigmentation (Fig. 35–3) consists of brown-black macules, 1 to 5 mm in diameter, which look like

**TABLE 35–2. Inherited Hamartomatous Polyposis Syndromes: Clinical Characteristics**

| SYNDROME | LOCATION OF POLYPS | EXTRAINTESTINAL ABNORMALITIES | RISK OF CANCER |
|---|---|---|---|
| Juvenile polyposis | Mainly colon; also small intestine | — | Colon—small |
| Peutz-Jeghers syndrome | Small intestine; also colon and stomach | Pigmented spots of lips, mouth, and hands | Gastrointestinal cancer and ovarian tumors |
| Cowden's syndrome | Colon and stomach | Lipomas, papillomas, multiple other hamartomas | Breast and thyroid cancer |

freckles and vary in number and distribution. They usually appear during infancy or early childhood and commonly involve the lips and oral mucosa; they may also be found on the hands, feet, digits, tongue, eyelids, or perineum.[32, 33] Although the hyperpigmentation on the lips is the most reliable finding, these, like cutaneous lesions, tend to fade over time. In addition, lip pigmentation is not uncommon in persons without Peutz-Jeghers syndrome. Unlike the skin pigmentation, mucosal lesions like those involving the gingiva persist and are thus more helpful for diagnosis.[23]

Multiple polyps are found in more than 90% of cases,[33] especially in older persons, although solitary polyps have been described. They vary in number and distribution, sometimes involving the entire gastrointestinal tract. The tumors are frequently present in the small bowel, particularly in the jejunum. In decreasing order of frequency, they can be found in the colon, stomach, duodenum, and appendix.[33] Rarely, polyps occur in the nasopharynx and the urinary bladder.[28]

## *Pathology*

The polyps in patients with Peutz-Jeghers syndrome are sessile or pedunculated, varying in size from 1 to 3 cm. Histologically (Fig. 35–4), the polyps are hamartomatous and consist of a glandular epithelium with prominent branching bands of smooth muscle within the lamina propria.[4] Unlike juvenile polyps, the lamina propria of Peutz-Jeghers syndrome polyps appears normal.

## *Diagnosis and Management*

Approximately one third of persons with Peutz-Jeghers syndrome are diagnosed during childhood or adolescence.[33] The commonest presenting complaint is abdominal pain, which has been reported to occur in as many as 87% of pediatric patients.[32] Symptoms usually appear during adolescence, although they have been reported in young children[34] and infants.[35] The abdominal pain is commonly colicky, intermittent, and related to recurrent intussusception, which rarely causes complete obstruction and usually reduces spontaneously.[36] Microcytic, hypochromic anemia secondary to chronic gastrointestinal blood loss is encountered. However, in contrast with children with juvenile polyposis, anemia is a far more common finding.[33]

The potential of polyps in Peutz-Jeghers syndrome to undergo malignant transformation has been much debated. Earlier literature probably overestimated malignant transformation because of the unusual histologic findings, especially the admixture of glandular tissue with smooth muscle elements interpreted as tumor invasion. As the hamartomatous nature of these tumors was recognized, the cancerous potential was considered negligible.[37] Although this is now generally accepted, hamartomatous polyps in patients with Peutz-Jeghers syndrome have been discovered to contain areas of adenoma and carcinoma.[38] In addition, gastrointestinal cancer has been reported in patients with Peutz-Jeghers syndrome, usually in those with stomach or duodenal involvement.[30] Small intestinal and colonic adenocarcinoma have also been noted.[39] Moreover, breast cancer,[40, 41] ovarian and cervical tumors,[42] sex cord tumors,[43, 44] and Sertoli cell tumors[45] have been described. In one series, malignancy developed in 15 patients with Peutz-Jeghers syndrome (gastrointestinal carcinoma, four; nongastrointestinal, 10; and multiple myeloma, one). With the use of relative risk analysis, it was concluded that persons with Peutz-Jeghers syndrome have a risk that is 18 times greater for cancer than that in the general population.[40] Thus, although the risk is considerably less than is seen with other inherited polyposis syndromes, the risk of malignancy is substantial in Peutz-Jeghers syndrome.[40, 46]

When the diagnosis of Peutz-Jeghers syndrome is considered based on family history and clinical findings, the gastro-

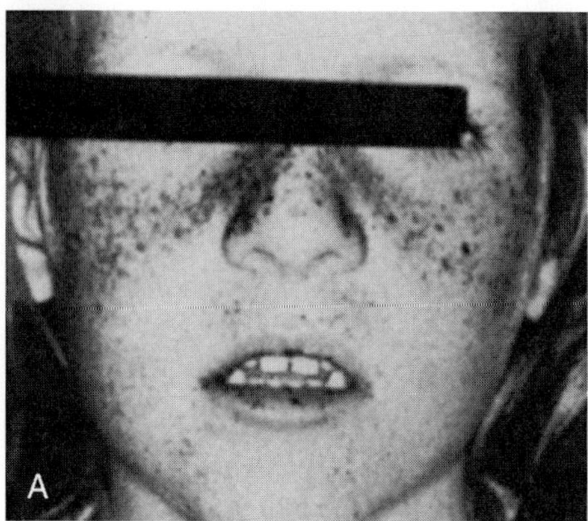


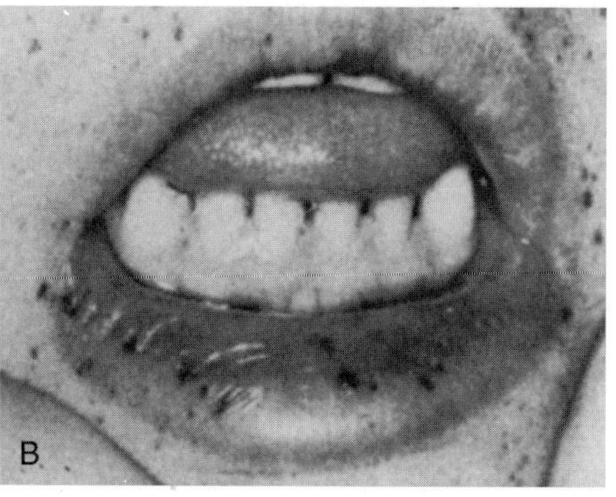


**FIGURE 35–3.** Mucocutaneous pigmentation in Peutz-Jeghers syndrome. *A,* Brown-black macules are distributed over the face and lips of a 5-year-old patient. *B,* The pigmented lesions are seen involving the lips and crossing the vermilion border. (From Yosowitz P, Hobson R, Ruymann F. Am J Dis Child 1974;128:709–712, with permission. Copyright 1974, American Medical Association.)

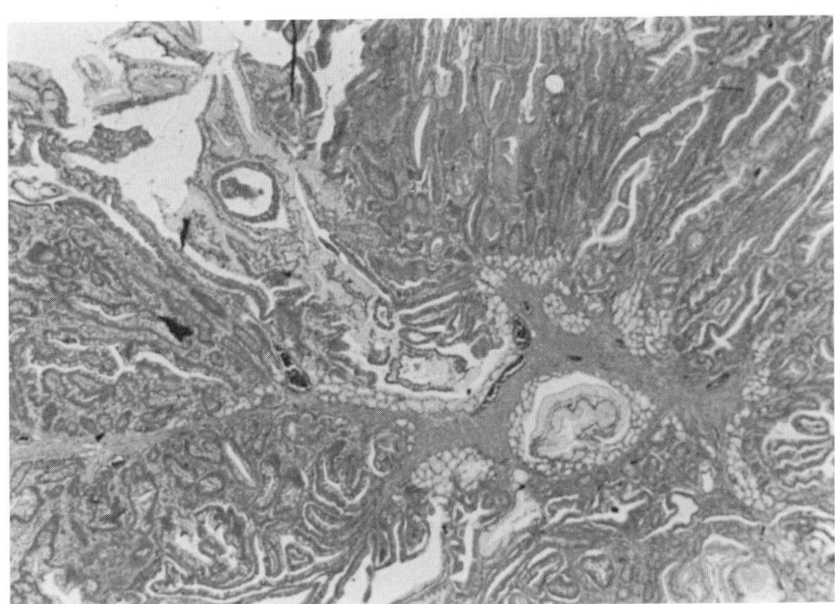

**FIGURE 35–4.** Peutz-Jeghers syndrome. Low-power photomicrograph (× 25) of Peutz-Jeghers polyp demonstrates the typical branching bands of smooth muscle surrounded by glandular epithelium.

intestinal tract must be thoroughly investigated. Upper gastrointestinal contrast studies may identify larger polyps in the stomach, the duodenum, and the small intestine (Fig. 35–5). Similarly, air-contrast barium enema or flexible colonoscopy delineates polyps in the large bowel. Conservative management is advocated in the treatment of patients with Peutz-Jeghers syndrome.[23, 30] Bed rest, mild sedation, and nasogastric suction usually suffice during an episode of intussusception. If bowel obstruction is suspected, surgical intervention should not be delayed. Because the subsequent development of polyps may require further surgical procedures, as many polyps as possible should be removed. Surgery should be considered also in patients with significant gastrointestinal bleeding or with frequent episodes of abdominal pain. Because of the apparent higher risk for malignant transformation, surgical or endoscopic removal of gastric (especially fundus) and duodenal polyps is recommended.[30, 34] Moreover, female patients should have regular pelvic examinations.

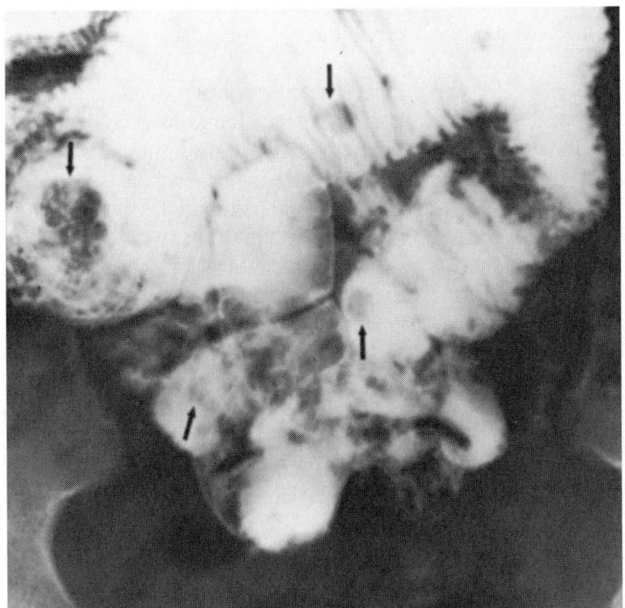

**FIGURE 35–5.** This barium contrast study demonstrates the presence of several polyps in the small intestine *(arrows)* of a child with Peutz-Jeghers syndrome.

## Cowden's Syndrome

Cowden's syndrome is characterized by multiple hamartomatous lesions of ectodermal, mesodermal, and endodermal origin. The mucocutaneous lesions are the most characteristic extraintestinal feature of this syndrome and include hyperkeratotic papillomas of the lips, tongue, and nares.[47] This polyposis syndrome with orocutaneous hamartomas is considered an autosomal-dominant disorder that usually presents in the second or third decade of life.[48] Polyps occur throughout the gastrointestinal tract but are commonest in the colon and stomach.[48] All colonic polyps have been characterized as hamartomatous.[49] The frequency of gastrointestinal cancer is apparently not increased in patients with this disorder. There is a high incidence of breast involvement in women; most of the lesions are fibrocystic or fibroadenomatous, but ductal carcinomas have been reported.[50] Thyroid disease is present in many patients, usually in the form of nodular hyperplasia or follicular adenoma of the thyroid.[50] The gene for Cowden's syndrome has been localized to chromosome 10.[51]

## INHERITED ADENOMATOUS POLYPOSIS SYNDROMES

The inherited adenomatous polyposis syndromes include familial polyposis coli, Gardner's syndrome, and Turcot's syndrome (see Table 35–1). All have an autosomal-dominant inheritance pattern, except for Turcot's syndrome, and are characterized by the development of hundreds of gastrointestinal polypoid lesions that invariably undergo malignant transformation. The syndromes are distinguished by the location of the polyps and the presence of extraintestinal abnormalities.

## Familial Polyposis Coli

Familial polyposis coli is an autosomal-dominant disease that occurs in approximately 1 in 10,000 live births. *Polyposis coli* is a misnomer, because polyps have been discovered in the stomach and the small intestine.[52]

### *Clinical Characteristics*

The adenomatous polyps usually appear in the second or third decade of life. Younger patients initially have a small number of polyps, but familial polyposis coli is characterized by the gradual development of thousands of sessile colonic polyps throughout its length (Table 35–3). As in Gardner's syndrome, colorectal cancer should be considered inevitable in the natural history of familial polyposis coli. Malignant change occurs in polyps but also can develop in surrounding mucosa that may appear normal to the endoscopist.[53]

The adenomatous polyposis syndromes cannot always be categorized exclusively as either familial polyposis coli or Gardner's syndrome. When carefully sought, even extraintestinal manifestations, such as mandibular osteomas and upper gastrointestinal polyps, can be seen in most patients with familial polyposis coli.[54] Adenomatous polyps may be found in the ileum, duodenum, periampullary region, papilla of Vater, and antrum.[55, 56, 57] Thus, it has become difficult to argue that familial polyposis coli and Gardner's syndrome are not varied expressions of a single disease entity.

### *Pathology*

In familial polyposis coli, the polyps are small, usually less than 5 mm in diameter (Fig. 35–6A), and histologically identical to the polyps of Gardner's syndrome. Their surface is often divided into "lobules" by interconnecting clefts in the apex of the polyp. The glands are lined by elongated epithelial cells with hyperchromatic nuclei, and mucin content is generally diminished (Fig. 35–6B). Numerous mitotic figures are commonly noted.

## Genetics and Cancer

Recently, alteration of gene structure and expression has been noted in familial polyposis coli and Gardner's syndrome. Specifically, there is a mutation in the APC (adenomatous polyposis coli) gene on chromosome 5 that inactivates the gene and leads to inhibition of apoptosis and proliferation of epithelial cells.[58, 59] Allelic deletions and mutations may occur on several chromosomes, implicating mutational activation of an oncogene and loss of tumor suppressor genes in the development of colon cancer.[60, 61] In general, findings suggest that an inherited susceptibility to colonic adenomas and colorectal cancer is responsible for the adenoma-dysplasia-carcinoma sequence.[62]

### *Diagnosis and Management of Adenomatous Polyposis*

New clinical guidelines were reported recently for the identification and monitoring of adults and children at risk for malignancy.[63] Many authors believe that surveillance of patients with asymptomatic familial polyposis should begin during adolescence.[64] However, other authors advocate a more aggressive approach and recommend an evaluation of the gastrointestinal tract by the end of the first decade of life.[65] This recommendation is based on the fact that malignant changes in patients with multiple colonic polyposis have been reported before age 9 years. Moreover, the incidence of colon cancer in children with adenomatous polyposis younger than 13 years of age was reported to be 6.5%.[66] In a large review of 75 patients, four children (5.3%) were documented to have carcinomatous changes at the time of initial evaluation.[67] In general, flexible sigmoidoscopy should be considered in all individuals at risk, beginning at 12 years of age and every year until age 40 years, at which time the frequency of surveillance may be decreased to every 3 years.[63] Diagnosis of familial polyposis coli is based on the presence of more than 100 adenomatous polyps in the colon. Surgery is generally required for polyps larger than 5 mm in diameter, because the risk of advanced cancer is higher for polyps of that size than for smaller ones.[68] When there are six to nine polyps per square centimeter, the malignant potential of familial adenomatous polyposis is highly significant. Children in this category should be operated on before age 15 years; otherwise, the timing of colectomy is controversial, and no markers are available to predict malignant transformation of adenomas. All family members should be carefully examined. Research advances, such as the protein truncation assay to identify the APC mutation,[69] will eventually be used clinically to identify children at risk for colon cancer. Physicians who order genetic tests must be prepared, however, to offer their patients genetic counseling.[70]

Colonoscopy is completed early in the evaluation, because it allows for identification of these small sessile lesions,

**TABLE 35–3. Inherited Adenomatous Polyposis Syndromes: Clinical Characteristics**

| SYNDROME | LOCATION OF POLYPS | EXTRAINTESTINAL ABNORMALITIES | RISK OF CANCER |
|---|---|---|---|
| Familial polyposis coli | Colon; also ileum, duodenum, ampulla, and gastric antrum | Osteomas of mandible | Colon, small intestine—marked |
| Gardner's syndrome | Colon; small intestine, ampulla, and stomach | Osteomas of mandible, skull, and long bones; lipomas; fibromas; desmoid tumors | Colon, small intestine—marked |
| Turcot's syndrome | Colon | Brain tumors | Colon—marked; medulloblastoma, glioma |

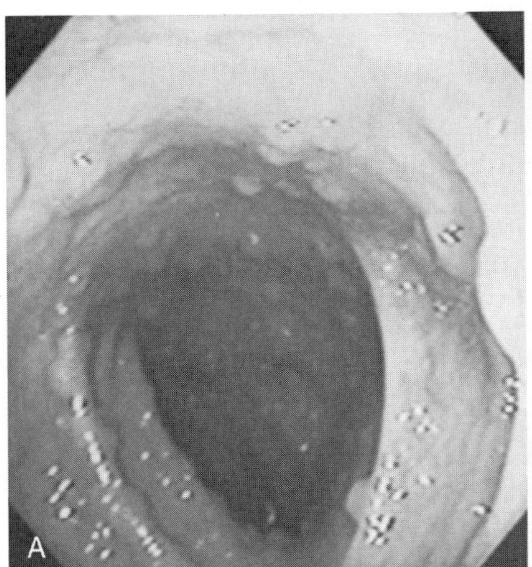


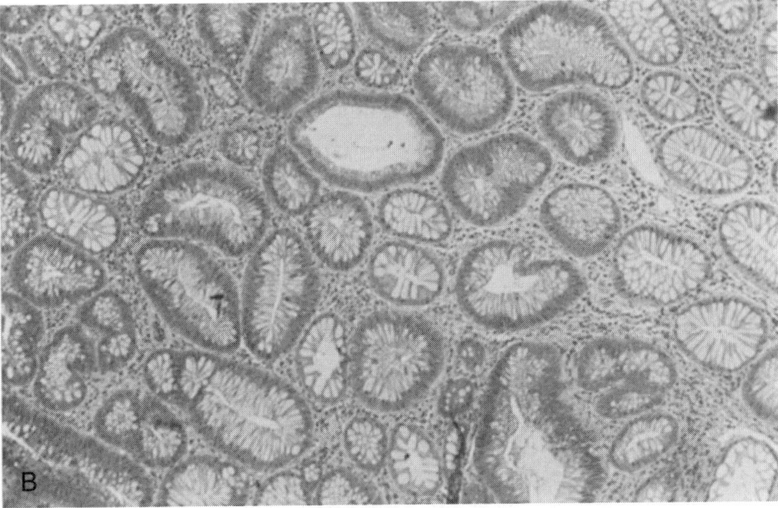


**FIGURE 35–6.** Familial polyposis coli. *A,* Multiple, small, sessile polyps noted at the time of colonoscopy. *B,* This photomicrograph (× 100) of a polyp demonstrates the tightly packed, proliferating adenomatous epithelium with hyperchromatic nuclei and mucin depletion. The small amount of lamina propria is free of inflammation.

which may be overlooked on barium studies, and provides tissue acquisition for histologic review. Children with documented adenomatous polyposis should be examined at least annually. Patients who manifest the polyposis gene require total colectomy; this usually occurs in late adolescence or young adulthood.

The ileal pouch–anal anastomosis is considered superior to the ileoanal or ileorectal anastomosis, although some surgeons believe the latter two procedures are satisfactory for children.[71] Ideally, the procedure should eliminate the need for ileostomy and ensure intestinal continuity and continence. Ileoanal anastomosis is preferable to the ileorectal anastomosis procedure, because the risk for future carcinoma is eliminated and there is no need for regular sigmoidoscopic reexaminations. The advantages of the ileorectal procedure include a better chance for anorectal continence and a shorter convalescence after major surgery. Some investigators advocate ileorectal anastomosis when no adenomatous polyps are discovered in the rectum.

Finally, because of the possibility of carcinoma of the ampulla of Vater, duodenum, and antrum in patients with familial adenomatous polyposis, it is imperative to conduct regular surveillance of the upper gastrointestinal tract in all of these patients, even after surgical extirpation of the large intestine.[72]

## Gardner's Syndrome

### *Clinical Characteristics*

Gardner's syndrome is characterized by the triad of gastrointestinal polyps, osteomas, and soft tissue tumors. The polyps are numerous (usually more than 1,000) and at times appear to carpet the intestinal mucosa. They are almost exclusively small (2 to 5 mm) and sessile, although occasional pedunculated lesions are encountered. The polyps were initially reported to involve only the colon; however, studies have demonstrated that they often occur in the stomach, the duodenum, and, less commonly, other parts of the small intestine.[73, 74] The upper gastrointestinal polyps are usually asymptomatic until they are large, when bleeding and bowel obstruction can become manifest. Histologically, adenomas are typically found in the gastric antrum and the duodenum, especially in the periampullary region. Jejunal and ileal polyps are, histologically, adenomas or focal lymphoid hyperplasia. In general the risk of malignant transformation of gastric and small intestinal polyps is negligible; however, duodenal tumors have a high proclivity for malignancy.[64]

Bony abnormalities include osteomas, which do not develop until the second decade of life, and thickening of the long bones. The osteomas most commonly involve the skull, including the calvaria, the maxilla, and the mandible. The soft tissue lesions are usually epidermoid cysts, which are often misdiagnosed as sebaceous cysts. They are usually found on the head, neck, and trunk. Subcutaneous fibromas, which commonly involve the scalp, shoulders, arms, and back, and desmoid tumors are sometimes noted. The desmoid tumors, also referred to as *diffuse mesenteric fibromatosis,* are a particularly serious complication, because they occur intra-abdominally and lead to intestinal, vascular, and ureteral obstruction.[75]

Other extraintestinal malformations of Gardner's syndrome include dental abnormalities, such as odontomas, dentiginous cysts, and supernumerary teeth. These lesions are usually detected by panoramic radiography of the teeth and mandible. Hyperpigmentation of the retinal epithelium was reported in patients with Gardner's syndrome.[76] The retinal pigmentation is a specific and sensitive early clinical marker for Gardner's syndrome and familial polyposis coli in persons at risk for these diseases.[76, 77] This syndrome has also been associated with carcinoma of the pancreas and the ampulla of Vater,[78] in addition to hepatoblastoma.[79]

### *Diagnosis*

Many patients initially seek medical attention because of known affected relatives. However, when the syndrome is not suspected, rectal bleeding, diarrhea, and abdominal pain are frequent presenting complaints; mucoid rectal discharge occurs less frequently. Interestingly, and in contrast with the familial hamartomatous polyposis syndromes, intussusception is rarely a problem in Gardner's syndrome.[80] Constitutional symptoms and signs, such as anorexia, weight loss, and weakness, may be the presenting manifestations of occult malignancy. Although colonic polyps generally appear during the first two decades of life, they have been documented from 8 months to 72 years of age.[65] Polyps usually do not produce symptoms until 10 years after their appearance, a fact that underscores the importance of identifying people at risk. The significance of adenomatous polyposis syndromes, including Gardner's syndrome, relates to the inevitable malignant transformation, which usually is not detected until 10 years after polyps are identified and approaches 100% by age 55 years in untreated cases.[64]

### Turcot's Syndrome

Turcot's syndrome represents the association of familial adenomatous polyposis and neural tumors. The initial report described two cases of familial polyposis in siblings who both developed cerebral tumors—a medulloblastoma and a glioblastoma.[81] This syndrome is a rare autosomal recessive disorder;[82] the diagnosis should be restricted to patients with familial polyposis associated with medulloblastomas or gliomas.[83] It is an example of a pluripotential gene mutation that also predisposes to neural malignancy.[83] Patients with Turcot's syndrome are frequently adolescents, and they present with symptoms attributable to either intestinal or neural tumors. In general, colon cancer may occur at an earlier age in this syndrome.[84] Already described in patients with the other familial adenomatous polyposis syndromes, hypertrophy of the retinal pigment epithelium was reported in a young patient with Turcot's syndrome.[85]

## NONINHERITED POLYPOSIS DISORDERS

### Lymphoid Polyposis

#### Clinical Characteristics

Nodular lymphoid hyperplasia, or aggregates of lymphoid follicles, gives rise to submucosal nodules in the intestines of children (Table 35–4). These lymphoid polyps are small (1- to 5-mm), sessile, umbilicated protrusions that typically are noted in the distal colon, although they may be seen throughout the intestinal tract. They probably represent a response of intestinal lymphoid tissue to chemical, infectious, or traumatic stimulation.[86] An association has been described with dysgammaglobulinemia,[87] especially when the lymphoid polyps are limited to the small intestine. It has also been noted in Hirschsprung's disease complicated by enterocolitis[88] and in children with inflammatory bowel disease.[89]

Lymphoid hyperplasia is generally considered a benign, self-limited entity, probably representing a normal response of lymphoid tissue in children. Although controversial, it may be a source of rectal bleeding when the lymphoid polyps are friable and associated with overlying ulcers.[90]

#### Diagnosis and Management

The radiologic and endoscopic appearance of nodular lymphoid hyperplasia may be confused with those of the familial polyposis syndromes. The lymphoid polyps are distinguished from adenomatous polyps by their central umbilication. Histologically, nodular lymphoid hyperplasia consists of lymphoid follicles with enlarged germinal centers composed of mature lymphocytes. Lymphoid polyps involving the terminal ileum have been reported in association with familial polyposis coli and Gardner's syndrome, and they may lead to confusion with the diagnosis of Crohn's disease of the ileum. Symptoms associated with lymphoid polyps usually regress spontaneously, unless the polyps are a lead point for intussusception.

### Inflammatory Polyposis

Inflammatory polyps, or pseudopolyps, are noted in all forms of severe colitis, especially during the regenerative and healing phase of inflammation. They are small, usually less than 1 cm in diameter, although they may be large, irregular, and solitary, mimicking a malignant mass. Inflammatory polyps should always be differentiated from colon carcinoma, especially in patients who have had inflammatory bowel disease for more than 10 years.[91] The estimated cumulative incidence of colon carcinoma in patients with ulcerative colitis is approximately 5% at 20 years and 12% at 25 years. Only recently has the magnitude of risk been appreciated for Crohn's colitis. It is now believed that for similar duration and extent of colon disease, the increased incidence of colon cancer is equivalent for both ulcerative and Crohn's colitis.[63] Surveillance colonoscopy

**TABLE 35–4. Noninherited Polyposis: Clinical Characteristics**

| DISORDERS | LOCATION AND TYPE OF POLYPS | EXTRAINTESTINAL ABNORMALITIES | RISK OF CANCER |
|---|---|---|---|
| Nodular lymphoid polyposis | Colon: lymphoid hyperplasia | — | — |
| Inflammatory polyposis | Colon: pseudopolyps | — | Colon (e.g., with ulcerative colitis or Crohn's colitis) |
| Cronkhite-Canada syndrome | Colon, small intestine: hamartomas | Skin hyperpigmentation, alopecia, dystrophic nails | Gastrointestinal cancer—small |
| Ruvalcaba-Myhre-Smith syndrome | Colon: hamartomas | Pigmentation of glans penis, mental retardation, macrocephaly | — |

should begin in patients with pancolitis after 8 years of symptoms and in patients with left-sided colitis after 15 years of symptoms. Repeat surveillance colon examinations should be performed every 1 to 2 years. If unequivocal dysplasia is found, colectomy is indicated. Colectomy should also be considered for patients who do not comply with surveillance and for adolescents with a long history of inflammatory disease.[63] Histologically, inflammatory cells and granulation tissue are noted first; later, the polyp may consist of normal mucosa. Other diseases that can give rise to inflammatory polyps include amebiasis[92] and chronic bacterial infections.

## Cronkhite-Canada Syndrome

Juvenile polyps occur throughout the gastrointestinal tract in the Cronkhite-Canada syndrome. This noninherited syndrome is rare in children; extraintestinal signs include alopecia, onychodystrophy, and brown macular lesions of the skin.[93] Severe malabsorption is present in most adult patients, and the prognosis is poor because of complications of protein-losing enteropathy and malnutrition.[93] A child with infantile Cronkhite-Canada syndrome was reported who, after removal of multiple polyps, died following surgery for intussusception.[94]

Adenomatous epithelium has been reported in the hamartomatous polyps of patients with Cronkhite-Canada syndrome, which may confer a risk of malignant transformation. Gastrointestinal carcinomas have occurred in 5% of these patients.[95]

## Ruvalcaba-Myhre-Smith Syndrome

The Ruvalcaba-Myhre-Smith syndrome is a rare entity characterized by macrocephaly, pigmented penile lesions, and intestinal polyps.[96] Additional associated features include café au lait spots; ocular abnormalities, for example, posterior embryotoxon; subcutaneous lipomas; psychomotor retardation; and a unique lipid storage disease.[97–99] The intestinal polyps primarily involve the colon, although they are also found in the terminal ileum. Upper gastrointestinal polyps have not been reported. These polyps occur during childhood, initially manifested by rectal bleeding and abdominal pain related to intussusception. Recurrent intussusception, just as in Peutz-Jeghers syndrome, has necessitated subtotal colectomy in some patients.[99] Histologically, the polyps are hamartomatous; malignant transformation has not been observed.[98]

## REFERENCES


1. Mestre JR: The changing pattern of juvenile polyps. Am J Gastroenterol 1986;81:312–314.
2. Cynamon HA, Milov DE, Andres JM: Diagnosis and management of colonic polyps in children. J Pediatr 1989;114:593–596.
3. Van Driel MF, Zwiers W, Grond J, et al: Juvenile polyps at the site of a ureterosigmoidostomy: report of five cases. Dis Colon Rectum 1988;31:553–557.
4. Cooper HS: Intestinal neoplasms. In Sternberg SS (ed): Diagnostic Surgical Pathology. New York, Raven Press, 1989, pp 1017–1026.
5. Friedman CJ, Fechner RE: A solitary juvenile polyp with hyperplastic and adenomatous glands. Dig Dis Sci 1982;27:946–948.
6. Stemper TC, Kent TH, Summers RW: Juvenile polyposis and gastrointestinal carcinoma: a study of a kindred. Ann Intern Med 1975;83:639–646.
7. Beacham CH, Shields HM, Raffensperger EC, et al: Juvenile and adenomatous gastrointestinal polyposis. Am J Dig Dis 1978;23:1137–1143.
8. Goodman ZD, Yardley JH, Milligan FD: Pathogenesis of colonic polyps in multiple juvenile polyposis. Cancer 1979;43:1906–1913.
9. O'Riordain DS, O'Dwyer PJ, Cullen AF, et al: Familial juvenile polyposis coli and colorectal cancer. Cancer 1991;68:889–892.
10. Rosen P, Baratz M: Familial juvenile colonic polyposis with associated colon cancer. Cancer 1982;49:1500–1503.
11. Morson BD: Genesis of colorectal cancer. Clin Gastroenterol 1976;5:505–525.
12. Baptist SJ, Sabatini MT: Coexisting juvenile polyps and tubulovillous adenoma of colon with carcinoma in situ: report of a case. Hum Pathol 1985;16:1161–1163.
13. Longo WE, Touloukian RJ, West AB, et al: Malignant potential of juvenile polyposis coli. Dis Colon Rectum 1990;33:980–984.
14. Jass JR, Williams CB, Bussey HJ, et al: Juvenile polyposis: a precancerous condition. Histopathology 1988;13:619–630.
15. Elitsur Y, Koh SJ, Moshier JA, et al: Ornithine decarboxylase and tyrosine kinase activity in juvenile polyps of childhood. Pediatr Res 1995;38:574–578.
16. Giardiello FM, Hamilton SR, Kem SE, et al: Colorectal neoplasia in patients with juvenile polyposis or juvenile polyps. Arch Dis Child 1991;66:971–975.
17. Coburn MC, Pricolo VE, DeLuca FG, et al: Malignant potential in intestinal juvenile polyposis syndromes. Ann Surg Oncol 1995;2:386–391.
18. Whitelaw SC, Murday YA, Tombinson IPM, et al: Clinical and molecular features of the hereditary mixed polyposis syndrome. Gastroenterology 1997;112:327–334.
19. Giardiello FM, Hamilton SR: Hereditary mixed polyposis syndrome: a zebra or a horse dressed in pinstripes? Gastroenterology 1997;112:643–645.
20. Nugent KP, Talbot IC, Hodgson SV, et al: Solitary juvenile polyps: not a marker for subsequent malignancy. Gastroenterology 1993;105:698–700.
21. Gathright, JB, Cofer TW: Familial incidence of juvenile polyposis coli. Surg Gynecol Obstet 1974;138:185–188.
22. Grotsky HW, Rickert RK, Smith WD, et al: Familial juvenile polyposis coli: a clinical and pathologic study of a large kindred. Gastroenterology 1982;82:494–501.
23. Erbe RW: Current concepts in genetics: inherited gastrointestinal-polyposis syndromes. N Engl J Med 1976;294:1101–1104.
24. LeLuyer B, LeBihan M, Metayer P, et al: Generalized juvenile polyposis in an infant: report of a case and successful management by endoscopy. J Pediatr Gastroenterol Nutr 1985;4:128–134.
25. Sachatello CR, Hahn IS, Carrington CB: Juvenile gastrointestinal polyposis in a female infant: report of a case and review of the literature of recently recognized syndrome. Surgery 1974;75:107–114.
26. Sachatello CR, Pickren JW, Grace JT: Generalized juvenile gastrointestinal polyposis. Gastroenterology 1970;58:699–708.
27. Watanabe A, Nagashima H, Motoi M, et al: Familial juvenile polyposis of the stomach. Gastroenterology 1979;77:148–151.
28. Peutz JLA. On a very remarkable case of familial polyposis of the mucous membranes, of the intestinal tract and nasopharynx accompanied by peculiar pigmentations of the skin and mucous membrane. Ned Tijdschr Geneeskd 1921;10:134–146.
29. Jeghers H, McKusick VA, Katz KH: Generalized intestinal polyposis and melanin spots of the oral mucosa, lip and digits: a syndrome of diagnostic significance. N Engl J Med 1949;241:1031–1036.
30. Dozois RR, Judd ES, Dahlin DC, et al: The Peutz-Jeghers syndrome: is there a predisposition to development of intestinal cancer? Arch Surg 1969;98:509–517.
31. McAllister AJ, Richards KF: Peutz-Jeghers syndrome: experience with 20 patients in 5 generations. 1977;134:717–720.
32. Wenzl JE, Bartholomew LG, Hallenbeck GA, et al: Gastrointestinal polyposis with mucocutaneous pigmentation in children (Peutz-Jeghers syndrome). Pediatrics 1961;28:655–661.
33. Bartholomew LG, Dahlin DC, Waugh JM: Intestinal polyposis associated with mucocutaneous melanin pigmentation (Peutz-Jeghers syndrome). Gastroenterology 1957;32:434–451.

34. Yosowitz P, Hobson R, Ruyman F: Sporadic Peutz-Jeghers syndrome in early childhood. Am J Dis Child 1974;128:709–712.
35. Morens DM, Garvey SP: An unusual case of Peutz-Jeghers syndrome in an infant. Am J Dis Child 1975;129:973–976.
36. MGH Case Records (Case 24–1975). N Engl J Med 1975;292:1340–1345.
37. Bussey HJR, Veale AMO, Morson BC: Genetics of gastrointestinal polyposis. Gastroenterology 1978;74:1325–1330.
38. Miller LJ, Bartholomew LG, Dozois RR, et al: Adenocarcinoma of the rectum arising in a hamartomatous polyp in a patient with Peutz-Jeghers syndrome. Dig Dis Sci 1983;28:1047–1051.
39. Dodds WJ, Schulte WJ, Hensley GT, et al: Peutz-Jeghers syndrome and gastrointestinal malignancy. Am J Roentgenol 1972;115:374–377.
40. Giardiello FM, Welsh SB, Hamilton SR, et al: Increased risk of cancer in the Peutz-Jeghers syndrome. N Engl J Med 1987;316:1511–1514.
41. Trau H, Schewach-Millet M, Fisher BK, et al: Peutz-Jeghers syndrome and bilateral breast carcinoma. Cancer 1982;50:788–792.
42. Dozois RR, Kempers RD, Dahlin DC, et al: Ovarian tumors associated with the Peutz-Jeghers syndrome. Ann Surg 1970;172:233–238.
43. Dubois RS, Hoffman WH, Krishnan TH, et al: Feminizing sex cord tumor with annular tubules in a boy with Peutz-Jeghers syndrome. J Pediatr 1982;101:568–571.
44. Solh HM, Azoury RS, Najjar SS: Peutz-Jeghers syndrome associated with precocious puberty. J Pediatr 1983;103:593–595.
45. Cantu JM, Rivera H, Ocampo-Campos R, et al: Peutz-Jeghers syndrome with feminizing Sertoli cell tumors. Cancer 1980;46:223–228.
46. Spigelman AD, Murday V, Phillips RK: Cancer and the Peutz-Jeghers syndrome. Gut 1989;30:1588–1590.
47. Lloyd KM, Dennis M: Cowden's disease: a possible new syndrome complex with multiple system involvement. Ann Intern Med 1963;58:136–143.
48. Weinstock JV, Kawanishi H: Gastrointestinal polyposis with orocutaneous hamartomas (Cowden's disease). Gastroenterology 1978;74:890–895.
49. Carlson GJ, Nivatvongs S, Snover DC: Colorectal polyps in Cowden's disease (multiple hamartoma syndrome). Am J Surg Pathol 1984;8:763–770.
50. MGH Case Records (Case 24-1987). N Engl J Med 1987;316:1531–1540.
51. Nelen MR, Padberg GW, Peeters EA: Localization of the gene for Cowden disease to chromosome 10q 22-23. Nat Genet 1996;13:114–116.
52. Bulow S: Colorectal polyposis syndromes. Scand J Gastroenterol 1984;19:289–293.
53. Deschner EE, Lipkin M: Proliferative patterns in colonic mucosa in familial polyposis. Cancer 1975;35:413–418.
54. Utsunomiya J, Nakamura T: The occult osteomatous changes in the mandible in patients with polyposis coli. Br J Surg 1975;62:45–51.
55. Tonelli F, Nardi F, Bechi P, et al: Extracolonic polyps in familial polyposis coli and Gardner's syndrome. Dis Colon Rectum 1985;28:664–668.
56. Iida M, Yao T, Itoh H, et al: Endoscopic features of adenoma of the duodenal papilla in familial polyposis of the colon. Gastrointest Endosc 1981;27:6–8.
57. Sarre RG, Frost AG, Jagelman DG, et al: Gastric and duodenal polyps in familial adenomatous polyposis: a prospective study of the nature and prevalence of upper gastrointestinal polyps. Gut 1987;28:306–314.
58. Bodmer WF, Bailey CJ, Bussey HJR, et al: Localization of the gene for familial adenomatous polyposis on chromosome 5. Nature 1987;328:614–616.
59. Leppert M, Dobbs M, Scambler P, et al: The gene for familial polyposis coli maps to the long arm of chromosome 5. Science 1987;238:1411–1412.
60. Vogelstein B, Fearon ER, Hamilton SR, et al: Genetic alterations during colorectal-tumor development. N Engl J Med 1988;319:529–532.
61. Ahnen DJ: Lessons from the genetics of colon cancer. Scand J Gastroenterol 1990;175:(Suppl)166–176.
62. Cannon-Albright LA, Skolnick MH, Bishop T, et al: Common inheritance of susceptibility to colonic adenomatous polyps and associated colorectal cancers. N Engl J Med 1988;319:533–537.
63. Winawer SJ, Fletcher RH, Miller L, et al: Colorectal cancer screening: clinical guidelines and rationale. Gastroenterology 1997;112:594–642.
64. Boman BM, Levin B: Familial polyposis. Hosp Pract 1986;21:155–170.
65. Naylor EW, Lebenthal E: Early detection of adenomatous polyposis coli in Gardner's syndrome. Pediatrics 1979;63:222–226.
66. Reed TE, Neel JV: A genetic study of multiple polyposis of the colon. Am J Hum Genet 1955;7:236–263.
67. Abramson DJ: Multiple polyposis in children: a review and a report of a case in a six year old child who had associated asthma and nephrosis. Surgery 1967;61:288–301
68. Bartram CL, Thornton A: Colonic polyp patterns in familial polyposis. Am J Roentgenol 1984;142:305–308.
69. Powell SM, Petersen GM, Krush AJ, et al: Molecular diagnosis of familial adenomatous polyposis. N Engl J Med 1993;329:1982–1987.
70. Giardiello FM, Brensinger JD, Petersen GM, et al: The use and interpretation of commercial APC gene testing for familial adenomatous polyposis. N Engl J Med 1997;336:823–827.
71. Odigwe L, Sherman PM, Filler R, et al: Straight ileoanal anastomosis and ileal pouch–anal anastomosis in the surgical management of idiopathic ulcerative colitis and familial polyposis in children: follow up and comparative analysis. J Pediatr Gastroenterol Nutr 1987;6:426–429.
72. Jagelman DG, DeCosse JJ, Bussey HJR: Upper gastrointestinal cancer in familial adenomatous polyposis. Lancet 1988;1:1149–1150.
73. Watanabe H, Enjoji M, Yao T, et al: Gastric lesions in familial adenomatosis coli. Hum Pathol 1978;9:269–283.
74. Burt RW, Rikkers LF, Gardner EJ: Villous adenoma of the duodenal papilla presenting as necrotizing pancreatitis in a patient with Gardner's syndrome. Gastroenterology 1987;92:532–535.
75. Richards RC, Rogers SW, Gardner EJ: Spontaneous mesenteric fibromatosis in Gardner's syndrome. Cancer 1981;47:597–601.
76. Traboulsi EI, Krush AJ, Gardner EJ, et al: Prevalence and importance of pigmented ocular fundus lesions in Gardner's syndrome. N Engl J Med 1987;316:661–667.
77. Traboulsi EI, Maumenee IH, Krush AJ, et al: Congenital hypertrophy of the retinal pigment epithelium predicts colorectal polyposis in Gardner's syndrome. Arch Ophthalmol 1990;108:525–526.
78. Schnur PL, David E, Brown PW, et al: Adenocarcinoma of the duodenum and the Gardner syndrome. JAMA 1973;223:1229–1232.
79. Krush AJ, Traboulsi EI, Offerhaus JA, et al: Hepatoblastoma, pigmented ocular fundus lesions and jaw lesions in Gardner's syndrome. Am J Med Genet 1988;29:323–332.
80. Bussey HJR: Familial Polyposis Coli: Family Studies, Histopathology, Differential Diagnosis, and Results of Treatment. Baltimore, Johns Hopkins University Press, 1975, p 69.
81. Turcot J, Despres J-P, St Pierre F: Malignant tumors of the central nervous system associated with familial polyposis of the colon. Dis Colon Rectum 1959;2:465–468.
82. Baughman FA, List CF, Williams JR, et al: The glioma-polyposis syndrome. N Engl J Med 1969;281:1345–1346.
83. Jarvis L, Bathwist N, Mohan D, et al: Turcot's syndrome: a review. Dis Colon Rectum 1988;31:907–914.
84. Itoh H, Ohsato K: Turcot's syndrome and its characteristic colonic manifestation. Dis Colon Rectum 1985;28:399–402.
85. Munden PM, Sobol WM, Weingeist TA: Ocular findings in Turcot syndrome (glioma-polyposis). Ophthalmology 1991;98:111–114.
86. McNicholas T, Brereton RJ, Raafat F: Lymphoid polyps of the rectum. J Pediatr Gastroenterol Nutr 1985;4:297–302.
87. Hermans PE, Huizenga KA, Hoffman HN, et al: Dysgammaglobulinemia associated with nodular lymphoid hyperplasia of the small intestine. Am J Med 1966;40:78–89.
88. Shannon R, Vickers TH: Multiple colonic polyposis and Hirschsprung's disease. Aust J Surg 1967;37:108–113.
89. Ament ME, Ochs HD, Davis SD: Structure and function of the gastrointestinal tract in primary immune deficiency syndrome. Medicine 1973;52:227–248.
90. Kaplan B, Benson J, Rothstein F, et al: Lymphonodular hyperplasia of the colon as a pathologic finding in children with lower gastrointestinal bleeding. J Pediatr Gastroenterol Nutr 1984;3:704–708.
91. Teague RH, Read AE: Polyposis in ulcerative colitis. Gut 1975;16:792–795.
92. Berkowitz O, Bernstein LH: Colonic pseudopolyps in association with amebic colitis. Gastroenterology 1975;68:786–789.
93. Daniel ES, Ludwig SL, Lewin KJ, et al: The Cronkhite-Canada syndrome: an analysis of the pathologic features and therapy in 55 patients. Medicine 1982;61:293–309.
94. Schart GM, Becker JHR, Laage NJ: Juvenile gastrointestinal polyposis or the infantile Cronkhite-Canada syndrome. J Pediatr Surg 1986;21:953–954.
95. Katayama Y, Kimura M, Konn M: Cronkhite-Canada syndrome associated with a rectal cancer and adenomatous changes in colonic polyps. Am J Surg Pathol 1985;9:65–71.

96. Ruvalcaba RHA, Myhre S, Smith DW: Sotos syndrome with intestinal polyposis and pigmentary changes of the genitalia. Clin Genet 1980;18:413–416.
97. DiLiberti JH, Weleber RG, Budden S: The Ruvalcaba-Myhre-Smith syndrome. Am J Med Genet 1983;15:491–495.
98. DiLiberti JH, D'Agostino AN, Ruvalcaba RHA, et al: A new lipid storage myopathy observed in individuals with the Ruvalcaba-Myhre-Smith syndrome. Am J Med Genet 1984;18:163–167.
99. Gretzula JC, Hevia O, Schachner LS, et al: Ruvalcaba-Myhre-Smith syndrome. Pediatr Dermatol 1988;5:28–32.

Chapter 36

# Neonatal Necrotizing Enterocolitis

*Robert M. Kliegman*

Neonatal necrotizing enterocolitis (NEC) is a disease of unknown origin that predominantly affects premature infants in level II, or more often level III, neonatal intensive care units during the infants convalescence from the common cardiopulmonary disorders associated with prematurity.[1–6] NEC is the most common and most serious acquired gastrointestinal disorder among hospitalized preterm neonates and is associated with significant acute and chronic morbidity and mortality.[1] Indeed, NEC is the most common cause of gastrointestinal perforation (followed by isolated idiopathic-focal intestinal perforation) and acquired short bowel syndrome among patients in the neonatal intensive care unit.[1, 7] It has been estimated that in the United States there are approximately 2,000 to 4,000 cases of NEC annually.[1, 8] NEC is one of the most common nosocomial neonatal diseases and in 1993 dollars cost the State of Washington approximately $74,000 per patient.[5, 6]

## EPIDEMIOLOGY

NEC is a disease that affects premature infants during their convalescence from other diseases of immaturity.[1, 9] It is unusual to see NEC during the acute phase of respiratory distress syndrome, hypoxic-ischemic encephalopathy (birth asphyxia), heart failure from congenital heart disease or patent ductus arteriosus, and other acute neonatal disease processes.[1, 10] Although NEC is noted predominantly in premature neonates, approximately 10% of cases occur in nearly full-term or full-term infants whose preceding risk factors have included polycythemia, cyanotic heart disease (usually with angiographic catheterization studies), chronic diarrhea, or a prior anatomic obstructive gastrointestinal malformation (volvulus or gastroschisis).[1, 11]

NEC occurs predominantly in neonates after the onset of enteral alimentation, as 95% of affected infants have been fed for various amounts of time.[1, 12, 13] NEC usually develops during the first 2 weeks of life in relatively well neonates who have been fed normally, but it may be delayed for 90 days in low–birth weight infants given nothing by mouth for long periods.[1] NEC tends to develop later among infants whose birth weights were less than 1,000 g. Thus, the more immature the infant at birth the later the possible onset of NEC. Such data suggest that immaturity of gastrointestinal function is a major risk factor.[1, 9, 14] Many case-control studies have suggested that immaturity is the only readily identifiable risk factor for the development of NEC.[1, 6] Immature function of host defense, gastrointestinal motility, digestion, healing, and mucosal integrity (permeability), and circulation may contribute to the pathogenesis of NEC (see later).[14–16]

The incidence of NEC varies among neonatal intensive care units, and some units have no cases. The overall incidence varies from 3% to 5% of all neonatal intensive care admissions.[1] The incidence among very low–birth weight (less than 1,500 g) infants who survive long enough to be fed approaches 10% to 15%. The incidence is greatest among infants between 500 and 750 g at birth (13% to 20%); it declines to approximately 1% to 3% among infants larger than 1,750 g.[1, 4] The baseline incidence is influenced by periodic outbreaks or epidemics of NEC that become superimposed on an endemic case background. Because infants between 500 and 750 g at birth represent a very small proportion of infants in neonatal intensive care units (less than 10% of all births), the mean birth weight of infants affected with NEC is between 1,350 and 1,500 g and the mean gestational age is between 30 and 32 weeks.

There is no association between NEC and sex, race (other than the increased incidence of low birth weight among blacks), and inborn or transport status.[1] NEC has very rarely been reported in successive pregnancies and among siblings in multiple gestations. Because twins and triplets are often born prematurely, they seem to be over-represented among cases of NEC.[1, 17] In contrast to what would be expected, the incidence of NEC among twins appears to be higher in the well, first-born twin rather than in the second twin, who usually has a lower Apgar score and a more complicated hospital course.

NEC is a disease of surviving neonates. Most affected patients are considered "gainers and growers" who, prior to the onset of NEC, had few if any manifestations of gastrointestinal dysfunction and few apparent sequelae of the previous diseases of prematurity from which they had been recovering.[9, 10] In many but not all instances, the affected preterm infants had respiratory distress syndrome days to weeks before the onset of NEC. With the advent of surfactant therapy for respiratory distress syndrome, more infants may survive this disorder and are now at risk for NEC during their convalescence.[10]

Because NEC is seen in premature infants, many factors associated with prematurity were thought to be risk factors for NEC. These were related to diseases, procedures, or complications that may produce gastrointestinal ischemia, infection, or altered digestion. Mucosal injury following a combination of these risk factors was thought to produce NEC. Ischemic risk factors included birth asphyxia, respiratory distress syndrome, hypoxia, hypotension, patent ductus arteriosus, polycythemia, anemia, umbilical arterialization, catheter, and exchange transfusion. Because these risk factors were identified as part of a profile among affected infants, they were thought to contribute to the pathogenesis of NEC. Although each may contribute to mucosal injury, case-control studies suggest that these processes are equally prevalent among affected patients and unaffected controls.[1] Therefore, these risk factors merely describe the low–birth weight population and are no longer thought to be direct contributing factors in the pathogenesis of NEC (see later). Epidemiologic investigations emphasize that the predominant risk factor is prematurity, with associated immature host defense and gastrointestinal function.

## PATHOLOGY

Traditionally, the pathologic appearance of NEC has demonstrated varying features of inflammation and coagulation necrosis.[18] The latter has been interpreted as being due to ischemia, but evidence also suggests that inflammatory mediators can produce lesions with coagulation necrosis similar to that following ischemia.[19]

Most tissue specimens from patients with NEC are obtained at autopsy in fatal cases or by surgical resection after gastrointestinal perforation.[18] There are a few studies that examined rectal mucosal biopsies in patients with mild NEC (not fatal, not requiring resection).[1] These latter studies, however, may not reveal a complete picture because (1) more severe NEC is a transmural process, involving all four layers of the bowel wall; (2) mild cases may not represent more severe disease in terms of etiology (mild NEC may represent an allergic-inflammatory process characterized by epithelial or lamina propria eosinophilic infiltration, a finding not usually observed in surgical pathology); and (3) NEC often involves the terminal ileum, ileocecal area, and ascending colon, and rarely only the rectal mucosa. Alternatively, the eosinophilia noted in the rectal mucosal biopsies may represent the early initiation phase of the illness, which later becomes masked by complicating peritonitis, secondary bacterial invasion, and neutrophilic infiltration. In addition, eosinophilic infiltrates may not always suggest allergic processes and may be a nonspecific gastrointestinal response.

Superficial inspection of affected resected surgical or autopsy tissue reveals mucosal ulceration, hemorrhage, edema, and submucosal or subserosal gas-filled cysts typical of pneumatosis intestinalis (Fig. 36–1). Approximately 50% of infants have involvement of both the small and large intestine (distal ileum and proximal colon), 25% have only colon disease, and 25% only ileal lesions.[1, 18] Involvement of the jejunum, the stomach, or the entire length of bowel from the ligament of Treitz to the rectum is less common; the latter is present in fatal cases of NEC (also known as *pan-NEC* or *NEC totalis*). Approximately equal numbers of infants have either continuous segments of involvement or skip lesions.

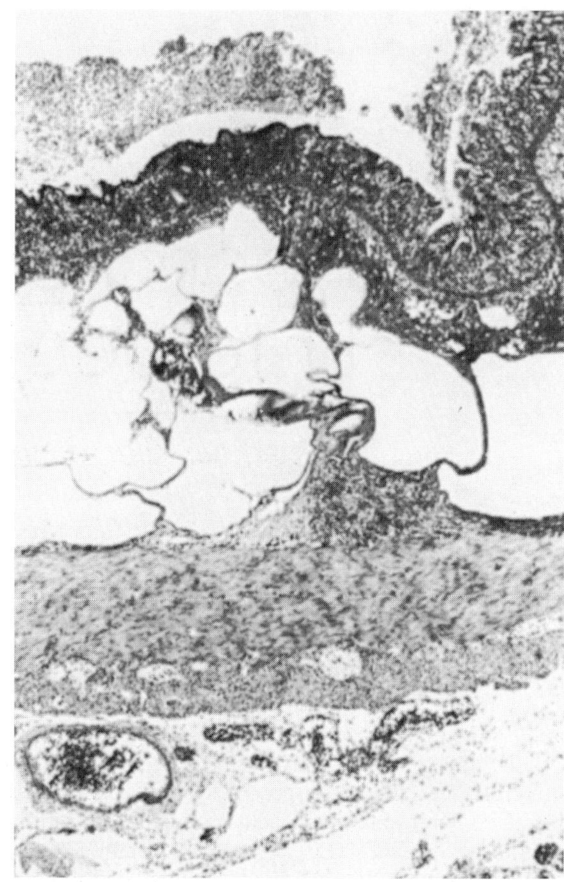

**FIGURE 36–1.** Microscopic evidence of severe submucosal gas-filled cysts (pneumatosis intestinalis) in a preterm infant with NEC. Note the marked hemorrhage throughout the bowel wall and the inflammatory exudate on the surface of the mucosa. Hematoxylin-eosin stain, ×56. (Courtesy of Beverly Dahms, MD.)

Histologic examination of resected tissue reveals coagulation necrosis in approximately 90%, inflammation in approximately 90%, and the presence of eosinophils (15%), ulceration (75%), hemorrhage (75%), peritonitis (70%), bacterial overgrowth (70%), and reparative process (70%).[18] Pneumatosis intestinalis is present in only 50% of pathology specimens.

Coagulation necrosis is the predominant lesion in most specimens.[1, 18] Coagulation necrosis, when present with inflammatory lesions, is often observed in an alternating manner in adjacent microscopic fields. Inflammatory changes include acute and chronic signs of inflammation, including serositis, peritonitis, inflammatory pseudomembranes, crypt abscesses, and bacterial or fungal overgrowth. When coagulation necrosis is present with signs of inflammation, the coagulative process is often the dominant lesion. Resected tissue also demonstrates extensive apoptosis, enterocyte expression of the inducible isozyme of nitric oxide synthase (iNOS), and the presence of interferon-γ. The latter is a known inducer of iNOS.

Large-vessel thrombi are unusual autopsy findings in the mesenteric arteriole system of patients with NEC.[1, 18] Small-vessel thrombi are present in 30% but may represent secondary phenomena or autopsy artifacts.

Interestingly, reparative processes of both acute and chronic types are noted in over 50% of cases.[18] Such reparative changes include focal epithelial regeneration, granulation tissue formation, and fibrosis. The latter two processes are usually noted in the mucosal and submucosal layers but occasionally extend into the muscularis. Such fibrotic processes may later be associated with development of strictures in recovering infants.

## PATHOGENESIS

Early theories of the pathogenesis of NEC proposed a relationship between gastrointestinal ischemia, enteral alimentation, and micro-organisms.[1] Although the precise contributions of these variables remain ill-defined, a multifactorial pathogenesis involving these risk factors plus immature gastrointestinal function and immature host defense mechanisms seems possible for the initiation and subsequent propagation of NEC (Figs. 36–2, 36–3).[1, 2]

### Hypoxic-Ischemic Injury

Potential alterations of mesenteric blood flow may occur at the large-vessel arterial level and may be associated with redistribution of systemic blood flow or may be within the gastrointestinal system itself with redistribution of local mucosal blood flow.[1, 2, 21–24] The possible systemic alterations may be associated with global hypoxia, asphyxia, exchange transfusion, arterial runoff lesions such as a patent ductus arteriosus, shock, or anemia. Local alterations of the mucosal circulation may be associated with less severe perturbations of these systemic factors plus those local changes occurring during enteral alimentation, polycythemia, intestinal distention, or luminal exposure to bacterial toxins or inflammatory mediators. Potential events may be initiated during the prenatal period (cocaine exposure, placental insufficiency with intrauterine growth retardation) or may occur after birth.[23, 24] Infants exposed to cocaine prenatally may be at higher risk for the development of NEC. Although they tend to have higher birth weights and greater gestational age than others at risk for NEC, they develop NEC sooner and have fewer traditionally identifiable risk factors. This suggests some circulatory role of in utero gastrointestinal ischemia secondary to cocaine's known vascular effects, which may produce fetal vasoconstriction.[23] Further evidence linking prenatal intestinal ischemia and NEC among intrauterine growth–retarded infants can be demonstrated by absent or reversed diastolic blood flow detected by fetal Doppler ultrasonography.[24] In most cases this reduced blood flow would not have been identified without ultrasonography, suggesting that fetal mesenteric ischemia often goes undetected.

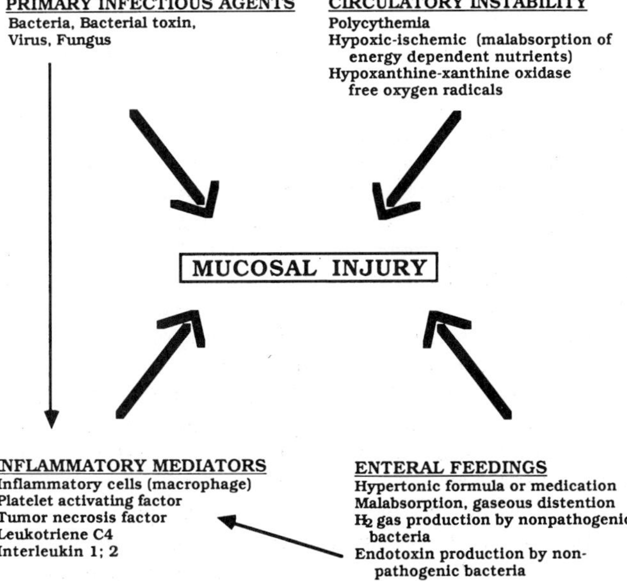


**FIGURE 36–2.** Hypothetical contributory variables that may initiate intestinal mucosal injury leading to necrotizing enterocolitis. (From Polin R, Fox W: Neonatal and Fetal Medicine: Physiology and Pathophysiology. Philadelphia, WB Saunders, 1992, with permission.)

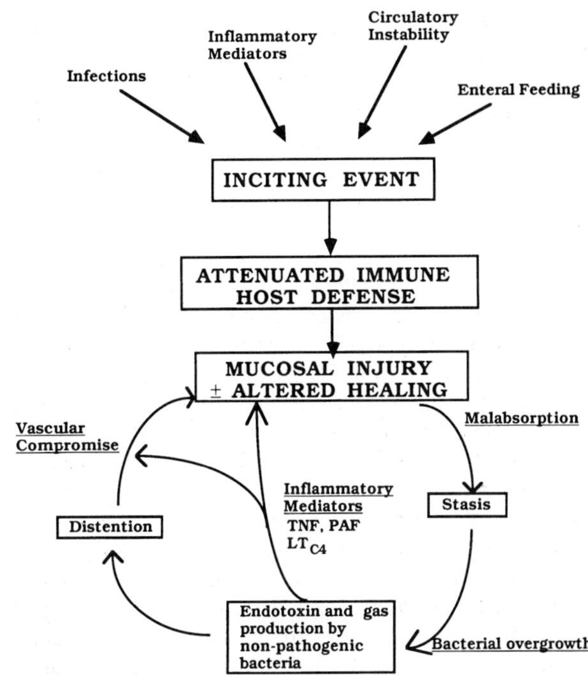


**FIGURE 36–3.** Hypothetical cycles of primary events and secondary propagating factors for neonatal intestinal mucosal injury that may produce necrotizing enterocolitis. (Adapted from Polin R, Fox W: Neonatal and Fetal Medicine: Physiology and Pathophysiology. Philadelphia, WB Saunders, 1992, with permission.)

The regulation of postnatal mesenteric blood flow is complex and not well-studied. Autoregulation of regional blood flow is determined by responses to nutrients and autocrine effects of various locally produced gut hormones.[1, 16] These effects may be modified by disease states, the autonomic and central nervous systems, and systemic processes producing vasoconstriction or hypotensive reduction of local tissue blood flow.

Regional intestinal hyperemia in response to local enteral nutrients is associated with increased local mucosal blood flow, oxygen delivery, oxygen consumption, and oxygen extraction. Oxygen-derived metabolic processes support aerobic energy–requiring intestinal mechanisms such as mucosal active transport, secretion, motility, digestion, macromolecule synthesis, and cell growth.[1, 16, 21] The postprandial intestinal mucosal hyperemia of adults is due to selective vasodilataion of the mesenteric artery and is regulated by central and local mechanisms (local hormones, nutrients). It is possible that an imbalance between oxygen delivery and oxygen consumption, together with inability to augment oxygen extraction (flow-dependent model), predisposes the immature intestine to hypoxic mucosal injury during alimentation. Such hypoxic mucosal injury may alter energy-dependent processes, produce malabsorption, mucosal ulceration, and increased mucosal permeability, and predispose to secondary bacterial invasion. Alternatively, postischemia reperfusion injury may further embarrass mucosal integrity and function, thus perpetuating the mucosal injury.

Experiments in mature and immature models support each of these hypotheses as possible mechanisms for mucosal injury.[1] Nonetheless there is a paucity of evidence to suggest that episodes of identifiable hypoxic-ischemic events contribute to the pathogenesis of NEC in most infants.[1] Of all the suggested ischemic risk factors for NEC, only polycythemia, exchange transfusion, and possibly exposure to cocaine are associated with the later development of NEC.[1]

## Enteral Alimentation

Because 95% of infants with NEC have been fed enterally before its onset, enteral alimentation has been proposed as a contributing factor in NEC.[12, 13] Various hypotheses propose that it is the composition of the milk, the rate of milk volume increments, the immaturity of gastrointestinal motility, absorptive, or host defense processes, or other variables (osmolality) that contribute to the pathogenesis of NEC.[1, 12, 13]

Human milk reduces the risk for NEC.[9, 25, 26] Animal models support a role for the breast milk macrophage, but human data suggest that immunoglobulins, specifically IgA, may have a protective advantage. Indeed, both enterally administered IgA and human milk may reduce the incidence of NEC.[26] Human milk may also reduce allergic reactions while enhancing digestion and absorption of normal nutrients. Although studies have demonstrated a protective effect of human milk, others have been confounded by milk preparation methods that may destroy the immunoprotective components of the milk. Evidence suggests that even pasteurized human milk is effective in reducing the incidence of NEC in premature infants.[25]

The volume of milk fed to infants may also predispose the patient to NEC.[12, 13] Excessively rapid increments of milk feeding may overcome the infant's intestinal absorptive capability especially in the presence of altered motility, resulting in malabsorption. Malabsorbed carbohydrates contribute to enhanced intestinal bacterial gas production, resulting in abdominal distention.[1, 27] High intraluminal pressure from gaseous distention may reduce mucosal blood flow, producing secondary intestinal ischemia.[9] In addition, dissection of bacterial gas products from the intestinal lumen may produce pneumatosis intestinalis or, if gas enters the portal venous system, hepatic venous gas may be evident. Analysis of gas from the intestinal lumen and cysts of pneumatosis intestinalis reveals a profile typical of intestinal bacterial fermentation of malabsorbed carbohydrates (e.g., hydrogen, methane, carbon dioxide).[1] Breath hydrogen excretion has been proposed as a method to support the diagnosis of NEC.[28]

Earlier hypotheses had suggested that giving patients at risk nothing by mouth might reduce the incidence of NEC. Delayed feeding for asphyxiated infants or those with umbilical arterial or venous catheters and respiratory distress syndrome has not consistently reduced the incidence of NEC.[1] In fact, delayed feeding may do more harm than good by increasing the risk of intestinal mucosal atrophy, cholestatic jaundice, osteopenia of prematurity, and hyperalimentation-related complications.[1]

Large-volume milk feedings, increased too rapidly during the feeding schedule, may place undue stress on a previously injured or immature intestine. Feeding increments in excess of 20 to 30 mL/kg per 24 hours have been associated with increased risk of NEC in at least two studies.[12, 13] Two other studies have demonstrated the safety of 30- to 35-mL/kg per 24 hours feeding increments.[29, 30] Such information should temper enthusiasm for excessively rapid feeding protocols for low–birth weight infants. It suggests that daily increments should be based on the clinical examination, evidence of feeding intolerance, and a recommended volume increment below 20 to 35 mL/kg per 24 hours.

Hypertonic formula and enteric medications may have direct adverse effects on mucosal blood flow and intestinal motility. Subsequent injury may predispose to NEC.[1] Alternatively, direct pharmacologic effects of an agent on systemic host defense (vitamin E) or regional blood flow (indomethacin) may result in mucosal injury, increasing the risks for NEC in susceptible neonates.[22]

## Infectious-Inflammatory Agents

There are multiple epidemiologic investigations that have provided circumstantial or direct evidence to suggest that NEC is associated with one or more microbiologic agents.[1] NEC has been reported to occur in epidemics or clustered episodes due to an identifiable enteric pathogen; more often no identifiable agent is discovered.[1, 9] When no agent is identifiable it may be due to the unculturable nature of the pathogen (e.g., Whipple's disease agent). Using a probe for the 165 ribosomal RNA to identify unculturable agents, these pathogens were found to be no more common in affected or unaffected patients.[31] The suspicion of a transmissible agent is corroborated by the observation that epidemics abate following the institution or reinforcement of specific infectious disease–control measures (gowning, gloving, nurse cohorts, and especially careful hand washing).[1] Epidemics have been associated with recovery of no specific agent and with the recovery of a single pathogen such as *Escherichia coli, Klebsiella, Salmonella, Staphylococcus epidermidis, Clostridium butyricum,* coronavirus, rotavirus, and enteroviruses.[1, 4] In the future, the more sensitive molecular biology techniques such as the polymerase chain reaction may be helpful in identifying agents. This method detects small amounts of viral or bacterial DNA or RNA that other culture and antigen (enzyme-linked immunosorbent assay) methods have failed to identify.[32] For example, in many older children with rotavirus diarrhea reverse transcriptase–polymerase chain reaction identifies rotavirus RNA when standard antigen immunoassays are negative.[32]

Additional evidence suggesting that NEC is due to an infectious agent includes the observation of related infantile diarrheal illnesses within a community or among personnel in the neonatal intensive care unit.[1] Furthermore, there are many similarities between NEC (pathology, symptoms, immature susceptibility) and many enterotoxemias of young animals and humans. Such enteric toxin–mediated illnesses may be due to *Clostridium, S. epidermidis,* or other toxin-producing enteric pathogens.[33, 34] Alternatively, endotoxin production by the "normal" gram-negative enteric flora may predispose the immature intestine to mucosal injury if endotoxin production exceeds elimination.[9, 20, 35] In addition trancytosis (crossing of epithelial cells by *E. coli,* etc.) could initiate this process; *E. coli* from patients with NEC have this capacity in animal models.[36] Endotoxin stimulates host inflammatory cells to produce various mediators such as tumor necrosis factor and platelet-activating factor.[20] Both of these and other inflammatory cytokines can initiate or propagate the pathologic process characterized by coagulation necrosis, inflammation, increased vascular permeability, edema, hemorrhage, local thrombosis, and platelet consumption. The resulting cytokine mediator–induced thrombocytopenia, neutropenia, hypotensive-hypovolemic shock (third space fluid losses), metabolic acidosis, and hemorrhagic diarrhea are quite similar to the clinical manifestations of NEC in human neonates.

The blood culture is positive in 20% to 30% of patients with NEC.[1, 4] Reports of the responsible bacteremic pathogens before 1980 demonstrated a predominance of *E. coli* and *Klebsiella.*[1] Current reports of agents producing bacteremia in patients with NEC suggest that *S. epidermidis* is the most common blood isolate, followed by the gram-negative organisms noted in earlier studies.[4] It remains to be determined whether the organisms recovered in blood or peritoneal cultures are the primary pathogens or secondary invading organisms that gain access to the circulation or peritoneum through a markedly compromised and damaged mucosa.

### Unifying Hypothesis of Pathophysiology

The predominant risk factor for NEC is prematurity, *not* the associated diseases of premature infants. Nonetheless, multiple potentially adverse events may produce mucosal injury, the net result being manifest as NEC. Figure 36–2 provides potential initiating events, and Figure 36–3 identifies additional pathologic factors that may propagate NEC once mucosal injury exceeds the immature host's ability to repair the process. Although it is hoped that one microbiologic agent or other process will be found to be responsible for NEC, it is more probable that NEC is a final common pathway for an immature intestinal response to injury.[9, 10] Indeed, NEC is a common cause of the systemic inflammatory response syndrome (SIRS) in neonates. If pneumonia can be caused by different bacteria, fungi, parasites, and viruses, it is equally tenable that NEC is caused by a select group of neonatal enteric pathogens or other pathologic processes all acting on an immature intestine.

## CLINICAL MANIFESTATIONS

Early signs and symptoms of NEC are often nonspecific and include subtle signs of the "sepsis syndrome" and more specific but equally subtle signs of gastrointestinal disease.[1] Nonspecific extra gastrointestinal manifestations include apnea, bradycardia, lethargy, temperature instability (hypothermia or the need to increase the Isolette temperature to maintain normal body temperature), cyanosis, mottling, cool extremities, and acidosis.[1] More specific but not diagnostic gastrointestinal manifestations are related to ileus, third space fluid losses, local coagulopathy, and intestinal hemorrhage. Gastrointestinal signs, and symptoms include abdominal distention, abdominal tenderness, emesis, increased gastric residual volume, hematemesis, hematochezia, bright red blood from the rectum, absent bowel sounds, abdominal guarding, and diarrhea. The latter is an uncommon isolated manifestation of NEC. As the disease progresses in severity, there is disseminated intrasvascular coagulation, hypotensive (septic and hypovolemic) shock, ascites, peritonitis, and intestinal perforation. Focal findings may include erythematous streaking of the anterior abdominal wall around the umbilicus and the course of the subcutaneous umbilical vein, and erythema with a mass in the right lower quadrant, representing a local perforation, with matted bowel forming a local abscess.

Disease stage should be classified as noted in Table 36–1 (modified Bell's criteria). Stage I represents subclinical (no diagnostic radiographic or ultrasonographic signs) NEC or another gastrointestinal or systemic disturbance. Stage II and III NEC are documented disease. Progression from one stage to another usually occurs within 24 to 48 hours after onset of symptoms. Once stabilized, patients with NEC rarely progress to another stage; most episodes of perforation occur at presentation (stage IIIB) or among patients with stage IIIA that progresses to stage IIIB. Perforation usually occurs within 48 to 72 hours of the onset of disease manifestations in patients with stage IIIA NEC. The modified Bell's staging criteria are also useful in comparing cases of NEC in the literature.

## DIAGNOSIS

The diagnosis of NEC is confirmed by the radiographic presence of pneumatosis intestinalis or hepatic venous gas (Figs 36–4 and 36–5). Gastrointestinal perforation (pneumoperitoneum; Figs 36–6 and 36–7) is strong evidence for NEC, but the diagnosis must then be confirmed by histopathologic evidence (see Pathology).

Hepatic venous gas and ascites may also be demonstrated by abdominal ultrasonography, and inapparent pneumatosis intestinalis may become more evident by performing a contrast enema.[1, 37–39] Nonetheless, except under unusual circumstances (to rule out volvulus), contrast studies are not needed to determine the diagnosis of NEC. Ancillary laboratory evaluations may reveal thrombocytopenia with or without evidence of disseminated intravascular coagulation, anemia,

**TABLE 36–1. Modified Bell's Staging Criteria for Neonatal Necrotizing Enterocolitis**

| | STAGE | SYSTEMIC SIGNS | INTESTINAL SIGNS | RADIOLOGIC SIGNS | TREATMENT |
|---|---|---|---|---|---|
| IA | Suspected NEC | Temperature instability, apnea, bradycardia, lethargy | Elevated pregavage residuals, mild abdominal distention, emesis, guaiac-positive stool | Normal or intestinal dilatation; mild ileus | NPO, antibiotics for 3 days pending cultures, gastric decompression |
| IB | Suspected NEC | Same as IA | Bright red blood from rectum | Same as IA | Same as IA |
| IIA | Definite NEC, mildly ill | Same as IA | Same as IA and IB plus diminished or absent bowel sounds ± abdominal tenderness | Intestinal dilatation, ileus, pneumatosis intestinalis | Same as IA plus NPO, antibiotics for 7–10 days if examination is normal in 24–48 hr |
| IIB | Definite NEC, moderately ill | Same as IIA plus mild metabolic acidosis and mild thrombocytopenia | Same as IIA plus definite abdominal tenderness, ± abdominal cellulitis, or right lower quadrant mass, absent bowel sounds | Same as IIA ± portal vein gas, ± ascites | Same as IIA plus NPO, antibiotics for 14 days, $NaHCO_3$ for acidosis, volume replacement |
| IIIA | Advanced NEC, severely ill, bowel intact | Same as IIB plus hypotension, bradycardia, severe apnea, combined respiratory and metabolic acidosis, DIC, neutropenia, anuria | Same as IIB plus signs of generalized peritonitis, marked tenderness, distention, and abdominal wall erythema | Same as IIB, definite ascites | Same as IIB plus as much as 200 mL/kg fluids, fresh frozen plasma, inotropic agents, intubation, ventilation therapy, paracentesis; surgical intervention if patient fails to improve with medical management within 24–48 hr |
| IIIB | Advanced NEC, severely ill, bowel perforated | Same as IIIA, sudden deterioration | Same as IIIA, sudden increased distention | Same as IIB plus pneumoperitoneum | Same as IIIA plus surgical intervention |

From Kliegman R: Necrotizing enterocolitis. In Burg FD, Ingelfinger JR, Wald ER, Polin RA (eds): Gellis & Kagan's Current Pediatric Therapy, Philadelphia, 15th ed. WB Saunders, 1996, with permission.

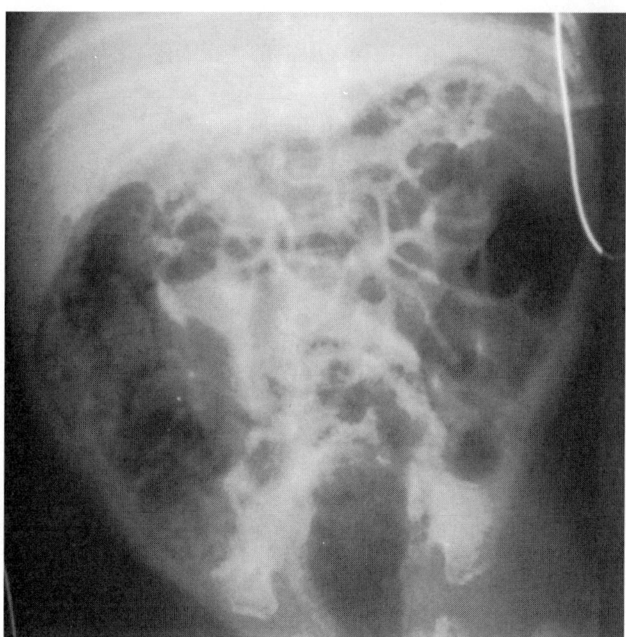

**FIGURE 36–4.** Abdominal roentgenogram demonstrating distended loops of small and large bowel, the bubble appearance of pneumatosis intestinalis predominantly in the right lower quadrant, and portal venous gas over the liver. (Courtesy of Stuart Morrison, MD.)

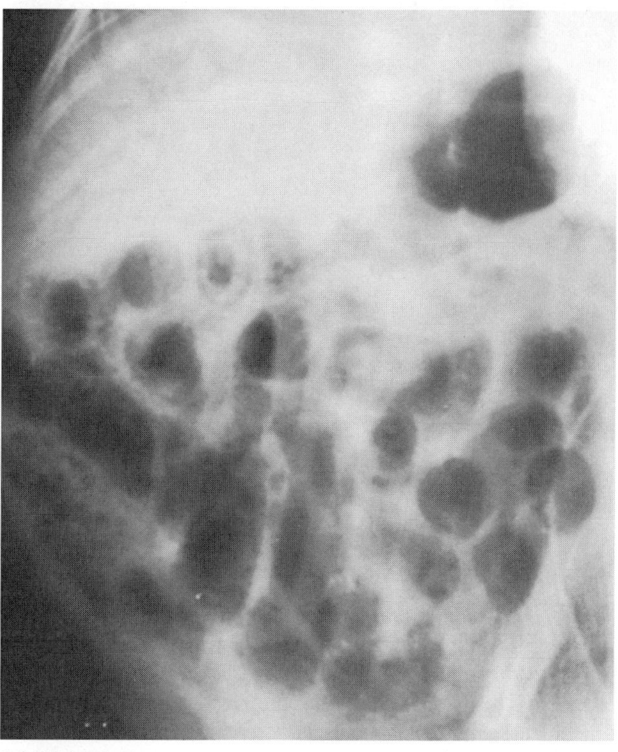

**FIGURE 36–5.** Abdominal roentgenogram demonstrating distention, pneumatosis intestinalis, and marked hepatic venous gas. (Courtesy of Stuart Morrison, MD.)

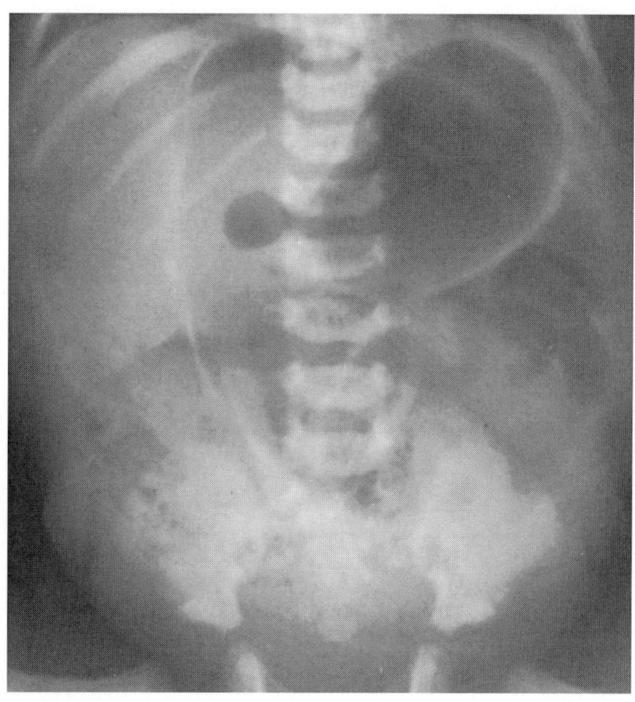

**FIGURE 36–6.** Abdominal roentgenogram demonstrating less pneumatosis intestinalis, marked distention, and pneumoperitoneum as evident by the line appearing between the liver and lower midline region depicting the falciform ligament of the umbilical vein. Note hazy, less clear area over the liver representing free gas in the abdomen. Pneumoperitoneum in patients with NEC represents intestinal perforation. (Courtesy of Stuart Morrison, MD.)

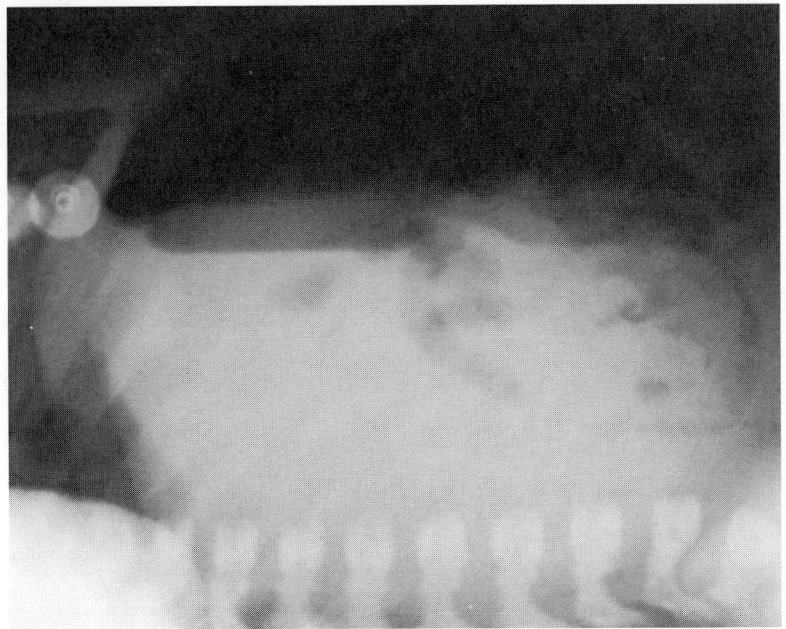

**FIGURE 36–7.** Cross-table lateral view most often to demonstrate pneumoperitoneum due to intestinal perforation in patients with NEC. Note the free gas in the abdomen above the liver and beneath the anterior abdominal wall. (Courtesy of Stuart Morrison, MD.)

neutropenia, metabolic acidosis from septic or hypovolemic shock, respiratory acidosis from increased intra-abdominal pressure and poor diaphragm excursion, elevated breath hydrogen excretion, and radiographic signs of ileus, an isolated dilated intestinal loop, or ascites.[1] The differential diagnosis of NEC is outlined in Table 36–2.

## PREVENTION

NEC may not be completely eliminated, but certain interventions have been demonstrated to lower the incidence. Oral administration of an IgA-IgG preparation has been demonstrated to reduse the incidence of NEC; however, intravenous administration of IgG (IVIG) has not affected the incidence of NEC.[26] The oral preparation (73% IgA, 26% IgG) reduced the incidence of NEC among recipients to zero, whereas control patients had an incidence of 7%. Further study is needed to determine whether this protocol can be generalized to other neonatal intensive care units.

Human milk was demonstrated to reduce the incidence of NEC among preterm infants.[40]

Prenatal and postnatal administration of corticosteroids has also been demonstrated to lower the incidence.[41] Steroids enhance lung maturation and are thought to accelerate intestinal maturation, thus potentially reducing the "immaturity" factor in the pathogenesis of NEC. Neonates received 2 mg/kg of dexamethasone every 12 hours for two doses. Postnatal steroids, independent of antenatal steroids, were effective in reducing the incidence of NEC in one investigation.[41]

Finally, although never demonstrated in a randomized trial, judicious slow enteral feeding protocols (no volume increments exceeding 20 to 35 mL/kg per 24 hours) may reduce the occurrence of NEC.[12, 13] There is sufficient circumstantial evidence from multiple case-control studies to suggest that slow feeding protocols are associated with a lower incidence of NEC. Furthermore, careful attention to the clinical appearance of the child and to signs of feeding intolerance (distention, hematochezia, larger gastric residuals, emesis) also may be beneficial in identifying infants with earlier-stage NEC.[1]

**TABLE 36–2. Differential Diagnosis of Neonatal Necrotizing Enterocolitis**

| |
|---|
| **Systemic Disease** |
| Sepsis with ileus |
| Pneumothorax dissecting to the abdomen, producing pneumoperitoneum |
| Hemorrhagic disease of the newborn |
| Swallowed maternal blood |
| Postasphyxia bowel necrosis |
| **Gastrointestinal Disease** |
| Volvulus |
| Malrotation |
| Pseudomembranous colitis |
| Hirschsprung's colitis |
| Intussusception |
| Umbilical arterial thromboembolism |
| Spontaneous isolated, focal bowel perforation |
| Hepatic-splenic-adrenal hemorrhage |
| Stress ulcer |
| Meconium ileus |
| Milk protein allergy |

## THERAPY (Table 36–3)

NEC has a wide spectrum of severity. The mildest enteritis form manifests as hemorrhagic colitis; the more fulminant state is similar to that noted in patients with gram-negative septic shock, commonly referred to as SIRS.

Abdominal distention is a universal feature of NEC. Significant abdominal distention may reduce the mesenteric arterial perfusion pressure, thus exacerbating a previously compromised intestinal blood flow. Models of the effects of increased intra-abdominal pressure have reported such adverse consequences as increased systemic vascular resis-

**TABLE 36–3. Approach to Management of Patients with Necrotizing Enterocolitis**

| ABNORMALITY | INTERVENTIONS | GOALS |
|---|---|---|
| Presumed infection | Broad-spectrum antibiotics | Eradicate infection |
| Peritonitis/intestinal perforation | Antibiotics plus surgery or paracentesis with drain placement | Eradicate nidus of infection; remove necrotic bowel, ascites |
| Intestinal distention/ileus | NPO; nasogastric tube drainage, paracentesis | Decrease intestinal gas production; remove intestinal secretions; decompress abdomen |
| Hypotension | Volume expansion, vasopressor agents | Restore gestational and postnatal age-appropriate blood pressure |
| Hypoperfusion/oxygen delivery | Volume expansion, vasopressor and inotropic agents; mechanical ventilation, oxygen, packed red blood cell transfusions | Hemoglobin 12–14 g/dL<br>Oxygen saturation >95%<br>Normal blood lactate level (pH)<br>Normal cardiac index |
| Organ system dysfunction | Volume expansion, vasopressor and inotropic agents; mechanical ventilation, oxygen; packed red blood cells, platelet, fresh frozen plasma transfusion; diuretics, dialysis-hemofiltration | Normalize or reverse abnormalities:<br>*Renal:* urine output, BUN, creatinine<br>*Hepatic:* bilirubin, coagulopathy, albumin<br>*Pulmonary:* alveolar-arterial gradient, hypercapnia<br>*Cardiac:* blood pressure, cardiac index<br>*CNS:* level of consciousness<br>*Hematologic:* correct anemia, disseminated intravascular coagulopathy (if active bleeding) |
| Poor nutritional intake | Parenteral alimentation (central or peripheral) | Reverse catabolism; improve nitrogen balance and healing; prevent hypoglycemia |

From Kliegman R: Necrotizing enterocolitis. In Burg FD, Ingelfinger JR, Wald ER, Polin RA (eds): Gellis & Kagan's Current Pediatric Therapy, 15th ed. Philadelphia, WB Saunders, 1996.

tance, decreased cardiac output, decreased urine output, and "apparent" hypovolemia.[42–44] Surgical decompression of increased intra-abdominal pressure in human adults restores systemic arterial oxygenation, cardiac output, and urine production within 15 minutes of the procedure.[42]

Increased intra-abdominal pressure in patients with NEC is due to the development of tense ascites, marked intestinal gas production, stasis (ileus), and inflammatory fluid exudation with hemorrhage into the lumina of the small and large intestines. It is imperative to reduce abdominal distention with nasogastric tube placement and no further formula feeding (NPO). The decompression tube should be the largest that the patient can tolerate. On occasion, paracentesis or placement of an intra-abdominal drain under local anesthesia has been helpful in stage III disease. Finally, if the patient fails to respond to medical management within 24 to 48 hours of the onset of illness, exploratory laparotomy can result in abdominal decompression by removing of necrotic tissue and inflammatory exudate (see Table 36–3).

The associated bacteremia in approximately 20% to 30% of patients with NEC is probably not the primary cause of the disease. Nonetheless, appropriate antimicrobial therapy must be directed against these bacteria, even when the bacteremia is due to bowel injury and secondary bacterial invasion. Patients with both NEC and bacteremia usually have more severe disease and higher mortality.[1] Although the precise antibiotic regimen for the treatment of NEC has not been determined, there is evidence that the clinician must remain flexible, as there has been an apparent change in the pathogens recovered in patients with NEC.[1, 4, 45, 46] This may reflect a bacterial shift in the fecal colonization of premature infants in the last two decades. Nonetheless, the changing pattern of the agents recovered during bacteremia requires close scrutiny and appropriate modification of antimicrobial therapy. Traditional antimicrobial treatment of NEC employs systemic administration of a semisynthetic penicillin (ampicillin, ticarcillin) and an aminoglycoside (gentamicin, kanamycin). Evidence suggests a beneficial response with the use of vancomycin and cefotaxime.[47] Vigilant attention to the microbiology of blood, fecal, and peritoneum cultures in patients with NEC is needed for appropriate modification of antibiotic therapy (see Table 36–1 for duration of antimicrobial therapy). Perforation with subsequent bacterial peritonitis is best managed surgically. Little is published about the antimicrobial therapy of neonatal peritonitis. Experience among adults suggests that *E. coli Bacteroides* species are more dominant than the enterococcus or *S. epidermidis.*[48, 49] Therefore, an aminoglycoside and an extended-spectrum penicillin (piperacillin), or clindamycin and an aminoglycoside are the suggested combination.

The treatment of severe NEC manifested as SIRS is not unlike that of other causes of bacteremia-associated hypotension. Endotoxin-stimulated production of inflammatory mediators such as bradykinin, tumor necrosis factor, or platelet-activating factor results in increased vascular permeability, large transcapillary fluid loss, increased pulmonary artery pressure with hypoxia, lactic acidosis, and hypotension. Hypermetabolism increases oxygen requirements. Once stabilized from the septic shock state, all patients require parenteral nutrition while NPO. Fluid losses plus the initial vasodilatation increase water and electrolyte requirements. Despite rapid killing of bacteria by antibiotics, the diverse effects of bacterial products (endotoxin, etc.) are still evident. The net result is a markedly reduced cardiopulmonary ability to meet the oxygen requirements of the peripheral tissues.[50–52]

Septic shock progresses through two important phases. The early phase is characterized by a pink, warm state with hyperventilation, increased cardiac output, decreased systemic vascular resistance, and a narrow arteriovenous oxygen difference. The latter observation is due to maldistribution of oxygen to tissue beds; those tissues with a greater oxygen requirement remain hypoxic. The second phase of septic shock is characterized by cyanosis, mottling, cold extremities, oliguria, narrow pulse pressure, and decreased cardiac output with markedly increased systemic vascular resistance.

The decreased cardiac output in septic shock (and NEC) may be due to pooling of blood and fluid in the capacitance peripheral vessels and loss of fluid in third spaces as well as a specific myocardial dysfunction characteristic of severe bacteremic states. The myocardial depression is not due to ischemia but rather to various mediators released as a response to inflammation and hypotension. Circulatory failure results in a flow-limited ability to provide the oxygen necessary to support energy metabolism (local tissue oxygen consumption). Circulatory failure causes tissue hypoxia and metabolic (lactic) acidosis. Some of the cellular defects of oxygen utilization may not be due to hypoxia-ischemia alone. Tumor necrosis factor produced during endotoxemia has various metabolic consequences that may interfere with mitochondrial oxygen utilization.[50]

Methods used to treat septic shock must take into consideration the linear relationship between oxygen delivery and local tissue oxygen consumption.[50] This flow-dependent relationship can be improved by restoring the circulating blood volume (preload) with fluid resuscitation and by improving myocardial contractility with inotropic-sympathomimetic agents.

An acute "adult" respiratory distress–like syndrome (ARDS) may be observed in patients with NEC. This is due in part to inflammatory or vasoactive mediators producing noncardiogenic pulmonary edema. Hypoxia is exacerbated by increased pulmonary artery pressure, abdominal distention with reduced diaphragmatic excursion, and myocardial contractile failure. Adequate oxygen delivery is closely dependent on appropriate ventilator management of patients with NEC. Methods that improve oxygen delivery also reduce local lactate production and improve metabolic acidosis. A successful outcome in patients with septic shock is related to the ability of the therapeutic measures to improve cardiac output. In addition to support for the failing circulation, careful attention must be given to the pulmonary problems associated with NEC.

The application of these principles to the therapy of NEC must emphasize judicious use of fluid resuscitation. If fluid administration is unsuccessful in restoring perfusion and urine production or correcting the metabolic acidosis, inotropic drugs (dopamine, dobutamine) can be used to improve oxygen delivery by improving myocardial contractility and occasionally by vasodilation. The administration of inotropic, vasodilator, or vasopressor agents must be carefully titrated against peripheral perfusion, blood pressure, urine production, metabolic acidosis, and central venous pressure if available. The therapeutic balance between vasopressor (myocardial contractility) agents and vasodilatation (afterload reduction) is often difficult to achieve but may be benefited by additional fluid therapy.

Future therapy of NEC or septic shock–like states may need to take into consideration the effects of the various inflammatory mediators (e.g., cytokines, prostaglandins) associated with tissue injury. Various blocking agents of these mediators and anti-inflammatory drugs have produced encouraging results in experimental models of endotoxemia or septic shock. Nonetheless, it is possible that the mediator-induced damage is already irreversible by the time the patient presents with hypotensive septic shock. It is most likely that therapy directed against these mediators must be initiated early in the course of the disease, before irreversible tissue injury occurs.

Intestinal perforation is an indication for exploratory laparotomy. In certain high-risk, unstable patients (often less than 1000 g), paracentesis and placement of a drain under local anesthesia has been performed.[53–56] In many patients managed with paracentesis and a drain, exploratory laparotomy is necessary 24 to 72 hours later. Additional indications for surgery include progressive clinical deterioration despite aggressive medical management (see Table 36–3) and in the convalescent stages for the resection of strictures and enteric fistulas.[57]

Surgical management should attempt to preserve as much viable bowel as possible, resecting only the most obviously necrotic and gangrenous tissue. In circumstances of NEC totalis, a high diverting jejunostomy is recommended—and a second laparotomy within 48 to 72 hours if the patient remains critically ill—to determine if what previously looked like nonviable tissue was actually viable.[53, 58] This approach may avoid massive resection and the subsequent development of the short gut syndrome.[58]

For patients with minimal and well-defined disease some surgeons recommend that primary anastomosis be performed after resection of dead bowel, at the time of the initial laparotomy.[59] Such patients should be observed carefully for development of strictures (at the anastomosis site and at other sites) or recurrent NEC. Strictures may present with signs of obstruction (emesis, obstipation, abdominal distention), sepsis, or gastrointestinal bleeding.

## REFERENCES


1. Kliegman RM, Walsh MC: Neonatal necrotizing enterocolitis: pathogenesis, classification and spectrum of disease. Curr Prob Pediatr 1987;17:213–288.
2. Kosloske AM: A unifying hypothesis for pathogenesis and prevention of necrotizing enterocolitis. J Pediatr 1990;117:S68–S74.
3. Holman RC, Stehr-Green JK, Zelasky MT: Necrotizing enterocolitis mortality in the United States, 1979–85. Am J Publ Health 1989;79:987–989.
4. Palmer SR, Biffin A, Gamsu HR: Outcome of neonatal necrotising enterocolitis: results of the BAPM/CDSC surveillance study, 1981–1984. Arch Dis Child 1989;64:388–394.
5. Andrews J, Anderson G, Han C, Neff J: The use of disease-specific conditions as risk adjusters in capitated payment systems. Arch Pediatr Adolesc Med 1997;151:236–242.
6. Gaynes R, Edwards J, Jarvis W, et al: National Nosocomial Infections Surveillance System. Nosocomial infections among neonates in high-risk nurseries in the United States. Pediatrics 1996;98:357–361.
7. Grosfeld J, Molinari F, Chaet M, et al: Gastrointestinal perforation and

peritonitis in infants and children: experience with 179 cases over ten years. Surgery 1996;120:650–656.

8. Jason JM: Infectious disease–related deaths of low birth weight infants, United States, 1968 to 1982. Pediatrics 1989;84:296–303.
9. Kliegman RM: Models of the pathogenesis of necrotizing enterocolitis. J Pediatr 1990;117:S2–S5.
10. Kliegman RM: Neonatal necrotizing enterocolitis: bridging the basic science with the clinical disease. J Pediatr 1990;117:833–835.
11. Eggli KD, Loyer E, Anderson K: Neonatal pneumatosis cystoides intestinalis caused by volvulus of the mid-intestine. Arch Dis Child 1989;64:1189–1190.
12. Anderson DM, Kliegman RM: The relationship of neonatal alimentation practices to the occurrence of endemic necrotizing enterocolitis. Am J Perinatol 1991;18:62–67.
13. Zabielski PB, Groh-Wargo SL, Moore JJ: Necrotizing enterocolitis: feeding in endemic and epidemic periods. J Parenteral Enteral Nutr 1989;13:520–524.
14. Udall JN: Gastrointestinal host defense and necrotizing enterocolitis. J Pediatr 1990;117:S33–S43.
15. Morriss FH, Moore M, Gibson T, et al: Motility of the small intestine in preterm infants who later have necrotizing enterocolitis. J Pediatr 1990;117:S20–S23.
16. Aynsley-Green A, Lucas A, Lawson GR, et al: Gut hormones and regulatory peptides in relation to enteral feeding, gastroenteritis, and necrotizing enterocolitis in infancy. J Pediatr 1990;117:S24–S32.
17. Powell RW, Dyess DL, Luterman A, et al: Necrotizing enterocolitis in multiple-birth infants. J Pediatr Surg 1990;25:319–321.
18. Ballance WA, Dahms BB, Shenker N, et al: Pathology of neonatal necrotizing enterocolitis: a ten-year experience. J Pediatr 1990;117:S6–S13.
19. Caplan MS, Hsueh W: Necrotizing enterocolitis: role of platelet activating factor, endotoxin, and tumor necrosis factor. J Pediatr 1990;117:S47–S51.
20. Ford HR, Sorrells DL, Knisely AS: Inflammatory cytokines, nitric oxide, and necrotizing enterocolitis. Semin Pediatr Surg 1995;5:155–159.
21. Nowicki P: Intestinal ischemia and necrotizing enterocolitis. J Pediatr 1990;117:S14–S19.
22. Coombs RC, Morgan MEI, Durbin GM, et al: Gut blood flow velocities in the newborn: effects of patent ductus arteriosus and parenteral indomethacin. Arch Dis Child 1990;65:1067–1071.
23. Lopez SL, Taeusch HW, Findlay RD, Walther FJ: Time of onset of necrotizing enterocolitis in newborn infants with known prenatal cocaine exposure. Clin Pediatr 1995;34:424–429.
24. Craigo S, Beach M, Harvey-Wilkes K, D'Alton M: Ultrasound predictors of neonatal outcome in intrauterine growth restriction. Am J Perinatol 1996;13:465–471.
25. Hoy C, Millar MR, MacKay P, et al: Quantitative changes in faecal microflora preceding necrotising enterocolitis in premature neonates. Arch Dis Child 1990;65:1057–1059.
26. Eibl MM, Wolf HM, Furnkranz H, et al: Prevention of necrotizing enterocolitis in low-birth-weight infants by IgA-IgG feeding. N Engl J Med 1988;319:1–7.
27. Clark DA, Miller MJS: Intraluminal pathogenesis of necrotizing enterocolitis. J Pediatr 1990;117:S64–S67.
28. Cheu HW, Brown DR, Rowe MI: Breath hydrogen excretion as a screening test for the early diagnosis of necrotizing enterocolitis. Am J Dis Child 1989;143:156–158.
29. Caple JI, Armentrout DC, Huseby VD, et al: The effect of feeding volume on the clinical outcome in premature infants. Pediatr Res 1997;41:229A.
30. Rayyis S, Ambalavanan N, Wright L, Carlo W: Randomized trial of "slow" versus "fast" feeding advancement in very low birth weight infants. Pediatr Res 1997;41:172A.
31. Millar MR, Linton CJ, Cade A, et al: Application of 16S rRNA gene PCR to study bowel flora of preterm infants with and without necrotizing enterocolitis. J Clin Microbiol 1996;34:2506–2510.
32. Wilde J, Yolken R, Willoughby R, et al: Improved detection of rotavirus shedding by polymerase chain reaction. Lancet 1991;337:323–326.
33. Scheifele DW: Role of bacterial toxins in neonatal necrotizing enterocolitis. J Pediatr 1990;117:S44–S46.
34. Rotbart HA, Johnson ZT, Reller LB: Analysis of enteric coagulase-negative staphylococci from neonates with necrotizing enterocolitis. Pediatr Infect Dis J 1989;8:140–142.
35. Fink MP, Cohn SM, Lee PC, et al: Effect of lipopolysaccharide on intestinal intramucosal hydrogen ion concentration in pigs: evidence of gut ischemia in a normodynamic model of septic shock. Crit Care Med 1989;17:641–646.
36. Panigrahi P, Bamford P, Horvath K, et al: *Escherichia coli* transcytosis in a caco-2 cell model: implications in neonatal necrotizing enterocolitis. Pediatr Res 1996;40:415–421.
37. Buras R, Guzzetta P, Avery G, et al: Acidosis and hepatic portal venous gas: indications for surgery in necrotizing enterocolitis. Pediatrics 1986;78:273–277.
38. Brill PW, Olson SR, Winchester P: Neonatal necrotizing enterocolitis: air in Morison pouch. Radiology 1990;174:469–471.
39. Weinberg B, Peralta VE, Diakoumakis EE, et al: Sonographic findings in necrotizing enterocolitis with paucity of abdominal gas as the initial symptom. Mt Sinai J Med 1989;56:330–333.
40. Dugdale AE: Breast milk and necrotising enterocolitis. Lancet 1991;337:435.
41. Halac E, Halac J, Begue EF, et al: Prenatal and postnatal corticosteroid therapy to prevent neonatal necrotizing enterocolitis: a controlled trial. J Pediatr 1990;117:132–138.
42. Cullen DJ, Coyle JP, Teplick R, et al: Cardiovascular, pulmonary, and renal effects of massively increased intra-abdominal pressure in critically ill patients. Crit Care Med 1989;17:118–121.
43. Richards WO, Scovill W, Baekhyo S, et al: Acute renal failure associated with increased intra-abdominal pressure. Ann Surg 1983;197:183–187.
44. Celoria G, Steingrub J, Dawson JA, et al: Oliguria from high intraabdominal pressure secondary to ovarian mass. Crit Care Med 1987;15:78–79.
45. Rotbart H, Levin M: How contagious is necrotizing enterocolitis? Pediatr Infect Dis 1983;2:406–413.
46. Scheifele DW, Bjornson GL, Dyer RA, et al: Delta-like toxin produced by coagulase-negative staphylococci is associated with neonatal necrotizing enterocolitis. Infect Immun 1987;55:2268–2273.
47. Scheifele DW, Ginter GL, Olsen E, et al: Comparison of two antibiotic regimens for neonatal necrotizing enterocolitis. J Antimicrob Chemother 1987;20:421–429.
48. Gorbach SL: Intraabdominal infections. Clin Infect Dis 1993;17:961–967.
49. Montravers P, Gauzit R, Muller C, et al: Emergence of antibiotic-resistant bacteria in cases of peritonitis after intraabdominal surgery affects the efficacy of empirical antimicrobial therapy. Clin Infect Dis 1996;23:486–494.
50. Rackow EC, Astiz ME, Weil MH: Cellular oxygen metabolism during sepsis and shock: the relationship of oxygen consumption to oxygen delivery. JAMA 1988;259:1989–1993.
51. Natanson C, Danner RL, Elin RJ, et al: Role of endotoxemia in cardiovascular dysfunction and mortality: *Escherichia coli* and *Staphylococcus aureus* challenges in a canine model of human septic shock. J Clin Invest 1989;83:243–251.
52. Carcillo JA, Pollack MM, Ruttimann UE, et al: Sequential physiologic interactions in pediatric cardiogenic and septic shock. Crit Care Med 1989;17:12–16.
53. Albanese CT, Rowe MI: Necrotizing enterocolitis. Semin Pediatr Surg 1995;4:200–206.
54. Horwitz JR, Lally KP, Cheu HW, et al: Complications after surgical intervention for necrotizing enterocolitis: a multicenter review. J Pediatr Surg 1995;30:994–999.
55. Korones S: No survival among 20 infants $<$ 1000 g with NEC stage 3 for whom surgical management was limited to peritoneal drainage: a six-year experience (1990–1995). Pediatr Res 1997;41:159A.
56. Ahmed T, Moore A: Early laparotomy improve survival in necrotizing enterocolitis (NEC). Pediatr Res 1997;41:135A.
57. Stringer MD, Cave E, Puntis WL, et al: Enteric fistulas and necrotizing enterocolitis. J Pediatr Surg 1996;31:1268–1271.
58. Luzzatto C, Previtera C, Boscolo R, et al: Necrotizing enterocolitis: late surgical results after enterostomy without resection. Eur J Pediatr Surg 1996;6:92–94.
59. Ade-Ajayi N, Kiely E, Drake D, et al: Resection and primary anastomosis in necrotizing enterocolitis. J R Soc Med 1996;89:385–388.

Chapter 37

# Appendicitis

Peter A. Mattei, Richard J. Stevenson, and Moritz M. Ziegler

Acute appendicitis is the most common abdominal surgical emergency in childhood. In addition, many more patients with right lower quadrant pain are evaluated by pediatric surgeons to "rule out" appendicitis every day. More than 80,000 children undergo appendectomy each year in the United States. Despite this extensive collective clinical experience, two very important facts remain: many normal appendices are found at appendectomy, and at least one third of all cases of acute appendicitis in children are diagnosed after the appendix has perforated. There is no single diagnostic study that can confirm or exclude acute appendicitis in a reliable and cost-effective way. It remains, therefore, a significant cause of illness and potentially serious morbidity in the pediatric population.

Although acutely suppurative and typically lethal right lower quadrant processes attributed to inflammation of the cecum were described in medieval times, acute appendicitis appears to be a disease of modern Western civilization, perhaps related to dietary factors.[1] Melier, in 1827, described several cases of perforated acute appendicitis, which he ascribed to obstruction of the appendiceal lumen with fecal matter.[1] He went on to describe in detail the typical presentation and natural history of classic acute appendicitis. However, because Melier was publicly and viciously ridiculed by Dupuytren, the premier surgeon in France at the time, the concept remained obscure. It was not until 1886, when Reginald Fitz published his treatise entitled *Perforating Inflammation of the Vermiform Appendix: With Special Reference to its Early Diagnosis and Treatment,* that the modern era of surgical management of acute appendicitis began. Reports of successful operation soon became commonplace, and during the early 20th century appendectomy was the most commonly performed operative procedure in the United States.

The true function of the appendix is not known, nor have any effects been attributed to its absence or removal. The appendix is a blind pouch of variable length and position that arises from the cecum at the point at which the taeniae converge. The majority of appendices (approximately 65%) occupy a retrocecal position; the remainder are intraperitoneal, most commonly in the pelvis.[2] Further anatomic variability arises from the uncommon variations in cecal position.

## PATHOPHYSIOLOGY

The pathogenesis of acute appendicitis was elucidated and confirmed in clinical experiments by Wangensteen and Dennis in 1939.[3] The sequence of events, beginning with the earliest clinical manifestations of appendiceal colic and ending in selected cases with frank rupture and peritonitis, is thought to begin with obstruction of the appendiceal lumen. The mucosa of the obstructed appendix continues to secrete and, as the lumen progressively fills with mucus, the intraluminal pressure gradually rises. This leads to the earliest manifestations of acute appendicitis, namely colicky periumbilical abdominal pain and nausea. Meanwhile, luminal bacteria proliferate and invade the wall of the appendix, resulting in suppuration, serosal exudate, local inflammatory change, and, potentially, bacteremia. As the pressure within the organ continues to rise, the wall tension eventually exceeds capillary perfusion pressure. This results in ischemic necrosis of the appendiceal wall and either circumferential gangrene or localized perforation. Subsequent clinical manifestations are determined by the speed of progression and local reactive changes. In some cases, the perforation is effectively walled off and produces a phlegmon or abscess, manifesting clinically as an "appendiceal mass." In others, there is frank peritoneal soilage and purulent ascites.

The stage at which the progression of acute appendicitis is recognized and arrested by surgical intervention determines the clinicopathologic stage of the disease. *Simple* or "early" appendicitis is often diagnosed by histopathologic study only, since the appendix may appear grossly normal or have minimal findings such as hyperemia or induration at the tip. *Suppurative* appendicitis is recognized by congestion and marked edema of the organ and the mesoappendix. Typically, an adherent fibrinous exudate and signs of local inflammation in adjacent organs or omentum are present. *Gangrenous* appendicitis is characterized by focal areas or circumferential necrosis of the wall of the appendix. There may be purulent ascites and areas of near-perforation. *Perforated* or *ruptured* appendicitis is the end result of ischemic necrosis of the wall. Again, depending on the degree of local reaction to the process, this stage is manifested either by frank peritonitis or by a walled-off abscess.

The microbiology of acute appendicitis is that of the

normal colonic flora. The infectious process is typically polymicrobial, and both aerobes and anaerobes play important roles. The most common isolates are *Escherichia coli* and *Klebsiella*, but *Streptococcus, Pseudomonas, Enterobacter, Bacteroides,* and occasionally clostridial species are also seen.[4]

## DIAGNOSIS

Since its earliest description, the emphasis for the optimal management of appendicitis has been on its early diagnosis and treatment. The diagnosis is still based primarily on clinical grounds, namely the history and physical examination, and there is currently no laboratory or imaging study that can reliably confirm or rule out the diagnosis in children. Although the classic presentation of acute appendicitis is well described and easily recognized, many patients, including most children, do not present with an obvious clinical picture. In addition, many children present with signs and symptoms suggestive of acute appendicitis when another condition is the cause.

## CLINICAL HISTORY

The initial symptom is usually abdominal pain. The initial colicky and vague abdominal pain is caused by distention of the appendix, a hollow viscus. These pain impulses are transmitted by visceral afferent sympathetic fibers and are referred to the 10th somatic dermatome. This is perceived as a cramping pain in the periumbilical region that quickly becomes constant and progressive. A history of pain worsened by bumps during the car ride to the hospital is very nonspecific.

Nausea and vomiting are common symptoms that in most cases follow the onset of pain. Anorexia is also very common but not an absolute sign in the pediatric population. Bowel hypermotility manifested by diarrhea can also occur, mimicking gastroenteritis. This latter finding is more common when appendiceal perforation causes irritation and inflammation of the sigmoid colon.

As the inflammation progresses and involves the serosa of the appendix and the peritoneum of the abdominal wall, the pain shifts to the right lower quadrant. This shift results from the involvement of somatic afferent pain fibers, which also accounts for the very localized and often exquisite tenderness noted on physical examination. The most common point of maximal tenderness was described by McBurney in 1889 as being located two thirds of the distance along a line between the umbilicus and the anterior superior iliac spine.

Given the variability of anatomic location and presentation of the illness, any child with focal tenderness, regardless of location, should be considered potentially to have acute appendicitis. In very rare cases, the location of the appendix is truly ectopic owing to nonrotation of the colon (left upper quadrant) or situs inversus (left lower quadrant). An inflamed appendix in the retrocecal or retrocolic position may produce flank pain or right upper quadrant tenderness. The pain may also be referred to other locations as a result of inflammation of adjacent organs. Bladder wall irritation can cause symptoms suggestive of a urinary tract infection and may also result in microscopic pyuria. Periureteral inflammation can cause pain referred to the inguinal region or testis, and rectal irritation can cause tenesmus or diarrhea.

The temporal progression of symptoms is also important. It is unusual and often difficult to make the diagnosis of acute appendicitis within the first 12 hours of the illness. In cases of rapidly progressive gangrenous appendicitis, the overall clinical condition and the physical findings may be so worrisome and suggestive of acute appendicitis that operation is recommended within 24 hours after the onset of symptoms. Similarly, symptoms that are present for more than 72 hours suggest either another disease process or a well-localized perforation or phlegmon associated with appendicitis.

## PHYSICAL EXAMINATION

On physical examination, the child with acute appendicitis is typically ill-appearing and anorexic, often walking slowly and hunched forward and lying very still on the examination table. A low-grade fever and mild tachycardia often are present early in the disease process and may worsen as the illness progresses and dehydration becomes more evident.

The most important physical finding is focal abdominal tenderness. The child should be asked to point to the area of maximal pain, and this area should be the last to be examined. Although mild diffuse tenderness can often be elicited, the diagnosis of appendicitis is suggested by exquisite focal tenderness. In some cases this can be elicited only by very deep palpation, particularly in cases of early appendicitis. Involuntary guarding and rigidity of the abdominal musculature is common but may be subtle. There are localized peritoneal signs in most cases, manifested by tenderness to gentle percussion or elicited by other maneuvers such as a heel-strike or a shake of the bed. Other maneuvers include having the patient jump off the examining table or hop up and down. Rovsing's sign—tenderness in the right lower quadrant elicited by palpation or percussion in the left lower quadrant—may also be useful. The practice of testing for "rebound tenderness" by deep palpation and sudden release is less useful. Not only can the pain be excruciating, but the finding of tenderness by this method is nonspecific and may be elicited with equal frequency in normal patients.

The other well-known findings, such as the psoas sign and the obturator sign (elicited by forced extension and by internal rotation at the hip, respectively), are commonly described but rarely useful. They lack specificity.

The digital rectal examination is an essential part of the physical examination in cases of suspected appendicitis. It is rare, however, that important clinical decisions are made solely on the basis of findings on rectal examination. The examination is more useful in pelvic appendicitis, which occurs in only one third of cases. The finding of focal tenderness or a tender mass suggestive of acute appendicitis is rarely recognized in the absence of other suggestive physical findings. We use rectal examination in selected cases in which the information has a high probability of being helpful—most notably in cases in which the physical findings are suggestive but equivocal, when an abscess is suspected, or to palpate the cervix or adnexae when formal vaginal examination is contraindicated.

Perforated and gangrenous appendicitis are more likely to be found more than 48 hours after the onset of symptoms. Either is more likely to occur in very young children. The diagnosis is suggested by high fever, severe dehydration, severe regional peritonitis, diffuse peritonitis, marked abdominal distention, or tender fluctuance on rectal examination.

## LABORATORY EVALUATION

Laboratory findings are rarely helpful in the diagnosis of appendicitis. Although the leukocyte count can be increased in acute appendicitis, an elevated leukocyte count has a sensitivity of only 80% to 85%, meaning that the count is normal in as many as 20% of cases.[5–7] Furthermore, the specificity of an elevated leukocyte count is as low as 50%. The finding of a left shift may be slightly more accurate, but it is rarely more useful than a thorough history and physical examination. Urinalysis can be helpful in equivocal cases to rule out ureteral calculus or cystitis, but it should be noted that appendiceal inflammation adjacent to the bladder or ureter can cause mild microscopic pyuria or hematuria. A urine pregnancy test should be performed in a every adolescent female presenting with possible appendicitis to rule out ectopic pregnancy as a cause of the presenting symptoms and to rule out coincidental intrauterine pregnancy before radiologic examination or general anesthesia is performed.

Radiologic studies can be helpful for the diagnosis of some cases of appendicitis. Plain abdominal radiographs may reveal a fecalith or a focal right lower quadrant ileus suggestive of acute appendicitis. They should be obtained only in clinically equivocal cases or to rule out bowel obstruction or constipation as potential causes of abdominal pain. Barium enema may reveal failure of the appendiceal lumen to fill with contrast material, suggesting the diagnosis, but this finding is nonspecific and the test is considered impractical for routine use. Many published studies suggest that ultrasound can improve the diagnostic accuracy in acute appendicitis.[8, 9] In practical terms, however, ultrasound can provide only minimal improvement over the history and physical examination. Nevertheless, we have found ultrasound to be useful in adolescent girls, in whom gynecologic processes such as rupture of an ovarian cyst can mimic appendicitis. Computed tomography (CT) may be slightly more accurate than ultrasound, but it is more impractical. Studies have suggested that a high-resolution CT scan of the lower abdomen, specifically looking at the appendix, may be highly accurate in the diagnosis of appendicitis and more cost-effective than selective negative laparotomy.[10–12] This observation remains to be proved in the pediatric age group.

In summary, the diagnosis of acute appendicitis is made on the basis of clinical criteria. A compatible history and suggestive examination (i.e., focal tenderness) warrant operative exploration in most cases. It cannot be overstated that not all cases of acute appendicitis exhibit the signs and symptoms described here. Likewise, no clinical finding can rule out appendicitis with certainty, including the absence of anorexia. Laboratory studies and radiologic examinations rarely help in the decision whether to operate. Perhaps the most useful tool in equivocal cases is careful observation and serial examination. In the appropriate clinical setting, serial observation may be accurate and cost-effective. Patients are given nothing by mouth, are hydrated intravenously, and undergo serial examination by the same experienced clinician. The period of observation typically is 2 to 12 hours. Because it is distinctly unusual for acute appendicitis to resolve without treatment or for another condition to mimic the natural history of appendicitis over such a time period, it usually becomes obvious whether acute appendicitis is likely. It is very rare for acute appendicitis to progress to perforation during such a period of observation.

## DIFFERENTIAL DIAGNOSIS

There are many conditions that can mimic appendicitis. Gastroenteritis is very common and can manifest with a clinical picture suggestive of appendicitis. Vomiting and diarrhea are more prominent and usually precede the abdominal pain in gastroenteritis, and focal pain and tenderness usually are not present or are transient. Often there is a history of infected contacts. A period of observation usually allows differentiation of gastroenteritis from acute appendicitis. Constipation can produce abdominal pain, vomiting, and low-grade fever. There is often no clinical history of constipation, but examination supplemented by abdominal films may confirm the presence of massive amounts of stool. It should be cautioned that constipation is a common coincidental finding and its presence does not rule out appendicitis. Mesenteric adenitis is painful lymphadenopathy in the setting of pharyngitis or upper respiratory infection, and it can almost perfectly mimic appendicitis. The diagnosis is one of exclusion, sometimes aided by radiologic techniques. Urinary tract infections can cause lower abdominal pain, fever, and dysuria, but rarely can the focal tenderness of acute appendicitis be accounted for by such an infection. Likewise, the pyuria sometimes associated with appendicitis is typically very mild. Pelvic inflammatory disease can be confirmed in the acute setting in most cases by gynecologic examination and cervical smear. Ultrasound examination may confirm pyosalpinx or tubo-ovarian abscess. Ovarian cysts, especially when ruptured or hemorrhagic, are often suggested by the history and lack of gastrointestinal complaints. Ultrasound examination can confirm the diagnosis in some cases, but others require exploration or laparoscopy. Ovarian torsion is also suggested by a history of extreme pain of very abrupt onset, and patients typically present with a tender mass in the pelvis. Ultrasound can be a useful diagnostic adjunct if it is undertaken without delay. Meckel's diverticulitis can be indistinguishable from acute appendicitis, but in most cases it also requires operation. It is mandatory that the ileum be examined in its entirety whenever a normal appendix is found at appendectomy. Intussusception occasionally manifests in a manner suggestive of appendicitis, but it is uncommon in children older than 3 years of age. The diagnosis is suggested by a history of intermittent pain, the presence of blood in the stool, and the absence of focal tenderness. If intussusception is suspected, a diagnostic air enema should be performed immediately.

Certain medical conditions can also produce right lower quadrant pain, the most important being pneumonia and meningitis. A chest radiograph or lumbar puncture should be considered in the appropriate clinical setting. Acute cholecystitis, pancreatitis, duodenal ulcer, and acute ileitis are rare in children, but each can clinically resemble appendicitis. Sickle cell crisis can pose a difficult clinical dilemma, but it typically involves a fall in the hematocrit and a history of similar previous episodes. Serial examination is very useful in this setting. An uncommon but sometimes vexing diagnostic problem arises in patients with malignancy who are treated with cytotoxic drugs and present with right lower quadrant pain. Perityphlitis is a nonsuppurative inflammatory process involving the cecum and ascending colon that can be difficult to differentiate from appendicitis. An abdominal CT scan or ultrasound examination is a helpful adjunct in this situation.

## TREATMENT

Children who present for surgical consultation with possible acute appendicitis generally fall into three categories. In some the diagnosis is thought to be unlikely in favor of another specific diagnosis or gastroenteritis. The parents of these children should be warned that appendicitis cannot be ruled out with 100% certainty and that if the symptoms progress (increasing pain, vomiting, fever) the child should be re-examined. This is especially true when the patient presents within 12 hours after the onset of pain. The second group includes those with a compatible history and a physical examination consistent with acute appendicitis. These patients should be prepared for operation on an urgent basis. There are others whose history or physical examination is equivocal for acute appendicitis; the diagnosis must be seriously entertained, but the criteria for immediate operation are not satisfied. These patients should undergo observation and serial assessment, preferably by the same examiner. Our practice is to give such patients nothing by mouth, maintain intravenous hydration, and avoid analgesics other than acetaminophen. Those who improve are fed and discharged. Patients who fail to improve or whose clinical or laboratory picture is clearly evolving into one more consistent with acute appendicitis undergo operation.

## OPERATIVE TREATMENT

Early appendectomy is the therapeutic goal for acute appendicitis. The pursuit of this goal necessitates that in some equivocal cases a normal appendix will be found at operation in an attempt to avoid delay and possible gangrene or rupture. With straightforward cases, the operation should be performed with minimal delay. In some cases of gangrene or rupture, aggressive preoperative resuscitation with intravenous fluids is necessary and intravenous antibiotics should be started immediately. Rarely should operation be delayed for longer than 4 hours.

A right lower quadrant transverse muscle-splitting incision is preferred, the placement of which is facilitated by palpation of the abdomen after the induction of anesthesia. The incision can be extended as necessary. The appendix should be removed in all cases, if possible, including "normal" appendices and those that are difficult to locate or identify because of rupture and abscess. In rare instances, removal is not possible or it is thought to be unsafe, in which case the suppurative process should be controlled with drainage and debridement and the patient should be scheduled for interval appendectomy in 4 to 6 weeks. In very rare cases it may be necessary to remove all or part of the cecum if the inflammatory process has rendered the colon nonviable. An alternate technique in this situation is tube cecostomy; the tube can be removed after several days, with spontaneous closure of the fistula. The stump of the amputated appendix should be ligated securely. Some surgeons prefer to invert the stump with permanent suture after ligation of the base with absorbable suture. Others cauterize the exposed mucosa of the stump. Usually, the wound can be closed primarily in a layered fashion, even in the presence of perforation or gangrene. Some situations of gross contamination warrant either primary closure with drainage or packing of the wound with secondary healing. Delayed primary closure is yet another option in selected cases.

In the event that the appendix appears normal, appendectomy should still be done. Any peritoneal fluid encountered should be examined for evidence of purulence or blood. A thorough examination of the right lower quadrant can usually be performed without extending the incision. The distal 2 to 3 feet of ileum should be inspected for a Meckel's diverticulum or terminal ileitis. Mesenteric adenitis can sometimes be recognized as well. The ovary and salpinx should be palpated or inspected for cysts or pus. Despite these maneuvers, a cause for the pain is often not identified. Nevertheless, the majority of these patients report resolution of their symptoms after appendectomy.

Patients who have been ill for longer than 5 days or who have a palpable mass on presentation should undergo ultrasound examination for possible abscess. Those who are not systemically ill are candidates for antibiotics, percutaneous drainage, and interval appendectomy after 4 to 6 weeks, assuming that they continue to improve.

Laparoscopic appendectomy is a safe and effective alternative to traditional open appendectomy. Laparoscopy may be especially useful in equivocal cases, particularly when gynecologic pathology is suspected. As of yet, unanswered questions about laparoscopic appendectomy include its cost-effectiveness as well as its clinical effectiveness.

Most children after appendectomy in the absence of appendiceal perforation or gangrenous change, are able to tolerate a diet and be discharged on the first postoperative day. They usually resume full activity in 2 to 4 weeks.

## ANTIBIOTICS

All patients with the diagnosis of acute appendicitis should receive broad-spectrum antibiotic therapy before operation. Those with nonruptured appendicitis need only a prophylactic antibiotic schedule. This includes a minimum of one preoperative dose and typically one or two postoperative doses. Those with ruptured appendicitis or gangrenous appendicitis with purulent ascites should receive a minimum of 7 to 10 days of intravenous antibiotics to minimize the risk of postoperative abscess formation.

For nonruptured appendicitis, we currently favor single-drug therapy with a broad-spectrum cephalosporin that covers anaerobes (e.g., cefotetan). For ruptured or gangrenous appendicitis with purulent ascites, we use ampicillin/sulbactam and gentamicin; this regimen is started preoperatively in cases of suspected perforation. We add additional coverage (e.g., ceftazidime) if intraoperative cultures grow *Pseudomonas* or *Enterobacter* species.

In cases of ruptured appendicitis, patients are discharged from the hospital when their ileus has resolved and they are tolerating a regular diet, typically by postoperative day 5. They finish a full course of intravenous antibiotics at home with the help of home nursing specialists. They are followed up in 7 to 10 days and are evaluated for signs or symptoms of intra-abdominal abscess. Most patients have a complete blood count and undergo rectal examination. If an abscess is suspected, they undergo a screening CT examination of the abdomen.

## COMPLICATIONS

The most common complication after appendicitis is wound infection. These typically manifest within 7 days of operation with redness, tenderness, fever, fluctuance or drainage. Most require opening of the wound to allow evacuation of a subcutaneous abscess. Antibiotic therapy is often added, but in the absence of spreading cellulitis or systemic illness it probably is not necessary.

Intra-abdominal abscess most often occurs after ruptured or gangrenous appendicitis, but it can occur after milder cases as well. Abscesses most often occur in the pelvis but can be found anywhere in the abdomen. Patients usually present with malaise, nausea, and signs of an ileus. The leukocyte count is elevated, and a fluctuant mass may be palpated on rectal examination. The diagnosis is confirmed by abdominal CT scan. Early, small, or inaccessible abscesses can be treated with a longer course of intravenous antibiotics, but most abscesses require drainage. Many are accessible by percutaneous drainage in the radiology suite. Others are suitable for transrectal drainage. Rarely, laparotomy may be necessary to drain large or multiple abscesses.

Complications of perforated appendicitis with peritonitis also include small bowel obstruction secondary to adhesions. Girls with perforated appendicitis have an increased risk of infertility as adults.

The mortality rate of uncomplicated appendicitis is negligible. It is increased for ruptured appendicitis, especially in infants and those with underlying illnesses or immunodeficiency, but overall it remains quite low.

## CHRONIC APPENDICEAL PAIN

Chronic abdominal pain secondary to appendiceal pathology manifests in one of three ways. *Chronic appendicitis* describes any type of long-term appendiceal pain. From a histopathologic standpoint, chronic appendicitis implies an inflamed appendix infiltrated with chronic inflammatory mononuclear white cells. True chronic appendicitis is rare. *Recurrent appendicitis* is a product of low-grade appendicitis, with its familiar associated symptomatology, which resolves. When the inflammation subsides, the resulting fibrosis indelibly documents the preceding insult. Such fibrosis, as evidence of remote appendicitis, occurs in approximately 5% of incidental appendectomies. *Appendiceal colic (appendiceal cramping)* is by far the most common type of chronic appendiceal pain. Complete, unrelieved obstruction of the appendiceal lumen most often produces acute appendicitis. Partial or intermittent complete obstruction of the lumen results in appendiceal colic. Specific entities that may compromise the lumen of the appendix include circumferential fibrosis, fecalomas, and kinks. Additionally, lymphoid hyperplasia and carcinoid tumors may expand the wall of the appendix, compromising its lumen. Once the lumen is narrowed, internal foreign debris (seeds, vegetable matter) and even *Enterobius* (pinworms) may compound the problem.

Spasm of the obstructed appendix manifests clinically as colic. The magnitude of discomfort may be as severe as that noted with ureteral or biliary colic. If the material obstructing the appendiceal lumen is extruded, there is immediate and complete relief of symptoms. However, the pathology responsible for luminal narrowing remains, and the process of entrapment of foreign material is likely to repeat. The pain associated with complete luminal obstruction may be so severe that it encourages the unwary physician to make the erroneous diagnosis of perforated appendicitis. However, in this situation there usually is no fever, and the leukocyte count is within normal limits. As luminal pressure increases, necrosis of the appendix and associated nerves ensues. The colic, once severe, abates and the patient may appear dramatically improved.

The severity and periodicity of appendiceal colic is extremely variable. The pain may be severe and unrelenting for days; in such situations the appendix is invariably removed. In other cases, the pain may be severe but only for a brief period. Unless such episodes are witnessed by a physician, the patient may be destined for months or even years of sporadically presenting pain until the appendix is removed. Almost as significant as severe colic is the more mild form that recurs sporadically every few weeks or months. The academic, physical, social, and psychological consequences of such pain over the long term may be profound.

### History

Appendiceal colic is episodic and of variable intensity, duration, and periodicity. The patient is visibly uncomfortable and often writhing in pain. When the discomfort is more severe, the patient moves about holding the lower abdomen. The painful crises are virtually identical. The patient becomes pensive, pallor is evident, the eyes appear sunken. Occasionally flushing is noted, the skin is clammy, or there is frank diaphoresis. Headaches may be reported, and the colicky episodes may precipitate a migraine. The most severe appendiceal colic may precipitate lightheadedness or even syncopal attacks.

Patients very frequently feel nauseated when experiencing colic. With more severe pain, reflexive vomiting (dry heaves) occurs, as with ureteral or biliary colic. Nausea and vomiting are noted in association with the pain. Of most importance is the postprandial exacerbation of appendiceal colic. This usually occurs within 5 to 30 minutes after eating. In general, patients describe the discomfort as periumbilical in location. With more several colic, the discomfort may be described as being in the right lower quadrant.

As the duration of appendiceal colic increases, the incidence of associated complaints increases. School absenteeism and performance as well as social and athletic participation fall. Apathy and lethargy become more pronounced. Initial beliefs that the problem is organic in nature are replaced by parental doubt that the pain is real. Lastly, there may be documentation of weight loss, since eating exacerbates the pain.

## Physical Examination

If the history is classic for appendiceal colic, then the physical examination will probably confirm the diagnosis. The most important fact to remember is that the patient must be experiencing colic for the physical examination to be obviously positive. Pressure on an appendix that is in spasm accentuates the pain, leading to accurate identification of the location of the appendix. This point of maximal tenderness is reproducible. A rectal examination offers little information with regard to appendiceal colic. One needs to be alert for complaints of right flank, back, hip, or leg pain. A previously inflamed appendix that is scarred and tethered in the right gutter or iliac fossa may be responsible for such discomfort, especially when the appendix is in spasm. Patients with appendiceal colic generally are afebrile, but recurrent appendicitis may coexist with appendiceal colic, and intermittent febrile episodes may be reported. Histopathologic examination of the appendix documents fibrosis with acute inflammation in this situation.

Laboratory studies are usually ordered to exclude other diagnoses that may be responsible for abdominal pain. With regard to appendiceal colic, the leukocyte count usually is normal. It may be elevated if there is associated inflammation. A normal urinalysis is mandatory. A pregnancy test is essential in girls of appropriate age. An abdominal radiograph is of little value but may be diagnostic if a fecalith is present or if there is retained barium in the appendix after a previous contrast study. An abdominal-pelvic ultrasound study is useful to exclude pathology in other organ systems (the ovaries). However, documentation of an ovarian cyst does not necessarily exclude the diagnosis of appendiceal colic.

## Management

The patient presenting with severe appendiceal colic, as verified by a classic history and physical examination, should undergo an expedited appendectomy. An ultrasound examination in a female may be reassuring but is usually normal. The patient with a long history of appendiceal colic and extensive work-up deserves an urgent appendectomy. If the appendiceal colic is mild and of short duration, a 1- to 2-week period of observation is indicated. During this period, the diagnosis is secured with serial examinations, and diagnoses such as gastroenteritis and mesenteric adenitis are excluded. A pelvic ultrasound examination in a female patient is advised. Occasionally a patient presents with a classic history yet point tenderness on a physical examination has never been verified. In this situation it is incumbent on the physician to make arrangements for examination of the patient when the pain is present. Rarely, a patient with abdominal pain presents with confusing signs and symptoms, yet an appendectomy resolves the complaints. Occasionally, during operative exploration for abdominal pain, a normal-appearing appendix is discovered and is not removed. However, a normal external examination of the appendix at laparotomy or laparoscopy cannot ensure that the appendiceal lumen is not occluded. Therefore, in such a circumstance the "normal" appendix should be removed.

If the approach suggested is carefully followed, patients with appendiceal colic can be accurately identified in an expedited manner, and unnecessary laboratory and radiologic studies can be minimized. An appendectomy in this group of patients may be expected to provide relief of pain in more than 95% of patients.

## REFERENCES

1. Ravitch MM: Appendicitis: history. In Welch KJ, Randolph JG, Ravitch MM: Pediatric Surgery. Chicago, Year Book Medical Publishers, 1986, p 989.
2. Skandalakis JE, Gray SW, Ricketts R: The colon and rectum. In Skandalakis JE, Gray SW: Embryology for Surgeons, 2nd ed. Baltimore, Williams & Wilkins, 1994, p 242–281.
3. Kottmeier PK: Appendicitis. In Welch KJ, Randolph JG, Ravitch MM: Pediatric Surgery. Chicago, Year Book Medical Publishers, 1986, p 989–995.
4. Roberts JP: Quantitative bacterial flora of acute appendicitis. Arch Dis Child 1988;63:536–540.
5. Eriksson S, Granstrom L, Olander B, Pira U: Leukocyte elastase as a marker in the diagnosis of acute appendicitis. Eur J Surg 1995;161:901–905.
6. Izbicki JR, Knoefel WT, Wilker DK, et al: Accurate diagnosis of acute appendicitis: a retrospective and prospective analysis of 686 patients. Eur J Surg 1992;158:227–231.
7. Ko YS, Lin LH, Chen DF: Laboratory aid and ultrasonography in the diagnosis of appendicitis in children. Acta Paediatr Sin 1995;36:415–419.
8. Rioux M: Sonographic detection of the normal and abnormal appendix. AJR Am J Roentgenol 1992;158:773–778.
9. Wade DS, Morrow SE, Balsara ZN, et al: Accuracy of ultrasound in the diagnosis of acute appendicitis compared with the surgeon's clinical impression. Arch Surg 1993;128:1039–1046.
10. Rao PM, Rhea JT, Novelline RA, et al: Helical CT technique for the diagnosis of appendicitis. Radiology 1997;202:139–144.
11. Lane MJ, Katz DS, Ross BA, et al: Unenhanced helical CT for suspected acute appendicitis. AJR Am J Roentgenol 1997;168:405–409.
12. Balthazar EJ, Birnbaum BA, Yee J: Acute appendicitis: CT and US correlation in 100 patients. Radiology 1994;190:31–35.

Chapter 38

# Intussusception in Infants and Children

*Karen W. West and Jay L. Grosfeld*

Intussusception is a frequent cause of bowel obstruction in children younger than the age of 2 years and remains one of the most common surgical emergencies in infancy and childhood. The initial description of the invagination of one segment of bowel into another was made by Paul Barbette in the late 1600s,[1] and the first successful surgical reduction was described by Sir Jonathan Hutchinson in 1871.[2] This detailed report given before the Medico-Chirurgical Society described symptoms of crampy, intermittent abdominal pain in a toddler for a month, associated with vomiting, bloody stools, and the eventual prolapse of the ileum out the rectum. Attempts at reduction using chloroform anesthesia, dangling the child by the feet, and administering simultaneous enemas were unsuccessful, but laparotomy was pursued in spite of the moribund condition of the child. The bowel was found to be viable and was safely reduced. Scattered reports of hydrostatic reduction had appeared earlier in the literature, but Ravitch standardized and popularized the hydrostatic barium reduction techniques in the 1930s.[3] Early diagnosis and therapeutic intervention are aimed at preventing the patient morbidity and mortality noted in these early reports.

## ETIOLOGY

Intussusception is a process that occurs when a proximal segment of bowel (intussusceptum) telescopes into a more distal segment (intussuscipiens) dragging the associated mesentery with it. As edema develops, venous and lymphatic congestion leads to the "currant-jelly stools" (blood mixed with mucus), and vascular compromise is possible.

Seventy-five percent to 90% of the cases of ileocolic intussusception are idiopathic, with no identifiable lead point observed. Most episodes occur in otherwise healthy and well-nourished children with a male predominance. Sixty percent of the patients are younger than one year of age, and 80% of the cases occur before the second birthday.[3–5] Seasonal variation has been reported corresponding to the peak season for gastroenteritis, although this varies in larger series. Thirty percent of the children may experience otitis media, "flu-like illness," or an upper respiratory tract infection before the onset of symptoms associated with an intussusception. Viremia is thought to accentuate the lymphatic tissues in the intestinal tract, resulting in hypertrophy of Peyer's patches in the lymphoid-rich terminal ileum, which may act as a leadpoint for ileocolic intussusception. Although adenovirus and rotavirus have been implicated in the etiology of intussusception, the results of viral studies vary from one institution to another and may depend on methods of detection.[6–9] Using histochemical staining techniques, hypertrophic Peyer's patches were located in only 31% of the studied surgical specimens.[10] Additionally, *Yersinia enterocolitica* infections have been associated with rare cases of childhood intussusception.[11, 12]

In a minority of cases (2% to 10%) a pathologic lead point is identified. Lead points occur more commonly in older children (older than 5 years) and include small bowel lymphomas, Meckel's diverticulum, duplication cysts, various polyps (e.g., those occurring in Peutz-Jeghers syndrome), juvenile vascular malformations such as hemangiomas, inverted appendiceal stumps, and even *Ascaris lumbricoides* (Table 38–1).[13–15] Small bowel intussusception may follow an episode of Henoch-Schönlein purpura, with the bowel wall hematoma acting as the lead point.[15] Patients with cystic fibrosis have an increased risk of developing an intussusception particularly after an episode of dehydration and meconium ileus equivalent syndrome.[16] In the latter cases, the thick, inspissated stool may act as the lead point for the process. Additionally, the older child with repeated episodes of upper respiratory tract infections and a concomi-

**TABLE 38–1. Pathologic Lead Points in 19 of 209 Patients with Idiopathic Intussusception (J.W. Riley Hospital for Children)**

| | |
|---|---|
| Meckel's diverticulum | 6 |
| Bowel wall hematoma | 4 |
| Non-Hodgkin's lymphoma | 2 |
| Hamartomatous polyps | 2 |
| Submucosal hemangioma | 1 |
| Carcinoid tumor | 1 |
| Juvenile polyp | 1 |
| *Ascaris lumbricoides* | 1 |
| Appendix (cystic fibrosis) | 1 |

tant intussusception should have a sweat chloride determination as part of the evaluation.

Rarely, nonobstructive small bowel–small bowel intussusception may be associated with celiac disease and may be related to the disordered motility, excessive secretions, or bowel wall weakness found in this entity.[17, 18] Obstructing intussusception can be identified in patients with Crohn's disease who develop abdominal pain and bilious emesis unassociated with a previous surgical exploration.[19, 20] There have also been a few reports of familial intussusception not associated with hereditary polypoid conditions.[21] Cases of ileocolic intussusception have also been noted in children with hemolytic uremic syndrome.[22]

## CLINICAL PRESENTATION AND PHYSICAL EXAMINATION

Intussusception usually is characterized by the sudden onset of intermittent crampy abdominal pain accompanied by screaming, inconsolable crying, and a "drawing-up" of the legs toward the abdomen. The episodes become more frequent and may be followed by initially clear gastric emesis. Bilious emesis may develop as the obstruction progresses. In between the painful episodes, the child may act very appropriate for his or her age. Sixty percent of our patients had been evaluated for gastroenteritis by an office-based physician or in an emergency room setting at least once prior to referral for diagnosis.[7, 15] As the process progresses, *increasing lethargy* may develop and can be mistaken for early meningitis or sepsis until clear spinal fluid is obtained following lumbar puncture. The classically described triad of pain, a palpable sausage-shaped abdominal mass, and currant-jelly stools is seen in only 15 to 20% of patients at the time of presentation.[7, 15] In our series of 209 patients, the most frequent symptoms initiating referral included emesis (82%), abdominal pain (75%), rectal bleeding (currant-jelly stools, gross blood, or Hematest-positive stool) (75%), a palpable abdominal mass (65%), and lethargy or sepsis (40%). The currant-jelly stools (composed of mixed blood and mucus) result from the venous congestion of the involved bowel.[7] The sausage-shaped abdominal mass can usually be palpated in the right upper quadrant with an empty void noted in the right lower quadrant. In three patients in our series, the intussusceptum could be palpated on rectal examination at the time of admission. Abdominal tenderness is caused by distended loops of bowel stretching the visceral peritoneum as the intermittent obstruction develops. Evidence of peritonitis is rare, because the potentially necrotic intussusceptum is within the initially viable intussuscipiens. As the enveloping distal bowel remains distended, necrosis and perforation are possible.

Unusual presentations of intussusception in neonatal patients have been reported. Intrauterine intussusception is associated with the development of intestinal atresia and can rarely be associated with a lead point as a Meckel's diverticulum.[22, 23] When associated with a history of constipation and intussusception in the newborn period, the diagnosis of long segment Hirschsprung's disease or intestinal neuronal dysplasia should be considered.[24, 25] If the intussusception develops postnatally in the premature infant, the diagnosis is most often confused with the more common condition of necrotizing enterocolitis.[26, 27] Symptoms in reported cases included marked abdominal distention, bilious emesis, and blood per rectum without radiographic evidence of pneumatosis intestinalis or signs of systemic toxicity. The diagnosis is delayed (up to 19 days in reported series) and usually considered when the intestinal obstruction does not resolve. Attempts at hydrostatic reduction are associated with an increased incidence of colonic perforations in this group of patients, and early surgical treatment is warranted as soon as the diagnosis is confirmed.

## DIAGNOSIS AND NONOPERATIVE TREATMENT

A high index of suspicion coupled with early diagnosis of intussusception may obviate the need for surgical intervention. The electrolyte pattern depends on the duration of symptoms, degree of dehydration, and the frequency of vomiting. Laboratory findings usually show an elevated white blood cell count (commonly >10,000 mm$^3$). Erect and recumbent plain abdominal radiographs are obtained and often demonstrate a variety of findings, including a nonspecific bowel gas pattern, an ileus, the presence of a soft tissue mass, an empty sigmoid or rectum, a clearly obstructive small bowel pattern, or rarely, free air consistent with a bowel perforation in cases with delayed diagnosis.

A nasogastric tube is inserted and intravenous fluid resuscitation is initiated before obtaining radiologic studies to confirm the diagnosis and attempting reduction of the intussusception. Once the infant's condition is stable and adequate hydration is assured, sedation may be safely used (if required) prior to attempted reduction (Table 38–2). Because intussusception represents an intestinal obstruction, most surgeons routinely administer broad-spectrum antibiotics before any reduction attempts. When possible, the surgeon should be present to observe the actual procedure, and the operating room staff is also notified so that the transition from the radiology suite to the surgical theater is expeditious in instances in which the hydrostatic reduction of the intussusception is unsuccessful.

### Barium Enema Reduction

The "gold standard" procedure for diagnosis and treatment of idiopathic ileocolic intussusception remains the hydrostatic barium enema popularized by Ravitch in the early 1930s. The risk of bowel perforation during the procedure varies from 1% to 3% depending on the series reviewed.[3, 4, 15, 28, 29] Precautions include maintaining the height of the barium column at no more than 3 feet above the infant's

**TABLE 38–2. Suggested Sedation Protocol for Reduction Attempts**

| | |
|---|---|
| Secobarbital | 1.0 mg/kg IM |
| Morphine (>1 year) | 0.1 mg/kg IM |
| Meperidine | 1.0 mg/kg IM |
| Promethazine | 0.5 mg/kg IM |

chest, limiting the constant hydrostatic pressure to periods of no more than 5 minutes, and avoidance of excessive abdominal manipulation during the procedure. The presence of an intraluminal colonic mass with a "coiled spring" appearance confirms the diagnosis of intussusception. A satisfactory reduction is noted when the intussusception passes retrograde through the ileocecal valve and there is free reflux of barium into the last 2 feet of the distal ileum (Fig. 38–1). If significant progress in moving the intussusceptum proximally is noted, reduction can be attempted again. The supplemental use of glucagon, which relaxes colonic smooth muscle, has not been effective in a randomized multi-center double-blind study of 30 patients. This study reported no difference between the successful rate of reduction in children receiving a placebo or glucagon.[30, 31] Hydrostatic barium enema reduction is successful in 50% to 80% of cases, depending largely on the duration of symptoms and the referral pattern of the institution.[5, 9, 15, 32, 33] The success rate is reduced if symptoms have been present longer than 48 hours (50%) versus less than 48 hours (70%). Bowel perforations are documented in 0.5% to 2.4% of the attempted reduction studies.[15, 33–35] When perforation is noted, it often occurs at the point of the uninvolved intussuscipiens (usually the transverse colon) when no excessive pressure has been used during the procedure. The mesenteric vascular arcade system between the ileocolic and right colic vessels may be incomplete in some children, and the arterial supply to the transverse colon may be compromised before the region ever becomes involved as the actual intussusceptum. As the back pressure from venous and lymphatic obstruction exceeds the arterial inflow pressure, full-thickness necrosis of the surrounding bowel wall can occur with minimal hydrostatic pressure during the radiologic studies. This group of children tend to be younger than 6 months of age, are ill for more than 72 hours, and have evidence of a complete bowel obstruction noted on the initial abdominal radiographs.[12, 34, 35] In these high-risk cases, the barium study should be used only to confirm the diagnosis without attempting therapeutic reduction. In our last 209 patients with intussusception, two perforations occurred during attempted hydrostatic reduction (both in the transverse colon), and one child presented with free intraperitoneal air and was found to have a transverse colon perforation at laparotomy.

## Air Reduction

Air reduction techniques have gained popularity as an alternative to the barium or water-soluble hydrostatic methods.[36] The initial reports concerning air reduction were published in 1897, but large series were not reported until 1959.[37] With this method, the buttocks are securely taped together, and a catheter with an anal seal device allows for the controlled insufflation of the colon with air under fluoroscopic guidance. Precautions taken during the procedure include using a maximum insufflating pressure of less than 120 mm Hg, limiting reduction attempts to 3 minutes' duration, and using three successive attempts. Reflux of air into the terminal ileum and the disappearance of the mass at the ileocecal valve document a successful reduction (Fig. 38–2). If the completeness of reduction is questioned, the air study can be repeated or water-soluble contrast can be instilled to confirm the free retrograde flow of material into the small bowel.[38] Using the air reduction technique in more than 6,000 patients, Jinzhe and associates from China reported successful reduction of intussusception in 95% of cases; other reports document a somewhat lower reduction rate.[39–42] The perforation rate varies from 0.14% to 0.2% (compared with 0.5–2.4% with hydrostatic techniques).[38–41] Additional advantages of air reduction include lower radiation exposure and decreased patient cost. When perforations are noted (free air on an upright or lateral decubitus abdominal radiograph obtained at the end of the procedure), the colonic wall tears are smaller than those observed with the hydrostatic barium techniques, peritoneal spillage tends to be minimal, and barium peritonitis is avoided. In instances

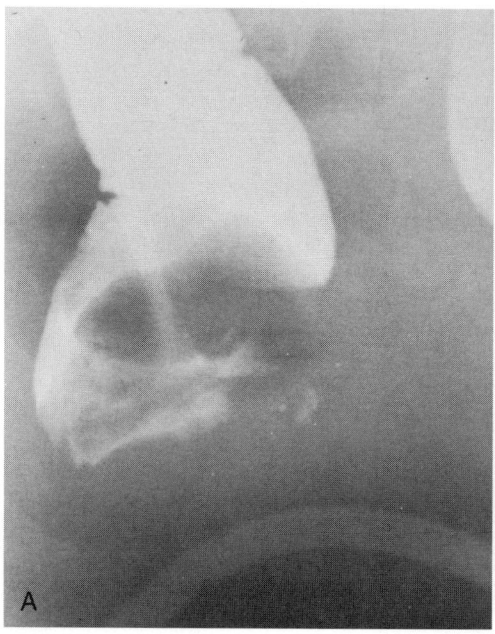


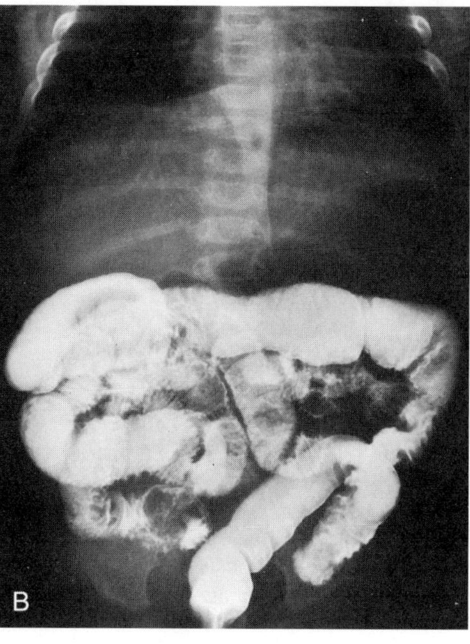


**FIGURE 38–1.** *A,* As an example of incomplete reduction of the intussusception, there is no free flow of barium into the small bowel noted on this study. *B,* Complete reduction is ensured with free flow of contrast flowing into the several feet of terminal ileum.

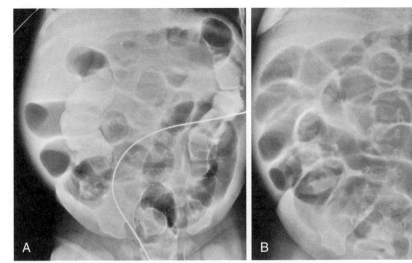

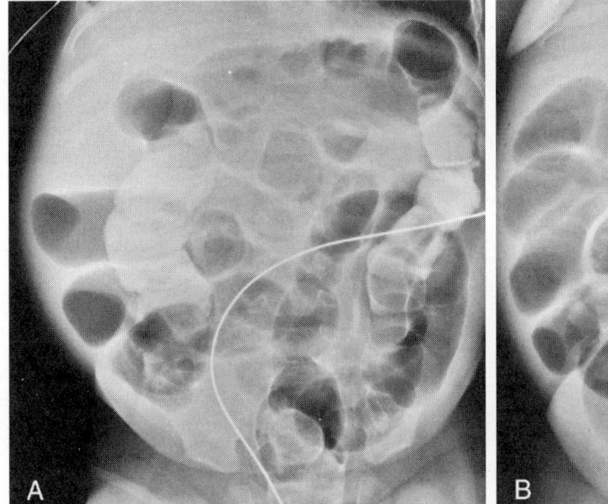


**FIGURE 38–2.** *A,* Using water-soluble contrast, the diagnosis of an ileocolic intussusception is confirmed in this 8-month-old with dilated and proximal small bowel loops. *B,* Reduction of the intussusceptum noted with the retrograde insufflation of air in the terminal ileum.

of perforation, if the amount of free intraperitoneal air compromises the cardiorespiratory status of the patient during the transfer to surgery, needle decompression of the abdomen can be safely accomplished.

In the clinically stable patient, a delayed second attempt (up to 3 hours later) can be attempted with an initial partial reduction and may be successful in half the cases in avoiding laparotomy.[36, 43, 44] These second attempts have been performed both in the radiology suite and in the operating room under a general anesthesia.

## Ultrasound-Guided Reduction

Ultrasonography can be a sensitive diagnostic treatment tool when used in conjunction with hydrostatic reduction or insufflation techniques.[45, 46] The diagnostic findings include a tubular or pseudokidney appearance of the mass in longitudinal views and a "doughnut" or "target" appearance in the transverse images.[47] The echogenic central area with the concentric circles represents the intussusception; the edematous wall of the intussusception is noted by the surrounding lucency (Fig. 38–3). The invaginated mesentery will appear echogenic as well.[43]

Hydrostatic reduction of the intussusception under ultrasound guidance has gained popularity as well.[33] In this method, water-soluble medium is used, and satisfactory reduction is noted with the disappearance of the intussusceptum at the ileocecal valve, retrograde flow of contrast into the small bowel, and the collapse of the previously distended right colon.[48, 49]

Ultrasound-guided water enema (USWE) is another technique used in the treatment of intussusception. The water height may be 4 to 5 feet above the table to generate a pressure of 120 mm Hg at the level of the intussusception, and ultrasound is used to monitor the reduction process.[50] Successful reduction is confirmed by the findings of water and bubbles in the terminal ileum, a water-distended terminal ileum, and the absence of the previous intussusception on the post-evacuation ultrasound images. Two to three attempts lasting 5 to 10 minutes are often required.[51]

In a series of 46 patients matched for age and duration of symptoms, the hydrostatic use of isotonic Hartmann's solution was successful in reducing 71% of the intussusceptions as compared with 55% in the barium enema group. Hartmann's solution may be able to more completely surround the intussusception, creating a more constant pressure head and allowing for the higher reduction rates noted. Three (11.6%) recurrences were noted in the ultrasound-guided group.[52]

## Post-Reduction Clinical Course

After the successful reduction of an ileocolic intussusception, temperature elevation higher than 38°C is often noted. Fever may result from the release of endotoxin, cytokines (tumor necrosis factor [TNF], interleukin [IL] -1, -6), or

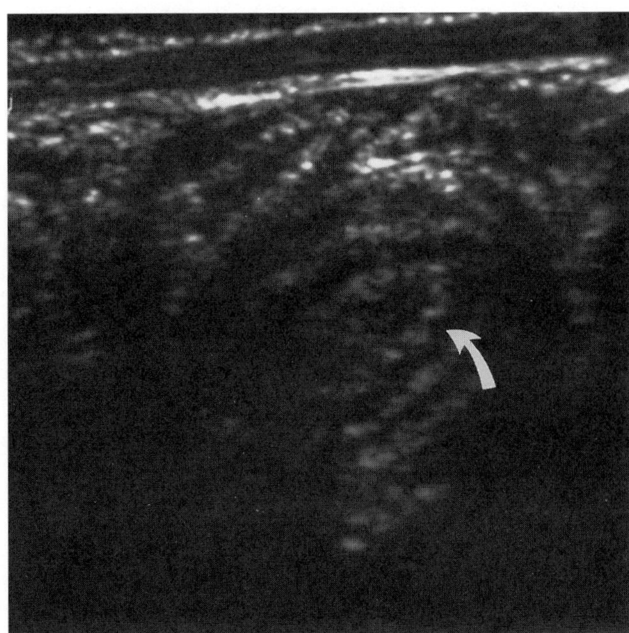

**FIGURE 38–3.** The ultrasound appearances of an intussusception is seen in cross section as a doughnut with concentric circles in the echodense center *(arrow).*

bacterial translocation. The incidence of positive blood cultures during and after nonsurgical reduction is very low.[53] Nasogastric suction is maintained until bowel function has returned and a normal bowel movement is passed. Feedings are advanced as tolerated, and most patients may be discharged from the hospital within 24 to 36 hours of reduction.[54] Recurrent intussusception may be noted in 8% to 12% of patients after radiologic reduction and may occur during the initial hospitalization or months later (4 hours to 2 years in our series).[15] If abdominal pain returns, a repeat diagnostic study is performed.[55]

## SURGICAL THERAPY

In children who have evidence of free peritoneal air on admitting abdominal radiographs, signs of peritoneal irritation, and prolonged symptoms (>5 days) at the time of clinical presentation, no attempt at hydrostatic barium reduction is made, and operation is planned after appropriate intravenous fluid resuscitation and the administration of broad-spectrum antibiotics.[12] In some patients in whom the radiologic reduction techniques have been unsuccessful, a complete reduction of the intussusception is noted at the time of laparotomy in 7% to 10% of reported cases.[12, 22, 33, 34] This may result from the relaxation of smooth muscles during induction of general anesthesia and spontaneous reduction of the intussusception. This may also represent cases of spontaneous reduction not related to anesthesia, because spontaneous reduction has been noted during ultrasound examinations.[55] In patients with spontaneous reduction at the time of laparotomy, the appendix is removed and the abdomen closed. If the mass is still present, the bowel is mobilized to allow identification of the site of intussusception. Manual reduction is attempted with the intussusceptum carefully being milked or squeezed proximally. If the mass cannot be completely reduced, a right hemicolectomy with end-to-end anastomosis is performed. Bowel resection may be necessary in 15% to 41% of cases in various reported series. When a pathologic lead point is identified, resection of the lesion is accomplished. When colonic perforations are encountered, the decision to perform a primary bowel anastomosis or temporary double-barrel ostomies depends on the hemodynamic status of the patient, extent of fecal soiling, and surgeon preference. Postoperative complications encountered include fever, prolonged ileus, wound infection, and intra-abdominal abscess (in cases of transverse colon perforations) (Table 38–3).

The incidence of recurrent intussusception after surgical reduction is extremely low, varying from 0% to 3%.[12, 33, 34] Significant patient morbidity, extended lengths of stay (Table 38–4), and increased hospital costs result from delay in diagnosis and referral for definitive treatment. Mortality, when it occurs, is related to sepsis, peritonitis, and hemodynamic instability.

**TABLE 38–3. Postoperative Complications in 209 Cases of Idiopathic Intussusception**

| | |
|---|---|
| Fever >38.5°C | 81 |
| Ileus >7 days | 9 |
| Wound infection | 9 |
| Pneumonia | 4 |
| Urinary tract infection | 2 |
| Ostomy stenosis | 2 |
| Wound dehiscence | 2 |
| Intra-abdominal abscess | 2 |
| Small bowel obstruction | 1 |

**TABLE 38–4. Length of Hospitalization Related to Type of Therapy for Intussusception**

| METHOD | MEAN DAYS | RANGE |
|---|---|---|
| Air reduction | 1.5 | 1–2 |
| Hydrostatic barium reduction | 1.5 | 1–4 |
| Intraoperative manual reduction | 4.2 | 2–29 |
| Bowel resection | 6.2 | 4–47 |

## POSTOPERATIVE INTUSSUSCEPTION

Postoperative intestinal obstruction is a well-recognized complication of abdominal surgery and is usually due to the formation of adhesions. A less well recognized cause is postoperative intussusception (POI), which differs from its idiopathic counterpart in its clinical presentation.[56, 57] In the patient with POI, the most frequent symptoms include bilious emesis, abdominal distention, and irritability.[57–66] Most episodes occur in the first postoperative week (contrasted with obstruction secondary to adhesions, in which symptoms present more than 14 days after surgery), and 75% of the children will have a return of bowel function after their initial procedure when the symptoms of an obstruction develop (Table 38–5). Abdominal radiographs reveal multiple air-fluid levels and a stepladder bowel pattern consistent with a mechanical small bowel obstruction. Over a 21-year period at J.W. Riley Hospital for Children (Indianapolis, IN), 48 patients with postoperative intussusception were encountered (Table 38–6). Seventeen of the children underwent the initial operative procedure for complications of gastroesophageal reflux or disordered esophageal motility. Fifteen of these children were neurologically impaired and included infants with Smith-Lemli-Opitz and Cornelia de Lange syndromes. As in most other series concerning POI, pathologic lead points were rarely found and accounted for

**TABLE 38–5. Initial Surgical Procedures Preceding Postoperative Intussusception (47 Cases)**

| | |
|---|---|
| Foregut motility | |
| Nissen fundoplication | 17 |
| Gastropexy | 1 |
| Heller myotomy | 1 |
| Neurocristopathy | |
| Neuroblastoma | 5 |
| Hirschsprung's disease | 5 |
| Small bowel resection | 5 |
| Inguinal herniorrhaphy | 3 |
| Urinary tract reconstruction | 3 |
| Thoracic procedures | 2 |
| Ventral hernia | 2 |
| Nephrectomy | 1 |
| Hepatic resection | 1 |
| Ventriculoatrial shunt | 1 |

**TABLE 38–6. Location of Lesion in Various Forms of Intussusception**

| | IDIOPATHIC (209 PATIENTS) | POSTOPERATIVE (48 PATIENTS) |
|---|---|---|
| Ileocolic | 195 | 5 |
| Ileo-ileal | 5 | 34 |
| Colocolic | 6 | 1 |
| Jejunojejunal | 3 | 6 |
| Jejunoileal | 0 | 2 |

only 3% of cases.[57–61] Although the etiology of POI is unknown, postulated causes of the invagination include a suture line, tumor implants on the bowel wall, appendiceal stumps, and Miller-Abbott tubes being removed with the balloon inflated. Other proposed causes for this form of intussusception include serosal damage during the previous operative procedure, which can lead to lymph node hypertrophy and may then act as a subsequent lead point for the process.[59, 67] Perhaps the serosal exudate may become fixed as an adhesion and prevents the spontaneous reduction of the small bowel intussusception that is often observed to occur spontaneously at the time of laparotomy.[65] Children with underlying conditions associated with disordered esophageal motility (e.g., gastroesophageal reflux, achalasia) may be at higher risk for POI.[57, 58, 63] A central nervous system component has also been implicated in this process, with the observation that stimulation of the premotor cortex in the brain of a *Macaca mulatta* primate model can induce the occurrence of a small bowel intussusception.[68] Other neuroendocrine factors have also been suggested, because children with neural crest abnormalities (Hirschsprung's disease, achalasia of the esophagus, and neuroblastoma) also appear to be at a greater risk for the occurrence of POI.[57, 58, 66]

Unlike infants and children with idiopathic ileocolic intussusception, diagnostic contrast studies are not as helpful in this group of patients because most cases of POI occur in the small bowel (see Table 38–6).[57, 58] In our experience, only five of the patients had the intussusceptum at the ileocecal valve, and the hydrostatic barium enema was successful in reducing the lead point in only three children. One child with Hirschsprung's disease had a right-sided colostomy, and the contrast was administered retrograde through the colostomy stoma to reduce the ileocecal lesion.[58] The most common opinion in the literature is that contrast studies are not helpful unless the diagnosis is uncertain and can be used to differentiate adynamic ileus from a mechanical obstruction. Laparotomy performed early in the clinical course of POI can obviate the need for segmental bowel resection and bowel anastomosis because most lesions can be manually reduced. Four of 41 children in this series required bowel resection. All four cases occurred more than 10 years ago, had a duration of symptoms ranging from 10 to 21 days (mean, 17), and had associated bacteremia or required mechanical ventilatory support and muscular paralysis after the initial surgical procedure. The postoperative complications encountered in POI patients included fever higher than 38.5°C (10), wound infection (4), pneumonia (4), prolonged ileus (4), urinary tract infection (2), and bacteremia (1). There were no deaths in this group of patients. As in the treatment of the more common idiopathic variety of intussusception, a prompt laparotomy prevents bowel necrosis and reduces the overall morbidity and mortality.

## REFERENCES


1. Barbette P: Oeuvres Chirurgiques et Anatomiques. Geneva, Francois Miege, 1674, p 522.
2. Hutchinson J: A successful case of abdominal section for intussusception. Proc R Med Chir Soc 1873;7:195–196.
3. Ravitch MM, McCune RM: Reduction of intussusception by hydrostatic pressure: an experimental study. Bull Johns Hopkins 1948;82:550–552.
4. Ravitch MM: Intussusception in infancy and childhood. N Engl J Med 1958;259:1058–1064.
5. Rosenkrantz JG, Cox JA, Silverman FN, et al: Intussusception in the 1970's: Indication for operation. J Pediatr Surg 1977;12:367–373.
6. Konno T, Suzuki H, Kutsuzawa T, et al: Human rotavirus infection in infants and young children with intussusception. J Med Virol 1982;2:265–269.
7. Mulcahy DL, Kamath KR, deSilva LM, et al: A two part study of the aetiological role of rotavirus in intussusception. J Med Virol 1982;9:51–55.
8. Nicholas JC, Ingrand D, Fortier B, et al: A one year urological survey of acute intussusception in childhood. J Med Virol 1982;9:267–271.
9. Freund H, Hurvitz H, Schiller M: Etiologic and therapeutic aspects of intussusception in childhood. Am J Surg 1977;134:272–274.
10. Montgomery EA, Pokek EJ: Intussusception, adenovirus, and children: a brief reaffirmation. Hum Pathol 1994;25:169–174.
11. Burchfield DJ, Rawlings D, Hamrick HJ: Intussusception associated with *Yersinia enterocolitica* gastroenteritis. Am J Dis Child 1983;137:803–804.
12. Hervás JA, Alberti P, Bregante JI, et al: Chronic intussusception associates with *Yersinia enterocolitica* mesenteric adenitis. J Pediatr Surg 1992;27:1591–1592.
13. Danis RK: Lymphoid hyperplasia of the ileum—always a benign disease? Am J Dis Child 1974;127:656–658.
14. Ein SH: Leading points in childhood intussusception. J Pediatr Surg 1976;11:209–211.
15. West KW, Stephens B, Vane DW, et al: Intussusception: current management in infants and children. Surgery 1987;102:781–787.
16. Holsclaw DS, Rocmans C, Shwachman H: Intussusception in patients with cystic fibrosis. Pediatrics 1971;48:51–58.
17. Ruoff M, Lindner AE, Marshak RH: Intussusception in sprue. AJR 1968;104:525–528.
18. Valletta EA, Mastella G: Incidence of celiac disease in a cystic fibrosis population. Acta Paediatr Scand 1989;78:784–785.
19. Cohen DM, Conard FU, Treem WL, Hyams JS: Jejunojejunal intussusception in Crohn's disease. J Pediatr Gastroenterol Nutr 1992;14(1):101–103.
20. Knowles MC, Fishman EK, Kuhlman JE, et al: Transient intussusception in Crohn's disease: CT evaluation. Radiology 1989;170:814.
21. Stringer MD, Homes SJK: Familial intussusception. J Pediatr Surg 1992;27:1436–1437.
22. Gherardi GJ, Fisher JH: Atresia of the small intestine produced by intussusception in utero. N Engl J Med 1961;264:229–231.
23. Senocak ME, Büyükpamakcu N, Hicsönmez A: Ileal atresia due to intrauterine intussusception caused by Meckel's diverticulum. Pediatr Surg Int 1990;5:64–66.
24. Kugelman A, Bader D, BarMaor JA, et al: Neonatal intussusception as a presenting sign of Hirschsprung's disease. Pediatr Surg Int 1996;11:500–501.
25. Till H, Schmittenbecher PP, Schmidt A, et al: Ileocolic intussusception: an unusual complication in a newborn with intestinal neuronal dysplasia. Pediatr Surg Int 1996;11:574–576.
26. Mooney DP, Steinthorsson G, Shorter NA: Perinatal intussusception in premature infants. J Pediatr Surg 1996;31:695–697.
27. Iuchtman M, Iurman S, Levin M: Neonatal intussusception diagnosed as necrotizing enterocolitis. Am J Perinat 1995;12:245–246.
28. Ravitch MM, McCune RM: Intussusception in infants and children. J Pediatr 1950;37:153–173.
29. Hirschsprung H: Et Tilfaelde at Subakut Tarminvagination. Hospitals-Tidende. 1976;3:321–322.
30. Hoy GR, Dunbar D, Boles ET: The use of glucagon in the diagnosis

and management of ileocolic intussusception. J Pediatr Surg 1977;6:939–944.
31. Franken EA, Smith WL, Chernish SM, et al: The use of glucagon in hydrostatic reduction of intussusception: a double blind study of 30 patients. Radiology 1983;146:687–689.
32. Lynn HB: Intussusception. In Holder TM, Ashcraft KW (eds): Pediatric Surgery, 5th ed. Philadelphia, WB Saunders, 1980, pp 438–444.
33. Bolia A: Case report: diagnosis and hydrostatic reduction of an intussusception under ultrasound guidance. Clin Radiol 1985;36:655–657.
34. Mercer S, Carpenter B: Mechanism of perforation occurring in the intussusception. Can J Surg 1982;25:481–483.
35. Ein SH, Mercer S, Humphrey A, et al: Colon perforation during attempted barium enema reduction of intussusception. J Pediatr Surg 1981;16:313–315.
36. Guo JB, Ma X, Ahou Q: Results of air pressure enema reduction of intussusception: 6,396 cases in 13 years. J Pediatr Surg 1986;21:1201–1203.
37. Fiorito ES, Recalde Cuestas LA: Diagnosis and treatment of acute intestinal intussusception with controlled insufflation of air. Pediatrics 1959;24:241.
38. Stringer DA, Ein SH: Pneumatic reduction: advantages, risks, and indications. Pediatr Radiol 1990;20:475.
39. Jinzhe Z, Yenxia W, Linchi W: Rectal inflation reduction of intussusception in infants. J Pediatr Surg 1986;21:30–32.
40. Hedlund GL, Johnson FJ, Strife JS: Ileocolic intussusception: extensive reflux of air preceding pneumatic reduction. Radiology 1990;174:187–189.
41. Shiels WE, Bisse GS, Kirks DR: Simple device for air reduction of intussusception. Pediatr Radiol 1990;20:472–473.
42. Palder SB, Ein SH, Stringer DA, et al: Intussusception: barium or air? J Pediatr Surg 1991;26:271–275.
43. Ein SH, Stephens CA: Intussusception: 354 cases in 10 years. J Pediatr Surg 1971;6:16–27.
44. Saxton V, Katz M, Phelan E, Beasley SW: Intussusception: a repeat delayed gas enema increases the nonoperative reduction rate. J Pediatr Surg 1994;29:588–589.
45. Stringer MD, Pablot SM, Breveton RJ: Paediatric intussusception. Br J Surg 1992;79:867–876.
46. Danemas A, Alton DJ: Intussusception issues and controversies related to diagnosis and reduction. Radiol Clin North Am 1996;34:743–756.
47. Swischuk LE, Hayden CK, Boulden T: Intussusception: indications for ultrasonography and an explanation of the doughnut and pseudokidney signs. Pediatr Radiol 1985;15:388–391.
48. Morrison SC, Stork E: Documentation of spontaneous reduction of childhood intussusception by ultrasound. Pediatr Radiol 1990;20:358–359.
49. Swischuk LE, Stansbury SD: Ultrasonographic detection of free peritoneal fluid in uncomplicated intussusception. Pediatr Radiol 1991;21:350–351.
50. Rohrschneider WK, Troge J: The post reduction donut sign. Pediatr Radiol 1994;24:156–160.
51. Choi SO, Park WH, Woo SK: Ultrasound guided water enemas: an alternative method of nonoperative treatment of childhood intussusception. J Pediatr Surg 1994;29:498–500.
52. Chan KL, Saing H, Peh WCG, et al: Childhood intussusception: ultrasound guided Hartmann's solution hydrostatic reduction or barium enema reduction? J Pediatr Surg 1997;32:3–6.
53. Somekh E, Serour F, Goncalves D, et al: Air enema for reduction of intussusception in children: risk of bacteremia. Radiology 1996;200:217–218.
54. Ein SH, Polder SB, Alton DJ, et al: Intussusception: toward less surgery? J Pediatr Surg 1994;29:433–435.
55. Prerio A, Donnell SC, Paraskevopoulou C, et al: Indications for laparotomy after hydrostatic reduction for intussusception. J Pediatr Surg 1993;28:1154–1157.
56. Wayer ER, Campbell JB, Burrington JD, et al: Management of 344 children with intussusception. Radiology 1973;107:597–601.
57. Mollitt DL, Ballantine TVN, Grosfeld JL: Postoperative intussusception in infancy and childhood: analysis of 119 cases. Surgery 1979;86:402–408.
58. West KW, Stephens B, Rescorla FJ, et al: Postoperative intussusception: experience with 36 cases in children. Surgery 1988;104:781–787.
59. Ein SH, Ferguson JN: Intussusception: the forgotten postoperative obstruction. Arch Dis Child 1982;57:788–790.
60. McGovern JB, Gross RE: Intussusception as a postoperative complication. Surgery 1968;63:507–513.
61. Cox JA, Martin CW. Postoperative intussusception. Arch Surg 1973;106:263–266.
62. Stevenson EO, Hays DM, Snyder WH: Postoperative intussusception in infants and children. Am J Surg 1967;113:562–567.
63. Jolley SG, Tunell WP, Hoelzer DJ, Smith EI: Postoperative small bowel obstruction in infants and children: a problem following Nissen fundoplication. J Pediatr Surg 1986;21:407–409.
64. Dudgeon DL, Hays DM: Intussusception complicating the therapy of malignancy in childhood. Arch Surg 1972;105:52–56.
65. Shaw A, Francois E: An unusual case of postoperative intussusception. Surgery 1966;59:455–457.
66. Cohen MO, Baker M, Grosfeld JL, et. al: Postoperative intussusception in children with neuroblastoma. Br J Radiol 1982;55:197–200.
67. Nissan S, Levy E: Intussusception in infancy caused by hypertrophic Peyer's patches. Surgery 1966;59:1108–1110.
68. Watts JW, Fulton JF: Intussusception—the relationship of the cerebral cortex to intestinal motility in the monkey. N Engl J Med 1934;210:883–896.

# Chapter 39

# Inguinal Hernia and Hydrocele

*Frederick Alexander*

Inguinal hernia is one of the more common surgical problems of infancy and childhood. It occurs in 0.8% to 4.4% of children[1]; however, in premature infants the incidence may increase to 30%, depending on the length of gestation.[2] The peak incidence occurs in the neonatal period, when the defect is also most likely to cause symptoms, usually related to incarceration and strangulation. The incidence declines with age but remains approximately six times higher in boys than in girls.[3]

Inguinal hernia usually manifests as an intermittent bulge in the groin that may extend into the scrotum or labia major with crying or straining. These findings contrast with the fluctuant scrotal swelling that is characteristic of a hydrocele. Because congenital inguinal hernias and hydroceles share a common origin (a patent processus vaginalis), they may be difficult to distinguish clinically and may occur together. Further, their management relative to the timing of surgery and contralateral exploration remains a point of controversy.

## HISTORY

Hernias were described in ancient times, but not until the early 19th century was the anatomy of the inguinal canal accurately described. Bassini[4] was the first author to describe the successful use of high ligation of the hernia sac in combination with anatomic repair in 1887. This concept was modified in 1899 by Ferguson,[5] who advocated incision of the external oblique fascia to improve surgical exposure. In 1950, Potts and coworkers[6] recommended simple high ligation and removal of the hernia sac for routine hernia repair in children, and this procedure has become the standard of care.

## EMBRYOLOGY AND PATHOGENESIS

The processus vaginalis is a tubular extension of the peritoneal membrane that passes through the internal ring and into the scrotum during the third month of gestation. This membrane surrounds the testis and gubernaculum and probably contributes to testicular descent in the seventh month of gestation by downward transmission of intra-abdominal pressure.[7] The processus vaginalis usually is obliterated some time after testicular descent is complete, although the timing and mechanism of closure are unknown. Failure of the processus vaginalis to obliterate is the most common cause of inguinal hernia and hydrocele in infants and children. However, autopsy studies have shown that the processus vaginalis may remain patent in a larger number of asymptomatic children and adults,[8, 9] suggesting that other factors also may be involved. For example, an increase in abdominal pressure or fluid may play an important role in the clinical development of a hernia or a hydrocele. Ascites from any cause, or placement of a ventriculoperitoneal shunt or a peritoneal dialysis catheter in a formerly asymptomatic patient, frequently leads to the development of a clinical hernia or hydrocele.

## CLINICAL PRESENTATION

Incomplete obliteration of the processus can lead to a variety of clinical presentations (Fig. 39–1). Closure of the processus may occur at any point between the internal ring and the scrotum, leading to various degrees of herniation into the inguinal canal. The processus vaginalis may remain open into the scrotum, forming a complete inguinal hernia. The processus vaginalis may close incompletely along its longitudinal axis, leading to fluid accumulation in the scrotum or a hydrocele. If the processus remains open sufficiently to allow bidirectional movement of fluid, the result is a *communicating hydrocele*, which usually fluctuates in size. Late obliteration of the processus may entrap fluid within the tunica vaginalis surrounding the testis, resulting in a *noncommunicating hydrocele.*

Usually the child with a hernia presents with a history of intermittent pain or swelling of the groin. Incarceration occurs when a segment of intestine becomes entrapped within the hernia sac. Incarceration often produces bilious vomiting and obstipation and is a common cause of small bowel obstruction in infants and children who have not had prior surgery. Therefore, an incarcerated inguinal hernia should be highly suspected in any child with signs of intestinal

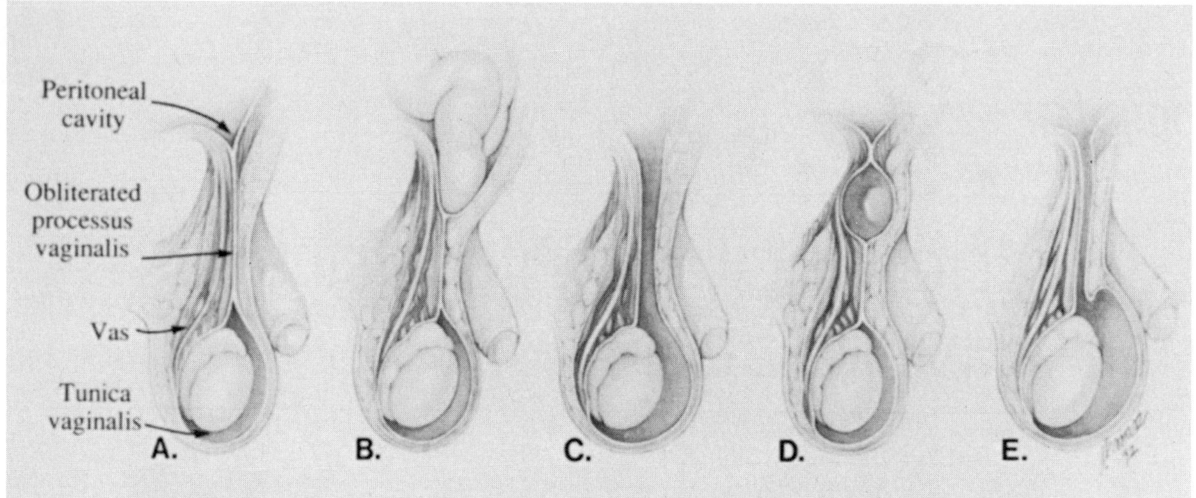


**FIGURE 39–1.** Spectrum of anatomic abnormalities of the processus vaginalis. *A,* Normal anatomy. *B,* Inguinal hernia. *C,* Complete hernia. *D,* Hydrocele of the cord. *E,* Communicating hydrocele.

obstruction. When incarceration leads to diminished circulation within the herniated viscus, strangulation with ischemic necrosis may result. In its late stages, strangulation may produce erythema and edema overlying a tender groin mass. In contrast, children with hydroceles usually present with asymptomatic scrotal swelling.

Examination of a child for inguinal hernia or hydrocele may be facilitated by placing the child in an upright position or by encouraging straining or coughing. The scrotum may be inverted into the distal inguinal canal over the thumb or forefinger in order to detect a groin mass. Manual palpation of the groin and scrotum often reveals the significant findings described previously. It is important to palpate both testicles within the scrotum, because an undescended or retractile testis may often pose as a groin mass. Usually, gentle pressure applied bimanually in a cephalad and posterior direction results in sudden reduction of an inguinal hernia. Reduction of the hernia may be confirmed by simultaneous palpation of the contralateral groin, which should feel absolutely symmetric after reduction of the hernia.

Transillumination is the hallmark of a hydrocele, and hydroceles frequently fluctuate in size, becoming less prominent at night when the child is sleeping. If scrotal swelling is reduced by gentle caudal pressure, leaving the scrotum decompressed and symmetric with the contralateral side, then the presence of a hydrocele has been confirmed. Occasionally it may be difficult to distinguish between an incarcerated hernia and a loculated hydrocele of the cord, particularly in premature or neonatal infants. Both conditions may transilluminate and may be irreducible; however, a hydrocele of the cord is otherwise asymptomatic, whereas an incarcerated hernia is usually tender and associated with intestinal symptoms. Failure to reduce a hernia after administration of intramuscular morphine sulfate or meperidine, or a plain radiographic film of the abdomen that reveals signs of small bowel obstruction or a gas bubble below the inguinal ligament, indicate an incarcerated hernia. If the clinician is unable to distinguish an incarcerated hernia (Fig. 39–2) from a loculated hydrocele, surgical exploration is recommended.

In some instances, a bulge in the groin is seen by the parents or pediatrician but is not apparent on examination. In this setting, the findings of thickening of the cord at the ring or an associated hydrocele may suggest the presence of a hernia. Otherwise, the surgeon may accept the diagnosis based on the description or may re-evaluate the child during a second visit.

## MANAGEMENT

Inguinal hernias should be repaired promptly after the diagnosis is made to prevent incarceration. Although the overall risk of incarceration is unknown, this risk is much higher during the first year of life. Rowe and Clatworthy[10] found that two thirds of incarcerated hernias occur in children younger than 1 year of age and that two thirds of these children required surgical reduction. Given proper technique and adequate sedation, most children may now undergo manual reduction and thus avoid the anesthetic hazards of emergency surgical reduction.

If manual reduction is easily and promptly accomplished, the child may be discharged and scheduled for elective outpatient surgery. In the more difficult cases, successful manual reduction should be followed by admission and subsequent elective hernia repair before discharge from the hospital. In those infants and children with hernias who are hospitalized for unrelated severe or life-threatening problems, hernia repair is best deferred until the primary problem is resolved. In premature infants, repair is often deferred until just before discharge from the neonatal intensive care unit, so that the child may be observed closely for postoperative apnea and bradycardia.

Hydrocele, in contrast to inguinal hernia, frequently resolves spontaneously during the first 2 years of life. Noncommunicating hydroceles in infancy often resolve spontaneously, and even communicating hydrocele may resolve during the first 12 to 18 months of life (Fig. 39–3). Therefore, in the absence of a hernia, it is prudent to observe a hydrocele for at least 18 months before recommending surgical repair. If the hydrocele shows no signs of resolution

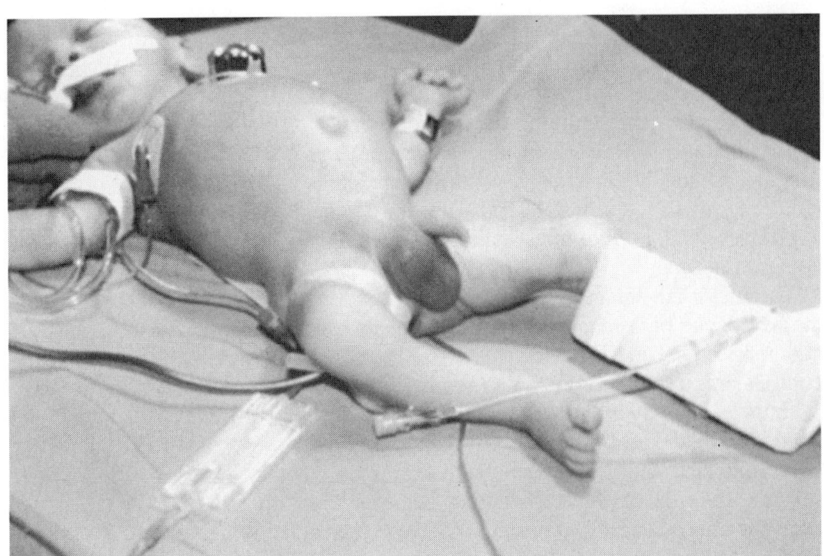

**FIGURE 39–2.** Typical appearance of an incarcerated hernia in a premature infant before surgical reduction and repair.

between 18 and 24 months of life, then surgical repair should be recommended. Since a persistent hydrocele in this setting is most likely to be communicating, the repair must be performed through the groin and must include a high ligation of the processus vaginalis. The distal portion of the hydrocele sac should be trimmed with care so as not to injure the testis or structures of the cord.

Surgical repair of hernias and hydroceles in children is usually performed under general anesthesia as an outpatient procedure. A transverse skin incision is made within the skin crease, midway between the symphysis pubis and the anterior iliac crest. This incision is carried down through Scarpa's fascia, exposing the external oblique fascia. The external oblique is then opened, exposing the inguinal canal and the structures of the cord. At this point, the cremasteric muscle is gently separated, exposing the hernia sac, which always lies anterior to the structure of the cord. The hernia sac is gently dissected away from the structures of the cord and is then divided and traced to its origin at the internal ring, where it is ligated and amputated. The distal sac may be trimmed but not completely removed, because removal is unnecessary and even hazardous. In a premature infant, or in any child with an associated undescended testicle, orchiopexy must be performed in connection with the hernia repair. Sliding hernias are rare in children and may include the appendix, salpinx, or Meckel's diverticulum (Littre's hernia) as part of the hernia sac. In this situation, the structure must be carefully dissected away from the wall of the sac before high ligation is performed. When exploration is carried out for incarceration, the incarcerated viscera should be carefully inspected for signs of ischemic necrosis and, if none are found, subsequently reduced. As a general rule, if an incarcerated hernia can be manually reduced successfully before surgery, it is unnecessary to inspect the intestine at the time of the subsequent hernia repair.

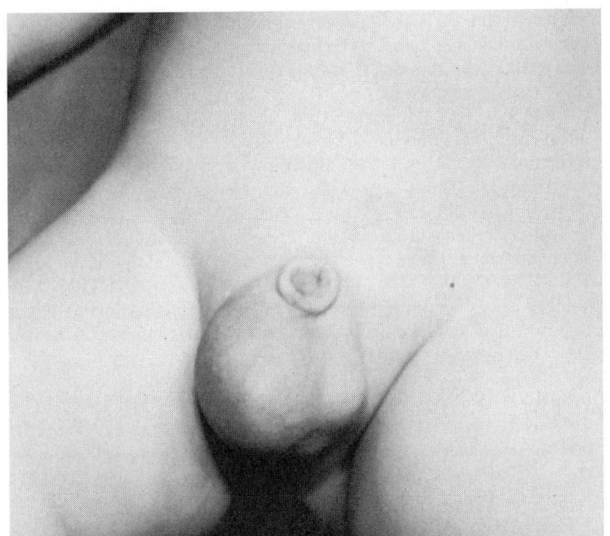

**FIGURE 39–3.** Typical appearance of a hydrocele, which frequently regresses by 2 years of age.

There has been considerable controversy regarding the issue of contralateral exploration. Many surgeons[11–13] have reported a high incidence of contralateral inguinal hernia or patent processus vaginalis when routine contralateral groin exploration is carried out in children with a unilateral, clinically apparent inguinal hernia. For example, Gilbert and Clatworthy[14] concluded that it was justifiable to perform a bilateral inguinal hernia repair in any healthy infant or child with a unilaterally apparent hernia, irrespective of age, sex, or side involved.

On the other hand, Sparkman,[15] in a large review, found that although a contralateral patent processus vaginalis may be found in 50% to 60% of all infants and children, unilateral hernia repair was followed by the subsequent development of a contralateral hernia in only 15% to 20% of the operated group. Bock and Sobye[16] reported only a 15% incidence of contralateral hernia in a group of 174 children who underwent unilateral hernia repair and were monitored for 27 to 36 years. More recently, Given and Rubin reported a 5.6% occurrence of contralateral hernia after unilateral hernia repair in 904 children.[17] Surana and Puri[18] found that a contralateral hernia developed in 10% of 165 infants (aged 1 week to 6 months) an average of 6 months after unilateral hernia repair. Finally, in a review of 2,764 infants and children,

Rowe and colleagues[19] found a contralateral patent processus vaginalis in 63% within 2 months, and 41% at 2 years of age. From these reports, it would appear that the contralateral processus vaginalis obliterates near the time of birth in approximately 40% of cases, and during the first 2 years of life in another 20%. After 2 years of age, almost 40% of children still have a contralateral patent processus vaginalis, but fewer than half of these children develop a clinically apparent hernia.

The major advantage of routine contralateral exploration is the avoidance of a second operation, with its associated cost and risk of anesthesia. The major disadvantages of routine contralateral exploration include the possibility of a technical mishap leading to infertility (a minimal risk in experienced hands) and increased cost and postoperative pain.

A number of studies[16, 20, 24–26] have examined whether age, sex, or the side of the hernia may be used to predict the need for contralateral exploration. Of these factors, only age has any relation to the risk of development of a contralateral hernia. Bock and Sobye[16] found that 47% of children whose primary hernia was repaired before the age of 1 year developed a contralateral hernia, compared with only 11% of those whose primary hernia was repaired after the first year of life. These data suggest that routine contralateral exploration may be justified during the first year of life, but not in older children. Several studies[16, 20] have shown a slightly increased risk of contralateral hernia when the clinically apparent hernia appears on the left side as compared with the right; however, these findings are disputed by other studies in which little or no difference was found.[24, 25] Finally, Bock and Sobye[16] found that the incidence of contralateral hernia in girls who underwent unilateral hernia repair was only 8%. Therefore, sex and the side of the clinical hernia may not reliably predict the existence of a contralateral hernia.

Some surgeons have advocated the use of laparoscopy to evaluate the contralateral processus vaginalis. Laparoscopy is quick and safe, and it requires no additional incisions. Its chief advantage is that it is much more accurate than clinical examination in determining patency of the contralateral processus vaginalis. However, most reports[21–23] indicate a patency rate of 30% to 40%, which greatly overestimates the actual risks of occurrence of a contralateral clinical hernia.

## COMPLICATIONS

According to Rowe and Lloyd,[27] the overall rate of complications after elective hernia repair is approximately 2%, increasing to 19% after repair of incarcerated hernia. With continued technical improvements and advances in pediatric anesthesia and neonatal intensive care, the incidence of perioperative complications should approach 1% or less. The risk of postoperative complications is higher in the premature infant, in whom intraoperative and postoperative respiratory complications are directly related to anesthetic care. Postoperative apnea caused by immaturity of the diaphragm or intercostal muscle or abnormal responses to hypoxia and hypercapnia is not uncommon in premature infants. Therefore, Rowe and Lloyd[27] recommended that premature infants with inguinal hernia undergo repair before they are discharged from the neonatal unit, allowing them to be closely monitored after surgery. Premature infants younger than 1 year of age who develop inguinal hernia while at home should be admitted for overnight observation after inguinal hernia repair, and the use of apnea monitors in this group of patients is highly recommended.

## REFERENCES


1. Bronsther B, Abrams MW, Elboim C: Inguinal hernias in children: a study of 1,000 cases and review of the literature. J Am Med Womens Assoc 1972;27:522–525.
2. Harper RG, Garcia A, Sia C: Inguinal hernia: a common problem of premature infants weighing 1,000 grams or less at birth. Pediatrics 1975;56:112–115.
3. Holder TM, Ashcraft KW: Groin hernias and hydroceles. In Holder TM, Ashcraft KW (eds): Pediatric Surgery. Philadelphia, WB Saunders, 1980, pp 594–608.
4. Bassini E: Nuovo metodo per la cura radicale dell'ernia inguinale. Atti Congr Assoc Med Ital Pavia 1889;2:179–182.
5. Ferguson AH: Oblique inguinal hernia: typical operation for its radical cure. JAMA 1899;33:6–14.
6. Potts WJ, Riker WL, Lewis JE: The treatment of inguinal hernia in infants and children. Ann Surg 1950;132:566–576.
7. Shrock P: The processus vaginalis and gubernaculum. Surg Clin North Am 1971;51:1263–1268.
8. Morgan EH, Anson BJ: Anatomy of region of inguinal hernia: the internal surface of parietal layers. Q Bull Northwester Univ Med School 1942;16:20–37.
9. Snyder WH Jr, Greaney EM Jr: Inguinal hernia. In Welch KJ, Ravitch MM, O'Neill JA, et al (eds): Pediatric Surgery, 2nd ed. Chicago, Year Book Medical Publishers, 1969, pp 692–700.
10. Rowe MI, Clatworthy HW: Incarcerated and strangulated hernias in children. Arch Surg 1970;101:136–139.
11. McLaughlin CW Jr, Kleager C: Management of inguinal hernia in infancy and early childhood. Am J Dis Child 1956;92:266–271.
12. Mueller B, Rader G: Inguinal hernia in children. Arch Surg 1956;73:595–596.
13. Rothenberg RE, Barnett T: Bilateral herniotomy in infants and children. Surgery 1955;37:947–950.
14. Gilbert M, Clatworth HW Jr: Bilateral operations for inguinal hernia and hydrocele in infancy and childhood. Am J Surg 1959;97:255–259.
15. Sparkman RS: Bilateral exploration in inguinal hernia in juvenile patients. Surgery 1962;51:393–406.
16. Bock JE, Sobye JV: Frequency of contralateral hernia in children. Acta Chir Scand 1970;136:707–709.
17. Given JP, Rubin SZ: Occurrence of contralateral inguinal hernia following unilateral repair in a pediatric hospital. J Pediatr Surg 1989;24:963–965.
18. Surana R, Puri P: Is contralateral exploration necessary in infants with unilateral inguinal hernia? J Pediatr Surg 1993;28:1026–1027.
19. Rowe MI, Copelson LW, Clatworthy HW: The patent processus vaginalis and the inguinal hernia. J Pediatr Surg 1969;4:102–107.
20. Clausen EG, Jake RJ, Bingley FM: Contralateral inguinal exploration of unilateral hernia in infants and children. Surgery 1958;44:735–740.
21. Holcomb GW, Morgan WM, Brock JW: Laparoscopic evaluation for contralateral patent processus vaginalis: part II. J Pediatr Surg 1996;31:1170–1173.
22. Pellegrin K, Bensard DD, Karrer FM, et al: Laparoscopic evaluation of contralateral patent processus vaginalis in children. Am J Surg 1996;172:602–605.
23. Wulkan ML, Wiender ES, VanBalen N, Vescio P: Laparoscopy through the open ipsilateral sac to evaluate presence of contralateral hernia. J Pediatr Surg 1996;31:1174–1176.
24. Kiesewetter WB, Parenzan L: When should hernia in the infant be treated bilaterally? JAMA 1959;171:287–290.
25. Fischer R, Mumenthaler A: 1st bilateral herniotomic bei Saiiglingen und Klein Kindern mit einseitiger Leistenhernia angezeigt? Helv Chir Acta 1957;24:346–350.
26. Wright JE: Inguinal hernia in girls: desirability and dangers of bilateral exploration. Aust Paediatr 1982;18:55–57.
27. Rowe MI, Lloyd DA: Inguinal hernia. In Welch KJ, Randolph JA, Ravitch MM, et al (eds): Pediatric Surgery, 3rd ed. Chicago, Year Book Medical Publishers, 1986, pp 779–793.

# Chapter 40

# Meckel's Diverticulum and Other Omphalomesenteric Duct Remnants

*Marshall Z. Schwartz*

The omphalomesenteric duct, or vitelline duct, represents remnants of the embryonic yolk sac. The persistence of portions of this in utero structure results in the most common postnatal anomalies of the gastrointestinal tract. The most frequently occurring residual of the yolk sac is a diverticulum arising from the antimesenteric border of the distal ileum, which has come to be known as Meckel's diverticulum. Knowledge of omphalomesenteric duct remnants is important because the complications related to these structures are numerous and may be life-threatening.

## HISTORY

An unusual diverticulum of the small intestine was first described in 1658 by Hildanus[1] and again described in 1672 by Lavater.[2] Ruysch[3] illustrated this anomaly in 1701. However, it was not until the early 19th century that Sir Johann Freidrich Meckel first published his observations on the anatomy and embryology of this ileal diverticulum.[4] As a result of this landmark paper, this anomaly bears his name.

## INCIDENCE

It is estimated that a remnant of the embryonic yolk sac remains in 1% to 4% of all infants, making this the most common congenital gastrointestinal anomaly.[5–9]

The distribution and frequency of omphalomesenteric duct remnants is shown in Table 40–1. Among Meckel's diverticula found incidentally at surgery or at autopsy, the sex ratio is approximately equal.[5] However, it appears that pathology related to a Meckel's diverticulum more frequently develops in males than in females, with a ratio of 3:1.[5, 10] This is related, in part, to a male preponderance of intussusception from a Meckel's diverticulum acting as the lead point. Although the incidence of omphalomesenteric duct remnants (especially Meckel's diverticulum) is high, the risk for development of symptoms from these anomalies is relatively low. According to Soltero and Bill,[7] the risk of developing a complication from a Meckel's diverticulum is approximately 4%. Development of symptoms from a Meckel's diverticulum appears to be more likely in childhood: 80% of all surveyed patients requiring surgery were younger than 10 years of age, and almost half of these patients were younger than 2 years of age.[11, 12]

## EMBRYOLOGY AND ANATOMY

During the first and second weeks after fertilization, the yolk sac arises from and dominates the ventral surface of the embryo. The embryo is sustained by the nutrient-filled yolk sac until the placental unit is established. A portion of the yolk sac becomes incorporated into the ventral wall of the primitive gut. Shortly thereafter, the connection between the embryo and the yolk sac narrows and lengthens to develop into the omphalomesenteric or vitelline duct. Be-

**TABLE 40–1. Distribution and Frequency of Omphalomesenteric Duct Remnants**

| | PERCENTAGE OF CASES | |
|---|---|---|
| TYPE OF REMNANT | Moses[9] (N = 1,605) | Soderlund[6] (N = 413) |
| Meckel's diverticulum | 82 | 86 |
| Patent omphalomesenteric duct | 6 | 2.4 |
| Solid cord | 10 | — |
| Umbilical remnant | 1 | 1.2 |
| Cystic remnant | 1 | 0.24 |

tween the fifth and seventh weeks of gestation, the omphalomesenteric duct attenuates, involutes, and separates from the intestine.[5] Just before this separation, the epithelium of the yolk sac develops an appearance similar to that of the gastric lining.[5] Partial or complete failure of involution of the omphalomesenteric duct results in various residual structures, depending on the stage at which this process fails to progress. That portion of the omphalomesenteric duct that does not become atretic persists and grows and develops along with the remainder of the gastrointestinal tract. Persistent patency of the omphalomesenteric duct is determined by the 10th week of gestation.[5] If the distal end of the omphalomesenteric duct remains attached to the umbilical cord, a fistula results (Fig. 40–1*A*). If the distal end retracts from the umbilicus, a diverticulum results (Fig. 40–1*D*). The diverticulum may remain attached to the undersurface of the umbilicus by a solid cord, either as a residual from the yolk sac (Fig. 40–1*C*) or the vitelline vessels (Fig. 40–1*B*).

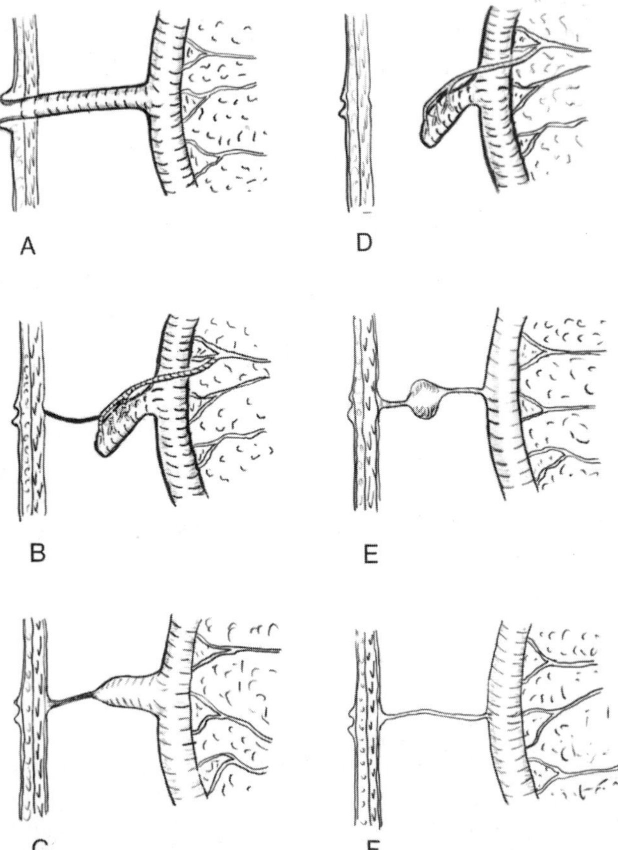


**FIGURE 40–1.** Illustrated are some of the more common abnormalities that result from the embryonic yolk sac, as follows: *A,* Patent omphalomesenteric duct representing a communication from the terminal ileum to the umbilicus. *B,* Meckel's diverticulum with a patent right vitelline artery as blood supply to the Meckel's diverticulum and a residual of the vitelline artery illustrated as a cord to the undersurface to the umbilicus. *C,* Meckel's diverticulum with a cord connecting the tip of the Meckel's diverticulum to the undersurface of the umbilicus. The cord (band) represents the distal residual of the omphalomesenteric duct. *D,* Typical appearance of a Meckel's diverticulum with persistence of the vitelline artery. *E,* Involution of the proximal and distal ends of the omphalomesenteric duct with residual cord or band and central preservation of the omphalomesenteric duct resulting in a mucosa-lined cyst. *F,* Intraperitoneal band from the ileum to the undersurface of the umbilicus representing involution without resolution of the omphalomesenteric duct.

There are many abnormalities that result from remnants of the embryonic yolk sac. The numerous variations can be generally categorized as in the following sections.

## Patent Omphalomesenteric (Vitelline) Duct

A patent omphalomesenteric (vitelline) duct represents a persistent connection between the distal ileum and umbilicus and accounts for 2.5% to 6% of the spectrum of omphalomesenteric duct remnants.[6, 9] Males predominate by a ratio of 5:1.[6] Ectopic gastric mucosa is identified in approximately one third of the patients with a complete fistula.[6] Clinical presentation of this anomaly usually occurs in the first 1 to 2 weeks of life. After the natural atrophy and separation of the umbilical cord stump, drainage from the umbilicus occurs that has the appearance of intestinal contents. Inspection of the umbilicus reveals either an opening or a polypoid mass, which represents a limited prolapse of the patent omphalomesenteric duct. Confirmation of the diagnosis can be made by injection of contrast material into the opening of the sinus tract with resultant drainage of the contrast agent into the distal small intestine. Complications of a patent omphalomesenteric duct include prolapse through the umbilicus of the patent duct only or the duct and the attached ileum. This can lead to increased intestinal drainage through the opening or to a partial intestinal obstruction. Partial prolapse of the duct or ileum has been mistaken for an umbilical polyp and amputated, with significant adverse sequelae.

## Meckel's Diverticulum

The congenital abnormality of Meckel's diverticulum is the most common of the embryonic yolk sac remnants and represents at least 80% of all these anomalies.[6, 9] The diverticulum contains all three layers of the intestinal wall and is typically located within 40 to 50 cm of the ileocecal valve.[13] However, this distance is related to the age of the patient at the time of diagnosis. Meckel's diverticulum develops in a variety of shapes and lengths. The diverticulum originates from the antimesenteric border of the bowel and is typically 3 to 6 cm in length and slightly smaller than the diameter of the small intestine (Fig. 40–2). However, it can have a wide base, and the length can range from only 1 or 2 cm to more than 6 cm. Occasionally, a Meckel's diverticulum is attached to the undersurface of the umbilicus, to another portion of the abdominal wall, or to another segment of bowel by a fibrous cord. Of considerable significance is the presence of ectopic tissue within a Meckel's diverticulum. Although most Meckel's diverticula are lined with ileal mucosa, gastric, duodenal, and colonic mucosa have been described.[13] In addition, bile duct mucosa and ectopic pancreatic tissue have also been demonstrated in Meckel's diverticula.[13] Numerous studies have indicated that in symptomatic patients 40% to 80% of Meckel's diverticula contain ectopic tissue.[14–17] In most of these cases the ectopic tissue

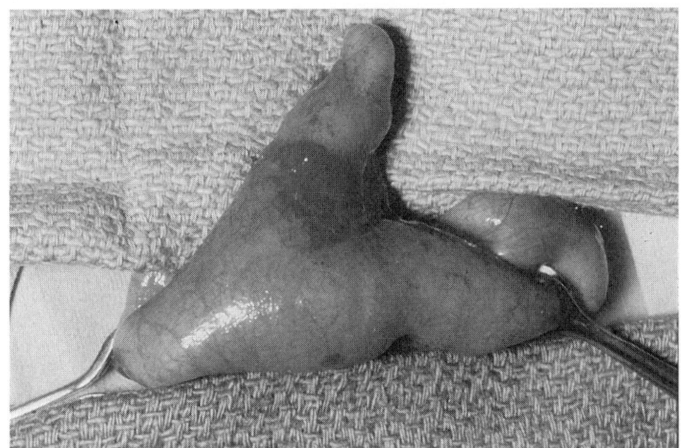

**FIGURE 40–2.** Typical appearance of a Meckel's diverticulum.

is gastric mucosa, with pancreatic tissue being the second most common finding.

### Omphalomesenteric Cyst

Involution of the omphalomesenteric duct at the umbilicus and at the ileal end can result in a mucosa-lined, cystic mass in either the intraperitoneal (see Fig. 40–1*E*) or the preperitoneal space. These cysts contain all three layers of the small intestine. Presentation of these cysts results from infection (particularly with preperitoneal cysts) or obstruction (with intraperitoneal cysts).

### Omphalomesenteric Duct Remnants at the Umbilicus

Omphalomesenteric duct remnants at the umbilicus are uncommon but, when present, they usually are identifiable within the first 1 to 2 weeks of life. Their presence usually is not evident until the umbilical stalk has atrophied and fallen off. What remains is a polypoid mass covered by mucosa at the umbilicus or a limited sinus that ends blindly. Omphalomesenteric duct remnants at the umbilicus are frequently confused with umbilical granulomas. Umbilical sinuses usually become evident because of persistent drainage at the umbilicus. The drainage is small in amount and does not have the typical appearance of intestinal contents. Treatment for both lesions is excision.

### Omphalomesenteric Band

An omphalomesenteric band results from involution of the omphalomesenteric duct but without disappearance of the tissue. As a result, a solid cord connecting the ileum to the undersurface of the umbilicus results (see Fig. 40–1*F*). This abnormality usually becomes evident as the cause of an intestinal obstruction. Diagnosis of these bands usually is made at the time of surgical exploration, either as an incidental finding or as a cause of a bowel obstruction.

### Vitelline Blood Vessel Remnants

Occlusion but failure of involution of vitelline blood vessel remnants also results in a fibrous cord within the peritoneal cavity. It may extend from the ileum or a Meckel's diverticulum to the undersurface of the umbilicus (see Fig. 40–1*B* and *F*). This remnant becomes clinically evident when it produces intestinal obstruction as a result of the twisting of a segment of a small intestine around the band.

## CLINICAL PRESENTATION

### Hemorrhage

Intermittent and painless bleeding per rectum is the most common presentation of a Meckel's diverticulum and therefore the most common presentation of all the variations of yolk sac remnants. The cause of the bleeding is peptic ulceration at the junction of the ectopic gastric mucosa and normal ileal mucosa. Acid production by the gastric mucosal parietal cells is not neutralized because of the absence of duodenal bicarbonate; thus, a "marginal" ulcer develops at the junction of the gastric and ileal mucosa. There is no relation between bleeding from a Meckel's diverticulum and *Helicobacter pylori*.[18] The bleeding can be excessive and dramatic if the erosion is at the site of the embryonic vitelline artery (see Fig. 40–1*B*). Although this bleeding may be massive, it usually is self-limiting because of contraction of the splanchnic vessels in response to hypovolemia. According to a study by Rutherford and Akers,[19] children younger than 2 years of age presenting with hemorrhage secondary to a Meckel's diverticulum had an average hemoglobin level of 6.6 mg/dL, whereas older children had an average hemoglobin level of 8.8 mg/dL. The typical appearance of the stool in patients with a bleeding Meckel's diverticulum is that of bright red blood, characterized as "current jelly" or "brick red" in appearance. Bleeding from a Meckel's diverticulum can also occur in an intermittent and less dramatic fashion, evidenced by tarry stools.

### Intestinal Obstruction

Complete or partial small bowel obstruction is the next most common clinical manifestation of a Meckel's diverticulum or other intraperitoneal omphalomesenteric duct remnant. The mechanism of obstruction can be by intraperitoneal bands, intussusception, internal herniation, or volvulus. The most common mechanism of obstruction is intussusception of a Meckel's diverticulum. The clinical presentation is similar to that of idiopathic intussusception. Most patients with this phenomenon are males, and it is most likely to appear in older children.[6] Other causes of intestinal obstruction usually are related to an intraperitoneal band as a residual of the omphalomesenteric duct itself or of the vessels associated with the duct. As noted previously, this fibrous band or cord can extend from a Meckel's diverticulum or from the antimesenteric border of the ileum itself. The presentation is typical of any patient with small bowel obstruction. The onset of bilious vomiting and abdominal distention is usually the heralding sign. Rarely is the cause of the partial or complete intestinal obstruction determined preoperatively in these patients. Obstruction can lead to strangulation, a life-threatening complication.

## Meckel's Diverticulitis

A Meckel's diverticulum can become the site of acute inflammation. The clinical presentation is almost identical to that of acute appendicitis. Rarely is the diagnosis of Meckel's diverticulitis made preoperatively. It is usually made at the time of exploration for acute appendicitis when a normal appendix is found, but only if the surgeon searches for a Meckel's diverticulum. As is the case with appendicitis, perforation in Meckel's diverticulitis occurs in approximately one third of cases.[7, 20] The mechanism of Meckel's diverticulitis is usually obstruction similar to appendicitis but may be peptic ulceration resulting in perforation. Apparently a more chronic form occurs, referred to as *Meckel's ileitis*, which can mimic the signs and symptoms of Crohn's disease.[21] Andreyev and colleagues[21] noted a higher incidence of Meckel's diverticulum in patients with Crohn's disease, but the significance of this finding is unknown.

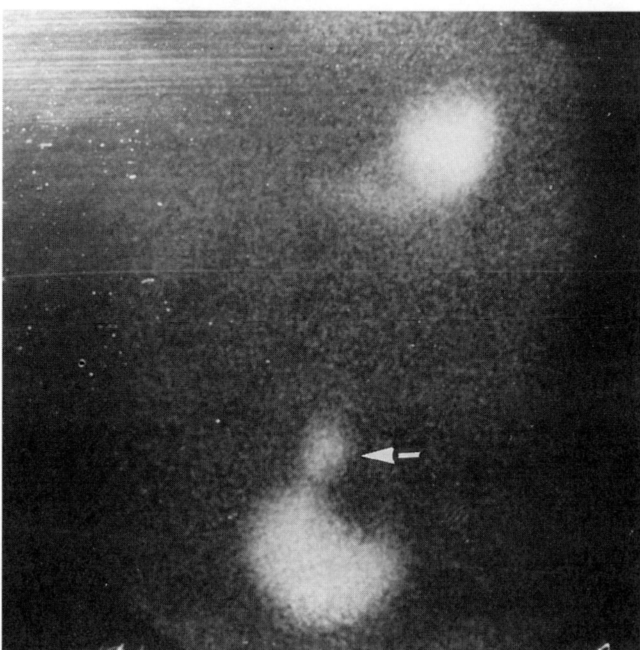

**FIGURE 40–3.** Typical appearance of a positive Meckel's scan with an area of increased uptake above the area of the bladder in the lower midabdomen *(arrow)*.

# DIAGNOSIS

Diagnosis of omphalomesenteric duct remnants depends on the clinical presentation. As noted previously, diagnosis of umbilical abnormalities usually can be made from the physical examination. In the absence of symptoms, diagnosis of a Meckel's diverticulum generally is not indicated. It is only when a Meckel's diverticulum or other intraperitoneal remnant of an omphalomesenteric duct produces symptoms that diagnosis becomes relevant. In an infant or child who presents with significant painless rectal bleeding, the presence of a Meckel's diverticulum should always be considered, although confirmation can be very difficult. Standard abdominal radiographs are of no value in the diagnosis of bleeding from a Meckel's diverticulum. Barium contrast studies, such as an upper gastrointestinal series with small bowel follow-through, rarely make the diagnosis of a Meckel's diverticulum.

In 1967 Harden and associates[22] described a technique using intravenous technetium 99m ($^{99m}$Tc) pertechnetate to visualize gastric mucosa, which has an affinity for this isotope. Because the cause of bleeding from a Meckel's diverticulum is most often ectopic gastric mucosa, Jewett and colleagues[14] applied this technique in 1970, and the study has now come to be known as a *Meckel's scan* (Fig. 40–3). The technique was further refined after it was noted that certain substances can enhance the visualization of the ectopic gastric mucosa; they include pentagastrin, glucagon, and histamine $H_2$ receptor blockers.[23–25] It was initially thought that the uptake of the $^{99m}$Tc isotope was by the gastric parietal cells. However, it was later demonstrated that the mucus-secreting cells of the gastric mucosa are responsible for the uptake.[26, 27] The availability of the Meckel's scan has significantly aided in the diagnosis of painless rectal bleeding in infants and children. However, this study has limitations, with a sensitivity of 85% and specificity of 95%.[23, 26] Therefore, a bleeding Meckel's diverticulum is not always visualized with this technique.

Superior mesenteric angiography has been used in patients with suspected bleeding from a Meckel's diverticulum.[28] The diagnosis is based on the demonstration of a branch of the ileocolic artery that represents a remnant of the right vitelline artery (see Fig. 40–1*B*). However, this study is rarely if ever indicated in the diagnosis of a Meckel's diverticulum.

An additional study that has been helpful in certain cases uses $^{99m}$Tc-labeled red blood cells. This nuclear medicine technique is not specific for a Meckel's diverticulum, but it can be used for localizing the site of bleeding in patients with intermittent and relatively low rates of bleeding.[29] Successful use of an in vitro, commercially available labeling kit has been reported.[30]

In patients who present with intestinal obstruction from an omphalomesenteric duct remnant, the cause of the obstruction is rarely determined preoperatively. Intussusception of a Meckel's diverticulum can produce symptoms and signs of intestinal obstruction or more vague symptoms. Diagnosis of this event can be difficult. Ultrasonography and computed tomography can be successful in visualizing an inverted Meckel's diverticulum.[31] Patients with obstruction from a Meckel's diverticulum require prompt surgical exploration to relieve the obstruction. Patients with inflammation of a Meckel's diverticulum also require prompt surgical exploration. Most often these patients undergo abdominal exploration with the preoperative diagnosis of appendicitis. However, one differentiating factor may be the presence of significant free intraperitoneal air. This radiographic finding is exceptionally rare in patients with perforated appendicitis, but it is not unusual in those patients with perforation of a Meckel's diverticulum. Laparoscopic surgery offers a new way to diagnose the presence of an omphalomesenteric duct remnant. However, it is routine to place the initial access port through the umbilicus, and there have been reports of injury to the bowel as a result of an omphalomesenteric duct remnant attached to the umbilicus.[32]

## TREATMENT

### Meckel's Diverticulum

Symptomatic Meckel's diverticula should always be removed. The surgical approach is generally through a right lower quadrant transverse incision. Adequate preoperative resuscitation with intravenous fluid and (if indicated) packed red blood cell transfusion is necessary. If the presenting problem is hemorrhage, the extent of the resection will depend on the extent of ectopic gastric mucosa within the Meckel's diverticulum. In general, the ectopic gastric mucosa is limited to the distal portion of the Meckel's diverticulum. However, in some circumstances the ectopic mucosa extends to the junction of the ileum or even into the ileum. Laparoscopy has been reported to be successful for both the diagnosis and surgical excision of a Meckel's diverticulum.[33, 34] In my opinion, this is not applicable in young children or when a bowel resection along with excision of the Meckel's diverticulum is indicated.

The surgical approach for intussusception induced by a Meckel's diverticulum is similar to that for the idiopathic variety. However, it is unusual for the cause of the intussusception to be known before laparotomy. The index of suspicion that a lead point is present should increase in children older than 2 to 3 years of age. If at exploration a Meckel's diverticulum is identified as the lead point, it should be excised.

Postoperative complications are uncommon after excision of a Meckel's diverticulum. Although a leak at the site of ileal closure and infection (either intraperitoneal or wound) can occur, these complications should not occur in more than 2% of cases.

Symptomatic Meckel's diverticula should be removed with care to avoid narrowing the ileal lumen. In the absence of ectopic tissue or a narrow base, asymptotic Meckel's diverticula do not need to be incidentally removed. An area of ongoing controversy is the approach to a Meckel's diverticulum found incidentally at the time of laparotomy for another reason. Some authors believe that a Meckel's diverticulum should always be removed when found.[5, 19, 35, 36] This is based on the potential risks of the complications of bleeding, perforation, obstruction, and the development of neoplasms. Those authors opposed to incidental diverticulectomy point to the low lifetime risk of development of symptoms related to the presence of a Meckel's diverticulum[11] and the risk of postoperative complications.[7, 37, 38]

### Patent Omphalomesenteric Duct

A patent omphalomesenteric duct should always be surgically excised from the junction of the umbilicus to its junction with the ileum. Care should be taken to remove all portions of the communication at the umbilicus to avoid subsequent complications.

### Omphalomesenteric Cyst

Frequently omphalomesenteric cysts manifest as an infected mass beneath the umbilicus. As previously noted, they are either preperitoneal or intraperitoneal. These cystic remnants can get quite large during the course of an infection, and an effort at excision at that time may be inappropriate. Incision and drainage followed by cyst excision after the infection has resolved would diminish the risk for complications.

## REFERENCES


1. Fabricius Hildanus: Opera observationum et curationum medico-chirurgicarum, quae extant omina, etc. Francof., J Beveri, 1646.
2. Lavater JH: De Εντεροπεριστολη seu intestinorum compressione. Basilae, 1672.
3. Ruysch F: Opera Omnia. Amsterdam, Jansson-Waesberg, 1757.
4. Meckel JF: Ueber die Divertikel am Darmkanal. Arch Physiol 1809;9:421–453.
5. Gray SW, Skanddalakis JE: Embryology For Surgeons. Philadelphia, WB Saunders, 1972, pp 156–167.
6. Soderlund S: Meckel's diverticulum, a clinical and histologic study. Acta Chir Scand Suppl 1959;118:1–233.
7. Soltero MJ, Bill AH: The natural history of Meckel's diverticulum and its relations to incidental removal. Am J Surg 1976;132:168–173.
8. Collins DC: A study of 50,000 specimens of the human vermiform appendix. Surg Gynecol Obstet 1955;101:137–145.
9. Moses WR: Meckel's diverticulum. N Engl J Med 1947;237:118–122.
10. Androulakis JA, Gray SW, Lionakis B, et al: The sex ratio of Meckel's diverticulum. Am Surg 1969;35:455–460.
11. Amory RA: Meckel's diverticulum. In Welch KJ, Randolph JG, Ravitch MM, et al (eds): Pediatric Surgery, 4th ed. Chicago, Year Book Medical Publishers, 1986, pp 859–867.
12. Gross RE: The Surgery of Infancy and Childhood. Philadelphia, WB Saunders, 1953, pp 212–220.
13. Yammaguchi M, Takeuchi S, Awazu S: Meckel's diverticulum: investigation of 600 patients in Japanese literature. Am J Surg 1978;136:247–249.
14. Jewett TC Jr, Duszynski DO, Allen JE: The visualization of Meckel's diverticulum with $^{99m}$Tc-pertechnetate. Surgery 1970;68:567–570.
15. Wansbrough RM, Thompson S, Leckey RG: Meckel's diverticulum: a 42-year review of 273 cases at the Hospital for Sick Children, Toronto. Can J Surg 1957;1:15–20.
16. Kiesewetter WB: Meckel's diverticulum in children. Arch Surg 1957;75:914–919.
17. Ludtke FE, Mende V, Kohler H, et al: Incidence and frequency of complications and management of Meckel's diverticulum. Surg Gynecol Obstet 1989;169:537–542.
18. Bemelman WA, Bosma A, Wiersman PH, et al: Role of *Helicobacter pylori* in the pathogenesis of complications of Meckel's diverticula. Eur J Surg 1993;159:171–175.
19. Rutherford RB, Akers DR: Meckel's diverticulum: a review of 148 pediatric patients, with special reference to the pattern of bleeding and to mesodiverticular vascular bands. Surgery 1966;59:618–626.
20. Seagram CGF, Louche RE, Stephens CA, et al: Meckel's diverticulum: a 10-year review of 218 cases. Can J Surg 1968;11:369–373.
21. Andreyev HJ, Owen RA, Thompson I, et al: Association between Meckel's diverticulum and Crohn's disease: a retrospective review. Gut 1994;35:788–790.
22. Harden RMcG, Alexander WD, Kennedy I: Isotope uptake and scanning of stomach in man with $^{99m}$Tc-pertechnetate. Lancet 1967;1:1305–1307.
23. Anderson GF, Sfakianakis G, King DR, et al: Hormonal enhancement of technetium-99m pertechnetate uptake in experimental Meckel's diverticulum. J Pediatr Surg 1980;15:900–905.
24. Khettery J, Effmann E, Grand RJ, et al: Effect of pentagastrin, histamine, glucagon, secretin, and perchlorate on the gastric hoarding of $^{99m}$Tc pertechnetate in mice. Radiology 1976;120:629–631.
25. Treves S, Grand RJ, Eraklis AJ: Pentagastrin stimulation of technetium 99m uptake by ectopic gastric mucosa in a Meckel's diverticulum. Radiology 1978;128:711–712.

26. Cooney DR, Duszynski DO, Camboa E, et al: The abdominal technetium scan (a decade of experience). J Pediatr Surg 1982;17:611–619.
27. Keramidas DC, Coran AG, Zaleska RW: An experimental model for assessing the radiopertechnetate diagnosis of gastric mucosa in Meckel's diverticulum. J Pediatr Surg 1974;9:879–883.
28. Okazaki M, Higashihara H, Yamasaki S, et al: Arterial embolization to control life-threatening hemorrhage from a Meckel's diverticulum. AJR Am J Roentgenol 1990;154:1257–1258.
29. Winzelberg GG, McKusick KA, Strauss HW, et al: Evaluation of gastrointestinal bleeding by red blood cells labeled *in vivo* with technetium 99m. J Nucl Med 1979;20:1080–1086.
30. Kwok CG, Lull RJ, Yen CK et al: Feasibility of Meckel's scan after RBC gastrointestinal bleeding study using in vitro labeling technique. Clin Nucl Med 1995;20:959–961.
31. Pantongrag-Brown L, Levine MS, Elsayed AM, et al: Inverted Meckel's diverticulum: clinical radiologic and pathologic findings. Radiology 1996;199:693–696.
32. Westcott CJ, Westcott RJ, Kerstein, MD: Perforation of a Meckel's diverticulum during laparoscopic cholecystectomy. South Med J 1995;88:661.
33. Schier F, Hoffman K, Waldschmidt J: Laparoscopic removal of Meckel's diverticula in children. Eur J Pediatr Surg 1996;6:38–39.
34. Sanders LE: Laparoscopic treatment of Meckel's diverticulum. Surg Endosc 1995;9:724–727.
35. Arnold JF, Pellicane JV: Meckel's diverticulum: a ten-year experience. Am Surg 1997;63:354–355.
36. Cullen JJ, Kelly KA, Moir CR, et al: Surgical management of Meckel's diverticulum: an epidemiologic, population-based study. Ann Surg 1994;220:564–568.
37. Kashi SH, Lodge JP: Meckel's diverticulum: a continuing dilemma? J R Col Surg Edinb 1995;40:392–394.
38. Mackey WC, Dinen P: A fifty-year experience with Meckel's diverticulum. Surg Gynecol Obstet 1983;156:56–64.

# Chapter 41

# Hirschsprung's Disease

Michael D. Klein and Randall S. Burd

## HISTORY

While Frederick Ruysch described what was probably a case of Hirschsprung's disease in 1691,[1] Harald Hirschsprung defined this syndrome with his report of two cases in 1887.[2] Ehrenpreis, in 1946, concluded that it was the distal bowel that was contracted that was abnormal.[3] Zuelzer and Wilson correlated the absence of ganglion cells with the syndrome that same year.[4] In 1948, Swenson published his observations, which agreed with those of Ehrenpreis but were based on manometric studies.[5] Swenson, however, went a giant step farther by performing an operation to resect the abnormal distal segment that corrected the problem.

## PATHOPHYSIOLOGY

The ganglion cells in the myenteric plexus of Auerbach and the submucosal plexus of Meissner, which were formerly intramural ganglia of the parasympathetic nervous system, are now classed as elements of an independent enteric nervous system (ENS).[6] The ENS is acted on by the central nervous system through the autonomic nervous system, which is made up of the sympathetic and parasympathetic nervous systems, which still have their own actions on the bowel. Neurochemical and endocrine substances have been measured in both the ganglionic and aganglionic bowel in Hirschsprung's disease and are summarized in Table 41–1.

In Hirschsprung's disease, ganglion cells are absent from the affected bowel. The resultant lack of parasympathetic (or enteric nervous system) stimulation leads to decreased relaxation of the intestinal sphincters. Unopposed sympathetic activity leads to increased intestinal tone.

The current theory of the pathophysiology of Hirschsprung's disease includes an absence of the inhibitory neurons of the ENS, which contain nitric oxide and vasoactive intestinal polpeptide. Normal colon has abundant nerve fibers staining for nicotinamide-adenine dinucleotide phosphate diaphorase (which represents nitric oxide synthase) whereas the aganglionic colon does not.[7–10] In addition to the contraction of abnormal bowel with loss of peristalsis, there is also a loss of the rectosphincteric reflex, so that a bolus presented to the rectum does not result in relaxation of the internal sphincter. This reflex appears to require the presence of normally innervated bowel above the rectum.[11] The aganglionic colon relaxes in response to nitric oxide,[12] but the internal sphincter does not. Cyclic guanosine monophosphate (produced by nitric oxide) relaxes both. Thus in the internal anal sphincter, the defect may be not only a lack of nitric oxide but also a lack of substrate for nitric oxide to produce cyclic guanosine monophosphate.[13]

The non-neural microenvironment has also been implicated in the etiology of Hirschsprung's disease.[14] Glial protein,[15] interstitial cells of Cajal,[16] smooth muscle cells,[17] and basal laminae[18] have all been reported to be abnormal in the aganglionic bowel.

## EMBRYOLOGY

The embryology of Hirschsprung's disease is still attributed to a failure of neural crest cells to migrate caudad along the vagus and enter the bowel wall. There is now, however, some evidence that there is also cranial migration of nerve cells from the sacral origins of what we still call the parasympathetic nervous system.[19] There is also some evidence that these embryologic events may have an immunologic origin.[20, 21]

## INCIDENCE AND GENETICS

Hirschsprung's disease has been estimated to occur in approximately 1:5000 live births with no racial predilection.[22–25] The male-to-female ratio found among patients with rectosigmoid disease is approximately 4:1, while the ratio is approximately 2:1 among patients with total colonic aganglionosis.[26] Although a family history of Hirschsprung's disease is found in 6% to 8% of patients,[27–30] more than 50% of patients with total colonic aganglionosis have an affected relative.[31] The risk of developing Hirschsprung's disease in siblings has been estimated at 4% and increases as the length of the aganglionic segment becomes more extensive.[32]

The gene for Hirschsprung's disease has been mapped to a locus between D10S208 and DS10S196 on chromosome 10q11.[2, 33] Hirschsprung's disease has also resulted from mutations of the *RET* gene (associated with multiple endocrine neoplasia types IIa and IIb) and the endothelin receptor type B gene on chromosome 13q22.[34] It has been estimated that as many as 80% of cases of Hirschsprung's disease are

**TABLE 41–1. Neurotransmitters in Hirschsprung's Disease**

| NEUROTRANSMITTER | NO CHANGE IN AGANGLIONIC BOWEL | INCREASED IN AGANGLIONIC BOWEL | DECREASED IN AGANGLIONIC BOWEL |
|---|---|---|---|
| Epinephrine | + | | |
| Dopamine | + | | |
| Alpha-adrenergic receptors | + | | |
| Neuron-specific enolase | + | | + |
| Protein S-100 | + | | + |
| Adrenergic neurotransmitters | | + | + |
| Responsiveness to acetylcholine | | + | + |
| Acetylcholin esterase (AChE) | | + | |
| Acetylcholine (ACh) | | + | |
| Neuropeptide Y | | + | |
| Vasoactive intestinal polypeptide (VIP) | | | + |
| Substance P | | | + |
| Gastrin-releasing peptide | | | + |
| Encephalin | | | + |
| Metenkephalin | | | + |
| Peptide histidine-leucine | | | + |
| Bombesin-like intestinal peptide | | | + |
| Pituitary adenylate cyclase-activating polypeptide | | | + |
| D7 immunoreactive protein (a Schwann cell antigen) | | | + |
| Nitric oxide synthase | | | + |
| Cyclic guanosine monophosphate | | | + |
| Endocrine cells | | + | |
| Chromogranin a | | + | |
| Synaptophysin | | + | |
| 5-Hydroxytryptamine | | + | |
| Peptide YY | | + | |
| Somatostatin | | + | |
| Neurofilament | | | + |
| Glial fibrillary acid protein | | | + |

due to genetic mutations and that these are autosomal dominant although with incomplete penetrance.[35]

Additional congenital problems are found in 11% to 30% of patients with Hirschsprung's disease.[14] The risk of anomalies appears to be higher the longer the length of the aganglionic segment. The most common association is with trisomy 21, which occurs in 4% to 13% of patients.[23, 30, 31, 36–39] Cardiac anomalies occur in 38% to 60% of patients with trisomy 21 and only 2% to 6% of unaffected patients.[25, 38, 39] Other associated anomalies include Waardenburg's syndrome, Smith-Lemli-Opitz syndrome, Ondine's curse, Von Recklinghausen's syndrome, type D brachydactyly, and multiple endocrine neoplasia type IIa.[40–45]

## CLINICAL PRESENTATION

The age at diagnosis of Hirschsprung's disease is younger than 1 month in 41% to 64% of patients, 1 month to 1 year in 21% to 35%, and older than 1 year in 15% to 26% of patients.[28, 30, 31, 37, 46] The diagnosis of Hirschsprung's disease is increasingly being made in the newborn period.[47] Only 4% to 8% of infants presenting with Hirschsprung's disease are premature.[26, 30, 37] A family history of this disease can be elicited in 3% to 17% of patients.[28, 30, 31, 37]

The clinical presentations of Hirschsprung's disease differ depending on the patient's age. The features of this disease in the newborn period include abdominal distention (32–90%), vomiting (18–67%), constipation (23%), and failure to pass meconium within the first 48 hours of life (37–51%).[30, 37] A bowel movement in the first 48 hours of life does not rule out Hirschsprung's disease.[47] Newborns often present with a clinical picture consistent with an acute intestinal obstruction including abdominal distention and bilious vomiting (see Chapter 12). Other infants may have infrequent stools and/or diarrhea with abdominal distention that is relieved by rectal stimulation or enemas. The diagnosis of Hirschsprung's disease should be considered in any infant with an unexplained perforation of the cecum or appendix.[48]

Some infants may have constipation that initially resolves and then subsequently recurs after several days to weeks. In older infants and children, the clinical features at presentation include constipation (68%), abdominal distention (64%), vomiting (37%), and a retrospective history of delayed passage of meconium (40%).[37] Constipation is a more common presenting symptom in older infants and children than in neonatal patients, in whom vomiting occurs more frequently. Because Hirschsprung's disease is a congenital anomaly, patients who appear in childhood or adolescence with Hirschsprung's disease in retrospect have had previous evidence of gastrointestinal dysfunction, including delayed passage of meconium, failure to thrive, or chronic constipation. Children with Hirschsprung's disease can be differentiated from patients with functional constipation by the absence of significant encopresis and frequently by the presence of abdominal distention and malnutrition.

## DIAGNOSIS

Although 85% of patients with Hirschsprung's disease have aganglionic bowel limited to the rectosigmoid area,

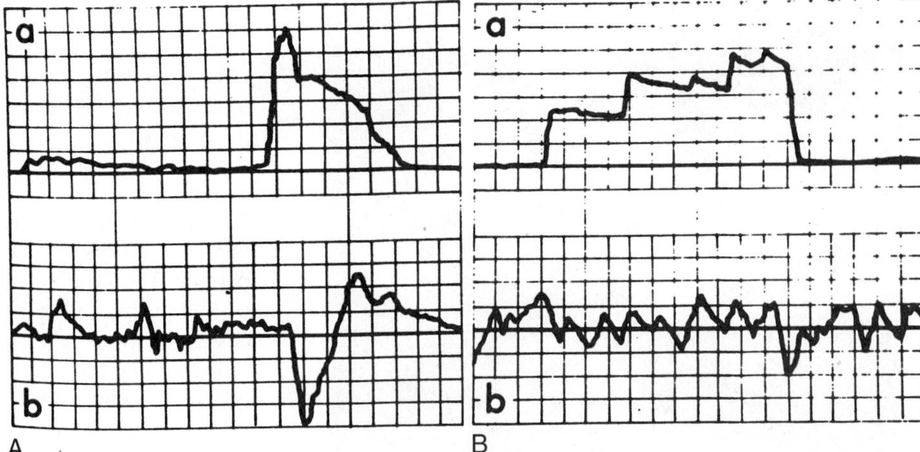


FIGURE 41–1. Pressure tracing from internal sphincter (b) and distending rectal balloon (a). *A*, Normal reflex with decrease in internal sphincter pressure as balloon is inflated. *B*, Abnormal reflex with no change in internal sphincter pressure as balloon is inflated.

many patients have longer segment or total colon involvement. With long-segment disease, patients usually present in the newborn period with intestinal obstruction. The barium enema may very well be nondiagnostic, and one must think of the diagnosis and perform a rectal biopsy.

## Manometry

By 12 days of life, the normal rectosphincteric reflex is present.[49] When a balloon is distended in the rectal ampulla, the internal sphincter relaxes and the external sphincter contracts. At an appropriate time, cortical input then relaxes the external sphincter so that defecation can occur. In Hirschsprung's disease, when a balloon is distended in the rectal ampulla, the pressure at the internal sphincter increases (Fig. 41–1). This abnormality of the rectosphincteric reflex is as much a part of Hirschsprung's disease as is the absence of ganglion cells.[50] The abnormal neurochemistry underlying the abnormality of the rectosphincteric reflex is similar to that in the rest of the affected bowel.[51] The findings on anorectal manometry are so characteristic that anorectal manometry has been used to establish the diagnosis in many centers.[52] Although some small series report no false-positive or false-negative results,[53–55] in large series the false-positive and false-negative rates are 5% and 25%, respectively.[56] Most of the errors are made in the newborn period.[57]

## Barium Enema

The rectum is normally the largest part of the large bowel (although occasionally the cecum may be just as large). In Hirschsprung's disease the rectum is small and may have tertiary (or uncoordinated) contraction waves noted. Thus, one should look at a lateral film taken during the filling phase of an unprepared barium enema to make the diagnosis. A previous rectal examination can obviate this finding. Other radiographic features of Hirschsprung's disease include the presence of a transition zone where the narrow aganglionic bowel joins the dilated ganglionic bowel and delayed evacuation on a plain film taken 24 hours later (Fig. 41–2). In total-colon Hirschsprung's disease there may be no transition zone, but often the colon is small and appears shortened with rounded flexures (Fig. 41–3), although the radiographic features are certainly variable.[58]

In constipated infants and children, Taxman and associates[59] found that 80% of infants with histologic aganglionosis had a barium enema that they interpreted as Hirschsprung's disease and 29% of those whose barium enema suggested

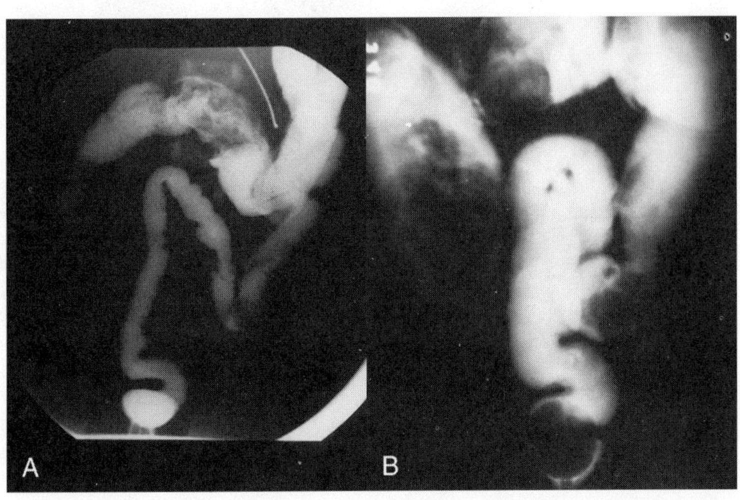


FIGURE 41–2. Barium enema showing small rectum and transition zone. *A*, Newborn with splenic flexure transition zone. *B*, Older child with low sigmoid transition zone. The finding of a small rectum is more subtle.

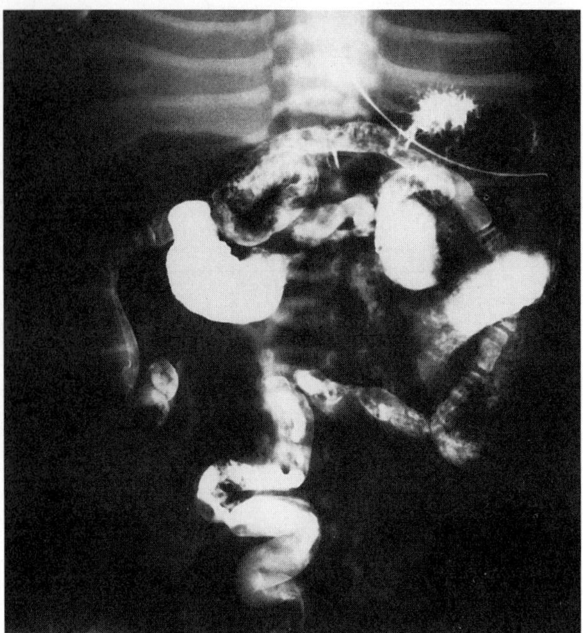

**FIGURE 41–3.** Barium enema of patient with total-colon Hirschsprung's disease. Contrast medium not in colon is from an initial upper gastrointestinal study for malrotation. Colon is shortened, and flexures are rounded.

Hirschsprung's disease had ganglion cells on biopsy. Kekomaki and coworkers[60] found a 10% error rate for barium enema. We found that barium enema was diagnostic in 92% of a series of newborns.[47]

## Suction Rectal Biopsy

Because the level of aganglionosis is the same in both the myenteric and submucosal plexuses, it is possible to make the diagnosis of Hirschsprung's disease by sampling only the submucosal plexus. This can be done with no anesthesia and few complications with a suction biopsy apparatus, introduced by Noblett,[61] that pulls some mucosa and submucosa into a small hole in the side of a metal capsule. The suction biopsy has the advantage that there is no full-thickness scar on the rectal wall when the surgeon is attempting to dissect the mucosa from the muscular coat of the bowel in a Soave procedure. Complications with this procedure are unusual, but perforations have occurred.[62] Andrassy and associates[63] in 444 patients and Lake and colleagues[64] in 168 patients reported no false-positive results and no false-negative results. For many, however, the procedure is not perfect. The specimen from the suction rectal biopsy varies in adequacy, and some have found that only in 80% of cases is sufficient tissue obtained.[65] Some pathologists have thought that the suction rectal biopsy is more difficult to interpret because the ganglia in the submucosal plexus are not as well identified. For this reason they rely on the acetylcholinesterase stain introduced by Meier-Ruge and coworkers.[66] In Hirschsprung's disease the regular neural network is absent and is replaced by hypertrophic nerves with no network.[67] They accompany blood vessels into the bowel wall.[68] These hypertrophic nerves are responsible for increased acelylcholinesterase in the aganglionic bowel (Fig. 41–4).

Park and associates[69] found a 97% accuracy using suction rectal biopsy and acetylcholinesterase staining while the same specimens with hematoxylin-eosin staining had only a 74% accuracy. Athow and coworkers found that the acetylcholinesterase-stained rectal suction biopsy specimen gave misleading results 10% of the time.[70]

## Full-Thickness Rectal Biopsy

Full-thickness rectal biopsy is considered the gold standard for the diagnosis of Hirschsprung's disease. It requires general anesthesia and some skill when performed in a newborn. Interpretation of the biopsy is not always straightforward. There is always a short segment above the anal valves where there are no ganglion cells, then they are infrequent, and by 3 cm they are normal. Nerves are present when there are no ganglion cells as they precede the ganglia (Fig. 41–5). Stratified squamous epithelium is present in the lower anal canal and on the lower surface of the anal valves.

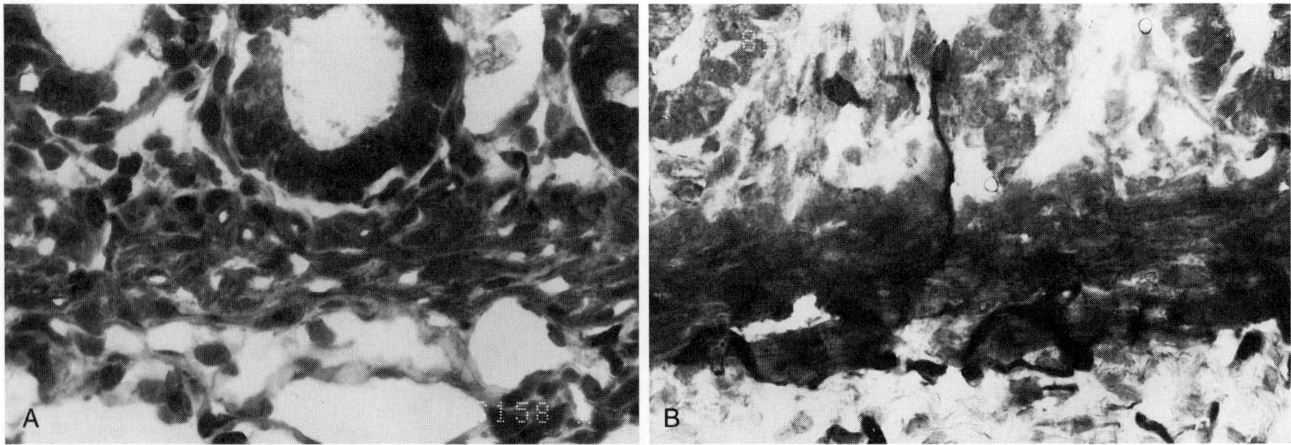


**FIGURE 41–4.** Photomicrograph of rectal biopsy specimen with silver nitrate staining. *A,* Normal ganglionic bowel does not stain for acetylcholine esterase. *B,* Hypertrophic nerves in aganglionic bowel stain for acetylcholine esterase (very dark areas).

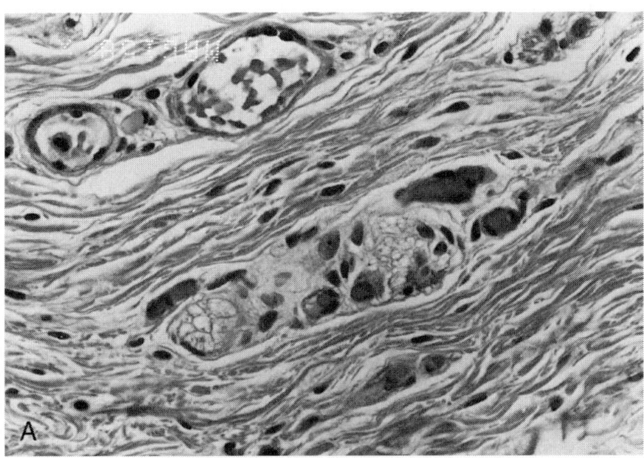


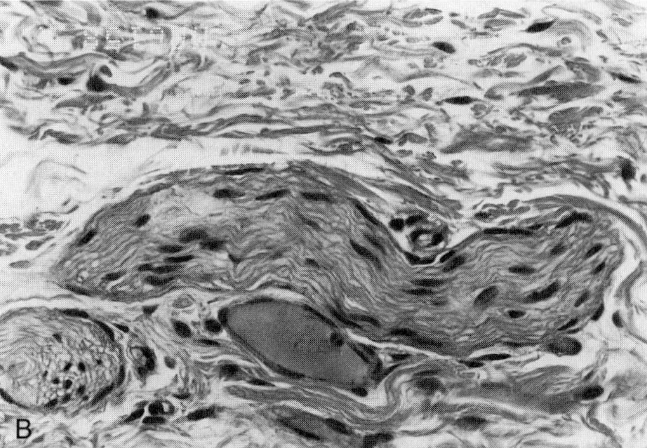


**FIGURE 41–5.** Photomicrograph of full-thickness rectal biopsy. *A*, Normal specimen with ganglion cells and few or no nerves. *B*, Specimen from a patient with Hirschsprung's disease. There are no ganglion cells, and there are hypertrophic nerves.

On the upper surface of the valves the epithelium is stratified columnar epithelium, and it changes to colonic mucus-secreting epithelium with crypts at a variable distance (about 2.3 mm). Finding the intermediate epithelium on biopsy indicates the biopsy specimen was taken from a hypoganglionic area. The specimen should be taken 1 to 2 cm above the anal valves in infants and at 3 to 4 cm above the valves in older children.[71, 72]

Although a suction rectal biopsy is less expensive and less painful than a barium enema, it is hazardous and unrewarding in the child older than 6 months to 1 year old. If the child does have constipation, the mucosa has usually become thick and engorged with blood vessels so that hemorrhage is a likely complication and it is much less likely that submucosa will be obtained. A barium enema will usually give the diagnosis, which can then be confirmed with a full-thickness biopsy and frozen section at the time of proposed colostomy. If symptoms persist despite a normal barium enema and appropriate treatment for constipation, one should consider ultra-short-segment Hirschsprung's disease (although we are not sure of the clinical importance of this entity). In ultra-short-segment Hirschsprung's disease, anorectal manometry is characteristic, showing absence of the normal rectosphincteric reflex, but normal ganglion cells are present througout the colon and anorectum.[73] Ganglion cells are normally absent this close to the anus, but some of the neurochemical features now associated with Hirschsprung's disease such as a lack of nitric oxide synthase–containing neurons have been demonstrated in the short segment.[74]

## DIFFERENTIAL DIAGNOSIS

In patients older than 3 months of age, the differential diagnosis usually includes only functional constipation. Patients with functional constipation may have encopresis or abdominal pain as presenting complaints. Active withholding may be obvious. Often there is a clear history of a period of normal bowel movements before the onset of bowel problems. On physical examination the perineum and underwear may be soiled and there is stool right down on the perineum. In Hirschsprung's disease there is rarely an unassisted bowel movement and defecatory problems usually have been present since birth. On physical examination, the rectum is small and contracted and stool is palpable only at the tip of the examining finger if at all.

In the newborn the differential diagnosis is somewhat longer. The presentation is usually that of intestinal obstruction: abdominal distention, emesis (often bilious), and failure to pass stool. Plain films reveal multiple distended loops of bowel so that other causes of low small bowel or colonic obstruction need to be considered: ileal atresia or stenosis, meconium ileus, intestinal duplication, colonic atresia, and incarcerated inguinal hernia. The barium enema is usually characteristic. Other forms of low small bowel obstruction in the newborn usually demonstrate a microcolon and have no transition zone. Small left colon syndrome and meconium plug syndrome probably represent the same underlying abnormality. This illness presents as multiple distended loops of bowel, often in the infant of a diabetic mother. Barium enema shows a small left colon with a transition zone to more dilated proximal colon, but it is differentiated from Hirschsprung's disease because the rectum is still the largest part of the large bowel. Usually the barium enema is curative and normal bowel movements follow.[75]

Other causes of functional bowel obstruction that affect the ENS and present with symptoms very similar if not identical to those of Hirschsprung's disease are less common. Intestinal neuronal dysplasia is characterized by hyperganglionosis rather than an absence of enteric ganglia. It has been reported in combination with Hirschsprung's disease.[76, 77] Other diagnoses include hypoganglionosis and microcolon-megagcystis-intestinal hypoperistalsis syndrome. In this latter syndrome, ganglia and nerve elements appear normal on electron microscopy, but severe degenerative changes are seen in the longitudinal and circular muscle layers.

## SURGICAL THERAPY

The general principle of operations for Hirschsprung's disease is to place bowel with normal peristalsis at the anus and to eliminate the tonic contraction of the internal sphincter. Swenson's first operative approach fulfilled the first principle by a total resection of aganglionic bowel from an abdominal approach staying on the wall of the rectum to avoid injury to nerves to the genitourinary organs. The diseased bowel is then everted out the anus and resected. Ganglionic bowel is then drawn through the very short anal stump and anastomosed on the perineum to the most distal anal canal. Swenson reported 200 patients treated with his operation in 1957 with good results.[78] In 1964 he reported to the American Surgical Association[79] that some of the patients had postoperative enterocolitis and occasionally some would have multiple episodes of enterocolitis. This could often be treated with internal sphincterotomy. He therefore reported in this paper a revision of the original operative procedure that provided for a resection of the colon anteriorly to 1.5 to 2 cm from the mucocutaneous junction and posteriorly to 1 cm from the mucocutaneous junction, thus doing a partial internal sphincterectomy. The Swenson procedure is currently the least popular but is still performed with excellent results (Fig. 41–6).[80, 81]

Another approach was reported in 1960 by Bernard Duhamel[82] (modified by Martin in 1967[83]). In this procedure, the ganglionic bowel is pulled down behind the aganglionic distal rectum and then anastomosed to it in a side-to-side fashion so that the anterior wall of the neorectum contains aganglionic tonically contracted bowel and the posterior wall contains normally contracting ganglionic bowel. The aganglionic bowel above the side-to-side anastomosis is resected. In at least one series there were fewer complications related to stenosis but more episodes of postoperative enterocolitis with this procedure.[26]

In 1964, Franco Soave[84] developed a third procedure (modified by Boley in 1968[85]) in which only the rectal mucosa is stripped out distally and the ganglionic bowel is pulled through the residual muscular cuff and then anastomosed to the anus at the columns of Morgagni. The presence of the remaining muscular cuff guides the ganglionic bowel precisely through the mechanisms of continence.

For many years the patient with Hirschsprung's disease required a colostomy at the time of diagnosis to allow the proximal bowel to recover from its dilated state before a pull-through procedure could be performed. Now diagnosis is made earlier, the proximal bowel is usually not so greatly dilated, and the primary pull-through or one-stage procedure is gaining in popularity. If the diagnosis can be made reliably, any of the three operations can be performed in a healthy full-term newborn.[81, 86]

The most recent innovation in the surgery of Hirschsprung's disease is the performance of the procedure using minimally invasive or laparoscopic techniques.[87] It may be that this approach will eventually be both less expensive and have less morbidity, although it is not yet clear that this is the case.

For children with long-segment or total-colon Hirschsprung's disease, water absorption can be improved by using the Martin modification of the Duhamel procedure and making a longer side-to-side anastomosis so that more colonic mucosa will be in the fecal stream.[88] Boley has described doing a Soave procedure and then anastomosing a long segment of aganglionic colon to the pulled-through ileum above the pelvic brim.[89, 90] Still others report that the Soave procedure with no modification is effective treatment for long-segment disease.[91]

When aganglionosis involves the entire intestine there is frequently little that can be offered other than total parenteral nutrition at home. There are no reports of intestinal transplantation for this problem. Ziegler and colleagues have reported some amelioration with a long myectomy of the involved bowel.[92]

Treatment for ultra-short-segment Hirschsprung's disease is a longitudinal posterior anorectal myectomy that essentially performs a sphincterectomy. The specimen can be examined to see if there is a definite transition zone low in the anus.

## ENTEROCOLITIS

Enterocolitis is a significant cause of morbidity and mortality in children with Hirschsprung's disease. Because this entity can occur any time during the treatment of these patients, it is important for all physicians treating patients with Hirschsprung's disease to recognize the signs and symptoms of enterocolitis and to initiate early and aggressive therapy when it occurs. Patients with enterocolitis initially present with abdominal distention, explosive diarrhea, vom-

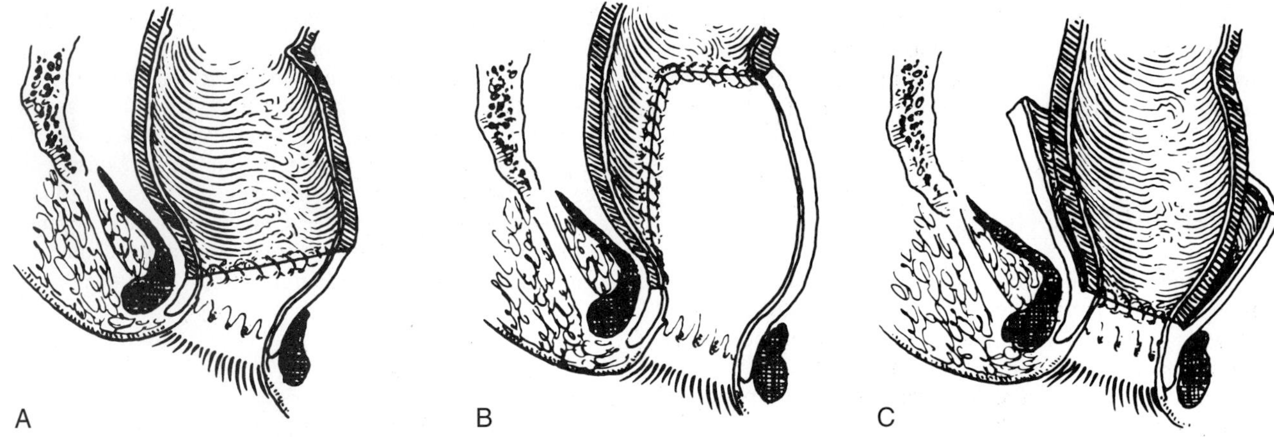


**FIGURE 41–6.** Operative procedures for the treatment of Hirschsprung's disease. *A*, Swenson procedure. *B*, Duhamel-Martin procedure. *C*, Soave-Boley procedure.

iting, fever, lethargy, rectal bleeding, colonic perforation, and/or shock.[93–95] They often have an explosive release of stool after rectal examination. In some patients, the initial presentation of Hirschsprung's enterocolitis may be mild and easily mistaken for viral gastroenteritis. Some patients may quickly become quite ill and even die unexpectedly despite aggressive attempts at resuscitation.[96] Laboratory studies may demonstrate electrolyte loss, hypoalbuminemia, metabolic acidosis, hemoconcentration, and/or leukocytosis. Abdominal radiograph findings (Fig. 41–7) may include small bowel or colonic dilatation, air-fluid levels, and gaseous intestinal distention with an abrupt cutoff at the level of the pelvic brim.[97]

Enterocolitis most often occurs after definitive pull-through procedure, 6% to 33% in some reports.[98] It is the initial presentation of Hirschsprung's disease in 10% to 24% of patients. Although the mortality associated with preoperative enterocolitis exceeded 30% in early reports,[99–101] later studies have described a mortality of 0% to 27%. After diverting enterostomy, 2% to 10% of patients can present with enterocolitis. Although enterocolitis occurs less commonly during this stage of treatment, patients with a diverting colostomy still need to be followed closely and treated aggressively when enterocolitis occurs.

Despite extensive experimental and clinical study, the etiology of Hirschsprung's enterocolitis has yet to be established. It is likely that it is multifactorial and that immunologic, microbial, and mechanical variables each contribute to the pathophysiology of this disease process. Several microbial agents have been suggested as etiologic agents in this disease, including *Clostridium difficile* and its toxin, enteropathogenic *Escherichia coli*, and rotavirus.[102–104] Enterocolitis has been associated with *C. difficile* pseudomembranous colitis even in the absence of antibiotic use.[105] Mechanical factors that may contribute to the onset of enterocolitis include the hypertonicity of the anal sphincter associated with Hirschsprung's disease, anal anastomotic stricture, cuff stenosis after the Soave pull-through procedure, and retained aganglionic segment. It has been hypothesized that mechanical factors may cause obstruction at the anal level leading to proximal intestinal dilatation with increased bacterial invasion.[96]

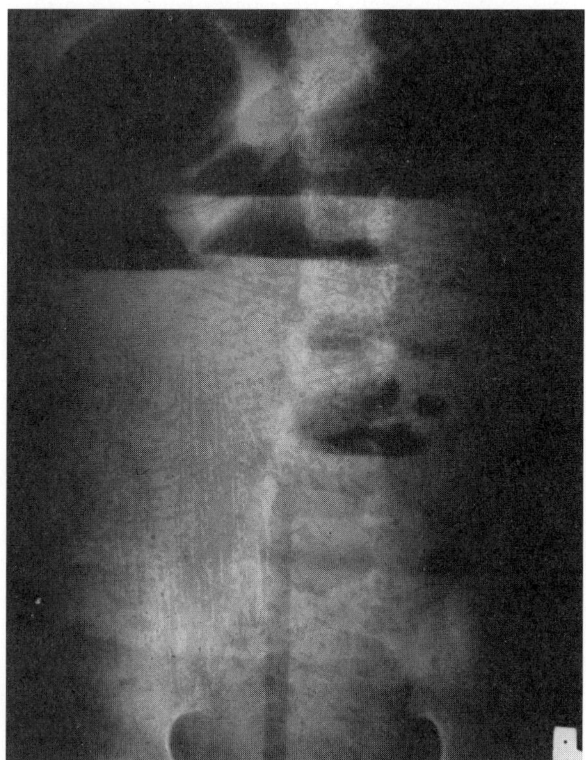

**FIGURE 41–7.** Plain film of a patient with Hirschsprung's enterocolitis.

To prevent the development of potentially life-threatening episodes of enterocolitis, parents should be educated about the signs and symptoms of enterocolitis and the need for rapid treatment should these occur. In addition to close follow-up of patients at risk for enterocolitis, severe enterocolitis may be avoided by rectal irrigations initiated at first symptoms or signs.

Hospitalization is recommended for any patient in whom enterocolitis is suspected. Patients with enterocolitis should be given nothing by mouth and undergo nasogastric decompression and intravenous hydration. A rectal decompression tube should be placed to open the hypertonic anal sphincter and decompress the distal intestinal segment. Stool samples should be sent for bacterial culture, assay for *C. difficile* toxin, and rotavirus testing. Abdominal radiographs should be obtained to help establish the diagnosis and exclude other potential causes of symptoms. Enterocolitis should be differentiated from viral gastroenteritis and postoperative complications including small bowel obstruction from adhesions, bowel perforation, anal anastomotic stricture, and constipation. An attempt should be made to evacuate any retained stool or air by using normal saline rectal irrigations. These patients should receive broad-spectrum intravenous antibiotics directed at enteric organisms. The addition of vancomycin to the rectal irrigation should be considered when *C. difficile* is suspected as a pathogen.

Patients with recurrent enterocolitis should be evaluated for a surgically correctable lesion that may be contributing to this disease. Previous pathologic specimens obtained at the time of the pull-through procedure should be re-examined to confirm the presence of ganglion cells in the pull-through segment. Rectal biopsy should be considered in patients with recurrent enterocolitis to rule out the rare occurrence of acquired aganglionosis. Procedures directed at relieving functional or mechanical obstruction may decrease the incidence of recurrent enterocolitis and should be considered in these patients. The procedure performed should be based on the findings observed on intestinal contrast study and the results of the rectal biopsy and may include anal dilatation under anesthesia, sphincterotomy, myectomy, revision of the pull-through procedure, or diverting enterostomy.

## Long-Term Results

Mishalany and Wooley[106] studied in detail a select group of 62 patients who had all three classic operations 1 to 30 years postoperatively. Half of the patients who had either the Duhamel or the Soave procedure and one third of those who had the Swenson procedure considered their stooling pattern normal; the rest complained of either loose stools or constipation. Half the patients from any of the three operative groups considered themselves completely continent. Enterocolitis occurred in 50% of patients after the Swenson procedure, in 33% after the Soave procedure, and in 21% after the Duhamel procedure.

In 1989, Sherman and colleagues reviewed 880 patients who underwent the Swenson procedure by pediatric surgeons in seven cities in Europe and North America.[107] The postoperative mortality was 2.4% and was related to Down syndrome, age, and leak at the colonic anastomosis. Follow-up averaged 10.3 years. There was no urinary incontinence or impotence. Fifty-two percent of the patients had some complication, either early or late enterocolitis. Rectal stricture occurred in 8%, usually requiring dilatation only. Temporary incontinence occurred in 13%. Twenty-two percent had postoperative enterocolitis. Ninety percent of the patients reported normal bowel habits, and 95% had no soiling.

At the James Whitcomb Riley Children's Hospital in Indianapolis, the mortality for Hirschsprung's disease was 6%.[30] Enterocolitis occurred in 18%. Long-term follow-up was available in 103 patients who had the Duhamel procedure. Sixty-five percent had normal bowel function, 27% required occasional enemas or stool softeners, and 8% had severe constipation or soiling. Bowel problems improved with time. Fifty-eight percent of patients were normal at less than 5 years, and 88% were normal at more than 15 years.

At the Children's Hospital of Michigan in Detroit, the incidence of postoperative enterocolitis is 0.67 episode per patient.[26] This is greatest with the Duhamel procedure (0.95), less with the Swenson procedure (0.60), and least with the Soave procedure (0.38). The complication rate, however (excluding enterocolitis and including stenosis requiring dilatation), was greater for the Soave (20%) than for the Duhamel (15%) procedures. Mortality has decreased from 19% in the 1960s to 6% in the 1980s, indicating that Hirschsprung's disease is still a life-threatening problem.

Marty and coworkers[31] reviewed 135 patients treated for Hirschsprung's disease at Primary Children's Medical Center in Salt Lake City between 1971 and 1993. The mortality rate was 6%, although only 3% was related to Hirschsprung's disease (enterocolitis). Postoperative complications occurred in 16%, and 27% experienced postoperative enterocolitis. Thirty-two percent reported some soiling postoperatively, and in 13% this was a severe problem. The severe soiling was 7% after the Soave procedure and 12% after the Duhamel procedure. There was no urinary incontinence or impotence.

Moore and associates interviewed 178 of the 330 patients operated for Hirschsprung's disease between 1957 and 1990 at the Red Cross Children's Hospital in Capetown, South Africa.[108] Only 5% were less than the third percentile for weight. Eight percent had developmental delay, with no specific cause being identified in 5 of the 9 patients. Of those in school, all but 18% were doing satisfactorily and only 6% had behavioral disturbances. Postoperative enterocolitis occurred in 11%. Constipation, sexual dysfunction, and micturition disturbances were much less after the Soave procedure compared with the Swenson and Duhamel procedures but were present in less than 10% in all cases. Full continence was present in 75%, and 22% had some leakage (usually at night).

Clearly not all patients are permanently cured by the current procedures for Hirschsprung's disease. We have always been suspicious that there might be neurochemical abnormalities proximal to the absence of ganglion cells that accounted for at least some of the postoperative problems. Kobayashi and associates[77] studied the proximal resection margin in 31 patients operated on for Hirschsprung's disease. Neuronal dysplasia was found in 10 patients, all of whom had persistent bowel problems, such as enterocolitis, soiling, or constipation. Only 4 of the 21 patients with normal findings at the resection margin had persistent bowel symptoms. Hirschsprung's disease remains an area of challenge for both surgeons and scientists.

## REFERENCES

1. Ruysch F: Observationum anatomiae-chirurgicarum centuria. Amsterdam, 1691. Cited in Leenders E, Sieber WK: Congenital megacolon observation by Frederick Ruysch—1691. J Pediatr Surg 1970;5:1–3.
2. Hirschsprung H: Stuhltragheit neugeborener in folge von Dilatation und Hypertrophie des Colons. Jarb Kinderheilkd 1887;27:1.
3. Ehrenpreis TH: Megacolon in the newborn: a clinical and roentgenological study with special regard to the pathogenesis. Acta Chir Scand 1946;94:1–116.
4. Zuelzer WW, Wilson JL: Functional intestinal obstruction on a congenital neurogenic basis in infancy. Am Dis Child 1948;75:40.
5. Swenson O, Bill A: Resection of rectum and rectosigmoid with preservation of sphincter for benign spastic lesions producing megacolon: experimental study. Surgery 1948;24:212.
6. Goyal RK, Hirano I: The enteric nervous system. N Engl J Med 1996;334:1106–1115.
7. Larsson LT, Shen Z, Ekblad E, et al: Lack of neuronal nitric oxide synthase in nerve fibers of aganglionic intestine: a clue to Hirschsprung's disease. J Pediatr Gastroenterol Nutr 1995;20:49–53.
8. Hanani M, Louzon V, Udassin R, et al: Nitric oxide–containing nerves in bowel segments of patients with Hirschsprung's disease. J Pediatr Surg 1995;30:818–822.
9. Kobayashi H, O'Briain DS, Puri P: Lack of expression of NADPH-diaphorase and neural cell adhesion molecule, NCAM, in colonic muscle of patients with Hirschsprung's disease. J Pediatr Surg 1994;29:301–304.
10. Vanderwinden JM, De Laet MH, Schiffmann SN, et al: Nitric oxide synthase distribution in the enteric nervous system of Hirschsprung's disease. Gastroenterology 1993;105:969–973.
11. Nagasaki A, Ikeda K, Suita S: Postoperative sequential anorectal manometric study of children with Hirschsprung's disease. J Pediatr Surg 1980;15:615–619.
12. Omita R, Munakata K, Kurosu Y, et al: A role of nitric oxide in Hirschsprung's disease. J Pediatr Surg 1995;30:437–440.
13. VanderWall KJ, Bealer JF, Adzick NS, et al: Cyclic GMP relaxes the internal anal sphincter in Hirschsprung's disease. J Pediatr Surg 1995;30:1013–1016.
14. Kato H, Yamamoto T, Yamamoto H, et al: Immunocytochemical characterization of supporting cells in the enteric nervous system in Hirschsprung's disease. J Pediatr Surg 1990;25:514–519.
15. Kawana T, Nada O, Ikeda K, et al: Distribution and localization of glial fibrillary acidic protein in colons affected by Hirschsprung's disease. J Pediatr Surg 1989;24:448–452.
16. Vanderwinden JM, Rumessen JJ, Liu H, et al: Interstitial cells of Cajal in human colon and in Hirschsprung's disease. Gastroenterology 1996;111:901–910.
17. Langer JC, Betti PA, Blennerhassett MG: Smooth muscle from aganglionic bowel in Hirschsprung's disease impairs neuronal development in vitro. Cell Tissue Res 1994;276:181–186.
18. Parikh DH, Tam PK, Van Velzen D, et al: Abnormalities in the distribution of laminin and collagen type IV in Hirschsprung's disease. Gastroenterology 1992;102:1236–1241.
19. Vaos GC: Quantitative assessment of the stage of neuronal maturation in the developing human fetal gut—a new dimension in the pathogenesis of developmental anomalies of the myenteric plexus. J Pediatr Surg 1989;24:920–925.
20. Hirobe S, Doody DP, Ryan DP, et al: Ectopic class II major histocompatibility antigens in Hirschsprung's disease and neuronal intestinal dysplasia. J Pediatr Surg 1992;27:357–363.

21. Kobayashi H, Hirakawa H, Puri P: Overexpression of intercellular adhesion molecule-1 and MHC class II antigen on hypertrophic nerve trunks suggests an immunopathologic response in Hirschsprung's disease. J Pediatr Surg 1995;30:1680–1683.
22. Ikeda K, Goto S: Diagnosis and treatment of Hirschsprung's disease in Japan: an analysis of 1628 patients. Ann Surg 1984;199:400–405.
23. Goldberg EL: An epidemiological study of Hirschsprung's disease. Int J Epidemiol 1984;13:479–485.
24. Spouge D, Baird PA: Hirschsprung disease in a large birth cohort. Teratology 1985;32:171–177.
25. Russell MB, Russell CA, Niebuhr E: An epidemiological study of Hirschsprung's disease and additional anomalies. Acta Paediatr 1994;83:68–71.
26. Klein MD, Philippart AI: Hirschsprung's disease: three decades' experience at a single institution. J Pediatr Surg 1993;28:1291–1294.
27. Moore SW, Rode H, Millar AJ, et al: Familial aspects of Hirschsprung's disease. Eur J Pediatr Surg 1991;1:97–101.
28. Fortuna RS, Weber TR, Tracy TF Jr, et al: Critical analysis of the operative treatment of Hirschsprung's disease. Arch Surg 1996;131:520–525.
29. Engum SA, Petrites M, Rescorla FJ, et al: Familial Hirschsprung's disease: 20 cases in 12 kindreds. J Pediatr Surg 1993;28:1286–1290.
30. Rescorla FJ, Morrison AM, Engles D, et al: Hirschsprung's disease: evaluation of mortality and long-term function in 260 cases. Arch Surg 1992;127:934–942.
31. Marty TL, Seo T, Matlak ME, et al: Gastrointestinal function after surgical correction of Hirschsprung's disease: long-term follow-up in 135 patients. J Pediatr Surg 1995;30:655–658.
32. Badner JA, Sieber WK, Garver KL, et al: A genetic study of Hirschsprung disease. Am J Hum Genet 1990;46:568–580.
33. Fewtrell MS, Tam PKH, Thomson AH, et al: Hirschsprung's disease associated with a deletion of chromosome 10(q11.2q21.2): a further link with the neurocristopathies? J Med Genet 1994;31:325–327.
34. Tam PK, Gould SJ, Martucciello G, et al: Ret protein in the human fetal rectum. J Pediatr Surg 1996;31:568–571.
35. Online Mendelian Inheritance in Man (OMIM), Johns Hopkins University, Baltimore, MD. MIM Number: 142623 Hirschsprung Disease; HSCR: 10/23/1996 and 600155 Hirschsprung Disease-2; HSCR2: 2/1/1996.
36. Teitelbaum DH, Qualman SJ, Caniano DA: Hirschsprung's disease: identification of risk factors for enterocolitis. Ann Surg 1988;207:240–244.
37. Jung PM: Hirschsprung's disease: one surgeon's experience in one institution. J Pediatr Surg 1995;30:646–651.
38. Quinn FM, Surana R, Puri P: The influence of trisomy 21 on outcome in children with Hirschsprung's disease. J Pediatr Surg 1994;29:781–783.
39. Caniano DA, Teitelbaum DH, Qualman SJ: Management of Hirschsprung's disease in children with trisomy 21. Am J Surg 1990;159:402–404.
40. el-Halaby E, Coran AG: Hirschsprung's disease associated with Ondine's curse: report of three cases and review of the literature. J Pediatr Surg 1994;29:530–535.
41. Attie T, Till M, Pelet A, et al: Exclusion of RET and Pax 3 loci in Waardenburg-Hirschsprung disease. J Med Genet 1995;32:312–313.
42. Blank RD, Sklar CA, Dimich AB, et al: Clinical presentations and RET protooncogene mutations in seven multiple endocrine neoplasia type 2 kindreds. Cancer 1996;78:1996–2003.
43. Clausen N, Andersson P, Tommerup N: Familial occurrence of neuroblastoma, von Recklinghausen's neurofibromatosis, Hirschsprung's agangliosis and jaw-winking syndrome. Acta Paediatr Scand 1989;78:736–741.
44. Stannard VA, Fowler C, Robinson L, et al: Familial Hirschsprung's disease: report of autosomal dominant and probable recessive X-linked kindreds. J Pediatr Surg 1991;26:591–594.
45. Cass DT, Hutson J: Association of Hirschsprung's disease and mullerian inhibiting substance deficiency. J Pediatr Surg 1992;27:1596–1599.
46. Joseph VT, Sim CK: Experience in the surgical management of Hirschsprung's disease Ann Acad Med Singapore 1987;16:518–526.
47. Klein MD, Coran AG, Wesley JR, et al: Hirschsprung's disease in the newborn. J Pediatr Surg 1984;19:370–374.
48. Newman B, Nussbaum A, Kirkpatrick JA Jr: Bowel perforation in Hirschsprung's disease AJR Am J Roentgenol 1987;148:1195–1197.
49. Holschneider AM, Kellner E, Streibl P, et al: The development of anorectal continence and its significance in the diagnosis of Hirschsprung's disease. J Pediatr Surg 1976;11:151–156.
50. Blair GK, Murphy JJ, Fraser GC: Internal sphincterotomy in post-pull-through Hirschsprung's disease. J Pediatr Surg 1996;31:843–845.
51. Kobayashi H, Hirakawa H, Puri P: Abnormal internal anal sphincter innervation in patients with Hirschsprung's disease and allied disorders. J Pediatr Surg 1996;31:794–799.
52. Yokoyama J, Kuroda T, Matsufugi H, et al: Problems in diagnosis of Hirschsprung's disease by anorectal manometry. Prog Pediatr Surg 1989;24:49–58.
53. Lopez-Alonso M, Ribas J, Hernandez A, et al: Efficiency of the anorectal manometry for the diagnosis of Hirschsprung's disease in the newborn period. Eur J Pediatr Surg 1995;5:160–163.
54. Tamate S, Shiokawa C, Yamada C, et al: Manometric diagnosis of Hirschsprung's disease in the neonatal period. J Pediatr Surg 1984;19:285–288.
55. Vela AR, Rosenberg AJ: Anorectal manometry: a new simplified technique. Am J Gastroenterol 1982;77:486–490.
56. Holschneider AM, Kraeft H: The value and reliability of anorectal electromanometry. Z Kinderchir 1981;33:25–38.
57. Meunier P, Marechal JM, Mollard P: Accuracy of the manometric diagnosis of Hirschsprung's disease. J Pediatr Surg 1978;13:411–415.
58. DeCampo JF, Mayne V, Boldt DW, et al: Radiologic findings in total aganglionosis coli. Pediatr Radiol 1984;14:205–209.
59. Taxman TL, Yulish BS, Rothstein FC: How useful is the barium enema in the diagnosis of infantile Hirschsprung's disease? Am J Dis Child 1986;140:881–884.
60. Kekomaki M, Rapola J, Louhimo I: Diagnosis of Hirschsprung's disease. Acta Pediatr Scand 1979;68:893–897.
61. Noblett HR: A rectal suction biopsy tube for use in the diagnosis of Hirschsprung's disease. J Pediatr Surg 1969;4:406–409.
62. Rees BI, Azmy A, Nigam M, et al: Complications of rectal suction biopsy. J Pediatr Surg 1983;18:273–275.
63. Andrassy RJ, Isaacs H, Weitzman JJ: Rectal suction biopsy for the diagnosis of Hirschsprung's disease. Ann Surg 1981;193:419–424.
64. Lake BD, Puri P, Nixon HH, et al: Hirschsprung's disease: an appraisal of histochemically demonstrated acetylcholinesterase activity in suction rectal biopsy specimens as an aid to diagnosis. Arch Pathol Lab Med 1978;102:244–247.
65. Challa VR, Moran JR, Turner CS, et al: Histologic diagnosis of Hirschsprung's disease: the value of concurrent hematoxylin and eosin and cholinesterase staining of rectal biopsies. Am J Clin Pathol 1987;88:324–328.
66. Meier-Ruge W, Lutterbeck PM, Herzog B, et al: Acetylcholinesterase activity in suction biopsies of the rectum in the diagnosis of Hirschsprung's disease. J Pediatr Surg 1972;7:11–17.
67. Miura H, Ohi R, Tseng SW, et al: The structure of the transitional and aganglionic zones of Auerbach's plexus in patients with Hirschsprung's disease: computer-assisted three-dimensional reconstruction study. J Pediatr Surg 1996;31:420–426.
68. Tam PK, Boyd GP: Origin, course, and endings of abnormal enteric nerve fibers in Hirschsprung's disease defined by whole-mount immunohistochemistry. J Pediatr Surg 1990;25:457–461.
69. Park WH, Choi SO, Kwon KY, et al: Acetylcholinesterase histochemistry of rectal suction biopsies in the diagnosis of Hirschsprung's disease. J Korean Med Sci 1992;7:353–359.
70. Athow AC, Filipe MI, Drake DP: Problems and advantages of acetylcholinesterase histochemistry of rectal suction biopsies in the diagnosis of Hirschsprung's disease. J Pediatr Surg 1990;25:520–526.
71. Aldridge RT, Campbell PE: Ganglion cell distribution in the normal rectum and anal canal: a basis for the diagnosis of Hirschsprung's disease by anorectal biopsy. J Pediatr Surg 1968;3:475–490.
72. Hoffman S, Orestano F: Histology of the myenteric plexus in relation to rectal biopsy in congenital megacolon. J Pediatr Surg 1967;2:575–577.
73. Neilson IR, Yazbeck S: Ultrashort Hirschsprung's disease: myth or reality? J Pediatr Surg 1990;25:1135–1138.
74. Moore BG, Singaram C, Eckhoff DE, et al: Immunohistochemical evaluations of ultrashort-segment (Hirschsprung's) disease: report of three cases. Dis Colon Rectum 1996;39:817–822.
75. Philippart AI, Reed JO, Georgeson KE: Neonatal small left colon syndrome: intramural not intraluminal obstruction. J Pediatr Surg 1975;10:733–740.
76. Briner J, Oswald HW, Hirsig J, et al: Neuronal intestinal dysplasia—clinical and histochemical findings and its association with Hirschsprung's disease. Z Kinderchir 1986;4:282–286.

77. Kobayashi H, Hirakawa H, Surana R, et al: Intestinal neuronal dysplasia is a possible cause of persistent bowel symptoms after pull-through operation for Hirschsprung's disease. J Pediatr Surg 1995;30:253–259.
78. Swenson O: Follow-up on 200 patients treated for Hirschsprung's disease during a 10-year period. Ann Surg 1957;146:706.
79. Swenson O: Partial internal sphincterectomy in the treatment of Hirschsprung's disease. Ann Surg 1964;160:540–550.
80. Sherman JO, Snyder ME, Weitzman JJ, et al: A 40-year multinational retrospective study of 880 Swenson procedures. J Pediatr Surg 1989;24:833–838.
81. Carcassonne M, Morisson-Lacombe G, Letourneau JN: Primary corrective operation without decompression in infants less than three months of age with Hirschsprung's disease. J Pediatr Surg 1982;17:241–243.
82. Duhamel B: A new operation for the treatment of Hirschsprung's disease. Arch Dis Child 1960;35:38.
83. Martin LW, Caudill DR: A method for elimination of the blind rectal pouch in the Duhamel operation for Hirschsprung's disease. Surgery 1967;62:951.
84. Soave F: A new surgical technique for treatment of Hirschsprung's disease. Surgery 1964;56:1007–1014.
85. Boley SJ: An endorectal pullthrough operation with primary anastomosis for Hirschsprung's disease. Surg Gynecol Obstet 1968;127:353–357.
86. So HB, Schwartz DL, Becker JM, et al: Endorectal "pull-through" without preliminary colostomy in neonates with Hirschsprung's disease. J Pediatr Surg 1980;15:470–471.
87. Georgeson KE, Fuenfer HH, Hardin WD: Primary laparoscopic pull-through for Hirschsprung's disease in infants and children. J Pediatr Surg 1995;38:1017–1022.
88. Heath AL, Spitz L, Milla PJ: The absorptive function of colonic aganglionic intestine: are the Duhamel and Martin procedures rational? J Pediatr Surg 1985;20:34–36.
89. Boley SJ: A new operative approach to total aganglionosis of the colon. Surg Gynecol Obstet 1984;159:481–484.
90. Kimura K, Nishijima E, Muraji T, et al: Extensive aganglionosis: further experience with the colonic patch graft procedure and long-term results. J Pediatr Surg 1988;23:52–56.
91. Jordan FT, Coran AG, Wesley JR: Modified endorectal procedure for management of long-segment aganglionosis. Ann Surg 1981;194:70–75.
92. Ziegler MM, Royal RE, Brandt J, et al: Extended myectomy-myotomy: a therapeutic alternative for total intestinal aganglionosis. Ann Surg 1993;218:504–511.
93. Ethalaby E, Coran A, Blane C, et al: Enterocolitis associated with Hirschsprung's disease: a clinical-radiological characterization based on 168 patients. J Pediatr Surg 1995;30:76–83.
94. Carneiro P, Brereton R, Drake D, et al: Enterocolitis in Hirschsprung's disease. Pediatr Surg Int 1992;7:356–360.
95. Surana R, Quinn F, Puri P: Evaluation of risk factors in the development of enterocolitis complicating Hirschsprung's disease. Pediatr Surg Int 1994;9:234–236.
96. Marty T, Matlak M, Hendrickson M, et al: Unexpected death from enterocolitis after surgery for Hirschsprung's disease. Pediatrics 1995;96:118–121.
97. Blane C, Elhalaby E, Coran A: Enterocolitis following endorectal pull-through procedure in children with Hirschsprung's disease. Pediatr Radiol 1994;24:164–166.
98. Foster P, Cowan G, Wrenn E Jr, et al: Twenty-five years' experience with Hirschsprung's disease. J Pediatr Surg 1990;25:531–534.
99. Bill A Jr, Chapman N: The enterocolitis of Hirschsprung's disease: its natural history and treatment. Am J Surg 1962;103:70.
100. Swenson O, Sherman J, Fisher J: Diagnosis of congenital of megacolon: an analysis of 501 patients. J Pediatr Surg 1973;8:587–594.
101. Kleinhaus S, Boley S, Sheran M, et al: Hirschsprung's disease: a survey of the members of the Surgical Section of the American Academy of Pediatrics. J Pediatr Surg 1979;14:588–597.
102. Wilson-Storey D: Microbial studies of enterocolitis in Hirschsprung's disease. Pediatr Surg Int 1994;9:248–250.
103. Thomas D, Fernie D, Bayston R, et al: Enterocolitis in Hirschsprung's disease: a controlled study of the etiologic role of *Clostridium difficile*. J Pediatr Surg 1986;21:22–25.
104. Brearly S, Armstrong G, Nairn R, et al: Pseudomembranous colitis: a lethal complication of Hirschsprung's disease unrelated to antibiotic usage. J Pediatr Surg 1987;22:257–259.
105. Soave F: Endorectal pull-through: 20 years experience. J Pediatr Surg 1985;20:568–579.
106. Mishalany HG, Wooley MM: Postoperative functional and manometric evaluation of patients with Hirschsprung's disease. J Pediatr Surg 1987;22:443–446.
107. Sherman JO, Snyder ME, Weitzman JJ, et al: A 40-year multinational retrospective study of 880 Swenson procedures. J Pediatr Surg 1989;24:833–838.
108. Moore SW, Albertyn R, Cywes S: Clinical outcome and long-term quality of life after surgical correction of Hirschsprung's disease. J Pediatr Surg 1996;31:1496–1501.

# Chapter 42

# Imperforate Anus

*Alberto Pẽna*

The term *imperforate anus* is a misnomer that is commonly used to refer to a spectrum of anorectal malformations, ranging from a small defect that requires a minor operation and results in an excellent prognosis to complex malformations with a high incidence of associated defects requiring sophisticated and specialized surgical procedures. Since the mid-1980s, significant advances have been achieved in the field of pediatric surgery that allow a better anatomic reconstruction of these defects, preserving other important pelvic structures. Yet, at least 30% of all patients born with these defects still have fecal incontinence even after a technically correct surgical repair, and another 30% also have other functional defecation problems, mainly constipation and various degrees of occasional soiling.[1, 2] These malformations occur in about 1:4000 to 1:5000 newborns.[3–5] The chance of having a second child affected by this type of defect is about 1%.[6–8]

## CLASSIFICATION AND DESCRIPTION OF DEFECTS

A classification presented here (Fig. 42–1) is based on therapeutic and prognostic facts as well as frequency of associated defects. It was designed to help the clinician to increase the index of suspicion and to establish therapeutic priorities.

### Perineal Fistula

The rectum opens into the perineum anterior to the center of the sphincter, into a usually stenotic orifice. In male patients, the perineum may exhibit other features that help in recognition of this defect, such as a prominent midline skin bridge (known as "bucket handle" malformation) or a subepithelial midline raphe fistula that looks like a black ribbon because it is full of meconium. These features are externally visible and help in the diagnosis of a perineal fistula. This is the most benign of anorectal defects. Fewer than 10% of these children have an associated urologic defect, and 100% of them achieve bowel control after proper treatment.[1, 2] The operation used to repair these malformations is a relatively simple anoplasty; it usually is performed during the neonatal period without a protective colostomy. All other anorectal defects are treated with a protective colostomy before the main repair.

### Rectal Atresia

In this defect, the patient is born with an externally normal-looking anus, but an attempt to take the rectal temperature discloses an obstruction located 1 to 2 cm above the mucocutaneous junction of the anus. The sphincter mechanism in these patients is normal, as is the sacrum. Associated defects are almost nil. The prognosis is excellent, and 100% of these patients achieve bowel control.[1, 2] The repair includes an operation called posterior sagittal anorectoplasty, which can be done 1 month after the child is born.

### Imperforate Anus Without Fistula

In these cases, the rectum ends blindly, without a fistula, approximately 1 to 2 cm above the perineum. The sacrum

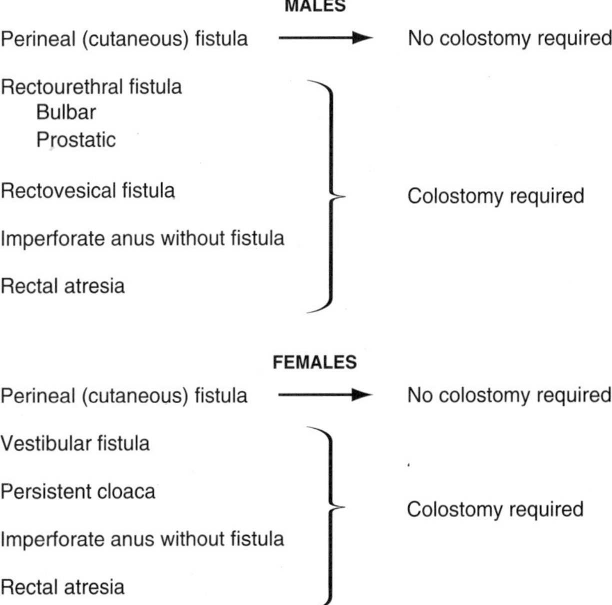


**FIGURE 42–1.** Classification (males and females).

and sphincter mechanism are usually good, and about 80% of these patients achieve bowel control after the main repair.[1,2] Approximately 50% of patients with this defect have Down syndrome. Conversely, 95% of patients with Down syndrome who have an anorectal malformation have this specific type.

### Vestibular Fistula

This is the most common defect in female patients. The rectum opens into the vestibule of the female genitalia, which is the wet area located outside the hymen. Rectum and vagina share a very thin common wall. The sacrum and sphincters are usually of good quality. Approximately 93% of these patients achieve bowel control after surgery.[1,2] About 30% of them have associated urologic defects.[9]

### Rectourethral Fistula

This is by far the most common defect in male patients. The rectum communicates with the posterior urethra through a narrow orifice (fistula). This fistula may be located in the lower posterior urethra (bulbar fistula) or in the upper posterior urethra (prostatic fistula). Eighty-five percent of patients with rectourethral bulbar fistula achieve fecal continence after the main repair, but only 60% of those with rectoprostatic fistula do so.[1,2] About 30% of patients with bulbar urethral fistula have associated urologic defects,[9] as do 60% of patients with rectoprostatic fistula.[9] The quality of the sacrum usually is good in the former case but frequently is abnormal in the latter. These patients are operated on after 1 month of life.

### Rectobladderneck Fistula

This is the highest defect seen in male patients. The rectum opens into the bladderneck. Ninety percent of these patients have significant associated urologic defects,[9] and only 15% achieve bowel control after the main repair.[1,2] The sacrum usually has poor quality. In these patients, the repair includes a posterior sagittal approach plus a laparotomy to reach a very high rectum.

### Cloaca

This is by far the most complex problem seen in female patients. This defect is defined as a malformation in which rectum, vagina, and urethra are fused together into a single common channel that opens into a single orifice in the perineum. This orifice is located where the normal urethra would be. The prognosis varies depending on the quality of the sacrum and the length of the common channel. Most patients with a common channel longer than 3 cm require intermittent catheterization after the main repair in order to empty the bladder. About 50% of these patients have voluntary bowel movements. On the other hand, if the common channel is shorter than 3 cm, 20% of the patients require intermittent catheterization to empty the bladder and about 70% of the patients have voluntary bowel movements.[1,2,10]

Ninety percent of patients with cloaca have an important associated urologic problem.[9] This may represent a serious urologic emergency that the clinician should recognize early in life, in order to detect and treat an obstructive uropathy.

More than 60% of these patients also have hydrocolpos, which is a very distended, tense, giant vagina that may compress the opening of the ureters, provoking bilateral megaureters.[10] A significant number of these patients also have massive vesicoureteral reflux. At birth these patients require the opening of a colostomy and, frequently, some sort of urinary diversion to take care of the obstructive uropathy. After 3 months of life, they undergo a large operation during which the three main structures (rectum, vagina, and urethra) are separated and placed in their normal locations.

## ASSOCIATED DEFECTS

The most common defects associated with anorectal malformations are urologic. The frequency of these associations has already been described. The next most common associated defects are those of the spine and sacrum. The quality of the sacrum has a direct relation to the prognosis for bowel and urinary control. A very hypoplastic sacrum or an absent sacrum correlates directly with fecal and urinary incontinence.

Another significant group of patients have gastrointestinal defects, including esophageal atresia, duodenal atresia, or other kinds of atresia in the intestinal tract. Approximately 10% of patients have some form of cardiac malformation.

## EARLY MANAGEMENT AND DIAGNOSIS

When a child is born with an anorectal malformation, two main questions must be answered within the first 24 hours of life: (1) Does the infant need a colostomy, or can the malformation be repaired with an anoplasty? and (2) Does the infant have an associated defect (most likely urologic or cardiac) that endangers life and requires immediate treatment?

The higher and more complex the anorectal defect, the greater the chance of a dangerous associated defect. Figures 42–2 and 42–3 show the decision-making algorithms used in the early management of these newborns.

All infants with anorectal malformations should have an abdominal and pelvic ultrasound examination during the first hours of life. These simple tests can exclude hydronephrosis, megaureters, and hydrocolpos. If the study results are normal, no further urologic evaluations are required. If the patient has any of these conditions, further urologic evaluation may be required. An echocardiogram can also be performed during the first hours of life. The perineum must be meticulously evaluated, because it provides a series of clues that help to answer the questions listed previously. The presence of a midline groove with two well-formed buttocks and a conspicuous anal dimple is a good prognostic sign indicating that the patient probably has a rather low type of malformation. One should always look for the presence of a

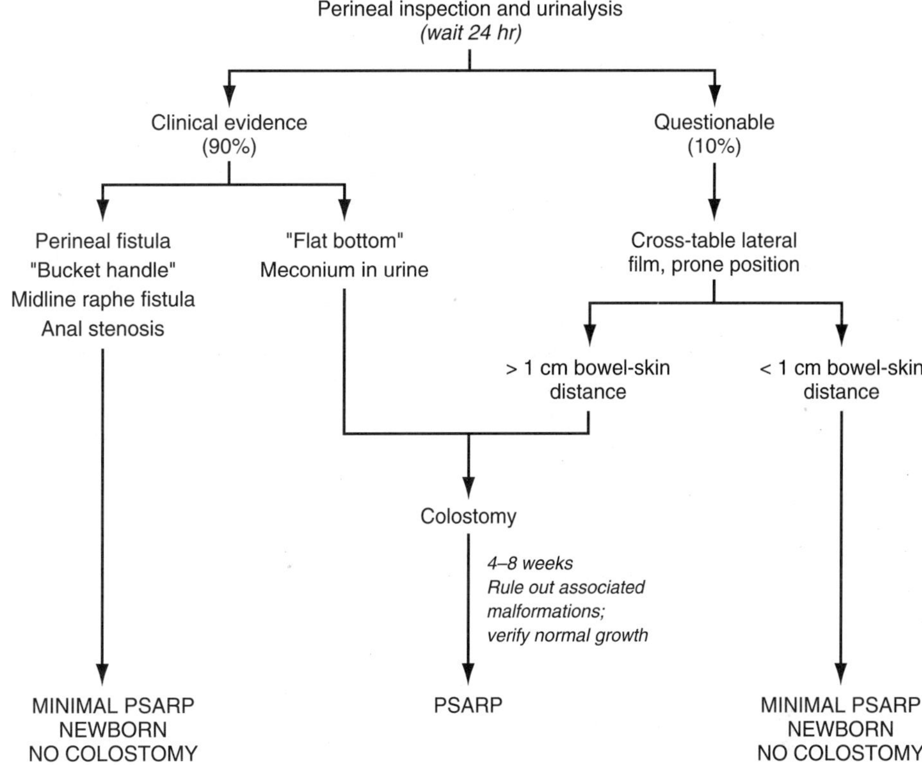


**FIGURE 42–2.** Decision-making algorithm (males). PSARP, posterior sagittal anorectoplasty.

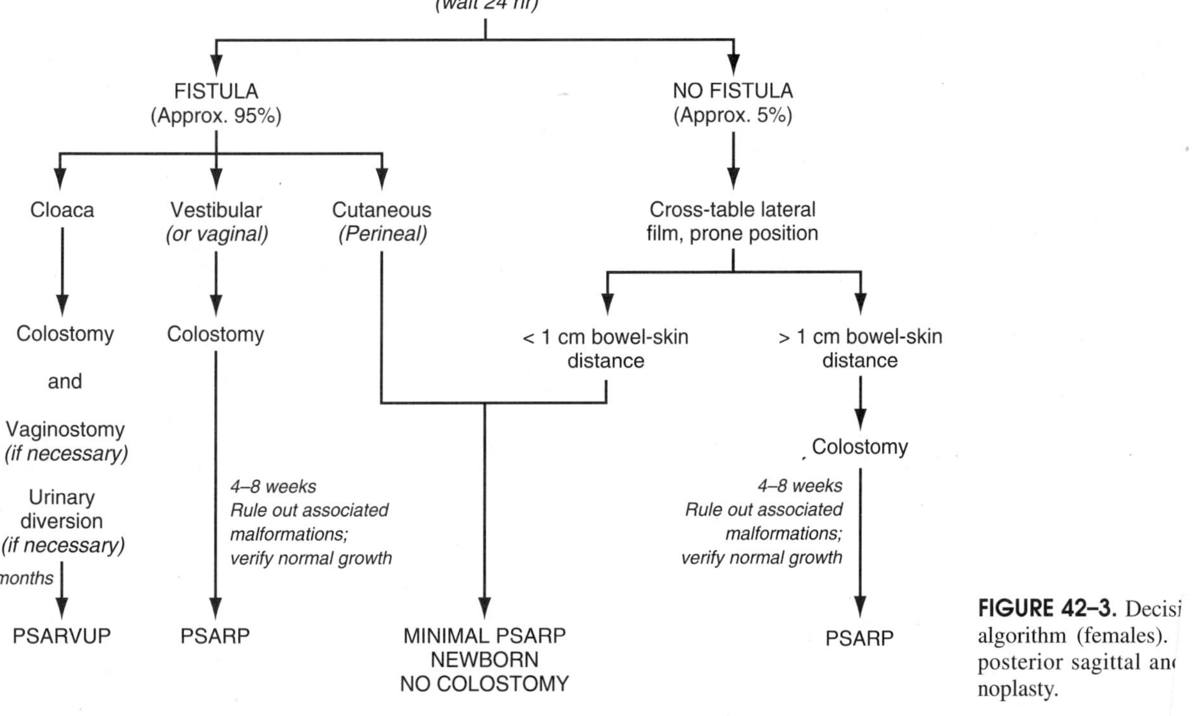


**FIGURE 42–3.** Decisi[...] algorithm (females). [...] posterior sagittal an[...]noplasty.

perineal fistula, which sometimes is extremely small. On the other hand, a flat bottom (no midline groove and absence of an anal dimple) occurs in infants with very high defects. An ultrasound study of the lower spine must also be done in the first few days of life to rule out the presence of tethered cord, which is associated with a very high type of anorectal malformation with poor prognosis.[11]

When a child is born with an anorectal malformation, the abdomen is not distended. During the following 18 to 24 hours, the abdomen becomes distended and the intraluminal pressure of the bowel significantly increases, forcing the meconium through the lowest part of the rectum, which is surrounded by the sphincter mechanism. One must expect the meconium to pass through a fistula, usually after 18 to 24 hours. The golden rule in the early diagnosis of these children is to wait at least 18 to 24 hours before making a decision. Male infants need a urinalysis to look for traces of meconium. A piece of gauze placed on the tip of the penis may filter the meconium when the infant voids, making the diagnosis of a rectourinary fistula, and this is an indication to open a colostomy. A tiny perineal fistula may remain unnoticed, and after 20 to 24 hours a drop of meconium may become evident. The presence of meconium in the perineum or an obvious perineal fistula establishes the diagnosis of perineal fistula, which can be treated with an anoplasty and without a colostomy.

In about 5% of all patients, a perineal fistula cannot be found, there is no evidence of cloaca, there is no evidence of vestibular fistula, and no meconium in the urine is found. In such cases the patient may have an imperforate anus without fistula. To confirm this, a cross-table lateral film with the child in prone position and the pelvis elevated is taken with a lead marker located in the anal dimple. The location of the rectum full of gas can be radiologically detected, and the distance between the rectum and the perineum can be measured. If that distance is longer than 1 cm, the infant needs a colostomy and most likely has an imperforate anus without fistula. If the rectum is closer than 1 cm to the perineum, the patient probably has a perineal fistula that was undetected and can be treated with an anoplasty.

## MAIN REPAIR

### Anoplasty

An anoplasty is a small operation performed with the patient in prone position and the pelvis elevated. A newborn does not require any bowel preparation. The operation takes about 30 to 45 minutes but requires many meticulous and delicate maneuvers to avoid potential damage to important continence structures.

An older child with an untreated perineal fistula usually comes for treatment with severe fecal impaction and megasigmoid. These patients require a full bowel preparation before the operation, and after the procedure they also need parenteral nutrition and fasting for several days to avoid potential infection.

### Posterior Sagittal Anorectoplasty

Most anorectal malformations can be repaired by using a posterior midsagittal approach between the buttocks. The rationale behind this operation is that the entire sphincter mechanism can be divided in the midline to avoid nerve damage. An electric stimulator is used to determine the precise limits of the sphincter. The goal of the operation is to separate the rectum from the genitourinary tract, to dissect it enough to reach the perineum and to place it within the limits of the sphincter mechanism. Sometimes the rectum is so dilatated that some degree of tapering is needed to achieve these goals. In 10% of male patients, it is necessary to open the abdomen in addition to the posterior sagittal approach to reach a rectum that is located extremely high in the abdomen (rectobladderneck fistula).[1, 2] In such cases, the posterior sagittal procedure is started and the surgeon creates a path immediately behind the urinary tract, through which the rectum is to be pulled down. A rubber tube is placed in the desired tract, the patient is turned to the supine position, the abdomen is opened, the rectum is separated from the bladderneck, and then the rectum is anchored to the rubber tube, which is found in the retroperitoneal space. The rubber tube is pulled down, bringing with it the rectum, which is then placed within the limits of the sphincter mechanism and anastomosed to the perineum.

About 40% of female patients born with a cloaca also need a laparotomy to reach a very high rectum, a very high vagina, or both. In these cases, the operation is called posterior sagittal anorectovaginourethroplasty. These are very specialized, delicate, demanding operations that have as a goal the anatomic reconstruction of the rectum, urethra, and vagina.[10]

## FUNCTIONAL SEQUELAE

### Elements Required for Bowel Control

In order to have bowel continence, it is necessary to have three main elements: sensation, sphincters, and normal rectosigmoid motility.

#### *Sensation*

The most important sensation useful for bowel control resides in the anal canal, from a few millimeters above the pectinate line to the anal verge. In that area, it is possible for the patient to discriminate among gas, liquid, and solid contents, and even to discern changes in temperature.[12] There is another type of sensation that resides in the rectum and is elicited when the rectum is distended, which supposedly stretches the voluntary muscles that surround the rectum. This type of sensation is vague and is called proprioception. The rectal mucosa has no sensation; the proprioception receptors reside in the voluntary muscle that surrounds the rectum.[13]

#### *Sphincters*

There are two types of sphincters. First is the voluntary external sphincter mechanism, represented by a funnel-like voluntary muscle structure that inserts in the middle portion of the pelvic rim and extends all the way down to the skin surrounding the rectum and anus. The internal sphincter is a more controversial structure defined as a thickening of the circular layer of the smooth muscle in the lowest part of the intestine. This is an involuntary sphincter.

## *Rectosigmoid Motility*

Normal rectosigmoid colonic motility is extremely important for bowel control. Under normal circumstances, the rectosigmoid acts likes a reservoir. It catches all the solid stool that comes from the rest of the colon. Once a day or every other day, depending on the person's habit, the rectosigmoid gives signs of trying to empty by pushing the fecal contents toward the anal canal. The contact of the rectal contents with the anal canal gives the person the necessary information to know the nature of the rectal contents. Depending on the surrounding social circumstances, the person may elect to relax the voluntary sphincter or to contract it. Once the decision is made to empty the rectosigmoid, the voluntary sphincter is relaxed, and the next wave of peristaltic contraction empties the rectosigmoid.

Children with anorectal malformations have deficiencies in all three of these main elements of bowel control. The sensation that resides in the anal canal exists only in those with anorectal malformations in which an anal canal is present. There is only one specific defect with that characteristic; it is called rectal atresia and occurs in only 1% of all cases.[1, 2] These patients have a normal looking anus with an atresia located 1 or 2 cm above the anal verge. All other patients with anorectal malformations are born with no anal canal or with a very abnormal one. Therefore, one cannot expect a very precise discrimination in these children. On the other hand, all of them have different degrees of proprioception, usually good enough to be toilet trained provided the prognosis for their type of defect is good. The presence of a solid piece of stool moving in the rectum is perceived by the patient in a rather vague manner but is strong enough to give the alert signal to defecate. Liquid stool is more difficult to sense.

The internal sphincter in children with anorectal malformations is a matter of debate and, in addition, there is no scientific evidence that such a structure exists or is preserved after surgical repair of these defects. Postoperative manometric studies attempting to elicit the presence of an internal sphincter have yielded controversial results, but most of them indicate that there is no such structure.[14, 15] The voluntary sphincter mechanism has different degrees of hypodevelopment in children with anorectal malformations. In very severe cases of very high defects there is basically no evidence or trace of the sphincter, whereas in patients with perineal fistula the sphincter is almost normal. Finally, rectosigmoid motility in children with anorectal malformations is very abnormal. If the surgical technique includes preservation of the rectosigmoid, these children usually experience constipation, which is the clinical manifestation of rectosigmoid hypomotility. They do not have the capacity to empty the rectum in a massive way but rather keep passing small amounts of stool throughout the day. The severity of this disorder varies from minimal to very severe, the latter resulting in fecal impaction.

Patients for whom the operative technique included resection of the rectosigmoid do not have a reservoir. They have a tendency to pass rather liquid stools constantly day and night, the worst type of incontinence. This was the result with endorectal techniques, which are very rarely used today.

## **Fecal Incontinence**

The most feared sequela in children with anorectal malformations is fecal incontinence. At least 30% of all children with these defects have this devastating problem.[1, 2]

The general goals in the management of children with anorectal malformations are to anatomically reconstruct all malformations, to monitor the patients on a long-term basis taking care of their functional disturbances, and to provide the optimal circumstances for them to maintain bowel control if possible. For those patients who were born with a defect with a poor prognosis, a bowel management program must be provided so that they can stay clean and socially acceptable. Some patients who were born with a defect that has a good prognosis reach 3 years of age and still do not have bowel control. In these cases, the bowel management program is provided on a temporary basis, and every year during summer vacation the child is given the opportunity to become toilet trained again.

The bowel management program used for children with fecal incontinence consists of teaching the family to clean the colon once a day and, subsequently, to manipulate the diet and sometimes to administer medications to keep the colon quiet for 24 hours between enemas. With this plan, patients remain completely clean. The colon is cleaned every day by the parents with the use of enemas. The type and quality of the enemas vary, depending on the type of colon that the patient has. Some patients have giant megasigmoids and therefore require large-volume enemas. Some patients retain the enemas because they have severe hypomotility of the colon. In such cases, it is necessary to use some form of hyperosmotic fluid (increased sodium chloride concentration) or phosphate to provoke a bowel movement and avoid enema retention.

The bowel management program is implemented over a period of 1 week. A nurse clinician teaches the parents how to clean the colon. Some children respond to a small phosphate enema and others require high colonic irrigations. The contrast enema performed at the initiation of the program provides a clue to determine the volume and type of enema that the patient requires, but it is still a process of trial and error.

Fecally incontinent constipated patients require only a large enema to stay completely clean, 24 hours per day. In retrospect, the fact that they are constipated helps them to remain clean in between enemas. The emphasis in this group of patients is the use of large enemas.

There is another group of patients who have fecal incontinence and a tendency to diarrhea and who were operated on with a technique that included resection of the original rectosigmoid. The main problem in their bowel management is to keep the colon quiet between enemas. The colon is easy to clean because it is not dilatated, and yet liquid stool that comes from the cecum runs very fast to the rectum and in a few hours the patient passes stool again. Therefore, in this group of patients, the emphasis is on a very constipating diet and administration of medication to decrease colonic peristalsis. The contrast enema permits diagnosis of such a type of colon. This bowel management program has been successful in 90% of the cases in my experience.[2]

Once the patient responds to the bowel management program and remains completely clean for 24 hours, the patient and family are given the option of an operation called Malone procedure (continent appendicostomy).[16] It consists of connecting the cecal appendix to the umbilicus so as to be able to administer enemas through it in an antegrade fashion. A one-way valve mechanism is created between the appendix and the cecum to avoid stool leakage and allow catheterization. The patient can self-administer an enema while sitting on the toilet. This operation is favored by teenaged patients who want to gain some autonomy and independence and do not like to receive enemas from their parents.

For those patients who have already lost their appendix for whatever reason, one can create a new appendix from the wall of the cecum and use it as previously described. This operation is called continent neoappendicostomy.

## Soiling

Seventy percent of all patients who were born with anorectal malformations have voluntary bowel movements, but almost 50% of them still soil their underwear occasionally. Further examination of these patients, including contrast enema, reveals that most of them have chronic fecal impaction; in other words, the soiling often represents overflow pseudoincontinence. Reasonable use of laxatives and bulk-forming agents may help to eliminate this type of soiling in most of these patients. When the soiling is significant enough to interfere with the social life of the patient, then it is preferable to implement the bowel management program previously described.

## Constipation

Constipation is the most common problem in children with anorectal malformations who have undergone an operation in which the original rectum was preserved. The rectosigmoid in these patients behaves like an excessively large and quiet reservoir that does not have the capacity to empty as well as in a normal individual. Constipation is a self-aggravating and self-perpetuating disorder. If the rectum is not emptied every day by some mechanism, it accumulates stool and becomes larger (megarectum), resulting in decreased or ineffective peristalsis. This provokes more constipation, creating a vicious circle.

The worst final sequela from constipation is overflow pseudoincontinence. This occurs in severely constipated children (i.e., those with chronic impaction). They constantly pass small amounts of stool as an overflow phenomenon. Sometimes patients who were born with benign anorectal defects with good functional prognosis do not achieve fecal continence, simply because they have overflow pseudoincontinence secondary to chronic fecal impaction.

The problem of constipation correlates directly with the degree of rectal dilatation that the patient had originally. Some malformations include more severe megarectum than others. The lower the defect, the greater the megarectum and the worse the constipation. Patients with higher defects (and therefore poorer prognosis for functional bowel control) have less constipation.[2] Other factors, such as the type of colostomy, also influence the degree of megarectum. Loop colostomies sometimes allow the passage of stool from proximal to distal colon, provoking a severe megarectum, and for that reason they are contraindicated. Patients with transverse colostomies develop a more severe megarectum and more constipation. Patients who are born with perineal fistulas and are not treated early in life develop a very severe megarectum and eventually have overflow pseudoincontinence. Every effort should be made at prevention, but when megarectum is present, the patient should receive enough laxatives to empty the rectum every day.

## Urinary Incontinence

Male patients with anorectal malformations almost never have urinary incontinence unless they have an absent sacrum, a severe dysplastic sacrum, or nerve damage occurring during the main repair of the malformation.[2] Female patients who are born with a cloaca frequently have an incapacity to empty the bladder and require a program of intermittent catheterization. Leakage of urine because of a lack of bladderneck strength is very unusual in patients with anorectal malformations. These patients have an atonic type of megabladder. Only 20% of the patients born with a cloaca with a common channel shorter than 3 cm require intermittent catheterization,[2, 10] and 70% of those with a common channel longer than 3 cm require this type of maneuver to remain dry and clean.

## REFERENCES

1. Pēna A: Posterior sagittal anorectoplasty: results in the management of 332 cases of anorectal malformations. Pediatr Surg Int 1988;3:4–104.
2. Pēna A: Anorectal malformations. Semin Pediatr Surg 1995;4:35–47.
3. Brenner EC: Congenital defects of the anus and rectum. Surg Gynecol Obstet 1915;20:579–588.
4. Santulli TV: Treatment of imperforate anus and associated fistulas. Surg Gynecol Obstet 1952;95:601–614.
5. Trusler GA, Wilkinson RH: Imperforate anus: a review of 147 cases. Can J Surg 1962;5:169–177.
6. Anderson RC, Read SC: The likelihood of recurrence of congenital malformations. Lancet 1954;74:175–176.
7. Cozzi F, Wilkinson AW: Familial incidence of congenital anorectal anomalies. Surgery 1968;64:669–671.
8. Murken JD, Albert A: Genetic counseling in cases of anal and rectal atresia. Prog Pediatr Surg 1976;9:115–118.
9. Rich MA, Brock WA, Pēna A: Spectrum of genitourinary malformations in patients with imperforate anus. Pediatr Surg Int 1988;3:110–113.
10. Pēna A: The surgical management of persistent cloaca: results in 54 patients treated with a posterior sagittal approach. J Pediatr Surg 1989;24:590–598.
11. Levitt M, Patel M, Rodriguez G, et al: The tethered cord in patients with anorectal malformations. J Pediatr Surg 1997;32:462–468.
12. Duthie HL, Gairns FW: Sensory nerve endings and sensation in the anal region of man. Br J Surg 1960;206:585–595.
13. Goligher JC, Hughes ESR: Sensibility of the rectum and colon: its role in the mechanism of anal continence. Lancet 1951;1:543–548.
14. Stephens FD, Smith ED: Anatomy and function of the normal rectum and anus. In Stephens FD, Smith ED: Anorectal Malformations in Children. Chicago, Year Book Medical Publishers, 1987, pp 14–32.
15. Hedlund H, Pēna A: Does the distal rectal muscle in anorectal malformations have the functional properties of a sphincter? J Pediatr Surg 1990;25:985–989.
16. Malone PS, Ransley PG, Kiely EM: Preliminary report: the antegrade continent enema. Lancet 1990;336:1217–1218.

Chapter 43

# Congenital Anomalies of the Midgut

*John R. Gosche and Robert J. Touloukian*

The distal duodenum, jejunum and ileum, cecum and vermiform appendix, ascending colon, and proximal half of the transverse colon are derived from the midgut. Errors in the normal embryonic development of the midgut result in a number of congenital anomalies, which include (1) errors of rotation and fixation, (2) atresias and stenoses, (3) duplications, (4) persistence of vestigial structures, and (5) defects of innervation and motility.[1] The first three of these conditions are discussed in this chapter.

Many anomalies of the midgut present in the first days or weeks of life. Some, however, may not produce symptoms until later in life. In addition, the symptoms these anomalies cause may be vague and nondescript. It is important, therefore, to consider the possibility that a congenital anomaly may be the origin of symptoms, even in an older child or adult, so that the correct diagnosis can be made and appropriate treatment instituted.

## NORMAL EMBRYOLOGY

The midgut begins as a straight endodermal tube. In the early embryo, the midgut is connected to the yolk sac on its ventral aspect. Dorsally, the midgut is attached by a mesentery through which courses the superior mesenteric artery. During the fourth and fifth weeks of development the midgut undergoes a period of rapid growth. By the sixth week of gestation the rapidly growing midgut, along with the enlarging liver, exceed the capacity of the abdominal cavity. Therefore, the midgut herniates into the umbilical cord early in the sixth week of gestation. This "physiologic" herniation continues until approximately the 10th week of gestation.

During fetal development, the midgut undergoes 270 degrees of rotation in a counterclockwise direction around its axis, the superior mesenteric artery. The process of rotation and fixation is generally discussed in three stages (Fig. 43–1).[2] The first stage of rotation occurs during the period of physiologic herniation and results in an initial 90 degrees of counterclockwise rotation. The second stage occurs as the intestine returns to the abdominal cavity during the 10th week of gestation. The midgut returns from the umbilicus in an orderly sequence: the proximal midgut returns first and passes behind the superior mesenteric artery toward the left upper quadrant. The distal midgut returns last and becomes situated anterior to the superior mesenteric artery in an epigastric location. At the completion of the second stage of rotation, the proximal midgut has rotated 270 degrees counterclockwise and the distal midgut counterclockwise about 180 degrees. The third stage of rotation begins at the 11th week of gestation and continues until just before birth. During this stage, the proximal colon lengthens and the cecum descends into the right iliac fossa. In addition, the mesenteries of the duodenum and the distal midgut fuse with the parietal peritoneum of the dorsal abdominal wall. This fusion anchors the proximal and distal ends of the midgut, resulting in a broad base of attachment for the small bowel mesentery.

## ANOMALIES OF INTESTINAL ROTATION

### Incidence

The true incidence of anomalies of intestinal rotation is not known. Many cases remain asymptomatic throughout life, and thus are never detected. Kantor[3] has reported nonrotation of the colon in 0.2% of patients studied by barium enema. The majority of patients who develop symptoms related to an anomaly of rotation present within the first month of life.[4] Most anomalies of rotation affect males more frequently than females.[5, 6] Reversed rotation, however, is more common in females.[7]

### Classification and Embryology

Anomalies of midgut rotation and fixation represent a spectrum with a multitude of intermediate stages. Rotational anomalies, however, have been grouped according to similar derangements in the rotational process and the stage of rotation during which that derangement occurred.[6]

Derangements of the first and third stages of rotation are infrequent. A defect in the first stage of rotation is associated with extroversion of the cloaca.[6] Anomalies of the third stage of rotation cause failure of elongation of the cecum, so that the cecum remains in the right upper quadrant. Failure of fixation of the distal midgut also results in varying degrees of ileocecal mobility.

The majority of anomalies of midgut rotation reflect derangements of the second stage of rotation. These anomalies have been grouped by Dott,[6] as representing nonrotation, reversed rotation, and malrotation. Of these anomalies, nonrotation is most common (Fig. 43–2).[8] Nonrotation reflects complete failure of the second stage of rotation. Nonrotation is thought to be the result of laxity of the umbilical ring, which allows reduction en masse of the midgut from the umbilicus during the 10th week of fetal life.[6] With nonrotation, the intestinal tract occupies the same position in the abdomen as in an 8-week embryo (i.e., the small intestine is located to the right of the midline and the colon is on the left).

Reversed rotation of the midgut loop is rare, accounting for only 4% of rotational anomalies.[9] This defect most frequently presents in adults.[7] In reversed rotation, the midgut rotates 180 degrees clockwise during the second stage of rotation, resulting in a net 90 degrees of clockwise rotation. Two variants of reversed rotation have been described, the *retroarterial colon type* and the *liver and entire colon ipsilateral type* of reversed rotation.[10] In the more common retroarterial colon type of reversed rotation (Fig. 43–3), the cecum passes through the root of the mesentery behind the superior mesenteric artery, and the duodenum lies anterior to the superior mesenteric vessels. In the rare liver and entire colon ipsilateral type of reversed rotation, both the duodenum and colon are located anterior to the mesenteric vessels.

Malrotation of the midgut loop, according to the nomenclature of Dott,[6] refers to "irregular defects of rotation." Unfortunately, in common usage the term *malrotation* may refer to any anomaly of midgut rotation. Thus, this group of anomalies of rotation is more accurately called *anomalies of mixed rotation*[10] or of *incomplete rotation.*[11] Anomalies of mixed rotation occur when the proximal midgut fails to rotate around the mesenteric vessels during the second stage of rotation. The distal midgut, however, rotates 90 degrees in a counterclockwise direction. As a result, the jejunum and ileum remain to the right of the superior mesenteric artery and the cecum comes to lie in the subpyloric region.

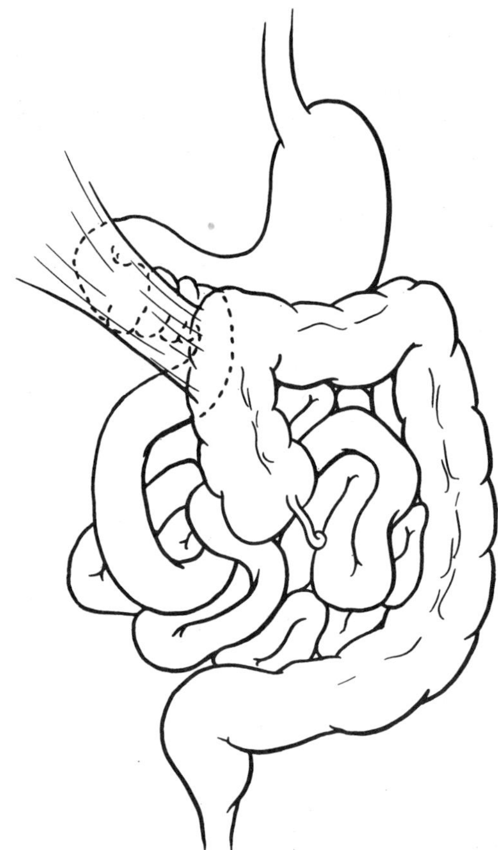

**FIGURE 43–2.** Nonrotation of the midgut. All of the small bowel lies to the right of the superior mesenteric artery, and all of the colon lies to the left. (From Oldham KT, Colobani PM, Foglia RP (eds): Surgery of Infants and Children, Philadelphia, Lippincott-Raven, 1997, p 1232, with permission.)

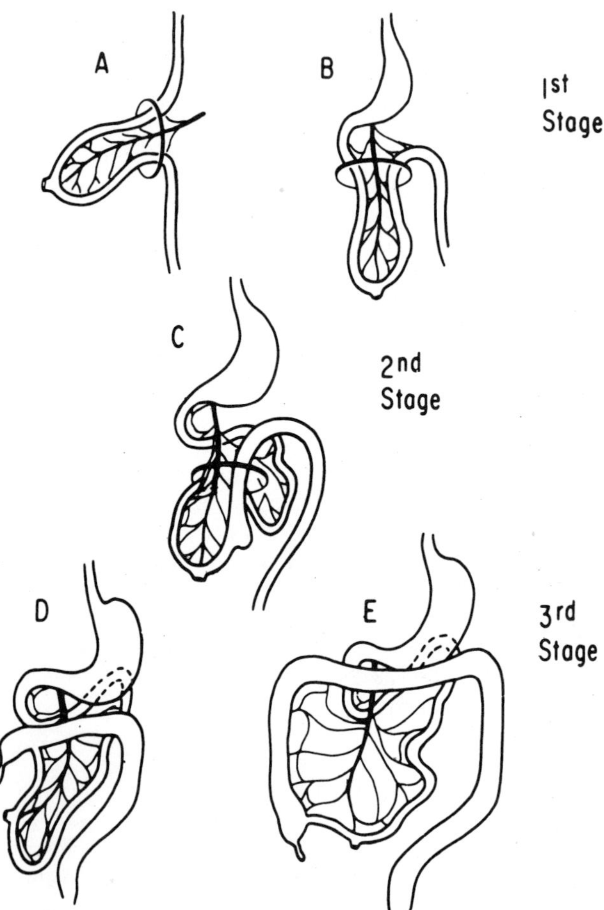


**FIGURE 43–1.** Illustration of normal intestinal rotation: *(A)* Sixth week of gestation, *(B)* 8th week of gestation, *(C)* 9th week of gestation, *(D)* 11th week of gestation, *(E)* 12th week of gestation. (From Filston HC, Kirks DR: Malrotation—the ubiquitous anomaly. J Pediatr Surg 1981;16 (suppl 1):616, with permission.)

## Associated Anomalies

Some 30% to 60% of patients with defects in intestinal rotation have an associated anomaly.[4, 12, 13] Some degree of

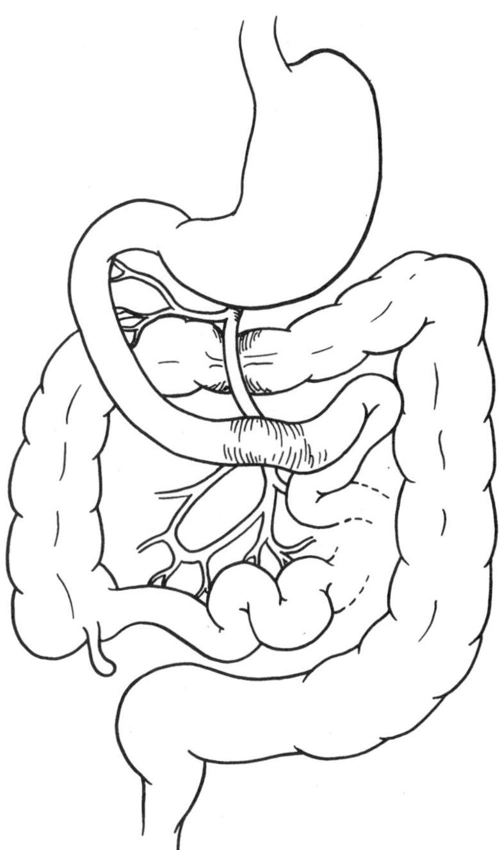

**FIGURE 43–3.** Retroarterial colon type of reversed rotation. The colon crosses dorsal to the superior mesenteric vessels, and the duodenum passes ventrally. (From Oldham KT, Colombani PM, Foglia RP (eds): Surgery of Infants and Children, Philadelphia, Lippincott-Raven, 1997, p 1233, with permission.)

incomplete rotation is found in nearly every infant with a congenital diaphragmatic hernia or an abdominal wall defect. Rotational defects also occur in a third to half of infants with duodenal atresia[4, 11] and in a third of infants with jejunoileal atresia.[4] Other gastrointestinal anomalies associated with anomalies of midgut rotation include Hirschsprung's disease, esophageal atresia, biliary atresia, annular pancreas, meconium ileus, intestinal duplications, mesenteric cysts, Meckel's diverticulum, and imperforate anus.[4, 11, 12, 14] Anomalies of rotation also occur in 15% of children with intestinal pseudo-obstruction.[15]

Abnormalities of intestinal rotation and fixation also coexist with *heterotaxia,*[16] an abnormal arrangement of body organs different from situs solitus (normal) or complete situs inversus. Gastrointestinal anomalies associated with heterotaxia include a midline liver, malpositioned stomach, anomalies of intestinal rotation and fixation, and a nonretroperitoneal pancreas. Major cardiac anomalies and asplenia or polysplenia are also common.

## Presentation

Anomalies of intestinal rotation and fixation result in a narrowed base of attachment for the small bowel mesentery. This narrowed mesenteric pedicle predisposes the midgut to twisting (volvulus), which can obstruct the mesenteric vessels and cause intestinal ischemia (Fig. 43–4). Acute midgut volvulus is most often encountered in the newborn period[11] but can occur in older children and adults.[17, 18] The most common symptom associated with acute midgut volvulus is vomiting of acute onset, usually bilious. Other common signs and symptoms of acute midgut volvulus include abdominal distention, crampy abdominal pain, abdominal tenderness, and passage of blood or mucosal tissue from the rectum. If the ischemic process is allowed to progress, patients develop signs of peritonitis and hypovolemic shock. Older children and adults frequently have a history that suggests previous intermittent episodes of partial volvulus with recurring colicky abdominal pain associated with bilious emesis.

Anomalies of rotation can also cause chronic midgut volvulus. In these patients, partial volvulus of long-standing results in venous and lymphatic obstruction, which can lead to altered intestinal motility and absorption. These patients may present with failure to thrive, chronic abdominal pain, nausea, vomiting, and diarrhea. Other symptoms include constipation, intermittent apnea, solid food intolerance, obstructive jaundice, and chylous ascites.[19, 20] Failure to suspect this diagnosis has resulted in diet manipulation and even psychiatric evaluation.[12]

Anomalies of midgut rotation can also cause acute or chronic obstruction of the duodenum. In some patients, duodenal obstruction is the result of midgut volvulus. Duodenal obstruction, however, can also occur in the absence of volvulus. In these patients, peritoneal bands (Ladd's bands) between a malpositioned cecum in the subpyloric region and the peritoneum over the right flank cross the second or third portion of the duodenum and obstruct it by external compression or by kinking it. Patients with duodenal obstruction may present with a history of forceful, bilious emesis. Patients with chronic duodenal obstruction may also have a history of failure to gain weight and intermittent colicky abdominal pain. Upper abdominal distention with visible gastric peristaltic waves may be noted on physical examination.

## Diagnostic Studies

In patients who present with bilious vomiting of acute onset and peritoneal signs, no further diagnostic studies are indicated. In these patients, delaying surgical intervention for results of contrast studies to confirm malrotation could miss the opportunity to prevent irreversible intestinal ischemic injury.

Plain abdominal radiographs of patients with anomalies of midgut rotation are frequently nondiagnostic. In patients who present with acute duodenal obstruction, plain films may reveal gastric or duodenal distention, with or without distal intraluminal air. In older patients the diagnosis of an anomaly of intestinal rotation may be suggested by an abnormal colon gas pattern. In patients with acute midgut volvulus, abdominal radiographs may be unremarkable; however, they may also reveal a "gasless" abdomen or findings consistent with intestinal obstruction.

For patients who present with vague or less acute symptoms, additional diagnostic studies are required. An upper

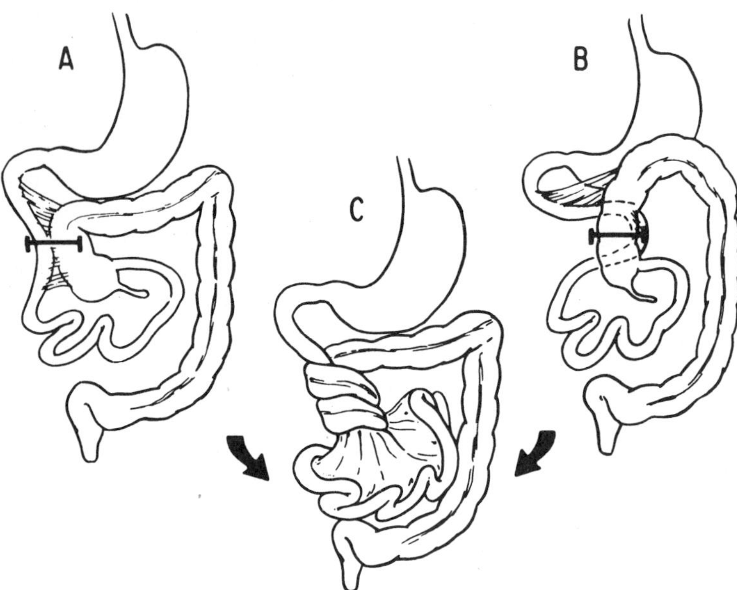


**FIGURE 43–4.** Pathophysiology of midgut volvulus *(C)* with malrotation *(A)* or incomplete rotation *(B)*. (From Filston HC, Kirks DR: Malrotation—the ubiquitous anomaly. J Pediatr Surg 1981;16 (suppl 1):616, with permission.)

gastrointestinal contrast examination with delineation of the duodenojejunal junction is usually diagnostic. Findings on upper gastrointestinal contrast studies that are diagnostic of malrotation include abnormal position of the ligament of Treitz, obstruction of the second, or third portion of the duodenum (often with a beak, spiral, or corkscrew appearance; Fig. 43–5), and proximal jejunal loops that are located to the right of the midline.[2] Occasionally, upper gastrointestinal contrast findings are equivocal. In these patients, further diagnostic information can be gained from delayed images that demonstrate the site of the ileocecal junction, or the position of the cecum can be determined by barium enema. The finding of an abnormally positioned cecum or ileocecal junction in the right upper quadrant or to the left of the midline on contrast examination of the colon supports a diagnosis of malrotation. The diagnostic accuracy of barium enema examination alone is limited, however, since the cecum is positioned normally in as many as 30% of patients with malrotation.[21] In addition, a high-riding or mobile cecum can occur in the absence of a rotational anomaly.[4]

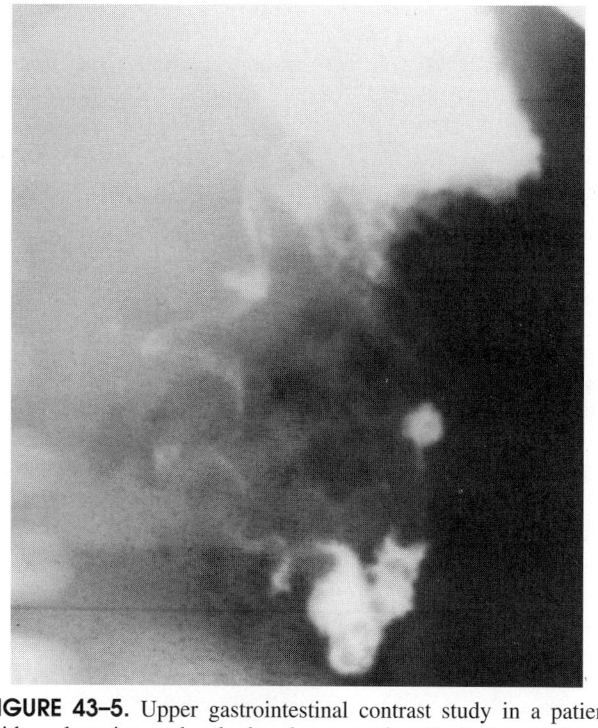

**FIGURE 43–5.** Upper gastrointestinal contrast study in a patient with malrotation and volvulus demonstrating "coiled spring" appearance of the duodenum. (Courtesy of Marc S. Keller, MD, Yale–New Haven Children's Hospital.)

Recently ultrasonography has been used to detect rotational anomalies. Ultrasound findings that suggest the diagnosis of malrotation with volvulus include duodenal obstruction, thickened bowel loops to the right of the spine, and peritoneal fluid.[22] In addition, a superior mesenteric vein located to the left of the superior mesenteric artery is highly suggestive of malrotation.[23] A normal relationship of the superior mesenteric vessels, however, does not exclude malrotation.[24]

## Treatment

Patients who present with evidence of midgut volvulus and peritonitis should be fluid resuscitated and then taken "emergently" to the operating room. Patients who present with less acute symptoms should undergo operative correction at the earliest possible opportunity. The reason for urgency is the inability of diagnostic studies to exclude midgut volvulus.[25]

Occasionally, anomalies of midgut rotation are diagnosed in patients beyond the neonatal period who are asymptomatic. Previously it was felt that after their second birthday patients with asymptomatic malrotation had little risk of volvulus, so surgical intervention was not recommended. Multiple reports, however, indicate that patients of all ages with an anomaly of rotation can develop volvulus, even without pre-existing symptoms.[12, 25] Thus, at present, surgical treatment is recommended for any patient with an anomaly of rotation, regardless of age or symptoms.

The classic surgical procedure for midgut volvulus is Ladd's operation, which includes several important steps: (1) evisceration of the entire midgut and inspection of the mesenteric root; (2) derotation of volvulus, if present (usually in a counterclockwise direction); (3) division of peritoneal bands (Ladd's bands) that overlie and compress the duodenum; (4) dissection of the mesenteric pedicle to broaden its base of attachment; (5) appendectomy; and (6) placement of the mobilized cecum into the left lower quadrant. At the completion of the operation, the entire small intestine is positioned in the abdomen to the right of the midline with the large intestine on the left. This orientation results in maximal widening of the mesenteric root. Adhesions that develop contribute to the very low incidence of recurrent volvulus. Some surgeons have advocated suture fixation of the duodenum and cecum to further decrease the risk of recurrent midgut volvulus[26]; however, a comparative study of the late results with fixation versus no fixation has shown no benefit for suture fixation.[27]

## Outcome

The operative mortality associated with correction of malrotation is directly related to the presence and extent of intestinal necrosis. The mortality rate for patients without necrosis is approximately 1%.[28] In contrast, the mortality rate for patients with necrosis approaches 50%. The most common late complication of Ladd's procedure is adhesive bowel obstruction.[20] Recurrent volvulus following Ladd's procedure is uncommon,[29] and probably is the result of incomplete division of Ladd's bands.[25]

Most series report partial or complete resolution of symptoms in nearly 100% of patients.[17, 19, 20] However, a few patients have persistent vomiting, diarrhea, and intolerance to enteral feeding. In these patients, intestinal dysmotility may be the cause of persistent symptoms.[30]

# ATRESIA AND STENOSIS

## Incidence

Atresias and stenoses are the most common congenital anomalies of the midgut. *Atresia* refers to a complete obstruction of the lumen of the gut; *stenosis* is an incomplete obstruction. Atresia is more common than stenosis (10:1 in the duodenum, 20:1 in the jejunum and ileum). The incidence of midgut atresia is approximately 1 in 2,710 live births.[31] Jejunoileal atresia usually occurs more frequently than duodenal atresia[32]; however, in some series duodenal and jejunoileal atresia occur with nearly equal frequency.[33] Jejunoileal atresias are equally distributed throughout the jejunum and ileum. Multiple atresias are found in as many as in 20% of patients.[34] Colonic atresia is least common, accounting for fewer than 10% of all atresia cases.[35]

## Embryology and Pathogenesis

The embryonic origins are different for duodenal atresia and jejunoileal atresia. In the duodenum, atresia results from failure of recanalization of a solid stage of duodenal development. Between the fifth and seventh weeks of gestation rapidly proliferating epithelial cells plug the lumen of the primitive duodenum.[36] By the eighth week, vacuoles appear in the epithelial plug, which coalesce and enlarge so that by the 10th week the duodenal lumen has been re-established. Failure of the duodenal lumen to recanalize by a critical point during development triggers resorption and replacement of the duodenum by mesenchyme.[37]

In contrast, in the small intestine and colon an intestinal ischemic event leads to atresia. Proposed mechanisms of intestinal ischemia in utero include volvulus, internal hernia, intussusception, obstruction with perforation, and constriction of the mesentery in a tight abdominal wall defect. Evidence in support of an ischemic cause of intestinal atresia includes macroscopic evidence of a vascular accident (in 30% to 40% of infants with atresia),[34] the frequent occurrence of a V-shaped mesenteric defect, often with deficiency of the mesenteric arcade, at the site of an atresia,[38] and the presence of bile and squamous epithelium in the lumen distal to the point of obstruction.[38] The latter finding suggests that the atresia developed after the solid stage of duodenal development (fifth to seventh weeks),[36] because bile is not secreted until the 11th week of gestation and the fetus does not swallow amniotic fluid until the 12th week. Atresias have also been produced in animals by devascularizing a segment of the gut.[39]

## Classification

Congenital duodenal obstructions can be classified as being either intrinsic or extrinsic, partial or complete, and preampullary or postampullary. Postampullary obstructions are four times more common than preampullary ones.[40] Intrinsic obstructions may take the form of a diaphragm of mucosa and submucosa without involvement of the muscularis, or the site of the narrowing may involve all layers of the duodenal wall. When all layers of the duodenal wall are involved in an atresia, the blind ends of the duodenum may be connected by a fibrous cord, or they may be separated by a variable gap. In a compiled series of 503 patients with duodenal obstruction,[40] complete atresia was present in 245 patients, an obstructing duodenal diaphragm in 206, and duodenal stenosis in 50.

Jejunoileal and colonic atresia can be classified according to a scheme suggested by Grosfeld and coworkers (Fig. 43–6).[41] Type I atresias are obstructions caused by an intraluminal diaphragm. They account for 32% of cases in one series.[42] In type I atresias the outer muscle coats of the proximal and distal segment remain in continuity. In types II and III, all layers of the bowel wall are involved in the atresia. In type II atresias (26% of cases[42]), the two blind ends of the bowel are attached by a fibrous cord. There are two forms of type III atresia. Type IIIa atresia (15%) is complete separation of the bowel ends, usually accompanied by a V-shaped mesenteric defect. Type IIIb (also referred to as *apple-peel atresia* or *Christmas tree deformity*) is proximal atresia with wide separation of the bowel ends, associated with absence of the distal superior mesenteric artery. In type IIIb atresias the distal ileum receives its blood supply by retrograde perfusion via the ileocolic artery. Type IIIb

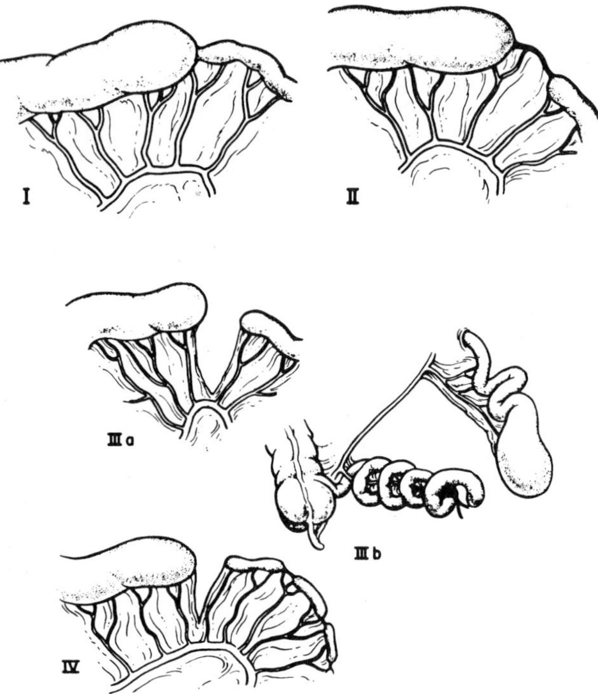


**FIGURE 43–6.** Suggested classification of jejunoileal atresia: type I, mucosal; type II, atretic ends separated by fibrous cord; type IIIa, atretic ends separated by V-shaped mesenteric gap; type IIIb, "apple peel" atresia; type IV, multiple atresias. (From Grosfeld JL, Ballantine TVN, Shoemaker R: Operative management of intestinal atresia and stenosis based on pathologic findings. J Pediatr Surg 1979;14(3):369, with permission.)

atresias account for fewer than 5% of all atresias.[43] Type IV is multiple atresias and accounts for approximately 17% of cases.[42] Individual atresias in a patient with type IV atresia may be type I, type II, or type IIIa.

## Associated Anomalies

Approximately 50% of patients with duodenal atresia have an additional associated anomaly.[40] The most common of these is Down syndrome, which occurs in about 30% of patients. Other frequently reported anomalies include congenital heart defects, malrotation, esophageal atresia with or without tracheoesphageal fistula, imperforate anus, genitourinary anomalies, and skeletal deformities.

In contrast, major anomalies occur less frequently in patients with jejunoileal or colonic atresia. The most common of these anomalies are abnormalities that might have been the cause of intestinal ischemia. Among these are malrotation, meconium ileus, volvulus, and gastroschisis. Extragastrointestinal anomalies associated with jejunoileal atresia include cardiovascular, pulmonary, and renal malformations, Down syndrome, and skeletal deformities.

## Presentation

Nearly all patients with atresia come to attention in the first days of life because of bowel obstruction. The most common symptom is vomiting, which is usually bilious. Another common presenting symptom is abdominal distention. Abdominal distention is usually more severe and occurs in a larger percentage of patients with distal atresias; however, upper abdominal distention occurs in 30% of patients with duodenal atresia.[40] Other presenting symptoms associated with midgut atresias include failure to pass meconium (prevalence 50% with duodenal atresia,[40] 70% with ileal atresia[44]) and indirect hyperbilirubinemia (30% with duodenal[40] or proximal jejunal atresia,[44] 20% with ileal atresia[44]).

Some cases of atresia are detected on prenatal ultrasound examination, usually for evaluation of maternal polyhydramnios. Polyhydramnios is most frequently associated with proximal intestinal obstructions (45% with duodenal atresia,[40] 32% with proximal jejunal atresia[44]) but also occurs in approximately 20% of patients with more distal atresias.[44] Another frequent obstetrical complication associated with intestinal atresia is premature delivery (50% with duodenal atresia,[40] 38% with jejunal atresia, and 25% with ileal atresia). Infants with proximal atresias frequently are also small for gestational age, probably owing to inability to absorb swallowed amniotic fluid.[45]

Patients with intestinal stenosis typically present with symptoms similar to those observed in patients with atresia. The onset of symptoms, however, may be delayed by weeks or even months, depending on the degree of stenosis. Occasionally, patients with stenosis present only with feeding difficulties or failure to thrive.

## Diagnostic Studies

In most patients the diagnosis is obvious on plain abdominal radiographs. The radiographic finding of an air-filled, dilated stomach and proximal duodenum ("double-bubble" sign) without air in the distal bowel loops (Fig. 43–7), is diagnostic of duodenal obstruction, but not necessarily of duodenal atresia. In patients with proximal atresias, plain abdominal radiographs demonstrate a few dilated, air-filled loops of bowel with air-fluid levels. In patients with distal obstructions abdominal radiographs demonstrate multiple dilated, air-filled bowel loops. Other findings on plain abdominal radiographs can include extraluminal air, intraperitoneal calcifications suggesting meconium peritonitis, or absence of air-fluid levels with a "soap-bubble" appearance of the meconium suggesting meconium ileus.

In a patient with radiographic evidence of a duodenal obstruction, the most important diagnosis to consider is malrotation with midgut volvulus. In this situation, an upper gastrointestinal contrast study, with or without a barium enema, may help to rule out malrotation that requires emergent surgery.

In a patient with radiographic evidence of a distal obstruction, the differential diagnosis includes ileal and colon atresia, meconium ileus, Hirschsprung's disease, meconium plug syndrome, and small left colon syndrome. A contrast study of the colon can help to make the correct diagnosis. In addition, for some patients the contrast enema itself is therapeutic. A contrast study of the colon can also rule out concurrent colonic atresia in a patient with proximal obstruction.

In patients with stenoses, when the diagnosis is not obvi-

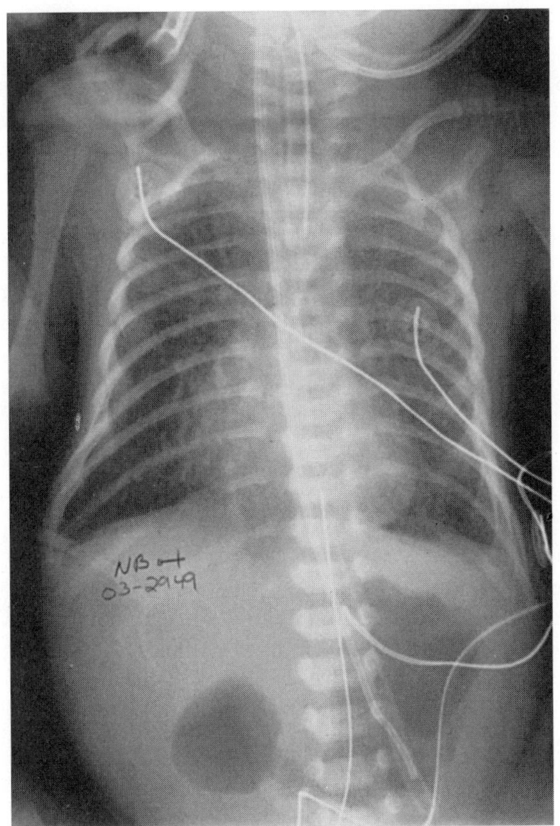

**FIGURE 43–7.** Double bubble in a patient with duodenal atresia. (Courtesy of Craig Mitchell, DO.)

ous from plain abdominal radiographs an upper gastrointestinal contrast study with small bowel follow-through may help to establish the diagnosis.

## Treatment

Correction of an atresia requires surgical intervention. The goal of the operation is to remove or bypass the cause of the obstruction. In patients with duodenal atresia with separation of the duodenal ends, intestinal continuity may be reestablished by anastomosing the proximal duodenum to the distal duodenum or to a loop of jejunum. In a patient with duodenal obstruction due to a web, the obstruction can often be relieved by excising the web.

In cases of jejunoileal or colonic atresia, the problem in reestablishing intestinal continuity is the marked discrepancy in diameters of the proximal and distal bowel segments. In general, attempts to simply anastomose the dilated proximal segment to the narrow distal segment result in a high incidence of functional obstruction owing to poor peristalsis in the dilated proximal segment.[32, 46] When only a short segment of the proximal bowel is markedly dilated, the dilated segment can be resected and the two ends anastomosed. In other cases, however, there may be a long segment of markedly dilated proximal intestine or the bowel may be shorter than normal. In these patients, the dilated proximal intestine can be narrowed by tapering[47] or by plication,[48] preserving bowel length.

The presence of an additional obstruction should be sought in every patient with atresia. This can be done by passing a catheter into the bowel and irrigating the lumen to ensure free flow of fluid into the distal intestine.

## Outcome

Reported survival rates for patients with uncomplicated midgut atresias approach 100%. Primary causes of death include major associated anomalies, pulmonary disease, and sepsis.[33, 42] Some patients with multiple atresias and most patients with type IIIb atresias have short-bowel syndrome. For this latter group, survival is only 53%.[43]

# INTESTINAL DUPLICATIONS

## Incidence

Duplications of the alimentary tract are rare. In one series, only two were identified in more than 11,000 autopsies.[49] Intestinal duplications can occur at any level of the alimentary tract from the mouth to the anus, but they most frequently occur in association with the midgut (Fig. 43–8). The majority of alimentary tract duplications present in childhood, usually before 1 year of age.[50] Duplications of the midgut occur in boys and girls with equal frequency, though in some series boys outnumber girls.[51, 52]

## Embryology and Pathogenesis

The embryonic basis of alimentary tract duplications is unknown; however, a number of theories have been pre-

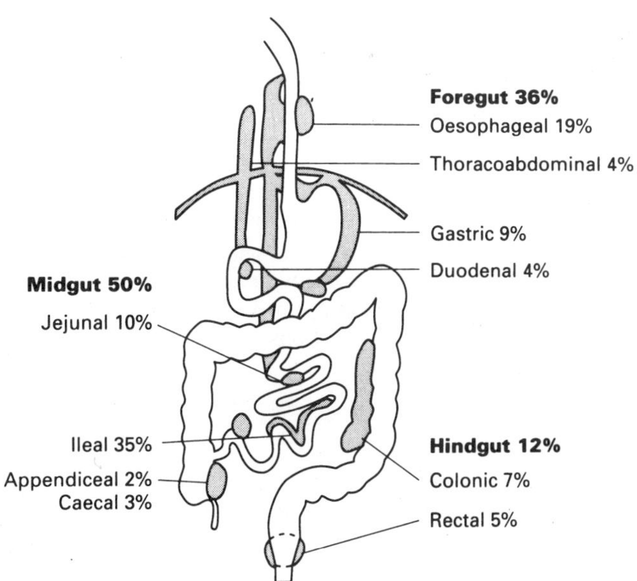


**FIGURE 43–8.** Distribution of a collected series of 495 alimentary tract duplications in 455 patients. (From Stringer MD, Spitz L, Abel R, et al: Management of alimentary tract duplication in children. Br J Surg 1995;82:77, with permission.)

sented to explain them. One theory suggests that duplications arise from intestinal diverticula that occur in human and other animal embryos[53] at an early stage of development. Another theory is that duplications occur as a result of a defect in recanalization of a solid cord stage of intestinal development.[54]

The most widely accepted theory of origin is persistence of the neurenteric canal. According to this theory, duplications occur as a result of persistence of adhesions between the ectoderm and the endoderm at the level of the primitive pit. These adhesions cause a diverticulum of the bowel, which becomes pinched off to form a duplication. Persistence of the neurenteric canal also results in splitting of the notocord, which could explain the frequent occurrence of vertebral anomalies in patients with thoracic and some abdominal duplications.

Another theory is that some hindgut duplications are a form of partial twinning. This theory is supported by the frequent finding of duplications of the genitourinary tract and genitalia in patients with tubular hindgut duplications.

Finally, duplications may also result from an ischemic event in utero.[55] This cause is suggested by the observation that some duplications are associated with atresias of the intestine. According to this theory, if, after an ischemic event, a segment of intestine maintains adequate blood flow to prevent necrosis, that intestinal remnant may survive to become a duplication.

## Classification

Duplications can be either cystic or tubular. Duplications have a seromuscular wall similar to that of the adjacent intestine and are lined by mucosa of endodermal origin. Duplications of the midgut are nearly always located on the mesenteric side of the native bowel and usually share a common muscle wall with the adjacent bowel. The majority of midgut duplications are cystic. Cystic duplications seldom communicate with the neighboring bowel, and the mucosal lining nearly always resembles that of the neighboring intestine. Tubular duplications can also occur in the midgut, and can vary in length from a few centimeters to nearly the full length of the small intestine. Tubular duplications are more likely to have a communication with the adjacent bowel, and approximately 25% contain heterotopic (gastric) mucosa. About 10% of patients with duplications of the small bowel have additional duplications.

## Presentation

Midgut duplications often are asymptomatic and are detected on physical examination as a mobile, cystic mass in the abdomen. Duplications, however, can cause obstruction by compressing the adjacent bowel or by causing intussusception or volvulus. Duplications can also cause chronic abdominal pain owing to gradual enlargement and stretching of the wall of the duplication. Acute abdominal pain can be the result of bleeding into the duplication, perforation of a peptic ulcer in a duplication with heterotopic gastric mucosa, or inflammation. Duplications containing gastric mucosa can also cause acute or chronic gastrointestinal blood loss.

## Diagnostic Studies

Duplications are occasionally detected prenatally as a fluid-filled mass in the thorax or abdomen. Ultrasonography is the most useful test for detecting or confirming the presence of an intra-abdominal duplication. Ultrasound findings that suggest a duplication include a sonolucent or echogenic cystic mass close to the bowel with an echogenic inner rim (mucosa).[56] Intra-abdominal duplications can also be identified by contrast studies as a filling defect that compresses the intestinal lumen, or occasionally a duplication fills with contrast medium when there is a communication with the native bowel. Furthermore, duplications that contain gastric mucosa can sometimes be detected by technetium scintigraphy.

## Treatment

For most cystic duplications, the preferred treatment is resection of the duplication along with the adjacent bowel. Some cystic duplications, however, lie close to vital structures. Complete resection of these duplications risks injuring these stuctures. In such cases, treatment options include (1) partial resection with mucosal stripping of the residual duplication and (2) drainage of the duplication into the adjacent bowel or through a Roux-en-Y limb of intestine.

Tubular duplications can be more challenging. In some cases, the duplication is short and can be resected completely with the adjacent intestine. More often, however, resection of the entire duplication with associated bowel would result in excessive loss of intestinal length. Some reports suggest that these duplications can be managed by anastomosing the distal end of the duplication to the native bowel[57]; however, some tubular duplications have ectopic gastric mucosa, so this approach risks subsequent bleeding or perforation from peptic ulcers. Another option is to strip the mucosal lining from the entire duplication, leaving only the muscle wall intact.[58]

## Outcome

With early recognition and treatment, survival should approach 100%. The principal causes of death are severe associated anomalies and postoperative complications.[52] Duplications that persist into adult life can become a site of neoplastic degeneration.[59]

## REFERENCES

1. Trier JS, Winter HS: Anatomy, embryology, and developmental abnormalities of the small intestine and colon. In Sleisenger MH, Fordtran JS (eds): Gastrointestinal Disease: Pathophysiology, Diagnosis, Management, 4th ed, Vol 2. Philadelphia, WB Saunders, 1989, p 1011.
2. Frazer JE, Robbins RH: On the factors concerned in causing rotation of the intestine in man. J Anat Physiol 1915;50:75–110.
3. Kantor JL: Anomalies of the colon: their roentgen diagnosis and clinical significance. Resume of ten years' study. Radiology 1934;23:651–662.
4. Filston HC, Kirks DR: Malrotation—the ubiquitous anomaly. J Pediatr Surg 1981;16:614–620.
5. Snyder WH, Chaffin L: Embryology and pathology of the intestinal

tract: Presentation of 40 cases of malrotation. Ann Surg 1954;140:368–379.
6. Dott NM: Anomalies of intestinal rotation: their embryology and surgical aspects with report of five cases. Br J Surg 1923;11:251–286.
7. Berardi RS: Anomalies of midgut rotation in the adult. Surg Gynecol Obster 1980;151:113–124.
8. Bill AH: Malrotation of the intestine. In Ravitch MM, Welch KJ, Benson CD, et al (eds): Pediatric Surgery. Chicago, Year Book, 1979, p 912.
9. Borghol M, Holdswort H: Reversed rotation of the midgut in an adult. Acta Chir Scand 1987;153:395–397.
10. Estrada RL: Anomalies of Intestinal Rotation and Fixation. Springfield Ill, Charles C Thomas, 1958.
11. Rescorla FJ, Shedd FJ, Grosfeld JL, et al: Anomalies of intestinal rotation in childhood: analysis of 447 cases. Surgery 1990;108:710–716.
12. Stewart DR, Colodny AL, Daggett WC: Malrotation of the bowel in infants and children: a 15 year review. Surgery 1976;79:716–720.
13. Kieswetter WB, Smith JW: Malrotation of the midgut in infancy and childhood. Arch Surg 1958;77:483–491.
14. Ford EG, Senac MO, Srikanth MS, et al: Malrotation of the intestine in children. Ann Surg 1992;215:172–178.
15. Vargas JH, Sachs P, Ament ME: Chronic intestinal pseudo-obstruction syndrome in pediatrics. Results of a national survey by members of the North American Society of Pediatric Gastroenterology and Nutrition. J Pediatr Gastroenterol Nutr 1988;7:323–332.
16. Chang J, Brueckner M, Touloukian RJ: Intestinal rotation and fixation abnormalities in heterotaxia: early detection and management. J Pediatr Surg 1993;28:1281–1284.
17. Maxson RT, Franklin PA, Wagner CW: Malrotation in the older child: surgical management, treatment and outcome. Am Surg 1995;61:135–138.
18. von Flüe M, Herzog U, Ackerman C, et al: Acute and chronic presentation of intestinal nonrotation in adults. Dis Colon Rectum 1994;37:192–198.
19. Powell DM, Otherson HB, Smith CD: Malrotation of the intestines in children: the effect of age on presentation and therapy. J Pediatr Surg 1989;24:777–780.
20. Spigland N, Brandt ML, Yazbeck S: Malrotation presenting beyond the neonatal period. J Pediatr Surg 1990;25:1139–1142.
21. Slovis TL, Klein MD, Watts FB: Incomplete rotation of the intestine with a normal cecal position. Surgery 1980;87:325–330.
22. Leonidas JC, Magid N, Soberman N, et al: Midgut volvulus in infants: diagnosis with US. Radiology 1991;179:491–493.
23. Weinberger E, Winters WD, Lidell RM, et al: Sonographic diagnosis of intestinal malrotation in infants: importance of relative positions of the superior mesenteric vein and artery. AJR Am J Roentgenol 1992;159:825–828.
24. Dufour D, Delaet MH, Dassonville M, et al: Midgut malrotation, the reliability of songraphic diagnosis. Pediatr Radiol 1992;22:21–23.
25. Seashore JH, Touloukian RJ: Midgut volvulus. An ever present threat. Arch Pediatr Adolesc Med 1994;148:43–46.
26. Brennom WS, Bill AH: Prophylactic fixation of the intestine for midgut nonrotation. Surg Gynecol Obstet 1974;138:181–184.
27. Stauffer UG, Herrmann P: Comparison of late results in patients with corrected intestinal malrotation with and without fixation of the mesentery. J Pediatr Surg 1980;15:9–12.
28. Messineo A, MacMillan JH, Palder SB, et al: Clinical factors affecting mortality in children with malrotation of the intestine. J Pediatr Surg 1992;27:1343–1345.
29. Andrassy RJ, Mahour GH: Malrotation of the midgut in infants and children. A 25-year review. Arch Surg 1981;116:158–160.
30. Coombs RC, Buick RB, Gornall PG, et al: Intestinal malrotation: the role of small intestinal dysmotility in the cause of persistent symptoms. J Pediatr Surg 1991;26:553–556.
31. Ravitch MM, Barton BA: The need for pediatric surgeons as determined by the volume of work and the mode of delivery of surgical care. Surgery 1974;76:754–763.
32. Nixon HH, Tawes R: Etiology and treatment of small intestinal atresia: analysis of a series of 127 jejunoileal atresias and comparison with 62 duodenal atresias. Surgery 1971;69:41–51.
33. Rescorla FJ, Grosfeld JL: Intestinal artesia and stenosis: analysis of survival in 120 cases. Surgery 1985;98:668–676.
34. Cywes S, Davies MRQ, Rode H: Congenital jejuno-ileal atresia and stenosis. S Afr Med J 1980;57:630–639.
35. Benson CD, Lotfi MW, Brough AJ: Congenital atresia and stenosis of the colon. J Pediatr Surg 1968;3:253–257.
36. Tandler J: Zur Entwicklungsgeschichte des menschlichen Duodenums in frühen Embryonalstadium. Morphol Jahrb 1900;29:187–216.
37. Boyden EA, Cope JG, Bill AH: Anatomy and embryology of congenital intrinsic obstruction of the duodenum. Am J Surg 1967;114:190–202.
38. Louw JH: Jejunoileal atresia and stenosis. J Pediatr Surg 1966;1:8–23.
39. Louw JH, Barnard CN: Congenital intestinal atresia. Observations on its origin. Lancet 1955;2:1065–1067.
40. Fonkalsrud EW, deLorimier AA, Hays DM: Congenital atresia and stenosis of the duodenum. Pediatrics 1969;43:79–83.
41. Grosfeld JL, Ballantine TVN, Shoemaker R: Operative management of intestinal atresia and stenosis based on pathologic findings. J Pediatr Surg 1979;14:368–375.
42. Touloukian RJ: Diagnosis and treatment of jejunoileal atresia. World J Surg 1993;17:310–317.
43. Seashore JH, Collins FS, Markowitz RI, et al: Familial apple peel jejunal atresia: surgical, genetic and radiological aspects. Pediatrics 1987;80:540–544.
44. deLorimier AA, Fonkalsrud EW, Hays DM: Congenital atresia and stenosis of the jejunum and ileum. Surgery 1969;65:819–827.
45. Surana R, Puri P: Small intestinal atresia: effect on fetal nutrition. J Pediatr Surg 1994;29:1250–1252.
46. Louw JH: Resection and end-to-end anastomosis in the management of atresia and stenosis of the small bowel. Surgery 1967;62:940–950.
47. Thomas CG: Jejunoplasty for the correction of jejunal atresia. Surg Gynecol Obstet 1969;129:545–546.
48. deLorimier AA, Harrison MR: Intestinal plication in the treatment of atresia. J Pediatr Surg 1983;18:734–737.
49. Potter EL: Pathology of the fetus and the infant, 2nd ed. Chicago, Year Book, 1961, p 367.
50. Grosfeld JL, O'Neill JA, Clatworthy HW: Enteric duplications in infancy and childhood. Ann Surg 1970;172:83–90.
51. Ildstad ST, Tollerud DJ, Weiss RG, et al: Duplications of the alimentary tract. Clinical characteristics, preferred treatment, and associated malformations. Ann Surg 1988;208:184–189.
52. Stringer MD, Spitz L, Abel R, et al: Management of alimentary tract duplications in children. Br J Surg 1995;82:74–78.
53. Lewis FT, Thyng FW: The regular occurrence of intestinal diverticula in embryos of the pig, rabbit and man. Am J Anat 1907;7:505–519.
54. Bremer JL: Diverticula and duplications of the intestinal tract. Arch Pathol 1944;38:132–140.
55. Favara BE, Franciosi RA, Akers DR: Enteric duplications. Thirty seven cases: a vascular theory of pathogenesis. Am J Dis Child 1971;122:501–506.
56. Kangarloo H, Sample WF, Hansen G, et al: Ultrasonic evaluation of abdominal gastrointestinal tract duplication in children. Radiology 1979;131:191–194.
57. Holcomb GW, Gheissari A, O'Neill JA, et al: Surgical management of alimentary tract duplications. Ann Surg 1989;209:167–174.
58. Iyer CP, Mahour GH: Duplications of the alimentary tract in infants and children. J Pediatr Surg 1995;30:1267–1270.
59. Orr MM, Edwards AJ: Neoplastic change in duplications of the alimentary tract. Br J Surg 1975;62:269–274.

Chapter 44

# Anterior Abdominal Wall Defects

William P. Tunell

## HISTORY

Omphalocele was described as an abdominal wall defect by Ambrose Paré in the mid-16th century.[1] The modern distinction of omphalocele as a defect into the umbilical cord and of gastroschisis as a defect lateral to the umbilical cord was made in 1953 by Moore and Stokes.[2] Any chronology of gastroschisis before that time, and in some instances after 1953, contains a mixture of what is currently described as omphalocele or gastroschisis.

The first successful repair of an omphalocele was that reported by Hey in 1803, and D.E. Watkins reported the first successful repair of a gastroschisis in 1943.[3, 4] R.E. Gross published the first series of such cases successfully operatively repaired in 1948.[5] Little success was reported for those patients identified as having gastroschisis until the 1960s. In that decade, care for abdominal wall defects improved in three distinct but correlated areas. The first was the development of modern ventilation for infants; the second, the development by Dudrick and associates of total parenteral nutrition as a practical means of feeding children; and the third, the development by Shuster, and then by Allen and Wrenn, of enlargement of the abdominal wall to augment cavity volume with the use of plastic sheeting.[6–8] These three innovations, with improved anesthesia and antibacterial care, allowed the survival of neonates needing ventilatory support, nutritional supplementation, and abdominal wall enhancement.

## DEFINITIONS

Omphalocele and gastroschisis, although paired as abnormalities of the anterior abdominal wall are probably separate entities. In omphalocele, the intestines and other viscera are covered by a membrane or sac, or, alternately, they herniate into the umbilical cord. This condition differs from umbilical hernia in that the sac consists of an inner lining of peritoneum and an outer layer of amnion, and is not covered with skin as in an umbilical hernia. Omphaloceles vary in size from small defects, appearing to be simply a large umbilical cord, to extensive defects of the abdominal wall (Figs. 44–1 and 44–2). The abdominal wall defect in gastroschisis is lateral to a normal umbilical cord and is usually smaller than 4 cm in diameter; there is no sac, and the midgut and stomach herniate through this abdominal wall defect, which is characteristically to the right of the umbilical cord (Fig. 44–3).

## PATHOLOGY

The incidence and descriptions of omphalocele and gastroschisis were comingled before the modern description of these entities by Moore and Stokes in 1953.[2] Although they both represent defects of the abdominal wall, omphalocele is distinguished by a membrane consisting of external amnion and internal peritoneum with intervening mesenchyme; the umbilical cord inserts into this membrane. The size of the defect is variable, ranging from a few centimeters in diameter, containing a knuckle or a few loops of bowel—essentially a herniation into the cord—to an absence of the principal portions of the abdominal wall, with the defect membrane enclosing bowel, liver, and, in some instances, retroperitoneal organs (see Fig. 44–1). Omphalocele sacs frequently are intact at the time of delivery, although some are ruptured, often in patients with multiple congenital anomalies.

Gastroschisis, a small defect usually located to the right of an intact umbilical cord, has no sac, and the varying length of extruded bowel is adherent, thickened, and shortened. This alteration is thought to be determined by the length of exposure.[9] Histologic examination shows the bowel to be normal, although sometimes with atresia or mummification, which is thought to occur secondary to vascular compromise caused by the small defect itself or by volvulus of the bowel.[10–12] The "peel" or bowel membrane is an inflammatory process that includes deposited collagen and sometimes a lanugo or vernix. Normal bowel wall layers are present.[13] Malrotation occurs frequently in moderate- and large-sized omphaloceles and almost invariably in gastroschisis.

In addition to the specific anatomic differences between gastroschisis and omphalocele, the incidence of coexisting

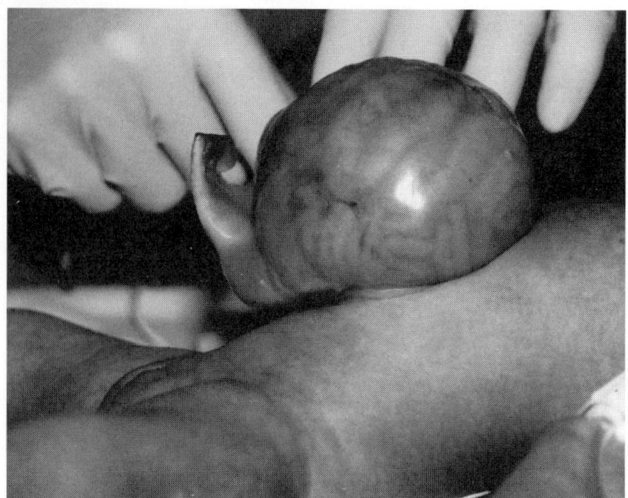

**FIGURE 44–1.** Omphalocele. Note cord origination from sac.

congenital anomalies further differentiates these two entities. Prematurity is more common in patients born with gastroschisis, but other anomalies are much more common in those children with omphalocele.[14, 15] The morbidity and mortality in patients born with gastroschisis is largely related to technical issues and to the presence or absence of intestinal atresia or damage. Morbidity and mortality in omphalocele, on the other hand, is substantially determined by the presence or absence of major congenital anomalies, particularly including those of cardiovascular and chromosomal origin.[16, 17] Although descriptively omphaloceles have been described as small (<4 cm) or large (>4 cm) in diameter, with attendant differences in closure and postoperative care, a more useful classification considers (1) those patients who have an omphalocele without a syndrome, in whom mortality can be anticipated to be less than 5% and (2) those with omphalocele associated with inferior and superior ventral defects or with a syndrome, in whom the expected mortality is 50% or greater.[16, 18]

## INCIDENCE AND DEMOGRAPHICS

The live birth incidence of omphalocele and gastroschisis is difficult to determine. Practical issues confounding these

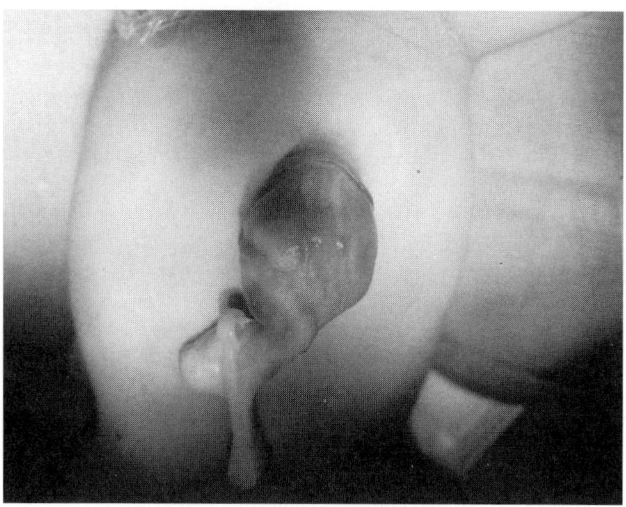

**FIGURE 44–2.** Omphalocele. Small defect.

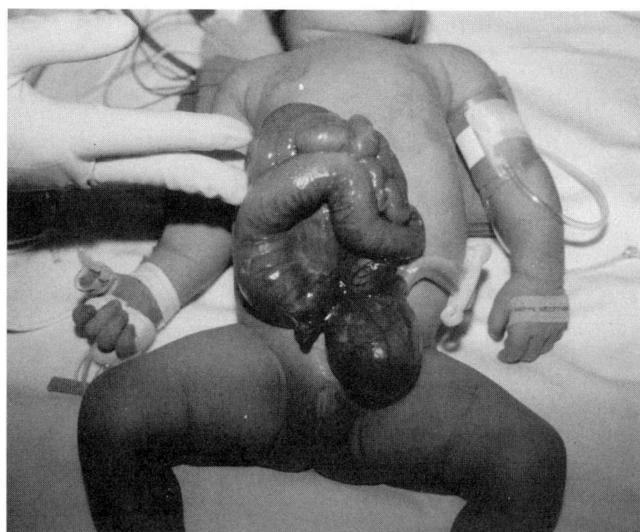

**FIGURE 44–3.** Gastroschisis. Note cord to left of defect and extra-abdominal bowel and bladder with no sac.

determinations are (1) the likelihood that gastroschisis was underreported as a specific anomaly before the 1970s; (2) statistical determination from birth registries, which include stillbirths; and (3) termination of pregnancies after ultrasound identification of these anomalies. For example, Calzolari and associates indicated that in Europe termination of pregnancy occurred in approximately one third of cases in which abdominal wall defects were identified.[19] Nevertheless, statistics from Europe and the United States report an incidence of approximately 1 in 4,000 live births for these two anomalies.[19–21] Omphalocele was more commonly reported until the 1970s; currently, there is an increasing proportion of gastroschisis.[22]

Demographics demonstrate that advancing maternal age and familial occurrence increase the incidence of these abnormalities.[23]

## EMBRYOLOGY AND PATHOGENESIS

The abdominal wall is derived from cephalic, caudal, and lateral folds, well demarcated by the third week of gestation. Each of these folds is composed of somatic layers, which form the abdominal wall, and splanchnic layers, which enclose the foregut, midgut, and hindgut during the third and fourth weeks of gestation. The midgut enlarges more rapidly than does the body of the embryo, filling the yolk sac. The extraembryonic coelom (a large opening from the midgut, which is connected to the yolk sac and referred to as the omphalomesenteric duct) continues to decrease in size throughout gestation. By the 10th and 11th weeks, development of the abdominal wall is sufficient to allow the return of the midgut into the embryonic coelom where rotation and subsequent fixation take place. Current theory suggests a teratogenic event, occurring during the first 3 weeks of gestation, that prevents return of the bowel to the abdomen, resulting in failure of latent embryonic fold development. This failure, in turn, results in an omphalocele. Likewise, failure of closure of the cephalic folds leads to anomalies of the upper coelosomia, including sternal defects. Finally, failure of caudal fold development results in extrophy of the bladder, and in extreme cases, extrophy of the cloaca.[15, 24]

Skandalakis and colleagues noted that gastroschisis is an enigmatic clinical entity; its cause is elusive.[24] A number of potential teratogens, maternal demographic (age) factors, and other risk factors have been implicated to explain gastroschisis. Based on the myriad of differences between gastroschisis and omphalocele, it is likely that they represent separate entities.[25] Nevertheless, both involve herniation of abdominal contents outside the abdominal wall and are considered "abdominal wall defects." The most plausible explanation for gastroschisis is that of Shaw, who postulated a mechanical event with rupture of the umbilical cord and extrusion of bowel outside the amniotic sac—this without the presumed teratogenic event preventing primary return of the midgut to the abdominal cavity, as in omphalocele.[26] This theory would explain the anatomic finding of uncovered bowel in gastroschisis while leaving intact mechanisms suggesting that teratogenesis may cause the multiple congenital anomalies seen in patients with omphalocele.

The most remarkable difference between omphalocele and gastroschisis is the occurrence of other congenital anomalies in omphalocele. Chromosomal abnormalities appear in approximately one third of patients with omphalocele, and cardiac malformations in up to 50%. Gastroschisis, however, is infrequently accompanied by congenital anomalies. Principal problems for these children are intestinal shortening and thickening secondary to exposure to the amniotic fluid and atresias of intestine. It is believed that the irritating effects of the amniotic fluid on the bowel begin at about 30 weeks' gestation, the time when renal function and urine production begins.[9] The "peel" that develops is inflammatory and is not associated with abnormalities of the muscle, bowel, or ganglion cells.[13] Atresia occurs in 10% to 15% of patients with gastroschisis and is believed to result from a constriction of the midgut by the abdominal wall at the point of exit and entrance to the abdominal cavity of the midgut, or by a volvulus of the midgut external to the abdominal wall. This constriction or volvulus of the midgut at the abdominal wall may explain the occurrence of "disappearing gastroschisis" with subsequent healing of the abdominal wall.[10, 11, 27]

## ANTEPARTUM CARE

### Diagnosis

A final diagnosis of abdominal wall defect is made with birth and observation. Prenatally, increased levels of maternal serum alpha-fetoprotein provide a clue pointing toward congenital abnormality.[28] The common use of ultrasound during pregnancy allows the diagnosis of an abdominal wall defect in most infants.[29, 30] Although the abdominal cavity of the fetus can be imaged on ultrasonography by 10 weeks after the mother's last menstrual period, it is when the fetal intestine normally returns to the abdomen (by 13 weeks) that the diagnosis is made. On ultrasonography, the presence of a smooth outline with an echogenic sac from which the umbilical cord is seen to arise provides the diagnosis of omphalocele, whereas a more irregular defect with no echogenic covering and a visualized umbilical cord at some distance from the defect suggest gastroschisis (Figs. 44–4 and 44–5). Ultrasonography has proved to be an accurate determinant of abdominal wall defects and of the presence of omphalocele or gastroschisis. Particularly in the case of omphalocele, ultrasonography may identify other congenital abnormalities, stimulating the use of amniocentesis or other diagnostic techniques to prepare for parental counseling and for patient care[30–33] (Fig. 44–6).

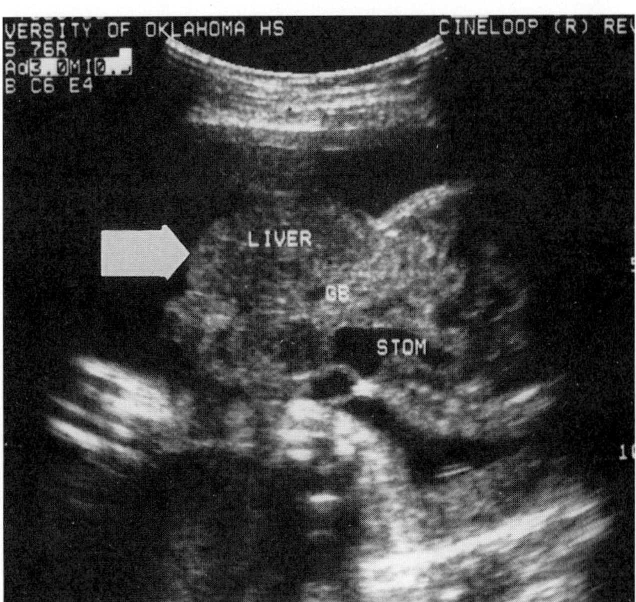


**FIGURE 44–4.** Omphalocele *(arrow)*. Ultrasound examination at 33 weeks.

### Fetal Management

The presence of an abdominal wall defect, particularly omphalocele, with other associated abnormalities, is considered in the counseling of families concerning termination of

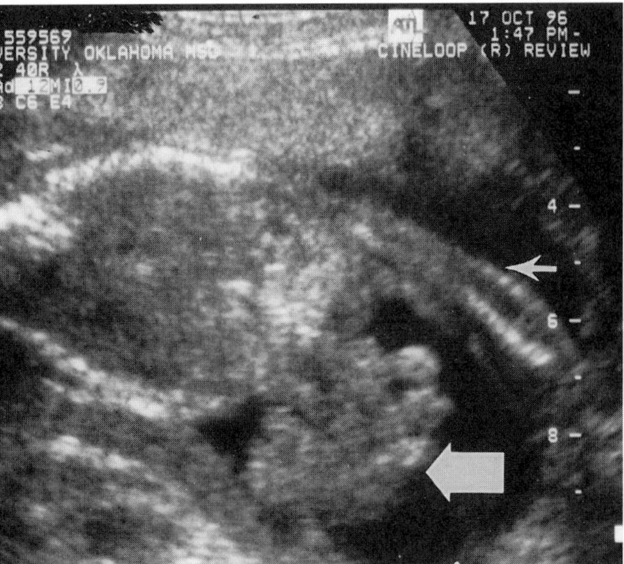


**FIGURE 44–5.** Ultrasound examination showing gastroschisis with cord *(thin arrow)* adjacent to extra-abdominal bowel *(thick arrow)*.

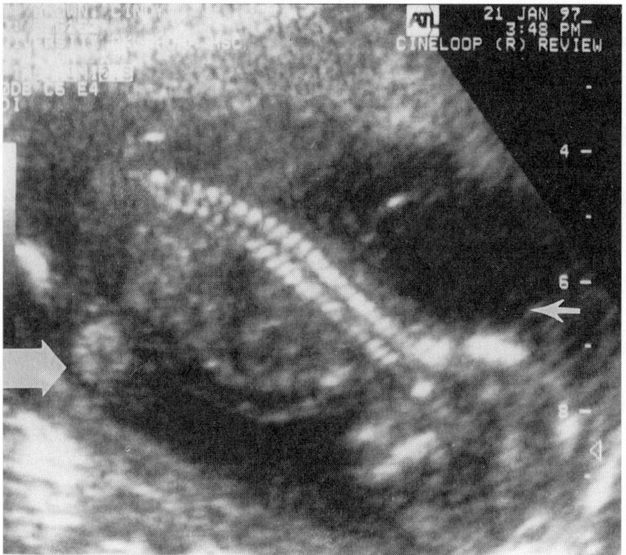


**FIGURE 44–6.** Ultrasound study showing omphalocele *(thick arrow)* and cervical cystic hygroma *(thin arrow)* in a patient with hydrops and fetal death.

pregnancy. If pregnancy is continued, determination of the best method of fetal management must be made. This includes mode of delivery and provision for care of a child with coexisting anomalies. If life-threatening abnormalities are absent, the size of the defect, dilatation of the bowel, and degree of mural thickening in the gastroschisis, and defect size and contents in the omphalocele, as demonstrated on sonography, allow the physician to make timely and accurate estimates of the care that is likely to be required by the infant at birth.[34–36]

The duration of an imageable gastroschisis—that is, the length of exposure to amniotic fluid—does not alter the mortality rate in this disease.[36] Small bowel dilatation in excess of 11 mm in diameter is a predictor of postnatal bowel complications[37] (Fig. 44–7). A progression recognized with sequential ultrasonography is that of the "disappearing gastroschisis." This disappearance is associated with atresias of the jejunum and colon at the presumed points of exit and entrance of bowel to the coelomic cavity. This may be seen postnatally as a "healed gastroschisis," with a normal umbilical stalk and with atresias of the jejunum and colon adjacent to this stalk[10, 11, 27] (Fig. 44–8).

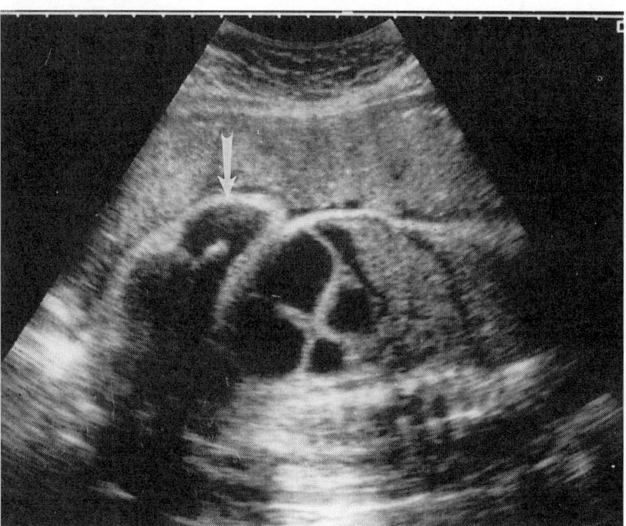

**FIGURE 44–7.** Ultrasound study showing omphalocele with dilated bowel *(arrow)* in a patient delivered with atresia of the bowel.

## Mode of Delivery

The ideal mode of delivery for infants with abdominal wall defect is controversial. It was suggested by Moore that the early elective delivery of patients with omphalocele or gastroschisis, when lung maturity is demonstrated, improves survival.[38] Although not unanimous, most reports demonstrate no advantage to cesarean section at term in so far as determining morbidity and mortality for these infants.[39–42] Vaginal delivery seems atraumatic. Nevertheless, an elective delivery, presumably by cesarean section, during the routine workday, makes all of the facilities of a children's hospital available for the sick neonate. There seem to be no demonstrable differences in survival between omphalocele and gastroschisis related to early ultrasound diagnosis or method of delivery; differing survival is related to the underlying disease process and health.[31, 40]

# TREATMENT CONSIDERATIONS

## Operative Treatment

An orderly plan of treatment can be established with the parents when the diagnosis is made antenatally and then instituted with birth of the child. Ideally, one has the opportu-

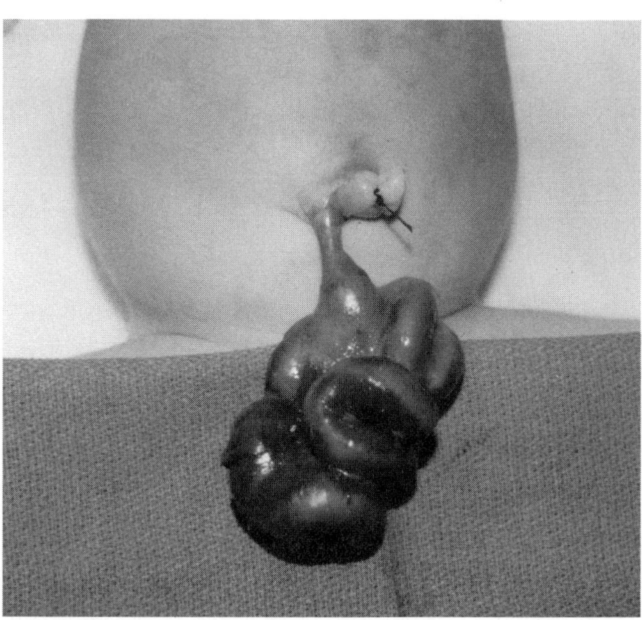

**FIGURE 44–8.** "Nearly healed" gastroschisis. There is a normal cord with exiting lateral vascular stalk. There is no bowel continuity, and internal proximal jejunal and distal colonic obstruction is present.

nity to meet and counsel the parents prenatally and then, postnatally but preoperatively, to discuss with them the previously established plan, making alterations based on evaluation of the child at birth. The closure of gastroschisis is an emergency, and the infrequency of associated congenital anomalies makes emergency repair feasible in most infants. On the other hand, with an omphalocele, unless it is ruptured, there is the opportunity for a period of at least hours for preoperative evaluation and refinement of planning. It is useful to obtain ultrasonic definition of the status of the renal and cardiac systems before closure; although urgent treatment may not be altered, "forewarned is forearmed."

Certain problems are common to these patients. A distended gastrointestinal tract is an impediment to closure or alternate management of the abdominal wall. A nasogastric tube should be placed for gastrointestinal tract decompression. Conservation of body heat is important; in addition to the usual neonatal management in radiant warmers, the omphalocele sac or extruded bowel in gastroschisis should be supported with a plastic film and wrapped with a dry, bulky, sterile dressing. Antibiotics and intravenous hydration should be begun. The hydration scheme described by Mollitt and associates for gastroschisis, but also applicable to omphalocele, has proved useful.[43] In this scheme, colloid solution (20 mL/kg) is administered intravenously, followed by lactated Ringer's solution (hypotonic saline solution with potassium) to provide a total volume of 120 to 125 mL/kg in the first 24 hours. Photographs of omphalocele and particularly gastroschisis are very dramatic when compared with postoperative results; therefore, preoperative and postoperative photography is recommended, even if instant prints, to be kept for both the chart and the family.

## Intraoperative Treatment

Intraoperative observations and measurements in omphalocele and gastroschisis closure are important for successful postoperative ventilation and perfusion. Central venous, right heart, venacaval, intragastric, and inspiratory inhalation pressures have been suggested as useful measures in the successful management of abdominal wall defects during surgery.[44] End-tidal carbon dioxide monitoring, available in most pediatric operating rooms, is accurate in assessing the prospective ability to ventilate patients postoperatively and to maintain blood volume and urinary output.[45] This predicts the ability to manage the increased intra-abdominal pressure that occurs inevitably with either primary or sequentially staged closure of the abdominal wall.

# SPECIFIC MANAGEMENT

## Gastroschisis

Most patients with gastroschisis can safely undergo primary repair (Fig. 44–9). In a minority of patients with difficult reduction through the existent gastroschisis defect, a right lateral extension provides a laparotomy-like incision, which can be repaired after bowel reduction. Although a variety of techniques have been described for augmentation of the abdominal wall in gastroschisis, the wall is not small, and reports indicate an increasing proportion of patients undergoing primary closure.[46, 47] Barring bowel atresia, it can be expected that most gastroschisis patients will undergo primary repair. I advocate a "stuff and stretch" technique, whereby the loops of gastroschisis bowel are gently insinuated into the abdominal cavity. This bowel reduction allows a more natural dilation of the abdominal wall, over a period of 1 or 2 days, than can be obtained by intraoperative manual stretching. When considerations of ventilation and venous return are thought not to be tolerable, gastroschisis can be controlled by the application of a silo and then closed, much like the reduction of an omphalocele.[8, 48] This technique is not necessary in most patients.[49, 50]

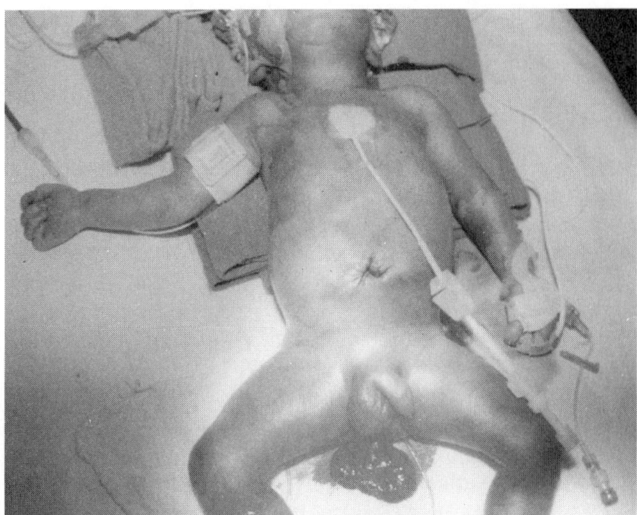

**FIGURE 44–9.** Primary closure of gastroschisis.

## Primary Operative Treatment of Omphalocele

A report by Gross in 1948, of a series of patients with large omphaloceles successfully managed by mobilization and closure of skin flaps, led to a series of advances in treatment for these patients.[5] The successful treatment has been simplified to primary fascial closure of small and medium-sized omphaloceles, a clinical situation not unlike the closure of the abdominal wall in a patient with gastroschisis.[51] Closure follows inspection of the abdominal cavity and correction, as appropriate, of malrotation or Meckel's diverticulum, the two common intra-abdominal gastrointestinal anomalies found in omphalocele. If a portion of liver is within an omphalocele sac that can otherwise be closed primarily, that portion of liver will be intimately attached to the peritoneal lining of the omphalocele sac. This peritoneum should not be disturbed but should be left in place on the liver surface. Inversion of the amniotic sac with closure of the abdominal wall layers over the sac has been reported,[52] but this technique excludes abdominal exploration of the peritoneal cavity with its attendant benefits.

## Delayed Primary Closure (With a Silo)

Large omphaloceles, sufficient in size to preclude a primary repair without causing respiratory insufficiency, interference with venacaval blood return, reduction of renoarterial blood flow, or necrosis of a "too tight" abdominal wall, have been treated with expansion of the abdominal cavity by the application of Silastic sheeting in the form of a silo, followed by gradual reduction of the extra-abdominal contents into the abdominal cavity over a period of days.[7, 8, 14, 35] This gradual approximation of abdominal wall layers is preferable to a skin flap closure with secondary repair of the abdominal wall, since the herniation of abdominal contents after skin closure may make secondary repair almost as difficult as primary repair, albeit in a somewhat larger child.

The use of synthetic materials to temporarily enlarge the abdominal cavity permitting a staged reduction of the omphalocele was first suggested by Shuster in 1967.[7] The current technique of applying Silastic sheets in an extracoelomic fashion with gradual reduction of the contents was popularized by Allen and Wrenn in 1969.[8] Silastic sheeting that has been sewn to the border of the fascial defect of the abdominal cavity to create an extra-abdominal pouch or silo is gradually reduced by daily compression of the silo contents into the abdominal cavity, thereby enlarging the abdominal musculature and permitting final closure of the fascia. Most moderate to large omphalocele defects can be reduced to secondary closure within 2 to 4 days. A number of mechanical devices have been described for this technique, but I prefer the sequential reduction of silo contents into the abdominal cavity with approximation of the sheeting by several sterile safety pins—like squeezing toothpaste out of a tube into a jar (Fig. 44–10). Since these patients almost invariably are being ventilated, they can be sedated and given analgesia in the neonatal intensive care unit for this procedure, with final fascial closure being reserved for the operating room at the appropriate time.

### Nonoperative Treatment

Occasionally a huge omphalocele sac is best treated by scarification of the intact omphalocele sac while there is growth of the abdominal wall and of the patient. Each of the drying or scarifying agents (e.g., merbromin, povidone-iodine, silver nitrate) has its own deficiencies and complications and should be used only in the situation where it is crucial to avoid an operation in the neonatal period.[53]

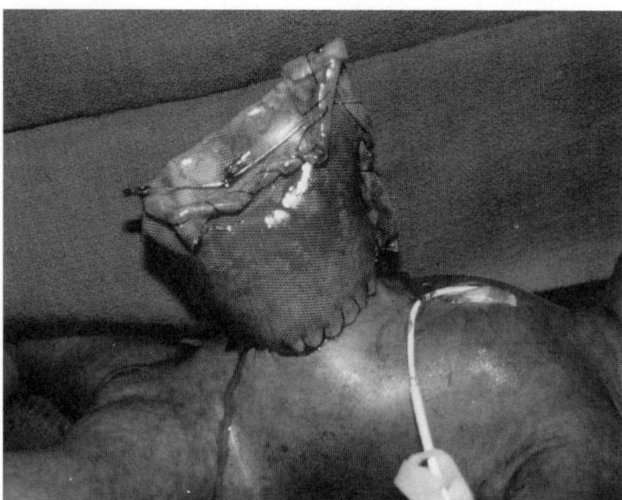

**FIGURE 44–10.** Omphalocele. Delayed, staged closure using Silastic sheeting (silo). Gradual reduction in neonatal care unit has begun, with sterile safety pins used to roll sheeting.

## POSTOPERATIVE CARE

Modern techniques of ventilation in the neonatal unit, satisfactory management of infections, and the provision of adequate nutrition, typically with central venous alimentation, are crucial in caring for patients with abdominal wall defects. The advent in the mid-1960s of infant pressure ventilators, and later of infant volume ventilators, for use in neonatal patients made possible many of the operative and postoperative manipulations of the abdominal wall that are necessary and used in the care of these infants. In 1965, the development by Dudrick and associates of a method of adequate intravenous nutrition by means of central venous access allowed for sequential planning and unhurried care without practical fear of starvation.[6] Other technical issues, such as provision of adequate glucose intake, antibiotic administration, and adequate fluid intake, are also eased by this means.

## MANAGEMENT OF INTESTINAL ATRESIA

A specific complication of gastroschisis is the presence of intestinal atresias. These often originate at the site of exit or entrance of the bowel from the abdominal wall, presumably because of pressure on the mesentery or bowel. Although an occasional case (e.g., proximal jejunal atresia) may lend itself to a primary anastomosis, for most of these patients bowel exteriorization (with ostomies) and a secondary closure is the preferred treatment.[54] The patient with atresias must be treated to conserve intestinal length; the patient with multiple bowel atresias presents a particularly difficult problem. Several ingenious schemes for preservation of bowel length have been described, including a "shishkabob" technique whereby areas of membranous atresia are stented with indwelling Silastic catheters, creating numerous intrinsic small bowel anastomoses while conserving bowel length.[55]

## FOLLOW-UP OF ABDOMINAL WALL DEFECTS

Long-term results for children born with omphalocele or gastroschisis have been addressed in a number of studies; the results are tabulated well into adult life.[17, 56–58] Survival of those with omphalocele is, in large measure, related to coexisting congenital anomalies; with gastroschisis, survival is related to the existence of bowel atresia. Most long-term studies have concentrated on the presence or absence of "good health" or disabilities and on bowel function. As reported to examiners, most survivors of gastroschisis consider their health to be good. Both Lindham[57] and Tunell and colleagues[14] reported satisfaction of patients and their families with their general health and a feeling of sameness with their peers. Nevertheless, almost 50% of respondents who had gastroschisis noted their small stature, and most suggested some resulting impairment in interpersonal relationships. These issues should be dealt with in pediatric care. Patients with omphalocele infrequently report concerns of bodily stature. Dissatisfaction with disfiguring scars of the abdominal wall is variable.[14] By report, the seeking of corrective procedures for appearance is uncommon, although many patients express concern for the absence of a navel.[14, 57] Omphalocele may necessitate surgery for coexisting congenital anomalies, usually in the perioperative period or shortly thereafter. Long-term follow-up of omphalocele suggests that later surgery is infrequently needed for congenital anomalies.[14] Gastroschisis, on the other hand, may require reoperative surgery for correction of residual bowel disease caused by bowel atresia. Atresia, whether treated by stomas by primary resection and anastomosis, requires reoperation in 25% of cases, either for reclosure of stomas or for subsequent bowel obstruction.[14] A number of authors have noted the resolution with time of intra-abdominal adhesions. The surgical correction of these intestinal complications is straightforward and is determined by the degree of illness of the patient. A diminishing number of patients have been observed to require reoperative surgery as time passes after neonatal repair. It is uncommon for children reaching school age to require additional surgical intervention.[14, 59]

Although most patients have no gastrointestinal problems, some complain of recurrent abdominal pain and frequent stooling. It has been uncommon for these children to have a specific diagnosis or to require specific medical care.[14, 59] Radiographic studies have shown a return to normal bowel function after correction of omphalocele or gastroschisis.[60] History and radiographic examination usually reveal no alteration from normal except for malrotation. Specifically, it can be expected that functional bowel absorption and radiographic bowel appearance for length will have returned to normal by 1 year of age.[60] In the absence of intestinal obstruction, no specific therapy is warranted in these children with varying abdominal complaints.

Because many patients with omphalocele and, particularly, with gastroschisis, have prolonged periods of total parenteral nutrition, cholestasis and subsequent cirrhosis of the liver will develop in some. This subject has been poorly studied. No hard data are available, and it is likely that treatment parallels that of cholestasis, jaundice, and cirrhosis caused by total parenteral nutrition in other circumstances. Although many of these patients, particularly those with gastroschisis, have small stature, most, including those with large omphaloceles, report no restriction in normal activities with their peers.[14] An increased incidence of gastroesophageal reflux has been noted in both gastroschisis and omphalocele on follow-up.[61, 62]

The expected follow-up observations in these children, then, are (1) general normal activities and health; (2) a preschool incidence of bowel obstruction in appropriate patients; (3) a tendency for recurrent abdominal hernias after abdominal wall reconstruction; (4) an increased incidence of gastroesophageal reflux after repair of abdominal wall defects; and (5) generally good health, with care to be determined by the individual patient, not by predictable postoperative disability.

## REFERENCES


1. Paré A: The Works of That Famous Chirurgeon. In Cates TH, Young R (eds): book 24. London, 1634, p 59.
2. Moore TC, Stokes GE: Gastroschisis: report of two cases treated by a modification of the Gross operation for omphalocele. Surgery 1953;33:112–120.
3. Hey W: Practical Observations in Surgery. London, Cadell and Davies, 1803, p 266.
4. Watkins DE: Gastroschisis. Va Med Q 1943;70:42–44.
5. Gross RE: A new method for surgical treatment of large omphalocele. Surgery 1948;24:277–292.
6. Wilmore DW, Groff DB, Bishop HC, et al: Total parenteral nutrition in infants with catastrophic gastrointestinal anomalies. J Pediatr Surg 1969;4:181–189.
7. Schuster SR: A new method for the staged repair of large omphalocele. Surg Gynecol Obstet 1967;125:837–840.
8. Allen RG, Wrenn EL Jr: Silon as a sac in the treatment of omphalocele and gastroschisis. J Pediatr Surg 1969;4:3–8.
9. Tibboel D, Raine P, McNee M, et al: Developmental aspects of gastroschisis. J Pediatr Surg 1986;21:865–869.
10. Grosfeld JL, Clatworthy HW Jr: Intrauterine midgut strangulation in a gastroschisis defect. Surgery 1970;67:519–521.
11. Johnson N, Lilford RJ, Irving H, et al: The vanishing bowel: case report of bowel atresia following gastroschisis. Br J Obstet Gynaecol 1991;98:214–215.
12. Anueden-Hertzberg L, Gauderer MWL: Paraumbilical intestinal remnant, closed abdominal wall and midgut loss in a neonate. J Pediatr Surg 1996;31:862–863.
13. Amoury RA, Beatty EC, Wood WG: Histology of the intestine in human gastroschisis: relationship to intestinal malformation. J Pediatr Surg 1988;23:950–956.
14. Tunell WP, Puffinbarger NK, Tuggle DW, et al.: Abdominal wall defects in infants: survival and implications for adult life. Ann Surg 1995;221:525–528.
15. Randolph JG: Omphalocele and gastroschisis: different entities, similar therapeutic goals. South Med J 1982;75:1517–1519.
16. Moore TC: Gastroschisis and omphalocele: clinical differences. Surgery 1977;82:561–568.
17. Yazbeck S: Abdominal wall development defects and omphalomesenteric remnants. In Roy CC, Silverman A, Alagille D (eds): Pediatric Clinical Gastroenterology, 4th ed. St. Louis, Mosby-Yearbook, 1995, pp 130–134.
18. Knight PJ, Sommer A, Clatworthy HW Jr: Omphalocele: a prognostic classification. J Pediatr Surg 1981;16:599–604.
19. Calzolari E, Volpato S, Bianchi F, et al: Omphalocele and gastroschisis: a collaborative study of five Italian congenital malformation registries. Teratology 1993;47:47–55.
20. Torfs CP, Velie EM, Oechsli FW, et al: A population-based study of gastroschisis: demographic, pregnancy, and lifestyle risk factors. Teratology 1994;50:44–53.
21. Tan KH, Kilby MD, Whittle MJ, et al: Congenital anterior abdominal wall defects in England and Wales 1987–1993: retrospective analysis of OPCS data. BMJ 1996;313:903–906.
22. Puffinbarger NK, Taylor DV, Stevens RJ: Gastroschisis: a birth defect seen in increasing numbers in Oklahoma? J Okla State Med Assoc 1995;88:291–294.
23. Werler MM, Mitchell AA, Shapiro S: Demographic, reproductive, medical, and environmental factors in relation to gastroschisis. Teratology 1992;45:353–360.
24. Skandalakis JE, Gray SW, Ricketts R: The anterior body wall. In Skandalakis JE, Gray SW (eds): Embryology for Surgeons, 2nd ed. Baltimore, Williams & Wilkins, 1994, pp 571–575.
25. Kluth D, Lambrecht W: The pathogenesis of omphalocele and gastroschisis: an unsolved problem. Pediatr Surg Int 1996;11:62–66.
26. Shaw A: The myth of gastroschisis. J Pediatr Surg 1975;10:235–244.
27. Pinette MG, Pan Y, Pinette SG, et al: Gastroschisis followed by absorption of the small bowel and closure of the abdominal wall defect. J Ultrasound Med 1994;13:719–721.
28. Palomaki GE, Hill LE, Knight GJ, et al: Second-trimester maternal serum alpha-fetoprotein levels in pregnancies associated with gastroschisis and omphalocele. Obstet Gynecol 1988;71:906–909.
29. Walkinshaw SA, Renwick M, Hebisch G, et al: How good is ultrasound in the detection and evaluation of anterior abdominal wall defects? Br J Radiol 1992;65:298–301.
30. Sermer M, Benzie RJ, Pitson L, et al: Prenatal diagnosis and management of congenital defects of the anterior abdominal wall. Am J Obstet Gynecol 1987;156:308–312.
31. Fisher R, Attah A, Partington A, et al: Impact of antenatal diagnosis

on incidence and prognosis in abdominal wall defects. J Pediatr Surg 1996;31:538–541.
32. Bahlmann F, Merz E, Weber G, et al: Prenatal diagnosis and management of gastroschisis and omhalocele. Pediatr Surg Int 1996;11:67–71.
33. Burge DM, Ade-Ajayi N: Adverse outcome after prenatal diagnosis of gastroschisis: the role of fetal monitoring. J Pediatr Surg 1997;32:441–444.
34. Touloukian RJ, Hobbins JC: Maternal ultrasonography in the antenatal diagnosis of surgically correctable fetal abnormalities. J Pediatr Surg 1980;15:373–377.
35. Nakayama DK, Harrison MR, Gross BH, et al: Management of the fetus with an abdominal wall defect. J Pediatr Surg 1984;19:408–413.
36. Bond SJ, Harrison MR, Filly RA: Severity of intestinal damage in gastroschisis: correlation with prenatal sonographic findings. J Pediatr Surg 1988;23:520–525.
37. Babcook CJ, Hedrick MH, Goldstein RB, et al: Gastroschisis: can sonography of the fetal bowel accurately predict postnatal outcome? J Ultrasound Med 1994;13:701–706.
38. Moore TC: The role of labor in gastroschisis bowel thickening and prevention by elective pre-term and pre-labor cesarean section. Pediatr Surg Int 1992;7:256–259.
39. Bethel CAI, Seashore JH, Touloukian RJ: Cesarean section does not improve outcome in gastroschisis. J Pediatr Surg 1989;24:1–4.
40. Sipes SL, Weiner CP, Sipes DR II, et al: Gastroschisis and omphalocele: does either antenatal diagnosis or route of delivery make a difference in perinatal outcome? Obstet Gynecol 1990;76:195–199.
41. Moretti M, Khoury A, Rodriquez J, et al: The effect of mode of delivery on the perinatal outcome in fetuses with abdominal wall defects. Am J Obstet Gynecol 1990;163:833–838.
42. Sakala EP, Erhard LN, White JJ: Elective cesarean section improves outcomes of neonates with gastroschisis. Am J Obstet Gynecol 1993;169:1050–1053.
43. Mollitt DL, Ballantine TVN, Grosfeld JL: A critical assessment of fluid requirements in gastroschisis. J Pediatr Surg 1978;13:217–219.
44. Yaster M, Buck JR, Dudgeon DL, et al: Hemodynamic effects of primary closure of omphalocele/gastroschisis in human newborns. Anesthesiology 1988;69:84–88.
45. Puffinbarger NK, Taylor DV, Tuggle DW, et al: End-tidal carbon dioxide for monitoring primary closure of gastroschisis. J Pediatr Surg 1996;31:280–282.
46. Filston HC: Gastroschisis: primary fascial closure. The goal for optimal management. Ann Surg 1982;197:260–264.
47. Canty TG, Collins DL: Primary fascial closure in infants with gastroschisis and omphalocele: a superior approach. J Pediatr Surg 1983;18:707–712.
48. Schwartz MZ, Tyson KRT, Milliorn K, et al: Staged reduction using a silastic sac is the treatment of choice for large congenital abdominal wall defects. J Pediatr Surg 1983;18:713–719.
49. Ein SH, Rubin SZ: Gastroschisis: primary closure or Silon pouch. J Pediatr Surg 1980;15:549–552.
50. Chang PY, Yeh ML, Sheu JC, et al: Experience with the treatment of gastroschisis and omphalocele. J Formos Med Assoc 1992;91:447–451.
51. Girvan DP, Webster DM, Shandling B: The treatment of omphalocele and gastroschisis. Surg Gynecol Obstet 1974;139:222–224.
52. Stringel G, Blocker SH: Omphalocele closure: surgical technique with preservation of the amniotic sac. J Pediatr Surg 1986;12:1081–1083.
53. Nuchtern JG, Baxter R, Hatch EI Jr: Nonoperative initial management versus Silon chimney for treatment of giant omphalocele. J Pediatr Surg 1995;30:771–776.
54. Gornall P: Management of intestinal atresia complicating gastroschisis. J Pediatr Surg 1989;24:522–524.
55. El Shafie M, Rickham PP: Multiple intestinal atresias. J Pediatr Surg 1970;5:655–659.
56. Berseth CL, Malachowski N, Cohn RB, et al: Longitudinal growth and late morbidity of survivors of gastroschisis and omphalocele. J Pediatr Gastroenterol Nutr 1982;1:375–379.
57. Lindham S: Long-term results in children with omphalocele and gastroschisis: a follow-up study. Z Kinderchir 1984;39:164–167.
58. Swartz KR, Harrison MW, Campbell JR, et al: Long-term follow-up of patients with gastroschisis. Am J Surg 1986;151:546–549.
59. Larsson LT, Kullendorff CM: Late surgical problems in children born with abdominal wall defects. Ann Chir Gynaecol 1990; 79:23–25.
60. Touloukian RJ, Spackman TJ: Gastrointestinal function and radiographic appearance following gastroschisis repair. J Pediatr Surg 1971;6:427–434.
61. Blane CE, Wesley JR, DiPietro MA, et al: Gastrointestinal complications of gastroschisis. AJR Am J Roentgenol 1985;144:589–591.
62. Fasching G, Huber A, Uray E, et al: Late follow-up in patients with gastroschisis: gastroesophageal reflux is common. Pediatr Surg Int 1996;11:103–106.

Chapter 45

# Neoplasms of the Gastrointestinal Tract

Steven K. Bergstrom

Although tumors of the gastrointestinal tract are uncommon in childhood, a wide spectrum of lesions is seen, ranging from benign isolated polyps of the colon to more aggressive lymphomas, carcinomas, and soft tissue tumors. They may be seen as isolated occurrences or a component of syndromes such as familial polyposis coli. Although children do not usually present with the gastrointestinal tumors typically seen in adults, the symptoms of disease are somewhat generic. There may be a palpable mass, bleeding, pain, intestinal obstruction, or even failure to thrive. Once evaluation points to a mass lesion somewhere in the gastrointestinal system, consultation with the pediatric oncologist and pathologist is essential. Even though no more than 5% of the tumors prove to be malignant, careful handling of any biopsy specimen or solid tissue mass may prove to be critical to the diagnostic evaluation. Samples of a lymphoma, for example, should be processed routinely for cell surface markers and studied for cytogenetics, and by histology and electron microscopy. Similar studies may be necessary for other malignancies as well. Such an evaluation not only contributes to the staging evaluation of the child but can also significantly influence the choice of a specific treatment plan.

In this chapter tumors of the gastrointestinal tract are discussed based on pathology and anatomic location.

## LYMPHOID TUMORS

Lymphoproliferative disorders represent a spectrum of diseases ranging from self-limited enlargement of normal lymphoid follicles to invasive malignant lymphoma. This array of disorders, which can be associated with inherited or acquired immunodeficiency, provide insight into the interactions between infectious agents, chromosomal abnormalities, and the immune system.

### Benign Lymphoid Hyperplasia

Lymphoid hyperplasia is generally a reactive process that results in enlargement of the normal lymphoid follicles of the intestinal submucosa. Histologic examination shows these to be normal, polyclonal cell populations that retain the normal architecture of the nodule. Focal disease has been described in the small intestine, particularly the distal ileum, appendix, and in children the rectum.[1] More extensive involvement of the stomach or the small intestine may be associated with dysgammaglobulinemia, in which the lymphoid hyperplasia appears to be compensatory. An underlying infectious process (e.g., *Giardia*) can lead to follicular enlargement. Lymphoid hyperplasia of the small intestine and the rectum has been associated with intussusception and prolapse, respectively.[2, 3] Rectal lymphoid hyperplasia can also present with rectal bleeding. Treatment is generally symptomatic and related to the extent of disease induced by the presence of the hyperplasia.

### Lymphomas

Malignant lymphoid disease, be it Hodgkin's disease or non-Hodgkin's lymphoma, frequently involves the abdomen. Hodgkin's disease rarely presents with symptoms associated with the gastrointestinal tract, although enlargement of the aortic and mesenteric nodes may displace the bowel. Non-Hodgkin's lymphomas, particularly of the small, noncleaved cell type, have frequently been associated with the gastrointestinal tract and warrant special consideration. The evaluation of a child with a lymphoma is detailed in Table 45–1.

### Non-Hodgkin's Lymphoma

Non-Hodgkin's lymphoma accounts for about 7% of all malignancies in children.[4] Greater than 90% of these childhood tumors may be classified into one of three categories: small noncleaved cell lymphomas, large cell lymphomas, and lymphoblastic lymphomas.[5]

Small noncleaved cell lymphomas, including Burkitt's lymphoma, represent the largest group of gastrointestinal lymphomas of children. These tumors may or may not express B cell characteristics (Table 45–2). They may arise in several locations in the gastrointestinal tract. Gastric Burkitt's lymphoma with pancreatic infiltration but no local

**TABLE 45–1. Evaluation of Child with Lymphoma**

Complete blood count
Liver and renal chemistries
Lactate dehydrogenase
Uric acid
Calcium and phosphorus
Serum electrolytes
Quantitative immunoglobulins
Tissue biopsy
  Immunologic surface markers
  Hematoxylin and eosin slides
  Electron micrographs
Bone marrow aspirate and biopsy
Lumbar puncture with cytology
Chest radiograph and (if abnormal) computed tomography
Abdominal-pelvic ultrasound
Gallium-67 scan

lymph node involvement has been described in an adolescent boy.[6] Ileocolic lymphoma appears to be the commonest site in the gastrointestinal tract of children.[7] A case of what appeared to be a classic benign rectal polyp but instead was a localized non-Hodgkin's lymphoma has been described.[7]

The tumor consists of sheets of small, round, blue cells. Infiltrating histiocytes give the characteristic, although not pathognomonic, "starry-sky" pattern. Much of the current understanding of these tumors began in equatorial Africa, where Burkitt observed that their occurrence among native Africans coincided with the distribution of malaria-causing mosquitoes.[8] Further observations led to an association with Epstein-Barr virus (EBV) infections and with a chromosomal abnormality, the t(8;14) translocation.[9]

The nature of small noncleaved cell lymphomas in American children differs in many respects from those seen in Africa. Both frequently present with abdominal involvement, but the familiar jaw presentation seen in African children is rare among the sporadic cases seen in the Western world. Also, underlying EBV infection is seen in fewer than 15% of sporadic Burkitt's (American) whereas more than 90% of endemic (African) cases show evidence of viral involvement.[10]

The t(8;14) translocation has been seminal in our understanding of the underlying mechanisms of cell dysregulation in Burkitt's lymphoma. This brings the immunoglobulin heavy chain gene enhancer, found on chromosome 14, into juxtaposition with the *MYC* gene, found on chromosome 8.[11, 12] The *MYC* gene participates in regulation of progression of the cell through the cell cycle.[13] Changes in the expression of the *MYC* gene are thought to result in the malignancy. While the contribution of EBV and malaria to the malignant transformation of Burkitt's lymphoma remains to be demonstrated, it is likely that the resulting B cell mutagenesis and T cell immunosuppresion that accompany these diseases give rise to a pool of rapidly multiplying B lymphocytes, in which the chromosomal abnormalities are more likely to occur.

**TABLE 45–2. Common Types of Childhood Non-Hodgkin's Lymphoma**

| | |
|---|---|
| **Lymphoblastic** | **Diffuse Large Cell** |
| Usually T (thymocyte) | Usually B (immunoblastic) |
| Some pre-B | Some B (follicular) |
| **Small, Noncleaved Cell** | Rare T |
| Usually B | |

Non-Hodgkin's lymphoma is 60 times more common among patients with acquired immunodeficiency syndrome (AIDS) than in the general population of the United States.[14] Of these tumors, most are Burkitt's lymphoma, and a small number are immunoblastic (large cell) lymphoma.[15] Patients usually present with advanced-stage disease, frequently with extranodal involvement. Successful treatment is often complicated by pre-existing pancytopenias and the predisposition for opportunistic infections.

Inherited as well as iatrogenic immunosuppression is associated with a similar increase in the incidence of non-Hodgkin's lymphoma. Among the inherited conditions associated with this increase are ataxia-telangiectasia, Wiskott-Aldrich syndrome, Bloom's syndrome, severe combined immunodeficiency syndrome (SCIDS), and common variable immunodeficiency.[16] Drug-induced immunosuppression, seen in solid organ and bone marrow transplant recipients, has also been associated with an increased incidence of non-Hodgkin's lymphomas.[16]

Large cell lymphomas represent a diverse group of lymphoid malignancies that vary tremendously in their clinical course, morphologic appearance, immunophenotypic characteristics, and associated chromosomal abnormalities. A subgroup, the immunoblastic lymphomas, related to small noncleaved cell lymphomas in their B cell origin. These tumors may present in almost any site, including primary visceral involvement. The anaplastic large cell lymphomas, which express Ki-1 (CD30) antigen, may be seen in the skin, bone, or soft tissue.

The lymphoblastic lymphomas, which may present with hepatosplenomegaly, only rarely involve the structures of the gastrointestinal tract.[17] These tumors frequently present with mediastinal enlargement and many express T cell phenotype. In patients with more than 25% blasts in the bone marrow, the diagnosis of acute lymphoblastic leukemia (ALL) is made, but the two diagnoses are parts of the spectrum of a single disease.

The chronic inflammatory response to *Helicobacter pylori* infection has been associated with the development of non-Hodgkin's lymphoma of the stomach in adults and children.[18] Lymphoid abnormalities associated with *H. pylori* infection range from benign hyperplasia of mucosa-associated lymphoid tissue (MALT) to high-grade lymphoma.[19, 20] Lesions may demonstrate polyclonal or monoclonal antigen receptor gene rearrangements, suggesting a progression of the disorder from chronic inflammation to a neoplastic process. Treatment of these lesions remains controversial. Eradication of the organism with bismuth and antibiotics has proven only partially effective;[21] however, regression of MALT lesions has been reported with this therapy.[22–24] Malignant disease ranging from MALT lymphoma, which is generally limited to the mucosal layers, to high-grade non-Hodgkin's lymphoma involving deeper tissues has been treated as are other non-Hodgkin's lymphomas, with aggressive surgery and multiagent chemotherapy. The efficacy of these treatments, and the prognosis for children with the disease, have yet to be determined in clinical trials (see Chapter 18).

### *Treatment and Survival*

The application of multi-agent chemotherapy, pioneered in the treatment of Hodgkin's disease, has led to revolutionary advances in the therapy and survival of children with non-Hodgkin's lymphoma. These advances have been most dramatic in patients with small, noncleaved cell tumors. The use of cyclophosphamide, vincristine, methotrexate, and prednisone (COMP),[25] and then more intensive regimens based on the $LSA_2$-$L_2$ protocol of Memorial-Sloan Kettering Cancer Center[26] demonstrated the curative potential of intensive, multi-agent therapy for Burkitt's lymphoma. Most current treatment protocols for small, noncleaved cell lymphoma are based on intensive, multi-agent chemotherapy, including cyclophosphamide and methotrexate, given over a relatively short time. Complete surgical excision of limited abdominal disease has been shown to play an important curative role.[27] Survival rates of 85% to 95% have allowed clinicians to focus on reducing the amount of treatment-related morbidity, especially anthrocycline-related cardiomyopathy, and sterility associated with cyclophosphamide.[28, 29] More extensive disease, including extensive bone marrow involvement (B cell ALL), has been shown to respond to aggressive chemotherapy as well. Long-term survival rates of 75% to 85% have been demonstrated with the current generation of protocols used to treat extensive small noncleaved cell tumors.[30, 31]

A subgroup of the large cell lymphomas, the immunoblastic lymphomas, also appear to respond reasonably well to chemotherapy used in Burkitt's lymphoma.[32] For anaplastic large cell lymphomas, further intensification of therapy, including autologous or allogeneic bone marrow transplant, has been shown to improve long-term survival.

Lymphoblastic lymphoma therapy differs in both intensity and duration from that used in Burkitt's lymphoma. Most current regimens involve variations of drugs used in the $LSA_2$-$L_2$ protocol, administered in a fashion similar to therapy for ALL over 18 to 36 months.[33–35] Patients with limited disease have an excellent prognosis, although the optimal length of therapy for these patients has yet to be determined. Patients with a large tumor burden, particularly in the mediastinum, are at increased risk of relapse. While a majority of patients, 65% to 75%, are cured of their disease, these figures have not improved in more than a decade.

## POLYPS

Benign polyps are, overall, the most common tumors of the lower gastrointestinal tract in children (see Chapter 35). These polyps may be divided into four groups: juvenile, hamartomatous, inflammatory fibroid, and lymphoid polyps.

Malignant adenomas of the colon, either solitary or multiple, may be seen, usually in connection with familial polyposis. Although three separate clinical syndromes have been described (familial polyposis coli, Gardner's syndrome, and Turcot's syndrome), they share many clinical and pathologic features that make them difficult to distinguish. All three represent autosomal-dominant inherited diseases, and adenomatous polyposis is a common feature of them all.

Lynch's syndrome, or hereditary nonpolyposis colorectal carcinoma (HNPCC), is another hereditary syndrome associated with colorectal carcinoma and also with nongastrointestinal tumors of the endometrium, stomach, and urinary tract.[36] While generally seen in patients older than 20 years, a report of a 13-year-old patient with a family history of HNPCC who developed adenocarcinoma of the transverse colon underscores the potential early appearance of tumors in these families.[37] Colon tumors are more likely to be located proximal to the splenic flexure. The genes involved belong to the family of DNA mismatch repair genes and are inherited in an autosomal-dominant manner. A prospective study among adults in Finland suggests that patients with this syndrome may have a better prognosis than those with sporadic colorectal cancer.[38]

## NEURAL TUMORS

Gastrointestinal involvement with von Recklinghausen's disease is not unusual: approximately 25% of patients with von Recklinghausen's disease manifest gastrointestinal symptoms, including recurrent abdominal pain, bleeding, or symptoms of obstruction. Tumors, as well as hyperplasia of the neuronal elements of the gastrointestinal tract, have been described in these patients and may be the cause of gastrointestinal symptoms.[39] These include neurofibromas, leiomyomas, neuroepitheliomas, and ganglioneuromas. Malignant transformation occurs in about 10% of these tumors. The most common gastrointestinal sites for tumors in von Recklinghausen's disease include jejunum, stomach, and ileum; duodenum, colon, and mesentery are less often involved.

## CARCINOID TUMORS

Carcinoid tumors are epithelial tumors that can contain endocrinologically active argentaffin cells. A number of these tumors, both benign and malignant, have been reported in the gastrointestinal tracts of children, usually in the esophagus, stomach, and large and small bowel. Most of them are benign tumors of the appendix, where they are generally discovered as an incidental finding after surgery for acute appendicitis (Table 45–3). A large series of patients with appendiceal carcinoid tumors reported by Parkes and coworkers showed a strong preponderance of females among children.[40] Although invasion of the muscularis was noted in some of these cases, no metastatic disease was seen, and follow-up showed no recurrence. Field and associates reviewed 19 cases of carcinoid tumor, 16 involving the appendix.[41] A single case of a 15-year-old patient with a 2-cm lesion in the ileum and multiple hepatic nodules was included in the series. This patient also had symptoms of carcinoid syndrome, with flushing and respiratory difficulties. Chow and colleagues reported four cases of malignant carcinoid tumors in children.[42] The primary site of the tumor was reported in two of these cases: ileum and transverse colon; three showed evidence of widespread metastases; and the fourth invaded the bowel wall. None of these patients had symptoms associated with carcinoid syndrome, nor were elevated serotonin metabolites detected. Three succumbed to their disease, and a fourth remained alive at the time of the report. Among the patients who received therapy, doxorubi-

**TABLE 45–3. Locations and Types of Gastrointestinal Tumors**

| | COMMON | UNCOMMON |
|---|---|---|
| Carcinoid | Appendix | Ileum<br>Colon<br>Stomach |
| Tongue and mouth | Benign remnants<br>Thyroid<br>Hemangioma<br>Cyst | Carcinoma<br>Rhabdomyosarcoma |
| Esophagus | Benign lesions<br>Cyst<br>Duplication<br>Lipoma<br>Hamartoma | Leiomyoma<br>Carcinoma |
| Stomach | Benign lesions<br>Polyps<br>Duplication<br>Teratoma<br>Lipoma | Leiomyoma<br>Leiomyosarcoma<br>Leiomyoblastoma<br>Rhabdomyosarcoma<br>Adenocarcinoma |
| Small intestine | Lymphoma | Leiomyoma<br>Leiomyosarcoma<br>Carcinoma |
| Large intestine | Colorectal carcinoma | Leiomyoma<br>Leiomyosarcoma<br>Hemangioma<br>Lymphoma |
| Pancreas | Endocrine tumors<br>Insulinoma<br>Vipoma<br>Glucagonoma<br>Gastrinoma | Serous adenoma<br>Mucinous adenoma<br>Pancreaticoblastoma<br>Pancreatic carcinoma |
| Biliary tract | Rhabdomyosarcoma | Carcinoma |
| Retroperitoneum | Rhabdomyosarcoma<br>Wilms' tumor<br>Lymphoma<br>Neuroblastoma<br>Ovarian germ cell tumor<br>Primitive neuroectodermal tumor | — |

cin, cyclophosphamide, actinomycin D, and vincristine were used.[43]

## TUMORS OF THE TONGUE AND MOUTH

Tumors of the tongue and mouth are uncommon in children and infants (see Table 45–3). Carcinoma of the tongue has been reported in an adolescent and in a neonate.[44, 45] A series of 23 children with squamous cell lesions of the lips or tongue was published by Moore, but almost all patients were adolescents.[46] Squamous cell carcinoma of the tongue has been reported in association with Fanconi's anemia[47] and as a second malignancy in a child treated for ALL.[48] Two infants with rhabdomyosarcoma of the tongue presented as newborns with botryoid-type lesions.[49, 50] It appears the majority of lesions in this site are benign and often represent embryonic remnants, including lingual thyroid glands, hemangiomas, or cysts. When lesions arc large enough, even benign ones can compromise the airway. Nasopharyngeal carcinomas may extend into the oral cavity. These tumors are the second most common carcinoma of childhood. They arise outside the gastrointestinal tract and are not covered in this discussion.[51, 52]

## ESOPHAGEAL TUMORS

Benign, rather than malignant, tumors predominate in the esophagus. Intramural cysts are common; only rarely have intramural or intraluminal solid lesions been reported.[53, 54] More commonly, duplications, lipomas, or hamartomas have been noted (see Table 45–3).

Leiomyoma of the esophagus was reported by Bourque and associates in two children.[55] The authors were also able to locate a total of 18 other patients, whose combined mean age was 14 years. More than 35% of these children had involvement of the entire esophagus. As expected, patients presented with dysphagia, vomiting, dyspnea, retrosternal pain, or coughing. Simple radiographic studies may be misleading and can suggest the misdiagnosis of achalasia. Endoscopy is essential and helps plan for a difficult surgical procedure, which usually involves resection. Carcinomas of the esophagus are rare in children. Attempts have been made to associate these lesions with caustic ingestion, as in adults.[56–58] These squamous cell lesions have been diagnosed anywhere from 13 to 71 years after the initial insult. Two fatal cases of adenocarcinoma in older children with Barrett's esophagitis were reported by Hoeffel and colleagues.[59] Another patient with Barrett's had been followed closely with esophagoscopy and biopsy, received aggressive surgical therapy, and achieved long-term disease-free survival.[60] Other examples of similar carcinomatous lesions were not associated with specific esophageal disorders.[61–63]

## GASTRIC TUMORS

A vast array of benign tumors of the stomach have been seen in children (see Table 45–3). Various types of polyps, duplications, ectopic pancreatic tissue, leiomyomas, hemangiopericytomas, carcinoid tumors, and lipomas can be found in children of various ages.[64–67] Benign gastric teratomas are well-documented in the pediatric literature. They are most often seen in newborns and predominantly in males.[68–72] Although teratomas in other sites are frequently found to contain malignant components, it appears that such components are rarely seen in gastric teratomas.[73, 74] All these tumors may present with similar clinical signs, including mass effect, bleeding, and gastric obstruction.

Muscle tumors of the stomach range from benign leiomyoma to malignant rhabdomyosarcoma and leiomyosarcoma.[75] Over half of the smooth muscle tumors were malignant. The leiomyosarcomas can invade locally and in remote sites such as the liver.[67, 76] They may be particularly difficult for pathologists to distinguish from benign leiomyomas. Thus, generously wide surgical margins that may require subtotal gastrectomy are preferred. Several children with epithelioid leiomyomas (leiomyoblastoma) who were treated successfully with surgery have also been reported.[77–79] None of these children had associated pulmonary chondrohamartomas, which have been associated with these tumors and may be mistaken for distant metastases.[80] Reports of two fatal cases of gastric rhabdomyosarcoma, which had associated neck metastases, emphasize the need to consider the stomach a potential primary site of this malignancy.[81, 82]

Although two newborn infants have been reported with adenocarcinoma of the stomach, this tumor, so common in adults, is very rare in children.[83] There may be an association between severe immunodeficiency syndromes and adenocarcinoma of the stomach. These include ataxia-telangiectasia, common variable immunodeficiency, and isolated immunoglobulin A (IgA) deficiency.[84] Chronic infection with *H. pylori* has also been associated with gastric adenocarcinoma in adults. Most cases, however, appear to be sporadic in older children.[85–87] Surgical management of these malignant tumors must be aggressive. The precise roles, if any, for chemotherapy and radiation therapy remain to be determined, but experience with etoposide, doxorubicin, and cisplatin in the adult population suggests they may be useful in children.

## SMALL INTESTINAL TUMORS

As previously mentioned, gastrointestinal lymphomas are most common in the small intestine (see Table 45–3). It is also true that in children, lymphomas are the commonest tumor in this site. Lymphoid hyperplasia and carcinoid tumors are the next most common tumors. As one would expect, tumors in this site commonly lead to intussusception, intestinal obstruction, and bleeding. They also cause nonspecific symptoms such as abdominal pain, vomiting, and diarrhea.

Smooth muscle tumors are found in this site and in the stomach. These lesions include duodenal and jejunal leiomyomas and duodenal and ileal leiomyosarcomas.[88–92] It would appear that complete surgical resection is the most reliable therapy for these malignant tumors; most children who undergo subtotal surgical treatment of these tumors eventually succumb to the sarcomatous lesions. A relationship of these tumors to infection with human immunodeficiency virus (HIV) has been described.[16, 93, 94] The precise relationship of this viral infection with the cause of the tumors remains to be determined.

A case of granulocytic sarcoma of the ileum with local lymph node metastases was treated with allogeneic bone marrow transplantation.[95] This approach may have a role for the other refractory gastrointestinal malignancies. Other malignancies that have been treatment enigmas include the adenocarcinomas; however, these tumors appear in the small bowel less often than in the stomach or colon.[52, 96] Several cases of hemangiomas in the small intestine have been noted, with expected bleeding complications.[97, 98]

## COLORECTAL TUMORS

Tumors of the large bowel and rectum follow the same general histologic patterns discussed in the sections covering the more proximal anatomic sites (see Table 45–3). Colorectal carcinoma is not only the most common carcinoma of children but, after primary liver tumors, the most common true gastrointestinal malignancy.[52, 99] Ulcerative colitis, familial polyposis, Turcot's syndrome, Gardner's syndrome, and HPNCC are conditions that predispose to colon carcinoma.[100–104] Children who have undergone ureterocolic anastomoses for conditions such as exstrophy of the bladder have a several thousandfold greater risk of developing adenocarcinoma at the surgical site.[105]

Colorectal carcinoma is more common in males. It may occur more frequently in the Mississippi Valley in the United States, where investigators have attempted to correlate the incidence with exposure to herbicides and pesticides.[106, 107] In addition, there may be a higher incidence in young blacks.[100] These tumors often produce increased amounts of the carcinoembryonic antigen (CEA) or CA 19-9 (another carcinoma membrane marker), which allows easier follow-up during and after therapy. Children infrequently have lesions in the rectum[108]; in fact, there appears to be a shift from lesions on the left side of the colon (seen in adults) to a more even distribution throughout the colon in children.[52, 109] Abdominal pain, which may be vague, is often the presenting complaint. Sometimes there are signs of obstruction or bleeding. Children and adolescents tend to present with more advanced disease than adults.[110–112] In fact, the majority have Dukes' stage D disease. It is not uncommon for peritoneal, lymph node, omental, liver, ovary, or distant metastases to be present at diagnosis. Almost one third of these young patients have the mucinous variant of adenocarcinoma, which may represent a more poorly differentiated form with a worse prognosis.[112]

Surgery should attempt complete resection. If lesions are too large or involve critical structures, preoperative radiotherapy and/or chemotherapy may be indicated. Various agents have been used in adults, with limited success; however, inadequate tumor removal is ultimately associated with a grim prognosis.[52, 100]

Other tumors that may be encountered in the large intestine or rectum are those of smooth muscle or vascular origin. Leiomyosarcomas have been reported, including several in neonates.[113–115] In addition, leiomyomas and leiomyosarcomas have been seen in HIV-infected children.[16, 94, 95] Finally, intestinal hemangiomas presenting both as a single mass lesion and as diffuse colonic hemangiomatosis have been reported in young infants.[116, 117]

## PANCREATIC TUMORS

Pancreatic tumors are, fortunately, rare in children.[118, 119] They may be of endocrine origin, benign cystic origin, or malignant (see Table 45–3). Because of their retroperitoneal location, some become rather extensive before diagnosis. The functioning endocrine tumors may produce insulin, vasoactive intestinal peptide, glucagon, gastrin, or somatostatin.[120–124] Most of these tumors are small, solitary, nonmalignant lesions that come to attention because of associated endocrine symptoms. Even the malignant varieties present with overproduction of substances such as insulin rather than because of mass effect or metastatic disease (see Chapter 56).[120] Benign cysts of the pancreas are also rare.[120, 125] These lesions can be rather large and may produce symptoms by compressing surrounding structures. The serous adenomas are truly benign and do not require aggressive surgical removal. On the other hand, the mucinous cysts have malignant potential and must be resected.[125] Benign pseudocysts occur in children. There is a single report of a primitive neuroectodermal tumor (PNET) arising in the pancreas of an adolescent.[126] This tumor displayed the characteristic t(11;12) chromosomal translocation of PNETs.

Pancreatoblastoma (infantile carcinoma of the pancreas) usually arises in the head of the pancreas and is an encapsulated tumor that must be distinguished from true pancreatic carcinoma.[127, 128] The undifferentiated appearance of the tumors may suggest a neuroblastoma or even an islet cell tumor. Pancreatoblastoma may produce alpha-fetoprotein, CEA, or alpha$_1$-antitrypsin.[129–131] These tumors may represent fetal rests from the ventral anlage of the pancreas. Surgical removal is often possible and leads to an excellent prognosis. One case of a recurrence in the liver has been noted.[120]

Pancreatic carcinoma, which is rare in children, may have the same grim prognosis as in adults.[132, 133] This tumor has been diagnosed in an infant as young as 3 weeks of age,[134] but in a series of 38 cases reviewed by Welch[135] the mean age was just over 9 years. The tumors tend to arise in the head or body of the pancreas.[136] There may be lymph node or liver involvement. Surgery usually necessitates pancreaticoduodenectomy. In the few cases when surgery was subtotal and adjunctive chemotherapy and radiotherapy were employed, the experience was similar to that in adults, with fatal outcome.[120, 137]

## BILIARY TRACT TUMORS

Biliary tract tumors have been described in children (see Table 45–3).[138–142] When such lesions are discovered, they usually have already spread to the liver or adjacent lymph nodes. Such a diagnosis should be considered in all patients who present with extrahepatic biliary obstruction. Adenocarcinoma may develop in the wall of a choledochal cyst (see Chapter 48).[140] The prognosis for carcinomatous tumors of the biliary tree is, unfortunately, thought to be similar to that in adults. Unless there can be surgical removal of all tumor, survival is very poor.

In children and adolescents, the most common tumor in these sites is rhabdomyosarcoma. Lesions may be seen in the biliary ducts or in the gallbladder itself.[141, 142] In a review of 33 total cases reported in the literature, only seven patients were alive 7 to 42 months after diagnosis.[142] Most children had tumors originating in the common bile duct. Ruymann and colleagues reported on 10 additional cases of this tumor that were collected from almost 1,700 children enrolled in the Intergroup Rhabdomyosarcoma Study during an 11-year period.[143] Seven of the patients had common bile duct disease, three had extension into the liver, and three had lymph node spread. These patients were all treated with combined modality therapy involving extirpating or debulking surgery (seven patients), chemotherapy (10 patients), or radiotherapy (seven patients). Four children were long-term survivors. Thus, aggressive multimodal therapy may play a critical role in this rare tumor.

## RETROPERITONEAL TUMORS

Sarcomas, usually rhabdomyosarcomas, are the most frequently encountered tumors involving the retroperitoneum.[143, 144] These tumors are often quite large at diagnosis, and more than one third of patients already have distant metastatic disease. Critical vascular structures or organs are often caught in the large primary tumor, making complete resection difficult or impossible. The prognosis with chemotherapy and radiation therapy remains dismal when primary surgical treatment is less than complete. The use of aggressive second-look procedures after cytoreduction with these other modalities may improve survival for these difficult to treat children. Other retroperitoneal tumors are listed in Table 45–3.

## REFERENCES

1. Byrne WJ, Jimenez JF, Euler AR, et al: Lymphoid polyp (focal lymphoid hyperplasia) of the colon in children. Pediatrics 1982;69:598–600.
2. Ranchod M, Lewin KJ, Dorfman RF: Lymphoid hyperplasia of the gastrointestinal tract: a study of 26 cases and review of the literature. Am J Surg Pathol 1978;2:383–400.
3. Rambaud JC, De Saint-Louvent P, Marti R, et al: Diffuse follicular lymphoid hyperplasia of the small intestine without primary immunoglobulin deficiency. Am J Med 1982;73:125–132.
4. Ross JA, Severson RK, Pollock BH, et al: Childhood cancer in the United States: a geographical analysis of cases from the pediatric cooperative clinical trials group. Cancer 1996;77:201–207.
5. Sandlund JT, Downing JR, Crist WM: Non-Hodgkin's lymphoma in childhood. N Engl J Med 1996;334:1238–1248.
6. Olinici CD, Vasiu R: Gastric Burkitt's lymphoma: case report and review of the literature. Morphol Embryol (Bucur) 1990;36:39–41.
7. Pais RC, Hammami A, Kim H, et al: Non-Hodgkin's lymphoma presenting as a rectal polyp in a child. J Pediatr Surg 1990;25:1280–1282.
8. Burkitt DP: Geographical distribution. In Burkitt DP, Wright DH (eds): Burkitt's Lymphoma. Edinburgh, Churchill Livingstone, 1970, pp 186–197.
9. Zech L, Haglund U, Nilsson K: Characteristic chromosomal abnormalities in biopsies and lymphoid cell lines from patients with Burkitt and non-Burkitt lymphoma. Int J Cancer 1976;17:47–56.
10. Shad A, Magrath I: Malignant non-Hodgkin's lymphomas in children. In Pizzo PA, Poplack DG (eds): Principles and Practice of Pediatric Oncology, 3rd ed. Philadelphia, Lippincott-Raven, 1997, pp 545–587.
11. Taub R, Kirsh I, Morton C, et al: Translocation of the c-myc gene into the immunoglobulin heavy chain locus in human Burkitt lymphoma and murine plasmacytoma cells. Proc Natl Acad Sci USA 1982;79:7837–7841.
12. Dalla-Favera R, Bregni M, Erikson J, et al: Human c-myc oncogene is located on the region of chromosome 8 that is translocated in Burkitt lymphoma cells. Proc Natl Acad Sci USA 1982;79:7824–7827.
13. Packham G, Cleveland JL: Ornithine decarboxylase is a mediator of c-Myc–induced apoptosis. Mol Cell Biol 1994;14:5741–5747.
14. Beral V, Peterman T, Berkelman R, et al: AIDS-associated non-Hodgkin's lymphoma. Lancet 1991;337:805–809.
15. Mueller BU, Pizzo PA: Cancer in children with primary or secondary immunodeficiencies. J Pediatr 1995;126:1–10.
16. Ioachim HL: The opportunistic tumors of immune deficiency. Adv Cancer Res 1990;54:301–317.
17. Sandlund JT, Hutchison RE, Crist WM: Non-Hodgkin's lymphoma. In Fernbach DJ, Vietti TJ (eds): Clinical Pediatric Oncology, 4th ed. St. Louis, Mosby–Year Book, 1991, pp 337–353.
18. Ashorn P, Lahde PL, Ruuska T, et al: Gastric lymphoma in an 11-year old boy: a case report. Med Pediatr Oncol 1994;22:66–67.
19. Nakamura S, Yao T, Aoyagi K, et al: *Helicobacter pylori* and primary gastric lymphoma. A histopathologic and immunohistochemical analysis of 237 patients. Cancer 1997;79:3–11.
20. Sorrentino D, Ferraccioli GF, DeVita S, et al: B-cell clonality and infection with *Helicobacter pylori:* implications for development of gastric lymphoma. Gut 1996;38:837–840.
21. Sherman PM, Hunt RH. Why guidelines are required for the treatment of *Helicobacter pylori* infection in children. Clin Invest Med 1996;19:362–367.

22. Nagashima R, Takeda H, Maeda K, et al: Regression of duodenal mucosa-associated lymphoid tissue lymphoma after eradication of *Helicobacter pylori.* Gastroenterology 1996;111:1674–1678.
23. Cammarota G, Tursi A, Montalto M, et al: Prevention and treatment of low-grade B cell primary gastric lymphoma by anti–*H. pylori* therapy. J Clin Gastroenterol 1995;21:118–122.
24. Bayerdorffer E, Neubauer A, Rudolph B, et al: Regression of primary gastric lymphoma of mucosa-associated lymphoid tissue after cure of *Helicobacter pylori* infection. MALT lymphoma study group. Lancet 1995;345:1591–1594.
25. Ziegler JL: Treatment results of 54 American patients with Burkitt's lymphoma are similar to the African experience. N Engl J Med 1977;297:75–80.
26. Wollner N, Burchenal JH, Lieberman PH, et al: Non-Hodgkin's lymphoma in children: a comparative study of two modalities of therapy. Cancer 1976;37:123–134.
27. Murphy SB, Fairclough DL, Hutchison RE, et al: Non-Hodgkin's lymphomas of childhood: an analysis of the histology, staging, and response to treatment of 338 cases at a single institution. J Clin Oncol 1989;7:186–193.
28. Murphy SB, Hustu HO, Rivera G, et al: End results of treating children with localized non-Hodgkin's lymphoma with a combined modality approach of lessened intensity. J Clin Oncol 1983;1:326–330.
29. Link MJ, Donaldson SS, Berard CW, et al: Results of treatment of childhood localized non-Hodgkin's lymphoma with combination chemotherapy with or without radiotherapy. N Engl J Med 1990;322:1169–1174.
30. Patte C, Phillip T, Rodary C, et al: High survival rate in advanced-stage B-cell lymphomas and leukemias without CNS involvement with a short intensive polychemotherapy: results from the French Pediatric Oncology Society of a randomized trial of 216 children. J Clin Oncol 1991;9:123–132.
31. Schwenn MR, Blattner SR, Lynch E, et al: HiC-COM: a 2-month intensive chemotherapy regimen for children with stage III and IV Burkitt's lymphoma and B cell acute lymphoblastic leukemia. J Clin Oncol 1991;9:133–138.
32. Hutchison RE, Berard CW, Shuster JJ, et al: B cell lineage confers a favorable outcome among children and adolescents with large-cell lymphoma: a Pediatric Oncology Group study. J Clin Oncol 1995;13:2023–2032.
33. Anderson JR, Jenkins RDT, Wilson JF, et al: Long-term follow-up of patients treated with COMP or LSA2-L2 therapy for childhood non-Hodgkin's lymphoma: a report of CCG-551 from the Children's Cancer Group. J Clin Oncol 1993;11:1024–1032.
34. Hvidala EV, Berard C, Callihan T, et al: Lymphoblastic lymphoma in children—a randomized trial comparing LSA2-L2 with the A-COP+ therapeutic regimen: a Pediatric Oncology Group study. J Clin Oncol 1988;6:26–33.
35. Patte C, Kalifa C, Flamant F, et al: Results of the LMT81 protocol, a modified LSA2-L2 protocol with high dose methotrexate, on 84 children with non–B cell (lymphoblastic) lymphoma. Med Pediatr Oncol 1992;20:105–113.
36. Lynch HT, Lynch JF: The Lynch syndromes. Curr Opin Oncol 1993;5:687–696.
37. Faragher IG, Cox CJ, Stevenson A: Hereditary non-polyposis colorectal cancer (Lynch syndrome I) in a 13 year old male. Aust NZ J Surg 1993;63:494–496.
38. Sankila R, Aaltonen LA, Jaervinen HJ, et al: Better survival rates in patients with MLH-1-associated hereditary colorectal cancer. Gastroenterology 1996;110:682–687.
39. Feinstat T, Tesluk H, Schuffler MD: Megacolon and neurofibromatosis: a neuronal intestinal dysplasia. Case report and review of the literature. Gastroenterology 1984;86:1573–1579.
40. Parkes SE, Muir KR, al Sheyyab M, et al: Carcinoid tumours of the appendix in children 1957-1986: incidence, treatment, and outcome. Br J Surg 1993;80:502–504.
41. Field JL, Adamson LF, Stoeckle HE: Review of carcinoids in children. Pediatrics 1962;29:953–960.
42. Chow CW, Sane S, Campbell PE: Malignant carcinoid tumors in children. Cancer 1982;49:802–811.
43. Moertel CG, Hanley JA: Combination chemotherapy trials in metastatic carcinoid tumor and the malignant carcinoid syndrome. Cancer Clin Trials 1979;2:327–334.
44. Frank LW, Enfield CD, Miller AJ: Carcinoma of the tongue in a newborn child: report of a case. Am J Cancer 1936;26:775–777.
45. Patel DD, Dave RI: Carcinoma of the anterior tongue in adolescence. Cancer 1976;37:917–921.
46. Moore C: Visceral squamous cancer in children. Pediatrics 1958;21:573–581.
47. Somers GR, Tabrizi SN, Tiedemann K, et al: Squamous cell carcinoma of the tongue in a child with Fanconi anemia: a case report and review of the literature. Pediatr Pathol 1995;15:597–607.
48. Morehead JM, Parsons DS, McMahon DP: Squamous cell carcinoma of the tongue occurring as a subsequent malignancy in a 12-year-old acute leukemia survivor. Int J Pediatr Otorhinolaryngol 1993;26:89–94.
49. Telleschi S: Unusual pathology and cytological peculiarities of so-called botryoid sarcoma (congenital botryoid sarcoma of the tongue and infantile uterine botryoid sarcoma with rupture of the organ and hemoperitoneum). Arch Vecchi Anat Pathol 1970;56:671–705.
50. Leibert PS, Stool SE: Rhabdomyosarcoma of the tongue in an infant. Results of combined radiation and chemotherapy. Ann Surg 1973;178:621–624.
51. Pratt CB, George SL, Green AA, et al: Carcinomas in children: clinical and demographic characteristics. Cancer 1988;61:1046–1050.
52. McWhirter WR, Stiller CA, Lennox EL: Carcinomas in childhood: a registry-based study of incidence and survival. Cancer 1989;63:2242–2246.
53. Totten RS, Stout AP, Humphreys GH, et al: Benign tumors and cysts of the esophagus. J Thorac Surg 1953; 25:606–622.
54. Watson RR, O'Connor TM, Weisel W: Solid benign tumors of the esophagus. Ann Thorac Surg 1967;4:80–91.
55. Bourque MD, Spigland N, Bensoussan AL, et al: Esophageal leiomyoma in children: two case reports and review of the literature. J Pediatr Surg 1989;24:1103–1107.
56. Leape LI, Ashcraft KW, Scarpelli DG, et al: Hazard to health—liquid lye. N Engl J Med 1971;284:578–581.
57. Kinnman J, Shin HI, Wetteland P: Carcinoma of the esophagus after lye corrosion. Acta Chir Scand 1968;134:489–493.
58. Appelqvist P, Salmo M: Lye corrosion carcinoma of the esophagus. Cancer 1980;45:2655–2658.
59. Hoeffel JC, Nihoul-Fekete C, Schmitt M: Esophageal adenocarcinoma after gastroesophageal reflux in children. J Pediatr 1989;115:259–261.
60. Hassall E, Dimmick JE, Magee JF: Adenocarcinoma in childhood Barrett's esophagus: case documentation and the need for surveillance in children. Am J Gastroenterol 1993;88:282–288.
61. Stephan BH: Zur Casuistik der Dysphagie bei Kindern (Sarcoma oesphagei bei einem 4 jahrigen Knaben). Jahrb Kinderheilkd 1990;30:354–359.
62. Soni NK, Chatterji P: Carcinoma of the esophagus in an eight-year-old child. J Laryngol Otol 1980;94:327–329.
63. Shahi UP, Sudarsan, Dattagupta S, et al: Carcinoma of the oesophagus in a 14 year old child: report of a case and review of the literature. Trop Gastroenterol 1989;10:225–228.
64. Landing BH, Martin LW: Tumors of the gastrointestinal tract and pancreas. Pediatr Clin North Am 1959;6:413–426.
65. Murphy S, Shaw K, Blanchard H: Report of three gastric tumors in children. J Pediatr Surg 1994;29:1202–1204.
66. Yannopoulos K, Stout AP: Smooth muscle tumors in children. Cancer 1962;15:958–971.
67. Quinn FMJ, Brown S, O'Hara D: Hemangiopericytoma of the stomach in a neonate. J Pediatr Surg 1991;26:101–102.
68. Nandy AK, Sengupta P, Chatterjee SK, et al: Teratoma of the stomach. J Pediatr Surg 1974;9:563–564.
69. Cairo MS, Grosfeld JL, Weetman RM: Gastric teratoma: unusual cause for bleeding of the upper gastrointestinal tract in the newborn. Pediatrics 1981;67:721–724.
70. Purvis JM, Miller RC, Blumenthal BI: Gastric teratoma: first reported case in a female. J Pediatr Surg 1979;14:86–87.
71. Senocak ME, Kale G, Buyukpamukcu N, et al: Gastric teratoma in children including the third reported female case. J Pediatr Surg 1990;25:681–684.
72. Matias IC, Huang YC: Gastric teratoma in infancy: report of a case and review of world literature. Ann Surg 1973;178:631–636.
73. Balik E, Tyncyurek M, Sayan A, et al: Malignant gastric teratoma in an infant. Z Kinderchir 1990;45:383–385.
74. Goetsch SJ, Hadley GP: Hodgkin's disease following successful treatment of gastric teratoma in a neonatal female. Pediatr Pathol 1995;15:455–461.
75. Wurlitzer FP, Mares AJ, Isaacs H, et al: Smooth muscle tumors of the

stomach in childhood and adolescence. J Pediatr Surg 1973;8:421–427.

76. Johnson H, Hutter JJ, Paplanus SH: Leiomyosarcoma of the stomach: results of surgery and chemotherapy in an eleven-year-old girl with liver metastases. Med Pediatr Oncol 1980;8:137–142.
77. Rogers BB, Grishaber JE, Mahoney DH, et al: Gastric leiomyoblastoma (epithelioid leiomyoma) occurring in a child: a case report. Pediatr Pathol 1989;9:79–85.
78. Luzzatto C, Galligioni A, Candiani F, et al: Gastric leiomyoblastoma in childhood—a case report and review of the literature. Z Kinderchir 1989;44:373–376.
79. Hamazoe R, Shimizu N, Nishidoi H, et al: Gastric leiomyoblastoma in childhood. J Pediatr Surg 1991;26:225–227.
80. Tisell L-E, Angervall L, Dahl I, et al: Recurrent and metastasizing gastric leiomyoblastoma (epithelioid leiomyosarcoma) associated with multiple pulmonary chondro-hamartomas. Cancer 1978;41:259–265.
81. Templeton AW, Heslin DJ: Primary rhabdomyosarcoma of the stomach and esophagus. Am J Roentgenol Radium Ther Nucl Med 1961;86:896–899.
82. Mahour GH, Isaacs H, Chang L: Primary malignant tumors of the stomach in children. J Pediatr Surg 1980;15:603–608.
83. Siegel SE, Hays DM, Romansky S, et al: Carcinoma of the stomach in childhood. Cancer 1976;38:1781–1784.
84. Fraser KJ, Rankin JG: Selective deficiency of IgA immunoglobulins associated with carcinoma of the stomach. Aust Ann Med 1970;19:165–167.
85. McGill TW, Downey EC, Westbrook, et al: Gastric carcinoma in children. J Pediatr Surg 1993;28:1620–1621.
86. Goto S, Ikeda K, Ishii E, et al: Carcinoma of the stomach in a 7 year old boy: a case report and a review of literature on children under 10 years of age. Z Kinderchir 1984;39:137–140.
87. Schwartz MG, Sgaglione NA: Gastric carcinoma in the young: overview of the literature. Mt Sinai J Med 1984;51:720–723.
88. Freeman J: Leiomyoma of small bowel: a case report. J Pediatr Surg 1979;14:477–478.
89. Riggle KP, Boeckman CR: Duodenal leiomyoma: a case report of hematemesis in a teenager. J Pediatr Surg 1988;23:850–851.
90. Gamoudi A, Hechiche M, Khattech R, et al: Leiomyosarcome primitif de l'intestin grele chez l'enfant. Arch Pediatr 1996;3:566–568.
91. Marshall DG, Kim F: Leiomyosarcoma of the duodenum. J Pediatr Surg 1987;22:1007–1008.
92. McGrath PC, Neifeld JP, Kay S, et al: Principles in the management of pediatric intestinal leiomyosarcomas. J Pediatr Surg 1988;23:939–941.
93. Chadwick EG, Connor EJ, Hanson IC, et al: Tumors of smooth muscle origin in HIV infected children. JAMA 1990;263:3182–3184.
94. McLoughlin LC, Nord KS, Joshi VV, et al: Disseminated leiomyosarcoma in a child with acquired immune deficiency syndrome. Cancer 1991;2618–2621.
95. Kowal-Vern A, Johnson FL, Trujillo Y, et al: Granulocytic sarcoma of the ileum treated by bone marrow transplantation. Am J Pediatr Hematol Oncol 1991;13:34–38.
96. Kabra SK, Kumar CL, Mathur M, et al: Adenocarcinoma of small bowel. Indian J Pediatr 1990;27:987–989.
97. Basaklar AC: Haemangioma of the gastrointestinal tract in children. Z Kinderchir 1990;45:114–116.
98. Hansen U, Boesgaard S, Andersen J: Cavernous hemangioma of the jejunum: long-standing anaemia in a child. Acta Paediatr Scand 1990;79:1124–1127.
99. Rao BN, Pratt CB, Fleming ID, et al: Colon carcinoma in children and adolescents: a review of 30 cases. Cancer 1985;55:1322–1326.
100. Wilcox HR, Beattie JL: Carcinoma complicating ulcerative colitis during childhood. Am J Clin Pathol 1956;26:778–786.
101. Kottmeier PK, Clatworthy HW: Intestinal polyps and associated carcinomas in childhood. Am J Surg 1975;110:709–716.
102. Sherlock P, Lipkin M, Winawer SJ: Predisposing factors in carcinoma of the colon. Adv Intern Med 1975;20:121–150.
103. Turcot J, Despies JP, St. Pierre F: Malignant tumors of the central nervous system associated with familial polyposis of the colon. Report of two cases. Dis Colon Rectum 1959;2:465–468.
104. Gardner EJ: Follow-up study of a family group exhibiting dominant inheritance for a syndrome including intestinal polyps, osteomas, fibromas, and epidermal cysts. Am J Hum Genet 1962;14:376–390.
105. Eraklis AJ, Folkman MJ: Adenocarcinoma at the site of ureterosigmoidostomies for exstrophy of the bladder. J Pediatr Surg 1978;13:730–734.
106. Pratt CB, Rivera G, Shanks E, et al: Colorectal carcinoma in adolescents: Implications regarding etiology. Cancer 1977;40:2464–2472.
107. Caldwell GG, Cannon SB, Pratt CB, et al: Serum pesticide levels in childhood colorectal carcinoma. Cancer 1981;48:774–778.
108. Redkar RG, Kulkarni BK, Naik A, et al: Colloid carcinoma of rectum in an 11 year old child. J Postgrad Med 1993;39:218–219.
109. Abrams JS, Reines HD: Increasing incidence of right-sided lesions in colorectal cancer. Am J Surg 1979;137:522–526.
110. Hoerner MT: Carcinoma of the colon and rectum in persons under twenty years of age. Am J Surg 1958;96:47–53.
111. Griffin PM, Liff JM, Greenberg RS, et al: Adenocarcinomas of the colon and rectum in persons under 40 years old. Gastroenterology 1991;100:1033–1040.
112. Brown RA, Rode H, Hillar AJW, et al: Colorectal carcinoma in children. J Pediatr Surg 1992;27:919–921.
113. Ein SH, Beck AR, Allen JE: Colon sarcoma in the newborn. J Pediatr Surg 1979;14:455–457.
114. Kriss N: Leiomyosarcoma of the colon in an infant: case report and review. Am J Roentgenol Radium Ther Nucl Med 1960;84:540–545.
115. Nagaya M, Tsuda M, Ishiguro Y: Leiomyosarcoma of the transverse colon in a neonate: a rare cause of meconium peritonitis. J Pediatr Surg 1989;24:1177–1180.
116. Leighton DM, Benghanem T, Montagne JP, et al: A case of rectal bleeding in infancy. Aust Radiol 1990;34:89–90.
117. Ibarguen E, Sharp HL, Snyder CL, et al: Hemangiomatosis of the colon and peritoneum: case report and management discussion. Clin Pediatr 1988;27:425–430.
118. Jaksic T, Yaman M, Thorner P, et al: A 20-year review of pediatric pancreatic tumors. J Pediatr Surg 1992;27:1315–1317.
119. Grosfeld JL, Vane DW, Rescorla FJ, et al: Pancreatic tumors in childhood: analysis of 13 cases. J Pediatr Surg 1990;25:1057–1062.
120. Rich RH, Dehner LP, Okinaga K, et al: Surgical management of islet-cell adenoma in infancy. Surgery 1978;84:519–526.
121. Garces LY, Drash A, Kenny FM: Islet cell tumors in the neonate. Pediatrics 1968;41:789–796.
122. Brenner RW, Sank LI, Kerner MB, et al: Resection of a vipoma of the pancreas in a 15-year-old girl. J Pediatr Surg 1986;21:983–985.
123. Wilson SD, Ellison EH: Total gastric resection in children with the Zollinger-Ellison syndrome. Arch Surg 1965;91:165–173.
124. Gundersen AE, Janis JF: Pancreatic cystadenoma in childhood: report of a case. J Pediatr Surg 1969;4:478–481.
125. Logan SE, Voet RL, Tompkins RK: The malignant potential of mucinous cysts of the pancreas. West J Med 1982;136:157–162.
126. Canner DB, Hruban RH, Pitt HA, et al: Primitive neuroectodermal tumor arising in the pancreas. Mod Pathol 1994;7:200–204.
127. Klimstra DS, Wenig BM, Adair CF, et al: Pancreatoblastoma: a clinicopathologic study and review of the literature. Am J Surg Pathol 1995;19:1371–1389.
128. Horie A, Yano Y, Kotoo Y, et al: Morphogenesis of pancreatoblastoma, infantile carcinoma of the pancreas. Cancer 1977;39:247–254.
129. Iseki M, Suzuki T, Koizumi Y, et al: Alpha-fetoprotein–producing pancreatoblastoma. Cancer 1986;57:1833–1835.
130. Ohaki Y, Misugi K, Fukuda J, Et al: Immunohistochemical study of pancreatoblastoma. Acta Pathol Jpn 1987;37:1581–1590.
131. Buchino JJ, Castello FM, Nagaraj HS: Pancreatoblastoma, a histochemical and ultrastructural analysis. Cancer 1984;53:963–969.
132. Moynan RW, Neerhout RC, Johnson TS: Pancreatic carcinoma in childhood. J Pediatr 1964;65:711–720.
133. Tsukimoto I, Watanabe K, Lin JB, et al: Pancreatic carcinoma in children in Japan. Cancer 1973;31:1203–1207.
134. Robey G, Daneman A, Martin DJ: Pancreatic carcinoma in a neonate. Pediatr Radiol 1983;13:284–286.
135. Welch KJ: The pancreas. In Ravich MM, Randolph JG, Rowe MI, et al (eds): Pediatric Surgery, 3rd ed. Chicago, Year Book, 1984, pp 1090–1096.
136. Taxy JB: Adenocarcinoma of the pancreas in childhood. Cancer 1976;37:1508–1518.
137. Carmprodon R, Quentanilla E: Successful long-term results with resection of pancreatic carcinoma in children: Favorable prognosis for an uncommon neoplasm. Surgery 1984;95:420–426.
138. Kelly TR, Chamberlain TR: Carcinoma of the gallbladder. Am J Surg 1982;143:737–741.
139. Fujiwara Y, Ohizumi T, Kakizaki G, et al: Case of a congenital choledochal cyst associated with carcinoma. J Pediatr Surg 1976;11:587–588.

140. Nagaraj HS, Kmetz DR, Leitner C: Rhabdomyosarcoma of the bile ducts. J Pediatr Surg 1977;12:1071–1074.
141. Mihara S, Matsumoto H, Tokunaga F, et al: Botryoid rhabdomyosarcoma of the gallbladder in a child. Cancer 1982;49:812–818.
142. Ruymann FB, Raney RB, Crist WM, et al: Rhabdomyosarcoma of the biliary tree in childhood: a report from the Intergroup Rhabdomyosarcoma Study. Cancer 1985;56:575–581.
143. Crist WM, Raney RB, Tefft M, et al: Soft tissue sarcomas arising in the retroperitoneal space in children: a report from the Intergroup Rhabdomyosarcoma Study (IRS) Committee. Cancer 1985;56:2125–2132.
144. Jaques DP, Coit DG, Hajdu SI, et al: Management of primary and recurrent soft-tissue sarcoma of the retroperitoneum. Ann Surg 1990;212:51–59.

# Chapter 46

# Other Diseases of the Small Intestine and Colon

*Samuel A. Kocoshis*

## ACRODERMATITIS ENTEROPATHICA

### Etiology and Pathogenesis

Acrodermatitis enteropathica, an autosomal-recessive disorder, is characterized by reduced transport of zinc across small intestinal mucosa.[1] Proposed mechanisms suggested by experimental evidence include defective prostaglandin synthesis,[2] abnormal phospholipid production,[3] aberrant tryptophan metabolism,[4] and depletion of a pancreatic zinc-binding ligand.[5] When grown in tissue culture, fibroblasts from acrodermatitis enteropathica patients appear to take up zinc normally at low zinc concentrations[6]; however, at higher concentrations, the affinity (Km) for zinc is normal, but the transport velocity ($V_{max}$) is decreased.[7]

### Clinical Manifestations

Patients are generally symptomatic by 3 to 18 months of age. They display profuse, watery diarrhea, weight loss, anorexia, and a characteristic dermatitis.[8] Skin lesions are most prominent at mucocutaneous junctions such as the perianal and perioral regions and on hands and feet, flexural areas, and areas exposed to friction. Lesions may be open sores or hyperkeratotic, scaly, erythematous eruptions. Stomatitis or cheilitis may accompany the skin lesions. Keratitis or xerophthalmia may also appear, as can alopecia or onychodystrophy.

### Laboratory Abnormalities

The hallmark of the disorder is zinc deficiency, but the total body zinc level may be difficult to ascertain by measuring serum levels,[8] which mainly reflect albumin-bound zinc, which may be depressed in hypoproteinemic states. Thus, an abnormally low serum zinc level (less than 6 mol/L) is significant only when serum albumin levels are normal. Early enthusiasm for measuring hair or nail zinc levels has waned because these levels correlate poorly with clinical signs of zinc deficiency; however, a low serum zinc level combined with clinical features of deficiency can be accepted as evidence for acrodermatitis.[8] It should be remembered that large diarrheal zinc losses[9] or inadequate zinc supplementation in parenteral nutrition[10] can lead to secondary zinc deficiency.

Because zinc functions to stimulate T cell activation, immunoglobulin (Ig) production, and phagocytosis of bacteria, zinc deficiency may result in abnormal results on tests of immune function.[11–13]

Furthermore, because zinc is a major cofactor for many intracellular enzymes, zinc deficiency is customarily associated with very low levels of alkaline phosphatase, gamma-glutamyl transpeptidase, and 5-nucleotidase.[14]

### Treatment and Prognosis

The minimum daily zinc requirement of 15 mg must be exceeded by 8- or 10-fold. Thus, a daily dose of 100 mg of zinc usually corrects all of the manifestations of acrodermatitis enteropathica.[15] Extra supplementation must be maintained through puberty for males and throughout life for females.[15]

## PNEUMATOSIS INTESTINALIS

### History, Pathophysiology, and Epidemiology

According to Heng and coworkers,[16] pneumatosis intestinalis was recognized as early as 1730 by DuVernoi. Bang, in the second half of the 19th century, carefully described the disorder in humans.[16]

The two most popular etiologic theories are the mechanical theory and the bacterial theory.

The mechanical theory proposes that gas dissects directly into the intestinal wall from the intestinal lumen or lung.[17] Obstruction of the gastrointestinal (GI) tract increases luminal pressure, which leads to dissection of gas either through an intestinal mucosal break or directly through the mediastinal root.[18] Ruptured pulmonary alveoli can also permit air to track along blood vessels and bronchi to the mediastinum, through the diaphragmatic crura, and along the mesenteric root into the intestinal wall. Favoring this theory is gas analysis of cysts from patients with pulmonary disease that show a composition identical to that of alveolar air.[19]

The bacterial theory holds that bacteria enter the submucosa through breaks and form gas there. This finding is supported by the finding of elevated breath hydrogen level in many patients with pneumatosis and the observation that a large enteral carbohydrate load is associated with pneumatosis in patients with already damaged intestine.[20]

It is very likely that one or the other mechanism is responsible among individual subsets of patients with pneumatosis. Patients of all ages can develop this disorder, and the male-female ratio is about 3:1. Very rarely, a familial association has been observed.[21] Associated conditions include neonatal necrotizing enterocolitis,[22] pulmonary disorders such as cystic fibrosis,[23] ischemic bowel disease,[24] intestinal pseudo-obstruction,[25] inflammatory bowel disease,[26] and infection with cytomegalovirus.[27] Pneumatosis has also been seen in immunosuppressed transplant recipients.[28, 29]

### Clinical Manifestations

Pneumatosis may involve any portion of the GI tract from esophagus to anus. Some patients have no symptoms, but on other occasions (as with necrotizing enterocolitis) patients present with abdominal distention and septic shock. Diarrhea, rectal bleeding, abdominal pain, tenesmus, and constipation have all been reported. Physical findings may include abdominal distention, hypoactive bowel sounds, and palpable rectal cysts on digital examination.

### Laboratory and Radiographic Findings

The subset of patients with pneumatosis of a bacterial cause have an elevated breath hydrogen level.[20] Other laboratory findings are very nonspecific but may include leukocytosis, anemia, and hypoproteinemia.

Radiographically, abdominal plain films,[30] abdominal sonography,[31] or computed tomography (CT)[32] will reveal intramural and intramesenteric gas. Rupture of cysts into peritoneum results in pneumoperitoneum. Portal venous gas develops in the severest cases.

### Histology

Three patterns of cystic change are common.[33] The microvesicular form consists of 10- to 100-μm spaces within the lamina propria. The cystic form has larger cysts in the submucosa or subserosa. A layer of macrophages lines the cyst walls. The diffuse type of cystic change has a spongy character that contrasts with the discrete cysts of other forms. There is no lining of cyst walls in "diffuse" cystic change.

### Therapy

The most effective therapy is to eradicate the underlying condition. Antibiotics directed against anaerobes are reportedly effective.[34] Administration of oxygen in quantities sufficient to raise the $Pa_{O_2}$ to 200 mm Hg has also been successfully employed.[35] Surgical resection should be performed only when necrotic bowel must be removed.[36]

## ISCHEMIC BOWEL DISEASE

### Etiology and Pathogenesis

Bowel ischemia is produced by arterial occlusion, venous occlusion, and nonocclusive low-flow states. Even though ischemic bowel disease is relatively uncommon among children, small intestinal or colonic ischemia can result from a wide variety of pediatric conditions. These conditions cause ischemia by obstructing superior mesenteric arterial flow, restricting superior mesenteric venous return, or impeding superior and inferior mesenteric flow to the colon (Table 46–1). Regardless of the underlying condition, ischemia occurs only when a combination of factors interact to overcome the abundant collateral blood flow that supplies both the small and large intestines. Generally, rapid occlusion of a single large vessel leads to almost immediate opening of collaterals[36]; however, after prolonged obstruction, persistent, generalized small vessel vasoconstriction may exacerbate vascular insufficiency.[37] Important, if ill-understood, factors that alter intestinal blood flow include preferential flow to higher-priority organs during conditions of low cardiac output,[38] local changes in vasoactive peptide levels,[39] and alterations in sympathetic nervous system tone.[39, 40]

In addition to endogenous factors, certain exogenous pharmacologic agents may predispose to intestinal ischemia. Chief among them are digoxin,[41] ergot alkaloids,[42] and estrogens.[43] When a vessel is acutely occluded, a predictable chain of events is initiated.[44] The bowel deprived of blood goes into spasm but after a while becomes hypoperistaltic owing to impaired muscle function. Blood from collaterals extravasates into the submucosa to produce "thumbprints," mucosal cysts develop, and intramural gas is produced. When the ischemia persists, the serosal surface eventually ruptures to produce a perforation.

### Clinical Manifestations

The patient with chronic mesenteric arterial insufficiency may experience classic abdominal angina.[44] Long pain-free periods are associated with fasting, but 20 to 30 minutes after meals, crampy or colicky periumbilical abdominal pain occurs that lasts as long as several hours. Weight loss ensues despite absence of diarrhea or steatorrhea. A striking paucity of abdominal findings belies the seriousness of the condition.

Bowel long subjected to arterial insufficiency tends to heal with stricture formation.[45] When strictures have formed, symptoms of partial or complete bowel obstruction appear.

Acute interruption of mesenteric flow has much more catastrophic consequences.[44, 46] The patient initially experiences colicky periumbilical pain that rapidly worsens, becomes generalized, and eventually leads to peritoneal findings, including exquisite abdominal pain on movement. The pain is accompanied by ileus and bilious vomiting. Patients experience hematemesis or pass "currant jelly" stools when

**TABLE 46–1. Disorders Associated with Ischemic Bowel Disease in Children**

| MESENTERIC ARTERIAL INSUFFICIENCY | | MESENTERIC VENOUS THROMBOSIS | ISCHEMIC COLITIS |
|---|---|---|---|
| **Large Vessel Disease** | **Small Vessel Disease** | | |
| Congenital constrictive mesenteric bands | Amyloidosis | Antithrombin III deficiency | Ascariasis |
| Congenital mesenteric artery aneurysm or arteriovenous malformation | Repair of coarctation of aorta | Ascariasis | Drug-induced |
| Septic emboli from bacterial endocarditis | Drug-induced | Hepatic cirrhosis | Digoxin |
| Ehlers-Danlos syndrome | Digoxin | Factor V Leyden mutation | Ergot alkaloids |
| Pancreatitis | Ergot alkaloids | Intra-abdominal sepsis | Oral contraceptives |
| Liver transplantation with hepatic artery "steal" | Oral contraceptives | Oral contraceptives | Necrotizing enterocolitis of infancy |
| Mycotic emboli from fungal sepsis | Thiazides | Pancreatectomy | Schistosomiasis |
| Umbilical artery catheterization | Necrotizing enterocolitis of infancy | Pancreatitis | Sigmoid volvulus |
| | Vasculitis | Paroxysmal nocturnal hemoglobinuria | Strangulated hernia |
| | Degos' disease | Protein C deficiency | Surgical compromise of inferior mesenteric artery |
| | Dermatomyositis | Schistosomiasis | Vasculitis |
| | Hemolytic-uremic syndrome | Sickle cell anemia | Degos' disease |
| | Henoch-Schönlein purpura | Splenectomy | Dermatomyositis |
| | Hepatitis | Thrombocytosis | Hemolytic-uremic syndrome |
| | Inflammatory bowel disease | Variceal sclerotherapy | Henoch-Schönlein purpura |
| | Periarteritis nodosa | | Hepatitis |
| | Polymyositis | | Inflammatory bowel disease |
| | Systemic lupus erythematosus | | Periarteritis nodosa |
| | | | Polymyositis |
| | | | Systemic lupus erythematosus |

mucosal necrosis is severe. Fever (often with temperatures to 39°C or 40°C) and vascular collapse appear in advanced cases.

Patients with mesenteric venous thrombosis commonly experience abdominal pain, but the pain is nonspecific and poorly localized.[47, 48] Most patients experience vomiting, diarrhea, and occult rectal bleeding. Because enteric protein loss can be profound, these patients sometimes present with peripheral edema or ascites. When the thrombosis is acute, progression to peritonitis may be rapid.

Signs and symptoms of ischemic colitis are no different from those of ulcerative colitis. The patient experiences crampy, left lower quadrant abdominal pain with concomitant bloody diarrhea. Typically, the volume of blood loss is insufficient to produce adverse hemodynamic or hematologic consequences.

## Laboratory, Radiographic, Endoscopic, and Histologic Diagnosis

No specific laboratory findings accompany arterial or venous insufficiency. Patients may experience leukocytosis or anemia, and acute-phase markers may appear in serum.[49] Chronic insufficiency can lead to protein-losing enteropathy reflected by hypoproteinemia, hypoalbuminemia, and elevated fecal alpha$_1$-antitrypsin concentrations.[45] Steatorrhea or carbohydrate malabsorption is sometimes present.[45]

Sickle cell disease, thrombocytosis, liver disease, schistosomiasis, and abdominal sepsis are clinically obvious causes of pediatric mesenteric venous thrombosis. When these diagnoses have been excluded, patients should undergo evaluation for paroxysmal nocturnal hemoglobinuria and other hypercoagulable states such as factor V mutation or deficiency of protein C, protein S, or antithrombin III.

The plain abdominal film usually is not helpful in patients with mesenteric arterial insufficiency[50]; however, abdominal CT, which is the most valuable diagnostic modality,[44, 47, 51] may show thickened small bowel folds and a herringbone pattern of ulceration. Long-standing insufficiency may lead to single or multiple discrete strictures. Small bowel mucosa is also thickened and may show evidence of intramural hemorrhage in patients with mesenteric venous thrombosis. In ischemic colitis, thumbprinting of the colon is often quite evident.[44, 51] Abnormalities are most commonly found at the splenic flexure and sigmoid colon, which are watershed areas farthest from the superior and inferior mesenteric arterial supplies. A small bowel series may show similar findings but provides less information overall than does CT.[44, 50]

Early angiography has been advocated for adults with mesenteric atherosclerotic disease, but it may be meddlesome in children, who are much more likely to have small vessel disease than large vessel occlusion. Angiography may reveal venous thrombosis during the delayed phase or simply delayed emptying of arterial arcades[44]; however, angiography is seldom helpful in patients with colonic ischemia. Magnetic resonance angiography shows promise for the future.[47] In the patient with suspected mesenteric venous thrombosis, ultrasonography is helpful.[52]

Upper or lower GI tract endoscopy reveals patchy mucosal hemorrhage and ulcerations that extend into the submucosa when the process is of long standing. The rectum is spared in 94% of patients with ischemic colitis.

Histologic changes encompass a range of severity and bowel wall depth, depending on the type and severity of ischemia.[53] Acute, complete obstruction produces superficial necrosis quickly followed by full-thickness necrosis. In nonocclusive ischemia, necrosis may be confined to the mucosa and submucosa, sparing muscularis propria. Edema and vascular congestion are quite prominent in venous occlusion but also occur in arterial occlusion. Specimens from patients with vasculitis due to collagen-vascular disease may reveal arteritis, with or without medial fibrosis or medial necrosis. Fibrin thrombi may occlude the vessel walls. Leukocytoclasis is also characteristic.[53] Iron stains reveal extensive mucosal iron deposition in ischemic colitis when the vascular insult occurred remotely and a reparative process is taking place.

### Treatment

Vasodilators such as papaverine, although used in adults with large vessel disease,[44] probably have no place in the management of children, whose ischemia is usually due to vasculitis. However, a course of anticoagulants should be considered for children with venous thrombosis and hypercoagulable states.

Of course, correction of dehydration and acidosis and treatment of underlying predisposing conditions should be initiated, but patients with peritoneal signs are candidates for laparotomy and possibly segmental bowel resection. If the viability of bowel is in question, the surgeon may elect to perform diverting enterostomies and a subsequent second-look operation.

## RADIATION ENTERITIS

### Radiation Biology and Epidemiology

Radiation-induced enteropathy has been recognized since 1897.[54] Despite refinements in delivery of ionizing radiation over the past century, the disorder persists to this day. Authors vary in their diagnostic criteria for radiation enteritis, and many series fail to include those children who die early in the course of radiation therapy. These impediments notwithstanding, the prevalence figures generally quoted are approximately 2% to 25%[55–57]; however, one series suggests that 70% of patients suffer changes in bowel habits after pelvic irradiation.[58]

The total doses of radiation required to produce clinical damage in 5% of adult patients in 5 years (TD 5/5) or 50% of adult patients in 5 years (TD 50/5) range from 6,000 to 7,500 centigrays (cGy; 1 cGy = 1 rad) for the esophagus, 4,500 to 5,000 for the stomach, 4,500 to 6,500 for small bowel and colon, and 5,500 to 8,000 for the rectum.[59] Factors that predispose to chronic enteropathy include high radiation dose, ongoing chemotherapy, large areas of intestine residing within the pelvis (as seen in females and the elderly), previous surgery, and peripheral vascular disease.[60]

Some authors suggest that children are more resistant to chronic enteritis than are adults.[61, 62] The paucity of complications in children may instead be due to the lower radiation doses they receive. In contrast to adults with relatively radioresistant carcinoma, most pediatric patients with neuroblastoma, Wilms' tumor, or Hodgkin's lymphoma receive less than 3,600 cGy.[59] Pediatric patients with pelvic rhabdomyosarcoma may receive a maximum of 6,000 cGy to the pelvis.[59]

### Pathogenesis

The adverse effects of radiation on the bowel may be categorized as acute or chronic injury. Acute injury has a direct cytotoxic effect on replicating epithelial cells.[63] The mechanism of cell destruction begins with free-radical generation and subsequent alterations of DNA structure. DNA transcription and protein synthesis subsequently cease.[64] Generally, the small bowel is more sensitive than the colon to acute injury.[64] Chronic damage leads to submucosal fibrosis and obliteration of small blood vessels and lymphatics.[65] In many respects, this entity resembles chronic ischemic enteritis.

### Clinical Features

During radiation therapy, acute injury produces abdominal cramps, diarrhea, and vomiting in 67% to 100% of patients.[57, 58] Symptoms resolve within 6 weeks of cessation in most patients, but damage is severe enough in 20% to mandate reduction of radiation dose.[66] The severity of acute symptoms is directly related to the development of chronic enteritis.[67]

Symptoms of chronic enteritis usually appear within 6 to 24 months after therapy[68]; however, a number of patients develop their first symptoms many years later. The most common presentation is small bowel obstruction with bilious vomiting, abdominal distention, and abdominal pain.[69] Fistulas, leading to diarrhea, may also develop. Free or confined perforation with abscess formation may complicate the course. A separate entity, radiation proctocolitis, produces bloody diarrhea, crampy abdominal pain, and tenesmus.[70]

### Laboratory, Radiographic, and Histologic Diagnosis

Laboratory findings are neither diagnostically sensitive nor specific, but lactose malabsorption,[71] steatorrhea, vitamin $B_{12}$ malabsorption, and bile salt wasting are common in acute injury.[72]

The laboratory findings described may also be present in chronic injury; in addition, the patient often experiences small intestinal bacterial overgrowth secondary to stasis or fistula.[72] Secondary lymphangiectasia results in protein-losing enteropathy characterized by depressed serum proteins, lymphopenia, elevated fecal $alpha_1$-antitrypsin levels, and lymphocytes in the stool.

Contrast radiography may reveal thickened folds, adhesions, mucosal effacement, fistula, and luminal narrowing.[73]

Histologic changes include subtotal villus atrophy,[63] mucosal ulceration, bowel wall necrosis, and lymphangiectasia.[74]

Vasculitis may also be seen, and vascular morphology may be altered by hyaline-ring thickening of arteriolar walls.[63] Inflammatory cells may infiltrate the intima of vessels, and intraluminal thrombi may form.[65]

### Treatment

When large doses of pelvic irradiation are anticipated, exclusion of the bowel from the field using a surgically placed Vicryl sling has proven to be quite effective.[75]

During the acute phase, low-residue, low-lactose diets

are often helpful.[76] Various authors have also successfully employed prostaglandin synthetase inhibitors,[77] corticosteroids,[78] sulfasalazine,[79] and elemental diets.[78] A multicenter, double-blind, placebo-controlled trial of mesalamine for acute radiation enteritis showed only marginal benefit.[80] An animal study suggests that prophylactic administration of prostaglandin $E_1$ minimizes intestinal damage.[81]

Chronic enteritis is more difficult to control, and trials of elemental diets, steroids, sulfasalazine, cholestyramine, and other antibiotics have met with variable results.[72, 74] Patients with malnutrition despite adequate intake should receive parenteral nutrition.

Surgical resection and fistulectomy are often necessary. Wide resection, rather than limited surgery, is recommended by Galland and Spencer.[68] Ideally, anastomoses should be made between segments of bowel that have escaped the radiation field. Some surgeons bypass, rather than resect, involved bowel loops.[82] Others, however, feel just as strongly that, when possible, excision is preferable to bypass because bypassed bowel is still at risk for perforation and fistulization.[68]

## HEMOLYTIC-UREMIC SYNDROME

### Epidemiology

First described by von Gasser and colleagues in 1955,[83] the triad of microangiopathic hemolytic anemia, thrombocytopenia, and acute renal failure, known as *hemolytic-uremic syndrome,* has a worldwide distribution. It is the most common cause of acute renal failure in children.[84] It usually appears in children younger than 10 years, has a peak incidence in children 1 to 2 years of age,[85–88] and is rarely seen in older children or adults.[89] It appears to be common in Argentina,[90] South Africa,[91] and the Pacific coast of North America,[85, 92] but the overall incidence seems to be increasing in many other regions.[85–88] The current incidence is about 7 per 100,000[93] in North America and 3 per 100,000 in Europe.[94]

Prognosis tends to be better for the "epidemic" form[86] than the sporadic form.[95] The worst prognosis is for the autosomal-recessive familial form.[96] An extraordinarily large percentage of cases are preceded by infection with verotoxin-producing *Escherichia coli* O157:H7[85, 89, 97–101]; thus it is most often diagnosed in the summer months. Recent epidemiologic studies document infection with *E. coli* O157:H7 among 64% of patients with hemolytic-uremic syndrome from Vancouver, Canada,[98] 58% from Seattle, Washington,[99] 23% from Great Britain,[100] 7.5% from Toronto, Canada,[97] and 2% from Buenos Aires, Argentina.[101] Other bacteria,[101] viruses,[102] or parasites are also associated. For example, 55% of Argentinian children with hemolytic-uremic syndrome have evidence of antecedent *Shigella* infection.[101] Other predisposing factors include administration of antiviral vaccines to children[103] and cancer chemotherapeutic agents to adults.[104]

Many of the bacteria associated with hemolytic-uremic syndrome produce cytotoxins. Indeed, there is a striking similarity between *E. coli* O157:H7 verotoxin and Shiga toxin produced by *Shigella dysenteriae.*[105]

Blood group $P_1$ predisposes to postenteropathic hemolytic-uremic syndrome because the terminal disaccharide on the $P_1$ antigen acts as a verotoxin receptor.[106]

### Pathogenesis

The pathologic events of "typical" hemolytic-uremic syndrome are initiated by intravascular platelet activation that, in turn, is precipitated by endothelial cell damage (Fig. 46–1). Evidence supporting platelet activation includes loss of platelet nucleotide into plasma,[107] hyporesponsiveness to platelet-aggregating agents,[108] and alterations in platelet-produced growth factors.[109]

Endothelial damage may occur by direct bacterial cytotoxin–induced cytolysis,[105] by systemic endotoxin release,[110] by cell membrane lipid peroxidation,[111] or by immune complex–mediated damage.[112] Release of platelet-aggregating factor,[113] selectins,[114] cell adhesion molecules,[114] or factor VIII multimers[115] is probably a secondary process.

Prostacyclin depletion is commonly observed in hemolytic-uremic syndrome, but this may be an epiphenomenon.[116] The role of nitric oxide (NO) is controversial, with NO enhancing vascular injury[117] but inhibiting platelet aggregation.[118] A schematic diagram of the proposed pathogenic mechanism is shown in Figure 46–1.

### Clinical Features

A prodromal gastroenteritis precedes about 95% of epidemic hemolytic-uremic syndrome cases.[84, 89–91] In 75% of those cases, diarrhea is bloody.[49, 84, 90, 91] Diffuse abdominal pain and vomiting are also common. At times, peritoneal signs are prominent, leading to exploratory laparotomy.[119, 120] As gastrointestinal symptoms improve about 1 week into the course, there is sudden onset of extreme pallor, easy bruising, oliguria, and sometimes anasarca.[90]

### Radiologic, Endoscopic, and Laboratory Findings

Barium enemas are frequently requested in the emergency department at the time of presentation to rule out intussus-

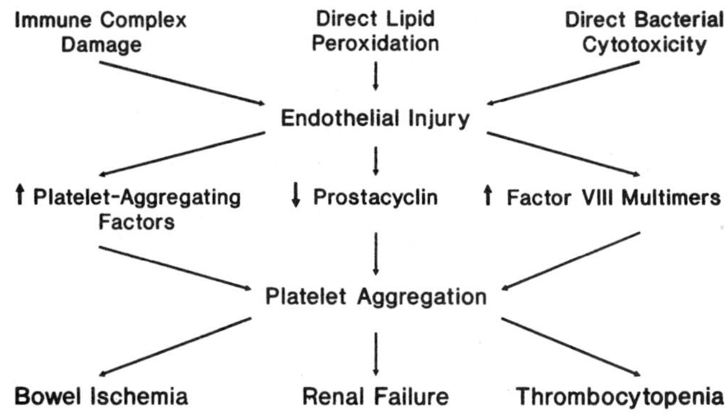


**FIGURE 46–1.** Proposed pathogenesis of hemolytic-uremic syndrome. Increased platelet aggregation antedates the development of thrombocytopenia, ischemic bowel disease, and renal failure, which characterize this disorder.

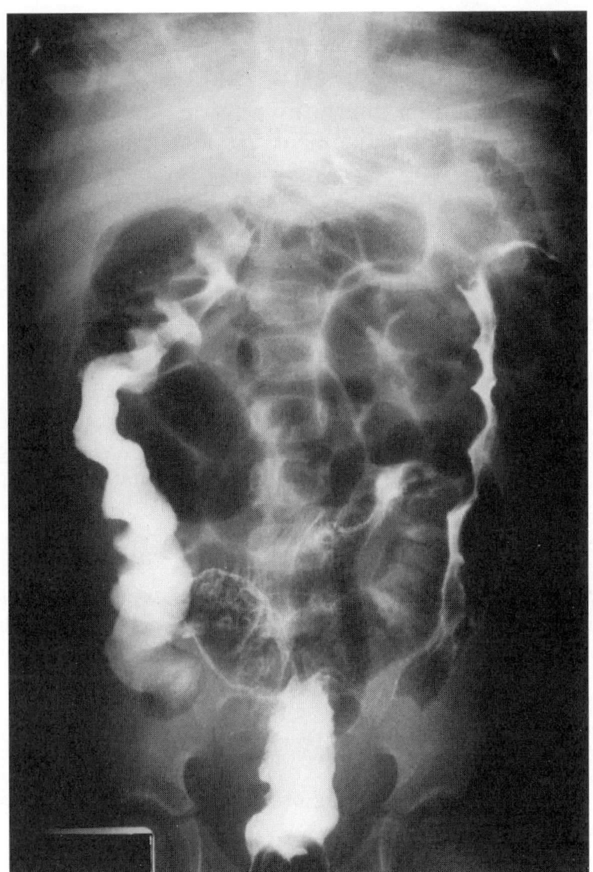

**FIGURE 46–2.** Extensive colonic "thumbprinting" in a patient who presented with bloody diarrhea associated with *E. coli* O157:H7 infection. The thumbprints represent submucosal hemorrhages throughout the colon. (Courtesy of Richard Towbin, MD.)

ception. Findings of thumbprinting (Fig. 46–2), mucosal irregularity, and ulceration are consistent with an ischemic process.[116]

Endoscopic findings are nonspecific, and the mucosa usually appears hyperemic, edematous, and friable.[121]

Histologic appearance may vary from that of nonspecific colitis to that of ischemic bowel disease.[121]

Stool culture may reveal enteric pathogens such as *Campylobacter, Yersinia, Salmonella,* or *Shigella.* Of these four, *Shigella* organisms are most likely to be found.[101] Stools should also be cultured for coliforms—specifically, strains that do not ferment sorbitol. *E. coli* O157:H7 is the most common of these associated with hemolytic-uremic syndrome.[85–89, 97–101] Although some sorbitol-fermenting strains of *E. coli* produce "Shiga-like" toxin and do induce hemorrhagic colitis, they are less commonly found than is *E. coli* O157:H7. Cultures taken during the first 6 days of enteritis are more likely to be positive than those taken later.[122] Searching for fecal verotoxin by DNA probes also improves yield.[101]

As the enteritis improves, hemoglobin concentration falls precipitously, to the range of 5 to 6 g/dL, and red cells are morphologically abnormal. Fragments, burr cells, helmet cells, and other bizarre forms appear. Thrombocytopenia is present in 92% of patients, and coagulopathy in 85%.[85, 90, 91]

Oliguric acute renal failure occurs in 64% to 92% of patients, who sometimes develop hypertension or azotemia.[84, 90, 91] Elevation of serum aminotransferases has been reported in more than half of patients, and pancreatitis affects 21%.[123]

### Complications

Small bowel and colon perforation (often occurring during peritoneal dialysis) are recognized complications.[119] Intussusception has also been reported. Intestinal strictures or fistulas are potential late complications. Severe pancreatitis may lead to exocrine or endocrine pancreatic insufficiency.[123] Renal thrombotic microangiopathy produces glomerulosclerosis and chronic renal failure in 6% of children with the epidemic form[124] and in 60% with the sporadic form.[84, 90, 91] Central nervous system complications such as encephalopathy, seizures, and stroke may be seen.

### Treatment

Patients with severe gastrointestinal symptoms should receive bowel rest and parenteral nutrition. Broad-spectrum antibiotics should be considered for children with fulminant colitis, but benefits should be weighed against the theoretical risk of increasing cytotoxin release from dying bacteria. Red cell transfusions, fluid restriction, and diuretics constitute the cornerstone of supportive therapy. Azotemia or electrolyte imbalance may necessitate peritoneal dialysis or hemodialysis. The risks of hemodialysis in the face of coagulopathy should be weighed against the risks of peritoneal dialysis in the face of bowel ischemia.[119]

A large controlled series has failed to show benefit from anticoagulant therapy,[125] but some data favor plasmapheresis[126] or plasma transfusions[127] for selected patients. Caution in transfusing anti-T-negative plasma is mandated by the high incidence of circulating T (Thomsen-Friedenreich) antigen among patients with hemolytic-uremic syndrome.[128]

A novel experimental approach yet to be tried in humans is the administration of monoclonal antibodies, which bind to platelet glycoprotein receptors, thus inhibiting platelet aggregation.[129]

## HENOCH-SCHÖNLEIN PURPURA

### History and Epidemiology

Henoch-Schönlein purpura is a systemic vasculitis characterized by a purpuric rash that was probably first described in 1801 by Heberden.[130] Thirty-one years later, Schönlein carefully described the rash as purpura and recognized that the rash and associated arthritis constituted a distinct clinical syndrome.[131] In 1874, Henoch, one of Schönlein's students, noted that gastrointestinal symptoms accompanied the rash.[132] Later he reported the association between nephritis and the syndrome.[133]

This entity is distributed worldwide and can affect persons of any age[134]; however, 75% of patients are younger than 7 years, and the median age at onset is 4 years.[135] There is a 2:1 male predominance, and the majority of cases occur in winter and early spring.[135] Almost all pediatric cases are preceded by a viral[136–138] or bacterial[139] illness or by a vaccination.[140] Some adult cases are associated with lymphoma,[141] prostate cancer,[142] and other neoplasms.[143] Drugs such as salicylates, phenacetin, penicillin, erythromycin, and quinidines have also been implicated.[140]

## Pathogenesis

Central to the pathogenic process is deposition of immunoglobulin A (IgA) immune complexes upon postcapillary venules throughout the body after presentation of some unknown antigen.[144] The alternate complement pathway is activated, resulting in depletion of plasma C3 and deposition of C3 in immune complexes. The fact that the classical pathway is not activated is proved by the development of Henoch-Schönlein purpura in C2-deficient persons.[145] Whether excessive IgA production or diminished degradation takes place is not known.

## Clinical Features

Skin involvement is invariable.[135] Discrete, red, "palpable purpura" develops, principally on the buttocks, lower extremities, and distal upper extremities (Fig. 46–3). Rarely, the rash involves the face and upper trunk as well. Lower extremity edema is quite common, and scrotal, facial, or scalp edema less common.[135] GI tract involvement is also very common and usually appears no sooner than 1 week before the rash or 1 week later.[135, 146–148] Occasionally it precedes the rash by several weeks. Patients usually experience diffuse abdominal pain, vomiting, and hematochezia.[135]

Joint pain and overt pauciarticular arthritis occur in more than half of affected patients. The knees and ankles are the joints most often involved.

Renal manifestations such as overt hematuria and proteinuria occur in 30% to 40% of patients.[135] At times the renal involvement is severe enough to produce hypertension or the nephrotic syndrome. Central nervous system vasculitis may produce headaches and personality changes ranging from emotional lability to stupor and seizures.[149] Pancreatitis,[150] cholecystitis,[151] pulmonary hemorrhage,[152] ureteral obstruction,[153] orchitis,[148] and myocardial infarction[154] have all been reported. Intussusception occurs in about 2% of affected children with abdominal pain. Bowel perforation and small bowel stricture are much less common.[155]

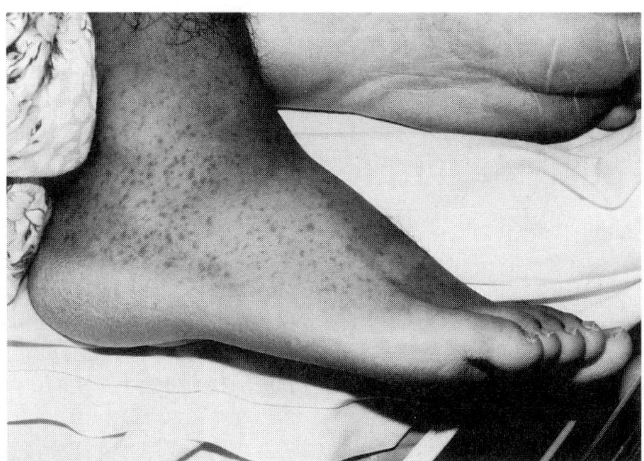

**FIGURE 46–3.** Showers of 2- to 4-mm palpable purpura that appeared on the lower extremities of a teenager who had been complaining of diffuse abdominal pain and diarrhea for 1 week before their appearance. The presence of purpura in this distribution confirmed the diagnosis of Henoch-Schönlein purpura.

## Laboratory, Radiographic, Endoscopic, and Histologic Findings

About 75% of patients have leukocytosis and an elevated sedimentation rate, but GI bleeding is rarely severe enough to produce anemia.[135] Platelet counts are generally normal, despite the presence of purpura. Microscopic hematuria and proteinuria are seen in nearly half of patients.[135] Immunologic abnormalities include elevation of serum IgA, deficiency in serum C3, and presence of circulating immune complexes in serum.[144, 145] Additionally, circulating antineutrophil cytoplasmic antibodies are present in a large percentage of patients.[156] An important indicator of poor prognosis is depletion of circulating factor XIII.[157]

Barium enema, a small bowel series, or abdominal CT may reveal findings identical to those of any ischemic process—namely, coarsening of folds, spiculations of bowel wall, and thumbprinting.[158]

Endoscopy displays purpuric lesions of the small bowel and colon that are similar to those on the skin.[159] In addition, punctate hemorrhages and aphthoid lesions may be seen.

Biopsy of bowel or skin reveals leukocytoclastic vasculitis. Immunohistochemical stains show selective IgA and C3 deposition on the wall of venules and the mesangium of renal glomeruli, a finding that differentiates Henoch-Schönlein purpura from other vasculitides.[144] Renal biopsy findings traverse a spectrum of severity from focal glomerulonephritis to glomerular crescent formation and necrotizing arteriolitis, which carry a poor prognosis.[135]

## Treatment and Prognosis

Corticosteroids do not alter the course of either the skin disease or the renal process, but an anecdotal report from 1960 suggests a salutary effect on GI symptoms.[135] More recent retrospective analysis casts doubt on the efficacy of corticosteroids. At best, steroids seem to shorten the GI course by only 1 to 2 days.[147] The decision to embark on a course of corticosteroids should be tempered by the concern that symptoms of perforation or intussusception may be masked by the medication.

Although corticosteroids do not alter the course of renal insufficiency, case reports have suggested that azathioprine may be effective therapy.[160] Results of renal transplantation have been disappointing because at least 75% of patients experience a relapse in the transplanted kidney.[161] Plasmapheresis may induce a temporary drop in serum IgA levels with symptomatic improvement, but symptoms tend to recur within a few days after cessation of therapy.[162] Administration of factor XIII to patients with depressed serum levels seems to ameliorate symptoms and shorten the symptomatic period.[163, 164]

Generally, Henoch-Schönlein purpura carries a good prognosis: complete resolution of central nervous system, gastrointestinal, and renal disease is the rule in more than 90% of patients.[135] Rarely, signs and symptoms wax and wane. Some 2% to 4% of children develop renal insufficiency warranting dialysis.[161]

## AMYLOIDOSIS

### Nomenclature

The current classification of amyloidoses subdivides them into the following six categories: (1) primary (lacking an intercurrent disease); (2) associated with myeloma; (3) secondary (associated with infection or collagen-vascular disease); (4) familial; (5) local (confined to one organ); and (6) amyloidosis of aging.[165] This classification takes into account the pathogenesis of the disorder and the biochemical structure of individual amyloids.

### Epidemiology

The overall prevalence of primary and secondary amyloidosis is probably less than 0.15%, and most cases are seen in adults.[166] Amyloidosis does occasionally affect children on hemodialysis[167] or those who have familial Mediterranean fever,[168] long-standing juvenile rheumatoid arthritis,[169] cystic fibrosis,[170] Crohn's disease,[171] autoimmune enteropathy,[172] or glycogenosis.[173] In developing countries it has been seen in young people with long-standing tuberculosis[174] or leprosy.[175]

### Pathogenesis and Biochemistry

The pathogenesis of amyloidosis remains unknown, but a large amount of data is available on the biochemistry of amyloid. A working hypothesis can therefore be proposed for amyloid deposition. Amyloid A (AA) predominates in inflammatory diseases and in familial Mediterranean fever.[176] It is composed of 76 amino acids and has a molecular weight of 8,500. A soluble protein (SAA) of 160,000 displays N-terminal homology with AA, and its production is markedly enhanced during inflammation.[177] However, elevated SAA does not always lead to amyloidosis.[178] A second substance, amyloid-enhancing factor, also produced by inflammation in susceptible persons, catalyzes the proteolytic conversion of SAA to AA.[179] The site of synthesis is not known, but electron microscopy suggests that reticuloendothelial cells both synthesize and degrade amyloid.[179]

### Clinical Findings

Although amyloidosis may produce peripheral neuropathy, respiratory disease, cardiac conduction defects or cardiac failure, renal failure, or hepatomegaly with portal hypertension, this discussion is confined to GI manifestations. Some 70% to 85% of patients with secondary amyloidosis have GI involvement. Symptoms are produced by one of three mechanisms.[180, 181] First, amyloid deposits may produce gastric outlet or small bowel obstruction.[182] Second, diffuse infiltration of the bowel wall may impair motility. Finally, infiltration around blood vessels produces bowel ischemia.[180] The symptoms of GI amyloidosis may therefore be those of obstruction (vomiting and abdominal distention), steatorrhea (copious and frequent stools, weight loss, and nutrient deficiencies), or intestinal ischemia (abdominal pain and GI bleeding).

### Radiographic, Endoscopic, and Histologic Findings

Although single-contrast radiography may miss subtle findings, double-contrast small bowel series may reveal innumerable 1- to 3-mm granularities, 3- to 4-mm nodules, or 4- to 10-mm polypoid lesions.[183] Irregular folds or multiple erosions may also be seen. Endoscopy also reveals excrescences or erosions in any region of the GI tract from tongue to rectum. Endoscopic abnormalities are most common in the duodenum (75%) and least common in the esophagus (16%).[181] Gastric lesions are present in 70% of patients, and colonic lesions in 54%.[181]

Histologic examination—more sensitive than endoscopy—reveals submucosal and mucosal amyloid deposits in 100% of duodenal biopsy specimens, 95% of gastric ones, and 91% of colonic and 72% of esophageal specimens.[181] Diagnostic sensitivity is decreased unless the specimen includes ample submucosa. Conversely, sensitivity can be increased by staining specimens with Congo red and inspecting them under a polarizing microscope to display the green birefringence of amyloid.[184]

### Treatment

A variety of therapeutic agents have been employed in attempts to decrease antigenic stimulation, inhibit amyloid synthesis, prevent amyloid deposition, or enhance amyloid mobilization. None has been unequivocally successful. Corticosteroids appear to have no effect on the progression of disease.[185] Results of vitamin C therapy are also disappointing.[186]

The use of alkylating agents in primary amyloidosis is controversial,[187, 188] but survival of patients with juvenile rheumatoid arthritis and secondary amyloidosis appears to be appreciably lengthened when chlorambucil is employed in oral doses of 0.1 mg/kg/day.[189] Pharmacotherapy also unquestionably modifies the course of familial Mediterranean fever. Colchicine reduces the frequency of pain episodes and prevents amyloid deposition.[190]

Surgery to resect ischemic bowel may be necessary if amyloidosis has produced mesenteric vascular occlusion.[191]

## BEHÇET'S DISEASE

### History and Epidemiology

Behçet, a Turkish dermatologist, first described the constellation of oral and genital ulceration and iritis in 1937.[192]

After his original report, GI ulceration, central nervous system vasculitis, arthritis, thrombophlebitis, skin lesions, and cardiovascular abnormalities were recognized as components of the same entity.[193] The prevalence is 0.3 to 10 per 100,000, and there is a 3:1 male predominance.[194] The disorder is much more common in Japan, Turkey, and countries along the ancient "Silk Road" than in the United States or Europe.[195, 196] The strong ethnic predisposition has led some to apply the term *Behçet's disease* only to cases from endemic areas, cases from Europe or North America being termed *Behçet's syndrome.*[196] The disease most often presents in the third decade of life, but pediatric cases are being recognized with greater frequency. Human leukocyte antigen (HLA) type B27 is associated with the arthritis of Behçet's disease, B12 with the mucocutaneous lesions, and B51 with the iritis.[194, 197] An even stronger association is with a specific triplet repeat polymorphism in the transmembrane region of the major histocompatibility complex (MHC) class I–related gene (MICA gene).[198] This polymorphism is seen in 75% of Japanese patients.

## Pathogenesis

The pathogenesis of Behçet's disease is unknown, but infectious causes have been proposed. Candidate microorganisms include herpes simplex virus, *Streptococcus sanguis,* and atypical mycobacteria.[199] A tantalizing hypothesis based on experimental evidence is the molecular mimicry theory.[199] Heat shock proteins of *S. sanguis* and *Mycobacterium* possess striking homology with human heat shock protein. Repeated exposure to them results in the development of a reactive T cell epitope directed against the human protein. The proliferative response of gamma-delta T cell receptor lymphocytes of Behçet's patients to a specific peptide fraction of heat shock protein supports this hypothesis.[199] Consistent findings among Behçet's patients are increased leukocyte migration and increased leukocyte superoxide generation. Whether these are central to pathogenesis or an epiphenomenon is unclear.[200]

## Clinical Features

Aphthous ulceration of the mouth and genitalia is present in 60% to 98% of patients with Behçet's disease. Mouth ulcers are quite small. They are covered by pseudomembrane and surrounded by a red margin. The genital ulcers, identical in appearance to mouth ulcers, are located on the scrotum or vulva. Skin lesions include erythema nodosum and sterile pustules. Although 80% of adults have anterior and posterior uveitis, only 21% of pediatric patients have this finding.[201] In contrast, GI involvement is more common among children. Superficial thrombophlebitis, deep vein thrombosis, and arterial occlusion may affect any extremity. The arthritis is a nonmigratory, nondeforming polyarticular type.[194]

Neurologic symptoms include peripheral neuropathies, cranial nerve palsies, dementia, and seizures. Meningoencephalitis with cerebrospinal fluid pleocytosis may occur.[202] GI symptoms are identical to those of inflammatory bowel disease. GI involvement includes the right colon in 50% of children, ileum in 25%, and distal colon in 25%. Patients have pain, diarrhea, and sometimes hematochezia. Fistulas and perforation are common. The 12% of patients with esophageal ulceration experience dysphagia.[201]

## Diagnosis

No biochemical, radiographic, endoscopic, or histologic findings are pathognomonic. Indeed, many cases described in the literature share features with Crohn's disease, including discontinuous distribution of lesions, ileal involvement, and giant cell granulomas.[201] However, the GI ulcers of Behçet's disease tend to be deep and flask-shaped.[203, 204] They are devoid of giant cell change.

The Japanese Behçet Disease Research Committee has defined clinical criteria for the diagnosis.[205] The presence of four major criteria (iritis, oral ulceration, genital ulceration, and skin changes) satisfies the requirement for complete Behçet's disease. The presence of two major findings and two of the three minor ones (arthritis, bowel disease, and neurologic findings) constitutes a diagnosis of incomplete Behçet's disease.

## Treatment

Corticosteroids have produced variable results, but other immunosuppressants, such as chlorambucil and cyclosporine, have been employed with some success.[202] Successful therapy with colchicine has also been reported. More recently, excellent results have been reported with cyclosporine A and tacrolimus.[197] Pentoxifylline, an antagonist of tumor necrosis factor and a suppressor of neutrophil superoxide generation, has also shown promise.[206]

# DEGOS' DISEASE

## History and Epidemiology

Kohlmeier first described this disorder in 1941, but he considered it an atypical form of thromboangiitis obliterans.[207] Degos, Delort, and Tricot, in their publications of 1942[208] and 1948,[209] characterized it as a distinct clinicopathologic entity. Very few cases have been reported. Most patients have been in their second or third decade of life, but the age range is 3 weeks to 65 years.[210, 211] The male-female ratio is 3:1,[210, 211] and Degos' has been reported in a family.[212]

## Pathogenesis

Degos' disease is a unique obliterative (but not necrotizing) endarteritis that affects small to medium-sized vessels. The pathogenesis is unknown, and all attempts to implicate a particular virus or specific immunologic mechanism have been unsuccessful.[210] However, the discovery of anticardiolipin antibodies and circulating lupus anticoagulant links it to other collagen-vascular diseases.[213] Additionally, there is evidence for increased platelet adhesiveness that can be corrected by antiplatelet drugs.[214, 215]

### Clinical Features

The hallmark of Degos' disease is the development of 1- to 3-mm cutaneous papules that appear singly or in crops of as many as several dozen.[210] They are found predominantly over the upper trunk and arms. Face, scalp, hands, and feet are generally spared. The lesions begin as pinkish, round papules that umbilicate and become depressed within a few days. Finally, the lesions atrophy to become depressed, porcelain-white ovals that may be covered by a fine scale. The margin is often telangiectatic. Most patients develop skin lesions before abdominal symptoms, but occasionally abdominal symptoms antedate the rash.[216, 217]

Identical lesions appear throughout the GI tract and can be identified on the mucosal surface by endoscopy or on the serosal surface by laparoscopy or laparotomy.[211] At least two thirds of patients experience intermittent bouts of diffuse, severe abdominal pain that tends to improve spontaneously if perforation has not occurred.[210] There is a strong propensity, however, for spontaneous, minute perforations that sometimes can be seen endoscopically.[211] Regardless of multiple intestinal surgeries, the majority of patients die of abdominal sepsis or peritonitis within 2 years after diagnosis.[217] Other viscera such as heart, kidneys, bladder, liver, pancreas, and lungs may be affected, but such involvement seldom produces symptoms.[210]

Seventeen percent of patients experience neurologic involvement, multiple small infarctions eventually leading to encephalomalacia.[216, 218] Approximately 8% of patients develop severe, progressive dementia.[218]

### Histologic Diagnosis

Skin biopsy specimens reveal hyperkeratotic, atrophic epidermis; dyscellular basal layer; and avascular, acellular dermis.[210] The margins of lesions exhibit numerous ectatic blood vessels.[210]

Arteriolar changes seen in the skin are also present in intestine and other organs.[211] Arteriolar lumina are occluded by proliferating endothelial cells and thrombi.[210] The vessel walls are thickened by edema but do not become necrotic.

### Therapy

A variety of agents such as corticosteroids, cyclophosphamide, sulfonamides, iodohydroxyquinolone, and other antibiotics have been used—without success.[210]

Heparin, phenformin, and ethylestrenol have been employed to increase fibrinolysis, but these also appear ineffective.[210] Two case reports suggest efficacy of aspirin plus dipyridamole in the face of increased platelet adhesiveness.[214, 215]

## DERMATOMYOSITIS

### Epidemiology

The incidence of dermatomyositis ranges from 1 per million[219] to 2.2 per 100,000 (in Israel[220]). The incidence is 7 to 10 times higher in North American and South African blacks than among whites.[219] The disorder has a worldwide distribution, and its greatest incidence among children is in 10- to 14-year-olds.[219, 220] A second peak is seen in 45- to 64-year-olds.[219, 220] One report suggests that most patients present in late winter and early spring,[221] but those results have been disputed.[222] A few reports of familial dermatomyositis have appeared.[223] The clinical course and autoantibody pattern of juvenile dermatomyositis are different enough from those of the adult variant to categorize it as a discrete entity.[224] HLA types B8, DR3,[225] and DQA1*0501[226] are present with greater than expected frequency among children with dermatomyositis.

### Pathogenesis

The etiology of dermatomyositis is unknown, but the current working hypothesis is that affected patients experience an immune response to a virus. Serologic evidence implicates coxsackievirus B[221] and other enteroviruses,[227] but data are far from convincing. A variety of autoantibodies are present, but none are specific for the disorder.[228] Compared with the adult form of the disease, the juvenile form is associated with a higher prevalence of antinuclear antibodies but a lower prevalence of muscle-specific (JO-1 and mi-2) antibodies.[229]

### Clinical Features

The rash is the most consistent finding in the majority of cases, but muscle weakness predominates in others.[230] The skin rash has three salient features (Fig. 46–4).[231] First, a heliotrope facial rash may be quite prominent. This rash consists of periorbital erythroderma with swollen eyelids, resembling a sunburn. The second prominent feature is Gottron's patch, an elevated, bluish-red papule overlying the knuckles. Several papules may overlie fingers or toes. The third feature is telangiectasia overlying the proximal nail folds. Calcinosis of soft tissues accompanies long-standing disease.[232]

Muscle weakness is symmetric and involves the proximal muscles. Subtle difficulty appears in motor skills such as placing objects on high shelves, phonating, or climbing steps.[233] Progression is slow, but eventually the weakness becomes quite apparent to the casual observer.

GI symptoms are prominent in as many as one third of patients.[224, 232–236] Most complain of dysphagia due to weakness of esophageal striated muscle.[224, 232, 234] Furthermore, mesenteric vasculitis may produce intestinal ulcerations and multiple GI tract perforations. Abdominal pain may be a prominent symptom in this subset of patients. A malabsorption syndrome has also been reported in occasional patients.[237]

### Laboratory Findings

No specific laboratory tests exist, but several are extremely helpful. Serum muscle enzymes (creatine kinase, lactate dehydrogenase, aldolase, and aspartate aminotransfer-

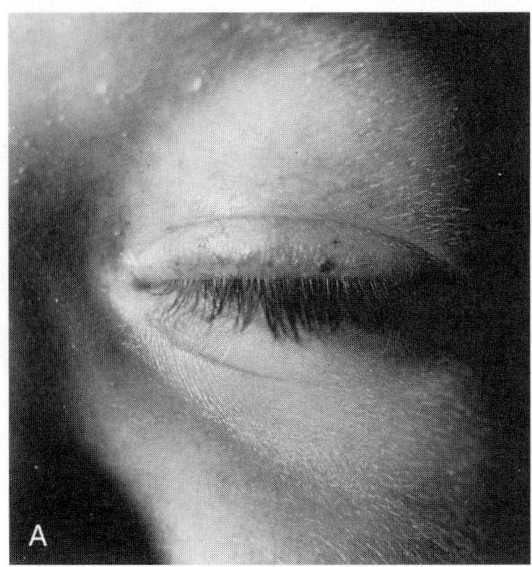


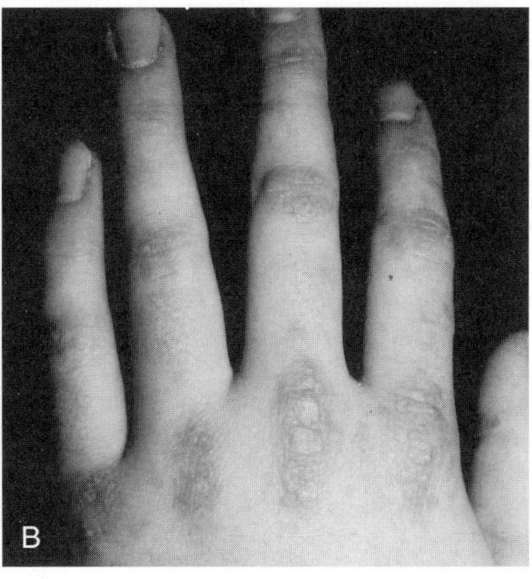


**FIGURE 46–4.** *A,* Heliotrope rash of dermatomyositis with violaceous discoloration of eyelids. *B,* Gottron's patches, which are erythematous, scaly areas overlying the metacarpophalangeal joints of both hands. (Courtesy of Bernard Cohen, MD.)

ase) are likely to be moderately elevated.[238] In addition, serum levels of cytokine inhibitors rise and fall as disease activity waxes and wanes.[239]

Electromyographic abnormalities are also present. Muscle irritability and spontaneous activity at rest are common. In addition, about half of patients display fibrillation and early full recruitment with moderate activity. High-frequency discharges are seen in about 20% of patients. Biopsy of involved muscle reveals a focal inflammatory myopathy.[233, 238]

The vasculitis of this disorder affects capillaries, arterioles, and venules. Inflammation may be absent or present, and the most consistent finding is reticulotubular endothelial inclusions.[240]

### Treatment and Prognosis

Prednisone at a dose of 1 to 2 mg/kg/day unquestionably improves the course of childhood dermatomyositis.[224, 238] For corticosteroid-refractory or steroid-dependent cases, azathioprine,[241] cyclophosphamide,[242] methotrexate,[243] and hydroxychloroquine[244] have been employed, with positive results. Intravenous immunoglobulin given monthly at doses of 2 g/kg body weight divided over 3 to 5 days seems to be efficacious in open trials.[224, 245]

Long-term prognosis is favorable in the majority of cases.[224, 228, 238] Seventy-five percent of patients are left with no sequelae, and only 15% to 25% experience long-term muscle weakness or loss of function.[224, 228, 238] Only 5% to 10% of patients die of complications, but bowel perforation is a common cause of death and must be diagnosed early to permit a satisfactory surgical outcome.[235, 236]

## SOLITARY RECTAL ULCER SYNDROME AND COLITIS CYSTICA PROFUNDA

### History and Pathogenesis

Solitary rectal ulcer syndrome and colitis cystica profunda were thought to be unrelated processes throughout the 18th, 19th, and first half of the 20th centuries. However, in 1967, Wayte and Helwig[246] noted a striking histologic similarity between biopsy specimens from nine patients with colitis cystica profunda and those of four additional patients with solitary rectal ulcers reported by Haskell and Rovner in 1965.[247] Madigan and Morson confirmed the histologic similarity of the two disorders.[248]

Visualization of external or internal rectal prolapse in a large percentage of patients with both disorders has led to a working theory of the pathogenesis.[249, 250] Presumably, mucosal prolapse of the anterior rectum leads to stretching of blood vessels, trauma to the mucosa, thickening of the muscularis mucosae, ulceration, and (in colitis cystica profunda) implantation of surface epithelium into the submucosa. Rectal electromyographic and manometric studies have confirmed that patients with both disorders frequently experience abnormal expulsion dynamics.[251] They contract, rather than relax, their external sphincters with voluntary defecatory effort. This abnormality leads to excessive intrarectal pressure during defecation. Presumably, the increased pressure initiates the sequence of events delineated previously.

### Epidemiology

In Ireland, where the most extensive epidemiologic studies have been performed, the incidence is 1 case per 100,000.[252] Although most patients reported in the literature are adults, children are unquestionably affected. Females appear to be at somewhat greater risk than males.

### Clinical Features

Symptoms are variable, but 70% to 89% of patients pass bright red blood from the rectum.[253, 254] Other symptoms include mucoid rectal discharge, diarrhea, constipation, crampy abdominal pain, tenesmus, and proctalgia. Bleeding can be severe enough to require transfusion. Rare patients also experience rectal obstruction.

### Endoscopic Features

The anus may be patulous, and Valsalva's maneuver may produce internal prolapse of the anterior rectal wall.[254] The mucosa can be hyperemic, edematous, or friable.[254] In colitis cystica profunda, endoscopic ultrasound delineates submucosal cysts.[255]

The solitary ulcer syndrome is a misnomer, as more than half of patients have multiple ulcers.[254, 256] The ulcer or ulcers range from a few millimeters to several centimeters in diameter. Most are located between 5 and 18 cm from the anal verge. Polypoid lesions are seen in some patients with the solitary rectal ulcer syndrome. Patients with colitis cystica profunda should, by definition, lack ulcers; however solitary rectal ulcer and colitis cystica profunda are probably the same entity in different phases of evolution, and ulceration can coexist with multiple firm nodules studding the bowel wall in colitis cystica profunda.[257]

### Histologic Features

Because many diagnostic entities could explain the sigmoidoscopic findings of solitary rectal ulcer and colitis cystica profunda, all patients should undergo biopsy of ulcerated areas and of intact mucosa to search for the pathognomonic histologic features of these syndromes. Biopsy examination reveals "fibromuscular obliteration" of the lamina propria.[253, 254] This finding rules out idiopathic inflammatory bowel disease even in the face of acute and chronic inflammation. A second feature of solitary rectal ulcer syndrome and colitis cystica profunda that distinguishes them from inflammatory bowel disease is the presence of submucosal mucus-filled cysts up to 2 cm in diameter.[253, 254]

### Treatment

Conservative medical management with stool softeners or mineral oil sometimes reduces bleeding[253, 254]; however, refractory cases may require one of the many available surgical options—among them, anterior proctopexy, posterior proctopexy, and mucosal sleeve resection with rectal wall plication.[257] Strictures have been successfully treated by endoscopic balloon dilation.[258] In the unlikely event of severe bleeding or obstruction, diverting colostomy may be necessary.[259]

## MALAKOPLAKIA

### History and Epidemiology

This rare disorder was first described in the urinary tract by Michaelis and Gutmann in 1902.[260] Subsequently involvement elsewhere was identified, and in 1965 Terner and Lattes reported a case of GI malakoplakia.[261] Since that time, only a handful of GI tract cases have been reported,[262–268] but despite the rarity of this disorder, some generalizations can be made. It occurs with equal frequency in males and females, and the age range is 6 weeks to 88 years. It may be confined to the GI tract or may also involve testis, prostate, epididymis, endometrium, broad ligament, vagina, retroperitoneum, adrenal gland, brain, bone, tonsil, or conjunctiva.[269] It may be a primary phenomenon or associated with other pathologic entities such as collagen-vascular disease, ulcerative colitis, adenocarcinoma, or immunodeficiency.[265] It has also been reported after solid organ transplantation in patients receiving immunosuppressant drugs.[267]

### Pathogenesis

Though the pathogenesis remains unknown, work by Lou and Teplitz[270] and by Abdou and coworkers[271] suggests that phagocyte bacterial killing is impaired. Therefore, gram-negative bacteria aggressively attack the epithelium of a number of tubular organs. Reports of malakoplakia associated with paracoccidioidomycosis imply that fungi may produce similar lesions.[268]

### Clinical Features

Most patients experience diarrhea, gross rectal bleeding, and abdominal pain.[262, 266] Weight loss and fever may predominate, or the lesions may produce intestinal obstruction. Some patients develop fistulas or confined perforations with pelvic abscesses.[266] In occasional patients who are asymptomatic, the lesions are found incidentally.

The lesions may be unifocal, multinodular, or masslike with involvement of adjacent organs.[263] Sixty percent of cases are located in the left colon; others are confined to right colon, cecum, or ileocecal region. The stomach is affected in about 10% of cases, and the most common type of fistula is gastrocolic.[263]

### Endoscopic and Histologic Appearance

Grossly, the lesions are soft, slightly raised, umbilicated, bright yellow plaques.[267] A multinodular variant consists of multiple 3- to 4-mm polypoid nodules. The histologic lesions are composed of sheets of histiocytes with small, eccentric nuclei. They contain pathognomonic, target-shaped, calcified cytoplasmic inclusions called Michaelis-Gutmann bodies.[267] Numerous coliform bacteria and digested bacterial remnants are present within lysosomes.[267]

### Treatment

Some patients have responded symptomatically to trimethoprim-sulfamethoxazole[266] or to bethanechol[271] (which facilitates bacterial killing). Reduction of immunosuppression has helped transplant recipients[267]; however, patients with fistulas require surgical excision. Patients with associated malignancy usually succumb, but isolated malakoplakia is sometimes compatible with long-term survival.[266]

## TYPHLITIS

### History and Epidemiology

The term *typhlitis* was first employed by Wagner and associates[272] in 1970 to describe a necrotizing colitis that involves the cecum and possibly the ileum or several regions of the colon. It is identical to the ileocecal syndrome or neutropenic enteropathy. Most reported cases affect neutropenic pediatric patients with leukemia,[272–274] but it has also been seen in patients with other forms of neutropenia[275] or immune deficiency[275] and in solid organ transplant recipients.[276] Though considered rare by some, it is present at the time of death in 10% to 25% of leukemia patients who come to autopsy.[272, 273] Thus, it may be the terminal event in a significant number of fatal leukemias. The gender distribution appears to be approximately equal.[273, 274] The majority of cases have been reported in children, but as chemotherapy regimens for adults become more aggressive, its incidence in adults also appears to be increasing.[277] It appears to be more common in patients with myelocytic leukemia than in those with lymphocytic leukemia.[274] The use of cytosine arabinoside, daunomycin, or VP-16 appears to be an associated risk factor.[274]

### Pathogenesis

The pathogenesis of this disorder is unknown, but Prolla and Kirsner[278] have postulated that the sequence of events is initiated by a breakdown in the mucosal barrier due to chemotherapy or to leukemic infiltrates. Subsequently, bacteria invade the bowel wall, proliferate because of neutropenia, and produce endotoxin that further damages mucosa.

### Clinical Features

According to Katz and colleagues,[273] 78% of patients have abdominal pain and distention. The pain is usually in the right lower quadrant but may be more diffuse. Bright red rectal bleeding was not observed in early reports,[272] but more recent reports describe it in about one third of patients.[273, 274] Vomiting, diarrhea, and upper GI tract bleeding occur less frequently. Fever is noted in nearly all patients, and 14% experience respiratory distress.

### Anatomic Distribution

At autopsy, disease is confined to the cecum and appendix in only 22% of patients, whereas the cecum is involved in conjunction with the ileum, and sometimes the ascending colon, in 51%.[273] Discrete ulcerations extending throughout the colon are seen in 27% of autopsy specimens.[273]

### Laboratory Findings

Almost all patients have absolute neutrophil counts less than 1,500 per mm$^3$, and 78% have counts less than 500 per mm$^3$.[272–274]

Blood cultures taken when the patient is symptomatic are almost always positive for gram-negative bacteria or *Staphylococcus aureus*.[273, 274] Fungal sepsis is also quite common: 16% of antemortem blood cultures grow *Candida, Aspergillus,* or *Cryptococcus* organisms.[273, 274]

Stool cultures rarely yield specific pathogens, but stool is frequently positive for *Clostridium difficile* toxin.[274] A positive clostridial toxin assay need not imply pathogenicity, because clostridial colitis is usually left-sided rather than right-sided.

### Radiographic, Endoscopic, and Histologic Findings

Plain films and barium enema examination may show evidence of ileus, small bowel obstruction, pneumatosis coli, thickened bowel wall, cecal deformity, or "nonfilling" of the cecum.[279, 280] However, the preferred diagnostic modality is ultrasonography[281] or CT.[282] Thickened bowel wall may be visualized, and the progression or regression of the process can be followed with serial sonographic or tomographic examinations.

Under most circumstances endoscopy need not be performed because of the excellent resolution of radiography in the right colon. When the left colon is predominantly involved and clostridial toxin assay is negative, endoscopy should be considered to rule out cytomegalovirus enteritis[283]; however, the benefits should be weighed against the risk of endoscopy in a neutropenic, possibly thrombocytopenic patient. When endoscopy is performed, it may reveal multiple colonic ulcers or a large, discrete area of cecal necrosis and ulceration. Biopsy material should be sent not only for microscopy but also for bacterial, fungal, and viral culture.

A histologic picture of superficial cecal ulceration and hemorrhagic mucosal necrosis is characteristic.[272–274] Blood vessels may be infiltrated by bacteria or fungal elements. Adjoining tissue is histologically normal.

### Treatment

Typhlitis is not uniformly fatal if aggressive antibiotic treatment and supportive care are provided.[273, 274] Fluid depletion and electrolyte imbalance should be corrected. Antibiotics with a broad enough spectrum to cover *S. aureus,* coliforms, and anaerobes should be administered. If a patient fails to "defervesce" after 72 hours of antibacterial therapy, antifungal coverage should be considered.

Authors' thinking differs about the timing of surgery and what type of operation to perform in this group of patients. Some would operate when patients experience local peritoneal irritation or when pneumatosis intestinalis is radiographically evident.[284] Most would await the onset of generalized peritonitis. Even some cases of severe GI hemorrhage have been managed nonoperatively. Surgical techniques cover a spectrum from cecostomy and drainage to right hemicolectomy and ileocolostomy.[284] Operative mortality ranges from 8% to 50%,[285] as compared with an overall mortality rate of less than 8% for patients managed medically.[274]

## COLLAGENOUS COLITIS AND LYMPHOCYTIC COLITIS

### History, Epidemiology, and Pathogenesis

Collagenous colitis, first described by Lindstrom in 1976,[286] and lymphocytic colitis, subsequently described by

Read's group in 1980,[287] share many features. They are both common to middle-aged patients with watery diarrhea, and evolution from lymphocytic to collagenous colitis has been reported.[288, 289] Differences do exist. The 80% female predominance of collagenous colitis is not true of microscopic colitis. Furthermore, autoantibodies and a specific HLA phenotype are more often seen in lymphocytic colitis than in collagenous colitis.[288] Both disorders are rare in children, but a handful of cases have been reported in pediatric patients.[290]

## Clinical Characteristics

Both collagenous and lymphocytic colitis patients present with watery, nonbloody diarrhea and crampy abdominal pain.[288, 289] Nausea and vomiting sometimes occur, and many patients lose weight. About 10% of collagenous colitis patients have rheumatoid arthritis, 10% have thyroid disease, and 10% have sprue.[291] There appears to be a strong association between use of nonsteroidal anti-inflammatory agents and collagenous colitis.[291] The frequency of sprue among lymphocytic colitis patients has not been determined, but as many as 30% of sprue patients have lymphocytic colitis.[292] Other autoimmune processes may coexist with lymphocytic colitis.[293]

## Laboratory, Radiographic, and Endoscopic Findings

Most patients do not experience anemia or leukocytosis, but the erythrocyte sedimentation rate may be mildly elevated in both disorders.[288, 289] Steatorrhea is sometimes present, and white blood cells are sometimes present in stools. By definition, barium enema and colonoscopy findings are normal.

## Histologic Features

Collagenous colitis and lymphocytic colitis are both characterized by an inflammatory infiltrate of the lamina propria.[288, 289] While eosinophils, plasma cells, and mast cells contribute to the infiltrate of both collagenous and lymphocytic colitis, lymphocytes predominate in both. Additionally, lymphocytes infiltrate both crypt and surface epithelium. A thickened subepithelial layer of type I or type III collagen is typical of collagenous colitis.

## Differential Diagnosis

Inflammatory bowel disease, irritable bowel syndrome, and surreptitious laxative abuse should be considered in the differential diagnosis of both disorders.

## Treatment and Prognosis

Some patients respond to discontinuation of nonsteroidal agents.[288] Others respond to cholestyramine, bismuth subsalicylate,[288] or 5-aminosalicylic acid therapy. Finally, 1 mg/kg/day of prednisone helps the majority of patients.[288] Medications can sometimes be tapered and discontinued without symptomatic recurrence; however, some patients require intermittent courses of steroids for many years to keep symptoms under control.

## REFERENCES


1. Atherton DJ, Muller DPR, Aggett PJ, Harries JT: A defect in zinc uptake by jejunal biopsies in acrodermatitis enteropathica. Clin Sci 1979;56:505–507.
2. Evans GW, Johnson PE: Defective prostaglandin synthesis in acrodermatitis enteropathica. Lancet 1997;1:52.
3. Cunnane SC, Krieger I: Long chain fatty acids in serum phospholipids in acrodermatitis enteropathica before and after zinc treatment: a case report. J Am Coll Nutr 1988;7:249–250.
4. Krieger I, Cash R, Evans GW: Picolinic acid in acrodermatitis enteropathica: evidence for a disorder of tryptophan metabolism. J Pediatr Gastroenterol Nutr 1984;3:62–68.
5. Casey CE, Hambidge KM, Walravens PA: Zinc binding in human duodenal secretions. J Pediatr 1979;95:1008–1010.
6. Ackland, ML, Danks DM, McArdle HJ: Zinc transport by fibroblasts from patients with acrodermatitis enteropathica. Biol Trace Elem Res 1989;22:257–263.
7. Grider A, Young EM: The acrodermatitis enteropathica mutation transiently affects zinc metabolism in human fibroblasts. J Nutr 1996;126:219–224.
8. VanWouwe JP: Clinical and laboratory diagnosis of acrodermatitis enteropathica. Eur J Pediatr 1989;149:2–8.
9. Castillo-Duran C, Vial P, Uauy R: Trace mineral balance during acute diarrhea in infants. J Pediatr 1988;113:452–457.
10. Wolman SL, Anderson GH, Marliss EB, Jeejeebhoy KN: Zinc in total parenteral nutrition: requirements and metabolic effects. Gastroenterology 1979;76:458–467.
11. Allen JJ, Kay EN, McClain CJ: Severe zinc deficiency in humans. Association with a reversible T-lymphocyte dysfunction. Ann Intern Med 1981;95:154–157.
12. Fraker PJ, Jardieu P, Cook J: Zinc deficiency and immune function. Arch Dermatol 1987;123:1699–1701.
13. Peretz A, Cantinieaux B, Neve J, et al: Effects of zinc supplementation on the phagocytic functions of polymorphonuclear cells in patients with inflammatory rheumatic diseases. J Trace Elem Electrolytes Health Dis 1994;8:189–194.
14. Sanstead HH: Understanding zinc: recent observations and interpretations. J Lab Clin Med 1994;124:322–327.
15. Aggett PJ: Clinical zinc deficiency: an overview. In Kruse-Jarres JD, Scholmerich J (eds): Zinc and Diseases of the Digestive Tract. Boston, Kluwer Academic, 1997, pp 37–35.
16. Heng Y, Schuffler MD, Haggitt RC, Rohrman CA: Pneumatosis intestinalis: a review. Am J Gastroenterol 1995;90:1747–1758.
17. Keyting W, McCarver R, Kovarik J, et al: Pneumatosis intestinalis: a new concept. Radiology 1961;76:733–741.
18. Steinnon O: Pneumatosis intestinalis in the newborn. Am J Dis Child 1951;81:651–653.
19. McGregor J, McKinnon D: Intestinal interstitial emphysema (pneumatosis cystoides intestinalis). Gastroenterology 1958;36:75–76.
20. Levitt M, Olsson S: Pneumatosis cystoides intestinalis and high breath $H_2$ excretion: insights into the role of $H_2$ in this condition. Gastroenterology 1995;108:1560–1565.
21. Underwood J, Finnis D, Scott W: Pneumatosis coli: a familial association. Br J Surg 1978;65:64–65.
22. Engel R, Virnig N, Hunt C, et al: Origin of mural gas in necrotizing enterocolitis. Pediatr Res 1973;7:292.
23. Hernanz-Schulman M, Kirkpatrick JJ, Shwachman H, et al: Pneumatosis intestinalis in cystic fibrosis. Radiology 1986;160:497–499.
24. Scott J, Miller W, Urso M, et al: Acute mesenteric infarction. Radiology 1971;113:269–279.
25. Tak P, Van Duinen C, Bun P, et al: Pneumatosis cystoides intestinalis in intestinal pseudo-obstruction. Resolution after therapy with metronidazole. Dig Dis Sci 1992;37:949–954.
26. John A, Dickey K, Fenwick J, et al: Pneumatosis intestinalis in patients with Crohn's disease. Dig Dis Sci 1992;37:813–817.

27. Day D, Ramsay N, Letourneau J: Pneumatosis intestinalis after bone marrow transplantation. AJR Am J Roentgenol 1988;151:85–87.
28. Ammons M, Bauling P, Weil R: Pneumatosis cystoides intestinalis with pneumoperitoneum in renal transplant patients on cyclosporine and prednisone. Transplant Proc 1986;18:1868–1870.
29. Janssen D, Kalayoglu M, Solinger H: Pneumatosis cystoides intestinalis following lactulose and steroid treatment in a liver transplant patient with an intermittently enlarged scrotum. Transplant Proc 1987;19:2949–2952.
30. Marshak R, Lindner A, Maklansky D: Pneumatosis cystoides coli. Gastrointest Radiol 1977;2:85–89.
31. Vernacchia F, Jeffery R, Laing F, et al: Sonographic recognition of pneumatosis intestinalis. AJR Am J Roentgenol 1985;145:51–52.
32. Connor R, Jones B, Fishman E, et al: Pneumatosis intestinalis: role of computed tomography in diagnosis and management. J Comput Assist Tomogr 1984;8:269–275.
33. Pieterse A, Leong Y, Rowland R: The mucosal changes and pathogenesis of pneumatosis cystoides intestinalis. Hum Pathol 1985;16:683–688.
34. Ellis B: Symptomatic treatment of primary pneumatosis coli with metronidazole. Br Med J 1980;280:763–764.
35. Mirables M, Hinojosa J, Alonso J, et al: Oxygen therapy in pneumatosis coli. Dis Colon Rectum 1983;26:458–460.
36. Boley SJ, Treiber W, Winslow PR, et al: Circulatory response to acute reduction of superior mesenteric arterial flow (abstract). The Physiologist 1969;12:180.
37. Boley SJ, Regan JA, Tunick PA, et al: Persistent vasoconstriction—a major factor in nonocclusive mesenteric ischemia. Curr Top Surg Res 1971;3:425–433.
38. Haglund U, Abe T, Ahren C, et al: The intestinal mucosal lesions in shock. I. Studies on the pathogenesis. Eur Surg Res 1976;8:435–447.
39. Granger D, Richardson P, Kvietys P, Mortillaro N: Intestinal blood flow. Gastroenterology 1980;78:837–863.
40. Nowicki PT, Caniano DA, Szaniazlo K: Effect of intestinal denervation on intestinal vascular response to severe arterial hypoxia in newborn swine. Am J Physiol 1987;253:G201–G205.
41. Shanbour LL, Jacobson ED: Digitalis and the mesenteric circulation. Am J Dig Dis 1972;17:826–828.
42. Stillman A, Weinberg M, Mast W, Palpant S: Ischemic bowel disease attributable to ergot. Gastroenterology 1977;72:1336–1337.
43. Bernardino M, Lawson T: Discrete colonic ulcers associated with oral contraceptives. Dig Dis Sci 1976;21:503–506.
44. Scholz FJ: Ischemic bowel disease. Radiol Clin North Am 1993; 31(6):1197–1218.
45. Huizinga WK, Nirmul D, Domingo Z, Ngakane H: Late presentation of small-bowel injury—hypoproteinemia, anaemia and obstruction. A report of 2 cases. South Afr Med J 1988;73:251–252.
46. Ottinger L: Mesenteric ischemia. N Engl J Med 1982;307:535–537.
47. Rhee RY, Gloviczki P: Mesenteric venous thrombosis. Surg Clin North Am 1997;77(2):327–339.
48. Anane-Sefah JC, Blair E, Reckler S: Primary mesenteric venous occlusive disease. Surg Gynecol Obstet 1975;141:740–742.
49. DeLaney HM: Prognostic factors in infarction of the intestine. Surg Gynecol Obstet 1972;135:253–256.
50. Tomchick S, Wittenberg J, Ottinger LW: The roentgenographic spectrum of bowel infarction. Radiology 1970;96:249–260.
51. O'Connell TX, Kadell B, Tompkins RK: Ischemia of the colon. Surg Gynecol Obstet 1976;142:337–342.
52. Milley VE, Berland LL: Pulsed Doppler duplex sonography and CT of portal vein thrombosis. AJR Am J Roentgenol 1985;145:73.
53. Morson BC, Dawson IMP: Gastrointestinal Pathology, 2nd ed. Oxford, Blackwell, 1979, pp 380–398.
54. Walsh D: Deep tissue traumatism from roentgen ray exposure. Br Med J 1987;2:272–273.
55. Manson GR, Guernse JM, Hanks GE, Nelson TS: Surgical therapy for radiation enteritis. Oncology 1968;22:241–257.
56. Roswit B, Malsky SJ, Reid CB: Severe radiation injuries of the stomach, small intestine, colon and rectum. Am J Roentgenol Radium Ther Nucl Med 1972;114:460–475.
57. Donaldson SS, Jundt S, Ricour C, et al: Radiation enteritis in children. A retrospective, clinicopathologic correlation, and dietary management. Cancer 1975;35:1167–1178.
58. Newman A, Katsaris J, Blendis LM, et al: Small intestinal injury in women who have had pelvic radiotherapy. Lancet 1973;2:1471–1473.
59. Rubin P, Casarett G: A direction for clinical radiation pathology: the tolerance dose. In Vaeth JM (ed): Frontiers of Radiation Therapy and Oncology, Vol 16. Baltimore, University Park Press, 1972, pp 1–16.
60. DeCosse JJ, Rhodes RS, Wentz WB, et al: The natural history and management of radiation induced injury of the gastrointestinal tract. Ann Surg 1969;170:369–384.
61. Loughlin KR, Retik AB, Weinstein HJ, et al: Genitourinary rhabdomyosarcoma in children. Cancer 1989;63:1600–1606.
62. Mauch P, Tarbell N, Weinstein H, et al: Stage IA and IIA supradiaphragmatic Hodgkin's disease: prognostic factors in surgically staged patients treated with mantle and paraaortic irradiation. J Clin Oncol 1988;6:1576–1583.
63. Trier JS, Browning TH: Morphological response of the mucosa of the human small intestine to x-ray exposure. J Clin Invest 1966;45:194–204.
64. Quastlar H: The nature of intestinal radiation death. Radiation Res 1956;4:303–320.
65. Carr ND, Pullen BR, Haselton PS, et al: Microvascular studies in human radiation bowel disease. Gut 1984;25:448–454.
66. Joslin CA, Smith CW, Malik A: The treatment of cervix cancer using high activity Co-60 sources. Br J Radiol 1972;45:257–270.
67. Buchler DA, Kline JC, Peckham BM, et al: Radiation reactions in cervical cancer therapy. Am J Obstet Gynecol 1971;111:745–750.
68. Galland RB, Spencer J: Natural history and surgical managment of radiation enteritis. Br J Surg 1987;74:742–747.
69. Galland RB, Spencer J: The natural history of clinically established radiation enteritis. Lancet 1985;1:1257–1258.
70. Bosch A, Frias Z: Complications after radiation therapy for cervical carcinoma. Acta Radiol (Ther) (Stockh) 1977;16:53–62.
71. Strykker JA, Mortel R, Hepner GW: The effect of pelvic irradiation on lactose absorption. Radiat Oncol Biol Phys 1978;4:859–863.
72. Yeoh E, Horowitz M: Radiation enteritis. Br J Hosp Med 1988;39:498–504.
73. Mendelson RM, Nolan DJ: The radiological features of chronic radiation enteritis. Clin Radiol 1985;36:141–148.
74. Wellwood JM, Jackson BT: The intestinal complications of radiotherapy. Br J Surg 1973;60:814–818.
75. Meric F, Hirschl RB, Mahboubi S, et al: Prevention of radiation enteritis in children using a pelvic mesh sling. J Pediatr Surg 1994;29:917–921.
76. Bounous G, LeBel E, Shuster J, et al: Dietary protection during radiation therapy. Strahlentherapie 1975;149:476–482.
77. Mennie AT, Dalley VM, Dinneen LC, et al: Treatment of radiation-induced gastrointestinal distress with acetylsalicylate. Lancet 1975;2:942–943.
78. Loiudice TA, Lang JA: Treatment of radiation enteritis: a comparison study. Am J Gastroenterol 1983;78:481–487.
79. Rauch K, Weiland H: Behandlung der radiogenen Kolitis mit Salicylazosulfapyridin (Azulfidine). Strahlungtherapie 1972;143:660–663.
80. Resbeut M, Marteau P, Cowen D, et al: A randomized double blind placebo controlled multicenter study of mesalazine for the prevention of acute radiation enteritis. Radiother Oncol 1997;44:59–63.
81. Delaney JP, Bonsack ME, Felemovicius I: Misoprostol in the intestinal lumen protects against radiation injury of the small bowel. Radiat Res 1994;137:405–409.
82. Swann RW, Fowler WC, Boronow RC: Surgical management of radiation injury to the small intestine. Surg Gynecol Obstet 1976; 142:325–327.
83. von Gasser C, Gautier E, Steck A, et al: Hämolytisch-urämische Syndrome. Bilaterale Nierenrindennekrosen bei akuten erworbenen hämolytischen Anamien. Schweiz Med Wschr 1955;85:905–909.
84. Kaplan BS, Proesmans W: The hemolytic uremic syndrome of childhood and its variants. Semin Hematol 1987;24:148–160.
85. Kinney JS, Gross TP, Porter CC, et al: Hemolytic-uremic syndrome: a population-based study in Washington, DC and Baltimore, Maryland. Am J Public Health 1988;78:64–64.
86. Tarr PL, Neill MA, Allen J, et al: The increasing incidence of the hemolytic-uremic syndrome in King County, Washington: lack of evidence for ascertainment bias. Am J Epidemiol 1989;129:582–586.
87. Martin DL, MacDonald KL, White KE: The epidemiology and clinical aspects of the hemolytic-uremic syndrome in Minnesota. N Engl J Med 1990;33:1161–1167.
88. Rowe PC, Orrbine E, Wells GA, et al: Epidemiology of hemolytic-uremic syndrome in Canadian children from 1986 to 1988. J Pediatr 1991;119:218–224.
89. Neill MA, Agosti J, Rosen H: Hemorrhagic colitis with *Escherichia*

*coli* O157:H7 preceding adult hemolytic uremic syndrome. Arch Intern Med 1985;145:2215–2217.
90. Gianantonio CA, Vitacco M, Mendilaharzu F, et al: The hemolytic-uremic syndrome. Nephron 1973;11:174–192.
91. Kaplan JBS, Katz J, Krawitz S, et al: An analysis of the results of therapy in 67 cases of the hemolytic-uremic syndrome. J Pediatr 1971;78:420–425.
92. Lieberman E: Hemolytic-uremic syndrome. J Pediatr 1972;80:1–16.
93. Siegler RL, Povia AT, Christofferson RD, et al: A 20-year population-based study of hemolytic-uremic syndrome in Utah. Pediatrics 1994;94:35–40.
94. Hall S, Glickman M: The British Pediatric Surveillance Unit. Arch Dis Child 1988;63:344–346.
95. Drummond KN: Hemolytic uremic syndrome—then and now. N Engl J Med 1985;312:116–118.
96. Kaplan BS, Chesney RW, Drummond KN: Hemolytic uremic syndrome in families. N Engl J Med 1975;292:1090–1093.
97. Karmali MA, Petric M, Lim C, et al: The association between hemolytic uremic syndrome and infection by verotoxin-producing *Escherichia coli.* J Infect Dis 1985;151:775–782.
98. Gransden WPR, Damm MAS, Anderson JD, et al: Further evidence associating hemolytic uremic syndrome with infection by verotoxin-producing *Escherichia coli* O157:H7. J Infect Dis 1986;154:522–524.
99. Neill MA, Tarr PI, Clausen C, et al: *Escherichia coli* O157:H7 as the predominant pathogen associated with the hemolytic uremic syndrome: a prospective study in the Pacific Northwest. Pediatrics 1987;80:37–40.
100. Scotland SM, Rowe B, Smith HR, et al: Vero cytotoxin–producing strains of *Escherichia coli* from children with haemolytic uraemic syndrome and their detection by specific DNA probes. J Med Microbiol 1988;25:237–243.
101. Lopez EL, Diaz M, Grinstein S, et al: Hemolytic uremic syndrome and diarrhea in Argentine children: the role of Shiga-like toxins. J Infect Dis 1989;160:469–475.
102. Ray C, Tucker VL, Harris DJ, et al: Enterovirus associated with the hemolytic-uremic syndrome. Pediatrics 1970;46:378–388.
103. Mathieu H, LeClerc F, Habib R, et al: Etude clinique et biologique de 37 observations de syndrome hemolytique et uremique. Arch Franc Pediat 1969;26:369–390.
104. Gradishar WJ, Vokes EE, et al: Chemotherapy-related hemolytic-uremic syndrome after the treatment of head and neck cancer. Cancer 1990;66:1914–1918.
105. O'Brien AD, Holmes RK: Shiga and shiga-like toxins. Microbiol Rev 1987;51:206–220.
106. Taylor CM, Milford DV, Rose PE, et al: The expression of blood group P1 in post-enteropathic haemolytic uraemic syndrome. Pediatr Nephrol 1990;4:59–61.
107. Walters MDS, Levin M, Smith C, et al: Intravascular platelet activation in the hemolytic uremic syndrome. Kidney Int 1988;33:107–115.
108. Fong JSC, Kaplan BS: Impairment of platelet aggregation in the hemolytic uremic syndrome. Evidence for platelet "exhaustion." Blood 1982;60:564–569.
109. Levin M, Stroobant P, Walters MDS, et al: Platelet derived growth factors as possible mediators of vascular proliferation in the sporadic haemolytic uremic syndrome. Lancet 1986;2:830–833.
110. Koster F, Levin J, Walker L, et al: Hemolytic uremic syndrome after shigellosis: relation to endotoxemia and circulating immune complexes. N Engl J Med 1978;298:927–933.
111. O'Regan S, Chesney RW, Kaplan BS, et al: Red cell membrane phospholipid abnormalities in the hemolytic uremic syndrome. Clin Nephrol 1980;15:14–17.
112. Furase A, Hattori S, Matusda I: A case of hemolytic uremic syndrome with high concentration of circulating immune complexes in the initial stage. Int J Pediatr Nephrol 1983;4:123–126.
113. Monnens L, Van de Meer W, Langenhuysen C, et al: Platelet aggregating factor in the epidemic form of hemolytic uremic syndrome in childhood. Clin Nephrol 1985;24:135–137.
114. Inward CD, Pall AA, Adu D, et al: Solùble circulating cell adhesion molecules in haemolytic uremic syndrome. Pediatr Nephrol 1995;9:574–578.
115. Moake JL, Byrnes JJ, Troll JH, et al: Abnormal VIII: von Willebrand factor patterns in the plasma of patients with the hemolytic-uremic syndrome. Blood 1984;64:592–598.
116. Remuzzi G, Misiani R, Marchesi D, et al: Haemolytic uraemic syndrome: deficiency of plasma factor(s) regulating prostacyclin activity? Lancet 1978;2:871–872.
117. Mulligan MS, Hevel JM, Marletta MA, et al: Tissue injury caused by deposition of immune complexes is L-arginine dependent. Proc Natl Acad Sci USA 1991;88:6338–6342.
118. Westberg G, Shultz PJ, Ray L: Exogenous nitric oxide prevents endotoxin-induced glomerular thrombosis in rats. Kidney Int 1994;46:711–716.
119. Whitington PF, Friedman AL, Chesney RW: Gastrointestinal disease in the hemolytic-uremic syndrome. Gastroenterology 1979;76:728–733.
120. Brandt MI, O'Regan S, Rousseau E, et al: Surgical complications of the hemolytic-uremic syndrome. J Pediatr Surg 1990;25:1109–1112.
121. Berman W Jr: The hemolytic-uremic syndrome: initial clinical presentation mimicking ulcerative colitis. J Pediatr 1972;81:275–278.
122. Tarr PI, Neill MA, Clausen CR, et al: *Escherichia coli* O157:H7 and the hemolytic uremic syndrome: importance of early cultures in establishing the etiology. J Infect Dis 1990;162:553–556.
123. Grodinsky S, Telmesani A, Robson WL, et al: Gastrointestinal manifestations of hemolytic uremic syndrome: recognition of pancreatitis. J Pediatr Gastroenterol Nutr 1990;11:518–524.
124. Gordjani N, Sutor A, Zimmerhackl LB, et al: Hemolytic uremic syndromes in childhood. Semin Thromb Hemost 1997;23(3):281–293.
125. Van Damme Lombaerts R, Proesmans W, Van Damme B, et al: Heparin plus dipyridamole in childhood hemolytic-uremic syndrome: a prospective, randomized study. J Pediatr 1988;113:913–918.
126. Defreyn JG: Plasmapheresis in the haemolytic-uraemic syndrome in chldren. Br Med J 1981;282:1667–1668.
127. Loirat C, Sonsino E, Hinglais N, et al: Treatment of the childhood haemolytic uraemic syndrome with plasma. Pediatr Nephrol 1988;2:279–285.
128. McGraw ME, Lendon M, Stevens RF, et al: Haemolytic uraemic syndrome and the Thomsen-Friedenreich antigen. Pediatr Nephrol 1989;3:135–139.
129. Taylor SB, Coller BS, Chang ACK, et al: 7E3 $F(ab')_2$, a microsomal antibody to the platelet GP, IIb/IIIa receptor protects against microangiopathic hemolytic anemia and microvascular thrombotic renal failure in baboons treated with C4b binding protein and a sublethal infusion of *E. coli.* Blood 1997;89:4078–4084.
130. Rook A: Heberden's cases of anaphylactoid purpura. Arch Dis Child 1958;33:271–272.
131. Schonlein JL: Allgemeine und Specielle Pathologie und Therapie. Freiburg, Etlinger, 1837, pp 48–49.
132. Henoch E: Uber eine eigenthumliche form von purpura. Klin Wchnschr 1874;11:641–643.
133. Henoch E: Neunter Aschnitt III. Die hämorrhagische diatheses purpura. In Vorlesung uber Kinderdandkeiten. Berlin, Hirschwald, 1895, p 847.
134. Cream JJ, Gumpel JJ, Peachey RDG: Schönlein-Henoch purpura in the adult. Q J Med 1970;39:461–484.
135. Allen DM, Diamond LK, Howell DA: Anaphylactoid purpura in children (Schönlein-Henoch syndrome). Am J Dis Child 1960;99:833–854.
136. Maggiore G, Martini A, Grifco D: Hepatitis B virus infection and Schönlein-Henoch purpura. Am J Dis Child 1984;138:681–682.
137. Garty BZ, Danon YL, Nitzan M: Schönlein-Henoch purpura in children (Schönlein-Henoch syndrome). Am J Dis Child 1985;139:547.
138. Lefrere J, Courouce A, Soulier J, et al: Henoch-Schönlein purpura and human parvovirus infection. Pediatrics 1986;78:183–184.
139. Bywaters EG, Isdale I, Kempton JJ: Schönlein-Henoch purpura: evidence for a group A beta-hemolytic streptococcal aetiology. Q J Med 1957;26:161–175.
140. Ackroyd MD: Allergic purpura, including purpura due to foods, drugs, and infections. Am J Med 1953;14:605–632.
141. Gagliano RS, Costanzi JJ, Beathard GA, et al: The nephrotic syndrome associated with neoplasia: an unusual paraneoplastic syndrome. Report of a case and review of the literature. Am J Med 1976;60:1026–1031.
142. Garcias VA, Her HW: Henoch-Schönlein purpura associated with cancer of the prostate. Urology 1982;19:155–158.
143. Mitchell DM: Relapse of Henoch-Schönlein purpura associated with lung carcinoma. J R Soc Med 1979;72:614–615.
144. Stevenson JA, Leong LA, Cohen AH, et al: Henoch-Schönlein purpura: simultaneous demonstration of IgA deposits in involved skin, intestine, and kidney. Arch Pathol Lab Med 1982;106:192–195.
145. Fauci AS, Haynes BF, Katz P: The spectrum of vasculitis: clinical, pathologic, immunologic and therapeutic considerations. Ann Intern Med 1978;80:660–676.
146. Glasier CM, Siegel MK, McAlister WH, et al: Henoch-Schönlein

syndrome in children: gastrointestinal manifestations. Am J Roentgenol 1981;136:1081–1085.
147. Rosenbloom ND, Winter HS: Steroid effects on the course of abdominal pain in children with Henoch-Schönlein purpura. Pediatrics 1987;79:1018–1021.
148. Katz S, Borst M, Seekri I, et al: Surgical evaluation of Henoch-Schönlein purpura: experience with 110 children. Arch Surg 1991;126:849–854.
149. Belman A, Leicher C, Moshe S, et al: Neurologic manifestations of Schönlein-Henoch purpura: report of three cases and review of the literature. Pediatrics 1985;75:687–692.
150. Branski D, Gross V, Gross-Kieselstein E, et al: Pancreatitis as a complication of Henoch-Schönlein purpura. J Pediatr Gastroentrol 1982;1:275–276.
151. Case 14-1980: Case records of the Massachusetts General Hospital: weekly clinicopathological exercises. N Engl J Med 1980;302:853–858.
152. Olson JC, Kelly KJ, Pan CG, et al: Pulmonary disease with hemorrhage in Henoch-Schönlein purpura. Pediatrics 1992;89:1177–1181.
153. Powell JM, Ware H, Williams G: Recurrent ureteric obstruction in association with Henoch-Schönlein purpura. Postgrad Med J 1987;63:699–701.
154. Delhumeau A, Cavellat JF, Granry JC, et al: Cardiac tamponade in rheumatoid purpura. Ann Franc Anesth Reanim 1982;1:183–185.
155. Lombard KA, Shah PC, Thrasher TV, et al: Ileal stricture as a late complication of Henoch-Schönlein purpura. Pediatrics 1986;77:396–398.
156. Wall Blake AWL, Lobatto SS, Jonges L, et al: IgA antibodies directed against cytoplasmic antigens of polymorphonuclear leukocytes in patients with Henoch-Schönlein purpura. Adv Exp Med Biol 1987;216B:1593–1598.
157. Kamitsumji H, Tani K, Yasui M, et al: Activity of blood coagulation factor XIII as a prognostic indicator in patients with Henoch-Schönlein purpura. Eur J Pediatr 1987;146:519–523.
158. Rodriquez-Erdmann F, Levitan R: Gastrointestinal and roentgenological manifestations of Henoch-Schönlein purpura. Gastroenterology 1968;54:260–264.
159. Tomomasa T, Hsu JY, Itoh K, et al: Endoscopic findings in pediatric patients with Henoch-Schönlein purpura and gastrointestinal symptoms. J Pediatr Gastroenterol Nutr 1987;6;725–729.
160. Dosa S, Caerns SA, Mallich NP, et al: Relapsing Henoch-Schönlein syndrome with renal involvement in a patient with an IgA monoclonal gammopathy—a study of the results of immunosuppresssant and cytotoxic therapy. Nephron 198;26:145–148.
161. Hasegawa A, Kawamura T, Ito H, et al: Fate of renal grafts with recurrent Henoch-Schönlein purpura nephritis in children. Transplant Proc 1989;21:2130–2133.
162. Kauffmann RH, Houwert DA: Plasmaphoresis in rapidly progressive Henoch-Schönlein glomerulonephritis and the effect on circulating IgA immune complexes. Clin Nephrol 1981;16:155–160.
163. Utani A, Ohta M, Shinya A, et al: Successful treatment of adult Henoch-Schönlein purpura with factor XIII concentrate. J Am Acad Dermatol 1991;24:438–442.
164. Fukui H, Kamitsuiji H, Nagao T, et al: Clinical evaluation of a pasteurized factor XIII concentrate administration in Henoch-Schönlein purpura. Thromb Res 1989:56:667–675.
165. Kyle R, Bayrd E: Amyloidosis. Medicine 1975;54:271–299.
166. Cohen AS: Amyloidosis. In McCarty DJ (ed): Arthritis and Allied Conditions, 4th ed. Philadelphia, Lea & Febiger, 1989, pp 1273–1293.
167. Bardin T, Zingraff J, Shirahame T, et al: Hemodialysis associated amyloidosis and beta-2 microglobulin: a clinical and immunohistochemical study. Am J Med 1987;83:419–424.
168. Kocak H, Besbas N, Saatci U, et al: Amyloidosis in children with familial Mediterranean fever. Turk J Pediatr 1989;31:281–287.
169. David J: Amyloidosis in juvenile chronic arthritis. Clin Exp Rheumatol 1991;9:73–78.
170. Travis WD, Castile R, Vawter G, et al: Secondary (AA) amyloidosis in cystic fibrosis. A report of three cases. Am J Clin Pathol 1986;85:419–424.
171. Kahn E, Markowitz J, Simpser E, et al: Amyloidosis in children with inflammatory bowel disease. J Pediatr Gastroenterol Nutr 1989;8:447–453.
172. Pearson RD, Swenson I, Schenk EA, et al: Fatal multisystem disease with immune enteropathy heralded by juvenile rheumatoid arthritis. J Pediatr Gastroenterol Nutr 1989;8:259–265.
173. Kikuchi M, Haginoya K, Miyabayashi S, et al: Secondary amyloidosis in glycogen storage disease type Ib. Eur J Pediatr 1990;149:344–345.
174. Looi LM: The pattern of amyloidosis in a Malaysian patient population. Histopathology 1991;18:133–141.
175. Ponce P, Ramos A, Ferreira ML, et al: Renal involvement in leprosy. Nephrol Dial Transplant 1989;4:81–84.
176. Husby G, Sletten K, Michaelson TE, et al: Amyloid fibril protein subunit, "protein AS": distribution in tissue and serum in different clinical types of amyloidosis including that associated with myelomatosis and Waldenström's macroglobulinemia. Scand J Immunol 1973;2:395–404.
177. Linke RP, Sipe JD, Pollock PS, et al: Isolation of low–molecular weight serum component antigenically related to an amyloid fibril protein of unknown origin. Proc Natl Acad Sci USA 1974;72:1473–1475.
178. Sipe JD, Vogel SN, Sztein MB, et al: The role of interleukin I on acute phase serum amyloid A (SAA) and serum amyloid P (SAP) biosynthesis. Ann NY Acad Sci 1982;389:137–150.
179. Kisilevsky R, Boudreau L: Kinetics of amyloid deposition I. The effects of amyloid-enhancing factor and splenectomy. Lab Invest 1983;48:53–59.
180. Gilat T, Revach M, Sohar E: Deposition of amyloid in the gastrointestinal tract. Gut 1969;10:98–104.
181. Tada S, Iida M, Iwashita A, et al: Endoscopic and biopsy findings of the upper digestive tract in patients with amyloidosis. Gastrointest Endosc 1990;36:10–14.
182. Jensen K, Raynor S, Rose SG, et al: Amyloid tumors of the gastrointestinal tract: a report of two cases and review of the literature. Am J Gastroenterol 1985;80:784–786.
183. Tada S, Iida M, Matsui T, et al: Amyloidosis of the small intestine: findings on double-contrast radiographs. Am J Roentgenol 1991;156:741–744.
184. Bennhold H: Eine spezifische Amyloidfarbung mit Kongorot. Munch Med Wochenschr 1922;69:1537–1538.
185. Stoeber E: Corticosteroid treatment of juvenile chronic polyarthritis over 22 years. Eur J Pediatr 1976;121:141–147.
186. Baltz ML, Caspi D, Glatthaar B, et al: The failure of ascorbic acid therapy to alter the induction or remission of murine amyloidosis. Clin Exp Immunol 1984;57:657–662.
187. Buxbaum JN, Hurley ME, Chuba J, et al: Amyloidosis of the AL type. Clinical, morphologic and biochemical aspects of the response to therapy with alkylating agents and prednisone. Am J Med 1979;67:867–878.
188. Gertz MA, Kyle RA, Greipp PR: Response rates and survival in primary systemic amyloidosis. Blood 1991;77:257–262.
189. David J, Youjiouka O, Ansell BM: Amyloidosis in juvenile chronic arthritis: a morbidity and mortality study. Clin Exp Rheumatol 1993;11:85–90.
190. Zemer D, Pras M, Sohar E, et al: Colchicine in the prevention and treatment of the amyloidosis of familial Mediterranean fever. N Engl J Med 1986;314:1001–1005.
191. O'Doherty DP, Neoptolemos JP, Wood VF: Place of surgery in the management of amyloid disese. Br J Surg 1987;74:83–88.
192. Behçet H: Uber rezidivierende Aphthose, durch ein Virus verusaschte Geschwure am Mund, am Auge and an den Genitalien. Dermatol Wochenschr 1937;105:1152–1157.
193. Mason RM, Barnes CG: Behçet's syndrome with arthritis. Ann Rheum Dis 1969;28:95–102.
194. Chajek T, Fainaru M: Behçet's disease. Report of 41 cases and a review of the literature. Medicine 1975;54:179–196.
195. O'Duffy JD: Summary of international symposium on Behçet's disease. J Rheumatol 1978;5:229–233.
196. Sahane T: New perspective on Behçet's disease. Int Rev Immunol 1997;14:89–96.
197. Mochizuki M: Immunotherapy for Behçet's disease. Int Rev Immunol 1997;14:49–66.
198. Mizuki N, Ota M, Kimura M, et al: Triplet repeat polymorphism in the transmembrane region of the MICA gene: a strong association of six GCT repetitions with Behçet's disease. Proc Natl Acad Sci USA 1997;94:1298–1303.
199. Lehner T: The role of heat shock protein, microbial and autoimmune agents in the aetiology of Behçet's disease. Int Rev Immunol 1997;14:21–32.
200. Yamashita N: Hyperreactivity of neutrophils and abnormal T cell homeostasis: a new insight for the pathogenesis of Behçet's disease. Int Rev Immunol 1997;14:11–19.

201. Stringer DA, Cleghorn GJ, Durie PR, et al: Behçet's syndrome involving the gastrointestinal tract—a diagnostic dilemma in childhood. Pediatr Radiol 1986;16:131–134.
202. Arbesfeld SJ, Kurban AK: Behçet's disease. New perspectives on an enigmatic syndrome. J Am Acad Dermatol 1988;19:767–779.
203. Watanabe I, Kuwabara N, Fukada Y: Histopathological studies in intestinal Behçet's disease. Stomach Intest 1979;7:903–913.
204. Chong SKF, Wright VM, Nishigame T, et al: Infantile colitis: a manifestation of intestinal Behçet's syndrome. J Pediatr Gastroenterol Nutr 1988;7:622–627.
205. Lakhanpal S, Tani K, Lie JT, et al: Pathological features of Behçet's syndrome. A review of Japanese autopsy registry data. Hum Pathol 1985;16:790–795.
206. Yasui K, Ohta K, Kobayashi M, et al: Successful treatment of Behçet's disease with pentoxifylline. Ann Intern Med 1996;124(10):801–893.
207. Kohlmeier W: Multiple Hautnekrosen bei Thrombangitis obliterans. Arch Dermatol Syphilol 1941;181:783–792.
208. Degos R, Delort J, Tricot R: Dermatite papulo-squameuse atrophiante. Bull Soc Franc Dermatol Syphilol 1942;49:148–150.
209. Degos R, Delort J, Tricot R: Papulose atrophiante maligne (syndrome cutaneo-intestinal). Bull Mem Soc Med Hôp Paris 1948;64:803–806.
210. Snow JL, Muller SA: Degos syndrome: malignant atrophic papulosis. Semin Dermatol 1995;14(2):99–105.
211. Casparie MK, Meyer JWR, vanHuystee BEW, et al: Endoscopic and histopathologic features of Degos' disease. Endoscopy 1991;23:231–233.
212. Habbema L, Kisch LS, Starink TM: Familial malignant atrophic papulosis (Degos' disease)—additional evidence for heredity and a benign course (letter). Br J Dermatol 1986;114:134–135.
213. Englert HJ, Hawkes CH, Boey ML, et al: Degos' disease: association with anticardiolipin antibodies and the lupus anticoagulant. Br Med J 1984;289:576.
214. Stahl D, Thomsen K, Hou-Jensen K: Malignant atrophic papulosis. Arch Dermatol 1978;114:1687–1689.
215. Drucker CR: Malignant atrophic papulosis: response to antiplatelet therapy. Dermatologica 1990;180:90–92.
216. Case 44-1980: Case records of the Massachusetts General Hospital: weekly clinicopathologic exercises. N Engl J Med 1980;303:1103–1111.
217. Black MM: Malignant atrophic papulosis (Degos's disease). Int J Dermatol 1976;15:405–411.
218. Horner FA, Myers GJ, Stumpf DA, et al: Malignant atrophic papulosis (Kohlmeier-Degos disease) in childhood. Nerology 1976;26:317–321.
219. Medsger TA Jr, Dawson WN, Masi AT: The epidemiology of polymyositis. Am J Med 1970;48:715–723.
220. Benbassat J, Geffel D, Zlotnick A: Epidemiology of polymyositis-dermatomyositis in Israel. Isr J Med Sci 1980;16:197–200.
221. Christensen ML, Pachman LM, Maryjowski MC: Antibody to coxsackie-B virus: increased incidence in sera from children with recently diagnosed juvenile dermatomyositis (abstract). Arthritis Rheum 1983;26:S24.
222. Koch MJ, Brody JA, Gillespie MM: Childhood polymyositis: a case-control study. Am J Epidemiol 1976;104:627–631.
223. Harati Y, Niakan E, Bergman EW: Childhood dermatomyositis in monozygotic twins. Neurology 1986;36:721–723.
224. Pachman LM: An update on juvenile dermatomyositis. Curr Opin Rheumatol 2994;7:437–441.
225. Friedman JM, Pachman LM, Maryjowski ML, et al: Immunogenetic studies of juvenile dermatomyositis: HLA-DR antigen frequencies. Arthritis Rheum 1983;26:214–216.
226. Reed AM, Sterling JD: Association of the DQA0*0501 allele in multiple racial groups with juvenile dermatomyositis. Hum Immunol 1995;44:131–135.
227. Rosenberg NL, Rotbart HA, Abzug MJ, et al: Evidence for a novel picornavirus in human dermatomyositis. Ann Neurol 1989;26:204–209.
228. Pachman LM, Friedman JM, Maryjowski-Sweeney ML, et al: Immunogenetic studies of juvenile dermatomyositis: III. Study of antibody to organ-specific and nuclear antigens. Arthritis Rheum 1985;28:151–157.
229. Feldman BM, Reichlin M, Laxer RM, et al: Clinical significance of specific autoantibodies in juvenile dermatomyositis. J Rheumatol 1996;23:1794–1797.
230. Spenser CH, Hanson V, Singsen BH, et al: Course of treated juvenile dermatomyositis. J Pediatr 1984;105:399–408.
231. Everett MA, Curtis AC: Dermatomyositis. Arch Intern Med 1957;100:70–76.
232. Miller LC, Michael AF, Kim Y: Childhood dermatomyositis: clinical course and long-term follow-up. Clin Pediatr 1987;26:561–566.
233. Norins AI: Juvenile dermatomyositis. Med Clin North Am 1989;73:1193–1209.
234. Metheny JA: Dermatomyositis: a vocal and swallowing disease entity. Laryngoscope 1978;88:147–161.
235. Magill HL, Hixson SD, Whitington D, et al: Duodenal perforation in childhood dermatomyositis. Pediatr Radiol 1984;14:28–30.
236. Schullinger JN, Jacobs JC, Berdon WE: Diagnosis and management of gastrointestinal perforations in childhood dermatomyositis with particular reference to perforations of the duodenum. J Pediatr Surg 1984;20:521–524.
237. Transfeldt EE, Morley JE, Segal F, et al: Polymyositis as a cause of malabsorption. A case report. S Afr Med J 1977;151:176–168.
238. Pachman LM: Juvenile dermatomyositis. Pediatr Clin North Am 1986;33:1097–1117.
239. Prieur AM, Dayer A, Roux-Lombard P, et al: Levels of cytokine inhibitors: a possible marker of disease activity in childhood dermatomyositis and polymyositis. Clin Exp Rheumatol 1997;15:211–214.
240. Boylan RC, Sokoloff L: Vascular lesions in dermatomyositis. Arthritis Rheum 1960;3:379–386.
241. Benson MD, Aldo MA: Azathioprine therapy in polymyositis. Arch Intern Med 1973;132:547–551.
242. Miller G, Heckmatt JZ, Dubowitz V: Drug treatment of juvenile dermatomyositis. Arch Dis Child 1983;58:445–450.
243. Metzger AL, Bohan A, Goldberg LS: Polymyositis and dermatomyositis: combined methotrexate and corticosteroid therapy. Ann Intern Med 1974;81:182–189.
244. Olson NY, Lindsley CB: Adjunctive use of hydroxychloroquine in childhood dermatomyositis. J Rheumatol 1989;16:1545–1547.
245. Vedanarayan V, Subramony S, Ray LI, et al: Treatment of childhood dermatomyositis with high dose intravenous immunoglobulin. Pediatr Neurol 1995;13:336–339.
246. Wayte DM, Helwig EB: Colitis cystica profunda. Am J Clin Pathol 1965;48:159–169.
247. Haskell B, Rovner H: Solitary ulcer of the rectum. Dis Colon Rectum 1965;8:333–336.
248. Madigan MR, Morson BC: Solitary ulcer of the rectum. Gut 1969;10:871–881.
249. Kuijpers MC, Shreve RH, Hoedemakers HTC: Diagnosis of functional disorders of defecation causing the solitary rectal ulcer syndrome. Dis Colon Rectum 1986;29:126–129.
250. Goei R, Baeten C, Arends JW: Solitary rectal ulcer syndrome: findings at barium enema study and defecography. Radiology 1988;163:303–306.
251. Womack NR, Williams NS, Mist JHH, et al: Anorectal function in the solitary rectal ulcer syndrome. Dis Colon Rectum 1987;30:319–323.
252. Martin CJ, Parks TG, Biggart JD: Solitary rectal ulcer syndrome in Northern Ireland 1971–1980. Br J Surg 1981;68:744–747.
253. Levine DS: "Solitary" rectal ulcer syndrome: are "solitary" rectal syndrome and "localized" colitis cystica profunda analogous syndromes caused by rectal prolapse? Gastroenterology 1987;92:243–253.
254. Niv Y, Bat L: Solitary rectal ulcer syndrome—clinical, endoscopic, and histological spectrum. Am J Gastroenterol 1986;48:486–491.
255. Petritsch W, Hinterleitner TA, Aichbicher B, et al: Endosonography in colitis cystica profunda and solitary rectal ulcer syndrome. Gastrointest Endosc 1996;44:746–751.
256. Hershfield NB, Langevin JE, Kelly JK: Endoscopic and histologic features of the solitary rectal ulcer syndrome (SRUS). Gastrointest Endosc 1984;30:162.
257. Guest CB, Reznick RK: Colitis cystica profunda: review of the literature. Dis Colon Rectum 1989;32:983–988.
258. Over H, Ulher A, Baysal C, et al: Endoscopic balloon dilation of strictures complicating solitary rectal ulcer syndrome. Endoscopy 1997;29:427–429.
259. Stavorovsky M, Weintraub S, Ratan J, et al: Successful treatment of a benign solitary rectal ulcer by temporary diverting sigmoidostomy: report of a case. Dis Colon Rectum 1977;20:347–350.
260. Michaelis L, Gutmann C: Uber Einschlusse in Blasentumoren. Ztschr Klin Med 1902;47:208–215.
261. Terner JY, Lattes R: Malakoplakia of colon and retroperitoneum. Am J Clin Pathol 1965;44:20–31.
262. Sanusi ID, Tio FO: Gastrointestinal malacoplakia: report of a case and a review of the literature. Am J Gastroenterol 1974;62:356–365.

263. Nakabayashi H, Ito T, Izutsu K: Malakoplakia of the stomach: report of a case and review of the literature. Arch Pathol Lab Med 1978;102:136–139.
264. Chaudhry AP, Saigal KP, Intengan M, et al: Malakoplakia of the large intestine found incidentally at necropsy: light and electron microscopic features. Dis Colon Rectum 1979;22:73–81.
265. McClure J: Malakoplakia of the gastrointestinal tract. Postgrad Med J 1981;57:95–103.
266. Harfi HA, Akhtar M, Subayti YA, et al: Gastrointestinal malacoplakia in children. Clin Pediatr 1985;24:423–428.
267. Rull R, Grande L, Garcia-Valdecasas JC, et al: Malakoplakia in the gastrointestinal tract of a liver transplant patient. Transplantation 1995;59:1492–1494.
268. Rocha N, Suguima EH, Maia D, et al: Intestinal malakoplakia associated with paracoccidioidomycosis: a new association. Histopathology 1997;30:79–83.
269. Scheiner C, Dor AM, Basbous D, et al: La malacoplasie: formes anatomo-cliniques, revue de la littérature, à propos de 15 observations personnelles. Arch Anat Pathol 1975;23:199–208.
270. Lou TY, Teplitz C: Malakoplakia: pathogenesis and ultrastructural morphogenesis—a problem of altered macrophage response. Hum Pathol 1974;5:191–207.
271. Abdou NI, NaPombejara C, Sagawa A, et al: Malakoplakia: evidence for monocyte lysosmal abnormality correctable by cholinergic agonist in vitro and in vivo. N Engl J Med 1977;297:1413–1419.
272. Wagner ML, Rosenberg HS, Fernbach DJ, et al: Typhlitis: a complication of leukemia in childhood. Am J Roentgenol 1970;109:341–350.
273. Katz JA, Wagner ML, Gresik MV, et al: Typhlitis: an 18-year experience and postmortem review. Cancer 1990;65:1041–1047.
274. Slous MM, Flynn RM, Kaste SC, et al: Typhlitis in children with cancer: a 30-year experience. Clin Infect Dis 1993;17:484–490.
275. Merine DS, Fishman EK, Jones B, et al: Right lower quadrant pain in the immunocompromised patient: CT findings in 10 cases. AJR Am J Roentgenol 1987;149:1177–1179.
276. Matalo NM, Garfinkle SE, Wolfman EF Jr: Intestinal necrosis and perforation in patients receiving immunosuppressive drugs. Am J Surg 1976;132:753–754.
277. Keidan RD, Fanning J, Gatenby RA, et al: Recurrent typhlitis: a disease resulting from aggressive chemotherapy. Dis Colon Rectum 1989;32:206–209.
278. Prolla JC, Kirsner JB: The gastrointestinal lesions and complications of leukemias. Ann Intern Med 1964;61:1084–1103.
279. Abramson SJ, Berdon WE, Baker DH: Childhood typhlitis: its increasing association with acute myelogenous leukemia. Radiology 1983;146:61–64.
280. Taylor AJ, Dodds WJ, Gonyo JE, et al: Typhlitis in adults. Gastrointest Radiol 1985;10:363–369.
281. Teefey SA, Montana MA, Goldfogel GA, et al: Sonographic diagnosis of neutropenic typhlitis. Am J Radiol 1987;149:731–733.
282. Williams GW, Rauch RF, Kelvin FM, et al: CT detection of typhlitis. J Comput Asst Tomogr 1985;9:363–365.
283. Proujansky R, Orenstein SR, Kocoshis SA, et al: Cytomegalovirus gastroenteritis after liver transplantation. J Pediatr 1988;113:700–703.
284. Skibber JM, Matter GJ, Pizzo PA, et al: Right lower quadrant pain in young patients with leukemia. Ann Surg 1987;206:711–716.
285. Meyerovitz MF, Fellows KE: Typhlitis: a cause of gastrointestinal hemorrhage in children. Am J Radiol 1984;143:833–835.
286. Lindstrom C: "Collagenous colitis" with watery diarrhea. A new entity? Pathol Eur 1976;11:87–89.
287. Read NW, Krejs GJ, Read MG, et al: Chronic diarrhea of unknown origin. Gastroenterology 1980;78:264–271.
288. Bogomoletz WV: Collagenous, microscopic and lymphocytic colitis. An evolving concept. Virchows Arch 1994;424:573–579.
289. Jackson K: Are collagenous colitis and lymphocytic colitis distinct syndromes? Dig Dis 1995;13:301–311.
290. Gremse DA, Boudreaux CW, Manci EA: Collagenous colitis in children. Gastroenterology 1993;104:906–909.
291. Bohr J, Tysk C, Eriksson S, et al: Collagenous colitis: a retrospective study of clinical presentation and treatment in 163 patients. Gut 1996;39:846–851.
292. Wolber R, Owen D, Freeman H: Colonic lymphocytosis in patients with celiac sprue. Hum Pathol 1990;21:1092–1096.
293. Giardiello F, Lazenby AJ, Bayless TM, et al: Lymphocytic (microscopic) colitis. Clinicopathologic study of 18 patients and comparison to collagenous colitis. Dig Dis Sci 1989;34:1730–1738.

SECTION FIVE

# THE LIVER AND BILE DUCTS

Chapter 47

# Neonatal Hepatitis

Constantinos G. Siafakas and Maureen M. Jonas

Neonatal hepatitis is a syndrome of symptoms, signs, and hepatic histology that includes many types of neonatal liver disease of infectious, genetic, toxic, and metabolic origin. The term *neonatal hepatitis* is often used interchangeably with *neonatal cholestasis* because of the prominent conjugated hyperbilirubinemia that is present in most of these disorders. The designation *idiopathic neonatal hepatitis* describes the neonatal liver disease for which no specific cause can be ascertained. The incidence ranges from 1 in 4,800 to 1 in 9,000 live births.[1] Idiopathic neonatal hepatitis/cholestasis and extrahepatic biliary atresia account for 60% to 70% of all cases of neonatal cholestasis.[2]

Cholestasis is defined physiologically as a reduction in canalicular bile flow, clinically as the accumulation in the blood and extrahepatic tissues of substances normally excreted in bile, and histologically by evidence of bile stasis in hepatocytes and bile ducts.[3] During the neonatal period, infants are susceptible to cholestasis resulting from a variety of insults, including infections, drugs, and ischemia.[4] Many of these insults produce a stereotypical histologic response of the immature liver which has been called "neonatal hepatitis." Factors predisposing the neonate to cholestasis are summarized in Table 47–1.

## EVALUATION AND DIFFERENTIAL DIAGNOSIS

The major diagnostic goals are differentiation between intrahepatic and extrahepatic disorders, detection of potentially treatable diseases, and recognition of complications of cholestasis for which medical therapy may improve quality of life and outcome. The physician evaluating an infant with neonatal hepatitis/cholestasis is confronted with a long list of diagnostic possibilities (Table 47–2). Therefore, a stepwise approach is required (Table 47–3). Metabolic causes of neonatal cholestasis are discussed in Chapter 49.

**TABLE 47–1. Factors Predisposing the Neonate to Cholestasis**

| |
|---|
| Quantitative differences in bile acids |
| Reduced bile acid pool size |
| Increased basal serum bile acid levels |
| Decreased intraluminal bile acid level |
| Differences in bile acid metabolism |
| Reduced bile acid secretion rate |
| Inefficient hepatic uptake, intracellular binding, or transport of bile acids |
| Absence of a lobular gradient for bile acid uptake |
| Decreased conjugation, sulfation, and glucuronidation of bile acids |
| Decreased ileal absorption of bile acids |
| Qualitative differences in bile acids |

From Balistreri WF: Fetal and neonatal bile acid synthesis and metabolism: clinical implications. J Inherit Metab Dis 1991;14:459–477, with kind permission from Kluwer Academic Publishers.

A careful history, including family history as well as prenatal and postnatal course, and a detailed physical examination, looking for hepatic and extrahepatic abnormalities, are essential components of the initial assessment. Poor feeding and vomiting may guide to a metabolic disorder, whereas the presence of a murmur of peripheral pulmonic stenosis, vertebral anomalies, and posterior embryotoxon are highly suggestive of Alagille syndrome. Congenital infections are often associated with low birth weight, microcephaly, and chorioretinitis.

Examination of the stools may be helpful. Persistently acholic stools are strongly suggestive of biliary obstruction, but this finding is not specific to extrahepatic biliary atresia since it is seen in patients with severe intrahepatic cholestasis.

Serum bilirubin fractionation must be performed in any infant with prolonged jaundice. A conjugated bilirubin level higher than 2.0 mg/dL (34 μmol/L) or a fraction greater than 20% of an elevated total bilirubin level defines cholestasis.

No single test has been found to reliably differentiate intrahepatic from extrahepatic cholestasis. Elevated aminotransferase concentrations are indicative of hepatocellular damage, whereas elevations of alkaline phosphatase, 5′-nucleotidase or γ-glutamyl transpeptidase (GGTP) indicate biliary injury or obstruction. However, low or normal GGTP levels are seen in some cholestatic conditions. Poor hepatic function at birth may indicate a process that began prenatally, such as infection or inborn errors of metabolism.

Ultrasonography is helpful in the detection of choledochal cysts, biliary stones, abdominal masses, and ascites. It may also provide information about liver size and texture. Nonvisualization of the gallbladder on a fasting study is suggestive of, but not diagnostic for, biliary atresia. Hepatobiliary scintigraphy may be useful in differentiating extrahepatic obstruction from intrahepatic cholestasis. To enhance biliary secretion, phenobarbital is administered for 5 days before the test at a dose of 3 to 5 mg/kg per day. In intrahepatic disorders, the uptake of tracer often is delayed secondary to

**TABLE 47–2. Disorders Associated with Neonatal Hepatitis/Cholestasis**

**Anatomic Abnormalities**

Extrahepatic biliary atresia
Choledochal cyst
Bile duct stenosis
Neonatal sclerosing cholangitis
Spontaneous perforation of common bile duct
Cholelithiasis
Masses or neoplasia

**Idiopathic Neonatal Hepatitis/Cholestasis**

**Infections**

Viral
- Cytomegalovirus
- Herpes viruses (simplex, herpes-6 virus)
- Rubella virus
- Enteroviruses
- Hepatotropic viruses (A,B,C,D,E)
- Human immunodeficiency virus
- Adenovirus
- Parvovirus
- Reovirus type 3

Bacterial
- Syphilis
- Bacterial sepsis, urosepsis
- Listeriosis
- Tuberculosis

Parasitic
- Toxoplasmosis

**Familial Intrahepatic Cholestasis Syndromes**

Alagille syndrome
Nonsyndromic paucity of the interlobular bile ducts
Progressive familial intrahepatic cholestasis
Benign recurrent intrahepatic cholestasis
Miscellaneous familial cholestatic syndromes

**Metabolic Disorders**

Disorders of carbohydrate metabolism
- Galactosemia
- Hereditary fructose intolerance
- Glycogen storage disease type IV

Disorders of amino acid metabolism
- Tyrosinemia
- Hypermethioninemia

Disorders of lipid metabolism
- Gaucher's disease
- Niemann-Pick disease
- Wolman's disease
- Cholesteryl ester storage disease

Disorders of bile acid synthesis
- 3β-Hydroxy-$\Delta^5$-C27-steroid dehydrogenase/isomerase deficiency
- $\Delta^4$-3-oxosteroid 5β-reductase deficiency

Peroxisomal disorders
- Zellweger's syndrome (cerebrohepatorenal syndrome)

Disorders of oxidative phosphorylation

Disorders of urea cycle
- Arginase deficiency

Miscellaneous metabolic disorders
- Alpha$_1$-antitrypsin deficiency
- Cystic fibrosis
- Neonatal iron storage disease

**Cholestasis Associated with Total Parenteral Nutrition**

**Miscellaneous Causes of Neonatal Hepatitis/Cholestasis**

Vascular disorders of the liver
Drug hepatotoxicity
Inspissated bile syndrome
Ischemia
Endocrine disorders
Chromosomal disorders
Neonatal lupus erythematosus
Neonatal histiocytosis

**TABLE 47–3. Diagnostic Evaluation of the Neonate with Hepatitis/Cholestasis**

**Initial Evaluation**

History, physical examination
Stool examination for color
Bilirubin fractionation
Bacterial cultures of blood and urine
Liver enzymes: aminotransferases, alkaline phosphatase, 5′-nucleotidase, γ-glutamyl transpeptidase
Assessment of synthetic liver function: serum albumin, glucose, ammonia, cholesterol, prothrombin time
Urinalysis including reducing substances

**Secondary Evaluation**

Ultrasonography
Serology for viral hepatitides, HIV, TORCH infections, VDRL test
Viral cultures (e.g., herpes simplex)
Ophthalmologic examination (chorioretinitis, embryotoxin)
Sweat chloride determination
Metabolic tests
- Urine and serum for amino acids
- Urine for organic acids
- Urine for bile acids, fasting serum bile acid level
- Red blood cell galactose-1-phosphate uridyl transferase
- Serum alpha$_1$-antitrypsin level and Pi type
- Serum iron and ferritin

Radiographs of the long bones and skull for congenital infections
Assessment of the patency of the extrahepatic biliary tree
- Duodenal intubation or string test for bilirubin
- Hepatobiliary scintigraphy
- Percutaneous or endoscopic cholangiography

Percutaneous liver biopsy
Exploratory laparotomy and intraoperative cholangiography

hepatocellular dysfunction, but excretion into the intestine can be seen eventually. In biliary atresia, uptake of the tracer usually is rapid but excretion is absent even with prolonged imaging. However, because biliary excretion of the radioactive substance may not be detected in cases of severe intrahepatic cholestasis, some clinicians find this test less helpful.

Histologic examination of the liver is the most reliable means of determining the diagnosis in neonatal cholestasis. It is estimated that interpretation by experienced pathologists provides the correct diagnosis in approximately 95% of cases,[5] although some diseases such as extrahepatic biliary atresia or alpha$_1$-antitrypsin deficiency may not manifest characteristic histologic changes early in their course. Other methods to assess the patency of the extrahepatic biliary tree, such as duodenal intubation, string tests, and percutaneous or endoscopic cholangiography, may be of some use in defined clinical settings. Exploratory laparotomy with intraoperative cholangiography should not be delayed in those patients in whom all clinical, biochemical, and histologic data support the diagnosis of biliary atresia. If extrahepatic obstruction is excluded, a wedge hepatic biopsy should be performed (see Chapter 48).

Multiple diagnostic algorithms have been proposed to select those infants who are surgical candidates. Alagille, in a series of 288 infants with cholestasis, used clinical, biochemical, and histologic findings to differentiate intrahepatic from extrahepatic cholestatic disorders.[6] He found that features associated more frequently with *intrahepatic* cholestasis were low birth weight (mean, 2,700 versus 3,200 g); male gender; presence of congenital anomalies; later onset of acholic stools (mean, 30 versus 16 days); and pigmented stools within 10 days of admission (79% versus 26%). Infants with *extrahepatic* disease had a greater incidence of liver enlargement (87% versus 53%) and the histologic findings of portal fibrosis (94% versus 47%) and bile ductular proliferation (86% versus 30%).

## Giant Cell Hepatitis

*Giant cell hepatitis* is a general term applied when large multinucleated cells are found on histologic examination of the liver. It is not a specific diagnosis and may be associated with a variety of disorders. The origin and mechanisms of giant cell formation are not clear. Hepatocytes,[7] peripheral blood monocytes,[8] Kupffer cells (tissue macrophages),[9] and oval cells[10] have been suggested as the origin of the giant cells. Giant cells are large, active cells, as indicated by their increased number of nuclei, numerous mitochondria, prominent rough endoplasmic reticulum, and lysosomal proliferation.[11] Whether these cells originate from cell fusion or cell division is debated.[9, 12] Their function and role are not well established. Giant cell transformation is a common response of the infantile liver to heterogeneous insults.

# CONGENITAL INFECTIONS

The neonate with a congenital infection may present with cholestatic jaundice, hepatomegaly, and increased aminotransferase levels. These may be the predominant features, or they may be part of a multi-system illness. Numerous agents—viral, bacterial, and protozoal—have been implicated in congenital infections associated with hepatitis.

## Viral Infections

### *Cytomegalovirus*

Cytomegalovirus (CMV), a herpesvirus, is the most common cause of congenital infection.[13] Primary CMV infection acquired during pregnancy is associated with a 30% to 40% risk of neonatal infection. It can be transmitted to the infant transplacentally, at delivery, or postnatally from maternal saliva or milk, as well as iatrogenically from blood transfusions.[14]

Clinically apparent disease occurs in only 10% to 15% of infected infants. Signs in the newborn include intrauterine growth retardation, microcephaly, periventricular intracranial calcifications, psychomotor retardation, deafness, and thrombocytopenia. Hepatosplenomegaly with conjugated hyperbilirubinemia and mild elevation of aminotransferase levels is common.[15] Hepatic calcifications may be noted. Hepatic histologic findings include multinucleated giant cells, hepatitis, cholangitis, fibrosis, and extramedullary hematopoiesis.[15] The presence of CMV immunoglobulin M (IgM) antibody in the newborn may suggest congenital infection. CMV infection is confirmed by isolation of the virus from urine or from the upper respiratory tract within the first 2 weeks of life. The diagnosis is confirmed by the presence of large intranuclear inclusion bodies in the bile duct epithelium, hepatocytes or Kupffer cells, or cytoplasmic inclusions in hepatocytes.[15, 16] The polymerase chain reaction (PCR) has been used to detect CMV DNA directly from liver tissue.[17]

Treatment of congenital CMV infection includes the use of ganciclovir and CMV immune globulin.[18] The liver injury usually resolves if the patient survives the neurologic injury.[19, 20]

### *Herpes Simplex Virus*

The herpes simplex viruses (HSV1 and HSV2) may be transmitted vertically, either in utero or perinatally, as the result of ascending infection or contact with cervicovaginal secretions. Postnatal transmission sources include parents or personnel with nongenital lesions caring for infants and infected infants in the same nursery. Approximately 90% of congenital herpes infections are caused by HSV2.[21] Primary maternal infection (especially late in gestation), prolonged rupture of membranes, prematurity, and skin trauma (e.g., fetal scalp monitoring) are factors that increase the risk of neonatal HSV disease.[22]

Perinatal HSV infection is manifested in three syndromes with different presentations: skin, eye, mouth disease; central nervous system disease; and disseminated HSV disease. Hepatitis is often part of the disseminated disease,[23] and it usually is severe, with jaundice, hepatomegaly, coagulopathy, and gastrointestinal bleeding. Liver histologic findings include multifocal necrosis with characteristic intranuclear hepatocyte inclusions.[24] Multinucleated giant cells may be present. Diagnosis is confirmed by isolation of virus from the skin or mucous membranes, by acute and convalescent serology,[22] or by detection of viral DNA by PCR.[25] Culture of liver tissue obtained by biopsy may reveal the virus, but the diagnosis can be made earlier on the basis of the characteristic morphologic findings. Immunohistochemistry has been used to confirm the diagnosis in liver tissue specimens. Prognosis is ominous without treatment. Early parenteral administration of acyclovir decreases both mortality and morbidity.[26]

### *Rubella*

Congenital infection with rubella occurs transplacentally, and more severe consequences result from infection earlier in gestation. Common manifestations of congenital infection are ophthalmologic, cardiac, and neurologic abnormalities; mental retardation; and sensorineural deafness. Hepatic involvement is common[27] and may range from an early presentation with jaundice, hepatosplenomegaly, and transient cholestasis to a late anicteric hepatitis. Hepatosplenomegaly is a consistent feature and may persist until the end of the first year or even later.[28] Mononuclear infiltrates in the portal tracts, intralobular fibrosis, and extramedullary hematopoiesis are typical histologic features, and giant cell transformation, cholestasis, and bile duct proliferation may be seen.[28] The diagnosis of neonatal infection is confirmed by isolation of the virus from nasopharyngeal or other body fluids, demonstration of rubella IgM antibody at birth, or a postnatal increase in the infant's IgG titer with stable or decreasing maternal IgG titer. The widespread use of rubella vaccine has resulted in a marked decrease in the incidence of congenital rubella.

### Enteroviruses

Transmission of the nonpolio enteroviruses (coxsackieviruses, echoviruses, and others) may occur during the prenatal, intrapartum, or perinatal period. In 60% of cases there is a history of viral-like syndrome with fever during the last 2 weeks of pregnancy.[29] Infants appear healthy in the first days of life before they develop fever, lethargy, poor feeding, and diarrhea. Hepatitis and jaundice are the most common manifestations. In most cases the course is benign and self-limited. However, progressive hepatic failure with markedly increased aminotransferase levels, disseminated intravascular coagulation, and massive hepatic necrosis have been reported with infections of coxsackievirus group B or echovirus types 6, 11,[30] 14,[28] and 19.[31] Therapy is supportive. Intravenous immune globulin has been used to treat life-threatening neonatal enteroviral infections.

### Hepatitis A

Hepatitis A virus is transmitted via the fecal-oral route. It is not a common cause of neonatal hepatitis. It is believed that the neonate may become infected if the mother has acute hepatitis within the last 2 weeks of pregnancy.[32] The first case of intrauterine transmission, confirmed by identification of hepatitis A IgM in fetal blood, was reported in 1996.[33] Acquisition of the virus by blood transfusion also has been reported in the neonatal period.[34] Although the infant may be given intramuscular immune serum globulin shortly after birth if the mother has onset of symptoms in the period from 2 weeks before to 1 week after delivery, the efficacy of this intervention has not been established.[32] Breast-feeding is not restricted, and isolation from the mother is not recommended.[35] In infants, the infection may be asymptomatic or may produce a gastroenteritis-like syndrome. One report documented the development of hepatic necrosis in a premature infant during the course of acute hepatitis A infection.[36] No specific treatment is available.

### Hepatitis B

In the United States, Canada, and western Europe, neonatal hepatitis B is uncommon. However, in certain densely populated areas, such as the Far East and Africa, and in isolated groups such as Eskimos in Alaska, there is a high rate of vertical transmission of hepatitis B virus (HBV).

Mothers who either are chronic carriers of HBV or have acute infection during the third trimester of pregnancy may transmit the virus to their infants.[37] It is speculated that infants are infected during passage through the birth canal or early in infancy, via transmucosal or transcutaneous contact, swallowing of maternal blood, or swallowing of vaginal secretions.[38] There is evidence of in utero infection in approximately 5% of cases. The risk of vertical transmission is highest when the mother is seropositive for both hepatitis B surface antigen ($HB_sAg$) and e antigen ($HB_eAg$) or has high serum HBV DNA levels.[39] In contrast, infants born to anti-HBe–positive mothers, although at low overall risk for HBV acquisition, may develop fulminant hepatitis. Some of these cases have been attributed to viral mutants.[40] Infants born to HBsAg-positive mothers demonstrate serologic or clinical evidence of HBV infection 1 to 4 months after birth. The diagnosis usually is confirmed by detection of $HB_sAg$ and anti-HBc. The majority of perinatally infected neonates are asymptomatic, and acute icteric hepatitis is rare. Ninety percent or more of infants infected in the newborn period become chronically infected.[41]

### Hepatitis C

Accumulating evidence indicates that hepatitis C virus (HCV) can be transmitted perinatally.[42, 43] Initial studies indicated that maternal-infant transmission occurred predominantly in the context of maternal coinfection with human immunodeficiency virus (HIV).[44] However, subsequent reports documented that perinatal infection is possible even without HIV coinfection.[42] In one large study, 5.6% of infants born to anti-HCV–seropositive mothers became positive for HCV RNA; this increased to 10% in infants of HCV RNA–positive mothers.[43]

HCV infection in the newborn usually is asymptomatic. Some infected infants, however, may have mild to moderate aminotransferase elevation. The frequency and timing of chronic hepatitis, cirrhosis, and hepatocellular carcinoma after HCV infection in the newborn are unknown.

In most instances, second-generation enzyme-linked immunosorbent assay (ELISA) and recombinant immunoblot assay are used as the diagnostic tests for antibody to HCV. The American Academy of Pediatrics recommends that infants born to HCV-infected women be tested by anti-HCV after 12 months of age, after maternally-derived antibody has disappeared.[45] The PCR technique is particularly useful for the diagnosis of perinatally acquired HCV[46] before 12 months, but its routine use is not recommended.

### Hepatitis D

Hepatitis delta virus is a single-stranded RNA virus, infection with which requires concomitant infection with HBV. Perinatal transmission is possible[47] but uncommon.

### Hepatitis E

Vertical transmission of hepatitis E virus (HEV) has been described. In one report, six of eight infants born to mothers infected with HEV in the third trimester had clinical, serologic, or virologic evidence of HEV infection. Most of them had anicteric hepatitis, but one was icteric at birth. Two of these infants died within 24 hours, and one was found to have massive hepatic necrosis.[48]

### Human Immunodeficiency Virus

The vertical transmission rate of HIV varies from 14% to 40%.[49] Hepatosplenomegaly is a common early manifestation of the disease in infants (more than 90% of pediatric cases).[50] Cholestatic hepatitis has been reported as the first manifestation of HIV infection in children as young as 5 months of age.[51]

ELISA and Western blot testing for HIV-specific antibodies to the core and envelope regions have limited value in the diagnosis of vertically acquired infection because of transplacental transfer. Uninfected infants may retain maternal antibody in the circulation through 18 months of age.

Therefore, virologic studies (culture and PCR) and the immune complex–dissociated p24 assay are extremely important for the early identification of infected infants.[49] Hepatobiliary manifestations of HIV infection outside the neonatal period are discussed in Chapter 31.

### Other Viral Agents

Parvovirus B19, the etiologic agent of erythema infectiosum (fifth disease), has been associated with severe in utero infection causing hydrops fetalis, cholestasis, bile duct proliferation, prominent periportal fibrosis, and hemosiderin deposition in hepatocytes and Kupffer cells.[52] Human herpesvirus 6, the cause of roseola infantum (exanthem subitum, sixth disease), has been associated with cholestasis, neonatal hepatitis, giant cell transformation,[53] and fatal fulminant hepatitis.[54] Adenovirus can cause hepatitis in the neonate and in immunosuppressed children. Fatal cases with massive hepatic necrosis have been reported.[55] There are isolated cases of infantile paramyxovirus hepatitis manifesting as syncytial giant cell or autoimmune-like chronic active hepatitis.[56]

## Bacterial Infections

### Syphilis

Transmission of the spirochete *Treponema pallidum* can occur either transplacentally or at delivery through contact with a genital lesion. Congenital infection can occur at any time in gestation, but the risk of fetal infection increases as termination of pregnancy is approached. There are two characteristic clinical syndromes of congenital syphilis: early (within the first 2 years) and late.

Hepatitis and hepatosplenomegaly are manifestations of early congenital syphilis. Jaundice may be the predominant feature within the first 24 hours. Laboratory findings include conjugated hyperbilirubinemia and elevated aminotransferases.[57] Fulminant hepatitis has been associated with death in a few patients.[58]

Characteristic histologic findings are centrilobular mononuclear infiltrates with portal and interstitial fibrosis.[28] Other histologic patterns may be seen, such as neonatal hepatitis with giant cell transformation, nonspecific hepatitis with portal inflammation and portal fibrosis, or even completely normal histology in the presence of heavy infiltration by treponemes.[28] Extramedullary hematopoiesis is seen in both liver and spleen. Gumma, lesions characterized by a central zone of necrosis surrounded by a dense infiltrate of lymphocytes, plasma cells, histiocytes, epithelioid cells, and giant cells, are seldom seen in early congenital syphilis.[28]

The treatment is penicillin administered parenterally. Aminotransferase concentrations may remain elevated for months after treatment.[57] Although treatment may arrest or eradicate the infection, the prognosis depends on the damage done before initiation of therapy.

### Other Bacterial Infections

Bacteremia and urosepsis are well documented causes of jaundice in the newborn period,[59] and jaundice may be the earliest manifestation of sepsis. Hepatomegaly occurs in 40% to 60% of patients; aminotransferase levels are normal or mildly increased.[28] The most commonly reported agent is *Escherichia coli*. Genitourinary evaluation is mandatory, although anatomic urinary abnormalities are infrequently found. Histologic examination of the liver reveals nonspecific findings of periportal inflammation, Kupffer cell hyperplasia, and moderate cholestasis.[28] The pathogenesis of bacterial sepsis–associated cholestasis is not clear. Hepatocellular damage and enhanced hemolysis causing overload of the immature liver function are among the factors considered. Endotoxin, a complex lipopolysaccharide of the outer membrane of the bacterial cell wall, has been implicated in the pathogenesis of hepatocellular injury. The lipid moiety appears to be the toxic agent; it has similar structure in all Enterobacteriaceae species. It is speculated that this moiety inhibits the activity of $Na^+,K^+$-ATPase, interfering with bile flow at the canalicular level.[60]

Direct bacterial infections of the hepatic parenchyma are very uncommon in the newborn infant. The exception is septicemia caused by *Listeria monocytogenes*, in which hepatic manifestations are always present. *Listeria* is acquired transplacentally or at delivery from infected cervicovaginal secretions. Two histologic forms have been described: diffuse hepatitis and, more commonly, demarcated areas of necrosis or microabscesses that contain pleomorphic gram-positive bacilli.[61] Other rare bacterial infections of the liver in newborns include tuberculosis, tularemia, typhoid fever, and brucellosis. Pyogenic abscesses, usually associated with umbilical catheterization, are most often caused by *Staphylococcus aureus* or *E. coli*.

## Parasitic Infections

### Toxoplasmosis

*Toxoplasma gondii* is an obligate intracellular protozoan parasite that can cross the placenta and infect the fetus. Congenital infection occurs primarily as a result of acute maternal infection during pregnancy, either by ingestion of cysts in undercooked meat or by direct contact with feces of infected animals such as cats or kittens. A minority of cases result from reactivated disease in pregnant immunosuppressed women, especially those infected with HIV. The risk of transmission is estimated to be 15% in the first trimester, 30% in the second trimester, and 60% in the third trimester.[62] Severe clinical disease is observed in fetuses infected in the first trimester, whereas those infected in the second or third trimester have mild or subclinical disease at birth.[62] Treatment of acute infection during pregnancy with spiramycin has been shown to decrease the incidence of vertical transmission.[62]

The majority of infected infants have subclinical disease.[63] Clinical manifestations, when they occur, include microcephaly or hydrocephalus, intracranial calcifications, chorioretinitis, seizures, psychomotor retardation, thrombocytopenia, hepatosplenomegaly, and jaundice. Hepatitis may be the only clinical sign of disease.[62] Hepatic microcalcifications may be detected on plain abdominal radiographs. Liver histology is not specific and includes mononuclear periportal inflammation, canalicular bile duct stasis, and extramedullary hematopoiesis.[28]

The ELISA detecting toxoplasma IgM antibody has high sensitivity and specificity.[64] Pyrimethamine and sulfadiazine are synergistic and are the drugs most commonly used in the treatment of infants with documented infection.[65]

## FAMILIAL INTRAHEPATIC CHOLESTASIS SYNDROMES

Familial intrahepatic cholestasis syndromes are generally included in the differential diagnosis of the neonatal hepatitis syndrome. They are presumed to be of genetic origin because they tend to occur in families or in isolated inbred populations and have onset in infancy or childhood. Although they are grouped together arbitrarily because they have similar features, many of these disorders are not completely characterized, and the pathogenetic mechanisms may be unrelated. As each entity is better defined, the designation of familial intrahepatic cholestasis undergoes revision. Comparative features of these syndromes are listed in Table 47–4.

### Alagille Syndrome and Nonsyndromic Paucity of the Interlobular Bile Ducts

Alagille syndrome, or arteriohepatic dysplasia, is also called syndromic paucity of interlobular bile ducts. It is the most common of the familial intrahepatic cholestatic syndromes.[66] In its classic form, five typical features are seen: chronic cholestasis, bone defects (usually butterfly vertebrae), congenital heart disease (usually peripheral pulmonic stenosis), ophthalmologic findings (posterior embryotoxon), and typical facies (frontal bossing, pointed chin, deep set and widely spaced eyes).

Nonsyndromic paucity of interlobular bile ducts includes patients with the typical hepatic histologic findings who do not have the somatic abnormalities associated with Alagille syndrome. Alagille syndrome and nonsyndromic paucity are described more extensively in Chapter 48.

### Progressive Familial Intrahepatic Cholestasis

Progressive familial intrahepatic cholestasis (PFIC) comprises a heterogeneous group of intrahepatic cholestatic disorders with progressive hepatocellular damage. Byler's disease is the best defined type of PFIC.[67] It is inherited in an autosomal recessive pattern. A locus for Byler's disease has been mapped to chromosome 18.[68] At least two further types of PFIC have been proposed but not yet clearly defined.[69, 70] The pathogenesis of PFIC is unknown, but several theories have been postulated.[70–72]

Patients with PFIC are of normal birth weight and present with pruritus and jaundice within the first 3 to 6 months of life. Initially the jaundice may be episodic, but the biochemical cholestasis persists, and eventually the patient becomes permanently icteric. In rare instances, the cholestasis is preceded by profuse watery diarrhea.[73] Physical examination usually reveals mild to moderate hepatomegaly. Serum bile acid, bilirubin, and alkaline phosphatase are elevated. In most types of PFIC, the biochemical profile differs from that of other forms of cholestasis in that serum GGTP, which may be two to three times normal initially, becomes normal. Serum cholesterol usually is normal as well.

The hepatic histology early in the course may show hepatocanalicular cholestasis, giant cell transformation, and ballooning of hepatocytes around terminal hepatic venules. Paucity of interlobular bile ducts and bile duct epithelial degeneration are prominent findings. With progression, fibrosis is initially centrilobular and later causes central to portal bridging. A characteristic pattern consists of diffuse stellate and lacy lobular fibrosis, severe cholestasis, and pseudoacinar transformation of hepatocytes.[74]

The diagnosis of PFIC is made by the following criteria: (1) progressive intrahepatic cholestasis resulting in permanent jaundice and liver injury for which all other known causes of cholestasis have been excluded; (2) normal extrahepatic bile ducts by cholangiography; (3) normal number of interlobular bile ducts on liver histology, although early in the course paucity may be seen; (4) mild or no elevation of serum GGTP and cholesterol levels (except rarely[70]); and (5) absence of extrahepatic abnormalities.[71, 75]

Complications include fat-soluble vitamin deficiencies, growth retardation, delay in sexual maturation, infections related to cholestasis, cholelithiasis, and chronic pancreatitis.[71, 76] Hepatocellular carcinoma may develop in children with advanced cirrhosis, even before 3 years of age.[71]

PFIC is generally refractory to medical therapy. Prompt surgical management with partial diversion of the bile flow may arrest progression of hepatic fibrosis and improve pruritus, school attendance, and growth.[77] Liver transplantation is reserved for patients who have cirrhosis at the time of presentation. Post-transplantation recurrence has not been reported.

### Benign Recurrent Intrahepatic Cholestasis

Benign recurrent intrahepatic cholestasis (BRIC) is a form of relapsing cholestasis that does not progress to chronic liver disease or cirrhosis. The first episode often occurs in childhood, although rarely during infancy, but the age of onset may be as young as 2 weeks.[66] The possibility of such early onset, and some important similarities with PFIC, merit mention of BRIC under the category of neonatal cholestasis. Both autosomal recessive[78] and autosomal dominant inheritance of variable penetrance[79] have been described. The gene has been mapped to chromosome 18,[80] to the same region as Byler's disease.[68] The current hypothesis for the cause of cholestasis in both disorders is disturbance in hepatocellular bile acid secretion.[72] It is proposed that in Byler's disease a homozygous mutation completely disrupts bile acid secretion.[68] Individuals with BRIC presumably have a less severe genetic defect and experience symptoms only under conditions of extreme stress, such as pregnancy or illness. Patients with BRIC are normal both clinically and biochemically between the cholestatic bouts. During attacks, patients present with severe pruritus followed by jaundice, weight loss, and abdominal pain. The duration of the episode is also variable, from 2 weeks to 2 years.[81] Serum GGTP levels typically are normal.

**TABLE 47–4. Clinical Features of the Familial Intrahepatic Cholestasis Syndromes**

| CHARACTERISTIC | ALAGILLE SYNDROME | NONSYNDROMIC PAUCITY | PFIC/BYLER'S DISEASE | BRIC | NORWEGIAN CHOLESTASIS | NORTH AMERICAN INDIAN CHOLESTASIS | GREENLAND ESKIMO CHOLESTASIS |
|---|---|---|---|---|---|---|---|
| Age at onset | <3 mo | <3 mo | 3–12 mo | Any age | <3 mo | <3 mo | <3 mo |
| Associated findings | Cardiac, eye, bone, kidney abnormalities | None | None | None | Lymphedema | Telangiectasia of the cheeks | Thrombocytosis, subcutaneous bleeding |
| Recurrent cholangitis | No | No | Yes | Yes | Yes | No | No |
| GGTP | Elevated | Elevated | Normal | Normal | Elevated | Elevated | Not reported |
| Cholesterol | Elevated | Elevated | Normal | Normal | Elevated | Normal | Normal |
| Early biopsy | Paucity of bile ducts | Paucity of bile ducts | Cholestasis, giant cells | Cholestasis | Giant cells | Giant cells | Centrizonal cholestasis |
| Late biopsy | Biliary cirrhosis | Biliary cirrhosis | Centrizonal or portal fibrosis | Cholestasis | Portal fibrosis | Cirrhosis | Centrizonal fibrosis |
| Course | Cholestasis often improves | Progressive | Progressive | Benign | Usually benign | Progressive | Progressive |
| Inheritance | Autosomal dominant | No pattern | Autosomal recessive | Autosomal recessive and dominant | Autosomal recessive | Autosomal recessive | Autosomal recessive |

BRIC, benign recurrent intrahepatic cholestasis; GGTP, γ-glutamyl transpeptidase; PFIC, progressive familial intrahepatic cholestasis; TORCH, toxoplasmosis, other infections, rubella, cytomegalovirus infection, and herpes simplex; VDRL, Venereal Disease Research Laboratory.

Modified from Reily CA: Familial intrahepatic cholestatic syndromes. Semin Liver Dis 1997;7:119–133, with permission, Thieme Medical Publishers, Inc.

### Miscellaneous Familial Cholestatic Syndromes

A number of familial, presumably genetic, syndromes of childhood intrahepatic cholestasis have been described in ethnic populations. Whether they are variants of a single disorder, expressed in geographically different kindreds, or clinically similar but genetically distinct diseases has not been elucidated.

Norwegian cholestasis has been reported in patients of Norwegian extraction and is characterized by lymphedema of the lower extremities and recurrent bouts of intrahepatic cholestasis that begin within the first 3 months of life.[82–84] North American Indian cholestasis is restricted to a tribe of native North Americans from northwestern Quebec.[85] Patients often present with neonatal cholestasis, and a striking feature is the presence of telangiectasias of the cheeks ("paper-money skin"). Greenland Eskimo cholestasis also is limited to a well-defined ethnic group.[86] The patients present at birth or within the first 3 months of life with permanent jaundice and pruritus. The cholestasis is progressive. Other laboratory findings include thrombocytosis and low to normal levels of cholesterol and triglycerides.

## NEONATAL CHOLESTASIS ASSOCIATED WITH TOTAL PARENTERAL NUTRITION

There are three distinct but overlapping hepatobiliary syndromes associated with total parenteral nutrition (TPN). Gallbladder sludge and gallstones may occur at any age but are rarely symptomatic. Older children and adults may develop hepatic steatosis or steatohepatitis.[87] In infants, the typical complication is cholestasis or cholestatic hepatitis.[88]

The incidence of cholestasis associated with TPN varies from 7% to 50%.[88–90] The frequency increases with younger gestational age, lower birth weight, and longer duration of TPN.[90] Most cases occur from 2 to 10 weeks after the initiation of TPN, and 90% of infants develop cholestasis within 13 weeks.[90]

### Clinical and Laboratory Findings

TPN-associated liver injury is characterized by hepatomegaly and jaundice. The first biochemical abnormality is an increase in the serum bile acid concentration. The most widely accepted laboratory indicator is a rising conjugated bilirubin level in a patient who has received TPN for at least 2 weeks.[91] In a series of 308 patients, alkaline phosphatase was reported to rise first, followed by alanine aminotransferase (ALT) and then bilirubin.[92] The ALT concentration peaked between the second and fourth week of continuous TPN and then declined, whereas the bilirubin and alkaline phosphatase concentrations continued to increase and remained elevated over the duration of TPN. GGTP appears to be a sensitive indicator of the cholestasis.[93]

Patients who cannot be fed enterally and require continued TPN despite cholestasis may develop cirrhosis.[94] These patients usually have received TPN for longer than 20 months.[95] Extreme short bowel syndrome may shorten this period to as little as 6 months.[96] Infants with necrotizing enterocolitis have a seven-fold increased risk for cholestasis. Hepatitis without cholestasis is not associated with progressive liver disease.[97] Hepatocellular carcinoma has been reported even in noncirrhotic patients.[98, 99]

Hemolytic anemia and administration of furosemide appear to act synergistically in the development of cholelithiasis in infants receiving TPN.[100]

### Histologic Findings

The histologic changes of TPN-associated liver disease are nonspecific and variable and evolve over time. The major components are centrilobular cholestasis, mild periportal inflammation, steatosis, and progressive portal fibrosis. The degree of histologic cholestasis may not correlate with the serum bilirubin values.[101] Biliary cirrhosis may eventually develop.[94]

### Pathogenesis

A single cause for TPN-associated cholestasis has not been identified. Factors that have been associated with TPN-related liver disease include immaturity of the enterohepatic circulation, perinatal insults, toxins, nutrient deficiency, contaminants, substrate imbalance, absence of enteral intake, and infection.[89, 90, 102] Potential pathogenetic mechanisms for TPN-associated cholestatic hepatitis are listed in Table 47–5.

### Management

When biochemical evidence of cholestasis or hepatocyte injury is found, other causes of liver disease should be excluded. Avoidance of TPN, when possible, is the best approach. In cases in which its use is mandatory, it is important to use enteral alimentation as soon as possible, even if only for partial or minimal feeding. Discontinuation of TPN before development of frank cirrhosis results in substantial improvement in the histologic changes in the

**TABLE 47–5. Potential Pathogenetic Mechanisms of TPN-Associated Cholestatic Hepatitis**

- Immature bile acid metabolism[157,158]
- Injury to the liver from bacterial endotoxins[159] and/or toxic bile acids[160] as a result of bacterial overgrowth
  - Hypochlorhydria
  - Slow gastric emptying[161]
  - Diminished small bowel motility[162]
  - Decreased secretion of hormones with trophic and promotility effects[163,164]
- Nutrient deficiencies
  - Taurine[165]
  - Carnitine
  - Glutamine[109]
  - Essential fatty acids
  - Trace minerals[166]
- Excess amino acid administration[103]
- Absence of enteral intake[89,90]
- Infection[89,90]

liver.[94] If use of TPN is necessary, then cyclic administration with a period of rest and enteral feeding may be helpful.

Energy and nitrogen delivered by TPN should be sufficient to achieve positive nitrogen balance and catch-up growth. Amino acids or dextrose in excess may be hepatotoxic.[103] Dosages of trace elements (e.g., copper, manganese) that are excreted via the biliary tree should be adjusted in TPN solutions for patients with cholestatic liver disease.

Antibiotics active against anaerobic bacteria, such as metronidazole, seem to prevent cholestasis, especially in patients with short bowel syndrome.[104] Ursodeoxycholic acid appears to be a promising choleretic agent, but the studies performed so far in TPN-associated cholestasis have included only small numbers of patients.[105] Phenobarbital has been ineffective in treating or preventing cholestasis in infants.[106]

Administration of gastrointestinal hormones is another potential intervention. Intravenous infusion of cholecystokinin, a peptide hormone that increases bile flow, promotes the motility of the biliary tract and gallbladder emptying and relaxes the sphincter of Oddi. It has resulted in reversion of TPN-associated cholestasis in some neonates who had undergone gastrointestinal operations.[107] Addition of glucagon to TPN solutions has prevented hepatic steatosis in rats.[108] Glutamine has also been shown to prevent intestinal atrophy.[109] Surgical irrigation of the biliary tree has been used successfully to relieve persistent TPN-associated cholestasis.[110] Finally, liver transplantation is the ultimate treatment for end-stage liver disease.

## MISCELLANEOUS CAUSES OF NEONATAL HEPATITIS/CHOLESTASIS

### Vascular Disorders of the Liver

Vascular disorders are an unusual cause of the neonatal hepatitis syndrome, but patients with these disorders may present with conjugated hyperbilirubinemia and elevated aminotransferase and alkaline phosphatase concentrations. Two major categories of vascular disorders—hemangiomas and vascular malformations—have been distinguished, based on the cellular biology and natural history of the lesions.[111] True hemangiomas exhibit rapid neonatal growth and slow involution, whereas vascular malformations grow in proportion to the child and fail to regress. Hepatic hemangiomas may be solitary or multiple, involving both lobes. Multiple hepatic hemangiomas are usually associated with cutaneous hemangiomas[112] or diffuse neonatal hemangiomatosis involving the brain, lungs, and gastrointestinal tract.[113] Patients commonly present within the first 6 months of life.[114] Single large or multiple hemangiomas may cause hepatomegaly, obstructive jaundice, congestive heart failure, anemia, or thrombocytopenia with or without the Kasabach-Merritt syndrome. Less common presenting features include intestinal obstruction, portal hypertension, and intestinal bleeding from the tumor.[115]

Hepatic arteriovenous malformations are less common than hemangiomas and result in similar clinical presentations. Ultrasonography of hepatic hemangiomas shows nodules of heterogeneous or decreased echogenicity, whereas magnetic resonance imaging (MRI) displays discrete parenchymal lesions. Dilated hepatic arteries and veins are found on both ultrasound and MRI studies of hepatic arteriovenous malformations (flow voids on MRI), and arteriovenous shunting is seen with Doppler examination.[114]

Hepatic hemangiomas invariably regress late in infancy, but they can be life-threatening during the proliferative phase, with a mortality rate of 30% to 80%.[114] Pharmacologic therapy with corticosteroids and interferon alfa-2a has been used for symptomatic hepatic hemangiomas, large asymptomatic lesions, and extensive multiple hemangiomas that might cause congestive heart failure. The response rate to corticosteroids has ranged from 18% to 70%, and that to interferon has been reported to be as high as 85%.[114] Hepatic artery embolization can be useful for temporary control of life-threatening congestive heart failure or before resection of a solitary liver hemangioma that is unresponsive to pharmacologic therapy. Combined embolization and resection is advised for symptomatic arteriovenous malformations, because they do not regress with time.[114]

Infantile hemangioendothelioma is the most common benign liver tumor in children and the most common liver tumor in the first year of life. In 87% of cases it is detected before the age of 6 months.[116] Clinical presentation includes an abdominal mass, failure to thrive, fever, jaundice, congestive heart failure, and the Kasabach-Merritt syndrome. Anemia, hyperbilirubinemia, and elevated aspartate aminotransferase are usually present. Serum alpha-fetoprotein is normal. Complete resection of the tumor, if possible, is the treatment of choice. For large single or multifocal tumors, hepatic artery ligation or embolization, often in association with corticosteroids, has been successful.

Other vascular disorders of the liver are rarely described in neonates. These include veno-occlusive disease (obstruction of the intrahepatic venules) and Budd-Chiari syndrome (noncardiogenic obstruction of the main hepatic veins or of the suprahepatic inferior vena cava).[117, 118]

### Drug Hepatotoxicity

Neonatal cholestasis has been reported after administration of chloral hydrate,[119] pancuronium bromide,[120] and erythromycin estolate.[121] Di-2-ethylhexyl phthalate, a plasticizer found in the tubing for extracorporeal membrane oxygenation (ECMO) has been implicated in the pathogenesis of cholestasis seen in infants supported with ECMO.[122] Isolated reports describe infantile hepatitis caused by halothane and phenobarbital.[123] Veno-occlusive disease has been reported in a breast-fed infant whose mother drank herbal tea.[118]

### Inspissated Bile Syndrome

Inspissated bile syndrome is a term that was first used to describe conjugated hyperbilirubinemia in fetal erythroblastosis.[124] The liver histology in those infants was similar to that seen in neonatal hepatitis. Rh-incompatibility (see Chapter 8) and cystic fibrosis (see Chapter 54) are currently the most common causes of inspissated bile syndrome.

The clinical presentation of cystic fibrosis–associated liver disease in infancy includes hepatomegaly and cholestatic jaundice with acholic stools that may linger for months.[125]

Biliary obstruction in neonates with cystic fibrosis has been attributed to inspissation of mucus in the bile ducts.[126]

## Ischemia

The liver is somewhat protected from major hemodynamic disturbances by its dual blood supply, two thirds of which comes from the portal vein and the remainder from the systemic circulation through the hepatic artery.[127] Under normal conditions, oxygen and nutrients in blood decrease from periportal (zone 1) to pericentral (zone 3) areas. Therefore, the pericentral zone is more susceptible to hypoxia/ischemia as it occurs in cardiorespiratory arrest, congestive heart failure, shock, asphyxia, seizures, or profound dehydration.[128] Ischemic hepatic injury may occur without recognition or documentation of the preceding hypotensive episode.[129]

Ischemic hepatitis or "shock liver" is characterized by marked increase in aminotransferase levels, within 24 to 48 hours after the insult, followed by a return to normal levels over a period of several days to 1 week.[130] The aminotransferase levels may reach 10,000 IU/L, but typically the alkaline phosphatase concentration is normal. Serum creatinine phosphokinase (CPK) and creatinine may be elevated, indicating hypotensive damage to other organs. Hepatomegaly, jaundice, and coagulopathy may develop. The diagnosis can usually be made on clinical and biochemical grounds. Liver biopsy is not recommended because it may cause further complications in those patients who are usually very ill with multi-system disease. The prognosis is determined predominantly by the underlying disease.[130]

The liver may also be affected by chronic cardiac disorders. In chronic left-sided heart failure, hepatic ischemia is usually associated with reduced cardiac output and subsequent hypotension, but the clinical and biochemical findings may be subtle.[131] Right-sided heart failure results in hepatic congestion. This is manifested by tender hepatomegaly and slow increases in the aminotransferase, alkaline phosphatase, and GGTP levels. Histologically, sinusoidal dilatation and congestion with necrosis of pericentral (zone 3) hepatocytes is seen. Congenital heart disease, such as coarctation of the aorta or hypoplastic left heart syndrome, may be associated with severe hepatic necrosis.[132, 133]

## Endocrine Disorders

Congenital hypothyroidism is associated with neonatal jaundice in approximately 20% of cases.[134] Jaundice may be the presenting symptom, and it is prolonged if the hypothyroidism is left untreated. Hyperbilirubinemia usually is unconjugated in primary congenital hypothyroidism. In contrast, neonatal conjugated hyperbilirubinemia has been reported in association with hypopituitarism[135] and septo-optic dysplasia (de Morsier's syndrome).[136] This syndrome consists of absence of the septum pellucidum, optic nerve hypoplasia, and secondary hypopituitarism of hypothalamic origin. Signs of hypopituitarism in the neonatal period include hypoglycemia, jaundice, hepatomegaly, and micropenis in males. Conjugated bilirubin, aminotransferase, and alkaline phosphatase levels are increased. Histologic changes in the liver include multinucleated giant cells, cholestasis without bile duct proliferation, and minimal portal fibrosis.[137] Delay in diagnosis and treatment may result in prolonged cholestasis, progressing to significant permanent hepatic injury and even cirrhosis.[138] Prompt recognition and treatment with hormone replacement result in resolution of cholestasis. The pathogenesis of cholestasis in hypopituitarism is not clear. It is speculated that cholestasis develops secondary to lack of the trophic hormones, such as growth hormone and cortisol, which modulate bile acid synthesis and flow.[137, 139]

Cholestasis has also been reported in infants with primary adrenal insufficiency.[137]

## Chromosomal Disorders

Neonatal hepatitis syndrome and extrahepatic biliary atresia have been reported in association with trisomy 17–18 syndrome (trisomy E)[140] and trisomy 21 (Down syndrome).[141] The mechanism is unknown.

Transient myeloproliferative disorder, an acute leukemia-like disorder that may affect neonates with Down syndrome, has been associated with diffuse hepatic fibrosis and obstructive jaundice.[142] Histologically, there is excessive extramedullary hematopoiesis but multinucleated giant cells are absent. The prognosis is poor.

## Neonatal Lupus Erythematosus

Cholestasis has been reported in infants with neonatal lupus erythematosus.[143] The infant may manifest jaundice and hepatosplenomegaly. Hepatic histology may demonstrate giant cell transformation, extramedullary hematopoiesis, and ductular proliferation. Paucity of interlobular bile ducts has also been reported. It is speculated that maternal autoantibodies that pass to the fetus transplacentally are involved in the pathogenesis of the liver injury. Cholestasis usually resolves by 9 months, provided that severe liver damage has not occurred.[143]

## Other Causes

The causes of neonatal cholestasis are further discussed in Chapters 48 and 49.

# COMPLICATIONS AND MANAGEMENT OF NEONATAL HEPATITIS/CHOLESTASIS

The complications of cholestasis are common to all of the disorders. They are caused by reduction in intraluminal bile acids, which results in malabsorption of fat- and lipid-soluble vitamins; retention of the constituents of bile, such as bile acids, bilirubin, and cholesterol, which results in pruritus and xanthomas; and progressive hepatocellular damage, which leads to portal hypertension and liver failure. The complications of cholestasis are listed in Table 47–6. The management of cholestasis is directed first toward specific treatment of the underlying disorder.

Medical management of cholestasis may be needed during

**TABLE 47–6. Complications of Chronic Cholestasis**

- Malabsorption and malnutrition
  - Steatorrhea
  - Growth failure
  - Fat-soluble vitamin deficiencies
  - Mineral and trace element deficiencies
- Retention of constituents of bile (bile acids, cholesterol)
  - Pruritus
  - Xanthomas
  - Jaundice
- Hepatic fibrosis/cirrhosis
  - Portal hypertension, variceal bleeding
  - Ascites
- End-stage liver disease

recovery from some of the treatable conditions. This medical management includes treatment of fat malabsorption and its consequences, as well as expectant therapy for the complications of chronic cholestatic hepatic injury (Table 47–7). Steatorrhea, almost always present in children with severe cholestasis, is a major cause of malnutrition. Other conditions that are associated with malnutrition in these infants include altered metabolism of glucose and amino acids,[144] increased resting energy expenditure,[145] recurrent infections,[146] anorexia,[145] and early satiety secondary to compression of abdominal viscera by the enlarged liver/spleen or ascites. The combination of long-chain triglyceride malabsorption and inadequate intake may lead to essential fatty acid deficiency causing further growth failure, dry scaly rash, thrombocytopenia, and impaired immune function.[147]

**TABLE 47–7. Management of the Complications of Chronic Cholestasis**

**Malabsorption and Malnutrition**

- Supply adequate calories: 125–150% of RDA
- Supply adequate protein
- Decrease dietary long-chain fats
- Supply medium-chain triglycerides as fat source
- Supply essential fatty acids (corn oil, safflower oil, macrolipid emulsion)
- Supplement fat-soluble vitamins (see Table 47–8)
- Supply water-soluble vitamins at 200% of RDA
- Correct or prevent mineral and trace element deficiencies:
  - Elemental calcium, 25–100 mg/kg/day;
  - Phosphate, 25–50 mg/kg/day;
  - Zinc, 1.0 mg/kg/day;
  - Selenium, 1–2 μg/kg/day
  - Magnesium, 1–2 mEq/kg/day

**Retention of Constituents of Bile**

- Ursodeoxycholic acid, 15–30 mg/kg/day in two doses
- Cholestyramine, 0.25–0.5 g/kg/day in three doses
- Rifampin, 10 mg/kg/day in two doses

**Fibrosis/Cirrhosis**

- Portal hypertension, variceal bleeding
  - Infusion of vasopressin, octreotide
  - Variceal sclerotherapy, band ligation
  - Balloon tamponade of varices
  - Portosystemic shunt surgery
  - Prophylactic or therapeutic propranolol
- Ascites
  - Limitation of sodium intake
  - Aldosterone antagonist (spironolactone)
  - Loop diuretic
  - Albumin infusions
  - Large-volume paracentesis

**End-stage Liver Disease**

- Liver transplantation

RDA, recommended dietary allowance.

Bile acids are necessary for effective intraluminal long-chain triglyceride absorption and for micellar solubilization of lipid-soluble vitamins (A, D, E, and K). In addition, vitamin A and E esters require hydrolysis by pancreatic or intestinal esterases that are bile acid dependent. Therefore, supplementation with at least two to four times the recommended dietary allowances of these vitamins is necessary (Table 47–8). Signs of deficiency as well as toxicity of these vitamins should be monitored periodically by measurement of serum levels of vitamin A, E, and 25-hydroxy vitamin D; calcium; phosphorus; and prothrombin time. The ratio of serum vitamin E to total serum lipids is more reliable in assessing vitamin E status, since elevated lipid levels during cholestasis allow vitamin E to partition into the plasma lipoproteins, artificially raising the serum vitamin E concentration. A water-soluble formulation of vitamin E, D-α-tocopheryl polyethylene glycol succinate (TPGS), is a prodrug; vitamin E linked to polyethylene glycol is passively absorbed by the intestinal epithelium. It has been shown to increase the absorption of other lipid-soluble chemicals.[148]

Hyperlipidemia, xanthomas, and pruritus associated with cholestasis can cause significant morbidity. The pathogenesis of pruritus has not been clearly established. Although originally thought to be caused by the retention of bile acids, there is more recent evidence that impaired clearance of endogenous opiates with cholestasis results in elevated serum levels, with activation of central nervous system receptors.[149, 150] The nonabsorbable anion exchange resins cholestyramine and colestipol exert their effect by binding bile acids intraluminally, increasing their fecal excretion and interrupting the enterohepatic circulation. The diminished return of bile acids to the liver stimulates the conversion of cholesterol to bile acids, resulting in reduction of toxic bile acids in the liver and lowering of serum cholesterol.[151, 152] Potential side effects of these agents are hyperchloremic metabolic acidosis, worsening steatorrhea, and intestinal obstruction caused by inspissation of the drug. Cholestyramine should not be mixed with formula or given at the same time as oral vitamin supplements, and it should be followed by administration of extra fluid.[153]

Phenobarbital increases bile acid–independent flow[154] and decreases the bile acid pool, but the sedative effect of the drug and its alteration of the metabolism of many other drugs are limiting factors for its use. Rifampin provides relief from pruritus in some children with chronic cholestasis.[155] Ursodeoxycholic acid, a natural hydrophilic bile acid, has ameliorated pruritus, improved the biochemical markers of cholestasis, and improved the nutritional state. Proposed mechanisms of action include displacement of toxic hydrophobic bile acids from the bile acid pool and intracellular space, reduction in intestinal bile acid reabsorption, and induction of bicarbonate-rich hypercholeresis and bile acid excretion. It also stabilizes and protects against membrane destruction and mitochondrial injury induced by hydrophobic bile acids.[156]

A review of the treatment of end-stage liver disease and its complications can be found in Chapters 51 and 52.

**TABLE 47–8. Recommendations for Supplementation of Fat-Soluble Vitamins in Cholestatic Liver Disease**

| VITAMIN | DEFICIENCY | SUPPLEMENT | DOSAGE |
|---|---|---|---|
| Vitamin A | Night blindness, pigmentary retinopathy, xerophthalmia, keratomalacia, poor growth | Water-miscible retinol | 5,000–25,000 IU/day |
| Vitamin D | Rickets, osteomalacia, cranial bossing, epiphyseal enlargement, persistently open anterior fontanelle | Vitamin D<br>25-OH vitamin D<br>1,25-$(OH)_2$ vitamin D | 1,200–5,000 IU/day<br>3–5 μg/kg/day<br>0.05–0.2 μg/kg/day |
| Vitamin E | Ataxia, areflexia, ophthalmoplegia, retinal abnormalities, loss of proprioception and vibratory sense, peripheral neuropathy | D-α-Tocopheryl polyethylene glycol succinate (TPGS) | 15–25 IU/kg/day |
| Vitamin K | Coagulopathy, hemorrhagic manifestations | Mephyton ($K_1$)<br>Aquamephyton (intramuscularly) | 2.5 mg twice per week<br>2–5 mg every 3–4 weeks |

## REFERENCES


1. Dick MC, Mowat AP: Hepatitis syndrome in infancy: an epidemiological survey with 10-year follow up. Arch Dis Child 1985;60:512–516.
2. Balistreri WF: Neonatal cholestasis: lessons from the past, issues for the future. Semin Liver Dis 1987;7:61–66.
3. Kasai M: Treatment of biliary atresia with special reference to hepatic porto-enterostomy and its modifications. Prog Pediatr Surg 1974;6:5–52.
4. Balistreri WF: Fetal and neonatal bile acid synthesis and metabolism: clinical implications. J Inherit Metab Dis 1991;14:459–477.
5. Ferry DG, Selby ML, Udall J, et al: Guide to early diagnosis of biliary obstruction in infancy: review of 143 cases. Clin Pediatr (Phila) 1985;24:305–311.
6. Alagille D: Cholestasis in the first three months of life. Prog Liver Dis 1979;16:471–485.
7. Andres JM, Darby BR, Walter WA: The effect of *E. coli* endotoxin in the developing rat liver: II. Immunohistochemical localization of alpha-fetoprotein in rat liver multinucleated giant cells. Pediatr Res 1983;17:1017–1020.
8. Postlethwaite AE, Jackson BJ, Beachey EH, et al: Formation of multinucleated giant cells from human monocyte precursors: mediation by a soluble protein from antigen and mitogen-stimulated lymphocytes. J Exp Med 1982;155:168–178.
9. Pulford K, Souhami RL: Cell division and giant cell formation in Kupffer cell cultures. Clin Exp Immunol 1980;42:67–76.
10. Germain L, Noel M, Gourdeau H, et al: Promotion of growth and differentiation of rat ductular oval cells in primary culture. Cancer 1987;59:310–316.
11. Schaffner F, Popper H: Morphologic studies in neonatal cholestasis with emphasis in giant cells. Ann N Y Acad Sci 1963;111:358–374.
12. Shulman LN, Robinson SH: Origin of multinucleated giant cells in long-term diffusion chamber cultures. Proc Soc Exp Biol Med 1982;170:359–362.
13. Hanshaw JB: Congenital cytomegalovirus infection. Pediatr Ann 1994;23:124–128.
14. Reynolds DW, Stagno S, Hosty TS, et al: Maternal cytomegalovirus excretion and perinatal infection. N Engl J Med 1973;289:1–5.
15. McCracken GH Jr, Shinefield HR, Cobb K, et al: Congenital cytomegalovirus inclusion disease: a longitudinal study of 20 patients. Am J Dis Child 1969;117:522–539.
16. Ahlfors K, Ivarsson SA, Harris S, et al: Congenital cytomegalovirus infection and disease in Sweden and the relative importance of primary and secondary maternal infections. Scand J Infect Dis 1984;16:129–137.
17. Brainard JA, Greenson JK, Vesy CJ, et al: Detection of cytomegalovirus in liver transplant biopsies: a comparison of light microscopy, immunohistochemistry, duplex PCR and nested PCR. Transplantation 1994;57:1753–1757.
18. Nigro G, Scholz H, Bartmann U: Ganciclovir therapy for symptomatic congenital infection in infants: a two-regimen experience. J Pediatr 1994;124:318–322.
19. Berenberg W, Nankervis G: Long-term follow up of cytomegalic inclusion disease in infancy. Pediatrics 1970;46:403–410.
20. Binder ND, Buckmaster JW, Benda GI: Outcome for fetus with ascites and cytomegalovirus infection. Pediatrics 1988;82:100–103.
21. Hutto C, Arvin A, Jacobs R, et al: Intrauterine herpes simplex virus infections. J Pediatr 1987;110:97–101.
22. Whitley RJ: Herpes simplex virus. In Remington JS, Klein JO (eds): Infectious Diseases of the Fetus and Newborn Infant. Philadelphia, WB Saunders, 1990, pp 282–305.
23. Hanshaw JB: Herpesvirus hominis infections in the fetus and the newborn. Am J Dis Child 1973;126:546–555.
24. Raga J, Chrystal V, Cooradia HM: Usefulness of clinical features and liver biopsy in diagnosis of disseminated herpes simplex infection. Arch Dis Child 1984;59:820–824.
25. Cone RW, Hobson AC, Palmer J, et al: Extended duration of herpes simplex virus DNA in genital lesions detected by the polymerase chain reaction. J Infect Dis 1991;164:757–760.
26. Whitley R, Arvin A, Prober C, et al: A controlled trial comparing vidarabine with acyclovir in neonatal herpes virus infection. N Engl J Med 1991;324:444–449.
27. Dudgeon JA: Congenital rubella. J Pediatr 1975;87:1078–1086.
28. Watkins JB, Sunaryo FP, Berezin SH: Hepatic manifestations of congenital and perinatal disease. Clin Perinatol 1981;8:467–480.
29. Modlin JF: Perinatal echovirus infection: insights from a literature review of 61 cases of serious infection and 16 outbreaks in nurseries. Rev Infect Dis 1986;8:918–925.
30. Modlin JF: Fatal echovirus 11 disease in premature neonates. Pediatrics 1980;66:775–780.
31. Philip AG, Larson EJ: Overwhelming neonatal infection with echo 19 virus. J Pediatr 1973;82:391–397.
32. Stevens CE, Krugman S, Szmuness W, et al: Viral hepatitis in pregnancy: a problem for the clinician dealing with the infant. Pediatr Rev 1980;2:121–125.
33. Leikin E, Lysikiewicz A, Garry D, et al: Intrauterine transmission of hepatitis A virus. Obstet Gynecol 1996;88:690–691.
34. Noble RC, Kane MA, Reeves SA, et al: Post-transfusion hepatitis A in a neonatal intensive care unit. JAMA 1984;252:2716–2721.
35. American Academy of Pediatrics: Hepatitis A. In Peter G (ed): Red Book: Report of the Committee on Infectious Diseases. Elk Grove Village, IL, American Academy of Pediatrics, 1997, pp 237–246.
36. Balaraman V, Wilson CM, Nakamura KT, et al: Severe neonatal hepatitis A (HAV) infection in the newborn. Pediatr Res 1991;29:279A.
37. Tong MJ, Thursby MW, Lin JH, et al: Studies on the maternal-infant transmission of the viruses which cause acute hepatitis. Gastroenterology 1981;80:999–1004.
38. Boxall EH: Breast feeding and hepatitis B (letter). Lancet 1975;2:979.
39. Beasley RP, Trepo C, Stevens CE, et al: E antigen and vertical transmission of hepatitis B antigen. Am J Epidemiol 1977;105:94–98.
40. Carman WF, Hadziyannis S, Karayiannis P, et al: Association of the precore variant of HBV with acute fulminant hepatitis. In Hollinger F, Lemon S (eds): Viral Hepatitis and Liver Disease. Baltimore, Williams & Wilkins, 1991, pp 216–219.
41. Stevens CE, Beasley RP, Tsui JJ, et al: Vertical transmission of hepatitis B in Taiwan. N Engl J Med 1975;292:771–774.
42. Thaler MM, Park CK, Landers DV, et al: Vertical transmission of hepatitis C virus. Lancet 1991;338:17–18.
43. Ohto H, Terazawa S, Sasaki N, et al: Transmission of hepatitis C virus from mothers to infants. N Engl J Med 1994;330:744–750.
44. Giovanninni M, Tagger A, Ribero ML, et al: Maternal-infant transmission of hepatitis C virus and HIV infection: a possible interaction (letter). Lancet 1990;335:1166.
45. American Academy of Pediatrics: Hepatitis C. In Peter G (ed): Red Book: Report of the Committee on Infectious Diseases. Elk Grove Village, IL, American Academy of Pediatrics, 1997, p 263.

46. Brechot C: Polymerase chain reaction for the diagnosis of viral hepatitis B and C. Gut 1993;34(suppl 2):S39–S34.
47. Zanetti AR, Ferrons P, Magliano EM: Perinatal transmission of the hepatitis B virus and of the HBV-associated delta agent to offspring in northern Italy. J Med Virol 1982;9:139–148.
48. Khuroo MS, Kamili S, Jameal S: Vertical transmission of hepatitis E virus. Lancet 1995;345:1025–1026.
49. Luzuriaga K, Sullivan JL: Pathogenesis of vertical HIV-1 infection: implications for intervention and management. Pediatr Ann 1994;23:159–166.
50. Shannon KM, Ammann AJ: Acquired immunodeficiency syndrome in childhood. J Pediatr 1985;106:332–342.
51. Persaud D, Bangaru B, Greco A, et al: Cholestatic hepatitis in children infected with the human immunodeficiency virus. Pediatr Infect Dis J 1993;12:492–498.
52. Metzman R, Anand A, DeGiulio PA, et al: Hepatic disease associated with intrauterine parvovirus B 19 infection in a newborn premature infant. J Pediatr Gastroenterol Nutr 1989;9:112–114.
53. Tajiri H, Nose O, Baba K, et al: Human herpesvirus-6 infection with liver biopsy in neonatal hepatitis. Lancet 1990;335:863.
54. Asano Y, Yoshikawa T, Suga S, et al: Fatal fulminant hepatitis in an infant with human herpesvirus-6 infection. Lancet 1990;335:862–863.
55. Abzug MJ, Levin MJ: Neonatal adenovirus infection: four patients and review of the literature. Pediatrics 1991;87:890–896.
56. Phillips MJ, Blendis LM, Poucell S, et al: Syncytial giant-cell hepatitis: sporadic hepatitis with distinctive pathological features, a severe clinical course, and paramyxoviral features. N Engl J Med 1991;324:455–460.
57. Long WA, Ulshen MH, Lawson EE: Clinical manifestations of congenital syphilitic hepatitis: implications for pathogenesis. J Pediatr Gastroenterol Nutr 1984;3:551–555.
58. Oppenheimer EH, Hardy JB: Congenital syphilis in the newborn infant: clinical and pathological observations in recent cases. Johns Hopkins Med J 1971;129:63–82.
59. Bernstein J, Brown AK: Sepsis and jaundice in early infancy. Pediatrics 1962;29:873–882.
60. Utili R, Abernathy CO, Zimmerman HJ: Cholestatic effects of *Escherichia coli* endotoxin on the isolated perfused rat liver. Gastroenterology 1976;70:248–253.
61. Becroft DMO, Farmer K, Seddon RJ, et al: Epidemic listeriosis in the newborn. BMJ 1971;3:747–751.
62. Desmonts G, Gouvreur J: Congenital toxoplasmosis: a prospective study of the offspring of 542 women who acquired toxoplasmosis during pregnancy. Pathophysiology of Congenital Disease, Perinatal Medicine: Sixth European Congress, Stuttgart, 1979. New York, Thieme Publishers, 1979.
63. Alford CA Jr, Stagno S, Reynolds DW: Congenital toxoplasmosis: clinical laboratory and therapeutic considerations with special reference to subclinical disease. Bull N Y Acad Med 1974;50:160–181.
64. Naot Y, Desmonts G, Remington J: IgM enzyme-linked immunosorbent assay test for the diagnosis of congenital toxoplasma infection. J Pediatr 1981;98:32–36.
65. McAuley J, Boyer K, Patel D, et al: Early and longitudinal evaluations of treated infants and children and untreated historical patients with congenital toxoplasmosis: the Chicago collaborative treatment trial. Clin Infect Dis 1994;18:38–72.
66. Riely CA: Familial intrahepatic cholestatic syndromes. Semin Liver Dis 1987;7:119–133.
67. Clayton RJ, Iber FL, Reubner BH, et al: Fatal familial intrahepatic cholestasis in an Amish kindred. J Pediatr 1965;67:1026–1028.
68. Carlton VE, Knisely AS, Freimer NB: Mapping of a locus for progressive familial intrahepatic cholestasis (Byler's disease) to 18q21–q22, the benign recurrent intrahepatic cholestasis region. Hum Mol Genet 1995;4:1049–1053.
69. Strautnieks SS, Kagawalla AF, Tanner MS, et al: Locus heterogeneity in progressive familial intrahepatic cholestasis. J Med Genet 1996;33:833–836.
70. Deleuze JF, Jacquemin E, Dubuisson C, et al: Defect of multidrug-resistance 3 gene expression in a subtype of progressive familial intrahepatic cholestasis. Hepatology 1996;23:904–908.
71. Whitington PF, Freese DK, Alonso EM, et al: Progressive familial intrahepatic cholestasis (Byler's disease). In Lentze M Jr (ed): Paediatric Cholestasis. Lancaster, UK, Kluwer Academic Publishers, 1992, pp 165–180.
72. Jacquemin E, Dumont M, Bernard O, et al: Evidence for defective bile acid secretion in children with progressive familial intrahepatic cholestasis (Byler's disease). Eur J Pediatr 1994;153:424–428.
73. Winklhofer-Roob BM, Shmerling DH, Soler R, et al: Progressive idiopathic cholestasis presenting with profuse watery diarrhea and recurrent infections (Byler's disease). Acta Paediatr 1992;81:637–640.
74. Alonso EM, Snover DC, Montag A, et al: Histologic pathology of the liver in progressive familial intrahepatic cholestasis. J Pediatr Gastroenterol Nutr 1994;18:128–133.
75. Soubrane O, Gauthier F, Victor DD, et al: Orthotopic liver transplantation for Byler's disease. Transplantation 1990;50:804–806.
76. Odievre M, Goutier M, Hadchouel M, et al: Severe familial intrahepatic cholestasis. Arch Dis Child 1973;48:806–812.
77. Emond JC, Whitington PF: Selective surgical management of progressive familial cholestasis. J Pediatr Surg 1995;30:1635–1641.
78. de Koning TJ, Sandkuijl LA, De Schryver JE, et al: Autosomal-recessive inheritance of benign recurrent intrahepatic cholestasis. Am J Med Genet 1995;57:479–482.
79. Brenard R, Geubel AP, Benhamou JP: Benign recurrent intrahepatic cholestasis: a report of 26 cases. J Clin Gastroenterol 1989;11:546–551.
80. Houwen RH, Baharloo S, Blankenship K, et al: Genome screening by searching for shared segments: mapping a gene for benign recurrent intrahepatic cholestasis. Nat Genet 1994;8:380–386.
81. de Pagter AGF, van Berge Henegouen GP, ten Bokkel Huinink JA, et al: Familial benign recurrent intrahepatic cholestasis: interrelation with intrahepatic cholestasis of pregnancy and from oral contraceptives? Gastroenterology 1976;71:202–207.
82. Aagenaes O: Hereditary recurrent cholestasis with lymphoedema. Acta Paediatr Scand 1974;63:465–471.
83. Sharp HL, Krivit W: Hereditary lymphedema and obstructive jaundice. J Pediatr 1971;78:491–496.
84. Aagenaes O, Henriksen PE, Sorland S: Hereditary neonatal cholestasis combined with vascular malformations. In Beienberg S (ed): Liver Diseases in Infancy and Childhood. Baltimore, Williams & Wilkins, 1976, pp 199–206.
85. Weber AM, Tuchweber B, Yousef I, et al: Severe familial cholestasis in North American Indian children: clinical model of microfilament dysfunction? Gastroenterology 1981;81:653–662.
86. Nielsen IM, Ornvold K, Jacobsen BB, et al: Fatal familial cholestatic syndrome in Greenland Eskimo children. Acta Paediatr Scand 1986;75:1010–1016.
87. Quigley EMM, Morsh MN: Hepatobiliary complications of total parenteral nutrition. Gastroenterology 1993;104:286–301.
88. Postuma R, Trevenen CL: Liver disease in infants receiving total parenteral nutrition. Pediatrics 1979;63:110–115.
89. Bell RL, Ferry GD, Smith EO, et al: Total parenteral nutrition related cholestasis in the infant. JPEN J Parenter Enteral Nutr 1986;10:356–359.
90. Beale EF, Nelson RM, Bucciarelli RL, et al: Intrahepatic cholestasis associated with parenteral nutrition in premature infants. Pediatrics 1979;64:342–347.
91. Vileisis RA, Inwood RJ, Hunt CE: Prospective control study of parenteral nutrition-associated cholestatic jaundice: effect of protein intake. J Pediatr 1980;96:893–897.
92. Clarke PJ, Ball MJ, Kettlewell MGW: Liver function tests in patients receiving total parenteral nutrition. JPEN J Parenter Enteral Nutr 1991;15:54–59.
93. Whitington PF: Cholestasis associated with total parenteral nutrition in infants. Hepatology 1985;5:693–696.
94. Dahms BB, Halpin TC: Serial liver biopsies in parenteral nutrition–associated cholestasis of early infancy. Gastroenterology 1981;81:136–144.
95. Briones ER, Iber FL: Liver and biliary tract changes and injury associated with total parenteral nutrition: pathogenesis and prevention. J Am Coll Nutr 1995;14:219–228.
96. Ito Y, Shils M: Liver dysfunction associated with long term total parenteral nutrition in patients with massive bowel resection. JPEN J Parenter Enteral Nutr 1985;9:11–17.
97. Balistreri WF, Bore KE: Hepatobiliary consequences of parenteral hyperalimentation. Prog Liver Dis 1989;9:567–600.
98. Vileisis RA, Sorensen K, Gonzalez-Crussi F, et al: Liver malignancy after total parenteral nutrition. J Pediatr 1982;100:88–90.
99. Patterson K, Kapur SP, Chandra RS: Hepatocellular carcinoma in a noncirrhotic infant after prolonged parenteral nutrition. J Pediatr 1985;106:797–800.

100. Whitington PF, Black DD: Cholelithiasis in premature infants treated with parenteral nutrition and furosemide. J Pediatr 1980;97:647–649.
101. Bernstein J, Chang CH, Brough AJ, et al: Conjugated hyperbilirubinemia in infancy associated with parenteral alimentation. J Pediatr 1977;90:361–367.
102. Dosi PC, Raut AJ, Chellaih BP, et al: Perinatal factors underlying neonatal cholestasis. J Pediatr 1985;106:471–474.
103. Moss RL, Das JB, Ansari G, et al: Hepatobiliary dysfunction during total parenteral nutrition is caused by infusate, not the route of administration. J Pediatr Surg 1993;28:391–396.
104. Capron JP, Gineston JL, Herve MA, et al: Metronidazole in prevention of cholestasis associated with total parenteral nutrition. Lancet 1983;1:446–447.
105. Spagnuolo MI, Iorio R, Vegnente A, et al: Ursodeoxycholic acid for treatment of cholestasis in children on long-term total parenteral nutrition: a pilot study. Gastroenterology 1996;111:716–719.
106. Gleghorn EE, Merritt RJ, Subramanian N, et al: Phenobarbital does not prevent total parenteral nutrition associated cholestasis in noninfected neonates. JPEN J Parenter Enteral Nutr 1986;10:282–283.
107. Rintala RJ, Lindahl H, Pohjavuori M: Total parenteral nutrition–associated cholestasis in surgical neonates may be reversed by intravenous cholecystokinin: a preliminary report. J Pediatr Surg 1995;30:827–830.
108. Li S, Nussbaum MS, McFadden DW, et al: Addition of glucagon to total parenteral nutrition (TPN) prevents hepatic steatosis in rats. Surgery 1990;104:350–357.
109. Grant J, Snyder P: Use of L-glutamine in TPN. J Surg Res 1988; 44:506–513.
110. Rintala RJ, Lindahl H, Pohjavuori M, et al: Surgical treatment of intractable cholestasis associated with total parenteral nutrition in premature infants. J Pediatr Surg 1993;28:716–719.
111. Mulliken JB, Glowaski J: Hemangiomas and vascular malformations in infants and children: a classification based on endothelial characteristics. Plast Reconstr Surg 1982;69:412–422.
112. Berman B, Lim HW-P: Concurrent cutaneous and hepatic hemangiomata in infancy: report of a case and review of the literature. J Dermatol Surg Oncol 1978;4:869–873.
113. Stenninger E, Schollin J: Diffuse neonatal hemangiomatosis in a newborn child. Acta Paediatr 1993;83:102–104.
114. Boon LM, Burrows PE, Paltiel HJ, et al: Hepatic vascular anomalies in infancy: a twenty-seven-year experience. J Pediatr 1996;129:346–354.
115. Larcher VF, Howard ER, Mowat AP: Hepatic haemangiomata: diagnosis and management. Arch Dis Child 1981;56:7–14.
116. Selby DM, Stocker TJ, Waclawiw MA, et al: Infantile hemangioendothelioma of the liver. Hepatology 1994;20:39–45.
117. McClead RE, Birken G, Wheller JJ, et al: Budd-Chiari syndrome in a premature infant receiving total parenteral nutrition. J Pediatr Gastroenterol Nutr 1986;5:655–658.
118. Roulet M, Laurine R, Rivier L: Hepatic venoocclusive disease in newborn infant of a woman drinking herbal tea. J Pediatr 1988;112:433–436.
119. Lambert GH, Muraskas J, Anderson CL, et al: Direct hyperbilirubinemia associated with chloral hydrate administration in the newborn. Pediatrics 1990;86:277–281.
120. Freeman J, Lesko SM, Mitchell AA, et al: Hyperbilirubinemia following exposure to pancuronium bromide in newborns. Devel Pharmacol Therapeut 1990;14:209–215.
121. Krowchuk D, Seashore JH: Complete biliary obstruction due to erythromycin estolate administration in an infant. Pediatrics 1979;64:956–958.
122. Shneider B, Maller E, Marter LV, et al: Cholestasis in infants supported with extracorporeal membrane oxygenation. J Pediatr 1989;115:462–465.
123. Roberts EA: Drug induced liver disease in children. In Suchy F (ed): Liver Disease in Children. St Louis, Mosby, 1994, pp 523–549.
124. De Wolf-Peeters C, Moens-Bullens AM, Van Assghe A, et al: Conjugated bilirubin in foetal liver in erythroblastosis. Lancet 1969;1:471.
125. Taylor WF, Qaqundah B: Neonatal jaundice associated with cystic fibrosis. Am J Dis Child 1972;123:161–162.
126. Fitz JG, Basavappa S, McGill J, et al: Regulation of membrane chloride currents in the rat bile duct epithelial cells. J Clin Invest 1993;91:319–328.
127. Lautt WW, Greenwall CV: Conceptual review of the hepatic vasculature. Hepatology 1987;7:952–963.
128. Kanel GC, Ucci A, Kaplan MM: A distinctive perivenular hepatic lesion associated with heart failure. Am J Clin Pathol 1980;73:235–239.
129. Rawson JS, Achord JL: Shock liver. South Med J 1985;78:1421–1425.
130. Garland JS, Werlin SL, Rice TB: Ischemic hepatitis in children: diagnosis and clinical course. Crit Care Med 1988;16:1209–1212.
131. Cohen JA, Kaplan MM: Left-sided heart failure presenting as hepatitis. Gastroenterology 1978;74:583–587.
132. Weinberg AG, Bolande G: The liver in congenital heart disease: effects of infantile coarctation of the aorta and the hypoplastic left syndrome in infancy. Am J Dis Child 1970;119:390–393.
133. Shiraki K: Hepatic cell necrosis in the newborn: a pathologic study of 147 cases with particular reference to congenital heart disease. Am J Dis Child 1970;119:395–400.
134. Weldon AP, Danks DM: Congenital hypothyroidism and neonatal jaundice. Arch Dis Child 1972;47:469–471.
135. Herman SP, Baggenstoss AH, Cloutier MD: Liver dysfunction and histologic abnormalities in neonatal hypopituitarism. J Pediatr 1975;87:892–895.
136. Kaufman FR, Costin G, Thomas W: Neonatal cholestasis and hypopituitarism. Acta Paediatr Scand 1984;59:787–798.
137. Leblanc A, Odievre M, Hadchouel M: Neonatal cholestasis and hypoglycemia: possible role of cortisol deficiency. J Pediatr 1981;99:577–579.
138. Sheehan AG, Martin SR, Stephure D, et al: Neonatal cholestasis, hypoglycemia and congenital hypopituitarism. J Pediatr Gastroenterol Nutr 1992;14:426–430.
139. Layden TJ, Boyer JL: The effect of thyroid hormone on bile flow and Na, K-ATPase activity in liver plasma membranes enriched in bile canaliculi. J Clin Invest 1976;57:1009–1018.
140. Alpert LI, Strauss L, Hirschhorn K: Neonatal hepatitis and biliary atresia associated with trisomy 17–18 syndrome. N Engl J Med 1969;280:16–20.
141. Puri P, Guiney EJ: Intrahepatic biliary atresia in Down's syndrome. J Pediatr Surg 1975;10:423–424.
142. Miyauchi J, Ito Y, Kawano T, et al: Unusual diffuse liver fibrosis accompanying transient myeloproliferative disorder in Down's syndrome: a report of four autopsy cases and proposal of a hypothesis. Blood 1992;80:1521–1527.
143. Laxer RM, Roberts EA, Gross KR: Liver disease in neonatal lupus erythematosus. J Pediatr 1989;116:238–242.
144. Cascino A, Cangiano C, Calcaterra V, et al: Plasma aminoacids imbalance in patients with liver disease. Am J Dig Dis 1978;23:591–598.
145. Goulet OJ, de Ville de Goyet J, Otte JB, et al: Preoperative nutritional evaluation and support for liver transplantation in children. Transplant Proc 1987;19:3249–3255.
146. Sokol RJ: Medical management of neonatal cholestasis. In Balistreri WF, Stocker JT (eds): Pediatric Hepatology. Philadelphia, Hemisphere Publishing, 1990, pp 41–76.
147. Hansen AE, Wiese HF, Boelihe AN, et al: Role of linoleic acid in infant nutrition. Pediatrics 1963;31:171–192.
148. Argao E, Heubi J, Hollis B, et al: D-Alpha tocopherol polyethylene glycol-1000 succinate (TPGS) enhances absorption of vitamin D in chronic cholestatic liver disease of infancy and childhood. Pediatr Res 1992;31:146–150.
149. Swain MG, Rothman RB, Xu H, et al: Endogenous opioids accumulate in plasma in a rat model of acute cholestasis. Gastroenterology 1992;103:630–635.
150. Rapaport SI, Klee WA, Pettigrew KD, et al: Entry of opioid peptides into the CNS. Science 1980;207:84–86.
151. Gillespie DA, Vickers CR: Pruritus and cholestasis: therapeutic options. J Gastroenterol Hepatol 1993;8:168–173.
152. Grundy SM, Ahrens EH, Salen G: Interruption of the enterohepatic circulation of bile acids in man: comparative effects of cholestyramine and ileal exclusion on cholesterol metabolism. J Lab Clin Med 1971;78:94–121.
153. Lloyd-Still JD: Cholestyramine therapy and intestinal obstruction in infants. Pediatrics 1977;89:626–627.
154. Stiehl A, Thaler MM, Admirad WH: The effects of phenobarbital on bile salts and bilirubin in patients with intrahepatic and extrahepatic cholestasis. N Engl J Med 1972;286:858–861.
155. Cynamon HA, Andres JM, Iafrate RP: Rifampin relieves pruritus in children with cholestatic liver disease. Gastroenterology 1990;98:1013–1016.

156. Balistreri WF: Bile acid therapy in pediatric hepatobiliary disease: the role of ursodeoxycholic acid. J Pediatr Gastroenterol Nutr 1997;24:573–589.
157. Ballatori N, Clarkson TN: Developmental changes in the biliary excretion of methyl-mercury and glutathione. Science 1982;216:61–63.
158. Balistreri WF, Novak DA, Farrell MK: Bile acid metabolism, total parenteral nutrition and cholestasis. In Lebenthal E (ed): Total Parenteral Nutrition: Indications, Utilization, Complications and Pathophysiological Considerations. New York, Raven Press, 1986, p 319.
159. Berg RD: Bacterial translocation from the gastrointestinal tract. J Med 1992;23:217–244.
160. Kakis G, Yousef IM: Pathogenesis of lithocholic acid and taurolithocholic acid induced intrahepatic cholestasis in rats. Gastroenterology 1978;75:595–607.
161. MacGregor IL, Wiley ZD, Lavigne ME, et al: Slowed rate of gastric emptying of solid food in man by high caloric parenteral nutrition. Am J Surg 1979;138:652–654.
162. Ducrotte P, Koning E, Guillemat F, et al: Jejunal motility during cyclic total parenteral nutrition. Gut 1989;30:815–819.
163. Greenberg GR, Wolman SL, Christofides ND, et al: Effect of total parenteral nutrition on gut hormone release in humans. Gastroenterology 1981;80:988–993.
164. Lucas A, Bloom SR, Aynsley-Green A: Metabolic and endocrine consequences of depriving preterm infants of enteral nutrition. Acta Paediatr Scand 1983;72:245–249.
165. Jarvenpaa AL, Rassin DL, Kuitunen P, et al: Feeding the low-birth-weight infant: III. Diet influences bile acid metabolism. Pediatrics 1983;72:677–683.
166. Merritt RJ: Cholestasis associated with total parenteral nutrition. J Pediatr Gastroenterol Nutr 1986;5:9–22.

# Chapter 48

# Biliary Atresia and Neonatal Disorders of the Bile Ducts

*Philip Rosenthal*

## BILIARY ATRESIA

Biliary atresia is defined as an idiopathic, serious disorder affecting the newborn that results in complete obliteration of the biliary tract.[1] The resultant obstruction to bile flow causes cholestasis and progressive fibrosis with end-stage cirrhosis. The progressive, inflammatory process observed in biliary atresia affects the extrahepatic biliary tree as well as the intrahepatic biliary tree. Thus, the previous designation "extrahepatic biliary atresia" is more appropriately referred to as simply "biliary atresia." It is estimated that biliary atresia affects 1 in 15,000 live births with a slight predominence in girls.[2] Biliary atresia can result in the development of end-stage liver disease within the first year of life and remains the leading indication for liver transplantation in children.[3]

Two forms of biliary atresia have been recognized.[1, 4, 5] The embryonic or fetal type of biliary atresia occurs in 10% to 35% of cases and is the less commonly observed presentation. In this form there is early onset of neonatal cholestasis and no jaundice-free interval between the end of physiologic jaundice of the newborn and the onset of the cholestasis. This form of biliary atresia is often associated (10–20%) with congenital malformations, suggesting that the insult occurs prenatally. Congenital anomalies include the laterality sequence (polysplenia, cardiovascular defects, asplenia, abdominal situs inversus, intestinal malrotation, and vascular malformations of the portal vein and hepatic artery) or isolated anomalies of the gastrointestinal, urinary, or cardiac systems. Bile duct remnants are rarely seen at the time of exploratory laparotomy. Although these associated anomalies may suggest a genetic influence, no cases of familial biliary atresia with the laterality sequence have been recognized.

The more common perinatal type that occurs in 65% to 90% of cases usually presents at 4 to 8 weeks of life with persistent cholestasis and jaundice. These affected children have a benign initial history, having been born full-term with a normal birth weight and passing normally pigmented meconium stools. Often, after physiologic jaundice passes, there may be a short period of a jaundice-free interval. Stools that are usually normally pigmented after meconium passage become progressively more acholic (chalky, white, lacking bile pigment) as the process evolves. At exploratory laparotomy, remnants of a previous bile duct structure may be found in the hepatoduodenal ligament.

### Pathogenesis

The etiologic mechanism(s) for biliary atresia remain(s) enigmatic. Several proposed hypotheses have been contemplated over the years, but none alone seems to explain the disease process clinically observed.

Because the disease occurs so early in the perinatal period a genetic factor being causal or contributory must be considered. Biliary atresia is not thought to be inherited. While there are case reports of biliary atresia occurring in families, there are also reports of HLA identical twins who are discordant for biliary atresia.[6–8] In one study, HLA-B12 was found more commonly then expected in children with biliary atresia without other associated anomalies.[9] Preliminary data from my own group have suggested an increased incidence of HLA-Cw4/7 in children with biliary atresia.[10] Additionally, the HLA-Cw7 locus has also been observed more frequently in adults with primary sclerosing cholangitis.[11]

The less common embryonic or fetal type of biliary atresia associated with the laterality sequence and splenic malformations might be considered a prime candidate for a gene defect. Although left-right asymmetry is genetically controlled, there have been no reports of familial cases of biliary atresia with the laterality sequence.

Other mechanisms to explain the progressive destruction of the bile ducts in biliary atresia include the possibility of ischemia or toxic injury. These have been considered less likely candidates because no abnormal bile acids have been discovered and no single environmental toxin has been linked to biliary atresia in humans.

Several studies have investigated immunologic causes for biliary atresia.[12, 13] In these theories, the possibility of abnormal HLA class I molecules on the biliary epithelium or abnormal expression of inflammatory adhesion molecules such as ICAM-1 has been proposed. Preliminary work has demonstrated the presence of antineutrophil cytoplasmic antibodies (ANCA) in the serum of children with biliary atresia.[14] ANCA positivity in adults with hepatic disorders has been associated with primary sclerosing cholangitis and autoimmune liver disease.

A defect in the development of the biliary system in the fetus has been proposed to explain biliary atresia. Failure of the normal remodeling process at the hepatic hilum with persistence of fetal bile ducts is an attractive hypothesis to explain at least some cases of biliary atresia. In fact, a mouse model (the *inv* mutation on mouse chromosome 4) of biliary atresia has been reported.[15] In this model, there is abnormal development of the common bile duct, jaundice, complete abdominal situs inversus, and death within the first week of life. These anomalies of left-right symmetry, polysplenia, and preduodenal portal vein are similar to the findings of some children with the fetal type of biliary atresia.

Studies directed at the development of the intrahepatic bile ducts have been performed by Desmet and others.[5, 16, 17] Using anticytokeratin antibodies, it was found that the intrahepatic bile ducts appear to arise from primitive hepatocytes that undergo a phenotypical switch (metaplasia) to form ductular cells. Evidence of bile ductular replication in normal fetal livers was not found. In contrast, in the livers of children with biliary atresia, we observed both bile ductular metaplasia and proliferation. The arrest in the remodeling of the ductular cells such that a lumen does not form has been referred to as a "ductal plate malformation" and may explain some cases of biliary atresia.

A vascular insult during hepatobiliary development has been postulated as a potential cause of biliary atresia because of the finding of thickened, tortuous, and dilated arteries in the biliary remnant of some infants with biliary atresia.[18] No additional reports of this finding have occurred.

The role of viral infections in the etiology of biliary atresia has been frequently hypothesized. Reports of an association with cytomegalovirus, Epstein-Barr virus, and rubella have been made, but these common infections may be coincidental findings.[19, 20] In the 1980s reovirus type 3, which causes an obliterative cholangiopathy in weanling mice, was purported to be a potential infectious etiologic agent because children with biliary atresia tended to have serologic reactivity to this virus.[21–23] Unfortunately, further studies including those with molecular techniques have failed to substantiate this association.[24–27] More recently, studies focusing on an association of biliary atresia with rotavirus have been reported.[28, 29] Rotavirus group A causes biliary obstruction in a weanling mouse model. Preliminary reports of rotavirus group C in the stools, liver, and serum of children with biliary atresia require further verification.

## Diagnosis

A combination of laboratory, imaging, and histologic studies aids in establishing the diagnosis and differentiating biliary atresia from the extensive list of causes of neonatal cholestasis.[30] Because several studies have documented that successful reestablishment of bile flow is dependent on early surgical intervention,[31–33] it is imperative that an orderly, efficient, and cost-effective work-up proceed rapidly. The first step in the evaluation is to recognize the possibility of neonatal cholestasis and to fractionate the serum bilirubin. *A conjugated hyperbilirubinemia in a newborn is always pathologic and deserving of investigation.* Other laboratory studies include determination of serum transaminases, alkaline phosphatase, albumin, and prothrombin time, which may be of serial value in following the progression of the disease process but have no discriminatory value.

Ultrasonography is noninvasive and of significant screening value. An ultrasound examination may be helpful in detecting the presence of a choledochal cyst, presence and size of the gallbladder and extrahepatic common bile duct, or identification of anomalies such as polysplenia or preduodenal portal vein.

A simple and inexpensive test of biliary excretion can be achieved by serial observation of the stools by a trained observer. Description of the stool color by the parents is not acceptable because many parents misinterpret acholic stools for pale yellow or tan. The use of nuclear hepatobiliary scans (Fig. 48–1) or duodenal bile sampling via a string device (Fig. 48–2) or actual duodenal aspiration after phenobarbital pretreatment to induce bile flow may also aid in determining patency of the extrahepatic biliary tree.[34, 35] Unfortunately, severe intrahepatic cholestasis from numerous etiologic causes may result in false-positive nuclear hepatobiliary scans.

Endoscopic retrograde cholangiopancreatography (ERCP) has been advocated by some investigators as a helpful adjunct in the evaluation.[36, 37] The technical challenge to ac-

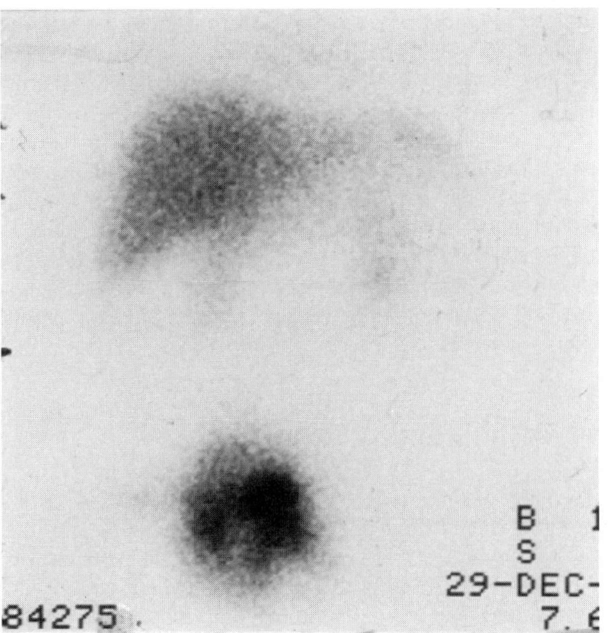


**FIGURE 48–1.** Hepatobiliary nuclear scan from an infant with conjugated hyperbilirubinemia and acholic stools. (From Rosenthal P: Pediatric liver disease. In Hyman PE [ed]: Gastroenterology and Hepatology—The Comprehensive Visual Reference, Vol 4, Pediatric GI Problems. Philadelphia, Current Medicine, 1997, with permission.)

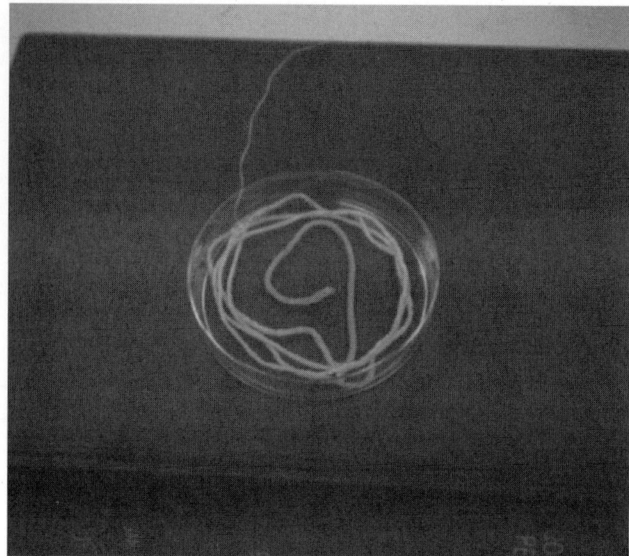

**FIGURE 48–2.** A string test from an infant with conjugated hyperbilirubinemia and history of acholic stools. Note the yellow pigmented bile-stained distal end of the string. (From Rosenthal P: Pediatric liver disease. In Hyman PE [ed]: Gastroenterology and Hepatology—The Comprehensive Visual Reference, Vol 4, Pediatric GI Problems. Philadelphia, Current Medicine, 1997, with permission.)

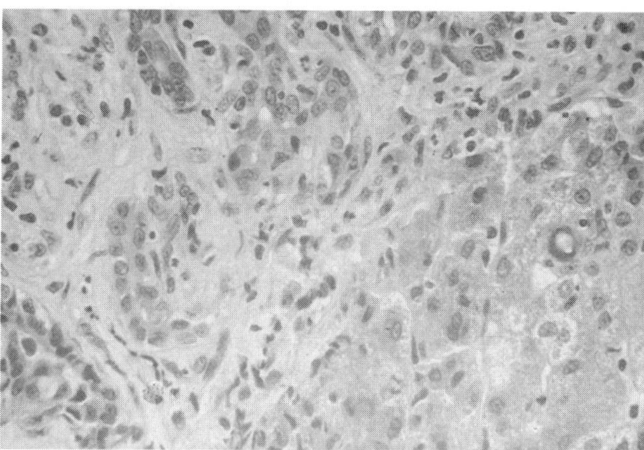

**FIGURE 48–3.** Percutaneous liver biopsy from a child with biliary atresia. Note the cholestasis characterized by bilirubinostasis and bile plugs. Other findings characteristic of biliary atresia include parenchymal giant cells, extramedullary hematopoiesis, ductular proliferation, and lymphocytic infiltration in the portal tracts and polymorphonuclear cells between the ductules. With continued cholestasis, portal and periportal fibrosis develop, proceeding to bridging fibrosis and cirrhosis if uncorrected. Hematoxylin-eosin stain, original magnification × 450. (From Rosenthal P: Pediatric liver disease. In Hyman PE [ed]: Gastroenterology and Hepatology—The Comprehensive Visual Reference, Vol 4, Pediatric GI Problems. Philadelphia, Current Medicine, 1997, with permission.)

complish this procedure in such small infants, and the need for certainty that the inability to demonstrate flow into the liver is not due to technical difficulties, make this procedure less universally applicable.

A percutaneous liver biopsy affords a reliable and accurate diagnostic means of establishing the diagnosis. Liver biopsy affords a diagnostic accuracy of close to 95% if an adequate sample is obtained and a skilled hepatopathologist examines the tissue. The histologic hallmarks of biliary atresia include bile ductular proliferation, canalicular and hepatocyte bile stasis, and periportal edema and fibrosis (Fig. 48–3).

If the initial diagnostic evaluation suggests biliary atresia, then exploratory laparotomy with intraoperative cholangiography is the next step. An attempt is made to inject contrast medium into the gallbladder if present. Patency must be established not just in the extrahepatic ductal system but also into the intrahepatic ducts because biliary atresia may occur at different anatomic levels. If biliary atresia is indeed present, then surgical therapy can proceed.

## Surgical Therapy

Excision of the atretic extrahepatic biliary tree, identification of a ductal remnant at the porta hepatis, and then anastomosis of a bowel segment to this ductal remnant form the basis for the Kasai portoenterostomy, which with several modifications has become the standard surgical procedure for the initial management of the child with a diagnosis of biliary atresia (Fig. 48–4).[31, 33, 38, 39] If performed early (in infants younger than 2 months of age), the Kasai portoenterostomy may successfully re-establish bile flow in up to 80% of infants. Unfortunately, re-establishment of bile flow alone does not guarantee long-term success. Predictors of poor outcome include white race, presence of cirrhosis on initial biopsy, absence of bile ducts at the liver hilum, and severe intrahepatic cholestasis. Approximately one third of children undergoing Kasai portoenterostomy do poorly soon after surgery and require liver transplantation within the first year of life, one third require liver transplants by their teenage years, and one third do reasonably well with varying degrees of liver disease.

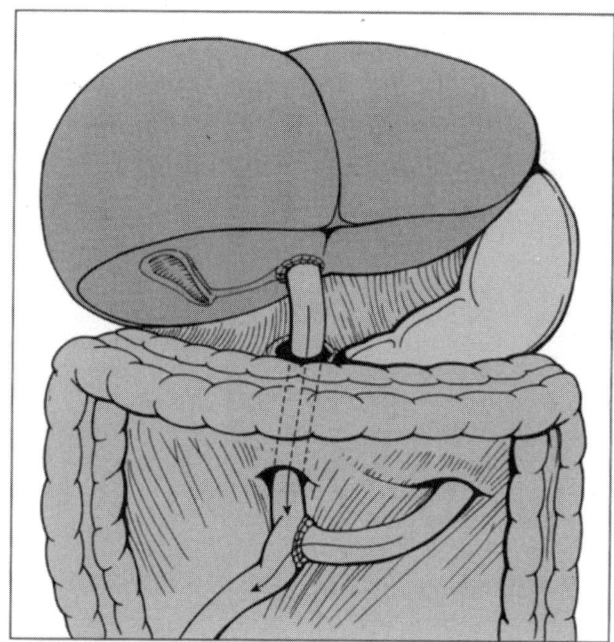

**FIGURE 48–4.** Kasai portoenterostomy for biliary atresia. (Adapted from Altman RP: Recent developments in hepatobiliary surgery. Pediatr Ann 1977;6:90, with permission.)

Biliary atresia is the leading indication for pediatric liver transplants in the United States and accounts for one half of all liver transplantation in children.[3] In the past, there was much debate as to the order of surgical procedures for the child with biliary atresia.[40–42] Currently, it is widely accepted that the Kasai portoenterostomy should be the primary surgical procedure. Multiple attempts at revising an unsuccessful Kasai portoenterostomy are discouraged because they are rarely successful and complicate later liver transplantation. Liver transplantation is appropriate therapy for the child with a failed Kasai portoenterostomy. Evidence of a failed Kasai procedure includes progressive cholestasis, hepatocellular decompensation, or development of portal hypertension and subsequent bleeding. The lack of donor organ availability particularly in the young child with biliary atresia has significantly hampered the ability to care for these sick children. Advances in surgical techniques to improve the donor organ pool for these children include the development of reduced-size liver transplant techniques, split-liver transplants, and living-related liver transplants.[43] Using these procedures has resulted in a significant decline in waiting list mortality for these children. Survival rates for children after liver transplantation for biliary atresia are in the 90% range in many centers (see Chapter 52).

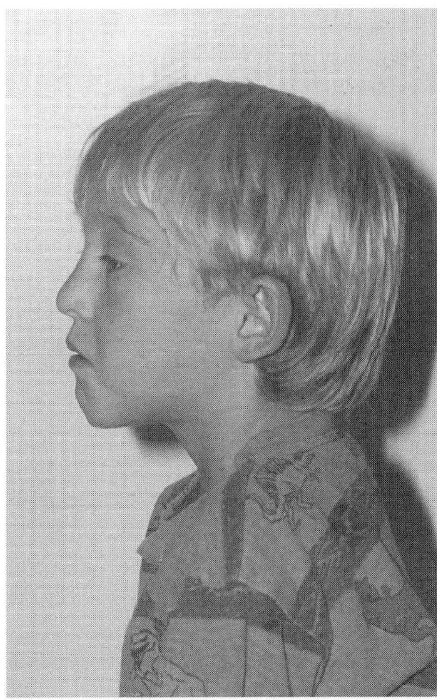

**FIGURE 48–5.** Typical facies associated with Alagille syndrome. Note frontal bossing, deep-set eyes, bulbous tip of the nose, and pointed chin. (From Rosenthal P: Pediatric liver disease. In Hyman PE [ed]: Gastroenterology and Hepatology—The Comprehensive Visual Reference, Vol 4, Pediatric GI Problems. Philadelphia, Current Medicine, 1997, with permission.)

## ALAGILLE SYNDROME

Alagille syndrome (arteriohepatic dysplasia, intrahepatic biliary hypoplasia, syndromic paucity of interlobular bile ducts) refers to a multisystemic disorder that has been recognized in all races throughout the world.[44, 45] It may be the most common of the familial intrahepatic cholestatic syndromes.

### Pathogenesis

There is good evidence to suggest that Alagille's syndrome is a hereditary disorder, being autosomal dominant with variable penetrance. Many cases appear to be sporadic, suggesting spontaneous mutations. Work suggests that some patients with Alagille syndrome have a deletion in the short arm of chromosome 20,[46–51] particularly in human Jagged1 gene.[51a]

### Diagnosis

The classic syndrome consists of five characteristics: (1) chronic cholestasis associated with pruritus and hypercholesterolemia and paucity of interlobular bile ducts on liver biopsy; (2) congenital heart disease (peripheral pulmonic stenosis being the most common); (3) bone defects including butterfly vertebrae and hemivertebrae and a lack of the progression of the interpedicular distance; (4) eye findings (especially posterior embryotoxon); and (5) typical facies including frontal bossing, deep-set eyes, bulbous tip of the nose, and pointed chin (Fig. 48–5). Not all patients with Alagille syndrome display all of the classic findings, making diagnosis in some patients difficult.[44, 45, 52–54]

The liver disease associated with Alagille syndrome may be highly variable. Jaundice during the first 6 weeks of life may be associated with Alagille syndrome with hepatic involvement. The cholestasis may be so severe that biliary atresia may need to be considered. With time, the jaundice may actually improve. However, severe cholestasis may persist, with intolerable pruritus and skin infections and lichenification the result. Exceedingly high cholesterol levels may lead to xanthomas, which can be quite debilitating (Fig. 48–6). Fat and fat-soluble vitamin malabsorption is noted. There are reports of hepatocellular carcinoma occurring in Alagille syndrome patients with cirrhosis.[55, 56]

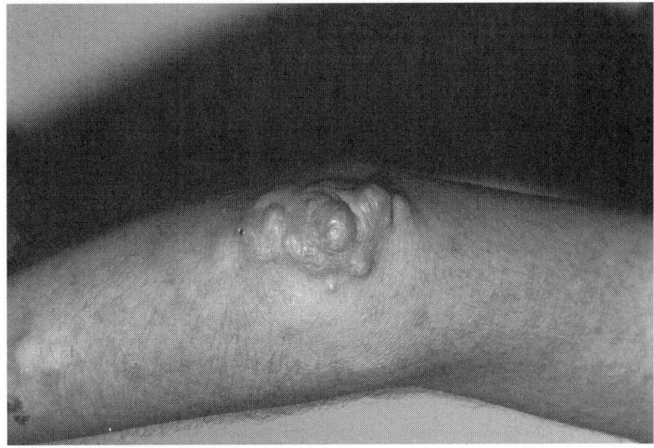

**FIGURE 48–6.** Severe xanthomas in a 7-year-old boy with Alagille syndrome. (From Rosenthal P: Pediatric liver disease. In Hyman PE [ed]: Gastroenterology and Hepatology—The Comprehensive Visual Reference, Vol 4, Pediatric GI Problems. Philadelphia, Current Medicine, 1997, with permission.)

The cardiovascular system may also be affected in patients with Alagille syndrome, with peripheral pulmonic stenosis being the most frequently encountered abnormality.[57] Other associated cardiac abnormalities have included tetralogy of Fallot, septal defects, and coarctation of the aorta. The cardiac disease in Alagille syndrome may be more clinically significant than the liver disease.

Renal disease may also be observed often late in the course of the disease, presumed secondary to prolonged hyperlipidemia and resulting in a membranous nephropathy affecting the glomeruli and tubules.[58, 59] Other congenital renal defects reported include reduplication of the renal pelvis, interstitial fibrosis, juvenile nephronophthisis, medullary cysts, and single kidney.

Skeletal abnormalities associated with Alagille syndrome include the classic butterfly vertebrae.[60] Other reported deformities include hemivertebrae, incomplete spina bifida, shortening of the distal phalanges, short ulna, and a lack of the normal progressive widening of the interpedicular distance down the lumbar spine. A seronegative polyarticular arthritis may also be observed in some cases.[61] Many of the bony abnormalities observed in Alagille syndrome cause little clinical symptomatology for the patient. However, significant osteopenia from poor vitamin D and calcium absorption due to the severe cholestasis may result in pathologic bone fractures in many of these children.

Ophthalmologic findings also occur in Alagille syndrome.[62] Most common is posterior embryotoxon, a thickening of Schwalbe's line, which does not interfere with vision. Other associated findings include Axenfeld's anomaly (strands observed in the iris that if connected to the posterior embryotoxon can result in glaucoma). Vitamin A and/or E deficiency may result in retinal pigmentary changes with resultant night blindness or tunnel vision. High myopia and keratoconus have also been observed, and many of these children require eyeglasses for correction.[63]

In some patients with Alagille syndrome pancreatic insufficiency has been recognized.[64, 65] Although the etiology of this pancreatic insufficiency is unknown, Alagille syndrome children with diarrhea not on the basis of cholestasis should be evaluated for pancreatic insufficiency.

Dermatologic problems associated with Alagille syndrome have predominantly been the result of the severe cholestasis. Lichenification from chronic pruritus and xanthomata from elevated cholesterol levels may be commonly observed.[66] Reports of photosensitivity and porphyric rashes have also been documented.[67]

Reports of recurrent otitis media and hearing deficits have been made in association with Alagille syndrome. An unusual finding has been the complete or partial absence of the posterior semicircular canal in some Alagille syndrome patients.[68]

Neurologic abnormalities including mental retardation were initially considered significantly associated with Alagille syndrome in early reports. Subsequently, it has been recognized that vitamin deficiencies, in particular that of vitamin E, may have been responsible for this clinical association. Most patients with Alagille syndrome have normal or above-normal intelligence. Central nervous system vascular abnormalities have been reported in a few patients with Alagille syndrome.[52, 64, 69] These have included intracranial hemorrhages, Arnold-Chiari malformation, and a complete occlusion of the internal carotid arteries with collateral formation.

### Therapy

Most therapy required for Alagille syndrome focuses on dealing with the complications of cholestasis.[70, 71] Severe fat and fat-soluble vitamin malabsorption often requires vitamins A, D, E, and K supplementation. Infants may require specialized formulas with medium-chain triglycerides as the major fat component. Some children with Alagille syndrome benefit from continuous feedings via nasogastric tube or gastrostomy tube. This allows for increased calories for children who may be unable to physically eat the required calories needed for growth because of severe malabsorption.

The pruritus associated with Alagille syndrome may be exceedingly difficult to manage. Potentially useful medications include bile salt–binding resins such as cholestyramine, rifampin, and either phenobarbital or ursodeoxycholic acid.[72]

The surgical biliary diversion procedure often used for other intrahepatic cholestatic syndromes is not effective in Alagille syndrome.[73] A small percentage of children with Alagille syndrome progress to end-stage liver disease and benefit from liver transplantation.[43, 74] Liver transplantation may also be indicated for patients with Alagille syndrome with intractable itching unresponsive to medical therapy, portal hypertension, and growth failure.

## PROGRESSIVE FAMILIAL INTRAHEPATIC CHOLESTASIS (BYLER'S SYNDROME/DISEASE)

Progressive familial intrahepatic cholestasis (PFIC) refers to a more heterogeneous group then Alagille syndrome. In this diagnosis, there are two subtypes: PFIC type 1, in which patients have normal serum gamma glutamyl transpeptidase, and type 2, in which patients have elevated serum gamma glutamyl transpeptidase activity.[75] The original description of these disorders included four Dutch Amish sibships each named Byler with a disorder of progressive intrahepatic cholestasis.[76] Byler's syndrome begins in infancy, is progressive, and leads to fibrosis, cirrhosis, and death unless liver transplantation is performed.[77]

There is no elevation or only a modest elevation in serum gamma glutamyl transpeptidase and cholesterol levels. No associated abnormalities are noted in other organ systems. Byler's syndrome differs from other childhood cholestatic disorders in that there is a profound and selective decrease in bile acid levels in bile.[78] Bile acid synthesis in these children is normal, suggesting a primary defect in canalicular bile acid transport. Because of the severe cholestasis, these children often suffer from severe pruritus and fat malabsorption, with concomitant rickets and growth failure. Surgical therapy in the form of a biliary diversion procedure in which a biliary-cutaneous fistula is created to allow bile to be collected in a stoma and to be discarded may have significant improvement in pruritus and histology if performed early in the course.[73, 79]

Byler's syndrome is hereditable. There is often a history of an affected sibling or consanguinity. A search for chromosomal segments in these children led to localization of the Byler's syndrome gene to chromosome 18. Recent work suggests that the gene for Byler's syndrome is at the same region of chromosome 18 as the gene for benign recurrent intrahepatic cholestasis (BRIC) (see later).[80] The data suggest that Byler's syndrome and BRIC may be allelic disorders resulting from different mutations in the same gene.

For children with progressive liver disease leading to hepatic failure, liver transplantation is a viable option. Byler's disease has not recurred in the transplanted liver, suggesting that liver replacement replaces the defect permanently.[81] Because hepatocellular carcinoma has been reported in Byler's syndrome, surveillance is warranted and consideration of liver transplantation before this development may be justified.[82–84]

## BENIGN RECURRENT INTRAHEPATIC CHOLESTASIS

As the name implies, BRIC refers to a disorder of recurrent episodes of cholestasis with a normal extrahepatic biliary tree that can mimic extrahepatic biliary obstruction.[85, 86] Recently, the mode of inheritance of BRIC has been elucidated from study of a Dutch kindred. The inheritance is compatible with an autosomal recessive pattern.[87] Genetic analysis has demonstrated a defect in chromosome 18 responsible for this disorder. Furthermore, localization of the gene has shown that the gene for BRIC is allelic to the gene for Byler's syndrome.[80]

Episodes may vary greatly in duration and age at onset. There is no progression to cirrhosis and no consequences of chronic liver disease. The cholestasis may be severe with pruritus, restlessness, and weight loss lasting from weeks to months. Laboratory studies demonstrate typical findings of cholestasis, with elevations of serum alkaline phosphatase, bile acids, and cholesterol but, similar to Byler's syndrome, a normal serum gamma glutamyl transpeptidase level.

## NONSYNDROMIC PAUCITY

Several different causes may be responsible for a paucity of intrahepatic bile ducts in infants in which syndromic causes have been excluded.[88, 89] These disorders may be categorized into infectious, chromosomal, and metabolic abnormalities. Congenital infections (rubella, syphilis, hepatitis B, cytomegalovirus) have been associated with intrahepatic bile duct paucity. Chromosomal defects include partial trisomy 11, monosomy X, and trisomy 18 and 21, which have been associated with bile duct paucity as well as with biliary atresia. Alpha$_1$-antitrypsin deficiency may result in bile duct paucity in association with a neonatal hepatitis and portends a poor prognosis. Other metabolic disorders with this finding include cystic fibrosis, Zellweger's (cerebrohepatorenal) syndrome, prune belly syndrome, and hypopituitarism.

Chronic hepatobiliary disease may also terminate in bile duct paucity. Children with biliary atresia with re-establishment of bile flow by Kasai portoenterostomy may develop a paucity of intrahepatic bile ducts in the late stages of disease. Immunologically mediated disorders such as primary sclerosing cholangitis, primary biliary cirrhosis, graft-versus-host disease after bone marrow transplantation, and chronic rejection after liver transplantation can lead to bile duct paucity.[90, 91]

## CHOLEDOCHAL CYST

Choledochal cysts occur in girls four times more frequently than in boys, with an estimated incidence of 1 in 13,000 to 2 million live births. It is more frequently observed in Asians, and about half of the cases are diagnosed during infancy.[92, 93]

Choledochal cysts have been categorized into several different types.[94] Type I, which is the most common type encountered, consists of a diffuse enlargement of the common bile duct. Types II and III affect the extrahepatic bile ducts. Type II consists of a diverticular cyst, and type III consists of a choledochocele. Type IV consists of multiple intrahepatic and extrahepatic cysts. Type V is also referred to as Caroli's disease, which is considered a ductal plate malformation resulting in intrahepatic dilatation of the biliary tree.

The etiology of choledochal cysts remains an enigma. One theory suggests a defect in the junction of the common bile duct and the pancreatic duct, which allows pancreatric fluid to reflux into the common duct causing injury.[95–97] Whereas the anatomy and finding of amylase in choledochal cysts support this theory, the presence of prenatal choledochal cysts on ultrasound examination in the first trimester raises questions about the likelihood of injury of pancreatic fluid reflux.[98]

Most patients with a choledochal cyst are recognized during infancy.[99, 100] The combination of jaundice and abdominal pain occurs much more frequently then in combination with the appreciation of an abdominal mass. Often fever, nausea, and vomiting are accompanying complaints on presentation.

Ultrasonography is a valued and preferred means of screening for a choledochal cyst (Fig. 48–7). Differentiation of a cystic structure that is not the gallbladder is an important consideration. If there is doubt after ultrasound examination, the use of nuclear hepatobiliary scans or computed tomography or magnetic resonance imaging may provide important discriminatory information.[101, 102] Ultimate diagnosis can be confirmed by an intraoperative cholangiogram at surgery.

Therapy for choledochal cysts is complete surgical excision.[103, 104] It has been well documented that the epithelial lining of choledochal cysts can undergo malignant transformation with time.[105, 106] Adenocarcinoma is the most common malignancy associated with retained choledochal cysts and often results in a poor outcome. In the past, many surgeons performed internal drainage procedures for choledochal cysts.[107] Many of these patients have been doing well with this procedure; however, the risk of malignancy is great enough to warrant revision and excision of the retained cyst.

## NEONATAL SCLEROSING CHOLANGITIS

Sclerosing cholangitis refers to a disorder with irregular narrowing of either the extrahepatic or the intrahepatic bile ducts. Although more common in adults, the diagnosis is

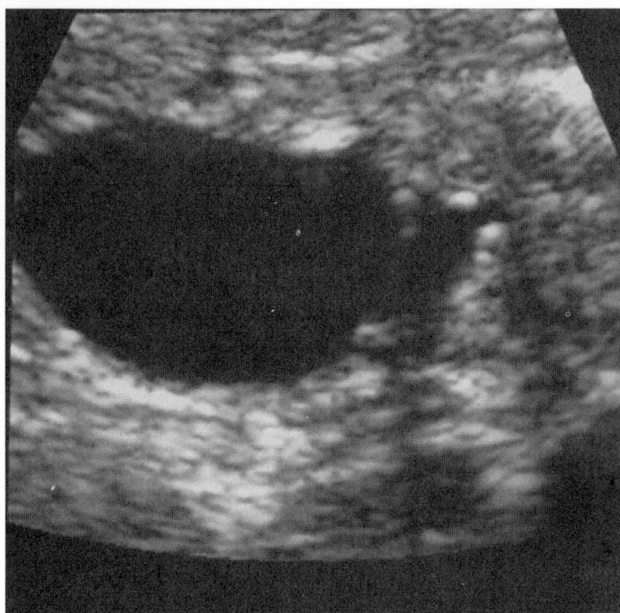

**FIGURE 48–7.** Ultrasonographic findings of a choledochal cyst in an infant with a conjugated hyperbilirubinemia and acholic stools. (From Rosenthal P: Pediatric liver disease. In Hyman PE [ed]: Gastroenterology and Hepatology—The Comprehensive Visual Reference, Vol 4, Pediatric GI Problems. Philadelphia, Current Medicine, 1997, with permission.)

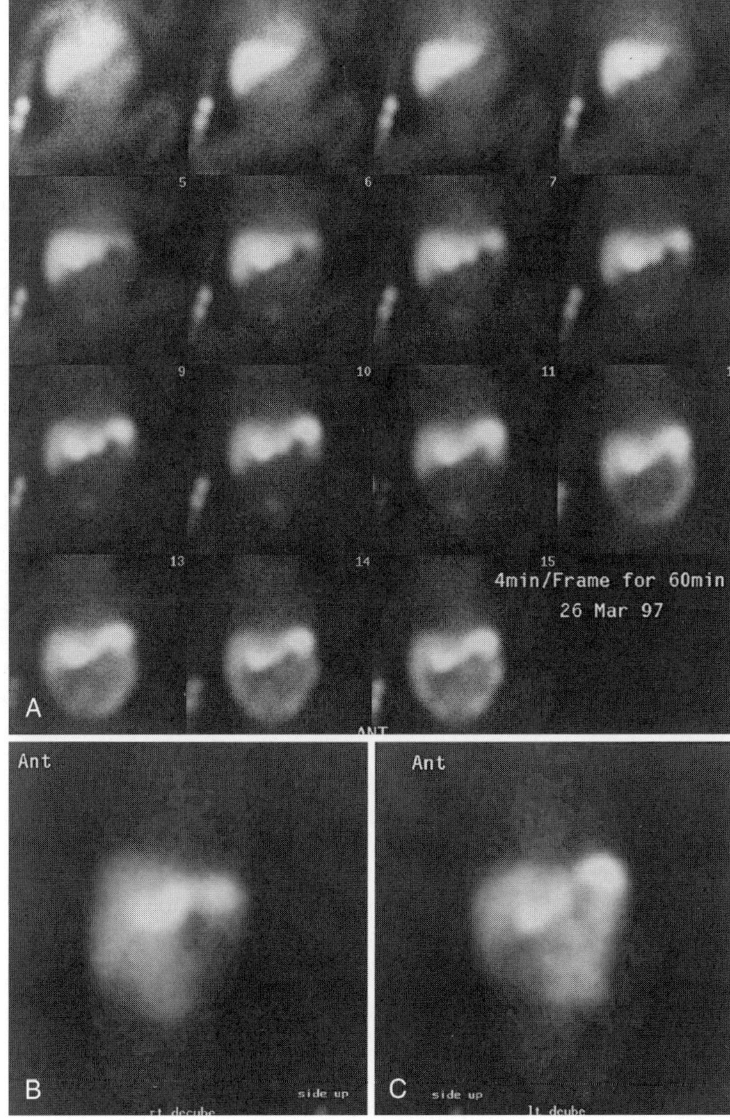


**FIGURE 48–8.** Nuclear hepatobiliary scan in an infant with spontaneous perforation of the bile duct. Note concentration of isotope in the liver followed by the presence of the isotope diffusely throughout the abdomen in later frames. *A*, Moving the patient from side to side in right *(B)* and left *(C)* decubitus positions confirms the isotope freely moves within the peritoneum. (Courtesy of Dr. William Bediger.)

confirmed by radiologic study and is often associated with other disorders such as ulcerative colitis. A neonatal form of sclerosing cholangitis has been reported in infants.[108, 109] Jaundice was observed within the first weeks of life. Liver histology revealed a cholangiopathy that progressed to a biliary cirrhosis between 2 and 9 years of age. Radiologic examination by percutaneous cholecystography disclosed abnormal intrahepatic and extrahepatic bile ducts with rarefaction of segmental branches, stenosis, and focal dilation. Clinical symptoms soon after birth suggest the possibility of an in utero onset. A history of consanguinity in many of these affected infants suggests an inherited basis for this disorder.

## SPONTANEOUS PERFORATION OF BILE DUCTS

Spontaneous perforation of the bile ducts is a rare but documented problem in the newborn that may present as a conjugated hyperbilirubinemia.[110–114] Although the cause is unknown, there is a predilection for the perforation to occur at the confluence of the cystic duct and the common bile duct, suggesting a particular susceptibility to weakness or injury at this site. Spontaneous perforation of the bile ducts occurs between 4 and 12 weeks of age. Infants may have lethargy, nonbilious vomiting, acholic stools, mild jaundice, dark urine, abdominal distention, and, rarely, an abdominal catastrophe. Serum biochemical tests reveal a mildly elevated conjugated hyperbilirubinemia. Nuclear hepatobiliary imaging (Fig. 48–8) and abdominal paracentesis may be helpful in establishing the diagnosis. Therapy requires surgical intervention in an attempt to repair the perforation if possible and to re-establish bile flow from the liver to the intestine while decompressing the biliary tree.

## REFERENCES


1. Balistreri WF, Grand R, Hoofnagle JH, et al: Biliary atresia: current concepts and research directions. Hepatology 1996;23:1682–1692.
2. Balistreri WF: Neonatal cholestasis—medical progress. J Pediatr 1985;106:171–184.
3. 1996 Annual Report of the U.S. Scientific Registry for Transplant Recipients and the Organ Procurement and Transplantation Network—Transplant Data: 1988–1995. UNOS, Richmond, VA, and the Division of Transplantation, Bureau of Health Resources Development, Health Resources and Services Administration, U.S. Department of Health and Human Services, Rockville, MD, p 81.
4. Schweizer P: Treatment of extrahepatic bile duct atresia: results and long-term prognosis after hepatic portoenterostomy. Pediatr Surg Int 1986;1:30–36.
5. Desmet VJ: Congenital diseases of intrahepatic bile ducts: variation on the theme "ductal plate malformation." Hepatology 1992;16:1069–1083.
6. Smith BM, Laberge JM, Schreiber R, et al: Familial biliary atresia in three siblings including twins. J Pediatr Surg 1991;26:1331–1333.
7. Moore TC, Hyman PE: Extrahepatic biliary atresia in one human leukocyte antigen identical twin. Pediatrics 1985;76:604–605.
8. Werlin S: Extrahepatic biliary atresia in one of twins. Acta Paediatr 1981;70:943.
9. Silveira TR, Salzano FM, Donaldson PT, et al: Association between HLA and extrahepatic biliary atresia. J Pediatr Gastroenterol Nutr 1993;16:114–117.
10. Rosenthal P, Woolf GM, Tyan DB: A striking association between HLA-C and biliary atresia. Gastroenterology 1995;108:A1158.
11. Moloney MM, Thomson LJ, Donaldson PT, et al: HLA Cw genotypes in primary sclerosing cholangitis: HLA Cw marks the telomeric limit of HLA-encoded susceptibility in PSC. Hepatology 1996;24:169A.
12. Screiber RA, Kleinman RE, Barksdale EM, et al: Rejection of murine cogenic bile ducts: model for immune-mediated bile duct disease. Gastroenterology 1992;102:924–930.
13. Dillon P, Belchis D, Tracy T, et al: Increased expression of intracellular adhesion molecules in biliary atresia. Am J Pathol 1994;145:263–267.
14. Vasiliauskas EA, Targan SR, Cobb L, et al: Biliary atresia—an autoimmune mediated disorder? Hepatology 1995;22:128A.
15. Yokoyama T, Copeland NG, Jenkins NA, et al: Reversal of left-right asymmetry: a situs inversus mutation. Science 1993;260:679–682.
16. Desmet VJ: Embryology of the liver and intrahepatic biliary tract, an overview of malformations of the bile duct. In McIntyre N, Benhamou J-P, Bircher J, et al (eds): The Oxford Textbook of Clinical Hepatology, Vol 1. Oxford, Oxford University Press, 1991, pp 497–519.
17. Cocjin J, Rosenthal P, Buslon V, et al: Bile ductule formation in fetal, neonatal, and infant liver compared with extrahepatic biliary atresia. Hepatology 1996;24:568–574.
18. Ho C-W, Shioda K, Shirasaki K, et al: The pathogenesis of biliary atresia: a morphological study of the hepatobiliary system and the hepatic artery. J Pediatr Gastroenterol Nutr 1993;16:53–60.
19. Hart MH, Kaufman SS, Vanderhoof JA, et al: Neonatal hepatitis and extrahepatic biliary atresia associated with cytomegalovirus infection in twins. Am J Dis Child 1991;145:302–305.
20. Chang M-H, Huan H-H, Huan E-S, et al: Polymerase chain reaction to detect human cytomegalovirus in livers of infants with neonatal hepatitis. Gastroenterology 1992;103:1022–1025.
21. Bangaru B, Morecki R, Glasser JH, et al: Comparative studies of biliary atresia in the human newborn and reovirus-induced cholangitis in weanling mice. Lab Invest 1980;43:456–462.
22. Phillips PA, Keast D, Papadimitiau JM, et al: Chronic obstructive jaundice induced by reovirus type 3 in weanling mice. Pathology 1969;1:193–203.
23. Morecki R, Glaser JH, Cho S, et al: Biliary atresia and reovirus type 3 infection. N Engl J Med 1982;307:481.
24. Dussaix E, Hadchouel M, Tardieu M, et al: Biliary atresia and reovirus type 3 infection. N Engl J Med 1984;310:658.
25. Brown WR, Sokol RJ, Levin MJ, et al: Lack of correlation between infection with reovirus 3 and extrahepatic biliary atresia or neonatal hepatitis. J Pediatr 1988;113:670–676.
26. Steele MI, Marshall CM, Lloyd RE, et al: Reovirus 3 not detected by reverse transcriptase-mediated polymerase chain reaction analysis of preserved tissue from infants with cholestatic liver disease. Hepatology 1995;21:697–702.
27. Rosenthal P: The association of reovirus 3 and biliary atresia: finally resolved? Am J Gastroenterol 1995;90:1895–1896.
28. Riepenhoff-Talty M, Shaekel K, Clark HF, et al: Group A rotaviruses produce extrahepatic biliary obstruction in orally inoculated newborn mice. Pediatr Res 1993;33:394–399.
29. Riepenhoff-Talty M, Gouvea V, Evans MJ, et al: Detection of group C rotavirus in infants with extrahepatic biliary atresia. J Infect Dis 1996;174:8–15.
30. Rosenthal P, Sinatra FR: Jaundice in infancy. Pediatr Rev 1989;11:79–86.
31. Kasai M: Treatment of biliary atresia with special reference to hepatic portoenterostomy and its modifications. Prog Pediatr Surg 1974;6:5–52.
32. Chandra RS, Altman RP: Ductal remnants in extrahepatic biliary atresia: a histopathologic study with clinical correlation. J Pediatr 1978;93:196–200.
33. Lally KP, Kanegaye J, Matsumura M, et al: Perioperative factors affecting the outcome following repair of biliary atresia. Pediatrics 1989;83:723–726.
34. Majd M, Reba RC, Altman RP: Hepatobiliary scintigraphy with $^{99m}$Tc-PIPIDA in the evaluation of neonatal jaundice. Pediatrics 1981;67:140–145.
35. Rosenthal P, Liebman WM, Sinatra FR, et al: String test in evaluation of cholestatic jaundice in infancy. J Pediatr 1985;107:253–255.
36. Lebwohl O, Waye JD: Endoscopic retrograde cholangiopancreatography in the diagnosis of extrahepatic biliary atresia. Am J Dis Child 1979;133:647–649.
37. Heyman MB, Shapiro HA, Thaler MM: Endoscopic retrograde cholangiography in the diagnosis of biliary malformations in infants. Gastrointest Endosc 1988;34:449–453.

38. Kasai M, Mochizuki I, Ohkohchi N, et al: Surgical limitations for biliary atresia: indication for liver transplantation. J Pediatr Surg 1989;24:851–854.
39. Laurent J, Gauthier F, Bernard O, et al: Long-term outcome after surgery for biliary atresia: study of 40 patients surviving for more than 10 years. Gastroenterology 1990;99:1793–1797.
40. Lilly JR: Biliary atresia and liver transplantation: the National Institutes of Health point of view. Pediatrics 1984;74:159–160.
41. Lilly JR: The National Institutes of Health point of view. Pediatrics 1985;75:802–803.
42. Lilly JR, Hall RJ, Altman RP: Liver transplantation and Kasai operation in the first year of life: therapeutic dilemma in biliary atresia. J Pediatr 1987;110:561–562.
43. Rosenthal P, Podesta L, Sher L, et al: Liver transplantation in children. Am J Gastroenterol 1994;89:480–492.
44. Watson GH, Miller V: Arteriohepatic dysplasia: familial pulmonary arterial stenosis with neonatal liver disease. Arch Dis Child 1973;48:459–466.
45. Alagille D, Odievre M, Gautier M, et al: Hepatic ductular hypoplasia associated with characteristic facies, vertebral malformations, retarded physical, mental and sexual development, and cardiac murmur. J Pediatr 1975;86:63–71.
46. Schnittger S, Hoefers C, Heidemann P, et al: Molecular and cytogenetic analysis of an interstitial 20p deletion associated with syndromic intrahepatic ductular hypoplasia (Alagille syndrome). Hum Genet 1989;83:239–244.
47. Anad F, Burn J, Matthews D, et al: Alagille syndrome and deletion of 20p. J Med Genet 1990;27:729–737.
48. Zhang F, Deleuze J-F, Aurias A, et al: Interstitial deletion of the short arm of chromosome 20 in arteriohepatic dysplasia (Alagille syndrome). J Pediatr 1990;116:73–77.
49. Hol FA, Hamel BC, Geurds MP, et al: Localization of Alagille syndrome to 20p11.2-p12 by linkage analysis of a three-generation family. Hum Genet 1995;95:687–690.
50. Desmaze C, Deleuze JF, Dutrilaux AM, et al: Screening of microdeletions of chromosome 20 in patients with Alagille syndrome. J Med Genet 1992;29:233–235.
51. Rand EB, Spinner NB, Piccoli DA, et al: Molecular analysis of 24 Alagille syndrome families identifies a single submicroscopic deletion and further localizes the Alagille region within 20p12. Am J Hum Genet 1995;57:1068–1073.
51a. Oda T, Elkahloun AG, Pike BL, et al: Mutations in the human Jagged1 gene are responsible for Alagille syndrome. Nat Genet 16:235–242.
52. Alagille D, Estrada A, Hadchouel M, et al: Syndromic paucity of interlobular bile ducts (Alagille syndrome or arteriohepatic dysplasia): review of 80 cases. J Pediatr 1987;110:195–200.
53. Hoffenberg EJ, Narkewicz MR, Sondheimer JM, et al: Outcome of syndromic paucity of interlobular bile ducts (Alagille syndrome) with onset of cholestasis in infancy. J Pediatr 1995;127:220–224.
54. Deleuze JF, Dhorne-Pollet S, Pollet N, et al: Alagille syndrome in 1995: clinical and genetic data. Gastroenterol Clin Biol 1995;19:587–596.
55. Kaufman SS, Wood RP, Shaw BW Jr, et al: Hepatocarcinoma in a child with the Alagille syndrome. Am J Dis Child 1987;141:698–700.
56. Rabinovitz M, Imperial JC, Schade RR, et al: Hepatocellular carcinoma in Alagille syndrome: a family study. J Pediatr Gastroenterol Nutr 1989;8:26–30.
57. Silberbach M, Lashley D, Reller MD, et al: Arteriohepatic dysplasia and cardiovascular malformations. Am Heart J 1991;127:695–699.
58. Tolia V, Dubois RS, Watts FB Jr, et al: Renal abnormalities in paucity of interlobular bile ducts. J Pediatr Gastroenterol Nutr 1987;6:971–976.
59. Hyams JS, Bergman MM, Davis BH: Tubulointerstitial nephropathy associated with arteriohepatic dysplasia. Gastroenterology 1983; 85:430–434.
60. Rosenfield NS, Kelley MJ, Jensen PS, et al: Arteriohepatic dysplasia: radiologic features of a new syndrome. AJR 1980;135:1217–1223.
61. Berman MD, Ishak KG, Schaefer ER: Syndromic hepatic ductular hypoplasia (arteriohepatic dysplasia): a clinical and hepatic histologic study of three patients. Dig Dis Sci 1981;26:485–497.
62. Johnson BL: Ocular pathologic features of arteriohepatic dysplasia. Am J Ophthalmol 1990;110:504–512.
63. Ricci B, Lepore D, Iossa M, et al: Anomalies oculaires dans le syndrome d'Alagille. J Fr Ophthalmol 1991;14:481–485.
64. Schwarzenberg SJ, Grothe RM, Sharp HL, et al: Long-term complications of arteriohepatic dysplasia. Am J Med 1992;93:171–176.
65. Chong SKF, Lindridge J, Moniz C, et al: Exocrine pancreatic insufficiency in syndromic paucity of interlobular bile ducts. J Pediatr Gastroenterol Nutr 1989;9:445–449.
66. Doutre M-S, Beylot C, Couzigou P, et al: Lichen amyloidosis in Alagille syndrome. Arch Dermatol 1991;127:1590–1592.
67. Poh-Fitzpatrick MB, Zaider E, Sciales C: Cutaneous photosensitivity and coproporphyrin abnormalities in the Alagille syndrome. Gastroenterology 1990;99:831–835.
68. Okuno TH, Shibahara Y, Hashida Y, et al: Temporal bone histopathologic findings in Alagille syndrome. Arch Otolaryngol Head Neck Surg 1990;116:217–220.
69. Levin S, Zarvos P, Milner S, et al: Arteriohepatic dysplasia: association of liver disease with pulmonary arterial stenosis as well as facial and skeletal abnormalities. Pediatrics 1980;66:876–883.
70. Argao EA, Heubi JE, Hollis W, et al: D-α-Tocopherol polyethylene glycol-1000 succinate enhances the absorption of vitamin D in chronic cholestatic liver disease of infancy and childhood. Pediatr Res 1992;31:146–150.
71. Sokol RJ, Guggenheim MA, Iannaccone ST, et al: Improved neurologic function after long-term correction of vitamin E deficiency in children with chronic cholestasis. N Engl J Med 1985;313:1580–1586.
72. Balistreri WF, Al-Kader HH, Ryckman FC, et al: Ursodeoxycholic acid therapy in paediatric patients with chronic cholestasis. In Lentze M, Reichen J (eds): Paediatric Cholestasis: Novel Approaches to Treatment. Lancaster, England, Kluwer Academic Publishers, 1992, pp 333–343.
73. Whitington PR, Whitington GL: Partial external diversion of bile for the treatment of intractable pruritus associated with intrahepatic cholestasis. Gastroenterology 1988;95:130–136.
74. Marino IR, ChapChap P, Esquivel O, et al: Liver transplantation for arteriohepatic dysplasia (Alagille syndrome). Transpl Int 1992;5:61–64.
75. Whitington PF, Freese DK, Alonso EM, et al: Clinical and biochemical findings in progressive familial intrahepatic cholestasis. J Pediatr Gastroenterol Nutr 1994;18:134–141.
76. Clayton RJ, Iber FL, Ruebner BH, et al: Byler disease: fatal familial intrahepatic cholestasis in an Amish kindred. Am J Dis Child 1969;117:112–124.
77. Alonso EM, Snover DC, Montag A, et al: Histologic pathology of the liver in progressive familial intrahepatic cholestasis. J Pediatr Gastroenterol Nutr 1994;18:128–133.
78. Jacquemin E, Dumont M, Bernard O, et al: Evidence for defective bile acid secretion in children with progressive familial intrahepatic cholestasis (Byler disease). Eur J Pediatr 1994;153:424–428.
79. Emond JC, Whitington PF: Surgical management of progressive familial intrahepatic cholestasis. J Pediatr Surg 1995;30:1635–1641.
80. Carlton VEH, Knisely AS, Freimer NB: Mapping of a locus for progressive familial intrahepatic cholestasis (Byler's disease) to 18q21-q22, the benign recurrent intraheptic cholestasis region. Hum Mol Genet 1995;4:1049–1053.
81. Soubrane O, Gauthier F, DeVictor D, et al: Orthotopic liver transplantation for Byler disease. Transplantation 1990;50:804–806.
82. Dahms BB: Hepatoma in familial cholestatic cirrhosis of childhood. Arch Pathol Lab Med 1979;103:30–33.
83. Ugarte N, Gonzalez-Crussi F: Hepatoma in siblings with progressive familial cholestatic cirrhosis of childhood. Am J Clin Pathol 1981;76:172–177.
84. Quillin SP, Brink JA: Hepatoma complicating Byler disease. AJR 1992;159:432–433.
85. Summerskill WHJ, Walshe JM: Benign recurrent intrahepatic obstructive jaundice. Lancet 1959;2:686–690.
86. Brenard R, Geubel AP, Benhamou JP: Benign recurrent intrahepatic cholestasis: a report of 26 cases. J Clin Gastroenterol 1989;11:546–551.
87. DeKoning TJ, Sandkuijl LA, De Schryver JE, et al: Autosomal recessive inheritance of benign recurrent intrahepatic cholestasis. Am J Med Genet 1995;57:479–482.
88. Kahn E, Daum F, Markowitz J, et al: Nonsyndromic paucity of interlobular bile ducts: light and electron microscopic evaluation of sequential liver biopsies in early childhood. Hepatology 1986;6:890–901.
89. Dimmick JE: Intrahepatic bile duct paucity and cytomegalovirus infection. Pediatr Pathol 1993;13:847–852.

90. Wiesner RH, Ludwig J, van Hoek B, et al: Current concepts in cell-mediated hepatic allograft rejection leading to ductopenia and liver failure. Hepatology 1991;14:721–729.
91. Shulman HM, Sharma P, Amos D, et al: A coded histologic study of hepatic graft-versus-host disease after human bone marrow transplantation. Hepatology 1988;8:463–470.
92. Yamaguchi M: Congenital choledochal cyst: analysis of 1,433 patients in the Japanese literature. Am J Surg 1980;140:653–657.
93. Kim SH: Choledochal cyst: survey by the surgical section of the American Academy of Pediatrics. J Pediatr Surg 1981;16:402–407.
94. Todani T, Watanabe Y, Narusue M, et al: Congenital bile duct cysts: classification, operative procedures, and review of thirty-seven cases including cancer arising from choledochal cyst. Am J Surg 1977;134:263–269.
95. Babbitt DP, Starshak RJ, Clement AR: Choledochal cyst: a concept of etiology. AJR 1973;119:57–62.
96. Okada A, Nakamura T, Higaki J, et al: Congenital dilatation of the bile duct in 100 instances and its relationship with anomalous junction. Surg Gynecol Obstet 1990;17:291–298.
97. Wood WJJ, Trump DS: Pancreaticobiliary common channel associated with common duct stricture. J Pediatr Surg 1986;21:738–740.
98. Schroeder D, Smith L, Prain HC: Antenatal diagnosis of choledochal cyst at 15 weeks' gestation: etiologic implications and management. J Pediatr Surg 1989;24:936–938.
99. Sherman P, Kolster E, Davies C, et al: Choledochal cysts: heterogeneity of clinical presentation. J Pediatr Gastroenterol Nutr 1986;5:867–872.
100. Kasai M, Asakura Y, Taira Y: Surgical treatment of choledochal cyst. Ann Surg 1970;172:844–851.
101. Camponovo E, Buck JL, Drane WE: Scintigraphic features of choledochal cyst. J Nucl Med 1989;30:622–628.
102. Gupta RK, Kakar AK, Jena A, et al: Magnetic resonance in obstructive jaundice. Australas Radiol 1989;33:245–251.
103. Mc Whorter GL: Congenital cystic dilatation of the bile and pancreatic ducts. Arch Surg 1939;38:397–411.
104. Lilly JR: Total excision of choledochal cyst. Surg Gynecol Obstet 1978;146:254–256.
105. Todani T, Watanabe Y, Toki A, et al: Carcinoma related to choledochal cysts with internal drainage operations. Surg Gynecol Obstet 1987;164:61–64.
106. Yoshida H, Itai Y, Minami M, et al: Biliary malignancies occurring in choledochal cysts. Radiology 1989;173:389–392.
107. Alonso-Lej F, Rever WBJ, Pessagno DJ: Congenital choledochal cyst, with a report of 2 and analysis of 94 cases. Int Abstr Surg 1959;108:1–30.
108. Amedee-Manesme O, Bernard O, Brunelle F, et al: Sclerosing cholangitis with neonatal onset. J Pediatr 1987;111:225–229.
109. Baker AJ, Portmann B, Westaby D, et al: Neonatal sclerosing cholangitis in two siblings: a category of progressive intrahepatic cholestasis. J Pediatr Gastroenterol Nutr 1993;17:317–322.
110. Kolbe A, Beaver BL, Rosenbaum R, et al: Diagnosis of spontaneous perforation of the biliary tract in the newborn. J Pediatr Surg 1986;21:1139–1142.
111. Lilly JR, Weintraub WH, Altman RP: Spontaneous perforation of the extrahepatic bile ducts and bile peritonitis in infancy. Surgery 1974;75:664–673.
112. Prevot J, Babut JM: Spontaneous perforations of the biliary tract in infancy. Prog Pediatr Surg 1970;1:187–208.
113. Howard ER, Johnston DI, Mowat AP: Spontaneous perforation of common bile duct in infants. Arch Dis Child 1976;51:883–886.
114. Fitzgerald RJ, Parbhoo R, Guiney EJ: Spontaneous perforation of bile ducts in neonates. Surgery 1978;83:303–305.

# Chapter 49

# Metabolic Disorders of the Liver

*Jeffrey H. Teckman and David H. Perlmutter*

## ALPHA$_1$-ANTITRYPSIN DEFICIENCY

Alpha$_1$-antitrypsin (α1-AT) deficiency occurs in 1 of every 1,600 to 1,800 live births,[1] but prospective natural history studies indicate that only 10% to 15% of the affected population develop clinically significant liver disease.[2, 3] A substantial number of α1-AT–deficient individuals develop destructive lung disease and emphysema beginning in the third decade of life. Cigarette smoking markedly increases the rate and severity of this destructive lung disease.

### Clinical Manifestations

α1-AT deficiency is associated with features of the neonatal hepatitis syndrome (Table 49–1). Typically, the infant is evaluated in the first 8 weeks of life for jaundice or hepatomegaly and is found to have elevated levels of conjugated bilirubin and transaminases. Only 25% of these infants develop clinically significant liver disease. In some cases, this is manifested by poor growth and progressive liver failure; in other cases, there is slow progression of liver disease over several years. The remaining 75% of the infants who are discovered in the neonatal period may have elevated transaminase concentrations for many years but never develop significant liver disease.[2] Follow-up studies of infants diagnosed at birth in a nationwide prospective screening study have shown that more than 85% have persistently normal serum transaminase levels with no evidence of liver dysfunction.[3]

**TABLE 49–1. Clinical and Diagnostic Features of Alpha$_1$-Antitrypsin Deficiency**

| | |
|---|---|
| **Clinical Manifestations** | |
| Infancy | Prolonged obstructive jaundice<br>Mild transaminase elevation<br>Symptoms of cholestasis |
| Early childhood | Mild transaminase elevation<br>Severe liver dysfunction possible |
| Late childhood/adolescence | Portal hypertension<br>Severe liver dysfunction |
| Adulthood | Chronic hepatitis<br>Cryptogenic cirrhosis<br>Portal hypertension<br>Hepatocellular carcinoma<br>Premature pulmonary emphysema |
| **Diagnostic Features** | Reduced serum α1-AT level (10–15% normal)<br>Abnormal mobility of α1-AT serum protein in isoelectric focusing (PiZ-type)<br>Periodic acid–Schiff–positive, diastase-resistant globules in hepatocytes |

α1-AT deficiency may also manifest later in childhood or early in adolescence with complications of portal hypertension, such as ascites, edema, esophageal/gastric variceal bleeding, or hypersplenism. In adults, α1-AT deficiency can cause chronic hepatitis, cirrhosis, and/or hepatocellular carcinoma.[4] On clinical grounds alone, it may be difficult to distinguish between α1-AT deficiency and other chronic liver diseases, including autoimmune hepatitis, drug-induced hepatitis, chronic viral hepatitis, and Wilson's disease.

It is well established in the literature that homozygous PiZZ α1-AT deficiency alone can explain the liver disease in each of these clinical situations. It is not clear whether the heterozygous PiZ α1-AT state by itself can account for clinically significant liver disease of any kind. In most cases, other causes, such as autoimmune or viral hepatitis, provide an explanation for liver injury in the heterozygote.[1]

### Diagnosis

The diagnosis of α1-AT deficiency is based on the phenotype of the α1-AT protein that is present in a patient's serum, as determined by isoelectric focusing or by agarose electrophoresis at acidic pH. The determination of the α1-AT level in a patient's serum should not be the sole basis of the diagnosis, because α1-AT is an acute phase reactant and therefore may be transiently elevated even in PiZZ patients during the host response to tissue injury or inflammation.

The diagnosis of PiZZ α1-AT deficiency can be substantiated by the characteristic histologic appearance of periodic acid–Schiff–positive, diastase-resistant globules in the endoplasmic reticulum (ER) of hepatocytes. However, this finding alone, or its absence, is not regarded as diagnostic, because the globules can be difficult to detect in the first few months of life and because similar structures can be observed in PiMM individuals with other liver disease. The liver biopsy may also be characterized by a variable degree of cholestasis, hepatocellular necrosis, inflammatory cell infiltrate, bile duct epithelial cell destruction, and periportal fibrosis or cirrhosis. In some cases, there is bile duct proliferation; in a few, there is paucity of intrahepatic bile ducts.

### Pathogenesis

The mutant α1-AT Z molecule is characterized by a single nucleotide substitution of lysine for glutamic acid at codon 342. It is synthesized normally but is retained early in the secretory pathway in the ER. Structural studies have shown that the mutant α1-AT Z molecule folds very slowly, leading to accumulation of an intermediate that has a tendency to polymerize, presumably within the ER.[5–7]

In contrast to the pathogenesis of lung injury in α1-AT deficiency, which involves an uninhibited proteolytic attack on lung elastin,[8] there is no evidence that the pathophysiology of liver injury in this condition is caused by a deficiency of elastase inhibitory capacity. Most evidence favors the concept that the accumulation of α1-AT in the ER is directly related to liver cell injury. Experiments in transgenic mice carrying the mutant Z α1-AT allele have provided direct experimental support for this "accumulation theory." These mice have intrahepatocytic globules of α1-AT and develop liver disease and, ultimately, hepatocellular carcinoma.[9, 10] Because there are normal levels of α1-AT and presumably other anti-elastases in these animals, as directed by the endogenous murine genes, liver injury cannot be attributed to diminished serum or tissue levels of α1-AT.

Several studies have indicated that PiZZ individuals who are "protected" from liver disease are able to degrade the mutant α1-AT Z molecules that are retained in the ER.[11] The mechanism for ER degradation appears to be complex, requiring at least several general steps.[12] The studies also provide evidence that PiZZ individuals who are "susceptible" to liver disease have a lag in ER degradation and that different steps in the ER degradation pathway can be altered in a single susceptible individual.

### Management

In most infants and children with α1-AT deficiency, clinically significant liver disease never develops. Even children with cholestasis in the first 6 months have a low likelihood (less than 25%) of developing clinical liver disease.[2]

There is no specific therapy for liver disease associated with α1-AT deficiency; clinical care primarily involves supportive management for liver dysfunction and prevention of complications. Progressive liver dysfunction and failure in children has been treated by orthotopic liver transplantation with survival rates approaching 90% at 1 year and 80% at 5 years.[13, 14] Patients with α1-AT deficiency and emphysema have undergone replacement therapy with purified and recombinant plasma α1-AT, administered either intravenously or by intratracheal aerosol.[15, 16] All patients with α1-AT deficiency should be advised to avoid cigarette smoking.

Several novel types of gene therapy, such as homologous recombination for targeted gene disruption and use of ribozymes for targeted RNA destruction, are theoretically attractive strategies for treatment of liver disease in α1-AT deficiency, because they would prevent the synthesis of the mutant α1-AT Z protein and its ER retention. Studies have also shown that trans-splicing of ribozymes can emend a mutant transcript and that chimeric oligonucleotides composed of DNA and modified RNA can correct mutant transcripts.[17, 18]

## HEREDITARY TYROSINEMIA

There has been a remarkable series of advances in understanding hereditary tyrosinemia type I. Several molecular defects in the fumarylacetoacetate hydrolase (FAH) gene have been characterized, an animal model in which the FAH gene is deleted has been identified, and a potential drug therapy has been tested. Although long-term results are not yet available, treatment with the drug 2-(2-nitro-4-trifluoromethylbenzoyl)-1,3-cyclohexanedione (NTBC) has completely arrested the progression of hereditary tyrosinemia in many cases.

### Clinical Manifestations

Hereditary tyrosinemia type I is characterized by progressive liver failure, renal tubular dysfunction, and hypophosphatemic rickets. It is an autosomal recessive defect that is most prevalent in French-Canadian descendants of Quebec.[19] There is wide variability among affected persons in clinical severity of disease. In the acute form of the disease, the infant (3 to 4 months of age) may be referred for evaluation because of poor growth, irritability, and vomiting. In some cases, an enlarged liver or enlarged kidneys are palpated by the general pediatrician at a routine visit. Diarrhea and a cabbage-like odor are occasionally noted. Bruising and nosebleeds may be evident. Although one is always concerned about the possibility of more devastating manifestations of the bleeding diathesis, such as intracranial hemorrhage, these are not usually observed at the time of the initial clinical presentation. Ascites and edema may be noted. If untreated, the disorder results in liver failure within 6 to 8 months.

In the chronic form, hepatic dysfunction and hypophosphatemic rickets are present. Patients with this form of the disease may also develop neurologic crises that resemble those of acute intermittent porphyria.[20] These are abrupt episodes of peripheral neuropathy with severe pain, extensor hypertonia, vomiting or paralytic ileus, and muscle weakness, occasionally necessitating mechanical ventilation. These crises presumably result from competitive inhibition of δ-aminolevulinic acid dehydratase by succinylacetone, a metabolite of tyrosine degradation that accumulates in hereditary tyrosinemia. There is an increased susceptibility to hepatocellular carcinoma even within the first 1 to 5 years of life.

Laboratory evaluation includes a markedly prolonged prothrombin time, with only mild elevation of liver enzymes and conjugated bilirubin. The plasma tyrosine and methionine concentrations are increased to a level in excess of that associated with chronic liver disease, and the alpha-fetoprotein concentration is elevated to an even greater extent than that associated with other forms of neonatal hepatitis. Abnormalities in the urine are consistent with proximal renal tubular insufficiency. Imaging of the intra-abdominal organs usually shows increased echogenicity of the liver and enlargement and increased echogenicity of kidney, sometimes with nephrocalcinosis. Liver biopsy specimens are notable for hepatocellular inflammation and necrosis, fatty infiltration, pseudoacinar formation, and marked nodular regeneration.

## Diagnosis

The diagnosis is established by elevated urine succinylacetone, absent or decreased FAH in liver tissue, or skin fibroblasts. Prenatal diagnosis based on elevation of amniotic fluid succinylacetone had a sensitivity of approximately 94% and a specificity of 100% in a study of 64 pregnancies.[19]

## Pathogenesis

This disorder is caused by a deficiency of FAH,[21–23] an enzyme that catalyzes the last step in tyrosine degradation.[24, 25] A total of seven different mutations in the FAH gene have been identified in affected patients.[26, 27] The most severe defects, with the absence of FAH mRNA and protein, are associated with the acute form of the disease, early onset, and the highest levels of alpha-fetoprotein in serum.[28]

Deficiency of FAH activity presumably results in the accumulation of fumarylacetoacetate and maleylacetoacetate and the formation of succinylacetoacetate and succinylacetone (Fig. 49–1). Succinylacetone is thought to be the most toxic intermediate that accumulates. It can inhibit renal tubular transport of glucose and amino acids,[29] which may explain the renal tubular insufficiency observed in patients with this disorder. It is a structural analogue of δ-aminolevulinic acid and a competitive inhibitor of δ-amino acid dehydratase.[30] This last property explains the characteristic increased levels of δ-aminolevulinic acid and symptoms of acute intermittent porphyria in affected patients.

Several studies have shown that FAH deficiency causes a hepatorenal syndrome similar to hereditary tyrosinemia in the C14CoS albino mouse.[31–34] Moreover, Kelsey and colleagues showed that the introduction of a wild-type FAH transgene into albino deletion mutant mice reversed the hepatorenal phenotype.[33]

In a very important study, Kvittingen and associates showed that there is reversion of the genetic defect in regions within the liver of tyrosinemic patients.[35] In these regions there is FAH activity and correction of a mutant adenine-thymidine (AT) nucleotide pair to the wild-type guanine-cytosine (GC) sequence. The mechanism for this self-induced genetic correction is unknown.

## Treatment

Many children with hereditary tyrosinemia undergo liver transplantation. If considered before the development of hepatocellular carcinoma, transplantation appears to have a salutary effect on both the renal and the liver disease. Dietary restriction of phenylalanine and tyrosine is instituted while the infant awaits the availability of a donor liver. This diet must be carefully monitored. If the restriction is too severe, the infant can develop growth failure, anorexia, and lethargy as a result of phenylalanine-tyrosine deficiency. Rank and coworkers used hematin to treat the neurologic crises.[36] The rationale for this intervention is the capacity of hematin to inhibit aminolevulinic acid synthase and the production of δ-aminolevulinic acid during the time that the patient awaits liver transplantation.

In 1992, Lindstedt and colleagues published a report[37] in which five patients were treated successfully with NTBC.

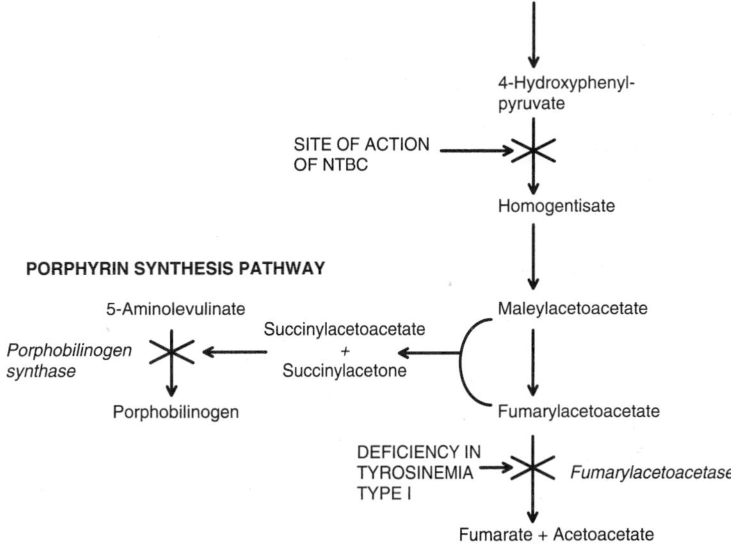


**FIGURE 49–1.** Tyrosine degradation pathway. A block in the last step of the tyrosine degradation pathway is caused by deficient activity of the enzyme fumarylacetoacetase in tyrosinemia type I. This leads to the overproduction of alternative metabolites, succinylacetoacetate and succinylacetone, which in turn inhibit the pathway for porphyrin synthesis. NTBC blocks tyrosine degradation at its second step, thereby preventing production of these toxic substances.

This compound was developed as an insecticide but, on the basis of its structural similarity to tyrosine, was later found to be a potent inhibitor of 4-hydroxyphenylpyruvate dioxygenase. The hypothesis of this therapeutic trial was that inhibition of the dioxygenase would prevent accumulation of maleylacetoacetate and fumarylacetoacetate and their saturated, presumably toxic, derivatives succinylacetoacetate and succinylacetone. Over 7 to 9 months, treatment was associated with marked improvement in clinical, histologic, and biochemical abnormalities. There were no side effects, although the patients were carefully monitored for neurologic, ocular, and cutaneous signs. A marked reduction in concentrations of alpha-fetoprotein suggested that the treatment abolished the marked tendency for nodular liver regeneration.

The results of treatment with NTBC for 92 patients with tyrosinemia showed that 87% were doing well after more than 1 year.[38] Patients with severe liver disease improved dramatically with NTBC treatment, but six patients with acute liver failure did not improve and had to undergo liver transplantation or died. NTBC also had a significant effect in the FAH murine model of tyrosinemia.[39] However, the correction was not complete. Mutant mice accumulated succinylacetone levels to an intermediate level, and some developed hepatocellular carcinoma. This may mean that patients with tyrosinemia will also develop hepatocellular carcinoma after long intervals, even while taking NTBC.

Studies have shown that transplanted hepatocytes can repopulate the diseased liver of the FAH mouse.[40] Replication of the transplanted hepatocytes occurs only when there is injury/regeneration in the liver—that is, it ceases when NTBC is given to the FAH mouse. The results suggest that it may be possible to use hepatocyte transplantation techniques to treat hereditary tyrosinemia, and perhaps other metabolic liver diseases in which the defect is cell autonomous.

## MITOCHONDRIAL DEFECTS

Inherited deficiencies of several mitochondrial enzymes can be associated with liver disease. These are usually defects in the respiratory chain that result in uncoupling of oxidative phosphorylation. In most cases, the clinical picture is dominated by neurologic and neuromuscular involvement with lactic acidosis.

### Mitochondrial Respiratory Chain Defects

The affected infant is often first identified because of poor Apgar scores, jaundice, lethargy, and even coma in the first week of life. There may be disordered eye movement and ataxia. Hepatomegaly and ascites are sometimes present. Laboratory studies show moderately elevated transaminases, hyperbilirubinemia, hypoalbuminemia, prolonged prothrombin time, hypoglycemia, hyperammonemia, and severe lactic acidosis. Because the pyruvate concentration is only mildly elevated, the ratio of lactate to pyruvate is significantly increased.[41–44] Levels of 3-hydroxybutyrate are increased to a greater extent than those of acetoacetate, resulting in a ratio of 3-hydroxybutyrate to acetoacetate greater than 2.0. Liver biopsy shows microvesicular and macrovesicular fat, glycogen depletion, and cholestasis. There may be fibrosis or even cirrhosis. The mitochondria are characterized by swelling, pleomorphism, inclusions, and decreased cristae on electron microscopic examination of liver biopsy specimens.[45] In most of these cases there is a 90% to 95% reduction in cytochrome C oxidase levels in liver tissue and sometimes muscle, but in other cases enzyme levels are normal in muscle and lymphocytes. Some of the infants die from liver failure or sepsis within the first week of life. In several patients a deficiency in succinate:cytochrome C reductase has been associated with a slightly later onset, 2 to 3 months of age.[46] An even more delayed form of the disease has also been described.[47] Onset ranged from 2 to 18 months of age, and the disease was characterized by liver enlargement, jaundice, and variable neurologic involvement. Hepatic failure developed later. A few patients presented with only myoclonus epilepsy and later died from liver failure. These patients had minimal elevation of lactic acid and minimal liver histologic abnormalities at onset and were initially thought to have Alpers' disease (see later discussion).

### Mitochondrial Depletion Syndrome

This is an autosomal recessive defect in which there is depletion of mitochondrial DNA in liver and muscle.[48–51] It is thought to involve a nuclear gene defect that impairs mitochondrial DNA replication. Hypotonia, vomiting, and liver failure develop within the first 3 months of life. The liver is enlarged, and a myopathy may be present. Increased serum transaminases, lactic acidosis, and ketonuria are present. Liver biopsy indicates the presence of steatosis. Levels of all the respiratory chain enzymes are decreased in liver and, to a lesser extent, in muscle, presumably reflecting the decrease in mitochondrial DNA in liver and muscle. There is no decrease in enzymes or mitochondrial DNA in heart, kidney, or brain. The infants die by 3 to 7 months of age.

### Alpers' Disease (Progressive Neuronal Degeneration of Childhood with Liver Disease)

This disease is characterized by diffuse cerebral degeneration with developmental delay, progressive seizures, vomiting, and liver failure.[52–56] Its onset is usually between 6 months and 2 years of age with developmental delay and refractory seizures. The child is hypotonic, failing to thrive, and vomiting. Valproic acid is often used to treat the seizure disorder and is later implicated in the evolving hepatic dysfunction.[56] Liver involvement usually is first indicated by hyperbilirubinemia and prolongation of the prothrombin time. Liver enzymes are mildly elevated. The liver disease often progresses very rapidly, with fatal liver failure within 4 to 6 weeks. In milder cases, the liver biopsy shows mild periportal inflammation with focal hepatocyte necrosis, microvesicular fat, and portal fibrosis. In more severe cases, the liver is characterized by lobular collapse, bile duct proliferation, and micronodular cirrhosis at postmortem examination. If the child does not have liver involvement, the clinical picture is dominated by progressive neurologic degeneration with death by 4 to 5 years of age. Neuropathologic examination shows generalized loss of gray matter with swollen, dense mitochondria. Studies have suggested that there is a defect in NADH:ubiquinone oxidoreductase in patients with Alpers' disease.[57, 58]

### Mitochondrial Genomic Deletion Syndromes

These syndromes were initially described by Pearson and coworkers as refractory sideroblastic anemia with exocrine pancreatic insufficiency.[59] They are now known to be multisystem diseases with large-scale deletions and rearrangements of the mitochondrial genome.[60–62] The disorder manifests in infancy with failure to thrive, poor feeding, vomiting, diarrhea, developmental delay, muscle weakness, and metabolic acidosis with markedly increased levels of lactic acid. Some patients have ophthalmoplegia. Liver involvement is characterized by elevated liver enzymes, hyperbilirubinemia, prolonged prothrombin time, and hepatomegaly. A number of these patients die within the first 3 years of life from liver failure.[61] The diagnosis is established by Southern blot analysis of genomic DNA using mitochondrial DNA probes.

There is no effective therapy for mitochondrial genomic deletion syndromes or for the other mitochondrial defects discussed in this section. Because multiple systems are involved and because severe disease develops very early in infancy, there have been no reports of organ replacement therapy in these patients. There have been several suggestions in the literature for supportive therapy, including a low-carbohydrate diet.[60]

## FATTY ACID OXIDATION DEFECTS

Defects in mitochondrial fatty acid oxidation have been associated with a number of liver diseases, including fatal familial hepatic steatosis, recurrent Reye's syndrome, acute fatty liver of pregnancy (AFLP), and acute liver failure. Patients with these disorders may present in infancy with myopathy, cardiomyopathy, hepatomegaly, elevated transaminases, hypoglycemia, and lethargy after fasting or during an intercurrent respiratory illness. Liver involvement usually takes the form of diffuse macrovesicular steatosis, mild to moderate increase in transaminases, normal bilirubin, normal or mildly prolonged prothrombin time, and mild hyperammonemia. In addition to hypoglycemia, metabolic derangements include elevated plasma free fatty acids, mild to moderate lactic acidosis, and marked hyperuricemia. Apnea and sudden infant death syndrome have occurred. Rhabdomyolysis, myoglobinuria, and elevated serum creatinine phosphokinase may be present. Urinary organic acid assays show the presence of dicarboxylic acids. Plasma levels of carnitine are low, but there is elevation in acylcarnitine and accumulation of specific acylcarnitines. The diagnosis of these defects may require analysis of acylcarnitine conjugates in urine and plasma by fast atom bombardment mass spectroscopy, measurement of enzyme activity in cultured skin fibroblasts,[63] and sophisticated molecular diagnostic assays.[64]

Treatment centers on the immediate institution of intravenous dextrose at a rate sufficient to inhibit fatty acid oxidation. Avoidance of fasting is a very important part of preventing acute illness in patients with this type of defect. Frequent feedings or even gastrostomy tube feedings may be required. Although carnitine supplementation is an important part of the treatment of the carnitine transport defects, it is not clear that it benefits patients with other fatty acid oxidation defects.

### Long-Chain 3-Hydroxyacyl–Coenzyme A Dehydrogenase (LCHAD) Deficiency

As with the other specific defects in fatty acid oxidation, patients with LCHAD deficiency present in the first year of life with a severe, sometimes fatal, episode of hypoketotic hypoglycemia, hepatic steatosis, cardiomyopathy, and hypotonia. These infants have prominent peaks of long-chain 2-hydroxydicarboxylic acids in their urine.[65–67] Most of the affected infants have lactic acidosis, increased serum creatinine phosphokinase levels, and low serum carnitine levels, although normal levels of serum carnitine and acylcarnitine do not exclude this diagnosis. LCHAD deficiency may cause cholestatic liver disease and even fulminant liver failure in early infancy.[67] It now appears that AFLP and the syndrome of hypertension, hemolysis, elevated liver enzymes, and low platelets of pregnancy (HELLP) may be caused by carriage of a fetus with LCHAD deficiency.[64, 66, 68, 69] AFLP is a rare disease characterized by late third-trimester anorexia, vomiting, jaundice, severe coagulopathy, hepatic coma, and sometimes death. There is a characteristic infiltration of liver by microvesicular fat. Most of the recent work on this disorder indicates that the mothers are heterozygous carriers and that AFLP develops only when they bear a child homozygous for LCHAD deficiency. It is believed that toxic metabolites generated in the fetal liver precipitate the metabolic effects on the mother's liver.

LCHAD is also known as the trifunctional enzyme because it catalyzes the last three steps in mitochondrial beta-oxidation of long-chain substrates—the dehydrogenase, ketothiolase, and enoylhydratase steps. It is a multimeric protein with four $\alpha$- and four $\beta$-subunits. Most of the patients with LCHAD deficiency who have been studied have deficient dehydrogenase activity and mutations in the $\alpha$-subunit.[64, 67]

### Other Specific Fatty Acid Oxidation Defects

Although fatty infiltration causing liver enlargement may be found in almost all of the other defects in fatty acid oxidation, liver dysfunction usually is not a major part of these disorders. A Reye-like syndrome with vomiting, hypoglycemia, and coma; sudden unexplained death; dilated or hypertrophic cardiomyopathy; and skeletal myopathies are usually the major problems in these disorders. These defects include deficiencies of medium-chain acyl–coenzyme A (CoA) dehydrogenase (MCAD), long-chain acyl-CoA dehydrogenase (LCAD), short-chain acyl-CoA dehydrogenase (SCAD), carnitine palmitoyl transferase (CPT), and hydroxymethyl glutaryl (HMG)-CoA lyase.[70] The major characteristics of each of these defects are listed in Table 49–2.

## REYE'S SYNDROME

Reye's syndrome is a disease characterized by a severe noninflammatory encephalopathy with fatty infiltration of the liver.[71] There is usually a prodromal viral illness, but shortly after apparent recovery pernicious vomiting, low-grade fever, and encephalopathy develop. Liver involvement is characterized by elevated transaminases, hyperammonemia, and, in some cases, hypoglycemia. There is fatty infiltration of the liver with alteration in the structure of the mitochondria. Liver involvement usually is transient, and the clinical picture is dominated by the effects of cerebral edema. The cause of Reye's syndrome is unknown, but there has been a dramatic decline in the number of cases since the administration of aspirin to infants and children has been discouraged. Most of the evidence favors the pathophysiologic concept that this syndrome requires genetic susceptibility and exposure to an environmental toxin such as aspirin, hypoglycin A in the unripe Akee fruit as described in Jamaican vomiting sickness,[72] or the *Bacillus cereus* toxin.[73] One study showed that patients with MCAD deficiency (resembling Reye's syndrome) do not have the hepatic mitochondrial abnormalities that frequently are seen in Reye's syndrome.[74]

## PEROXISOMAL DISORDERS

Abnormalities in peroxisomes or in peroxisomal enzymes cause a recently recognized group of genetic disorders (Table 49–3). The best described of these disorders, Zellweger's cerebrohepatorenal syndrome, consists of facial dysmorphism, hypotonia, seizures, failure to thrive, and liver disease.[75] Infants with this syndrome survive only a few months. There is often abnormal calcification of the patella and other apophyseal cartilage, a lesion referred to as chondrodysplasia punctata. Congenital anomalies of the heart, particularly septal defects and conotruncal malformations, may be present. The central nervous system involvement is characterized by developmental delay, profound hypotonia, refractory seizures, apnea, and aspiration syndromes. There are malformations of the brain, including cerebellar heterotopia, pachymicrogyria, olivary hypoplasia, partial agenesis of the corpus callosum, hypoplasia of the cerebellar vermis, and septo-optic dysplasia. Involvement of the kidneys usually causes only generalized aminoaciduria and proteinuria but, in some cases, can cause severe renal insufficiency. Liver disease may be suspected only by enlargement of the liver on examination, but some infants already have elevated serum transaminases, coagulopathy, and hypoalbuminemia in the neonatal period. Liver involvement progresses to liver failure in most of the infants with this syndrome who survive beyond the neonatal period. Liver biopsy shows lobular disarray, focal liver cell necrosis, cholestasis, siderosis, bridging fibrosis, and even frank cirrhosis. Electron microscopy usually shows absence of peroxisomes, but there are a few genetic variants that are clinically and biochemically identical to Zellweger's syndrome in which there are peroxisomal membrane ghosts[76] or even intact peroxisomes.[77] There are also variants in which peroxisomes are present in normal numbers in clusters of hepatocytes but are absent from 90% of hepatocytes in the liver biopsy specimen, so-called peroxisome mosaicism.[78, 79] Abnormal mitochondrial morphology is also present, with tubular cristae, paracrystalline inclusions, and dark staining.

Laboratory studies show elevated transaminases, elevated conjugated bilirubin, prolonged prothrombin time, increased serum iron, decreased serum cholesterol, proteinuria, and generalized aminoaciduria. There are increased levels of very-long-chain fatty acids (VLCFAs), pipecolic acid, phytanic acid, and dicarboxylic acids and decreased levels of plasmalogens (e.g., platelet-activating factor). Serum levels of normal bile acids are markedly decreased, whereas abnormal bile acid intermediates accumulate in the liver. Levels of docosahexaenoic acid and related essential polyunsaturated fatty acids are severely decreased.

The pathogenesis of liver injury in Zellweger's syndrome is unknown. Increased levels of hydrogen peroxide, unsaturated VLCFAs, and abnormal bile acid intermediates, which are metabolized aberrantly in the peroxisome-deficient liver, have been considered potentially hepatotoxic. Studies have suggested that defects in peroxisomal assembly factor-1[80, 81] and in the PTS1 peroxisomal import receptor[82, 83] account for some of the cases of Zellweger's syndrome.

The diagnosis of Zellweger's syndrome can generally be made by measuring plasma levels of VLCFAs. The absolute level of C26:0 VLCFA and the ratio of C26:0 to C22:0 VLCFA are markedly increased in Zellweger's syndrome.

A number of other disorders can mimic Zellweger's syndrome. In infantile Refsum's disease, neurologic dysfunction is less severe but hepatomegaly and hepatic dysfunction are common. Patients with rhizomelic chondrodysplasia punctata also have liver disease. Like patients with Zellweger's syndrome, these patients have diminished serum levels of red blood cell plasmalogens, and a liver biopsy specimen usually shows absence of peroxisomes. Patients with Refsum's disease may be distinguished by their increased phytanic acid levels. Rhizomelic chondrodysplasia punctata usually is suggested by dysmorphic and skeletal features on initial presentation. However, it can be difficult to distinguish this condition from Conradi's syndrome and from the congenital rubella syndrome, both of which can manifest with arthrogryposis multiplex, calcific epiphyseal stippling, and hepatic injury associated with abnormal peroxisomes and peroxisomal metabolic abnormalities.[84] Neonatal and X-linked adrenoleukodystrophy also can mimic Zellweger's syndrome. Several studies have contributed to the elucidation of the pathogenesis of these two disorders. Watkins and colleagues showed that the peroxisomal bifunctional enzyme is deficient in neonatal adrenoleukodystrophy.[85] Mosser and associates used positional cloning to map the gene for X-linked adrenoleukodystrophy to a 70-kd transmembrane protein involved in peroxisome biogenesis. This protein, PMP70, has structural features[86] characteristic of a family of transporters that bind ATP, including the cystic fibrosis transmembrane conductance regulator.

A consortium of investigators has recently subdivided the

## TABLE 49–2. Major

| DEFICIENCY | HEPATIC FAILURE | FASTING COMA | HEPATIC STEATOSIS | CARDIOMY |
|---|---|---|---|---|
| LCHAD | + | + | + | |
| MCAD | – | + | + | |
| LCAD | – | + | + | |
| SCAD | – | + | + | |
| CPT I | – | + | + | |
| CPT II (mild) | – | + | + | |
| CPT II (severe) | – | + | + | |
| HMG-CoA lyase | – | + | + | |

+, present; –, absent.

## TABLE 49–3. Manifestations of Disorders of Peroxisome Biogenesis

| FEATURE | ZELLWEGER'S SYNDROME | INFANTILE REFSUM'S DISEASE | NEONATAL ADRENOLEUKODYSTROPHY | HYPERPIPECOLIC ACIDEMIA | RHIZOMELIC CHONDRODYSPLASIA PUNCTATA |
|---|---|---|---|---|---|
| Dysmorphism | + | + | +/– | – | ++ |
| Central nervous system disease | ++ | + | ++ | + | + |
| Liver disease | ++ | ++ | + | + | + |
| Renal dysfunction | +/– | – | +/– | – | – |
| Bone abnormalities | + | – | +/– | – | ++ |
| Abnormal serum fatty acids | + | + | + | + | +/– |
| Survival | <1 yr | 10 yr | 2 mo–20 yr | 2–3 yr | Variable |
| Peroxisomes | Usually absent | Usually absent | Usually absent | Absent or deranged | Present but deranged |

+, present; ++, prominent; –, absent; +/–, variable.

peroxisomal defects into two groups, the single peroxisomal enzyme deficiencies and the assembly deficiencies.[87, 88]

Treatment of peroxisomal disorders is largely supportive. Nutritional repletion may require gastrostomy tube feedings. Special attention is given to supplementation of fat-soluble vitamins. Anticonvulsants are a major part of the supportive treatment regimen. Dietary restriction of phytanic acid and phytol, which appears to work well in adult Refsum's disease, is not clearly beneficial in the other peroxisomal disorders. Treatment with clofibrate or with a mixture of triolein and trierucin (Lorenzo's oil) has also garnered mixed results. Bone marrow transplantation worked well in one patient with X-linked adrenoleukodystrophy.[89] Ursodeoxycholic acid treatment may also be beneficial in some patients.[90]

## GAUCHER'S DISEASE

Gaucher's disease is an autosomal recessive deficiency in the lysosomal enzyme glucocerebrosidase.[91] The accumulation of globosides and gangliosides in macrophages is responsible for the disease manifestations (Table 49–4).

### Clinical Aspects

Type 1 Gaucher's disease, also called chronic, non-neuronopathic Gaucher's disease, is the most common phenotype. Its incidence in the general population is low, but in Ashkenazi Jews it is approximately 1 in 800 to 1,000 live births.[91] Affected persons with a few known mild mutations often are not diagnosed until the third decade of life or later, whereas children with severe mutations may not reach adulthood.[91, 92] These patients usually are first discovered with a combination of painless splenomegaly, anemia, and leukopenia. Hepatomegaly and elevated serum transaminases are common, but hepatic failure is rare.[93] Occasionally, there is cirrhosis and portal hypertension. As the disease progresses, enlargement of the liver and spleen may become great enough to lead to mechanical complications within the abdomen, local pain, dyspareunia, early satiety at meals, and splenic infarction. Bleeding or easy bruising is also common in type 1 Gaucher's. This is usually a result of thrombocytopenia from splenic sequestration or marrow infiltration, but it can sometimes be independent of the platelet count. The most common serious complications are skeletal, with osteoporosis and osteolysis leading to pain and pathologic fractures.[94] These may occur episodically in bone crises, especially in children and adolescents. Bone deformity and joint dysfunction can result. The skin of affected patients often has a yellow-brown appearance, especially on the face and legs, that can deepen quickly with minimal sun exposure.[95]

In type 2, acute neuronopathic Gaucher's disease, there is less heterogeneity among patients and no ethnic predilection. The patients are usually first discovered at 3 months of age with splenomegaly and by 6 months of age have symptoms of neurologic dysfunction. The triad of strabismus, trismus, and retroflexion of the head is common. Hepatomegaly develops, and early signs of hepatic dysfunction can occur. A severe ichthyosis-like skin disorder can occur.[96] Progressive spasticity, dysphagia, decreased spontaneous movement, and seizures lead to the further complications of aspiration pneumonia and respiratory failure. Death is common before 1 year of age and almost always occurs before 2 years of age.[97]

Type 3 or subacute neuronopathic Gaucher's disease is a rare disorder that has variable systemic features similar to those of type 2 disease but with an onset of neurologic symptoms several years later and a slower progression. Approximately one half of the children develop neurologic symptoms in the first decade of life.[97] Hepatosplenomegaly and moderate serum transaminase elevations are discovered in early childhood. Later, patients develop ataxia, spastic paraparesis, seizures, and dementia. Supranuclear ophthalmoplegia is present in almost all cases. Bone disease is usually less debilitating than in type 1 disease, and hepatic dysfunction is less advanced.[98] Histopathologically, the disorder is characterized by Gaucher cells. These are lipid-laden histiocytic cells that are abundant in the spleen, hepatic sinusoids, bone marrow, and lymph nodes; near alveolar capillaries; in the walls of other blood and lymph vessels, and in many tissues.[97] These cells have an eccentric nucleus and diffuse, lightly eosinophilic striations of the cytoplasm ("wrinkled tissue paper" appearance). Hepatic histology is similar in the three types of Gaucher's disease. Gaucher cells, derived from Kupffer cells, are found in aggregates scattered through the parenchyma but often are concentrated around the central vein. The central vein may be compressed. The sinusoids may also be narrowed and obscured.[93] There are fibrous bands around aggregates of Gaucher cells. In some instances, pericentral fibrosis can lead to a pattern of micronodular cirrhosis.

Conventional plain films or magnetic resonance imaging may show the classic flaring of the distal femur, the Erlenmeyer-flask deformity, or marrow replacement.[97] Laboratory evaluation is characterized by elevated plasma levels of acid phosphatase, lysozyme, angiotensin-converting enzyme, and β-hexosaminidase. A marked increase in plasma chitotriosidase activity may correlate well with the activity of Gaucher's disease.[99]

### Diagnosis

A bone marrow biopsy specimen showing Gaucher-like cells is strongly suggestive, but the definitive diagnostic test is measurement of the glucocerebrosidase activity in blood leukocytes, fibroblasts, or urine.[100] Enzymatic assays also can be used in cells from amniocentesis or chorionic villus sampling to allow for prenatal diagnosis.

### Pathogenesis

Molecular analysis and diagnosis in Gaucher's disease has been made possible by the discovery of the glucocerebrosidase gene (approximately 7.25 kb) on chromosome 1q2.1.[101, 102] More than 60 different mutations of this gene have been discovered in Gaucher's alleles, but mutations have not yet been characterized in a significant number of the known alleles.[91]

It has been suggested that determinants of phospholipid traffic and intralysosomal pH modify the disease phenotype by influencing the activity of the residual glucocerebrosidase.[103] Mutations that lead to changes in the glucocerebrosi-

**TABLE 49–4. Manifestations of Gaucher's and Niemann-Pick Lipidoses**

| | GAUCHER'S DISEASE | | | NIEMANN-PICK DISEASE | | |
|---|---|---|---|---|---|---|
| **FEATURE** | **Type 1** | **Type 2** | **Type 3** | **Type A** | **Type B** | **Type C** |
| Onset | Childhood<br>Adulthood | Infancy | Childhood | Infancy | Childhood<br>Adolescence | Infancy<br>Childhood |
| Central nervous system involvement | − | + | + | + | − | + |
| Hepatosplenomegaly | + | + | + | + | + | + |
| Pulmonary involvement | +/− | − | +/− | +/− | + | − |
| Bone involvement | + | − | + | +/− | +/− | − |
| Cherry-red macula | − | − | − | + | + | − |
| Survival | 6 yr–adult | 2 yr | 10–40 yr | 2–3 yr | 10 yr–adult | 20 yr |
| Ethnic predilection | Ashkenazic | Panethnic | Panethnic, Swedish | Panethnic, Ashkenazic | Panethnic, Ashkenazic | Panethnic, Nova Scotia, Colorado |
| Molecular defect | Glucocerebrosidase | Glucocerebrosidase | Glucocerebrosidase | Acid sphingomyelinase | Acid sphingomyelinase | Cholesterol processing |

+, present; −, absent, +/−, variable.

dase cofactor, saposin C, have also been implicated in a Gaucher-like disease phenotype.[104] An animal model for Gaucher's disease has been created by targeted disruption of the mouse glucocerebrosidase gene.[105, 106]

## Treatment

Splenectomy has been a mainstay of management for thrombocytopenia or complications of hypersplenism. Partial splenectomy was introduced when it was suggested that splenectomy, in some patients, worsened disease symptoms at other sites in the body.[107] Bone complications have been managed with various orthopedic procedures and with careful surveillance for osteomyelitis. Aminohydroxypropylidene biphosphonate administration has been suggested for improved bone mineralization, and steroids have been used in pilot studies to treat bone crises.[108, 109] Attempts at liver transplantation for the rare patient with liver failure caused by Gaucher's disease have led to recurrence of severe liver disease as the normal donor liver became repopulated with Gaucher-type Kupffer cells from the recipient.[110] Specific enzyme replacement therapy for Gaucher's disease has become possible by modifying the carbohydrate side chain of glucocerebrosidase so that it is delivered to the lysosome of tissue macrophages via the mannose receptor.[111–113] The enzyme preparations, originally purified from placenta (alglucerase [Ceredase]) and now in a recombinant form (imiglucerase [Cerezyme]), have been shown to be effective in type 1 and type 3 patients in reducing organomegaly, improving anemia and thrombocytopenia, improving macrophage antimicrobial function, and reducing bone complications. Studies have also shown arrest of neurologic deterioration in type 3 Gaucher's disease[113] and restoration of catch-up growth in growth-retarded children.[114, 115]

Bone marrow transplantation has been used sporadically in the treatment of Gaucher's disease. Although the specific indications are unclear and initial morbidity is significant, successful engraftment appears to reduce or eliminate symptoms in some type 1 patients.[116]

# NIEMANN-PICK DISEASE

Niemann-Pick disease (NPD) types A and B are lysosomal storage disorders resulting from the deficient activity of acid sphingomyelinase (ASM), which leads to the intracellular accumulation of sphingomyelin and other lipids (see Table 49–4). NPD type C is now known to result from an unrelated defect in cholesterol processing and is considered separately from types A and B.[117, 118]

## Niemann-Pick Disease Types A and B

The NPD type A phenotype is relatively uniform, with marked hepatosplenomegaly developing within the first few months of life, often with moderate lymphadenopathy. Microcytic anemia and thrombocytopenia usually follow within the first year. Muscle weakness and hypotonia occur early, leading to feeding difficulties and poor growth. By 8 to 12 months of age, psychomotor retardation becomes progressive, with loss of developmental milestones. Cardiac function usually is normal, and respiratory difficulties are minimal, although diffuse abnormalities visible on chest radiographs often appear before 1 year of age as the Niemann-Pick (NP) cells infiltrate the lungs (see later discussion). Ophthalmologic examination reveals the characteristic cherry-red macula in about one half of patients within the first 2 years, although visual impairment is rare. Examination of the bone marrow shows NP cell infiltration, but bone deformity is uncommon. Death by 2 to 3 years of age usually occurs in a setting of severe neurologic deterioration and emaciation with nutritional deficiency syndromes such as osteoporosis, hepatomegaly, and muscle spasticity. The skin may develop an orange-brown to yellow discoloration. Xanthomas can occur.

NPD type B is more variable in clinical presentation and has a less characteristic rate of progression. Asymptomatic hepatomegaly or splenomegaly, or both, may be detected within the first few years of life. In mild cases, the disorder may not be recognized until adulthood.[119] Thrombocytopenia or pancytopenia can result from splenic sequestration. Liver disease can progress to cirrhosis and portal hypertension in severely affected persons. Infiltration of alveoli by NP cells may begin in childhood and often can be detected by diffuse nodular or reticular patterns on chest radiographs. Clinically significant decreases in pulmonary function can occur by the late second decade of life.

The NP cell can be distinguished from the altered cells found in other diseases, such as Gaucher's disease, by histologic or histochemical analysis. NP cells usually have one nucleus that is surrounded by cytoplasm crowded with lipid droplets.[117] NP cells seen in bone marrow preparations may have characteristic blue inclusions, which has given rise to the term "sea-blue histiocytes."

Liver involvement may be uneven, with abnormal-appearing Kupffer cells in the sinuses early in the disease and abnormal hepatocytes with NP cell infiltration of portal areas late in the course. Hepatic fibrosis can occur.[120]

The biochemical defect in NPD types A and B has been identified as deficient activity of ASM, an enzyme that degrades the phospholipid components of various cellular organelles, myelin, and other structures. Without this activity, cholesterol, sphingomyelin, and other lipids accumulate in the lysosomes of affected cells. Various reports have correlated residual activity with disease severity, indicating 0% to 2% of normal activity remaining in type A patients and 2% to 10% in type B patients.[117] Defective alleles encoding the ASM gene are inherited in an autosomal recessive fashion, giving asymptomatic heterozygous carriers of a defective gene approximately 70% of normal enzyme activity. The human ASM gene has been cloned and is located on chromosome 11p15.1.[121, 122]

Although the occurrence of NPD is panethnic, there is a predilection among persons of Ashkenazi Jewish ancestry. A large number of mutations of various types have been identified, including point mutations and deletions, and phenotype-genotype correlations are beginning to be made. In general, mutations that are predicted to produce a truncated polypeptide or a full-length construct that appears to have no enzymatic activity are associated with more severe type A disease.[117] A murine model of ASM deficiency has been generated by selective targeting of the mouse ASM gene, which produces a neuropathic phenotype.[123, 124]

Definitive diagnosis is made by analysis of specific enzyme activity in peripheral blood leukocytes, cultured fibroblasts, or lymphoblasts, or by molecular genetic DNA analysis. Prenatal diagnosis by enzyme or DNA analysis of cultured cells from amniocentesis or chorionic villus sampling is also possible.[117]

There is no specific treatment for NPD type A or B. Bone marrow transplantation has been performed in a number of patients, but no change in neurologic status has been reported in any of the type A patients.[117] Data on long-term success in type B patients are lacking. Orthotopic liver transplantation has met with limited success and has not altered disease progression in other areas.[125]

### Niemann-Pick Disease Type C

NPD type C is a highly variable clinical syndrome related to an intracellular defect in cholesterol processing, although the exact nature of the defect is still unknown. The most common presentation of NPD type C is as neonatal liver disease with hepatosplenomegaly, conjugated hyperbilirubinemia, and elevation of serum transaminases.[126] Liver synthetic function usually is normal. Hepatomegaly may regress, but splenomegaly often remains. In rare cases, ascites may be present and liver disease can progress to portal hypertension and death.[127]

By 3 to 6 years of age, affected children commonly begin to manifest neurologic symptoms of ataxia, developmental delay, seizures, dysarthria, poor fine motor skills, dystonia, and learning problems. In some children who escape detection as neonates, a retrospective history of prolonged infantile jaundice can be elicited from the parents. The most common neurologic finding is supranuclear ophthalmoplegia, especially in the vertical direction. Late in the first decade of life cognitive decline often accelerates, gross motor function deteriorates, and respiratory complications can occur. Dementia or other psychiatric disturbances appear. Death in the teenage years usually follows.

Histopathologic examination of the liver during the neonatal involvement is variable but usually reveals some combination of cholestasis, lobular inflammation, portal edema, and multinucleated giant cell transformation. In some cases fibrosis is prominent, especially as a result of hepatocyte collapse.[126, 127] So-called activated Kupffer cells can be seen in addition to classic NP cells.

The molecular lesion causing NPD type C is inherited in an autosomal recessive fashion and appears to lead to the lysosomal sequestration of endocytosed cholesterol. Fibroblast complementation studies suggest that at least two different lesions may be responsible for the cholesterol trafficking errors.[127, 128] Genetic analysis has shown that at least the majority of patients have a lesion linked to chromosome 18p.[129]

The definitive diagnosis is based on determinations of the rate of cholesterol esterification in cultured patient fibroblasts.[130, 131] Fibroblast ASM activity may be moderately decreased as an epiphenomenon, but it is not as low as in NPD type A or B.

There is no specific treatment of NPD type C, other than supportive measures such as nutritional support and antiepileptic drugs. Suggestions that a low-cholesterol diet or cholesterol-lowering medications such as lovastatin may slow the progression of the disease have so far not been supported by pilot study data.[132] Liver transplantation does not appear to slow the neurologic deterioration.[117]

## GALACTOSEMIA

Galactosemia is a syndrome of liver disease, failure to thrive, and developmental delay in infants that is caused by deficiency in galactose-1-phosphate uridyltransferase (GALT) and the resulting block in the metabolism of galactose, one of the monosaccharide constituents of the milk sugar lactose.[133, 134]

### Clinical Aspects

The most common clinical manifestation of galactosemia is failure to thrive in infancy. Weight loss and vomiting are seen in approximately half of patients, usually within several days of starting lactose.[135, 136] Diarrhea is also common. Jaundice, ascites, hepatomegaly, and/or splenomegaly may develop and can progress to cirrhosis and severe liver dysfunction if galactose intake continues. Hemolytic anemia can occur, and cataracts may develop within the first 6 months of life. Lethargy, hypotonia, difficulty feeding, and developmental delay can also occur. Affected infants may be discovered during an episode of *Escherichia coli* sepsis.[137] However, it is not known whether galactosemia truly predisposes infants to gram-negative sepsis by a disease-specific mechanism.

Laboratory evaluation shows hepatic dysfunction with elevated serum transaminases and hyperbilirubinemia. Elevated blood galactose, hyperchloremic metabolic acidosis, and, rarely, hypoglycemia may also be seen. Renal tubular dysfunction may be manifested initially by albuminuria and later by aminoaciduria and galactosuria.[133, 134] Anemia with microscopic evidence of hemolysis may be present.

### Diagnosis

The diagnosis of galactosemia is often suggested by the presence of reducing substance in the urine (as measured by Clinitest tablet) in the absence of glucose in the urine (as measured by commercially available glucose oxidase assay). However, the detection of galactosuria by these determinations is insensitive and nonspecific. Poor lactose intake or intermittent excretion of excess galactose can be responsible for false-negative results. False-positive results are observed in patients with severe liver disease or after certain medications are administered. Specific diagnosis relies on determination of red blood cell GALT activity.[134] Prenatal diagnosis can be made by the enzymatic assay of tissue from amniocentesis or chorionic villus sampling.[138] In recent years the majority of patients have been recognized by newborn screening programs, which are administered in 44 states in the United States and in many other countries.[139]

## Treatment

The mainstay of treatment for galactosemia is the elimination of all forms of galactose intake. Soy and protein hydrolysate formulas that are lactose free are substituted for breast milk or lactose-containing formula. The institution of a galactose-free diet results in a rapid regression of vomiting, diarrhea, and hepatic dysfunction. There is improvement in growth and development. Cataracts regress and renal tubular dysfunction resolves on the restricted diet.

Later in childhood, treatment involves elimination of dairy products and foods containing milk or lactose as additives. Studies have also suggested that galactose is present in fruits, vegetables, grains, and meats.[140] This may explain the residual defects in mental functioning that have been identified in these patients in long-term studies.[141] These defects include speech dyspraxia, delays in language skill acquisition, mental retardation, short attention span, social withdrawal, abnormalities of visual perception, ataxia, and even mental retardation. Almost all affected females exhibit some form of ovarian dysfunction. Primary or secondary amenorrhea can result, although pregnancies have been reported.[136, 141]

## Molecular Pathogenesis

The GALT enzyme is a 379-amino-acid, 43- to 44-kd polypeptide encoded by a 4-kb gene on chromosome 9.[142, 143] A variety of mutations that are inherited in an autosomal recessive fashion have been identified. In general, alleles associated with disease have a very low level of enzymatic activity, 2% to 7% of normal.[134] The metabolic defect in galactosemia is shown in Figure 49–2.

Galactitol is an end product of metabolism produced from a portion of the accumulated galactose and is considered a major factor in cataract formation. There are data suggesting that glucose can be converted to galactose by other pathways and that such pathways are responsible for the neurologic defects in patients who abstain from galactose.[144]

## HEREDITARY FRUCTOSE INTOLERANCE

Hereditary fructose intolerance (HFI) is caused by the deficiency of fructose-1,6-bisphosphate aldolase (aldolase B).[145, 146] This is one of a group of enzymes that convert fructose to intermediates of the glycolytic-gluconeogenic pathway (Fig. 49–3) which can then be metabolized to glucose or glycogen or used for energy.[146]

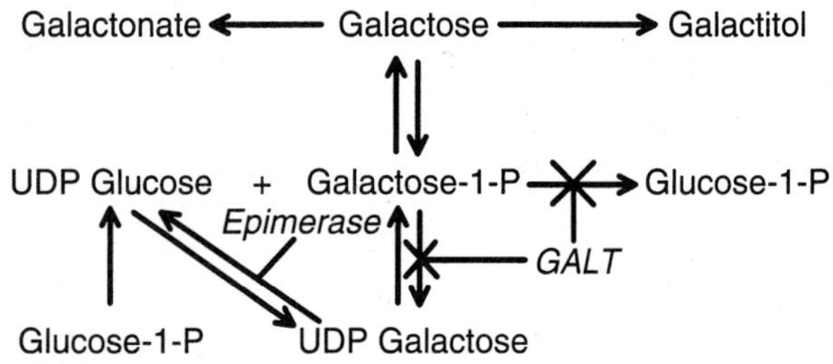


**FIGURE 49–2.** Galactose metabolism. Ingested galactose 3 phosphorylated to galactose-1-phosphate (galactose-1-P) and then converted to uridine diphosphate (UDP) galactose and glucose-1-phosphate (glucose-1-P) by galactose-1-phosphate uridyltransferase (GALT), the enzyme affected in galactosemia. In the absence of GALT activity, alternative pathways overproduce the potentially toxic metabolites galactonate and galactitol.

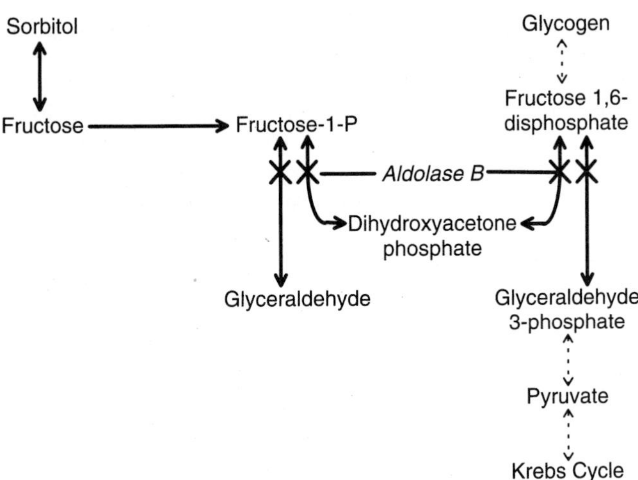


**FIGURE 49–3.** Fructose metabolism. Ingested fructose can be metabolized to glycogen or to products of the Krebs cycle. An important step is catalyzed by the enzyme, aldolase B. Deficiency of aldolase B activity in HFI leads to accumulation of fructose-1-phosphate, which, in turn, triggers a variety of cellular derangements.

## Clinical Aspects

Individuals with HFI are completely healthy unless or until they ingest food containing fructose or more complex molecules that contain fructose as a subunit (e.g., sorbitol, sucrose). Symptoms may be observed acutely if infants are fed a sucrose-containing formula. Otherwise, children commonly present when fructose-containing baby foods are introduced or when they are weaned from breast milk. Often vomiting and other gastrointestinal symptoms are present, including diarrhea, abdominal pain, feeding difficulties, fever, jaundice, extreme fussiness, episodes of trembling, and pallor. Occasionally, after large doses of fructose, an infant experiences convulsions and coma.[147] Some infants exhibit hypoglycemia during acute episodes. If exposed to fructose chronically, the infant may develop hepatomegaly, edema, ascites, splenomegaly, and failure to thrive. Nutritional deficiency states such as rickets may develop. Laboratory abnormalities are in keeping with the nonspecific nature of the symptoms and the target organ dysfunction. Most common are elevated serum transaminases, prolonged prothrombin time, hyperbilirubinemia, hypoproteinemia, hypokalemia, and hypophosphatemia. In the urine, reducing substances, protein, amino acids, organic acids, and specifically fructose are all increased. Hypoglycemia, anemia, and thrombocytopenia also can occur. In some children the only manifestation of HFI is poor growth and hepatomegaly.[148] Presumably, these children are getting a low dose of fructose on a chronic basis or have a milder defect in the aldolase B gene. Occasionally HFI is diagnosed in adolescents or adults. These persons develop specific aversions to foods containing fructose or sucrose and have unusual feeding behaviors, such as eating only the peel but not the pulp of fruit. They also have a very low incidence of dental caries, which are known to be produced by sucrose.[149, 150]

Histopathologically, the liver may exhibit steatosis, necrosis of scattered hepatocytes, and intralobular or periportal fibrosis progressing to cirrhosis.[146, 147] Electron microscopic evaluation suggests a florid lysosomal reaction to intracellular deposits of fructose-1-phosphate with polymorphous, electron-dense cytoplasmic inclusions in concentric membranous arrays.[146]

The metabolic pathogenesis of the symptoms of acute fructose ingestion in HFI has been examined in vitro, in animals, in healthy controls, and in affected patients.[146] Acute fructose intake in HFI results in accumulation of fructose-1-phosphate in liver, kidney, and small intestine due to the inability of aldolase B to further metabolize this intermediate.[151] This leads to a cascade that depletes the intracellular milieu of inorganic phosphate and adenosine triphosphate (ATP). Protein synthesis and other cellular functions are disrupted. Hypoglycemia is caused by temporary impairment in hepatic glycogenolysis and gluconeogenesis.[151]

## Diagnosis

Definitive diagnosis should be determined by enzyme assay on liver tissue.[146] The intravenous fructose tolerance test has been discouraged by many investigators who have observed severe toxic effects during the study.

## Treatment

Treatment of acute episodes in HFI involves supportive care to correct metabolic derangements and complications. This may take the form of intravenous fluid and glucose, blood products to treat coagulopathy and bleeding, and, later, vitamins and nutritional support to restore growth.[146] Long-term management focuses on scrupulous avoidance of foods and medicines containing fructose. This requires a high degree of vigilance, because various forms of fructose (e.g., sorbitol) are commonly used as food additives. Long-term abstinence leads to gradual reduction in hepatomegaly, reversal of organ dysfunction, normal intellectual function, and catch-up growth.[147, 148]

## Molecular Genetics

The aldolase B gene occupies approximately 14.5 kb on chromosome 9q21.3–q22.2 and encodes a 364-amino-acid polypeptide.[152, 153] Alleles deficient in activity are inherited in an autosomal recessive fashion, and therefore only homozygotes manifest the disease phenotype. More than 20 different mutations of various types and 5 different polymorphisms have been described.[154]

# GLYCOGEN STORAGE DISEASE

Glycogen storage disease (GSD) results from deficiencies in specific enzymes of the glycogenolytic system and is associated with accumulation of glycogen in tissues, especially liver, skeletal muscle, and, in one case, cardiac muscle.[155] More than 10 forms have been reported, each with distinct clinical features. Types I, III, IV, and VI predominantly affect the liver (Table 49–5).

Type I GSD, or glucose-6-phosphatase deficiency, was initially considered a single clinical entity. It is now known that at least two clinical entities, types Ia and Ib, exist. Glucose-6-phosphatase is comprised of at least six different polypeptides.[156] A catalytic subunit spans the membrane of the ER six times.[157] The other five polypeptides include a polypeptide stabilizing protein (SP) that transports glucose-6-phosphate (T1), two polypeptides that transport phosphate (T2), and a glucose transporter (T3), also known as GLUT-7. Mutations in the gene for the catalytic subunit result in inactive enzyme and GSD type Ia.[158–161] In type Ib GSD, normal phosphatase activity is present in fully disrupted liver microsome preparations but not in intact microsomal vesicles. This disorder is believed to involve a defect in the T1 translocase. There is also a type Ic GSD in which the T2 translocase is thought to be defective.[161] Although a type Ia SP GSD was thought to involve defects in SP, a mutation in the catalytic subunit has been identified in a patient with type Ia SP GSD.[161]

In classic Ia GSD, infants are short but chubby, with doll-like faces; poorly developed, flabby musculature; abdominal distention; and hepatomegaly. They are most commonly recognized because of hypoglycemia and metabolic acidosis caused by high circulating levels of lactic acid. Laboratory evaluation may also indicate the presence of elevated triglyceride and uric acid concentrations. Liver enzymes usually are not elevated, and liver biopsy specimens are remarkable only for evidence of increased glycogen. These patients may develop adenomas and carcinomas of the liver. They also develop nephrolithiasis and progressive renal dysfunction.[162, 163] Determination of glycogen content and glucose-6-phosphatase activity in liver provides a definitive diagnosis.

The prognosis for patients with type Ia GSD has improved dramatically since the introduction of nocturnal nasogastric infusion of glucose[164] and oral cornstarch therapy.[165, 166] The latter regimen is based on slow degradation by amylase, which allows maintenance of normal blood glucose level for up to 6 hours. In most cases, affected infants are given oral cornstarch therapy when they reach an age at which small, frequent feedings of infant formula are no longer feasible. Targeted mutagenesis of glucose-6-phosphatase has been used to generate an animal model of type Ia GSD[167] that should allow testing of new treatment strategies.

In type Ib GSD, patients have the additional burden of recurrent infections as a result of neutropenia and neutrophil dysfunction.[168] Recurrent pneumonia, oral mucositis, perianal abscesses, and inflammatory lesions of the bowel may dominate the clinical picture.[169] The introduction of recombinant human granulocyte colony-stimulating factor has greatly improved the lives of several patients.[170]

In type III GSD, the glycogen debranching enzyme is deficient.[171] This enzyme is a polypeptide of about 165,000 kd that is encoded by a gene (approximately 85 kb) on chromosome 1.[172] Mutations in this gene have been demonstrated in several patients.[173] During infancy these patients are often difficult to distinguish clinically from patients with type I GSD. However, they usually do not develop acido-

**TABLE 49–5. Glycogen Storage Diseases**

| TYPE | ENZYME DEFICIENCY | TISSUE INVOLVED | SYMPTOMS |
|---|---|---|---|
| Ia | Glucose-6-phosphatase (von Gierke's disease) | Liver, kidney, intestine | Visceromegaly, "doll face"<br>Lactic acidosis, hypoglycemia, hyperlipidemia |
| Ib | Translocase (T1 defect) | Liver | Recurrent infections<br>Visceromegaly, "doll face"<br>Lactic acidosis, hypoglycemia, hyperlipidemia |
| Ic | Translocase (T2 defect) | Liver | Visceromegaly, "doll face"<br>Lactic acidosis, hypoglycemia, hyperlipidemia |
| III | Amylo-1,6-glucosidose (debrancher enzyme) | Liver, muscle, heart | Hepatomegaly, no hypoglycemia<br>Some hypotonia and cardiomegaly |
| IV | Amylo-1,4-1,6-transglucosidose (brancher enzyme) | Generalized | Hepatosplenomegaly<br>Progressive cirrhosis and liver failure<br>Death in childhood |
| VI | Liver phosphorylase | Liver | Hepatomegaly, no acidosis<br>No hypoglycemia |
| IX | Liver phosphorylase-kinase | Liver | Hepatomegaly, no acidosis<br>No hypoglycemia, usually not progressive |

sis, hyperuricemia, or hypertriglyceridemia. Abnormalities include increased serum transaminases, mild hepatocellular necrosis, and portal fibrosis on liver histologic examination. Occasionally these patients develop cirrhosis, portal hypertension, or even hepatocellular adenoma and carcinoma.[174, 175] Several patients have responded well to liver transplantation. In others with type III GSD, the hepatomegaly tends to recede and progressive muscle weakness and wasting develop as the patient reaches adulthood. Definitive diagnosis may be established by enzyme activity measurements in muscle, liver, skin fibroblasts, and sometimes erythrocytes.

Type IV GSD is characterized by deficiency in the glycogen branching enzyme.[176] Several types of defects in this gene have been identified in affected children,[177] manifesting in progressive liver dysfunction, hypotonia, growth failure, and delayed development. Liver failure is common in the first 3 to 5 years of life. The diagnosis can be made by enzyme assays on leukocytes and skin fibroblasts as well as liver and muscle biopsies.

Liver transplantation has been used successfully to treat patients with GSD type IV.[178] The observation that amylopectin deposits in the hearts of two of these patients resorbed after orthotopic liver transplantation provided the first evidence that donor cells could migrate from a liver graft into other host tissues, so-called systemic microchimerism.[179]

Type VI GSD has been diagnosed in asymptomatic children with hepatomegaly and is thought to represent a genetically heterogeneous deficiency in liver phosphorylase or phosphorylase b kinase.[155] However, one patient with phosphorylase b kinase deficiency has developed severe liver disease and cirrhosis.[180]

## WILSON'S DISEASE

Wilson's disease is a progressive disorder characterized by abnormalities of the motor system, psychiatric symptoms, and hepatic disease resulting in cirrhosis. A specific defect in copper transport (Fig. 49–4) results in progressive accumulation of copper in target tissues.[181]

### Clinical Aspects

Wilson's disease, also known as hepatolenticular degeneration, can have a variety of presentations from childhood through middle age, including predominantly hepatic symptoms, predominantly neurologic symptoms, or both. Liver injury is present at the time of diagnosis in approximately 50% of patients.[182] In the typical case, a teenager presents with malaise and abdominal pain and is found to have a number of signs and symptoms of liver dysfunction, including hepatomegaly with or without splenomegaly, jaundice, ascites, or gastrointestinal bleeding as a result of portal hypertension. The liver is the predominant or sole organ involved in approximately one third of affected persons. Serum transaminases are often mildly elevated but can be normal. Occasionally, Wilson's disease manifests as acute

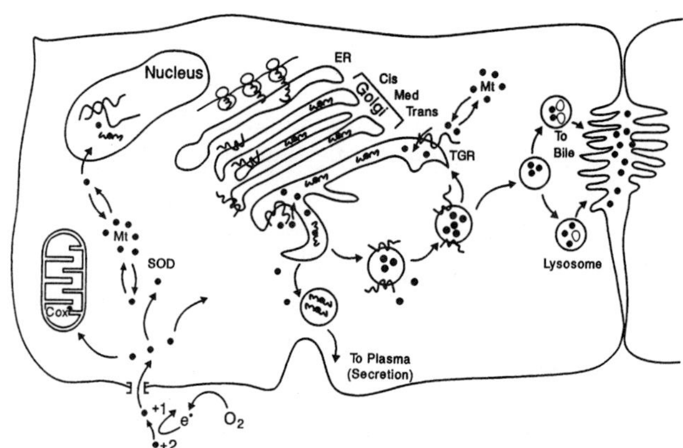


**FIGURE 49–4.** Model of copper metabolism within the hepatocytes. Potential fate of copper (●) is shown. The wild type ATPase is shown as a transmembrane protein with multiple membrane-spanning domains, and ceruloplasmin as shown as a luminal molecule. ER, endoplasmic reticulum; TGR, trans-Golgi reticulum; Mt, mitochondria; SOD, superoxide dismutase; COX, cytochrome oxidase. (From Harris AL, Gitlin JD: Genetic and molecular basis for copper toxicity. Am J Clin Nutr 1996;63:836S-841S with permission.)

hepatic failure, which can be accompanied by an acute, life-threatening hemolytic anemia.[183, 184]

Approximately one third of patients present with neuropsychiatric symptoms alone, and often at a somewhat later age than those with predominant hepatic involvement. Motor symptoms are common, including dystonia, weakness, choreiform movements, tremors, dysarthria, and gait disturbances. Headaches can be a prominent complaint. Common psychiatric disturbances range from mild decreases in social functioning or school performance to acute psychosis. Other tissues and organs can also be involved; for example, there may be primary proximal and distal renal tubular dysfunction, sometimes with renal calculi.[185] Endocrine abnormalities of glucose intolerance, hypoparathyroidism, and amenorrhea have been described. Complaints of joint pain and stiffness are not uncommon and can be associated with degenerative changes of the large joints and spine. Osteoporosis can occur.[186] Kayser-Fleischer rings, a yellow-brown deposition of copper in the Descemet membrane at the limbus of the cornea, are observed in 70% of children and in almost all affected adults. The absence of Kayser-Fleischer rings does not exclude the diagnosis of Wilson's disease, and similar structures may sometimes be observed in patients with other liver disease.[187]

Pathologic changes in the liver early in the course of the disease include cytoplasmic macrovesicular and microvesicular lipid droplets, ballooning and glycogenation of nuclei, pleomorphic alteration of mitochondria, and increased specific stains for copper in cytoplasm and, later, in lysosomes. Progressive fibrosis and cirrhosis then develop, with minimal hepatocyte death unless there is an episode of acute hepatic failure with massive or submassive hepatic necrosis.[188] Copper overload in the brain can occur, commonly in the lenticular nuclei, basal ganglia, cerebellum, and pons. Neuronal edema and inflammation with neuronal loss and reactive gliosis may be evident. Laboratory evaluation may reveal increased urinary copper, increased copper content of liver tissue, and decreased serum concentrations of the copper transport protein, ceruloplasmin.

### Genetic and Molecular Pathogenesis

Wilson's disease is an autosomal recessive disease with an approximate incidence for homozygotes of 1 in 30,000 persons. The gene was originally linked to chromosome 13q,[189] and later the cDNA was cloned and sequenced.[190–193] The gene product appears to be a membrane-bound copper transporter with P-type ATPase activity. It is highly homologous to the copper transporter that is mutated in Menkes' disease, another disorder of copper metabolism.[194–196] Some preliminary evidence suggests that the protein is localized in the ER or trans-Golgi. The defective gene is thought to be necessary for the transport of copper to intracellular sites required for incorporation into copper-binding proteins. For instance, copper is not efficiently incorporated into ceruloplasmin to allow for secretion into the blood and is not efficiently incorporated into other copper-binding proteins to allow for excretion into bile. The defect results in a partial reduction in biliary excretion of copper; for this reason, it is a relatively long time before copper accumulation in the liver becomes significant. Eventually, copper overflows into other tissues, such as corneas, brain, kidneys, bones, joints, and cardiac muscle.[194–198]

Approximately 50 mutations of various types have been described in the Wilson's disease gene. Preliminary genotype-phenotype correlations indicate that some mutations resulting in no functional gene product could lead to earlier-onset liver disease, and other specific alleles are associated with the late-onset, neurologic presentation of Wilson's disease.[199]

### Diagnosis

Laboratory evaluation shows decreased serum ceruloplasmin, elevated nonceruloplasmin serum copper, and elevated urine copper concentrations. Definitive diagnosis is made by elevated hepatic copper levels if liver biopsy is possible.[200] In children, it may be difficult to diagnose Wilson's disease without a hepatic copper determination because serum ceruloplasmin levels can be normal, Kayser-Fleischer rings can be absent, and 24-hour urinary copper levels can be only minimally elevated. In one study, the serum ceruloplasmin level was less than 20 mg/dL in 73% of patients with Wilson's disease, urinary copper excretion was elevated in 88%, hepatic copper was elevated in 91%, and Kayser-Fleischer rings were detected in 55% of patients at time of diagnosis.[201] Once an index patient within a family has been diagnosed, all of the siblings should be investigated for subclinical disease, which should be amenable to immediate institution of treatment.

### Treatment

All of the tissue injury caused by Wilson's disease can be stabilized by chelation therapy. D-Penicillamine is the safest and most effective drug. It can be taken orally and is generally well tolerated.[202, 203] In patients with hypersensitivity to penicillamine, trientine or zinc can be used.[202] Orthotopic liver transplantation may be necessary if fulminant liver failure develops before penicillamine has elicited a positive effect.[204, 205] Several animal models of Wilson's disease are now available.[206–213]

## NEONATAL HEMOCHROMATOSIS

Neonatal hemochromatosis, also called neonatal iron storage disease, is a rare disorder of unknown origin. Neonatal hemochromatosis usually follows a course that is fatal in days to weeks and is manifested by liver failure with fibrosis and tissue siderosis. Although the pattern of hemosiderin deposition is similar to that seen in hereditary hemochromatosis, the two disorders are not genetically related.[214]

### Clinical Aspects

Infants with neonatal hemochromatosis usually are recognized at birth, or hours thereafter, with hypoglycemia, hypoalbuminemia, edema, ascites, thrombocytopenia, and severe bleeding. The pregnancy may be characterized by prematurity or intrauterine growth retardation.[215, 216] Fetal death in utero, oligohydramnios, and polyhydramnios have been reported. Hepatomegaly may be mild to moderate. Liver disease rapidly progresses to severe liver failure. Serum alpha-fetoprotein levels usually are high. Anemia, heart failure, and portal hypertension may be present. Death is the result in almost all cases.

Histopathologic examination of the liver often is not possible before necropsy because of uncorrectable coagulopathy. The liver usually is small and fibrotic. Hepatocellular loss is severe, leading to reticulin collapse and focal nodular regeneration or pseudoacinar transformation. Marked perisinusoidal fibrosis is common. Cholestasis, giant cell transformation, and moderate to marked siderosis of hepatocytes are evident.[215, 216] Much less hemosiderin is present in other hepatic cell types. Proliferation of bile ducts and fatty infiltration can be seen. Hemosiderin deposits usually are present in the pancreas, myocardium, adrenal cortex, and thyroid, but the reticuloendothelial system is spared.

### Genetics and Pathophysiology

The pathogenesis of neonatal hemochromatosis is unknown. Both sporadic cases and affected siblings have been reported, and both autosomal recessive and autosomal codominant modes of inheritance have been suggested.[214, 215, 217–219] One long-term follow-up study of first-degree relatives of affected children failed to detect any abnormalities in iron handling. It is unclear whether the primary defect is one of fetoplacental iron metabolism or whether some other primary liver disease leads to a secondary alteration in iron trafficking.[220, 221] It is possible that multiple types of injury could produce this same clinical phenotype.

### Diagnosis

Often it is not possible to safely perform liver biopsy in these unstable infants. Determination of serum transferrin saturation and ferritin levels may be helpful. Some authorities use biopsy of the lower lip to look for iron staining of the minor salivary glands[222] or magnetic resonance imaging to obtain evidence of increased tissue iron. Magnetic resonance imaging also has been used successfully for prenatal diagnosis.[214]

### Treatment

The outcome of general supportive care in neonatal hemochromatosis has been dismal. Various proposals for prenatal or neonatal iron depletion (phlebotomy) or chelation have been discussed but rarely tried. Several patients have been treated with deferoxamine alone without success.[214, 223] An abstract has described the use of so-called antioxidant cocktails, which include various doses of *N*-acetylcysteine, α-tocopherol, selenium, prostaglandin E, and deferoxamine.[224] There is an initial report of three survivors using this approach. Liver transplantation has been performed successfully in a small number of cases, but the long-term prognosis is unknown.[225, 226] There has been one report of a possible recurrence of neonatal hemochromatosis in a transplanted liver.[227]

## LIVER DISEASE ASSOCIATED WITH DEFECTS IN BILE ACID METABOLISM

In the last decade several inborn errors of bile acid synthesis have been shown to cause progressive cholestatic liver disease in infants. A defect in 3β-hydroxysteroid dehydrogenase/isomerase in a Saudi Arabian family was first described in 1987.[228] Four siblings with cholestasis from birth were found to have $\Delta^4$-3-oxosteroid 5β-reductase deficiency in 1988.[229]

### 3β-Hydroxy-C27-Steroid Dehydrogenase/Isomerase Deficiency

In this deficiency, the infant develops progressive cholestasis by 3 months of age, jaundice, steatorrhea, and fat-soluble vitamin deficiency. Examination is remarkable for hepatomegaly.[230] The serum transaminase and conjugated bilirubin levels are increased, but gamma glutamyl transpeptidase and serum bile acids are normal. Liver biopsy shows hepatitis with giant cells, canalicular plugs, and bile stasis. Urinary bile acid analysis is characterized by the presence of sulfate and glycosulfate conjugates of dihydroxy- and trihydroxy-cholenoic acids, indicating that there is a defect in the second step in the primary bile acid synthetic pathway. Liver injury is thought to be a consequence of poor bile flow and accumulation of toxic bile acid intermediates. If the condition is left untreated, the infant develops cirrhosis and liver failure. Treatment with chenodeoxycholic acid or ursodeoxycholic acid is associated with almost complete resolution of liver disease.[231–233]

### $\Delta^4$-3-Oxosteroid 5β-Reductase Deficiency

Infants with this disorder present in the neonatal period with jaundice, pale stools, dark urine, and poor weight gain. The serum transaminases are mildly elevated, and the prothrombin time prolonged. Serum levels of alkaline phosphatase and gamma glutamyl transpeptidase are mildly elevated. Liver biopsies show lobular disarray with pseudoacinar formation, giant cell transformation, bile stasis, and extramedullary hematopoiesis. There is a striking lack of microvilli at the canalicular epithelium, and the canaliculi are slit-like in appearance on electron microscopy. Atypical bile acids, specifically oxo- and allo-derivatives, are found in urine and serum, indicating a defect at the fourth step in bile acid synthesis. Immunoblot analysis has shown that $\Delta^4$-3-oxosteroid 5β-reductase is absent in the liver of these patients.[234] The pathophysiology of liver injury is not known but presumably involves accumulation of the atypical bile acid intermediates. Treatment with the hyperchloretic bile acid ursodeoxycholic acid is associated with improvement in clinical, biochemical, and histologic abnormalities if it is initiated before significant liver injury develops.[235] More than 14 other patients with this deficiency have been described.[236] Among these patients were four infants previously carrying a diagnosis of neonatal iron storage disease, raising the possibility that iron storage associated with the defect in bile acid secretion contributes to liver damage.

## REFERENCES


1. Teckman JH, Qu D, Perlmutter DH: Molecular pathogenesis of liver disease in α1-antitrypsin deficiency. Hepatology 1996;24:1504–1516.
2. Sveger T: Liver disease in α1-antitrypsin deficiency detected by screening of 200,000 infants. N Engl J Med 1976;294:1216–1221.
3. Sveger T, Eriksson S: The liver in adolescents with α1-antitrypsin deficiency. Hepatology 1995;22:514–517.
4. Erikson S, Carlson J, Velez R: Risk of cirrhosis and primary liver cancer in α1-antitrypsin deficiency. N Engl J Med 1989;314:736–739.
5. Lomas DA, Evans DL, Finch JJ, et al: The mechanism of Z α1-antitrypsin accumulation in the liver. Nature 1992;357:605–607.
6. Sidhar SK, Lomas DA, Carrell RW, et al: Mutations which impede loop-sheet polymerization enhance the secretion of human α1-antitrypsin deficiency variants. J Biol Chem 1995;270:8393–8396.
7. Yu M-H, Lee KN, Kim J: The Z type variation of human α1-antitrypsin causes a protein folding defect. Nat Struct Biol 1995;2:363–367.
8. Crystal RG: α1-Antitrypsin deficiency, emphysema and liver disease: genetic basis and strategies for therapy. J Clin Invest 1990;95:1343–1352.
9. Dycaico JM, Grant SGN, Felts K, et al: Neonatal hepatitis induced by α1-antitrypsin: a transgenic mice model. Science 1988;242:1404–1412.
10. Geller SA, Nichols WS, Kim SS, et al: Hepatocarcinogenesis is the sequel to hepatitis in Z #2 α1-antitrypsin transgenic mice: histopathological and DNA ploidy studies. Hepatology 1994;19:389–397.
11. Wu Y, Whitman I, Molmenti E, et al: A lag in intracellular degradation of mutant α1-antitrypsin correlates with the liver disease phenotype in homozygous PiZZ α1-antitrypsin deficiency. Proc Natl Acad Sci U S A 1994;91:9014–9018.
12. Qu D, Teckman TH, Omura S, et al: Degradation of mutant secretory protein, α1-antitrypsin Z, in the endoplasmic reticulum requires proteasome activity. J Biol Chem 1996;271:22791–22795.
13. Filipponi F, Soubrane O, Labrousse F, et al: Liver transplantation for end-stage liver disease associated with alpha-1-antitrypsin deficiency in children: pretransplant natural history, timing and results of transplantation. J Hepatol 1994;20:72–78.
14. Casavilla FA, Reye J, Tzakis A, et al: Liver transplantation for neonatal hepatitis as compared to the other two leading indications for liver transplantation in children. Hepatology 1994;21:1035–1039.
15. Wewers MD, Casolaro MA, Sellers SE, et al: Replacement therapy for α1-antitrypsin deficiency associated with emphysema. N Engl J Med 1987;316:1055–1062.
16. Hubbard RC, McElvaney NG, Sellers SE, et al: Recombinant DNA-produced α1-antitrypsin administered by aerosol augments lower respiratory tract antineutrophil elastase defense in individuals with α1-antitrypsin deficiency. J Clin Invest 1989;84:1349–1354.
17. Cole-Strauss A, Yoon K, Xiang Y, et al: Correction of the mutation responsible for sickle cell anemia by an RNA-DNA oligonucleotide. Science 1996;273:1385–1389.
18. Sullenger BA, Cech TR: Ribozyme-mediated repair of defective mRNA by targeted trans-splicing. Nature 1994;371:619–621.
19. Goldsmith LA, Laberge C: Tyrosinemia and related disorders. In Scriver CR, Beaudet AL, Sly WS, Valle D (eds): The Metabolic Basis of Inherited Disease, 6th ed. New York, McGraw-Hill, 1989, pp 547–562.
20. Mitchell G, Larochelle J, Lambet M, et al: Neurologic crisis in hereditary tyrosinemia. N Engl J Med 1990;32:432–437.
21. Scriver CR, Perry JRT, Lasley L, et al: Neonatal tyrosinemia in the Eskimo: results of protein polymorphism. Pediatr Res 1977;11:411–416.
22. Lindbald B, Lindstedt S, Steen G: On the enzymatic defects in hereditary tyrosinemia. Proc Natl Acad Sci U S A 1977;74:4641–4645.
23. Kvittingen EA, Brodtkorb E: The pre- and post-natal diagnosis of tyrosinemia type I and the detection of the carrier state by assay of fumarylacetoacetase. Scand J Clin Lab Invest 1986;46:35–40.
24. Tanguay RM, Valet JP, Lescault A, et al: Different molecular basis for fumarylacetoacetate hydrolase deficiency in the two clinical forms of hereditary tyrosinemia (type I). Am J Hum Genet 1990;47:308–316.
25. Kvittingen EA, Halorsen S, Jellum E: Deficient fumarylacetoacetate fumarylhydrolase activity in lymphocytes and fibroblasts from patients with hereditary tyrosinemia. Pediatr Res 1983;14:541–544.
26. Phaneuf D, Lambert M, Laframbosie R, et al: Type I hereditary tyrosinemia: evidence for molecular heterogeneity and identification of a causal mutation in a French Canadian patient. J Clin Invest 1992;90:1185–1192.
27. Grompe M, Al-Dhalimy M: Mutations of the fumarylacetoacetate hydrolase gene in four patients with tyrosinemia, type I. Hum Mutat 1993;2:85–93.
28. Kvittingen EA, Rootwelt H, Van Dam T, et al: Hereditary tyrosinemia type I: lack of correlation between clinical findings and amount of immunoreactive fumarylacetoacetase protein. Pediatr Res 1992;31:43–46.
29. Roth KS, Spencer PD, Higgins ES, et al: Effects of succinylacetone on methyl α-D-glucoside uptake by the rat renal tubule. Biochim Biophys Acta 1985;820:140–146.
30. Sassa S, Kappas A: Hereditary tyrosinemia and the heme biosynthetic pathway: profound inhibition of α-aminolevulinic acid dehydratase activity by succinylacetone. J Clin Invest 1983;71:625–634.
31. Klebig ML, Russell LB, Rinchik EM: Murine fumarylacetoacetate hydrolase (FAH) gene is disrupted by a neonatally lethal albino deletion that defines the hepatocyte-specific development regulation 1 (HSDR-1) locus. Proc Natl Acad Sci U S A 1992;89:1363–1367.
32. Grompe M, Al-Dhalimy M, Finegold M, et al: Loss of fumarylacetoacetate hydrolase is responsible for the neonatal hepatic dysfunction phenotype of lethal albino mice. Genes Dev 1993;7:2298–2307.
33. Kelsey G, Ruppert S, Beerman F, et al: Rescue of mice homozygous for lethal albino deletions: implications for an animal model for the human liver disease tyrosinemia type I. Genes Dev 1993;7:2285–2297.
34. Holdener BC, Magnuson T: A mouse model for human hereditary tyrosinemia I. Bioessays 1994;16:85–87.
35. Kvittingen EA, Rootwell H, Berger R, et al: Self-induced correction of the genetic defect in tyrosinemia type I. J Clin Invest 1994;94:1657–1661.
36. Rank JM, Pascaul-Leone A, Payne W, et al: Hematin therapy for the neurologic crisis of tyrosinemia. J Pediatr 1991;118:136–139.
37. Lindstedt S, Holme E, Lock EA, et al: Treatment of hereditary tyrosinemia type I by inhibition of 4-hydroxyphenylpyruvate dioxygenase. Lancet 1992;340:813–817.
38. Holme E, Lindstedt S, Lock EA: Treatment of tyrosinemia type I with an enzyme inhibitor (NTBC). Int Pediatr 1995;10:41–43.
39. Grompe M, Lindstedt S, Al-Dhalimy M, et al: Pharmacological correction of neonatal lethal hepatic dysfunction in a murine model of hereditary tyrosinemia type I. Nat Genet 1995;10:453–460.
40. Overturf K, Al-Dhalimy M, Tanguay R, et al: Hepatocytes corrected by gene therapy are selected in vivo in a murine model of hereditary tyrosinemia type I. Nat Genet 1996;12:266–273.
41. Boustany RN, Aprille JR, Halperin J, et al: Mitochondrial cytochrome deficiency presenting as a myopathy with hypotonia, external ophthalmoplegia, and lactic acidosis in an infant and as fatal hepatopathy in a second cousin. Ann Neurol 1983;14:462–470.
42. Cormier V, Rustin P, Bonnefont J-P, et al: Hepatic failure in disorders of oxidative phosphorylation with neonatal onset. J Pediatr 1991;119:951–954.
43. Fayon M, Lamircau T, Bioulac-Sag P, et al: Fatal neonatal liver failure and mitochondrial cytopathy: an observation with antenatal ascites. Gastroenterology 1992;103:1332–1335.
44. Vilaseca MA, Briones P, Ribes A, et al: Fetal hepatic failure with lactic acidemia: Fanconi syndrome and defective activity of succinate:cytochrome c reductase. J Inherit Metab Dis 1991;14:285–288.
45. Bioulac-Sage P, Parrot-Roulaud F, Mazat JP, et al: Fetal neonatal liver failure and mitochondrial cytopathy (oxidative phosphorylation deficiency): a light and electron microscopic study of liver. Hepatology 1993;18:839–846.
46. Birch-Mackin MA, Shepherd JM, Watmough NJ, et al: Fatal lactic acidosis in infancy with a defect of complex III of the respiratory chain. Pediatr Res 1989;25:553–559.
47. Cormier-Dairre V, Chretien D, Rustin P, et al: Neonatal and delayed

onset liver involvement in disorders of oxidative phosphorylation. J Pediatr 1997;130:817–822.
48. Mazziota MRM, Ricci E, Bertini E, et al: Fatal infantile liver failure associated with mitochondrial DNA depletion. J Pediatr 1992;121:896–901.
49. Mazziotta MRM, Ricci E, Bertini E, et al: Fatal infantile liver failure associated with mitochondrial DNA depletion. J Pediatr 1992;121:896–901.
50. Maaswinkel-Mooij PD, Van den Bogert C, Scholte HR, et al: Depletion of mitochondrial DNA in the liver of a patient with lactic acidemia and hypoketotic hypoglycemia. J Pediatr 1996;128:679–683.
51. Bakker HD, Scholte HR, Dingemans KP, et al: Depletion of mitochondrial deoxyribonucleic acid in a family with fatal neonatal liver disease. J Pediatr 1996;128:683–687.
52. Alpers BJ: Diffuse progressive degeneration of the gray matter of the cerebrum. Arch Neurol Psychiatry 1931;25:469–505.
53. Wilson DC, McGibben D, Hicks EM, et al: Progressive neuronal degeneration of childhood (Alpers' syndrome) with hepatic cirrhosis. Eur J Pediatr 1993;152:260–262.
54. Harding BN, Egger J, Portmann B, et al: Progressive neuronal degeneration of childhood with liver disease: a pathological study. Brain 1986;109:181–206.
55. Narkewicz MR, Sokol RJ, Beckwith B, et al: Liver involvement in Alpers disease. J Pediatr 1991;119:260–267.
56. Bicknese AR, May W, Hickey WF, et al: Early childhood hepatocerebral degeneration misdiagnosed as valproate hepatotoxicity. Ann Neurol 1992;32:767–775.
57. Tulimius MH, Holme E, Kristiansson B, et al: Mitochondrial encephalomyopathies in childhood: I. Biochemical and morphologic investigations. J Pediatr 1991;119:242–250.
58. Tulimius MH, Holme E, Kristiansson B, et al: Mitochondrial encephalomyopathies in childhood: II. Clinical manifestations and syndromes. J Pediatr 1991;119:251–259.
59. Pearson HA, Lobel JS, Kocoshis SA, et al: A new syndrome of refractory sideroblastic anemia with vacuolization of marrow precursors and exocrine pancreatic dysfunction. J Pediatr 1979;95:976–984.
60. Johns DR: Mitochondrial DNA and disease. N Engl J Med 1995;333:638–644.
61. Rotig A, Cormier V, Slanche S, et al: Pearson's marrow-pancreas syndrome: a multisystem mitochondrial disorder in infancy. J Clin Invest 1990;86:1601–1608.
62. Bernes SM, Bacino C, Prezant TR, et al: Identical mitochondrial DNA deletion in mother with progressive external ophthalmoplegia and son with Pearson marrow-pancreas syndrome. J Pediatr 1993;123:598–602.
63. Bennett MJ: The laboratory diagnosis of inborn errors of mitochondrial fatty acid oxidation. Ann Clin Biochem 1990;27:519–531.
64. Sims HF, Brackett JC, Powell CK, et al: The molecular basis of pediatric long-chain 3-hydroxyacyl-CoA dehydrogenase deficiency associated with maternal acute fatty liver of pregnancy. Proc Natl Acad Sci U S A 1995;92:841–845.
65. Rocchiccioli F, Wanders RJA, Aubourg P, et al: Deficiency of long-chain 3 hydroxyacyl-CoA dehydrogenase: a cause of lethal myopathy and cardiomyopathy in early childhood. Pediatr Res 1990;28:657–662.
66. Jackson S, Bartlett K, Lund J, et al: Long-chain 3-hydroxyacyl CoA dehydrogenase deficiency. Pediatr Res 1991;29:406–410.
67. Tyni T, Palotie A, Viinikka L, et al: Long-chain 3-hydroxyacyl-coenzyme A dehydrogenase deficiency with the G1582C mutation: clinical presentation of thirteen patients. J Pediatr 1997;130:67–76.
68. Schoeman MN, Batey RG, Wilcken B: Recurrent acute fatty liver of pregnancy associated with a fatty-acid oxidation defect in the offspring. Gastroenterology 1991;100:544–548.
69. Treem WR, Rinaldo P, Hale DE, et al: Acute fatty liver of pregnancy and long-chain 3-hydroxyacyl-coenzyme A dehydrogenase deficiency. Hepatology 1994;19:339–345.
70. Treem WR: Inborn defects in mitochondrial fatty acid oxidation. In Suchy FJ (ed): Liver Disease in Children. St. Louis, Mosby–Year Book, 1994, pp 852–887.
71. Reye RDK, Morgan G, Baral J: Encephalopathy and fatty degeneration of the viscera: a disease entity in childhood. Lancet 1963;2:749–752.
72. Tanaka K, Ikeda Y: Hypoglycin and Jamaican vomiting sickness. Prog Clin Biol Res 1990;321:167–194.
73. Mahler H, Pasi A, Kramer JM, et al: Fulminant liver failure in association with the emetic toxin of *Bacillus cereus*. N Engl J Med 1997;336:1142–1148.
74. Treem WR, Witzleben CA, Picolli DA, et al: Medium-chain and long-chain acyl CoA dehydrogenase deficiency: clinical, pathologic, and ultrastructural differentiation from Reye's syndrome. Hepatology 1986;6:1270–1278.
75. Moser HW: Peroxisomal disease. Adv Pediatr 1989;36:1–38.
76. Santos MJ, Imanaka T, Shio H, et al: Peroxisomal membrane ghosts in Zellweger syndrome: aberrant organelle assembly. Science 1988;239:1536–1538.
77. Suzuki Y, Shimozawa N, Orii T, et al: Zellweger-like syndrome with detectable hepatic peroxisomes: a variant form of peroxisomal disorder. J Pediatr 1988;113:841–845.
78. Mandel H, Espeel M, Roels F, et al: A new type of peroxisomal disorder with variable expression in liver and fibroblasts. J Pediatr 1994;125:549–555.
79. Espeel M, Mandel H, Poggi F, et al: Peroxisome mosaicism in the livers of peroxisomal deficiency patients. Hepatology 1995;22:497–504.
80. Tsukamoto T, Miura S, Fujiki V: Restoration by a 35kd-membrane protein of peroxisome assembly in a peroxisome-deficient mammalian cell mutant. Nature 1991;350:77–81.
81. Shimozawa N, Tsukamoto T, Suzuki Y, et al: A human gene responsible for Zellweger syndrome that affects peroxisome assembly. Science 1992;255:1132–1134.
82. Wiemer EAC, Nuttley WM, Bertolaet BL, et al: Human peroxisomal targeting signal-1 receptor restores peroxisomal protein import in cells from patients with fatal peroxisomal disorders. J Cell Biol 1995;130:51–65.
83. Dodt G, Braverman N, Wong C, et al: Mutation in the PTS1 receptor gene, *PXR1*, define complementation group 2 of the peroxisome biogenesis disorders. Nat Genet 1995;9:115–125.
84. Pike MG, Applegarth DA, Dunn GH, et al: Congenital rubella syndrome associated with calcific epiphyseal stippling and peroxisomal dysfunction. J Pediatr 1990;116:86–94.
85. Watkins PA, Chen WW, Harris CJ, et al: Peroxisomal bifunctional enzyme deficiency. J Clin Invest 1989;83:771–777.
86. Mosser J, Douar A-M, Sarde C-O, et al: Putative X-linked adrenoleukodystrophy gene shares unexpected homology with ABC transporters. Nature 1993;361:726–730.
87. Moser AB, Rasmussen M, Naidu S, et al: Phenotype of patients with peroxisomal disorders subdivided into sixteen complementation groups. J Pediatr 1995;127:13–22.
88. Gartner J, Moser H, Valle D: Mutations in the 70-kd peroxisomal membrane protein gene in Zellweger syndrome. Nat Genet 1992;1:16–23.
89. Aubourg P, Blanche S, Jambaque I, et al: Reversal of early neurologic and neuroradiologic manifestations of X-linked adrenoleukodystrophy by bone marrow transplantation. N Engl J Med 1990;322:1860–1866.
90. Setchell KDR, Bragetti P, Zimmer-Nechemias L, et al: Oral bile acid treatment and the patient with Zellweger's syndrome. Hepatology 1992;15:198–207.
91. Beutler E: Gaucher's disease as a paradigm of current issues regarding single gene mutations of humans. Proc Natl Acad Sci U S A 1993;90:5384–5390.
92. Sibille A, Eng CM, Kim S-J, et al: Phenotype/genotype correlations in Gaucher disease type I: clinical and therapeutic implications. Am J Hum Genet 1993;52:1094–1101.
93. James SP, Stromeyer FW, Chang C, et al: Liver abnormalities in patients with Gaucher's disease. Gastroenterology 1981;80:126–133.
94. St Owens DW, Teitelbaum SL, Kohn AJ, et al: Skeletal complications of Gaucher's disease. Medicine (Baltimore) 1985;64:310–322.
95. Goldbatt J, Beighton P: Cutaneous manifestations of Gaucher's disease. Br J Dermatol 1984;111:331–334.
96. Sidransky E, Fartosch M, Lee RE, et al: Epidermal abnormalities may distinguish type 2 from type 1 and type 3 Gaucher's disease. Pediatr Res 1996;39:134–141.
97. Grabowski GP, Saul HM, Wenstrup RJ, et al: Gaucher's disease: a prototype for molecular medicine. Crit Rev Oncol Hematol 1996;23:25–55.
98. Dahl N, Hiliborg PO, Olofsson A: Gaucher disease (Norrbottnian type III): probable founders identified by genealogical and molecular studies. Hum Genet 1993;92:513–515.
99. Hollok CEM, van Weely S, van Oers MHM, et al: Marked elevation of plasma chitotriosidase activity. J Clin Invest 1994;93:1288–1292.
100. Barringer JA, Rice E, Sakallah SA, et al: Enzymatic and molecular diagnosis of Gaucher's disease. Genetic Testing 1985;15:899–913.

101. Tsuji S, Choudory PV, Martin BM, et al: Nucleotide sequence of cDNA containing the complete coding sequence for human lysosomal glucocerebrosidase. J Biol Chem 1986;261:50–53.
102. Sorge J, West C, Westwood B, et al: Molecular cloning and nucleotide sequence of human glucocerebrosidase cDNA. Proc Natl Acad Sci U S A 1985;82:7289–7293.
103. Van Weely S, van den Berg M, Barringer JA, et al: Role of pH in determining the cell-type specific residual activity of glucocerebrosidase in type I Gaucher disease. J Clin Invest 1993;191:1167–1175.
104. O'Brien JS, Kishimoto Y: Saposin proteins: structure, function and role in human lysosomal storage disorder. FASEB J 1991;5:300–308.
105. Tybulewicz VLJ, Tremblay ML, La Marca ME, et al: Animal model of Gaucher's disease from targeted disruption of the mouse glucocerebrosidase gene. Nature 1992;357:407–410.
106. Willemsen R, Tybulewicz VLJ, Sidransky E, et al: A biochemical and ultra-structural evaluation of the type 2 Gaucher mouse. Mol Chem Neuropathol 1995;24:179–192.
107. Beutler E: Gaucher disease. Adv Genet 1995;32:17–49.
108. Ostlere L, Warner T, Meunier PJ, et al: Treatment of type I Gaucher's disease affecting bone with aminohydroxypropylidene bisphosphonate (pamidronate). Q J Med 1991;79:503.
109. Cohen IJ, Kornreich L, Mekhmandarov S, et al: Effective treatment of painful bone crises in type I Gaucher's disease with high dose prednisolone. Arch Dis Child 1996;75:218–222.
110. Carlson DE, Busuttil RW, Giudici TA, et al: Orthotopic liver transplantation in the treatment of complications of type I Gaucher's disease. Transplantation 1990;49:1192.
111. Barton NW, Brady RO, Dambrosia JM, et al: Replacement therapy for inherited enzyme deficiency: macrophage-targeted glucocerebrosidase for Gaucher's disease. N Engl J Med 1991;324:1464.
112. Zimran A, Elstein D, Levy-Lahad E, et al: Replacement therapy with imiglucerase for type I Gaucher's disease. Lancet 1995;2:1479–1480.
113. Rosenthal DI, Doppelt SH, Mankin HJ, et al: Enzyme replacement therapy for Gaucher disease: skeletal responses to macrophage-targeted glucocerebrosidase. Pediatrics 1995;96:629–637.
114. Kaplan P, Mazur A, Manor O, et al: Acceleration of growth in children with Gaucher's disease after treatment with alglucerase. J Pediatr 1996;129:149–153.
115. Beutler E: The cost of treating Gaucher's disease. Nature Med 1996;2:523–524.
116. Ringden O, Groth CG, Erikson A, et al: Ten years' experience of bone marrow transplantation for Gaucher's disease. Transplantation 1995;59:864–870.
117. Schuchman EH, Desnick RJ: Niemann-Pick disease types A and B: acid sphingomyelinase deficiencies. In Scriver CR, Beaudeut AC, Sly WS, Valle D (eds): The Metabolic Basis of Inherited Disease, 6th ed. New York, McGraw-Hill, 1989, pp 2601–2624.
118. Weisz B, Spirer Z, Reif S: Niemann-Pick disease: newer classification based on genetic mutations of the disease. Adv Pediatr 1994;41:415–526.
119. Tassoni JP, Fawaz KA, Johnson DE: Cirrhosis and portal hypertension in a patient with adult Niemann-Pick disease. Gastroenterology 1991;100:567–671.
120. Takahashi T, Akiyama K, Tomihara M, et al: Heterogeneity of liver disorder in type B Niemann-Pick disease. Hum Pathol 1997;28:385–388.
121. Quintern LE, Schuchman EH, Levran O, et al: Isolation of cDNA clones encoding human acid sphingomyelinase: occurrence of alternatively processed transcripts. EMBO J 1989;8:2469–2473.
122. Schuchman EH, Suchi M, Takahashi T, et al: Human acid sphingomyelinase: isolation, nucleotide sequence, and expression of the full-length and alternatively spliced cDNAs. J Biol Chem 1991;266:8531–8539.
123. Otterbach B, Stoffel W: Acid sphingomyelinase-deficient mice mimic the neurovisceral form of human lysosomal storage disease (Niemann-Pick disease). Cell 1995;81:1053–1061.
124. Horinouchi K, Erlich S, Perl DP, et al: Acid sphingomyelinase deficient mice: model of types A and B Niemann-Pick disease. Nat Genet 1995;10:288–293.
125. Gartner JC, Bergman I, Malatack JJ, et al: Progressional neurovisceral storage disease with supranuclear ophthalmoplegia following orthotopic liver transplantation. Pediatrics 1996;77:104–109.
126. Kelly DA, Portmann B, Mowat AP, et al: Niemann-Pick disease type C: diagnosis and outcome in children, with particular reference to liver disease. J Pediatr 1993;123:242–247.
127. Schiffmann R: Niemann-Pick disease type C: from bench to bedside. JAMA 1996;276:561–564.
128. Steinberg SJ, Mondal D, Fensom AH: Co-cultivation of Niemann-Pick disease type C fibroblasts belonging to complementation groups alpha and beta stimulated LDL-derived cholesterol esterification. J Inherit Metab Dis 1996;19:769–774.
129. Carstea ED, Polymeropoulos MH, Parker CC, et al: Linkage of Niemann-Pick disease types C to human chromosome 18. Proc Natl Acad Sci U S A 1993;90:2002–2004.
130. Kopitz J, Harzer K, Kohlschutter A, et al: Methylamine accumulation in cultured cells as a measure of the aqueous storage compartment in the laboratory diagnosis of genetic lysosomal diseases. Am J Med Genet 1996;63:198–202.
131. Vanier MT, Duthel S, Rodriguez-Lafrasse C, et al: Genetic heterogeneity in Niemann-Pick C disease: a study using somatic cell hybridization and linkage analysis. Am J Hum Genet 1996;58:118–125.
132. Patterson MV, Di Bisceglie AM, Higgins JJ, et al: The effect of cholesterol-lowering agents on hepatic and plasma cholesterol in Niemann-Pick disease type C. Neurology 1993;43:61–64.
133. Mason HH, Turner ME: Chronic galactemia. Am J Dis Child 1935;50:359–362.
134. Segal S, Berry GT: Disorder of galactose metabolism. In Scriver CR, Beaudet AC, Sly WS, Valle D (eds): The Metabolic Basis of Inherited Disease. New York, McGraw-Hill, 1995, pp 957–1000.
135. Hsia D Y-Y, Walker FA: Variability in the clinical manifestations of galactosemia. J Pediatr 1961;159:872–883.
136. Schweitzer S, Shin Y, Jakobs C, et al: Long-term outcome in 134 patients with galactosemia. Eur J Pediatr 1993;152:36–43.
137. Levy HL, Sape SJ, Glick VE, et al: Sepsis due to *Escherichia coli* in neonates with galactosemia. N Engl J Med 1997;297:823.
138. Jakobs C, Kleijer WJ, Allen J, et al: Prenatal diagnosis of galactosemia. Eur J Pediatr 1995;154:S33–S36.
139. Schweitzer S: Newborn mass screening for galactosemia. Eur J Pediatr 1995;154:S37–S39.
140. Gross KC, Acosta PB: Fruits and vegetables are a source of galactose: implications in planning the diets of patients with galactosemia. J Inherit Metab Dis 1991;14:253.
141. Waggoner DD, Buist NRM, Donnell GN: Long-term prognosis in galactosemia: results of a survey of 350 cases. J Inherit Metab Dis 1990;13:802–818.
142. Reichardt JKV, Berg P: Cloning and characterization of a cDNA encoding human galactose-1-phosphate uridyltransferase. Mol Biol Med 1988;5:107–122.
143. Leslie ND, Immerman EB, Flach JE, et al: The human galactose-1-phosphate uridyltransferase gene. Genomics 1992;14:474–480.
144. Gitzelmann R: Galactose-1-phosphate in the pathophysiology of galactosemia. Eur J Pediatr 1995;154:S45–S49.
145. Cox TM: Aldolase B and fructose intolerance. FASEB J 1994;8:62–71.
146. Gitzelmann R, Steinmann B, van den Berghe G: Disorders of fructose metabolism. In Scriver CR, Beaudet AC, Sly WS, Valle D (eds): The Metabolic Basis of Inherited Disease. New York, McGraw-Hill, 1995, p 905.
147. Odievre M, Gentil C, Gautier M, et al: Hereditary fructose intolerance in childhood: diagnosis, management, and course in 55 patients. Am J Dis Child 1978;132:605–608.
148. Mock DM, Perman JA, Thaler MM, et al: Chronic fructose intoxication after infancy in children with hereditary fructose intolerance: a cause of growth retardation. N Engl J Med 1983;309:764.
149. Howarth D: Sugar intake and dental caries. Lancet 1983;1:827.
150. Swales JD, Smith ADM: Adult fructose intolerance. Q J Med 1966; 35:455–460.
151. Boesiger P, Buchli R, Meier D, et al: Changes of liver metabolite concentrations in adults with disorders of fructose metabolism after intravenous fructose by $^{31}P$ magnetic resonance spectroscopy. Pediatr Res 1994;36:436–440.
152. Cross NC, Tolan DR, Cox TM: Catalytic deficiency of human aldolase B in hereditary fructose intolerance caused by a common missense mutation. Cell 1988;53:881–885.
153. Tolan DR, Penhoet EE: Characterization of the human aldolase B gene. Mol Biol Med 1988;3:245–264.
154. Ali M, Cox TM: Diverse mutations in the aldolase B gene underlie the prevalence of HFI. Am J Hum Genet 1995;56:1002–1005.
155. Hers M-G, VanHoof F, DeBarsy T: Glycogen storage disease. In Scriver CR, Beaudet AL, Sly WS, Valle D (eds): The Metabolic Basis of Inherited Disease. New York, McGraw-Hill, 1989, pp 425–452.

156. Burchell A: The molecular basis of type 1 glycogen storage disease. Bioessays 1992;14:395–400.
157. Lei K-J, Pan C-J, Liu J-L, et al: Structure-function analysis of human glucose-6-phosphatase, the enzyme deficient in glycogen storage disease type 1a. J Biol Chem 1995;270:11882–11886.
158. Lei K-J, Shelly LL, Pan C-J, et al: Mutations in the glucose-6-phosphatase gene that cause glycogen storage disease type 1a. Science 1993;262:580–593.
159. Shelly LL, Lei K-J, Pan C-J, et al: Isolation of the gene for murine glucose-6-phosphatase, the enzyme deficient in glycogen storage disease type 1a. J Biol Chem 1993;268:21482–21485.
160. Lei K-J, Pan C-J, Shelly LL, et al: Identification of mutations in the gene for glucose-6-phosphatase, the enzyme deficient in glycogen storage disease type 1a. J Clin Invest 1994;93:1994–1999.
161. Lei K-J, Shelly LL, Lin B, et al: Mutations in the glucose-6-phosphatase gene are associated with glycogen storage disease type 1a and 1aSP but not 1b and 1c. J Clin Invest 1995;95:234–240.
162. Chen Y-T, Coleman RA, Scheinman JI, et al: Renal disease in type I glycogen storage disease. N Engl J Med 1988;318:7–11.
163. Chen Y-T, Scheinman JI, Park HK, et al: Amelioration of proximal renal tubular dysfunction in type 1 glycogen storage disease with dietary therapy. N Engl J Med 1990;323:590–593.
164. Greene HL, Slonim AE, O'Neill JA, et al: Continuous nocturnal intragastric feeding for management of type I glycogen storage disease. N Engl J Med 1992;326:1666–1669.
165. Chen Y-T, Cornblath M, Sidbury JB: Cornstarch therapy in the I glycogen storage disease. N Engl J Med 1984;310:171–175.
166. Wolfsdorf JI, Keller RJ, Landy H, et al: Glucose therapy for glycogenosis type 1 infants: comparison of intermittent uncooked cornstarch and continuous overnight glucose feedings. J Pediatr 1990;117:384–391.
167. Lei K-J, Chen H, Pan C-J, et al: Glucose-6-phosphatase dependent substrate transport in the glycogen storage disease type-1a mouse. Nat Genet 1996;13:203–209.
168. McCawley LJ, Korchak HM, Douglas SD, et al: In vitro and in vivo effects of granulocyte colony stimulating factor on neutrophils in glycogen storage disease type 1b: granulocyte colony-stimulating factor therapy corrects the neutropenia and the defects in respiratory burst activity and $Ca^{2+}$ mobilization. Pediatr Res 1994;35:84–90.
169. Couper R, Kapelushink J, Griffith AM: Neutrophil dysfunction in glycogen storage disease Ib: association with Crohn's like colitis. Gastroenterology 1991;100:549–554.
170. Schroten H, Roesler J, Briedenbach T, et al: Granulocyte and granulocyte-macrophage colony-stimulating factor for treatment of neutropenia in glycogen storage disease type Ib. J Pediatr 1991;119:745–754.
171. Ding J-H, de Barsy T, Brown BI, et al: Immunoblot analyses of glycogen debranching enzyme in different subtypes of glycogen storage disease type III. J Pediatr 1990;116:95–100.
172. Yhang B-Z, Ding J-H, Enghild JJ, et al: Molecular cloning and nucleotide sequence of cDNA encoding human muscle glycogen debranching enzyme. J Biol Chem 1992;267:9294–9299.
173. Shen J, Bao Y, Liu H-M, Lee P, et al: Mutations in exon 3 of the glycogen debranching enzyme gene are associated with glycogen storage disease type III that is differentially expressed in liver and muscle. J Clin Invest 1996;98:352–357.
174. Markowitz AJ, Chen Y-T, Muenzer J, et al: A man with type III glycogenosis associated with cirrhosis and portal hypertension. Gastroenterology 1993;105:1882–1885.
175. Haagsma EB, Smit GPA, Niezen-Koning KE, et al: Type IIIb glocygen storage disease associated with end-stage cirrhosis and hepatocellular carcinoma. Hepatology 1997;25:537–540.
176. Thon VM, Khalil M, Cannon JF: Isolation of human glycogen branching enzyme cDNAs by screening complementation in yeast. J Biol Chem 1993;268:7509–7513.
177. Bao Y, Kishnani P, Wu J-Y, et al: Hepatic and neuromuscular forms of glycogen storage disease type IV caused by mutations in the same glycogen-branching enzyme gene. J Clin Invest 1996;97:941–948.
178. Selby R, Starzl TE, Yunis E, et al: Liver transplantation for type IV glycogen storage disease. N Engl J Med 1991;324:39–42.
179. Starzl TE, Demetris AJ, Trucco M, et al: Chimerism after liver transplantation for IV glycogen storage disease and type I Gaucher's disease. N Engl J Med 1993;328:745–749.
180. Kagalwalla AF, Kagalwalla YA, Ajaji SA, et al: Phosphorylase b kinase deficiency glycogenosis with cirrhosis of the liver. J Pediatr 1995;127:602–605.
181. Walshe JM: Treatment of Wilson's disease: the historical background. Q J Med 1996;89:553–555.
182. Dobyns WB, Goldstein NP, Gordon H: Clinical spectrum of Wilson's disease (hepatolenticular degeneration). Mayo Clin Proc 1989;54:35–42.
183. McCullough AM, Fleming RC, Thistle JL, et al: Diagnosis of Wilson's disease presenting as fulminant hepatic failure. Gastroenterology 1983;84:161–167.
184. McCall JT, Dickson RE: Diagnosis of Wilson's disease presenting as fulminant hepatic failure. Gastroenterology 1983;84:161–167.
185. Wiebers DD, Wilson DM, McLeod RA, et al: Renal stones in Wilson's disease. Am J Med 1979;67:249–254.
186. Golding DN, Walshe JM: Arthropathy of Wilson's disease. Ann Rheum Dis 1977;36:99–111.
187. Schilsky ML: Wilson's disease: genetic basis of copper toxicity and natural history. Semin Liver Dis 1996;16:83–95.
188. Strickland GT, Leu M-L: Wilson's disease: clinical and laboratory manifestations in 40 patients. Medicine (Baltimore) 1975;54:113–137.
189. Frydman M, Bonne-Tamir B, Farrer LA, et al: Assignment of the gene for Wilson's disease to chromosome 13: linkage to the esterase D locus. Proc Natl Acad Sci U S A 1985;82:1819–1821.
190. Petrukhin K, Fischer SG, Pirastu M, et al: Mapping, cloning and genetic characterization of the region containing the Wilson's disease gene. Nat Genet 1993;5:338–343.
191. Tanzi RE, Petrukhin K, Chemov I, et al: The Wilson's disease gene is a copper transporting ATPase with homology to the Menkes disease gene. Nat Genet 1993;5:344–350.
192. Bull PC, Thomas GR, Rommens JM, et al: The Wilson's disease gene is a putative copper transporting P-type ATPase similar to the Menkes gene. Nat Genet 1993;5:327–336.
193. Yamaguchi Y, Heiny ME, Gitlin JD: Isolation and characterization of a human liver cDNA as a candidate gene for Wilson's disease. Biochem Biophys Res Commun 1993;197:271–277.
194. Harris ZL, Gitlin JD: Genetic and molecular basis for copper toxicity. Am J Clin Nutr 1996;63:836S–841S.
195. Cox DW: Molecular advances in Wilson's disease. Prog Liver Dis 1996;14:245–264.
196. Yuan DS, Stearman R, Dancis A, et al: The Menkes/Wilson's disease gene homologue in yeast provides copper to a ceruloplasmin-like oxidase required for iron uptake. Proc Natl Acad Sci U S A 1995;92:2632–2636.
197. Chowrimootoo GF, Ahmed HA, Seymour CA: New insights into the pathogenesis of copper toxicosis in Wilson's disease: evidence for copper incorporation and defective canalicular transport of caeruloplasmin. Biochem J 1996;315:851–855.
198. Davis W, Chowrimootoo GF, Seymour CA: Defective biliary copper excretion in Wilson's disease: the role of caeruloplasmin. Eur J Clin Invest 1996;26:893–901.
199. Thomas GR, Forbes JR, Roberts EA, et al: The Wilson's disease gene: spectrum of mutations and their consequences. Nat Genet 1995;9:210–217.
200. Perman JA, Werlin SL, Grand RJ, et al: Laboratory measures of copper metabolism in the differentiation of chronic active hepatitis and Wilson's disease in children. J Pediatr 1979;94:564–568.
201. Steindl P, Frenci P, Dienes HP, et al: Wilson's disease in patients presenting with liver disease: a diagnostic challenge. Gastroenterology 1997;113:212–218.
202. Brewer GJ: Practical recommendations and new therapies for Wilson's disease. Drugs 1995;50:240–249.
203. Santos S, Ermelinda E, Sarles J, et al: Successful medical treatment of severely decompensated Wilson's disease. J Pediatr 1996;128:285–287.
204. Diaz J, Acosta F, Canizares F, et al: Does orthotopic liver transplantation normalize copper metabolism in patients with Wilson's disease? Trans Proc 1995;27:2306–2309.
205. Gaurino M, Stracciari A, D'Alessandro R, et al: No neurological improvement after liver transplantation for Wilson's disease. Acta Neurol Scand 1995;92:405–408.
206. Yoshida MC, Masuda R, Sasaki M, et al: New mutation causing hereditary hepatitis in the laboratory rat. J Hered 1987;78:361–365.
207. Li Y, Togashi Y, Sato S, et al: Spontaneous hepatic copper accumulation in Long-Evans Cinnamon rats with hereditary hepatitis. J Clin Invest 1991;87:1858–1861.
208. Kang J-H, Togashi Y, Kasai H, et al: Prevention of spontaneous hepatocellular carcinoma in Long-Evans Cinnamon rats with heredi-

tary hepatitis by the administration of D-penicillamine. Hepatology 1993;18:614–620.

209. Muramatsu Y, Yamada T, Miura M, et al: Wilson's disease gene is homologous to hts causing abnormal copper transport in Long-Evans Cinnamon rats. Gastroenterology 1994;107:1189–1192.
210. Maramatsu Y, Yamada T, Moralejo DH, et al: The rat homologue of Wilson's disease gene was partially deleted at the 3′ end of its protein-coding region in Long-Evans Cinnamon mutant rats. Res Commun Mol Pathol Pharmacol 1995;89:421–424.
211. Murata Y, Yamakawa E, Iizuka T, et al: Failure of copper incorporation into ceruloplasmin in the Golgi apparatus of LEC rat hepatocytes. Biochem Biophys Res Commun 1995;209:349–355.
212. Suzuki KT: Disordered copper metabolism in LEC rats, an animal model of Wilson disease: roles of metallothionein. Res Commun Mol Pathol Pharmacol 1995;89:221–240.
213. Theophilos MB, Cox DW, Mercer JF: The toxic milk mouse is a murine model of Wilson's disease. Hum Mol Genet 1995;5:1619–1624.
214. Knisely AS: Neonatal hemochromatosis. Adv Pediatr 1992;39:383–403.
215. Barnard JA, Manci E: Idiopathic neonatal iron storage disease. Gastroenterology 1991;101:1420–1427.
216. Bothwell TH, Charlton RW, Motulsky AG: Hemochromatosis. In Scriver CR, Beaudet AC, Sly WS, Valle D (eds): The Metabolic Basis of Inherited Disease. New York, McGraw-Hill, 1995, pp 2237–2258.
217. Hoogstraten J, de Sa DJ, Knisely AS: Fetal liver disease may precede extrahepatic siderosis in neonatal hemochromatosis. Gastroenterology 1990;98:1699–1701.
218. Clayton PT: Delta$^4$-3-oxosteroid 5-beta-reductase deficiency and neonatal hemochromatosis. J Pediatr 1994;125:845–846.
219. Schoenlebe J, Buyon JP, Zitelli BJ, et al: Neonatal hemochromatosis associated with maternal autoantibodies against Ro/SS-A and La/SS-B ribonucleoproteins. Am J Dis Child 1993;147:1072–1075.
220. Hardy L, Hansen JL, Kushner JP, et al: Neonatal hemochromatosis: genetic analysis of transferrin-receptor, H-apoferritin, and L-apoferritin loci and of the human leukocyte antigen class I region. Am J Pathol 1990;137:149–153.
221. Knisely AS, Grady RW, Kramer EE, et al: Cytoferrin, maternofetal iron transport, and neonatal hemochromatosis. Am J Clin Pathol 1989;92:755–759.
222. Knisely AS, O'Shea PA, Stocks JF, et al: Oropharyngeal and upper respiratory tract mucosal-gland siderosis in neonatal hemochromatosis: an approach to biopsy diagnosis. J Pediatr 1988;113:871–874.
223. Jonas MM, Kaweblum YA, Fojaco R: Neonatal hemochromatosis: failure of deferoxamine therapy. J Pediatr Gastroenterol Nutr 1987;6:984–988.
224. Shamieh I, Kibort PK, Suchy FJ, et al: Antioxidant therapy for neonatal iron storage disease (NISD) (abstract). Pediatr Res 1993;33:109a.
225. Rand EB, McClenathan DT, Whitington PF: Neonatal hemochromatosis: report of successful orthotopic liver transplantation. J Pediatr Gastroenterol Nutr 1992;15:325–329.
226. Lund DP, Lillehei CW, Kevy S, et al: Liver transplantation in newborn liver failure: treatment for neonatal hemochromatosis. Trans Proc 1993;25:1068–1071.
227. Egawa H, Berquist W, Garcia-Kennedy R, et al: Rapid development of hepatocellular siderosis after liver transplantation for neonatal hemochromatosis. Transplantation 1995;62:1511–1513.
228. Clayton PT, Leonard JV, Lawson AM, et al: Familial giant cells hepatitis associated with synthesis of 3$\beta$,7$\alpha$-dihydroxy- and 3$\beta$,7$\alpha$,12$\alpha$-trihydroxy-5-cholenoic acids. J Clin Invest 1987;79:1031–1038.
229. Setchell KDR, Suchy FJ, Welsh MB, et al: $\Delta^4$-3-Oxosteroid 5$\beta$-reductase deficiency described in identical twins with neonatal hepatitis: a new inborn error in bile acid synthesis. J Clin Invest 1988;82:21478–2157.
230. Jacquemin E, Setchell KDR, O'Connell NC, et al: A new cause of progressive intrahepatic cholestasis: 3$\beta$-hydroxy-C27-steroid dehydrogenase/isomerase deficiency. J Pediatr 1994;125:379–384.
231. Horslen SP, Lawson AM, Malone M, et al: 3$\beta$-hydroxy-$\Delta^5$-C27-steroid dehydrogenase deficiency, effect of chenodeoxycholic acid therapy on liver histology. J Inherit Metab Dis 1992;15:38–46.
232. Ichimiya H, Egestad B, Nazer H, et al: Bile acids and bile alcohols in a child with hepatic 3$\beta$-hydroxy-$\Delta^5$-C27-steroid dehydrogenase deficiency: effects of chenodeoxycholic acid treatment. J Lipid Res 1991;32:839–841.
233. Ichimiya H, Nazer H, Gunasekaran T, et al: Treatment of chronic liver disease caused by 3$\beta$-hydroxy-$\Delta^5$-C27-steroid dehydrogenase deficiency with chenodeoxycholic acid. Arch Dis Child 1990;65:1121–1124.
234. Russell DW, Setchell KDR: Bile acid biosynthesis. Biochemistry 1992;31:4737–4749.
235. Daugherty CC, Setchell KDR, Heubi JE, et al: Resolution of biopsy alterations in three siblings with bile acid treatment of an inborn error of bile acid metabolism ($\Delta^4$-3-oxosteroid 5$\beta$-reductase deficiency). Hepatology 1993;18:1096–1101.
236. Shneider BL, Setchell KDR, Whitington PF, et al: $\Delta^4$-3-Oxosteroid 5$\beta$-reductase deficiency causing neonatal liver failure and hemochromatosis. J Pediatr 1994;124:234–238.

# Chapter 50

# Acute and Chronic Hepatitis

*Jonathan S. Evans*

Historically, hepatitis has most often referred to liver disease caused by viruses, especially the hepatitis A and B viruses. Etymologically, however, hepatitis is defined as any inflammatory liver injury regardless of cause. Recent discoveries in the field of molecular biology and microbiology have greatly expanded the "hepatitis alphabet" and our understanding of these diseases. New questions have also been raised, and the body of information has become more complex.

The information presented in this chapter concentrates on those viruses that primarily affect the liver (the "hepatotropic" viruses) but also includes a discussion of other systemic viral infections that may result in hepatitis and a discussion of chronic autoimmune hepatitis. Other causes of hepatitis (e.g., chemical and nonviral infectious agents) are listed to provide the reader with a comprehensive differential diagnosis.

## EVALUATION AND DIAGNOSIS OF THE CHILD WITH HEPATITIS

Hepatitis in pediatric patients can result from a large and diverse number of causes and clinically can present with a variety of signs and symptoms. The evaluation may be subdivided into the assessment of the clinical presentation, serologic testing and imaging, and histopathologic examination. A list of the most common differential diagnoses of pediatric hepatitis is provided in Table 50–1.

### Clinical Presentation

Some children with hepatitis may be asymptomatic and the disease is "discovered" fortuitously while they are being investigated for an unrelated illness or during a routine well-child examination. This would be a typical presentation for hepatitis A, B, or C, especially in very young children. Other children may present with frank signs of cirrhosis and/or hepatic failure (e.g., autoimmune hepatitis). In between these two extremes lie an infinite variety of presentations. Many of these children will complain of a variety of nonspecific prodromal symptoms, including fever, fatigue, malaise, anorexia, or nausea. In these cases the child may receive a preliminary diagnosis of viral illness. If the chief complaint is jaundice or dull right upper quadrant pain, then the evaluation is more easily directed toward the possibility of hepatitis. Some children may present initially with extrahepatic manifestations (e.g., the urticarial rash or migratory arthritis of hepatitis B) that can be misleading.

A detailed history should include the possibility of hepatitis and endeavor to determine the possible etiologic agent (e.g., exposure to hepatotoxic drugs) and mode of transmission (e.g., intravenous drug abuse, family history of inherited or acquired liver disease). A complete physical examination should look for the presence of scleral, mucosal, or cutaneous icterus; hepatosplenomegaly; ascites; edema; clubbing; petechiae; ecchymosis; spider angiomas; or mental state changes. Nonhepatic causes of hepatitis should also be looked for such as signs of congestive heart failure and joint disease.

### Serologic Testing and Imaging

Blood tests have become the basis on which the diagnosis of hepatitis and the determination of its cause are made. Often the child's history and clinical examination will provide important clues and guidelines in the choice of appropriate tests. For example, testing for gonorrhea may be all that is indicated in an adolescent female with signs and symptoms of salpingitis and hepatitis (Fitz-Hugh-Curtis syndrome).

Imaging studies such as ultrasonography or computed tomography have become important tools in the evaluation of patients with liver dysfunction. They may identify patients with hepatic abscess or nonhepatic causes of hepatitis (e.g., Budd-Chiari syndrome). They must be ordered judiciously and are not indicated in all patients.

### Histopathologic Examinations

Histologic examination of liver tissue is an important adjunct in the evaluation of children with hepatitis. It is not

**TABLE 50–1. Causes and Differential Diagnosis of Hepatitis in Children**

- Infectious
  - Hepatotropic viruses
    - HAV
    - HBV
    - HCV
    - HEV
    - HDV
    - HGV
    - Hepatitis non A–G viruses
  - Viruses causing systemic infections including hepatitis:
    - Adenovirus
    - Arbovirus
    - Coxsackievirus
    - Cytomegalovirus
    - Enterovirus
    - Epstein-Barr virus
    - "Exotic" viruses (e.g., yellow fever)
    - Herpes simplex virus
    - Human immunodeficiency virus
    - Paramyxovirus
    - Rubella
    - Varicella zoster
    - Other
  - Nonviral causes
    - Abscess
    - Amebiasis
    - Bacterial sepsis
    - Brucellosis
    - Fitz-Hugh-Curtis syndrome
    - Histoplasmosis
    - Leptospirosis
    - Tuberculosis
    - Other
- Autoimmune
  - Chronic autoimmune hepatitis
  - Other (e.g., systemic lupus erythematosus, juvenile rheumatoid arthritis)
- Metabolic
  - $Alpha_1$-antitrypsin deficiency
  - Glycogen storage disease
  - Tyrosinemia
  - Wilson's disease
  - Other
- Neoplasia
- Chemical
  - Iatrogenic/drug induced (e.g., acetaminophen)
  - Environmental (e.g., pesticides)
- Anatomic
  - Choledochal duct cyst
  - Biliary atresia
  - Other
- Hemodynamic
  - Shock
  - Congestive heart failure
  - Budd-Chiari syndrome
  - Other
- Idiopathic
  - Sclerosing cholangitis
  - Reye's syndrome
  - Other

required in all patients, especially for those in whom the etiologic diagnosis is known and who are expected to have a good prognosis. However, in cases when the etiology and/or the outcome is uncertain, examination of liver tissue may be critical in the determination of diagnosis and prognosis. Repeat biopsies may be helpful in some instances, especially in children with chronic hepatitis, but the time intervals need to be carefully chosen based on the diagnosis and clinical progression. Guidelines for the histopathologic interpretation of liver biopsy specimens in children with viral and autoimmune hepatitis are provided in Table 50–2.

## HEPATOTROPIC VIRUSES

### Hepatitis A

#### *Biology and Pathogenesis*

The virus responsible for hepatitis A (hepatitis A virus [HAV]) is a 27-nm, nonenveloped, spherical endovirus with a single-stranded RNA genome.[1] Humans are the only natural host, although certain primates can be experimentally infected.[2] Hepatitis is the result of direct cytolytic and immune-mediated activities of HAV.[3]

#### *Epidemiology*

Hepatitis A is widespread and can be found throughout the world. The incidence of HAV in the United States is approximately 25,000 cases per year[4]; however, this is an underestimate because most cases are asymptomatic and do not come to medical attention. HAV is spread primarily by the fecal-oral route from an infected individual. The disease may be acquired from direct fecal contact (e.g., daycare centers) or indirectly through ingestion of contaminated water or food (e.g., the Minnesota frozen strawberry epidemic of 1997).[5] There is no known carrier state. Parenteral transmission has been described but is rare.[6, 7]

High rates of HAV infection have been clearly associated with low socioeconomic status both in the United States and other countries.[8, 9] In developing nations, under poor living conditions HAV, like other enteroviral infections, is a childhood disease. In these countries, 92% to 100% of 18-year olds show serologic evidence of past infection.[9] In developed countries the disease is acquired at a later age (20% by age 20, 50% by age 50 in the United States). It could be argued that because the disease is more severe in older patients, it poses a greater health problem in these countries.[2, 8, 9]

Favorable conditions for endemic infections include crowding, poor sanitation, and poor personal hygienic practices. Specific risk factors include contact with another infected person (26% of cases), homosexuality (15%), foreign travel (14%), contact with children attending a daycare center (11%), and illicit drug use (10%). In 40% of cases no risk factor can be identified.[2] Well-documented high-risk areas include households with an infected individual, prisons, military camps, residential centers for the disabled, and daycare centers.

Daycare centers are likely settings for transmission, especially if they have a large proportion of young children with orocentric behaviors or those not yet toilet trained. Under these conditions the disease usually comes to medical attention from either an infected adult staff member or an infected older household contact rather than the asymptomatic daycare vector.[10, 11]

#### *Clinical Course and Outcomes*

The clinical and serologic course of a typical HAV infection is shown in Figure 50–1. The average incubation period

**TABLE 50–2. Histopathologic Guidelines for Viral and Autoimmune Hepatitis**

| TYPE | INFLAMMATION | | | PORTAL LYMPHOID AGGREGATES | STEATOSIS | MALLORY BODIES | BILE DUCT DAMAGE |
|---|---|---|---|---|---|---|---|
| | Portal | Periportal | Lobular | | | | |
| HAV | 1+ | 1+ | ± | – | – | – | – |
| HBV | 2+ | 2+ | 2+ | ± | – | – | – |
| HCV | 2+ | 1+ | 1+ | 2+ | 2+ | 1+ | 2+ |
| HDV | 2+ | 2+ | 2+ | ± | – | – | – |
| HEV | 1+ | 1+ | ± | – | – | – | – |
| HGV | 2+ | 1+ | 1+ | 2+ | 2+ | 1+ | 2+ |
| EBV | 2+ | 1+ | 2+ | 1+ | – | – | – |
| CMV | 1+ | ± | – | ± | – | – | – |
| AIH | 3+ | 3+ | 3+ | 1+ | – | – | 1+ |

HAV: Hepatitis A virus often causes periportal inflammation, possible pericentral cholestasis but without significant lobular inflammation.
HBV: Hepatitis B virus causes lymphocytic inflammation in and around the portal area; with increasing severity inflammation and/or necrosis extends toward the centrolobular area.
HCV: The characteristic histology of HCV is portal inflammation with lymphoid aggregates often disproportionate to the minimal lobular inflammation. Steatosis and mild bile duct injury are common.
HDV: HDV is essentially indistinguishable from HBV, although some studies have suggested higher levels of inflammation and more rapid progression to cirrhosis.
HEV: The minimal information available for HEV infection suggests it is similar to HAV.
HGV: Very little information is available regarding the primary pathology of HGV infection. Preliminary information suggests it is commonly a co-infection with HCV, but in such patients the histology is the same as HCV alone.
EBV: Epstein-Barr viral infection in infectious mononucleosis typically causes a diffuse lymphocytic infiltrate in the sinusoids. Any part or all of the lobule may be affected.
CMV: In immunocompetent individuals cytomegalovirus produces a mononucleosis-like picture with characteristic intracytoplasmic and nuclear inclusions. In the neonatal period giant cell transformation occurs. In immunocompromised individuals inflammation may be minimal and necrosis is variable.
AIH: Autoimmune hepatitis often produces a severe necroinflammatory injury with dense mononuclear infiltration of portal tracts and periportal areas. Plasma cells may be conspicuous.

Prepared with assistance of Ken Barwick, M.D.

is 28 days (range, 14–49 days).[12, 13] Fecal shedding can occur for 2 to 3 weeks before and for 1 week after the onset of jaundice. It is during this period and while the patient is asymptomatic that the virus is most likely to be transmitted. Serum aminotransferase elevations may persist for several months and rarely for as long as a year.[2]

The clinical expression of HAV infection is age dependent, and there are no pathognomonic clinical signs that allow it to be differentiated from other forms of viral hepatitis. Infants are more likely to be asymptomatic ("anicteric hepatitis") whereas the majority of adults will develop clinically evident hepatitis ("icteric hepatitis")[10, 11, 14] Only 1 of 12 young children are likely to develop jaundice.[15] Children are more likely than adults (60% vs. 20%) to have diarrhea, often leading to the mistaken diagnosis of infectious gastroenteritis.

The outcome of hepatitis A infection in general is excellent. There are no reported cases of chronic HAV infection. Most complications are rare, and the fatality rate from fulminant hepatitis in children younger than 14 years of age is 0.1%, as compared with 1% in adults older than 40.[2, 5] The complications and extraintestinal manifestations of HAV infection are outlined in Table 50–3.[16–26]

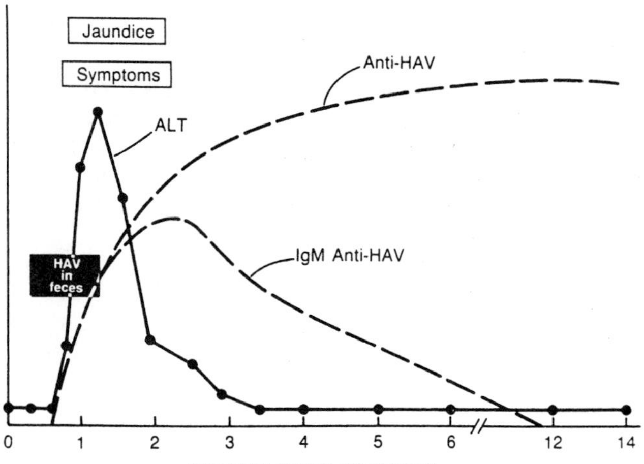

**FIGURE 50–1.** Typical clinical and serologic course of symptomatic hepatitis A. (From Hoofnagle JH, Di Bisceglie AM: Serologic diagnosis of acute and chronic viral hepatitis. Semin Liver Dis 1991;11:73–83, with permission.)

## *Diagnosis*

The diagnosis of HAV infection may be suspected if the child becomes symptomatic, but it is confirmed by specific serologic markers. These include anti-HAV IgG and IgM (Table 50–4). Anti-HAV is present at the onset of disease,

**TABLE 50–3. Complications of HAV Infection**

| COMPLICATION | COMMENTS | REFERENCE |
|---|---|---|
| Prolonged jaundice | May last 12 weeks; pruritus is frequent | 16 |
| Relapse | 3–20% of cases; most often a single benign episode | 17, 18 |
| Meningoencephalitis | | 19, 20 |
| Arthritis/rash | | 21, 22, 23 |
| Cryoglobulinemia | | 22 |
| Pancreatitis | | 24 |
| Autoimmune hepatitis | Rare | 23, 25 |
| Fulminant hepatitis | 0.1% in children | 26 |

**TABLE 50–4. Serologic Markers of Viral Hepatitis**

| VIRUS | MARKER | DEFINITION | METHOD | SIGNIFICANCE |
|---|---|---|---|---|
| HAV | Anti-HAV | Total antibodies to HAV | RIA/EIA | Current or past infection |
| | Anti-HAV-IgM | IgM antibody to HAV | RIA/EIA | Current or recent infection |
| HBV | HBsAg | Hepatitis B surface antigen | RIA/EIA | Ongoing HBV infection or carrier state |
| | Anti-HBS | Antibody to HBsAg | RIA/EIA | Resolving or past infection<br>Protective immunity<br>Immunity from vaccination |
| | HBeAg | Nucleocapsid derived Ag | RIA/EIA | Active infection<br>High infectivity |
| | Anti-HBe | Antibody to HBeAg | RIA/EIA | Resolving or past infection |
| | HBV DNA | HBV viral DNA | PCR | Active infection<br>Correlates with disease activity<br>Loss indicates resolution |
| | HBcAg | Core Ag of HBV | | Can be detected in liver only<br>Sensitive indication of replication |
| | Anti-HBc | Antibody to HBcAg | RIA/EIA | Ongoing or past infection |
| HCV | Anti-HCV | Antibody to multiple HCV antigens | ELISA<br>RIBA | Current or past HCV infection<br>More specific confirms positive ELISA |
| | HCV-RNA | HCV viral RNA | PCR | Active infection |
| HDV | Anti-HDV | IgG/IgM to HDV antigen | EIA/RIA | Acute or chronic infection |
| | Anti-HDV IgM | IgM to HDV antigen | EIA/RIA | Acute infection |
| HEV | Anti-HEV IgM | IgM to HEV protein | EIA | Early HEV infection |
| | Anti-HEV IgG | IgG to HEV protein | | Late HEV infection |
| HGV | HGV-RNA | RNA of HGV | PCR | Current infection |

and anti-HAV IgG persists for life (see Fig. 50–1). Commercial assays are sensitive and specific ways to measure total anti-HAV (IgG, IgM, and IgA). A positive anti-HAV test indicates acute infection, immunity from past infection, passive antibody acquisition (e.g., transfusion, serum immune globulin infusion), or vaccination. The diagnosis of acute or recent HAV infection in the presence of a positive anti-HAV requires measurement of anti-HAV IgM. Anti-HAV IgM is present at the onset of disease but persists for only 3 to 12 months. Detection of HAV antigen in stool and HAV-RNA in stool, liver, and sera of infected individuals is rarely required.[27]

## Hepatitis B

### *Biology and Pathogenesis*

The etiology of "transfusion hepatitis" was first described in 1965 as a protein detected in the serum of an Australian aborigine ("the Australia antigen")[28] and then visualized with electron microscopy in 1970. It appeared as a 42-nm diameter spherical virus.[29] Hepatitis B virus (HBV) is a member of the hepadnavirus family (*hepa*totropic *DNA* viruses). It is the only member of this family capable of causing hepatitis in humans and nonhuman primates.

The structure of the intact virus (the Dane particle) shows a double-shelled organism. The external shell, or envelope, expresses "the Australia antigen," now called hepatitis B surface antigen (HBsAg). An inner shell termed the *core* or *nucleocapsid* expresses a second antigen: hepatitis B core antigen (HBcAg). The presence of a viral shell has been associated with parenteral transmission, the development of chronicity, and carcinoma.[30] Inside the core resides the viral genome, a reverse transcriptase (DNA polymerase), and a third antigen, hepatitis B e antigen (HBeAg). The clinical significance of these three antigens is described in Table 50–4.

The HBV genome is a double-stranded DNA circle with a unique single-stranded area. It is 3200 nucleotide bases in length.[30] Viral replication, in a fashion similar to retroviruses, involves reverse transcription of an intermediate RNA template.[31]

Mutations of the HBV genome have been described and may determine outcomes such as the development of a fulminant course, latency, or response to treatment.[32–34] A single individual may be infected with multiple strains. Two groups of mutants have been described: pre-core mutants and pre-S/S mutants.

Pre-core mutant strains are responsible for "e-minus" HBV infections when HBeAg is absent, the result of a single point mutation causing a premature stop codon. HBV-DNA and anti-HBe remain detectable. E-minus infections can be responsible for a more severe course or outbreaks of fulminant hepatitis.[32, 35] This contrasts to "wild type" (i.e., absence of mutation) infections in which lack of detectable HBeAg signifies mild disease or a carrier state.

The pre-S1, S2, and S genes are responsible for envelope protein synthesis, including HBsAg. These mutants have been found in chronic HBV carriers who are HBsAg negative. This has raised concerns regarding safety and screening of blood supplies. These carriers do have detectable HBV-DNA, HBeAg, and anti-HBs antibody.[34, 36] The clinical significance of HBV mutations in pediatric liver disease is unclear because the study of these mutations is still ongoing and pediatric reports are rare.[37, 38]

Although HBV can infect other organs, such as the spleen, kidneys, or pancreas, its replication has been demonstrated only in the liver.[39, 40] Replication produces not only complete viruses but also smaller 22-nm spherical and variable-length (50–1,000 nm) filamentous particles. These latter particles are rich in HBsAg and are thought to be incomplete viral coats. All three forms can be detected in the blood.

Clinical expression of HBV is polymorphic and is thought to be determined by the body's immune response to infection rather than a direct cytotoxic effect of the virus. The factors that determine a specific response, whether it be viral eradication, chronic persistent infection, or fulminant hepatitis, are still ill defined.

Study of the pathogenesis of chronically acquired HBV infection is ongoing. It is thought that neonates are predisposed to chronic HBV infection, the result of their immature immune systems. This is supported by the observation that these children most often demonstrate little, if any, hepatic inflammatory injury. It has been shown that the passive transplacental transfer of anti-HBc IgG may interfere with the recognition of HBcAg on the hepatocyte by cytotoxic T-cells.[41] Additionally, two studies have shown that in both humans and transgenic mice, HBeAg crosses the placental barrier and may induce immune tolerance.[42, 43] This tolerance is achieved through neonatal T-cell unresponsiveness to HBeAg and HBcAg, both antigens sharing similar amino acid sequences.

## *Epidemiology*

Hepatitis B is a major health problem throughout the world: 300 million people are infected chronically, with 250,000 deaths annually.[44] In the United States, the incidence has declined by 55% since 1985 and is now approximately 14,000 new cases per year.[4] The true incidence of childhood infections is unknown because 85% to 90% of infections in this age group are asymptomatic.[44]

The development of a chronic carrier state is the most important consequence of childhood infection.[45] Ten percent of initial infections across all age groups will become chronic carriers. Even though children younger than age 5 represent only 1% to 3% of all HBV infections in the United States, they account for 30% of all chronic infections.[4, 44] The epidemiology of hepatitis B is strongly influenced by age, geographic location, and mode of transmission.

**AGE.** The age at the time of initial infection influences both the development of symptoms and chronicity. A 1985 study by McMahon and associates[46] followed 1,280 seronegative Eskimos in an endemic area of Alaska for 5 years. Their results, summarized in Table 50–5, show that the age of infection is inversely related to the development of an asymptomatic infection and the development of a chronic infectious state. These results have been confirmed by others and underline the significant influence of age on the epidemiology of HBV infections.[44, 47, 48]

Age at the time of initial infection is believed to be the most important factor affecting prevalence. In areas where prevalence rates are high the disease is acquired perinatally or at a very young age when it is most likely to become persistent. Chronically infected individuals represent a persistent reservoir for infection and contribute significantly over their life spans to the maintenance of high endemicity. In areas of low endemicity the infection is acquired in young or later adulthood and is less likely to become chronic and generate high prevalence rates.

**TABLE 50–5. HBV Infection: The Role of Age on the Development of Clinically Evident Hepatitis and Chronicity***

| AGE (YR) | NO. TESTED | CLINICAL HEPATITIS (%) | CHRONIC INFECTION (%) |
|---|---|---|---|
| 0–4 | 21 | 10 | 29 |
| 5–9 | 61 | 10 | 16 |
| 10–19 | 58 | 10 | 7 |
| 20–29 | 22 | 14 | 14 |
| >30 | 27† | 33 | 8 |

*Based on 189/1,280 (15%) Yupik eskimos who seroconverted for HBV infection between 1971–1976.

†n = 26 for those tested for chronicity.

Adapted from McMahon BJ, Wallace LM, Alward DB, et al: Acute hepatitis B infection: relation of age to the clinical expression of disease and subsequent development of the carrier state. J Infect Dis 1985;151:599–603, with permission from University of Chicago Press.

**GEOGRAPHY OF HBV.** Hepatitis B virus has a worldwide distribution, but prevalence rates vary significantly from areas of high endemnicity, mainly in developing countries, to areas of low endemicity in developed countries (Fig. 50–2).[44] Small pockets of high prevalence exist and may be associated with ethnic minorities (e.g., Alaskan Yupik Eskimos). In a mobile society it is important to recognize these geographic differences because it is not unusual to care for patients emigrating from areas of high endemicity.

**MODE OF TRANSMISSION.** There are no environmental reservoirs (e.g., food, water) for HBV transmission such as are found in HAV infections. Also, there are no natural animal reservoirs and humans are the principal source of HBV infection. The traditional route of transmission is parenteral through contaminated transfused blood products or intravenous drug abuse. Transmission may also occur percutaneously or transmucosally from exposure to blood or other contaminated body fluids. Although HBsAg has been found in virtually every body fluid (e.g., feces, bile, breast milk, sweat, tears, vaginal secretions, urine), only blood, semen, and saliva have been shown to contain infectious HBV particles.[49] Transmission from infected human bites has been documented whereas transmission from feces has not.[50, 51] The lack of fecal-oral transmission and the types of close contact required for transmission probably explain the infrequent appearance of epidemics.

The route of acquisition within the pediatric population can be divided into three relevant age groups: perinatal, infancy-childhood, and adolescent–young adult.

Each year in the United States, 22,000 HBsAg-positive mothers give birth. Selective prenatal screening, based on the identification of known risk factors, is difficult and has shown an unacceptably low sensitivity (<50%).[44] The failure of selective prenatal screening has prompted recommendations for universal HBV screening of all pregnant women to identify at-risk newborns. The risk of perinatal or vertical transmission can be further defined by the mother's full serologic profile: mothers who are HBeAg positive have the highest rates of transmission (70–90%) whereas infants of mothers who are HBsAg positive but HBeAg negative carry a lower risk (10–67%).[52 54] The presence of anti-HBe antibody in an HBsAg-positive mother does not always confer

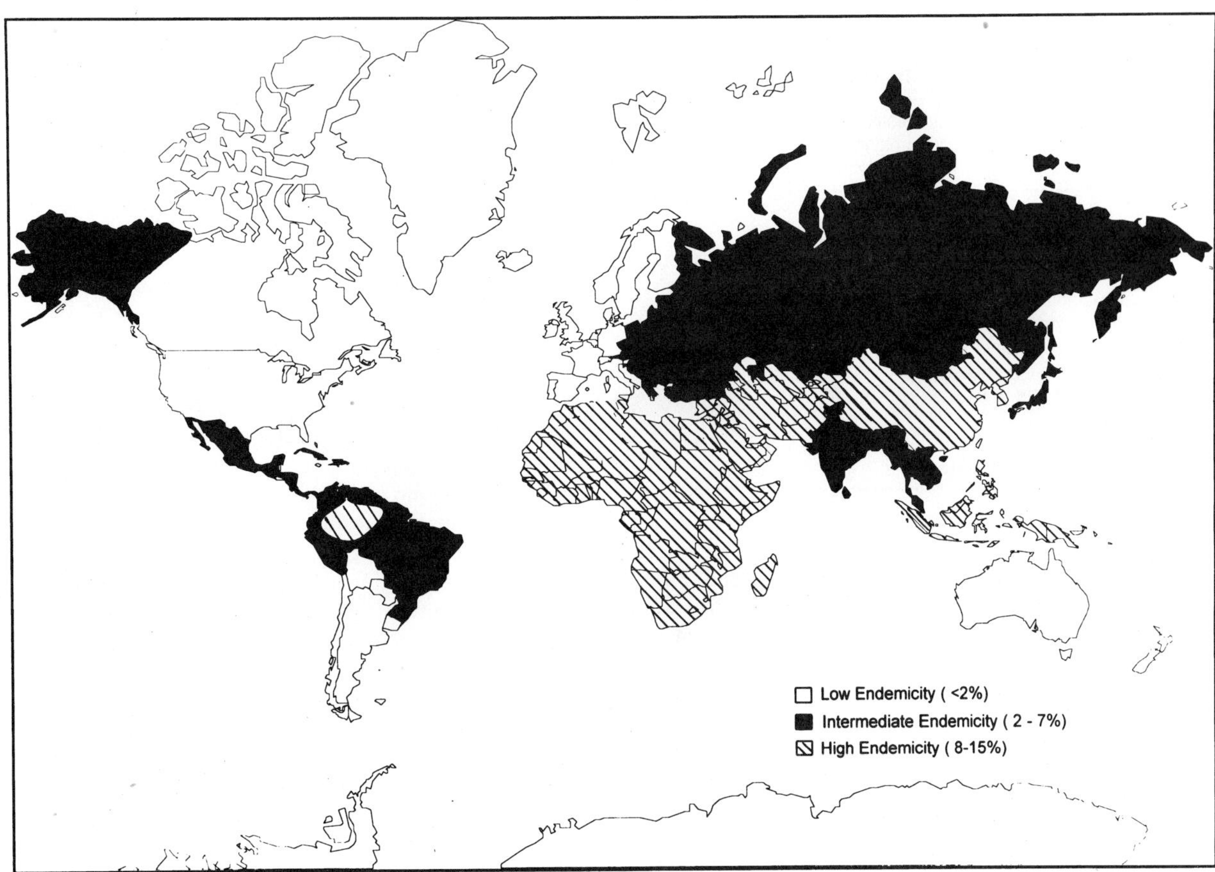


**FIGURE 50–2.** Geographic distribution of hepatitis B. (Adapted from Margolis HS, Alter MJ, Hadler SC: Evolving epidemiology and implications for control. Semin Liver Dis 1991;11:84–92, with permission.)

safety to her child: even though in most instances it signifies resolving disease, it may in rare cases of mutant strains predispose the newborn to fulminant hepatitis.[55–58]

Acute maternal infection during the third trimester carries the highest risk of perinatal transmission.[47] In utero infections are rare but have been described.[59] Perinatal acquisition is thought to occur during the birthing process because infection in newborns cannot be detected serologically for the first 1 to 3 months of age. It is postulated that during birth the infant comes into contact with infected maternal body fluids (most likely blood), although whether the virus crosses through the infant's mucosal membranes, intestinal tract, or minor skin abrasions is still not known.

Infants and children who do not become infected perinatally from their HBsAg-positive mothers still remain at high risk of infection during their first 5 years of life.[60–62] This risk has been estimated in Asian children at 60% if the mother is HBeAg positive and 40% if she is HBeAg negative.[60] Transmission in these instances was found to occur horizontally between children within the same family.[62] HBsAg can be detected in breast milk, but whether infection can be transmitted through ingested breast milk or from swallowed maternal blood from injured nipples is unclear.[58]

High rates of early childhood infection have been reported in certain well-defined populations. These include Alaskan Eskimos, Pacific Islanders, and infants of first-generation immigrants from areas with high or intermediate endemicity (see Fig. 50–2).[44] Children of southeast Asian immigrants to the United States for example carry a 7% to 13% rate of infection even if the mother is HBsAg negative.[61, 62]

Available data suggest that the risk of HBV transmission within the daycare setting, either between children or between caregivers and children, is low.[4, 63, 64] Current recommendations allow HBV-infected children to attend daycare unless they have other medical conditions or behaviors that would increase the risk of transmission.[64]

Nine percent of all cases of acute HBV reported to the Centers for Disease Control and Prevention occur in adolescents and young adults between 10 and 19 years of age.[4] In 60% of reported cases, no source of infection can be found. However, among the 40% with a reported source of infection, 50% of these are from sexual contact and 47% from intravenous drug abuse. The male-to-female ratio in adolescents is 0.7:1, but in adults it is 2:1.[4, 44] The reasons for this ratio reversal are unclear but perhaps reflect the earlier age of sexual activity in females.

The epidemiology of HBV infection allows the identification of certain high-risk groups, which are listed in Table 50–6.

## *Acute Hepatitis B*

**CLINICAL COURSE.** The clinical expression of acute HBV infection depends on the age at acquisition. The clini-

**TABLE 50–6. Groups at High Risk for HBV Infection**

| AGE | GROUP |
|---|---|
| <11 yr | Children of HBsAg-positive mothers (especially ages 0–5 yr)<br>Children of immigrants from highly endemic areas<br>Adoptees from highly endemic areas<br>Minority inner-city children<br>Household contacts of HBV carriers<br>Institutionalized children<br>Polytransfused children |
| >11 yr | Immigrants from highly endemic areas<br>Sexually active adolescents, especially if multiple partners<br>Intimate contacts of HBV carriers<br>Intravenous drug abusers<br>Homosexual males<br>Prisoners<br>Occupational exposure (e.g., health care)<br>Travelers to highly endemic areas |

cal course of a typically icteric and self-limited, acute HBV infection is portrayed in Figure 50–3. The incubation period ranges from 28 to 180 days (mean 80 days), after which the patient may develop a prodrome consisting of fever, anorexia, fatigue, malaise, and nausea. Also during this period the child may present with immune-mediated extrahepatic manifestations, including migratory arthritis, angioedema, and a maculopapular or urticarial rash. Papular acrodermatitis of childhood or Gianotti-Crosti syndrome has been associated with HBV and may become evident during this period. The syndrome includes a characteristic "lenticular, flat, erythematopapular" rash of the extremities, face, and buttocks and lymphadenitis associated with hepatitis.[65] It can be associated with other viral infections and is reported rarely in North America.[66] It is thought to be the result of circulating immune complexes.

After 1 to 2 weeks most of the prodromal symptoms subside and clinically evident hepatitis develops including, in many cases, jaundice, hepatosplenomegaly, and pruritus. Ongoing intense fatigue is a common complaint during this period. Symptoms may persist for up to 1 to 2 months and longer in a minority of patients.

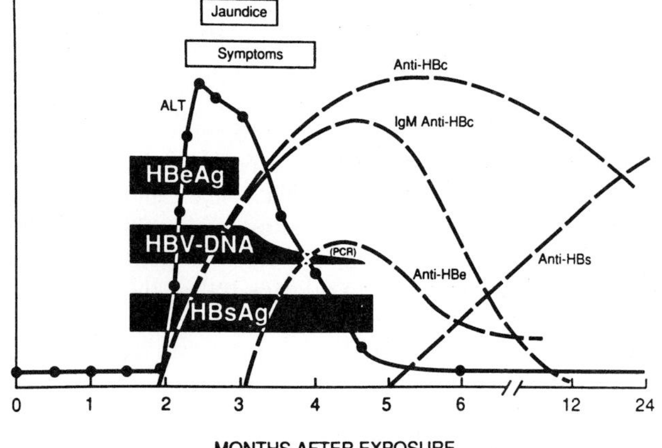


**FIGURE 50–3.** Typical clinical and serologic course of symptomatic acute hepatitis B. (From Hoofnagle JH, Di Bisceglie AM: Serologic diagnosis of acute and chronic viral hepatitis. Semin Liver Dis 1991;11:73–83, with permission.)

**OUTCOMES.** The potential outcomes of an acute HBV infection are outlined in Figure 50–4. The complications that may result from an acute infection with HBV include fulminant hepatitis or the persistence of infection. Chronic HBV infection is discussed later along with the development of hepatocellular carcinoma. Fulminant hepatitis and hepatic failure is covered in Chapter 52. Any child with an acute fulminant HBV infection or a biphasic course should be investigated for concomitant HDV co-infection (see later).

### *Chronic HBV Infection*

Chronic infection with HBV is defined as the persistence of circulating HBsAg for more than 6 months.[27] Anti-HBc and markers of viral replication (HBeAg and HBV DNA) are also usually present. Asymptomatic carriers are defined as individuals who are HBsAg positive but without evidence of clinical hepatitis or abnormal aminotransferase levels.

**CLINICAL COURSE.** Chronic HBV infections in children may present clinically in a variety of manners. Often it is suspected during the screening of asymptomatic children of HBV-positive mothers or other close household contacts. Other times the fortuitous discovery of elevated transaminase levels in a child evaluated for an unrelated illness may lead to the diagnosis. Rarely, it may present initially in a child who already has well-established cirrhosis and end-stage liver disease. Finally, chronic HBV infection should be included in the differential diagnosis of any child with hepatomegaly, jaundice, or other signs of liver disease. HDV superinfection should be suspected in any patient with stable, chronic HBV infection whose condition suddenly deteriorates (see later section on HDV).

**OUTCOMES.** The natural history of chronic HBV infection in children is still unclear and requires further study. In a Chinese study of 51 asymptomatic HBsAg-positive children followed for up to 4 years (mean, 30 months), persistent high levels of viral replication were found but were associated with mild and stable liver disease.[67] Over the study period, 7% cleared HBeAg but all continued to be HBsAg positive. In contrast, an Italian study observed 76 HBsAg-positive children for up to 12 years (mean, 5 years).[68] These researchers found that 70% of their study population lost serologic evidence of viral replication, with most of these (92%) normalizing their liver functions. Five patients became HBsAg negative. These results are more favorable than those of the earlier Chinese study but may reflect confounding variables, such as differing epidemiologic backgrounds. Other pediatric reports have described a 10% to 14% annual seroconversion rate from HBeAg to anti-HBe, progression of liver disease over a longer follow-up period, and reactivation of viral replication after conversion to anti-HBe status in some chronically infected children.[69–72] It is difficult, owing to the number of variables, to compare these studies and draw broad conclusions.

**CIRRHOSIS.** Several studies in children with chronic HBV infection have shown cirrhosis in 3% to 5% of initial liver biopsy specimens.[68, 73, 74] In chronically infected adults with cirrhosis the estimated 5-year survival rate is 50%.[75] Asymptomatic carriers of HBV with normal results of liver function tests carry little risk of developing cirrhosis.

**HEPATOCELLULAR CARCINOMA.** It is estimated that 320,000 new cases of hepatocellular carcinoma (HCC)

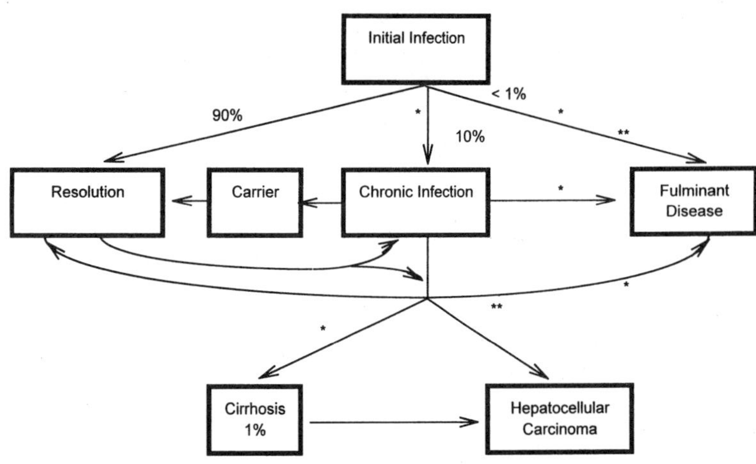


**FIGURE 50–4.** Potential outcomes of hepatitis B across all age groups.

occur worldwide each year.[76] This is an important complication from the pediatric perspective, not only because it is a major cause of childhood malignancy in certain parts of the world (e.g., Asia)[77] but also because the initial HBV infection in most patients with HCC occurs in childhood. Established risk factors for the development of HCC include chronic infection with HBV, long duration of infection, male gender, and the presence of cirrhosis.

HCC has been linked etiologically to chronic HBV infection, although the exact oncogenic mechanism remains unknown. This is supported by the discovery of HBsAg in resected neoplastic and non-neoplastic hepatic tissue[78, 79] and integration of HBV-DNA sequences into the tumor genome.[77, 79] Epidemiologic observations also support this association. Beasley and coworkers, for example, have shown that the relative risk of developing HCC is 223 times greater in HBsAg-positive adult males than in HBsAg negative controls.[80] Furthermore, it has been reported that incidence rates of HCC are higher in areas of high HBV endemicity (>15 cases/100,000 population/year) than in areas of low endemicity (<3 cases/100,000 population/year).[76]

The higher incidence of HBsAg positivity in the mothers than in the fathers of patients with HCC suggests that primary infection occurs perinatally or in early infancy.[81] This and other observations imply that the mean duration from primary infection to the development of HCC is 35 years.[82] Reported cases in children, some as young as 8 months, however, raise the issue of different oncogenic mechanisms than in adults.[83]

**EXTRAHEPATIC MANIFESTATIONS.** Circulating immune complexes including HBsAg/anti-HBs complexes are reported to be responsible for the appearance of extrahepatic manifestations. Essential mixed cryoglobulinemia, polyarteritis nodosa, and glomerulonephritis have been described in association with chronic HBV infection.[84–87]

## Diagnosis of Acute and Chronic Hepatitis B

Several serologic markers for HBV infection appear at different intervals, and their detection is necessary to confirm the diagnosis and determine the stage of infection. The diagnosis of chronic HBV infection is based on the persistence of appropriate markers for at least 6 months or on detection of these markers in a child who on initial presentation has historical or physical evidence of long-standing infection. This information is summarized in Figures 50–3 and 50–5 and Tables 50–4 and 50–7. Serum transaminase levels become elevated but are nonspecific. They begin to increase just before the development of symptoms and then peak, sometimes 20 times or greater than normal, with the development of jaundice.

HBsAg is the first serologic marker to appear and when sensitive assays are used may be detected within 1 to 2 weeks after exposure. It precedes the development of symptoms by an average of 4 weeks.[88] The presence of HBsAg indicates ongoing infection. Qualitative but not quantitative methods are used by most clinical laboratories because the amount of antigen does not correlate with disease activity nor with the presence of an acute or chronic infection.[27] Some symptomatic patients may have self-limited, acute

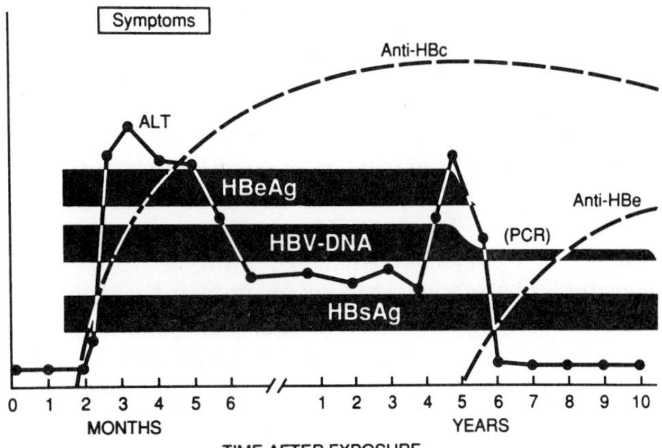


**FIGURE 50–5.** Typical clinical and serologic course of chronic hepatitis B. (From Hoofnagle JH, Di Bisceglie AM: Serologic diagnosis of acute and chronic viral hepatitis. Semin Liver Dis 1991;11:73–83, with permission.)

**TABLE 50–7. Guidelines for the Serologic Diagnosis and Staging of HBV Infections***

| HBsAg | HBeAg | ANTI-HBs | ANTI-HBc | ANTI-HBe | INTERPRETATION |
|---|---|---|---|---|---|
| + | ± | − | − | − | Early acute disease or carrier state |
| + | ± | − | + | − | Acute disease, chronic disease or carrier state |
| + | − | − | + | − | Late acute disease or carrier state |
| + | − | − | + | + | Early resolution or "e-minus" disease |
| − | − | − | + | − | Early resolution or "window" period |
| − | − | + | + | + | Resolution |
| − | − | + | + | − | Immunity from past infection |
| − | − | + | − | − | Immunity from HBV vaccine |

*Exceptions are described in the text.
HBV-DNA is of limited usefulness in this context except in limited circumstances (see text).

HBV infection without detectable HBsAg. These patients, up to 9% in some studies, have other detectable markers of infection.[88]

HBeAg appears virtually simultaneously, peaks, and then declines in parallel with HBsAg. It usually disappears before HBsAg. Adult patients who remain persistently positive for HBeAg for more than 10 weeks are likely to become chronically infected. HBeAg indicates a high level of viral replication and infectivity. Most patients with nondetectable HBeAg have either resolving, minimal, or no active liver disease.[27] Pre-core mutants of HBV do not express HBeAg; they may be responsible for a more severe course and, in some cases, fulminant disease (see earlier).

The third marker of disease to appear is HBV viral DNA (HBV-DNA), which appears with HBsAg, peaks with the onset of symptoms, and then declines. Its quantitative value is also useful in determining disease activity, "viral load," and potential response to therapy. HBcAg cannot be detected in the blood with commercially available techniques, but its detection in the liver using immunoperoxidase may be the most sensitive method to detect viral replication.[27] Anti-HBc is the fourth serologic marker to appear. It can usually be detected 3 to 5 weeks after the appearance of HBsAg but before the onset of symptoms and persists for life. Its detection indicates ongoing or past infection. It does not appear after HBV vaccination and can be helpful in distinguishing between immunity from vaccination and natural infection. A commercially available test for the detection of IgM antibodies to the core antigen (IgM anti-HBc) is available and may be helpful in some limited instances for the diagnosis of acute HBV infection.

Anti-HBs confers protective immunity and indicates resolving or past infection. In the majority of patients with self-limited infection it can be detected only after HBsAg becomes nondetectable. In a minority of patients with serum sickness–like symptoms (arthralgia, rash), it may appear before the onset of clinical symptoms.[89, 90] A "window" of variable duration has been described in some patients, during which HBsAg has disappeared and anti-HBs cannot yet be detected.[88] The measurement of anti-HBc may be helpful in these instances.

Antibody to HBeAg (anti-HBe) appears after HBeAg becomes undetectable and persists for 1 to 2 years after the resolution of hepatitis. It is an important marker indicating, in most cases, decreasing viral replication even though HBsAg may still be present.

## Hepatitis C

A third form of infectious hepatitis, not due to hepatitis A or B ("non-A, non-B hepatitis" [NANB]), was first recognized epidemiologically in 1974 and was linked to transfused blood products in 1975.[91, 92] In 1989, the cloned complementary DNA (cDNA) of RNA recovered from chimpanzees infected with post-transfusion NANB hepatitis was isolated.[93] This cDNA and its expressed antigen were linked etiologically to post-transfusion NANB hepatitis through the development of an antigen-antibody assay[94]; this long-suspected virus is now called the hepatitis C virus (HCV). This immunologic assay against HCV (anti-HCV) allowed the demonstration that HCV was the major cause of post-transfusion NANB and sporadic NANB hepatitis.[95] It was not until 1994 that HCV was first visualized using immunoelectron microscopy.[96]

### *Biology and Pathogenesis*

It has been suggested based on its physical properties and similarity to other viruses that HCV be considered a new genus within the flavivirus family. HCV is a 55-nm diameter lipid-enveloped virus with a 33-nm inner nucleocapsid. The genome is a linear, single-stranded, positive-sense RNA approximately 9,400 nucleotides in length. In vitro translation of the genome results in three structural and four nonstructural proteins.

The genome is highly susceptible to mutations, and comparison of different HCV isolates has shown nucleotide sequence variation confined to specific areas. This has allowed the identification of six major genotypes and a number of subtypes based on major and minor genomic differences.[97, 98] At this time, genotype determination remains a research tool and the study of the relevance of genotypes to clinical practice is ongoing. Genotype determination has already provided useful information in regard to prognosis and response to therapy. Types 1a, 1b, 2a, 2b, 3a, and 4a are known, for example, to be associated with more severe and progressive disease. Type 1b has been shown to be particularly resistant to antiviral therapy.[97, 99] Mapping of the geographic distribution of the known genotypes shows that types 1 (a and b) and 2 are the most prevalent genotypes in North America and Western Europe.[97, 99] This will have clinical significance for the development of effective vaccines.

The pathogenesis of hepatitis due to HCV continues to be studied, involving both immune-mediated and directly hepatopathic mechanisms of injury. The finding of autoantibodies in HCV-infected patients and activated B and T lymphocytes within hepatic lymphoid follicles suggests an immune-mediated mechanism,[100, 101] whereas the more severe progression found in immune-compromised patients supports a direct cytopathic effect.[102] The conditions that predispose to persistent HCV infection are unknown; however, it has been suggested that particular HCV genotypes or the presence of multiple genotypes may result in chronic infection.

## Epidemiology

The epidemiology of pediatric hepatitis C is poorly understood. The distribution of HCV, like that of HAV and HBV, is worldwide, but the prevalence rates appear to be evenly distributed, ranging from 0.3% to 1.5% when assessed among adult volunteer blood donors.[103] In the United States, 1993 incidence rates for NANB hepatitis were 1.86 per 100,000 population or approximately 150,000 new cases each year. Eight percent of cases occurred in patients younger than age 20.[4] The incidence of HCV-associated disease has been declining since 1989, which corresponds to the development of the first serologic screening tools.[104]

The majority of cases of NANB hepatitis in adults (50–90%) have been attributed to HCV.[103, 105, 106] Bortolotti and coworkers have compiled data to show that anti-HCV prevalence rates in children with NANB hepatitis are 60% to 65% in children with thalassemia, 59% to 95% in those with hemophilia, and 52% to 72% in survivors of leukemia.[107]

Although infection with HCV is far less common on a worldwide basis than infection with HAV or HBV, its propensity to become chronic has resulted in HCV becoming a major cause of chronic hepatitis. In the United States, it is responsible for 65% of all cases of chronic viral hepatitis and 35% of all cases of chronic liver disease and cirrhosis.[104]

There does not appear to be an epidemiologically relevant reservoir for HCV other than humans. The typical route of transmission is parenteral. Transmission may be divided into percutaneous (e.g., blood transfusions, intravenous drug abuse) and nonpercutaneous routes (e.g., intrafamilial, sexual).

**PERCUTANEOUS TRANSMISSION.** Historically, the transmission of HCV has been associated with the transfusion of blood and blood products. Improved donor screening and processing of transfused blood and blood products has resulted in a greatly reduced risk of acquiring post-transfusion NANB hepatitis. This risk has fallen from 3.8% per patient (or 4.5 cases per 1,000 units transfused) to 0.6% per patient (or 0.3 cases per 1,000 units transfused) as a result of policies to screen all donated blood for anti-HCV and surrogate markers.[108] Blood products such as factor concentrates have also been made safer through the development of improved inactivation procedures. However, the risk of acquiring HCV from contaminated blood cannot be eliminated completely. This is due in part to recently infected individuals who do not yet have detectable markers at the time of blood donation and also due to seronegative, asymptomatic carriers who have been implicated in up to 15% of HCV transmission from contaminated blood.[109]

In a study of 77 Italian and Spanish children, the most important risk factor (found in 60%) for acquiring HCV was transfusion during the neonatal period.[110] In a smaller number of American children reported to the Viral Hepatitis Surveillance Program,[4] 14% of all cases of HCV/NANB hepatitis were acquired from blood transfusions. The risk of acquiring HCV hepatitis increases with the total number of units transfused[108]; multiply transfused children with thalassemia, hemophilia, leukemia, or renal failure undergoing dialysis and bone marrow transplant recipients are at greatest risk.[111] Infected organ grafts have also been implicated in the transmission of HCV infections to transplant recipients.[112]

The proportion of cases attributable to intravenous drug abuse has been increasing and may be as high as 40%.[113] This is due in part to the declining risk of transmission from blood products but also to the increasing frequency of drug abuse. The prevalence of anti-HCV among intravenous drug abusers ranges from 60% to 90%.[103] Intravenous drug abuse in mothers also imposes a significant risk to their children: in one study this association was found in 6% of pediatric HCV cases.[110]

Occupational exposure in health care professionals occurs from percutaneous transmission of contaminated blood in instances of accidental needle stick. The risk of infection from a single needle stick from an HCV-RNA-positive patient is 10% and the disease is usually symptomatic.[113] Skin tattooing has become increasingly popular among adolescents and has been associated with the transmission of HCV.[114]

**NONPERCUTANEOUS TRANSMISSION.** This route of transmission pertains to all cases that cannot be attributed to percutaneous transfer of HCV. This includes cases of perinatal and sexual transmission, intrafamilial and occupational spread, and sporadic cases in which no mode of transmission can be found. Although transmission of HCV through contaminated blood has been well established, the role of other body fluids as vehicles of transmission has not. Several studies have failed to detect the presence of HCV-RNA in the semen, saliva, urine, stool, or vaginal secretions of patients with chronic HCV infection, leaving uncertainty surrounding the mechanism of transmission in cases of nonpercutaneously transmitted infection.[115, 116]

Perinatal or vertical transmission of HCV has been clearly documented, but in contrast to HBV it is an infrequent occurrence. After review of pertinent published data, Nowicki and Balistreri estimated that vertical transmission occurs in 7% of children born to seropositive mothers and the risk of transmission correlates with the mother's HCV-RNA titer.[113] There is also evidence to suggest that vertical transmission is enhanced by maternal co-infection with the human immunodeficiency virus (HIV).[117]

Intrafamilial spread of HCV can also occur: the prevalence within the family of an infected person has been assessed at 5% to 9%, 6 to 10 times greater than the general population.[113, 118] Transmission of HCV among institutionalized children is thought to be rare.[113] Occupational exposure of health care professionals not exposed to blood or blood products is low. The risk of infection among child care providers is also low, with a prevalence of anti-HCV reported in one study less than that in the general population.[118]

Sexual transmissions of HCV has been documented but at a low rate. The inefficiency of sexually transmitted HCV is thought to be due to the low viral load associated with HCV infection.[113] An increased risk of sexual transmission has been associated with an increased number of sexual partners, the presence of other sexually transmitted diseases (e.g., HIV), and anal receptive intercourse.

Sporadic or community-acquired HCV infections are defined as those cases in which there is no identifiable source of exposure. This occurs in 35% to 50% of cases and transmission is postulated to occur from inapparent percutaneous or nonpercutaneous transmission.[103, 119] In children, the proportion of sporadic cases has been reported to range from 15% to 80% in small groups of patients.[4, 110]

### Acute Hepatitis C

**CLINICAL COURSE.** Acute hepatitis due to HCV appears to be an uncommon presentation in childhood, with most cases diagnosed once the chronic state has already been well established.[107] This implies that the majority of initial HCV infections in children are asymptomatic. When it presents acutely, it cannot be distinguished on clinical grounds from other forms of viral hepatitis. Studies of experimental infections and post-transfusion hepatitis demonstrate that the incubation period ranges from 14 to 160 days with a mean of 50 days. Studies in adults show that the most common symptom is fatigue, with jaundice reported in only 25% of cases.[120]

Acute self-limited disease is the outcome in 15% to 50% of adults[27, 121]; the percentage of resolving disease in children is unknown. Some individuals infected with HCV experience multiple episodes of acute hepatitis. Results of primate experimentation have shown that "relapse" may be the result of reinfection with a different strain of HCV or lack of complete protective immunity resulting in reinfection (or reactivation) with a homologous strain.[122, 123]

**OUTCOMES AND COMPLICATIONS.** Evolution of acute HCV to fulminant hepatitis is rare, but co-infection with other hepatropic viruses (e.g., HBV) may accelerate progression.[113, 124] The most common complication of a primary infection with HCV is the development of a chronic infectious state.

### Chronic Hepatitis C

**CLINICAL COURSE.** In adults, 50% to 80% of primary HCV infections will become persistent and 10% or more will progress to clinically evident cirrhosis.[27, 104] Adult patients with chronic HCV infection who have now been followed for more than 20 years do not appear to suffer from an excess morbidity and mortality as a result of HCV liver disease.[104, 125]

The natural history of HCV disease in children remains ill defined. Our best understanding of chronic pediatric HCV comes from several European studies. In one study, HCV was found to be the major cause of cryptogenic cirrhosis, responsible for 14 cases in 33 children.[126] In another study, 77 HCV-seropositive children without underlying systemic disease were followed for a mean duration of 6 years.[110] At presentation only 22% were symptomatic, as manifested by asthenia, anorexia, or abdominal pain, with the remainder of patients discovered incidentally on routine blood tests for other illnesses. Four percent of patients had a history of intermittent jaundice, and approximately half presented with hepatomegaly. Only 32% at the time of diagnosis had histologic evidence of active liver disease. During the observation period the majority of children remained asymptomatic (81%); only 11 of 40 biopsied cases (27%) showed histologically active liver disease, and 2 patients were found to be cirrhotic. Only 6 of 57 studied children (10%) achieved a sustained biochemical remission. This study indicates that chronic HCV disease in children is usually asymptomatic, and histologically severe disease and cirrhosis are infrequent findings but spontaneous resolution is rare. It should be cautioned, however, that the study period in this report was of relatively short duration and that the epidemiologic and virologic differences between this population and other populations of children are not known.

**OUTCOMES AND COMPLICATIONS.** Similar to chronic HBV infection, an association between chronic hepatitis C and the development of HCC has been found. Retrospective studies support a slow, sequential progression from acute HCV infection to chronic hepatitis, cirrhosis, and finally the development of HCC. This progression occurs over a 30-year period.[127] Co-infection with HBV, the most common predisposing factor for the development of HCC may accelerate this progression.[128] Duration of infection is a significant risk factor, and children with long expected life spans can be considered at higher risk for the development of HCC. The development of cirrhosis in children with chronic hepatitis C has been described earlier.

Several extrahepatic complications of chronic HCV infection have now been well recognized. These include essential mixed cryoglobulinemia, glomerulonephritis, and porphyria cutanea tarda. Other complications that have been provisionally linked but still require confirmatory studies include polyarteritis nodosa, Sjögren's syndrome, lichen planus, and rheumatoid arthritis.[84]

One to 2 percent of adult patients with chronic hepatitis C have mixed essential (or type II) cryoglobulinemia, which is characterized by a recurring purpuric rash, nondeforming arthritis, and glomerulonephritis. Other symptoms include fatigue, headaches, neuropathy, and Raynaud's phenomenon.[129] The pathogenesis is unclear but appears to involve an immune-mediated vasculitis. Patients with chronic HCV infection may also have membranous and membranoproliferative glomerulonephritis, which may or may not be associated with cryoglobulinemia.[84] The renal disease of cryoglobulinemia may be manifested by nephrotic syndrome or progressive renal failure.

HCV infection may in some patients induce autoimmunity indistinguishable from chronic autoimmune hepatitis type II (anti-$LKM_1$, see later).[130, 131] It is hypothesized that in these patients HCV infection induces the production of autoantibody (anti-GOR) directed toward protein that is homologous to an HCV nucleocapsid protein. This type of autoimmunity is more likely to occur in older men[130] but has been documented in children.[132] It should be distinguished from those hyperglobulinemic patients with autoimmune hepatitis type I (antinuclear antibody positive) in whom positive anti-HCV is the result of a false-positive enzyme-linked immunosorbent assay (ELISA) and rarely confirmed by tests of higher specificity.[133]

### Diagnosis of Acute and Chronic Hepatitis C

Virus-specific serology is required for the accurate diagnosis of HCV infection. The serologic course of HCV disease is shown in Figure 50–6. Serum transaminase levels begin to rise with the development of symptoms and jaundice. They rise rapidly and then decline in a fashion that may be either monophasic and rapid or multiphasic with wide fluctuations and a more protracted course. The multiphasic pattern may portend more severe disease or progression to a chronic state.[103, 113] Assays for the detection of HCV antigens are not available, owing to the low concentrations of virus in the blood; diagnosis depends on the detection of antibodies to viral proteins (anti-HCV) and the viral genome (HCV-RNA) (see Table 50–4).

The original ELISA (i.e., ELISA-1) for anti-HCV detected nonprotective antibodies to a single nonstructural antigen. It suffered from poor sensitivity and specificity, with false-positive results noted in cases of hypergammaglobulinemia (e.g., autoimmune hepatitis) and rheumatoid arthritis. Also it rarely allowed the diagnosis of acute hepatitis C: its rise to detectable levels occurred on average 15 weeks and sometimes as late as a year after the onset of hepatitis.[27, 103] A second-generation test (ELISA-2) was developed. It detects antibodies to multiple, immunodominant, structural, and nonstructural proteins of HCV. It allows earlier detection of anti-HCV and improves both sensitivity and specificity.[134] A positive anti-HCV indicates current or past infection. A negative anti-HCV does not exclude infection in its early stages nor does it exclude past infection because it generally disappears in patients whose disease has resolved. Furthermore, 10% of patients with chronic hepatitis C will not have detectable anti-HCV. False-positive results may still occur, especially in patients with autoimmune disorders, and this lack of specificity has led to the development of a more specific but less sensitive recombinant immunoblot assay (RIBA) for anti-HCV. This test, now in its second generation (RIBA-2), also tests against multiple antigens and has a specificity of 98%. It is used as a confirmatory test in the presence of a positive ELISA anti-HCV. Improved higher generation anti-HCV tests continue to be developed, as are assays to detect anti-HCV IgM.

HCV-RNA is the earliest detectable marker in the blood of patients with hepatitis C. It can be detected during the incubation period, before the development of symptoms. Its detection is performed using polymerase chain reaction (PCR) techniques, which can detect as few as 1 to 10 molecules of nucleic acid.[27] Once found only in research institutions it is now becoming more accessible through commercial specialty laboratories. PCR testing for HCV-RNA is the only method available to directly assay the presence of HCV. Its presence is the most reliable measure of active infection[135] and in the absence of anti-HCV may be the only test to detect early, acute hepatitis C or infection in individuals who cannot mount an antibody response (e.g., immunocompromised patients). Persistence of HCV-RNA beyond 6 months indicates chronic infection, and its loss correlates with resolved disease. Quantitation of HCV-RNA may be helpful in determining the response to antiviral therapy (see later).

It is important but sometimes difficult to distinguish between chronic autoimmune hepatitis and chronic HCV infection. Patients with chronic hepatitis C may show autoimmune phenomena, and patients with autoimmune hepatitis and hyperglobulinemia may exhibit a false-positive anti-HCV. In one report, 64% of children with autoimmune hepatitis were positive for anti-HCV by ELISA.[136] It is therefore important to differentiate between these two entities. This involves specific diagnostic testing for autoimmune hepatitis (see later) and for HCV (e.g., anti-HCV by RIBA or HCV-RNA).[133]

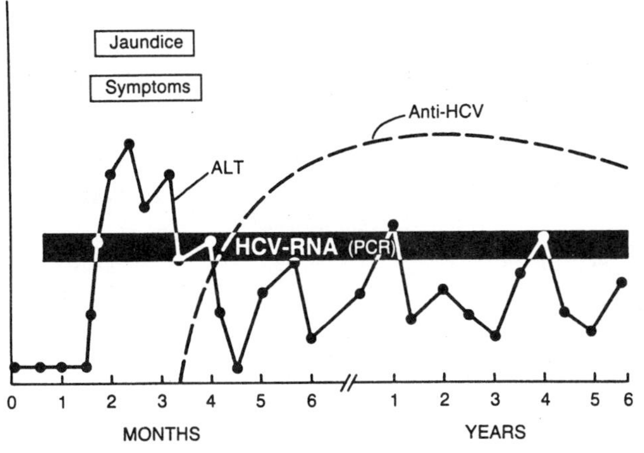


**FIGURE 50–6.** Typical clinical and serologic course of symptomatic acute hepatitis C. (From Hoofnagle JH, Di Bisceglie AM: Serologic diagnosis of acute and chronic viral hepatitis. Semin Liver Dis 1991;11:73–83, with permission.)

## Hepatitis Delta

The hepatitis D virus (HDV) is a small defective RNA virus that replicates and causes hepatitis only in individuals who are concurrently infected with HBV.[27] It was first detected in 1977 by Rizetto and colleagues using immunofluorescent staining of liver tissue from patients with chronic HBV infection.[137] A new nuclear antigen was discovered and named "δ," its associated antibody "anti-δ," and the purported virus to which this antigen belonged, the delta agent. Subsequent identification of this virus and its genome led to its final appellation: hepatitis D (or delta) virus.

### *Biology and Pathogenesis*

HDV is defined as an unclassified satellite virus of HBV. The complete viral particle is a 36- to 38-nm diameter hybrid, consisting of the δ antigen and a genome (HDV-RNA) surrounded by a coat composed of lipid and "borrowed" HBsAg. The genome is a single-stranded circular RNA molecule 1,700 nucleotides in length.

HDV can propagate only in HBV-infected individuals. The role of HBV may be to provide an envelope to HDV-RNA and δ antigen so complete viral particles can penetrate and infect adjacent cells. HDV must use the host cell's polymerase for replication, and it has been postulated that a function of the δ antigen is to alter the specificity of the host cell's polymerase, allowing transcription of the viral genome.[138]

The pathogenesis of HDV-related hepatic injury is incompletely understood. Although HDV has been shown to have a direct cytopathic effect on liver cells, this alone is inconsistent with the existence of a well-described HDV carrier

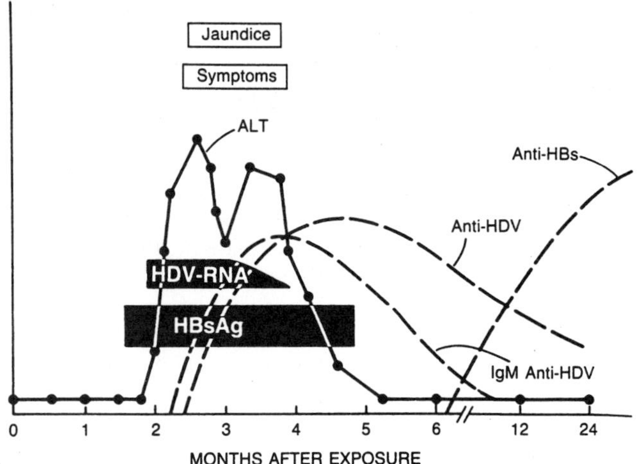


**FIGURE 50–7.** Typical clinical and serologic course of hepatitis D co-infection. (From Hoofnagle JH, Di Bisceglie AM: Serologic diagnosis of acute and chronic viral hepatitis. Semin Liver Dis 1991;11:73–83, with permission.)

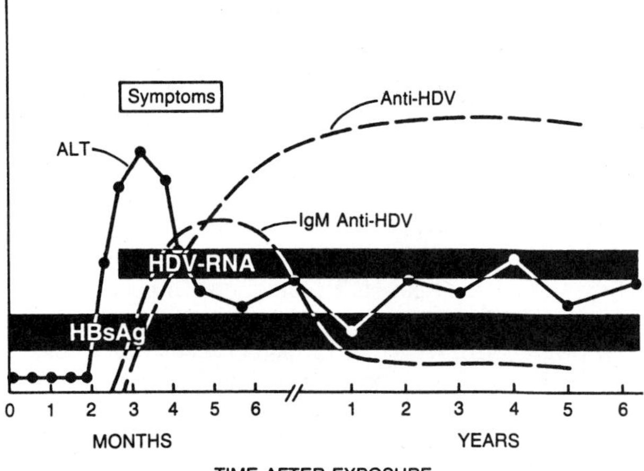


**FIGURE 50–8.** Typical clinical and serologic course of hepatitis D superinfection. (From Hoofnagle JH, Di Bisceglie AM: Serologic diagnosis of acute and chronic viral hepatitis. Semin Liver Dis 1991;11:73–83, with permission.)

state.[139, 140] Immune-mediated mechanisms of hepatocyte injury are also suspected.

## Epidemiology

Because HDV depends on HBV for its propagation its epidemiology is similar to that of HBV. Its distribution is worldwide, and humans are the only natural hosts; there are no environmental reservoirs. HDV is transmitted parenterally by both percutaneous and nonpercutaneous routes.

Hepatitis D can occur in three epidemiologic patterns: (1) as an endemic disease occurring in a large proportion of HBsAg carriers, (2) as epidemics in isolated communities of HBsAg carriers, and (3) in certain high-risk populations.[138] HDV is highly endemic in the Mediterranean basin, especially southern Italy, the Middle East, and northern Africa, where 20% to 40% of HBsAg carriers are also anti-HDV positive. Other areas of high endemicity include northern South America and Romania.[138, 141] HDV infection can also occur in epidemic form, usually in isolated populations of less developed countries. Repeated outbreaks of "Labrea fever" have been described in the Amazon basin: it affects children frequently and is often severe, with mortality rates reaching 10% to 20%.[138] Developed areas such as northern Europe and North America have low prevalence rates, and disease occurs mainly in high-risk groups of individuals (e.g., intravenous drug abusers and multitransfused patients). In these areas the anti-HDV prevalence rate is between 1% and 10% among HBsAg carriers.[142, 143] Pediatric disease appears to be infrequent in developed countries with low prevalence.

## Clinical Course and Outcomes

Hepatitis D may be both acute and chronic. Although it clinically resembles other forms of viral hepatitis, its course and prognosis tend to be more severe. It is important to distinguish two types of acute HDV infection: superinfection and co-infection.

Acute HDV co-infection is defined as simultaneous acquisition of both HDV and HBV. The clinical and serologic course of acute HDV co-infection is shown in Figure 50–7. This type of infection is often self-limited and leads to a chronic HDV infection in less than 5%.[144] Acute HDV superinfection is defined as the occurrence of HDV infection in an individual with chronic HBV infection. The ongoing persistence of HBsAg in these patients predisposes to the persistence of HDV, and the development of chronic HDV infection is noted in more than 75% of superinfections.[144] The clinical and serologic course of an acute HDV superinfection progressing to chronicity is shown in Figure 50–8. A comparison of acute HDV co-infections and superinfections is shown in Table 50–8.

The outcomes for both the acute and chronic forms of HDV infection are more severe than for HBV alone. The mortality rate from acute HDV infections ranges from 2% to 20%, as compared with less than 1% from acute HBV infections.[138] Cirrhosis may develop rapidly, within 2 years, in 15% and in 70% to 80% over the long term, as compared with 10% in chronic hepatitis B.[138]

Outcome studies of childhood HDV infections are few in number and patients; consequently, general conclusions cannot be drawn. In one study, HDV infection was associated

**TABLE 50–8. Comparison of HDV Co- and Superinfections**

| CHARACTERISTIC | CO-INFECTION | SUPERINFECTION |
|---|---|---|
| HBV infection | Acute | Chronic |
| HDV infection | Acute, transient | Acute to chronic |
| Acute mortality rate | 1–10% | 5–20% |
| Chronicity rate | <5% | >75% |
| HBsAg | +, transient | +, usually persists |
| IgM anti-HBc | + | − |
| Anti-HDV | ±, transient | +, usually persists |
| HDV-RNA | +, transient | +, usually persists |

Adapted from Hoofnagle JH: Type D (delta) hepatitis. JAMA 1989; 261:1321–1325, with permission. Copyright 1989, American Medical Association.

with more severe histopathology at presentation, and the hepatitis deteriorated in 38% of patients over 2 to 7 years.[145] In another study, 26% of children demonstrated histologic evidence of cirrhosis at presentation, but little deterioration was seen over a 5- to 12-year period of follow-up.[146]

### Diagnosis

HDV infection can occur only in individuals with concurrent HBV infection, and serologic markers for HBV must be present for diagnosis. HDV infection should be suspected in any HBV-infected patient who has a particularly severe, biphasic or fulminant initial presentation or who has had stable chronic disease and whose condition suddenly begins to deteriorate rapidly. HDV serologic markers are outlined in Table 50–4.

Detection of anti-HDV measures IgG and IgM antibodies to HDV-antigen. In acute HDV co-infection the disease is usually self-limited and anti-HDV titers are low and short lived. For this reason the diagnosis of acute HDV co-infection is often difficult and requires the measurement of acute and convalescent phase titers.[27] Acute HDV superinfections most often progress to a chronic state, and in these cases anti-HDV titers rise to high levels and persist. The differentiation between co-infection and superinfection can be further facilitated by the detection of anti-HBc IgM, a marker for acute HBV infection. A sensitive assay for anti-HDV IgM alone is available and may be helpful in the diagnosis of acute infection when the "conventional" anti-HDV is undetectable. Anti-HDV IgM can persist at low levels during chronic HDV infections. HDV-RNA and HDV-Ag assays in both serum and liver may be helpful in the diagnosis of acute and chronic HDV infections but are only available through research laboratories.

## Hepatitis E

Hepatitis E is a recently described disease for which little information is available. It has been reported only in specific geographic areas and rarely in children.

Epidemic NANB hepatitis was first confirmed as a distinct entity in 1982, and the responsible viral particles were identified in fecal material in 1983.[147, 148] The causative agent of epidemic NANB hepatitis was named hepatitis E virus (HEV) in 1988, and the complete genome was sequenced, with the subsequent development of diagnostic tests in the early 1990s.[149] Study of this disease is ongoing, and comprehensive reviews have been published.[150, 151]

### Biology and Pathogenesis

The virus responsible for HEV has a diameter of 32 nm; it is nonenveloped and has a single-stranded RNA genome 7,500 bases in length. Although it has morphologic similarities to calciviruses, its genome is dissimilar, and the virus remains unclassified. Nucleotide sequence homology among HEV isolates from different parts of the world indicate only one major genotype. The pathogenesis of hepatocellular injury caused by HEV awaits elucidation.

### Epidemiology

HEV infection can occur as a unimodal epidemic with a highly compressed incidence curve, as a more prolonged epidemic with multiple small peaks of incidence, or as sporadic cases occurring in endemic areas.[152] Transmission is fecal-oral, and epidemics are usually waterborne, occurring in many cases during the rainy season. Outbreaks have been described in India, China, Southeast and Central Asia, northern and eastern Africa, and Mexico. No confirmed cases have been reported from the United States or Canada, Western Europe, and the developed countries of Asia except in travelers returning from disease-prone areas.[151] Hepatitis E affects mainly adults, but isolated childhood infections have been reported.[152]

### Clinical Course and Outcomes

The incubation period for hepatitis E is 2 to 9 weeks (mean, 6 weeks).[150] The disease is acute and self-limited. Chronic liver disease or a carrier state has not been observed. Symptomatology is identical to the other forms of viral hepatitis, but fever (found in over 50% of patients) and arthralgia (in 30%) appear to be more common.[151] Symptoms and biochemical abnormalities usually resolve within 6 weeks. The proportion of asymptomatic infections is unknown. The outcome in general is excellent. Mortality rates are low (<1%), except in pregnant women in whom the mortality can reach 20%. Women in their third trimester are at particular risk, and miscarriages are frequent.[150, 151]

### Diagnosis

Recombinant HEV proteins are used to detect anti-HEV antibodies in the blood. An enzyme immunoassay (EIA) can be used to detect both IgG and IgM separately. The diagnosis of HEV infection is based on the detection of anti-HEV, but these tests are not usually available outside endemic areas.

## Hepatitis G

Hepatitis G presents an emerging story, the responsible virus having only recently been discovered. In 1995 three new viruses were identified, using PCR methodology, from primates infected with a human hepatitis virus. They were designated GB viruses (A through C) after the physician with the initials GB who developed a nontypable hepatitis in 1964. Subsequently, another virus isolated independently and designated hepatitis G virus (HGV) was found to be identical to GB-C virus. Although the recent literature regarding HGV has focused on adults and the population at large, the available information indicates that children are at risk from transfusion or community-acquired disease.

### Biology and Pathogenesis

HGV is a distant relative of HCV, sharing 25% nucleotide homology. It is a member of the flavivirus family and has a single-stranded RNA genome 9,400 bases in length.[153] HGV does not appear to replicate in the liver, raising the question of whether it is a true hepatotropic virus. The pathogenesis of hepatocellular injury is unknown, but HGV appears to cause mild disease and does not alter the course and severity of those patients co-infected with HCV.[154, 155]

### Epidemiology

Little is known about the epidemiology of hepatitis G, but transmission appears to be parenteral, with both post-transfusion and sporadic community-acquired cases being reported.[155–157] The prevalence of HGV in 500 randomly selected blood donors without hepatitis was 1.4%, and it was 23% in patients with post-transfusion–associated non-A, non-B, non-C hepatitis.[155] In community-acquired hepatitis, HGV has been found in 9% of non–A-E hepatitis patients.[157] Co-infection of HGV with cases of HAV, HBV, and HCV has been found in 25%, 32%, and 20%, respectively.[156]

### Clinical Course and Outcomes

Initial studies indicated that infection with HGV may be both acute and chronic or lead to fulminant hepatitis. In one study,[156] the clinical characteristics of acute infection were similar for patients with HGV alone and those with hepatitis A, B, C with or without co-infection with HGV. This same study also found that persistent infection after HGV is common but does not appear to cause significant clinical disease or to complicate the acute or chronic courses of hepatitis A, B, or C.

### Diagnosis

Reliable serum immunoassays for the detection of HGV are not yet available, and diagnosis of infection currently requires documentation of the presence of HGV-RNA by PCR.

## Hepatitis Non–A-E

In one study of 79 patients with post-transfusion–associated hepatitis, 10 (13%) failed to show evidence for any of the known hepatitis viruses.[155] It is clear that other, still to be identified, agents can be responsible for clinically evident hepatitis. Consequently, it can be expected, especially with further refinements in molecular biology techniques, that the "hepatitis alphabet" will continue to expand, as will our knowledge of infectious hepatitis. A virus tentatively designated hepatitis F virus has been recovered from the stool of a patient with hepatitis and transmitted to primates, but this finding awaits independent confirmation.[153]

# VIRUSES CAUSING SYSTEMIC INFECTION INCLUDING HEPATITIS

A large number of viral agents that cause generalized infections can also cause hepatitis. These infections are usually acute, are self-limited, and have an excellent prognosis. In most cases the hepatic component of the illness is clinically silent and the patient receives a diagnosis of "flulike" illness. A nonexhaustive list of etiologic agents is given in Table 50–1.

From a pediatric perspective three viral agents are clinically important, especially in the newborn and immunocompromised patient: Epstein-Barr virus (EBV), cytomegalovirus, and HIV.

## Epstein-Barr Virus

Epstein-Barr virus is a gamma herpesvirus in the family of Herpesviridae. It is the principal cause of infectious mononucleosis, but it is also responsible for significant disease in immunocompromised patients such as children with the acquired immunodeficiency syndrome (AIDS) or who have undergone organ transplantation. EBV has also been linked to the development of tumors and lymphoproliferative disorders, especially in the immunosuppressed post-transplant patient.

Infectious mononucleosis in otherwise healthy children is generally a mild disease.[158] In addition to generalized symptoms of malaise, fatigue, pharyngitis, and nausea, hepatitis is common, with hepatomegaly found in 10% to 15%. Serum transaminase levels are elevated in 80% of children, but jaundice becomes apparent in less than 5%. Major symptoms typically persist for 2 to 4 weeks and then gradually recede. The prognosis is generally excellent; and once the diagnosis is established, the hepatic component need only be followed clinically. Diagnosis is strongly suspected based on clinical findings of exudative pharyngitis, lymphadenopathy, hepatosplenomegaly, and peripheral atypical lymphocytosis. The diagnosis is confirmed by the detection of heterophil and/or EBV-specific antibodies. EBV, like other herpesviruses, establishes a persistent latent infection after the primary illness. In immunocompromised patients, and rarely in healthy individuals, a chronic active infection including hepatitis may occur.

## Cytomegalovirus

Cytomegalovirus (CMV) is the largest of the herpesviruses, with a diameter of 200 nm. Infection with cytomegalovirus can be acquired by intrauterine, perinatal, intrafamilial, or sexual transmission as well as by transfusion or organ transplantation.[159] CMV-DNA persists after primary infection and multiple reactivations can occur that are normally controlled by a host cell–mediated immune response. In immunocompetent individuals the primary infection and subsequent reactivations are generally asymptomatic but may be responsible for an infectious mononucleosis–type picture with mild hepatic involvement.

From a pediatric perspective congenital CMV infections and infections in immunocompromised children are especially important. In these instances a severe and/or chronic condition can ensue. Newborns with congenital CMV frequently have hepatic involvement, with hepatosplenomegaly in 60%, jaundice in 67%, and purpura in 13%.[160] The degree of jaundice is attributed to both the hepatitis and hemolytic anemia. The hepatitis may persist but rarely progresses to cirrhosis.[159]

The prototypical CMV infection in immunocompromised children occurs in those children who have received an organ transplant. In organ transplantation the source of infection is either the grafted organ, transfused blood products, or reactivation of a latent infection. CMV infection in this instance may cause hepatitis, which in the liver transplant patient for example may be difficult to distinguish from rejection or vascular compromise of the graft. In these children the infection may become persistent and lead to liver failure.[161]

Diagnosis is best established by isolation of CMV from urine, saliva, or biopsy tissues. It may also be isolated from other body secretions. Total antibodies against CMV may also be assayed, but results may be confounded in the polytransfused child and in the neonate from circulating "foreign" IgG antibodies. Antibodies directed against CMV may be helpful in diagnosing a primary infection by determining the presence of IgM and seroconversion from IgM to IgG. In limited instances PCR to detect the CMV genome may be helpful. In the presence of hepatitis, and when clinically indicated, characteristic intranuclear inclusion bodies can be found on histologic examination of liver biopsy specimens.

### Human Immunodeficiency Virus

AIDS is caused by the retrovirus HIV. The route of transmission is parenteral, and in children AIDS is usually acquired perinatally or as the result of blood transfusions. As a result of systematic screening of the blood supply, this latter route has become much less frequent. In adolescents and young adults the disease may be acquired through sexual contact and intravenous drug abuse with shared needles. HIV is strongly suspected to directly cause hepatic injury, but definitive evidence is lacking. Hepatitis in AIDS may also be caused by the drugs used to treat its manifestations and by opportunistic infections. These include the hepatotropic viruses B and C, CMV, EBV, *Mycobacterium* species, *Pneumocystis carinii,* and fungi. Evidence of liver disease can be found in over 90% of children but rarely results in injury to the point of causing coagulopathy and liver failure.[162, 163] Hepatic involvement, however, can contribute significantly to the child's general condition and outcome.

## AUTOIMMUNE HEPATITIS

### Definition and Classification

Autoimmune hepatitis (AIH), which has been described since the early 1950s, is a chronic necroinflammatory hepatitis of unknown etiology. It is characterized histologically by dense mononuclear cell infiltrates in the portal tracts and serologically by autoantibodies targeted against liver-specific and nonorgan-specific antigens.

Two types of AIH have been described: type I or classic (AIH-I) and type II or anti-LKM-1 autoimmune hepatitis (AIH-II). The distinction is made according to differing profiles of circulating autoantibodies (Table 50–9). A third type of autoimmune hepatitis, characterized by antibodies against soluble liver antigens, has been proposed (AIH-III).[164] It, however, has not been universally accepted, and many include this third type as a subset of AIH-I.[165]

**TABLE 50–9. Classification of Autoimmune Hepatitis (AIH)**

| TYPE | CHARACTERISTIC AUTOANTIBODIES | OCCASIONALLY PRESENT AUTOANTIBODIES |
|---|---|---|
| I. Classic AIH | Antinuclear<br>Anti–smooth muscle<br>Antiactin<br>Anti-asialoglycoprotein receptor | Antimitochondrial<br>Anti–soluble liver antigen<br>Anti–liver-pancreas protein<br>Antineutrophil cytoplasmic |
| II. Anti-LKM-I AIH | Anti-LKM-I<br>Anti-liver cytosol-I | Anti-liver cytosol*<br>Antinuclear* |

*Rare

Adapted from Krawitt EL: Autoimmune hepatitis. N Engl J Med 1996; 334:897–903, with permission. 

### Pathogenesis

A conceptual framework for the pathogenesis of AIH has been proposed and involves a genetically predisposed individual exposed to an environmental agent. This agent triggers an autoimmune response targeted against liver antigens and results in a chronic hepatic necroinflammatory response, leading to fibrosis and cirrhosis.[165]

The search for predisposing genetic factors has focused on the major histocompatibility complex on chromosome 6 and in particular on the HLA-DR region. Susceptibility to AIH has been linked to two histocompatibility genes: DR3 and DR4. It has been shown that the association with HLA-DR3 predisposes to more severe disease: it appears at an earlier age and results more frequently in liver transplantation.[166] A partial deficiency of the complement component C4, which is coded at the HLA-DR3 locus, has been described in some children with AIH. C4 plays a role in virus neutralization, and this type of deficiency may lead to the development of autoimmunity.[131]

The environmental triggers presumed to initiate autoimmune hepatitis are unknown, but several viral candidates have been proposed based on reported evidence. These include rubella,[167] Epstein-Barr virus,[168] and the hepatotropic viruses A, B, and C.[23, 169, 170] Interferon alfa (INF-$\alpha$) used for the treatment of chronic viral hepatitis has also been reported to trigger the development of AIH.[170]

The target antigen for AIH-I has not been identified, and none of the diagnostic autoantibodies for AIH-I appear to be pathogenic. Anti-LKM-1 antibodies recognize the cytochrome mono-oxygenase P450IID6 expressed on hepatocyte membrane surfaces, and this protein is suspected to be the pathogenic autoantigen in AIH-II.[164]

### Clinical Course and Outcomes

AIH affects both children and adults, with two peaks of incidence between 10 and 20 and 45 and 70 years of age.[131] AIH-I represents 80% of all cases in adults.[164] AIH-II usually affects children and young adults. It is common in young females, with three fourths of patients being female and half of the patients presenting between 10 and 20 years of age. Its course can be particularly severe and rapidly progressive.

Although AIH may present acutely, it always becomes chronic and it is not necessary to wait 6 months to confirm chronicity.[131] The clinical features are heterogeneous and cover the spectrum from asymptomatic patients in whom hepatitis is an incidental biochemical finding to patients with fulminant hepatitis and liver failure.[165] The differential diagnosis between AIH, acute viral hepatitis, and other acute or chronic liver disorders may be difficult.[171] There may be no correlation between the clinical findings, or lack thereof, and the often severe histologic lesion seen on liver biopsy.[165]

The clinical course in adults has been well described and appears to be benign in most cases.[164, 165] This does not appear to be the case for AIH presenting in childhood. A 20-year experience in 52 children with a median follow-up of 5 years has been reported.[172] The results of this study (Table 50–10) indicate that AIH-II presents at an earlier age, with a more severe initial presentation, including fulminant hepatitis, and a poorer response to immunosuppressive therapy. Long-term outcome between both groups, however, appears to be similar. A significant number of associated immune-related disorders have been found in patients and/or their first-degree relatives (21% and 40%, respectively), including inflammatory bowel disease, thyroiditis, and nephrosis. Bilirubin level and prothrombin time at initial presentation appeared to be good predictors of outcome. Similar results in children with AIH were reported in two other studies,[173, 174] but cirrhosis was present on biopsy in a larger proportion of patients (up to 89%), emphasizing the severity of this disease in the pediatric population.

## Diagnosis

The diagnosis of AIH in childhood must take into consideration clinical features, histologic appearance on liver biopsy, and the presence of detectable autoantibodies. A severe presentation with deep jaundice, dark urine, and coagulopathy along with accompanying immune-related disorders (e.g., thyroiditis, ulcerative colitis) may be important diagnostic clues, allowing the differentiation from other disorders with which it may be easily confused (e.g., hepatitis C). A histologic picture of severe necroinflammatory hepatocellular injury and dense portal triad mononuclear cell infiltrates is also helpful in differentiating AIH from viral hepatidites.

**TABLE 50–10. Characteristics, Clinical Course and Outcomes in 52 Children with Autoimmune Hepatitis (AIH) Followed for a Median of 5 Years**

| | AIH-I | AIH-II |
|---|---|---|
| **Demographics** | | |
| No. patients (%) | 32 (62) | 20 (38) |
| Females (%) | 24 (75) | 15 (75) |
| Age at diagnosis (range) | 10 yr (2–15) | 7 yr (0.3–19) |
| **Initial Presentation** | | |
| Acute hepatitis (%) | 16 (50) | 13 (65) |
| Insidious onset (%) | 12 (38) | 5 (25) |
| Hepatosplenomegaly (%) | 15 (47) | 8 (40) |
| Cirrhosis on biopsy (%) | 18/26 (69) | 5/13 (38) |
| Fulminant hepatitis (%) | 1 (3) | 5 (25) |
| **Response to Immunosuppressive Therapy** | | |
| Initial remission (%) | 31 (97) | 13 (65) |
| Stopped after 3 years (%) | 6 (19) | 0 (0) |
| Liver transplant | 2 | 2 |
| Deaths | 1 | 2 |

From Gregorio GV, Portmann B, Reid F, et al: Autoimmune hepatitis in childhood: a 20-year experience. Hepatology 1997;25:541–547, with permission.

Delineation of a patient's autoantibody profile is important for diagnostic, typing, and prognostic purposes (see Table 50–9). Patients with AIH-I typically present with circulating antinuclear, anti–smooth muscle, and antiactin antibodies. Although antiactin antibodies are more specific than anti–smooth muscle antibodies, testing for them is not performed in most clinical laboratories. In AIH-II, antibodies against liver-kidney microsome-1 (anti–LKM-1) are characteristically present. A large proportion of adult anti-LKM-1 patients will show positivity for markers of HCV infection. This association is rare in children, and most likely represents a reactivity different from the one found in AIH-II.[130, 131] In some patients with AIH-II, anti–liver cytosol-1 antibodies can be present alone or with anti–LKM-1. Several pediatric patients with this profile and asymptomatic disease have been described.[175]

Autoantibodies can be found in low titers in adults with a variety of nonautoimmune disorders. In children who are healthy or who have nonautoimmune diseases this situation is very rare, and the presence of autoantibodies even in low titers is sufficient for the diagnosis of AIH.[131] Some patients with all the features of autoimmune hepatitis but without detectable autoantibodies have been reported and are included in a group labeled as having "cryptogenic cirrhosis."[165]

Since its initial description, hyperproteinemia and hyperglobulinemia have been described in association with AIH. The hyperglobulinemia may lead to false-positive screening results for hepatitis C, but more specific HCV testing (see hepatitis C) and detection of non–organ-specific and liver-specific autoantibodies should result in the proper diagnosis.

# TREATMENT OF HEPATITIS

## Treatment of Acute Hepatitis

### *Acute-Phase Supportive Care*

Every child with hepatitis should receive the care necessary to ensure his or her comfort and an acceptable outcome. In most cases this requires supportive care only, as for example with hepatitis A or infectious mononucleosis in which the outcomes are generally excellent. General measures include adequate rest and diet, although these aspects of therapy have not been sufficiently studied in children. A balanced diet that prevents weight loss, dehydration, and nutritional deficiencies should be advocated. Strict bed rest is generally not required, but permitted levels of activity should take into account the child's general condition. The return to normal activities and school requires knowledge of the child's clinical status, the type of hepatitis (including mode of transmission and duration of infectivity), and local health regulations. For example, most school-age children with HBV infection can return to school as soon as they are physically able because they pose little threat of transmission. Young children with HAV infection, regardless of their general condition, however, should not return to daycare centers until their period of viral shedding has ended, which is 1 week after the onset of symptoms.[176]

Measures must also be undertaken to reduce the risk of spread during the period of infectivity, and these include educational measures directed toward the child's caregivers and contacts, reporting to local health authorities when required, and active and passive immunization when indicated. Appropriate follow-up should be carried out to confirm resolution.

### Antiviral Therapy

Antiviral therapy is not recommended for the treatment of acute hepatitis in immunocompetent hosts. Treatment has been advocated for immunocompromised children with evidence of acute EBV or CMV infection, including hepatitis. Acyclovir and gancyclovir have been used for the treatment of EBV infection but act only on the active and not on the latent phases of infection. The antiviral effect of gancyclovir for disease due to EBV is believed to be more prolonged on withdrawal than that of acyclovir.[177]

Gancyclovir has been used with success in immunocompromised children with active CMV. Induction therapy for 2 to 3 weeks is usually followed by prolonged maintenance therapy because viral excretion most usually recurs on cessation. CMV immune globulin derived from pooled plasma from adults selected for high CMV antibody titers has also been used in conjunction with an antiviral agent. Prospective studies of its efficacy in children are lacking. Treatment with currently available antiviral agents is also not recommended in the neonate with congenital CMV infection because no benefits have been found in this situation.

### Immunosuppressive Therapy

It was thought early on that immunosuppressive therapy with corticosteroids would hasten the recovery from acute viral hepatitis and curtail the progression of chronic viral hepatitis. However, prospective trials failed to demonstrate a beneficial effect and, in fact, suggested a more rapid progression, the development of chronic hepatitis, and other harmful outcomes.[121, 178–180] Immunosuppressive therapy is now contraindicated in the treatment of both acute and chronic viral hepatitis.

## Treatment of Chronic Hepatitis

Patients with chronic hepatitis require care and monitoring from physicians comfortable in evaluating and treating children with chronic liver disease. The frequency and depth of this care are dictated by the nature of the underlying injury, knowledge of its natural history correlated with the child's overall condition, and course. Until recently there was no specific therapy for the treatment of chronic viral hepatitis other than supportive care and prevention of spread. Perhaps as a consequence of our increasing recognition of the outcomes that may result from years of chronic infection, efforts have focused on specific therapies to suppress or eliminate the virus and resolve hepatic inflammation.

### Chronic Phase Supportive Care

Supportive care for the child with chronic hepatitis involves maintenance of long-term well-being, monitoring for the complications of chronic liver disease, and avoidance of any further hepatic injury. Many children with chronic hepatitis are diagnosed fortuitously and are asymptomatic. In these children there are no restrictions to activity and they may lead a normal lifestyle. Some children with stable disease and mild symptoms such as fatigue or poor appetite will require interventions commensurate with their disability to maintain nutritional status, normal schooling, and overall well-being. Other children, such as those with chronic AIH, may have labile disease, with frequent "flares" separated by disease-free periods of variable duration. These children will require early recognition of relapses with appropriate modification of their therapy. Patients with advanced disease and manifestations such as ascites or coagulopathy require aggressive therapy directed at the specific sequelae of long-term liver disease.

Children with chronic hepatitis should avoid all but the most necessary medications because some may further aggravate liver injury. Exposure to all environmental hepatotoxic agents (e.g., organophosphates) should also be carefully avoided.

### Immunosuppressive Therapy

Immunosuppressive therapy is contraindicated in individuals with chronic viral hepatitis (see earlier).

Chronic AIH, however, generally responds to immunosuppressive therapy, of which corticosteroids have become the mainstay. Immunosuppressive therapy for AIH can be divided into two phases: (1) induction of remission and (2) maintenance of remission. There are no widely accepted guidelines for initial dosage and withdrawal of immunosuppressive agents. One pediatric regimen begins with prednisolone, 2 mg/kg/day (maximum 60 mg), and is gradually decreased over a period of 4 to 6 weeks to the minimal dose able to maintain normal transaminase levels.[131] If excessive doses of corticosteroids are required to maintain normal transaminases, or if the child does not achieve remission, then azathioprine at a dose of 0.5 mg/kg/day is started. Based on the patient's response and presence or lack of drug-induced toxicity, the dose of azathioprine may be increased to 2 mg/kg/day. 6-Mercaptopurine, a related purine analogue, can be substituted for azathioprine at a lower dose and, in some cases, has facilitated induction of remission when azathioprine has failed.[181] Results of this treatment protocol are shown in Table 50–10. The time necessary to achieve normalization of transaminases can be prolonged. In this protocol, normalization was reached after a median of 0.5 year (range, 0.2 to 7) in AIH-I and 0.8 year (range, 0.2 to 3.2) in AIH-II.[131]

Immunosuppressive therapy may be withdrawn in some patients, allowing a prolonged "disease-free" period. Other children will require chronic, low-maintenance doses of corticosteroids and a purine analogue, alone or in combination, to maintain a state of remission. Alternate-day or pulsed corticosteroid regimens to concurrently maintain remission and avoid side effects of prolonged therapy have been disappointing.[165]

Forty percent of children will have at least one episode of relapse while on treatment, and many will progress to cirrhosis.[131] Poor indicators of response to therapy include cirrhosis at initial biopsy, diagnosis at a young age, long duration of disease, and presence of the HLA-B8 or DR3 phenotype.[165] When conventional therapy has failed, cyclosporine or tacrolimus has been tried; but published experience has been preliminary or anecdotal.[182–184] Patients with AIH who have failed medical therapy or who presented initially with end-stage liver disease have been referred for liver transplantation with success (see Chapter 52). The disease may recur after transplantation despite aggressive immunosuppression or several years after grafting when immunosuppression is reduced.[165]

### *Interferon Therapy*

The interferons are a family of naturally occurring glycoproteins that have been studied since the 1950s. They are secreted in response to viral infections and are part of our natural host defense system. There are three classes of interferon (IFN), depending on their cell of origin: α, β, and γ. Efforts to eliminate chronic viral hepatitis with interferon have focused on IFN-α, which can now be synthesized using recombinant DNA technology. There are two available forms of recombinant IFN-α: 2a and 2b. IFN-α 2b has been released commercially in the United States and is indicated for the treatment of chronic HBV and HCV infections in adults with compensated liver disease.

Early side effects of IFN-α include in almost all patients a flulike illness that lasts for 6 to 12 hours after each injection. Evening administration of IFN and treatment with acetaminophen allow most children to handle this without incident. Late-appearing complications occur in less than 2% of adults and are mainly infectious (e.g., pneumonia), hematologic (e.g., neutropenia), autoimmune (e.g., hepatitis), and psychiatric.[185, 186] Clinical trials are ongoing to investigate the effects of other interferons (e.g., hybrid-IFN) in the treatment of chronic viral hepatitis.[187]

**CHRONIC HEPATITIS B.** Treatment with interferon is based on the rationale that persistent infection with HBV involves a defective immunologic response to the virus including the decreased production of endogenous interferons and a diminished interferon-induced cellular activation.[188] Since the first report in 1976 of treatment with pharmacologic doses of interferon, a number of studies in adults using mainly IFN-α have been published. They have used a variety of treatment regimens in terms of dosage, length of treatment, and use of adjuvant therapies, such as "steroid priming."[188] Adult studies have shown that the greatest effectiveness was achieved at doses of 5 to 10 MU three times a week.[187] Most studies define a favorable response to therapy as the sustained loss of HBeAg and HBV-DNA and normalization of transaminases. In many patients who eventually clear HBeAg and HBV-DNA a transient increase in serum transaminase levels may occur between the first and third months of treatment. It is thought that this increase corresponds to activation of the host immune response and early clearance of HBV-DNA. Approximately half of "responders" will eventually clear HBsAg and acquire anti-HBs. Duration of therapy is variable, with at least 6 months in most studies. A short pretreatment trial of corticosteroids ("steroid priming") has been tried in a number of studies in an effort to increase the efficacy of IFN by creating an "immunologic rebound" on corticosteroid withdrawal. This approach has not been found to be beneficial except in those patients with normal serum transaminase levels before therapy.[188]

In adults, predictors of a beneficial response to treatment have been identified and include elevated serum aspartate aminotransferase levels (>twice normal) and low HBV-DNA levels (<200 pg/mL).[189] Other positive predictive factors include a short duration of infection, histologically active disease, and immunocompetency.[188] Our understanding of the benefits of IFN-α in the treatment of adults with chronic HBV infection is best summarized in a report by Wong and associates.[190] In this meta-analysis of 15 previously published randomized and controlled trials, the authors showed that 36% of 498 treated patients lost HBV-DNA and 32% lost HBeAg as compared with 339 controls who lost HBV-DNA and HBeAg in 16% and 12%, respectively.

The results of therapy in 330 children have now been reported in eight separate pediatric trials.[186, 187] Comparison of the study parameters among these studies has shown a great degree of variability. These parameters have included choice of the study population (European and Chinese children), IFN dosage regimen (range, 3–10 MU/m$^2$ subcutaneously, thrice weekly), and duration of therapy (range, 12–48 weeks). In the studies of European children, 36% of treated children (n = 124; range, 20–50%) lost HBeAg as compared with 14% of controls (n = 92; range, 9–25%). These results are comparable to those found in adults. In Chinese children the response rate was much lower: 9% in 72 treated children versus 5% in 42 controls. Genetic factors, the presence of mutant strains, perinatally acquired disease, and a long duration of infection in these Chinese children have all been postulated to justify these striking differences. The poorer response rate of Chinese children to IFN therapy is not well understood.

**CHRONIC HEPATITIS C.** IFN-α has also been used in the treatment of chronic HCV infections. Efficacy of IFN-α is defined biochemically as normalization of serum alanine aminotransferase and virologically as loss of serum HCV-RNA. These parameters are measured at two endpoints: at the end of treatment (end of treatment response [ETR]) and 6 months after treatment (sustained response [SR]). Based on these definitions, randomized clinical trials have demonstrated benefits of IFN-α in adult patients.[191] With treatment with 3 MU subcutaneously thrice weekly for 6 months, biochemical ETRs of 40% to 50% and virologic ETRs of 30% to 40% have been observed. Relapses are common, however, with SRs of only 15% to 20% and 10% to 20% for biochemical and virologic parameters, respectively.

Predictors of SR include short duration of infection, low HCV-RNA titers, absence of cirrhosis, and favorable genotype (e.g., types 2 and 3).[192] Nonresponders can be identified after 3 months of therapy by persistent elevations of serum alanine aminotransferase and HCV-RNA. In this situation, treatment can be stopped because the likelihood of a future favorable response is remote.[191] For patients who relapse biochemically during follow-up, re-treatment for 12 months has been associated with a biochemical ETR rate of 87% and an SR rate of 50%.[191] Some studies have advocated longer periods of treatment (e.g., 60 months) to achieve higher sustained response rates.[193]

The efficacy and safety of IFN-α in the treatment of children with chronic HCV has been reported in only a few studies. In a published pilot study, 12 Spanish HCV-RNA positive children were treated for 6 months with 3 MU/m$^2$ IFN thrice weekly for 6 months.[194] Eleven children completed the study, and the ETR was 36% and 72% for biochemical and virologic parameters, respectively. At 24 months, however, only 5 children (45%) had maintained a sustained response to therapy. IFN was well tolerated by the children in this study. In an Italian study,[195] 11 children were treated with 3 MU/m$^2$ of lymphoblastoid IFN-α three times per week for 12 months and compared with 10 controls. Five treated patients (45%) showed a biochemical response that occurred early (mean 3 weeks) and persisted until the end of follow-up at 30 months. Only 1 control exhibited a similar biochemical response. Virologic responses were demonstrated in all the biochemical responders and persisted to the end of follow-up. This study is particularly interesting in that no relapses in the treated children were noted; however, these findings await independent confirmation.

### *Other Antiviral Agents*

Research is ongoing in the quest to develop other efficacious and safe antiviral therapies. Agents that continue to be studied for use in human viral hepatitis include ribavirin, thymosins, and second-generation nucleosides such as famciclovir and lamivudine.

Ribavirin, a synthetic guanosine nucleoside analogue with antiviral properties, when administered in combination with IFN-α for the treatment of chronic HCV has been found to significantly improve sustained virologic response rates as compared with IFN-α alone. In one study, 43% of 277 patients treated with combination therapy for 48 weeks showed a sustained virologic response as compared with 19% of 278 patients treated with IFN-α alone.[196] Lamivudine, another nucleoside analogue, has been associated with substantial histologic improvement when given alone for 1 year to Chinese patients with chronic HBV.[197] These promising advances in the treatment of viral hepatitis await duplication in separately run pediatric trials.

## PREVENTION OF HEPATITIS

### Passive Immunization

The parenteral administration of immune globulin has been given to prevent occurrence of viral hepatitis in well-documented instances of exposure to infected individuals. Both serum immune globulin and disease-specific immune globulin (e.g., hepatitis B immunglobulin) have been given depending on the circumstance.

**HEPATITIS A.** Serum immune globulin can be given before exposure (e.g., travelers to endemic areas) or after exposure to an index case. The most frequent example in the latter situation occurs in the daycare setting or in household contacts. The recommended dose is 0.02 mL/kg body weight given as soon as possible but no more than 2 weeks after exposure. Exact dosing and administration regimens are provided elsewhere.[176, 198, 199]

**HEPATITIS B.** Hepatitis B serum immune globulin (HBIG) is prepared from pooled plasma from donors seropositive for anti-HBS. It has a high titer of anti-HBS (>1:100,000). Its protective value is excellent when given as soon as possible after exposure and persists for 3 to 6 months. Its effect is doubtful, however, when given more than 7 days after exposure. It is indicated for single instances of exposure, such as needle stick accidents, sexual contact, and perinatal exposure. It should be paired with HBV vaccine in cases of repeated or prolonged exposure, such as in health care employees, intimate household contacts, and neonates of infected mothers. A detailed discussion of HBV immunoprophylaxis is given in the American Academy of Pediatrics *Red Book*.[200]

**OTHER VIRUSES.** Exposure to hepatitis D should be treated the same as exposure to hepatitis B with HBIG.[198] CMV immune globulin derived from pooled plasma from adults selected for high CMV antibody titers is commercially available and can be used as prophylaxis in immunocompromised patients exposed to CMV. Reliable methods for passive immunization against the other hepatitis viruses have not been developed.

### Active Immunization

Active immunization involves inoculation with inactivated viral particles or live attenuated virus. The expected result is a persistent immune-mediated protective response against the targeted pathogen. Vaccines against HAV and HBV are now commercially available. Efforts to develop a vaccine against HCV have been hindered by its genetic heterogeneity and difficulties in the identification of neutralizing antibodies. Protection against HDV can be afforded by active immunization against HBV.

**HEPATITIS A VACCINE.** In 1995, the United States became the 41st country to license a vaccine against HAV. Two preparations are currently available, both prepared from formalin-inactivated virus grown in culture.[201] Dosages are prescribed in proprietary unit measurements with both pediatric and adult formulations available. Recommended schedules include two injections 6 to 12 months apart, with 99% of children developing protective levels of antibody.[199, 201, 202] The vaccine is safe, with no serious complications having been reported. The most frequent side effects reported in children are pain and tenderness at the injection site.[199, 202]

Routine immunization has been recommended for children living in communities with high hepatitis A rates and periodic outbreaks.[199, 202] Persons traveling to regions of endemic disease and those who belong to groups at high risk of acquiring HAV (see epidemiology of HAV) should also be immunized. Vaccines should replace serum immune globulin for use in pre-exposure cases and may be active in interrupting epidemics.[199] It may be reasonable in such situations to pair both active and passive immunization.

**HEPATITIS B VACCINE.** The first vaccine against hepatitis B was prepared from human plasma of chronic HBV carriers and released in the United States in 1982. It has since been replaced by recombinant vaccines prepared by introducing an HBsAg gene containing plasmid into baker's yeast *(Saccharomyces cerevisiae).* Recommended schedules involve three intradeltoid injections over a 6-month period.[199] Combination vaccines for children that will include the HBV vaccine are under development. The vaccine is considered very safe; rare complications include anaphylaxis and Guillain-Barré syndrome.[199] The vaccine induces the production of anti-HBs, and the vaccine manufacturers report protective titers in 95% to 99% of healthy children who receive the full schedule of injections.

Initial immunization policies in the United States targeted individuals at high risk such as newborns of seropositive mothers, illicit drug abusers, and homosexual males. However, it became apparent that this strategy was ineffective in reducing the incidence of hepatitis B and in 1991 the Centers for Disease Control and Prevention issued new recommendations.[203] This new three-part strategy recommended prevention of mother to infant transmission through prenatal testing of all pregnant women, universal vaccination of all infants and children by age 11, and immunization of adolescents and adults in high-risk groups such as teenagers with multiple sexual partners and homosexual males. These recommendations have only been partially implemented, and initial results are not yet known.

The long-term effectiveness of HBV vaccine, even in those who have lost detectable anti-HBs, does not support the administration of late booster doses; however, when exposure is clearly documented and titers are low, it is reasonable to administer HBIG and a booster dose of HBV vaccine.[202]

## REFERENCES


1. Feinstone S, Kapikian A, Purcell R: Hepatitis A: detection by immune electron microscopy of a virus-like antigen associated with acute illness. Science 1973;182:1026–1028.
2. Lemon SM: Type A viral hepatitis: new developments in an old disease. N Engl J Med 1985;313:1059–1067.
3. Siegl G, Weitz M: Pathogenesis of hepatitis A: persistent viral infection as basis of an acute disease? Microb Pathog 1993;14:1–8.
4. Centers for Disease Control and Prevention: Hepatitis Surveillance (report no. 56). Atlanta, GA, Centers for Disease Control and Prevention, 1996.
5. Hepatitis A associated with the consumption of frozen strawberries—Michigan 1997. MMWR 1997;46:288–289.
6. Hollinger FB, Khan NC, Oefinger PC, et al: Posttransfusion hepatitis type A. JAMA 1983;250:2313–2317.
7. Rosenblum LS, Villarino M, Nainan OV, et al: Hepatitis A outbreak in a neonatal intensive care unit: risk factors for transmission and evidence of prolonged viral excretion among preterm infants. J Infect Dis 1991;164:476–482.
8. Szmuness W, Dienstag JL, Purcell RH, et al: Distribution of antibody to hepatitis A antigen in adult urban populations. N Engl J Med 1976;295:755–759.
9. Szmuness W, Dienstag JL, Purcell RH, et al: The prevalence of antibody to hepatitis A antigen in various parts of the world. Am J Epidemiol 1977;106:392–398.
10. Benenson MW, Takafuji ET, Bancroft WH, et al: A military community outbreak of hepatitis type A related to transmission in a child care facility. Am J Epidemiol 1980;112:471–481.
11. Hadler SC, McFarland L: Hepatitis in day care centers. Rev Infect Dis 1986;8:548–557.
12. Havens WP: Infectious hepatitis. Medicine 1948;27:279–326.
13. Philip JR, Hamilton TP, Albert TJ: Infectious hepatitis outbreak with mai tai as the vehicle of transmission. Am J Epidemiol 1973;97:50–54.
14. Lednar WM, Lemon SM, Kirkpatrick JW, et al: Frequency of illness associated with epidemic hepatitis A virus infection in adults. Am J Epidemiol 1985;122:226–233.
15. Krugman S, Ward R, Giles J, et al: Infectious hepatitis: studies on the effect of gamma globulin on the incidence of inapparent infection. JAMA 1960;174:823–830.
16. Gordon SC, Reddy KR, Schiff L, et al: Prolonged intrahepatic cholestasis secondary to acute hepatitis A. Ann Intern Med 1984;101:635–637.
17. Glikson M, Galun E, Oren R, et al: Relapsing hepatitis A: review of 14 cases and literature survey. Medicine 1992;71:14–23.
18. Tong MJ, El Farra NS, Grew MI: Clinical manifestations of hepatitis A: recent experience in a community teaching hospital. J Infect Dis 1995;171(suppl) S15–S18.
19. Bromberg K, Newhall DN, Peter G: Hepatitis A and meningoencephalitis. JAMA 1982;247:815.
20. Brenningstal GN, Belani KK: Acute transverse myelitis and brainstem encephalitis associated with hepatitis A infection. Pediatr Neurol 1995;12:169–171.
21. Routenberg JA, Dienstag JL, Harrison WO, et al: Foodborne outbreak of hepatitis A: Clinical and laboratory features of acute and protracted illness. Am J Med Sci 1979;278:123–131.
22. Inman RD, Hodge M, Johnston ME, et al: Arthritis, vasculitis and cryoglobulinemia associated with relapsing hepatitis A infection. Ann Intern Med 1986;105:700–703.
23. Vento S, Garofano T, Di Perri G, et al: Identification of hepatitis A virus as a trigger for autoimmune chronic hepatitis type 1 in susceptible individuals. Lancet 1991;337:1183–1187.
24. Shrier LA, Karpen SJ, McEvoy C: Acute pancreatitis associated with acute hepatitis A in a young child. J Pediatr 1995;126:57–59.
25. Rahaman SM, Chira P, Koff RS: Idiopathic autoimmune hepatitis triggered by hepatitis A. Am J Gastroenterol 1994;89:106–108.
26. Masada CT, Shaw BW, Zetterman RK, et al: Fulminant hepatic failure with massive necrosis as a result of hepatitis A infection. J Clin Gastroenterol 1993;17:158–162.
27. Hoofnagle JH, Di Bisceglie AM: Serologic diagnosis of acute and chronic viral hepatitis. Semin Liver Dis 1991;11:73–83.
28. Blumberg BS, Alter H, Visnich S: A "new" antigen in leukemia sera. JAMA 1965;191:541–545.
29. Dane DS, Cameron CC, Briggs M: Virus-like particles in serum of patients with Australia-antigen associated hepatitis. Lancet 1970;2:695–698.
30. Miller RH: Comparative molecular biology of the hepatitis viruses. Semin Liver Dis 1991;11:113–120.
31. Summers J, Mason WS: Replication of the genome of a hepatitis B–like virus by reverse transcription of an RNA intermediate. Cell 1982;29:403–415.
32. Liang TJ, Hasegawa K Rimon N, et al: A hepatitis B mutant associated with an epidemic of fulminant hepatitis. N Engl J Med 1991;324:1705–1709.
33. Santantonio T, Jung MC, Monno L, et al: Long-term response to interferon therapy in chronic hepatitis B: importance of hepatitis B heterogeneity. Arch Virol 1993;8(suppl):171–178.
34. Carman WF, Zanetti AR, Karayiannis P, et al: Vaccine induced escape mutant of hepatitis B virus. Lancet 1990;336:325–329.
35. Naoumov NV, Schneider R, Grotzinger T, et al: Pre-core mutant hepatitis B virus infection and liver disease. Gastroenterology 1992;102:538–543.
36. Yamamoto K, Horikita M, Tsuda F, et al: Naturally occurring escape mutants of hepatitis B virus with various mutations in the S gene in carriers seropositive for antibody to hepatitis B surface antigen. J Virol 1994;68:2671–2676.
37. Raimondo G, Tanzi E, Brancatelli S, et al: Is the course of perinatal hepatitis B infection influenced by genetic heterogeneity of the virus? J Med Virol 1993;40:87–90.
38. Terazawa S Kojima M, Yamanaka T, et al: Hepatitis B virus mutants with pre-core region defects in two babies with fulminant hepatitis B virus and their mothers positive for antibody to hepatitis B e antigen. Pediatr Res 1991;29:5–9.
39. Honigwachs, J, Faktor O, Dikstein R, et al: Liver specific expression of hepatitis B virus is determined by the combined action of the core gene promoter and the enhancer. J Virol 1989;63:919–924.
40. Mason A, Wick M, White H, et al: Hepatitis B viral replication in diverse cell types during chronic hepatitis B infection. Hepatology 1993;18:781–789.
41. Pignatelli M, Waters J, Lever AML, et al: Cytotoxic T-cell responses to the nucleocapsid proteins of HBV in chronic hepatitis. J Hepatol 1987;4:15–21.

42. Milich DR, Jones JE, Hughes JL, et al: Is a function of the secreted HBe antigen to induce immunologic tolerance in utero? Proc Natl Acad Sci 1990;87:6599–6603.
43. Hsu HY, Chang MH, Hsieh KH, et al: Cellular immune response to HBcAg in mother-to-infant transmission of hepatitis B virus. Hepatology 1992;15:770–776.
44. Margolis HS, Alter MJ, Hadler SC: Hepatitis B: Evolving epidemiology and implications for control. Semin Liver Dis 1991;11:84–92.
45. Maynard JE: Hepatitis B: Global importance and need for control. Vaccine 1990;8(suppl):18–20.
46. McMahon BJ, Wallace LM, Alward DB, et al: Acute hepatitis B infection: relation of age to the clinical expression of disease and subsequent development of the carrier state. J Infect Dis 1985;151:599–603.
47. Tong MJ, Thursby M, Rakela J, et al: Studies of the maternal-infant transmission of the viruses which cause acute hepatitis. Gastroenterology 1981;80:999–1003.
48. Stevens CE, Beasley RP, Tsui J, et al: Vertical transmission of hepatitis B antigen in Taiwan. N Engl J Med 1975;292:771–774.
49. Alter HJ, Purcell JH, Gerin JL: Transmission of hepatitis B to chimpanzees by hepatitis B surface antigen-positive saliva and semen. Infect Immun 1977;16:928–933.
50. Center for Disease Control: Hepatitis transmitted from a human bite. MMWR Morbid Mortal Weekly Rep 1974;23:24.
51. Neefe JR, Stokes J, Rheinhold JG: Oral administration to volunteers of feces from patients with homologous serum hepatitis and infectious (epidemic) hepatitis. Am J Med Sci 1945;210:29–32.
52. Dupruy JM, Giraud P, Dupruy C, et al: Hepatitis B in children: II. Study of children born to chronic HBsAg carrier mothers. J Pediatr 1978;92:200–204.
53. Xu ZY, Liu CB, Francis DP, et al: Prevention of perinatal acquisition of hepatitis B virus carriage using vaccine: preliminary report of a randomized, double-blinded placebo-controlled and comparative trial. Pediatrics 1985;76:713–718.
54. Stevens CE, Neurath RA, Beasley RP, et al: HBeAg and anti-HBs detection by radioimmunoassay: correlation with vertical transmission of hepatitis B virus in Taiwan. J Med Virol 1979;3:237–241.
55. Heijtink RA, Boender PJ, Schalm SW, et al: Hepatitis B virus DNA in serum of pregnant women with HBsAg and HBeAg or antibodies to HBe. J Infect Dis 1984;150:462–470.
56. Sinatra FR, Shah P, Weissman JY, et al: Perinatal transmitted acute icteric hepatitis B in infants born to hepatitis surface antigen-positive and anti-hepatitis B e-positive mothers. Pediatrics 1982;70:557–560.
57. Beath SV, Boxall EH, Watson RM, et al: Fulminant hepatitis in infants born to anti-HBe hepatitis B carrier mothers. BMJ 1992;304:1169–1170.
58. Shimuzu H, Mitsuda T, Fujita S, et al: Perinatal hepatitis B infection caused by anti–hepatitis B e-positive maternal mononuclear cells. Arch Dis Child 1991;66:718–721.
59. Ohto H, Lin HH, Kawana T, et al: Intrauterine transmission of hepatitis B virus is closely related to placental leakage. J Med Virol 1987;21:1–6.
60. Beasley RP, Hwang LY: Postnatal infectivity of hepatitis B surface antigen-carrier mothers. J Infect Dis 1983;147:185–190.
61. Hurie MB, Mast EE, Davis JP: Horizontal transmission of hepatitis B virus infection to United States–born children of Hmong refugees. Pediatr 1992;89:269–273.
62. Franks AL, Berg CJ, Kane MA, et al: Hepatitis B infection among children born in the United States to Southeast Asian refugees. N Engl J Med 1989;321:1301–1305.
63. Shapiro CN, McCaig LF, Gensheimer KF, et al: Hepatitis B virus transmission between children in day care. Pediatr Infect Dis J 1989;8:870–875.
64. Hurwitz ES, Deseda CC, Shapiro CN, et al: Hepatitis infections in the day care setting. Pediatrics 1994;94:1023–1024.
65. Gianotti F: Papular acrodermatitis of childhood: an Australia antigen disease. Arch Dis Child 1973;48:794–799.
66. Draelos ZK, Hansen RC, James WD: Gianotti-Crosti syndrome associated with infections other than hepatitis B. JAMA 1986;256:2386–2388.
67. Lok ASF, Lai C-L: A longitudinal follow-up of asymptomatic hepatitis B surface antigen-positive Chinese children. Hepatology 1988;8:1130–1133.
68. Bortolotti F, Cadrobbi P, Crivellaro C, et al: Long-term outcome of chronic type B hepatitis in patients who acquire hepatitis B virus infection in childhood. Gastroenterology 1990;99:805–810.
69. Ruiz-Moreno M, Camps T, Aguado JG, et al: Serological and histological follow-up of chronic hepatitis B infection. Arch Dis Child 1989;64:1165–1169.
70. Moyes CD, Milne A, Waldon J: Liver function tests of hepatitis B carriers in childhood. Pediatr Infect Dis J 1993;12:120–125.
71. Mengoli M, Balli ME, Tomelli S, et al: Long-term outcome of chronic type B hepatitis in childhood. Arch Virol 1992;4(suppl):263–264.
72. Bortolotti F, Crivellar C, Brunetto MR, et al: Selection of a pre-core mutant of hepatitis B virus and reactivation of chronic hepatitis B acquired in childhood. J Pediatr 1993;123:883–885.
73. Zancan L, Chiaramonta M, Ferrarese N, et al: Pediatric HBsAg chronic liver disease and adult asymptomatic carrier status: two stages of the same entity. J Pediatr Gastroenterol Nutr 1990;11:380–384.
74. Bortolotti F, Calzia R, Cadrobbi P, et al: Liver cirrhosis associated with hepatitis B virus infection. J Pediatr 1986;108:224–227.
75. Weissberg JI, Andres LL, Smith CI, et al: Survival in chronic hepatitis B: an analysis of 379 patients. Ann Intern Med 1984;101:613–616.
76. Parkin DM, Laara E, Muir CS: Estimates of the worldwide frequency of sixteen major cancers in 1989. Int J Cancer 1988;41:184–197.
77. Chang M-H, Chen P-J, Chen J-Y, et al: Hepatitis B virus integration in hepatitis B virus-related hepatocellular carcinoma in childhood. Hepatology 1991;13:316–320.
78. Cheah P-L, Looi L-M, Lin H-P, et al: Childhood primary hepatocellular carcinoma and hepatitis B viral infection. Cancer 1990;65:174–176.
79. Giacchino R, Navone C, Giambortolomei G, et al: HBV-DNA related hepatocellular carcinoma occurring in childhood: Report of three cases. Dig Dis Sci 1991;8:1143–1146.
80. Beasley RP, Lin C-C, Hwang L-Y, et al: Hepatocellular carcinoma and hepatitis B virus: a prospective study of 22,707 men in Taiwan. Lancet 1981;2:1129–1132.
81. Larouze B, London WT, Saimot G, et al: Host responses to hepatitis B infection in patients with primary hepatic carcinoma and their families: a case-control study in Senegal, West Africa. Lancet 1976;2:534–538.
82. Steiner PE: Cancer of the liver and cirrhosis in trans-Saharan Africa and the United States of America. Cancer 1960:13:1085–1166.
83. Chung T, Tong MJ, Hwang B, et al: Primary hepatocellular carcinoma and hepatitis B infection during childhood. Hepatology 1987;7:46–48.
84. Willson RA: Extrahepatic manifestations of chronic viral hepatitis. Am J Gastroenterol 1997;92:4–17.
85. Hogg RJ: Hepatitis B surface antigenemia in North American children with membranous glomerulonephropathy. J Pediatr 1985;106:571–578.
86. Gower RG, Sausker WF, Kohler PF, et al: Small vessel vasculitis caused by hepatitis B virus immune complexes. J Allergy Clin Immunol 1978;62:222–228.
87. Levo Y, Gorevic PD, Kassab HJ, et al: Association between hepatitis B virus and essential mixed cryoglobulinemia. N Engl J Med 1977;296:1501–1504.
88. Hoofnagle JH, Seef LB, Bales ZB, et al: Serologic responses in hepatitis B. In Vyas GN, Cohen SN, Schmidt R (eds): Viral Hepatitis: A Contemporary Assessment of Etiology, Epidemiology, Pathogenesis and Prevention. Philadelphia: Franklin Institute Press, 1978, p 278.
89. Gocke DJ: Extrahepatic manifestations of viral hepatitis. Am J Med Sci 1975;270:49–52.
90. Willson RA: Extrahepatic manifestations of chronic viral hepatitis. Am J Gastroenterol 1997;92:4–17.
91. Prince AM, Brotman B, Grady GF, et al: Long-incubation post-transfusion hepatitis without serological evidence of exposure to hepatitis B serum. Lancet 1974;2:241–246.
92. Feinstone SM, Kapikian AZ, Purcell RH, et al: Transfusion-associated hepatitis not due to viral hepatitis type A or B. N Engl J Med 1975;292:767–770.
93. Choo Q-L, Kuo G, Weiner AJ, et al: Isolation of a cDNA clone derived from a blood-borne non-A, non-B viral hepatitis genome. Science 1989;244:359–362.
94. Kuo G, Choo Q-L, Alter HJ, et al: An assay for circulating antibodies to a major etiologic virus of human non-A, non-B hepatitis. Science 1989;244:362–364.
95. Alter HJ, Purcell RH, Shih JW, et al: Detection of antibody to hepatitis C virus in prospectively followed transfusion recipients with acute and chronic non-A, non-B hepatitis. N Engl J Med 1989;321:1494–1500.
96. Kaito M, Watanabe S, Tsukiyama-Kohara K, et al: Hepatitis C virus particles detected by immunoelectron microscopic study. J Gen Virol 1994;75:1755–1760.

97. Brechot C: Hepatitis C virus: molecular biology and genetic variability. Dig Dis Sci 1996;41(suppl):6–21.
98. Simmonds P: Variability of hepatitis C virus. Hepatology 1995;21:570–583.
99. Cooreman MP, Scoondermark-Van de Ven EM: Hepatitis C: Biological and clinical consequences of genetic heterogeneity. Scand J Gastroenterol 1996;31(suppl 218):106–115.
100. Mosnier JF, Degott C, Marcellin P, et al: The intraportal lymphoid follicle and its environment in chronic active hepatitis C: an immunohistochemical study. Hepatology 1993;17:366–371.
101. Pawlotsky JM, Yakia MB, Andre C, et al: Immunological disorders in C virus chronic active hepatitis: a prospective case-control study. Hepatology 1994;19:841–848.
102. Martin P, Di Bisceglie AM, Kassianides C, et al: Rapidly progressive non-A non-B hepatitis in patients with human immunodeficiency virus infection. Gastroenterology 1989;97:1559–1561.
103. Alter HJ: Descartes before the horse: I clone therefore I am: The hepatitis C virus in current perspective. Ann Intern Med 1991;115:644–649.
104. Di Bisceglie AM, Hoofnagle JH: Chronic viral hepatitis. In Zakim D, Boyer TD (eds): Hepatology: A Textbook of Liver Disease, 3rd ed. Philadelphia: WB Saunders, 1996, pp 1299–1329.
105. Aach RD, Stevens CE, Hollinger FB: Hepatitis C virus infection in post-transfusion hepatitis. N Engl J Med 1991;325:1325–1329.
106. Alter MJ, Hadler SC, Judson FN, et al: Risk factors for acute non-A, non-B hepatitis in the United States and association with hepatitis C infection. JAMA 1990;264:2231–2235.
107. Bortolotti F, Vajro P, Barbera C, et al: Hepatitis C in childhood: epidemiological and clinical aspects. Bone Marrow Transpl 1993;12(suppl 1):21–23.
108. Donahue JG, Munoz A, Ness PM, et al: The declining risk of post-transfusion hepatitis C virus infection. N Engl J Med 1992;327:369–373.
109. Katkov WN, Friedman LS, Cody H, et al: Elevated serum alanine aminotransferase levels in blood donors: the contribution of hepatitis C virus. Ann Intern Med 1991;115:882–884.
110. Bortolotti F, Jara P, Diaz C, et al: Posttransfusion and community-acquired hepatitis C in childhood. J Pediatr Gastroenterol Nutr 1994;18:279–283.
111. Romero R, Lavine JE: Viral hepatitis in children. Semin Liver Dis 1994;14:289–302.
112. Pereira BJ, Milford EL, Kirkman RL, et al: Transmission of hepatitis C virus by organ transplantation. N Engl J Med 1991;325:454–460.
113. Nowicki MJ, Balistreri WF: The hepatitis C virus: identification, epidemiology and clinical controversies. J Pediatr Gastroenterol Nutr 1995;20:248–274.
114. Ko YC, Ho MS, Chiang TA, et al: Tattooing as a risk of hepatitis C infection. J Med Virol 1992;38:288–291.
115. Hsu HH, Wright TL, Luba D, et al: Failure to detect hepatitis C virus genome in human secretions with the polymerase chain reaction. Hepatology 1991;14:763–767.
116. Fried MW, Shindo M, Fong T-L, et al: Absence of hepatitis C viral RNA from saliva and semen of patients with chronic hepatitis C. Gastroenterology 1992;102:1306–1308.
117. Weintrub PS, Veereman-Wauters G, Cowan MJ, et al: Hepatitis C virus infection in infants whose mothers took street drugs intravenously. J Pediatr 1991;119:869–874.
118. Jackson LA, Stewart LK, Solomon SL, et al: Risk of infection with hepatitis A, B, C, cytomegalovirus, varicella or measles in child care providers. Pediatr Infect Dis J 1996;15:584–589.
119. Alter MJ: Hepatitis C: a sleeping giant? Am J Med 1991; 91(suppl):112–115.
120. Alter HJ, Purcell RH, Holland PV, et al: Clinical and serologic analysis of transfusion associated hepatitis. Lancet 1975;2:838–841.
121. Seef LB: Diagnosis, therapy and prognosis of viral hepatitis. In Zakim D, Boyer TD (eds): Hepatology: A Textbook of Liver Disease, 3rd ed. Philadelphia: WB Saunders, 1996, pp 1067–1145.
122. Prince AM, Brotman B, Huima T, et al: Immunity in hepatitis C infection. J Infect Dis 1992;165:438–443.
123. Farci P, Alter HJ, Govindarajan S, et al: Lack of protective immunity against reinfection with hepatitis C virus. Science 1992;258:135s–139s.
124. Feray C, Gigou M, Samuel D, et al: Hepatitis C virus RNA and hepatitis B virus DNA in serum and liver of patients with fulminant hepatitis. Gastroenterology 1993;104:549–555.
125. Seef LB, Buskell-Bales Z, Wright EC, et al: Long-term mortality after transfusion-associated non-A, non-B hepatitis. N Engl J Med 1992;327:1906–1911.
126. Bortolotti F, Vajro P, Cadrobbi P, et al: Cryptogenic chronic liver disease and hepatitis C virus infection in children. J Hepatology 1992;15:73–76.
127. Kiyosawa K, Sodeyama S, Tanaka E, et al: Interrelationship of blood transfusion, non-A, non-B hepatitis and hepatocellular carcinoma: analysis by detection of antibody to hepatitis C virus. Hepatology 1990;12:671–675.
128. Colombo M, Choo QL, Del Ninno E: Prevalence of antibodies to hepatitis C virus in Italian patients with hepatocellular carcinoma. Lancet 1989;2:1006–1009.
129. Lunel F, Musset L, Cacoub P, et al: Cryoglobulinemia in chronic liver disease: role of hepatitis C virus and liver damage. Gastroenterology 1994;106:1291–1300.
130. Lunel F, Abuaf N, Frangeul L, et al: Liver/kidney microsome antibody type 1 and hepatitis C infection. Hepatology 1992;16:630–636.
131. Mieli-Vergani G, Vergani D: Progress in pediatric autoimmune hepatitis. Semin Liver Dis 1994;14:282–288.
132. Mackie FD, Peakman M, Yun M, et al: Primary and secondary liver/kidney microsomal autoantibody response following infection with hepatitis C virus. Gastroenterology 1994;106:1672–1675.
133. Fried MW, Draguesku JO, Shindo M, et al: Clinical and serological differentiation of autoimmune and hepatitis C virus-related chronic hepatitis. Dig Dis Sci 1993;38:631–636.
134. Alter HJ: New kit on the block: evaluation of second generation assays for detection of antibody to hepatitis C virus. Hepatology 1992;15:350–352.
135. Garson J, Tedder R, Briggs M, et al: Detection of hepatitis C viral sequences in blood donations by "nested" polymerase chain reaction and prediction of infectivity. Lancet 1990;335:1419–1422.
136. Alvarez F, Martres P, Maggiore G, et al: False-positive result of hepatitis C enzyme-linked immunosorbent assay in children with autoimmune hepatitis. J Pediatr 1991;119:75–77.
137. Rizzetto M, Canese MG, Arico S, et al: Immunofluorescence detection of a new antigen-antibody system (δ/anti-δ) associated with hepatitis B virus in liver and serum of HBsAg carriers. Gut 1977;18:997–1003.
138. Hoofnagle JH: Type D (delta) hepatitis. JAMA 1989;261:1321–1325.
139. Cole SM, Gowans EJ, MacNaughton TB, et al: Direct evidence for cytotoxicity associated with expression of hepatitis delta antigen. Hepatology 1991;13:845–851.
140. Gowans EJ, Bonnino F: Hepatitis delta pathogenicity. Prog Clin Biol Res 1993;382:243–250.
141. Hadler SC, Alcala de Monzon M, Bensabath B, et al: Epidemiology of hepatitis delta virus in less developed countries. Prog Clin Biol Res 1991;364:21–31.
142. Rizetto M, Purcell RH, Gerin JL: Epidemiology of HBV associated delta agent: geographical distribution of anti-delta and prevalence in polytransfused HBsAg positive carriers. Lancet 1980;1:1215–1218.
143. Lettau LA, McCarthy JG, Smith MH, et al: Outbreak of severe hepatitis due to delta and hepatitis B viruses in parenteral drug abusers and their contacts. N Engl J Med 1987;317:1256–1262.
144. Caredda F, Antinori S, Re T, et al: Course and prognosis of acute HDV hepatitis. Prog Clin Biol Res 1987;234:267–276.
145. Farci P, Barbera C, Navone C, et al: Infection with the delta agent in children. Gut 1985;26:4–7.
146. Bortolotti F, Di Marco V, Vajro P, et al: Long-term evolution of chronic delta hepatitis in children. J Pediatr 1993;122:736–738.
147. Tandon BN, Joshi YK, Jain SK, et al: An epidemic of non-A/non-B hepatitis in North India. Indian J Med Res 1982;75:739–744.
148. Balayan MS, Andjaparidze AG, Savinskaya SS, et al: Evidence for a virus in non-A/non-B hepatitis transmitted via the fecal-oral route. Intervirology 1983;20:23–28.
149. Reyes GR, Purdy MA, Kim JP, et al: Isolation of cDNA from the virus responsible for enterically transmitted non-A, non-B hepatitis. Science 1990;247:1335–1339.
150. Krawczynski K: Hepatitis E. Hepatology 1993;17:932–941.
151. Robinson WS: Biology of human hepatitis viruses. In Zakim D, Boyer TD (eds): Hepatology: A Textbook of Liver Disease, 3rd ed. Philadelphia: WB Saunders, 1996, pp 1146–1206.
152. Hyams KC, Purdy MA, Kaur A: Acute sporadic hepatitis E in Sudanese children: analysis based on a new Western blot assay. J Infect Dis 1992;165:1001–1005.
153. Miyakawa Y, Mayumi M: Hepatitis G virus: a true hepatitis or an accidental tourist? N Engl J Med 1997;336:795–796.

154. Bralet MP, Roudot-Thorval F, Pawlotsky JM, et al: Histopathologic impact of GB virus C infection on chronic hepatitis C. Gastroenterology 1997;112:188–192.
155. Alter HJ, Nakatsuji Y, Melpolder J, et al: The incidence of transfusion-associated hepatitis G virus infection and its relation to liver disease. N Engl J Med 1997;336:747–754.
156. Alter MJ, Gallagher M, Morris TT, et al: Acute non-A-E hepatitis in the United States and the role of hepatitis G infection. N Engl J Med 1997;336:741–746.
157. Rochling FA, Jones WF, Chau K, et al: Acute sporadic non-A, non-B, non-C, non-D, non-E hepatitis. Hepatology 1997;25:478–483.
158. Sumaya CV, Ench Y: Epstein-Barr virus infectious mononucleosis in children: I. Clinical and general laboratory findings. Pediatrics 1985;75:1003–1010.
159. Griffiths PD, Ellis DS, Zuckerman AJ: Other common types of viral hepatitis and exotic infections. BMJ 1990;46:512–532.
160. Bopanna SP, Pass RF, Stagno S, et al: Symptomatic congenital cytomegalovirus infection: neonatal mortality and morbidity. Pediatr Infect Dis J 1992;11:93–99.
161. Wiesner RH, Marin E, Porayko MK, et al: Advances in the diagnosis, treatment and prevention of cytomegalovirus infections after liver transplantation. Gastroenterol Clin North Am 1993;22:351–366.
162. Scott GB, Buck BE, Leterman JG: Acquired immunodeficiency syndrome in infants. N Engl J Med 1984;310:76–81.
163. Shannon KM, Amman AJ: Acquired immune deficiency syndrome in childhood. J Pediatr 1985;106:332–342.
164. Czaja AJ: Autoimmune hepatitis and viral infection. Gastroenterol Clin North Am 1994;23:547–566.
165. Krawitt EL: Autoimmune hepatitis. N Engl J Med 1996;334:897–903.
166. Scully LJ, Toze C, Sengar DP, et al: Early-onset autoimmune hepatitis is associated with a C4A gene deletion. Gastroenterology 1993;104:1478–1484.
167. Robertson DA, Zhang SL, Guy EC, et al: Persistent measles virus genome in autoimmune chronic active hepatitis. Lancet 1987;2:9–11.
168. Vento S, Guella L, Mirandola F, et al: Epstein-Barr virus as trigger for autoimmune hepatitis in susceptible individuals. Lancet 1995;346:608–609.
169. Bellary S, Sciano T, Hartman G, et al: Chronic hepatitis with combined features of autoimmune hepatitis and chronic hepatitis C. Ann Intern Med 1995;123:32–34.
170. Garcia-Buey L, Garcia-Monzon C, Rodriguez S, et al: Latent autoimmune hepatitis triggered during interferon therapy in patients with chronic hepatitis C. Gastroenterology 1995;108:1770–1708.
171. Paradis K, Alvarez F, Seidman E, et al: Pitfalls in the diagnosis of autoimmune hepatitis associated with liver and kidney microsomal proteins. J Pediatr Gastroenterol Nutr 1994;19:453–459.
172. Gregorio GV, Portmann B, Reid F, et al: Autoimmune hepatitis in childhood: a 20-year experience. Hepatology 1997;25:541–547.
173. Vajro P, Hadchouel P, Hadchouel M, et al: Incidence of cirrhosis in children with chronic hepatitis. J Pediatr 1990;117:392–396.
174. Maggiore G, Veber F, Bernard O, et al: Autoimmune hepatitis associated with antiactin antibodies in children and adolescents. J Pediatr Gastroenterol Nutr 1993;17:376–381.
175. Klein C, Philipp T, Greiner P, et al: Asymptomatic autoimmune hepatitis associated with anti-LC-1 autoantibodies. J Pediatr Gastroenterol Nutr 1996;23:461–465.
176. American Academy of Pediatrics. Hepatitis A. In Peter G (ed): 1994 Red Book: Report of the Committee on Infectious Diseases, 24th ed. Elk Grove Village, IL: American Academy of Pediatric, 1997 pp 237–246.
177. Lin JC, Smith MC, Pagano JS: Prolonged inhibitory effect of 9-(1,3-dihydroxy-2-popoxymethyl)guanine against replication of Epstein-Barr virus. J Virol 1984;50:50–55.
178. Dudley FJ, Scheuer PJ, Sherlock S: Natural history of hepatitis-associated antigen-positive chronic liver disease. Lancet 1972;2:1388–1393.
179. Lam KC, Lai CL, NG RP, et al: Deleterious effect of prednisolone in HBsAg positive chronic active hepatitis. N Engl J Med 1981;304:380–386.
180. Hoofnagle JH, Dusheiko GM, Schafer DF, et al: Reactivation of chronic hepatitis B virus infection by cancer chemotherapy. Ann Intern Med 1982;96:447–449.
181. Pratt DS, Flavin DP, Kaplan MM: The successful treatment of autoimmune hepatitis with 6-mercaptopurine after failure with azathioprine. Gastroenterology 1996;110:271.
182. Jackson LD, Song E: Cyclosporin in the treatment of corticosteroid resistant autoimmune chronic active hepatitis. Gut 1995;36:459–461.
183. Treem WR, Hyams JS: Cyclosporine therapy for gastrointestinal disease. J Pediatr Gastroenterol Nutr 1994;18:270–278.
184. Van Thiel DH, Wright H, Carroll P, et al: Tacrolimus: a potential new treatment for autoimmune chronic active hepatitis: results of an open-label preliminary trial. Am J Gastroenterol 1995;90:771–776.
185. Renault PF, Hoofnagle JH: Side effects of alpha interferon. Semin Liver Dis 1989;9:273–277.
186. Barbera C, Bortolotti F, Crivellaro C, et al: Recombinant interferon-α2a hastens the rate of HBeAg clearance in children with chronic hepatitis B. Hepatology 1994;20:287–290.
187. Jonas MM: Interferon-α for viral hepatitis. J Pediatr Gastroenterol Nutr 1996;23:93–106.
188. Perillo RP: Interferon in the management of chronic hepatitis B. Dig Dis Sci 1993;38:577–593.
189. Brook MG, Karayiannis P, Thomas HC: Which patients with chronic hepatitis B infection will respond to alpha-interferon? Hepatology 1989;10:761–763.
190. Wong DKH, Cheung AM, O'Rourke K, et al: Effect of alpha-interferon treatment in patients with hepatitis B e antigen-positive chronic hepatitis B. Ann Intern Med 1993;119:312–323.
191. Management of hepatitis C. NIH Consens Statement 1997 March 24–26;15(3):1–41.
192. Conjeevaram HS, Everhart JE, Hoofnagle JH: Predictors of a sustained beneficial response to interferon alpha therapy in chronic hepatitis C. Hepatology 1995;22:1326–1329.
193. Reichard O, Foberg U, Fryden A, et al: High sustained response rate and clearance of viremia in chronic hepatitis C after treatment with interferon-α2b for 60 weeks. Hepatology 1994;19:280–285.
194. Ruiz-Moreno M, Rua MJ, Castillo I, et al: Treatment of children with chronic hepatitis C with recombinant interferon-α: a pilot study. Hepatology 1992;16:882–885.
195. Iorio R, Pensati P, Porzio S, et al: Lymphoblastoid interferon alfa treatment in chronic hepatitis C. Arch Dis Child 1996;74:152–156.
196. Poynard T, Marcellin P, Niederau C, et al: Randomised trial of interferon α2b ribavirin for 48 weeks or for 24 weeks versus interferon α2b plus placebo for 48 weeks for treatment of chronic infection with hepatitis C virus. Lancet 1998;352:1426–1432.
197. Lai C-L, Chien R-N, Leung N, et al: A one-year trial of lamivudine for chronic hepatitis B. N Engl J Med 1998;339:61–68.
198. Immunization Practices Committee: Protection against viral hepatitis. MMWR Morbid Mortal Weekly Rep 1990;39:1–27.
199. Advisory Committee on Immunization Practices: Prevention of hepatitis A through active or passive immunization. MMWR Morbid Mortal Weekly Rep 1996;45:1–30.
200. American Academy of Pediatrics. Hepatitis B. In Peter G (ed): 1994 Red Book: Report of the Committee on Infectious Diseases, 24th ed. Elk Grove Village, IL: American Academy of Pediatrics, 1997 pp 247–260.
201. Bader TF: Hepatitis A vaccine. Am J Gastroenterol 1996;91:217–222.
202. Lemon SM, Thomas DL: Vaccines to prevent viral hepatitis. N Engl J Med 1997;336:196–204.
203. Immunization Practices Advisory Committee: The hepatitis B virus: a comprehensive strategy for eliminating transmission in the United States through universal childhood vaccination. MMWR Morbid Mortal Weekly Rep 1991;40:1–19.

# Chapter 51

# Portal Hypertension

*Benjamin L. Shneider*

The last 30 years have witnessed a tremendous increase in our knowledge of both the pathophysiology and treatment of portal hypertension. This is reflected in both the steady increase in publications related to portal hypertension and the increasing complex therapeutic options available to the practitioner. The interesting evolution to the modern age of the study of portal hypertension can be reviewed in Graham and Smith's description of the natural history of variceal hemorrhage.[1] Advances in the science of portal hypertension have occurred as the result of animal models and clinical studies. The nearly exclusive use of mature animals or adults in these studies potentially limits their applicability to pediatrics.

The purpose of this chapter is to review the principles of the pathophysiology of portal hypertension and apply them to the practice of pediatric hepatology. The complexities of the decisions that face the practitioner are reviewed, with empiric recommendations made based on the pediatric descriptive literature and adult randomized trials. Two of the more common causes of pediatric portal hypertension, extrahepatic biliary atresia (EHBA) and extrahepatic portal vein obstruction (EPVO), are used as examples at the two ends of the spectrum of pediatric portal hypertension, the former representing an example of an ongoing hepatobiliary disease associated with progressive hepatic dysfunction and the latter being an example of portal hypertension without hepatic parenchymal damage.

## PATHOPHYSIOLOGY OF PORTAL HYPERTENSION

It was not until the 1930s that there was agreement that the liver and not the spleen played a central role in the pathophysiology of portal hypertension.[2, 3] It now appears that there are at least two separate pathologic components of portal hypertension: an increase in resistance to blood flow through the liver (backward flow theory) and an increase in the volume of blood that flows through the liver (forward flow theory). The relative contributions of each of these components are not completely clear; they may change with time and may depend on the type of liver disease.

### Backward Flow Theory

Increased resistance to blood flow through the liver is central to the development of most forms of portal hypertension and can be subdivided according to the anatomic location of the increase in resistance (Fig. 51–1). Increased posthepatic resistance is relatively uncommon in pediatrics and is best exemplified by the Budd-Chiari syndrome, in which there is obstruction to hepatic blood flow at the level of the major hepatic veins or the suprahepatic inferior vena cava.[4] Budd-Chiari syndrome may sometimes be associated with hypercoagulable states, tumors, trauma, and abnormalities of the inferior vena cava. However, in most circumstances it is idiopathic, although increased prevalence in selected populations suggests either environmental or genetic influences in its pathogenesis.[5] Prehepatic obstruction, as exemplified by EPVO (Figs. 51–1 and 51–2), represents one of the most common causes of pediatric portal hypertension. Nearly 40% of a cohort of children treated for esophageal varix bleeding had EPVO.[6–10] In most circumstances, the pathophysiology of the formation of EPVO is unknown. Umbilical vein catheterization and sepsis have been associated with some cases of EPVO, although a causal relationship has not been demonstrated.[11, 12] A hypercoagulable state might also predispose to EPVO. Diminished levels of protein C, protein S, and antithrombin III have been measured in children with EPVO, but these findings appear to be secondary phenomena and not the primary cause of the thrombosis.[13] Congenital anatomic abnormalities may be one of the most important factors in the development of EPVO, especially in light of the high incidence of other associated congenital anomalies.[14–16]

In both pre- and posthepatic obstruction, the primary pathogenesis of the increase in resistance to portal blood flow is simply related to anatomic obstruction. This is in contrast to the more complex pathophysiology associated with intrahepatic obstruction. Increased intrahepatic resistance to portal blood flow as a result of intrinsic liver disease is best exemplified in pediatrics by EHBA (Fig. 51–3). Increased resistance to portal blood flow may occur by a number of mechanisms. Portal inflammatory processes most likely lead to some distortion of the portal microvasculature. Because resistance to flow is inversely related to the radius of the vascular lumen raised to the fourth power, small changes in diameter can lead to marked alterations in resistance. Hepatocyte swelling and deposition of collagen within the space of Disse may lead to similar compromise of the portal vascular lumen.[17, 18] Finally, contractile properties of

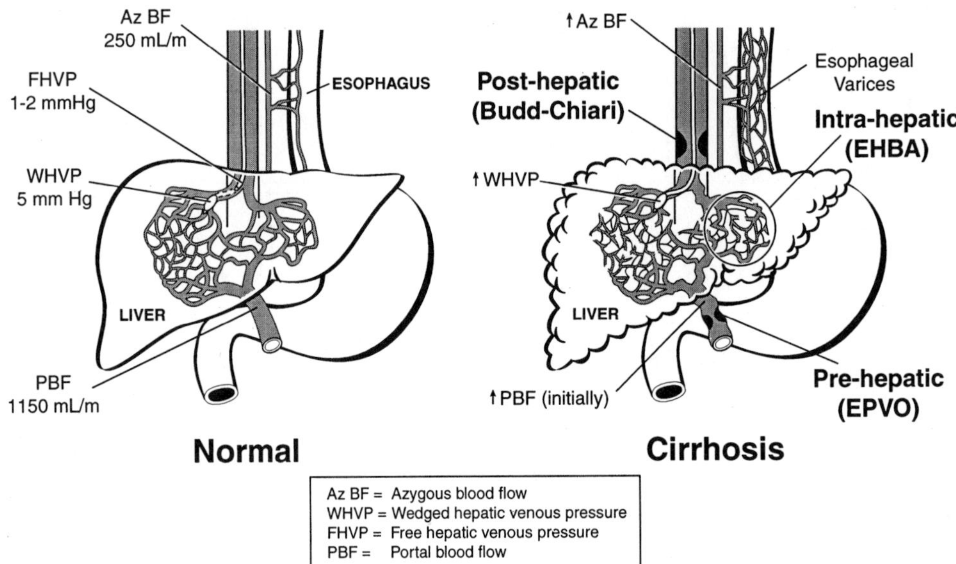


**FIGURE 51–1.** Diagram of the pathophysiology of portal hypertension and the method of measurement of the wedged hepatic venous pressure (WHVP) gradient. Normal adult parameters for hemodynamic measurements of the portal circulation are seen on the left. A balloon-tipped pressure-measuring catheter is seen in the hepatic vein. Changes in parameter measurements in portal hypertension are seen on the right. Obstruction can be post-, intra-, or prehepatic, as commonly seen in Budd-Chiari syndrome, extrahepatic biliary atresia (EHBA), or extrahepatic portal vein obstruction (EPVO), respectively. WHVP is increased in both EHBA and EPVO but not in Budd-Chiari syndrome. (Adapted from Roberts LR, Kamath PS: Pathophysiology and treatment of variceal hemorrhage. Mayo Clin Proc 1996;71:973–983, with permission.)

stellate cells in response to endothelins may lead to vasoconstriction of the hepatic microcirculation.[19]

## Forward Flow Theory

It is clear that changes in portal venous resistance cannot completely explain the development of portal hypertension. Investigations of a portal vein ligation model of portal hypertension have shown that the initial cause of increased portal pressure may be increased resistance to blood flow, but the development of portosystemic collaterals leads to a normalization of resistance without a commensurate reduction in portal pressure.[20] Analysis of hemodynamic parameters in this animal model reveals that an increase in portal venous inflow is the cause of the sustained portal hypertension. The increased portal venous inflow is mediated by both an increase in cardiac index and a reduction in splanchnic vascular resistance. This hyperdynamic circulation has been well described in cirrhotic adults and preliminarily characterized in children.[21] The clinical implications of these circulatory alterations are quite important, because correction of these derangements forms the basis of many of the current therapeutic approaches to the management of portal hypertension.

Parabiotic animal models provide good evidence that this hyperdynamic circulation is mediated by systemic factors.[22] A number of potential mediators have been proposed to induce the systemic vasodilatation seen in portal hypertension, including glucagon, prostaglandins, bile acids, adenosine, nitric oxide, tumor necrosis factor-α, and the calcitonin gene-related peptide.[23–29] It is possible that these factors act in a synergistic fashion.

## Collateral Circulation and the Formation of Esophageal Varices

Increased portal venous pressure, which results from increased portal venous resistance and blood flow, leads to the development of portosystemic collaterals as a means of decompression of the portal system (see Fig. 51–3). These collaterals lead to the development of esophageal and rectal varices. Pressure within the varices is directly related to the quantity of blood flowing through them, whereas their size is determined by both the pressure within the varix and the capacitance of the variceal wall. Once varices enlarge to a point where wall tension exceeds the strength of the varix, rupture occurs. Physiologically this seems to be related to an increase in portal pressure above 12 mm Hg, as measured by hepatic venous pressure gradients (see later).[30]

## Clinical Manifestations

The first manifestation of previously unrecognized portal hypertension is typically splenomegaly. Splenomegaly may be the initial presenting feature of EPVO, but it is usually noted on follow-up of patients with EHBA even after portoenterostomy. Other clinical scenarios that might suggest the presence of portal hypertension include gastrointestinal hemorrhage, ascites, protein-losing enteropathy, encephalopathy, hemorrhoids/anorectal varices, and hepatopulmonary syndrome.

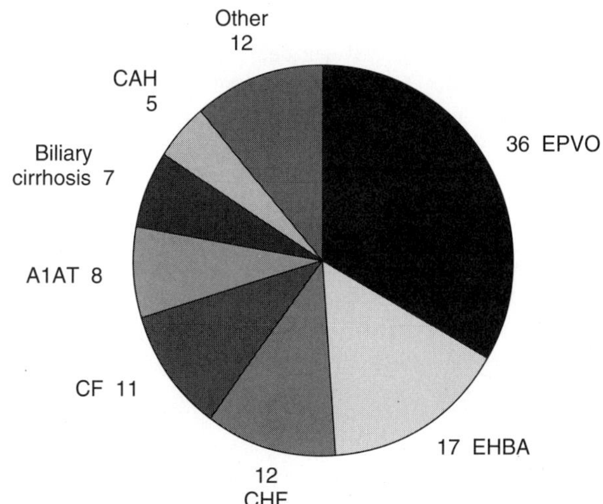


**FIGURE 51–2.** The etiology of portal hypertension leading to variceal hemorrhage in children. The causes of portal hypertension leading to variceal hemorrhage in a cohort of children from King's College Hospital, London, UK, are diagrammed. CF, cystic fibrosis; A1AT, alpha$_1$-antitrypsin deficiency; CAH, chronic active hepatitis; CHF, congenital hepatic fibrosis. (Adapted from Howard ER, Stringer MD, Mowat AP: Assessment of injection sclerotherapy in the management of 152 children with oesophageal varices. Br J Surg 1988;75:404–408, with permission.)

## MANAGEMENT OF PORTAL HYPERTENSION/CLINICAL DECISION-MAKING

### Diagnosis

A number of potential modalities exist to assess the status of esophageal varices, including barium radiography, ultrasonography, and upper endoscopy. Barium studies can detect relatively large varices but are unable to give additional clinically important information that may be obtained from either ultrasonography or upper endoscopy. Important anatomic information, especially with regard to patency of the extrahepatic portal vein, can be obtained by ultrasonography. Portal vein diameter, the ratio of the lesser omental thickness relative to the aorta, and maximal portal velocity all have been used to assess the severity of portal hypertension and the risk of esophageal varices.[31–33] The noninvasive nature of ultrasonography makes it attractive for use in pediatrics, although its value may be limited by sonographer expertise and general reliability of the procedure.[34] At this time, ultrasonography has an important role in defining vascular anatomy and as a screening tool for esophageal varices.[35]

Upper endoscopy is currently the best and most reliable method available for ascertaining whether esophageal varices are present. In addition, this technique provides information that may be indicative of the likelihood of variceal rupture and hemorrhage. Prospective analysis of adult patients has revealed that the variceal size, gastric varices, and congestive gastropathy all are independent predictors of bleeding.[36] The finding of red wale markings, cherry-red spots, and large blue varices may also indicate a higher risk of bleeding.[37] The importance of some of these features has been validated in children with EPVO.[11] Small or nonexistent varices may be found in some patients with suspected portal hypertension. Follow-up endoscopic studies may be advisable in these patients. The timing of that follow-up must be individualized for both the patient and underlying disease. A recent consensus workshop recommended yearly follow-up examinations in untreated adult patients, although this may be impractical and inappropriate for most pediatric patients.[38]

### Natural History

The natural history of EPVO can be relatively unpredictable, and protection from variceal hemorrhage seems to be related to the development of spontaneous portosystemic shunts (like gastrorenal or splenorenal shunts, see Fig. 51–3) and/or recanalization of the portal vein.[11, 39–41] Ten percent to 20% of patients with EPVO never have an episode of significant gastrointestinal hemorrhage. The majority of children who have variceal hemorrhage do so before the age of 10.[11] In patients with reasonable access to medical care, the first episode of hemorrhage is usually not fatal.[11, 39] Therefore, in the absence of extenuating circumstances (e.g., living in isolated areas or very poor social supports) or endoscopic evidence of very high risk of variceal hemorrhage, it does

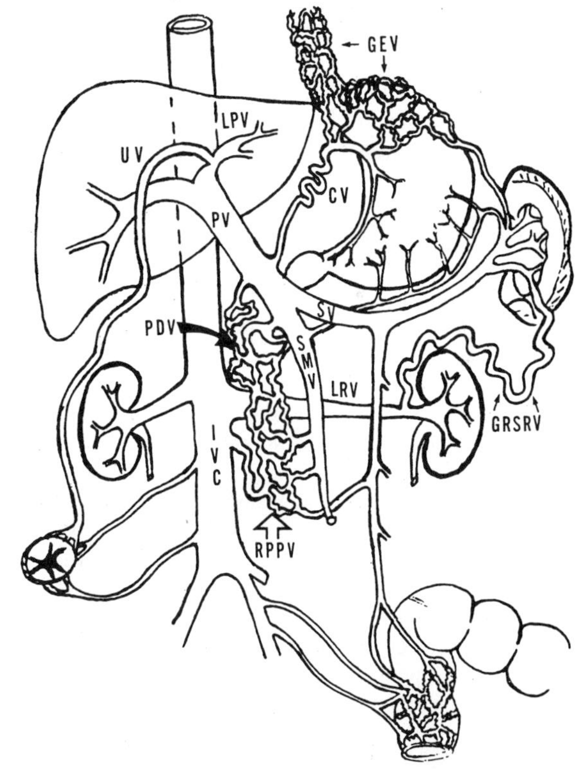


**FIGURE 51–3.** Portal venous anatomy and common portosystemic collaterals. CV, coronary vein (CV plus short gastric veins lead to GEV); GEV, gastroesophageal varices; GRSRV, gastrorenal-splenorenal veins; IVC, inferior vena cava; LPV, left branch of the portal vein; LRV, left renal vein; PDV, pancreaticoduodenal veins; PV, portal vein; RPPV, retroperitoneal-paravertebral veins; SMV, superior mesenteric vein; SV, splenic vein; UV, umbilical vein (to caput medusae). (From Subramanyam B, Balthazar E, Madamba M, et al: Sonography of portosystemic venous collaterals in portal hypertension. Radiology 1983;146:161–166, with permission.)

not seem to be advisable to consider prophylactic therapy for children with EPVO.

The natural history of portal hypertension in EHBA is quite dissimilar from that of EPVO. Portal hypertension, as determined by direct measurement at laparotomy, appears to be present at the time of portoenterostomy in many patients with EHBA.[42] Varices appear to develop in as many as 67% of patients who have undergone portoenterostomy for EHBA. Significant hemorrhage occurs in nearly 40% of these children with varices, typically before 5 years of age.[43] Portal hypertension and esophageal varix bleeding can lead to significant mortality and thus are important complications in children who ultimately undergo liver transplantation for EHBA.[44, 45] Even in long-term survivors of EHBA, complications of portal hypertension, including gastrointestinal bleeding and hepatopulmonary syndrome, are important sources of morbidity and mortality.[46, 47] The primary difference between EHBA and EPVO is the progressive hepatic disease associated with EHBA, which is secondary to ongoing intrahepatic disease, the variable response to portoenterostomy, and the effects of recurrent ascending cholangitis on the development of portal hypertension.

## Prophylactic Therapy

The results of prophylactic sclerotherapy in adults remain controversial, and there is limited but encouraging information regarding prophylactic variceal ligation.[48, 49] Given the invasive nature of these interventions, risk-to-benefit considerations preclude their routine prophylactic use in pediatrics at this time. In contrast, the relative safety and proven effectiveness of β-blocker therapy make it a plausible investigational approach to the prophylaxis of variceal hemorrhage in EHBA.[48, 50] Nonspecific β-blockers are felt to reduce portal hypertension by at least two distinct mechanisms. Competitive inhibition of $\beta_1$ receptors leads to a reduction in both inotropy and chronotropy, thereby blocking important mechanisms of the hyperdynamic circulation associated with the genesis of portal hypertension. Splanchnic blockade of $\beta_2$ receptors leads to unopposed β-adrenergic tone, an increase in splanchnic resistance, and thus a reduction in portal blood flow and pressure. Using a murine schistosomiasis model of portal hypertension, propranolol has been shown to prevent the development of portal hypertension.[51] The efficacy of β-blockers appears to be greater in individuals with portal hypertension who have not yet developed varices.[52]

Determining which children are at high risk for variceal hemorrhage is crucial. The degree of splenomegaly and endoscopic appearance of varices may give some indication as to the risk of bleeding.[11, 43] Fever, coughing, and aspirin administration have also been presumed to predispose to variceal hemorrhage.[53, 54] Interestingly, physical exercise has recently been shown to increase portal pressure in adults with cirrhosis.[55] Mounting information suggests that indirect measurements of portal pressure may yield clinically relevant information, especially concerning the risk of hemorrhage.[56] Portal pressure can be measured indirectly by examining the hepatic venous pressure gradient (HVPG), which is the difference between free and wedged hepatic pressures (see Fig. 51–3). Portal hypertension is defined as a HPVG higher than 6 mm Hg, and a level of 12 mm Hg seems to be a threshold for risk of variceal hemorrhage.[30] Two prospective longitudinal studies of primarily alcoholic cirrhotic patients have demonstrated that decreases in HVPG, either from abstinence or β-blocker therapy, are associated with a significant reduction in the risk of variceal hemorrhage.[57, 58] The utility of HVPG measurements in children will need to be addressed in research protocols. Although prophylactic treatment of esophageal varices in children is not currently the standard of care, rational arguments can be made for investigative trials of this approach, especially in children with progressive liver disease and evidence of high risk of hemorrhage.

## Urgent Management of Variceal Hemorrhage

Acute variceal hemorrhage represents a true emergency. The initial approach should include standard therapies of fluid resuscitation and correction of bleeding diathesis. Fluid administration should be done in a manner that maintains appropriate systemic blood pressure without overexpanding central blood volume, which can potentially increase portal pressure and worsen or reinduce variceal hemorrhage. Central venous pressure measurements can be quite helpful in assessing appropriateness of fluid administration. Nasogastric tube placement is critical in the management of variceal hemorrhage. Concerns regarding variceal trauma secondary to nasogastric tube placement are unwarranted. Nasogastric tube placement permits moment-to-moment assessment of hemorrhage rates. It also facilitates the removal of luminal blood, which otherwise can precipitate encephalopathy and has been shown to increase portal pressures secondary to increases in splanchnic blood flow.[59] Once the child is clinically stable, upper endoscopy should be performed to ascertain whether the hemorrhage is of variceal origin, because in many circumstances it is not and requires a substantially different therapeutic approach.[60]

Some episodes of variceal hemorrhage spontaneously terminate, although many do not. Persistent hemorrhage for longer than 12 hours or hemorrhage that requires the administration of red blood cells warrants the consideration of medical or surgical therapy. These therapies have not been rigorously tested in pediatrics, but meta-analysis of many trials in adults attests to their efficacy.[48] Most pediatric centers advocate an initial pharmacologic approach, which is based on agents that lead to acute splanchnic vasoconstriction (Table 51–1). Vasopressin is a potent vasoconstrictor and has the longest history of use in the treatment of acute variceal hemorrhage.[61] Its use is often compromised by side effects related to systemic vasoconstriction, including most importantly myocardial infarction and bowel ischemia. Coincident administration of nitroglycerin, or related compounds, has been used to ameliorate some of these problems. Terlipressin, a synthetic analogue of vasopressin, has a longer half-life than vasopressin, which permits bolus administration and may impart a better safety profile. Somatostatin and its longer-acting synthetic analogue, octreotide, act by inducing relatively selective splanchnic vasoconstriction. Both of these agents appear to have similar efficacy to vasopressin with significantly fewer side effects. Unlike va-

**TABLE 51–1. Pharmacologic Management of Acute Variceal Hemorrhage**

| AGENT | STANDARD ADULT REGIMEN | PEDIATRIC REGIMEN | REFERENCE |
|---|---|---|---|
| Vasopressin | 0.1 to 1 U/min IV | 0.3 to 1 U/kg/hr IV | 61 |
| Terlipressin | 1 to 2 mg IV q 2–4 hr | Unknown | |
| Somatostatin | 250 μg/hr IV | Unknown | |
| Octreotide | 25 to 50 μg/hr IV | 1 to 5 μg/kg/hr IV | 62 |

sopressin, their administration is extended beyond the acute phase in order to prevent early rebleeding. Preliminary reports of the use of octreotide in pediatrics have been presented.[62, 63] For all these agents, many practitioners favor the administration of a bolus equal to 1 hour's infusion prior to commencing the continuous infusion (initial bolus 1 μg/kg followed by continuous infusion of 1 μg/kg/hr). Pharmacologic therapy is usually successful in controlling acute variceal hemorrhage in children. Uncontrolled hemorrhage may necessitate other interventions, including endoscopic sclerotherapy or band ligation, transjugular intrahepatic portosystemic shunting, surgical portosystemic shunting, esophageal devascularization, or Sengstaken-Blakemore tube use (see later).

## Prevention of Recurrent Variceal Hemorrhage

Once the initial episode of variceal hemorrhage has been controlled, the issue of prevention of recurrent hemorrhage needs to be addressed. This assumes that there will be recurrent episodes, which is typically true in progressive diseases like EHBA, but may not necessarily be the case for relatively static disease like EPVO. A multitude of therapeutic options exist, including pharamacologic (β-blockers, nitrates), endoscopic (sclerotherapy, band ligation, clipping), radiologic (transjugular intrahepatic portosystemic shunting), and surgical (portosystemic shunting, esophageal transsection/devascularization, liver transplantation) approaches. The relative risks and benefits of each procedure must be considered along with the expected course of the liver disease in each child.

### *Pharmacologic Approaches*

The mainstay of pharmacologic approaches to prevent recurrent variceal hemorrhage is β-blocker therapy (as described earlier). Typically, β-blockers are administered at doses titrated to reduce resting heart rate by 25%.[64] Pooled analysis of 11 randomized studies indicates that β-blocker therapy is effective in reducing the risk of recurrent hemorrhage.[48] It appears that the major limitation of β-blocker therapy is an inadequate reduction in portal pressure in the majority of patients. In a prospective study, only 12% of patients had a reduction in HVPG levels to less than 12 mm Hg. Importantly, if HVPG was reduced below 12 mm Hg, recurrent hemorrhage was not observed.[57] Acute measurement of HVPG after starting β-blocker therapy may represent a means of identifying whether patients might need alternative, more invasive forms of management. Vasodilators, like isosorbide mononitrate, have been assessed as adjuncts to β-blocker therapy to enhance the reductions in HVPG.[65] Combined vasodilators and β-blockers have recently been assessed.[66] In addition, simple approaches like sodium restriction coupled with spironolactone therapy can reduce portal pressure.[67] Despite the inherent attractiveness of pharmacologic therapy of portal hypertension in children little clinical data exist.[50]

### *Endoscopic Approaches*

In contrast to the dearth of information about pharmacologic management of pediatric portal hypertension, a relative abundance of data exists regarding endoscopic approaches in children.[9, 10, 68–74] Injection sclerotherapy and variceal ligation are the primary endoscopic techniques that have been used in pediatrics (Fig. 51–4). In both techniques, thrombosis of the varix is induced and results in eradication of the risk of hemorrhage from that particular site. Sclerotherapy involves either intravariceal or paravariceal injection of irritating compounds, which cause either thrombosis in the esophageal varix or inflammatory responses around the varix.[75] Variceal ligation involves strangulation of the esophageal varix by the application of a rubber band around it. Sclerotherapy has been demonstrated in a number of adult trials to be effective in reducing both mortality and the risk of rebleeding.[48] A limited number of studies seem to indicate that variceal ligation may have equal or better efficacy than sclerotherapy with fewer complications.[76]

Comparison of cumulative data from four pediatric sclerotherapy reports including 268 children[8, 9, 68, 70] and four pediatric ligation reports including 53 children[10, 72–74] reveals similarities in the number of sessions required to eradicate varices (sclerotherapy 5.4 versus ligation 3.3), percentage of variceal eradication (sclerotherapy 89% versus ligation 78%), and percentage of patients rebleeding during therapy (sclerotherapy 38% versus ligation 23%). Long-term follow-up of pediatric ligation therapy is too short for meaningful comparisons. Follow-up data for a mean of 8.7 years in a group of patients with EPVO treated with sclerotherapy revealed recurrent varices in 31% of patients, which reflects the fact that this technique does not address the primary issues of the pathophysiology of portal hypertension.[77] Currently, sclerotherapy is the endoscopic therapeutic standard of care in pediatrics.[78] Ligation therapy has the potential to obviate or lessen some of the common complications that are associated with sclerotherapy, including fever, ulceration, and stricture formation.[79, 80] Current technologies for ligation require multiple passages of the endoscope, which introduces potential risks and makes general anesthesia necessary in most patients. Multiple rubber-band ligator devices or esophageal clipping apparatus may help circumvent this problem.[81, 82]

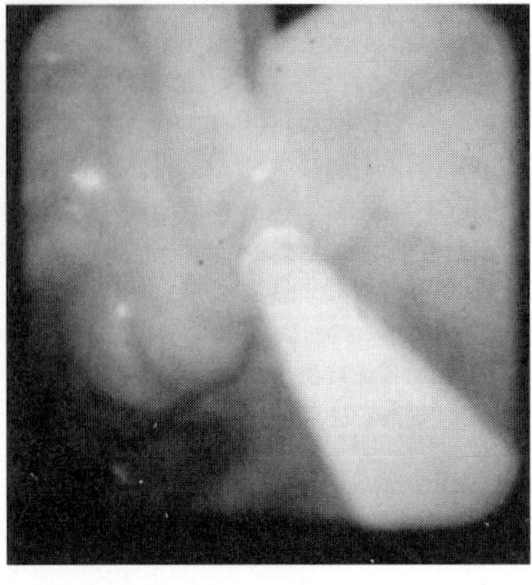

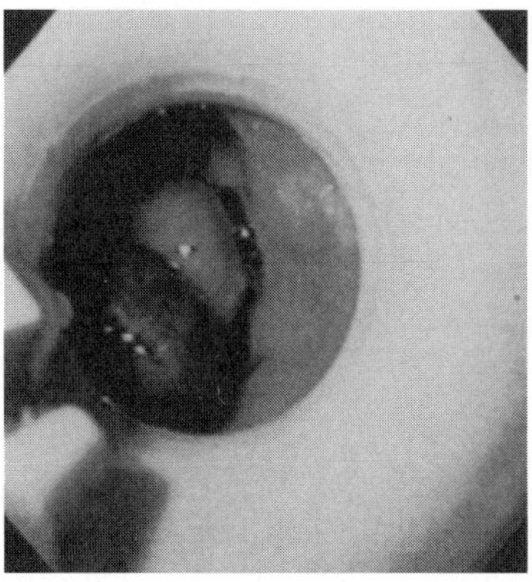

**FIGURE 51–4.** Endoscopic management of esophageal varices. Endoscopic views of sclerotherapy *(left)* and ligation *(right)* of esophageal varices. (From Sivak M: Endoscopic sclerotherapy of varices. In Silvis S [ed]: Therapeutic Gastrointestinal Endoscopy. New York, Igaku-Shoin Medical Publishers, 1984; and Fox V, Carr-Locke D, Connors P, et al: Endoscopic ligation of esophageal varices in children. J Pediatr Gastroenterol Nutr 1995;20:202–208, with permission.)

## Radiologic Approaches

Transjugular intrahepatic portosystemic shunting (TIPS) is a radiologic approach for temporarily decompressing esophageal varices[83] (Fig. 51–5). The technique involves the transjugular insertion of a catheter into the hepatic vein and creation of a stented intrahepatic shunt between branches of the hepatic and portal veins. It is a highly efficacious means of rapidly reducing portal hypertension and risk of variceal bleeding. In addition, it is quite useful in the management of resistant ascites. The major problems associated with TIPS are the development of encephalopathy and shunt stenosis or occlusion.[84] Pediatric applications of TIPS have been primarily in the context either of endoscopically unresponsive variceal hemorrhage, as a bridge to liver transplantation, or in selected patients whose clinical condition precludes other approaches.[85–88]

## Surgical Approaches

The two major surgical approaches to pediatric portal hypertension are portosystemic shunting and orthotopic liver transplantation. Liver transplantation is a definitive and effective method for managing portal hypertension but carries with it significant potential morbidity and mortality.[89] Recurrent variceal hemorrhage is often a complication in liver transplant candidates and is sometimes the primary indication for liver transplantation in pediatric patients.[60] In children with progressive end-stage hepatic disease like EHBA, liver transplantation is probably the surgical approach of

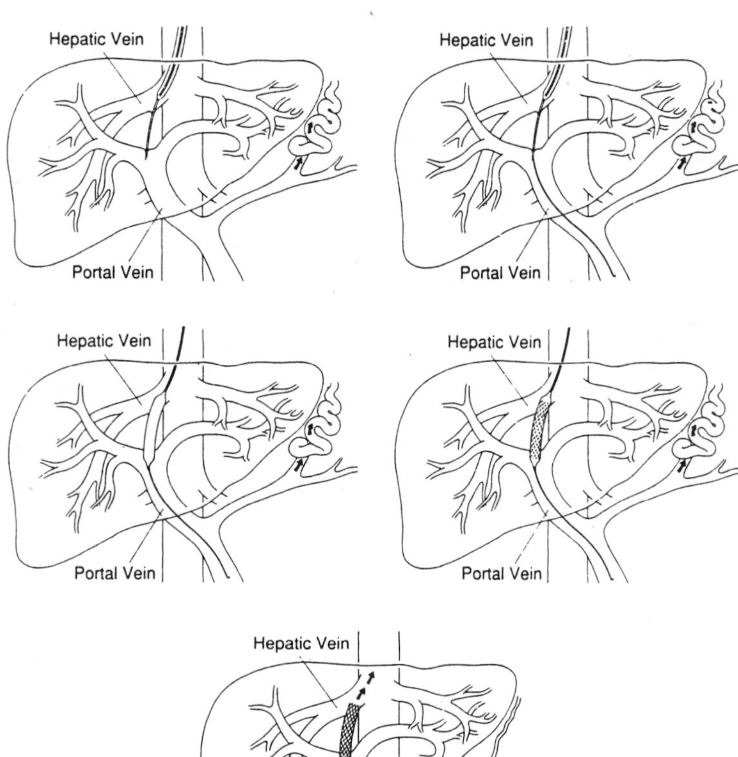


**FIGURE 51–5.** Technique of transjugular intrahepatic portosystemic shunting (TIPS). A catheter is inserted into the jugular vein and is advanced into the hepatic vein, where a needle is used to form a tract between the portal vein and the hepatic vein. This tract is then expanded with a balloon angioplasty catheter, and a stent is then placed, forming the permanent portosystemic shunt. (From Zemel G, Katzen B, Becker G, et al: Percutaneous transjugular portosystemic shunt. JAMA 1991;266:390–393, with permission.)

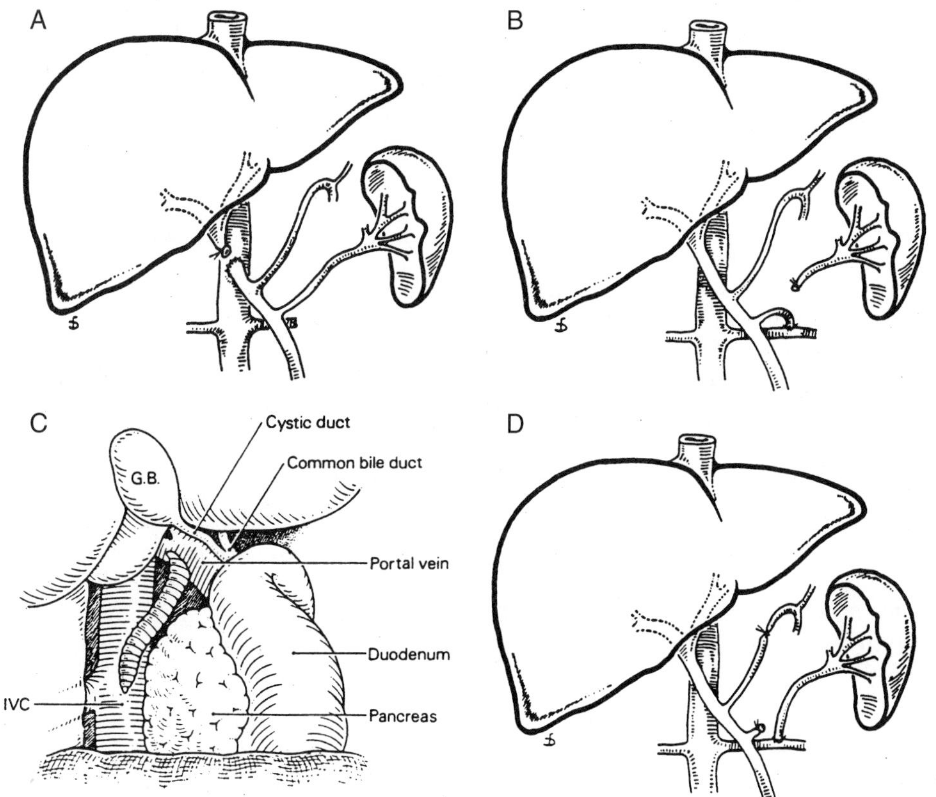


**FIGURE 51–6.** Types of portosystemic shunts. *A,* Portacaval end-to-side. *B,* Central splenorenal. *C,* Small diameter portacaval H-graft. *D,* Distal splenorenal. (From Sutton R, Shields R: The place of portosystemic shunting. In Blumgart LH [ed]: Surgery of the Liver and Biliary Tract. New York, Churchill Livingstone, 1994, with permission.)

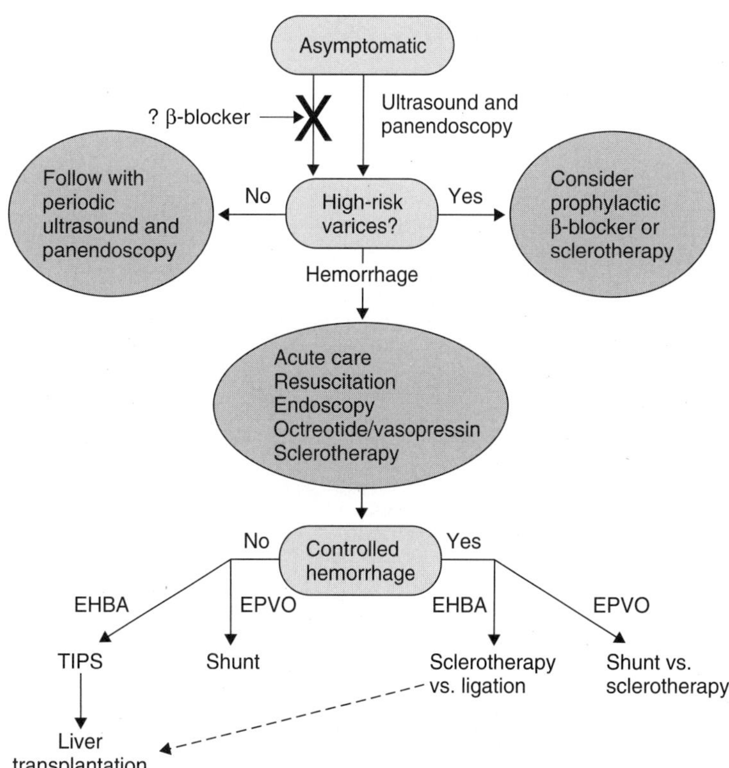


**FIGURE 51–7.** Algorithm for the management of portal hypertension in children.

choice, with TIPS being used as a bridge. EPVO is one of the most common causes of variceal hemorrhage in children and typically does not evolve into end-stage liver disease. As a result, portosystemic shunting has had an important role in its management.

Multiple procedures have been devised to surgically produce portosystemic shunts (Fig. 51–6). In all of these procedures, portal pressure and variceal blood flow are reduced by shunting portal blood past the liver into the systemic circulation. This is one of the most effective means of treating portal hypertension.[48] Unfortunately, the results are compromised by significant complications, including shunt dysfunction and hepatic encephalopathy.[90] Typically, some type of distal splenorenal shunt is used for pediatric patients. This procedure was initially developed in an effort to minimize the development of encephalopathy. Controversy exists as to whether it actually accomplishes this goal.[91] In spite of this, some version of a splenorenal shunt is most commonly used for the treatment of pediatric EPVO.[92–95] For EPVO, shunt surgery is well tolerated with no reports of hepatic encephalopathy in three major pediatric series.[93–95] Recurrent gastrointestinal hemorrhage occurred in only 10% of patients, all of whom had shunt malfunction or occlusion. A novel potential future approach to EPVO would be application of a jugular vein autograft between the portal vein and the intrahepatic portal vein.[96] Analysis of the relative merits of sclerotherapy versus portosystemic shunting for children with EPVO is complex.[94] The potential for the development of spontaneous portosystemic shunts argues in favor of sclerotherapy, whereas the superb efficacy of shunting procedures argues in their favor. A prospective trial of these two approaches is under way.[94]

## SUMMARY

The approach to the treatment of portal hypertension is summarized in Figure 51–7.

## REFERENCES


1. Graham DY, Smith JL: The course of patients after variceal hemorrhage. Gastroenterology 1981;80:800–809.
2. Larrabee RC: Chronic congestive splenomegaly and its relationship to Banti's disease. Am J Med 1934;188:745–760.
3. Rousselot LM: The role of congestion (portal hypertension) in so-called Banti's syndrome: a clinical and pathological study of thirty-one cases with late results following splenectomy. JAMA 1936;107:1788–1793.
4. Gentil-Kocher S, Bernard O, Brunelle F, et al: Budd-Chiari syndrome in children: report of 22 cases. J Pediatr 1988;113:30–38.
5. Safouh M, Shehata AH: Hepatic vein occlusion: disease of Egyptian children. J Pediatr 1965;67:415–422.
6. Thapa BR, Mehta S: Endoscopic sclerotherapy of esophageal varices in infants and children. J Pediatr Gastroenterol Nutr 1990;10:430–434.
7. Vane DW, Boles ET, Clatworthy HW: Esophageal sclerotherapy: an effective modality in children. J Pediatr Surg 1985;20:703–707.
8. Hill ID, Bowie MD: Endoscopic sclerotherapy for control of bleeding varices in children. Am J Gastroenterol 1991;86:472–476.
9. Howard ER, Stringer MD, Mowat AP: Assessment of injection sclerotherapy in the management of 152 children with oesophageal varices. Br J Surg 1988;75:404–408.
10. Price MR, Sartorelli KH, Karrer FM, et al: Management of esophageal varices in children by endoscopic variceal ligation. J Pediatr Surg 1996;31:1056–1059.
11. Alvarez F, Bernard O, Brunelle F, et al: Portal obstruction in children. I. Clinical investigation and hemorrhage risk. J Pediatr 1983;103:696–702.
12. Yadav S, Dutta AK, Sarin SK: Do umbilical vein catheterization and sepsis lead to portal vein thrombosis? A prospective, clinical, and sonographic evaluation. J Pediatr Gastroenterol Nutr 1993;17:392–396.
13. Dubuisson C, Boyer-Neumann C, Wolf M, et al: Protein C, protein S, and antithrombin III in children with portal vein obstruction. Hepatology 1995;108:A1059.
14. Odievre M, Pige G, Alagille D: Congenital anomalies associated with extrahepatic portal hypertension. Arch Dis Child 1977;52:383–385.
15. Ramirez RO, Sokol RJ, Hays T, Silverman A: Familial occurrence of cavernous transformation of the portal vein. J Pediatr Gastroenterol Nutr 1995;21:313–318.
16. Ando H, Kaneko K, Ito F, et al: Anatomy and etiology of extrahepatic portal vein obstruction in children leading to bleeding esophageal varices. J Am Coll Surg 1996;183:543–547.
17. Colman JC, Britton RS, Orrego H, et al: Relationship between osmotically induced hepatocyte enlargement and portal hypertension. Am J Physiol 1983;245:G382–G387.
18. Orrego H, Blendis LM, Crossley IR, et al: Correlation of intrahepatic pressure with collagen in the Disse space and hepatomegaly in humans and in the rat. Gastroenterology 1980;80:546–556.
19. Rockey D: The cellular pathogenesis of portal hypertension: stellate cell contractility, endothelin, and nitric oxide. Hepatology 1997;25:2–5.
20. Vorobioff J, Bredfeldt JE, Groszmann RJ: Hyperdynamic circulation in portal-hypertensive rat model: a primary factor for maintenance of chronic portal hypertension. Am J Physiol 1983;244:G52–G57.
21. Ismail-Zade IA, Trifonova NA, Razumovski AY, Stepanenko SM: Haemodynamic changes in children with portal hypertension during the postoperative period. Paediatr Anaesth 1995;5:311–317.
22. Benoit JN, Barrowman JA, Harper SL, et al: Role of humoral factors in the intestinal hyperemia associated with chronic portal hypertension. Am J Physiol 1984;247:G486–G493.
23. Pak JM, Lee SS: Glucagon in portal hypertension. J Hepatol 1994;20:825–832.
24. Bruix J, Bosch J, Kravetz D, et al: Effects of prostaglandin inhibition on systemic and hepatic hemodynamics in patients with cirrhosis of the liver. Gastroenterology 1985;88:430–435.
25. Kvietys PR, McLendon JM, Granger DN: Postprandial intestinal hyperemia: role of bile salts in the ileum. Am J Physiol 1981;241:G469–G477.
26. Lee SS, Chilton EL, Pak J-M: Adenosine receptor blockade reduces splanchnic hyperemia in cirrhotic rats. Hepatology 1992;15:1107–1111.
27. Bomzon A, Blendis LM: The nitric oxide hypothesis and the hyperdynamic circulation in cirrhosis. Hepatology 1994;20:1343–1350.
28. Lopez-Talavera JC, Cadelina G, Olchowski J, et al: Thalidomide inhibits tumor necrosis factor alpha, decreases nitric oxide synthesis, and ameliorates the hyperdynamic circulatory syndrome in portal-hypertensive rats. Hepatology 1996;23:1616–1621.
29. Moller S, Bendtsen F, Schifter S, Henriken JH: Relation of calcitonin gene-related peptide to systemic vasodilatation and central hypovolaemia in cirrhosis. Scand J Gastroenterol 1996;31:928–933.
30. Garcia-Tsao G, Groszmann RJ, Fisher RL, et al: Portal pressure, presence of gastroesophageal varices and variceal bleeding. Hepatology 1985;5:419–424.
31. Kumari-Subaiya S, Gorvoy J, Phillips G, et al: Portal vein measurement by ultrasonography in patients with long-standing cystic fibrosis: preliminary observations. J Pediatr Gastroenterol Nutr 1987;6:71–78.
32. De Giacomo C, Tomasi G, Gatti C, et al: Ultrasonographic prediction of the presence and severity of esophageal varices in children. J Pediatr Gastroenterol Nutr 1989;9:431–435.
33. Kozaiwa K, Tajiri H, Yoshimura N, et al: Utility of duplex Doppler ultrasound in evaluating portal hypertension in children. J Pediatr Gastroenterol Nutr 1995;21:215–219.
34. Valletta EA, Loreti S, Cipolli M, et al: Portal hypertension and esophageal varices in cystic fibrosis, unreliability of echo-Doppler flowmetry. Scand J Gastroenterol 1993;28:1042–1046.
35. Rabinowitz SS, Norton KI, Benkov KJ, et al: Sonographic evaluaton of portal hypertension in children. J Pediatr Gastroenterol Nutr 1990;10:395–401.
36. Zoli M, Merkel C, Magalotti D, et al: Evaluation of a new endoscopic index to predict first bleeding from the upper gastrointestinal tract in patients with cirrhosis. Hepatology 1996;24:1047–1052.
37. Beppu K, Inokuchi K, Koyangi N, et al: Prediction of variceal hemorrhage by esophageal endoscopy. Gastrointest Endosc 1981;27:213–218.

38. de Franchis R: Developing consensus in portal hypertension. J Hepatol 1996;23:390–394.
39. Fonkalsrud EW, Myers NA, Robinson MJ: Management of extrahepatic portal hypertension in children. Ann Surg 1974;180:487–492.
40. Mitra SK, Kumar V, Datta DV, et al: Extrahepatic portal hypertension: a review of 70 cases. J Pediatr Surg 1978;13:51–54.
41. Webb LJ, Sherlock S: The aetiology, presentation and natural history of extra-hepatic portal venous obstruction. Q J Med 1979;192:627–639.
42. Kasai M, Okamoto A, Ohi R, et al: Changes of portal vein pressure and intrahepatic blood vessels after surgery for biliary atresia. J Pediatr Surg 1981;16:152–159.
43. Stringer MD, Howard ER, Mowat AP: Endoscopic sclerotherapy in the management of esophageal varices in 61 children with biliary atresia. J Pediatr Surg 1989;24:438–442.
44. Pettitt BJ, Zitelli BJ, Rowe MI: Analysis of patients with biliary atresia coming to liver transplantation. J Pediatr Surg 1984;19:779–784.
45. Tagge DU, Tagge EP, Drongowski RA, et al: A long-term experience with biliary atresia. Reassessment of prognostic factors. Ann Surg 1991;214:590–598.
46. Karrer FM, Price MR, Bensard DD, et al: Long-term results with the Kasai operation for biliary atresia. Arch Surg 1996;131:493–496.
47. Valayer J: Conventional treatment of biliary atresia: long-term results. J Pediatr Surg 1996;31:1546–1551.
48. D'Amico G, Pagliaro L, Bosch J: The treatment of portal hypertension: a meta-analytic review. Hepatology 1995;22:332–354.
49. Lay C-S, Tsai Y-T, Teg C-Y, et al: Endoscopic variceal ligation in prophylaxis of first variceal bleeding in cirrhotic patients with high-risk esophageal varices. Hepatology 1997;25:1346–1350.
50. Ozsoylu S, Kocak N, Yuce A: Propranolol therapy for portal hypertension in children. J Pediatr 1985;106:317–320.
51. Sarin SK, Groszmann RJ, Mosca PG, et al: Propranolol ameliorates the development of portal-systemic shunting in a chronic murine schistosomiasis model of portal hypertension. J Clin Invest 1991;87:1032–1036.
52. Escorsell A, Ferayorni L, Bosch J, et al: The portal pressure response to β-blockade is greater in cirrhotic patients without varices than in those with varices. Gastroenterology 1997;112:2012–2016.
53. Pinkerton JA, Holcomb GW, Foster JH: Portal hypertension in childhood. Ann Surg 1972;175:870–886.
54. Spence RAJ, Johnston GW, Odling-Smee GW, Rodgers HW: Bleeding oesophageal varices with longterm follow up. Arch Dis Child 1984;59:336–340.
55. Garcia-Pagan JC, Santos C, Barbera JA, et al: Physical exercise increases portal pressure in patients with cirrhosis and portal hypertension. Gastroenterology 1996;111:1300–1306.
56. Groszmann RJ: The hepatic venous pressure gradient: has the time arrived for its application in clinical practice? Hepatology 1996;24:739–741.
57. Feu F, Garcia-Pagan JC, Bosch J, et al: Relationship between portal pressure response to pharmacotherapy and risk of recurrent variceal hemorrhage in patients with cirrhosis. Lancet 1995;346:1056–1059.
58. Vorobioff J, Groszmann RJ, Picabea E, et al: Prognostic value of hepatic venous pressure gradient measurements in alcoholic cirrhosis: a 10 year prospective study. Gastroenterology 1996;111:701–709.
59. Chen L, Groszmann RJ: Blood in the gastric lumen increases splanchnic blood flow and portal pressure in portal-hypertensive rats. Gastroenterology 1996;111:1103–1110.
60. Sokal E, Van Hoorebeeck N, Van Obbergh L, et al: Upper gastrointestinal tract bleeding in cirrhotic children candidates for liver transplantation. Eur J Pediatr 1992;151:326–328.
61. Mowat AP: Liver Disorders in Childhood, 2nd ed. Boston, Butterworths, 1987.
62. Siafakas C, Fox VL, Klaes L, Nurko S: Treatment of severe gastrointestinal bleeding in children with octreotide. Gastroenterology 1996;110:A839.
63. Gokhale R, Alonso EM, Dean R, et al: Intravenous Octreotide Infusion in Treatment of Acute Variceal Bleeding in Children. North Chicago, American Society for Pediatric Gastroenterology and Nutrition, 1993.
64. Lebrec D, Poynard T, Hillon P, Benhamou J-P: Propranolol for prevention of recurrent gastrointestinal bleeding in patients with cirrhosis. N Engl J Med 1981;305:1371–1374.
65. Garcia-Pagan JC, Feu F, Bosch J, Rodes J: Propranolol compared with propranolol plus isosorbide-5-mononitrate for portal hypertension in cirrhosis. Ann Intern Med 1991;114:869–873.
66. Forrest EH, Bouchier IAD, Hayes PC: Acute hemodynamic changes after oral carvedilol, a vasodilating beta-blocker, in patients with cirrhosis. J Hepatol 1996;23:909–915.
67. Garcia-Pagan JC, Salmeron JM, Feu F, et al: Effects of low-sodium diet and spironolactone on portal pressure in patients with compensated cirrhosis. Hepatology 1994;19:1095–1099.
68. Maksoud JG, Goncalves MEP, Porta G, et al: The endoscopic and surgical management of portal hypertension in children: analysis of 123 cases. J Pediatr Surg 1991;26:178–181.
69. Hill ID, Bowie MD: Endoscopic sclerotherapy for control of bleeding varices in children. Am J Gastroenterol 1991;86:472–476.
70. Yachha SK, Sharma BC, Kumar M, Khanduri A: Endoscopic sclerotherapy for esophageal varices in children with extrahepatic portal venous obstruction: a follow up study. J Pediatr Gastroenterol Nutr 1997;24:49–52.
71. Hall RJ, Lilly JR, Stiegmann GV: Endoscopic esophageal varix ligation: technique and preliminary results in children. J Pediatr Surg 1988;23:1222–1223.
72. Fox VL, Carr-Locke DL, Connors PJ, Leichtner AM: Endoscopic ligation of esophageal varices in children. J Pediatr Gastroenterol Nutr 1995;20:202–208.
73. Nijhawan S, Patni T, Sharma U, et al: Endoscopic variceal ligation in children. J Pediatr Surg 1995;30:1455–1456.
74. Cano I, Urruzuno P, Medina E, et al: Treatment of esophageal varices by endoscopic ligation in children. Eur J Pediatr Surg 1995;5:299–302.
75. Sarin SK, Kumar A: Sclerosants for variceal sclerotherapy: a critical appraisal. Am J Gastroenterol 1990;85:641–649.
76. Stiegmann GV, Goff JS, Michaletz-Onody PA, et al: Endoscopic sclerotherapy as compared with endoscopic ligation for bleeding esophageal varices. N Engl J Med 1992;326:1527–1532.
77. Stringer MD, Howard ER: Longterm outcome after injection sclerotherapy for oesophageal varices in children with extrahepatic portal hypertension. Gut 1994;35:257–259.
78. Hassall E, Treem WR: To stab or strangle: how best to kill a varix? J Pediatr Gastroenterol Nutr 1995;20:121–124.
79. Proujansky R, Orenstein SR, Kocoshis SA: Patient and procedure variable associated with complications following variceal sclerotherapy in children. J Pediatr Gastroenterol Nutr 1991;12:33–38.
80. Broor SL, Lahoti D, Bose PP, et al: Benign esophageal strictures in children and adolescents: etiology, clinical profile, and results of endoscopic dilation. Gastrointest Endosc 1996;43:474–477.
81. Saeed ZA: The Saeed Six-Shooter: a prospective study of a new endoscopic multiple rubber-band ligator for the treatment of varices. Endoscopy 1996;28:559–564.
82. Ohnuma N, Takahashi H, Tanabe M, et al: Endoscopic variceal ligation using a clipping apparatus in children with portal hypertension. Endoscopy 1997;29:86–90.
83. Zemel G, Katzen BT, Becker GJ, et al: Percutaneous transjugular portosystemic shunt. JAMA 1991;266:390–393.
84. Stanley AJ, Jalan R, Forrest EH, et al: Longterm follow up of transjugular intrahepatic portosystemic stent shunt (TIPSS) for the treatment of portal hypertension: results in 130 patients. Gut 1996;39:479–485.
85. Kerns SR, Hawkins IF: Transjugular intrahepatic portosystemic shunt in a child with cystic fibrosis. AJR 1992;159:1277–1278.
86. Berger KJ, Schreiber RA, Tchervenkov J, et al: Decompression of portal hypertension in a child with cystic fibrosis after transjugular intrahepatic portosystemic shunt placement. J Pediatr Gastroenterol Nutr 1994;19:322–325.
87. Johnson SP, Leyendecker JR, Joseph FB, et al: Transjugular portosystemic shunts in pediatric patients awaiting liver transplantation. Transplantation 1996;62:1178–1181.
88. Cao S, Monge H, Semba C, et al: Emergency transjugular intrahepatic portosystemic shunt (TIPS) in an infant: a case report. J Pediatr Surg 1997;32:125–127.
89. Iwatsuki S, Starzl T, Todo S, et al: Liver transplantation in the treatment of bleeding esophageal varices. Surgery 1988;104:697–705.
90. Teres J, Bordas JM, Bravo D, et al: Sclerotherapy vs. distal splenorenal shunt in the elective treatment of variceal hemorrhage: a randomized controlled trial. Hepatology 1987;7:430–436.
91. Nussbaum MS, Schoettker PJ, Fischer JE: Comparison of distal and proximal splenorenal shunts: a ten-year experience. Surgery 1993;114:659–666.
92. Fonkalsrud EW: Surgical management of portal hypertension in childhood. Arch Surg 1980;115:1042–1045.
93. Alvarez F, Bernard O, Brunelle F, et al: Portal obstruction in children.

II. Results of surgical portosystemic shunts. J Pediatr 1983;103:703–707.
94. Mitra SK, Rao KLN, Narasimhan KL, et al: Side-to-side lienorenal shunt without splenectomy in noncirrhotic portal hypertension in children. J Pediatr Surg 1993;28:398–402.
95. Prasad AS, Gupta S, Kohli V, et al: Proximal splenorenal shunts for extrahepatic portal venous obstruction in children. Ann Surg 1994;219:193–196.
96. de Ville de Goyet J, Gibbs P, Claypuyt P, et al: Original extrahilar approach for hepatic portal revascularization and relief of extrahepatic portal vein hypertension related to late portal vein thrombosis after pediatric liver transplantation. Transplantation 1996;62:71–75.

Chapter 52

# Liver Failure and Transplantation

*Marsha H. Kay and Suzanne V. McDiarmid*

## HEPATIC FAILURE

Hepatic failure can be classified as fulminant or chronic. Fulminant hepatic failure (FHF) is defined as the development of signs of advanced liver failure such as hepatic encephalopathy in the absence of previous liver disease and is considered to be present if liver failure develops over a period of 8 weeks or less. Fulminant hepatic failure is further subclassified into acute (less than 2 weeks duration of symptoms) and subacute (symptoms from 2 to 8 weeks). Chronic liver failure is the development of advanced signs of liver disease with pre-existing liver disease.

There is no significant difference in the clinical presentation of FHF in children who recover spontaneously or those who die or require liver transplantation.[1] Without liver transplantation, FHF is associated with a very high mortality, especially cases of viral hepatitis.[2, 3] Some causes of FHF, such as acetaminophen overdose, are potentially reversible. It is difficult to predict, however, which patients will recover, and early listing for orthotopic liver transplantation (OLT) is necessary if evidence of liver failure develops. Mortality is due to complications of hepatic failure such as cerebral edema and infection. In those cases in which the cause is irreversible, OLT offers the only effective cure. Transplantation is discussed later in this chapter.

### Etiology

#### *Viral Hepatitis*

Hepatitis A, B, C, Δ, E, and non-A, non-B, non-C infections are important causes of acute liver failure and may be the cause in up to 50 % or more of patients with acute liver failure.[1, 3–8] The relative incidence of each varies based on patient age, geographic location, and risk factors for infection. It is anticipated that vaccination strategies and the ability to screen blood products will decrease the incidence of hepatitis A, B, C, and Δ infection causing acute hepatic failure. The survival from each type of infection varies, with highest survival rates with acute hepatitis A infection and lowest survival rates with non-A, non-B, non-C hepatitis in patients who have not received transplants.[9, 10] Patients with viral hepatitis die from the same mechanisms as patients with nonviral acute liver failure—cerebral edema, renal failure, coagulopathy, and infection.[11] The median survival following onset of grade 3 encephalopathy in patients with viral hepatitis who ultimately die is 4 to 5 days after hospital admission.[12] Survival in patients with viral hepatitis due to hepatitis A or B infection is influenced by coexisting complications. Survival rates without liver transplantation are 67% if cerebral edema or renal failure are absent, 50% in patients with isolated cerebral edema, and 30% with coexisting cerebral edema and renal impairment.[12]

In India and Asia, hepatitis E virus is an important cause of acute liver failure, especially in pregnant females. The reasons that pregnant women are susceptible are unknown. Hepatitis E virus has recently been identified as a cause of acute hepatic failure in the United States. Travelers to Mexico and other areas where the disease is endemic are at risk for infection.[13] Hepatitis E virus RNA levels in stool and serum are important in establishing the diagnosis (see Chapter 50).

#### *Drug Reactions*

In pediatric series, toxin- or drug-induced liver injury represents 15% to 20% of cases of FHF[1, 9] (Table 52–1). Liver toxicity due to medications may be dose related, as seen with acetaminophen, aspirin, azathioprine, and cyclosporine, or may represent an idiosyncratic reaction seen with valproic acid, phenytoin, isoniazid, chlorpromazine, and halothane.[14–16] Some medications such as methotrexate may result in chronic dose-related liver damage. With some toxic reactions, damage may not resolve after medication withdrawal. Before the availability of liver transplantation, the survival rate for patients developing FHF with grade 3 or 4 encephalopathy due to idiosyncratic drug reactions or halothane hepatitis was 12.5%, compared with 53% for other causes.[12]

The most common cause of drug-related FHF in adolescents and young adults is intentional acetaminophen overdose.[17] The median survival after acetaminophen ingestion for patients who ultimately die is 6 to 7 days, with a range

**TABLE 52–1. Medication-Related Hepatotoxicity by Histologic Findings**

| PATTERN OF INJURY | EXAMPLES OF DRUGS | FULMINANT LIVER INJURY |
|---|---|---|
| Zonal necrosis | Acetaminophen, carbon tetrachloride (centrilobular), halothane, cimetidine, ketoconazole, pemoline | Yes |
| Nonspecific hepatitis | Aspirin, semisynthetic penicillin analogues, retinoids, ketoconazole, isoniazid | Very rare |
| Viral hepatitis–like injury | Isoniazid, halothane, methyldopa, phenytoin, rifampin | Yes |
| Granulomatous hepatitis | Quinidine, allopurinol, sulfonamides, carbamazepine, hydralazine | Occasionally |
| Chronic hepatitis | Nitrofurantoin, methyldopa, isoniazid, sulfonamides | |
| Fibrosis | Methotrexate (liver function tests may be normal) | |
| Cholestasis | Erythromycin estolate (macrolide), nitrofurantoin, chlorpromazine, captopril, azathioprine (6-mercaptopurine), estrogens, anabolic steroids | Unlikely |
| Fatty liver | Ethanol, corticosteroids, (macrovesicular), tetracycline (microvesicular), valproic acid (microvesicular), amiodarone (phospholipidosis) | Possible with microvesicular, renal injury may worsen |
| Vascular lesions (thrombosis, VOD, portal hypertension, peliosis hepatis) | OCPs, chemotherapy, alkaloids, anabolic steroids | |
| Tumors (adenoma, focal nodular hyperplasia, carcinoma, angiosarcoma) | OCPs, androgens, vinyl chloride monomer | |

VOD, veno-occlusive disease; OCP, oral contraceptive pill.
Adapted from Bass NM, Ockner RK., Drug induced liver disease. In Zakim D, Boyer TD, editors. Hepatology, 2nd ed. Philadelphia: WB Saunders, 1990, pp. 754–791.

of 3 to 56 days.[12] The degree of aminotransferase elevation is highest after acetaminophen overdose when compared with other causes of FHF, although there is great variability.[12] Poor prognostic factors include the presence of cerebral edema, oliguric renal failure, and uncompensated metabolic acidosis. Patients without any of these factors may have survival rates up to 100%. The presence of cerebral edema alone decreases the survival rate to 71%; coexisting cerebral edema and renal failure decrease the survival to 53%. If uncompensated metabolic acidosis is present, the survival rate decreases to 7%.[12] Other causes of medication-induced liver failure are listed in Table 52–1.

### *Reye's Syndrome*

Reye's syndrome is characterized by acute encephalopathy and hepatic dysfunction. The cause is unknown but thought to relate to a disorder of mitochondrial function. A viral syndrome due to influenza or varicella often antedates the development of symptoms.[18] This is followed by vomiting, irritability, listlessness, evidence of cerebral edema, and severe hepatic dysfunction. Although aspirin administration may play an etiologic role, many cases not associated with aspirin have been reported. Liver function abnormalities consist of markedly elevated aminotransferase levels and prothrombin times, without a proportionate increase in serum bilirubin levels.[19] Ammonia levels may be elevated, and hypoglycemia may be present.[18, 19] Hepatomegaly may be present, and liver biopsy reveals a microvesicular steatosis, with swollen mitochondria on electron microscopy.[20] Management is directed to control of cerebral edema, while maintaining cerebral perfusion pressure.[21] There is a high case-fatality rate due to cerebral herniation and high morbidity rate if this disorder is unrecognized and appropriate management is not initiated. Patients who survive show rapid improvement in their liver function tests. Several inborn errors of metabolism such as medium- and long-chain acyl coenzyme A dehydrogenase deficiency and organic acidemias mimic Reye's syndrome in presentation.[20, 22, 23]

### *Wilson's Disease*

Children with Wilson's disease can present with symptoms characteristic of FHF or can present with cirrhosis. Wilson's disease is a frequent indication for OLT in pediatric patients with FHF.[24–26] Wilson's disease is characterized by decreased serum ceruloplasmin levels, elevated 24-hour urine copper, hemolytic anemia, the presence of Kayser-Fleischer rings (a discoloration of Descemet's membrane in the limbic area of the cornea seen by slit lamp examination), and renal and neurologic abnormalities. Serum ceruloplasmin levels may be elevated to normal levels in patients with Wilson's disease, and urinary copper excretion may be elevated in patients with liver failure from other causes. Urinary copper excretion after penicillamine challenge and an alkaline phosphatase–to–total bilirubin ratio of less than 2.0 may be helpful in differentiating Wilson's disease from other causes of FHF.[27, 28] The gene for Wilson's disease, inherited in an autosomal recessive manner, is located on chromosome 13.[29]

The most frequent causes of fulminant and chronic liver failure are indicated in Tables 52–2 through 52–5. A discussion of these is found in Chapters 48, 49, and 50.

## Manifestations of Liver Failure

### *Portal Hypertension*

Portal pressure, or hepatic venous pressure gradient (HVPG), is the difference between wedged hepatic pressure

**TABLE 52–2. Etiology of Fulminant Hepatic Failure in Neonates and Early Infancy**

| | CHARACTERISTICS | SELECTED REFERENCES |
|---|---|---|
| **Infectious** | | |
| CMV | May have hepatic calcifications | |
| EBV | Onset usually after 3 weeks of age | |
| Echovirus | Maternal fever, malaise, abdominal pain ante partum; onset at younger than 10 days of age; mimics HSV | 147, 148 |
| Hepatitis B | Onset at younger than 6 weeks of age; precore mutant may be important; measure HBV DNA | 6, 7, 149 |
| Herpesvirus | Skin and mucous membrane changes, pneumonitis, DIC, CNS and multi-organ disease, HSV PCR and culture | 150, 151 |
| Syphilis | First 4 weeks of life, hepatosplenomegaly, hepatic calcification, anemia, jaundice, RPR/FTA | 152 |
| **Metabolic** | | |
| Galactosemia | Decreased erythrocyte galactose-1-phosphate uridyltransferase, *E. coli* sepsis associated | |
| Hereditary fructose intolerance | Onset at 8–10 days of age if sucrose fed or shortly after weaning from breast feeding, aldolase B deficiency chromosome 9 | 153, 154 |
| Hereditary tyrosinemia | Renal tubular dysfunction and failure, coagulopathy, hypophosphatemic rickets, neurologic disease, defect in fumaryl acetoacetate hydrolase, increased urinary succinylacetone, treatment with NTBC (inhibits tyrosine metabolism), increased risk of hepatocellular cancer | 151, 155 |
| Mitochondrial disease | Hypoglycemia, severe lactic acidosis, fetal onset | 156, 157 |
| Neonatal hemochromatosis | Severe hypoalbuminemia, coagulopathy, hypoglycemia; iron deposition in liver, heart, intestine, pancreas, buccal mucosa; MRI may be diagnostic | 153 |
| Niemann-Pick disease type C | Presentation at infancy, childhood, or adolescence; severe hepatic dysfunction, psychomotor delay; bone marrow diagnostic; may progress despite OLT | 151 |
| Zellweger syndrome (cerebrohepatorenal syndrome) | Hypotonia, growth retardation, mental retardation, renal cortical cysts, hepatic dysfunction, increased urinary pipecolic acid, abnormal mitochondria liver, kidneys, brain | |

CMV, cytomegalovirus; CNS, central nervous system; DIC, disseminated intravascular coagulopathy; EBV, Epstein-Barr virus; FTA, fluorescent treponemal antibody; HBV, hepatitis B virus; HSV, herpes simplex virus; MRI, magnetic resonance imaging; NTBC, 2-(2-nitro-4-trifluoromethylbenzoyl)cyclohexane-1-3-dione; OLT, orthotopic liver transplantation; PCR, polymerase chain reaction; RPR, rapid plasma reagin.

and free hepatic venous pressure, which reflects inferior vena cava (IVC) pressure. The normal gradient should be less than 5 mm Hg. A gradient higher than this indicates portal hypertension. A gradient of more than 12 mm Hg indicates severe portal hypertension and is associated with an increased risk of variceal bleeding and the development of ascites in patients with chronic liver disease.

Patients with FHF do not invariably have evidence of severe portal hypertension such as ascites or splenomegaly, unlike the majority of patients with chronic liver failure.[11] Portal hypertension in patients with FHF is secondary to increased hepatic resistance to hepatic blood flow due to sinusoidal collapse and distortion of the liver cell architecture and microcirculation after extensive liver cell necrosis.[30] Although important prognostic information can be obtained by liver biopsy in acute liver injury, biopsy is associated with a high rate of complications and may not alter management. The development of ascites correlates with elevated HVPG even in patients with acute liver failure. Eighty percent of the patients with ascites have a HVPG of more than 12, whereas only 30% of the patients without ascites had a similar gradient.[30] The presence of ascites at admission is a poor prognostic factor in children with FHF who do not undergo a liver transplant.[9]

In patients with chronic liver failure, portal hypertension can be due to sinusoidal fibrosis and nodular regeneration in the liver. Other causes of portal hypertension in patients with chronic liver disease include massive infiltration of the liver parenchyma seen with amyloid or an oncologic disorder or outflow obstruction that is seen with veno-occlusive disease. Portal hypertension is associated with an increased risk of bleeding from esophageal varices in children with chronic liver disease. Endoscopic sclerotherapy, band ligation, and prophylactic β-blockade therapy are discussed elsewhere[31–40] (see Chapter 51).

## *Circulatory Changes*

Acute liver failure is associated with a hyperdynamic circulation—a high cardiac output and a decrease in systemic vascular resistance and mean arterial pressure.[30] Vasodilation may trigger activation of neurohumoral factors that result in sodium retention, extracellular fluid volume expansion, and the development of ascites.[30] Dilation of the splanchnic circulation will result in increased portal venous flow and increased portal pressure, especially in the context of increased hepatic vascular resistance.[30] The cause of systemic vasodilation may be the accumulation of vasoactive substances of splanchnic origin in the systemic circulation that are either metabolized by the normal liver or abnormally released during acute liver failure.[30]

Patients with chronic liver failure have elevated portal pressures and may have intravascular volume depletion, peripheral vasodilation, dilation of the splanchnic vascular bed, and arteriovenous shunting. Vigorous diuretic administration or therapeutic paracentesis may result in a further decrease in the circulating plasma volume, further reducing renal perfusion and increasing sodium retention.[41]

**TABLE 52–3. Etiology of Fulminant Hepatic Failure in Late Infancy and Childhood**

| | CHARACTERISTICS | SELECTED REFERENCES |
|---|---|---|
| **Infectious** | | |
| EBV | Measure EBV VCA IgM, and IgG; anti-EA to diagnose; no chronic hepatic disease | 158 |
| Hepatitis A | Serum HAV IgM | 54 |
| Hepatitis B, C, Δ, E | Measure HBV DNA, HCV RNA | 159, 160 |
| Hepatitis non-A, non-B, non-C | Togavirus–like particles found in some patients; may have acute liver failure and hemorrhagic necrosis following OLT | 161 |
| Varicella zoster | Very rare, cutaneous lesions, IV acyclovir and OLT | 162 |
| **Ischemia** | | |
| Congestive heart failure, pericardial tamponade, hepatic artery thrombosis | Arterial thrombosis may follow OLT and cause graft failure | |
| Budd-Chiari syndrome/ hepatic vein thrombosis | Ascites, retrograde portal flow, acute hepatocellular necrosis possible with acute occlusion, malignancy may be associated | 163 |
| Veno-occlusive disease | Nonthrombotic occlusion of small veins; occurs after pyrrolizidine alkaloid ingestion (bush tea), chemotherapy, transplantation, irradiation | 164 |
| **Malignancy** | Hemophagocytic lymphohistiocytosis, leukemia, lymphoma (Hodgkin's and non-Hodgkin's), hemangioendothelioma or lymphendothelioma, nephroblastoma | 151, 163, 165–168 |
| **Metabolic/Miscellaneous** | | |
| Autoimmune hepatitis | Anti-LKM or anti–smooth muscle antibody positive | 169 |
| Sickle cell disease | May be due to massive hepatic sickling | |
| **Toxin** (see also medications in Table 52–1) | | |
| Aflatoxin | *Aspergillus* sp. and other molds; contamination of nuts, corn, wheat, barley, rice, soybeans; increased prevalence in tropics | 170 |
| *Amanita phalloides* | Dose-related hepatic and renal toxicity; initially cholera-like watery diarrhea, later develop jaundice, encephalopathy, seizures, mortality high if encephalopathy present | 171 |
| Copper intoxication | May be due to tap water with high copper levels, histology resembles Indian childhood cirrhosis | 172 |
| Iron | Pathology due to mitochondrial damage | 173 |

EA, early antigen; EBV, Epstein-Barr virus; HAV, hepatitis A virus; HBV, hepatitis B virus; HCV, hepatitis C virus; IV, intravenous; LKM, liver-kidney microsomal; OLT, orthotopic liver transplantation; VCA, viral capsid antigen.

**TABLE 52–4. Etiology of Fulminant Hepatic Failure in Adolescents and Young Adults**

| | CHARACTERISTICS | SELECTED REFERENCES |
|---|---|---|
| **Infectious** | | |
| *Bacillus cereus* | Rhabdomyolysis associated, rapid development after exposure; toxin inhibits mitochondrial fatty acid oxidation; histology: microvesicular steatosis | 174 |
| Hepatitis A, B, C, Δ, E | See Table 52–3 | |
| Parvovirus | Aplastic anemia associated, parvovirus B19 DNA and anti-B19 ELISA diagnostic | 175 |
| **Metabolic/Miscellaneous** | | |
| Autoimmune hepatitis | Anti-LKM or anti–smooth muscle antibody positive | |
| Pregnancy | Presentation in third trimester, microvesicular steatosis, renal dysfunction, improved liver function after delivery if patient survives, high maternal and infant mortality | |
| Wilson's disease | Incidence, 1 in 30,000; elevated copper levels cornea, brain, kidneys, bones, joints, and cardiac muscle, severe Coombs'-negative hemolytic anemia | 155, 176 |
| See also causes in Table 52–3. | | |

ELISA, enzyme-linked immunosorbent assay; LKM, liver-kidney microsomal.

**TABLE 52–5. Etiology of Cirrhosis in Childhood**

| |
|---|
| Alagille's syndrome |
| Alpha$_1$-antitrypsin deficiency |
| Autoimmune disease |
| Biliary atresia |
| Byler's disease |
| Cryptogenic |
| Cystic fibrosis |
| Galactosemia |
| Glycogen storage disease type 4 |
| Hemochromatosis |
| Hepatic venous outflow obstruction |
| Budd-Chiari/veno-occlusive disease |
| Indian childhood cirrhosis |
| Inflammatory bowel disease |
| Sclerosing cholangitis |
| Medication |
| Protoporphyria (rare) |
| Total parenteral nutrition/intestinal bypass |
| Tyrosinemia |
| Viral hepatitis (B, C, Δ) |
| Wilson's disease |
| Zellweger's syndrome (cerebrohepatorenal syndrome) |
| Other miscellaneous |

## Electrolyte Changes and Renal Failure

Hypoglycemia (blood glucose <40 mg/dL) is due to depletion of hepatic glycogen stores and impaired gluconeogenesis with massive hepatic necrosis or end-stage liver disease.[42, 43] Contributing factors include elevated serum insulin concentrations, as a result of decreased hepatic insulin catabolism, and abnormal levels of glucagon and growth hormone. Hypoglycemia is more frequently a significant problem with FHF than with chronic hepatic failure. It is especially problematic in patients with Reye's syndrome and hereditary fructose intolerance. Neurologic changes due to hypoglycemia may be the initial presenting symptom in unsuspected hepatic failure.

Hyponatremia is frequently present in patients with acute and chronic liver disease because of decreased water excretion, increased renal sodium retention due to stimulation of the renin-angiotensin aldosterone system, and decreased activity of the sodium-potassium pump.[44] Hypokalemia often accompanies hyponatremia and may be due to renal losses and hyperaldosteronism. With severe renal impairment, hyperkalemia may develop. Other electrolyte abnormalities seen with acute or chronic liver failure include hypocalcemia and hypomagnesemia. Calcium levels should be corrected for corresponding albumin levels.

Renal failure is present in 40% of patients with acute liver failure and may be due to an imbalance between neurohumoral factors, renal vasoconstrictors, and vasodilators.[1, 30] Patients have marked renal vasoconstriction despite systemic vasodilation.[30] Plasma renin activity is typically increased and renal prostaglandin activity is decreased in patients with acute liver failure. An elevated serum creatinine at admission is a poor prognostic sign in patients with FHF due to acetaminophen overdose or other causes. Creatinine levels are significantly higher after acetaminophen overdose than with other causes of FHF.[10, 45, 46] Acidosis at admission is also a poor prognostic sign.[45] Acid-base disturbances may be present in up to 60% of children with FHF.[1] Acute tubular necrosis is present at autopsy in some children with FHF, although others appear to have "functional renal failure" with normal histology.[3]

Renal excretion of sodium is significantly decreased in patients with well-established cirrhosis and is an important pathophysiologic cause of ascites formation.[44] In addition to the development of hepatorenal syndrome characterized by redistribution of blood flow away from the renal cortex, renal changes in cirrhosis include glomerular sclerosis and membranoproliferative glomerulonephritis.[47–49] Acute tubular necrosis is also seen in patients with cirrhosis and is distinguished by a higher fractional excretion of sodium than seen with hepatorenal syndrome.

## Hepatic Encephalopathy and Cerebral Edema

**FULMINANT LIVER FAILURE.** Hepatic encephalopathy is graded from I to IV[50–52] (Table 52–6). In one pediatric series, encephalopathy developed within 3 weeks of the initial symptoms of hepatitis in 88% of children with FHF. The survival in many series of acute liver failure correlates directly with the degree of encephalopathy, with 60% survival with grade I, decreasing to 5% to 25% with grade IV disease.[3, 11] There is a rapid progression through the stages of encephalopathy in children with FHF, although in some cases there may be a transient improvement prior to the final deterioration.[3, 53] In pediatric series before the availability of OLT for FHF, the mean interval between the onset of encephalopathy and death was 4.2 to 8.4 days.[1, 3] The duration of encephalopathy does not correlate directly with survival owing to early deaths of nonsurvivors.[11] Jaundice of longer than 7 days' duration before the development of hepatic encephalopathy is associated with a poor outcome.[10] Severe encephalopathy may be associated with electrolyte disturbances and hypotension, making affected patients less suitable candidates for transplantation.[9] Because of the short interval between onset of encephalopathy and patient death in patients with FHF, rapid transfer to a center able to perform emergency liver transplantation and early listing is essential to improve patient survival.[9, 53] Even with early listing and successful transplantation, there may be neurologic sequelae in patients with advanced encephalopathy who undergo transplantation. Neurologic disease is a significant cause of post-transplant morbidity and mortality in patients receiving transplants for FHF.[1, 9, 54]

It is generally accepted that hepatic encephalopathy is due to ammonia-induced alteration of the brain neurotransmitter balance, especially at the astrocyte-neuron interface.[55] The specific mechanisms are still controversial. Several authors have postulated that activation of the gamma-aminobutyric acid (GABA)/benzodiazepine inhibitory neurotransmitter system plays an important role in the pathogenesis of hepatic encephalopathy. GABA, the principal inhibitory neurotransmitter of the brain, is normally generated in the intestinal tract and degraded in the liver. During liver failure, GABA may escape hepatic metabolism and induce an increase in the number of its own receptors.[53] An endogenous benzodiazepine agonist present in patients with liver failure may increase the inhibitory activity of GABA in patients with FHF. Intravenous administration of flumazenil, a benzodiaze-

TABLE 52–6. Stages of Hepatic Encephalopathy

| STAGE | CLINICAL MANIFESTATIONS | ASTERIXIS/ REFLEXES | NEUROLOGIC SIGNS | EEG CHANGES |
|---|---|---|---|---|
| Subclinical | None | Absent/normal | Abnormalities on psychometric testing and proton magnetic spectroscopy in older patients | Usually absent |
| I | Confused, mood changes, altered sleep habits, loss of spatial orientation, forgetfulness | Absent/normal | Tremor, apraxia, impaired handwriting | May be absent, or diffuse, slowing to theta rhythm, triphasic waves |
| II | Drowsy, inappropriate behavior, decreased inhibitions | Present/hyperreflexic | Dysarthria, ataxia | Abnormal, generalized slowing, triphasic waves |
| III | Child is stuporous but obeys simple commands; infant is sleeping but arousable | Present/hyperreflexic with positive Babinski sign | Muscle rigidity | Abnormal, generalized slowing, triphasic waves |
| IV | Child is comatose but arousable by painful stimuli (IVa) or does not respond to stimuli (IVb) | Absent | Decerebrate or decorticate | Abnormal, very slow delta activity |

EEG, electroencephalography.
Data from references 50, 52, 53, 177.

pine antagonist, has not been effective in reversing clinical or electrophysiologic brain abnormalities in children with FHF.[53] Other postulated mechanisms of hepatic encephalopathy include depletion of excitatory neurotransmitters such as norepinephrine or dopamine, production of false neurotransmitters such as octopamine, increased permeability of the blood-brain barrier allowing toxic substances access to the central nervous system, and astrocyte dysfunction.[56, 57]

Cerebral edema is frequently present in patients with FHF and hepatic encephalopathy, unlike patients with chronic hepatic encephalopathy.[53] Brain edema occurs in 45% or more of patients with FHF and is the major cause of morbidity and mortality.[1, 56] It may develop concurrently with other symptoms of hepatitis, or its development may be delayed.[3] Papilledema is usually absent in patients with FHF and cerebral edema, unlike patients with cerebral edema from other causes.

Cerebral blood flow adjusted for $CO_2$ levels (aCBF) correlates with cerebral swelling and mortality in patients with FHF. Patients with FHF may have hyperemia, normal flow, or decreased cerebral blood flow. Increased cerebral blood flow may be associated with cerebral swelling on computed tomography (CT) scan, but CT changes occur late and are absent in the majority of patients with increased intracranial pressure (ICP) by epidural monitoring.[58] The presence of cerebral edema is a worse prognostic sign than renal failure, gastrointestinal (GI) bleeding, or infection; only a bilirubin level higher than 20 mg/dL is a worse prognostic sign. In a series of children not undergoing liver transplantation for FHF, cerebral edema by CT scan was seen in 50% of nonsurvivors but never seen in survivors ($p = .02$).[9]

Epidural ICP monitors appear to be more effective than CT scanning to detect increased ICP in patients with FHF, and they appear to be safe even in patients with markedly prolonged coagulation studies without associated thrombocytopenia (platelets $<50 \times 10^9$/L). This type of monitor can identify rises in ICP not associated with clinical symptoms.[59] Complications of ICP monitoring include hemorrhage, infection, and cerebrospinal fluid leak.[60] Epidural monitors appear to be safer than subdural bolts or parenchymal monitors, which are associated with a higher rate of hemorrhage in patients with FHF.[60] Absolute ICP pressures may be less accurate with epidural monitors than with parenchymal monitors, but epidural monitors are still effective in measuring changes in ICP.[60]

**CHRONIC HEPATIC FAILURE.** Chronic hepatic encephalopathy may be present in up to 50% to 70% of patients with cirrhosis.[52] Episodes of encephalopathy usually have a precipitating event or are due to portosystemic shunting, for example after insertion of a transjugular intrahepatic portosystemic shunt (TIPS) for management of esophageal varices.[52, 61] Other precipitating factors include GI hemorrhage, infection, and hypokalemia, which increase ammonia production; systemic alkalosis, which increases diffusion of ammonia across the blood-brain barrier; and hypoxemia, hypotension, dehydration, and progressive parenchymal damage, which decrease hepatic metabolism.[52] Postulated contributing factors include decreased activity of urea cycle enzymes as a result of zinc depletion and manganese deposition in the basal ganglia.[52] Characteristic changes have been noted by proton magnetic resonance spectroscopy in patients with chronic cirrhosis without clinical evidence of hepatic encephalopathy, but further study will be required before determining whether they are a cause or effect of encephalopathy.[55, 57] There may be a long latency before changes of chronic hepatic encephalopathy are detectable by current neuropsychological and neurophysiologic testing methods such as psychometric testing, evoked potentials, and electroencephalographic procedures.[55, 57] In children without encephalopathy but with chronic liver disease, patients with early-onset liver disease (initial symptoms in the first year of life) have been found to have reduced intelligence quotient scores when compared with children with chronic liver disease of later onset.[62] This may be due to vulnerability of an infant's brain to metabolic abnormalities accompanying liver disease or to poor nutritional status, including vitamin E deficiency in young children with chronic liver disease.[62]

Although ammonia levels are typically elevated in patients with chronic hepatic encephalopathy, especially patients with portosystemic shunting, they correlate poorly with the degree of encephalopathy and are therefore not helpful in following the progression of encephalopathy.[52]

### *Pulmonary Disease*

Adult respiratory distress syndrome (ARDS) frequently complicates acute or chronic liver failure and is often irreversible despite medical therapy. ARDS is characterized by a combination of bilateral diffuse infiltrates on chest x-ray, decreased pulmonary compliance, and hypoxemia requiring supplemental oxygen. Sepsis appears to be an important risk factor for the development of ARDS in patients with liver failure; patients with liver failure may have impaired Kupffer cell function, normally responsible for detoxification of gut-derived bacteria and their products.[63] Although the prognosis of ARDS associated with liver failure is very poor, ARDS has been shown to rapidly resolve after successful liver transplantation.[63]

Pulmonary arteriovenous shunting with hypoxemia is frequently present in children with chronic liver disease and portal hypertension and may present with dyspnea on exertion or cyanosis.[64] This complication is more frequent in patients with biliary atresia and polysplenia syndrome, although it may be present in noncirrhotic patients with portal hypertension. Shunting is detected by measuring serial arterial blood gases while breathing room air and 100% oxygen, technetium $^{99m}$Tc macroaggregated albumin pulmonary scanning, measurement of the alveoloarterial $PO_2$ gradient, or contrast echocardiography.[64] This condition is reversible after liver transplantation.[64]

### *Coagulopathy*

The liver is responsible for the synthesis of factors II, V, VII, VIII, IX, and X. Reduced levels of these factors and other proteins important in coagulation reflect abnormalities of protein synthesis and impaired post-translational modification of vitamin K–dependent proteins (factors II, VII, IX, X; protein C, S). Factor VIII is synthesized in the liver and endothelial cells; levels are increased in acute and chronic liver disease, including FHF. A high concentration of factor VIII is a result of damaged vascular endothelial cells. The levels of all the other factors are typically decreased in liver disease, usually to an average of 20% or less of normal.[24]

Factor V, which is vitamin K independent, may be the most sensitive single indicator of outcome in FHF. A rapid decrease in the level of this factor, which has a half-life of 12 to 24 hours, reflects impaired synthesis due to rapidly developing liver damage.[45] Factor V levels are significantly decreased in nonsurvivors as compared with survivors.[1, 24] The degree of decrease varies with the cause of FHF. In children with FHF due to viral hepatitis or drug injury, factor V levels were significantly higher in survivors without liver transplant (28 ± 11%) than in children who died (13 ± 7%) or received a transplant (18 ± 5%) ($p < .01$).[1] In patients with acetaminophen overdose, admission levels less than 10% were 91% sensitive but only 55% specific in predicting fatal cases.[45] The specificity increased to 91% if the admission factor V level of less than 10% was combined with grade III or IV encephalopathy. Admission values of these factors could be used to select patients who would benefit from early listing for liver transplantation after acetaminophen overdose or other causes of FHF, while avoiding performing transplants on patients who would be expected to recover.[24] The levels can be rapidly assayed in coagulation laboratories.

The prothrombin time (PT) is an important prognostic sign in patients with fulminant and chronic hepatic failure and is used to determine the timing of listing for liver transplant[65] (Table 52–7). With intact vitamin K stores, the prothrombin time is a reliable indicator of hepatic synthetic capacity.[66] In children with FHF due to viral hepatitis or toxin injury, prothrombin times are usually less than 14% to 20% of normal.[1] In one pediatric series of FHF, only patients with a PT of less than 90 seconds survived, although 60% of nonsurvivors had PTs of less than 90 seconds.[3] In the case of acetaminophen overdose, the PT at admission is not helpful in differentiating survivors and nonsurvivors.[45] Fibrinogen levels are in the range of 0.8 g/L in children with FHF, and when associated with increased fibrinogen degradation products indicate fibrinolysis and disseminated intravascular coagulation.[1, 67]

Patients with coagulopathy secondary to liver disease may

**TABLE 52–7. Child-Turcotte Classification with Pugh Modification**

| | A | B | C |
|---|---|---|---|
| Serum bilirubin (mg/dL) | <2 | 2–3 | >3 |
| Serum albumin (g/dL) | >3.5 | 3–3.5 | <3 |
| Ascites | Absent | Easily controlled | Poorly controlled |
| Neurologic disorder | Absent | Minimal | Coma |
| Nutrition* | Excellent | Good | Poor |
| Prothrombin time (PT)* (seconds above control) | <4 | 4–6 | >6 |

*If a numerical score is assigned, either the PT or nutritional status should be included, but not both.

Data from Child CG III, Turcotte J: In Child CG III (ed): The Liver and Portal Hypertension. Philadelphia, WB Saunders, 1965; and Pugh RN, Murray-Lyon IM, Dawson JL, et al: Transection of the oesophagus for bleeding oesophageal varices. Br J Surg 1973;60:646–649.

be asymptomatic or may have bleeding from the GI tact, nasopharynx, retroperitoneum, tracheobronchial tree, genitourinary tract, or subcutaneous tissues or intracranial bleeding.[66] Bleeding may be intermittent or continuous.

### Abnormal Liver Function Tests and Liver Biopsy

**FULMINANT HEPATIC FAILURE.** At admission, the mean aminotransferase in pediatric FHF is in the range of 2500 IU/L, with a wide standard deviation (SD ± 2400).[1, 3] The extent of elevation varies based on the cause. In patients not undergoing liver transplantation, survivors have significantly higher admission aminotransferase levels than nonsurvivors (SGOT mean 5644 U/L, SGPT mean 3522 U/L versus SGOT 1092 U/L, SGPT 1004 U/L; $p = .02$).[9] Low transaminase values with an elevated bilirubin suggest ongoing liver deterioration rather than improvement. Mean total serum bilirubin values at admission are in the range of 23 mg/dL, with a wide standard deviation.[1] Serum aminotransferase levels and bilirubin levels are not helpful in differentiating survivors from nonsurvivors after acetaminophen overdose.[45] Serum albumin levels are frequently less than 3.5 g/dL in patients with FHF.

Liver biopsies performed in patients with FHF are classified into two types. Type 1 is characterized by extensive hepatocellular necrosis with collapse of the reticulin fibers, infiltration with lymphocytes and plasma cells, bile duct proliferation, and canalicular cholestasis.[43, 54] The necrosis may be diffuse or centrilobular, adjacent to the hepatic venule seen typically with acetaminophen overdose. Type 1 is seen with viral hepatitis, halothane hepatitis, acetaminophen toxicity, isoniazid toxicity, and *Amanita phalloides* poisoning. Type 2 is characterized by microvesicular fatty infiltration of the hepatocytes without nuclear displacement and is seen with pregnancy and with tetracycline, valproate, and pirprofen toxicity and is similar to the liver biopsies of patients with Reye's syndrome. [43]

Biopsy is infrequently helpful in establishing the cause of acute liver failure and may be dangerous in the setting of severe coagulopathy. Cases in which liver biopsy may help establish the diagnosis include neonatal hemochromatosis, although buccal biopsy is safer, and malignancy presenting as FHF. Transjugular liver biopsy has been advocated in patients with FHF as a safer alternative to percutaneous biopsy.[46] Extensive necrosis of the liver parenchyma indicates little chance of spontaneous recovery and should prompt immediate listing for OLT.[46]

**CHRONIC HEPATIC FAILURE.** Serum aminotransferase levels are normal in patients with end-stage liver disease and cirrhosis due to significant hepatocyte destruction, although they are increased in some patients. Serum bilirubin levels and gamma globulin levels are frequently increased. Gamma globulin levels may be particularly high in patients with autoimmune liver disease (see Chapter 50). Serum albumin levels are decreased and along with bilirubin levels are used to classify the severity of liver disease (see Table 52–7). Alkaline phosphatase levels are usually increased.[68]

In patients with cirrhosis, liver biopsy may be diagnostic, especially if special staining or quantitative methods are available to confirm the diagnosis. This is true in alpha$_1$-antitrypsin deficiency, hepatitis B infection, iron deposition, and Wilson's disease. However, the cause is often established by blood chemistries, and biopsy is used to determine the degree of parenchymal scarring. Cirrhosis is characterized by diffuse fibrosis of the liver with regenerating nodules.[69]

## Findings on Physical Examination

**FULMINANT HEPATIC FAILURE.** Patients with FHF often have rapidly progressing jaundice associated with nausea and malaise. The liver may be normal in size, enlarged, or small. Ascites may be present or absent. Splenomegaly does not necessarily accompany FHF. Hyperventilation and tachycardia may be present, especially with significant neurologic disease. Prolonged bleeding may be noted from venipuncture sites. Fetor hepaticus, a sweetish smell to the breath, may be present. Hepatic encephalopathy may antedate or follow other signs of hepatic failure.

**CHRONIC HEPATIC FAILURE.** Jaundice is a late feature of chronic liver disease, indicating significant hepatocellular destruction. The liver is usually not palpable, but if felt, is very firm. Other signs of cirrhosis include splenomegaly due to portal hypertension, ascites, caput medusae, fetor hepaticus, spider telangiectasias, petechiae, palmar erythema, white nails, clubbing, malnutrition, gynecomastia in males, and hypogonadism.[70] Hepatic encephalopathy has already been discussed. Patients with chronic liver disease due to specific causes have additional findings, such as Kayser-Fleischer rings in patients with Wilson's disease or posterior embryotoxon in patients with Alagille's syndrome. These are discussed in Chapters 47–49.

## Prognostic Factors

**FULMINANT HEPATIC FAILURE.** Younger age may be a good prognostic factor, with age younger than 15 years associated with an increased survival rate than age between 15 and 44 years or age older than 45.[4, 71] Survival rates in acute liver failure differ significantly based on the cause. In acute liver failure due to hepatitis B infection, younger age, negative HBsAg, positive anti-HBs, higher factor V concentrations, and elevated alpha fetoprotein levels are associated with a better outcome.[71] Negative hepatitis B surface antigen (HBsAg) levels and positive antibody to hepatitis B surface antigen titers are thought to reflect clearance and neutralization of serum HBsAg, as a result of an excessive immune response to HBsAg or cessation of HBsAg production secondary to massive destruction of hepatitis B virus (HBV)–infected hepatocytes.[71] The presence or absence of coma and aminotransferase levels are not good prognostic indicators.[10] Massive hepatocyte necrosis on liver biopsy is a poor prognostic indicator.[2, 46] The stage of hepatic encephalopathy discussed earlier is probably the most important prognostic indicator.[4, 46] Complications of FHF such as renal failure, ventilatory failure, and GI bleeding also decrease survival rates. In patients with FHF not caused by acetaminophen toxicity, a serum bilirubin level of more than 18mg/dL and PT INR (Prothrombin Time International Normalized Ratio) levels of more than 3.5, and especially more than 6.5, are associated with poor outcome.[46]

**CHRONIC LIVER FAILURE.** Patients with cirrhosis

are usually classified by the Child's scoring system, which incorporates serum bilirubin and albumin, the presence of ascites, or neurologic changes and the patient's nutritional status.[72, 73] A modified Child's-Pugh scale uses PT in place of nutritional status.[74] Each variable is assigned one point (see Table 52–7). In a large study of liver disease–related deaths, 1 year survival was 100% for patients with a Child's-Pugh score of 5 to 6, 80% for a score of 7 to 9, and 45% for a score of 10 to 15.[75] In addition to predicting short-term survival, this classification system is used to predict the likelihood of variceal bleeding and influences the timing of listing for liver transplantation. Other more extensive classification systems have been developed but do not appear to offer any significant advantage over the Child's-Pugh system.[75, 76]

## Management

Care of the patient with FHF may be optimized by hospitalization at a transplant center. Survival is significantly better in patients undergoing early rather than late transfer.[9] Although there is significant morbidity within the first few days of developing hepatic failure, those patients surviving the early stages of the disease benefit from the intensive care management and the ability to recognize and treat the developing signs of progressive liver failure.

### *Fluid Restriction and Treatment of Hypoglycemia and Hyponatremia*

Patients with liver failure have an increased glucose requirement, which can usually be satisfied by administration of dextrose 10% to 20% to maintain a serum glucose of more than 60 mg/dL. Higher concentrations of glucose are required for persistent or symptomatic hypoglycemia. Maintaining normal blood glucose levels is especially challenging in these patients who require fluid restriction because of total body sodium and fluid overload and frequently have hypokalemia due to diuretic therapy and impaired renal function.

In patients unable to take fluids orally, intravenous fluids are usually administered at a rate to replace insensible losses, while maintaining adequate blood glucose levels. Supplementation of intravenous fluids with calcium and magnesium is often required.[42, 43] Hyponatremia should not be corrected with hypertonic saline, which worsens hepatic encephalopathy and total body fluid overload. Potassium-sparing diuretics such as spironolactone are helpful in patients with ascites due to hyperaldosteronism.[44] Severe renal dysfunction may be associated with the development of hyperkalemia. In patients with chronic liver failure, a sodium-restricted diet is an important adjuvant to diuretic therapy.[41] Medication administration to patients with acute and chronic liver disease and renal impairment should be modified accordingly.

### *Nutrition*

Adequate nutritional intake is essential in patients with liver failure. Enteral nutrition is preferred. Infants are given formulas with a higher concentration of medium-chain triglycerides, which do not require incorporation into bile acid–containing mixed micelles for intestinal absorption.[77] Care should be taken to avoid formulas that predispose patients to essential fatty acid deficiency or dicarboxylic aciduria.[78] Patients with biliary tract obstruction should receive supplementation of fat-soluble vitamins (A, D, E, K) because of deficient bile acid reabsorption.[77, 79] Complications of fat-soluble vitamin deficiency include xerosis, night blindness, rickets, osteoporosis, peripheral neuropathy, ataxia, ophthalmoplegia, impaired immune function, and coagulopathy.[77, 79]

Patients with chronic liver disease and hepatic encephalopathy may benefit from oral protein restriction, but they may require a daily intake of 0.8 to 1.0 g/kg/day to maintain nitrogen balance.[80] Vegetable protein with increased fiber may have advantages when compared with animal protein.[52, 81] In patients with end-stage disease due to acute or chronic liver failure, parenteral nutrition may be required. The majority of patients with chronic liver failure tolerate parenteral nutrition solutions containing a standard amino acid mixture.[82] Branched chain amino acid (BCAA) solutions that have 35% BCAA compared with 14% to 25% in standard solutions have been advocated for patients with chronic liver failure and encephalopathy. Abnormalities have been noted in amino acid profiles in cirrhotics, and it has been hypothesized that decreased concentrations of BCAAs and increased concentrations of aromatic amino acids result in the production of false neurotransmitters.[52] Randomized controlled trials using BCAA solutions have noted a short-term beneficial effect on mental recovery from hepatic encephalopathy with conflicting results on case fatality rates.[82]

### *Management of Hepatic Encephalopathy: Fulminant Hepatic Failure*

The primary goal in patients with FHF is to keep intracranial pressure (ICP) lower than 25 mm Hg. Intracranial pressures lower than 25 mm Hg are associated with improved cerebral perfusion and a decreased risk of herniation. The cerebral perfusion pressure (CPP) should be higher than 40 to 50 mm Hg. CPP is the calculated difference between the mean arterial pressure (MAP) and the ICP.[66] Because of coagulation abnormalities, many patients will be unable to undergo invasive monitoring and will be monitored by CT scans instead of a bolt or epidural monitor.[58] Following ICP by CT is less reliable than using direct measurement.[58]

Methods to reduce ICP include elective intubation, mannitol infusion, and sodium and fluid restriction.[9]

### *Management of Chronic Hepatic Encephalopathy*

Approximately 50% of ammonia production is derived from the small intestine and 50% from the colon. Small intestinal ammonia production increases in relative importance after a meal, when amino acid metabolism and absorption result in increased ammonia production. Metabolism of dairy and vegetable proteins appears to produce less ammonia than animal protein. Other factors influencing intestinal nitrogen balance include accompanying carbohydrate malabsorption and increased dietary fiber.[83]

Lactulose (β-galactosidofructose) and lactitol (β-galactosidosorbitol), two nonabsorbable disaccharides administered to reduce ammonia levels, have been shown to be effective in diminishing signs of chronic hepatic encephalopathy, by their osmotic cathartic actions and other mechanisms.[52, 84, 85] Lactulose, like neomycin, has beneficial effects on small intestinal ammonia production by interfering with intestinal glutaminase, thereby inhibiting enterocyte glutamine uptake.[83] Lactulose's alteration of colonic bacterial metabolism can potentially interfere with one half of fasting ammonia production. Lactulose works by providing a carbohydrate energy source to colonic bacterial flora, thereby competitively decreasing bacterial metabolism of nitrogen-containing compounds and increasing incorporation of ammonia and amino acid nitrogen into an expanding bacterial mass excreted in the stool.[52, 83] Lactitol and lactose enemas are effective in patients unable to take disaccharides by mouth or via nasogastric tube.[86] It is helpful to discontinue lactulose administration before OLT, to reduce gaseous distention of the bowel.

Administration of purified soluble fiber pectin in cirrhotic patients also increases fecal nitrogen excretion, decreases urea production, inhibits bacterial ureolysis in the colon, and has been shown to have a beneficial effect in patients with hepatic encephalopathy.[83, 87] Other agents of demonstrated benefit in chronic hepatic encephalopathy include ornithine aspartate, sodium benzoate, and zinc, all important in ammonia detoxification.[52]

Poorly absorbed oral antibiotics such as neomycin are given to inhibit urease-containing colonic bacteria and inhibit proteolytic enzyme activity, thereby reducing ammonia production. These antibiotics may have other beneficial effects on bacterial metabolites that contribute to hepatic encephalopathy. When used in combination with lactulose, antibiotics with high efficacy against anaerobes such as metronidazole may reduce the efficacy of lactulose, which depends on bacterial metabolism. This can be monitored by an increase in fecal pH.[52] Oral neomycin and lactulose coadministration has additive beneficial effects.[83]

### *Infection*

*Candida albicans* is frequently an opportunistic pathogen in children and adults with fulminant hepatic failure.[3, 88] Bacterial infections are frequently due to staphylococcal disease and *Pseudomonas*. Indwelling catheters and procedures such as plasmapheresis increase the risk of infection. *Escherichia coli* sepsis and meningitis may occur in infants with galactosemia; streptococcus pneumonia peritonitis is a frequent cause of infection in patients with ascites. Patients with fulminant hepatic failure may fail to develop fever or leukocytosis with bacterial infection or may develop these complications without infection due to hepatic necrosis.[88] In some centers, routine surveillance cultures are performed. Intravenous antibiotics are administered as necessary but are not used prophylactically.

### *Treatment of Coagulopathy*

Vitamin K, 5 to 10 mg subcutaneously, is administered in patients with depleted hepatic stores but may be administered intravenously in patients with fulminant hepatic failure. The dose is 1 mg/kg/year of age/day for three consecutive days, and then every other day.[42] Fresh frozen plasma (FFP) may be administered in asymptomatic patients with a severe prolongation of their PT (>25 to 35 seconds) but is almost always used for patients with active bleeding with a prolonged PT and decreased factor V levels or before invasive procedures.[66] Administration of FFP increases the difficulty of following PT and factor V levels as prognostic indicators. Volumes of FFP administered may be limited by fluid overload.[66] Patients with a mild asymptomatic prolongation in clotting studies do not usually require therapy.

### *Charcoal Hemoperfusion and Plasmapheresis*

Early trials suggested that charcoal hemoperfusion would significantly improve survival in patients with fulminant hepatic failure. Charcoal is an effective adsorbent for a wide range of soluble molecules and toxins that accumulate in fulminant hepatic failure.[12] In controlled trials, charcoal hemoperfusion does not provide an additional benefit over specialized intensive care unit care. Plasmapheresis has been shown to have limited beneficial effect in children with fulminant hepatic failure and hepatic encephalopathy.[2, 56] Plasmapheresis should be initiated early in the course of hepatic failure to be of benefit.[2, 56] Complications of plasmapheresis include thrombocytopenia and catheter-related infections.[2]

### *Acetylcysteine*

Acetylcysteine replenishes depleted glutathione stores in acute acetaminophen overdose, thereby decreasing hepatotoxicity. If given more than 15 hours after overdose, this agent is thought to be ineffective. Continuous intravenous acetylcysteine administration has been shown to improve mean arterial blood pressures and oxygen consumption and extraction in patients with established fulminant hepatic failure when administered after the time frame when it would be useful to prevent acetaminophen-induced hepatotoxicity.[89] This effect may be due to stimulation of microcirculatory blood flow or by increasing the ability of the tissues to utilize oxygen.[90] Acetylcysteine administration appears to be most beneficial in FHF resulting from acetaminophen overdose but may be effective in FHF from other causes.[90]

## Outcome in Survivors

Children surviving fulminant hepatic failure typically do well if advanced encephalopathy does not develop. Although changes are frequently present on follow-up liver biopsy, clinical evidence of liver dysfunction is unusual.[3] Patients with advanced encephalopathy before transplant may have persistent neurologic sequelae after successful liver transplant.

# LIVER TRANSPLANTATION

Survival after liver transplantation has improved dramatically since the early 1980s, when cyclosporine use for liver transplantation became common. Between 1987 and 1994, the United Network of Organ Sharing (UNOS) database reported 5-year actuarial patient and graft survivals after pediatric OLT of 75.8% and 59.9%, respectively.[91] More recently, the combination of new immunosuppressive modalities with innovative surgical techniques has allowed pediatric 1-year survival rates to reach close to 90% in many large centers.[92–94]

## Indications

The indications for liver transplantation in children are listed in Tables 52–2 through 52–5 and 52–8.[95, 96] Biliary atresia is the most common indication for OLT in children.[97] Even with timely performance of a biliary drainage procedure, 75% of children with biliary atresia will require OLT, usually before age 5[98] (see Chapter 48). Other frequent indications for OLT include alpha$_1$-antitrypsin deficiency, Wilson's disease, fulminant hepatic failure, chronic active hepatitis with cirrhosis, neonatal hepatitis, autoimmune hepatitis, hepatoblastoma, and hepatocellular carcinoma[99, 100] (see Chapters 47 and 49). Hepatoblastoma has a more favorable prognosis than hepatocellular carcinoma after transplant. Although rare, urea cycle disorders such as ornithine transcarbamylase deficiency and Crigler-Najjar syndrome require OLT in early infancy to avoid profound central nervous system damage.[101, 102] Patients with hereditary tyrosinemia usually undergo OLT before 2 years of age to decrease the risk of developing hepatocellular carcinoma.[103]

## Time of Listing for Orthotopic Liver Transplantation

Children should be listed for OLT if one or more of the following criteria are present: intractable cholestasis, portal hypertension with variceal bleeding, multiple episodes of ascending cholangitis, impaired synthetic function, failure to thrive and malnutrition, intractable ascites, encephalopathy, unacceptable quality of life (e.g., school failure, intractable pruritus), and metabolic diseases for which liver transplantation will reverse life-threatening illness and prevent central nervous system damage. The contraindications to OLT in children are life-threatening, extrahepatic multi-organ system failure and disseminated sepsis. Malnutrition is an important predictor of morbidity and mortality pre- and post-transplant, and preoperative nutrition should be optimized.[104, 105] Children with cholestasis and malabsorption may require parenteral nutrition.

**TABLE 52–8. Other Indications for Liver Transplantation**

| | |
|---|---|
| Caroli's disease | Hyperoxaluria type 1 |
| Crigler-Najjar syndrome type 1 | Lipid storage disease |
| Disorders of bile acid metabolism | Neonatal hepatitis |
| Familial cholestasis syndromes | Organic acidemias |
| Familial hypercholesterolemia | Protein C deficiency |
| Glycogen storage disease IA | Sarcoma |
| Hemophilia A, B | Trauma |
| Hepatoblastoma | Urea cycle defects |
| Hepatocellular carcinoma | |

## Surgical Techniques

Recent advances in transplantation include *reduced liver grafting,* the left lobe or left lateral segment of a cadaveric liver is transplanted, the right side of the donor liver is discarded; *living-related transplantation,* the left lobe or left lateral segment of a parent or a relative is transplanted into the child; and *split liver grafting,* a cadaveric donor liver is surgically divided to create two viable grafts, the smaller left lateral segment for a small child, the right lobe for an adult or larger child.[106] These techniques have significantly reduced waiting time and pre-transplant morbidity of pediatric OLT candidates.[107] Split liver OLT increases the donor pool by allowing two recipients to benefit from one liver. Patient and graft survival rates for both the right and left lobes are approaching 80% to 90%. Living-related transplantation requires careful donor assessment. The success rate for the recipient is excellent, and donor morbidity and mortality is very low (one reported death in the world literature).[108] Despite increased technical difficulty, the complication rates of partial liver grafting have not been increased compared with cadaveric whole organ grafts.

## Surgical Complications

The most important complications are hepatic artery thrombosis (HAT), bleeding, biliary leaks, and bowel perforation. HAT has its highest incidence in young children and is the most common cause of pediatric graft loss.[109] The caliber of the hepatic artery anastomosis may be less than 2 mm. The application of microsurgical techniques in recent years has decreased the incidence of this complication from 15% to 2%.[110] Thrombosis occurs less frequently after partial liver grafting (larger donor artery) than with whole organs transplants from a small donor.[111] Thrombosis may present as fulminant hepatic failure, biliary leaks, relapsing septicemia with fever, or late-onset biliary strictures.[112] Biliary complications occur with thrombosis because the biliary system is dependent on the grafted hepatic artery. Because the presentation may be subtle, a high index of suspicion must be maintained. Diagnosis is by duplex ultrasonography or angiography. The majority of children with HAT require retransplantation.

Biliary leaks may occur either from the cut surface of a partial graft (a minor complication) or from disruption of the biliary anastomosis associated with HAT. The latter is a serious complication requiring urgent surgical repair and possibly retransplantation.[113] Bleeding in the early postoperative period is often associated with coagulopathy due to poor graft function. Bowel perforation is more common in children who have had prior abdominal surgery and has a high morbidity and mortality.[114] Disruption of vascular anastomoses and rupture of mycotic aneurysms are rare but life threatening.

## Immunosuppression

Immunosuppression after OLT is achieved primarily with either cyclosporine (CsA) (Sandimmune, Sandoz Pharmaceuticals, East Hanover, NJ) or tacrolimus (Prograf, Fujisawa

USA Inc., Deerfield, IL). Both drugs are calcineurin inhibitors and inhibit transduction signals for production of interleukin-2 (IL-2) and other cytokines important in rejection.[115] Both drugs are initially combined with low-dose prednisone; azathioprine is sometimes used in conjunction with cyclosporine. Neoral (Sandoz Pharmaceuticals, East Hanover, NJ) is a new microemulsion form of CsA with improved bioavailability.[109] Compared with cyclosporine, tacrolimus-based regimens have a decreased incidence of steroid-resistant chronic rejection and result in a lower cumulative steroid dose.[116, 117] The toxicity profiles of the two drugs are similar; both are nephrotoxic and neurotoxic.[118–120] Unlike cyclosporine, tacrolimus does not result in hirsutism and gingival hypertrophy. Tacrolimus is associated with an increased incidence of Epstein-Barr virus (EBV)–related post-transplant lymphoproliferative disease (PTLD).[121]

Starting doses of oral cyclosporine and tacrolimus are 10 to 20 mg/kg and 0.1 to 0.2 mg/kg, respectively.[122] Pediatric dose requirements are highly variable, frequently exceeding the mg/kg doses of adults. In the early post-transplant period, therapeutic levels of cyclosporine are 250 to 350 ng/mL and for tacrolimus are 10 to 15 ng/mL. Doses are reduced after 3 to 6 months to achieve levels of 150 to 200 ng/mL for cyclosporine and 5 to 8 ng/mL for tacrolimus. Successful steroid weaning has been reported for both cyclosporine- and tacrolimus-based regimens but is associated with a risk of rejection.[123–125]

OKT3 (Orthoclone OKT3, Ortho Biotech Inc., Raritan, NJ), a monoclonal antibody used to treat acute steroid-resistant rejection, is used less often with tacrolimus immunosuppression.[126] The major side effects of OKT3 are high fevers, pulmonary edema, and cardiovascular instability. The development of human anti-mouse antibodies limits its long-term use. Mycophenolate mofetil (CellCept, Roche Laboratories, Nutley, NJ), used for resistant rejection, reduces lymphocyte proliferation and can be used in conjunction with cyclosporine or tacrolimus.[127] Pediatric experience with this agent is limited.

## Rejection

Acute rejection occurs in 50% to 80% of pediatric OLT recipients, usually within the first 3 months after transplantation.[97] Early acute rejection is easily managed and does not have an impact on graft survival or mortality.[128] Signs and symptoms include fever, changes in bile color, increasing aminotransferases or bilirubin levels, back pain, and graft tenderness. Patients are frequently asymptomatic, with elevated aminotransferases noted on routine monitoring. Rejection should be confirmed by liver biopsy to exclude viral infection. Corticosteroid recycling is initiated with high-dose intravenous methylprednisolone for 3 to 7 days with a rapid taper to baseline oral steroid doses. Steroid-resistant rejection is treated by conversion to tacrolimus or a course of OKT3. Chronic rejection has a more ominous prognosis and may result in graft loss. Conversion to tacrolimus may be successful in reversing the process in up to 50% of children if initiated before established hyperbilirubinemia. The incidence of chronic rejection with cyclosporine is 10% to 15%, but less than 3% with tacrolimus. Late acute rejection and chronic rejection may be due to noncompliance with medication.

## Major Medical Complications

### Renal

Renal failure is unusual but is associated with a high morbidity and mortality.[129] Long-term nephrotoxic side effects of tacrolimus and cyclosporine are common and are associated with a significant decline in glomerular filtration rates.[130] Dehydration or administration of a nephrotoxic drug may precipitate acute renal failure. In order to minimize side effects, tacrolimus and cyclosporine levels should be kept as low as possible without precipitating rejection.

### Neurologic

Both tacrolimus and cyclosporine can cause pruritus, tremor, and headache; these effects are relatively mild and are dose related.[131] More serious problems include generalized seizures, often associated with hypomagnesemia, and white matter changes in the brain.[132, 133]

### Pulmonary

Prolonged ventilatory dependence may occur after transplant as a result of paralysis of the right diaphragm or from ongoing systemic complications such as sepsis and poor graft function. Pleural effusions, particularly right-sided, are very common and seldom require active management. Pulmonary infections may be viral, bacterial, fungal, or protozoal. Necrotizing pneumonitis due to adenovirus may be fatal.[134] Cytomegalovirus (CMV) and EBV pneumonitis also carry a high mortality. Pulmonary fungal infections are almost always fatal.

### Infectious Complications

Infection is the most common cause of death after transplant. Bacterial infections, particularly gram-negative septicemia, are most common in the early post-transplant period. Viral infections, particularly EBV and CMV, tend to occur later. Cytomegalovirus infection is most common between 4 and 12 weeks after transplant; EBV infection may be seen at any time. Fungal infections usually occur after the first 2 weeks and are frequently associated with complicated postoperative courses, particularly multiple abdominal surgeries. Systemic fungal infections, especially aspergillosis, carry a very poor prognosis.

After OLT, children are more susceptible to both common and opportunistic infections. Long-term prophylaxis against *Pneumocystis carinii* is recommended. Appropriate immunizations include pneumococcal vaccine, hepatitis A vaccine, and yearly influenza vaccination. Live vaccines such as the measles-mumps-rubella (MMR), varicella, or oral polio vaccines are contraindicated.[135]

### Gastrointestinal Complications

Diarrhea and poor feeding occur frequently after transplant. Infectious causes of diarrhea, especially *Clostridium difficile,* must be excluded. Both cyclosporine and tacrolimus can cause delayed gastric emptying, decreased appetite, and diarrhea. Gastrointestinal bleeding in the early postoperative period may be from the intestinal anastomosis. Later in the post-transplant period, PTLD must be ruled out.[136] Variceal bleeding postoperatively may be due to portal vein thrombosis. Bleeding from gastric or duodenal ulcers may also occur. Prophylactic $H_2$-blockade is recommended in the early post-transplant period. Symptomatic pancreatitis is an uncommon but potentially serious complication after transplantation; asymptomatic chemical pancreatitis is common and requires no specific therapy.

### Malignancy

Post-transplant lymphoproliferative disease ranges from a mild mononucleosis syndrome to malignant lymphoma. Eighty percent to 90% of PTLD in children is EBV-related and B cell in origin.[137] Risk factors include young age, primary EBV infection in the early post-transplant period, (e.g., an EBV-negative recipient receiving an EBV-positive graft), and increasing potency of immunosuppression. The incidence increases from 4% using cyclosporine, to 10% with OKT3, to 6% to 11% with primary tacrolimus, to 27% in children requiring conversion to tacrolimus.[108, 138–141] Mortality rates may be as high as 60% and are worst with monoclonal disease. Initial therapy is withdrawal of immunosuppression, which increases the risk of rejection. Other therapies include interferon, immunoglobulins, and chemotherapy.

### Growth and Development

The long-term effects of transplantation on growth, development, and intellectual capacity have not been determined. Growth impairment may occur even with successful graft function.[142–144] Intellectual function and school performance may also be impaired.[145, 146]

## Future Considerations

The ability to improve short- and long-term results of OLT in children will depend on the development of less toxic and more targeted immunosuppressive agents and the achievement of long-term, donor-specific tolerance. Until then, long-term monitoring of the effects of immunosuppression and strategies to potentiate growth and development are essential to the care of children after liver transplantation, whose life expectancy is continuously increasing.

**REFERENCES**


1. Devictor D, Tahiri C, Rousset A, et al: Management of fulminant hepatic failure in children—an analysis of 56 cases. Crit Care Med 1993;21:S348–S349.
2. Shin K, Nagai Y, Hirano C, et al: Survival rate in children with fulminant hepatitis improved by a combination of twice daily plasmapheresis and intensive conservative therapy. J Pediatr Gastroenterol Nutr 1989;9:163–166.
3. Psacharopoulos HT, Mowat AP, Davies M, et al: Fulminant hepatic failure in childhood: an analysis of 31 cases. Arch Dis Child 1980;55:252–258.
4. Trey C, Lipworth L, Davidson CS: Parameters influencing survival in the first 318 patients reported to the fulminant hepatic failure surveillance study (abstract). Gastroenterology 1970;58:306.
5. Zacarias J, Brinck P, Cordero J, Velasco M: Etiologies of fulminant hepatitis in pediatric patients in Santiago, Chile. Pediatr Infect Dis J 1987;6:686–687.
6. Dupuy JM, Frommel D, Alagille D: Severe viral hepatitis type B in infancy. Lancet 1975;1:191–194.
7. Chang MH, Lee CY, Chen DS, et al: Fulminant hepatitis in children in Taiwan: the important role of hepatitis B virus. J Pediatr 1987;111:34–39.
8. Alonso EM, Sokol RJ, Hart J, et al: Fulminant hepatitis associated with centrilobular hepatic necrosis in young children. J Pediatr 1995;127:888–894.
9. Rivera-Penera T, Moreno J, Skaff C, et al: Delayed encephalopathy in fulminant hepatic failure in the pediatric population and the role of liver transplantation. J Pediatr Gastroenterol Nutr 1997;24:128–134.
10. Frohburg E, Stolzel U, Lenz K, et al: Prognostic indicators in fulminant hepatic failure. Z Gastroenterol 1992;30:571–575.
11. Tandon BN, Joshi YK, Tandon M: Acute liver failure. Experience with 145 patients. J Clin Gastroenterol 1986;8:664–668.
12. O'Grady JG, Gimson AE, O'Brien CJ, et al: Controlled trials of charcoal hemoperfusion and prognostic factors in fulminant hepatic failure. Gastroenterology 1988;94:1186–1192.
13. Sallie R, Chiyende J, Tan KC, et al: Fulminant hepatic failure resulting from coexistent Wilson's disease and hepatitis E. Gut 1994;35:849–853.
14. Lee WM: Drug-induced hepatotoxicity [see comments]. N Engl J Med 1995;333:1118–1127.
15. Konig SA, Siemes H, Blaker F, et al: Severe hepatotoxicity during valproate therapy: an update and report of eight new fatalities. Epilepsia 1994;35:1005–1015.
16. Bashir RM, Lewis JH: Hepatotoxicity of drugs used in the treatment of gastrointestinal disorders. Gastroenterol Clin North Am 1995;24:937–967.
17. Makin AJ, Wendon J, Williams R: A 7-year experience of severe acetaminophen-induced hepatotoxicity (1987–1993). Gastroenterology 1995;109:1907–1916.
18. Osterloh J, Cunningham W, Dixon A, Combest D: Biochemical relationships between Reye's and Reye's-like metabolic and toxicological syndromes. Med Toxicol Adverse Drug Exp 1989;4:272–294.
19. Kutukculer N, Yagci RV: Our experience in Reye's syndrome (letter). J Pediatr Gastroenterol Nutr 1996;23:338–339.
20. Glasgow JF, Moore R: Reye's syndrome 30 years on. Br Med J 1993;307:950–951.
21. Jenkins JG, Glasgow JF, Black GW, et al: Reye's syndrome: assessment of intracranial monitoring. Br Med J (Clin Res Ed) 1987;294:337–338.
22. Smith ET Jr, Davis GJ: Medium-chain acylcoenzyme-A dehydrogenase deficiency. Not just another Reye syndrome. Am J Forensic Med Pathol 1993;14:313–318.
23. Hou JW, Chou SP, Wang TR: Metabolic function and liver histopathology in Reye-like illnesses. Acta Paediatr 1996;85:1053–1057.
24. Devictor D, Desplanques L, Debray D, et al: Emergency liver transplantation for fulminant liver failure in infants and children. Hepatology 1992;16:1156–1162.
25. Rela M, Heaton ND, Vougas V, et al: Orthotopic liver transplantation for hepatic complications of Wilson's disease. Br J Surg 1993;80:909–911.
26. Terajima H, Tanaka K, Okajima K, et al: Timing of transplantation and donor selection in living related liver transplantation for fulminant Wilson's disease. Transplant Proc 1995;27:1177–1178.
27. Martins da Costa C, Baldwin D, Portmann B, et al: Value of urinary copper excretion after penicillamine challenge in the diagnosis of Wilson's disease. Hepatology 1992;15:609–615.
28. Berman DH, Leventhal RI, Gavaler JS, et al: Clinical differentiation of fulminant Wilsonian hepatitis from other causes of hepatic failure. Gastroenterology 1991;100:1129–1134.
29. Frydman M, Bonne-Tamir B, Farrer LA, et al: Assignment of the gene for Wilson disease to chromosome 13: linkage to the esterase D locus. Proc Natl Acad Sci U S A 1985;82:1819–1821.
30. Navasa M, Garcia-Pagan JC, Bosch J, et al: Portal hypertension in acute liver failure. Gut 1992;33:965–968.
31. Anonymous: Prophylaxis of first hemorrhage from esophageal varices by sclerotherapy, propranolol or both in cirrhotic patients: a random-

ized multicenter trial. The PROVA Study Group. Hepatology 1991;14:1016–1024.
32. Howard ER, Stringer MD, Mowat AP: Assessment of injection sclerotherapy in the management of 152 children with oesophageal varices. Br J Surg 1988;75:404–408.
33. Fox VL, Carr-Locke DL, Connors PJ, Leichtner AM: Endoscopic ligation of esophageal varices in children [see comments]. J Pediatr Gastroenterol Nutr 1995;20:202–208.
34. Hassall E, Treem WR: To stab or strangle: how best to kill a varix? (editorial; comment). J Pediatr Gastroenterol Nutr 1995;20:121–124.
35. Teres J, Bosch J, Bordas JM, et al: Propranolol versus sclerotherapy in preventing variceal rebleeding: a randomized controlled trial. Gastroenterology 1993;105:1508–1514.
36. Fardy JM, Laupacis A: A meta analysis of prophylactic endoscopic sclerotherapy for esophageal varices. Am J Gastroenterol 1994;89:1938–1948.
37. Pagliaro L, D'Amico G, Sorensen TI, et al: Prevention of first bleeding in cirrhosis. A meta-analysis of randomized trials of nonsurgical treatment. Ann Intern Med 1992;117:59–70.
38. Groszmann RJ, Bosch J, Grace ND, et al: Hemodynamic events in a prospective randomized trial of propranolol versus placebo in the prevention of a first variceal hemorrhage. Gastroenterology 1990;99:1401–1407.
39. Poynard T, Cales P, Pasta L, et al: Beta-adrenergic-antagonist drugs in the prevention of gastrointestinal bleeding in patients with cirrhosis and esophageal varices. An analysis of data and prognostic factors in 589 patients from four randomized clinical trials. Franco-Italian Multicenter Study Group. N Engl J Med 1991;324:1532–1538.
40. Anonymous: Prediction of the first variceal hemorrhage in patients with cirrhosis of the liver and esophageal varices. A prospective multicenter study. The North Italian Endoscopic Club for the Study and Treatment of Esophageal Varices. N Engl J Med 1988;319:983–989.
41. Sherlock S, Dooley J: Ascites. In Sherlock S, Dooley J (eds): Diseases of the Liver and Biliary System, 10th ed. Oxford, Blackwell Science, 1997, pp 119–134.
42. Russell GJ, Fitzgerald JF, Clark JH: Fulminant hepatic failure. J Pediatr 1987;111:313–319.
43. Jones EA, Schafer DF: Fulminant hepatic failure. In Zakim D, Boyer TD (eds): Hepatology: A Textbook of Liver Disease, 2nd ed. Philadelphia, WB Saunders, 1990, pp 460–492.
44. Wyllie R, Arasu TS, Fitzgerald JF: Ascites: pathophysiology and management. J Pediatr 1980;97:167–176.
45. Pereira LM, Langley PG, Hayllar KM, et al: Coagulation factor V and VIII/V ratio as predictors of outcome in paracetamol induced fulminant hepatic falure: relation to other prognostic indicators. Gut 1992;33:98–102.
46. Donaldson BW, Gopinath R, Wanless IR, et al: The role of transjugular liver biopsy in fulminant liver failure: relation to other prognostic indicators. Hepatology 1993;18:1370–1376.
47. Crawford DH, Endre ZH, Axelsen RA, et al: Universal occurrence of glomerular abnormalities in patients receiving liver transplants. Am J Kidney Dis 1992;19:339–344.
48. Noble-Jamieson G, Thiru S, Johnston P, et al: Glomerulonephritis with end-stage liver disease in childhood. Lancet 1992;339:706–707.
49. Newell GC: Cirrhotic glomerulonephritis: incidence, morphology, clinical features, and pathogenesis. Am J Kidney Dis 1987;9:183–190.
50. Rogers EL, Rogers MC: Fulminant hepatic failure and hepatic encephalopathy. Pediatr Clin North Am 1980;27:701–713.
51. Rogers EL: Hepatic encephalopathy. Crit Care Clin 1985;1:313–325.
52. Riordan SM, Williams R: Treatment of hepatic encephalopathy. N Engl J Med 1997;337:473–479.
53. Devictor D, Tahiri C, Lanchier C, et al: Flumazenil in the treatment of hepatic encephalopathy in children with fulminant liver failure. Intensive Care Med 1995;21:253–256.
54. Masada CT, Shaw BW Jr, Zetterman RK, et al: Fulminant hepatic failure with massive necrosis as a result of hepatitis A infection. J Clin Gastroenterol 1993;17:158–162.
55. Schenker S, Butterworth R: NMR spectroscopy in portal-systemic encephalopathy: are we there yet? Gastroenterology 1997;112:1758–1761.
56. Riviello JJ Jr, Halligan GE, Dunn SP, et al: Value of plasmapheresis in hepatic encephalopathy. Pediatr Neurol 1990;6:388–390.
57. Laubenberger J, Haussinger D, Bayer S, et al: Proton magnetic resonance spectroscopy of the brain in symptomatic and asymptomatic patients with liver cirrhosis. Gastroenterology 1997;112:1610–1616.
58. Munoz SJ, Robinson M, Northrup B, et al: Elevated intracranial pressure and computed tomography of the brain in fulminant hepatocellular failure. Hepatology 1991;13:209–212.
59. Keays RT, Alexander GJ, Williams R: The safety and value of extradural intracranial pressure monitors in fulminant hepatic failure. J Hepatol 1993;18:205–209.
60. Blei AT, Olafsson S, Webster S, Levy R: Complications of intracranial pressure monitoring in fulminant hepatic failure. Lancet 1993;341:157–158.
61. Rossle M, Haag K, Ochs A, et al: The transjugular intrahepatic portosystemic stent-shunt procedure for variceal bleeding. N Engl J Med 1994;330:165–171.
62. Stewart SM, Uauy R, Kennard BD, et al: Mental development and growth in children with chronic liver disease of early and late onset. Pediatrics 1988;82:167–172.
63. Doyle HR, Marino IR, Miro A, et al: Adult respiratory distress syndrome secondary to end stage liver disease—successful outcome following liver transplantation. Transplantation 1993;55:292–296.
64. Barbe T, Losay J, Grimon G, et al: Pulmonary arteriovenous shunting in children with liver disease. J Pediatr 1995;126:571–579.
65. O'Grady JG, Alexander GJ, Hayllar KM, Williams R: Early indicators of prognosis in fulminant hepatic failure. Gastroenterology 1989;97:439–445.
66. Munoz SJ: Difficult management problems in fulminant hepatic failure. Semin Liver Dis 1993;13:395–413.
67. Sherlock S, Dooley J: The haematology of liver disease. In Sherlock S, Dooley J (eds): Diseases of the Liver and Biliary System, 10th ed. Oxford, Blackwell Science, 1997, pp 43–62.
68. Sherlock S, Dooley J: Hepatic cirrhosis. In Sherlock S, Dooley J (eds): Diseases of the Liver and Biliary System, 10th ed. Oxford, Blackwell Science, 1997, pp 371–384.
69. Lefkowitch JH: Pathologic diagnosis of liver disease. In Zakim D, Boyer TD (eds): Hepatology: A Textbook of Liver Disease, 2nd ed. Philadelphia, WB Saunders, 1990, pp 711–734.
70. Sherlock S, Dooley J: Hepato-cellular failure. In Sherlock S, Dooley J (eds): Diseases of the Liver and Biliary System, 10th ed. Oxford, Blackwell Science, 1997, pp 73–85.
71. Bernuau J, Goudeau A, Poynard T, et al: Multivariate analysis of prognostic factors in fulminant hepatitis B. Hepatology 1986;6:648–651.
72. Sherlock S, Dooley J: The portal venous system and portal hypertension. In Sherlock S, Dooley J (eds): Diseases of the Liver and Biliary System, 10th ed. Oxford, Blackwell Science, 1997, pp 135–180.
73. Child CGI, Turcotte JG: Surgery and portal hypertension. In Child CGI (ed): The Liver and Portal Hypertension. Philadelphia, WB Saunders, 1964, pp 1–85.
74. Pugh RN, Murray-Lyon IM, Dawson JL, et al: Transection of the oesophagus for bleeding oesophageal varices. Br J Surg 1973;60:646–649.
75. Infante-Rivard C, Esnaola S, Villeneuve JP: Clinical and statistical validity of conventional prognostic factors in predicting short-term survival among cirrhotics. Hepatology 1987;7:660–664.
76. Christensen E, Schlichting P, Fauerholdt L, et al: Prognostic value of Child-Turcotte criteria in medically treated cirrhosis. Hepatology 1984;4:430–435.
77. Kaufman SS, Murray ND, Wood RP, et al: Nutritional support for the infant with extrahepatic biliary atresia. J Pediatr 1987;110:679–686.
78. Wu PY, Edmond J, Morrow JW, et al: Gastrointestinal tolerance, fat absorption, plasma ketone and urinary dicarboxylic acid levels in low-birth-weight infants fed different amounts of medium-chain triglycerides in formula. J Pediatr Gastroenterol Nutr 1993;17:145–152.
79. Sokol RJ: Fat-soluble vitamins and their importance in patients with cholestatic liver diseases. Gastroenterol Clin North Am 1994;23:673–705.
80. Uribe M, Conn HO: Dietary management of portal-systemic encephalopathy. In Conn HO, Bircher J (eds): Hepatic Encephalopathy: Syndromes and Therapies. Bloomington, IL: Medi-Ed Press, 1994, pp 331–349.
81. Bianchi GP, Marchesini G, Fabbri A, et al: Vegetable versus animal protein diet in cirrhotic patients with chronic encephalopathy. A randomized cross-over comparison. J Intern Med 1993;233:385–392.
82. Naylor CD, O'Rourke K, Detsky AS, Baker JP: Parenteral nutrition with branched-chain amino acids in hepatic encephalopathy. A meta-analysis. Gastroenterology 1989;97:1033–1042.
83. Weber FL Jr: Lactulose and combination therapy of hepatic encepha-

lopathy: the role of the intestinal microflora. Dig Dis 1996;14(suppl 1):53–63.
84. Salerno F, Moser P, Maggi A, et al: Effects of long-term administration of low-dose lactitol in patients with cirrhosis but without overt encephalopathy. J Hepatol 1994;21:1092–1096.
85. Riggio O, Balducci G, Ariosto F, et al: Lactitol in prevention of recurrent episodes of hepatic encephalopathy in cirrhotic patients with portal-systemic shunt. Dig Dis Sci 1989;34:823–829.
86. Uribe M, Campollo O, Vargas F, et al: Acidifying enemas (lactitol and lactose) vs. nonacidifying enemas (tap water) to treat acute portal-systemic encephalopathy: a double blind randomized clinical trial. Hepatology 1987;7:639–643.
87. Hermann R, Shakoor T, Weber FL Jr: Beneficial effects of pectin in chronic hepatic encephalopathy (abstract). Gastroenterology 1987;92:1795.
88. Rolando N, Harvey F, Brahm J, et al: Prospective study of bacterial infection in acute liver failure: an analysis of fifty patients. Hepatology 1990;11:49–53.
89. Keays RT, Gove C, Forbes A, et al: Use of late *N*-acetyl cysteine in severe paracetamol overdose. Gut 1989;30:A1512.
90. Harrison PM, Wendon JA, Gimson AE, et al: Improvement by acetylcysteine of hemodynamics and oxygen transport in fulminant hepatic failure. N Engl J Med 1991;324:1852–1857.
91. Anonymous: 1996 Annual Report of the U.S. Scientific Registry for Transplant Recipients and the Organ Procurement and Transplantation Network Transplant Data 1988–1995. Rockville, MD, U.S. Department of Health and Human Services, Richmond, VA, UNOS, and the Division of Transplantation, Bureau of Health Resources Development, Health Resources and Services Administration, 1996.
92. Emond JC, Heffron TG, Kortz EO, et al: Improved results of living-related liver transplantation with routine application in a pediatric program. Transplantation 1993;55:835–840.
93. Rogiers X, Malago M, Gawad KA, et al: One year of experience with extended application and modified techniques of split liver transplantation. Transplantation 1996;61:1059–1061.
94. Goss J, Yersiz H, Shackleton C, et al: In situ splitting of the cadaveric liver for transplantation. Transplantation 1997;64:871–877.
95. Zitelli BJ, Gartner JC, Malatack JJ, et al: Pediatric liver transplantation: patient evaluation and selection, infectious complications, and life-style after transplantation. Transplant Proc 1987;19:3309–3316.
96. Whitington PF, Balistreri WF: Liver transplantation in pediatrics: indications, contraindications, and pretransplant management. J Pediatr 1991;118:169–177.
97. Busuttil RW, Seu P, Millis JM, et al: Liver transplantation in children. Ann Surg 1991;213:48–57.
98. Otte JB, de Ville de Goyet J, Reding R, et al: Sequential treatment of biliary atresia with Kasai portoenterostomy and liver transplantation: a review. Hepatology 1994;20:41S–48S.
99. Rivera-Penera T, Gugig R, Davis J, et al: Outcome of acetaminophen overdose in pediatric patients and factors contributing to hepatotoxicity. J Pediatr 1997;130:300–304.
100. Koneru B, Flye MW, Busuttil RW, et al: Liver transplantation for hepatoblastoma. The American experience. Ann Surg 1991;213:118–121.
101. Todo S, Starzl TE, Tzakis A, et al: Orthotopic liver transplantation for urea cycle enzyme deficiency. Hepatology 1992;15:419–422.
102. Sokal EM, Silva ES, Hermans D, et al: Orthotopic liver transplantation for Crigler-Najjar type I disease in six children. Transplantation 1995;60:1095–1098.
103. Weinberg AG, Mize CE, Worthen HG: The occurrence of hepatoma in the chronic form of hereditary tyrosinemia. J Pediatr 1976;88:434–438.
104. Moukarzel AA, Najm I, Vargas J, et al: Effect of nutritional status on outcome of orthotopic liver transplantation in pediatric patients. Transplant Proc 1990;22:1560–1563.
105. Shepherd RW, Chin SE, Cleghorn GJ, et al: Malnutrition in children with chronic liver disease accepted for liver transplantation: clinical profile and effect on outcome. J Paediatr Child Health 1991;27:295–299.
106. Broelsch CE, Emond JC, Thistlethwaite JR, et al: Liver transplantation, including the concept of reduced-size liver transplants in children. Ann Surg 1988;208:410–420.
107. de Ville de Goyet J, Hausleithner V, Reding R, et al: Impact of innovative techniques on the waiting list and results in pediatric liver transplantation. Transplantation 1993;56:1130–1136.
108. Inomata Y, Tanaka K, Egawa H, et al: The evolution of immunosuppression with FK506 in pediatric living-related liver transplantation. Transplantation 1996;61:247–252.
109. Dunn SP, Cooney GF, Kulinsky A, et al: Absorption characteristics of a microemulsion formulation of cyclosporine in de novo pediatric liver transplant recipients. Transplantation 1995;60:1438–1442.
110. Inomoto T, Nishizawa F, Sasaki H, et al: Experiences of 120 microsurgical reconstructions of hepatic artery in living related liver transplantation. Surgery 1996;119:20–26.
111. Stevens LH, Emond JC, Piper JB, et al: Hepatic artery thrombosis in infants. A comparison of whole livers, reduced-size grafts, and grafts from living-related donors. Transplantation 1992;53:396–399.
112. Tzakis AG, Gordon RD, Shaw BW Jr, et al: Clinical presentation of hepatic artery thrombosis after liver transplantation in the cyclosporine era. Transplantation 1985;40:667–671.
113. Peclet MH, Ryckman FC, Pedersen SH, et al: The spectrum of bile duct complications in pediatric liver transplantation. J Pediatr Surg 1994;29:214–219; discussion 219–220.
114. Shaked A, Vargas J, Csete ME, et al: Diagnosis and treatment of bowel perforation following pediatric orthotopic liver transplantation. Arch Surg 1993;128:994–998; discussion 998–999.
115. Groth CG, Ohlman S, Gannedahl G, Ericzon BG: New immunosuppressive drugs in transplantation. Transplant Proc 1993;25:2681–2683.
116. Tzakis AG, Reyes J, Todo S, et al: Two-year experience with FK 506 in pediatric patients. Transplant Proc 1993;25:619–621.
117. McDiarmid SV, Busuttil RW, Ascher NL, et al: FK506 (tacrolimus) compared with cyclosporine for primary immunosuppression after pediatric liver transplantation. Results from the U.S. Multicenter Trial. Transplantation 1995;59:530–536.
118. Fung JJ, Alessiani M, Abu-Elmagd K, et al: Adverse effects associated with the use of FK 506. Transplant Proc 1991;23:3105–3108.
119. McDiarmid SV, Colonna JO 2d, Shaked A, et al: A comparison of renal function in cyclosporine- and FK-506-treated patients after primary orthotopic liver transplantation. Transplantation 1993;56:847–853.
120. Mueller AR, Platz KP, Bechstein WO, et al: Neurotoxicity after orthotopic liver transplantation. A comparison between cyclosporine and FK506. Transplantation 1994;58:155–170.
121. Cox KL, Lawrence-Miyasaki LS, Garcia-Kennedy R, et al: An increased incidence of Epstein-Barr virus infection and lymphoproliferative disorder in young children on FK506 after liver transplantation. Transplantation 1995;59:524–529.
122. Esquivel CO, So SK, McDiarmid SV, et al: Suggested guidelines for the use of tacrolimus in pediatric liver transplant patients (letter). Transplantation 1996;61:847–848.
123. Dunn SP, Falkenstein K, Lawrence JP, et al: Monotherapy with cyclosporine for chronic immunosuppression in pediatric liver transplant recipients. Transplantation 1994;57:544–547.
124. McDiarmid SV: Special considerations for pediatric immunosuppression after liver transplantation. In Busuttil RW, Klintmalm GB (eds): Transplantation of the Liver. Philadelphia, WB Saunders, 1996, p 250.
125. Superina R, Acal L, Bilik R, Zaki A: Growth in children after liver transplantation on cyclosporine alone or in combination with low-dose azathioprine. Transplant Proc 1993;25:2580.
126. McDiarmid SV, Busuttil RW, Terasaki P, et al: OKT3 treatment of steroid-resistant rejection in pediatric liver transplant recipients. J Pediatr Gastroenterol Nutr 1992;14:86–91.
127. Young CJ, Sollinger HW: RS-61443: a new immunosuppressive agent. Transplant Proc 1994;26:3144–3146.
128. Dunn SP, Billmire DF, Falkenstein K, et al: Rejection after pediatric liver transplantation is not the limiting factor to survival (discussion). J Pediatr Surg 1994;29:1141–1143.
129. Ellis D, Avner ED, Starzl TE: Renal failure in children with hepatic failure undergoing liver transplantation. J Pediatr 1986;108:393–398.
130. McDiarmid SV, Ettenger RB, Hawkins RA, et al: The impairment of true glomerular filtration rate in long-term cyclosporine-treated pediatric allograft recipients. Transplantation 1990;49:81–85.
131. Eidelman BH, Abu-Elmagd K, Wilson J, et al: Neurologic complications of FK 506. Transplant Proc 1991;23:3175–3178.
132. Thompson CB, June CH, Sullivan KM, Thomas ED: Association between cyclosporin neurotoxicity and hypomagnesaemia. Lancet 1984;2:1116–1120.
133. Lopez OL, Martinez AJ, Torre-Cisneros J: Neuropathologic findings in liver transplantation: a comparative study of cyclosporine and FK 506. Transplant Proc 1991;23:3181–3182.

134. Michaels MG, Green M, Wald ER, Starzl TE: Adenovirus infection in pediatric liver transplant recipients. J Infect Dis 1992;165:170–174.
135. Anonymous: Recommendations of the Advisory Committee on Immunization Practices (ACIP): use of vaccines and immune globulins for persons with altered immunocompetence. MMWR Morb Mortal Wkly Rep 1993;42:1.
136. Cao S, Cox K, Esquivel CO, et al: Posttransplant lymphoproliferative disorders and gastrointestinal manifestations of Epstein-Barr virus infection in children following liver transplantation. Transplantation 1998;66:851–856.
137. Rustgi VK: Epstein-Barr viral infection and posttransplantation lymphoproliferative disorders. Liver Transplant Surg 1995;1:100.
138. Renard TH, Andrews WS, Foster ME: Relationship between OKT3 administration, EBV seroconversion, and the lymphoproliferative syndrome in pediatric liver transplant recipients. Transplant Proc 1991;23:1473–1476.
139. Reding R, Wallemacq PE, Lamy ME, et al: Conversion from cyclosporine to FK506 for salvage of immunocompromised pediatric liver allografts. Efficacy, toxicity, and dose regimen in 23 children. Transplantation 1994;57:93–100.
140. McDiarmid SV, Wallace P, Vargas J, et al: The treatment of intractable rejection with tacrolimus (FK506) in pediatric liver transplant recipients. J Pediatr Gastroenterol Nutr 1995;20:291–299.
141. Cacciarelli TV, Esquivel CO, Cox KL, et al: Oral tacrolimus (FK506) induction therapy in pediatric orthotopic liver transplantation. Transplantation 1996;61:1188–1192.
142. Moukarzel AA, Najm I, Vargas J, et al: Prediction of long-term linear growth following liver transplantation. Transplant Proc 1990;22:1558–1559.
143. Urbach AH, Gartner JC, Malatack JJ, et al: Linear growth following pediatric liver transplantation. Am J Dis Child 1987;141:547–549.
144. Sarna S, Sipila I, Jalanko H, et al: Factors affecting growth after pediatric liver transplantation. Transplant Proc 1994;26:161–164.
145. Zitelli BJ, Miller JW, Gartner JC Jr, et al: Changes in life-style after liver transplantation. Pediatrics 1988;82:173–180.
146. Stewart SM, Uauy R, Waller DA, et al: Mental and motor development, social competence, and growth one year after successful pediatric liver transplantation. J Pediatr 1989;114:574–581.
147. Modlin JF: Fatal echovirus II disease in premature neonates. Pediatrics 1980;66:775–780.
148. Halfon N, Spector SA: Fatal echovirus type II infections. Am J Dis Child 1981;135:1017–1020.
149. Hsu HY, Chang MH, Lee CY, et al: Precore mutant of hepatitis B virus in childhood fulminant hepatitis B: an infrequent association. J Infect Dis 1995;171:776–781.
150. Greenes DS, Rowitch D, Thorne GM, et al: Neonatal herpes simplex virus infection presenting as fulminant liver failure. Pediatr Infect Dis J 1995;14:242–244.
151. Bhaduri BR, Mieli-Vergani G: Fulminant hepatic failure: pediatric aspects. Semin Liver Dis 1996;16:349–355.
152. Herman TE: Extensive hepatic calcification secondary to fulminant neonatal syphilitic hepatitis. Pediatr Radiol 1995;25:120–122.
153. Shneider BL: Neonatal liver failure. Curr Opin Pediatr 1996;8:495–501.
154. Cross NC, De Franchis R, Sebastio G, et al: Molecular analysis of aldolase B genes in hereditary fructose intolerance. Lancet 1990;335:306–309.
155. Teckman J, Permutter DH: Conceptual advances in the pathogenesis and treatment of childhood metabolic liver disease. Gastroenterology 1995;108:1263–1279.
156. Bioulac-Sage P, Parrot-Roulaud F, Mazat JP, et al: Fatal neonatal liver failure and mitochondrial cytopathy (oxidative phosphorylation deficiency): a light and electron microscopic study of the liver. Hepatology 1993;18:839–846.
157. Bakker HD, Van den Bogert C, Scholte HR, et al: Fatal neonatal liver failure and depletion of mitochondrial DNA in three children of one family. J Inherit Metab Dis 1996;19:112–114.
158. Shaw NJ, Evans JH: Liver failure and Epstein-Barr virus infection. Arch Dis Child 1988;63:432–433.
159. Kong MS, Chung JL: Fatal hepatitis C in an infant born to a hepatitis C positive mother. J Pediatr Gastroenterol Nutr 1994;19:460–463.
160. Rosh JR, Schwersenz AH, Groisman G, et al: Fatal fulminant hepatitis B in an infant despite appropriate prophylaxis. Arch Pediatr Adolesc Med 1994;148:1349–1351.
161. Fagan EA, Ellis DS, Tovey GM, et al: Toga virus-like particles in acute liver failure attributed to sporadic non-A, non-B hepatitis and recurrence after liver transplantation. J Med Virol 1992;38:71–77.
162. Tojimbara T, So SK, Cox KL, et al: Fulminant hepatic failure following varicella-zoster infection in a child. A case report of successful treatment with liver transplantation and perioperative acyclovir. Transplantation 1995;60:1052–1053.
163. Kinmond S, Carter R, Skeoch CH, Morton NS: Nephroblastoma presenting with acute hepatic encephalopathy. Arch Dis Child 1990;65:542–543.
164. Boyer TD: Portal hypertension and bleeding esophageal varices. In Zakim D, Boyer TD (eds): Hepatology: A Textbook of Liver Disease, 2nd ed. Philadelphia, WB Saunders, 1990, pp 572–615.
165. Devictor D, Tahiri C, Fabre M, et al: Early pre-B acute lymphoblastic leukemia presenting as fulminant liver failure. J Pediatr Gastroenterol Nutr 1996;22:103–106.
166. Conway EE Jr, Santorineou M, Mitsudo S: Fulminant hepatic failure in a child with acute lymphoblastic leukemia. J Pediatr Gastroenterol Nutr 1992;15:194–197.
167. Woolf GM, Petrovic LM, Rojter SE, et al: Acute liver failure due to lymphoma. A diagnostic concern when considering liver transplantation. Dig Dis Sci 1994;39:1351–1358.
168. Gunasekaran TS, Hassall E, Dimmick JE, Chan KW: Hodgkin's disease presenting with fulminant liver disease. J Pediatr Gastroenterol Nutr 1992;15:189–193.
169. Maggiore G, Porta G, Bernard O, et al: Autoimmune hepatitis with initial presentation as acute hepatic failure in young children. J Pediatr 1990;116:280–282.
170. Lye MS, Ghazali AA, Mohan J, et al: An outbreak of acute hepatic encephalopathy due to severe aflatoxicosis in Malaysia. Am J Trop Med Hyg 1995;53:68–72.
171. Zimmerman HJ, Lewis JH: Chemical- and toxin-induced hepatotoxicity. Gastroenterol Clin North Am 1995;24:1027–1045.
172. Baker A, Gormally S, Saxena R, et al: Copper-associated liver disease in childhood. J Hepatol 1995;23:538–543.
173. Kozaki K, Egawa H, Garcia-Kennedy R, et al: Hepatic failure due to massive iron ingestion successfully treated with liver transplantation. Clin Transplant 1995;9:85–87.
174. Mahler H, Pasi A, Kramer JM, et al: Fulminant liver failure in association with the emetic toxin of Bacillus cereus. N Engl J Med 1997;336:1142–1148.
175. Langnas AN, Markin RS, Cattral MS, Naides SJ: Parvovirus B19 as a possible causative agent of fulminant liver failure and associated aplastic anemia. Hepatology 1995;22:1661–1665.
176. Walia BN, Singh S, Marwaha RK, et al: Fulminant hepatic failure and acute intravascular haemolysis as presenting manifestations of Wilson's disease in young children. J Gastroenterol Hepatol 1992;7:370–373.
177. Schafer DF, Jones EA: Hepatic encephalopathy. In Zakim D, Boyer TD (eds): Hepatology: A Textbook of Liver Disease, 2nd ed. Philadelphia, WB Saunders, 1990, pp 447–460.

Chapter 53

# Diseases of the Gallbladder

Mark A. Gilger

Gallbladder disease in children is perceived as rare and invariably associated with underlying hemolytic disease, but neither of these perceptions is true. Hemolytic disease predisposes children to gallstones, but there is an increasing likelihood of finding other associated conditions such as prematurity, necrotizing enterocolitis, and cystic fibrosis or conditions necessitating total parenteral nutrition (TPN). Since the advent of ultrasonography, "incidental" or "silent" gallstones are now being detected more often in children, even in utero.

## EPIDEMIOLOGY OF GALLSTONE DISEASE

Approximately 20 million adults in the United States have gallstones, and approximately 300,000 cholecystectomies are performed yearly.[1] Predominantly a disease of adulthood, gallstone disease ranges in prevalence from 4% to 11% in Western societies, with wide variations along racial and ethnic lines.[2–8] The incidence in adults is approximately 1% to 3%.[9] The incidence of gallstone disease is influenced by age, sex, culture, ethnicity, and a variety of medical factors,[6, 10–14] and it varies geographically. For instance, members of the Masai tribe of East Africa, whose bile is only half saturated with cholesterol, do not develop gallstones, whereas the Pima Indians of Arizona have an 80% prevalence.[5, 15] Investigations into gallstone formation using a mouse model suggest that genetic factors, such as presence of a gene Lith1, may determine susceptibility to gallstone formation.[16]

The earliest reported case of cholelithiasis in a child was by Gibson in 1737.[17] Attempts to estimate the frequency of childhood gallstones included an extensive review of 5,037 cases in 1959, in which a prevalence of 0.15% in children younger than 16 years of age was noted.[18] The prevalence of gallbladder disease in children since the 1960s appears to be increasing.[19–24] In a review of 708 infants referred for cholestasis between 1970 and 1981, an incidence of 1.4% was found.[24] Other reports have noted that 4% of all cholecystectomies are performed in patients younger than 20 years of age.[25, 26] Unfortunately, no detailed estimates of the incidence and prevalence of gallstone disease exist for children.

In a review of 693 cases of childhood gallstones reported since 1968, early infancy and adolescence were the most common ages for diagnosis.[27] Infants younger than 6 months of age represented 10% of all cases in which the age was known. Children from 6 months to 10 years of age accounted for 21%, and adolescents (mostly female) 11 to 21 years of age represented 69% of all cases.[27] Most gallstones in children have an underlying predisposing condition, such as hemolytic disease, pregnancy, and TPN. Gallstones of infancy are typically found in "ill" infants receiving TPN. Stones found in children from the ages of 1 to 5 years are usually secondary to hemolysis, and stones found in adolescents are most likely associated with menarche, pregnancy, and the use of oral contraceptives.[27]

## PATHOPHYSIOLOGY OF GALLSTONE DISEASE

Bile is composed of five major components: water, bilirubin, cholesterol, bile pigments, and phospholipids. Lecithin is the primary phospholipid. Calcium salts and some proteins are minor components of bile. Stone formation occurs owing to the precipitation of the insoluble constituents of bile, which are cholesterol, bile pigments, and calcium salts. Gallstones are classically divided into either cholesterol stones or pigment stones (Table 53–1). Chemically pure gallstones are rare, and in any single stone the composition varies from the core to the crust. Most stones are "mixed" in composition, and the formation patterns of both cholesterol and pigment stones share many characteristics.

Cholesterol, the major sterol in bile, is nearly insoluble in water. It is made soluble in aqueous bile by aggregation with bile salts or lecithin. When cholesterol is no longer soluble, cholesterol monohydrate crystals precipitate from solution, a process known as *nucleation*.[28, 29]

The interplay among the major bile components cholesterol, lecithin, and bile salts is depicted in Figure 53–1. When the composition of bile lies in the micellar zone, the bile can solubilize additional cholesterol. As the cholesterol

**TABLE 53–1. Characteristics of Gallstones in Children**

| CHARACTERISTICS | CHOLESTEROL STONES | PIGMENT STONES: Black | PIGMENT STONES: Brown |
|---|---|---|---|
| Color | Yellow-white (often with dark core) | Black to brown | Brown to orange |
| Consistency | Hard<br>Crystalline<br>Layered | Hard, shiny<br>Crystalline | Soft, greasy<br>50% amorphous; rest crystalline, inorganic salts |
| Number and morphology | Multiple: 2–25 mm faceted, smooth<br>Solitary: 2–4 cm (~10%) round, smooth | Multiple: <5 mm<br>Irregular or smooth | Multiple: 10–30 mm<br>Round, smooth |
| Composition | Cholesterol monohydrate >50%<br>Glycoprotein<br>Calcium salts | Bile pigment polymer ~40%<br>Calcium carbonate or phosphate salts ~15%<br>Cholesterol ~5%<br>Mucin glycoprotein ~20% | Calcium bilirubinate ~60%<br>Calcium palmitate and stearate soaps ~15%<br>Cholesterol ~15%<br>Mucin glycoprotein ~10% |
| Radiopaque | No | Yes ~50% | No |
| Location | Gallbladder ± common bile duct | Gallbladder | Common bile duct, intrahepatic ducts |
| Clinical associations | Hyperlipidemia<br>Obesity<br>Clofibrate<br>Pregnancy<br>Birth control pills<br>Cystic fibrosis<br>Octreotide | Hemolytic anemia<br>Cirrhosis<br>Total parenteral nutrition<br>Ileal disease (after puberty)<br>Ceftriaxone | Bacterial infection (*Escherichia coli*)<br>Parasitic infection<br>Bile duct anomaly |
| Recurrent | Yes | No | Yes |
| Sex | Female >male | No difference | No difference |
| Age | Pubertal; increases with age | Any; increases with age | Any; increases with age |
| Bacteria | No | No | Yes (consistently found at core) |
| Soluble | Yes | No | No (minimally) |

Data from references 24, 53, and 54.

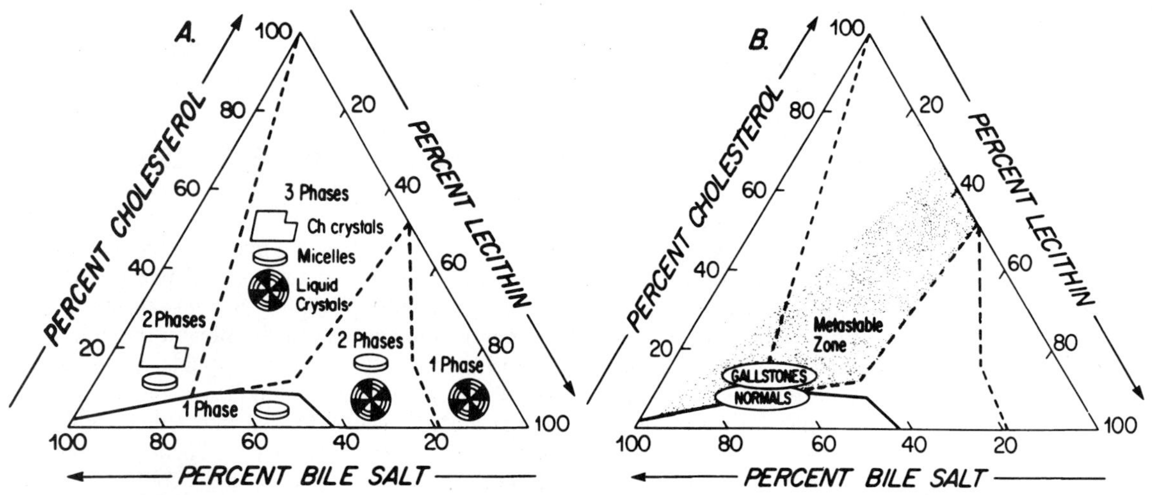


**FIGURE 53–1.** *A*, Triangular phase diagram showing phases present at equilibrium in biles of differing compositions. In the micellar zone (the area in the lower left of the triangle), all the cholesterol is held in solution as micelles. Biles with a composition outside the micellar zone, if allowed to come to equilibrium, would form liquid and/or solid cholesterol crystals (as depicted schematically in each of the zones). The micellar zone is larger for gallbladder bile (a 10% lipid solution shown here) than for hepatic bile (a 3% lipid solution not shown). *B*, Triangular phase diagram with schematic representations of ranges of lipid compositions found in gallbladder biles of normals and gallstone patients. Bile with a composition that falls in the metastable zone takes a prolonged time to come to equilibrium and thus appears to be stable. Excess cholesterol is "carried" in the metastable zone by cholesterol-rich unilamellar vesicles. The boundaries of the physiologically relevant metastable zone are approximate.[29] (From Carey MC, Cohen DE: Biliary transport of cholesterol in micelles and liquid crystals. In Paumgartner G, Stiehl A, Gerak W (eds): Bile Acids and the Liver. Lancaster, MTP Press, 1987, pp 287–300, with permission.)

concentration continues to increase, the likelihood of cholesterol crystallization, and hence gallstone formation, increases. A decrease in bile salt concentration or lecithin also predisposes to gallstones.

There appear to be three primary conditions that must be met to permit the formation of cholesterol gallstones.[30] First, the bile must be supersaturated with cholesterol, which then acts as the driving force behind crystal precipitation. Second, bile kinetics must be such as to allow nucleation, the transition to solid cholesterol crystals. Finally, gallbladder stasis must exist to allow agglomeration of cholesterol crystals into stones.[31] Two secondary conditions also appear to be critical in lithogenesis: gallbladder hypersecretion of mucus and excess arachidonyl lecithin (Fig. 53–2).[32–34]

Cholesterol supersaturation can result from the following conditions:

1. An increased delivery of cholesterol to the liver via increased lipoprotein (low-density lipoprotein and chylomicrons). This occurs in women secondary to estrogen or oral contraceptive use or to increased dietary cholesterol intake.[32, 35]
2. An increased endogenous cholesterol synthesis secondary to 3-hydroxy-3-methylglutaryl coenzyme A (HMG-CoA) reductase activity. Obesity and hypertriglyceridemia are causes of increased HMG-CoA reductase activity.[36, 37]
3. A decrease in 7-alpha-hydroxylase activity, thus decreasing the conversion of cholesterol to bile acids.[38] This defect occurs most commonly with increasing age.
4. A decrease in the conversion of cholesterol to cholesterol esters from inhibited acyl-CoA cholesterol acyltransferase activity (ACAT).[32] Progesterone, either pregnancy induced or exogenous, and clofibrate are examples of ACAT inhibitors.

The potential defects leading to cholesterol supersaturation are thus numerous and overlapping.

Nucleation is not as well understood as cholesterol supersaturation. Nucleation times are strikingly different between gallstone patients and control subjects. Gallbladder hypomotility seems to be involved in the crystallization process, because agitation prevents aggregation. Animal studies support hypomotility as an important causative factor.[39, 40] Technetium-99m-dimethyl iminodiacetic acid gallbladder emptying studies in adult gallstone patients have documented diminished gallbladder emptying after meals.[41]

Biliary sludge, or tumefacient sludge, a collection of mucus, calcium bilirubinate, and cholesterol crystals, appears to precede the formation of gallstones in animal models.[28, 29, 42] Mucin hypersecretion appears to be a primary event in sludge formation, and evidence suggests that prostanoids, such as arachidonyl lecithin, mediate the hypersecretion.[32–34] Mucin may serve as the nidus for nucleation and subsequent sludge formation owing to its hydrophobic domain, which binds phospholipid and cholesterol.[43]

Figure 53–2 summarizes the current understanding of the formation of cholesterol gallstones and, perhaps, of any gallstone. The process must have a supersaturated solution (either cholesterol or bilirubin pigment); a "still" environment, or gallbladder stasis; and crystal agglomeration or nucleation. The initial nucleating event creates the core of the stone, from which a self-perpetuating process ensues.

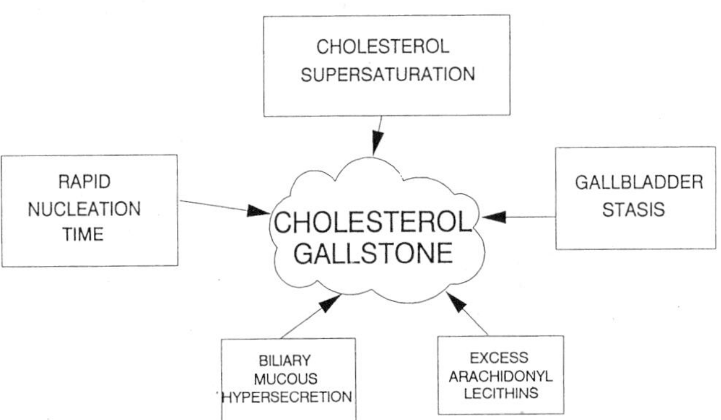


**FIGURE 53–2.** Current understanding of cholesterol gallstone formation. Cholesterol supersaturation is an essential prerequisite, which combined with a more rapid nucleation time and gallbladder stasis allows crystal formation. Excess biliary mucus provides a structural nidus for crystal growth, driven by increased dietary arachidonyl lecithins. (Adapted from Hay DW, Carey MC: Pathophysiology and pathogenesis of cholesterol gallstone formation. Semin Liver Dis 1990;10:159–170, with permission.)

## CHOLESTEROL STONES

Cholesterol gallstones are yellowish-white in appearance, hard, crystalline, and layered. They frequently have a brownish core, with a variety of substances found there, including calcium salts. "Rings" of protein (glycoproteins) and calcium salts (calcium bilirubinate, calcium hydroxyapatite, and calcium carbonate) form around the core, resulting in the layered appearance. The cholesterol content is higher than 50%, with minimal calcium salt content. This composition is not radiopaque; thus, the stones are rarely seen on plain film radiographs. Cholesterol stones form within the gallbladder and are frequently multiple, ranging in size from approximately 2 to 25 mm in diameter. The presence of cholesterol stones in the biliary tree is the result of migration. Cholesterol gallstones account for approximately 70% of all stones found in Western populations. The prevalence of cholesterol gallstones in children is unknown, but increases slowly with age in both sexes.[44] Pubertal changes, in particular early menarche, cause a dramatic increase in the incidence of cholesterol gallstones.[44, 45] This phenomenon has been attributed to the effect of estrogen and progesterone surges that occur during puberty; it has also been seen in pregnancy and with the use of oral contraceptives, although investigation suggests no relationship between oral contraceptives and gallstones.[46] Sex hormones appear to induce biliary stasis and cause cholesterol hypersecretion by the liver.[47] It remains unclear whether estrogen, the progestins, or a combination of both, are responsible. There clearly are genetic influences, with high prevalence rates seen in both children and adult Native Americans. Studies of the Pimas of Arizona have demonstrated the development of lithogenic bile containing excess cholesterol during adolescence.[45] Obesity has been shown to increase the likelihood of cholesterol gallstone formation, apparently from excessive hepatic cholesterol secretion secondary to increased cholesterol synthesis.[48]

Gallstones and gallbladder and biliary tract abnormalities

are frequently found in patients with cystic fibrosis, and they increase with age.[49] "Microgallbladders" have been identified in as many as 16% of adult cystic fibrosis patients radiologically and in 30% of patients at autopsy.[50] Common bile duct stenosis has been identified in 96% of cystic fibrosis patients with liver disease, resulting in enlarged gallbladders and elevated serum bile acid levels, which may predispose to gallstone formation.[49] Gallstones in cystic fibrosis patients appear secondary to excessive bile acid loss resulting in a reduced bile acid pool. The bile composition becomes abnormal, with a relative excess of cholesterol associated with the decrease in bile salts, thus making the bile lithogenic. The bile acid malabsorption and reduced bile salt pool respond to pancreatic enzyme therapy. Gallstones have not been found without pancreatic insufficiency.[51, 52]

## PIGMENT STONES

Pigment stones account for a much higher percentage of stones in prepubertal children, whereas cholesterol stones are predominant in adolescence and adulthood. Two types of pigment gallstones are found in children and are referred to as *black* and *brown.* In both black and brown stones, the pigment present is calcium bilirubinate, which interacts with mucin glycoproteins to form stones (see Table 53–1).[53]

*Black pigment stones* are black to dark brown in color and small (usually <5 mm), occur multiply, and are typically hard, shiny, and crystalline.[54] They are composed primarily of highly cross-linked polymers of bilirubin with mucin glycoproteins and calcium salts of phosphate and carbonate.[55, 56] The high concentration of calcium salts (as compared with brown and cholesterol stones) accounts for the 50% to 75% radiopacity seen on plain radiographs. Black stones typically form within the gallbladder and do not recur after resection. They are usually associated with hemolytic diseases, of which sickle cell disease and hereditary spherocytosis are the most common. The duration of the hemolytic disease appears to be a significant risk factor for stone formation. Children younger than 10 years of age with sickle cell disease have a 14% prevalence of stones, whereas children 11 to 20 years of age have a 36% prevalence. Older adults with sickle cell disease have more than a 50% prevalence.[57, 58] Other disease states, such as thalassemia, Wilson's disease, and mechanical shearing of erythrocytes associated with artificial heart valves, have all been associated with black pigment stones. Black pigment stones form within the gallbladder, and their presence in the common bile duct is the result of migration. Black stones are found in sterile bile and are not associated with infection.[59]

The formation of black stones results from altered gallbladder bile homeostasis and supersaturation of the bile. This process could occur by at least three mechanisms: an increase in bilirubin anions, an increase in unbound $Ca^{2+}$, and a decrease in factors that solubilize bilirubin and calcium.[54] An increase in bilirubin anions has been shown to occur secondary to hemolysis.[54, 60] Increased unbound calcium could occur secondary to increased plasma ionized calcium or to a decrease in calcium-binding agents, such as micellar bile salts and lecithin-cholesterol vesicles.[60] The decrease in the bile salt pool secondary to an interruption of the enterohepatic circulation as seen in ileal resection or the NPO status accompanying TPN could result in this phenomenon.

*Brown pigment stones* are brown to orange in color, soft, soaplike or greasy in texture, and commonly assume the shape of their origin, the common bile duct.[54] The stone color is derived from calcium bilirubinate, and their greasy texture belies a significant component of fat (calcium palmitate or stearate derived from lecithin).[61] The scarcity of calcium carbonate and phosphate accounts for their lack of opacity on radiography.[53] The cholesterol content ranges from 2% to 28%, which is higher than in black stones and allows in part for their increased solubility. The most distinct clinical feature of brown gallstones in both adults and children is the association with infection.[24, 62] These stones are a major public health problem in rural areas of Asian countries, where they are found secondary to parasitic infestation with such organisms as *Opisthorchis sinensis* and *Ascaris lumbricoides.*[63] They are an uncommon type of stone in Western society and are typically found in the common bile duct after cholecystectomy when the bile is infected. Urinary tract infections may predispose to stone formation in early childhood.[64] In some 85% of cases, the bile grows *Escherichia coli.*[65] In children, especially infants, these stones can be seen in association with other organisms such as *Staphylococcus, Enterobacter, Citrobacter,*[62] and *Salmonella virchow.*[66] Infection with stasis results in excessive secretion of mucin, which may serve as the glycoprotein nidus for stone formation.[60] Bacteria also release beta-glucuronidase, phospholipase $A_1$, and conjugated bile salt hydrolase, which hydrolyze bilirubin glucuronides, lecithin, and conjugated bile salts, producing unconjugated bilirubin, free saturated fatty acids, lysolecithin, and free bile acids.[67] With the exception of lysolecithin, these products precipitate with calcium to form stones.[60] Biliary tree abnormalities, such as stenosis, also may predispose to brown stone formation.

## GALLSTONES IN INFANTS

Infants younger than 12 months of age may be predisposed to gallstone formation, as compared with older children[68] (Table 53–2). For example, the bile of infants is more dilute than that of older children, with a lower bile salt concentration, a shorter nucleation time, and a higher cholesterol saturation index.[68] These factors may help explain the increased tendency of infants to produce sludge and gallstones.[27] Table 53–2 demonstrates the likelihood (nearly one half of reported cases) for spontaneous resolution of gallstones during infancy.[69–71h] Such information deserves special consideration concerning therapeutic intervention in infants, and suggests that, unless symptomatic, gallstones during infancy do not require surgical intervention and often resolve without treatment.

## TOTAL PARENTERAL NUTRITION–ASSOCIATED STONES

The association between TPN and cholelithiasis is clearly established.[72] Gallstone formation in premature infants and neonates receiving TPN appears to have four stages: decreased hepatobiliary flow due to immaturity, stasis within

TABLE 53–2. Gallstones in Infancy (<12 Months Old)

| AUTHORS | NUMBER OF INFANTS | SPONTANEOUS RESOLUTION | SURGICAL TREATMENT† | PERSISTENT ASYMPTOMATIC | RECURRENCE |
|---|---|---|---|---|---|
| Keller (1985) | 5 | 5 | | | |
| Jacir (1986) | 4 | 3 | 1 | | |
| Jonas et al (1990) | 7 | 2 | 5 | | |
| Ljung et al (1992) | 5 | 1 | 1 | 3 | |
| Debray et al (1993) | 40 | 15 | 21 | 4 | 2 |
| Roman et al (1994) | 1 | 1 | | | |
| Johart (1995) | 2 | 1 | | 1 | |
| Monnerie (1995) | 1 | 1 | | | |
| Morad (1995)* | 15 | 8 | | | |
| Ishitani et al (1996) | 1 | | 1 | | |
| Stringer et al (1996) | 3 | 2 | | 1 | |
| Totals | 84 | 39 (46%) | 29 (35%) | 9 (11%) | 2 (2%) |

*Data on six patients not furnished.
†Includes therapeutic ERCP.
Data from references 69 to 71h.

the biliary tree, sludge formation, and finally, stone formation. Cholestasis, which increases with decreasing gestational age, is found in at least 50% of infants with a birth weight less than 1,000 gm.[73] After 2 months on TPN, 80% of infants have cholestasis.[73] This predisposition to cholestasis in infancy is multifactorial. Bile acid transport, bile secretion, and basal and stimulated bile salt flow rates all are immature.[73a, 74] Bile salt–dependent and –independent flow are decreased, approximating only 50% of that in adults.[72, 73a] The absence of oral feeding reduces the enterohepatic circulation of bile acids.[72] Fasting also inhibits the release of gut and biliary tree hormones, such as cholecystokinin, gastrin, secretin, motilin, and glucagon. The formation of echogenic, thick, "molasses-like" biliary sludge within the gallbladder has been documented in both adults and children receiving TPN.[72, 75, 76] Serial ultrasound examinations of adults receiving continuous TPN infusion show sludge formation increasing from 6% of patients in the first week to 50% in the fourth week and 100% after 6 weeks.[77] Gallbladder enlargement may be the first physical sign of sludge formation in the infant. Stagnant bile in a dilated gallbladder provides an ideal milieu for the development of both acalculous cholecystitis and cholelithiasis. TPN-induced gallstones are pigment stones, typically black and usually found in the gallbladder. They often have a high calcium phosphate or carbonate content; however, stone analysis indicates that they are of a mixed bilirubin-cholesterol composition and perhaps belong to a special group of TPN-induced pigment stones.

## ILEAL DISEASE AND ILEAL RESECTION–ASSOCIATED STONES

The enterohepatic circulation constantly replenishes the bile acid pool, which in turn governs the rate of bile salt secretion. The terminal ileum serves as the site of nearly 98% of bile acid resorption. Terminal ileal disease, typically Crohn's disease, or surgical resection of the ileum can result in an interruption of this bile acid recycling. The bile salt pool is subsequently reduced, thus altering the balance of bile components and favoring cholesterol supersaturation and increased bile lithogenicity. The formation of gallstones secondary to ileal disease has been reported in both adults and children. However, it appears that ileal resection only increases the tendency to gallstone formation after puberty.[78] After puberty, cholesterol secretion increases, whereas bile salt secretion declines, predisposing to cholesterol supersaturation and, hence, stone formation.[78]

## DRUG-ASSOCIATED STONES

The use of several drugs, furosemide, octreotide, and ceftriaxone, has been associated with an increased tendency to form gallstones. In reported cases with furosemide, numerous other contributing factors, such as prematurity, sepsis, and small bowel disease, were also noted. Whether furosemide alone contributes to gallstone formation remains unclear.[78a]

Octreotide has a wide range of biologic activity, including several clinically useful applications such as treatment of secretory diarrhea, acromegaly, and gastroenteropancreatic endocrine tumors. Gallstone formation has been found in about half of patients receiving octreotide when used chronically.[79–81] It is believed that this may be related to octreotide-induced gallbladder stasis or a direct effect of octreotide on gallbladder absorption.[82]

Ceftriaxone can induce gallbladder concretions. Ceftriaxone is excreted in bile and has the ability to displace bilirubin from albumin-binding sites. Reports in both adults and children have noted biliary echo densities or sludge often causing symptoms of cholecystitis with right upper quadrant pain, nausea, and vomiting. Analysis of the sludge reveals high concentrations of a calcium salt of ceftriaxone, with traces of bilirubinate and cholesterol, thus resembling pigment stone composition.[83] Fasting and age older than 24 months are risk factors associated with this so-called "pseudolithiasis."[84] The process of bile concretion and the related symptoms are reversible when the drug is discontinued.[85]

Cyclosporine usage in children undergoing heart transplant and kidney transplant has been implicated in gallstone formation, possibly related to elevated drug levels and hepatic toxicity.[86, 87]

## SYMPTOMS OF GALLSTONE DISEASE

The classic symptom complex of right upper quadrant pain and vomiting is usually associated with stones only in older children and adolescents. Younger children tend to present with nonspecific symptoms. Jaundice is frequently encountered in "symptomatic" infants.[27] The most likely age for silent stones is infancy through the preschool years. Intolerance to fatty food is rarely reported in children. Fever is an unusual finding at any age, and, if present, indicates associated cholecystitis. Complications of gallstone disease include cholecystitis, choledocholithiasis, cholangitis, and gallbladder perforation, but these occur rarely in children. Pancreatitis has been identified in 8% of children with gallstone disease and may represent the most common complication in children.[88]

Laboratory evaluation is usually unrewarding. Occasional patients will have a leukocytosis as well as mildly elevated hepatic transaminase levels. Plain film radiography is more useful in children than in adults, because about 50% of stones in children are radiopaque. Ultrasonography is the diagnostic procedure of choice, because it is noninvasive, sensitive, and specific. The ultrasonography also allows examination of the surrounding abdominal viscera, such as the pancreas and the biliary tree. Oral cholecystography has been largely replaced by ultrasound, but it can occasionally be useful in the evaluation of gallbladder function. Endoscopic retrograde cholangiopancreatography (ERCP) is particularly useful in the evaluation of ductal stones. Percutaneous cholangiograms offer another approach but are seldom used in children.

## TREATMENT OF GALLSTONE DISEASE

Observation may be the most prudent treatment in infants with asymptomatic gallstone disease (see Table 53–2). As the infant ages, the hepatobiliary enzyme systems mature and the potential for spontaneous stone dissolution exists. Spontaneous stone resolution also has been observed in TPN-induced gallstones. In children for whom the duration of TPN is expected to be limited and the stones are asymptomatic, observation is indicated. However, in children who are chronically dependent on TPN, such as in Crohn's disease, pseudo-obstruction syndrome, and the short bowel syndrome, stones should be removed.[88a]

Gallstones in older children should be removed, because spontaneous resolution seldom occurs. Cholecystostomy is indicated for acute drainage of the gallbladder and perhaps in seriously ill patients for whom only simple stone extraction is needed. Laparoscopic cholecystectomy is rapidly becoming the surgical procedure of choice, in both adults and children.[89–91]

Options for nonsurgical treatment of gallstone disease continue to proliferate. Despite the growing popularity of medical therapy for adults, there is no such approved medical treatment for gallstones in children (Table 53–3). Two bile acids currently exist for oral gallstone dissolution: chenodeoxycholic acid (chenodiol) and ursodeoxycholic acid (ursodiol). Both agents occur naturally and are present in bile. Chenodiol works by inhibiting HMG-CoA reductase, which suppresses hepatic cholesterol synthesis.[92, 93] Side effects such as diarrhea and hepatotoxicity have limited its widespread use. The mechanism of action of ursodiol is similar to chenodiol, inhibiting HMG-CoA reductase, and additionally, blocking intestinal absorption of cholesterol.[92] It has no hepatotoxicity and is currently under experimental use in chronic cholestatic diseases for treatment of pruritus and fatigue in both adults and children.[93] Diarrhea is rarely encountered. Combination use of both chenodiol and ursodiol appears more effective and allows a 50% reduction in dosage with fewer side effects.[94] Drawbacks to the use of such therapy include the long duration of therapy, recurrence after stopping, low success rate, and high cost. Only cholesterol stones are amenable to this therapy, thereby limiting its use in children.

**TABLE 53–3. Treatment Alternatives for Gallstones in Children**

| TYPE | COMMENTS | APPROVED IN CHILDREN |
|---|---|---|
| Cholecystectomy | Method of choice in most cases | Yes |
| Cholecystostomy | Effective for acute gallbladder drainage (i.e., acalculous cholecystitis) | Yes |
| Laparoscopic cholecystectomy | Effective with severely ill patients, shortens hospitalization (e.g., cystic fibrosis) | Yes |
| ERCP | | |
| Basket removal | Bile duct stone removal | Yes |
| Mechanical basket lithotripsy | Stone crushing within bile ducts | No |
| Laser lithotripsy | Stone destruction within bile ducts (experimental) | No |
| ESWL | Limited experience (unpublished), only for cholesterol stones currently | No |
| Dissolution | | |
| Oral | Ursodeoxycholic acid and chenodeoxycholic acid | No |
| | Blocks HMG-CoA reductase, decreases cholesterol synthesis | |
| Contact | Methyl *tert*-butyl-ether (for cholesterol stones only) | No |
| | Bile acid EDTA (for pigment stones; experimental) | No |
| Preventive | | |
| Enteral feeds | Even small amounts during TPN decrease stone risk | Yes |
| Weight loss | For obesity—gradual weight loss | Yes |
| Lovastatin and simvastatin | Block HMG-CoA reductase, decrease cholesterol synthesis (experimental) | No |
| Cholecystokinin | Stimulates gallbladder contraction while NPO (experimental) | No |

EDTA, ethylene diaminetetraacetic acid; ERCP, endoscopic retrograde cholangiopancreatography; ESWL, extracorporeal shock-wave lithotripsy.

Extracorporeal shock-wave lithotripsy (ESWL) was first used successfully in humans to fragment renal calculi. ESWL generates high-amplitude pressure waves that are focused on the stone by computerized ultrasonography. Only symptomatic stones that are radiolucent can be treated with this method, again limiting its use in children. Best results are obtained with solitary stones, with success rates of 95% to 100% reported.[95] Oral dissolution therapy appears to be a rational addition to lithotripsy to achieve complete stone dissolution.[96] The two major complications of lithotripsy are cholecystitis and pancreatitis, reported in 1% to 2% of patients.[95, 96] Successful treatment of gallstones in children has been accomplished.[97, 98]

Cholesterol gallstones can be dissolved using methyl *tert*-butyl ether (MTBE). The procedure first requires placement of a percutaneous transhepatic catheter into a contrast-enhanced gallbladder. A greater than 95% success rate in stone dissolution has been reported.[99] Complications include leakage of the MTBE, causing nausea, vomiting, and duodenitis, and intravascular hemolysis if the MTBE enters the vascular system, which has limited its application in children.[99] Chemical dissolution of calcified cholesterol stones and brown pigment stones has been tried experimentally with bile acid ethylenediaminetetraacetic acid, but has shown only limited success.

The prevention of gallstones in children entails recognition of risk factors and an understanding of the pathophysiology of stone disease. The use of limited enteral feedings during TPN therapy, for example, stimulates gallbladder contraction, thus decreasing gallbladder stasis. Early use of pancreatic enzyme supplements in patients with cystic fibrosis decreases the propensity to stone formation. Informed use of contraceptives other than birth control pills, particularly in women with known gallstone risk factors, would seem advisable. Weight control in obese patients is advisable to decrease the risk of gallstone disease, but rapid weight loss programs in obese patients may actually promote gallstone formation secondary to increased bile cholesterol saturation and gallbladder stasis.[100, 101] Medical therapy with cholesterol-lowering agents, such as lovastatin and simvastatin, may be considered in high-risk patients, although no data exist for the use of this therapy in children (see Table 53–3).

## CHOLECYSTITIS

Cholecystitis is a disease that results from inflammation of the gallbladder, typically secondary to gallstone obstruction of the cystic duct. Cholecystitis may be acute or chronic. Most cholecystitis in children is chronic and is associated with gallstones. The presentation of "acute" cholecystitis in children most likely represents a significant episode of an ongoing process of gallbladder distention and mucosal damage that culminated in cholecystitis.

The pathophysiology of cholecystitis parallels that of gallstone formation, with gallbladder stasis as the initiating event. The stasis is usually secondary to obstruction of the cystic duct by a gallstone or to local edema secondary to a stone. Other causes include external compression of the cystic duct by swollen lymph nodes, torsion of the gallbladder, congenital ductal abnormalities, and trauma. The basis for the inflammation is unclear, although mechanical distention, ischemia, bacteria, and lysolecithins have been implicated.

The typical presenting symptom is right upper quadrant abdominal pain, occasionally radiating to the back and associated with vomiting. When distended and inflamed, the gallbladder lies on the anterior abdominal wall between the 9th and 10th costal cartilages, causing localized tenderness on palpation and giving rise to the diagnostic Murphy's sign. Jaundice and fever are seen in 25% to 30% of children and are more common in young infants. The onset of symptoms is usually over a period of 1 week, but lesser symptoms of biliary colic may occur over several years. The differential diagnosis should include hepatitis, hepatic abscess, tumor, gonococcal perihepatitis (Fitz-Hugh-Curtis syndrome), pancreatitis, appendicitis, peptic ulcer disease, pneumonia, pyelonephritis, and kidney stones.

Laboratory evaluation should include a complete blood count and differential; serum bilirubin, alkaline phosphatase or gamma-glutamyltransferase, serum aminotransferases, amylase levels; and urinalysis. Leukocytosis is frequently found. Elevated aminotransferase levels and mild hyperbilirubinemia are seen in 20% of patients. Elevated amylase levels are common even without pancreatitis. Marked elevation of the bilirubin, alkaline phosphatase, or gamma-glutamyltransferase levels may indicate stones in the biliary tree. The characteristic ultrasound finding is a discrete echo density indicating a stone, usually occupying a dependent position in the gallbladder, which changes or moves when the patient is moved and is associated with acoustic shadowing (Fig 53–3). Gallbladder dilation, a thickened gallbladder wall, the presence of sludge, and biliary tree anomalies also may be seen (Fig. 53–4). Cholescintigraphy can be helpful to evaluate gallbladder function, revealing normal hepatic uptake but nonvisualization of the gallbladder at 1 hour.[102] False-positive results may occur with prolonged fasting, TPN, and hepatocellular disease. Oral cholecystography is used less frequently, owing to several inherent drawbacks, such as failure to concentrate the dye (particularly if hyperbilirubinemia exists), a 6% to 8% false-negative rate, hypersensitivity to the dye, and radiation exposure.

Hospitalization with institution of intravenous fluids, cessation of oral feeding, gastric decompression, and analgesics is appropriate. Antibiotics are not needed in simple cases,

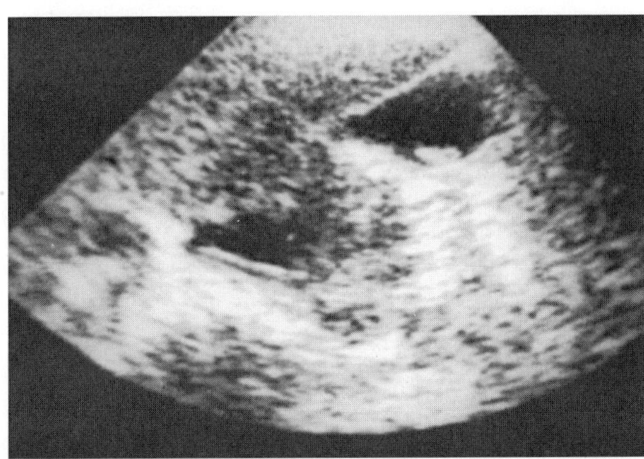

**FIGURE 53–3.** Ultrasound of gallstone within the gallbladder showing acoustic shadowing. (Courtesy of Dr. Robert V. Dutton.)

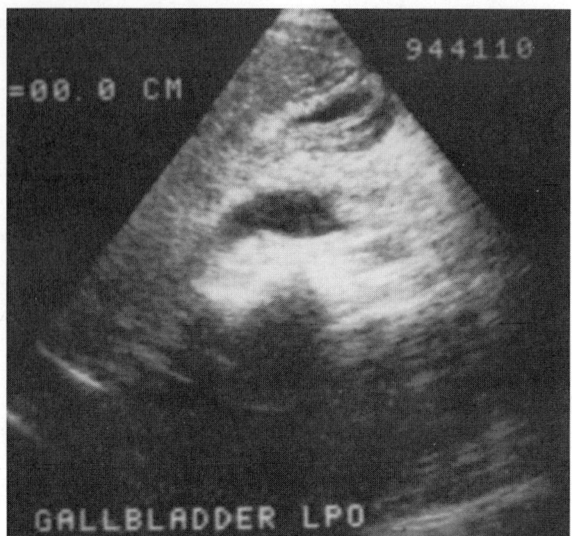


**FIGURE 53–4.** Ultrasound of dilated gallbladder with a thickened wall. (Courtesy of Dr. Robert V. Dutton.)

but if fever persists or the condition worsens, their use is indicated. Ampicillin, gentamicin, and clindamycin are a common combination used to cover enteric organisms and provide good biliary excretion. Cefoperazone also is a logical choice owing to its excellent biliary excretion and broad spectrum of bacterial sensitivity.

Cholecystectomy is the procedure of choice in calculous cholecystitis. In children with sickle cell disease, hypertransfusion should be performed prior to surgery. Cholecystostomy with stone removal can be done in those patients for whom a functioning gallbladder is important, such as in patients with Crohn's disease. Table 53–3 lists the possible treatment options in children.

Most cases of cholecystitis usually resolve over several days. Complications occur in 30% of cases and include gallbladder perforation, abscess, or empyema formation. When fever persists or exceeds 102°F and pain or tenderness worsens, perforation is likely. Such perforations typically occur in the fundus of the gallbladder. A local perforation may wall off as an abscess, extend into the peritoneum as peritonitis, or lead to a cholecystoenteric fistula. Surgical intervention with vigorous antibiotic support is essential.

Chronic obstruction of the cystic duct may lead to the interesting finding of the "milk of calcium" gallbladder or "limy bile" syndrome. In this situation, complete obstruction of the cystic duct leads to a hydropic gallbladder. Bile pigments are deconjugated to colorless compounds, and excess calcium is secreted, opacifying the bile to a white appearance both visually and radiographically. Calcium accumulating in the wall of the gallbladder secondary to chronic cystic duct obstruction may produce the "porcelain gallbladder." This condition appears secondary to chronic cholecystitis and in adults leads to carcinoma in as many as 50% of cases.[103]

## CHOLEDOCHOLITHIASIS (COMMON BILE DUCT STONES)

Common bile duct stones are an unusual occurrence in children. Most ductal stones in children are black pigment stones, although cholesterol stones have been found. Both of these types of stones originate from the gallbladder. Less common are brown pigment stones, which form within the common bile duct secondary to infection.[62] Most ductal stones in children are believed to lodge within the common bile duct because of congenital narrowing or stenosis.[104] The usual clinical presentation of common bile duct stones in children is jaundice, progressing to symptoms similar to those of cholecystitis. Right upper quadrant pain with fever is common.

Laboratory evaluation may reveal leukocytosis, elevated aminotransferase levels, and specific elevations of biliary tract enzymes such as alkaline phosphatase and gamma-glutamyltransferase. If fever is present, blood cultures may be positive. Abdominal ultrasound is indicated to detect the presence of stones or ductal dilation. Magnetic resonance cholangiography is a new diagnostic tool that is useful in viewing the biliary tree, especially if suspected stones are not detected by ultrasound.[105, 106]

The presence of fever requires broad-spectrum antibiotic coverage, as with cholecystitis. A dilated biliary tree with accompanying fever necessitates prompt surgical intervention, with drainage and stone removal. ERCP is an excellent tool for both diagnosis and therapy, including stone removal, dilation of a stenosis, or placement of a stent. The use of ERCP has become much more common in children, even infants.[107–109]

## ACALCULOUS CHOLECYSTITIS

Cholecystitis can occur without the presence of gallstones. This condition is rare in adults, but occurs with surprising frequency in pediatrics, usually in extremely ill children in intensive care units. The cause is not known but is associated with the immediate postoperative state, trauma, or burns. Sepsis from a variety of organisms, including *Leptospira,* group B streptococci, *Shigella, Salmonella,* and *E. coli,* has been associated with this condition, although no organism has emerged as definitive.[110] Because no obstructing stone is present, gallbladder stasis must play an important role. The stasis may be due to fever, dehydration, prolonged fasting, ileus, or TPN, which are common in the severely ill child.[110]

The clinical findings are usually fever, abdominal pain, and jaundice. Physical examination reveals a palpable abdominal mass, quite tender to touch. Laboratory studies are usually not helpful, but may reveal leukocytosis and elevated bilirubin levels. Diagnosis is aided by ultrasound identification of a large, distended gallbladder with a thickened wall and tenderness during the procedure (the ultrasonographic Murphy's sign). Biliary scintigraphy also is accurate, revealing normal liver uptake but no visualization of the gallbladder. Unfortunately, false-negative results of both ultrasound and scintigraphy occur in as many as 20% of cases when no stone is seen.[111]

In most instances, the treatment of choice is emergency laparotomy, with either cholecystostomy or cholecystectomy. Because the incidence of gallbladder gangrene is rare in children as compared with adults, simple drainage may be the method of choice. If gangrene is suspected on inspection of the gallbladder at laparotomy, resection is necessary.

## ACUTE HYDROPS OF THE GALLBLADDER

Hydrops of the gallbladder is characterized by distention but no inflammation. The distinction between acalculous cholecystitis and hydrops is therefore one of histology. Clinically, the differentiation of these two entities may be difficult. Most cases of acalculous cholecystitis are in severely ill patients, whereas hydrops tends to occur in a more benign setting, frequently involving a systemic vasculitis. The mucocutaneous lymph node syndrome (Kawasaki syndrome) is the commonest cause of gallbladder hydrops.[112] Hydrops also has been associated with other vascular disorders, such as Sjögren's disease, systemic sclerosis, and Henoch-Schönlein purpura, as well as nephrotic syndrome, familial Mediterranean fever, mesenteric adenitis, leptospirosis, Epstein-Barr virus, and bacterial infection with *Staphylococcus* and *Streptococcus*.[110, 113, 114] The cause is unknown, although local lymph node enlargement around the cystic duct and local vasculitis causing gallbladder ischemia are possibilities.

The clinical presentation is acute right upper quadrant abdominal pain, nausea, and vomiting. Examination reveals upper abdominal tenderness, often with a palpable mass. Diagnosis is aided by ultrasound findings of a distended gallbladder with normal wall thickness and no echo densities. Biochemical studies are usually of little help. Surgical consultation should be obtained in all cases of suspected hydrops, although surgical intervention is rarely indicated. Medical management is supportive, with vigilant surgical observation. The development of fever or an increasingly tender abdomen suggests perforation and requires surgery. Most cases show steady resolution over about 2 weeks, with no known long-term sequelae.

## UNUSUAL DISEASES OF THE GALLBLADDER

Carcinoma of the gallbladder has been reported in children, but is rare.[115] In adults, gallbladder carcinoma is usually associated with gallstones. Although commoner than carcinoma in children, benign gallbladder tumors also are rare. Adenomatous polyps have been described associated with Peutz-Jeghers syndrome.[116]

Adenomyomatosis, or hyperplastic gallbladder, denotes hyperplasia of the mucous membrane, thickening of the muscularis, and deep diverticular formations known as *Rokitansky-Aschoff sinuses*.[48] Odd deformities of the gallbladder, such as the phrygian cap, fish-hook anomaly, and Hartmann's pouch, are associated with adenomyomatosis of the gallbladder.[1] The cause of the hyperplasia is unknown, although increased intraluminal gallbladder pressure has been implicated. No specific symptoms have ever been attributed to this condition; therefore, no specific therapy is advised.

Cholesterolosis is characterized by accumulation of cholesterol esters in the mucosa and submucosa of the gallbladder. After resection, these areas are visible as yellow spots on a red mucosal background, giving the appearance of a strawberry, thus the term *strawberry gallbladder*. Occasionally, these areas enlarge and become polypoid, leading to cystic duct obstruction. Typically though, no symptoms are directly attributed to this condition, and thus no therapy is indicated. If symptoms do occur, cholecystectomy is indicated.

Metachromatic leukodystrophy, or sulfatide lipidosis, is an autosomal recessive disorder of sphingolipid metabolism. The biochemical defect in this disorder is the inability to degrade sphingolipid sulfatide or galactose-3 sulfate ceramide. The absence or deficiency of the lysosomal enzyme arylsulfatase A results in the accumulation of sulfatide in both neural and non-neural tissues, in particular the gallbladder. Gallstones have been reported in association with this disorder. The cause may involve gallbladder hypomotility secondary to sulfatide accumulation in the wall of the gallbladder or sulfatide granules serving as "seeds" for gallstone formation.[117]

Polypoid gastric heterotopia in the gallbladder is extremely rare in children, consisting of polyps within the gallbladder with ectopic gastric mucosa.[118] Gallbladder polyps are usually asymptomatic and occur in association with other diseases such as Crohn's disease, Peutz-Jeghers syndrome, or leukodystrophy.[119, 120] The presence of ectopic gastric mucosa may allow acid secretion, causing mucosal inflammation leading to cholecystitis.

Gallstones have been noted in pseudohypoaldosteronism,[121] presumed secondary to dehydration and electrolyte abnormalities. Wildervanck's syndrome (cervico-oculo-acoustic syndrome) also has been found to include gallstones,[122] although the cause is unknown.

## REFERENCES

1. Way LW, Sleisenger MH: Cholelithiasis: chronic and acute cholecystitis. In Sleisenger MH, Fordtran JS (eds): Gastrointestinal Disease: Pathophysiology, Diagnosis, Management. Philadelphia, WB Saunders, 1989, p 1691.
2. Holland C, Heaton KH: Increasing frequency of gallbladder operations in the Bristol area. Br Med J 1972;3:672.
3. Friedman GD, Kamel WB, Dawber TR: The epidemiology of gallbladder disease: observations in the Framingham Study. J Chron Dis 1966;19:273.
4. The Coronary Drug Project Research Group: the Coronary Drug Project: design, methods and baseline results. Circulation 1973;47 (Suppl 1):1.
5. Sampliner RE, Bennet PH, Comess LJ, et al: Gallbladder disease in the Pima Indians: demonstration of high prevalence and early onset by cholecystography. N Engl J Med 1970;283:1358.
6. Bainton D, Davies GT, Evans KT, et al: Gallbladder disease: prevalence in a South Wales industrial town. N Engl J Med 1976; 294:1147.
7. Maurer KR, Everhart JE, Exxati TM, et al: Prevalence of gallstone disease in Hispanic populations in the United States. Gastroenterology 1989;96:487.
8. Bates GC, Brown CH: Incidence of gallbladder disease in chronic hemolytic anemia (spherocytosis). Gastroenterology 1952;21:104.
9. Barbara L, Festi D, Frabboni R, et al: Incidence and risk factors for gallstone disease: the Sirmione study (abstract). Hepatology 1988;8:1256.
10. Barker DJP, Gardner MJ, Power C, et al: Prevalence of gallstones at necropsy in nine British towns: a collaborative study. Br Med J 1979;2:1389.
11. Bateson MC, Bouchier IAD: Prevalence of gallstones in Dundee: necropsy study. Br Med J 1975;4:4271.
12. Layde PM, Vessey MP, Yeatles D: Risk factors for gallbladder disease: a cohort study of young women attending family planning clinics. J Epidemiol Commun Health 1982;36:274.
13. Lindstrom CG: Frequency of gallstone disease in a well-defined Swedish population: a prospective necropsy study in Malmo. Scand J Gastroenterol 1977;12:341.
14. Rome Group for the Epidemiology and Prevention of Cholelithiasis

(GREPCO): prevalence of gallstone disease in an Italian adult female population. Am J Epidemiol 1984;119:796.
15. Biss K, Ho KJ, Mikkelson B, et al: Some unique biologic characteristics of the Masai of East Africa. N Engl J Med 1971;284:694.
16. Khanuja B, Cheah YC, Hunt M, et al: Lithil, a major gene affecting cholesterol gallstone formation among inbred strains of mice. Proc Natl Acad Sci USA 1995;92:7729–7733.
17. Gibson J: An extraordinary large gallbladder and hydropic cystis: medical essays and observations. Philos Soc Edin 1737;2:352.
18. Glenn F: 25-year experience in the surgical treatment of 5037 patients with non-malignant biliary tract disease. Surg Gynecol Obstet 1959; 109:591–606.
19. Andrassy RJ, Treadwell TA, Ratner, IA, et al: Gallbladder disease in children and adolescents. Am J Surg 1976;132:10.
20. Shafer AD, Ashley JV, Goodwin CD, et al: A new look at the multifactorial etiology of gallbladder disease in children. Am Surg 1983;49:314.
21. Lau GE, Andrassy RJ, Mahour GH: A 30-year review of the management of gallbladder disease at a children's hospital. Am Surg 1983;49:411.
22. Henschue CI, Littlewood-Teele R: Cholelithiasis in children: recent observations. J Ultrasound Med 1983;2:481.
23. Holcomb GW: Gallbladder disease. In Welch KJ, Randolph JA Jr, Rowe MI ed: Pediatric Surgery, Vol 2. Chicago, Year Book Publications, 1986, p 1060.
24. Descos B, Bernard O, Brunelle F, et al: Pigment gallstones of the common bile duct in infancy. Hepatology 1984;4:678.
25. Calabrese C, Pearlman DM: Gallbladder disease below the age of 21 years. Surgery 1971;70:413.
26. Honore LH: Cholesterol cholelithiasis in adolescent females. Arch Surg 1980;114:62.
27. Friesen CA, Roberts CC: Cholelithiasis: clinical characteristics in children, case analysis and literature review. Clin Pediatr 1989; 28:294.
28. Holan KR, Holzbach RT, Hermann RE, et al: Nucleation time: a key factor in the pathogenesis of cholesterol gallstone disease. Gastroenterology 1979;77:611–617.
29. Donovan JM, Carey MC: Separation and quantitation of cholesterol "carriers" in bile. Hepatology 1990;12:945–1045.
30. Carey MC: Formation of cholesterol gallstones: the new paradigms. In Paumgartner G, Stiehl A, Gerok W (eds): Trends in Bile Acid Research. Dordrecht, Kluwer Academic Publishers, 1989, pp 259–281.
31. Forgacs IC: Pathogenesis of cholesterol gallstone disease: the motility defect. In Northfield T, Jazrawi R, Zentler-Munro P (eds): Bile Acids in Health and Disease. Dordrecht, Kluwer Academic Publishers, 1988, pp 135–153.
32. Carey MC, Cahalane MC: Whither biliary sludge? Gastroenterology 1988;95:508–523.
33. Booker ML, Scott TE, LaMorte WW: Effect of dietary cholesterol on phosphatidylcholines and phosphatidylethanolamines in bile and gallbladder mucosa in the prairie dog. Gastroenterology 1989;97:1261–1267.
34. Kajiyama G, Kubota S, Sasaki H, et al: Lipid metabolism in the development of cholesterol gallstones in hamsters: I. Study on the relationship between serum and biliary lipids. Hiroshima J Med Sci 1980;29:133–141.
35. Lee DWT, Gilmore CJ, Bonorris G, et al: Effect of dietary cholesterol on biliary lipids in patients with gallstones and normal subjects. Am J Clin Nutr 1985;42:414–420.
36. Angelin B, Backman L, Einarsson K, et al: Hepatic cholesterol metabolism in obesity: activity of microsomal 3-hydroxy-3-methylglutaryl coenzyme A reductase. J Lipid Res 1981;23:770–773.
37. Ahlberg J, Angelin B, Bjorkhem I, et al: Hepatic cholesterol metabolism of normal and hyperlipidemic patients with cholesterol gallstones. J Lipid Res 1979;20:107–115.
38. Einarsson K, Nilsel K, Leijd B, et al: Influence of age on secretion of cholesterol and synthesis of bile acids by the liver. N Engl J Med 1985;313:277–282.
39. Pellegrini CA, Ryan T, Broderick W, et al: Gallbladder filling and emptying during cholesterol gallstone formation in the prairie dog. Gastroenterology 1986;90:143–149.
40. Li YF, Weisbrodt NW, Moody FG, et al: Calcium-induced contraction and contractile protein content of gallbladder smooth muscle after high-cholesterol feeding of prairie dogs. Gastroenterology 1987;92:746–750.
41. Behar J, Lee KY, Thompson WE, et al: Gallbladder contraction in patients with pigment and cholesterol stones. Gastroenterology 1989;97:1479–1484.
42. Lee SP, Maher K, Nicholls JF: Origin and fate of biliary sludge. Gastroenterology 1988;94:170.
43. Smith BF: Human gallbladder mucin binds biliary lipids and promotes cholesterol crystal nucleation in model bile. J Lipid Res 1987;28:1088.
44. Nilsson S: Gallbladder disease and sex hormones. Acta Chir Scand 1966;132:275.
45. Bennion LJ, Knowler WC, Mott DM, et al: Development of lithogenic bile during puberty in Pima Indians. N Engl J Med 1979;300:873.
46. Vessey M, Painter R: Oral contraceptive use and benign gallbladder disease revisited. Contraception 1994;50:167–173.
47. Kern F, Everson GT: Contraceptive steroids in cholesterol in bile: mechanisms of actions. J Lipid Res 1987;28:828.
48. Warren KW, Williams CI, Tan EGC: Diseases of the gallbladder and bile ducts. In Schiff L, Schiff ER, eds: Diseases of the Liver. Philadelphia, JB Lippincott, 1987, pp 1289–1335.
49. Gaskin KJ, Waters DLM, Howman-Giles R, et al: Liver disease and common-bile-duct stenosis in cystic fibrosis. N Engl J Med 1988;318:340.
50. Isenberg J, L'Heureux PR, Warwick W, et al: Clinical observations on the biliary system in cystic fibrosis. Am J Gastroenterol 1976; 65:134.
51. Weber AM, Roy CC, Morin CL, et al: Malabsorption of bile acids in children with cystic fibrosis. N Engl J Med 1973;289:1001.
52. Watkins JB, Tercyak AM, Szczepanik P, et al: Bile salt kinetics in cystic fibrosis. Gastroenterology 1974;67:385.
53. Crowther RS, Soloway RD: Pigment gallstone pathogenesis: from man to molecules. Semin Liver Dis 1990;10:171.
54. Ostrow JD: The etiology of pigment gallstones. Hepatology 1984;4:215S.
55. Black BE, Carr SH, Ostrow JD, et al: Equilibrium swelling of pigment gallstones: evidence for network polymer structure. Biopolymers 1882;21:601.
56. Burnett W, Dwyer KR, Kennard CHL: Black pigment in polybilirubinate gallstones. Ann Surg 1981;193:331.
57. Sarnaik S, Slovis TI, Corbett DP, et al: Incidence of cholelithiasis in sickle cell anemia using the ultrasonic gray-scale technique. J Pediatr 1980;96:1005.
58. Lackman BS, Lazerson J, Stashak RJ, et al: The prevalence of cholelithiasis in sickle cell disease as diagnosed by ultrasound and cholecystography. Pediatrics 1979;64:501.
59. Tabata M, Nakayama F: Bacteria and gallstones: etiological significance. Dig Dis Sci 1981;26:218.
60. Cahalane MJ, Neubrand MW, Carey MC: Physical-chemical pathogenesis of pigment gallstones. Semin Liver Dis 1988;8:317.
61. Wosiewitz U, Schenk J, Sabinski F, et al: Investigations on common bile duct stones. Digestion 1983;26:43.
62. Treem WR, Malet PF, Gourley GR, et al: Bile and stone analysis in two infants with brown pigment gallstones and infected bile. Gastroenterology 1989;96:519.
63. Hikasa Y, Nagase M, Tanimura H, et al: Epidemiology and etiology of gallstones. Arch Jpn Chir 1980;49:555.
64. Hes FJ, de Jong TP, Bax NM, Houwen RH: Urinary tract infections and cholelithiasis in early childhood. J Pediatr Gastroenterol Nutr 1995;21:319–321.
65. Tabata M, Nakayama F: Bacteria and gallstones: etiological significance. Dig Dis Sci 1981;26:218.
66. Beiler HA, Kuntz C, Eckstein TM, Daum R: Cholecystolithiasis and infection of the biliary tract with *Salmonella virchow*—a very rare case in early childhood. Eur J Pediatr Surg 1995;5:369–371.
67. Akiyoshi T, Nakayama F: bile acid composition in brown pigment stones. Dig Dis Sci 1990;35:27–32.
68. Halpern Z, Vinograd Z, Laufer H, et al: Characteristics of gallbladder bile of infants and children. J Pediatr Gastroenterol Nutr 1996;23:147–150.
69. Stringer MD, Lim P, Cave M, et al: Fetal gallstones. J Pediatr Surg 1996;31:1589–1591.
70. Morad Y, Zin N, Merlob P: Incidental diagnosis of asymptomatic neonatal cholelithiasis: a case report and a literature review. J Perinatology 1995;15:314–317.
71. Debray D, Pariente P, Gauthier F, et al: Cholelithiasis in infancy: a study of 40 cases. J Pediatr 1993;122:385–391.
71a. Keller MS, Markle BM, Laffey PA, et al: Spontaneous resolution of cholelithiasis in infants. Radiology 1985;157:345.

71b. Jacir NN, Anderson KD, Eichelberger M, et al: Cholelithiasis in infancy: resolution of gallstones in three of four infants. J Pediatr Surg 1986;21:567.

71c. Jonas A, Yahav J, Fradkin A, et al: Choledocholithiasis in infants: diagnostic and therapeutic problems. J Pediatr Gastroenterol Nutr 1990;11:513–517.

71d. Ljung R, Ivarsson S, Nilsson P, Solvig J: Cholelithiasis during the first years of life: a case report and literature review. Acta Paediatr 1992;81:69–72.

71e. Roman B, Chiappa JL, Formantici F, et al: Neonatal choledocholithiasis: a case report. Pediatr Med Chir 1994;16:595–597.

71f. Johart G: Congenital cholelithiasis. Orv Hetil 1995;136:67–70.

71g. Monnerie JL, Soulard D: Cholelithiasis in infants with spontaneously favorable course. Arch Pediatr 1995;2:654–656.

71h. Ishitani MB, Shaul DB, Padua EA, McAlpin CA: Choledocholithiasis in a premature infant. J Pediatr 1996;128:853–855.

72. Suchy FJ, Mullick FG: Total parenteral nutrition-associated cholestasis. In Balistreri WF, Stocker JT (eds): Pediatric Hepatology. New York, Hemisphere Publishing, 1990, pp 29–40.

73. Beale EF, Nelson RM, Buccarelli RL, et al: Intrahepatic cholestasis associated with parenteral nutrition in premature infants. Pediatrics 1979;64:347.

73a. Suchy FJ, Bucavalas JC, Novak DA: Determinants of bile formation during development: ontogeny of hepatic bile acid metabolism and transport. Semin Liver Dis 1987;7:77.

74. Suita S, Ikeda K, Naito K, et al: Cholelithiasis in infants: association with parenteral nutrition. J Parenter Enteral Nutr 1984;8:569.

75. Enzenauer RW, Montrey JS, Barcia PJ, et al: Total parenteral nutrition cholestasis: a cause of mechanical biliary obstruction. Pediatrics 1985;76:905.

76. Lilly JR, Sokol RJ: On the bile sludge syndrome or is total parenteral nutrition cholestasis a surgical disease? Pediatrics 1985;76:992.

77. Benjamin DR: Hepatobiliary dysfunction in infants and children associated with long-term total parenteral nutrition: a clinicopathologic study. Am J Clin Pathol 1980;81:276.

78. Heubi JE, O'Connell NC, Setchell KD: Ileal resection/dysfunction in childhood predisposes to lithogenic bile only after puberty. Gastroenterology 1992;103:636–640.

78a. Callahan J, Haller JO, Cacciarelli AA, et al: Cholelithiasis in infants: association with total parenteral nutrition and furosemide. Pediatr Radiol 1982;143:437.

79. Trendle MC, Moertel CG, Kvois LK: Incidence and morbidity of cholelithiasis in patients receiving chronic octreotide for metastatic carcinoid and malignant islet cell tumors. Cancer 1996;79:830–834.

80. Redfern JS, Fortuner WJ II: Octreotide-associated biliary tract dysfunction and gallstone formation: pathophysiology and management. Am J Gastroenterology 1995;90:1042–1052.

81. McKnight JA, McCance DR, Sheridan B, Atkinson AB: Four years' treatment of resistant acromegaly with octreotide. Eur J Endocrinol 1995;132:429–432.

82. Moser AJ, Abedin MZ, Giurgiu DI, Roslyn JJ: Octreotide promotes gallbladder absorption in prairie dogs: a potential cause of gallstones. Gastroenterology 1995;108:1547–1555.

83. Park HZ, Lee SP, Schy AL: Ceftriaxone-associated gallbladder sludge. Gastroenterology 1991;100:1665.

84. Kong MS, Chen CY: Risk factors leading to ceftriaxone-associated biliary pseudolithiasis in children. Chang Keng i Hsueh–Chang Gung Medical J 1996;19:50–54.

85. Robertson FM, Crombleholme TM, Barlow SE, et al: Ceftriaxone choledocholithiasis. Pediatrics 1996;98:133–135.

86. Weinstein S, Lipsitz EC, Addonizio L, Stolar CJ: Cholelithiasis in pediatric cardiac transplant patients on cyclosporine. J Pediatr Surg 1995;30:61–64.

87. Pitcher GJ, Azmy AF: Cholelithiasis in paediatric renal transplant patients: implications for screening and management. Br J Urol 1996;78:316–317.

88. Reif S, Sloven DG, Lebenthal E: Gallstones in children: characteristics by age, etiology and outcome. Am J Dis Child 1991;146:105.

88a. Thompson JS: The role of prophylactic cholecystectomy in the short bowel syndrome. Arch Surg 1996;131:556–559.

89. Kim PC, Wesson D, Superina R, Filler R: Laparoscopic cholecystectomy versus open cholecystectomy in children: which is better? J Pediatr Surg 1995;30:971–973.

90. Holbling N, Pilz E, Feil W, Schiessel R: Laparoscopic cholecystectomy—a meta analysis of 23,700 cases and status of a personal patient sample. Wien Klin Wochenschr 1995;107:158–162.

91. Holcomb GW III, Naffis D: Laparoscopic cholecystectomy in infants. J Pediatr Surg 1994;29:86–87.

92. Salen G, Tint GS, Shefer S: Oral dissolution treatment of gallstones with bile acids. Semin Liver Dis 1990;10:181.

93. Leuschner U, Leuschner M, Sieratzki J, et al: Gallstone dissolution with ursodeoxycholic acid in patients with chronic active hepatitis and two years follow-up: a pilot study. Dig Dis Sci 1985;30:642.

94. Podda M, Zuin M, Battezzati M, et al: Efficacy and safety of a combination of chenodeoxycholic and ursodeoxycholic acid for gallstone dissolution: a comparison with ursodeoxycholic acid alone. Gastroenterology 1989;96:222.

95. Sackman M, Delius M, Sauerbruch T, et al: Shock-wave lithotripsy of gallbladder stones—the first 175 patients. N Engl J Med 1988;318:393.

96. Albert MB, Fromm H: Extracorporeal shock-wave lithotripsy of gallstones with the adjuvant use of cholelitholytic bile acids. Semin Liver Dis 1990;10:197.

97. Ziegenhagen DJ, Wedel S, Kruis W, Zehnter E: Successful extracorporeal lithotripsy of gallbladder stones in a 12 year old girl. Padiatrie und Padologie 1993;28:55–56.

98. Sokal EM, De Bilderling G, Clapuyt P, et al: Extracorporeal shockwave lithotripsy for calcified lower choledocholithiasis in an 18 month old boy. J Pediatr Gastroenterol Nutr 1994;18:391–394.

99. Thistle JL, Peterson BT, Bender CE, et al: Percutaneous dissolution of gallstones using methyl tert-butyl ether. Can J Gastroenterol 1990;4:625.

100. Weinsier RL, Wilson LJ, Lee J: Medically safe rate of weight loss for the treatment of obesity: a guideline based on risk of gallstone formation. Am J Med 1995;98:115–117.

101. Gebhard RL, Prigge WF, Ansel HJ, et al: The role of gallbladder emptying in gallstone formation during diet-induced rapid weight loss. Hepatology 1996;24:544–548.

102. Pare P, Shaffer EA, Rosenthall L: Nonvisualization of the gallbladder by 99mTc-HIDA cholescintigraphy as evidence of cholecystitis. Can Med Assoc J 1978;118:384.

103. Freund MC: Images in clinical medicine:porcelain gallbladder. N Engl J Med 1994;330:402.

104. Lilly JR: Common bile duct calculi in infants and children. J Pediatr Surg 1980;15:577.

105. Ishizaki Y, Wakayama T, Okada Y, Kobayashi T: Magnetic resonance cholangiography for evaluation of obstructive jaundice. Am J Gastroenterol 1993;88:2072–2077.

106. Meakem TJ, Schnall MD: Magnetic resonance cholangiography. Gastroentrol Clin North Am 1995;24:221–238.

107. Gilger MA: The role of ERCP in children. Pract Gastroenterol 1996;20:11–20.

108. Werlin SL: Endoscopic retrograde cholangiopancreatography in children. Gastrointes Endosc Clin North Am 1994;4:161–178.

109. Guelrud M, Mendoza S, Zager A: ERCP and endoscopic sphincterotomy in infants and children with jaundice due to common duct stones. Gastrointest Endosc 1992;39:450–453.

110. Ternberg JL, Keating JP: Acute acalculous cholecystitis: complication of other illnesses in childhood. Arch Surg 1975;110:543.

111. Shuman WP, Rogers JV, Rudd TG, et al: Low sensitivity of sonography and cholescintigraphy in acalculous cholecystitis. AJR Am J Roentgenol 1984;142:531.

112. Grisoni E, Fisher R, Izant R: Kawasaki syndrome: report of four cases with acute gallbladder hydrops. J Pediatr Surg 1984;19:9–11.

113. Amemoto K, Nagita A, Aoki S, et al: Ultrasonographic gallbladder wall thickening in children with Henoch-Schonlein purpura. J Pediatr Gastroenterol Nutr 1994;19:126–128.

114. Dinulos J, Mitchell DK, Egerton J, Pickering LK: Hydrops of the gallbladder associated with Epstein-Barr virus infection: a report of two cases and review of the literature. Pediatr Infect Dis J 1994;13:924–929.

115. Iwai N, Goto Y, Taniguchi H, et al: Cancer of the gallbladder in a 9-year-old girl. Kinderchir 1985;40:106.

116. Foster DR, Foster DBE: Gallbladder polyps in Peutz-Jeghers syndrome. Postgrad Med J 1980;56:373.

117. McKhann GM: Metachromatic leukodystrophy: clinical and enzymatic parameters. Neuropediatrics 1984;15(suppl):4.

118. Schimpl G, Schaffer G, Sorantin E, et al: Polypoid gastric heterotopia in the gallbladder: clinicopathological findings and review of the literature. J Pediatr Gastroenterol Nutr 1994;19:129–131.

119. Sears HF, Golden GT, Horseley J: Cholecystitis in childhood and adolescence. Arch Surg 1973;106:651–653.
120. Warfel KA, Hull MT: Villous papilloma of the gallbladder in association with leukodystrophy. Hum Pathol 1984;15:1192–1194.
121. Hanaki K, Ohzeki T, Itisuka T, et al: An infant with pseudohypoaldosteronism accompanied by cholelithiasis. Biol Neonate 1994;65:85–88.
122. Kose G, Ozkan H, Ozdamar F, et al: Cholelithiasis in cervico-oculo-acoustic (Wildervanck's) syndrome. Acta Paediatr 1993;82:890–891.

# SECTION SIX

# THE PANCREAS

# Chapter 54

# Cystic Fibrosis and Congenital Anomalies of the Exocrine Pancreas

*Robert J. Rothbaum*

A wide spectrum of anatomic and functional congenital disorders affects the pancreas of infants, children, and adolescents. Generally, exocrine pancreatic insufficiency constitutes one manifestation of an underlying systemic disorder such as cystic fibrosis or Shwachman's syndrome. Maldigestion and malabsorption are often major features of such disorders, but treatment does not correct other multiple disease–associated problems. In contrast, a congenital predisposition to pancreatitis often affects only the pancreas. Recurrent inflammation, however, may produce complications that alter overall health and lifestyle. This chapter reviews the multiple causes and course of congenital pancreatic diseases with an emphasis on the more commonly encountered clinical problems.

## CYSTIC FIBROSIS

Cystic fibrosis (CF) is an autosomal recessive disorder of cyclic adenosine monophosphate (cyclic AMP)–regulated chloride transport that results from a defect in the CF transmembrane regulator (CFTR). CFTR contains several domains: two ATP binding folds (NBD 1 and NBD 2), two membrane spanning domains, and one central or R-domain.[1] CFTR regulates chloride conductance and, consequently, water flow in the apical cell membrane of ductular cells. Alterations in CFTR function, therefore, affect electrolyte and water secretion in pancreatic duct cells, biliary epithelium, and bronchial glands, leading to abnormal secretory products and the major phenotypic manifestations of CF.

Based on chromosome 7, CF-related genetic mutations disrupt CFTR function through four potential mechanisms[2] (Fig. 54–1). Class I mutations produce premature termination signals. Little or no full-length CFTR protein results, eliminating CFTR function in affected epithelia. The most common mutation, delta F508, typifies class II mutants. This three base pair deletion eliminates a phenylalanine residue from the structure of CFTR. The resultant protein does not mature to its fully glycosylated form and is degraded rather than being transported to and inserted in the apical cellular membrane. This mutation alters almost 70% of CF genes; homozygosity accounts for approximately 50% of CF patients. In class III mutants, the protein is processed correctly but the chloride channel does not respond to intracellular ATP as a result of mutations in the NBD region. Because of mutations in the membrane-spanning domain, class IV mutants produce chloride channels with slightly altered properties. Various mutations do appear to cluster within different ethnic populations, but no mutation besides delta F508 accounts for more than 4% of the entire CF population.

Individuals with CF may be homozygous for a single mutation, but many are compound heterozygotes for two distinct mutations. Patients homozygous for class I and II mutations have a more severe defect associated with pancreatic insufficiency. Patients with class III and IV mutations produce CFTR with significant residual function and characterize a minority of patients with pancreatic sufficiency.

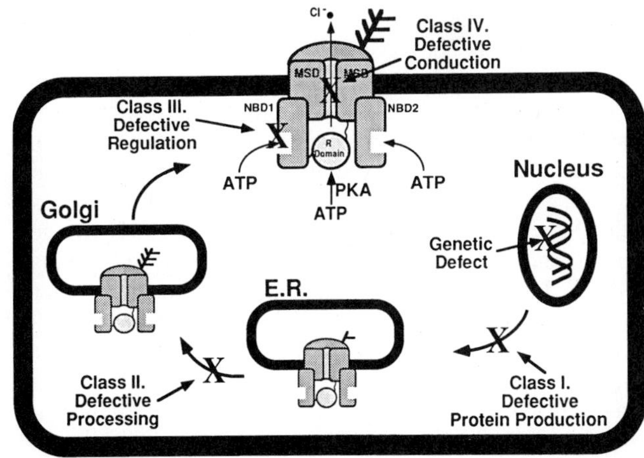


**FIGURE 54–1.** Diagram of four classes of mutations in CFTR with proposed mechanisms of dysfunction. (From Welsh M: Cystic fibrosis: approaches to therapy. Am J Gastroenterol 1994;89[8]:5101, with permission.)

An individual with one mutation associated with pancreatic insufficiency and a second mutation correlated with pancreatic sufficiency manifests the phenotype of the less severe mutation. The more functional CF gene is dominant.[2]

The degree of organ dysfunction engendered by a mutation in CFTR depends on both the nature of the mutation and the localization and level of expression of the gene in a particular organ.[3] The absence or dysfunction of CFTR results in diminished secretion of electrolytes and water by ductular epithelium. The concentration of macromolecules in the lumen of the affected duct increases significantly. Proteins precipitate into plugs, slow ductal flow, and produce duct obstruction. Thus, organs that produce secretions with a high protein concentration and slow ductular flow are most susceptible to damage from mutant CFTR.[3] Pancreas, epididymis and vas deferens, and, to a lesser extent, bile ducts represent vulnerable targets. Obstruction of small ducts prevents normal flow of pancreatic juice, seminal fluid, and bile, respectively. Pancreatic exocrine insufficiency, sterility, and biliary fibrosis result. In contrast, the sweat gland clearly has abnormal electrolyte and fluid flux as a result of mutant CFTR but, because of low protein concentration and high flow rate, does not sustain histologic damage.

The postnatal lung represents a special situation because of the requirement for macromolecules to move at an air-fluid interface through narrow passages. A decrease in water content of pulmonary secretions could thus lead to precipitation of secretory products in small airways. This represents the initial step in a cascade toward chronic obstructive pulmonary disease. In addition, dysfunction of CFTR and resultant high salt concentration in respiratory secretions may interfere with the naturally occurring, salt-dependent, antimicrobial activity of β-defensin. Diminished activity of β-defensin may allow the early bacterial colonization of CF airways and retard clearance of infection.[4]

## PANCREATIC DYSFUNCTION

### Basic Defects Associated with CFTR Dysfunction

CFTR is located in the apical cell membrane of centroacinar and intralobular duct cells in the pancreas.[5] Antibodies against CFTR do not localize to acinar cells. Presumably, the defect in chloride secretion in proximal ductular cells alters the electrochemical gradient promoting water and bicarbonate secretion from ductular cells. In addition, initial events in enzyme secretion require acidification of the acinar and duct lumen. Abnormal CFTR may alter this process, producing secondary defects in apical trafficking of zymogen granules and reducing solubilization of secretory proteins.[6] With low flow rates, protein-rich zymogen granule secretions may then become inspissated in the proximal ductules. Ductular obstruction limits the flow of bicarbonate-rich pancreatic juice into the duodenum, reducing the delivery of pancreatic enzymes below the level necessary for normal digestion. Kopelman and colleagues elegantly document these functional consequences: pancreatic secretions from CF patients are high in protein and low in water content at all levels of pancreatic function.[7] The low volume of secretions leads to an inadequate total amount of pancreatic enzyme within the intestinal lumen. The initial histologic abnormalities in the CF pancreas, intraluminal eosinophilic concretions and dilation of pancreatic ducts, correlate with the described functional abnormalities. Over time, acinar atrophy and fibrosis develop with notable ductular ectasia. Finally, total loss of acinar tissue and ductal obliteration occur. Islets of Langerhans remain relatively preserved.[8]

## DIAGNOSIS OF CYSTIC FIBROSIS

Pancreatic disease forms the basis of newborn screening tests for CF. Elevated circulating serum levels of immunoreactive trypsinogen or lipase are detectable in newborns with CF with and without exocrine insufficiency. In most individuals with CF, documentation of elevated chloride and/or sodium concentration in sweat still provides the cornerstone for diagnosis. Fifty to 100 mg of sweat is collected from skin maximally stimulated by pilocarpine iontophoresis. Sweat chloride concentration above 60 mEq/L is consistent with the diagnosis of CF. As an internal control, the sweat sodium concentration is usually within 10 to 15 mEq/L of the sweat chloride. The sweat test is accurate in patients of any age. In infants, however, collection of sufficient sweat may be difficult, and the differential between sweat chloride and sodium is often greater. Sweat potassium concentration is also elevated above normal and accounts for the difference. In some circumstances, molecular diagnostic techniques are used to identify specific mutations to confirm the diagnosis. Absence of two identifiable genetic mutations, however, does not exclude the diagnosis. More than 600 different mutations have been described, and genetic testing searches for the most common 20 or so mutations that account for approximately 90% of CF patients. Some CF patients possess unique mutations that are not detected by these routine analyses.

## CLINICAL EFFECTS OF EXOCRINE PANCREATIC INSUFFICIENCY

Approximately 85% of CF patients suffer exocrine pancreatic insufficiency. In approximately two thirds of infants with CF, pancreatic function is deficient at birth; about one-half the remainder develop exocrine insufficiency during the first few years of life.[9] Even patients with pancreatic sufficiency have lower rates of secretion of enzyme and bicarbonate than normal individuals.[7]

Exocrine pancreatic insufficiency results when less than 10% of normal pancreatic enzyme activity is present in the lumen of the proximal small bowel.[10] Up to 60% of ingested fat and 50% of ingested protein are not digested or absorbed. The caloric and protein losses prevent weight gain and growth or lead to weight loss. Most CF patients are diagnosed before 6 months of age, with deviation from normal rates of weight gain and growth providing the major indication for diagnostic testing. A decrease in subcutaneous fat stores produces accentuation of skin folds, and decreased muscle mass underlies hypotonia or delays major motor development. A characteristic syndrome of protein-calorie malnutrition afflicts 2- to 4-month-old infants with CF. They present with hypoalbuminemia, edema, and severe normochromic, normocytic anemia.[11] When initially described, these severely malnourished infants suffered a high mortality rate from the precipitous development of overwhelming pulmonary disease. With prompt recognition of this syndrome, nutritional rehabilitation begins early, resulting in survival and resumption of normal growth and development. Infants with CF who present with hypoalbuminemia now have no different prognosis than infants presenting with normal serum albumin.[12]

Chronic pulmonary disease can begin in young infants, presenting as tachypnea, cough, or wheezing. This early bronchiolitis often produces hyperexpansion on chest radiograph. Airways are colonized with *Staphylococcus aureus* or *Pseudomonas aeruginosa*. Viral infections, particularly respiratory syncytial virus, exacerbate airway inflammation and obstruction, potentiating bacterial infection.

Older infants and toddlers show slow weight gain and manifest diarrhea. Rectal prolapse is a key sign to suggest the diagnosis. Recurrent bouts of wheezing unresponsive to bronchodilator therapy and patchy pneumonias may occur. Also, refractory sinusitis or nasal polyps are not uncommon. The minority of patients with pancreatic sufficiency maintain normal growth parameters and may not present manifestations of pancreatic disease, respiratory tract disorders, or sterility that indicate the diagnosis until the second or third decade of life.

At the time of diagnosis, fat-soluble vitamin deficiencies are common in association with pancreatic insufficiency and steatorrhea. Vitamin A deficiency produces pseudotumor cerebri with sixth nerve palsy, irritability, and lethargy. Poor feeding or overt refusal to eat follows. Less commonly, dilation and tortuosity of the ureters with abnormalities of the ureteral epithelium predispose to urinary tract infection.[13] Vitamin K deficiency with resultant coagulopathy is common. Vitamin E lack is usually asymptomatic but is detectable by low serum vitamin E concentration. Vitamin D deficiency is rare, because of either subtle differences in absorption or compensatory synthesis of vitamin D within the skin.

## DIAGNOSIS OF EXOCRINE PANCREATIC INSUFFICIENCY

Because 85% of CF patients develop exocrine pancreatic insufficiency, patients newly diagnosed with CF are often presumed to have steatorrhea. Initial supportive evidence for inadequate pancreatic function includes (1) failure to gain weight or grow while consuming an age-appropriate diet, and (2) documentation of fat-soluble vitamin deficiencies. Exocrine pancreatic insufficiency can be documented more exactly with a variety of techniques (Table 54–1).[14] Many CF clinicians emphasize the importance of documentation of exocrine pancreatic insufficiency through a minimal evaluation of 72-hour fecal fat collection that demonstrates absorption of less than 90% of ingested fat.

**TABLE 54–1. Techniques to Establish Pancreatic Insufficiency**

| |
|---|
| Intraduodenal collection of pancreatic output during pancreatic stimulation with secretin-pancreozymin or liquid feeding. Bicarbonate, trypsin, and lipase content are analyzed in collected secretions. |
| Documentation of steatorrhea by quantitative comparison of fat excreted with fat ingested over a 72-hour period. Less than 90% absorption is abnormal. Abbreviated test by measurement of steatocrit in stool. |
| Examination of stool for fat globules using Sudan III staining and light microscopy. |
| Analysis of stool for chymotrypsin. |
| Measurement of serum level of para-aminobenzoic acid (PABA) after oral ingestion. |
| Determination of serum concentration of immunoreactive trypsinogen. |

These and other tests of exocrine pancreatic function are outlined in detail in Couper.[14]

## TREATMENT OF EXOCRINE PANCREATIC INSUFFICIENCY

Currently, no therapy exists to alter the function of CFTR in pancreatic duct cells and improve water and bicarbonate secretion. To reverse the lack of available pancreatic enzyme in the intestinal lumen, CF patients ingest exogenous or supplemental enzymes in the form of processed porcine pancreas. During the last 40 years, clinicians and investigators documented the effectiveness of and defined the limitations of supplemental pancreatic enzyme therapy. These clinical investigations often follow a similar outline: Study patients ingest various enzyme preparations and subsequently undergo balance studies to measure fat and/or protein absorption. Seventy-two-hour fecal fat collections are the gold standard. In these studies, fat absorption improved from 50% to 60% of ingested fat to 70% to 85% with exogenous enzyme supplementation.[15]

Most CF patients had marked improvement in absorption while taking early formulations of powdered supplemental enzymes, but a significant proportion did not have normal absorption or required large numbers of capsules. Enteric-coated, encapsulated enzymes were developed to protect the enclosed pancreatic enzymes from acid degradation in the stomach. These capsules contained beads of enzymes surrounded by an acid-resistant coating. The bead coating dissolved at pH 5 to 6, allowing for enzyme release in the proper environment for enzyme function in the proximal small bowel. This development allowed many patients to reduce the number of ingested capsules with improvement or maintenance of their fraction of absorbed fat and protein. Throughout the 1980s, most CF patients changed from powdered to enteric-coated enzymes. Controlled clinical studies and anecdotal reports of reduction in the number of capsules taken per meal and improvement in stool pattern and abdominal complaints proved impressive.[15] Even after the introduction of enteric-coated enzymes, a few CF patients had persistent steatorrhea. In an Italian CF center, Constantini and associates documented that approximately 25% of their CF patients continued to have fat absorption below 90% of ingested fat.[16]

Clinical investigators have formulated and proved several hypotheses to explain these limitations in enzyme effectiveness in CF.[17–24] To improve the efficacy of supplemental pancreatic enzymes, increase the absorption of ingested nutrients, and optimize nutritional state, clinicians attempted to ameliorate each of the potential factors limiting enzyme function. Table 54–2 outlines these approaches. Caregivers

**TABLE 54–2. Sequential Approach to Ameliorate Factors Limiting Enzyme Function**

| LIMITING FACTOR | POTENTIAL SOLUTION | EFFECTIVENESS |
|---|---|---|
| Gastric acidity destroys enzymes. | Enteric-coated beads in capsules | Improved absorption compared with powdered enzymes |
| Limited enzyme appears in proximal small bowel. | Increase enzyme dosage | No improvement in half of patients tested |
| Acid environment in small bowel prevents bead dissolution and enzyme function. | Reduce gastric acid secretion to increase pH in proximal bowel | Improves fat absorption in patients resistant to increase in enzyme dosage |
| Glycine-conjugated bile acids limit micelle formation. | Taurine supplementation and enrichment of bile acids | Variable success and not widely adopted |

first expected that ingesting more enzyme would increase the amount of enzyme available in the proximal small bowel and correct residual steatorrhea in refractory patients. In addition, several potent forces led to a progressive escalation of enzyme intake:

1. Clinicians recommended increased enzymes for various gastrointestinal symptoms without documenting persistent steatorrhea.
2. Patients became accustomed to increasing enzymes.
3. Manufacturers produced high-potency enzyme capsules. The maximal enzyme content of capsules increased from an average of 4,000 units of lipase/capsule to 10,000 units/capsule to 32,000 units/capsule. Patients could greatly increase their enzyme intake without raising the number of capsules ingested.
4. Licensing guidelines specified that the dosage state the minimum amount of enzyme contained without a potential maximum. Thus, patients may have been ingesting even greater amounts of enzyme than they anticipated.

Initially, asymptomatic hyperuricosuria or hyperuricemia represented the only apparent ill effects of high enzyme dosage. More recently, fibrosing colonopathy became associated with extremely high enzyme intake (>6,000 units lipase/kg/meal).[25, 26] Affected patients presented with crampy abdominal pain, vomiting, and plain abdominal films indicating partial distal bowel obstruction. Some patients reported blood-streaked diarrhea. Contrast enemas, colonoscopy, or resection demonstrated segmental colon narrowing with mucosal ulceration and marked submucosal fibrosis. Some patients improved with cessation of pancreatic enzyme supplements and provision of parenteral nutrition, but many required resection of damaged colon.[27, 28]

The exact pathophysiology that produced colon damage remains unclear, but the association with high enzyme intake was strong enough to initiate a recall of high-potency enzyme capsules from the commercial market. Also, the National Cystic Fibrosis Foundation delineated specific weight-based guidelines for dosing of supplemental pancreatic enzymes[26] (Table 54–3). In a small Australian study, Robinson and Sly showed that patients on high doses of supplemental enzymes could reduce their enzyme intake by an average of 50% (45 to 21 capsules per day) with no measured increase in fecal fat excretion.[29] Thus, CF patients on doses of pancreatic enzymes exceeding current recommendations should be considered candidates for enzyme reduction followed by objective documentation of fat absorption with fecal fat analysis.

When ingesting recommended doses of enzymes, approximately 75% of CF patients have adequately treated steatorrhea. The remaining 25% will most likely benefit from increasing intraluminal pH to promote enzyme release and activity. CF patients with resistant steatorrhea maintain a lower intraduodenal pH than patients with easily controlled fat malabsorption.[30] Robinson and several others demonstrated that reducing gastric acid secretion with $H_2$-receptor antagonists, proton pump inhibitors, or prostaglandin agonists improves fat absorption in CF patients with refractory steatorrhea.[31–33] This improvement occurs in association with an increase in intraluminal pH and in the proportion of intraluminal fat in the micellar phase. Presumably, the higher intraluminal pH allows for greater dissolution of the enteric coating, improves enzyme release, aids lipase activity, and augments micelle formation in the proximal small bowel. CF patients who previously had 90% or greater fat absorption on enzymes alone do not have further improvement with these adjunctive therapies.[32]

## DIET AND VITAMIN SUPPLEMENTATION IN CYSTIC FIBROSIS

CF patients should consume age-appropriate diets. For infants, breast feeding or standard infant formulas support normal weight gain and growth.[34] At times, specialized formulas containing hydrolyzed protein and medium-chain triglycerides are necessary. Weaning and the transition to table foods can progress along with developmental milestones. Intake of fat should be unrestricted in order to provide for maximal energy intake.

**TABLE 54–3. Current Recommended Dosages of Supplemental Pancreatic Enzymes in CF Patients**

| AGE | RECOMMENDED DOSAGES |
|---|---|
| Infant | 2,000 to 4,000 units lipase per 120 mL of formula or per breast feeding |
| Children age 4 yr or younger | 1,000 units lipase/kg/meal<br>500 units lipase/kg/snack |
| Children age 4 yr or older | 500 units lipase/kg/meal<br>250 units lipase/kg/snack |
| Adolescents and adults | Lower enzyme dosages may suffice because grams of fat intake/kg decrease with age. |

Maximum recommended dosage is 2,500 units lipase/kg/meal. Higher doses are not likely to improve effectiveness.

Oral fat-soluble vitamin supplementation is often recommended. Increased doses of multivitamin supplements may provide adequate amounts of vitamins A and D. Vitamins E and K must often be supplemented individually.[35] Water-soluble vitamins are not usually problematic. Table 54–4 lists currently recommended vitamin supplementation for CF patients.

## MONITORING OF EFFICACY OF SUPPLEMENTAL PANCREATIC ENZYME THERAPY

CF patients should follow normal rates of weight gain, growth, and maturation. Most clinicians accept the effectiveness of pancreatic enzymes if the patient achieves a normal nutritional state with an absence of significant gastrointestinal complaints. If resistant steatorrhea is suspected as the cause of persistent gastrointestinal complaints, then minor alterations in the pancreatic enzyme regimen may prove helpful. Enzyme effectiveness may be enhanced by simple measures: (1) change to a different enzyme preparation with different bead or microtablet size and different pH dissolution characteristics; (2) assess whether enzyme intake is well matched to fat intake; and (3) change the timing of enzyme intake from before eating to later in the meal. If these measures are not helpful, perform a 72-hour fecal fat collection to assess the degree of steatorrhea. If resistant steatorrhea is documented, add an $H_2$-receptor antagonist or proton pump inhibitor to the regimen.[36] Misoprostol has equal effectiveness but may produce abdominal cramps and diarrhea. If persistent steatorrhea is not demonstrated or if it persists after acid suppression, consider alternative diagnoses as potential causes of these resistant problems (Table 54–5).

Adequacy of vitamin dosages is confirmed by an absence of symptoms or findings referable to specific vitamin deficiencies and by annual biochemical testing. Vitamin K adequacy is assessed by measurement of prothrombin time and partial thromboplastin time. Serum levels of vitamin E reflect vitamin E stores. A normal ratio of serum vitamin A concentration to retinol-binding protein ensures vitamin A adequacy. Vitamin D nurtriture is assessed by measuring serum calcium, phosphorus, and 25-OH-vitamin D levels.

**TABLE 54–4. Vitamin Supplementation in Individuals with CF**

| VITAMIN | AMOUNT |
|---|---|
| **Infancy** | |
| Vitamin A | 1,500–3,000 units/day |
| Vitamin D | 400–800 units/day |
| Vitamin E | 25–50 IU/day |
| Vitamin K | 2–5 mg/wk |
| **Age 2–8 Years** | |
| Vitamin A | 3,000–5,000 units/day |
| Vitamin D | 400 IU/day |
| Vitamin E | 100–200 IU/day |
| Vitamin K | 10 mg/wk |
| **Adolescents** | |
| Vitamin A | Standard multivitamin preparation |
| Vitamin D | Same |
| Vitamin E | 200–400 IU/day |
| Vitamin K | 10 mg/wk |

**TABLE 54–5. Gastrointestinal Disorders in CF Patients**

| |
|---|
| **GI Conditions with Steatorrhea** |
| Giardiasis |
| Gluten-sensitive enteropathy |
| Intraluminal bile acid deficiency |
| Cholestatic liver disease |
| Ileal resection |
| Short gut syndrome |
| Blind loop with bacterial overgrowth |
| Portal hypertension |
| Diabetic enteropathy |
| **GI Conditions without Steatorrhea** |
| *Clostridium difficile* colitis |
| Disaccharide intolerance |
| Inflammatory bowel disease |
| Laxative use or abuse |
| Irritable bowel syndrome |
| Recurrent abdominal pain |
| Eating disorders |
| Fibrosing colonopathy |

GI, gastrointestinal.

Individuals with CF are also prone to the development of other specific nutritional deficiencies. Table 54–6 outlines multiple electrolyte, mineral, and trace element deficiencies in conjunction with their associated predisposing clinical factors. In contrast to infants, hypoalbuminemia in older children with CF is not usually indicative of protein undernutrition. In a study of 19 individuals with CF, aged 8 to 25 years, low concentrations of serum albumin resulted from dilution of a normal albumin mass due to fluid retention rather than from low rates of synthesis, increased catabolism, or high rates of enteric protein loss. The plasma volume expansion probably resulted from early congestive heart failure in association with progressive lung disease.[37]

## POTENTIAL PROBLEMS WITH GLOBAL NUTRITIONAL STATUS

Individuals with CF are vulnerable to generalized undernutrition. Energy consumption and energy loss through malabsorption can easily exceed energy intake. The resultant energy deficit limits weight gain and growth and may potentiate pulmonary dysfunction.

### Energy Intake

Current recommendations suggest that individuals with CF should consume approximately 120% of the recommended daily allowance for energy at all ages.[35] Several potential problems may prevent attainment of this goal. Pulmonary exacerbations with fever, cough, and tachypnea reduce appetite and intake. Behavioral feeding problems can confound efforts to maintain steady intake in toddlers and school-age children. With progressive pulmonary disease, anorexia and early satiety reduce ability to eat. Post-tussive emesis decreases net intake. In adolescence, depression and

**TABLE 54–6. Specific Nutritional Deficiencies Identified in Individuals with CF**

| NUTRIENT | USUAL AGE | CLINICAL SITUATION | FINDING |
|---|---|---|---|
| Energy | Any age | Poor weight gain | Low weight |
| Protein | Infancy | Soy or breast-fed infant | Hypoalbuminemia |
| Essential fatty acids | Infancy | Often present biochemically | Elevated tetrane/triene ratio |
| Vitamin K | Any age | Potentiated by liver disease | Prolonged PT and PTT |
| Vitamin E | Any age | Biochemical deficiency | Low serum vitamin E level |
| Vitamin A | Infancy | Usually present at time of diagnosis | Low vitamin A/RBP ratio |
| Vitamin D | Any age | Rare without concomitant liver disease | Low 25-OH-vitamin D level |
| Zinc | Infancy | Acrodermatitis-like rash | Low serum zinc |
| Sodium | Infancy | Infant diet low in sodium; ileostomy | Low hypochloremic alkalosis with hypokalemia |
| Magnesium | Adolescence | Prolonged aminoglycoside therapy | Hypomagnesemia |
| Selenium | Adolescence | Prolonged TPN without selenium supplement | Low serum selenium, high CPK |
| Calcium | Adolescence | Poor nutritional status | Osteoporosis, low bone density |
| Iron | Adolescence | Progressive lung disease or portal hypertension | Relative anemia |

CPK, creatine phosphokinase; PT, prothrombin time; PTT, partial thromboplastin time; RBP, retinol-binding protein; TPN, total parenteral nutrition.

overt eating disorders may occur. Intake of large amounts of medication may lead to early gastric filling. Intake need not be profoundly low to prevent normal weight gain. A caloric intake averaging 100 kcal/day below energy requirements produces weight loss of at least 1 kg/month. Low energy intake is the most common reason for failure to gain weight in individuals with CF.

## Energy Requirements

Total daily energy requirements include resting energy expenditure (basal metabolic rate), energy needed for digestion and absorption of food, energy required for activity, and energy demanded for tissue accretion or weight gain and growth. Increased energy expenditure may be an inherent part of CF. Shepherd and coworkers measured a 25% increase in total daily energy expenditure (TDEE) in infants with CF who did not have overt pulmonary disease when compared with normal infants.[38] Vaisman and colleagues documented a general increase in resting energy expenditure (REE) in children and adults with CF compared with values predicted by the Harris-Benedict equation.[39] Tomezsko and associates studied a more homogeneous group of 25 prepubertal children with CF.[40] In comparison to normal age-matched controls, the children with CF had an 8.5% increase in REE as kcal/kg/day and a 3.5% increase as kcal/kg of fat-free mass per day. Total daily energy expenditure was higher by 12%. Thus, the increase in TDEE could not be entirely explained by the increase in REE. The exact mechanism was unknown, but subtle pulmonary dysfunction or infection may be a contributing factor. In Vaisman's study, declining pulmonary function was associated with higher REE, but considerable variability existed at each level of lung function.[39] Tomezsko could not correlate energy expenditure with pulmonary function, although the severity of obstructive pulmonary disease was mild within the study population.[40] Increased work of breathing, metabolic alterations associated with infection, or medications may contribute to this increase in energy expenditure. For example, the beta agonist salbutamol increased resting energy expenditure by approximately 10% when inhaled by patients with CF.[41] Daily use of similar medications might, therefore, contribute to negative energy balance in susceptible individuals.

## Energy Losses

As described previously, approximately 25% of treated CF patients with pancreatic insufficiency have persistent significant steatorrhea. If intake is limited by one or more factors, then this caloric and protein loss may lead to energy deficiency and poor nutritional state. Manipulations of the enzyme regimen or initiation of acid suppression therapy will often improve the steatorrhea and promote resumption of weight gain. Murphy and coworkers demonstrated that stool energy losses in individuals with CF averaged 10% of total energy intake in comparison to 3.5% in controls.[42] The range in the patients with CF was from 5% to 20%. Stool lipid accounted for only 41% of the energy within the stool of patients with CF and 29% in controls. The substrate of the increased energy losses in patients with CF was not clear but could be related to increased loss of endogenous secretions, cellular debris, or bacterial flora. The authors suggested that more accurate energy balance studies might result from considering these total stool energy losses rather than just losses of fat.

## Effects of Undernutrition

Several studies examine the effect of undernutrition on metabolism and body composition in individuals with CF. In 1982, Miller and associates demonstrated that the weight deficit in undernourished CF patients consisted of deficits in both fat and lean body mass. In addition, muscle protein catabolism was markedly increased in comparison to healthy control children.[43] In 1987, Thompson and Tomas produced different findings using stable isotope studies of protein metabolism.[44] These investigators found no difference in whole body protein flux, synthesis, or catabolism between infection-free, well-nourished or mildly undernourished patients with CF and control children. The authors hypothesized that the previously reported results might have been confounded by ongoing pulmonary disease. Holt and coworkers attempted to delineate the effect of such pulmonary disease on metabolism in patients with CF. This group compared protein metabolism in children with CF with acute lung infection, patients with CF with stable lung disease, and healthy controls.[45] Protein synthesis was markedly decreased in the infected CF group in contrast to the other two groups. Protein catabolism was higher in the stable group of CF patients. Thus, CF patients appeared vulnerable to decreased protein accretion through periodic reductions in the rate of protein synthesis and continual accelerated rates of protein breakdown. Morton and colleagues attempted to document changes in net nitrogen balance during treatment of acute chest infection in a small group of CF patients. Rates of protein synthesis and degradation were higher at the peak of infection, but net nitrogen balance was near zero at the peak of and after antibiotic treatment of infection.[46]

Changes in metabolism and body composition may produce important functional changes in CF patients. In 1978, Kraemer and coworkers found that the degree of underweight of CF patients inversely correlated with survival.[47] Coates and associates then documented that exercise tolerance in CF patients appeared limited by nutritional state rather than by hypoxemia or hypercarbia.[48] Marcotte and colleagues also concluded that nutritional status was an important determinant of exercise tolerance in CF patients with advanced lung disease.[49] Because these limitations in exercise ability were independent of the degree of obstructive airway disease, a decrease in respiratory muscle mass, strength, and performance occurring as part of the overall decrement in lean body mass may represent the cause of the reduced exercise capability. Such functional and anatomic changes in diaphragmatic and other respiratory muscles are documented in patients suffering malnutrition from other causes besides CF.[8]

## Correction of Undernutrition

Several clinical studies demonstrate that energy and protein supplementation improves weight, nutritional status, and functional status in CF patients. Parsons and coworkers noted that energy intake in a small group of children with CF reached desired goals only when patients received aggressive oral nutritional supplementation. Increasing energy intake to 110% of recommended daily allowance led to a normal rate of weight gain in association with an increase in absorbed energy.[50] A further study documented a decrease in protein breakdown rate with no change in protein synthetic rate, resulting in increased nitrogen retention and net anabolism.[51] Shepherd and associates reproduced these findings in a similarly designed study.[52] Nutritional supplementation produced an increase in protein synthetic rate and in protein catabolic rate, but the net result was an increase in net protein deposition. Thus, the increase in body weight engendered by nutritional supplementation is likely to increase the essential compartment of lean body mass. In Shepherd's study, pulmonary function also improved to a modest degree.

Nutritional supplementation can be initiated with oral supplements, although ability and enthusiasm to maintain energy intake above that of a regular diet often fade.[53] Intravenous supplemental nutrition is effective but is costly, time-consuming, and carries multiple risks of metabolic imbalance and infection. Nasogastric or gastrostomy tube feedings are the most effective, least costly, and safest method of providing consistent nutritional supplementation. Weight, body image, and pubertal development all may improve. Strength and endurance may progress if the nutritional supplementation is coupled with a program of exercise or physical therapy. The exact feeding formulation and additional enzyme supplementation vary from CF center to CF center. Often, nighttime feedings are used to maintain a relatively normal daytime lifestyle. Such nutritional supplementation also reduces stress on the patient and family by relieving the constant need to encourage oral intake. The individual with CF can eat ad libitum without special efforts and continual reminders to eat more. Percutaneous placement of a gastrostomy tube button reduces the morbidity of tube placement and minimizes the alterations in body contour.

The length of time of nutritional supplementation may be an important determinant in achieving improvement in overall health. Bertrand and colleagues showed increased weight as a result of fat accretion, but no functional improvements in CF patients supplemented for 1 month.[54] The studies demonstrating greater effectiveness of nutritional supplementation continued for 6 to 12 months.[52, 53, 55] Once CF patients require aggressive nutritional supplementation, that requirement often persists unless there is major improvement in the degree of pulmonary impairment or resolution of other factors, such as depression, that are reducing voluntary intake.

## Pancreatitis

Approximately 1% of CF patients suffer recurrent episodes of acute pancreatitis. Pancreatitis may be the presenting manifestation of CF. Shwachman originally emphasized that CF patients with pancreatitis retained sufficient pancreatic exocrine function to avoid steatorrhea.[56] In his series, patients ranged in age from 14 to 30 years and presented with severe abdominal pain, vomiting, epigastric tenderness, and elevations of serum amylase and lipase typical of acute pancreatitis. Patients suffered an average of 3.5 attacks with a range of one to seven. A narrowed pancreatic duct was visualized by pancreatogram in two of three patients studied. Atlas and coworkers described recurrent pancreatitis in five younger CF patients; the youngest was aged 1 year.[57] Peripancreatic edema was evident on abdominal computed tomography in one patient. Imaging studies may, however, be normal. Systemic complications of pancreatitis and pseudocyst formation appear to be unusual in CF-related pancreatitis. In the few patients described, the acute illness spanned 2 to 7 days. Recurrent attacks of pancreatitis might be prevented or ameliorated by oral intake of supplemental pancreatic enzymes. Free trypsin in the lumen of the duodenum may provide negative feedback control to limit secretion of enzymes by the native pancreas.[58]

## HEPATOBILIARY DISEASE IN CYSTIC FIBROSIS

### Basic Defects Associated with CFTR Dysfunction in the Liver

CFTR is present in biliary epithelium but is not identifiable in hepatocytes.[59] Abnormal electrolyte and water flux across biliary epithelium might result in higher concentrations of macromolecules in bile. Biliary tract secretions would inspissate in small ductules; periportal inflammation would follow with the eventual development of focal fibrosis. Histopathologic findings consistent with this hypothesis are described in infants with CF.[60] Almost one third of infants with CF examined by biopsy or at autopsy had focal biliary fibrosis or mucous plugging of large intrahepatic ducts adjacent to the porta hepatis. In addition, some infants had mucous obstruction of extrahepatic bile ducts. Thus, the defect in CFTR function appears to produce microscopic and, possibly, macroscopic bile duct obstruction very early in life in some CF patients.

### Spectrum of Hepatic Dysfunction in CF

#### *Neonatal Cholestasis*

Approximately 5% of infants with CF develop neonatal cholestasis.[61, 62] From one quarter to one half of these infants suffer meconium ileus as newborns, and many require surgery.[62] In jaundiced infants with CF, bile plugs within bile canaliculi and intrahepatic bile ducts predominate, but biliary fibrosis, giant cell transformation, and intrahepatic paucity of bile ducts are also described.[62, 63] Hypoxemia, hypotension, bacterial or viral infection, and medications often accompany neonatal illness and surgery. In any newborn, transient cholestasis can follow these systemic problems. The infant with CF who has meconium ileus may undergo these exposures that predispose to neonatal cholestasis and thus is more likely to develop cholestasis than the infant with CF without neonatal illness. Neonatal cholestasis can persist for as long as 2 to 3 months but does not necessarily progress to chronic liver disease.[64]

#### *Asymptomatic Liver Disease*

Hepatic enlargement in CF is most often caused by hepatic steatosis. Untreated, malnourished CF patients may have generalized accumulation of fatty acids and triglycerides accounting for 50% of the liver weight.[65] The pathogenesis of steatosis is unclear but may be related to low levels of lipoproteins available for lipid transport from the liver. Steatosis is not a precursor of permanent liver damage and often regresses with improvement in nutritional state.

Asymptomatic elevation of serum transaminase or alkaline phosphatase levels represents the most common hepatic biochemical abnormality. At least 20% of CF patients experience elevations of serum enzymes.[66] Most often, no clinical symptoms or signs accompany these elevations. The potential to develop significant chronic liver disease is not evident from the magnitude or duration of elevation of serum enzyme levels. Possibly, these patients have focal but limited hepatic damage that is not sufficient to affect overall liver function or architecture.

#### *Cirrhosis*

Approximately 5% of CF patients develop multilobular, macronodular cirrhosis.[64, 66] Meconium ileus or its equivalent may be a predisposing factor.[67] Cirrhosis and portal hypertension develop silently and insidiously. A hard-edged, irregular liver and splenic enlargement are often first detected by careful physical examination between ages 4 and 14 years (mean, 8.7 years).[64] Superficial veins of the abdominal wall may be dilated and prominent. Digital clubbing and oxygen desaturation occur with cirrhosis even without significant parenchymal pulmonary disease.[68] Levels of serum transaminases and alkaline phosphatase are mildly elevated or normal. Liver synthetic function, evaluated with serum bilirubin, serum albumin, and coagulation studies, is initially normal. During the years after initial diagnosis, liver size may remain the same or decrease. As portal hypertension progresses, splenomegaly becomes more prominent.

The complications of portal hypertension (ascites and gastrointestinal hemorrhage) rather than liver synthetic failure threaten the health of the CF patient.[69–72] Portosystemic encephalopathy is uncommon.[73] Splenomegaly results in thrombocytopenia and leukopenia from hypersplenism, but these low counts do not usually contribute to clinical problems. Poor weight gain, slow growth, and delayed puberty may accompany cirrhosis and portal hypertension, but the mechanism is unclear. The management of complications of portal hypertension in the CF patient is similar to the treatment of these complications in other causes of cirrhosis. Portosystemic shunt procedures, variceal sclerotherapy, and variceal ligation have been applied to esophageal variceal bleeding.[74–76] Transjugular intrahepatic portosystemic shunting (TIPS) is now reported for refractory bleeding and intractable ascites.[77] Liver transplantation corrects liver synthetic dysfunction, cirrhosis, and portal hypertension without potentiating the development of further lung disease.[78] With relief of abdominal distention and improvement in muscle mass and strength, pulmonary function may actually improve after transplantation.

Ursodeoxycholic acid (UDCA) is a potent choleretic and hepatocyte protective agent. The increase in bile flow and cytoprotection could theoretically prevent bile duct obstruction and hepatocyte damage in CF-related liver disease. In uncontrolled trials, administration of UDCA to CF patients with elevated levels of transaminases or alkaline phosphatase produced a fall in those enzyme levels.[79] In addition, abnormal hepatobiliary scintigraphy improved with UDCA therapy, potentially indicating improved bile flow.[80] In a small controlled trial, O'Brien and associates substantiated the biochemical improvements but noted no change in hepatobiliary scrintigraphy in comparison with controls.[81] Because the development of cirrhosis is uncommon and difficult to detect with noninvasive measures, documentation that UDCA prevents the progression of liver dysfunction to cirrhosis is not currently available. No other therapy is available, however, to prevent the progression of CF-related liver disease. In usual clinical practice, therefore, many clinicians initiate UDCA therapy (10–30 mg/kg/day) in CF patients with early evidence of cirrhosis on physical examination or imaging studies.

## BILIARY TRACT DISEASE IN CYSTIC FIBROSIS

Asymptomatic microgallbladder is the most common biliary tract abnormality in CF.[82, 83] The gallbladder contains thick, colorless bile. Mucus-filled cysts are scattered beneath the mucosa. The cystic duct may be small or occluded, but hepatic and common bile duct obstruction does not occur.

Stern and colleagues described approximately 4% of CF patients developing symptomatic gallstones. The youngest patient was 4 years old, but 20 of the 24 patients were older than 16.[84] One patient, aged 26, had cholangiocarcinoma. CF gallstones are radiolucent but are not conventional cholesterol stones. Rather, recent analysis indicates the stones contain mostly calcium bilirubinate and protein.[85] No difference in biliary lipid concentrations is evident when CF patients with and without gallstones are compared. These findings may explain why treatment with ursodeoxycholic acid has not been effective in dissolving gallstones in CF patients.

Intrapancreatic compression of the common bile duct leading to distal duct obstruction has been hypothesized to contribute to the development of cirrhosis. Gaskin and coworkers studied a series of CF patients with and without clinical evidence of liver disease.[86] Fifty of the 61 patients with hepatomegaly or elevated serum transaminase levels had abnormal biliary excretion of radionucleotide on scintigraphic studies. Thirty patients underwent cholangiography with confirmation of distal common bile obstruction. The authors hypothesized that the bile duct compression led to obstruction and biliary fibrosis or cirrhosis. In two subsequent studies, however, O'Brien and colleagues and Nagel and associates found a far lower frequency of distal stricture of the common bile duct in CF patients with clinical liver disease.[87, 88] Although intrahepatic duct irregularities were common, only 1% of patients had documented distal abnormalities.

## INTESTINAL DISORDERS IN CYSTIC FIBROSIS

Strong, Boehm, and Collins localized CFTR mRNA expression to intestinal mucosal epithelium.[89] CFTR is expressed at relatively high levels in the duodenal mucosa, with expression decreasing steadily throughout the length of the small intestine. In all areas with expression, CFTR concentration is highest in crypt cells and diminishes in cells toward villous tips. Crypt cells secrete chloride in the normal intestine. Sodium follows and provides the driving force for water to enter the intestinal lumen. The presence of CFTR in crypt cells correlates with abnormalities in electrolyte flux documented in CF intestinal epithelia.[90] A disturbance in chloride crypt secretion is, therefore, likely to reduce hydration of intestinal secretions and predispose to intestinal obstruction.

Approximately 10% to 15% of newborns with CF present with neonatal meconium ileus or its complications.[91, 92] Viscous inspissated meconium produces distal small bowel obstruction with abdominal distention and bilious vomiting evident within several hours of birth. Small bowel ischemia and perforation may occur antenatally, resulting in meconium cyst, intestinal atresia, or intra-abdominal calcifications. In some infants, the intrauterine perforation seals spontaneously with restoration of intestinal continuity. A contrast enema filling the unused microcolon and refluxing into the distal small bowel outlines the filling defects of inspissated meconium and establishes the diagnosis[93] (Fig. 54–2). In addition, the hypertonic contrast medium may draw fluid into the intestinal lumen, dilute the persistent meconium, and mobilize the obstruction in 50% to 75% of affected infants. If the meconium ileus is complicated by intestinal perforation, fixed obstruction by atresia, meconium cyst, volvulus, or progressive illness due to resistant obstruction, laparotomy will be necessary.[94] The exact procedure will depend on the type of complication encountered.[93] Before the advent of contrast enema therapy, parenteral nutrition, and special neonatal surgical and anesthesia techniques, the perioperative mortality of meconium ileus was about 50%.[94, 95] By 1 year of age, up to 90% of patients died. The current mortality rate is in the range of 5%.

Not all infants with meconium obstruction syndromes have cystic fibrosis. Olsen and coworkers reviewed a series of infants with meconium plug syndrome, meconium ileus, and meconium peritonitis.[96] Meconium plug syndrome differs from meconium ileus. The initial symptoms and signs are similar, but the obstruction is in the colon, caused by mucous plugs. Contrast enema outlines the normal-caliber colon and generally mobilizes the inspissated plugs with relief of obstruction. In the Olsen series, 6 of the 25 infants with meconium plug syndrome had CF; one infant had aganglionosis; the remaining 18 appeared free of underlying disease. Of the 15 infants with meconium ileus, 12 had CF. Eight infants had meconium peritonitis; four had CF. Thus, meconium obstructive disease is not always indicative of CF, but the finding of distal small bowel or colon obstruction should prompt a sweat test.

### Meconium Ileus Equivalent or Distal Intestinal Obstruction Syndrome

In the late 1960s, Lillibridge and colleagues described older CF patients who suffered distal small bowel obstruction due to inspissated intestinal contents in the terminal ileum.[97] Originally labeled meconium ileus equivalent, this disorder has been renamed distal intestinal obstruction syndrome (DIOS). Lack of adherence to enzyme regimens and inadequate control of steatorrhea are potential contributing factors to DIOS.[98] Persistent steatorrhea exposes the distal ileum to unabsorbed fat, inducing secretion of neurotensin. Neurotensin slows intestinal motility, and such delays could underlie obstruction. Medications, particularly narcotic pain relievers and anticholinergics, can induce ileus and intraluminal obstruction. Also, CF patients suffering DIOS may have an inherent motility defect that predisposes to obstruction.[99]

DIOS presents with acute or chronic symptoms. The cardinal features include crampy abdominal pain (often in the right lower quadrant or lower abdomen), a palpable mass in the right lower quadrant, and decreased frequency of

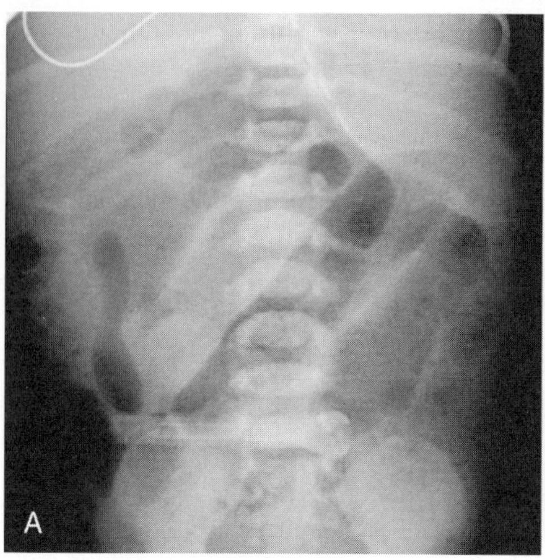


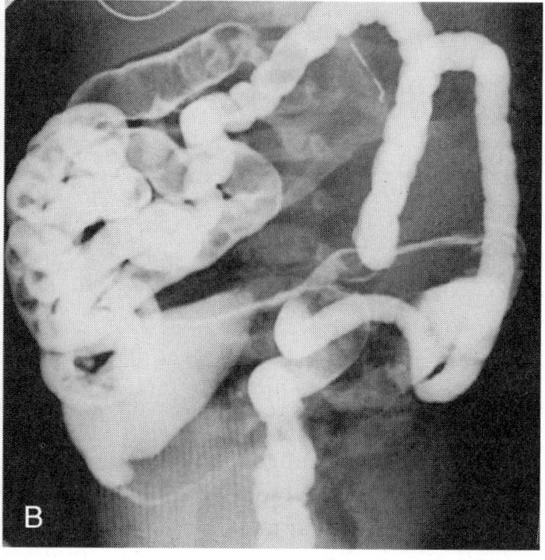


**FIGURE 54–2.** Neonatal meconium ileus. *A,* Multiple markedly dilated loops of bowel are evident on plain abdominal film. *B,* During hypaque enema, contrast medium fills the unused microcolon then refluxes into small bowel. Multiple intraluminal filling defects represent inspissated meconium. Contrast medium eventually fills more proximal dilated bowel segment in the right lower quadrant.

defecation. Abdominal distention and bilious vomiting, signs of actual or impending small bowel obstruction, may predominate. Approximately 10% of CF patients suffer this form of DIOS.[98] The patients are almost always older than age 5 years and are often older than age 15 years. In the more chronic form of DIOS, meals provoke colicky abdominal pain; anorexia becomes a method of avoiding pain. The attacks of pain may remit for weeks or months but return in association with right lower quadrant mass and relative constipation. In both forms of DIOS, abdominal plain films show bubbly fecal material in the right lower quadrant. Varying degrees of proximal bowel dilation are evident (Fig. 54–3).

Although DIOS is a common cause of abdominal pain in CF, other causes of partial or complete small bowel obstruction must be considered. Intussusception, appendicitis, and small bowel obstruction due to postoperative adhesions mimic the symptoms and signs of DIOS. If the classic historical, physical, and radiologic findings of DIOS are not present, then these alternative causes must be investigated.

Treatment of DIOS focuses on nonoperative relief of the distal small bowel obstruction. As in infants with meconium ileus, hypertonic, water-soluble contrast enema(s) can confirm the diagnosis and may dislodge inspissated material from the distal ileum. Attaining sufficient reflux of contrast into proximal dilated small bowel is sometimes problematic. Pain, abdominal distention, and dyspnea may limit success. If the course of DIOS is chronic of if there is no evidence of complete bowel obstruction, intestinal lavage with a balanced electrolyte solution represents an alternative therapy.[100] Lavage treatment provides a large volume of isotonic fluid flowing from the stomach to the distal small bowel to dilute the impacted material. Older CF patients may take sufficient lavage solution by mouth; younger patients often require an intragastric infusion through a nasogastric tube. The lavage continues until the rectal effluent is almost clear.

## SHWACHMAN'S SYNDROME

Shwachman's syndrome is the most common cause of exocrine pancreatic insufficiency besides cystic fibrosis, but it occurs much less frequently. Cystic fibrosis occurs in 1 in 2,500 live white births; Shwachman's syndrome occurs in 1 in 20,000 to 200,000 individuals. In 1964, Shwachman and colleagues described a small group of children with exocrine

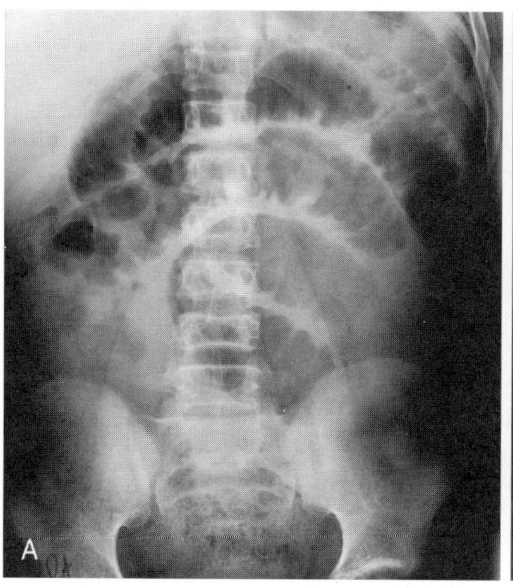


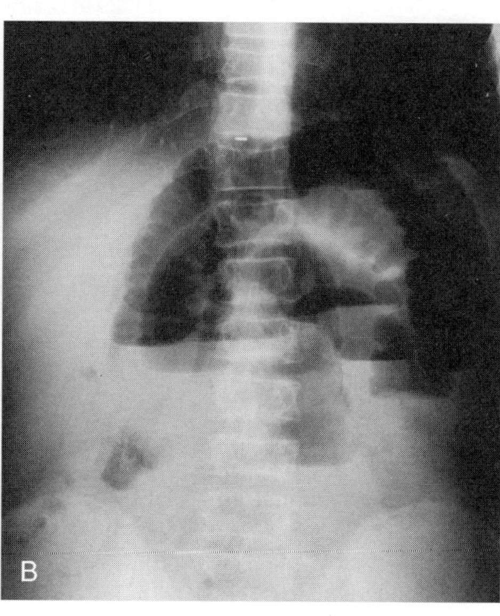


**FIGURE 54–3.** Abdominal plain films of DIOS. *A,* Abdominal flat plate demonstrates multiple dilated loops of small bowel. Bubbly fecal material is evident in the right lower quadrant and lower abdomen. *B,* Upright abdominal film demonstrates multiple air-fluid levels in dilated bowel, indicating small bowel obstruction.

pancreatic insufficiency, neutropenia, and short stature, delineating the major features of the syndrome.[101] Over the next few years, clinicians expanded the clinical manifestations, defining metaphyseal dysostosis, mild hepatic dysfunction, increased frequency of infections, and further hematologic abnormalities.[102, 103] Table 54–7 lists the current range of clinical abnormalities associated with Shwachman's syndrome.

The severity and timing of each clinical manifestation vary considerably within the population of Shwachman's syndrome patients. Exocrine pancreatic insufficiency and steatorrhea usually contribute to the initial clinical symptoms that prompt diagnosis. Fecal fat losses vary, however, between 3% and 60%, with a mean of 26% of ingested fat.[104] Between ages 4 and 8 years, the magnitude of steatorrhea decreases to a mean of 14%. After 8 years of age, fecal fat losses average 8% of intake. Pancreatic stimulation tests with duodenal drainage demonstrate that both lipase and trypsin output improve over this same time period.[104, 105] The exact reason for this improvement in pancreatic function is not clear. Hill and coworkers hypothesize that, similar to normal children, Shwachman's syndrome patients increase secretion of pancreatic enzymes with age as a result of growth of residual pancreatic tissue.[104]

Neutropenia is the most common hematologic abnormality in this syndrome, occurring in approximately 88% of patients.[105] The neutropenia may be intermittent or persistent. Patients with the persistently lowest neutrophil counts seem most prone to serious infection. In addition, clinical investigators delineate defects in neutrophil chemotaxis and surface adhesion that may contribute to the propensity for infection.[106–108] Although thrombocytopenia is the second most common hematologic abnormality, almost half of Shwachman's syndrome individuals have all three blood cell lines affected. This group appears most susceptible to the development of acute myelogenous leukemia (AML).[109, 110] In addition, patients who develop AML often have identifiable chromosomal structural abnormalities in their bone marrow. The overall risk of leukemia is unclear, but in one series of 21 patients identified and followed up over a 25-year period, five developed malignancy.[110]

During the latter half of the first year of life, growth velocity drops in Shwachman's syndrome patients, often resulting in length and weight below the fifth percentile for age. With treatment of the pancreatic insufficiency, growth velocity improves, but many patients parallel normal growth channels without rejoining normal percentiles.[105] Short stature occurs both with and without characteristic skeletal abnormalities. Symmetric metaphyseal dysostosis of the long bones occurs in 44% of patients but is not usually evident before age 6 years. Thoracic dystrophy, presenting as costochondral thickening, flaring of the lower ribs, or a narrow thoracic cage, appears in fewer patients and is most obvious in patients younger than age 2 years.

Clinicians direct the therapy of Shwachman's syndrome toward each of the individual manifestations. Early in life, patients take supplemental pancreatic enzymes to correct steatorrhea. With increasing age and improvement in pancreatic function, the need for exogenous enzymes may resolve. Fat-soluble vitamin status is monitored, and supplements are recommended as needed. Hematologic status is followed closely. There is controversy about the advisability and efficacy of treating the neutropenia with recombinant growth factors (G-CSF). Some clinicians now recommend periodic bone marrow examination to assess for premalignant changes. Growth rate is assessed, and if it is slow, additional causes of growth delay are investigated. Scattered Shwachman's syndrome patients with concomitant growth hormone deficiency have been noted (personal observation).

Shwachman's syndrome is an autosomal recessive disorder, but the exact etiologic genetic mutation has not been identified. Masuno and associates characterize a balanced translocation with break points on chromosomes 6 and 12 in a toddler with Shwachman's syndrome.[111] These investigators suggest that this finding indicates potential importance of genes close to the break points as candidate loci for Shwachman's syndrome. Further analyses of these and other loci are, however, clearly required.

**TABLE 54–7. Clinical Findings in Shwachman's Syndrome**

| |
|---|
| Exocrine pancreatic insufficiency |
| Neutropenia |
| Thrombocytopenia |
| Anemia |
| Short stature beginning in infancy |
| Metaphyseal dysostosis |
| Thoracic dystrophy |
| Increased frequency of infections |
| Elevated serum transaminases |
| Urologic abnormalities |
| Microscopic hematuria |
| Mild psychomotor retardation |
| Predisposition to leukemia |
| Nephrocalcinosis |
| Myocardial fibrosis |

## OTHER CAUSES OF PANCREATIC EXOCRINE INSUFFICIENCY

Multiple genetic and other syndromes contain exocrine pancreatic insufficiency as a clinical feature. Table 54–8 lists these syndromes and the associated documentation of the pancreatic disorder. In Johanson-Blizzard syndrome, infants with hypoplastic alae nasi, short stature, dental anomalies, and deafness develop hypoproteinemia and edema.[112, 113] Stool fat losses represent about 15% to 30% of intake. Pancreatic function studies document less than 0.1% of normal output of trypsin, lipase, and co-lipase.[114] In contrast, mean fluid secretion is similar to that of control subjects. Electrolyte secretion is not as depressed as in patients with CF. The pancreatic insufficiency thus appears to be caused by acinar failure rather than ductular dysfunction. With Alagille's syndrome, infants may have diarrhea and poor weight gain. Intraduodenal concentrations of lipase and bicarbonate are both low in symptomatic patients with Alagille's syndrome in comparison with disease controls.[115] Fecal fat losses have not been quantitated. A single reported patient constitutes the documentation of pancreatic insufficiency in congenital rubella.[116] In the Pearson syndrome, the mitochondrial enzyme defect produces lactic acidemia, bone marrow hypoplasia, and exocrine pancreatic insufficiency with mild steatorrhea.[117] Specific pancreatic function studies show absence of lipase and chymotrypsin secretion. Congenital defi-

**TABLE 54–8. Potential Causes of Exocrine Pancreatic Insufficiency**

| DIAGNOSIS | REPORTED PATIENTS | DEGREE OF STEATORRHEA | FUNCTIONAL ENZYME STUDY | NUTRITIONAL DEFICIENCY | SYNDROMATIC FEATURES | EFFECT OF THERAPY |
|---|---|---|---|---|---|---|
| Cystic fibrosis | 1:2,500 births | 40–50% | Marked reduction | Fat-soluble vitamin deficiency, global malnutrition | Pulmonary disease, elevated sweat chloride | Improved digestion and absorption |
| Shwachman's syndrome | 1:20,000 births | 10–50% | Low to absent | Not often detected | Neutropenia, short stature | Improved steatorrhea, persistent short stature |
| Jeune's thoracic dystrophy | <100 patients | >50% | Low | Not generally detected | Thoracic dystrophy | Unknown |
| Johanson-Blizzard syndrome | Approximately 35 patients | Severe | Absent | Hypoproteinemia | Hypothyroidism, short stature, hypoplastic alae nasi | Improved protein status |
| Pearson's syndrome | Very rare | Unknown | Marked reduction | Not described | Lactic acidosis, liver failure, sideroblastic anemia | Persistent liver disease and anemia |
| Congenital rubella | Single patient | 15% | Transient decrease | Low weight | Rubella virus | Improved function with time |
| Alagille's syndrome | 6 of 13 patients | Unknown | Low lipase, low bicarbonate | Low weight | Cholestasis, butterfly vertebrae, peripheral pulmonic stenosis | Improved weight, no acceleration in height |
| Congenital lipase deficiency | Isolated patients | Severe | Absent lipase | Not described | None | Improved fat absorption |
| Congenital co-lipase deficiency | Single patient | Severe | Absent co-lipase | Unknown | Consanguinity | Improved fat absorption |

ciencies of lipase and co-lipase secretion are rare but occur without evidence of other pancreatic or syndromic diagnoses.[118]

As in Shwachman's syndrome, growth retardation accompanies many of these genetic disorders, in both the presence and absence of steatorrhea. Pancreatic enzyme supplementation may reverse steatorrhea and improve undernutrition, but growth rate or other syndromic manifestations may not improve. Patients with Johanson-Blizzard or Jeune's syndrome improve their protein status but remain undersized.[113, 114, 119] Children with Alagille's syndrome show more rapid weight gain but not faster growth.[115] In the Pearson syndrome, refractory lactic acidosis and severe liver disease determine the dismal prognosis.[117] Thus, recognition and treatment of exocrine pancreatic insufficiency in these rare syndromes may not alter major components of the overall course.

## CONGENITAL STRUCTURAL ABNORMALITIES OF THE PANCREAS

The pancreas derives from dorsal and ventral buds developing from the foregut. The hepatobiliary system also arises from the ventral bud. At about the sixth to eighth week of embryologic development, the ventral pancreas rotates posterior to the duodenum, eventually residing inferior and posterior to the head of the dorsal pancreas. Parenchymal fusion occurs, but the two components can sometimes be identified anatomically or radiologically. The ventral pancreas is smaller than the dorsal and constitutes approximately 10% to 20% of the total parenchymal mass. In 90% of individuals, the ductal system fuses.[120] The ventral pancreatic duct usually becomes the outlet of the main pancreatic duct (duct of Wirsung), connecting to the adjacent axial duct of the larger dorsal pancreas. The remaining proximal duct (duct of Santorini) in the dorsal pancreas may regress to various degrees but may remain a functional drainage route through the minor papilla[121] (Fig. 54–4). The two reviews

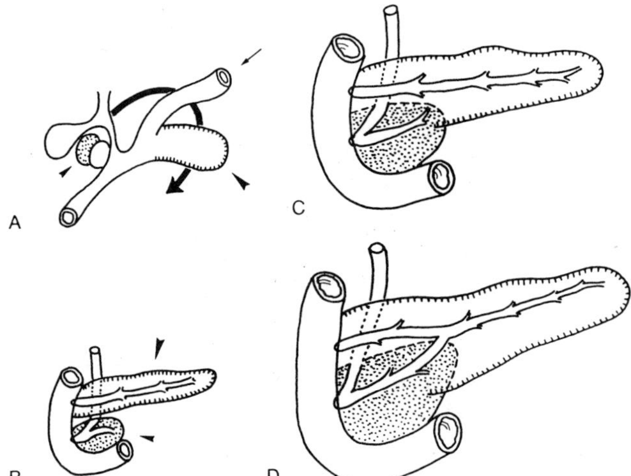


**FIGURE 54–4.** Development of the pancreas. *A,* The right ventral primordium *(small arrowhead)* moves backward and comes close to the posterior and inferior surface of the dorsal pancreatic primordium *(large arrowhead)* with the axial rotation of the foregut *(small arrow). B,* The dorsal pancreatic bud *(large arrowhead)* and the right ventral bud *(small arrowhead)* prior to their fusion. The left ventral bud has been obliterated. *C,* Parenchymal fusion of the dorsal bud and the right ventral bud. *D,* Anastomosis of the two ductal systems. (From Kozu T, Sude K, Toki F: Pancreatic development and anatomical variation. Gastrointest Endosc Clin North Am 1995;5[1]:1–30, with permission.)

cited here provide excellent descriptions and diagrams of this developmental process. Multiple anomalies of pancreatic anatomy and development have been described. Table 54–9 categorizes and lists the various abnormalities. The most commonly encountered clinical problems include pancreas divisum, annular pancreas, ectopic pancreas, and anomalous pancreaticobiliary junction.

Pancreas divisum is currently defined as a pancreas with two ductal systems that do not unite or communicate and that drain separately to the major and minor duodenal papillae.[121] The incidence of pancreas divisum has been reported from 0.5% to 11%. In most of these individuals, pancreatic juice from the larger dorsal pancreas flows out only through the minor papilla. Continuing debate centers on whether this situation predisposes to pancreatitis or pancreatic pain (see Chapter 55).

Annular pancreas is a malformation in which pancreatic tissue surrounds a portion of the descending duodenum. The exact etiology of this anomaly is not clear, but current theories suggest that the free end of the ventral bud is fixed and drawn around the right side of the duodenum, later fusing with the head of the pancreas and encircling the duodenum.[120] In children, duodenal obstruction is the most common presenting complaint. Frequently, other anomalies accompany annular pancreas, including intestinal malrotation, duodenal web or atresia, cardiac defects, and tracheoesophageal fistula. Both trisomy 21 and Rothmund-Thomson syndrome have been associated with annular pancreas.[122] In a series of adults, gastric outlet obstruction, pancreatitis, and pancreatic mass occur in association with this anomaly.[123] Often, annular pancreas is an incidental finding noted during an evaluation for gastrointestinal complaints unrelated to the pancreas.

Ectopic pancreatic rests most often lie along the greater curvature of the stomach in the antrum or prepyloric region.[124] This usually incidental finding is noted in 1% to 2% of autopsies. A smooth, 1- to 3-cm diameter, intramural bulge is noted on upper gastrointestinal x-ray series. At endoscopy, the mass is covered by normal gastric epithelium and contains a central umbilication. Histologically, the mass contains all of the cell types found in normal pancreatic tissue.[125] In about 5% of cases, the mass is within the pyloric canal and may produce intermittent gastrtic outlet obstruction. Nodules can occur in the duodenum but are usually smaller than 1 cm in diameter in the area above the ampulla of Vater. Although isolated cases of abdominal pain, neighboring ulceration, and gastric outlet obstruction are reported, most pancreatic rests remain asymptomatic and do not require specific intervention.[125–127]

Pancreaticobiliary maljunction describes a union of the pancreatic and biliary ducts outside the duodenal wall.[120] The exact form of the junction varies, but is always associated with choledochal cyst or congenital biliary dilation. This anomaly predisposes to the free flow of pancreatic juice into the extrahepatic bile duct and gallbladder because the intraductal pressure of the pancreatic duct exceeds that of the bile duct. Damage to the wall of the bile duct may occur, contributing to cystic dilatation. Patients may develop neoplasia of the biliary tract. In addition, some patients may develop biliary tract obstruction or pancreatitis as presenting features. Cholangiogram is required for diagnosis.

**TABLE 54–9. Anatomic Categorization of Congenital Pancreatic Anomalies**

| |
|---|
| Ventral/dorsal malfusion |
| Pancreas divisum |
| Isolated dorsal segment |
| Rotation/migration problems |
| Annular pancreas |
| Ectopic pancreas |
| Ectopic papillae |
| Quantitative underdevelopment |
| Agenesis |
| Hypoplasia |
| Duplication |
| Ductal |
| Accessory papilla |
| Atypical ductal configuration |
| Anomalous pancreaticobiliary junction |
| Cystic malformations |

*Acknowledgment*

I would like to acknowledge the perseverance and dedicated work of Jeanne M. Phelps in the preparation of this chapter.

## REFERENCES

1. Tsui L: The spectrum of cystic fibrosis mutations. Trends Genet 1992;8(11):392–398.
2. Welsh M: Cystic fibrosis: approaches to therapy. Am J Gastroenterol 1994;89(8):97–105.
3. Tizzano E, Buchwald M: CFTR expression and organ damage in cystic fibrosis. Ann Intern Med 1995;123(4):305–308.
4. Goldman M, Stolzenberg E, Zasloff M: Human β-defensin-1 is a salt-sensitive antibiotic in lung that is inactivated in cystic fibrosis. Cell 1997;88:553–560.
5. Marino C, Matovcik L, Gorelick F, Cohn J: Localization of the cystic fibrosis transmembrane conductance regulator in pancreas. J Clin Invest 1991;88:712–716.
6. Scheele G, Fukuoka S, Kern H, Freedman S: Pancreatic dysfunction in cystic fibrosis occurs as a result of impairments in luminal pH, apical trafficking of zymogen granule membranes, and solubilization of secretory enzymes. Pancreas 1996;12(1):1–9.
7. Kopelman H, Durie P, Gaskin K, et al: Pancreatic fluid secretion and protein hyperconcentration in cystic fibrosis. N Engl J Med 1985;312(6):329–334.
8. Shepherd RW, Cleghorn GJ: Cystic Fibrosis: Nutritional and Intestinal Disorders. Boca Raton, FL, CRC Press, 1989.
9. Bronstein M, Sokol R, Abman S, et al: Pancreatic insufficiency, growth, and nutrition in infants identified by newborn screening as having cystic fibrosis. J Pediatr 1992;120(4, part 1):533–540.
10. DiMagno EP, Go VL, Summerskill WH: Relations between pancreatic enzyme outputs and malabsorption in severe pancreatic insufficiency. N Engl J Med 1973;288:83–817.
11. Fleisher D, DiGeorge A, Barness L, Cornfeld D: Hypoproteinemia and edema in infants with cystic fibrosis of the pancreas. J Pediatr 1964;64(3):341–348.
12. Reisman J, Petrou C, Corey M, et al: Hypoalbuminemia at initial examination in patients with cystic fibrosis. J Pediatr 1989;115(5, part 1):755–758.
13. Keating J, Feigin R: Increased intracranial pressure associated with probable vitamin A deficiency in cystic fibrosis. Pediatrics 1970;46(1):41–46.
14. Couper R: Pancreatic function tests. In Watkins JB, Walker WA, Durie PR, et al (eds): Pediatric Gastrointestinal Disease. St. Louis, Mosby, 1996, pp 1621–1634.

15. George D, Mangos A: Nutritional management and pancreatic enzyme therapy in cystic fibosis patients: state of the art in 1987 and projections into the future. J Pediatr Gastroenterol Nutr 1988;7(suppl 1):S49–S57.
16. Constantini D, Padoan R, Curcio L, Guinta A: The management of enzymatic therapy in cystic fibrosis patients by an individualized approach. J Pediatr Gastroenterol Nutr 1988;7(1):536–539.
17. Regan PT, Malagelada JR, DiMagno EP, et al: Comparative effects of antacids, cimetidine, and enteric coating on the therapeutic response to oral enzymes in severe pancreatic insufficiency. N Engl J Med 1977;297:854–858.
18. Guarner L, Rodriguez R, Guarner F, Malagelada JR: Fate of oral enzymes in pancreatic insufficiency. Gut 1993;34:708–712.
19. Seal S, McClean P, Walters M, et al: Stable isotope studies of pancreatic enzyme release *in vivo.* Postgrad Med J 1996;72(suppl 2):S37–S38.
20. Layer P, Groger G: Fate of pancreatic enzymes in the human intestinal lumen in health and pancreatic insufficiency. Digestion 1993;54(suppl 2):10–14.
21. Youngberg CA, Berardi RR, Howatt WF, et al: Comparison of gastrointestinal pH in cystic fibrosis and healthy subjects. Dig Dis Sci 1987;32:472–480.
22. Darling P, Lepage G, Leroy C, et al: Effect of taurine supplements on fat absorption in cystic fibrosis. Pediatr Res 1985;19:578–582.
23. Layer P, Go VL, DiMagno EP: Fate of pancreatic enzymes during small intestinal aboral transit in humans. Am Physiol Soc 1986;251:G475–480.
24. Zerega J, Lerner S, Meyer JH: Duodenal instillation of pancreatic enzymes does not abolish steatorrhea in patients with pancreatic insufficiency. Dig Dis Sci 1988;33:1245–1249.
25. Smyth R, Van Velzen D, Smyth A, et al: Strictures of ascending colon in cystic fibrosis and high-strength pancreatic enzymes. Lancet 1994;343:85–86.
26. Borowitz D, Grand R, Durie P: Use of pancreatic enzyme supplements for patients with cystic fibrosis in the context of fibrosing colonopathy. Consensus Committee. J Pediatr 1995;127:681–684.
27. Schwarzenberg SJ, Wielinski CL, Shamieh I, et al: Cystic fibrosis-associated colitis and fibrosing colonopathy. J Pediatr 1995; 127(4):565–570.
28. Freiman J, FitzSimmons S: Colonic strictures in patients with cystic fibrosis: results of a survey of 114 cystic fibrosis care centers in the United States. J Pediatr Gastroenterol Nutr 1995;22:153–156.
29. Robinson P, Sly P: High dose pancreatic enzymes in cystic fibrosis. Arch Dis Child 1990;65(3):311–313.
30. Robinson P, Smith A, Sly P: Duodenal pH in cystic fibrosis and its relationship to fat malabsorption. Dig Dis Sci 1990;35:1299–1304.
31. Robinson P, Sly P: Placebo-controlled trial of misoprostol in cystic fibrosis. J Pediatr Gastroenterol Nutr 1990;11:37–40.
32. Carroccio A, Pardo F, Montalto G, et al: Use of famotidine in severe exocrine pancreatic insufficiency with persistent maldigestion on enzymatic replacement therapy. Dig Dis Sci 1992;37:1441–1446.
33. Zentler-Munro PL, Fine DR, Batten JC, Northfield TC: Effect of cimetidine on enzyme inactivation, bile acid precipitation, and lipid solubilization in pancreatic steatorrhea due to cystic fibrosis. Gut 1985;26:892–901.
34. Holliday KE, Allen JR, Waters DL, et al: Growth of human milk-fed and formula-fed infants with cystic fibrosis. J Pediatr 1991;118(1):77–79.
35. Consensus Conference in CF: Nutritional assessment and management. Am J Clin Nutr 1992;55(1):108–116.
36. Rothbaum R: Improving digestion in children with cystic fibrosis. Contemp Pediatr 1996;13(2):39–54.
37. Strober W, Peter G, Schwartz R: Albumin metabolism in cystic fibrosis. Pediatrics 1969;43(3):416–425.
38. Shepherd R, Holt T, Vasques-Velasquez L, et al: Increased energy expenditure in young children with cystic fibrosis. Lancet 1988;1:1300–1303.
39. Vaisman N, Pencharz P, Corey M, et al: Energy expenditure of patients with cystic fibrosis. J Pediatr 1987;111(4):496–500.
40. Tomezsko J, Stallings V, Kawchak A, et al: Energy expenditure and genotype of children with cystic fibrosis. Pediatr Res 1994;35(4):451–460.
41. Vaisman N, Levy L, Pencharz P, et al: Clinical and laboratory observations. J Pediatr 1987;111(1):137–139.
42. Murphy J, Wooton S, Bond S, Jackson A: Energy content of stools in normal healthy controls and patients with cystic fibrosis. Arch Dis Child 1991;66:495–500.
43. Miller M, Ward L, Thomas B, et al: Altered body composition and protein degradation in nutritionally growth-retarded children with cystic fibrosis. Am J Clin Nutr 1982;36:492–499.
44. Thompson G, Tomas F: Protein metabolism in cystic fibrosis: responses to malnutrition and taurine supplementation. Am J Clin Nutr 1987;46:606–613.
45. Holt T, Ward L, Francis P, et al: Whole body protein turnover in malnourished cystic fibrosis patients and its relationship to pulmonary disease. J Clin Nutr 1985;41:1061–1066.
46. Morton R, Hutchings J, Halliday D, et al: Protein metabolism during treatment of chest infection in patients with cystic fibrosis. Am J Clin Nutr 1988;47:214–219.
47. Kraemer R, Rudeberg A, Hadorn B, Rossi E: Relative underweight in cystic fibrosis and its prognostic value. Acta Pediatr Scand 1978;67:33–37.
48. Coates A, Boyce P, Muller D, et al: The role of nutritional status, airway obstruction, hypoxia, and abnormalities in serum lipid composition in limiting exercise tolerance in children with cystic fibrosis. Acta Paediatr Scand 1980;69:353–358.
49. Marcotte JE, Canny GJ, Grisdale R, et al: Effects of nutritional status on exercise performance in advanced CF. Chest 1986;90:375.
50. Parsons H, Beaudry P, Dumas A, Pencharz P: Energy needs and growth in children with cystic fibrosis. J Pediatr Gastroenterol Nutr 1983;2:44–49.
51. Parsons H, Beaudry P, Pencharz P: The effect of nutritional rehabilitation on whole body protein metabolism of children with cystic fibrosis. Pediatr Res 1985;19(2):189–192.
52. Shepherd R, Holt T, Thomas B, et al: Nutritional rehabilitation in cystic fibrosis: controlled studies of effects on nutritional growth retardation, body protein turnover, and course of pulmonary disease. J Pediatr 1986;109(5):788–794.
53. O'Loughlin E, Forbes D, Parsons H, et al: Nutritional rehabilitation of undernourished patients with CF. Am J Clin Nutr 1986;43:732–737.
54. Bertrand J, Morin C, Lasalle R, et al: Short-term clinical, nutritional, and functional effects of continuous elemental enteral alimentation in children with cystic fibrosis. J Pediatr 1984;104(1):41–46.
55. Skeie B, Askanazi J, Rothkopf M, et al: Improved exercise tolerance with long-term parenteral nutrition in cystic fibrosis. Crit Care Med 15(10):960–962.
56. Shwachman H, Lebenthal E, Khaw K: Recurrent acute pancreatitis in patients with cystic fibrosis with normal pancreatic enzymes. Pediatrics 1975;55(1):86–95.
57. Atlas A, Orenstein S, Orenstein D: Pancreatitis in young children with cystic fibrosis. J Pediatr 1992;120(5):756–759.
58. Slaff J, Jacobson D, Tillman C, et al: Protease-specific suppression of pancreatic exocrine secretion. Gastroenterology 1984;87:44–52.
59. Yang Y, Raper S, Cohn J, et al: An approach for treating the hepatobiliary disease of fibrosis by somatic gene transfer. Proc Natl Acad Sci U S A 1993;90:4601–4605.
60. Oppenheimer E, Esterly J: Hepatic changes in young infants with cystic fibrosis: possible relation to focal biliary cirrhosis. J Pediatr 1975;86(5):683–689.
61. Valman H, France N, Wallis P: Prolonged neonatal jaundice in cystic fibrosis. Arch Dis Child 1971;46:805–809.
62. Rosenstein BJ, Oppenheimer EH: Prolonged obstructive jaundice and giant cell hepatitis in an infant with cystic fibrosis. J Pediatr 1977;91(6):1022–1023.
63. Furuya K, Roberts E, Canny G, Phillips M: Neonatal hepatitis syndrome and paucity of interlobular bile ducts in cystic fibrosis. J Pediatr Gastroenterol Nutr 1991;12:127–130.
64. Psacharopoulos H, Howard E, Portmann B, et al: Hepatic complications of cystic fibrosis. Lancet 1981;2:78–80.
65. Lloyd-Still J: Textbook of Cystic Fibrosis. Boston, John Wright, PSG Inc., 1983.
66. Scott-Jupp R, Lama M, Tanner M: Prevalence of liver disease in cystic fibrosis. Arch Dis Child 1991;66:698–701.
67. Maurage C, Lenaerts C, Weber A, et al: Meconium ileus and equivalent are a factor for the development of cirrhosis: an autopsy study in cystic fibrosis. J Pediatr Gastroenterol Nutr 1989;9:17–20.
68. Barbe T, Losay J, Grimon G, et al: Pulmonary arteriovenous shunting in children with liver disease. J Pediatr 1995;126(4):571–579.
69. Stern R, Stevens D, Boat T, et al: Symptomatic hepatic disease in cystic fibrosis: incidence, course, and outcome of portal systemic shunting. Gastroenterology 1976;70(5):645–649.

70. Tyson K, Schuster S, Shwachman H: Portal hypertension in cystic fibrosis. J Pediatr Surg 1968;3(2):271–277.
71. Schuster S, Shwachman H, Toyama W, et al: The management of portal hypertension in cystic fibrosis. J Pediatr Surg 1977;12(2):201–206.
72. Doershuk C, Stern R: Spontaneous bacterial peritonitis in cystic fibrosis. Gut 1994;35(5):709–711.
73. Scully RE, Galdabini JJ, McNeely BU: Case records of the Massachusetts General Hospital. Case 34. N Engl J Med 1979;301(8):420–427.
74. Paquet K, Lazar A: Current therapeutic strategy in bleeding esophageal varices in babies and children and long-term results of endoscopic paravariceal sclerotherapy over twenty years. Eur J Pediatr Surg 1994;4(3):165–172.
75. Goenka A, Dasilva M, Cleghorn G, et al: Therapeutic upper gastrointestinal endoscopy in children: an audit of 443 procedures and literature review. J Gastroenterol Hepatol 1993;8(1):44–51.
76. Laine L, Cook D: Endoscopic ligation compared with sclerotherapy for treatment of esophageal variceal bleeding. Ann Intern Med 1995;123(4):280–287.
77. Kerns S, Hawkins I: Transjugular intrahepatic portosystemic shunt in a child with cystic fibrosis. AJR Am J Roentgenol 1992;159(6):1277–1278.
78. Noble-Jamieson G, Valente J, Barnes N, et al: Liver transplantation for cirrhosis in cystic fibrosis. Arch Dis Child 1994;71(4):349–352.
79. Galabert C, Montet J, Lecuire L, et al: Effects of ursodeoxycholic acid on liver function in patients with cystic fibrosis and chronic cholestasis. J Pediatr 1992;121(1):138–141.
80. Colombo C, Castellani M, Balistreri W, et al: Scintigraphic documentation of an improvement in hepatobiliary excretory function after treatment with ursodeoxycholic acid in patients with cystic fibrosis and associated liver disease. Hepatology 1992;15(4):677–684.
81. O'Brien S, Fitzgerald M, Hegarty J: A controlled trial of ursodeoxycholic acid treatment in cystic fibrosis-related liver disease. Eur J Gastroenterol Hepatol 1991;4(10):857–863.
82. Wilson-Sharp R, Irving H, Brown R, et al: Ultrasonography of the pancreas, liver, and biliary system in cystic fibrosis. Arch Dis Child 1984;59:923–926.
83. Quillin S, Siegel M, Rothbaum R: Hepatobiliary sonography in cystic fibrosis. Pediatr Radiol 1993;23:1–3.
84. Stern R, Rothstein F, Doershuk C: Treatment and prognosis of symptomatic gallbladder disease in patients with cystic fibrosis. J Pediatr Gastroenterol Nutr 1986;5(1):35–40.
85. Angelico M, Gandin C, Canuzzi P, et al: Gallstones in cystic fibrosis: a critical reappraisal. Hepatology 1991;14(5):768–775.
86. Gaskin K, Waters D, Howman-Giles R, et al: Liver disease and common bile duct stenosis in cystic fibrosis. N Engl J Med 1988;318(6):340–346.
87. O'Brien S, Keogan M, Casey M, et al: Biliary complications of cystic fibrosis. Gut 1992;33(3):387–391.
88. Nagel RA, Westaby D, Javaid A, et al: Liver disease and bile duct abnormalities in adults with cystic fibrosis. Lancet 1989;2(8677):1422–1425.
89. Strong T, Boehm K, Collins F: Localization of cystic fibrosis transmembrane regulator mRNA in the human gastrointestinal tract by *in situ* hybridization. J Clin Invest 1994;93:347–354.
90. Baxter PS, Wilson AJ, Read NW, et al: Abnormal jejunal potential difference in cystic fibrosis. Lancet 1989;1:464–466.
91. Rescorla F, Grosfeld J, West K, Vane D: Changing patterns of treatment and survival in neonates with meconium ileus. Arch Surg 1989;124(7):837–840.
92. Caniano D, Beaver B: Meconium ileus: a fifteen year experience with forty-two neonates. Surgery 1987;102(4):699–703.
93. Wagget J, Bishop H, Koop C: Experience with gastrografin enema in the treatment of meconium ileus. Pediatr Surg 1970;5(6):649–654.
94. Holsclaw DS, Eckstein HB, Nixon HH: Meconium ileus: a 20 year review of 109 cases. Am Dis Child 1965;109:101–113.
95. Gross K, Desanto A, Grosfeld J, et al: Intra-abdominal complications in cystic fibrosis.J Pediatr Surg 1985;20(4):431–435.
96. Olsen M, Luch S, Lloyd-Still J, Raffensperger J: The spectrum of meconium disease in infancy. J Pediatr Surg 1982;17(5):479–481.
97. Lillibridge C, Docter J, Eidelman S: Oral administration of *N*-acetyl cysteine in the prophylaxis of meconium ileus equivalent. J Pediatr 1967;71(6):887–889.
98. Rubenstein S, Moss R, Lewiston N: Constipation and meconium ileus equivalent in patients with cystic fibrosis. Pediatrics 1986;78(3):473–479.
99. Dalzell A, Heaf D: Oro-caecal transit time and intra-luminal pH in cystic fibrosis patients with distal intestinal obstruction syndrome. Acta Univ Carol Med 1990;36(4):159–160.
100. Koletzko S, Stringer D, Cleghorn G, Durie P: Lavage treatment of distal intestinal obstruction syndrome in children with cystic fibrosis. Pediatrics 1989;83(5):727–733.
101. Shwachman H, Diamond L, Oski F, Khaw K: The syndrome of pancreatic insufficiency and bone marrow dysfunction. J Pediatr 1964;65(5):645–663.
102. Aggett PJ, Cavanagh NPC, Matthew DJ, et al: Shwachman's syndrome. Arch Dis Child 1980;55:331–347.
103. Burke V, Colebatch J, Anderson C, Simons M: Association of pancreatic insufficiency and chronic neutropenia in childhood. Arch Dis Child 1966;42:147–153.
104. Hill R, Durie P, Gaskin K, et al: Steatorrhea and pancreatic insufficiency in Shwachman syndrome. Gastroenterology 1982;83:22–27.
105. Mack D, Forstner G, Wilschanski M, et al: Shwachman syndrome: exocrine pancreatic dysfunction and variable phenotypic expression. Gastroenterology 1996;111:1593–1602.
106. Ruutu P, Savilahti E, Repo H, Kosunen TU: Constant defect in neutrophil locomotion but decreasing susceptibility to infection in Shwachman syndrome. Clin Exp Immunol 1984;57:249–255.
107. Rothbaum R, Williams D, Daugherty C: Unusual surface distribution of concanavalin A reflects a cytoskeletal defect in neutrophils in Shwachman's syndrome. Lancet 1982;2:800–802.
108. Aggett PJ, Harries JT, Harvey B, Soothill JF: An inherited defect of neutrophil mobility in Shwachman syndrome. J Pediatr 1979;94(3):391–394.
109. Smith O, Hann I, Chessells J, et al: Haematological abnormalities in Shwachman-Diamond syndrome. Br J Haematol 1996;94:279–284.
110. Woods W, Roloff J, Lukens J, Krivit W: The occurrence of leukemia in patients with the Shwachman syndrome. J Pediatr 1981;99(3):425–428.
111. Masuno M, Imaizumi K, Nishimura G, et al: Shwachman syndrome associated with de novo reciprocal translocation t(6;12)(q16.2;q21.2). J Med Genet 1995;32:894-895.
112. Hurst J, Baraitser M: Johanson-Blizzard syndrome. J Med Genet 1989;26:45–48.
113. Johanson A, Blizzard R: A syndrome of congenital aplasia of the alae nasi, deafness, hypothyroidism, dwarfism, absent permanent teeth, and malabsorption. J Pediatr 1971;79(6):982–987.
114. Jones N, Hofley P, Durie P: Pathophysiology of the pancreatic defect in Johanson-Blizzard syndrome: a disorder of acinar development. J Pediatr 1994;125:406–408.
115. Chong S, Lindridge J, Moniz C, Mowat A: Exocrine pancreatic insufficiency in syndromic paucity of interlobular bile ducts. J Pediatr Gastroenterol Nutr 1989;9:445–449.
116. Donowitz M, Gryboski J: Pancreatic insufficiency and the congenital rubella syndrome. J Pediatr 1975;87(2):241–243.
117. Rotig A, Cormier V, Blanche S, et al: Pearson's marrow-pancreas syndrome. J Clin Invest 1990;86:1601–1608.
118. Figarella C, DeCaro A, Leupold D, Poley JR: Congenital pancreatic lipase deficiency. J Pediatr 1980;96(3, part 1):412–416.
119. Karjoo M, Koop E, Cornfeld D, Holtzapple P: Pancreatic exocrine enzyme deficiency associated with asphyxiating thoracic dystrophy. Arch Dis Child 1973;48:143–146.
120. Kozu T, Sude K, Toki F: Pancreatic development and anatomical variation. Gastrointest Endosc Clin North Am 1995;5(1):1–30.
121. Lehman GA, Sherman S: Pancreas divisum: diagnosis, clinical significance, and management alternatives. Gastrointest Endosc Clin North Am 1995;5(1):145–170.
122. Blaustein H, Stevens A, Stevens P, Grossman M: Rothmund-Thomson syndrome associated with annular pancreas and duodenal stenosis: a case report. Pediatr Dermatol 1993;10(2):159–163.
123. Urayama S, Kozarek R, Ball T, et al: Presentation and treatment of annular pancreas in an adult population. Am J Gastroenterol 1995;90(6):995–999.
124. Kilman W, Berk R: The spectrum of radiographic features of aberrant pancreatic rests involving the stomach. Radiology 1977;123:291–296.
125. Strobel C, Smith L, Fonkalsrud E, Isenberg J: Ectopic pancreatic tissue in the gastric antrum. J Pediatr 1978;92:586–588.
126. Jochmisen P, Shirazi S, Lewis J: Symptomatic ectopic pancreas relieved by surgical excision. Surg Gynecol Obstet 1981;153:49–52.
127. Besemann E, Auerbach S, Wolfe W: The importance of roentgenologic diagnosis of aberrant pancreatic tissue in the gastrointestinal tract. AJR Am J Roentgenol 1969;107(1):71–76.

# Chapter 55

# Pancreatitis

Steven L. Werlin

It has been estimated that between 5 and 10 cases of acute pancreatitis are seen at most large pediatric centers each year. Pancreatitis is being increasingly recognized in children, particularly in patients with multi-system disease. In adults, the most common causes of pancreatitis are alcoholism and biliary tract disease. Published pediatric series of children with pancreatitis contain relatively few patients.[1–6] The most common causes of pancreatitis in childhood are trauma, viral infection, multi-system disease, and congenital anomalies of the pancreatic duct. In many children no specific underlying cause can be identified. Unlike in adults, most children have a single, self-limited episode of pancreatitis. Except for hereditary pancreatitis and pancreatitis secondary to congenital malformations, few cases progress to chronicity.

## CLASSIFICATION

There have been many classification systems developed for pancreatitis. Although none are specific or entirely relevant for children, they provide a unifying vocabulary. The major purposes of classification are uniformity of terminology, prediction of outcome, and a basis for controlled clinical trials.

Acute pancreatitis is defined as an acute inflammatory process within the pancreas with variable involvement of localized tissues and remote organ systems.[7–9] Mild and severe acute pancreatitis are differentiated by the extent of local and systemic features. In mild pancreatitis, there is minimal organ dysfunction and eventual complete recovery. In severe pancreatitis, there is organ failure or local complications such as necrosis, abscess, or pseudocyst. Acute pancreatitis is distinguished from chronic pancreatitis by the absence of continuing inflammation, structural changes, and permanent impairment of exocrine or endocrine pancreatic function.

Chronic pancreatitis is a chronic inflammatory process that results in the destruction of exocrine pancreatic tissue, fibrosis, and, in some patients, loss of endocrine pancreatic function. Chronic pancreatitis may be associated with calcification and an irregular distribution of inflammation (chronic calcific pancreatitis), obstruction of the main pancreatic duct (chronic obstructive pancreatitis), or an uncommon chronic inflammatory pancreatitis that is characterized by fibrosis, mononuclear cell infiltrate and atrophy (chronic inflammatory pancreatitis).[7, 10]

## ACUTE PANCREATITIS

### Pathophysiology

Pancreatitis is a process of autodigestion caused by the premature activation of proenzymes to active digestive enzymes within the pancreas. The exact mechanisms that initiate the sequence of enzymatic reactions remain unknown, but several mechanisms have been proposed. The obstruction-secretion hypothesis suggests that pancreatic enzymes are activated when there is obstruction to the outflow of enzymes. The common channel theory attempts to explain pancreatitis in patients with gallstones by suggesting that obstruction at or near the ampulla results in reflux of bile acids into the pancreatic duct with intraductal zymogen activation and subsequent pancreatitis. A related hypothesis is the common channel theory that reflux of duodenal contents leads to activation of pancreatic enzymes. The hypotheses are supported by the finding that activated pancreatic enzymes into the pancreas mixed with bile produces pancreatitis in experimental animals. Pancreatitis can also be induced in dogs after creation of a closed loop duodenal obstruction, and there are occasional patients who develop pancreatitis in association with duodenal obstruction. Arguments against these obstructive hypotheses include the pressure gradient differential between the pancreatic duct and the duodenum (pancreatic duct pressure is greater than bile duct and duodenal pressure), normal sphincter of Oddi and pancreatic duct pressure in the majority of adult patients with chronic pancreatitis, and the absence of pancreatitis after ligation of the pancreatic duct or sphincteroplasty, which would enhance reflux into the duct of Wirsung. More recent data suggest that intracellular activation of zymogens may be the initiating event in pancreatitis.

Among the more than 20 proteins synthesized for export by the pancreas are phospholipase $A_2$, elastase, and a large number of proteases, including trypsin, chymotrypsin, and carboxypeptidase. The pancreas also synthesizes lysosomal hydrolases.[11–13] All of these enzymes are synthesized in the endoplasmic reticulum and then travel to the Golgi apparatus, where they are packaged. The lysosomal proteins are phosphorylated and then travel to the lysosomes. The exportable, zymogen proteins are packaged into condensing vacuoles that mature to become zymogen granules.

Mechanisms that protect the pancreas from autodigestion by these enzymes include storage in inactive form in membrane-bound zymogen granules. The granules themselves and the pancreatic acinar cell cytoplasm contain trypsin inhibitors. Active enzymes are not released into the acinar cell cytoplasm but directly into the ductal system after fusion of the zymogen granule membrane and the acinar cell membrane. Activation of proenzymes occurs in the intestinal lumen. Although trypsin can activate proenzymes, the cascade must be initiated by enterokinase, a brush border enzyme.

Experimental studies in laboratory animals have shown that during an episode of acute pancreatitis protein synthesis remains normal or is only slightly decreased.[14, 15] Secretion is decreased, but intracellular concentrations of exportable protein are markedly increased. Most investigators now believe that pancreatitis is induced after crinophagy or fusion of zymogen granule and lysosomal membranes and subsequent colocalization of lysosomal and zymogen granule proteins.[16–18] This is the usual mechanism of disposal of excess protein.

The lysosome activation of trypsinogen to trypsin is induced by the lysosomal enzyme, cathepsin B. Trypsin then activates other proteases, elastase, and phospholipase $A_2$. These activated enzymes then spill into the cytoplasm and leak into the interstitium through the basolateral membrane, initiating the autodigestive process. Once activated, these diverted secretions become proinflammatory. In summary, this theory has two implications. When acute pancreatitis occurs, at least initially, synthesis of protein must continue, but secretion is blocked and that activation of pancreatic hydrolases occurs within the acinar cell.

Although this secretory block or pancreastasis is considered an important event, there are data that demonstrate decreased synthesis of pancreatic enzymes and decreased levels and translation of mRNA transcripts for trypsinogen and chymotrypsinogen in an animal model of pancreatitis.[19]

The initial cell injury is caused by the release of activated enzymes and subsequent autodigestion of the gland and adjacent tissues. In experimental pancreatitis, lipase is by far the most toxic of the activated enzymes.[13] Elastase and phospholipase are less toxic, and trypsin is the least toxic of the enzymes tested. Thus, although activation of trypsin is required to start the cascade, trypsin itself is of relatively low toxicity.

The early pathologic findings in acute pancreatitis include edema and inflammation, which may be localized or diffuse.[10] Transformation from edematous to hemorrhagic pancreatitis with multisystem failure is caused by the extracellular discharge of elastase, phospholipase $A_2$, and hypochloric acid from activated phagocytes. Necrosis of the pancreas and peripancreatic tissue may be seen. Peripancreatic fat necrosis and vascular injury, including hemorrhage into the pancreas and retroperitoneum, and vascular thrombosis, occur in more severe cases.

## Pathophysiology of Systemic Effects

The cascade of events leading to pancreatitis begins with activation of trypsin and is followed by autoactivation of additional trypsin, which then activates other pancreatic enzymes. Early on, these proteins are bound to alpha$_1$-antiprotease and inactivated.[12, 17] The complex is then transferred to the proteinase inhibitor, alpha$_2$-macroglobulin. This complex is, in turn, phagocytosed by circulating macrophages and monocytes. This system is adequate in mild cases of pancreatitis. In severe cases, alpha$_2$-macroglobulin is depleted and the reticuloendothelial system is depressed. Activated inflammatory cells and free proteases then circulate and activate other enzyme systems that are responsible for the development of the systemic inflammatory response syndrome (SIRS), sepsis, and pancreatic necrosis and abscess. Activated agents include various vasoactive substances (kallikrein, thrombin), cytokines (interleukins, tumor necrosis factor), and enzymes (elastase, phospholipase $A_2$, trypsin, chymotrypsin). Neutrophil activation and the production of elastase and superoxide ions cause endothelial damage. Oxidative stress with depletion of glutathione is an early finding. Cellular injury compromises the ability to replenish the depleted stores of antioxidants. Studies have demonstrated that platelet activating factor, a pro-inflammatory mediator, has a major role in the pathogenesis of SIRS in a number of diseases, including acute pancreatitis.[20] The pathophysiology of acute pancreatitis is summarized in Figure 55–1.

## Etiology

In adults alcoholism and gallstones account for 60% to 80% of cases of acute pancreatitis. Acute pancreatitis in children is most commonly caused by trauma, multi-system disease, viral infection, and congenital anomalies of the ductal system or is idiopathic (Table 55–1).

### *Trauma*

Pancreatitis may follow blunt abdominal trauma such as automobile accidents and bicycle handlebar injuries.[21–24] The traumatic injury may vary from a minor hematoma with no parenchymal injury to ductal rupture and severe crush injury. The outcome usually depends on other associated injuries. Failure to recognize a ruptured duct may be the cause of considerable morbidity and even mortality. Pancreatitis resulting from child abuse and postoperative pancreatitis have gained increasing attention.[2] Pancreatitis has been reported after upper gastrointestinal endoscopy owing to duodenal hematoma formation.[25] Between 1% and 7% of children undergoing endoscopic retrograde cholangiopancreatography (ERCP) develop symptomatic pancreatitis, probably as a result of the irritative effect of the injected contrast material.[26, 27]

### *Multi-system Disease*

Acute pancreatitis is being increasingly recognized in association with multi-system diseases such as systemic lupus erythematosus,[28] Kawasaki disease,[29] hemolytic uremic syndrome,[30] and inflammatory bowel disease,[31] particularly Crohn's disease. Patients with the systemic immune response syndrome (SIRS) may develop pancreatitis during the course of their illness. Pancreatitis may follow solid organ and bone marrow transplantation.

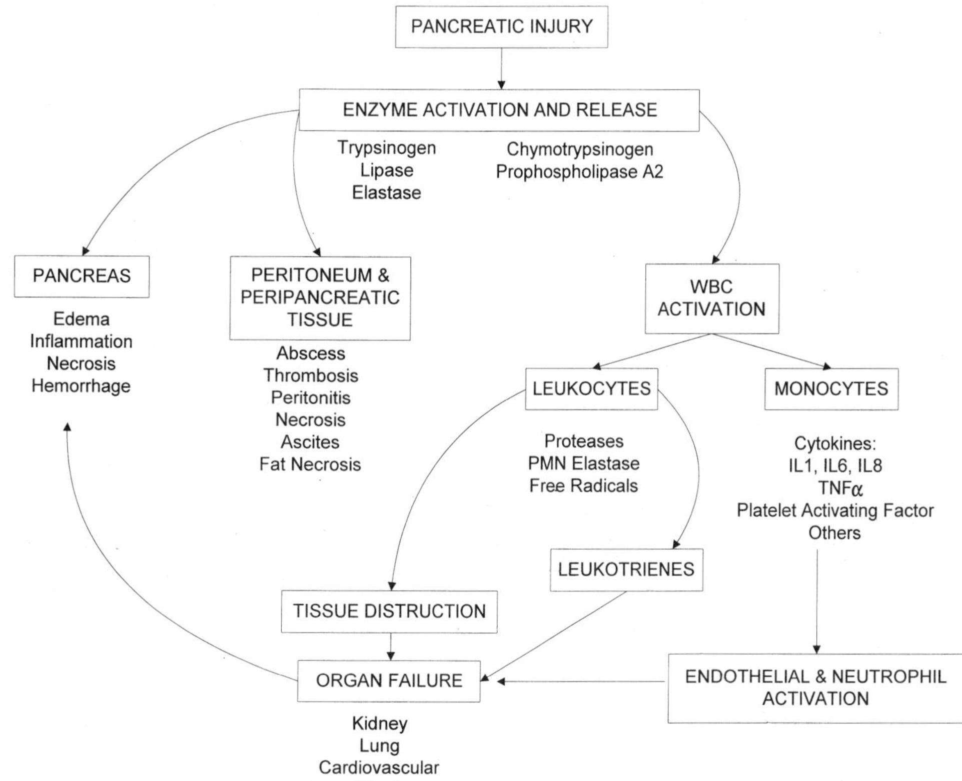


**FIGURE 55–1.** Pathophysiology of acute pancreatitis.

## *Drugs and Toxins*

Drugs are probably not a common cause of pancreatitis in children. Although a large number of pharmacologic agents have been associated with pancreatitis in adults, for most, proof of causality is weak and difficult to interpret because rechallenge has been done infrequently (see Table 55–1).[32–34] Complicating the situation is the fact that patients with complex diseases, which may themselves be associated with pancreatitis, are often treated with multiple therapeutic agents. For example, Crohn's disease is itself associated with pancreatitis but so are sulfasalazine, mesalamine, azathioprine, and 6-mercaptopurine.

Most reviews classify drugs as definite, probable, or possible causes of pancreatitis. Using the above scale, major reviews disagree about whether or not the following drugs are definite or probable causes of pancreatitis: metronidazole, vinca alkaloids, sulindac, 6-mercaptopurine, stibogluconate, and calcium.

## *Infection*

Pancreatitis may be caused by a number of infectious agents, particularly viruses.[35] The most common agents are mumps, hepatitis A, coxsackie B, cytomegalovirus (CMV) and varicella (see Table 55–1).

Reye's syndrome has been associated with pancreatitis.[36] However, many cases of Reye's syndrome are associated with varicella, a known cause of pancreatitis. Some cases of Reye's syndrome were probably acute crises of previously undescribed metabolic diseases such as organic acidemias, which are also now known to be associated with pancreatitis.[37–41]

Pancreatitis occurs in 50% to 70% of adult patients and has been reported in 17% of children with human immunodeficiency virus (HIV) infection.[42] This may be the result of drug toxicity (pentamidine, dideoxycytidine [DDI], trimethoprim-sulfamethoxazole) or infection with CMV, *Candida*, *Mycobacterium avium-intracellulare*, or other opportunistic agents. Although the development of pancreatitis in an HIV-infected child is a poor prognostic sign, it is only rarely the cause of significant morbidity or mortality.[43, 44]

## *Congenital Anomalies*

A variety of congenital, anatomic, partially obstructive anomalies of the pancreatobiliary tree have been described that may lead to obstructive pancreatitis. Such lesions include choledochal cyst, pancreas divisum, and other ductal anomalies. Some patients previously thought to have idiopathic pancreatitis have ductal anomalies, which can now be diagnosed because of the increased use of ERCP.[26, 27]

Pancreas divisum, the result of failure of normal fusion of the dorsal and ventral pancreatic anlage, occurs in 5% to 15% of the population.[45] As a result, the tail, body, and part of the head of the pancreas drain through the smaller accessory duct of Santorini rather than through the main duct of Wirsung. It has been proposed that relative obstruction of the accessory duct of Santorini may lead to the development of pancreatitis. In the 1% to 2% of cases where there is relative outflow obstruction, recurrent pancreatitis may de-

**TABLE 55–1. Etiology of Acute Pancreatitis in Children**

| | |
|---|---|
| **Drugs and Toxins** | **Obstructive** |
| Alcohol | Ampullary disease |
| L-Asparaginase | Ascariasis |
| Azathioprine | Biliary tract malformations |
| Cimetidine | Cholelithiasis and choledocholithiasis |
| Corticosteroids | Clonorchiasis |
| DDC | Duplication cyst |
| DDI | ERCP complication |
| Enalapril | Pancreas divisum |
| Erythromycin | Pancreatic ductal abnormalities |
| Estrogen | Postoperative |
| Furosemide | Sphincter of Oddi dysfunction |
| 6-Mercaptopurine | Tumor |
| Mesalamine | **Systemic Disease** |
| Methyldopa | Brain tumor |
| Pentamidine | Collagen vascular diseases |
| Scorpion bites | Cystic fibrosis |
| Sulfonamides | Diabetes mellitus |
| Sulindac | Head trauma |
| Tetracycline | Hemochromatosis |
| Thiazides | Hemolytic uremic syndrome |
| Valproic acid | Hyperlipidemia: types I, IV, V |
| **Hereditary Pancreatitis** | Hyperparathyroidism |
| **Infections** | Kawasaki disease |
| Coxsackie B virus | Malnutrition |
| Epstein-Barr virus | Organic acidemia |
| Hepatitis A, B | Periarteritis nodosa |
| Influenza A, B | Peptic ulcer |
| Leptospirosis | Renal failure |
| Malaria | Systemic lupus erythematosus |
| Measles | Transplantation: bone marrow, heart, liver, kidney, pancreas |
| Mumps | **Trauma** |
| Mycoplasma | Blunt injury |
| Rubella | Child abuse |
| Rubeola | Surgical trauma |
| Reye's syndrome: varicella, influenza B | Total body cast |

velop. The incidence of pancreatitis due to pancreas divisum is controversial (see Fig. 55–7).

Sphincter of Oddi dysfunction usually due to dyskinesia may cause pancreatic outflow obstruction.[46] The incidence of this condition in children is unknown. Diagnosis is made by manometry of the sphincter during ERCP. There is little experience with this technique in children, and the normal pressure profile of the sphincter of Oddi in children has not been defined.

### *Obstruction*

Choledocholithiasis, the most common cause of obstructive pancreatitis in adults, is far less common in children and occurs almost exclusively in patients with hemoglobinopathies, short gut syndrome, and in children receiving long-term total parenteral nutrition. It has been demonstrated that occult microlithiasis is a major cause of pancreatitis in adults.[47, 48] The incidence of microlithiasis in children is not known.

### *Metabolic and Systemic Diseases*

Acute pancreatitis is associated with a number of metabolic and systemic diseases, which are summarized in Table 55–1. Although rare causes of pancreatitis, these conditions must be considered in the appropriate clinical setting.

**CYSTIC FIBROSIS.** Pancreatitis occurs in 2% to 15% of patients with cystic fibrosis.[49–51] It may develop at any age, in both pancreatic sufficient and insufficient patients, and may be the presenting symptom. The pathophysiology of pancreatitis in cystic fibrosis patients is thought to be ductal obstruction due to thickened secretions.

**METABOLIC DISEASES.** Pancreatitis has been described in patients with a number of metabolic diseases, including branched chain organic acidemias,[38] propionic acidemia,[40] lactic acidosis,[41] glycogen storage disease type 1,[52] carnitine palmitoyltransferase II deficiency,[39] and homocystinuria.[53] Metabolic crises in these patients may be due to episodes of pancreatitis. Patients with previously undiagnosed metabolic disease may account for some of the cases of idiopathic pancreatitis. Although the pathogenesis of pancreatitis in these conditions is not known, it has been proposed that depletion of antioxidants and excess free radical formation may be factors.

**MALNUTRITION AND REFEEDING.** Malnutrition, refeeding after malnutrition, and anorexia nervosa are associated with acute pancreatitis.[54, 55] In severe malnutrition, the pancreatic acini become atrophic, but the cause of pancreatitis in these patients is not known.

**DIABETES MELLITUS.** Although hyperamylasemia is common in children with type 1 diabetes mellitus and ketoacidosis, it is usually due to elevation of salivary amylase. Acute pancreatitis may occur but is uncommon.

**HYPERLIPIDEMIA.** In adults, types I, IV, and V hyperlipidemias are associated with acute pancreatitis, which occasionally leads to chronic pancreatitis.[56] Adults with type V hyperlipidemia, the most common type, are frequently diabetic, obese, and hyperuricemic. The relationship of any of these factors to pancreatitis is not known.

**VASCULITIDES.** Pancreatitis is associated with many of the vasculitides, including systemic lupus erythematosus, periarteritis nodosa, Kawasaki disease, and Henoch-Schönlein purpura. In these patients, the pancreatitis is usually mild. Prognosis relates to the severity of the underlying disease.

**HEREDITARY PANCREATITIS.** The first episodes of hereditary pancreatitis can be indistinguishable from episodes of acute pancreatitis. Hereditary pancreatitis is discussed in detail later.

## Clinical Presentation and Course

Clinically, the child with acute pancreatitis has continuous, midepigastric and periumbilical abdominal pain (often radiating to the back, lower abdomen, or chest), vomiting, and frequently fever (Table 55–2).[57] Pain and vomiting are aggravated by eating. Pancreatic pain continues to progress after the first several hours. The patient appears acutely ill and is both restless and uncomfortable. The child may lie on his or her side curled in a knee-chest position. There may be mild jaundice and tachycardia. Bowel sounds are decreased or absent. The abdomen may be distended and is usually tender. The pain increases in severity for 24 to 48 hours. During this interval, vomiting may increase and the patient may require hospitalization for fluid and electrolyte therapy. The acute case is usually self-limited, and the prognosis is excellent.

**TABLE 55–2. Signs and Symptoms of Acute Pancreatitis**

| |
|---|
| **Common** |
| Abdominal pain |
| Abdominal tenderness |
| Nausea |
| Vomiting |
| Low-grade fever |
| Diminished or absent bowel sounds |
| Abdominal distention |
| **Less Common** |
| Hypotension |
| Grey Turner's sign |
| Cullen's sign |
| Renal failure |
| Respiratory distress |
| Fluid retention, ascites, pleural effusion |

In more severe cases, jaundice, ascites, and pleural effusions may occur. Severe acute pancreatitis is rare in children. In this life-threatening condition, the child is severely ill with intractable nausea, vomiting, and abdominal pain. The pancreas may become necrotic and transformed into an abscess. In these severe cases, Cullen's sign (bluish periumbilical discoloration) and Grey Turner's sign (bluish discoloration of the flanks) may be seen. In adults, mortality from shock, renal failure, infection, massive gastrointestinal bleeding, and other complications is between 20% and 50%. Predictors of a poor outcome include organ failure and severe metabolic abnormalities such as hyperglycemia, hypocalcemia, and hypoalbuminemia. The classification systems devised to predict the outcome of a severe case of pancreatitis in adults are usually not relevant to the pediatric patient.

## Diagnosis

The diagnosis of acute pancreatitis may be difficult. The symptoms of pancreatitis are nonspecific, and there is no single gold standard to establish the diagnosis. Ultrasonography and computed tomography (CT) are normal in as many as 30% of patients at the time of presentation.

Acute pancreatitis must be considered in the differential diagnosis of the child with sudden onset of abdominal pain and vomiting, particularly during the "non-gastroenteritis" season. The great majority of such patients do have routine illnesses. In children with recurrent pancreatitis, the first episodes are often attributed to gastroenteritis.

Because there is no reference standard test for the diagnosis of pancreatitis, a large number of individual tests have been recommended. The diagnosis of pancreatitis requires not only a high index of clinical suspicion but also careful interpretation of test results. The most widely used tests for the diagnosis of acute pancreatitis are the serum amylase and lipase assays.[58–60]

### *Amylase*

In pancreatitis, the serum amylase level is typically elevated within hours and remains elevated for 4 to 5 days. The specificity of the serum amylase level is highest when the level is increased at least threefold.

Both false-positive and false-negative results occur (Table 55–3). Approximately 20% of adults with acute pancreatitis have normal serum amylase levels.[61, 62] Adult patients with normal serum amylase level and pancreatitis usually have alcoholic pancreatitis (58%) or biliary lithiasis (18%), diagnoses that are uncommon in children.

A large number of nonpancreatic conditions have been associated with hyperamylasemia, such as diabetic ketoacidosis, abdominal surgical conditions, renal failure,[63] changes in burn patients,[64] and when there is an elevation of salivary amylase, such as may occur in mumps and in many other conditions (see Table 55–3).

Fractionation of serum amylase into the salivary and pancreatic components can be readily done in most clinical laboratories. Although elevation of serum pancreatic isoamylase is more specific than the serum amylase for the diagnosis of acute pancreatitis, it has not become a widely used test, probably because of the recent methodologic improvements for the measurement of the serum lipase. The amylase/creatinine clearance ratio has not proved to be of clinical value except in the diagnosis of macroamylasemia.

Macroamylasemia occurs in 1% of healthy persons and in 2.5% of adults with hyperamylasemia.[65] These patients have hyperamylasemia but not pancreatitis. Macroamylasemia occurs when amylase forms an enzymatically active complex that is too large for normal glomerular filtration. The diagnosis of macroamylasemia can be suspected when other tests for pancreatitis, including urinary amylase/creatinine clearance ratio, are normal in spite of an elevated serum amylase.

### *Lipase*

Measurement of serum lipase may be more specific than measurement of amylase for the diagnosis of acute pancreatitis. This test has been limited in the past by technical difficulties that have now been overcome. As with the serum amylase test, there are both false-positives and false-negatives. Specificity is increased when the serum lipase is increased at least threefold. Lipase is cleared by glomerular filtration but reabsorbed by the tubules. Thus, the lipase

**TABLE 55–3. Nonpancreatic Causes of Hyperamylasemia in Children**

| |
|---|
| **Pancreatic Amylase** |
| Biliary obstruction |
| Bowel obstruction |
| Perforated duodenal ulcer |
| Acute appendicitis |
| Mesenteric ischemia/infarction |
| Peritonitis |
| **Salivary Amylase** |
| Salivary: parotitis (mumps), trauma, surgery, salivary duct obstruction |
| Diabetic ketoacidosis |
| Anorexia nervosa, bulimia |
| Ovarian: malignancy, ruptured ectopic pregnancy, cysts |
| Malignancies |
| **Mixed or Unknown** |
| Renal failure |
| Head trauma |
| Burns |
| Postoperative |
| Macroamylasemia |

level, which rises within hours after the onset of pancreatitis, may remain elevated for 8 to 14 days, considerably longer than the serum amylase. After the first 24 hours of illness, the serum lipase level has a higher sensitivity than serum amylase level for the diagnosis of pancreatitis.[60]

### Other Tests

The roles of several other serum enzymes in the diagnosis of acute pancreatitis are being studied. Serum immunoreactive cationic trypsin (IRT) levels increase in acute pancreatitis and decrease in pancreatic insufficiency. Experience with this technique in children is still limited. Newer tests such as serum pancreatic elastase-1, fecal elastase,[66–67] phospholipase $A_2$, and urinary trypsinogen-2 are still under study. None of these tests has proved superior to measurement of serum amylase and lipase.

Transient mild hyperglycemia is common during the initial stages of an initial attack of pancreatitis. Hyperglycemia is thought to result from excess release of glucagon from the islet of Langerhans. Hypocalcemia can be detected in 30% to 50% of patients. Hypocalcemia is most frequent during the first few days of illness but rarely is associated with symptoms and usually requires no therapy. Acute pancreatitis associated with hyperparathyroidism may lead to normal serum calcium measurements during the course of pancreatitis.

Mild to moderate elevations in the serum aspartate aminotransferase level occur in approximately 50% of patients. Minor increases in the bilirubin level may also be noted secondary to compression to the intrapancreatic portion of the common bile duct. Significant elevations of the serum bilirubin or alkaline phosphatase level should raise the suspicion of obstruction of the biliary tree (gallstone).

Leukocytosis is common during the first few days of the disease. Moderate hypoproteinemia and hypoalbuminemia may be found, particularly after expansion of the vascular volume with intravenous fluids. Hyperlipemic serum should raise the suspicion of an underlying abnormality in lipid metabolism that may be associated with pancreatitis.

In adults, a number of tests have been shown to be helpful in predicting the severity of an episode of acute pancreatitis, including measurements of C-reactive protein (CRP), polymorphonuclear elastase, phospholipase $A_2$, and trypsinogen activation peptide.[68, 69] Of these only the CRP is widely available.

The plain abdominal radiograph may show a sentinel loop sign (distended small bowel loop adjacent to the pancreas), ileus, or colon cut-off sign (air in the splenic or hepatic flexure with absent distal colonic gas). Loss of the properitoneal fat line, indistinct psoas muscle margins, or generalized haziness may indicate more severe inflammation and ascites. None of these signs are unique to pancreatitis, and ultrasonography and CT are more sensitive and specific in establishing a diagnosis of pancreatitis.

Ultrasonography allows direct visualization of the pancreas without ionizing radiation and is the most frequently used radiographic technique in children with suspected pancreatitis. The sonographic findings of pancreatitis include diffuse or focal enlargement, poorly defined border, decreased echogenicity, a dilated pancreatic duct, or pseudocysts (Fig. 55–2). Ultrasonography may be normal, or the pancreas may be obscured by overlying bowel gas in 20% to 30% of patients with pancreatitis confirmed by other studies. Ultrasonography is also useful in the diagnosis of cholelithiasis and bile duct obstruction that may be associated with pancreatitis and is performed as an initial evaluation in most children.

Abdominal CT is usually reserved for more difficult patients or when the ultrasound yields unclear information. CT findings, including the presence of traumatic damage (Fig. 55–3), diffuse pancreatic enlargement, indeterminate pancreatic masses, pancreatic and extrapancreatic fluid collections, abscesses (Fig. 55–4), and hemorrhagic pancreatitis (Fig. 55–5), have been used to predict the outcome of adult patients with pancreatitis.[71] It is important to note that be-

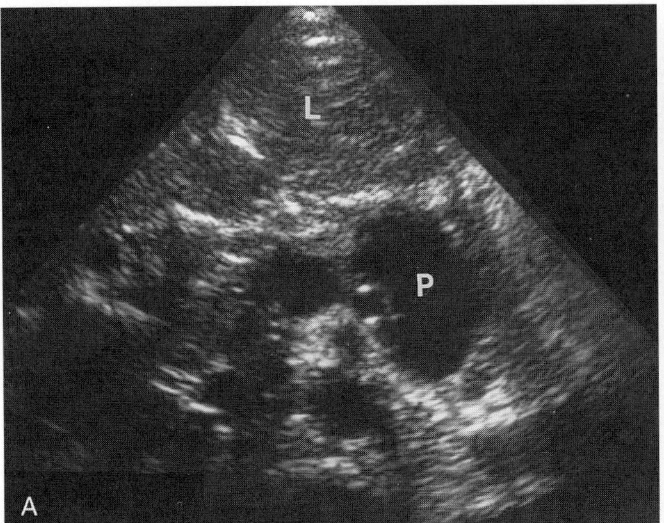


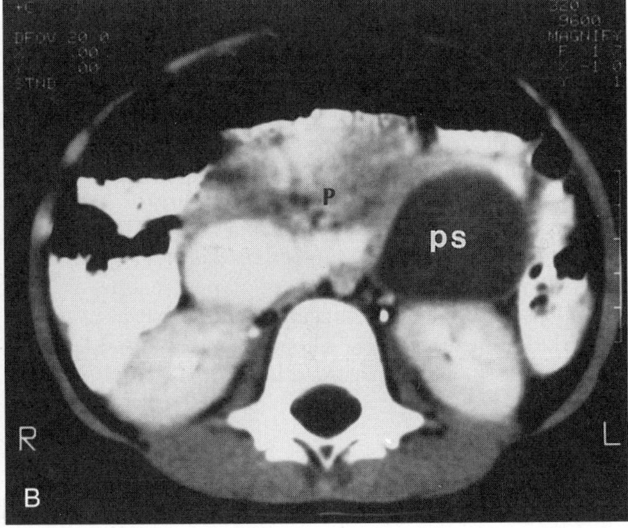


**FIGURE 55–2.** Pancreatic pseudocyst. *A*, Transverse sonogram shows a cystic mass in the tail of the pancreas (P). L, liver. *B*, CT scan demonstrates a cystic structure (PS) in the tail of the pancreas (P) elevating the tail of the pancreas. (Courtesy of John R. Sty, MD.)

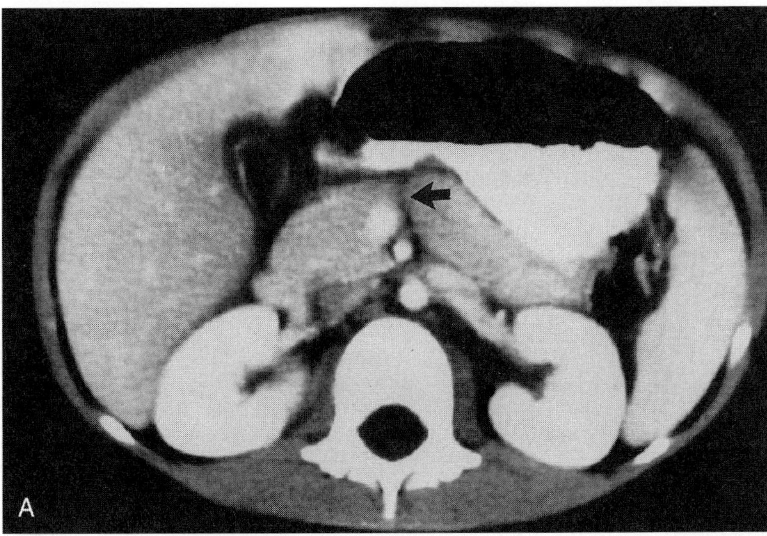


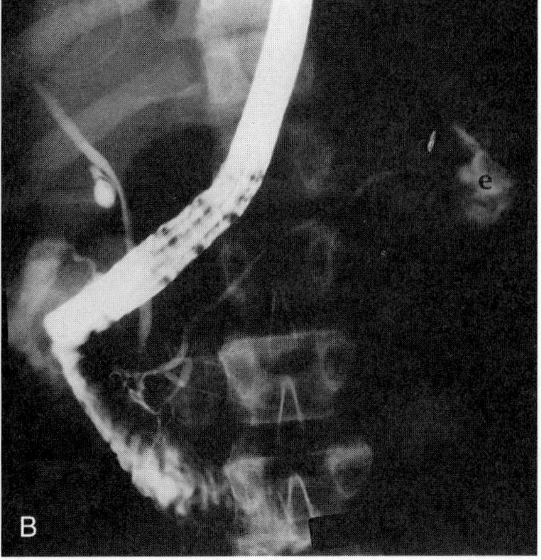


**FIGURE 55–3.** Ruptured duct. *A,* CT examination shows an enlarged linear low attenuation area at the neck of the pancreas *(arrow)*, compatible with a pancreatic laceration. (Courtesy of John R. Sty, MD.) *B,* ERCP examination showing extravasation at the pancreatic duct tail compatible with pancreatic duct laceration (e). (Courtesy of Andrew Taylor, MD.)

cause more than 20% of patients with acute pancreatitis have a normal CT examination, a normal examination does not exclude the diagnosis of pancreatitis.[68]

Magnetic resonance cholangiopancreatography and endoscopic ultrasonography are new techniques for the visualization of the pancreatobiliary ductal systems.[72–73] Limited experience suggests that these techniques may supplement or replace ERCP in the diagnosis or exclusion of ductal abnormalities in selected patients.

## Endoscopic Retrograde Cholangiopancreatography

ERCP is an accepted technique for the diagnosis and treatment of children with pancreatitis.[26, 27] ERCP is critical in the diagnosis of ductal anomalies that are frequently found in children with recurrent pancreatitis. Pancreas divisum can be detected only by pancreatography (see Fig. 55–7).

Diagnostic ERCP should be performed as part of the evaluation of children with pancreatitis that does not resolve after 1 month, recurrent pancreatitis (defined as two or more discrete episodes of pancreatitis), persistent elevation of pancreatic enzymes, the first episode of pancreatitis in a child with a family history of hereditary pancreatitis, pancreatitis following liver transplantation, and pancreatitis associated with cystic fibrosis. In adults ERCP has been shown to be important as part of preoperative evaluation of a nonresolving or enlarging pseudocyst or other pancreatic mass. ERCP performed during nonresolving traumatic pancreatitis may be helpful in identifying the need for endoscopic therapy or surgery.

It is now considered safe to perform ERCP during acute pancreatitis. ERCP and endoscopic sphincterotomy and stone extraction should be performed early in gallstone pancreatitis. When ERCP results are normal, a sample of bile should be aspirated and examined for cholesterol crystals. If crystals are seen, then cholecystectomy should be considered.

The complications of ERCP in children are similar to those that occur in adults. These include pancreatitis, pain requiring analgesia, cholangitis, ileus, fever, intramural dye

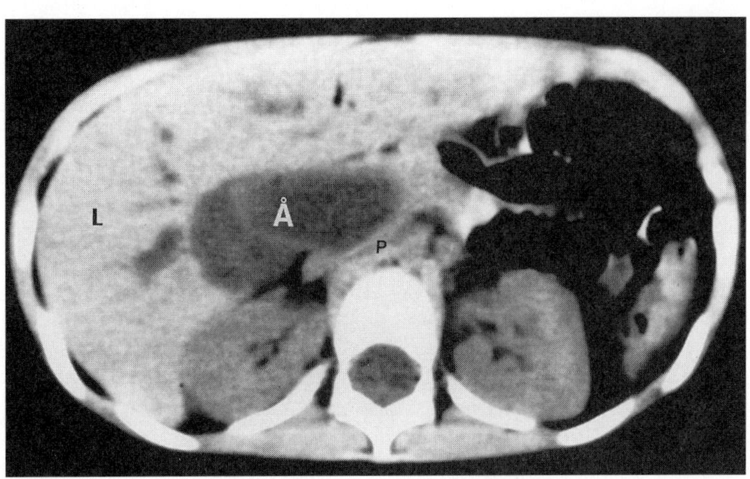


**FIGURE 55–4.** Pancreatic abscess. CT examination in a patient with severe pancreatitis showing a mass (A) in the region of the porta hepatis that represents an abscess in the head of the pancreas (P). L, liver. (Courtesy of John R. Sty, MD.)

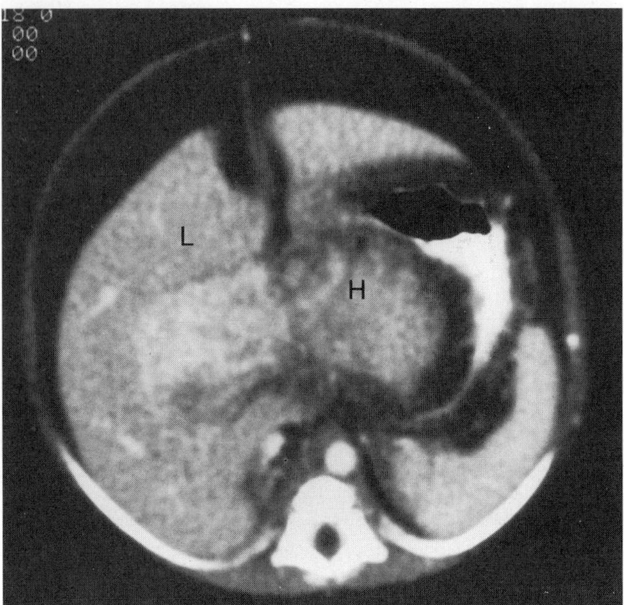


**FIGURE 55–5.** Hemorrhagic pancreatitis. Diffuse enlargement and high attenuation of the pancreas is compatible with hemorrhagic involvement of the pancreas in this patient with pancreatic ascites. H, hemorrhagic area; L, liver. (Courtesy of John R. Sty, MD.)

injection, and perforation. Because of the relatively large diameter of the endoscope and the positioning of the patient that may be required during ERCP, airway obstruction, decreased oxygen saturation, and bradycardia may occur in infants when conscious sedation is used. Reported complications in children have occurred in fewer than 5% of patients.

### Diagnostic Recommendations

Because the gland cannot be directly examined and because imaging studies may be normal, it is not always possible to be certain about the diagnosis. The initial evaluation of a patient with abdominal pain and suspected pancreatitis is determination of the serum amylase and lipase levels. Both tests are widely available. Although either may be normal or elevated in acute pancreatitis, it is rare for both to be falsely normal or falsely elevated. If either is elevated more than three times normal, the likelihood of pancreatitis is high. The difficulty occurs when only one of these two tests is elevated or if the elevation is less than three times normal. A search for extrapancreatic causes of enzyme elevation must then be done. Clinical judgment and radiographic evaluation are then required. A normal serum amylase level within 24 hours after the onset of acute abdominal pain argues strongly against the diagnosis of acute pancreatitis. The amylase may be normal if the patient has been ill for more than 2 days or has chronic pancreatitis.

A dynamic CT scan should be performed in patients with traumatic pancreatitis (ultrasonography is obtained to determine whether gallstones are present). A normal CT in a severely ill patient with suspected pancreatitis should suggest the possibility of extrapancreatic disease.

## Treatment

### Medical Therapy

Treatment of mild and moderate episodes of acute pancreatitis is supportive and expectant. The aims of therapy are to remove the initiating process when possible, halt the progression of disease, relieve pain, and restore homeostasis. Meperidine is given as necessary for pain control. Fluid and electrolyte balance is maintained. Nasogastric suction may reduce vomiting (but does not speed resolution of the underlying pancreatitis). Improvement usually occurs in 2 to 4 days. The patient with acute pancreatitis may be refed when clinical symptoms have resolved and the serum amylase level has returned to near normal. It must be remembered that the fall in the serum lipase level lags behind that of serum amylase. It is not necessary to wait until the lipase level has normalized to refeed the patient. Once the diagnosis of pancreatitis is made, only the serum amylase level needs to be followed. Surgery is rarely required.

Approximately 15% of patients with acute pancreatitis have a severe course. The mortality rate for severe pancreatitis associated with SIRS may be 20% to 50% in adults. In children, the mortality rate has been reported to be 21%, but these patients had multi-system disease that is often fatal when occurring without pancreatitis.[3] The cause of death may be difficult to determine.

The aims of treatment of severe disease in addition to those already mentioned include treatment of local, systemic, and septic complications.[68, 74] Homeostasis is maintained by the correction of hypocalcemia, anemia, hypoalbuminemia, electrolyte imbalances, and hypoxemia. Nutritional support with either total parenteral nutrition or jejunostomy is extremely important. The use of intravenous lipid in the patient with acute pancreatitis is safe. The treatment of severe acute pancreatitis is often prolonged.

A large number of medications have been used in an attempt to halt the progression of the autodigestive process within the pancreas and reduce pancreatic secretions. Controlled studies have shown that although antiproteases, such as aprotinin and gabexate, if given as pretreatment or concomitant treatment, reduce injury in experimental pancreatitis, they were of no benefit in clinical trials.[75] A controlled clinical trial suggested that lexipafant, a platelet-activating factor antagonist, significantly reduced the incidence of and improved recovery from multi-organ failure in a small group of adults with severe pancreatitis.[76] In several trials, somatostatin and its analogue octreotide have not been shown to be beneficial except after pancreatic resection.[77]

The early use of antibiotics has been generally discouraged, because most, but not all, investigators believe that they are of benefit only for the treatment of specific infection.[68, 78] Studies have suggested that intravenous cefuroxime or selective bowel decontamination with norfloxacin, amphotericin, and colistin may decrease mortality.[79]

Serial incremental dynamic bolus CT scanning, which is the best method for the detection of the presence, extent, and severity of pancreatic necrosis, is mandatory in the patient with severe pancreatitis in order to detect the development of necrotic and infected tissue (see Fig. 55–4).[80] CT-guided percutaneous culture will then allow the early detection of infection.

### *Surgical Treatment*

Surgical treatment of traumatic pancreatitis with ductal rupture may include repair or resection (see Fig. 55–3). At times, simple drainage is performed and definitive surgery is deferred until later.

Surgical treatment of severe pancreatitis includes debridement of necrotic and infected tissue.[80–83] Infection without abscess or necrosis does not usually require surgery. The emerging consensus appears to be that necrosectomy and local lavage or open management with planned re-exploration offers better survival than conventional therapy of resection plus drainage alone. Although the optimal timing of surgical intervention is not known, in one series, patients undergoing surgery within 2 weeks after the onset of pancreatitis all died, whereas 79% of patients undergoing surgical treatment after 2 weeks survived.

Today endoscopic stone removal rather than surgery is the acute treatment of choice for most cases of biliary pancreatitis. Cholecystectomy is performed electively after the acute episode resolves.

Accepted indications for surgical treatment include traumatic pancreatitis with disruption of a major duct, persistent severe biliary pancreatitis with an obstructing gallstone that cannot be removed endoscopically, infected pancreatic necrosis, and drainage of pancreatic abscess when percutaneous drainage has failed.[81–83] More controversial indications include persistent pancreatitis in spite of optimal medical therapy, clinical deterioration in the presence of multi-organ failure, and the presence of sterile pancreatic necrosis involving more than 50% of the gland.

### *Pancreatic Pseudocyst*

Pseudocyst formation is an uncommon sequela of pancreatitis. Pseudocysts are delineated by a fibrous wall in the lesser peritoneal sac that may enlarge or extend in almost any direction, thus producing a wide variety of symptoms. A pseudocyst is suggested when an episode of pancreatitis fails to resolve, when an abdominal mass develops after an episode of pancreatitis, or when pancreatitis recurs shortly after resolution. Clinical features may include pain, nausea, vomiting, and jaundice. The most useful diagnostic techniques are ultrasonography, CT scanning, and ERCP (see Fig. 55–2). Because of its ease, availability, and low cost, ultrasonography is the test of first choice. Sequential studies of patients with pancreatitis have demonstrated that pancreatic pseudocyst formation is more common than previously thought. Many are completely asymptomatic and resolve spontaneously. An ultrasound examination should routinely be performed 2 to 4 weeks after an episode of pancreatitis for evaluation of possible pseudocyst formation.

Pseudocysts smaller than 4 cm almost always resolve spontaneously. Treatment of pancreatic pseudocysts may be surgical, endoscopic, or by percutaneous drainage with a pig-tailed catheter.[84–87] If surgery is required, the pseudocyst must be allowed to mature for 4 to 6 weeks before drainage. A delay is not required before percutaneous or endoscopic drainage.

## CHRONIC PANCREATITIS

Unlike acute pancreatitis, which is defined by clinical criteria, chronic pancreatitis is typically defined by morphologic criteria. Chronic pancreatitis is the result of a continuing necroinflammatory process that causes irreversible scarring of both the acinar and ductular cells. The condition is dynamic, but progressive. The increased tissue damage after each flare may lead to exocrine and endocrine insufficiency. Whereas in acute pancreatitis the gland is normal before the attack and recovers, in chronic pancreatitis the gland is abnormal before the attack. Although acute pancreatitis only rarely leads to chronic pancreatitis, it may be clinically difficult to distinguish an attack of chronic pancreatitis from acute pancreatitis.

### Pathophysiology

There are two main pathologic forms of chronic pancreatitis, calcific and obstructive, and both are uncommon in children.[88, 89] Chronic calcifying pancreatitis, the form found in patients after chronic alcohol abuse, is found in about 95% of adults with chronic pancreatitis. In children, this form of pancreatitis occurs in patients with hereditary pancreatitis and tropical pancreatitis. The pancreas is hard, and calcifications can be palpated at surgery. Obstruction occurs when viscous plugs containing multiple proteins including digestive enzymes, mucopolysaccharides, and glycoproteins coalesce in the ductular lumen as a result of the secretion of high-protein, low-bicarbonate fluid. Calcium carbonate precipitates in the plugs forming intraductular stones.[90] It has also been proposed that toxic metabolites may play a major role in the development of the pancreatic injury.

Lithostathine, a glycoprotein, formerly called pancreatic stone protein, prevents precipitation of calcium salts in normal pancreatic fluid.[91] Both chronic ethanol intake and protein deficiency decrease synthesis of lithostathine. Lithostathine is poorly soluble and may precipitate when pancreatic fluid secretion or ductal alkalinization is impaired. Decreased levels of lithostathine with secondary formation of calcium calculi may be the common pathway in a variety of disorders leading to calcific pancreatitis.

Obstructive pancreatitis occurs when a major duct is occluded as the result of a congenital anomaly or an acquired lesion such as a tumor, fibrosis, or traumatic stricture. The pancreatic epithelium is inflamed and may be replaced by fibrous tissue. The ductal system remains relatively intact. Calcifications and protein plugs occur rarely.

Studies have demonstrated that free radicals and antioxidant deficiency may play important roles in the development and progression of chronic pancreatitis.[92]

### Etiology

Chronic pancreatitis is uncommon in children. In the developed world, most adult cases are due to chronic alcohol abuse or ductal obstruction (Table 55–4).

### Chronic Calcifying Pancreatitis

Hereditary pancreatitis is the second most common congenital pancreatic disorder after cystic fibrosis.[93] First de-

**TABLE 55–4. Etiology of Chronic Pancreatitis in Children**

| |
|---|
| **Obstructive** |
| Congenital ductal anomalies |
| Trauma |
| Sclerosing cholangitis |
| Idiopathic fibrosing pancreatitis |
| **Calcific** |
| Hereditary pancreatitis |
| Tropical pancreatitis |
| Cystic fibrosis |
| Hyperlipidemia |
| Hypercalcemia |
| **Miscellaneous** |
| Mitochondrial myopathy |
| Inflammatory bowel disease |
| Idiopathic |

scribed in 1952, hereditary pancreatitis is an autosomal dominant condition with 80% penetrance and variable expressivity. It has been described in more than 100 families. Unlike most cases of acute pancreatitis, pancreatitis in these patients progresses to chronicity. The hereditary pancreatitis gene has been mapped to the long arm of chromosome 7 and has been cloned.[94–96] In most kindreds, histidine substitutes for arginine on residue 117 of cationic trypsinogen. Cationic trypsin, which represents two thirds of the trypsin activity in normal pancreatic juice, has a tendency to autoactivate. Cleavage at this trypsin-sensitive site prevents autodigestion by activated trypsin. Loss of this cleavage site may permit autodigestion of the pancreas and initiate pancreatitis.

Pathologic findings include a shrunken, fibrotic, calcified pancreas, near complete acinar cell atrophy, ductal plugging, and extensive fibrosis. The islet cells are preserved.

Symptoms of recurrent episodes of acute pancreatitis often begin before age 10. Because of the family history, the diagnosis is usually apparent. Severe pain is accompanied by nausea and vomiting. Physical examination and clinical course are similar to those in acute pancreatitis of other causes, and resolution of the acute symptoms occurs in 4 to 8 days. Each episode is associated with increased tissue damage. The patient is well between episodes, and the symptom-free interval may be weeks or years. Finally, episodes resemble chronic pancreatitis. When chronic pancreatitis develops, amylase and lipase levels may be normal even during acute episodes. At CT or ultrasound, a shrunken, calcified pancreas with dilated ducts is seen. Dilated and strictured ducts, frequently with intraductal stones, are seen at ERCP (Fig. 55–6). After many years. pancreatic insufficiency commonly develops. Late complications of familial pancreatitis include diabetes, vascular thrombosis, and pancreatic and intra-abdominal carcinoma.

## Juvenile Tropical Pancreatitis

Juvenile tropical pancreatitis, the most common cause of chronic pancreatitis in children, is not seen in the developed world.[97] This condition develops from protein malnutrition. Patients with tropical pancreatitis consume large quantities of cassava root, which contains toxic cyanogenic glycosides. Clinically this condition is similar to other forms of chronic pancreatitis. Early attacks are similar to those of acute pancreatitis. Overt pancreatic insufficiency is uncommon because of the low-fat diet consumed in the parts of the world where tropical pancreatitis occurs.

## Chronic Obstructive Pancreatitis

### *Pancreas Divisum*

Pancreas divisum occurs in 5% to 15% of the general population and is the most common developmental anomaly of the pancreas.[45] As the result of failure of the dorsal and ventral pancreatic anlagen to fuse, the tail, body, and part of the head of the pancreas drain through the smaller accessory duct of Santorini rather than through the main duct of Wirsung. Although the clinical importance of this anomaly remains controversial, most investigators believe that pancreas divisum may be associated with recurrent pancreatitis, because of relative obstruction of the outflow of the ventral pancreas. Thus, patients may present with recurrent episodes of pancreatitis. The diagnosis can be made only by ERCP (Fig. 55–7).

The management of patients with pancreas divisum and recurrent pancreatitis remains controversial. A variety of surgical and therapeutic endoscopic procedures have been attempted with only mixed success; recent data suggest that in adults endoscopic sphincterotomy or surgical sphincteroplasty is beneficial in selected patients. Unfortunately, the long-term consequences of sphincterotomy in children are unknown.[98] We recommend endoscopic insertion of a stent into the minor papilla in children with recurrent pancreatitis and pancreas divisum. If episodes of pancreatitis stop occurring or occur only when the stent becomes dislodged or occluded, we recommend surgical sphincteroplasty.

### *Abdominal Trauma*

After abdominal trauma, unsuspected ductular damage can lead to strictures, pseudocyst formation, and chronic obstruction.[99]

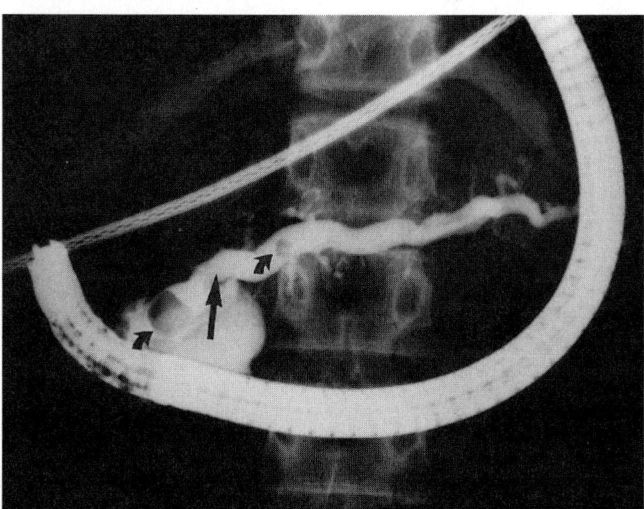

**FIGURE 55–6.** Familial pancreatitis. ERCP demonstrates a dilated pancreatic duct *(straight arrow)* and large concretions *(curved arrows)*. (Courtesy of Andrew Taylor, MD.)

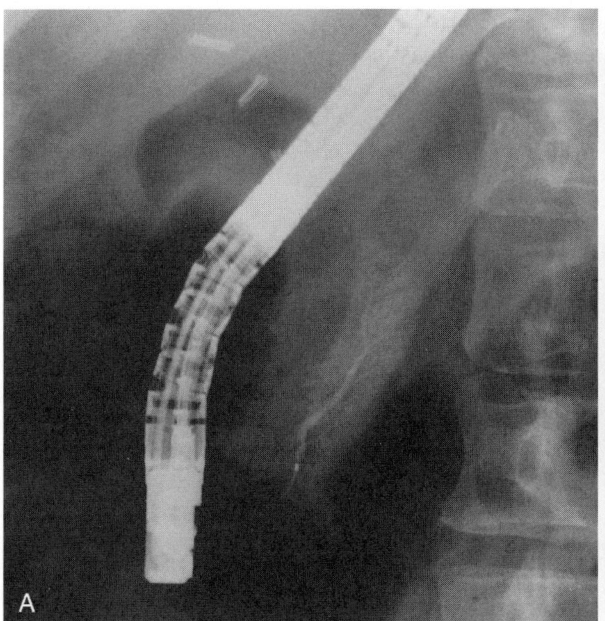


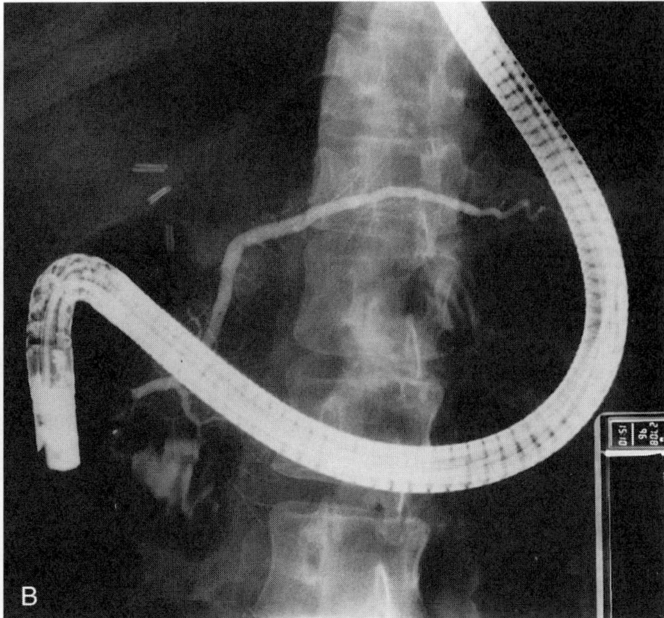


**FIGURE 55–7.** ERCP in pancreas divisum. *A,* Injection into the major papilla (Wirsung) filling only the ventral pancreas. *B,* In the same patient, injection into the minor papilla (Santorini) fills the dorsal pancreatic duct. (Courtesy of Andrew Taylor, MD.)

### *Idiopathic Fibrosing Pancreatitis*

Idiopathic fibrosing pancreatitis is a rare condition that may present with abdominal pain or obstructive jaundice caused by blockage of the common bile duct by the head of the pancreas.[100] In fibrosing pancreatitis, there is diffuse infiltration of the gland with dense fibrous tissue. Inflammation may or may not be present.

In children, it has been estimated that about one third of cases of chronic pancreatitis are idiopathic.

### *Other Causes*

Pancreatitis may develop in 30% of patients with hyperlipidemia type I, in 15% of patients with type IV, and 30% to 40% of patients with type V.[56] Because pancreatitis may itself cause transient hyperlipidemia, when the serum lipid level is elevated during an episode of pancreatitis, it must be remeasured after resolution. Acute pancreatitis secondary to hyperlipidemia does not occur unless the serum triglyceride level is more than 1000 mg/dL.

Additional conditions that have been associated with chronic pancreatitis include cystic fibrosis, alpha$_1$-antitrypsin deficiency, sclerosing cholangitis, and inflammatory bowel disease.

## Clinical Presentation and Course

Most patients with chronic pancreatitis present with repeated episodes of what appears to be acute pancreatitis. In patients without pain, pancreatic failure may occur with the insidious development of steatorrhea or diabetes.

Pain is the major cause of morbidity in chronic pancreatitis. The frequency of the episodes of pancreatitis is extremely variable but in most cases the severity and duration of the pain diminish over time. Symptomatic improvement may be correlated with a loss of pancreatic acinar mass and function. In calcific pancreatitis, the pain usually decreases with the development of pancreatic calcification, which may be associated with endocrine and exocrine failure. Exocrine failure does not occur until approximately 98% of the pancreatic reserve is lost.

Exocrine insufficiency leads to malabsorption, hyperphagia, and growth failure. Nutritional deficiencies, particularly of fat-soluble vitamins, vitamin $B_{12}$, and essential fatty acids, may develop. Fat malabsorption, which does not occur until lipase secretion is decreased by more than 97%, is accompanied by large, foul-smelling stools and crampy abdominal pain. Diabetes may occur but is usually not severe.

## Diagnosis

Chronic pancreatitis is readily diagnosed when a patient has a typical episode of pancreatitis and signs of chronicity are present on imaging studies. More typically, the patient presents with recurrent episodes of abdominal pain and vomiting and a serum amylase level or abdominal ultrasound is obtained. Some patients present with malabsorption and growth failure secondary to pancreatic insufficiency. Fat-soluble vitamin deficiency is uncommon.

**PANCREATIC ENZYMES.** During attacks of pain, the serum levels of amylase and lipase may be elevated or normal because of advanced destruction of the gland.

**ROUTINE LABORATORY TESTS.** Patients with chronic pancreatitis may have glucose intolerance, deficiency of fat-soluble vitamins, hypoalbuminemia, or elevated liver function tests.

**PANCREATIC FUNCTION TESTS.** Tests of pancreatic function are discussed in Chapter 54. These tests may measure pancreatic function directly or indirectly.

**RADIOLOGY.** When pancreatic calcifications are seen on plain abdominal radiographs, the diagnosis of chronic pancreatitis is confirmed. Ultrasonography and CT scanning are discussed earlier in the section on acute pancreatitis.[101]

**ENDOSCOPIC RETROGRADE CHOLANGIOPANCREATOGRAPHY.** ERCP is playing an increasing role in the diagnosis and management of patients with chronic pancreatitis. ERCP should be performed in newly diagnosed patients with chronic pancreatitis to confirm the diagnosis.[26, 27] In early disease, the ERCP may be normal. In advanced disease, the pancreatic ducts are beaded; there are areas of narrowing and dilatation (see Fig. 55–6). Acquired and congenital anomalies may be identified that are amenable to therapeutic maneuvers such as stricture dilatation, stone extraction, sphincterotomy, and insertion of endoprostheses. Preoperatively ERCP helps guide the surgeon.

## Treatment

**PAIN.** Pain control is an important but at times difficult component of therapy in children with chronic pancreatitis. The judicious use of non-narcotic and narcotic analgesics may be necessary.[102]

Pancreatic enzyme secretion is regulated by bile and proteases in the proximal intestine that inhibit the secretion of cholecystokinin (CCK), which stimulates pancreatic secretion.[103] This feedback inhibition is mediated by a trypsin-sensitive, CCK-releasing peptide that has been purified and sequenced.[104]

Patients with chronic pancreatitis have been given pancreatic enzyme supplements in an attempt to inactivate this peptide. This mode of therapy, which is commonly given to patients with chronic pancreatitis and pain, is not universally effective.

When medical therapy fails, endoscopic or surgical relief of ductal obstruction should be attempted.[105–107] Endoscopic sphincterotomy and insertion of endoprosthesis may alleviate the pain in many patients. Surgical drainage with the Puestow procedure may afford long-term pain relief. In this procedure, the pancreas and main pancreatic duct are sectioned longitudinally and oversewn with a segment of similarly fileted jejunum so that the pancreatic juice drains directly into the gut.

**MALABSORPTION.** Malabsorption is common in chronic pancreatitis, but the incidence in children is not known. The goals of treatment are improvement of both growth and absorption without increased pain. Before treatment is instituted, the degree of malabsorption should be documented with a fecal fat analysis. Enzyme replacement therapy is discussed elsewhere. A well-balanced diet with vitamin supplementation should be given.

**PSEUDOCYSTS.** Pseudocysts develop commonly in chronic pancreatitis. The diagnosis and treatment of pseudocysts are discussed earlier. A pseudocyst is best differentiated from a pancreatic abscess by CT. Untreated persistent pseudocysts may rupture into the peritoneal cavity, become infected, or erode into an adjacent viscus or blood vessel.

**BILIARY TRACT OBSTRUCTION.** Biliary tract obstruction may occur in idiopathic fibrosis pancreatitis, sclerosing cholangitis, cystic fibrosis, and hereditary pancreatitis. Relief of the obstruction may be done endoscopically or may require surgical therapy.

**DIABETES.** When diabetes mellitus occurs, it is usually mild and ketoacidosis is rare. Relatively low doses of insulin are required to maintain glycemic control. Hypoglycemia is common because of depressed glucagon secretion.

## REFERENCES

1. Hillemeier C, Gryboski JD: Acute pancreatitis in infants and children. Yale J Biol Med 1984;57:149–159.
2. Ziegler DW, Long JA, Philippart AI, et al: Pancreatitis in childhood. Ann Surg 1988;207:257–261.
3. Weizman Z, Durie PR: Acute pancreatitis in childhood. J Pediatr 1988;113:24–29.
4. Haddock G, Coupar G, Youngson GG, et al: Acute pancreatitis in children: a 15-year review. J Pediatr Surg 1994;29(6):719–722.
5. Yeung CY, Lee HC, Huang FY, et al: Pancreatitis in children—experience with 43 cases. Eur J Pediatr 1996;155:458–463.
6. Mathew P, Wyllie R, Caulfield M, et al: Chronic pancreatitis in late childhood and adolescence. Clin Pediatr (Phila) 1994;33:88–94.
7. Sarles H: Definitions and classifcations of pancreatitis. Pancreas 1991;6:470–474.
8. Bradley EL: A clinically based classification system for acute pancreatitis. Arch Surg 1993;128:586–590.
9. Klöppel G, Maillet B: Pathology of acute and chronic pancreatitis. Pancreas 1993;8(6):659–670.
10. Sarles H: Etiopathogenesis and definition of chronic pancreatitis. Dig Dis Sci 1986;31(9):91S–107S.
11. Keim V, Iovanna JL, Dagorn JC: The acute phase reaction of the exocrine pancreas. Digestion 1994;55:65–72.
12. Skaife P, Kingsnorth AN: Acute pancreatitis: assessment and management. Postgrad Med J 1996;72(847):277–283.
13. Niederau C, Fronhoffs K, Klonowski H, et al: Active pancreatic digestive enzymes show striking differences in their potential to damage isolated rat pancreatic acinar cells. J Lab Clin Med 1995;125(2):265–275.
14. Banerjee AK, Galloway SW, Kingsnorth AN: Experimental models of acute pancreatitis. Br J Surg 1994;81:1096–1103.
15. Lerch MM, Adler G: Experimental animal models of acute pancreatitis. Int J Pancreatol 1994;15(3):159–170.
16. Saluja A, Saluja M, Villa A, et al: Pancreatic duct obstruction in rabbits causes digestive zymogen and lysosomal enzyme colocalization. J Clin Invest 1989;84:1260–1266.
17. Bettinger JR, Grendell JH: Intracellular events in the pathogenesis of acute pancreatitis. Pancreas 1991;6(1):S2–S6.
18. Steer ML: How and where does acute pancreatitis begin? Arch Surg 1992;127:1350–1353.
19. Iovanna JL, Keim V, Michel R, et al: Pancreatic gene expression is altered during acute experimental pancreatitis in the rat. Am J Physiol 1991;261:G485–G489.
20. Kingsnorth AN: Platelet-activating factor. Scand J Gastroenterol 1996;31(suppl 219):28–31.
21. Smego DR, Richardson JD, Flint LM: Determinants of outcome in pancreatic trauma. J Trauma 1985;25(8):771–776.
22. Wilson RH, Moorehead RJ: Current management of trauma to the pancreas. Br J Surg 1991;78:1196–1202.
23. Ryan S, Sandler A, Trenhaile S, et al: Pancreatic enzyme elevations after blunt trauma. Surgery 1994;116:622–627.
24. Devière J, Bueso H, Baize M, et al: Complete disruption of the main pancreatic duct: endoscopic management. Gastrointest Endosc 1995;42(5):445–451.
25. Karjoo M, Luisiri A, Silberstein M, et al: Duodenal hematoma and acute pancreatitis after upper gastrointestinal endoscopy. Gastrointest Endosc 1994;40(4):493–495.
26. Brown CW, Werlin SL, Geenen JE, et al: The diagnostic and therapeutic role of endoscopic retrograde cholangiopancreatography in children. J Pediatr Gastrenterol Nutr 1993;17:19–23.
27. Werlin SL: Endoscopic retrograde cholangiopancreatography in children. Gastrointest Endosc Clin North Am 1994;4(1):161–178.
28. Huang JL, Huang CC, Chen CY, et al: Acute pancreatitis: an early manifestation of systemic lupus erythematosus. Pediatr Emerg Care 1994;10(5):291–293.

29. Lanting WA, Muinos WI, Kamani NR: Pancreatitis heralding Kawasaki disease. J Pediatr 1992;121:743–4.
30. Grodinsky S, Telmesani A, Robson WLM, et al: Gastrointestinal manifestations of hemolytic uremic syndrome: recognition of pancreatitis. J Pediatr Gastroenterol Nutr 1990;11(4):518–524.
31. Weber P, Seibold F, Jenss H: Acute pancreatitis in Crohn's disease. J Clin Gastroenterol 1993;17(4):286–291.
32. McArthur KE: Review article: drug-induced pancreatitis. Aliment Pharmacol Ther 1996;10:23–28.
33. Rünzi M, Layer P: Drug-associated pancreatitis: facts and fiction. Pancreas 1996;13(1):100–109.
34. Wilmink T, Frick TW: Drug-induced pancreatitis. Drug Safety 1996;14(6):406–423.
35. Parenti DM, Steinberg W, Kang P: Infectious causes of acute pancreatitis. Pancreas 1996;13(4):356–371.
36. Glassman M, Tahan S, Hillemeier C: Pancreatitis in patients with Reye's syndrome. J Clin Gastroenterol 1981;3:165–169.
37. Wilson WG, Cass MB, Søvik O: A child with acute pancreatitis and recurrent hypoglycemia due to 3-hydroxy-3-methylglutaryl-coa lyase deficiency. Eur J Pediatr 1984;142:289–291.
38. Kahler SG, Sherwood WG, Woolf D, et al: Pancreatitis in patients with organic acidemias. J Pediatr 1994;124:239–243.
39. Tein I, Christodoulou J, Donner E, et al: Carnitine palmitoyltransferase II deficiency: a new cause of recurrent pancreatitis. J Pediatr 1994;124:938–940.
40. Burlina AB, Dionisi-Vici C, Piovan S, et al: Acute pancreatitis in propionic acidaemia. J Inherit Metab Dis 1995;18:169–172.
41. Kishnani PS, Van Hove JLK, Shoffner JS, et al: Acute pancreatitis in an infant with lactic acidosis and a mutation at nucleotide 3243 in the mitochondrial DNA tRNALeu(UUR) gene. Eur J Pediatr 1996;155:898–903.
42. Murthy UK, DeGregorio F, Oates RP, et al: Hyperamylasemia in patients with the acquired immunodeficiency syndrome. Am J Gastroenterol 1992;87(3):332–336.
43. Miller TL, Winter HS, Luginbuhl LM, et al: Pancreatitis in pediatric human immunodeficiency virus infection. J Pediatr 1992;120(No. 2, part I):223–227.
44. Yabut B, Werlin SL, Havens P, et al: Endoscopic retrograde cholangiopancreatography in children with HIV infection. J Pediatr Gastroenterol Nutr 1993;17:19–23.
45. Lehman GA, Sherman S: Pancreas divisum. Gastrointest Endosc Clin North Am 1995;5(1):145–170.
46. Lehman GA, Sherman S: Sphincter of Oddi dysfunction. Int J Pancreatol 1996;20(1):11–25.
47. Ros E, Navarro S, Bru Conxita, et al: Occult microlithiasis in "idiopathic" acute pancreatitis: prevention of relapse by cholecystectomy or ursodeoxycholic acid therapy. Gastroenterology 1991;101:1701–1709.
48. Lee SP, Nicholls JF, Park HZ: Biliary sludge as a cause of acute pancreatitis. N Engl J Med 1992;326:589–93.
49. Masaryk TJ, Achkar E: Pancreatitis as initial presentation of cystic fibrosis in young adults: a report of two cases. Dig Dis Sci 1983;28(10):874–878.
50. Atlas AB, Orenstein SR, Orenstein DM: Pancreatitis in young children with cystic fibrosis. J Pediatr 1992;120:756–759.
51. Del Rosario JF, Putnam PE, Orenstein DM: Chronic pancreatitis in a patient with cystic fibrosis and clinical pancreatic insufficiency. J Pediatr 1995;126:951–952.
52. Kikuchi M, Hasegawa K, Handa I, et al: Chronic pancreatitis in a child with glycogen storage disease type 1. Eur J Pediatr 1991;150:852–853.
53. Collins JE, Brenton DP: Case report: pancreatitis and homocystinuria. J Inherit Metab Dis 1990;13:232–233.
54. Gryboski J, Hillemeier C, Kocoshis S, et al: Refeeding pancreatitis in malnourished children. J Pediatr 1980;97(3):441–443.
55. Rampling D: Acute pancreatitis in anorexia nervosa. Med J Aust 1982;2:194–195.
56. Toskes PP: Hyperlipidemic pancreatitis. Gastroenterol Clin North Am 1990;19(4):783–791.
57. Malferheiner P, Kemmer TP: Clinical picture and diagnosis of acute pancreatitis. Hepatogastroenterology 1991;38:97–100.
58. Sternby B, O'Brien JF, Zinsmeister AR, et al: What is the best biochemical test to diagnose acute pancreatitis?: a prospective clinical study. Mayo Clin Proc 1996;71:1138–1144.
59. Wong ECC, Butch AW, Rosenblum JL, et al: The clinical chemistry laboratory and acute pancreatitis. Clin Chem 1993;39(2):234–243.
60. Tietz NW, Shuey DF: Lipase in serum—the elusive enzyme: an overview. Clin Chem 1993;39(5):746–756.
61. Clavien PA, Robert J, Meyer P, et al: Acute pancreatitis and normoamylasemia. Ann Surg 1989;210(5):614–620.
62. Orebaugh SL: Normal amylase levels in the presentation of acute pancreatitis. Am J Emerg Med 1994;12(1):21–24.
63. Padilla B, Pollack VE, Pesce A, et al: Pancreatitis in patients with end-stage renal disease. Medicine 1994;73(1):8–20.
64. Ryan CM, Sheridan RL, Schoenfeld DA: Postburn pancreatitis. Ann Surg 1995;222(2):163–170.
65. Kleinman DS, O'Brien JF: Laboratory medicine—macroamylase. Mayo Clin Proc 1986;45(3)61:669–670.
66. Domínguez-Muñoz JE, Hieronymus C, Sauerbruch T, et al: Fecal elastase test: evaluation of a new noninvasive pancreatic function test. Am J Gastroenterol 1995;90(10):1834–1837.
67. Hedström J, Korvuo A, Kenkkimäki P, et al: Urinary trypsinogen-2 test strip for acute pancreatitis. Lancet 1996;347:729–731.
68. Carter DC: The modern management of acute pancreatitis. S Afr J Surg 1996;34(3):126–137.
69. Viedma JA, Pérez-Mateo M, Agulló J, et al: Inflammatory response in the early prediction of severity in human acute pancreatitis. Gut 1994;35:822–827.
70. Berrocal T, Prieto C, Pastor I, et al: Sonography of pancreatic disease in infants and children. Radiographics 1995;15:301–313.
71. Balthazar EJ, Ranson JHC, Naidich DP, et al: Acute pancreatitis: prognostic value of CT1. Radiology 1985;156:767–772.
72. Hirohashi S, Hirohashi R, Uchida H, et al: Pancreatitis: evaluation with MR cholangiopancreatography in children. Radiology 1997;203:411–415.
73. Sugiyama M, Atomi Y: Endoscopic ultrasonography for diagnosing anomalous pancreaticobiliary junction. Gastrointest Endosc 1997;45(3):261–267.
74. Fernandez-del Castillo C, Rattner DW, Warshaw AL: Acute pancreatitis. Lancet 1993;342:475–479.
75. Büchler M, Malfertheiner P, Uhl W, et al: Gabexate mesilate in human acute pancreatitis. Gastroenterology 1993;104:1165–1170.
76. Kingsnorth AN, Galloway SW, Formela LJ: Randomized, double-blind phase II trial of Lexipafant, a platelet-activating factor antagonist, in human acute pancreatitis. Br J Surg 1995;82:1414–1420.
77. McKay C, Baxter J, Imrie C: A randomized, controlled trial of octreotide in the management of patients with acute pancreatitis. Int J Pancreatol 1997;21(1):13–19.
78. Barie PS: A crtitical review of antibiotic prophylaxis in severe acute pancreatitis. Am J Surg 1996;172(suppl 6A):38S–43S.
79. Luiten EJ, Hop WCJ, Lange JF, et al: Controlled clinical trial of selective decontamination for the treatment of severe acute pancreatitis. Ann Surg 1995;222(1):57–65.
80. Bassi C: Infected pancreatic necrosis. Int J Pancreatol 1994;16(1):1–10.
81. D'Egidio A, Schein M: Surgical strategies in the treatment of pancreatic necrosis and infection. Br J Surg 1991;78:133–137.
82. McFadden DW, Reber HA: Indications for surgery in severe acute pancreatitis. Int J Pancreatol 1994;15(2):83–90.
83. Mier J, Luque-de León E, Castillo A, et al: Early versus late necrosectomy in severe necrotizing pancreatitis. Am J Surg 1997;173:71–75.
84. Jaffe RB, Arata JA, Matlak ME: Percutaneous drainage of traumatic pancreatic pseudocysts in children. AJR 1989;152:591–595.
85. Cremer M, Deviere J, Engelholm L: Endoscopic management of cysts and pseudocysts in chronic pancreatitis: long-term follow-up after 7 years of experience. Gastrointest Endosc 1989;35:1–9.
86. VanSonnenberg E, Wittich GR, Casola G, et al: Percutaneous drainage of infected and noninfected pancreatic pseudocysts: experience in 101 cases. Radiology 1989;170:757–761.
87. Gumaste VV, Dave PB: Editorial: pancreatic pseudocyst drainage—the needle or the scalpel? J Clin Gastroenterol 1991;13(5):500–505.
88. Steer ML, Waxman I, Freedman S: Review article: chronic pancreatitis. N Engl J Med 1995;332(22):1482–1490.
89. Mathew P, Wyllie R, Caulfield M, et al: Chronic pancreatitis in late childhood and adolescence. Clin Pediatr 1994;33:88–94.
90. Braganza JM: The pathogenesis of chronic pancreatitis. Q J Med 1996;89:243–250.
91. Geider S, Baronnet A, Cerini C, et al: Pancreatic lithostathine as a calcite habit modifier. J Biol Chem 1996;271(42):26302–26306.
92. Mathew P, Wyllie R, Van Lente F, et al: Antioxidants in hereditary pancreatitis. Am J Gastroenterol 1996;91(8):1558–1562.

93. Perrault J: Hereditary pancreatitis. Gastroenterol Clin North Am 1994;23(4):743–753.
94. Le Bodic L, Bignon JD, Raguénès O, et al: The hereditary pancreatitis gene maps to long arm of chromosome 7. Hum Mol Genet 1996;5(4):549–554.
95. Whitcomb DC, Gorry MC, Preston RA, et al: Hereditary pancreatitis is caused by a mutation in the cationic trypsinogen gene. Nat Genet 1996;14:141–145.
96. It takes a family (editorial). Nat Genet 1996;14(2):117–118.
97. Balakrishnan V, Sauniere JF, Harihan M, et al: Diet, pancreatic function, and chronic pancreatitis in South India and France. Pancreas 1988;3(1):30–35.
98. Lehman GA, Sherman S: Pancreas divism: diagnosis, clinical significance, and management alternatives. Gastrointest Endosc Clin North Am 1995;5:145–170.
99. Bradley EL III: Chronic obstructive pancreatitis as a delayed complication of pancreatic trauma. HPB Surg 1991;5:49–60.
100. Amerson JL, Ricketts RR: Idiopathic fibrosing pancreatitis: a rare cause of obstructive jaundice in children. Am Surg 1996;62(4):295–291.
101. Chen MH, Lee CH, WU CL, et al: Sonographic presentation of chronic pancreatitis complicated with acute duodenal obstruction in a battered child. J Clin Ultrasound 1994;22:334–337.
102. Banks PA: Management of pancreatic pain. Pancreas 1991;6(suppl 1):S52–S59.
103. Liddle RA: Regulation of cholecystokinin secretion by intraluminal releasing factors. Am J Physiol 1995;269:G319–G327.
104. Spannagel AW, Green GM, Guan D, et al: Purification and characterization of a luminal cholecystokinin-releasing factor from rat intestinal secretion. Proc Natl Acad Sci 1996;93:4415–4420.
105. Binmoeller KF, Jue P, Seifert H, et al: Endoscopic pancreatic stent drainage in chronic pancreatitis and a dominant stricture: long-term results. Endoscopy 1995;27:638–644.
106. Crombleholme TM, deLorimier AA, Way LW, et al: The modified Puestow procedure for chronic relapsing pancreatitis in children. J Pediatr Surg 1990;25(7):749–754.
107. Ponchon T, Bory RM, Hedelius F, et al: Endoscopic stenting for pain relief in chronic pancreatitis: results of a standardized protocol. Gastrointest Endosc 1995;42(5):452–456.

Chapter 56

# Secretory Neoplasms of the Pancreas

Hillel Naon and Daniel W. Thomas

Pancreatic neoplasms are exceedingly rare in children. The majority of childhood pancreatic tumors are benign endocrine neoplasms that secrete hormonally active peptides.[1, 2] A case of insulinoma was first described in 1927 by Wilder and colleagues[3] in an adult with a metastatic islet cell carcinoma and profound hypoglycemia. Islet cell adenoma in a neonate was described by Sherman[4] in 1947 and was the first reported case of a secretory type of pancreatic neoplasm in pediatrics. The focus in this chapter is on functioning neoplasms of the pancreas occurring in childhood.

Functioning pancreatic neoplasms are composed primarily of islet cells that elaborate various endocrine secretory products. More than 50% of pancreatic endocrine neoplasms are multihormonal. However, clinical manifestations are nearly always derived primarily from hypersecretion of only one of the hormones that is produced.[5–7] The diagnosis of pancreatic islet cell neoplasms with excessive hormone production depends on the recognition of clinical syndromes associated with autonomous endocrine product secretion. The pancreatic islet A cells secrete glucagon; the B cells secrete insulin; the D cells secrete somatostatin; the F cells secrete vasoactive intestinal polypeptide (VIP), substance P, and possibly secretin; and the G cells secrete gastrin.[7, 8] Pluripotent stem cells in the pancreatic duct epithelium called *nesidioblasts* give rise to the aforementioned differentiated islet cell types but may differentiate into neoplasms, producing ectopic hormones under aberrant conditions.[7, 9, 10]

The development of highly specific and sensitive radioimmunoassays for detection of circulating peptides in the blood has facilitated the recognition and diagnosis of hormone-secreting neuroendocrine tumors and their associated syndromes. In children, the most common secretory pancreatic neoplasm is insulinoma associated with B cell adenoma or hyperplasia. Zollinger-Ellison syndrome associated with gastrinoma, VIPoma (Verner-Morrison syndrome), and multiple endocrine neoplasia have been described in children.[11] Glucagonoma and somatostatinoma have not been reported in children.[11] Table 56–1 lists such tumors and their characteristics.

## MULTIPLE ENDOCRINE NEOPLASIA

Three distinct types of multiple endocrine neoplasms have been identified (MEN I, MEN IIA, and MEN IIB).[11a] MEN I, or Wermer's syndrome, is associated with islet cell tumors of the pancreas, hyperparathyroidism, and nonfunctional adenomas of the pituitary. The MEN II syndromes are not associated with pancreatic tumors but have thyroid (medullary carcinoma) and adrenal tumors (pheochromocytoma). MEN IIA, or Sipple's syndrome, is distinguished by its association with parathyroid hyperplasia; and MEN IIB is associated with multiple mucosal and alimentary tract neuromas. Each of these syndromes has autosomal dominant inheritance. MEN I and IIA usually occur in adults, whereas MEN IIB may present in childhood. Patients with MEN I may develop symptoms at any age, but the condition rarely presents in childhood or after the age of 60 years. Both sexes are affected with equal frequency.[12, 13] The disorder is inherited in a dominant mode with a high degree of penetrance.[14, 15] The MEN I gene has been mapped to chromosome 11[16] and the MEN II gene to chromosome 10.[16a] Evidence suggests that tumor formation is associated with loss of a specific gene, which possibly unmasks a recessive mutation at this locus. Genetic markers for MEN I will undoubtedly soon become available.[16]

The clinical manifestations of MEN I are heterogeneous and depend on the endocrine organ involved and the functional nature of the secretory neoplasm. An extensive review of 88 patients, 7 of whom were pediatric patients, by Ballard and coworkers[12] provided much of the early knowledge concerning the various features of MEN I, which include (1) parathyroid gland hyperfunction (84%), (2) pituitary neoplasms (65%), (3) adenomas and hyperplasia of the adrenal cortex (38%), (4) thyroid disease (19%) (thyrotoxicosis, thyroid carcinoma, and nonfunctioning adenomas), and (5) peptic ulcers (58%). Ulcers were multifocal in more than half of the patients. Some patients had watery diarrhea or bronchial carcinoids. Pancreatic neoplasms were found in more than 75% of all the patients with MEN I. These neoplasms were almost always multiple and consisted of both B cells, giving rise to insulinoma, and non-B cells, resulting in Zollinger-Ellison syndrome. Other associated neoplasms included glucagonoma, VIPoma, or somatostatinoma.

Genetic counseling and screening of family members with careful follow-up are important aspects in the management of patients with MEN I. Treatment of pancreatic neoplasms

TABLE 56–1. Secretory Neoplasms of the Pancreas

| NEOPLASM | HORMONE SECRETED | ISLET CELL TYPE | MAJOR CLINICAL FEATURES | % MALIGNANT | TREATMENT |
|---|---|---|---|---|---|
| Insulinoma (adenoma, hyperplasia, nesidioblastosis) | Insulin | B | Hypoglycemia | 10 | Diazoxide combined with frequent feedings, octreotide acetate, surgery |
| Gastrinoma | Gastrin | G | Peptic ulcers, diarrhea, acid secretion | 65 | Gastric acid antagonists/ blockers, surgery |
| VIPoma | VIP | F | Secretory diarrhea, hypokalemia, hypochlorhydria | 50 | Fluid and electrolyte replacement, octreotide acetate, steroids, surgery |
| Glucagonoma | Glucagon | A | Rash, stomatitis, diabetes | >75 | Octreotide acetate, surgery |

associated with MEN I is discussed later in this chapter in sections dealing with the specific types of secretory tumors.

Children with MEN IIB may have a distinctive phenotype with a marfanoid habitus, muscle wasting, growth failure, everted eyelids, thick lips, and multiple mucosal neuromas. Thickened lips and everted eyelids are secondary to the development of neuromas and tend to be more prominent over time.[16b] The importance of recognizing MEN IIB early is in the detection of medullary carcinoma of the thyroid, which tends to occur early in patients with MEN IIB with rapid metastasis.

The gastrointestinal manifestations of MEN IIB range from mild constipation to symptoms mimicking Hirschsprung's disease or episodes of frank pseudo-obstruction. Histologic examination demonstrates diffuse proliferation of nerves and ganglion cells throughout the small and large intestine. In children who have growth failure or physical stigmata of MEN IIB, rectal suction biopsy will demonstrate hyperplasia of nerve fibers. Serum calcitonin levels will confirm the diagnosis.

## INSULINOMA

Insulinomas, although rare, are the most common form of hormone-secreting tumors of the pancreas in children and adults.[17] These are discrete pancreatic endocrine neoplasms composed mainly or exclusively of B cells. Insulinomas have been recognized as a cause of inappropriate insulin secretion for more than half a century. Whipple[18] described the typical triad of symptoms associated with this syndrome: insulin shock with fasting, a fasting blood sugar of less than half normal, and relief of symptoms with the administration of glucose. Over 100 cases of insulinoma, including islet B cell adenoma and hyperplasia, were compiled by Tudor in the Childhood Disease Registry.[19] The number of reports has increased considerably since the radioimmunoassay for insulin became available for clinical use. Published cases of insulinoma indicate that an islet cell adenoma or hyperplasia may become manifest at any age during childhood, but there are two periods of peak incidence: (1) the neonatal period through the first year of life and (2) after age 4 years, with a peak from age 8 to 13 years.[13] Insulinomas are more frequent in females.[19, 20] Eighty percent are solitary neoplasms, and over 90% are benign.[19, 21] Malignant insulinomas are exceedingly rare in children.[2] Patients with insulinomas and the MEN I syndrome often have multiple insulinomas and are usually diagnosed at 15 to 25 years of age.[13] They account for about 10% of adult patients with insulinoma. In infants, diffuse adenomatosis or nesidioblastosis is frequently the cause of hyperinsulinemia.[22]

Insulinomas vary in size from lesions that are difficult to find even under dissection to huge tumors that are over 1500 g.[20] Ninety percent of insulinomas are less than 20 mm in diameter. Solitary tumors that are smaller than 5 mm in diameter are seldom associated with hypoglycemia.[20] They are usually encapsulated, firm, yellow-brown nodules that are histologically composed of cords and nests of well-differentiated B islet cells. Regardless of their size, insulinomas can be located anywhere in the pancreas and are rarely found outside the pancreas. Distinction between a benign or malignant insulinoma is difficult on the basis of histologic appearance alone.

The alpha chain of human chorionic gonadotropin (hCG-$\alpha$) was reported as a marker for malignancy in functioning endocrine neoplasms, including insulinomas.[23]

Because MEN I is the most common condition associated with multiple benign insulinomas, the presence of genetic markers for MEN I may alert the physician to the possibility of multiple insulinomas.[16]

Symptoms of hypoglycemia such as headaches, visual disturbances, confusion, weakness, sweating, and palpitations are characteristic; convulsions and coma are features of significant prolonged hypoglycemia. Most symptoms occur after fasting and are often confused with neurologic or psychiatric disease. The finding of hypoglycemia that can be provoked with fasting remains the keystone in the recognition of the possibility of an insulinoma. Significant hypoglycemia can be demonstrated after a 12-hour overnight fast in over 90% of cases of proven insulinoma.[20] Plasma insulin levels are inappropriately elevated during hypoglycemia. Patients with insulinoma have insulin-connecting peptide (C-peptide) concentrations that parallel the elevated plasma insulin levels. Normally, when insulin is cleared from its precursor proinsulin, the C-peptide is released into the portal vein at a 1:1 ratio with insulin. Because insulinoma cells often process proinsulin incompletely, the serum often has a high ratio of proinsulin to insulin.[20] In normal subjects, serum insulin concentrations decrease to less than 5 $\mu$U/mL when the blood sugar level falls to 40 mg/dL or lower, and the ratio of plasma insulin (in $\mu$U/mL) to serum glucose (in mg/dL) remains less than 0.3. In patients with insulinomas, the ratio is usually greater than 0.4 and increases with fasting.[24] Hypoglycemia in the absence of urinary ketones and the presence of low plasma β-hydroxybutyrate are consistent with the diagnosis of insulinoma.

It is often difficult to localize insulinomas once the diagnosis has been made on clinical and laboratory grounds. Noninvasive studies, such as computed tomography, ultrasonography, and magnetic resonance imaging, are usually helpful when the insulinoma is greater than 2 cm. Insulinomas that are less than 2 cm in diameter can be visualized preoperatively by endoscopic ultrasonography.[24, 25] The sensitivity of somatostatin receptor scintigraphy is less than 60% for insulinomas that express the somatostatin receptor subtype that can be recognized by the current radionuclide-labeled somatostatin analogue.[26] Selective arteriography is usually performed if the noninvasive studies are negative. A hypervascular insulinoma can be detected by selective arteriography in 50% to 80% of cases.[27] In patients with negative noninvasive studies and nondiagnostic arteriography, portal venous sampling of blood for insulin is performed before surgery. Tumors that cannot be identified preoperatively can be either palpated during surgery or detected by intraoperative ultrasonography.[28, 29]

The treatment of choice for insulinoma is surgical ablation, which carries an excellent prognosis in most infants and children. At surgery, the islet cell tumor is often pink and firmer than the surrounding gland. The tumor is usually discrete and well encapsulated. The majority of these neoplasms can be simply enucleated. If the neoplasm cannot be localized, distal pancreatectomy with careful examination of sequential frozen sections of the gland is advisable. Resection of more than 80% of the gland is rarely required.[11]

In patients with MEN I syndrome who have extensive microadenomatosis, a 95% subtotal pancreatectomy is needed to achieve a cure.[1] The residual pancreatic tissue mass is usually sufficient to maintain normal function. Transient hyperglycemia is frequent in the immediate postoperative period.[30, 31] Diabetes mellitus with refractory hyperglycemia and ketonemia may occur soon after massive subtotal pancreatectomy[31, 32] and can occur years after subtotal pancreatectomy.[33] Improved medical treatment has facilitated postponement of blind pancreatectomy until the tumor can be identified. Regularly scheduled feedings combined with diazoxide therapy can be used to manage some patients for a prolonged period of time. Octreotide acetate (Sandostatin, Sandoz Ltd, Basel, Switzerland) is an 8-amino-acid synthetic peptide that possesses pharmacologic effects similar to those of the native hormone somatostatin but has much longer duration of action. This drug effectively suppresses insulin release in approximately half the patients with insulinoma.[34] The agent most frequently used in the chemotherapy of malignant insulinoma is streptozotocin.[20]

## NESIDIOBLASTOSIS

Nesidioblastosis, or diffuse proliferation of nesidioblasts, was first described and named by Laidlaw in 1938.[35] Nesidioblasts, meaning islet builders, are cells that differentiate from the pancreatic duct epithelium to form pancreatic islets.

Two-hundred fifty-six cases of nesidioblastosis have been reported to date in the *Childhood Disease Registry.*[19] Since 1970, nesidioblastosis, sometimes also termed *neonatal hyperinsulinemic hypoglycemia,* has been diagnosed frequently in association with neonatal hypoglycemia.

The etiology of nesidioblastosis is unknown. Kloppel and Heitz[23] suggested that the histologic resemblance of pancreata with nesidioblastosis to those from immature fetuses occurred as a result of inappropriate control during the earliest phase of endocrine pancreatic development. A genetic component with an autosomal recessive inheritance pattern is suggested by the familial occurrence of neonatal nesidioblastosis and nesidioblastosis in familial endocrine adenomatosis.[22] Marks[20] suggested that, in addition to the natural immaturity of the endocrine pancreas shown by all infants, those with hyperinsulinemic hypoglycemia may have subtle differences in their intra-islet cellular relationships. Not only is the normal intra-islet relationship between the insulin-secreting B cells and the somatostatin-secreting D cells disturbed, but there is also a reduction in the total number of intra-islet D cells, which are thought to provide an inhibitory effect on insulin secretion. Unlike insulinomas, in which B cells appear to be unable to store and convert proinsulin to insulin efficiently, it seems that there is normal conversion of proinsulin into insulin in the B cells in cases of nesidioblastosis.

Clinically, hyperinsulinemic hypoglycemia is usually evident shortly after birth. Very rarely it presents after 3 months of age. Affected infants have the same broad spectrum of clinical manifestations as described for insulinoma and are equally refractory to medical therapy. They have a relatively high plasma insulin-to-glucose ratio.

The treatment of choice for neonatal hyperinsulinemic hypoglycemia is 95% pancreatectomy, which is successful in 80% to 90% of infants with nesidioblastosis.[36] Somatostatin analogue is used for preoperative management as well as in infants who fail surgery.[34, 36] Providing permanent brain damage from hypoglycemia has not occurred, the prognosis of nesidioblastosis is good. This condition may be familial, especially when associated with leucine-reactive hypoglycemia. Therefore, it is important to monitor newborn siblings of affected children.

## GASTRINOMA: ZOLLINGER-ELLISON SYNDROME

In 1955, Zollinger and Ellison[37] described one adult patient and a 16-year-old girl who presented with the triad of gastric hypersecretion, fulminant and intractable peptic ulcer disease, and a non–B cell neoplasm of the pancreas. The hormone produced by the pancreatic tumor in this syndrome was recognized as gastrin more than 10 years later.[38, 39]

Tumors producing gastrin may be associated with symptoms other than those of Zollinger-Ellison syndrome, such as diarrhea, steatorrhea, and malabsorption.[40] Gastrinomas can originate in organs other than the pancreas, but they occur in the pancreas more often than any other site. The duodenum is the second most common site of origin.[41, 42]

There are at least four major peptide forms of gastrin that differ in the length of their polypeptide chains but have identical C-terminal peptide amides. The C-terminal tetrapeptide amide has been shown to constitute the physiologically active site of the gastrin molecule.[43] Each of the peptide forms of the gastrin molecule exists in sulfated and nonsulfated forms, which appears to confer no differences in physiologic activity or potency of the molecule. The principal form of gastrin in gastrinoma is a heptadecapeptide (G-17), which contains 17-amino-acid residues.[44, 45]

Zollinger-Ellison syndrome can develop at any age. It occurs most frequently, however, between ages 35 and 65 years and is more common in men than in women. Forty-six cases of childhood gastrinomas are reported in the Childhood Disease Registry.[19] Forty-three cases occurred in boys. The youngest patient reported was a 5-year-old girl who also had Marden-Walker syndrome.[46] The age range of Zollinger-Ellison syndrome reported in children is 5 to 16 years. Thirty-seven children had documented neoplasms, and hyperplasia was observed in six. Sixty-five percent of the tumors were malignant. This is similar to the findings in adults, in whom 60% of the cases are malignant, most of the patients having liver metastases at the time of diagnosis.[47] Twelve cases of gastrinoma in childhood were associated with islet cell carcinoma.[19] Although many adult patients with Zollinger-Ellison syndrome have accompanying diseases, such as MEN I syndrome, similar cases have not been reported in the pediatric age group.[11]

Symptoms in Zollinger-Ellison syndrome are due to the high circulating serum gastrin levels, which cause proliferation of the gastric parietal cell mass and stimulation of excessive gastric acid secretion. Children with Zollinger-Ellison syndrome invariably have volumes of gastric secretions ranging from 600 to 2000 mL/day or more, with total acid production of 23 to 164 mEq/L.[48] Abdominal pain due to peptic ulcer disease is the most common clinical finding. Ulcers usually occur in the first portion of the duodenum or in the stomach. The ulcers are usually single but can be multiple. When multiple ulcers occur, they are frequently located not only in the first portion of the duodenum but also in the remainder of the duodenum or even the jejunum. Diarrhea is a frequent problem; it may precede ulceration in some patients or occur without ulcers in others. The diarrhea is due to the excessive amount of hydrochloric acid released into the duodenum. In addition to an osmotic diarrhea, the increased amounts of acid and pepsin entering the small bowel produce inflammatory changes of the intestinal mucosa. Steatorrhea is less common than diarrhea. Acidity of the duodenum and small intestine causes inactivation of pancreatic lipase, reduction of conjugated bile acids, and the previously mentioned mucosal damage.

The diagnosis of Zollinger-Ellison syndrome is based on the presence of gastric acid hypersecretion and hypergastrinemia.[49] Elevated fasting serum gastrin levels can also occur with massive small intestinal resection, pernicious anemia with gastric achlorhydria, renal failure, chronic gastritis, peptic ulcer disease, and antral G cell hyperplasia. Basal acid output of greater than 15 mEq/hr in the unoperated patient should prompt suspicion of gastrinoma. There is a smaller increase between basal acid output and pentagastrin-stimulated gastric acid secretion in patients with gastrinoma. This test by itself cannot establish or exclude the diagnosis of Zollinger-Ellison syndrome because of the overlap in values with normal and peptic ulcer patients. Acid output is difficult to measure after ulcer surgery because it is difficult to recover all the acid and because bile and pancreatic juice often reflux into the stomach. Therefore, decreased acid secretion after partial gastric resection does not exclude the diagnosis of Zollinger-Ellison syndrome.

By using radioimmunoassay for gastrin, the upper limit of normal is 100 to 150 pg/mL. Gastrin levels greater than 500 pg/mL in a patient with acid hypersecretion are diagnostic of gastrinoma.[49] Several provocative tests have been used to evaluate patients with possible gastrinoma, especially those who do not exhibit serum gastrin levels higher than 500 pg/mL. These tests use measurements of serum gastrin levels in response to intravenous secretin, calcium infusion, or ingestion of standard meal. The secretin stimulation test is by far the most valuable provocative test in identifying patients with Zollinger-Ellison syndrome.[49] Secretin, at a dose of 1 to 2 units per kilogram of body weight, is given intravenously over 30 to 60 seconds. Gastrin is measured in serum samples obtained before the injection of secretin and at 5-minute intervals thereafter for 30 minutes. In normal individuals and in patients with peptic ulcer disease, achlorhydria, or antral G cell hyperplasia, the infused secretin has little effect. In patients with Zollinger-Ellison syndrome, intravenous secretin induces a substantial and prompt increase of serum gastrin by at least 200 pg/mL, usually at 5 minutes, gradually returning to basal levels by 30 minutes. In patients with gastrinoma, intravenous calcium infusion causes an increase in serum gastrin of more than 400 pg/mL above the basal serum concentration. However, because this test does not add to the sensitivity or specificity of the secretin stimulation test and calcium infusion is potentially more hazardous, this test is not recommended. The third provocative test involves the feeding of a meal. In gastrinoma patients, serum gastrin levels increase little or not at all after a meal, but an increase in serum gastrin levels of more than 200% is observed in individuals with antral G cell hyperplasia.

Gastrinomas are difficult to find. In almost half the patients with clinical and laboratory evidence, the tumor cannot be identified at surgery.[42] Upper gastrointestinal series, computed tomography, magnetic resonance imaging, duodenography, selective angiography, and transhepatic portal venous sampling have been employed to locate gastrinomas preoperatively. It has been recommended that somatostatin receptor scintigraphy should be the initial imaging study of choice in patients with gastrinomas because of the test's high sensitivity and specificity, and its results may affect clinical management.[50]

Treatment of Zollinger-Ellison syndrome involves control of the effects of hypergastrinemia, in particular peptic ulcer disease, as well as surgical treatment of the tumor, which is often malignant. Treatment should be individualized. In selecting the best therapy, the biologic behavior of these neoplasms and the clinical manifestations in each patient must be taken into consideration. Histamine ($H_2$)-receptor antagonists are effective in reducing gastric acid secretion, producing relief from symptoms, and inducing ulcer healing in patients with Zollinger-Ellison syndrome. High-dosage cimetidine, usually four to eight times the dose used in the treatment of common duodenal ulcer, is often required.[11, 49] Ranitidine and famotidine are more potent $H_2$-receptor blockers than cimetidine. These drugs require a comparable increase in dosage from that used in treatment of common duodenal ulcer. The dose of $H_2$-receptor antagonist required to maintain a satisfactory reduction in gastric acid secretion can be assessed by measuring the basal gastric acid output during the hour immediately before the next scheduled dose. The goal is to reduce gastric acid output to less than 10 mEq/hr during this interval.[49] This approach is based on endoscopic evidence that duodenitis and ulceration are absent when acid secretion is kept below 10 mEq/hr.[51]

The most effective drugs in reducing gastric acid secretion and in inducing ulcer healing in patients with Zollinger-Ellison syndrome are omeprazole[52, 53] and lansoprazole, which inhibit the potassium-hydrogen pump located in the apical membrane of the gastric parietal cell. Risks associated with the long-term use of such medications in children are unknown. Data demonstrate that achlorhydria may lead to malabsorption of vitamin $B_{12}$ and iron, both of which require acid for optimum absorption.[54] In one study, researchers reported that 3% of patients with Zollinger-Ellison syndrome treated long term with omeprazole developed low serum vitamin $B_{12}$ levels.[55]

Complete surgical resection of the tumor should be performed when possible. Full surgical removal of gastrinoma with cure has been achieved in approximately 30% of all patients with Zollinger-Ellison syndrome.[56, 57] Forty percent of patients with sporadic gastrinoma who have no evidence of metastatic disease have occult neoplasms that are most often found in the duodenal wall and are frequently not greater than 2 mm in diameter.[43] These microgastrinomas can be detected only after duodenotomy and intraluminal exploration.[42] Pancreatic gastrinomas are not completely resectable in most cases. When a metastatic or nonresectable gastrinoma is present, control of the ulcer disease may be accomplished in most cases by treatment with acid production antagonists, in conjunction with parietal cell vagotomy,[58] and in some patients by total gastrectomy.[47, 59, 60] Total gastrectomy is not a preferred option in the management of gastric hypersecretion in patients with Zollinger-Ellison syndrome, except in the minority of patients who are noncompliant or who are unable to take medications.[61] There is no convincing evidence that tumor progression is influenced by gastrectomy.[62] The routine use of parietal cell vagotomy at the time of surgical exploration has been recommended, whereas the aggressive resections such as Whipple resections are not advised.[63] Success with chemotherapy using streptozotocin, 5-fluorouracil, and doxorubicin is limited.

## VIPOMA

Pancreatic cholera,[64] also called watery diarrhea, hypokalemia, and achlorhydria (WDHA) syndrome or Verner-Morrison syndrome,[65] is a secretory diarrheal disorder associated with pancreatic neoplasms. Secretory diarrhea in conjunction with a pancreatic islet non–B cell tumor in adults was first described by Verner and Morrison in 1958.[66] One of the patients they reported was a 19-year-old woman. It is now widely accepted that VIP is the principal mediator involved in the pathogenesis of the diarrhea.[67] In adults, about 50% of VIP-producing tumors are malignant and the remainder are due to pancreatic adenomas, hyperplasia, or nonpancreatic ganglioneuromas.[68] Most VIP-producing neoplasms in children are of neurogenic origin and include ganglioneuroblastomas, ganglioneuromas, and neuroblastomas.[19, 69, 70] Rare occurrences have been reported in association with neurofibromatosis and pheochromocytomas.[19] Sixty-four cases of childhood VIPoma have been reported.[19] Primary pancreatic islet cell lesions were evident in only two of these children. In 1979, Ghishan and coworkers[71] were the first to report on the association between sustained watery diarrhea and elevated levels of plasma VIP and pancreatic islet non–B cell hyperplasia. Their patient was a 3-month-old infant presenting with secretory diarrhea beginning at 2 weeks of age. After a 95% pancreatectomy, plasma VIP levels returned to normal. Brenner and associates[72] described a 15-year-old girl with massive watery and protein-losing diarrhea who was found to have an islet cell tumor secreting high levels of VIP. A subtotal pancreatectomy was needed to remove the tumor. There was no recurrence for up to 6 years later.

VIP is composed of 28 amino acids. Because the amino acid sequence of VIP is similar to those of secretin and glucagon,[73] it has endocrine functions similar to secretin, such as increased pancreatic bicarbonate excretion and inhibition of gastric acid secretion stimulated by pentagastrin and histamine. VIP also has a glucagon-like action of abnormal glucose tolerance. Additionally, the vasomotor action of VIP causes vasodilation in the systemic and splanchnic vascular beds. Evidence suggests that VIP stimulates cyclic adenosine monophosphate in intestinal epithelial cells, resulting in increased secretion of water and electrolytes into the small bowel that exceeds the normal absorptive capacity of the colon.[74] Localization of VIP is widespread throughout the body, being found normally in the ganglion cells of the autonomic nervous system, adrenal medulla, brain, bladder, and predominantly in the gastrointestinal tract.[75]

Clinically, the most prominent features of VIPoma are profuse diarrhea, hypochlorhydria, hypokalemia, and metabolic acidosis. Other described features include spontaneous cutaneous flushing, hypokalemic renal failure, reduced or absent gastric acid secretion, diabetes mellitus, hypomagnesemia, hypercalcemia, and excessive tearing.[75]

Diagnosis of VIPoma is made based on the clinical picture associated with increased plasma concentrations of VIP by radioimmunoassay. Confirmatory laboratory findings include hypokalemic acidosis, prerenal azotemia, and decreased gastric secretion. Catecholamine levels should be obtained. When the diagnosis of VIPoma has been confirmed, it is then necessary to determine whether the tumor is situated in the pancreas or in another location such as a paraspinal ganglioneuroma. Computed tomography and somatostatin receptor scintigraphy are indicated in the evaluation. If the pancreas remains the suspect organ, selective arteriography may localize the tumor. Transhepatic portal venous sampling for VIP may help localize the tumor preoperatively.[76] Surgical exploration is often necessary for diagnostic purposes. Confirmation of the diagnosis is made by the immunocytochemical detection of neuron-specific enolase, VIP in the neoplasm, and electron microscopy for secretory granules.[1, 68]

It is important that dehydration and electrolyte imbalance be corrected preoperatively. Many palliative agents for symptomatic relief have been used with some success and may allow time for further diagnostic studies to localize the tumor (Table 56–2). The most potent pharmacologic antagonist of VIPomas is octreotide acetate. This drug has been given successfully to patients with VIPoma to suppress peptide secretion and watery diarrhea.[34, 67] The mechanism

**TABLE 56–2. Treatment Regimens for VIPoma Syndromes**

| MODALITY | COMMENT |
|---|---|
| **Acute Supportive** | |
| Intravenous fluids | May require >6 L/day |
| Correct hypokalemia, metabolic acidosis | 350 mEq/day often required |
| **Peptide/Peptidomimetic** | |
| Somatostatin/Sandostatin | First-line symptomatic therapy.<br>Octreotide acetate is effective in the symptomatic improvement of the watery diarrhea syndrome in more than 90% of VIPoma patients. |
| **Pharmacotherapy** | |
| Corticosteroids<br>Alpha$_2$ agonists<br>Angiotensin II<br>Indomethacin<br>Lithium carbonate<br>Phenothiazines<br>Opiates<br>Propranolol<br>Calcium channel blockers<br>Aenylate cyclase inhibitors | All enhance absorption; corticosteroids most effective. All inhibit secretion; lithium carbonate and phenothiazines may be slightly more effective. All are only transiently effective. |
| **Surgery** | Considered as both definitive therapy and, when possible, debulking therapy |
| **Chemotherapy** | |
| Streptozotocin<br>5-Fluorouracil<br>Chlorozotocin<br>DTIC | Combination therapy is useful but does not produce a permanent remission.<br>Renal impairment can be very serious and is usually drug limiting. |

From O'Dorisio TM, Mekhjian HS, Gaginella TS: Medical Therapy of VIPomas. Endocrinol Metab Clin North Am 1989;18:549, with permission.

of action of this somatostatin analogue is to inhibit the release of VIP from the tumor and to inhibit intestinal secretion at the level of the enterocyte. The plasma concentrations of VIP in patients treated with octreotide acetate usually decline but normalize in only 30% of treated patients.[77] Although all patients treated with octreotide acetate responded initially with an improvement in their diarrhea and lower VIP plasma levels, some patients had a short-term effect. In other cases, a rebound situation was observed for the diarrhea as well as VIP levels.[77] In such cases, increased dosage of octreotide acetate in combination with steroids has proved to be helpful. Indomethacin may be useful in cases of VIPoma associated with elevated prostaglandin $E_2$ levels.[78] Other pharmacologic agents, including clonidine, phenothiazine, lithium carbonate, propranolol, and interferon, may be helpful in selected cases in which other therapies have failed.

The most definitive treatment of VIPoma is surgery. Because most VIPomas in children are of neurogenic origin, they are usually found in the adrenals or retroperitoneal area. Removal of the tumor with or without adjunctive chemotherapy is indicated. The infant with VIPoma reported by Ghishan and coworkers[71] died of sepsis after a 95% pancreatectomy. The histopathology consisted of non–B islet cell hyperplasia. The 15-year-old girl with VIPoma described by Brenner and associates[72] was found to have a large tumor of the body and tail of the pancreas. Microscopic examination revealed a tumor of islet cells. Because the tumor was found in one of 25 perisplenic lymph nodes and also in a small pancreatic vein, the diagnosis was islet cell carcinoma. Eighty-five percent distal pancreatectomy achieved complete cure in this case. Because the experience with primary pancreatic VIPoma is extremely limited in children, information concerning this type of pancreatic neoplasm is derived from the adult literature. This type of secretory neoplasm is usually found in the distal two thirds of the pancreas. Isolated, single tumors have been reported in 80% of the patients. About half of all VIPomas are benign. Twenty-five percent of the tumors consist of islet cell hyperplasia.[75] A complete cure can be expected with subtotal (85%) pancreatectomy for biopsy-proven islet cell hyperplasia.[1, 75] Excision of the primary malignancy, even in the presence of liver metastases, is indicated to reduce the bulk of the tumor for subsequent chemotherapy. The combination of 5-fluorouracil and streptozotocin is reported to have a response rate of 65%.[79]

## OTHER TUMORS

Glucagonoma and somatostatinoma have been reported only in adults. Glucagonoma is associated with increased levels of glucagon due to islet A cell tumors of the pancreas. Mallinson and colleagues[80] reported nine patients with pancreatic tumors who had a clinical complex consisting of diabetes mellitus, stomatitis, anemia, weight loss, diarrhea, and rash. Although the rash is not always present, it is the most characteristic feature of a glucagonoma. The rash is described as necrolytic with migratory erythema that most commonly involves the trunk, perineum, and thighs, but it can also involve the face and legs. As the erythematous rash spreads, central necrosis and scales appear. The etiology of the rash is uncertain but is directly related to the hyperglucagonemia. It is possible that the panhypoaminoacidemia induced by chronic hyperglucagonemia may be the cause of the dermatologic findings. The youngest patient reported with glucagonoma was a 19-year-old woman[81]; the average age of patients with glucagonoma is 56 years.[82, 83] Localization of the tumor is attempted by computed tomography, ultrasonography, liver scan, transhepatic portal venous sampling for glucagon, and arteriography if knowledge of the tumor vascular supply is desired before surgery. Somatostatin receptor scintigraphy is the best technique to visualize the tumor preoperatively. The majority of the tumors are found in the body and tail of the pancreas, are at least 3 cm in diameter, and have distinctive characteristics.[83] Surgery is the treatment of choice. Chemotherapy for metastatic glucagonomas includes streptozotocin, with or without 5-fluorouracil. Occasionally, dacarbazine (DTIC) is used.[84]

Somatostatinoma has been designated the *inhibitory syndrome* because of its physiologic and pharmacologic effects of suppression on insulin, glucagon, gastrin, and cholecystokinin release.[1] Clinical findings include diabetes, cholelithiasis, steatorrhea, indigestion, hypochlorhydria, and, occasionally, anemia.[85] The majority of tumors are found coincidentally at the time of cholecystectomy for cholelithiasis. However, the appearance of gallstones and steatorrhea in a diabetic patient should alert the physician to the remote possibility of somatostatinoma, necessitating exploration of the foregut organs for a tumor during the time of cholecystectomy. When found, the tumor is usually single, although it may metastasize to the liver. The diagnosis can be confirmed by radioimmunoassay for an increased plasma concentration of somatostatin. Treatment is surgical removal of the tumor. Chemotherapy consists of streptozotocin and 5-fluorouracil.[1]

## *Summary*

Secretory pancreatic tumors are rare in children. Most are benign, tend to grow slowly, and are difficult to localize. More advanced diagnostic techniques will make the diagnosis of such tumors much easier once the condition is suspected. The application of somatostatin receptor-scanning technique using a labeled analogue of octreotide as a radionuclide for the imaging of somatostatin receptor–positive tumors and their metastases proved to be highly successful.[26, 50, 86] This technique is based on evidence that the majority of endocrine neoplasms that respond to octreotide therapy do so because they have abundant somatostatin receptors. The development of other radionuclide-labeled somatostatin analogues that recognize other subtypes of the somatostatin receptors will further improve the usefulness of this technique. The ability to target receptors on tumor cells raises the possibility of selectively directed chemotherapy or radiation therapy for inoperable or advanced tumors.

## REFERENCES


1. Friesen SR: Update on the diagnosis and treatment of rare neuroendocrine tumors. Surg Clin North Am 1987;67:379–393.
2. Grosfeld JL, Clatworthy HW, Hamoudi AB: Pancreatic malignancy in children. Arch Surg 1970;101:370–375.
3. Wilder RM, Allan FN, Powell MH, et al: Carcinoma of islands of pancreas with hyperinsulinism and hypoglycemia. JAMA 1927;89:348–355.
4. Sherman H: Islet cell tumor of pancreas in a newborn infant. Am J Dis Child 1947;74:58–79.
5. Baylin SB, Mendelson G: Ectopic (inappropriate) hormone production by tumors: mechanisms involved and the biological and clinical implications. Endocr Rev 1980;1:45–77.
6. Polak JM, Bloom SR, Adrian TE, et al: Pancreatic polypeptide in insulinomas, gastrinomas, VIPomas and glucagonomas. Lancet 1976;1:328–330.
7. Larsson LI, Schwartz T, Lundgrist G: Occurrence of human pancreatic polypeptide in pancreatic endocrine tumors. Am J Pathol 1976;85:675–684.
8. Unger RH, Orci L: Glucagon and the cell: physiology and pathophysiology. N Engl J Med 1981;304:1518–1524.
9. Larson LI: Endocrine pancreatic tumors. Hum Pathol 1978;9:401–416.
10. Heitz PU, Kasper M, Polak JM, et al: Pancreatic endocrine tumors: immunocytochemical analysis of 125 tumors. Hum Pathol 1982;13:263–271.
11. Grosfeld JL, Vane DW, Rescorla FJ, et al: Pancreatic tumors in childhood. J Pediatr Surg 1990;25:1057–1062.
11a. Wick MJ: Clinical and molecular aspects of multiple endocrine neoplasia. Clin Lab Med 1997;17:39–57.
12. Ballard HS, Frame B, Hartsock RJ: Familial multiple endocrine adenoma–peptic ulcer complex. Medicine 1964;43:481–516.
13. Rasbach DA, Van Harden JA, Telander RL, et al: Surgical management of hyperinsulinism in the multiple endocrine neoplasia type 1 syndrome. Arch Surg 1985;120:584–589.
14. Wermer P: Genetic aspects of adenomatosis of the endocrine glands. Am J Med 1954;16:363–371.
15. Schimke RN: Genetic aspects of multiple endocrine neoplasia. Annu Rev Med 1984;35:25–31.
16. Larson C, Skogseid B, Oberg K, et al: Multiple endocrine neoplasia type I gene maps to chromosome 11 and is lost in insulinoma. Nature 1988;332:85–87.
16a. Gardner DG: Recent advances in multiple endocrine neoplasia syndromes. Adv Intern Med 1997;42:597–627.
16b. Griffiths AM, Mack DR, Byard RW, et al: Multiple endocrine neoplasia IIb: an unusual cause of chronic constipation. J Pediatr 1990;116:285–288.
17. Buchanan KD. Johnston CF, O'Hare MT, et al: Neuroendocrine tumors: a European review. Am J Med 1986;81(suppl 6B):14.
18. Whipple AO: Adenoma of islet cells with hyperinsulinism. Ann Surg 1935;101:1299–1355.
19. Tudor RB: Childhood Disease Registry. Bismarck, ND, Q & R Clinic, 1997.
20 Marks V: Hypoglycemia due to pancreatic causes. In Samols E (ed): The Endocrine Pancreas. New York, Raven Press, 1991, pp 207–227.
21. Liu TH, Tseng HC, Zhu Y, et al: Insulinoma: an immunocytochemical and morphologic analysis of 95 cases. Cancer 1985;56:1420–1429.
22. Aynsley-Green A, Polak JM, Bloom SR, et al: Nesidioblastosis of the pancreas: definition of the syndrome and management of the severe neonatal hyperinsulinemic hypoglycemia. Arch Dis Child 1981;56:496–508.
23. Kloppet G, Heitz PU: Pancreatic endocrine tumors. Pathol Res Pract 1988;183:155–168.
24. Palazzo L, Roseau G, Salmeron M: Endoscopic ultrasonography in the preoperative localization of pancreatic endocrine tumors. Endoscopy 1992;24:350–353.
25. Ueno N, Tomiyama T, Tano S, et al: Utility of endoscopic ultrasonography with color doppler function for the diagnosis of islet cell tumor. Am J Gastroenterol 1996;91:772–776.
26. Van Eijck C, Lambert S, Lemaire L, et al: The use of somatostatin receptor scintigraphy in the differential diagnosis of pancreatic duct cancers and islet cell tumors. Ann Surg 1996;224:119–124.
27. Boden G: Glucagonomas and insulinomas. Gastroenterol Clin North Am 1989;18:831–845.
28. Grant CS, Van Heerden J, Charboneau JW, et al: Insulinoma: the value of intraoperative ultrasonography. Arch Surg 1988;123:843–848.
29. Norton JA, Cromack DT, Shawker TH, et al: Intraoperative ultrasonographic localization of islet cell tumors: a prospective comparison to palpation. Ann Surg 1988;207:160–168.
30. Thomas CG, Underwood LE, Carney CN, et al: Neonatal and infantile hypoglycemia due to insulin excess: new aspects of diagnosis and surgical management. Ann Surg 1977;185:505–517.

31. Dunger DB, Burns C, Ghale GK, et al: Pancreatic exocrine and endocrine function after subtotal pancreatectomy for nesidioblastosis. J Pediatr Surg 1988;23:112–115.
32. Greene SA. Aynsley-Green A, Soltesz G, et al: Management of secondary diabetes mellitus after total pancreatectomy in infancy. Arch Dis Child 1984;59:356–359.
33. Labrune P, Lechevallier S, Rault M, et al: Diabetes mellitus 14 years after a subtotal pancreatectomy for neonatal hyperinsulinism. J Pediatr Surg 1990;25:1246–1247.
34. Maton PN: The use of the long-acting somatostatin analogue, octreotide acetate, in patients with islet cell tumors. Gastroenterol Clin North Am 1989;18:897–922.
35. Laidlaw GF: Nesidioblastoma, the islet cell tumor of the pancreas. Am J Pathol 1938;14:175–134.
36. Frake DL, Norton JA: The role of surgery in the management of islet cells tumors. Gastroenterol Clin North Am 1989;18:805–830.
37. Zollinger RM, Ellison EH: Primary peptic ulcerations of the jejunum associated with islet cell tumors of the pancreas. Ann Surg 1955;142:709–728.
38. Gregory RA. Grossman MI, Tracy HJ, et al: Nature of the gastric secretagogue in Zollinger-Ellison syndrome tumors. Lancet 1967;2:543–544.
39. Gregory RA, Tracy HJ, Agarwal KL, et al: Amino acid constitution of two gastrins isolated from Zollinger-Ellison tumor tissue. Gut 1969;10:603–608.
40. Ellison EH, Wilson SD: The Zollinger-Ellison syndrome: reappraisal and evaluation of 260 registered cases. Ann Surg 1964;160:512–530.
41. Creutzfeldt W, Arnold R, Creutzfeldt C, et al: Pathomorphologic, biochemical and diagnostic aspects of gastrinomas (Zollinger-Ellison syndrome). Hum Pathol 1975;6:47–76.
42. Thompson NW, Vinik Al, Eckhauser FE: Microgastrinomas of the duodenum: a cause for failed operations for the Zollinger-Ellison syndrome. Ann Surg 1989;209:396–404.
43. Tracy HJ, Gregory RA: Physiological properties of a series of synthetic peptides structurally related to gastrin 1. Nature 1964;204:935–977.
44. Dockray GJ, Taylor IL: Heptadecapeptide gastrin: measurement in blood by specific radioimmunoassay. Gastroenterology 1976;71:971–977.
45. Power DM, Bunnett N, Turner AJ, et al: Degradation of endogenous heptadecapeptide gastrin by endopeptidase 24.11 in the pig. Am J Physiol 1987;253:G33–G39.
46. Abe K, Niikawa N, Sasaki H: Zollinger-Ellison syndrome with Marden-Walker syndrome. Am J Dis Child 1979;133:735–738.
47. Thompson JC, Lewis BG, Wiener I, et al: The role of surgery in Zollinger-Ellison syndrome. Ann Surg 1983;197:594–605.
48. Schwartz DL, White JJ, Saulsbury F, et al: Gastrin response to calcium infusion: an aid to the improved diagnosis of Zollinger-Ellison syndrome in children. Pediatrics 1974;54:599–602.
49. Deveney CW, Deveney KE: Zollinger-Ellison syndrome (gastrinoma): current diagnosis and treatment. Surg Clin North Am 1987;67:411–423.
50. Termanini B, Gibril F, Reynolds J, et al: Value of somatostatin receptor scintigraphy: a prospective study in gastrinoma of its effect on clinical management. Gastroenterology 1997;112:335–347.
51. Raufman JP, Collins SM, Pandol SJ, et al: Reliability of symptoms in assessing control of gastric acid secretion in patients with Zollinger-Ellison syndrome. Gastroenterology 1983;84:108–113.
52. McArthur KE, Collen MJ, Maton PN, et al: Omeprazole: effective, convenient therapy for Zollinger-Ellison syndrome. Gastroenterology 1985;88:939–944.
53. Maton P, McArthur K, Wank S, et al: Long-term efficacy and safety of omeprazole in patients with Zollinger-Ellison syndrome. Gastroenterology 1986;90:1537.
54. Marcuard SP, Albernaz L, Khazanie PG: Omeprazole therapy causes malabsorption of cyanocobalamin (vitamin $B_{12}$). Ann Intern Med 1994;120:211–215.
55. Stewart CA, Termanini B, Gibril F, et al: Prospective study of the effect of long-term gastric acid antisecretory treatment on serum vitamin $B_{12}$ levels in patients with Zollinger-Ellison syndrome. Gastroenterology 1995;108:A226.
56. Wolfe MM, Jensen RT: Zollinger-Ellison syndrome: current concepts in diagnosis and management. N Engl J Med 1987;317:1200–1209.
57. Vogel SB, Wolfe MM, McGuigan JE, et al: Localization and resection of gastrinomas in Zollinger-Ellison syndrome. Ann Surg 1987;200:550–555.
58. Richardson CT, Peters MN, Feldman M, et al: Treatment of Zollinger-Ellison syndrome with exploratory laparotomy, proximal gastric vagotomy and $H_2$-receptor antagonists. Gastroenterology 1985;89:357–367.
59. Rothenberg RE, Radulescu OV, LaRaja RD, et al: The surgical treatment of the Zollinger-Ellison syndrome: an update. Am Surg 1987;53:573–574.
60. Vinik Al, Thompson N: Controversies in the management of Zollinger-Ellison syndrome. Ann Intern Med 1986;105:956–959.
61. Maton PN, Gardner JD, Jensen RT: Recent advances in the management of gastric acid hypersecretion in patients with Zollinger-Ellison syndrome. Gastroenterol Clin North Am 1989;18:847–863.
62. Morowitz DA, Levine AE: Malignant Zollinger-Ellison syndrome: remission of primary metastatic pancreatic tumor after gastrectomy: report of a case and review of the literature. Am J Gastroenterol 1986;81:471–473.
63. Jensen RT: Should the 1996 citation for Zollinger-Ellison syndrome read: "Acid-reducing surgery in, aggressive resection out"? Am J Gastroenterol 1996;91:1067–1070.
64. Matsumoto KK, Peter JB, Schultze RG, et al: Watery diarrhea and hypokalemia associated with pancreatic islet cell adenoma. Gastroenterology 1966;50:231–242.
65. Marks IH, Banks S, Louw JH: Islet cell tumor of the pancreas with reversible watery diarrhea and achlorhydria. Gastroenterology 1967;52:695–708.
66. Verner JV, Morrison AB: Islet cell tumor and a syndrome of refractory watery diarrhea and hypokalemia. Am J Med 1958;25:374–380.
67. O'Dorisio TM, Mekhjian HS, Gaginella TS: Medical therapy of VIPomas. Endocrinol Metab Clin North Am 1989;18:545–556.
68. Capella C, Polak JM, Buffa R, et al: Morphologic patterns and diagnostic criteria of VIP-producing endocrine tumors. Cancer 1983;52:1860–1874.
69. Jansen-Goemans A, Engelhardt J: Intractable diarrhea in a boy with vasoactive intestinal peptide-producing ganglioneuroblastoma. Pediatrics 1977;59:710–716.
70. Mitchell CH, Sinatra FR, Crast FW, et al: Intractable watery diarrhea, ganglioneuroblastoma and vasoactive intestinal peptide. J Pediatr 1976;89:593–595.
71. Ghishan FK, Soper RT, Nassif EG, et al: Chronic diarrhea of infancy: non-beta islet cell hyperplasia. Pediatrics 1979;64:46–49.
72. Brenner RW, Sank LI, Kemer MB, et al: Resection of a VIPoma of the pancreas in a 15-year-old girl. J Pediatr Surg 1986;21:983–985.
73. Mutt V: Isolation and structure of vasoactive intestinal polypeptide from various species. In Said SI (ed): Vasoactive Intestinal Peptide. New York, Raven Press, 1982, pp 1–10.
74. Racusen LC, Binder HJ: Alteration of large intestinal electrolyte transport by vasoactive intestinal polypeptide in the rat. Gastroenterology 1977;73:790–796,
75. Krejs GJ: VIPoma syndrome. Am J Med 1987;82(suppl 5B):37–48.
76. Parkman HP, Malet PF, Ogorek CP, et al: Preoperative localization of a vasoactive intestinal peptide–secreting tumor by transhepatic portal venous sampling. Am J Gastroenterol 1988;83:559–563.
77. Koelz A, Kraenzlin M, Gyr K, et al: Escape of the response to a long-acting somatostatin analogue (SMS 201–995) in patients with VIPoma. Gastroenterology 1987;92:527–531.
78. Jaffe BM, Kopen DF, DeSchryver-Kecskemeti K, et al: Indomethacin-responsive pancreatic cholera. N Engl J Med 1977;297:817–821.
79. Moertel CG, Hanley JA, Johnson LA: Streptozotocin alone compared with streptozotocin plus fluorouracil in the treatment of advanced islet cell carcinoma. N Engl J Med 1980;303:1189–1194.
80. Mallinson CN, Bloom SR, Warin AP, et al: A glucagonoma syndrome. Lancet 1974;2:1–5.
81. Riddle MC, Golper TA, Fletcher WS, et al: Glucagonoma syndrome in a 19-year-old woman. West J Med 1978;129:68–72.
82. Stacpoole PW: The glucagonoma syndrome: clinical features, diagnosis and treatment. Endocrinol Rev 1981;2:347.
83. Higgins GA, Recant L, Fischman AB: The glucagonoma syndrome: surgically curable diabetes. Am J Surg 1979;137:142–148.
84. Prinz RA, Badrinath K, Banerji M, et al: Operative and chemotherapeutic management of malignant glucagon-producing tumors. Surgery 1981;90:713–719.
85. Konomi K, Chijiiwa K, Katsuta T, et al: Pancreatic somatostatinoma: a case report and review of the literature. J Surg Oncol 1990;43:259–265.
86. Lamberts SWJ, Bakker WH, Reubi JC, Krennig EP: Somatostatin-receptor imaging in the localization of endocrine tumors. N Engl J Med 1990;323:1246–1249.

SECTION SEVEN

# NUTRITION

# Chapter 57

# Infant and Toddler Nutrition

*Donna K. Zeiter*

It has been estimated that 26% of infants are changed to formulas that do not contain cow's milk by 4 months of age.[1] Although some of these changes are in response to diagnosed disease processes, both parents and physicians may change the infant's formula in attempts to improve colic, fussiness, and diarrhea. Formula manufacturers seek to imitate human milk, the gold standard of infant food. Although the exact composition of human milk has not been defined, formulas are composed of carbohydrate, fat, protein, vitamins, and minerals in similar proportions to those found in human milk. The National Research Council's Recommended Dietary Allowances (RDAs) set the standards for these requirements (Tables 57–1 and 57–2). The Food and Drug Administration regulates the composition and manufacture of commercially prepared formulas in the United States.

## CLASSIFICATION OF FORMULA

### Human Milk

Many organizations, including the American Academy of Pediatrics, have position statements that human milk is the ideal form of nutrition for full-term infants.[2] In addition to providing a source of protein and energy, human milk also contains both cellular (T and B lymphocytes, leukocytes, and macrophages) and humoral (secretory IgA, lysozyme, lactoferrin) immunologic factors. The composition of human milk is dynamic, changing to meet the needs of each individual infant as the child develops.

Maternal secretion of human milk usually begins during the fifth month of pregnancy. After birth, larger amounts of milk are produced under the influence of prolactin. In the first 5 days after birth, human milk is referred to as colostrum and contains a large amount of minerals and proteins such as immunoglobulins. In the next 5 days, human milk becomes transitional, with increasing amounts of fat, lactose, and phosphorus until it is classified as mature.

#### *Composition*

**PROTEIN.** The protein concentration of human milk is relatively low (0.9 g/dL) compared with that found in proprietary formulas (25–30% less than that found in cow's milk). The concentration of protein required to promote growth in infants continues to be controversial. Alteration in amino acid patterns, elevated blood urea nitrogen levels, and increased urine urea nitrogen levels have been used to evaluate the adequacy or excess of protein found in various feeding regimens. As a result of this research, the protein content of proprietary formulas has decreased.[3] The European Society for Pediatric Gastroenterology and Nutrition (ESPGAN) has proposed a protein content of 1.8 to 2.8 g/100 kcal.[4] The Committee on Nutrition of the American Academy of Pediatrics suggests 1.8 to 4.5 g/100 kcal.[5]

Protein in human milk is provided as a predominance of whey to casein (65:35).[6] This whey-to-casein ratio varies over time, being 90:10 in early lactation, 60:40 with mature milk, and, ultimately, 50:50 by about the eighth month of lactation.[6] The whey protein fraction is primarily in the form of α-lactalbumins, which are considered to be less allergenic than the β-lactalbumins present in cow's milk. Other components of the whey fraction include lactoferrin (bacteriostatic, aids iron absorption), lysozyme (an antibacterial agent), immunoglobulins, albumin, enzymes, growth factors, and hormones. Whey protein provides the advantage of being more readily emptied from the stomach than casein-predominant formula because of smaller curd production and possibly improved digestibility.[7, 8] The casein in human milk is primarily in the form of β- and κ-casein (α-casein is the predominate form in cow's milk).[3] Casein phosphopeptides appear to improve calcium absorption by increasing intraluminal calcium solubility.[3]

The protein components of human milk and formula may affect intestinal motility. Both whey and casein proteins in human milk may be metabolized into opioid peptides, which can influence intestinal motility. Casein can lead to the formation of casomorphins or casoxins, whereas whey proteins lead to the formation of lactorphins. The lactorphins and casomorphins act as opioid agonists, whereas κ-casein derivatives, casoxins, act as opioid antagonists. Most studies involving the effects of these enteral components on intestinal motility have focused on β-casomorphins found in infant formula. β-Casomorphins, from casein suspensions, appear to slow gastric emptying in rats when compared with rats

## TABLE 57–1. Recommended Daily Dietary Allowances for Vitamins*

| | | WEIGHT† | | HEIGHT† | | FAT-SOLUBLE VITAMINS | | | | WATER-SOLUBLE VITAMINS | | | | | | |
|---|---|---|---|---|---|---|---|---|---|---|---|---|---|---|---|---|
| CATEGORY | AGE (YR) OR CONDITION | kg | lb | cm | in | A (μg RE)‡ | D (μg)§ | E (mg α-TE)‖ | K (μg) | C (mg) | Thiamine (mg) | Riboflavin (mg) | Niacin (mg NE)¶ | $B_6$ (mg) | Folate (μg) | $B_{12}$ (μg) |
| Infants | 0.0–0.5 | 6 | 13 | 60 | 24 | 375 | 7.5 | 3 | 5 | 30 | 0.3 | 0.4 | 5 | 0.3 | 25 | 0.3 |
| | 0.5–1.0 | 9 | 20 | 71 | 28 | 375 | 10 | 4 | 10 | 35 | 0.4 | 0.5 | 6 | 0.6 | 35 | 0.5 |
| Children | 1–3 | 13 | 29 | 90 | 35 | 400 | 10 | 6 | 15 | 40 | 0.7 | 0.8 | 9 | 1.0 | 50 | 0.7 |
| | 4–6 | 20 | 44 | 112 | 44 | 500 | 10 | 7 | 20 | 45 | 0.9 | 1.1 | 12 | 1.1 | 75 | 1.0 |
| | 7–10 | 28 | 62 | 132 | 52 | 700 | 10 | 7 | 30 | 45 | 1.0 | 1.2 | 13 | 1.4 | 100 | 1.4 |
| Males | 11–14 | 45 | 99 | 157 | 62 | 1000 | 10 | 10 | 45 | 50 | 1.3 | 1.5 | 17 | 1.7 | 150 | 2.0 |
| | 15–18 | 66 | 145 | 176 | 69 | 1000 | 10 | 10 | 65 | 60 | 1.5 | 1.8 | 20 | 2.0 | 200 | 2.0 |
| | 19–24 | 72 | 160 | 177 | 70 | 1000 | 10 | 10 | 70 | 60 | 1.5 | 1.7 | 19 | 2.0 | 200 | 2.0 |
| Females | 11–14 | 46 | 101 | 157 | 62 | 800 | 10 | 8 | 45 | 50 | 1.1 | 1.3 | 15 | 1.4 | 150 | 2.0 |
| | 15–18 | 55 | 120 | 163 | 64 | 800 | 10 | 8 | 55 | 60 | 1.1 | 1.3 | 15 | 1.5 | 180 | 2.0 |
| | 19–24 | 58 | 128 | 164 | 65 | 800 | 10 | 8 | 60 | 60 | 1.1 | 1.3 | 15 | 1.6 | 180 | 2.0 |
| Pregnant | | | | | | 800 | 10 | 10 | 65 | 70 | 1.5 | 1.6 | 17 | 2,2 | 400 | 2.2 |
| Lactating | 1st 6 mo | | | | | 1300 | 10 | 12 | 65 | 95 | 1.6 | 1.8 | 20 | 2.1 | 280 | 2.6 |
| | 2nd 6 mo | | | | | 1200 | 10 | 11 | 65 | 90 | 1.6 | 1.7 | 20 | 2.1 | 260 | 2.6 |

*The allowances, expressed as average daily intakes over time, are intended to provide for individual variations among most normal persons as they live in the United States under usual environmental stresses. Diets should be based on a variety of common foods to provide other nutrients for which human requirements have been less well defined.

†Weights and heights of Reference Adults are actual medians for the U.S. population of the designated age, as reported by NHANES II. The median weights and heights of those younger than 19 years of age were taken from Hamill PV, Drizd TA, Johnson CL, et al: Physical growth: National Center for Health Statistics percentiles. Am J Clin Nutr 1979;32(3):607–629. The use of these figures does not imply that the height-to-weight ratios are ideal.

‡Retinol equivalents: 1 retinol equivalent = 1 μg retinol or 6 μg beta-carotene.

§As cholecalciferol: 10 μg cholecalciferol = 400 IU vitamin D.

‖Alpha-tocopherol equivalents; 1 mg D-alpha tocopherol = 1 alpha-TE equivalent.

¶1 NE (niacin equivalent) is equal to 1 mg of niacin or 60 mg of dietary tryptophan.

Modified from The Harriet Lane Handbook: A Manual for Pediatric House Officers, 13th ed. St. Louis, Mosby, 1993.

**TABLE 57–2. Recommended Daily Dietary Allowances for Minerals***

| CATEGORY | AGE (YR) OR CONDITION | WEIGHT† kg | WEIGHT† lb | HEIGHT† cm | HEIGHT† in | AVERAGE ENERGY ALLOWANCE (kcal/kg) | MINERALS Calcium (mg) | Phosphorus (mg) | Magnesium (mg) | Iron (mg) | Zinc (mg) | Iodine (μg) | Selenium (μg) |
|---|---|---|---|---|---|---|---|---|---|---|---|---|---|
| Infants | 0.0–0.5 | 6 | 13 | 60 | 24 | 108 | 400 | 300 | 40 | 6 | 5 | 40 | 10 |
| | 0.5–1.0 | 9 | 20 | 71 | 28 | 98 | 600 | 500 | 60 | 10 | 5 | 50 | 15 |
| Children | 1–3 | 13 | 29 | 90 | 35 | 102 | 800 | 800 | 80 | 10 | 10 | 70 | 20 |
| | 4–6 | 20 | 44 | 112 | 44 | 90 | 800 | 800 | 120 | 10 | 10 | 90 | 20 |
| | 7–10 | 28 | 62 | 132 | 52 | 70 | 800 | 800 | 170 | 10 | 10 | 120 | 30 |
| Males | 11–14 | 45 | 99 | 157 | 62 | 55 | 1200 | 1200 | 270 | 12 | 15 | 150 | 40 |
| | 14–18 | 66 | 145 | 176 | 69 | 45 | 1200 | 1200 | 400 | 12 | 15 | 150 | 50 |
| | 19–24 | 72 | 160 | 177 | 70 | 40 | 1200 | 1200 | 350 | 10 | 15 | 150 | 70 |
| Females | 11–14 | 46 | 101 | 157 | 62 | 47 | 1200 | 1200 | 280 | 15 | 12 | 150 | 45 |
| | 15–18 | 55 | 120 | 163 | 64 | 40 | 1200 | 1200 | 300 | 15 | 12 | 150 | 50 |
| | 19–24 | 58 | 128 | 164 | 65 | 38 | 1200 | 1200 | 280 | 15 | 12 | 150 | 55 |
| Pregnant | | | | | | | 1200 | 1200 | 320 | 30 | 15 | 175 | 65 |
| Lactating | 1st 6 mo | | | | | | 1200 | 1200 | 355 | 15 | 19 | 200 | 75 |
| | 2nd 6 mo | | | | | | 1200 | 1200 | 340 | 15 | 16 | 200 | 75 |

*The allowances, expressed as average daily intakes over time, are intended to provide for individual variations among most normal persons as they live in the United States under usual environmental stresses. Diets should be based on a wide variety of common foods to provide other nutrients for which human requirements have been less well defined.

†Weights and heights of Reference Adults are actual medians for the U.S. population of the designated age, as reported by NHANES II. The median weights and heights of those younger than 19 years of age were taken from Hamill PV, Drizd TA, Johnson CL, et al: Physical growth: National Center for Health Statistics percentiles. Am J Clin Nutr 1979;32(3):607–629. The use of these figures does not imply that the height-to-weight ratios are ideal.

Modified from The Harriet Lane Handbook: A Manual for Pediatric House Officers, 13th ed. St. Louis, Mosby, 1993.

receiving whey protein suspension. This effect is reversed by naloxone.[9] β-Casomorphins also appear to enhance water and electrolyte absorption and may influence postprandial stimulation of insulin and somatostatin secretion.[3]

The amino acid pattern of human milk differs from cow's milk–based formula. Human milk has a lower content of phenylalanine and tyrosine, amino acids that are poorly metabolized in the newborn. Taurine, present in human milk, is believed to be important in the development of the retina as well as acting as a conjugate in bile salt formation.[10, 11] Infants fed proprietary formulas have relatively lower levels of taurine, which decline over time, primarily because cow's milk–based formulas have very little taurine initially, which is further depleted during processing.[3]

Processing of human milk appears to affect the activity of many of the bioactive proteins. The effect of heating on secretory IgA remains controversial, with one investigator demonstrating loss of activity above 62.5°C and another reporting intact secretory IgA after 5 seconds at 72°C.[12, 13] Bile salt–stimulated lipase loses activity at 50°C and serum-stimulated lipase has decreased activity at greater than 4°C.[3]

**CARBOHYDRATE.** The carbohydrate in human milk accounts for 40% to 50% of calories and is present primarily as lactose.[8] Human milk contains lactose at a concentration of 7 g/dL.[6] Human milk also contains over 100 different oligosaccharides.[14] The core structure is modified by the attachment of fucose and/or sialose monomers to various positions through the action of genetically determined fucosyltransferases and sialyltransferases. The most common oligosaccharides in human milk are lacto-*N*-tetraose, lacto-*N*-fucopentaose I, and lacto-*N*-fucopentaose II, compounds absent or present in only trace amounts in cow's milk. These oligosaccharides have a number of potential functions, including promoting growth of bifidobacteria, organisms that create an acid microenvironment in the bowel not favorable to pathogenic bacteria.[14] Oligosaccharides in human milk have also been found to interfere and inhibit bacterial adhesion to mucosal surfaces.[15, 16] Finally, oligosaccharides in human milk appear to contain structures that act as ligands for cell adhesion molecules, those molecules important in the interaction of the leukocyte with endothelial cells in the development of the inflammatory response.[14] Only human milk contains a high concentration of these oligosaccharides (neutral, fucosylated, and sialylated derivatives).[3] Cow's milk contains much lower concentrations of mainly the sialylated forms.

**FAT.** The lipid in human milk is highly unique, leading to improved absorption. Lipid provides approximately 50% of calories (approximately 3 g/dL). Human milk contains a bile salt–stimulated lipase that aids in digestion.[17] Human milk is high in palmitic, oleic, linoleic, and linolenic acids, which are important components of phospholipid involved in brain and red cell membranes.

## *Low Birth Weight*

Human milk may also be used in the feeding of low-birth-weight (LBW) infants. Studies have demonstrated that human milk may decrease the incidence of necrotizing enterocolitis in LBW infants, even when it forms only a portion of the diet.[18] However, there are a number of concerns that must be taken into account when deciding to feed LBW infants human milk. After the initial few weeks of feeding, human milk is not sufficient in protein for the growing LBW infant. Human milk does not contain sufficient calcium and phosphorus to meet the needs of LBW infants. Calcium needs of the LBW infant are 160 to 200 mg/kg/day, and human milk provides at the most 53 mg/kg/day. Phosphorus needs are estimated at 80 to 100 mg/kg/day, and human milk provides 25 to 26 mg/kg/day. Sodium content also declines through the first few weeks of feeding to 1.8 to 2.0 mEq/kg/day, which is lower than the estimated needs of 3 to 4 mEq/kg/day. Finally, the fat in human milk is not homogenized and may separate out and adhere to tubing if continuous tube feeding is required.[16]

To compensate for these deficiencies, human milk may be fortified with a human milk fortifier. Two currently available fortifiers are Human Milk Fortifier (Mead Johnson) and Similac Natural Care (Ross) (see later). Current practice is not to fortify human milk until the neonate is tolerating full volume feedings. These fortifiers will not only increase the caloric density of the breast milk but also provide the increased calcium, phosphorus, proteins, and vitamins needed by the LBW infant.

For both term and LBW infants, certain vitamins and minerals should be supplemented if human milk is the exclusive source of nutrition. For example, 400 IU of vitamin D is recommended to prevent rickets and promote bone mineralization. Iron, either as a supplement or as a fortified cereal, should be supplied to the breast-fed infant by 6 months.

A number of studies demonstrate the benefit of human milk feeding. Breast-fed infants, especially in the early months of life, have been shown to have a decreased incidence of gastrointestinal infections, respiratory infections, and otitis media.[2] Finally, one study does suggest that children who were previously breast fed had statistically higher intelligence quotients, although these conclusions remain controversial.[19]

### *Contraindications*

Despite all of the benefits, there are situations in which the feeding of human milk is contraindicated. Both cocaine and marijuana can be passed into breast milk with significant concentrations to affect the infant. In the United States, mothers with human immunodeficiency virus (HIV) infection are counseled not to breast feed; however, the risk of transmitting HIV infection to the infant is controversial. Some studies have not supported an increased risk of transmission.[20] However, additional studies have demonstrated a 29% risk of transmission in mothers with postpartum primary infection and 14% in mothers with established infection.[21] In the United States, where safe alternative formulas are readily available, breast feeding is not recommended when mothers are infected with HIV. Infants with the metabolic diseases of galactosemia should not be breast fed because of the lactose in human milk. Children with phenylketonuria need to be on phenylalanine-free diets.

## Cow's Milk–Based Formulas

Cow's milk–based formulas are most useful in the feeding of full-term infants without special nutritional needs or gastrointestinal problems or in the supplementation of infants on human milk. Although cow's milk–based formulas have been designed to mimic the composition of human milk, significant differences are present (Table 57–3).

Cow's milk formulas contain higher levels of protein than human milk (1.5–3.3 g/dL).[6] This protein has a whey-to-casein ratio of 20:80; however, manufacturers alter this ratio to mimic the 60:40 ratio found in human milk. The predominant whey protein in cow's milk is β-lactalbumin. Cow's milk formula has a greater concentration of phenylalanine and tyrosine and a lesser amount of cysteine and taurine than breast milk.[6]

The major carbohydrate in these formulas is lactose. Lactose is believed to enhance the absorption of calcium.[22] These formulas provide fat in the form of vegetable oils and C-16/C18 fatty acids. Fat is readily absorbed and provides approximately 50% of nonprotein calories.

## Soy-Based Formulas

All currently available soy-based formulas are lactose free (see Table 57–3). Soy-based formula is useful in infants who have primary congenital lactase deficiency, transient secondary lactase deficiency, in families who are vegetarians, or in infants with galactosemia. Although soy-based formulas are seen by some as the initial step when cow's milk protein allergy is suspected, approximately 30% of infants allergic to cow's milk will also be allergic to soy. Soy formula is contraindicated in infants with hypothyroidism who are being supplemented with L-thyroxine, because soy will bind the medication and prevent its absorption.[24]

Soy protein does not have as high a bioavailability as cow's milk and must be supplemented with methionine. Carbohydrate consists of glucose polymers, and some formulas contain sucrose. Fat is supplemented as vegetable oils and carnitine.

# SPECIAL FORMULAS

## Cow's Milk–Based Premature Formulas

Premature infants have decreased free water clearance; increased urinary losses of sodium, bicarbonate, and glucose; limited ability to acidify the urine and excrete ammonia; decreased glycogen stores; and increased needs of calcium and phosphate. Common premature formulas are shown in Table 57–3. The protein composition is designed to mimic human milk with a whey-to-casein ratio of 60:40 and supplies between 2.7 and 3.0 g/100 kcal. Carbohydrate is provided as a combination of glucose polymers and lactose (50:50). Glucose polymers or glucose polymers combined with lactose are better absorbed than lactose alone.[25] Glucose polymers facilitate the intestinal absorption of calcium.[25, 26] Fat in these formulas is a mixture of medium-chain triglyceride (MCT) and long-chain triglyceride (LCT) (approximately 50:50). MCT is absorbed through the enterocyte into the portal system and does not require emulsification with bile salts to the extent that LCT does. MCT does not require carnitine for its metabolism. However, studies have failed to confirm that MCT provides for improved nitrogen balance or increased growth.[27] As previously discussed, very-long-chain fatty acids are vital as structural components of cell membranes and are essential for brain growth and retinal development.[28–30] Premature formulas also contain increased vitamin A, vitamin D, calcium, phosphorus, and electrolytes.

### Premature Infant Follow-Up Formulas

Premature follow-up formulas are recommended for those ex-premature infants from 2 kg of weight to approximately 1 year of age (see Table 57–3). Protein is of intermediate composition and amount, with whey-to-casein ratio of 50:50 and approximately 2.6 g/100 kcal. Carbohydrate is provided as a 50:50 mixture of glucose polymers and lactose with an osmolality of approximately 290 mOsm. Fat is supplied as MCT and LCT; however, the ratio is now 25:75. Vitamin supplements are increased over standard infant formula.

The child should be taking less than or equal to 45 ounces to avoid vitamin D toxicity.[31] The formula supplies an intermediate amount of calcium and phosphorus and has been shown to lead to improved mineralization in these infants after discharge from the neonatal intensive care unit.[32]

### Protein Hydrolysate Formulas

Protein hydrolysate formulas (see Table 57–3) are indicated primarily in those situations when the infant is known to have milk protein allergy or galactosemia. Protein is predigested using proteolytic enzymes into peptides and free amino acid. These peptides are believed to be less allergenic than the intact protein; however, the peptides may continue to have molecular weights sufficient to cause an allergic response in some children (see Chapter 27).[33]

Carbohydrate composition is variable between formulas, with the majority having glucose polymers as the primary source. Fat may be supplied as long-chain or a combination of long-chain and medium-chain fatty acids.

### Crystalline Amino Acid Formulas

In those rare instances when even protein hydrolysate fails to prevent documented allergic bowel disease, an amino acid–based formula may be required (see Table 57–3). Formulas that may be used in infants 12 months or younger include Neocate and Pediatric Vivonex. Carbohydrate is 100% glucose polymers. Fat is provided as 95% LCT and 5% MCT.

### Lactose-Free Formulas

The use of a lactose-free formula is indicated in the setting of diagnosed primary or secondary lactose intolerance. Infants diagnosed with galactosemia need to be fed a lactose-free diet. A number of lactose-free formulas are available, including all of the soy protein–based formulas as well as one cow's milk–based preparation (see Table 57–3). Clinicians need to distinguish lactose malabsorption from cow's milk protein allergy.

### Low Carbohydrate Formulas

For those children with severe documented mucosal disease or those infants with glucose/galactose malabsorption, a carbohydrate modified formula may be indicated (see Table 57–3). These may be carbohydrate free or contain very low amounts. With these formulas, carbohydrate in the form of glucose polymers or fructose may be added gradually as tolerated, and an intravenous source of glucose is often provided while carbohydrate is enterally advanced.

### Metabolic Disease

For patients with defined inborn errors of metabolism, specialized formulas have been developed to bypass the enzymatic defects and provide sufficient energy and protein for growth. Table 57–4 contains a summary of different inborn errors of metabolism and their suggested infant formulas.

## SUPPLEMENTS AND ADDITIVES

### Human Milk Fortifier

Human milk fortifier is useful in very-low-birth-weight infants (<1500 g) and preterm infants who require higher calories or calcium and phosphorus. Usually, full enteral feeding is established before initiation of the supplementation. The powder form, Human Milk Fortifier (Mead Johnson), is dosed at 2 packets per 50 mL of human milk to concentrate calories to 24 cal/oz. Similac Natural Care (Ross) is a liquid preparation that when mixed 1 part fortifier to 1 part human milk provides 22 cal/oz. Both derive from cow's milk protein and have been modified to provide a whey-to-casein ratio of 60:40. Carbohydrate is provided as both glucose polymers and lactose. The powder does not contain any added fat; however, the liquid contains MCT. Both supplements provide improved calcium.

### Carbohydrate

For those patients on low-carbohydrate formulas or for those needing formula with a higher caloric density, carbohydrate may be supplemented using Polycose (Ross) or Moducal (Mead Johnson). Both products are hydrolysates of corn starch. Both powder forms provide an additional 3.8 kcal/g of product.

### Fat

In children receiving formula with low concentrations of long-chain fatty acids (Pediatric Vivonex, Portagen) or for infants who require very high caloric density, fat may be added to feedings through the use of safflower oil, MCT oil, or Microlipid. MCT oil is derived primarily from coconut oil and provides approximately 7.7 kcal/mL. Microlipid is derived from safflower oil and provides 4.5 kcal/mL.

### Protein

Protein may be added as a single component supplement through the use of Promod and Casec. Promod is derived

**TABLE 57–3. Infant Formula Analysis per 100 mL**

| FORMULA | kcal per oz | PROTEIN g | PROTEIN Type | PROTEIN % Cal | CARBOHYDRATE g | CARBOHYDRATE Type | CARBOHYDRATE % Cal | FAT g | FAT Type | FAT % Cal | Na (mEq) | K (mEq) | Ca (mg) | P (mg) | Fe (mg) | GASTROINTESTINAL SOLUTE LOAD (mOsm/L) |
|---|---|---|---|---|---|---|---|---|---|---|---|---|---|---|---|---|
| Human milk (mature) | 20 | 1.1 | 20% casein 80% whey | 6 | 7.2 | Lactose | 42 | 3.9 | Human milk fat | 52 | 0.8 | 1.3 | 28 | 14 | 0.03 | 290 |
| Human milk (premature) | 22 | 1.7 | 20% casein 80% whey | 9 | 8 | Lactose | 44 | 3.9 | Human milk fat | 48 | 1.3 | 1.4 | 28 | 16 | 0.1 | 290 |
| **Cow's Milk–Based Formula** | | | | | | | | | | | | | | | | |
| Cow's milk (whole) | 20 | 3.4 | 80% casein 20% whey | 21 | 4.8 | Lactose | 30 | 3.4 | Butterfat | 49 | 2.1 | 3.9 | 123 | 96 | 0.05 | 260 |
| Carnation Good Start | 20 | 1.6 | Whey | 9.8 | 7.4 | Lactose, malto-dextrin | 44 | 3.4 | Palm olein, safflower, coconut | 46 | 0.7 | 1.7 | 43 | 24 | 1.0 | |
| Enfamil 20 (with Fe) | 20 | 1.5 | Nonfat cow's milk, demineralized whey | 9 | 7.4 | Lactose | 44 | 3.6 | Coconut, soy oil, palm olein, sunflower oil | 48 | 0.8 | 1.86 | 53 | 36 | 0.5 (1.22) | 300 |
| Enfamil 24 (with Fe) | 24 | 1.8 | Nonfat cow's milk, demineralized whey | 9 | 8.3 | Lactose | 41 | 4.5 | Coconut, soy oil, palm olein, sunflower oil | 50 | 1.0 | 2.2 | 63 | 42 | 0.5 (1.5) | 360 |
| Similac 20 (with Fe) | 20 | 1.5 | Nonfat cow's milk | 9 | 7.2 | Lactose | 43 | 3.6 | Coconut and soy oil | 48 | 0.83 | 1.87 | 51 | 39 | 0.15 (1.2) | 300 |
| Similac 24 (with Fe) | 24 | 2.2 | Nonfat cow's milk | 11 | 8.5 | Lactose | 42 | 4.3 | Coconut and soy oil | 47 | 1.22 | 2.74 | 73 | 57 | 0.18 (1.5) | 380 |
| Similac PM 60/40 | 20 | 1.6 | Whey Sodium caseinate | 9 | 6.9 | Lactose | 41 | 3.8 | Coconut and soy oil | 50 | 0.7 | 1.5 | 38 | 19 | 0.15 | 280 |
| Lactofree | 20 | 1.5 | Milk protein isolate | 9 | 7.0 | Corn syrup solids | 42 | 3.7 | Palm, soy, coconut, oleic, sunflower oils | 49 | 0.9 | 1.9 | 55 | 37 | 1.2 | 200 |
| **Soy-Based Formula** | | | | | | | | | | | | | | | | |
| Isomil | 20 | 1.7 | Soy protein isolate | 10 | 6.9 | Corn syrup and sucrose | 41 | 3.7 | Soy and coconut oil | 49 | 1.3 | 1.9 | 71 | 51 | 1.22 | 240 |
| Prosobee | 20 | 2.0 | Soy protein isolate | 12 | 6.7 | Corn syrup solids | 40 | 3.5 | Coconut, soy oil, palm olein, sunflower oil | 48 | 1.0 | 2.1 | 71 | 56 | 1.22 | 200 |
| **Premature Infant Formula** | | | | | | | | | | | | | | | | |
| Enfamil Premature Formula (with Fe) | 20 | 2.0 | Demineralized whey, nonfat milk solids | 12 | 7.4 | Corn syrup solids, lactose | 44 | 3.4 | MCT 40%, soy oil 40%, coconut oil 20% | 44 | 1.1 | 1.8 | 111 | 56 | 0.17 1.22 | 260 |
| Enfamil Premature Formula 24 (with Fe) | 24 | 2.4 | Demineralized whey, nonfat milk solids | 12 | 9.0 | Corn syrup solids, lactose | 44 | 4.1 | MCT 40%, coconut and soy oils | 44 | 1.4 | 2.2 | 134 | 67 | 0.2 (1.5) | 310 |
| Similac Special Care | 20 | 1.8 | Nonfat cow's milk whey | 11 | 7.2 | Lactose and hydrolyzed corn starch | 42 | 3.7 | MCT 50%, coconut and soy oils | 47 | 1.3 | 2.2 | 122 | 61 | 0.25 | 250 |
| Similac Special Care 24 | 24 | 2.17 | Nonfat cow's milk and whey | 11 | 8.5 | Lactose and hydrolyzed corn starch | 42 | 4.4 | MCT 50%, coconut and soy oils | 47 | 1.5 | 2.7 | 146 | 73 | 1.5 | 300 |

| | | | | | | | | | | | | | | | |
|---|---|---|---|---|---|---|---|---|---|---|---|---|---|---|---|
| **Premature Follow-Up Formula** | | | | | | | | | | | | | | | |
| Neocare | 22 | 1.9 | Nonfat milk whey protein concentrate | 10 | 7.7 | Corn syrup solids, lactose | 41 | 4.1 | Soy, safflower oil, MCT, coconut oil | 49 | 1.1 | 2.7 | 78 | 46 | 1.3 | 290 |
| **Protein Hydrolysates** | | | | | | | | | | | | | | | |
| Alimentum | 20 | 1.9 | Hydrolyzed casein | 11 | 6.9 | Sucrose, modified tapioca starch | 41 | 3.8 | MCT 50%, safflower oil 40%, soy oil 10% | 48 | 1.3 | 2.0 | 71 | 51 | 1.2 | 370 |
| Nutramigen | 20 | 1.9 | Casein hydrolysate, amino acid premix | 11 | 7.4 | Corn syrup solids and corn starch | 44 | 3.4 | Corn oil | 45 | 1.4 | 1.9 | 63 | 42 | 1.22 | 320 |
| Pregestimil | 20 | 1.9 | Casein hydrolysate, cystine, tyrosine and tryptophan | 11 | 6.9 | Corn syrup solids, dextrose, corn starch | 41 | 3.8 | MCT 60%, corn oil 20%, safflower oil 20% | 48 | 1.15 | 1.9 | 63 | 42 | 1.27 | 320 |
| **Elemental Formula** | | | | | | | | | | | | | | | |
| Neocate | 20 | 2.1 | L-Amino acids | 12 | 7.9 | Corn syrup solids | 47 | 3.1 | Safflower oil, refined vegetable oils | 41 | 1.1 | 2.7 | 84 | 63 | 1.26 | 342 |
| **Carbohydrate Free** | | | | | | | | | | | | | | | |
| MJ3232A | 12.6 | 1.9 | Casein hydrolysate | 17 | 2.8 | Tapioca starch, mono- & di-saccharide free | 25 | 2.8 | MCT 40%, corn oil 13% | 57 | 1.3 | 1.9 | 63 | 42 | 1.26 | 250 (varies with added carbohydrate) |
| Ross Carbohydrate Free | 12 | 2.0 | Soy protein isolate | 20 | | Trace carbohydrate | | 3.6 | Coconut and soy oils | 80 | 1.3 | 1.9 | 70 | 50 | 0.15 | 74 |
| **High MCT** | | | | | | | | | | | | | | | |
| Portagen | 20 | 2.3 | Sodium caseinate | 14 | 7.7 | Corn syrup solids, sucrose, lactose | 46 | 3.1 | MCT 85%, corn oil 15% | 40 | 1.6 | 2.1 | 63 | 47 | 1.25 | 220 |
| **Fortifier** | | | | | | | | | | | | | | | |
| Human Milk Fortifier (per packet) | 3.5 (kcal per mL) | 0.2 | Reduced mineral whey and casein | 10 | 0.7 | Corn syrup solids and lactose | 77 | 0.01 | | 3 | 0.08 | 0.1 | 22.5 | 11.2 | 0 | 120 |

Modified from The Harriet Lane Handbook: A Manual for Pediatric House Officers, 13th ed. St. Louis, Mosby, 1993.

**TABLE 57–4. Diets for Inborn Errors of Metabolism**

| INBORN ERROR OF METABOLISM | FORMULA |
|---|---|
| Galactosemia | Isomil<br>Lactofree |
| Glutaric aciduria type 1 | Glutarex-1<br>XLYS, Try Analog |
| Homocystinuria | Hominex-1<br>Low Methionine Diet Powder<br>XMET Analog |
| Isovaleric acidemia (leucine catabolism defects) | I-Valex-1<br>XLEU Analog |
| Maple syrup urine disease | Ketonex-1<br>MSUD Analog<br>MSUD diet powder |
| Methylmalonic acidemia/propionic acidemia | Propimex-1<br>OS 1<br>XMET, THRE, VAL, ISOLEU Analog |
| Phenylketonuria | Phenex-1<br>Lofenalac<br>PKU 1 |
| Tyrosinemia type 1 | Tyromex-1<br>Low PHE/TYR diet powder<br>Tyr 1<br>XPHEN, TYR, MET Analog |
| Urea cycle disorders | Cyclinex-1<br>UCD 1<br>UCD 2 |

from whey protein and supplies 4.2 kcal/g. Casec is a calcium caseinate that provides 3.7 kcal/g of product.

## Enteral Nutrients

### Glutamine

Glutamine is the most abundant amino acid in the circulation and is vital in the transport of nitrogen throughout the body. This amino acid helps protect the body from the toxic effects of ammonia, acts in nitrogen transfer between different tissues of the body, provides a precursor for purine and pyrimidines, and is a primary fuel for rapidly dividing cells.[34, 35] The epithelium of the small intestine extracts a large amount of glutamine from both the lumen and the blood stream to utilize as fuel.[36] In the colon, glutamine is second only to ketone bodies, synthesized from short-chain fatty acids, as a metabolic substrate. In specific conditions such as trauma, sepsis, and bowel resection, the gut's demand for glutamine can increase above the body's ability to synthesize the amino acid, making glutamine a conditionally essential amino acid.[37]

Studies in the effects of enteral glutamine supplementation in adults are contradicting. In 1983, a study involving glutamine supplementation in adults undergoing surgery demonstrated improved nitrogen balance.[38] A later study involving trauma patients randomized to receive standard formula versus a formula enriched with glutamine demonstrated that the enriched formula was well tolerated but did not lead to any significant differences in glucose metabolism or nitrogen balance.[39]

In one study of very-low-birth-weight infants,[35] infants fed formula supplemented with glutamine, in addition to parenteral nutrition, had altered plasma amino acid levels after 2 weeks of supplementation. Infants fed the glutamine had a slower increase in plasma levels of most amino acids, including alanine, serine, and threonine. The investigators speculated that this alteration reflects increased uptake of these substrates by the liver and other tissues, with enhanced gluconeogenesis and incorporation into muscle protein.

Most foods in a regular diet contain 4% to 8% of the amino acids as glutamine. Enteral supplementation of glutamine is complicated by glutamine's short shelf-life and its decomposition into pyroglutamate and ammonia. However, glutamine will last at least 22 days at a temperature of 4°C in parenteral solutions.[40] It may also be administered as α-ketoglutarate or dipeptides. The utility and feasibility of adding the amino acid to formulas for use in stressed, very-low-birth-weight premature infants awaits further study.

### Nucleotides

Nucleotides are compounds consisting of a nitrogenous base, a ribose or deoxyribose sugar, and three phosphate groups. They are the building blocks of RNA and DNA and are vital components of carbohydrate, lipid, and protein metabolism.[41] Although human tissues have the capability of synthesizing nucleotides de novo, this synthesis entails a large energy cost. Salvage of these molecules from the degradation of nucleic acids may be more efficient. During times of stress, in rapidly dividing tissue, or in those tissues such as the intestinal mucosa where de novo synthesis of nucleotides is limited,[42] this de novo synthesis may be inadequate to meet needs. Therefore, investigators have classified nucleotides as being conditionally essential.[43]

Restriction of dietary nucleotides appears to decrease cell-mediated immunity by acting on the T helper/inducer cells, ultimately affecting antigen processing and lymphocyte proliferation.[44] Increased natural killer cell activity with nucleotide supplementation has been demonstrated in a study comparing infants fed a nucleotide-supplemented formula, breast-fed infants, and those receiving nonsupplemented formula.[45] Additional studies have demonstrated statistically higher titer antibody responses to diphtheria and *Haemophilus influenzae* type b (Hib) vaccines in infants receiving a nucleotide-supplemented formula than those receiving human milk or a control formula.[46]

Nucleotides appear to affect the intestinal environment by promoting the growth of bifidobacteria.[47] The nucleotide inosine appears to improve the reduction and release of iron from ferritin via the action of xanthine oxidase, leading to improved calcium absorption from the intestinal lumen.[48, 49] Nucleotides also appear to affect serum lipid levels, leading to a increase in high-density lipoproteins and lower levels of very-low-density lipoprotein.[50] Infants fed nucleotide-supplemented formula also have statistically lower linoleic acid plasma levels and increased omega-6 polyunsaturated fatty acids, suggesting that enteral nucleotides may influence the metabolism of linoleic acid to longer-chain fatty acids.[51]

Assuming nucleotides from nucleic acids can be digested, absorbed, and salvaged from human milk, 20% to 25% of daily nitrogenous needs may be provided this way.[47] Cow's milk–based infant formulas historically have not contained nucleotides at this significant level. In an attempt to improve the nutrition provided to formula-fed infants, many formulas are now supplemented with nucleotides.[47]

One study has demonstrated a statistically lower incidence of diarrheal disease in infants fed a nucleotide-supplemented formula compared with infants on a nonsupplemented formula.[52] However, the duration of diarrheal illness, the patterns of enteropathogens, or the incidence of other infections were not significantly different between the two groups.[52] In a recent prospective study of nucleotide supplementation in small-for-gestational-age infants, those on supplemental formula had a statistically higher weight and length at a 2-month evaluation. This improved growth persisted over the remainder of the 6-month follow-up period.[53] Head circumference growth tended to be better in the supplemented group but did not reach statistical significance.[53]

### *Docosahexaenoic and Arachidonic Acid*

The supplementation of formula with long-chain polyunsaturated fats, such as docosahexaenoic acid (DHA) and arachidonic acid (AA), remains controversial. Both DHA and AA are major phospholipid components of cell membranes in the retina and the brain. Studies using DHA-supplemented formula in preterm infants have demonstrated an improvement in visual acuity at 2 and 4 months of age over children receiving nonsupplemented formula; however, the difference was only temporary and not significant after 4 months.[54, 55] Additionally, two studies have suggested that preterm infants fed formulas supplemented with DHA had slower growth over the first 12 months of age.[56, 57]

In one study involving term infants, the supplementation of DHA and AA to the formula led to a statistically improved visual acuity at 2 months of age but did not maintain significance during 4-, 6-, 9-, or 12-month follow up.[57] A randomized prospective longitudinal study of healthy term infants fed human milk, formula without long-chain polyunsaturated fatty acids, formula with AA and DHA, or a formula with DHA alone failed to demonstrate any difference in growth or visual acuity over the 12-month study period.[58] In light of these studies, the decision to supplement infant formula with the long-chain polyunsaturated fats awaits further investigation.

## ENTERAL FEEDING AFTER AGE 12 MONTHS

Clinical situations requiring children to continue on higher calorie formula feeding after the age of 12 months include failure to thrive, gastrostomy tube feeding, cardiac disease, renal disease, chronic infection, and pulmonary disease. A number of formulas have been designed for these older infants after the first year (Table 57–5).

For those children able to tolerate cow's milk protein, commonly available formulas include PediaSure and Kindercal. Both of these formulas are lactose free. The fats are supplied as approximately 80% LCT and 20% MCT. Caloric density of both formulas is approximately 1 kcal/mL. PediaSure is also gluten free and is supplemented with taurine and carnitine. Neither formula is recommended for children younger than 12 months old.[59]

In those children who require a protein hydrolysate formula before 1 year and continue to have evidence of cow's milk or soy protein allergy, no specifically designed formula exists. Peptamen, although formulated for older individuals, may be used as an alternative formula. This is a whey protein hydrolysate with a caloric density of 1 kcal/mL. Fat is provided predominantly as 70% MCT.

For those children requiring an elemental diet consisting of amino acids due to food allergy, inflammation, short bowel syndrome, or severe malabsorption of any cause, formulas include Neocate One+, L-emental, and Pediatric Vivonex. Neocate One+ has the added benefits of being palatable and available in juice boxes. Pediatric Vivonex is also supplemented with glutamine, carnitine, and taurine.

## SPECIFIC CLINICAL PROBLEMS

### Lactose Malabsorption

Lactose is a disaccharide that is hydrolyzed into glucose and galactose by the enzyme lactase, a small bowel brush border enzyme. Unless there is intestinal mucosal injury or congenital lactase deficiency, children will have normal lactase activity until approximately 5 years of age for whites and 3 years of age for African Americans and Hispanic individuals. In some individuals, the lactase enzyme activity will then begin to decline (constitutional lactase deficiency). Even if this enzyme naturally declines in activity and individuals develop lactose malabsorption, few of these patients develop the symptoms of lactose intolerance (bloating, flatulence, abdominal cramping, and diarrhea).

Cases in which lactose malabsorption may develop in infancy include the preterm infant who has yet to develop full lactase activity, the rare infant with congenital lactase deficiency, or the more common secondary lactase deficiency. Lactase deficiency in infants requires investigation of underlying pathophysiology. Most commonly, lactase deficiency is linked to viral enteritis, giardiasis, celiac disease, or allergic enteropathy.

### Colic

Infantile colic is a syndrome defined by episodes of severe inconsolable crying that may last several hours each day. These episodes usually develop in the first 2 to 4 weeks of age and spontaneously resolve by the age of 3 to 4 months. A number of studies have estimated that 10% to 20% of infants are affected.[60, 61] Although some clinicians believe that lactose is involved in the development of colic, no link between the amount of lactose in formula and the amount of crying in normal infants has been demonstrated.[62]

It has been suggested that the symptoms of colic may be linked to irritable bowel syndrome as experienced by the infant.[63] Fiber supplementation, a treatment modality for irritable bowel in adults, was used in infant formula in one study. There was no statistically significant improvement in crying or fussiness with a higher-fiber formula.

Cow's milk or soy protein sensitivity has also been suggested as a cause of infantile colic. Although conflicting data have been published,[64–66] cow's milk/soy protein intolerance may account for between 9%[67] and 71%[68] of infants with colic. An empirical trial of a protein hydrolysate for-

**TABLE 57–5. Enteral Feeding Formula Analysis per Liter**

| FORMULA | kcal per oz | PROTEIN g | PROTEIN Type | PROTEIN % Cal | CARBOHYDRATE g | CARBOHYDRATE Type | CARBOHYDRATE % Cal | FAT g | FAT Type | FAT % Cal | Na (mEq) | K (mEq) | Ca (mg) | P (mg) | Fe (mg) | GASTROINTESTINAL SOLUTE LOAD (mOsm/L) |
|---|---|---|---|---|---|---|---|---|---|---|---|---|---|---|---|---|
| **Cow's Milk–Based** | | | | | | | | | | | | | | | | |
| Kindercal | 30 | 34 | Casein | 13 | 135 | Maltodextrin and sucrose | 50 | 44 | Canola, sunflower, and corn oils, MCT 20% | 37 | 1.6 | 3.4 | 85 | 85 | 1.06 | 310 |
| PediaSure | 30 | 29.6 | Sodium, caseinate, whey, protein concentrate | 12 | 110 | Hydrolyzed corn starch, sucrose | 44 | 50 | High oleic safflower oil 50%, soy oil 30%, MCT 20% | 44 | 16 | 34 | 970 | 800 | 14 | 345 |
| **Protein Hydrolysate** | | | | | | | | | | | | | | | | |
| Criticare HN | 30 | 36 | Hydrolyzed casein and amino acids | 14 | 208 | Maltodextrin, corn starch | 81.5 | 4.7 | Safflower oil | 4.5 | 27 | 34 | 530 | 350 | 9.5 | 650 |
| Peptamen Jr. | 30 | 30 | Hydrolyzed whey | 12 | 137.5 | Maltodextrin, corn starch | 55 | 38 | MCT oil, soy and canola oils | 33 | 20 | 34 | 1000 | 800 | 14 | 260 (unflavored) |
| Vital HN | 30 | 42 | Partially hydrolyzed whey, meat, soy, amino acids | 17 | 185 | Hydrolyzed corn starch, sucrose | 74 | 11 | Safflower oil, MCT 45% | 9 | 20 | 34 | 120 | 667 | 667 | 500 |
| **Elemental** | | | | | | | | | | | | | | | | |
| L-emental | 24 | 24 | 100% free amino acids | 12 | 130 | Maltodextrin, starch | 63 | 24 | MCT, soy oil | 25 | 17 | 31 | 970 | 800 | 10 | 360 |
| Neokate One+ | 30 | 25 | L-Amino acids | 10 | 146 | Maltodextrin, sucrose, corn syrup solids | 58 | 35 | Coconut oil, canola oil, high oleic safflower oil | 32 | 8.7 | 23.8 | 620 | 620 | 7.7 | Liquid: 835<br>Powder: 610 |
| Vivonex Pediatric | 24 | 30 | Free amino acids | 12 | 162.5 | Maltodextrin, corn starch | 63 | 30 | MCT, soy oil | 25 | 17 | 31 | 970 | 800 | 10 | 360 |

mula may be warranted in infants with severe colic.[69, 70] Parents should not be left with the impression that their child carries significant life-long food allergies.

## Low-Iron Formula

In 1989, the American Academy of Pediatrics' Committee on Nutrition published a statement concluding that there is "no role for the use of low-iron formulas in infant feeding."[71] Low-iron formulas are nutritionally deficient formulas because they do not supply the RDA for iron in infants. Iron deficiency anemia has been linked to adverse affects on development and behavior of children. Despite the lack of support in the literature, there continues to be a pervasive misconception implicating iron-containing formulas with colic, diarrhea, constipation, and vomiting. Multiple studies have shown no link between gastrointestinal symptoms and iron in both infants and adults.[72–74]

### REFERENCES


1. Forsyth BW, McCarthy PL, Leventhal JM: Problems of early infancy, formula changes and mothers' beliefs about their infants. J Pediatr 1985;106:1012–1017.
2. Lawrence PB: Breast milk: best source of nutrition for term and preterm infants. Pediatr Clin North Am 1994;41:925–941.
3. Rudloff S, Kunz C: Protein and nonprotein nitrogen components in human milk, bovine milk, and infant formula: quantitative and qualitative aspects in infant nutrition. J Pediatr Gastroenteral Nutr 1997;24:328–344.
4. ESPGAN Committee on Nutrition: Guidelines on infant nutrition: I. Recommendations for the composition of an adapted formula. Acta Paediatr 1977 (suppl 262):3–20.
5. American Academy of Pediatrics Committee on Nutrition: Commentary on breast-feeding and infant formulas, including proposed standards for formulas. Pediatrics 1976;57:278–285.
6. Redel CA, Shulman RJ: Controversies in the composition of infant formulas. Pediatr Clin North Am 1994;41:909–923.
7. Goedhart AC, Bindels JG: The composition of human milk as a model for the design of infant formulas: recent findings and possible applications. Nutr Res Rev 1994;7:1–23.
8. Garza C, Butte N, Goldman A: Human milk and infant formula. In Suskind RM, Lewinter-Suskind L (eds): Textbook of Pediatric Nutrition, 2nd ed. New York, Raven Press, 1993, pp 33–42.
9. Daniel H, Vohwinkel M, Rehner G: Effect of casein and β-casomorphins on gastrointestinal motility in rats. J Nutr 1990;120:252–257.
10. Lawrence R: Biochemistry of Human Milk in Breastfeeding: A Guide for the Medical Profession, 3rd ed. St. Louis, CV Mosby, 1989, pp 73–117.
11. Klish WJ: Special infant formulas. Pediatr Rev 1990;12(2):55–62.
12. Bjorksten B, Burman LG, de Chateau P, et al: Collecting and banking human milk: to heat or not to heat? BMJ 1980;281:765–769.
13. Goldblum RM, Dill CW, Albrecht TB, et al: Rapid high-temperature treatment of human milk. J Pediatr 1984;104:380–385.
14. Kunz C, Rudloff S: Biological functions of oligosaccharides in human milk. Acta Paediatr 1993;82:903–912.
15. Andersson B, Porras O, Hanson LA, et al: Inhibition of attachment of *Streptococcus pneumoniae* and *Haemophilus influenzae* by human milk and receptor oligosaccharides. J Infect Dis 1986;153:232–237.
16. Schanler RJ: Suitability of human milk for the low birthweight infant. Clin Perinatol 1995;22(1):207–221.
17. Innis SM: Human milk and formula fatty acids. J Pediatr 1992;120:S56–S61.
18. Lucas A, Cole TJ: Breast milk and neonatal necrotising enterocolitis. Lancet 1990;336:1519–1523.
19. Lucas A, Morley R, Cole T, et al: Breast milk and subsequent intelligence quotient in children born premature. Lancet 1992;339:261–264.
20. Halsey NA, Boulos R, Holt E, et al: Transmission of HIV-1 infection from mothers to infants in Haiti: impact on childhood mortality and malnutrition. JAMA 1990;264:2088–2092.
21. Dunn DT, Newell ML, Ades AE, Peckham CS: Risk of human immunodeficiency virus type 1 transmission through breastfeeding. Lancet 1992;340:585–588.
22. Zeigler EE, Foman SJ: Lactose enhances mineral absorption in infancy. J Pediatr Gastroenterol Nutr 1983;2:228–294.
23. Wicker Stoker T, Castle J: Special diets. In Walker WA, Watkins JB (eds): Nutrition in Pediatrics: Basic Science and Clinical Applications. Hamilton, Ontario, BC Decker, 1997, pp 761–789.
24. Chorazy PA, Himelhoch S, Hopwood NJ, et al: Persistent hypothyroidism in an infant receiving a soy formula: case report and review of the literature. Pediatrics 1994;96:148–150.
25. Schulman RJ, Feste A, Ou C: Absorption of lactose, glucose polymers, or combination in premature infants. J Pediatr 1995;127:626–631.
26. Stathos TH, Shulman RJ, Schanler RJ, Abrams SA: Effect of carbohydrates on calcium absorption in premature infants. Pediatr Res 1996;39(4 pt 1):666–670.
27. Sulkers EJ, Goudoever JB, Leunisse C, et al: Comparison of two preterm formulas with or without addition of medium-chain triglycerides (MCTs): I. Effects on nitrogen and fat balance and body composition changes. J Pediatr Gastroenterol Nutr 1992;15:34–41.
28. Uauy R, Hoffman DR, Birch EE, et al: Safety and efficacy of omega-3 fatty acids in the nutrition of very low birth weight infants: soy oil and marine oil supplementation of formula. J Pediatr 1994;124:612–620.
29. Luukkainen P, Salo MK, Nifkkari T: The fatty acid composition of banked human milk and infant formulas: the choices of milk for feeding preterm infants. Eur J Pediatr 1995;154:316–319.
30. Carlson SE, Werkman SH, Peeples JM, et al: Arachidonic acid status correlates with first year growth in preterm infants. Proc Natl Acad Sci U S A 1993;58:35–42.
31. Cox J: Recommendations for the use of Similac Neocare at Bronson Methodist Hospital. Ohio Neonatal Newsletter, Spring 1995.
32. Chan GM: Growth and bone mineral status of discharged very low birth weight infants fed different formulas or human milk. J Pediatr 1993;123:439–443.
33. Sampson HA, Bernhisel-Broadbent J, Yang E, Scanlon S: Safety of casein hydrolysate formula in cow milk allergy. J Pediatr 1991;118:520–525.
34. Hall JC, Heel K, McCauley R: Glutamine. Br J Surg 1996;83:305–312.
35. Roig JC, Meetze WH, Auestad N, et al: Enteral glutamine supplementation for the very low birthweight infant: plasma amino acid concentrations. J Nutr 1996;126:1115S–1120S.
36. Windmueller HG: Glutamine utilization by the small intestine. Adv Enzymol 1982;53:201–237.
37. Lacey JM, Wilmore DW: Is glutamine a conditionally essential amino acid? Nutr Rev 1990;48:297–309.
38. Long CL: Nutritional consideration of amino acid profiles in clinical therapy. In Blackburn GL, Grant JP, Young VR (eds): Amino Acids: Metabolism and Medical Applications. Boston, John Wright–PSG, 1983, pp 291–307.
39. Long CL, Nelson KM, DiRienzo DB, et al: Glutamine supplementation of enteral nutrition: impact on whole body protein kinetics and glucose metabolism in critically ill patients. JPEN J Parenter Enteral Nutr 1995;19:470–476.
40. Hornesby-Lewis L, Shike M, Brown P, et al: L-Glutamine supplementation in home total parenteral nutrition patients: stability, safety, and effects on intestinal absorption. JPEN J Parenter Enteral Nutr 1994;18:268–273.
41. Leach JL, Baxter JH, Molitor BE, et al: Total potentially available nucleosides of human milk by stage of lactation. Am J Clin Nutr 1995;61:1224–1230.
42. Savaiano DA, Clifford AJ: Adenine, the precursor of nucleic acids in intestinal cells unable to synthesize purines de novo. J Nutr 1981;111:1816–1822.
43. Rudolph FB: Symposium: Dietary nucleotides: a recently demonstrated requirement for cellular development and immune function. J Nutr 1994;124:1431S–1432S.
44. Carver JD: Dietary nucleotides: cellular immune, intestinal and hepatic system effects. J Nutr 1994;124:144S–148S.
45. Carver JD, Cox WI, Barness LA: Dietary nucleotide effects upon murine natural killer cell activity and macrophage activation. J Parenter Enteral Nutr 1990;14:18–22.
46. Pickering LD, Granoff DM, Erickson J, et al: Dietary modulation of the immune system by human milk (HM) and infant formula containing HM levels of nucleotides. Pediatr Res 1995;37:131A.

47. Quann R, Barness LA, Uauy R: Do infants need nucleotide supplemented formula for optimal nutrition? J Pediatr Gastroenter Nutr 1990;11:429–434.
48. Mazur A, Green S, Saha A, Carleton A: Mechanism of release of ferritin iron in vivo by xanthine oxidase. J Clin Invest 1958;37:1809–1817.
49. McMillan JA, Oski FA, Lourie G, et al: Iron absorption from milk, simulated human milk, and proprietary formulas. Pediatrics 1977;60:896–900.
50. Sanchez-Poza A, Pita ML, Martinez A, et al: Effects of dietary nucleotides upon lipoprotein pattern of newborn infants. Nutr Res 1986;6:763–771.
51. Gil A, Pita M, Martinez A, et al: Effect of dietary nucleotides on the plasma fatty acids in at-term neonates. Hum Nutr Clin Nutr 1986;40C:185–195.
52. Brunser O, Espinoza J, Araya M, et al: Effect of dietary nucleotide supplementation on diarrhoeal disease in infants. Acta Paediatr 1994;83:188–191.
53. Cosgrove M, Davies DP, Jenkins HR: Nucleotide supplementation and the growth of term small for gestational age infants. Arch Dis Child 1996;74:F122–F125.
54. Carlson SE, Werkman SH, Rhodes PG, Tolley EA: Visual acuity development in healthy preterm infants: Effect of marine oil supplementation. Am J Clin Nutr 1993;58:35–42.
55. Carlson SE, Werkman SH, Tolley EA: Effect on long chain n-3 fatty acid supplementation on visual acuity and growth of preterm infants with and without bronchopulmonary dysplasia. Am J Clin Nutr 1996;58:35–42.
56. Carlson SE, Cooke RJ, Werkman SH, Tolley EA: First year growth of preterm infants fed standard compared to marine oil n-3 supplemented formula. Lipids 1992;27:901–907.
57. Carlson SE, Ford AJ, Werkman SH, et al: Visual acuity and fatty acid status of term infants fed human milk and formulas with and without docosahexaenoate and arachidonate from egg yolk lecithin. Pediatr Res 1996;39:882–888.
58. Auestad N, Montalto MB, Hall RT, et al: Visual acuity, erythrocyte fatty acid composition, and growth in term infants fed formulas with long chain polyunsaturated fatty acids for one year. Pediatr Res 1997;41:1–10.
59. Pediatric Nutrition Formulary: Connecticut Children's Medical Center, Department of Clinical Nutrition Services, Hartford, CT, 1997.
60. Hide DW, Guyer BM: Prevalence of infant colic. Arch Dis Child 1982;57:559–560.
61. Forsyth BW, Leventhal JM, McCarthy PL: Mothers' perceptions of problems of feeding and crying behaviors. Am J Dis Child 1985;139:269–272.
62. Barr RG, Clogg LJ, Woolridge JA, et al: Carbohydrate change has no effect on infant crying behavior: a randomized controlled trial. Am J Dis Child 1987;141:391.
63. Treem WR, Hyams JS, Blankschen E, et al: Evaluation of the effect of a fiber-enriched formula on infant colic. J Pediatr 1991;119:695–701.
64. Jakobsson I, Lindberg T: Cow's milk proteins cause infantile colic in breast-fed infants: a double-blind crossover study. Pediatrics 1983;71:268–271.
65. Evans RW, Allardyce RA, Fergusson DM, Taylor B: Maternal diet and infantile colic in breast-fed infants. Lancet 1981;1:1340–1342.
66. Stahlberg M-R, Savilahti E: Infantile colic and feeding. Arch Dis Child 1986;61:1232–1233.
67. Lothe L, Lindberg T: Cow's milk whey protein elicits symptoms of infantile colic in colicky formula-fed infants: a double-blind crossover study. Pediatrics 1989;83:262–266.
68. Lothe L, Lindberg T, Jakobsson I: Cow's milk formula as a cause of infantile colic: a double-blind study. Pediatrics 1982;70:7–10.
69. Forsyth BW: Colic and the effect of changing formulas: A double-blind multiple-crossover study. J Pediatr 1989;115:521–526.
70. Hill DJ, Hudson IL, Sheffield LJ, et al: A low allergen diet is a significant intervention in infantile colic: results of a community-based study. J Allergy Clin Immunol 1995;96:886–892.
71. Committee on Nutrition. Iron fortified infant formulas. Pediatrics 1989;84:1114–1115.
72. Oski FA: Iron-fortified formulas and gastrointestinal symptoms in infants: A controlled study. Pediatrics 1980;66:168–170.
73. Reeves JD, Yip R: Lack of adverse side effects of oral ferrous sulfate therapy in 1 year old infants. Pediatrics 1985;75:352–355.
74. Kerr DS, Davidson S: Gastrointestinal intolerance to oral iron preparations. Lancet 1958;275:489.

# Chapter 58

# Nutritional Assessment

*Kathleen J. Motil, Sarah M. Phillips, and Claudia A. Conkin*

Nutritional assessment is an essential component of the history and physical examination of children with gastrointestinal disorders. Protein-energy malnutrition, linear growth failure, obesity, and iron deficiency anemia frequently complicate the clinical course of common gastrointestinal problems in childhood. The clinician should have an understanding of the normal and abnormal patterns of growth and the changes in body composition during childhood, as well as a working knowledge of the clinical and research techniques available to assess the nutritional status of the child. Technical skills to accurately perform a nutritional assessment and the ability to interpret the information obtained from the nutritional evaluation are crucial.

## EPIDEMIOLOGY OF NUTRITIONAL DISORDERS IN PEDIATRIC PATIENTS

Our clinical experience indicates that three nutritional disorders, protein-energy malnutrition (PEM), linear growth failure, and obesity, occur frequently in the practice of pediatric gastroenterology. Malnutrition and growth failure occur as a consequence of poor dietary intake in conjunction with loss of appetite and the presence of abdominal symptoms, increased intestinal losses secondary to diarrhea or malabsorption, and increased nutrient requirements associated with the inflammatory or infectious complications of gastrointestinal diseases. On the other hand, obesity is more likely to be identified in children who use medications such as corticosteroids, which may be prescribed for specific gastrointestinal disorders.

To determine the prevalence of common nutritional disorders in children, particularly those with gastrointestinal disorders, and to identify the clinical factors that placed these children at nutritional risk, nutritional assessments on newly hospitalized children and on children evaluated in our outpatient clinics were performed. Our survey documented that 44% (n = 288) of all patients (n = 655) had evidence of PEM, growth failure, or obesity. Of those children, 20% were acutely malnourished, 13% were obese, and 31% were chronically malnourished. Infants and toddlers, the age group most frequently admitted to the hospital, were at greatest risk for acute and chronic PEM. However, as a proportion of each age group, acute malnutrition, as well as obesity, was found most frequently among adolescents (Fig. 58–1), whereas chronic malnutrition was distributed evenly across all age groups, with an average prevalence of 30%. Gender or racial and ethnic differences did not influence the prevalence of PEM, growth failure, or obesity in these children. Although nutritional problems were identified across a broad spectrum of clinical disorders, children hospitalized with general pediatric problems that included failure to thrive were at greatest risk for acute malnutrition, whereas children diagnosed with gastrointestinal disease, followed by renal or cardiac disease (Fig. 58–2), were at greatest risk for chronic malnutrition.

In the outpatient setting, 35% (n = 221) of all children (n = 632) were diagnosed with PEM, growth failure, or obesity. Of those children with gastrointestinal disorders, 23% were acutely malnourished, 14% were obese, and 26% were chronically malnourished. The pattern of nutritional disorders among the children with gastrointestinal diseases paralleled the distribution of nutritional abnormalities of hospitalized children with respect to age, gender, and racial or ethnic features. These observations suggest that there is no single group of children in whom nutritional disorders prevail. Nevertheless, children with gastrointestinal diseases rank high with respect to the frequency of poor nutritional status among children with chronic illness.

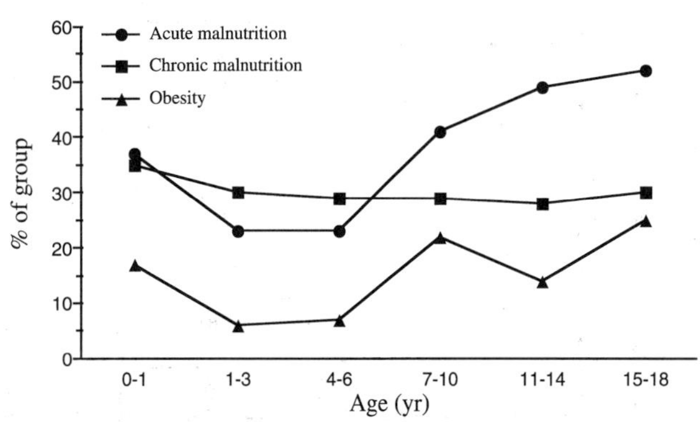


**FIGURE 58–1.** Prevalence of malnutrition and obesity by age in newly hospitalized children.

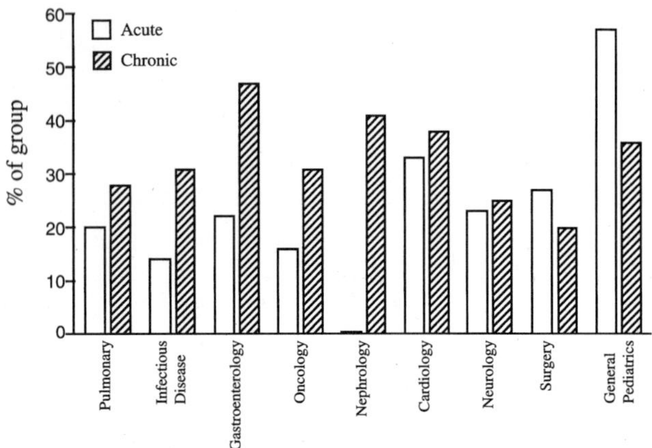


**FIGURE 58–2.** Prevalence of malnutrition by admitting diagnosis in newly hospitalized children.

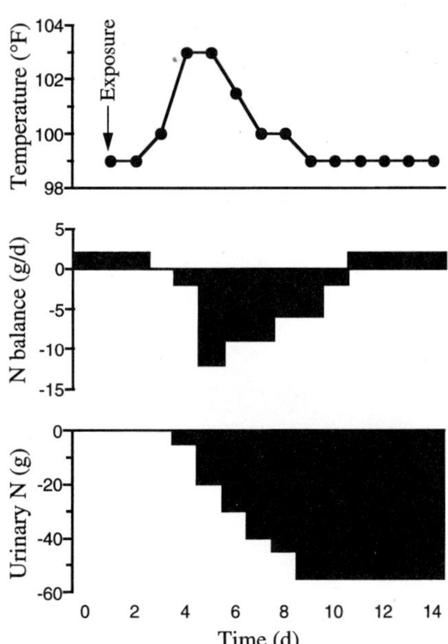


**FIGURE 58–4.** Consequences of a febrile illness on nitrogen balance. (Adapted from Beisel WR: Interrelated changes in host metabolism during generalized infectious illness. Am J Clin Nutr 1972;25:1254–1260, with permission.)

## CLINICAL SIGNIFICANCE OF NUTRITIONAL ASSESSMENT

Nutritional assessment is an important tool used in the clinical care of children with gastrointestinal disorders because it allows the clinician to characterize the patterns of growth and the changes in the body composition of the child in response to altered dietary intakes or poor appetite. For example, Figure 58–3 illustrates the changes in weight and body composition that occur during starvation in infancy.[1] In the healthy infant, 22% of body weight is composed of fat, 15% of protein, and 60% of body water. As the infant becomes progressively more malnourished, body weight loss occurs. The absolute amount of body fat, as well as the proportion of body fat that composes body weight, decreases markedly. The absolute amount of body protein also decreases, although the proportion of body protein stores relative to overall body weight is unchanged. The pattern of weight loss in the older child with chronic gastrointestinal disease may differ from that of the child with simple starvation. For example, children with Crohn's disease may have substantial weight deficits relative to their age-matched peers.[2] However, the absolute amount of lean body mass generally is reduced to a much greater extent than body fat. The significance of these changes in body composition is that a loss of 40% or more of body weight is associated with an increased risk of morbidity and mortality.

Nutritional assessment also is used to determine the changes in growth or body composition that occur in response to infectious or inflammatory processes concurrent with underlying disease. For example, a febrile illness promptly initiates a catabolic response that results in negative body nitrogen balance because of the increased urinary loss of body nutrients (Fig. 58–4).[3] Negative nitrogen balance persists until the febrile illness resolves. The cumulative urinary nitrogen losses are of significant magnitude and persist well beyond the period of the acute febrile illness. The recovery process may require as long as 3 weeks to replenish the depleted body stores. Failure to pay attention

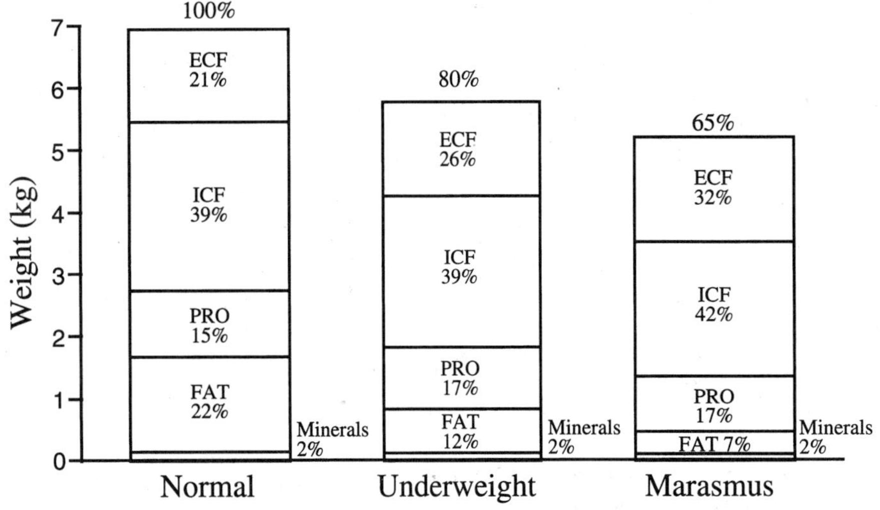


**FIGURE 58–3.** Changes in body composition during starvation in infancy. (Adapted from Viteri FE: Primary protein-energy malnutrition: clinical, biochemical, and metabolic changes. In Suskind RM [ed]: Textbook of Pediatric Nutrition. New York, Raven Press, 1981, pp 189–215, with permission.)

**TABLE 58–1. Normal Growth Rates in Children**

| AGE GROUP | HEIGHT VELOCITY | WEIGHT VELOCITY |
|---|---|---|
| Infancy (1st yr) | 25 cm/yr | 7 kg/yr |
| Toddler (2nd/3rd yr) | 11 cm/yr | 2.2 kg/yr |
| Preschool/school age | 6 cm/yr | 2.5 kg/yr |
| Adolescent | 3–4 cm/6 mo | 6–7 kg/6 mo |

to brief episodes of nutritional depletion leads to a vicious cycle in which the nutritional status of the child worsens with each repeated illness and becomes a factor contributing to morbidity.

## CLINICAL FEATURES OF NORMAL GROWTH AND BODY COMPOSITION IN CHILDREN

### Normal Patterns of Growth in Children

Growth is most rapid in healthy children during early infancy and adolescence (Table 58–1).[4] The average gain in length during the first year of life is 25 cm. This rate declines abruptly to 11 cm/yr during the second and third years, and then slows again to 6 cm/yr in the preschool- and school-age child. During the adolescent growth spurt, peak height velocities average 3 to 4 cm each 6 months in females and males, respectively, but may be as high as 5 to 6 cm every 6 months. The average gain in weight during the first year of life is 7 kg. This rate declines abruptly to 2.2 kg/yr in toddlers, then 2.5 kg/yr in the preschool- and school-age child. During the adolescent growth spurt, peak weight velocities average 3 kg per 6 months but may be as high as 6 to 7 kg per 6 months in females and males, respectively. Estimates of height and weight velocities are essential to quantify because these measurements predict the energy needs for normal growth. For example, if we estimate that the energy cost of tissue deposition averages 5.5 kcal/g and that tissue deposition is 75% lean and 25% fat, then an additional 15,200 kcal/yr is required to support the growth process in the preschool- and school-age child.[5]

### Normal Patterns of Body Composition in Children

The clinical features of body composition have been much more difficult to characterize because of the biologic complexity of the human body. From a theoretical perspective, the body has been represented as a two-compartment model or as multicompartment models.[6] In the two-compartment model, the body is divided into the fat mass and the fat-free mass (FFM) (Fig. 58–5). The fat mass is composed entirely of fat, as opposed to adipose tissue, which contains body fat and its supporting cellular and extracellular tissues. The FFM is composed of the lean body mass (LBM) plus the nonfat components of adipose tissue. In clinical practice, the two-compartment model is useful because of the ease with which body fat and FFM can be measured and the simplicity with which their changes during health and disease can be assessed. Nevertheless, the two-compartment model is subject to error because the methods used to measure body fat and FFM are based on the assumption that the chemical composition of these tissue stores remains constant across a broad range of ages and disease states.

New techniques that characterize multicompartment models of body composition have been developed to reduce the errors inherent in the two-compartment model.[6] The

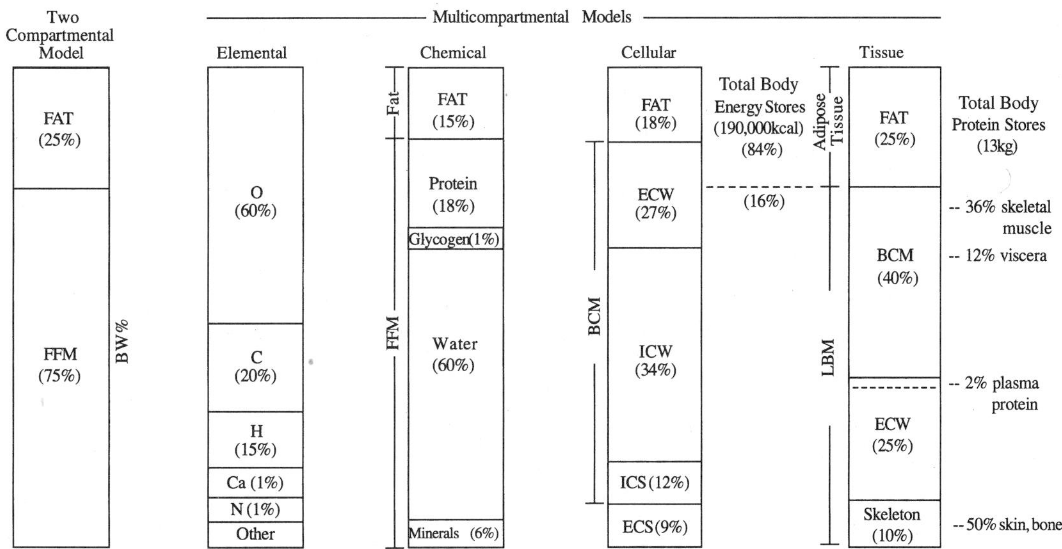


**FIGURE 58–5.** Multicompartment models of body composition. FFM, fat-free mass; BCM, body cell mass; ICW, intracellular water; ECW, extracellular water; ICS, intracellular solids; ECS, extracellular solids. (Adapted from Wang Z-M, Pierson RN, Heymsfield SB: The five-level model: a new approach to organizing body-composition research. Am J Clin Nutr 1992;56:19–28, with permission; and Heymsfield SB, Waki M: Body composition in humans: advances in the development of multicompartment clinical models. Nutr Rev 1991;49:97–108, with permission.)

multicompartment models derived from these techniques include elemental, chemical, cellular, and tissue models (see Fig. 58–5). The elemental model describes body composition in terms of the most common elements of the body (oxygen, carbon, hydrogen, nitrogen, calcium, phosphorus, sodium, potassium, and chloride), whereas the chemical model characterizes body composition on the basis of its water, mineral (osseous and nonosseous), and organic (protein, glycogen, and fat) components, and the cellular model describes the body on the basis of its cell mass and body water compartments. The tissue model provides the most useful information about body composition because it integrates the elemental, chemical, and cellular aspects of body composition into functional units that can be measured routinely in the clinical setting. For example, in this model the functional integrity of body fat can be measured by anthropometry and that of the viscera and skeletal muscle can be measured by serum albumin and 24-hour urinary creatinine excretion, respectively. Abnormalities in these clinical measurements suggest the presence of alterations in the functional adequacy of these compartments of the body and, hence, altered nutritional status.

The body composition of children from birth to 16 years of age, which has been derived from a multicompartment model, is summarized in Table 58–2.[7–9] The estimates of lean body mass and body fat increase with increasing age throughout childhood but vary at any given age depending on gender and race or ethnicity. These estimates serve as reference values for healthy children and may be useful comparative indices to assess the degree of nutritional deficits of children with gastrointestinal disorders.

## Methods to Measure Body Composition

Body composition can be determined from a number of direct (e.g., $^{18}O$ dilution) and indirect (e.g., total body electrical conductance [TOBEC]) methods, most of which, however, are carried out only in research facilities.[10] Direct methods quantify a specific component of the body, whereas indirect methods estimate body compartments on the basis of assumed relationships among body constituents. All of these methods have limitations, both theoretical and practical. In general, the estimates of body composition in children are highly dependent on their age, gender, and race or ethnicity.

Anthropometry is the method used routinely for estimating body composition in the clinical setting. A metal tape measure and calibrated skinfold calipers (Lange Skinfold Calipers, Cambridge Scientific Industries, Inc., Cambridge, MD) are the only instruments needed. In clinical practice, the

**TABLE 58–2. Body Composition of Healthy Children**

| GENDER | RACE/ETHNICITY | AGE (yr) | HEIGHT (cm) | WEIGHT (kg) | LEAN BODY MASS (kg) | FAT MASS (kg) |
|---|---|---|---|---|---|---|
| Female | Multiracial | Birth | 50 | 3.3 | 2.8 | 0.5 |
| | | 0.5 | 66 | 7 | 5.1 | 1.9 |
| | | 1 | 74 | 9 | 6.8 | 2.2 |
| | | 2 | 85 | 12 | 9.6 | 2.4 |
| | White | 4 | 107 | 18 | 14 | 4 |
| | | 8 | 127 | 28 | 20 | 7 |
| | | 12 | 151 | 44 | 30 | 12 |
| | | 16 | 164 | 56 | 38 | 15 |
| | African American | 4 | 106 | 18 | 14 | 4 |
| | | 8 | 133 | 33 | 23 | 9 |
| | | 12 | 157 | 54 | 36 | 16 |
| | | 16 | 162 | 63 | 40 | 21 |
| | Hispanic | 4 | 106 | 19 | 14 | 4 |
| | | 8 | 124 | 30 | 19 | 8 |
| | | 12 | 153 | 57 | 32 | 17 |
| | | 16 | 161 | 67 | 39 | 25 |
| Male | Multiracial | Birth | 52 | 3.5 | 3.0 | 0.5 |
| | | 0.5 | 68 | 8 | 6.0 | 2.0 |
| | | 1 | 76 | 10 | 7.8 | 2.2 |
| | | 2 | 87 | 13 | 10.5 | 2.5 |
| | White | 4 | 103 | 17 | 13 | 3 |
| | | 8 | 126 | 26 | 20 | 5 |
| | | 12 | 157 | 52 | 38 | 12 |
| | | 16 | 174 | 67 | 54 | 10 |
| | African American | 4 | 105 | 18 | 15 | 2 |
| | | 8 | 127 | 29 | 23 | 4 |
| | | 12 | 161 | 60 | 46 | 13 |
| | | 16 | 176 | 83 | 66 | 8 |
| | Hispanic | 4 | 99 | 16 | 12 | 1 |
| | | 8 | 127 | 30 | 21 | 4 |
| | | 12 | 158 | 56 | 39 | 9 |
| | | 16 | 172 | 69 | 54 | 6 |

Data from references 7 through 9.

upper-arm muscle circumference (or area) is determined most commonly because this value can be compared with reference standards to determine the degree of muscle wasting in children of various ages and gender.[11] Nevertheless, circumference measurements of the lower extremity may be helpful in situations when regional muscle wasting is present. The triceps skinfold thickness is the site most frequently selected as a measure of body fat because it can be compared with reference standards to determine the degree of obesity in children of various ages and gender.[11] However, no single skinfold site is entirely representative of the combined subcutaneous and deep fat stores of the body. Hence, a method that uses multiple skinfold thickness measurements, such as biceps, triceps, subscapular, and suprailiac sites, may provide a better estimate of body fat and its regional distribution.[12] Nevertheless, this method fails to incorporate measurements of the thigh and lower leg, sites that may contribute substantially to changes in body composition during periods of weight loss or gain. Accurate estimates of body fat mass using this method also are difficult to obtain in morbidly obese children or in children with generalized edema because of altered relationships between body tissue water and fat in these conditions.

All other body composition methods are, for practical purposes, limited to the research setting. In general, body fat and lean body mass can be measured by densitometry or derived from measures of total body water. Underwater weighing, the oldest method to determine body composition, is used to estimate body density by dividing the individual's actual weight by the weight lost while under water. This method assumes that the density of the FFM remains constant across a broad range of ages, an assumption known to be invalid, thereby requiring correction factors to determine the individual's body composition. Underwater weighing is not feasible in children because the child being weighed must be submerged totally under water and be able to hold his or her breath for a period of time to determine body density.

Total body water is measured directly by isotope dilution using the stable isotopes of deuterium ($^{2}H_2O$) or oxygen ($H_2{}^{18}O$)[13] and indirectly by TOBEC[14] or bioelectrical impedance analysis (BIA).[15] With TOBEC and BIA methods, total body water is estimated based on the principle that body fluids in lean tissue conduct a high-frequency electrical current more readily than body fat. Both of these methods require that the child rests quietly without movement for a short period of time, no small feat for a toddler or young child. BIA and TOBEC also are sensitive to changes in body shape. Because body shape varies among children of the same height, especially during growth, the measurement of body composition using these methods is imprecise.[16] Furthermore, because TOBEC and BIA are indirect methods, the instruments must be calibrated against an independent estimate of total body water such as isotope dilution. Once total body water has been determined, the FFM of the body must be calculated, based on the assumption that the hydration of lean tissue is constant across a broad range of ages and gender. Because this assumption is invalid, correction factors must be used to convert total body water to FFM.

Dual-energy x-ray absorptiometry has been developed to estimate FFM, body fat, and bone mineral density, a relative measure of bone mass.[17] In this method, the child is scanned with an x-ray source of two different energy levels, the difference in the absorption being proportional to the type of tissue scanned. Although the child is exposed to radiation, this technique is considered to be safe because the average radiation dose to the skin is 1 to 3 mrem per scan. Total body potassium counting is a method that measures the natural abundance of radioactive potassium ($^{40}K$) in the body.[18] $^{40}K$ emits a characteristic gamma ray that in turn serves as a marker for lean body mass, based on the assumption that the potassium content of the FFM remains constant with respect to tissue nitrogen content. This method is noninvasive and safe. Neutron activation analysis is a method in which exposure to a given dose of neutrons generates a known amount of radioactivity within a given mass.[19] The particular element being examined, such as nitrogen, calcium, or phosphorus, can be identified by the characteristic energy of the electromagnetic radiation it emits and its decay rate. Nevertheless, radiation exposure makes this technique generally prohibitive in children. Imaging techniques such as ultrasonography, computed tomography, and magnetic resonance imaging display a visual image of body fat and FFM throughout the body.[20] Although it is possible to estimate total body fat from these images, the inaccuracy of some of the methods, the high level of radiation exposure, and/or the cost and maintenance of the equipment preclude their use in children.

## INDICATIONS FOR NUTRITIONAL ASSESSMENT

A nutritional assessment is warranted if a child with newly diagnosed gastrointestinal disease meets screening criteria for the risk of developing PEM, growth failure, or obesity. This recommendation assumes that the child has not been evaluated previously by the physician and that the availability of accurate antecedent growth information is unlikely to be obtained. As a general guideline (1) any child whose height-for-age ratio is less than the 10th percentile is at risk for chronic malnutrition; (2) any child younger than 10 years of age whose weight-for-height ratio is less than the 10th percentile or any child age 10 or older whose weight-for-age ratio is less than the 10th percentile is at risk for acute malnutrition; and (3) any child younger than 10 years of age whose weight-for-height ratio is greater than the 90th percentile or any child 10 years of age or older whose weight-for-age ratio is greater than the 90th percentile is at risk for obesity (Table 58–3). These screening criteria do not imply categorically that the child has nutritional deficits but

**TABLE 58–3. Indications for Nutritional Assessment**

| CRITERIA (NCHS) | RISK |
|---|---|
| Height for age <10th percentile<br>Height velocity <5 cm/yr after 2 years of age | Chronic malnutrition |
| Weight for height (<10 yr) <10th percentile<br>Weight velocity <1 kg/yr (prepubertal)<br>Weight for age (≥10 yr) <10th percentile<br>Weight velocity (peak) <1 kg/6 mo (prepubertal) | Acute malnutrition |
| Weight for height (<10 yr) >90th percentile<br>Weight for age (≥10 yr) >90th percentile | Obesity |

NCHS, National Center for Health Statistics.

that children whose growth measurements plot at the extremes of the growth curves merit closer scrutiny to determine if nutritional deficits truly are present.

Serial height and weight measurements provide additional information on which nutritional risk can be identified. In this setting, a nutritional assessment is warranted if a child who is older than age 2 years fails to demonstrate appropriate linear or ponderal gains during a 6-month to 1-year interval. Thus, a height velocity less than 5 cm/yr after 2 years of age may be consistent with linear stunting or chronic malnutrition (see Table 58–3). A prepubertal weight velocity less than 1 kg/yr or a pubertal peak weight velocity less than 1 kg every 6 months may be consistent with acute malnutrition. In clinical practice, growth measurements are the most important factors for elucidating which children are at risk for nutritional disorders.

## COMPONENTS OF NUTRITIONAL ASSESSMENT

*Nutritional assessment* is defined as the comprehensive approach to characterizing quantitatively the nutritional status of the child.[21–23] A comprehensive nutritional assessment has four components: (1) dietary, medical, and medication history; (2) physical examination; (3) growth and anthropometric measurements; and (4) laboratory tests.

### Dietary History

A dietary history that determines the actual quality and quantity of the child's pattern of food consumption and the eating behaviors and beliefs of the family is an important component of the nutritional assessment. The physician should ask about the type of feeding that is provided to the child, the number of meals and snacks per day, the use of a special diet, the consistency with which vitamin and mineral supplements are given, food allergies, food intolerances or avoidances, and unusual feeding behaviors. Although the physician may review the child's dietary history by 24-hour recall, this method of analysis frequently is misleading. In general, a 3-day food record, performed while the infant or child is at home, is a more valid tool to quantify actual dietary intake. However, even in this setting, dietary intakes may be doubtful because anxious parents tend to overestimate or underestimate the child's food consumption depending on the nature of the nutritional problem. Despite these difficulties, every effort should be made to document the possibility that altered dietary intakes contribute to the child's nutritional problem. Once food records have been obtained, the help of a dietitian is invaluable in converting food servings into nutrient content using either the Atwater conversion factors (1 g of protein, carbohydrate, and fat equals 4, 4, and 9 kcal/g, respectively) to estimate the energy content of the diet or a computerized nutrient database to provide a more complete list of nutrient intakes. The estimate of the nutrient content of the diet should be compared with the age- and gender-specific Recommended Dietary Allowances, with the caveat that these standards meet the nutrient needs of nearly all healthy children but do not take into account the nutrient needs of children diagnosed with acute or chronic illness.[24]

The assessment of the dietary intake of infants with gastrointestinal illness should be rigorous because of the rapidity with which failure to thrive may develop in this age group. However, the assessment of the dietary intake of the breast-fed infant may be difficult to obtain because the feeding pattern of the nursing infant is highly variable. General guidelines to determine the adequacy of intake include the frequency and duration of breast feeding, the frequency of urination, and the infant's weight gain. The breast-fed infant generally nurses every 2 to 3 hours, or 8 to 12 times per day. The average duration of each nursing is 5 to 15 minutes per breast. As a rule, the breast-fed infant gains 30 g/day during the first 6 months of life.[4] The assessment of the dietary intake of the formula-fed infant is much easier to obtain than that of the breast-fed infant. General guidelines to determine the adequacy of the dietary intake include the frequency of feeding, the volume of milk consumed (150–180 $mL \cdot kg^{-1} \cdot day^{-1}$), the energy density of the formula, a comparison of the actual dietary energy intake with the Recommended Dietary Allowances for age,[24] and a weight gain of 30 g/day during the first 6 months of life.[4] In the presence of nutritional deficits, the physician should anticipate increased energy intakes in the range of 150 to 180 $kcal \cdot kg^{-1} \cdot day^{-1}$ and higher weight gains of 50 to 60 g/day to reverse the adverse nutritional consequences associated with gastrointestinal disorders.

The assessment of the dietary intake of children 2 years of age or older should follow the guidelines of the prudent diet.[25] Total daily fat intake should comprise less than 30% of total daily energy intake. Saturated and polyunsaturated fats should comprise less than 10% each of total daily energy intake. Cholesterol intake should be limited to 300 mg/day. Total daily carbohydrate intake should comprise 60% or more of total daily energy intake. Complex carbohydrates, such as starch, should comprise more than 50% and simple sugars should comprise less than 10% of the total daily energy intake. A high-fiber diet should be encouraged; a useful guideline is the child's age in years plus 5 equals the grams of fiber per day, where one serving of fruit, vegetable, or cereal each contains 2 to 3 g of fiber. Table salt should not be readily available. The diet should be nutritionally complete, include a variety of foods, and be adequate for normal growth and activity. In those conditions in which dietary modifications may be necessary to ameliorate bothersome gastrointestinal symptoms, careful attention to appropriate nutrient substitutes or supplements should be given to prevent specific nutrient deficiencies, imbalances, or toxicities.

A modification of the Food Guide Pyramid is the practical tool to assess the prudent diet across all age groups (Fig. 58–6).[26] The Food Guide Pyramid comprises five food groups: dairy, meat, vegetables, fruits, and grains. Children of all age groups should consume daily 3 to 4 servings of dairy products; 2 to 3 servings of meat, fish, poultry, or eggs; 3 to 5 servings of vegetables; 2 to 4 servings of fruits; and 6 to 11 servings of bread, rice, pasta, or cereals. Serving sizes for 7- to 10-year-old children approximate those for adults; serving sizes for 1- to 3- and 4- to 6-year-old children are proportionately less (Table 58–4). Fats and sugars should be used sparingly. Additional inquiry about "health foods," "junk foods," fad diets, and "popular" nutritional supplements should be included in this category.

The presence of acute or chronic gastrointestinal illness

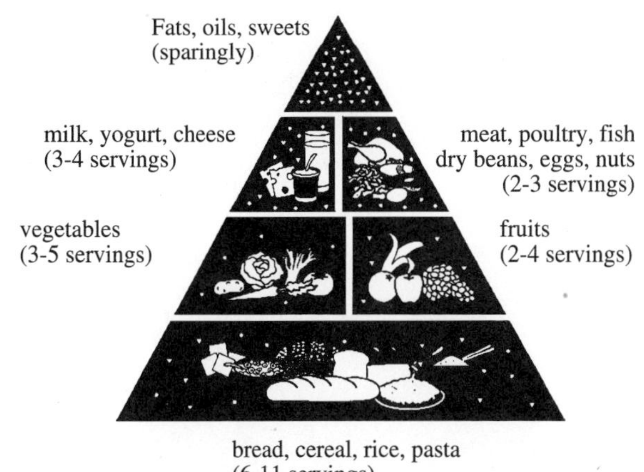


**FIGURE 58–6.** Food Guide Pyramid. (Adapted from U.S. Department of Agriculture: The Food Guide Pyramid. Home and Garden Bulletin, No. 252, 1992.)

generally has important implications for the nutritional management of the child. Medical factors that influence the child's nutritional status include the past and current status of the gastrointestinal illness, the expected course of the illness, and the effect of medical or surgical intervention on the child's nutrient intake and ultimate clinical outcome. Although nutrient deficiencies are the usual adverse outcome of poor clinical management, the physician should be aware of potential nutrient imbalances or toxicities from too-vigorous attempts to substitute or supplement individual nutrients in an effort to avoid nutrient deficiencies.[27]

## Physical Examination

Protein-energy malnutrition includes two clinical entities: marasmus and kwashiorkor. Marasmus is characterized by the wasting of muscle mass and the depletion of body fat stores, whereas kwashiorkor is characterized by generalized edema (anasarca) and flaky, peeling skin and rashes. Children with PEM may manifest a broad spectrum of clinical features. Children with malnutrition may be irritable or apathetic. The flag sign (i.e., loss of hair color) is associated with a period of malnutrition followed by recovery. Follicular hyperkeratosis and night blindness are characteristic of vitamin A deficiency. Weakness of the leg muscles, pedal edema, tachycardia, congestive heart failure, and seizures are associated with thiamine deficiency (beriberi). Angular stomatitis, cheilosis, and seborrheic dermatitis of the lips and nose are associated with riboflavin deficiency, whereas dry, cracked skin in areas exposed to sunlight, such as the neck, hands, and feet, is associated with niacin deficiency (pellagra). Weakness, nervousness, insomnia, a hypochromic, microcytic anemia, and seizures are associated with pyridoxine deficiency, whereas a macrocytic anemia is associated with folate and vitamin $B_{12}$ deficiency. A peripheral neuropathy, consisting of loss of vibratory sensation and proprioception, paresthesias, and motor weakness, is characteristic of vitamin $B_{12}$ deficiency. Petechiae and ecchymoses of the skin, hyperkeratotic hair follicles with red hemorrhagic halos, bleeding gums, and painful, subperiosteal bleeding of the lower extremities are consistent with vitamin C deficiency. Bone abnormalities, including craniotabes, frontal bossing of the skull, beading (rachitic rosary) of the rib cage, bowing of the shafts of the legs, and widening of the epiphysis of the radii at the wrists are features characteristic of vitamin D deficiency. A smooth tongue may be associated with multiple vitamin and mineral deficiencies, including riboflavin, pyridoxine, folate, vitamin $B_{12}$, and iron. Spooning and pallor of the nail beds also are associated with iron deficiency. Tetany and Chvostek's, Trousseau's, or Erb's signs are characteristic of calcium deficiency. Personality changes, muscle spasms, and seizures are associated with magnesium deficiency. Diarrhea, alopecia, and dermatitis localized to the perioral and perianal area are associated with zinc deficiency.

In clinical practice, it is uncommon to find many of the signs of severe malnutrition in children with acute or chronic gastrointestinal illnesses. In general, a combination of wasting and peripheral edema, signifying a combination of marasmus and kwashiorkor, is found most commonly. Nevertheless, the clinician should have a high index of suspicion for micronutrient deficiencies in the presence of these findings, particularly in children with malabsorptive or inflammatory disorders.

Obesity, on the other hand, is characterized by increased deposition of truncal and peripheral body fat. Increased fatness is associated with several other effects on growth, including increased lean body mass, increased height, advanced bone age, and the early onset of menarche. Obese children may be hypertensive and often display dysfunctional behaviors because of poor self-esteem. Morbid obesity is associated with orthopedic complications, including slipped capital femoral epiphysis and bowing of the tibia and femur, as well as respiratory problems, including sleep apnea and congestive heart failure. Whereas simple, exogenous obesity is a national epidemic, the obesity that occurs secondary to medications (e.g., prednisone) is more difficult to manage because these drugs ameliorate inflammatory conditions but lead to voracious appetites.

**TABLE 58–4. Daily Serving Sizes of Food**

| FOOD | AGE (yr) 1–3 | 4–6 | 7–10 |
|---|---|---|---|
| Milk, yogurt (c) | ½ | ¾ | 1 |
| Cheese (oz) | ½ | 1 | 1½ |
| Meat, poultry, fish (oz) | 1 | 1½ | 3 |
| Eggs | 1 | 1½ | 2 |
| Peanut butter (tbsp) | 1 | 2 | 3 |
| Vegetables—cooked or raw (c) | 3 tbsp | ⅓ | ½ |
| Fruits | | | |
| Canned (c) | 3 tbsp | ⅓ | ½ |
| Fresh (small) | ½ | 1 | 1 med |
| Juice (c) | ⅓ | ½ | ¾ |
| Bread (slice) | ½ | 1 | 1 |
| Dry cereal (c) | ½ | ¾ | 1 |
| Pasta, rice (c) | ⅓ | ½ | ¾ |

## Growth and Anthropometric Measurements

Growth measurements are the most important components of the nutritional assessment because normal growth patterns

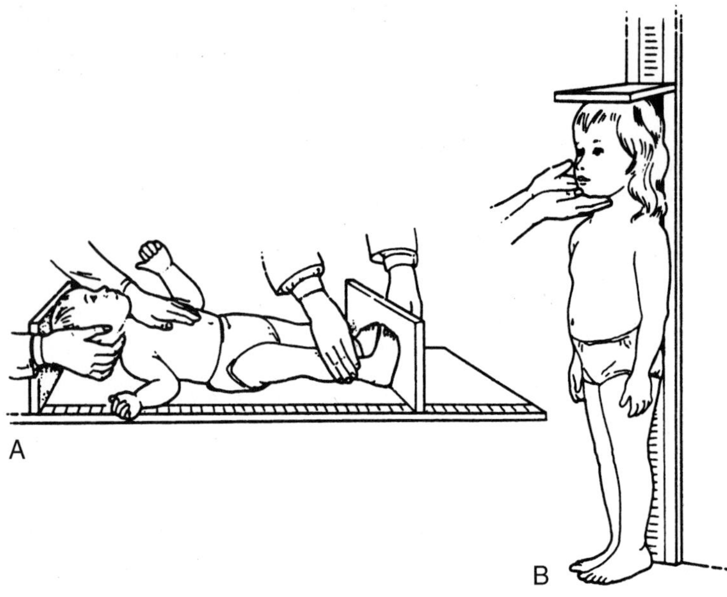


**FIGURE 58–7.** Technique for measuring *(A)* recumbent length or *(B)* height. (From Jelliffe DB: The assessment of the nutritional stature of the community. Geneva, World Health Organization, 1966, Monograph Series No. 53, with permission.)

are the gold standard by which physicians assess the health and well-being of the child. A normal growth pattern is not a guarantee of overall health, but the child with an atypical growth pattern is more likely to manifest the nutritional complications of gastrointestinal disease. Altered growth patterns are a relatively late consequence of nutritional insult. Thus, surveillance is an important component of the nutritional assessment of the child with gastrointestinal disease.

Height and weight measurements are the mainstay of the nutritional assessment of the child. These measurements inherently are not useful unless the physician is able to convert the absolute values to relative standards and to interpret correctly the information provided by the growth measurements.[4] The use of appropriate measurement techniques is essential to assess the adequacy of growth in children. The only appropriate way to measure length (Fig. 58–7*A*) or height (Fig. 58–7*B*) is to use a flat, horizontal or vertical surface with perpendicular surfaces at each end.[28] Weight measurements should be obtained on a scale that has been calibrated properly. The head circumference should be measured at the maximum diameter through the glabella and occiput (Fig. 58–8).[28] Growth measurements, including length or height, weight, and head circumference should be plotted on the National Center for Health Statistics (NCHS)

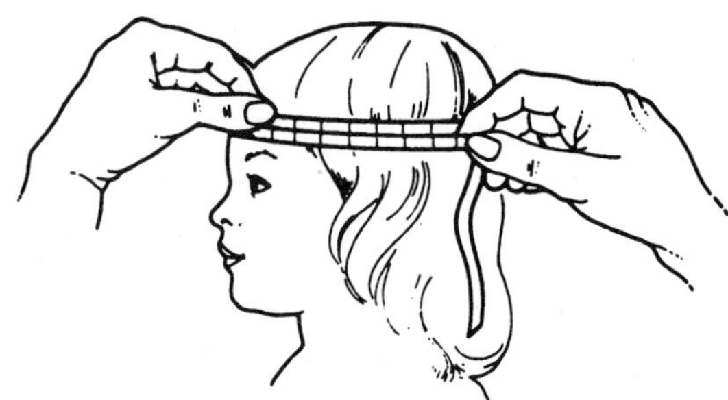

**FIGURE 58–8.** Technique for measuring head circumference. (From Jelliffe DB: The assessment of the nutritional stature of the community. Geneva, World Health Organization, 1966, Monograph Series No. 53, with permission.)

growth charts (Fig. 58–9).[4] Any length, height, or weight measurement that falls below the 5th percentile or crosses two major growth channels is considered to represent an abnormal growth pattern. Serial measurements must be obtained to determine if the growth pattern is truly abnormal or if these findings merely represent constitutional short stature or the rechanneling of normal growth curves. Radiographic studies of bone age[29] may help to clarify the presence of abnormal growth patterns because chronic undernutrition is one of the causes of delayed bone maturation and, hence, delayed linear growth.

Incremental growth charts that characterize height and weight velocities over a 6-month interval may be valuable in assessing the growth response of children with chronic illness.[30] Height velocity measurements may be the most sensitive measure to detect growth abnormalities early in the course of chronic gastrointestinal illnesses.[31] Any child older than 2 years of age whose height velocity is less than 5 cm/yr should be monitored carefully for progressive nutritional deficits (Fig. 58–10). Likewise, any prepubertal child whose weight velocity is less than 1 kg/yr, or any pubertal child whose peak weight velocity is less than 1 kg every 6 months, may be developing the nutritional complications of chronic illnesses (see Fig. 58–10).

Height and weight measurements can be converted to Z-scores, or values that represent standard deviations from the median height and weight values for age. Any child whose height or weight Z-scores are less than $-1.64$ (i.e., less than the 5th percentile) is considered to have an abnormal growth pattern; height and weight Z-scores more than 2 SD below the median are considered to represent significant nutritional abnormalities. Most clinicians do not use Z-scores routinely because growth abnormalities can be identified readily by plotting height and weight measurements on the growth charts. The use of Z-scores is particularly helpful when assessing growth information in the research setting.

The degree of acute and chronic malnutrition, characterized as ponderal wasting and linear stunting, respectively, can be assessed clinically using Waterlow criteria.[32, 33] This method assumes that during periods of nutritional deprivation, weight deficits occur initially, followed by length or height deficits. An arrest of head growth is spared unless compromised by severe starvation. The Waterlow criteria also assume that the expected height and weight measurements of the child fall along the 50th percentile of the growth curves. This assumption is necessary because prior height and weight measurements usually are not available when evaluating a child for the first time. Under these circumstances, the genetic growth potential of the child may not be known. The birth weight or the current head circumference percentile may provide a clue to the true growth potential of the child. Nevertheless, the genetic growth potential may be determined only in retrospect after aggressive nutritional intervention has been implemented.

Acute malnutrition, measured in terms of weight deficit, can be determined from the equation

$$\text{Weight deficit (\%)} = \frac{\text{Actual weight (kg)}}{\text{Expected weight (kg) for actual height}} \times 100$$

In this case, the expected weight measurement is determined by drawing a horizontal line from right to left between the child's measured height and the point at which the actual height measurement falls on the 50th percentile line, then connecting this point by means of a vertical line with the point at which the weight measurement falls on the 50th percentile line for a child of the same chronologic age (Fig. 58–11*A*).

Chronic malnutrition, measured in terms of a height or length deficit, can be determined from the equation

$$\text{Height deficit (\%)} = \frac{\text{Actual height (cm)}}{\text{Expected height (cm) at 50th percentile for chronologic age}} \times 100$$

In this case, the expected height is derived by plotting the height measurement at the 50th percentile for the child's actual chronologic age (Fig. 58–11*B*). However, if the child's true height potential has been documented previously from serial height measurements, then the adjusted value should be used to estimate the true height deficit.

The nutritional assessment of a malnourished child using Waterlow criteria is illustrated in Table 58–5. A child is considered to have first-, second-, or third-degree malnutrition if the weight-for-height estimate is less than 90%, 80%, or 70% of expected, respectively. Likewise, a child is considered to have first-, second-, or third-degree chronic malnutrition if the height-for-age estimate is less than 95%, 90%, or 85% of expected, respectively. The significance of these estimates is that they provide a useful guideline for the nutritional rehabilitation of the child with gastrointestinal disease. Thus, aggressive nutritional rehabilitation should be implemented by the oral route for first-degree acute and chronic malnutrition. Aggressive enteral refeeding using a nasogastric tube or button gastrostomy should be considered in the presence of second-degree malnutrition, whereas total parenteral nutrition may be required for third-degree malnutrition.

An alternative method to estimate the degree of acute malnutrition in children younger than 4 years of age is the McLaren criteria.[34] This method assumes that a malformation of the head, such as microcephaly, is not present. Acute malnutrition, measured in terms of the mid upper arm circumference and fronto-occipital (head) circumference ratio (MAC/FOC), can be determined from the equation

$$\text{MAC/FOC} = \frac{\text{Mid upper arm circumference (cm)}}{\text{Fronto-occipital head circumference (cm)}}$$

The child is considered to have first-, second-, or third-degree malnutrition if the MAC/FOC ratio is less than 0.31, 0.28, or 0.25, respectively (see Table 58–5). Although this method is used less frequently, the nutritional rehabilitation of the malnourished patient can be approached in the same fashion as that using the Waterlow criteria.

Conversely, the degree of obesity can be assessed using weight-for-height criteria or the body mass index. Weight-for-height estimates serve as the standard operational criteria where simple obesity is defined as a weight-for-height measurement greater than 120% of expected whereas morbid obesity is defined as a weight-for-height measurement greater than 140% of expected (see Table 58–5).[4] More recently, reference data for obesity, using the body mass index (kg/$m^2$), have been published for children.[35, 36] Using these criteria, obesity is defined as a body mass index greater than the 95th percentile (Tables 58–6 and 58–7). As in other methods used to assess body composition, the body mass index is age, gender, and race or ethnicity specific.

The most widely used anthropometric measurements are the mid upper arm circumference and the triceps skinfold thickness. The technique for measuring the mid upper arm circumference includes the following steps (Fig. 58–12): (1) the child's right arm should be flexed to a 90-degree angle; (2) the midpoint between the tip of the olecranon and acromion should be marked; (3) the child's arm should hang freely; and (4) the circumference of the arm should be measured to the nearest 0.1 cm at the midpoint with a flexible metal tape.[28] The technique for measuring the triceps skinfold thickness includes the following steps (Fig. 58–13): (1) the child's right arm should hang freely; (2) using the thumb and forefinger of the left hand, the upper arm skinfold (skin and fat minus the underlying muscle) should be pulled out 1 cm above midpoint; (3) using the right hand, the calipers should be applied 1 cm in depth at the measured midpoint; (4) the calipers should be released and the reading should be obtained to the nearest 1 mm as soon as the needle is steady; and (5) the average value of duplicate measurements should be recorded.[28] The mid arm circumference (MAC, cm), in conjunction with the triceps skinfold thickness (TSF, cm), can be used to estimate the midarm muscle circumference (MAMC, cm) as follows:[11]

$$\text{MAMC} = \text{MAC} - [\pi \cdot \text{TSF}]$$

where $\pi$ equals 3.1416. The values obtained for the arm muscle circumference and triceps skinfold thickness should be compared with reference values to assess the nutritional status of the child.[11] In general, values less than the 5th percentile for age are consistent with the diagnosis of acute malnutrition and values greater than the 90th percentile are consistent with the diagnosis of obesity.

Thigh and lower leg circumferences and skinfold thick-

*Text continued on page 736*

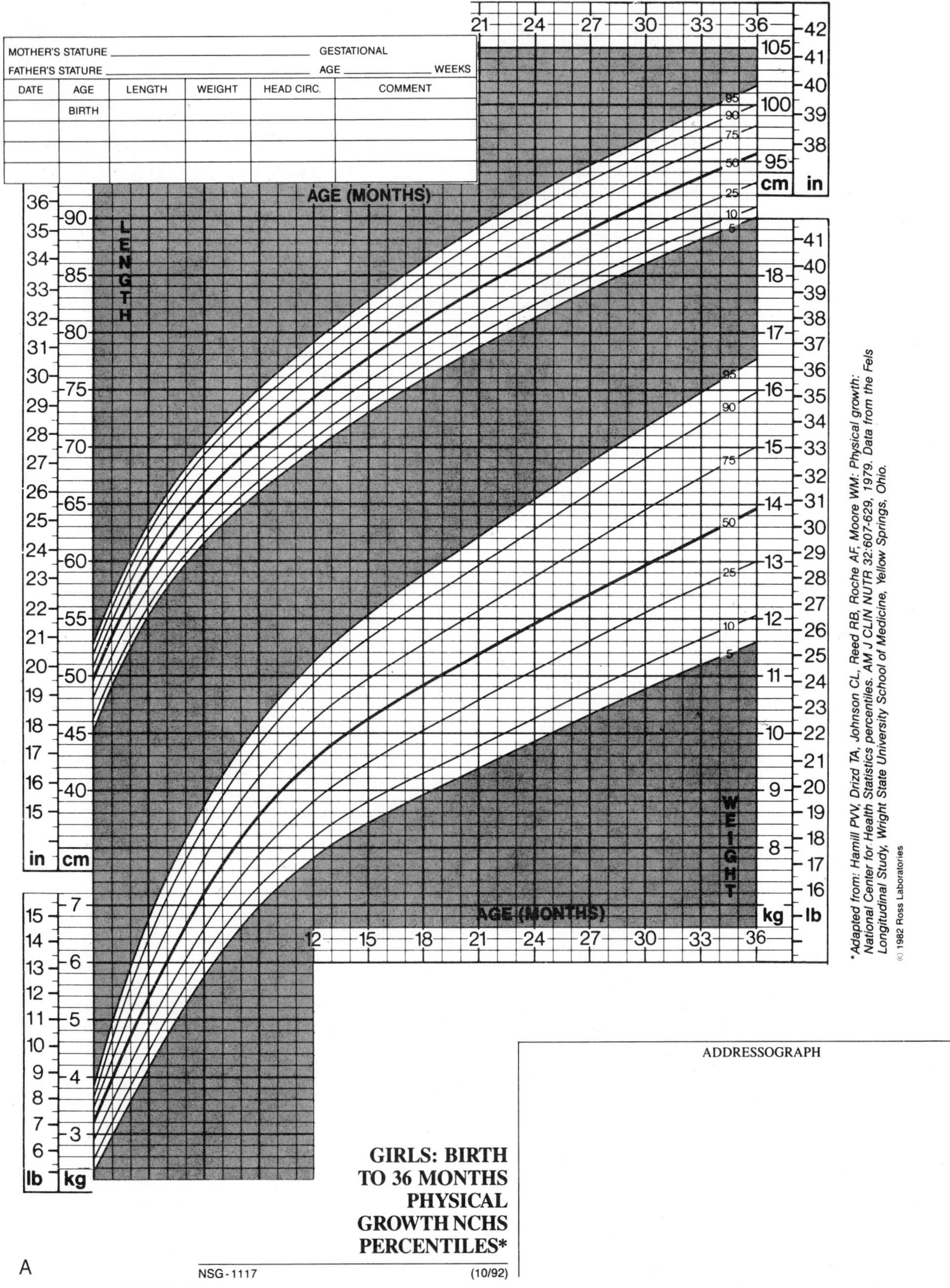


A

**FIGURE 58–9.** Physical growth NCHS percentiles. *A,* Girls, birth to 36 months. *B,* Girls, 2 to 18 years. *C,* Boys, birth to 36 months. *D,* Boys, 2 to 18 years. (*A–D,* Adapted from Hamill PVV, Drizd TA, Johnson CL, et al: NCHS growth charts, 1976. Monthly Vital Statistics Report. Health Examination Survey Data from the National Center for Health Statistics. [HRA]76-1120, vol 25, No 3, Supplement. Rockville, MD, U.S. Department of Health, Education, and Welfare, Public Health Service, Health Resources Administration, June 22, 1976.)

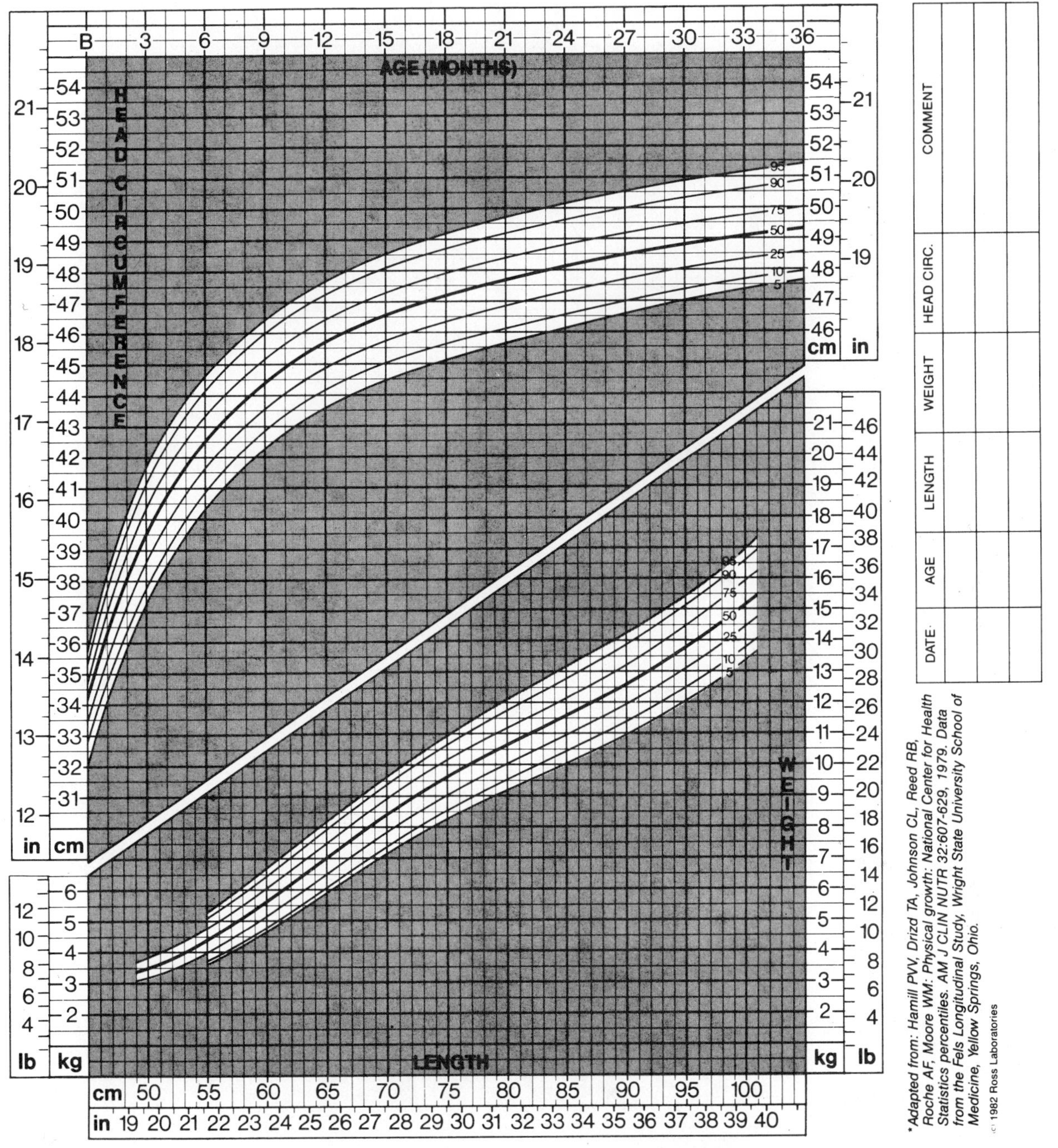


**GIRLS: BIRTH TO 36 MONTHS**
**PHYSICAL GROWTH**
**NCHS PERCENTILES***

NSG-1117 (10/92)

**FIGURE 58–9.** *Continued*

*Illustration continued on following page*

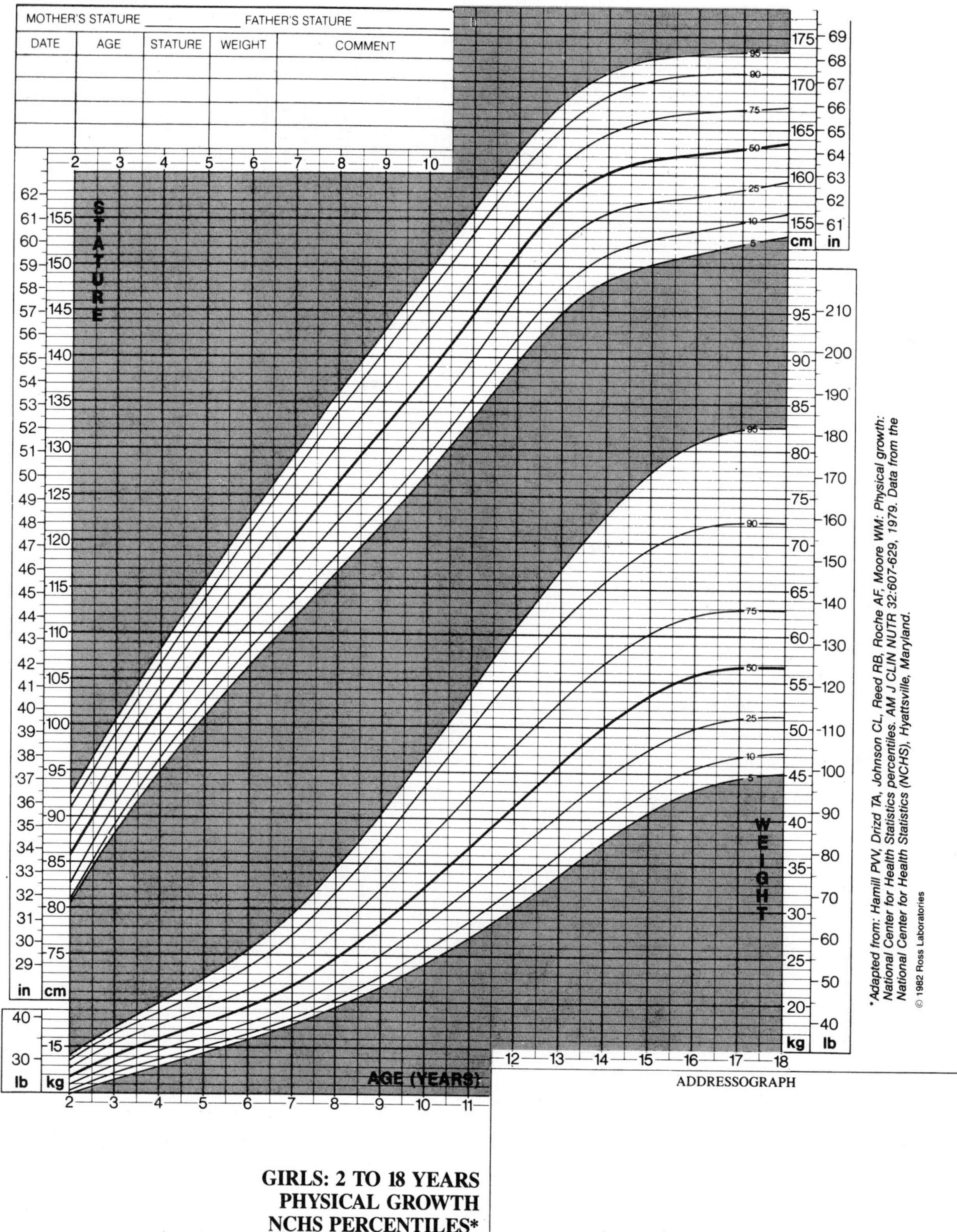
MOTHER'S STATURE
FATHER'S STATURE
DATE
AGE
STATURE
WEIGHT
COMMENT
STATURE
WEIGHT
AGE (YEARS)
in
cm
lb
kg
ADDRESSOGRAPH
GIRLS: 2 TO 18 YEARS
PHYSICAL GROWTH
NCHS PERCENTILES*
NSG-1116
(10/92)
*Adapted from: Hamill PVV, Drizd TA, Johnson CL, Reed RB, Roche AF, Moore WM: Physical growth: National Center for Health Statistics percentiles. AM J CLIN NUTR 32:607-629, 1979. Data from the National Center for Health Statistics (NCHS), Hyattsville, Maryland.
© 1982 Ross Laboratories

B

FIGURE 58–9. *Continued*

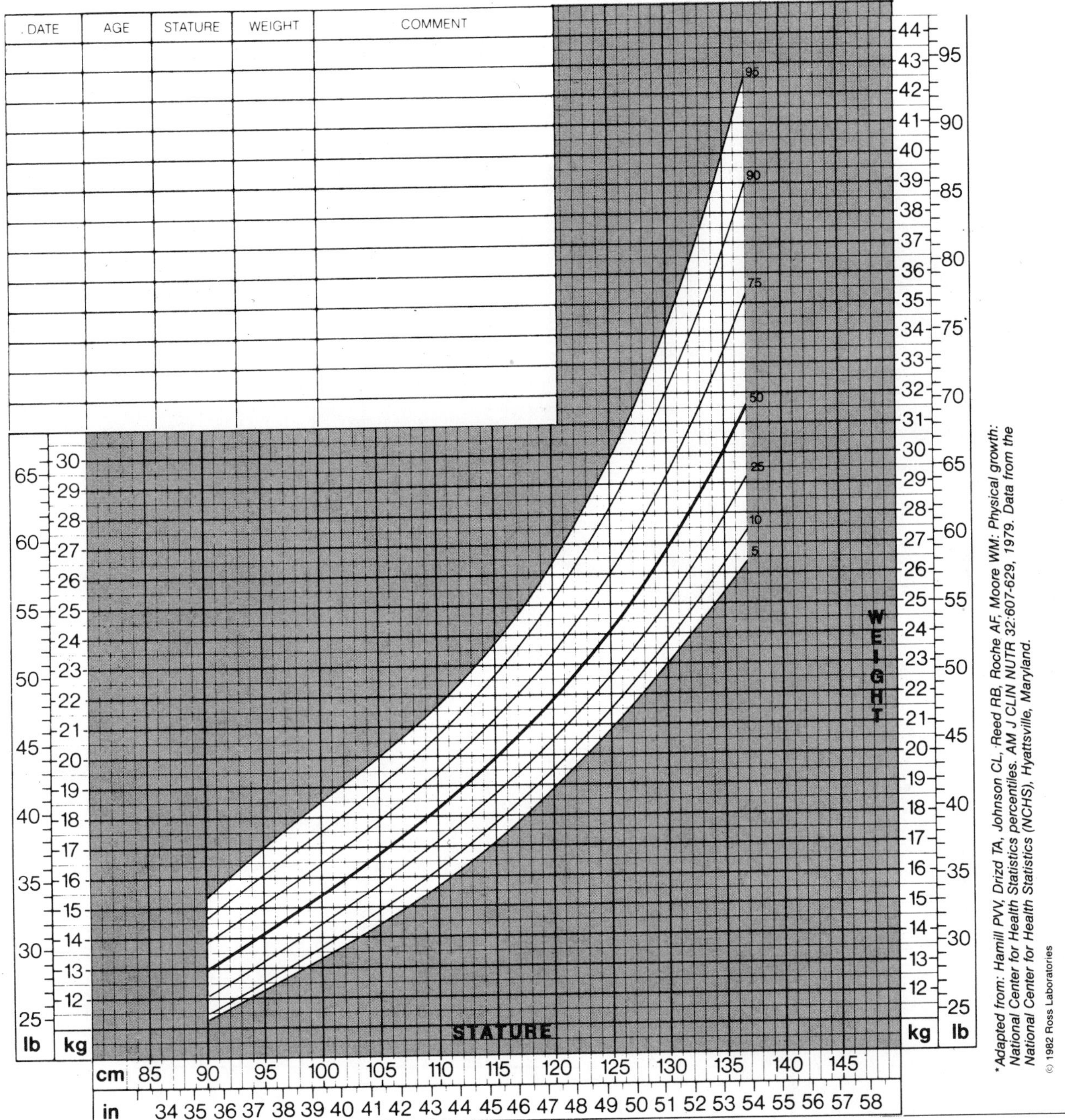


*Adapted from: Hamill PVV, Drizd TA, Johnson CL, Reed RB, Roche AF, Moore WM: Physical growth: National Center for Health Statistics percentiles. AM J CLIN NUTR 32:607-629, 1979. Data from the National Center for Health Statistics (NCHS), Hyattsville, Maryland.



**GIRLS: PREPUBESCENT PHYSICAL GROWTH NCHS PERCENTILES***

NSG-1116 (10/92)

**FIGURE 58–9.** *Continued*

*Illustration continued on following page*

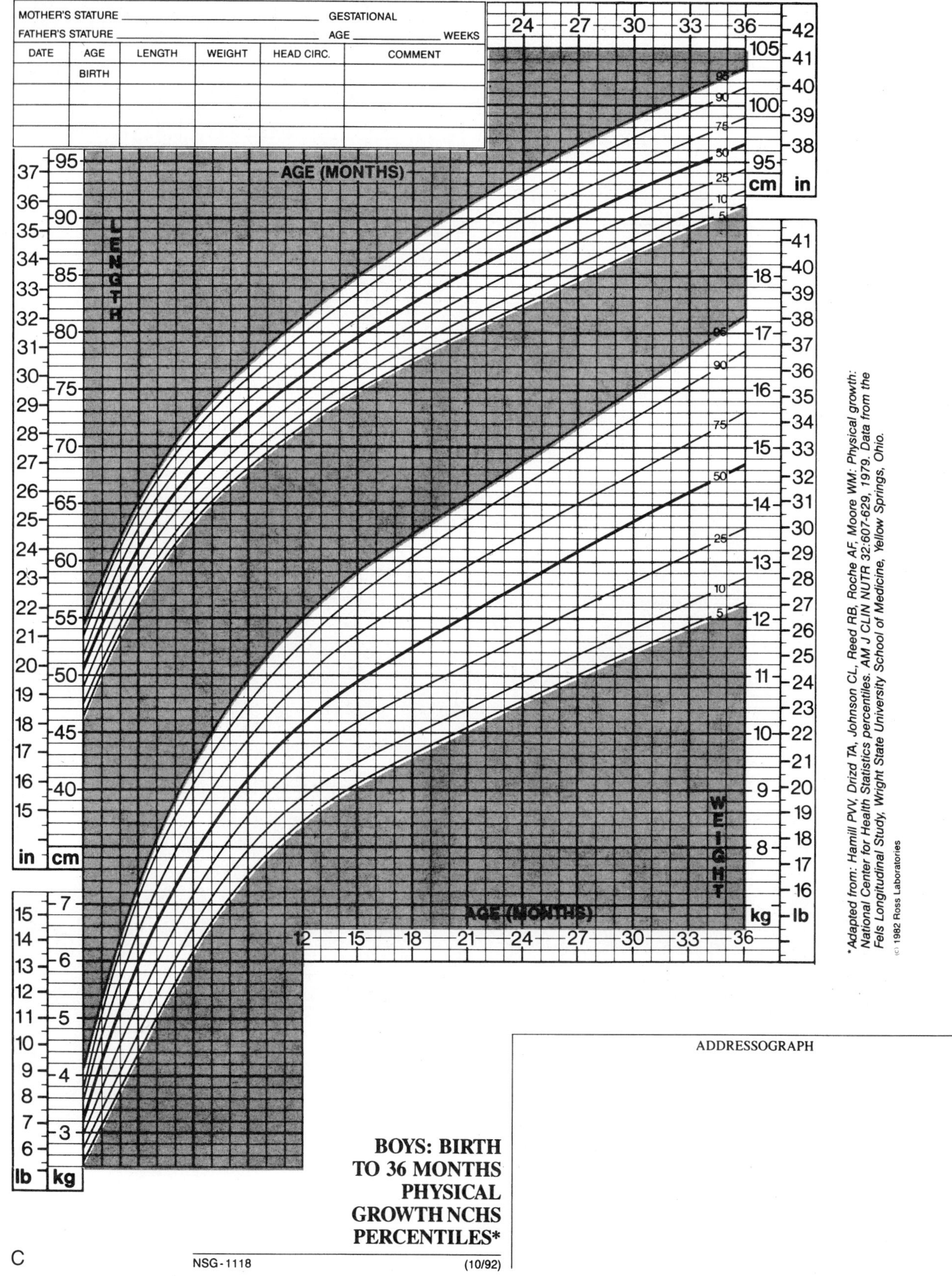

MOTHER'S STATURE
GESTATIONAL
FATHER'S STATURE
AGE
WEEKS
DATE
AGE
LENGTH
WEIGHT
HEAD CIRC.
COMMENT
BIRTH
AGE (MONTHS)
in
cm
lb
kg
ADDRESSOGRAPH
BOYS: BIRTH TO 36 MONTHS PHYSICAL GROWTH NCHS PERCENTILES*
NSG-1118
(10/92)
*Adapted from: Hamill PVV, Drizd TA, Johnson CL, Reed RB, Roche AF, Moore WM: Physical growth: National Center for Health Statistics percentiles. AM J CLIN NUTR 32:607-629, 1979. Data from the Fels Longitudinal Study, Wright State University School of Medicine, Yellow Springs, Ohio.
© 1982 Ross Laboratories

C

FIGURE 58–9. *Continued*

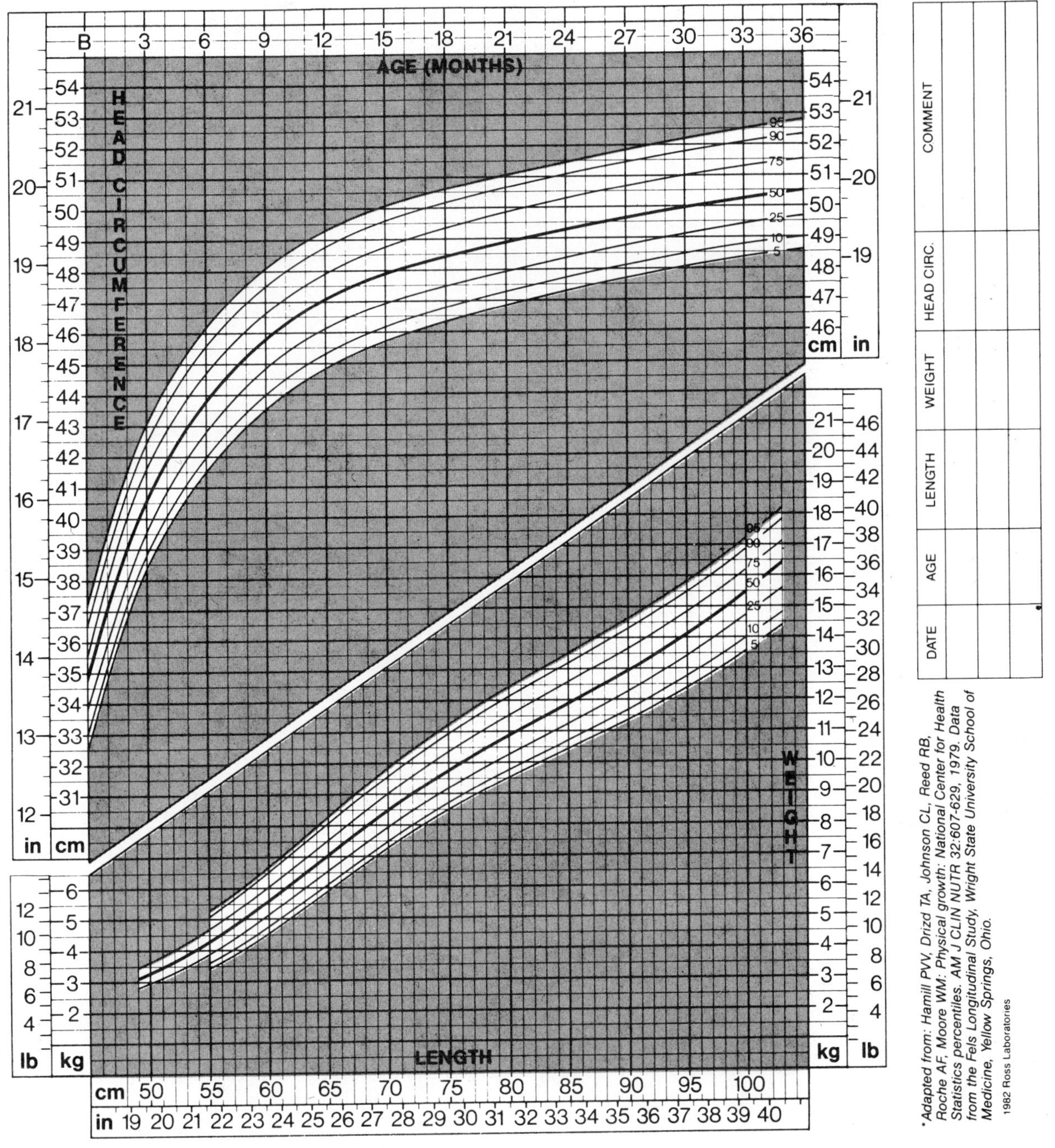


ADDRESSOGRAPH

**BOYS: BIRTH TO 36 MONTHS**
**PHYSICAL GROWTH**
**NCHS PERCENTILES***

NSG-1118 (10/92)

**FIGURE 58–9.** *Continued*

*Illustration continued on following page*

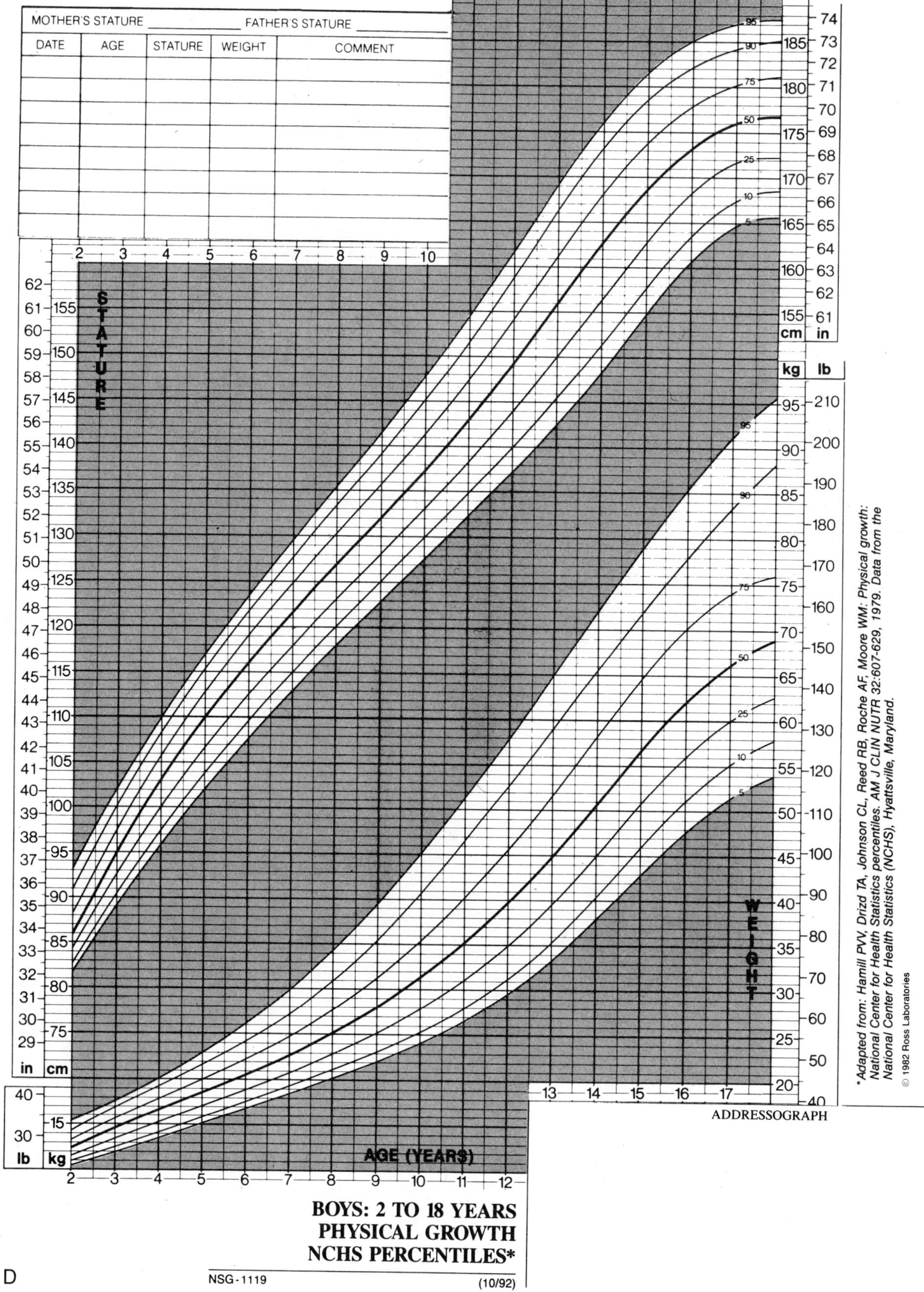


D

FIGURE 58–9. *Continued*

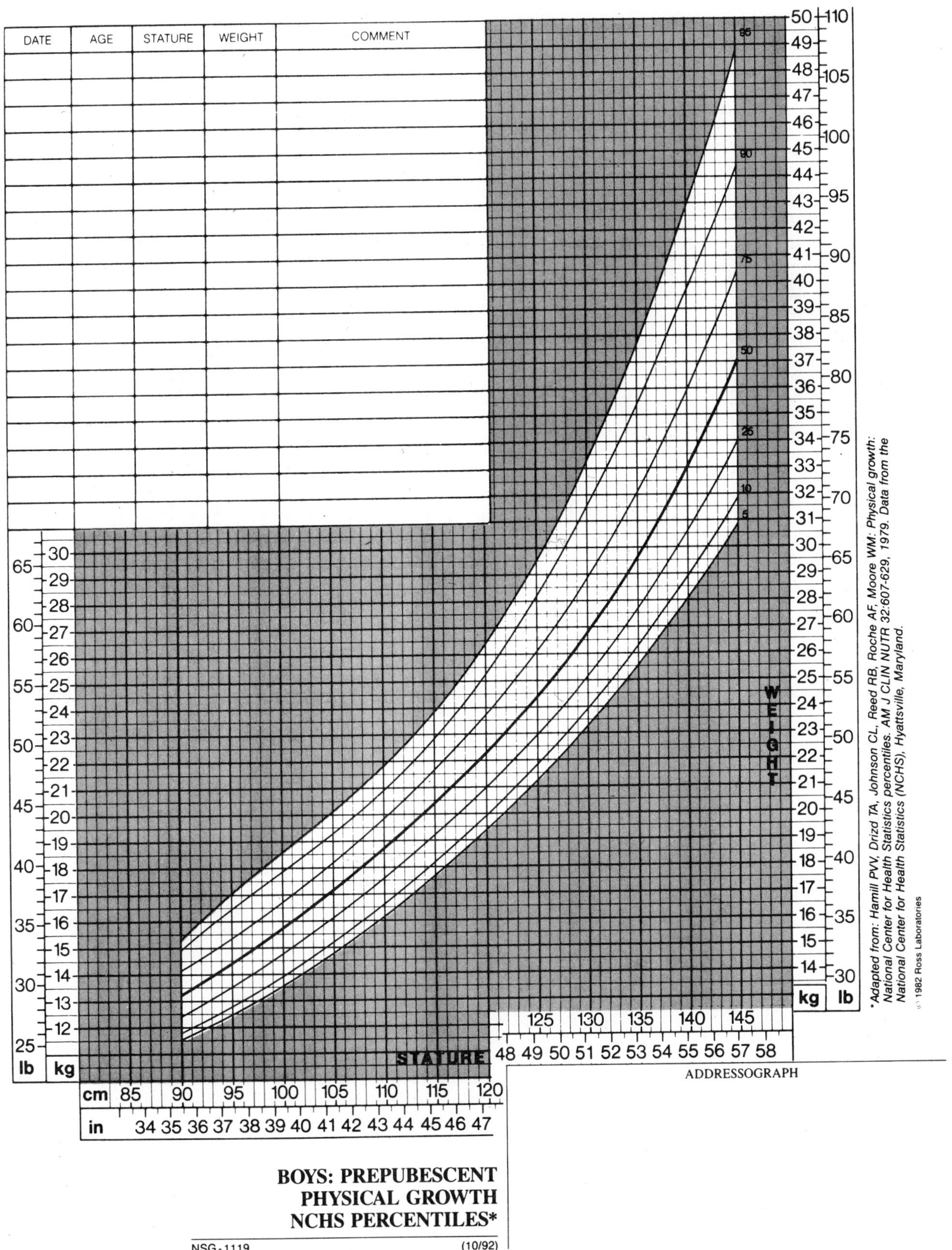


**FIGURE 58–9.** *Continued*

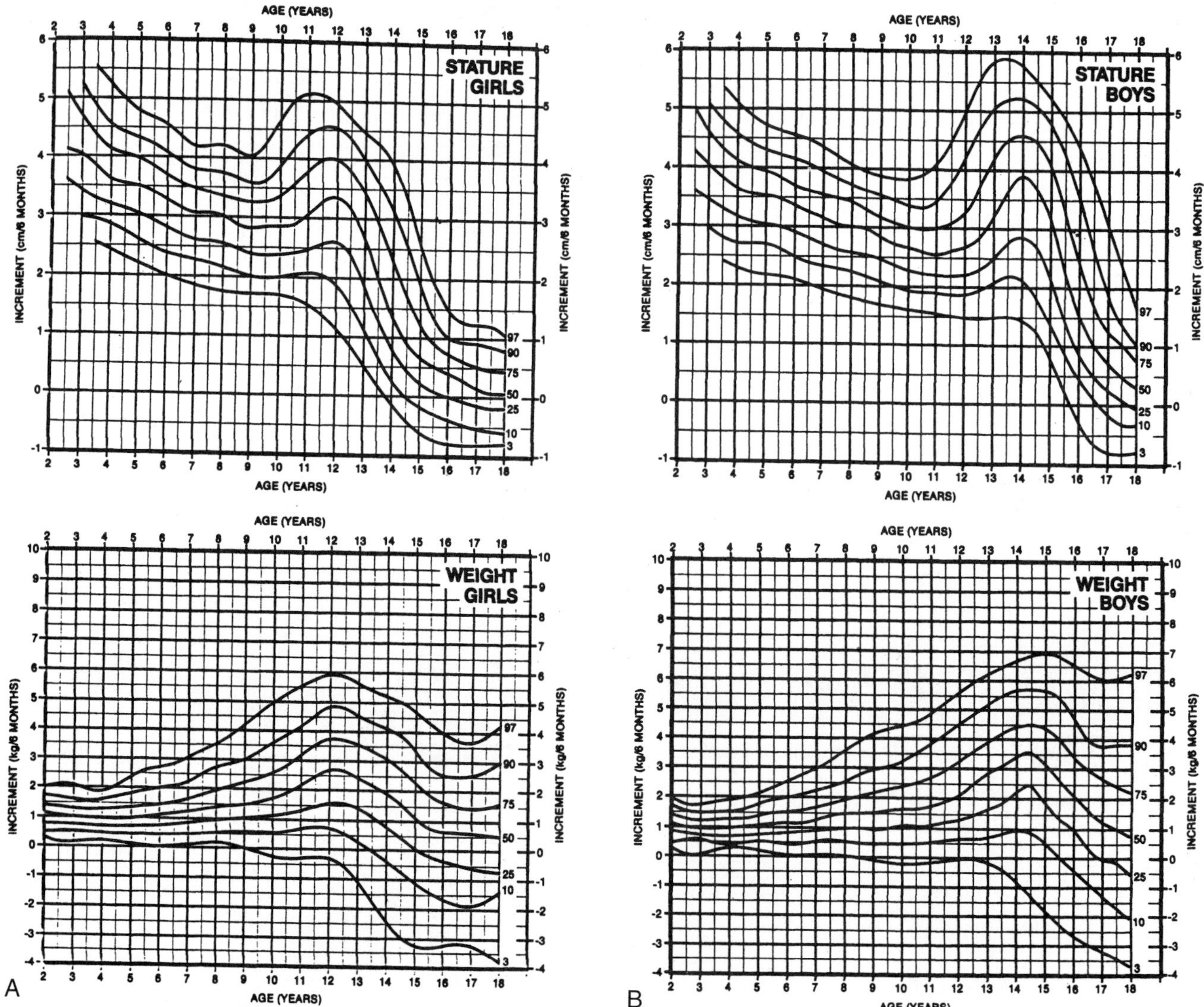


**FIGURE 58–10.** Incremental gain in stature and weight NCHS percentiles. *A,* Girls, 2 to 18 years. *B,* Boys, 2 to 18 years. (Adapted from Hamill PVV, Drizd TA, Johnson CL, et al: NCHS growth charts, 1976. Monthly Vital Statistics Report. Health Examination Survey Data from the National Center for Health Statistics. [HRA]76-1120, vol 25, No 3, Supplement. Rockville, MD, U.S. Department of Health, Education, and Welfare, Public Health Service, Health Resources Administration, June 22, 1976.)

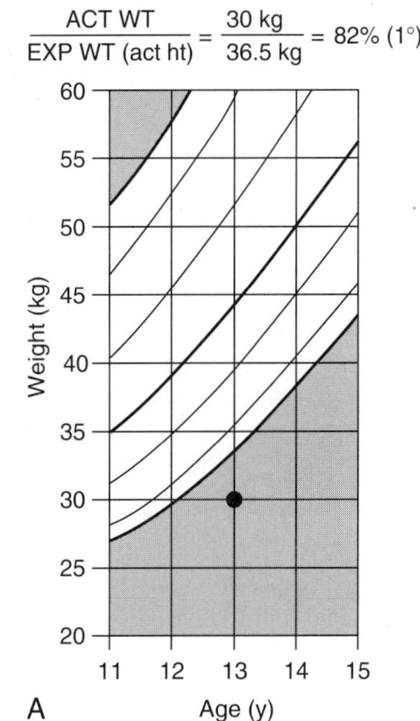


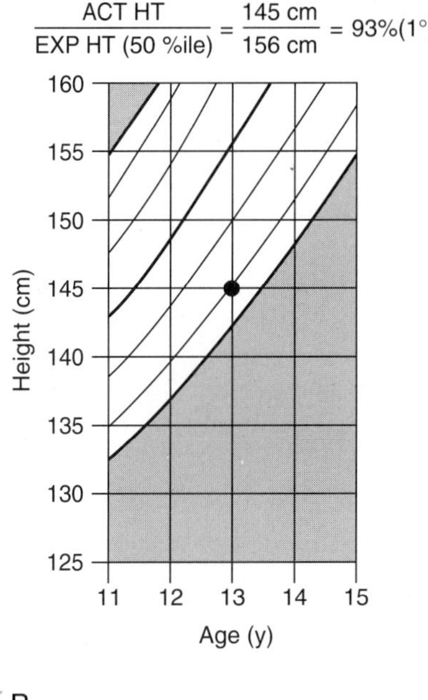


**FIGURE 58–11.** Clinical application of Waterlow criteria (see text for explanation).

**TABLE 58–5. Criteria for Malnutrition and Obesity**

| | DEGREE OF MALNUTRITION | | | | DEGREE OF OBESITY | | | |
|---|---|---|---|---|---|---|---|---|
| CRITERIA | 0 (Normal) | 1 (Mild) | 2 (Moderate) | 3 (Severe) | (Normal) | (Overweight) | (Obese) | (Morbid) |
| Weight for height (% expected) | ≥90 | <90 | <80 | <70 | ≤110 | >110 | >120 | >140 |
| Height for age (% expected) | ≥95 | <95 | <90 | <85 | | | | |
| MAC/FOC | ≥0.31 | <0.31 | <0.28 | <0.25 | | | | |

MAC, midarm circumference; FOC, fronto-occipital head circumference.
Data from references 32 through 34.

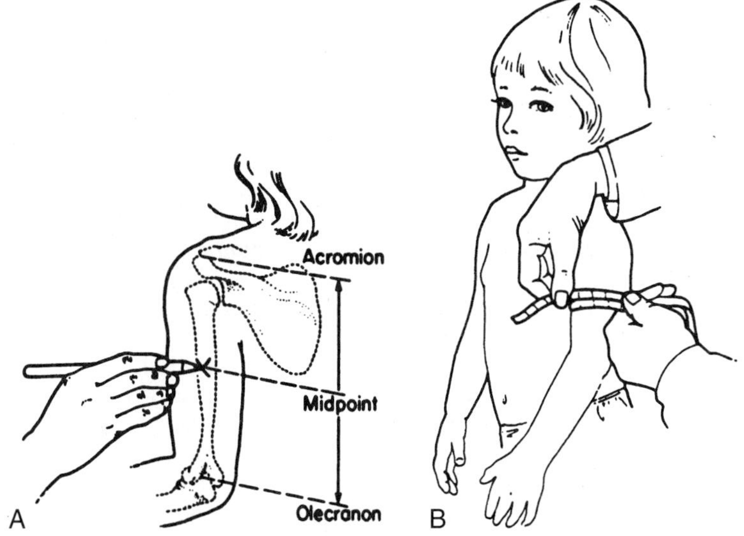


**FIGURE 58–12.** Technique for measuring mid upper arm length *(A)* and circumference *(B)*. (From Jelliffe DB: The Assessment of the Nutritional Stature of the Community. Geneva, World Health Organization, 1966, Monograph Series No. 53, with permission.)

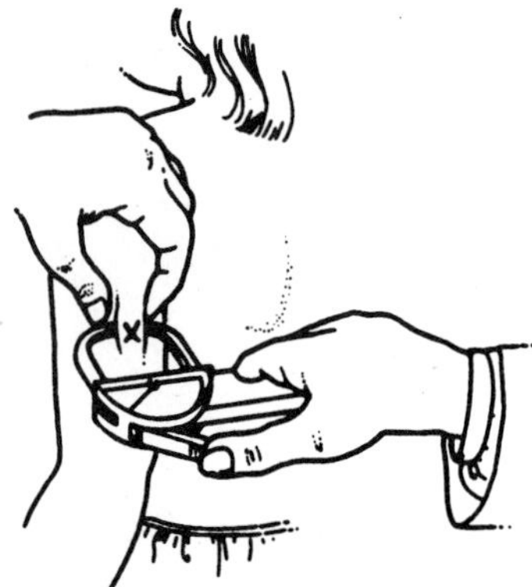

**FIGURE 58–13.** Technique for measuring triceps skinfold thickness. (From Jelliffe DB: The Assessment of the Nutritional Stature of the Community. Geneva, World Health Organization, 1966, Monograph Series No. 53, with permission.)

**TABLE 58–6. Body Mass Index ($kg/m^2$) for Children (1–5 yr)**

| GENDER | AGE (yr) | PERCENTILE | | |
|---|---|---|---|---|
| | | 5th | 50th | 95th |
| Males | 1 | 14.6 | 17.2 | 19.9 |
| | 2 | 14.4 | 16.5 | 19.0 |
| | 3 | 14.0 | 16.0 | 18.4 |
| | 4 | 13.8 | 15.8 | 18.1 |
| | 5 | 13.7 | 15.5 | 18.0 |
| Females | 1 | 14.7 | 16.6 | 19.3 |
| | 2 | 14.3 | 16.0 | 18.7 |
| | 3 | 13.9 | 15.6 | 18.3 |
| | 4 | 13.6 | 15.4 | 18.2 |
| | 5 | 13.5 | 15.3 | 18.3 |

Data from Hammer LD, Kraemer HC, Wilson DM, et al: Standardized percentile curve of body-mass index for children and adolescents. Am J Dis Child 1991;145:259–263.

nesses are secondary measurements that may be useful to assess the regional distribution of muscle wasting and loss or gain of peripheral body fat depots using the same calculations as described for the upper arm. In addition, four skinfold sites—biceps, triceps, subscapular, and suprailiac—have been measured collectively to provide a better estimate of body fat using the following age- and gender-specific equations:[12, 37]

| Gender | Age (yr) | Body Density *(y)* |
|---|---|---|
| Male | 2–18 | $y = [1.1315 + 0.0018\,(a - 2)] - \{0.0719 - [0.0006\,(a - 2) \cdot \log x]\}$ |
| Female | 2–10 | $y = [1.1315 + 0.0004\,(a - 2)] - \{0.0719 - [0.0003\,(a - 2) \cdot \log x]\}$ |
| | 11–18 | $y = [1.1350 + 0.0031\,(a - 10)] - \{0.0719 - [0.0003\,(a - 2) \cdot \log x]\}$ |

where $y$ equals body density, $a$ equals age (yr), $x$ equals the sum of the triceps, biceps, subscapular, and suprailiac skinfold thicknesses (mm), and

$$BF = \left(\frac{4.95}{y} - 4.5\right) \cdot 100$$

where BF equals the proportion (%) of body weight that is composed of body fat. The absolute body fat mass can be calculated as the multiple of BF and body weight, and the absolute lean body mass can be calculated as the difference between body weight and the absolute body fat mass. Although these measurements can be made readily in the clinical setting, anthropometric measurements may not provide substantially greater additional information about the nutritional status of the child than height and weight measurements.

## Laboratory Tests

Selected laboratory tests may be useful to assess the nutritional status of the child with gastrointestinal disease, although in the current era of managed care and cost containment, judicious use of these tools is warranted (Table 58–8). Laboratory tests may identify deficiencies before clinical findings are evident, may confirm the presence of selected nutrient deficiencies that are commonly associated with specific gastrointestinal entities, or may be helpful to monitor the clinical recovery from malnutrition when it occurs as a complicating feature of specific gastrointestinal diseases. Nevertheless, laboratory tests have limited usefulness over and above the clinical findings determined from growth and anthropometric measurements.

Malnutrition is associated with global nutrient deficits, but in general these deficiencies are not severe enough to be reflected in blood plasma or serum values. A complete blood cell count and serum ferritin level may be useful to confirm the diagnosis of iron deficiency anemia. Tests for urine specific gravity, serum electrolytes and carbon dioxide, or blood urea nitrogen (BUN) may be useful to determine the hydration, electrolyte, and acid-base status of the child. Low BUN or serum transthyretin levels suggest poor dietary intake of recent onset, whereas low albumin levels suggest poor dietary intake of long-standing duration. Low serum values of vitamin A, E, or 25-hydroxyvitamin D may be present in malabsorption disorders. Magnesium or zinc deficiencies may be found in chronic diarrheal illnesses. Elevated serum cholesterol and triglyceride levels, impaired glucose tolerance, and increased insulin levels may occur in conjunction with drug-associated obesity.

Although all laboratory tests may be of clinical importance, the most valuable tests of nutritional status in children with gastrointestinal disease are hemoglobin concentrations and red cell indices (mean corpuscular volume, mean corpuscular hemoglobin), as well as serum potassium, phosphorus, transthyretin, and albumin levels. Iron deficiency anemia is the most common nutritional anemia associated with chronic gastrointestinal diseases and should be assessed routinely. Hypochromic, microcytic, red cell morphology suggests iron deficiency anemia. Serum ferritin is the most sensitive measure of the adequacy of body iron status. Depressed serum folate levels may be the consequences of drug-nutrient interactions (e.g., sulfasalazine) or diffuse inflammation of the gastrointestinal tract. On the other hand, low vitamin $B_{12}$ levels occur in response to localized disease of the terminal ilium. Potassium and phosphorus are labile serum minerals that should be monitored carefully early in the course of aggressive nutritional rehabilitation of children with malnutrition. Serum potassium and phosphorus levels

**TABLE 58–7. Body Mass Index (kg/m²) for White and African American Children (6–18 yr)**

| | | PERCENTILE BY RACE | | | | | | | |
|---|---|---|---|---|---|---|---|---|---|
| | | White | | | | African American | | | |
| GENDER | AGE (yr) | *5th* | *50th* | *85th* | *95th* | *5th* | *50th* | *85th* | *95th* |
| Males | 6 | 12.93 | 14.62 | 16.52 | 17.75 | 12.68 | 14.49 | 16.83 | 18.58 |
| | 7 | 13.30 | 15.15 | 17.31 | 18.98 | 13.11 | 14.98 | 17.29 | 19.56 |
| | 8 | 13.67 | 15.70 | 18.10 | 20.22 | 13.54 | 15.49 | 17.76 | 20.51 |
| | 9 | 14.04 | 16.24 | 18.88 | 21.45 | 13.98 | 16.00 | 18.26 | 21.45 |
| | 10 | 14.42 | 16.79 | 19.67 | 22.66 | 14.41 | 16.53 | 18.78 | 22.41 |
| | 11 | 14.81 | 17.35 | 20.47 | 23.87 | 14.86 | 17.06 | 19.32 | 23.42 |
| | 12 | 15.21 | 17.93 | 21.28 | 25.01 | 15.36 | 17.61 | 19.85 | 24.39 |
| | 13 | 15.69 | 18.57 | 22.12 | 26.06 | 15.89 | 18.28 | 20.62 | 25.26 |
| | 14 | 16.16 | 19.25 | 22.97 | 27.02 | 16.43 | 18.94 | 21.54 | 26.13 |
| | 15 | 16.57 | 19.94 | 23.82 | 27.86 | 16.97 | 19.56 | 22.50 | 27.05 |
| | 16 | 17.00 | 20.63 | 24.63 | 28.69 | 17.51 | 20.19 | 23.45 | 27.95 |
| | 17 | 17.29 | 21.13 | 25.44 | 29.50 | 17.86 | 20.70 | 24.41 | 28.89 |
| | 18 | 17.50 | 21.46 | 26.08 | 29.89 | 18.05 | 21.09 | 25.06 | 29.35 |
| Females | 6 | 12.81 | 14.33 | 16.14 | 17.49 | 12.52 | 13.83 | 16.24 | 18.58 |
| | 7 | 13.18 | 15.00 | 17.16 | 18.93 | 12.88 | 14.55 | 17.36 | 19.56 |
| | 8 | 13.57 | 15.68 | 18.19 | 20.36 | 13.25 | 15.26 | 18.49 | 20.51 |
| | 9 | 13.96 | 16.35 | 19.21 | 21.78 | 13.63 | 15.98 | 19.64 | 21.45 |
| | 10 | 14.36 | 17.02 | 20.23 | 23.20 | 14.02 | 16.69 | 20.79 | 22.41 |
| | 11 | 14.76 | 17.69 | 21.24 | 24.59 | 14.41 | 17.39 | 21.96 | 23.42 |
| | 12 | 15.17 | 18.36 | 22.25 | 25.95 | 14.83 | 18.11 | 23.15 | 24.39 |
| | 13 | 15.59 | 18.91 | 23.13 | 27.07 | 15.33 | 18.78 | 24.41 | 25.26 |
| | 14 | 15.89 | 19.29 | 23.87 | 27.97 | 15.77 | 19.24 | 25.46 | 26.13 |
| | 15 | 16.21 | 19.69 | 24.28 | 28.51 | 16.20 | 19.67 | 26.04 | 27.05 |
| | 16 | 16.55 | 20.11 | 24.68 | 29.10 | 16.65 | 20.11 | 26.68 | 27.95 |
| | 17 | 16.76 | 20.39 | 25.07 | 29.72 | 16.92 | 20.45 | 27.38 | 28.89 |
| | 18 | 16.87 | 20.58 | 25.34 | 30.22 | 17.04 | 20.78 | 27.92 | 29.35 |

Data from Must A, Dallal GE, Dietz WH: Reference data for obesity: 85th and 95th percentiles of body mass index (wt/ht²) and triceps skinfold thickness. Am J Clin Nutr 1991;53:839–846.

may decline rapidly during the early refeeding period because of intracellular ion shifts and can lead to unwanted complications such as cardiac arrhythmias. Transthyretin, a rapidly turning-over protein with a half-life of 2 days, is a good predictor of the adequacy of the diet and serves to corroborate the details of the diet history obtained from the parent. If dietary intakes have been poor, serum transthyretin levels fall rapidly.[38] If adequate refeeding has been reinstituted, serum transthyretin levels will rise to low normal levels within 10 days after initiating nutritional therapy, whereas serum albumin, a slowly turning-over protein, may not be restored to normal levels for at least 3 weeks after nutritional therapy has commenced (Fig. 58–14).[39] On the other hand, the serum albumin level serves as a good predictor of gastrointestinal tolerance to enteral feedings,[40] with the likelihood that higher protein and energy intakes can be provided when serum albumin levels are greater than 30 g/L. The serum albumin level is also a good predictor of morbidity and mortality; when serum albumin levels fall below 10 to 15 g/L, the mortality rate of malnourished children approximates 40%.[41]

The assessment of specific nutrient deficiencies may be necessary in those gastrointestinal diseases in which malabsorption or inflammation is a prominent feature of the clinical course. Fat-soluble vitamin (A, D, E, K) levels should be monitored at 6-month to yearly intervals in children with malabsorption disorders such as cystic fibrosis and biliary atresia. In these conditions, low serum vitamin A, E, and 25-hydroxyvitamin D levels or a prolonged prothrombin time indicates the need for supplemental therapy. Serum folate and vitamin $B_{12}$ levels should be monitored at similar time intervals in children with gastrointestinal disorders that are associated with inflammatory processes of the terminal ileum (e.g., necrotizing enterocolitis, short gut syndrome, or Crohn's disease). Although water-soluble vitamin deficiencies have been described, the subclinical abnormalities that may occur in children with chronic gastrointestinal diseases remain difficult to diagnose and are of questionable significance.

## *Summary*

Nutritional assessment is an essential component of the evaluation of children with gastrointestinal diseases because the clinical course of these individuals frequently is complicated by nutritional disorders such as malnutrition, growth failure, drug-induced obesity, and iron deficiency anemia. Although a complete nutritional assessment includes a review of the diet history, physical examination, anthropometric measurements, and selected laboratory testing, accurate height and weight measurements, and their transformation to relative indices of overnutrition or undernutrition, serve as the mainstay of the nutritional assessment of the child with gastrointestinal disorders. The maintenance of a favorable nutritional status is essential to minimize disease-associated morbidity and enhance the child's quality of life.

**TABLE 58–8. Normal Values: Biochemical Measurements of Nutritional Status**

| TEST | AGE GROUP | | | |
|---|---|---|---|---|
| | **Birth–1 mo** | **1–12 mo** | **1–9 yr** | **9–18 yr** |
| **Protein** | | | | |
| Blood | | | | |
| Serum albumin (g/dL) | ≥2.5 | ≥3 | ≥3.5 | ≥3.5 |
| Retinol-binding protein (mg/dL) | 2–3 | 2–3 | 2–3 | 3–6 |
| Blood urea nitrogen (mg/dL) | 7–22 | 7–22 | 7–22 | 7–22 |
| Transthyretin (mg/dL) | 20–50 | 20–50 | 20–50 | 20–50 |
| Transferrin (mg/dL) | 170–250 | 170–250 | 170–250 | 170–250 |
| Urine | | | | |
| Creatinine/height index | >0.9 | >0.9 | >0.9 | >0.9 |
| 3-Methylhistidine (μmol/kg creatinine) | 253±78 | | | 126±32 |
| **Vitamin A** | | | | |
| Plasma retinol (μg/dL) | ≥30 | ≥30 | ≥30 | ≥30 |
| Plasma retinol-binding protein (mg/dL) | 2–3 | 2–3 | 2–3 | 2–3 |
| **Vitamin D** | | | | |
| 25-OH-$D_3$ (ng/mL) | ≥20 | ≥20 | ≥20 | ≥20 |
| **Riboflavin** | | | | |
| Red cell glutathione reductase stimulation (%) | <20 | <20 | <20 | <20 |
| **Vitamin $B_6$** | | | | |
| Red cell transaminases<br>Plasma pyridoxal phosphate<br>Xanthurenic acid excretion | Not readily available; not practical in children younger than 9 years of age | | | |
| **Folacin** | | | | |
| Serum folate (ng/mL) | >6 | >6 | >6 | >6 |
| Red blood cell folate (ng/mL) | >160 | >160 | >160 | >160 |
| **Vitamin K** | | | | |
| Prothrombin time (sec) | 11–15 | 11–15 | 11–15 | 11–15 |
| **Vitamin E** | | | | |
| Plasma α-tocopherol (mg/dL) | ≥0.7 | ≥0.7 | ≥0.7 | ≥0.7 |
| Red blood cell hemolysis (%) | ≤10 | ≤10 | ≤10 | ≤10 |
| **Vitamin C** | | | | |
| Plasma (mg/dL) | >0.2 | >0.2 | >0.2 | >0.2 |
| Leukocyte (μg/$10^8$ cells) | Difficult to perform on infants and children because of sample requirements | | | |
| **Thiamine** | | | | |
| Red blood cell transketolase stimulation (%) | >5 | >15 | >15 | >15 |
| **Vitamin $B_{12}$** | | | | |
| Serum vitamin $B_{12}$ (pg/mL) | ≥200 | ≥200 | ≥200 | ≥200 |
| Absorption test | Excretion of more than 7.5% of the orally ingested labeled vitamin $B_{12}$ | | | |
| **Iron** | | | | |
| Hematocrit (%) | 31 | 33 | 36 | 36 |
| Hemoglobin (g/dL) | >12 | >12 | >13 | >13 |
| Serum ferritin (ng/mL) | >10 | >10 | >10 | >10 |
| Serum iron (μg/dL) | >30 | >40 | >50 | >60 |
| Serum total iron-binding capacity (μg/dL) | 350–400 | 350–400 | 350–400 | 350–400 |
| Serum transferrin saturation (%) | >12 | >12 | >15 | >16 |
| Serum transferrin (mg/dL) | 170–250 | 170–250 | 170–250 | 170–250 |
| Erythrocyte protoporphyrin (μg/dL red blood cells) | <80 | <75 | <70 | <70 |
| **Zinc** | | | | |
| Serum zinc (μg/dL) | 80–120 | 80–120 | 80–120 | 80–120 |
| Erythrocyte zinc | Erythrocytes contain approximately 10 times more zinc than does plasma | | | |

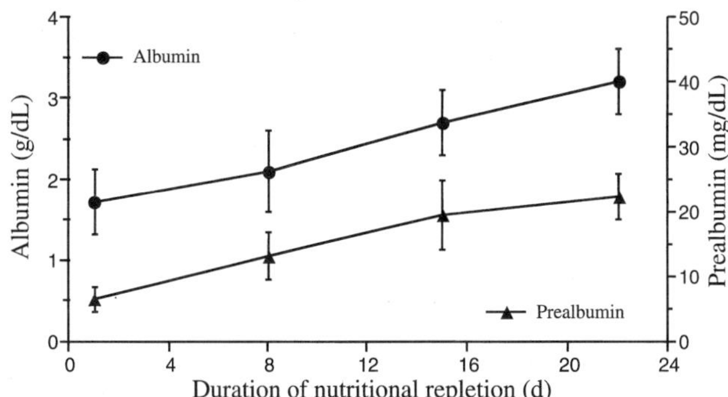


**FIGURE 58–14.** Response of serum albumin and prealbumin to refeeding in malnourished children. (Data from Helms RA, Dickerson RN, Ebbert ML, et al: Retinol-binding protein and prealbumin: useful measures of protein repletion in critically ill, malnourished infants. J Pediatr Gastroenterol Nutr 1986;5:586–592; and Ingenbleek Y, De Visscher M, De Nayer P: Measurement of prealbumin as index of protein-calorie malnutrition. Lancet 1972;2:106–109.)

*Acknowledgments*

The authors thank I. Tapper for secretarial support, L.A. Loddeke for editorial assistance, and A. Gillum for illustrations.

This work is a publication of the USDA/ARS Children's Nutrition Research Center, Department of Pediatrics, Baylor College of Medicine, Houston, TX, and has been funded in part with federal funds from the U.S. Department of Agriculture, Agricultural Research Service, under Cooperative Agreement Number 58-6250-1-003. The contents of this publication do not necessarily reflect the views or policies of the U.S. Department of Agriculture, nor does mention of trade names, commercial products, or organizations imply endorsement by the U.S. government.

## REFERENCES

1. Viteri FE: Primary protein-energy malnutrition: clinical, biochemical, and metabolic changes. In Suskind RM (ed): Textbook of Pediatric Nutrition. New York, Raven Press, 1981, pp 189–215.
2. Motil KJ, Grand RJ, Matthews DE, et al: Whole body leucine metabolism in adolescents with Crohn's disease and growth failure during nutritional supplementation. Gastroenterology 1982;82:1359–1368.
3. Beisel WR: Interrelated changes in host metabolism during generalized infectious illness. Am J Clin Nutr 1972;25:1254–1260.
4. Hamill PVV, Drizd TA, Johnson CL, et al: NCHS growth charts, 1976. Monthly Vital Statistics Report. Health Examination Survey Data from the National Center for Health Statistics. (HRA)76-1120, vol 25, No 3, Supplement. Rockville, MD, US Department of Health, Education, and Welfare, Public Health Service, Health Resources Administration, June 22, 1976.
5. Spady DW, Payne PR, Picou D, et al: Energy balance during recovery from malnutrition. Am J Clin Nutr 1976;29:1073–1088.
6. Wang Z-M, Pierson RN, Heymsfield SB: The five-level model: a new approach to organizing body-composition research. Am J Clin Nutr 1992;56:19–28.
7. Fomon SJ, Haschke F, Ziegler EE, et al: Body composition of reference children from birth to 10 years. Am J Clin Nutr 1982;35:1169–1175.
8. Ellis KJ, Abrams SA, Wong WW: Body composition of a young, multiethnic female population. Am J Clin Nutr 1997;65:724–731.
9. Ellis KJ: Body composition of a young multiethnic male population. Am J Clin Nutr 1997;66:1323–1331.
10. Klish WJ, Kretchmer N: Body composition measurements in infants and children. Columbus, OH, Ross Laboratories, 1989, pp 1–151.
11. Frisancho AR: New norms of upper limb fat and muscle areas for assessment of nutritional status. Am J Clin Nutr 1981;34:2540–2545.
12. Westrate JA, Devrenberg P: Body composition in children: proposal for a method for calculating body fat percentage from total body density or skinfold thickness measurements. Am J Clin Nutr 1989;50:1104–1115.
13. Schoeller DA, van Santen E, Peterson DW, et al: Total body water measurement in humans with $^{18}O$ and $^{2}H$ labeled water. Am J Clin Nutr 1980;33:2686–2693.
14. Fioritto M: Application of the TOBEC measurement for determining fat and fat-free mass of the human infant. In Klish WJ, Kretchmer N (eds): Body Composition Measurements in Infants and Children. Report of the 98th Ross Conference on Pediatric Research. Columbus, OH, Ross Laboratories, 1989, p 57.
15. Segal KR, Burastero S, Chun A, et al: Estimation of extracellular and total body water by multiple frequency bioelectrical-impedance measurement. Am J Clin Nutr 1991;54:26–29.
16. Forbes GB, Simon W, Amatruda JM: Is bioimpedance a good predictor of body composition change? Am J Clin Nutr 1992;56:4–6.
17. Lukaski HC: Soft tissue composition and bone mineral status: evaluation by dual-energy x-ray absorptiometry. J Nutr 1993;123:438–443.
18. Ellis KJ, Nichols BL: Body composition. Adv Pediatr 1993;40:159–184.
19. Heymsfield SB, Wang Z, Baumgartner RN, et al: Body composition and aging: a study by in vivo neutron activation analysis. J Nutr 1993;123:432–437.
20. Baumgartner RN, Rhyne RL, Garry PJ, et al: Imaging techniques and anatomical body composition in aging. J Nutr 1993;123:444–448.
21. Hubbard VS: Clinical assessment of nutritional status. In Walker WA, Watkins JB (eds): Nutrition in Pediatrics: Basic Science and Clinical Application, 2nd ed. Toronto, BC Decker, 1997, p 7.
22. Lo C: Laboratory assessment of nutritional status. In Walker WA, Watkins JB (eds): Nutrition in Pediatrics: Basic Science and Clinical Application, 2nd ed. Toronto, BC Decker, 1997, p 29.
23. Puig M: Body composition and growth. In Walker WA, Watkins JB (eds): Nutrition in Pediatrics: Basic Science and Clinical Application, 2nd ed. Toronto, BC Decker, 1997, p 44.
24. Food and Nutrition Board, National Research Council: Recommended Dietary Allowances, 10th ed. Washington, DC, National Academy of Sciences, 1989.
25. U.S. Department of Health and Human Services: Dietary Guidelines for Americans, 4th ed. Washington, DC, U.S. Government Printing Office, 1995.
26. U.S. Department of Agriculture: The Food Guide Pyramid. Home and Garden Bulletin, No. 252, 1992.
27. Herbert V: Toxicity of 25,000 IU vitamin A supplements in "health" food users. Am J Clin Nutr 1982;36:185–186.
28. Jelliffe DB: The assessment of the nutritional status of the community. Geneva, World Health Organization, 1966, Monograph Series No 53.
29. Greulich WW, Pyle SI: Radiographic Atlas of Skeletal Development of the Hand and Wrist, 2nd ed. Stanford, CA, Stanford University Press, 1959.
30. Roche AF, Himes JH: Incremental growth charts. Am J Clin Nutr 1980;33:2041–2052.
31. Kanof ME, Lake AM, Bayles TM: Decreased height velocity in children and adolescents before the diagnosis of Crohn's disease. Gastroenterology 1988;95:1523–1527.
32. Waterlow JC: Classification and definition of protein-calorie malnutrition. BMJ 1972;3:566–569.
33. Waterlow JC: Note on the assessment and classification of protein-energy malnutrition in children. Lancet 1973;2:87–89.
34. Kanawati AA, McLaren DS: Assessment of marginal malnutrition. Nature 1970;228:573–575.
35. Hammer LD, Kraemer HC, Wilson DM, et al: Standardized percentile curve of body-mass index for children and adolescents. Am J Dis Child 1991;145:259–263.
36. Must A, Dallal GE, Dietz WH: Reference data for obesity: 85th and 95th percentiles of body mass index (wt/ht$^2$) and triceps skinfold thickness. Am J Clin Nutr 1991;53:839–846.
37. Brook CGD: Determination of body composition of children from skinfold measurements. Arch Dis Child 1971;46:182–184.
38. Ingenbleek Y, De Visscher M, De Nayer P: Measurement of prealbumin as index of protein-calorie malnutrition. Lancet 1972;2:106–109.

39. Helms RA, Dickerson RN, Ebbert ML, et al: Retinol-binding protein and prealbumin: useful measures of protein repletion in critically ill, malnourished infants. J Pediatr Gastroenterol Nutr 1986;5:586–592.
40. Ford EG, Jennings M, Andrassy RJ: Serum albumin (oncotic pressure) correlates with enteral feeding tolerance in the pediatric patient. J Pediatr Surg 1987;22:597–599.
41. Waterlow JC: Protein-energy malnutrition: challenges and controversies. Proc Nutr Soc India 1991;37:59–87.

Chapter 59

# Parenteral and Enteral Nutrition

*Maria R. Mascarenhas, Andrew M. Tershakovec, and Virginia A. Stallings*

## PARENTERAL NUTRITION

Parenteral nutrition (PN) is the intravenous administration of nutrients necessary for the maintenance of life. These nutrients include dextrose, amino acids, fat, electrolytes, multivitamins, and trace elements. Clinicians caring for infants and children need to be concerned with the changing nutrient requirements with age; specialized needs of children; vascular access; the sometimes limited ability to handle large amounts of fluid, protein, fat, and carbohydrates; and nutritional therapeutics.[1] Guidelines have been developed for the use of nutrition support.[2]

### Indications

The enteral route is the one of choice for providing nourishment to any patient. It is only in those instances when a patient cannot receive some or all of his or her nutrition enterally that the parenteral route should be used. Every attempt must be made to start and advance the delivery of enteral nutrition when the patient's tolerance for enteral feeds improves. PN is therefore used in patients who cannot be fed enterally for 5 or more days and should be used to support the patient until recovery from the underlying condition has occurred. Appropriate indications include severe burns, liver failure, chemotherapy-induced emesis and feeding intolerance, after bone marrow transplantation or surgery, and severe diarrhea and malabsorption (Table 59–1). This is especially important in the patient with pre-existing malnutrition or with a chronic disease. PN may be used to supplement enteral intake in patients who have increased needs (e.g., patients with chronic diarrhea, malabsorption, short bowel syndrome, or cystic fibrosis) or who are unable to tolerate adequate enteral feeds to support themselves nutritionally. The use of supplemental PN should be considered when slow advancement of enteral feeds is anticipated. In addition to a supportive role, PN may be used to treat the underlying condition (e.g., chylothorax).

### Route of Administration

Parenteral nutrition can be administered via a central or peripheral venous route depending on the access available and the composition of the PN solution. Peripheral PN is generally used for patients whose nutritional status is normal, the anticipated period of inadequate enteral feedings is short (less than 2 weeks), and who have normal fluid requirements.[3] It is often difficult to maintain peripheral access for longer than 2 weeks or to deliver adequate calories with solutions containing 10% or 12.5% dextrose solutions. When hyperosmolar solutions with higher dextrose concentrations are administered through a peripheral intravenous line there is a risk of phlebitis and thrombosis. Solutions with high dextrose (>10–12.5% dextrose) and calcium concentrations may have increased risk for phlebitis. The concomitant administration of intravenous fat may help decrease these complications. Depending on the size of the vein, it may also not be possible to infuse large volumes or at a high rate. The central venous route is used for the administration of hypertonic solutions and for high infusion rates and chronic administration of PN solutions (more than 4 to 6 weeks).[4] This may be either a percutaneous intravenous central catheter line, a tunneled catheter (e.g., Broviac), or an implantable port (e.g., Portocath). It is recommended that the tip of the catheter be placed at the junction of the superior vena cava and right atrium. When femoral lines or umbilical venous catheters are used, the tip of the catheter should be placed above the level of the diaphragm.

Long lines or percutaneous intravenous central catheter lines are threaded into the heart through a peripheral vein. The success of their placement is dependent on the anatomy of the vein chosen (i.e., presence of valves and patency of vein) and experience of the person placing the lines. They have been used since the 1980s and are now quite popular because there are few limitations regarding their use related to age, gender, or diagnosis. They can remain in place for up to 1 year without complications. There is a low incidence of complications with percutaneous intravenous central catheter lines (less than 1% for infection, central vein thrombo-

**TABLE 59–1. Common Indications for Parenteral Nutrition**

- Prematurity
- Gastrointestinal tract
  - Congenital anomalies—atresia
  - Surgical disease—small bowel resection
  - Intractable diarrhea
  - Inflammatory bowel disease
  - Pseudo-obstruction syndrome
  - Liver failure
- Respiratory tract
  - Respiratory failure
  - Cystic fibrosis
- Hypermetabolic conditions
  - Sepsis
  - Burns
  - Major trauma
- Malignancy and bone marrow transplantation
- Cardiovascular
  - Congenital heart disease
  - Postoperative
- Miscellaneous
  - Inborn errors of metabolism
  - Chronic renal disease

sis, and catheter malposition). Additionally, cost savings are associated with the use of this type of catheter. Contraindications to the placement of percutaneous intravenous central catheter lines include dermatitis, cellulitis, and burns at or near the insertion site and previous ipsilateral venous thrombosis.

Patients receiving chronic PN benefit from the placement of a permanent central venous catheter or tunneled Silastic catheter (e.g., Broviac, Hickman, Portocath, and Groshong catheters) and subcutaneous ports.[5–7] These catheters are generally placed by a surgeon or an interventional radiologist using general anesthesia or conscious sedation. Tunneled catheters can be placed either via a cutdown or percutaneously and have a Dacron cuff located on the midportion of the catheter. This cuff stimulates the formation of dense fibrous adhesions, which anchor the catheter subcutaneously to prevent dislodgment of the catheter and also act as a barrier to bacteria migrating subcutaneously along the catheter surface. Sutures are needed to anchor the catheter at the exit site for several weeks after insertion to allow time for the formation of fibrous adhesions to the Dacron cuff.

Implantable ports are made of plastic or titanium with a compressed silicon disk that is designed for 1,000 to 2,000 insertions with a noncoring needle. They are inserted either percutaneously or by cutdown into the jugular, subclavian, or cephalic vein and placed in a subcutaneous pocket over the upper chest wall. There are smaller ports available that are primarily used for arm placement and for children. These ports are generally used in situations in which the catheter is only periodically accessed.

PN can also be delivered via peritoneal or hemodialysis catheters. Intradialytic PN is the administration of PN during dialysis.[8] PN solution can be infused during hemodialysis three times a week. This has been shown to be useful in those patients with end-stage renal disease not responding to oral nutritional intervention.

## Components of Parenteral Nutrition

### *Protein*

Protein in PN solutions is provided as crystalline amino acids.[9] Refinement in the protein source has generally eliminated previously common problems of metabolic acidosis and hyperammonemia. One gram of protein provides approximately 4 calories. There are several protein solutions available for use in infants, in children, and in special circumstances (e.g., hepatic and renal failure). Protein solutions used in infants differ from those used in children and adults in their amino acid composition. Certain amino acids considered nonessential in adults are essential in infants (i.e., cysteine, histidine, and tyrosine). In addition, lysine and arginine are considered semi-essential in infants. Trophamine (McGaw, Inc., Irvine, CA) is a commonly used protein solution in infants, including preterm infants. Its formulation was based on serum amino acid profiles of healthy 1-month-old breast-fed infants. Trophamine contains the essential amino acids taurine, tyrosine, and histidine in addition to aspartic acid, glutamic acid, and dicarboxylic acids. It differs from the adult formulations in that it contains tyrosine, taurine, and histidine, which the preterm infant requires. It also has a higher concentration of branched-chain amino acids and so may be advantageous for use in patients with chronic liver disease and cholestasis. In addition, branched-chain amino acid supplementation has been shown to improve nitrogen balance, protein synthesis, and immunocompetence in septic or trauma patients.[9]

Novamine (Clintec Nutrition Co., Deerfield, IL) is a standard protein formulation given to patients older than 6 months of age. It is available in 1% to 15% solution. The 15% solution is particularly useful in the fluid-restricted patient.

HepatAmine (McGaw, Inc., Irvine, CA) is a specialized amino acid formulation that contains increased amounts of branched-chain amino acids and reduced amounts of methionine and aromatic amino acids. It was designed for use in patients with severe liver failure and hepatic encephalopathy. However, studies have not demonstrated a clear beneficial survival effect in these patients.

Protein needs (in grams per kilogram of body weight) decline progressively with age and are higher in infants and children than in adults because of differing growth rates.[10] There are certain conditions when protein intake needs to be higher than normal, because of increased losses (protein-losing enteropathy) or increased needs (protein-calorie malnutrition, sepsis, inflammatory bowel disease). Protein can be safely administered on the first or second day of life in preterm infants.[11] Total protein needs can be provided on the day of initiation of PN, except in the infant with a very low birth weight (where goal protein intake can be achieved in 1 to 3 days), in critically ill patients with hepatic and renal insufficiency (not on dialysis), and in patients with disorders of protein metabolism. (See Tables 59–2 and 59–3 for guidelines for protein requirements and composition of commonly used protein solutions.)

Glutamine is a neutral amino acid that was originally considered to be nonessential but is currently classified as conditionally essential. Studies have shown improved nitrogen balance, immunocompetence and decreased sepsis, and maintenance of protein synthesis in postoperative patients. Glutamine has been shown to have a beneficial effect in patients with short bowel syndrome, those who have undergone bone marrow transplantation or trauma, and the critically ill.[12, 13] Glutamine supplementation has been shown to be safe in preterm infants.[14] It is not present in the currently

**TABLE 59–2. Protein Requirements During Parenteral Nutrition**

| | PROTEIN (g/kg/ day) |
|---|---|
| Preterm infants | 2.5–3.5 |
| Full-term infants | |
| Early infancy (birth–6 mo) | 2.5–3.0 |
| Late infancy (6–12 mo) | 2.0–2.5 |
| Children | |
| 1–6 yr | 1.0–2 |
| 7–10 yr | 1.0–2 |
| 11–18 yr | 0.8–2 |

available amino acid formulations and is unstable in solution, although this can be avoided by the use of glutamine dipeptides.

Carnitine is synthesized in the body from two essential amino acids, lysine and methionine, and is required for the transport of long-chain fatty acids into the mitochondria.[15] Supplementation of PN solutions in premature infants has been suggested to correct low free and acylcarnitine levels. Although hereditary carnitine deficiency responds to carnitine supplementation, it is not clear whether the low levels seen in premature infants[16] and patients with short bowel syndrome represent a true deficiency and need to be supplemented.

## *Carbohydrates*

Carbohydrate in PN is provided as dextrose and constitutes the main source of calories. Approximately 3.4 calories is obtained from 1 g of dextrose because of its formulation (monohydrate form) for intravenous use. Glucose delivery is usually expressed in milligrams per kilogram of body weight per minute, with neonates and infants generally requiring a glucose infusion rate of 5 to 12 mg/kg/min and older children one of 2 to 5 mg/kg/min. Glucose utilization in neonates has been shown to decrease when glucose delivery is 14 mg/kg/min and greater.[17] Only a 10% dextrose solution should be given through a peripheral vein because more concentrated dextrose solutions can result in osmolalities greater than 900 mOsm/L and an increased risk of phlebitis.[3] In special circumstances a 12.5% dextrose solution may be used peripherally with caution. Care must be taken to keep the delivery of carbohydrate calories at 50% to 60% of total caloric intake. Unbalanced macronutrient regimens may have a role in PN-associated liver disease. Excessive carbohydrate intake is related to hepatic steatosis and increased carbon dioxide production, which may increase ventilator dependency. Concomitant use of an insulin infusion will help with control of hyperglycemia while providing adequate calories. This is preferably used as a separate infusion as opposed to putting it in the PN solution, because the insulin can get adsorbed to the tubing, resulting in lower amounts being delivered to the patient. It is impossible to adjust the rate of insulin infusion without affecting caloric intake and glucose homeostasis when insulin is mixed with the PN solution.

## *Lipids*

Fat provides a concentrated form of both calories and essential fatty acids, which are required for prostaglandin and membrane lipid synthesis, brain and somatic growth, immune function, skin integrity, and wound healing. Con-

**TABLE 59–3. Composition of Commonly Available Amino Acid Solutions***

| | NOVAMINE | TROPHAMINE | HEPATAMINE | AMINOSYN RF |
|---|---|---|---|---|
| **Essential Amino Acids** | | | | |
| L-Isoleucine | 50 | 82 | 113 | 88 |
| L-Leucine | 69 | 140 | 138 | 139 |
| L-Lysine | 79 | 82 | 76 | 102 |
| L-Methionine | 50 | 33 | 13 | 139 |
| L-Phenylalanine | 69 | 48 | 13 | 139 |
| L-Threonine | 50 | 42 | 56 | 63 |
| L-Tryptophan | 17 | 20 | 8 | 31 |
| L-Valine | 64 | 82 | 105 | 101 |
| **Nonessential Amino Acids** | | | | |
| L-Alanine | 145 | 53 | 96 | |
| L-Arginine | 98 | 122 | 75 | 115 |
| L-Aspartic acid | 29 | 32 | | |
| L-Glutamic acid | 50 | 50 | | |
| L-Glycine | 69 | 68 | 113 | |
| L-Histidine | 60 | 38 | 100 | |
| L-Serine | 39 | 37 | 63 | |
| L-Histidine | 60 | 48 | 30 | 82 |
| L-Taurine | | 2.5 | | |
| L-Tyrosine | 3 | 23 | | |
| % Essential amino acids | 45% | 53% | 52% | 80% |
| % Nonessential amino acids | 55% | 47% | 48% | 20% |
| % Branched-chain amino acids | | 30% | 35% | 33% |

*Expressed as milligrams of amino acid per gram of protein.

From Darby M (ed): The Children's Hospital of Philadelphia Pharmacy Handbook and Formulary 1995–1997. Hudson, OH, Lexi-Comp, Inc., 1995, with permission.

**TABLE 59–4. Composition of Intralipid Emulsions**

| | 10% | 20% | 30% |
|---|---|---|---|
| Glycerol (g) | 22 | 22 | 22 |
| Egg phospholipids (g) | 12 | 12 | 12 |
| Soybean oil (g) | 100 | 200 | 300 |
| Kcal/mL | 1.1 | 2 | 3 |
| Osmolality (mOsm/L) | 300 | 350 | 310 |

Adapted from Bilodeau J, Poon C, Mascarenhas MR: Parenteral nutrition/care of central lines. In Altschuler SM, Liacouras CA (eds): Pediatric Gastroenterology. London, Churchill Livingstone, 1998, with permission.

ventional intravenous fat emulsions contain long-chain triglycerides and are usually made from soybean and safflower oils. Intralipid (10%, 20%, 30%) is a commonly used intravenous fat emulsion that contains soybean[18] (Table 59–4). The 20% emulsion is commonly used because it is relatively concentrated and because the patient receives lower amounts of phospholipids, which results in lower plasma triglycerides, cholesterol, and phospholipid levels. The 10% emulsion may produce hyperlipidemia because of its high phospholipid:triglyceride ratio and so is rarely used.[19, 20] Phospholipids are thought to inhibit lipoprotein lipase, the main enzyme responsible for intravenous fat clearance. The newly available 30% emulsion can only be used in a total nutrient admixture and cannot be infused alone into a peripheral vein.

The total daily dose of intravenous fat should be delivered over 24 hours, except when PN is cycled. There is no need to give a rest period. Continuous 24-hour infusions are better tolerated than intermittent infusions. Intravenous fat is usually started at a relatively low initial dosage and increased over 1 to 3 days if triglyceride clearance is within normal limits (see Table 59–5 for dosage).

When a PN regimen is planned, care must be taken to keep the percentage of total calories from fat in the range of 30% to 40% and never more than 60% of total calories (ketogenic diet). The maximum dose of intravenous fat in infants is 3 to 4 g/kg/day, and this decreases with age. Patients with hypertriglyceridemia who may not be able to tolerate intravenously administered fat need to get at least 0.5 to 1 g/kg of intravenous fat twice a week or 2% to 4% of calories as long-chain fat to meet essential fatty acid requirements. Essential fatty acid deficiency develops in patients who are not receiving any long-chain fat. This develops sooner in preterm infants (as little as 2 days) than in adults. Clinical signs of essential fatty acid deficiency include growth failure, flaky dry skin, alopecia, thrombocytopenia, increased infections, and impaired wound healing. An abnormal triene-to-tetraene ratio or abnormal fatty acid profile is diagnostic.

**TABLE 59–5. Guidelines for Intravenous Fat Administration***

| | PRETERM INFANTS | FULL-TERM INFANTS | OLDER INFANTS |
|---|---|---|---|
| Initial dose | 1–2 | 1–2 | 1–2 |
| Dose increments | 0.5–1 | 1 | 1 |
| Maximum dose† | 3–4 | 3–4 | 2–3 |

*Expressed as g/kg/day.
†Percentage of calories from fat should not exceed more than 50–60% of total caloric intake.

Newer intravenous fat formulations have been developed to prevent the complications seen with the conventional fat emulsions. These new formulations consist of structured lipids (medium- and long-chain triglycerides attached to a glycerol backbone), medium-chain triglyceride emulsions, and mixtures of long- and medium-chain triglyceride emulsions.[21–24] Emulsions of long- and medium-chain triglycerides and of just medium-chain triglycerides have been used in infants as well as in patients receiving PN at home.[25, 26] However, these new formulations are not available in the United States.

## *Electrolytes and Minerals*

Electrolyte requirements vary with age. Thus they are added to the PN solution in maintenance concentrations.[27] These requirements are derived from the Recommended Dietary Allowances (RDAs), with allowances made for the efficiency of absorption (see Table 59–6 for dosing guidelines). It is preferable to obtain baseline serum electrolyte values before ordering a PN solution and then add electrolytes accordingly. Other factors affecting electrolyte dosing include underlying illness, renal function, and medications. Periodic monitoring of serum electrolytes is required, especially in the critically ill and malnourished patient. In neonates and children with high calcium and phosphorus needs, the amounts added to a PN solution may be limited due to solubility issues. Increasing the amount of protein and adding cysteine (thereby lowering the pH of the solution) can allow the addition of higher amounts of calcium and phosphorus to the PN solution without causing precipitation. In instances in which the patient's calcium and phosphorus requirements cannot be added to the PN solution, a separate infusion of calcium or phosphorus may need to be given.

**TABLE 59–6. Intravenous Requirements (Daily) for Electrolytes and Minerals**

| | PRETERM | TERM | CHILDREN >1 yr |
|---|---|---|---|
| Sodium (mEq/kg/day) | 2–3 | 2–4 | 2–3 |
| Potassium (mEq/kg/day) | 2–3 | 2–3 | 2–3 |
| Chloride (mEq/kg/day) | 2–3 | 2–4 | 2–3 |
| Magnesium (mEq/kg/day) | 0.35–0.6 | 0.25–0.5 | 0.2–0.5 |
| Calcium (mEq/kg/day) | 3–4.5 | 3–4 | 1–2 |
| Phosphorus (mEq/kg/day) | 2.7–4 | 1.5–3 | 0.7–1.4 |
| Zinc (μg/kg/day) | 150 | <3 mo 250<br>>3 mo 100 | 50–200 |
| Copper (μg/kg/day) | 20 | 20 | 20 |
| Chromium (μg/kg/day) | 0.05–0.2 | 0.2 | 0.14–0.2 |
| Manganese (μg/kg/day) | 1–5 | 1–5 | 1–5 |
| Iron (mg/kg/day) (for patients >2 mo) | 0.2 | 0.1 | 0.1 |
| Selenium (μg/kg/day) | 2 | 2 | 2 |
| Molybdenum (μg/kg/day) | 0.2 | 0.25 | 0.25 |

From Darby M (ed): The Children's Hospital of Philadelphia Pharmacy Handbook and Formulary 1995–1997. Hudson, OH, Lexi-Comp, Inc., 1995, with permission.

### Vitamins

Recommendations for vitamin (fat- and water-soluble vitamin) requirements for infants, children, and adults are given in Table 59–7. PN vitamin recommendations are derived from these. There are currently two multivitamin (MVI) preparations used in the United States—pediatric and adult formulations. The pediatric MVI preparation was designed to meet the needs of preterm and term infants and children. It is used in infants and children up to 10 years of age.[27, 28] It is dosed on a per kilogram basis; preterm infants receive 40% of a vial per kilogram of body weight. The adult MVI preparation differs from the pediatric MVI preparation (generally has greater concentrations of the different vitamins per milliliter, except less vitamin D than pediatric MVI, and has no vitamin K). For children older than 10 years of age, the adult MVI is used with additional vitamin K. The dosing recommendations for vitamins take into account the losses associated with administration. For example, up to 40% of vitamin A may be lost because of adherence to the intravenous tubing. It has been shown that pyridoxine and riboflavin levels may be affected by light while the PN solution is hung at the patient's bedside (see Table 59–8 for vitamin requirements and composition of commonly available preparations).

### Trace Elements

In addition to the previously discussed components, iron, zinc, copper, chromium, manganese, selenium, and molybdenum need to be added to make the PN solution complete. These are dosed according to published guidelines.[27] We give all patients maintenance doses of iron (0.1 mg/kg/day) after 2 months of age, with the exception of chronically transfused patients (e.g., those with anemia and malignancies after bone marrow transplantation). Iron-deficient patients may receive additional amounts based on results of iron studies.

Additional zinc may be required in patients with zinc deficiency. Patients with poor wound healing, inflammatory bowel disease, and decubiti should have serum zinc levels evaluated. Low serum alkaline phosphatase levels may be indicative of zinc deficiency. Copper and manganese are excreted in bile and so may need to be removed from the PN solutions of patients with cholestatic liver disease, end-stage liver disease, and liver failure to prevent toxicity. Similarly, selenium and chromium are excreted in the urine, and it has been suggested that they be used with caution in the nondialyzed patient with renal failure. Serum levels of trace elements eliminated from PN solution need to be monitored. Molybdenum deficiency is extremely rare, and molybdenum need not be supplemented except in adolescent patients who have received 80% or more of their caloric requirements from PN for 3 to 6 months. Iodine is not added to PN solutions because patients usually receive enough iodine from unavoidable contamination of PN solutions and from topical administration of iodine-containing antiseptic solutions. Aluminum toxicity was relatively common in the past because previously used casein hydrolysate solutions were contaminated with aluminum. Currently, some calcium salts (e.g., calcium gluconate) may be contaminated with aluminum. Patients chronically dependent on PN should have aluminum levels monitored.

### Additives

Commonly used medications may be added to the PN solution if they are compatible with the PN solution (e.g., ranitidine, cimetidine). Patients with inborn errors of metabolism may need additional amounts of specific amino acids added. Hydrochloric acid may be added to PN solutions given to patients on extracorporeal membrane oxygenation (ECMO) to correct alkalosis. This has to be done through central access; when the patient comes off ECMO and PN is provided via peripheral access, the hydrochloric acid must be discontinued.

## Total Nutrient Admixtures

Total nutrient admixtures (TNA), also commonly known as 3-in-1 solutions, consist of formulations in which intravenous fat is added directly to the amino acid/dextrose solution, thereby obviating the need for separate infusion lines and pumps. This simplifies PN administration,[29] and is particularly useful in the home PN patient. However, in 1995, the Food and Drug Administration issued a safety alert after the death of two patients related to microvascular pulmonary thrombi containing calcium phosphate precipitates.[30] Several recommendations were made regarding the amounts of calcium and phosphorus added to the solution, order of addition, use of a filter, and so on.[31] With TNA it is difficult to meet the high calcium and phosphorus needs of neonates without resulting precipitation. The emulsion may also separate with high electrolyte concentration.

## Parenteral Nutrition Requirements

For infants up to 1 year of age, we use a per kilogram caloric requirement that decreases with age. Infants (including neonates) and children have a higher per kilogram caloric requirement when compared with adults, partly due to growth requirements.[10] We use the World Health Organization (WHO) equation for determining the needs of children older than 1 year of age.[32] This equation, which provides an estimate of resting energy expenditure (REE), is based on data from several thousand children and has been found to be accurate in children older than 1 year of age. The REE is then multiplied by a factor, depending on the activity level of the patient, and severity of underlying disease (Tables 59–9 through 59–11).

The energy needs of obese patients are best determined by the Schofield height-weight equation.[33] Increased needs and energy intake may be increased in a patient with head injury or sepsis. The paralyzed patient on a ventilator may have no physical activity and has lower energy needs.

It is important to provide not only calories but also protein in adequate amounts so that the patient is in positive nitrogen balance. Otherwise, the patient will utilize protein for energy. It should be remembered that a patient's enteral requirements are higher than parenteral requirements by 20% to account for the thermic effect of food and for the loss of some nutrients in the stool during the process of digestion and absorption.

Indirect calorimetry is increasingly available and is used

**TABLE 59–7. Food and Nutrition Board, National Academy of Sciences—National Research Council Recommended Dietary Allowances (Revised 1989)***

| CATEGORY | AGE (YR) OR CONDITION | WEIGHT† (kg) | WEIGHT† (lb) | HEIGHT† (cm) | HEIGHT† (in) | PROTEIN (g) | FAT-SOLUBLE VITAMINS: Vitamin A (μg RE)‡ | Vitamin D (μg)§ | Vitamin E (mg α-E)‖ | Vitamin K (μg) |
|---|---|---|---|---|---|---|---|---|---|---|
| Infants | 0.0–0.5 | 6 | 13 | 60 | 24 | 13 | 375 | 7.5 | 3 | 5 |
| | 0.5–1.0 | 9 | 20 | 71 | 28 | 14 | 375 | 10 | 4 | 10 |
| Children | 1–3 | 13 | 29 | 90 | 35 | 16 | 400 | 10 | 6 | 15 |
| | 4–6 | 20 | 44 | 112 | 44 | 24 | 500 | 10 | 7 | 20 |
| | 7–10 | 28 | 62 | 132 | 52 | 28 | 700 | 10 | 7 | 20 |
| Males | 11–14 | 45 | 99 | 157 | 62 | 45 | 1000 | 10 | 10 | 45 |
| | 15–18 | 66 | 145 | 176 | 69 | 59 | 1000 | 10 | 10 | 65 |
| | 19–24 | 72 | 160 | 177 | 70 | 58 | 1000 | 10 | 10 | 70 |
| | 25–50 | 79 | 174 | 176 | 70 | 63 | 1000 | 5 | 10 | 80 |
| | 51+ | 77 | 170 | 173 | 68 | 63 | 1000 | 5 | 10 | 45 |
| Females | 11–14 | 46 | 101 | 157 | 62 | 46 | 800 | 10 | 8 | 55 |
| | 15–18 | 55 | 120 | 163 | 64 | 44 | 800 | 10 | 8 | 60 |
| | 19–24 | 58 | 128 | 164 | 65 | 46 | 800 | 10 | 8 | 65 |
| | 25–50 | 63 | 138 | 163 | 64 | 50 | 800 | 5 | 8 | 65 |
| | 51+ | 65 | 143 | 160 | 63 | 50 | 800 | 5 | 8 | 65 |
| Pregnant | | | | | | 60 | 800 | 10 | 10 | 65 |
| Lactating | First 6 mo | | | | | 65 | 1300 | 10 | 12 | 65 |
| | Second 6 mo | | | | | 62 | 1200 | 10 | 11 | 65 |

*The allowances, expressed as average daily intakes over time, are intended to provide for individual variations among most normal persons as they live in the United States under usual environmental stresses. Diets should be based on a variety of common foods to provide other nutrients for which human requirements have been less well defined. See text (in original source) for detailed discussion of allowances and of nutrients not tabulated.

†Weights and heights of reference adults are actual medians for the U.S. population of the designated age, as reported by NHANES II. The median weights and heights of those younger than 19 years of age were taken from Hamill et al (1979) (see pages 16–17 [in original source]). The use of these figures does not imply that the height-to-weight ratios are ideal.

‡Retinol equivalents. 1 retinol equivalent (RE) = 1 μg retinol or 6 μg β-carotene. See text (in original source) for calculation of vitamin A activity of diets as retinol equivalents.

§As cholecalciferol. 10 μg cholecalciferol = 400 IU of vitamin D.

‖α-Tocopherol equivalents. 1 mg d-α tocopherol = 1 mg α-TE. See text for variation in allowances and calculation of vitamin E activity of the diet as α-tocopherol equivalent.

¶NE (niacin equivalent) is equal to 1 mg of niacin or 60 mg of dietary tryptophan.

From National Research Council: Recommended Dietary Allowances, 10th ed. Washington, DC, National Academy Press, 1989, with permission.

to measure energy needs. In our institution we can measure REE in nonventilated patients over 5 kg who are not receiving supplemental oxygen. Patients in the intensive care unit who have a pulmonary artery catheter can also have their REE calculated from cardiac output.[34]

## Formulating a Regimen

The first step in formulating a PN regimen is to decide on the patient's fluid requirements. These can be determined using body weight or surface area. Allowances must be made for ongoing losses (e.g., diarrhea, glycosuria, diuretic use, ventilator status, fever, phototherapy, or other conditions associated with increased fluid losses). Typical fluid requirements are 100 ml/kg for the first 10 kg of body weight with an additional 50 ml/kg for every kg above 10 kg. Patients who weigh more than 20 kg get 1500 mL plus 20 mL/kg for every kilogram above 20 kg. PN solution should not be used as replacement fluid for ongoing losses.

The next step is to determine the patient's goal calories and protein. Except in neonates, it is usually possible to start on goal protein on the first day. Depending on the patient's nutritional status (i.e., risk of refeeding syndrome), a patient can usually initially receive calories equaling the REE or 75% to 80% of goal calories and then have caloric delivery increased to goal calories over the next 2 to 3 days. A dextrose solution of 10% is used initially; and if it is tolerated and central access is present, then more concentrated dextrose solutions of up to 30% to 35% can be used. Once the carbohydrate and protein calories have been calculated, then the balance of calories is provided as intravenous fat starting at 1 to 2 g/kg/day. This may be increased over the next 2 to 3 days to goal calories if triglyceride clearance is acceptable. It is important to make sure that the final PN solution is balanced to prevent complications of overfeeding as well as excessive administration of protein, carbohydrate, and fat.

After a baseline chemistry panel is reviewed, appropriate amounts of electrolytes and mineral are added. Serum levels will need to be monitored and amounts adjusted accordingly in the PN solution (Table 59–12).

## Cyclic Parenteral Nutrition

This refers to the discontinuous administration of PN over a specified period of time resulting in a period each day during which the patient is not receiving any intravenous nutrition. Cyclic PN is usually initiated in the patient who is receiving a stable PN solution and who can tolerate large volumes of fluid and nutrients over a short period of time. The main advantage is the fact that the patient is free from all pumps and intravenous tubing, resulting in greater

**TABLE 59–7. Food and Nutrition Board, National Academy of Sciences—National Research Council Recommended Dietary Allowances (Revised 1989)*** *Continued*

| WATER-SOLUBLE VITAMINS | | | | | | | MINERALS | | | | | | |
|---|---|---|---|---|---|---|---|---|---|---|---|---|---|
| Vitamin C (mg) | Thiamine (mg) | Riboflavin (mg) | Niacin (mg NE)¶ | Vitamin $B_6$ (mg) | Folate (μg) | Vitamin $B_{12}$ (μg) | Calcium (mg) | Phosphorus (mg) | Magnesium (mg) | Iron (mg) | Zinc (mg) | Iodine (μg) | Selenium (μg) |
| 30 | 0.3 | 0.4 | 0.5 | 0.3 | 25 | 0.3 | 400 | 300 | 40 | 6 | 5 | 40 | 10 |
| 35 | 0.4 | 0.5 | 6 | 0.6 | 35 | 0.5 | 600 | 500 | 60 | 10 | 5 | 50 | 15 |
| 40 | 0.7 | 0.8 | 9 | 1.0 | 50 | 0.7 | 800 | 800 | 80 | 10 | 10 | 70 | 20 |
| 45 | 0.9 | 1.1 | 12 | 1.1 | 75 | 1.0 | 800 | 800 | 120 | 10 | 10 | 90 | 20 |
| 45 | 1.0 | 1.2 | 13 | 1.4 | 100 | 1.4 | 800 | 800 | 170 | 10 | 10 | 120 | 30 |
| 50 | 1.3 | 1.5 | 17 | 1.7 | 150 | 2.0 | 1200 | 1200 | 270 | 12 | 15 | 150 | 40 |
| 60 | 1.5 | 1.8 | 20 | 2.0 | 200 | 2.0 | 1200 | 1200 | 400 | 12 | 15 | 150 | 50 |
| 60 | 1.5 | 1.7 | 19 | 2.0 | 200 | 2.0 | 1200 | 1200 | 350 | 10 | 15 | 150 | 70 |
| 60 | 1.5 | 1.7 | 19 | 2.0 | 200 | 2.0 | 800 | 800 | 350 | 10 | 15 | 150 | 70 |
| 60 | 1.2 | 1.4 | 15 | 2.0 | 200 | 2.0 | 800 | 800 | 350 | 10 | 15 | 150 | 70 |
| 50 | 1.1 | 1.3 | 15 | 1.4 | 150 | 2.0 | 1200 | 1200 | 280 | 15 | 12 | 150 | 45 |
| 60 | 1.1 | 1.3 | 15 | 1.5 | 180 | 2.0 | 1200 | 1200 | 300 | 15 | 12 | 150 | 50 |
| 60 | 1.1 | 1.3 | 15 | 1.6 | 180 | 2.0 | 1200 | 1200 | 280 | 15 | 12 | 150 | 55 |
| 60 | 1.1 | 1.3 | 15 | 1.6 | 180 | 2.0 | 800 | 800 | 280 | 15 | 12 | 150 | 55 |
| 60 | 1.0 | 1.2 | 13 | 1.6 | 180 | 2.0 | 800 | 800 | 280 | 10 | 12 | 150 | 55 |
| 70 | 1.5 | 1.6 | 17 | 2.2 | 400 | 2.2 | 1200 | 1200 | 300 | 30 | 15 | 175 | 65 |
| 95 | 1.6 | 1.8 | 20 | 2.1 | 280 | 2.6 | 1200 | 1200 | 355 | 15 | 19 | 200 | 75 |
| 90 | 1.6 | 1.7 | 20 | 2.1 | 260 | 2.6 | 1200 | 1200 | 340 | 15 | 16 | 200 | 75 |

freedom of activity. Patients receiving 24-hour PN can be cycled to 10 to 12 hours/day by 4- to 6-hour reductions/day in time on PN. During the last hour of the infusion, the rate is cut in half to prevent hypoglycemia.[35, 36] Some patients may require tapering over 2 hours. Cyclic PN has been successfully used in children younger than 6 months of age,[37] although the limited ability of infants to tolerate fasting must be considered when changing to cycled PN.

## Monitoring

Monitoring patients on PN is very important. This consists of monitoring the appropriateness of the regimen using serum chemistries and growth parameters (see Table 59–12). Typically, one must check serum chemistries before starting a PN solution and then obtain daily laboratory values as the PN regimen is adjusted and after any changes in the regimen. Malnourished patients at risk for refeeding syndrome must be especially closely monitored. Once the patient is on a stable PN regimen then laboratory values need to be checked once a week. Patients on long-term PN solutions or with risk factors or increased losses or increased needs may need to have trace element and vitamin levels checked periodically.

## Complications

Complications related to the use of PN can be divided into three main categories: mechanical, infectious, and metabolic. With careful use of PN, these complications can be avoided or minimized[38, 39] (Table 59–13).

### *Mechanical Complications*

Mechanical complications seen with PN use include those associated with initial insertion of a central venous catheter

**TABLE 59–8. Daily Intravenous Vitamin Requirements, Recommendations, and Products**

| | PRETERM PER kg | TERM AND CHILD >1 yr | MVI PED | MVI 12 (5 mL) |
|---|---|---|---|---|
| A (retinol) (IU) | 700–1500 | 2300 | 2300 | 3300 |
| D (IU) | 40–160 | 400 | 400 | 200 |
| E (tocopherol) (IU) | 3.5 | 7 | 7 | 10 |
| C (mg) | 15–25 | 80 | 80 | 100 |
| Folate (μg) | 56 | 140 | 140 | 400 |
| Niacin (mg) | 4–6.8 | 17 | 17 | 40 |
| Riboflavin (mg) | 0.15–0.2 | 1.4 | 1.4 | 3.6 |
| Thiamine (mg) | 0.2–0.35 | 1.2 | 1.2 | 3 |
| $B_6$ (mg) | 0.15–0.2 | 1 | 1 | 4 |
| $B_{12}$ (μg) | 0.3 | 1 | 1 | 5 |
| Pantothenic acid (mg) | 1–2 | 5 | 5 | 15 |
| Biotin (μg) | 8 | 20 | 20 | 60 |
| K (mg) | 0.3 | 0.2 | 0.2 | —* |

*Patient receiving MVI 12 will get 0.2 mg/day of vitamin K.

From Darby M (ed): The Children's Hospital of Philadelphia Pharmacy Handbook and Formulary 1995–1997. Hudson, OH, Lexi-Comp, Inc., 1995, with permission.

**TABLE 59–9. Energy Requirements for Parenteral Nutrition in Preterm and Term Infants**

| | CALORIES (kcal/kg/day) |
|---|---|
| Preterm infants | 90–110 |
| Full-term infants | |
| Early infancy (0–6 mo) | 90–100 |
| Late infancy (6–12 mo) | 80–100 |

**TABLE 59–11. Disease Activity/Stress Factors***

| | |
|---|---|
| 1.1–1.3 | Well-nourished child at rest with mild-to-moderate stress or after minor surgery |
| 1.3–1.5 | Normal active child with mild-to-moderate stress, inactive child with severe stress (trauma, cancer, extensive surgery), or malnourished child requiring catch-up growth with minimal activity |
| 1.5–1.7 | Active child requiring catch-up growth or with severe stress |

*Estimated daily energy requirements = REE × disease activity/stress factor.

and subsequent use of the catheter. These include vessel puncture, arrhythmias, hemomediastinum, air embolism, pneumothorax, hemothorax, hydrothorax, intravascular and extravascular malpositioning, brachial plexus injury, and thrombosis.[40] Introduction of an air embolus can occur at the time of central venous catheter insertion, with defective catheters and with catheters with faulty connections. Symptoms of air embolism include shortness of breath, hypoxia, tachycardia, hypotension, and neurologic changes. Pneumothorax, hydrothorax, and hemothorax can occur at the time of central venous catheter placement or as a result of delayed catheter perforation due to erosion of the blood vessel. Intravascular malpositioning refers to coiled catheters, those in the right atrium or ventricle, or those placed in a peripheral vessel. If the catheter tip is positioned in the right atrium, arrhythmias can occur due to irritation of the myocardium. Extravascular malpositioning results when the catheter gets lodged in the pleural space, in the mediastinum, or outside the vascular space.

Catheter breakage and occlusion can occur with chronic use of central venous catheters. Small tears, pinholes, or breakage may occur in the Silastic material of the catheter. Damage to the septum of the implantable port may occur if an inappropriate needle is used, resulting in leakage of fluid into the surrounding tissue. Extravasation of fluid can also occur with tunneled catheters with fluid leaking into the surrounding tissue.

Catheter occlusion can occur as a result of an intramural thrombus, extraluminal fibrin sleeve, a mural thrombosis, or a buildup of precipitate from drugs or components of the PN solution. The occlusion can range from a withdrawal problem (inability to aspirate blood but fluids infuse without difficulty) to a complete occlusion when nothing can be infused through the catheter. The development of thrombi may occur as a result of a vascular injury during the catheter placement or from contact with the tip of the catheter. These thrombi can develop either within the catheter (intramural thrombi) or at the site of the vascular injury (mural thrombi). Over time, mural thrombi can become large veno-occlusive thrombi.

Fibrin sleeves also develop from the catheter's contact with blood. As with the development of a thrombus, platelets and fibrin adhere to the catheter, causing a "sleeve" to form that encapsulates the catheter.

Solutions used to flush the catheter are intended to maintain catheter patency and include heparin and normal saline. The results of prophylactic heparin therapy in PN solutions in preventing occlusion remain questionable with the risk of potential adverse effects and optimal dosage regimen unclear. Currently, a dose of 0.5 unit/mL and 1 unit/mL of PN solution is recommended for neonates and infants/children, respectively. With intraluminal blockages, urokinase, ethanol, hydrochloric acid, and sodium bicarbonate may be instilled in the catheter. Occasionally, a combination of fibrinolytic agents and guidewire manipulation is needed to restore patency. Embolization of occluding compounds may occur in such settings.

### *Infectious Complications*

The use of central venous catheters is frequently complicated by either local or systemic infections. These include sepsis (bacterial, fungal), line contamination, and infective thrombophlebitis. Common infectious agents are *Staphylococcus epidermidis, Staphylococcus aureus,* enterococci, gram-negative rods, and *Candida albicans.*[41] The majority of infections start with a local infection of the catheter site with the patient's own cutaneous flora invading the intracutaneous tract at the time that the catheter is placed or at sometime thereafter. Children with abnormal gastrointestinal tracts (i.e., short bowel syndrome) also have a significant incidence of gram-negative infection, presumably by blood invasion of bowel bacteria. In pediatric oncology patients, PN appears to increase the risk of central venous catheter

**TABLE 59–10. Estimated Daily Resting Energy Expenditure (kcal)**

| | AGE (yr) | | | |
|---|---|---|---|---|
| | 1–3 | 3–10 | 10–18 | 18–30 |
| Male | 60.9W − 54 | 22.7W + 495 | 17.5W + 651 | 15.3W + 679 |
| Female | 61.0W − 51 | 22.5W + 499 | 12.2W + 746 | 14.7W + 496 |

W, weight in kg.

Adapted from World Health Organization: Energy and protein requirements. Technical Report Series #724. Geneva, World Health Organization, 1985, p 71, with permission.

**TABLE 59–12. Parenteral Nutrition Monitoring Schedule**

**Laboratory Tests**

Baseline*: complete blood cell count, serum electrolytes, triglycerides, cholesterol, calcium, magnesium, phosphorus, alkaline phosphatase, total protein, albumin, blood urea nitrogen, creatinine, liver function tests, iron studies
Weekly: serum electrolytes, triglycerides, cholesterol, calcium, magnesium, phosphorus, alkaline phosphatase, total protein, albumin, liver function tests
Monthly: complete blood cell count, reticulocyte count, iron studies
Biannually: serum selenium, zinc; consider vitamin A, E, D (25-hydroxy), prothrombin/partial thromboplastin times, copper, and manganese (if cholestatic)

**Growth Measurement**

Weight: baseline, daily (patients <2 yr), every other day (patients >2 yr), twice weekly (adolescents)
Height length: baseline and every month
Head circumference: baseline and every month (patients <3 yr)
Arm anthropometrics: baseline and every month

*Additionally the following should be obtained after parenteral nutrition started and after changing doses: serum electrolytes, triglycerides, calcium, phosphorus, magnesium.

infections. The infection rate increased from 0.06/100 days to 0.5/100 days when PN was administered using Hickman-Broviac catheters.[42] Other risk factors include age, underlying disease, site of the central venous catheter, environmental factors, length of use, frequent line entry for blood drawing, and so on.[43] The majority (70–85%) of infections can be treated safely without line removal. Treatment consists of initial antibiotic therapy to cover common organisms pending cultures.[44] Once the organism has been identified, then the appropriate antibiotic is chosen and given for 7 to 14 days, depending on the clinical situation. Persistent fevers, positive blood cultures, and tunnel infections may require removal of the line. The Centers for Disease Control and Prevention has made recommendations for intravenous catheter care.[45]

### *Metabolic Complications*

Metabolic complications related to PN solution include electrolyte and mineral imbalances, hyperammonemia, hyperglycemia, hypoglycemia, bone disease, and cholestasis[46] (Table 59–14). Hyperammonemia was initially reported in infants who received casein hydrolysate containing PN solutions and is no longer noted with the currently available amino acid solutions. Hyperglycemia can occur with high infusion rates, especially in the presence of sepsis, trauma, and surgery. Hypoglycemia occurs when total parenteral nutrition (TPN) is abruptly stopped. Excessive glucose administration can lead to excessive carbon dioxide production and ventilator dependence. Rapid infusions of intravenous fat can result in hypertriglyceridemia and elevated free fatty acid levels due to saturation of lipoprotein lipase and subsequent accumulation of atypical lipoproteins. Hyponatremia can result from inadequate sodium intake, excessive free water, excess sodium loss, and renal disease. Hypernatremia can occur with excessive sodium intake and fluid restriction. Hyperkalemia may be noted with excessive intake and renal disease. Hypokalemia may result from increased losses and inadequate replacement or from increased requirements, as is seen with refeeding syndrome. Hypocalcemia occurs with osteopenia of prematurity, diuretics, excessive phosphate intake, severe vitamin D deficiency, inadequate calcium intake, and magnesium deficiency. Hypophosphatemia can result with refeeding syndrome, inadequate intake, use of amphotericin B, hypomagnesemia, and increased renal excretion of phosphorus. Hypomagnesemia occurs with decreased intake, increased losses (e.g., diarrhea, renal disease), and use of certain drugs (e.g., amphotericin B, cyclosporin A).

Hypertriglyceridemia occurs when there is decreased triglyceride clearance and is seen with excessive intravenous fat intake, sepsis, and overfeeding. Fat overload syndrome occurs with extremely high fat infusions over a short period. This is characterized by a decrease in oxygenation, thrombocytopenia, and tachypnea. If PN solutions without intravenous fat are administered, essential fatty acid deficiency can occur with deleterious effects on energy metabolism, membrane structure, prostaglandin synthesis, and fat tissue storage.

PN-related bone disease can occur in up to 3% of adult patients on long-term PN.[47–50] It is also seen in children receiving home PN. It is characterized by bone pain, pathologic fractures, and hypercalciuria. Symptoms usually improve after discontinuation of PN. The exact etiology is unknown, but possible factors include abnormal vitamin D metabolism, aluminum toxicity, hypercalciuria, inadequate phosphate administration, abnormal calcium-to-phosphorus ratio, and cycling of PN.

Refeeding syndrome occurs when malnourished patients receive aggressive nutritional rehabilitation via the enteral or parenteral intake.[51, 52] Patients with protein-calorie malnutrition commonly maintain normal serum electrolyte levels in the presence of intracellular depletion of these same electrolytes. Administration of carbohydrate calories results in stimulating insulin secretion, which drives phosphorus and potassium into the cell, with resultant hypokalemia, hypophosphatemia, and hypomagnesemia. Increased metabolic rate and anabolism further decrease potassium and phosphorus levels and also induce hypomagnesemia. Refeeding syndrome can be fatal if not recognized and treated appropriately. It is prudent to start calories at 75% of REE or at previously tolerated levels of calories and increase calories by 10% to 15% per day provided serum electrolyte

**TABLE 59–13. Common Complications of Parenteral Nutrition**

**Metabolic**

Electrolyte/mineral abnormalities
Glucose disturbances
Acid-base disorders
Hypertriglyceridemia
Metabolic bone disease
Refeeding syndrome
Hepatobiliary disease

**Mechanical**

Air embolism
Pneumothorax, hemothorax, hydrothorax
Perforation of an organ
Malposition—arrhythmias, cardiac tamponade, brachial nerve injury
Thrombosis/phlebitis
Extravasation

**Infectious**

Systemic or local
Bacterial or fungal

**TABLE 59–14. Electrolyte and Mineral Abnormalities During Parenteral Nutrition**

| ELECTROLYTE/ MINERAL ABNORMALITIES | ETIOLOGY | MANIFESTATIONS | TREATMENT/MANAGEMENT |
|---|---|---|---|
| Hypocalcemia | Inadequate calcium intake<br>Increased losses<br>Hypoparathyroidism<br>Pharmacotherapy (e.g., diuretics)<br>Excessive phosphate intake<br>Vitamin D deficiency<br>Magnesium deficiency<br>Hypoalbuminemia | Low serum calcium<br>Rickets of prematurity<br>Bone demineralization<br>Carpopedal spasm<br>Positive Chvostek's sign<br>Prolonged QT interval | Exogenous calcium replacement (i.e., separate infusion)<br>Maximize calcium supplementation in TPN solution (based on calcium and phosphate solubility) |
| Hyperkalemia | Excessive potassium intake<br>Renal insufficiency<br>Metabolic acidosis<br>Pharmacotherapy (e.g., potassium-sparing diuretics, amphotericin B) | Serum potassium >7 mEq/L<br>Cardiac arrhythmias | Decrease potassium in TPN<br>Treat symptomatic patients (e.g., glucose and insulin infusion) |
| Hypokalemia | Increased gastrointestinal losses<br>Diarrhea<br>Pharmacotherapy (e.g., diuretics, amphotericin B)<br>Alkalosis<br>Excessive renal losses<br>Refeeding syndrome<br>Insulin therapy<br>High dextrose infusion | Serum potassium <3.5 mEq/L<br>Lethargy<br>Muscle weakness or paralysis<br>Cardiac arrhythmias | Increase potassiumin TPN<br>Treat with separate potassium infusion |
| Hypermagnesemia | Excessive magnesium intake<br>Renal insufficiency | Serum magnesium >3 mg/dL<br>Hypotension<br>Respiratory depression | Restrict or decrease magnesium in TPN |
| Hypomagnesemia | Excessive losses (i.e., gastrointestinal)<br>Chronic diarrhea<br>Fistulas<br>Prolonged nasogastric suction<br>Pharmacotherapy (e.g., amphotericin B, aminoglycosides, chemotherapeutic agents) | Low serum magnesium<br>Numbness<br>Muscle weakness<br>Positive Chvostek's sign<br>Muscle spasm, tetany<br>Tachycardia<br>Seizure<br>Tremors | Increase magnesium in TPN |
| Hypernatremia | Excessive sodium intake<br>Dehydration<br>Inadequate fluid intake<br>Diabetes insipidus | Serum sodium >145 mEq/L | Restrict sodium in TPN<br>Increase fluid intake<br>Diuretic therapy (e.g., furosemide) to increase urinary sodium losses |

From Bilodeau J, Poon C, Mascarenhas MR: Parenteral nutrition/care of central lines. In Altschuler SM, Liacouras CA (eds): Pediatric Gastroenterology. London, Churchill Livingstone, 1998, with permission.

levels are normal and congestive heart failure or significant edema is not evident.

Hepatobiliary complications[53, 54] associated with PN can occur as early as 2 weeks after the initiation of PN. The earliest signs are elevated serum γ-glutamyltransferase and cholylglycine levels. The exact incidence is not known but may vary from 7.4% to 84%. The highest incidence occurs in the low-birth-weight premature infant with necrotizing enterocolitis, short bowel syndrome, multiple bouts of sepsis, and multiple periods of not being fed. The etiology is unknown, but the following factors have been implicated: excessive protein and carbohydrate intake, amino acid composition, relative carbohydrate-to-nitrogen imbalance, carnitine or taurine or serine deficiency, excessive phytosterol intake, essential fatty acid deficiency, bacterial overgrowth, and continuous delivery of PN. Adults on chronic PN appear to get steatosis, whereas neonates and children develop cholestasis, cirrhosis, and portal hypertension. Acalculus cholecystitis, biliary sludge, and gallstones can also be seen in patients on chronic PN. Ursodeoxycholic acid has been used to treat this hepatobiliary damage, but there have been no controlled trials. Prevention consists of the following measures: avoiding overfeeding and excessive protein and carbohydrate intake, cycling of PN, institution of some enteral feeds even if only trophic feeds, and discontinuation of copper and manganese from the PN solution (and, subsequently, monitoring of copper, ceruloplasmin, and manganese levels).

## Home Parenteral Nutrition

Home PN refers to the administration of PN solutions at home to patients who cannot maintain normal nutritional status with enteral feeds.[55] Patients usually receive a combination of some enteral and parenteral feeds, and every attempt is made to increase enteral feeds and wean PN. Patients have central access and are usually on 8 to 18 hours of cycled PN. Also used more commonly in older children and adults are TNA solutions for ease of administration.

## ENTERAL NUTRITION

The enteral pathway is the preferred route of nutritional delivery, is safer than PN, and is significantly less costly. Successful alimentation may be achieved using the oral route or utilizing a nasogastric, nasojejunal, gastrostomy, gastrojejunal, or jejunostomy feeding tube. The choice of the route depends on the primary medical problem and the clinical status of the child who is being supported. Defined formula diets provide flexibility in nutrient composition, caloric density, and osmolarity.

Patients who require nutritional support are suffering from either primary gastrointestinal disease or from the secondary gastrointestinal side effects of their primary disease. Studies after experimental intestinal resection[56–60] have shown that the return of normal gastrointestinal function is influenced by the delivery of intraluminal (i.e., alimentary tract) nutrients. Studies[61] of laboratory animals who were given identical nutritionally complete formulas either orally or through the parenteral route have shown that the mucosal weight of the gastrointestinal tract as well as the total protein and DNA content were all greater in the animals receiving enteral nutrition. The brush border enzymes, which are important in digestion, were also higher in those animals that were fed. It has been shown that exclusive PN results in decreased intestinal mucosal cell turnover and thereby a decreased height of the mucosal villi.[58, 59, 62] The infusion of small amounts of nutrients intraluminally similarly seems to have a protective and trophic effect on the intestinal mucosa.

From the metabolic view, there are several consequences that clearly relate to the pathway (enteral versus parenteral) of nutrition. After ingestion of a protein-containing meal, the cells of the intestinal mucosa absorb the protein as oligopeptides and free amino acids. The oligopeptides are hydrolyzed to amino acids within the epithelial cells, and then the amino acids are transported to the liver through the portal vein. Within the epithelial cells, glutamine and glutamic acid are metabolized, yielding alanine for the transport into the portal system. The liver metabolizes most amino acids during the first pass, with the exception of the branched-chain amino acids, which are catabolized primarily in the muscle, kidneys, adipose tissue, and brain. Studies of parenterally administered amino acids, especially branched chains,[61, 63] suggest that special careful attention needs to be paid to implications of parenteral versus enteral feeding. In patients with significant pathologic processes, such as burns or trauma, or who have undergone surgery, higher visceral protein levels, a decrease in stress-related hyperglycemia, reductions in energy expenditure, and greater decreases in elevated cytokine levels have been observed in patients receiving enteral nutrition, as opposed to PN.[64, 65] In addition, utilizing enteral nutrition stimulates the excretion of different substances (e.g., epidermal growth factor in saliva, bile, and pancreatic secretions), which may impact on gastrointestinal tract and other organ systems function.

Data suggest that a wide variety of substances (nucleotides, short-chain fatty acids, soluble fiber, glutamine) may have a positive effect on bowel function.[66–73] These may not be present in all formulas, or their concentration may vary widely between different products (see Chapter 57).

### Enteral Formulas

The large number of defined formula diets commercially available provides a number of alternative regimens from which to choose when children have special enteral needs. As a general rule, the least synthetic and least "predigested" or "elemental" formula that meets the patient's expected needs will be the safest and best formula. One of the few conditions that has been studied rather extensively relates to the use of enteral formulas in inflammatory bowel disease.[74]

It is important to consider the specific target age for the formula. If a formula is to be used for an age group it was not specifically made for, careful analysis of the macronutrient and micronutrient delivery to the child should be undertaken and appropriate supplementation provided to ensure a complete and balanced diet. Some supplements may be added directly to the formula, whereas others may not be stable in such a mixture. The ultimate impact on osmolality, absorption, and tolerance must be considered (see Chapter 57).

Pediatric formulas are generally designed to be "complete" (provide adequate macronutrients and micronutrients, assuming a certain volume of intake and subsequent absorption). Children with significantly decreased caloric needs (e.g., a child with cerebral palsy who is nonambulatory and dependent on enteral tube feedings) may not receive enough vitamins, electrolytes, minerals, other nutrients, or water due to his or her low caloric needs and small volume of formula actually ingested.

Formulas tend to be designed for infants or for children (generally 1 to 10 years of age). Although a greater range of pediatric formulas is now available, a much greater number of adult formulas exist. Older children and adolescents commonly receive adult enteral formulas.

One advantage of using formulas of known composition relates to the ease and accuracy in determining micronutrient delivery. However, calculating intake in this manner assumes normal absorption and utilization. For children with alterations in these processes (e.g., malabsorption, significant vomiting) it would be appropriate to monitor intake and actual serum levels of specific nutrients to gauge degree of absorption and potential need for supplementation. Using the simplest formula that meets the child's specific needs limits the potential of inducing other problems related to the formula chosen. For example, formulas with a very high caloric density or that are very "elemental" have relatively high osmolalities. Experience suggests that even the child without intrinsic gastrointestinal disease may begin to complain of gastrointestinal symptoms when the osmolality of the formula approaches 600 mOsm/L. This experience is consistent with that of investigators,[75] who have reported delayed gastric emptying when the osmolality of the duodenal contents is 560 mOsm/L.

Formulas should be used to take advantage of the physiologic properties of the constituents and address the specific needs or pathology of each child. For example, the protein content of the formula has been demonstrated to be directly proportional to its capacity to stimulate acid-secretion potential.[76] Gastrin release itself is related to the presence of specific amino acids and small peptides.[77] The administration of intragastric protein results in significant pancreatic stimulation, which can be minimized if the infusion is altered to become intrajejunal and the formula has a neutral pH.[78] The decreased pancreatic output that results suggests a possible explanation of the apparent efficacy of elemental formula diets in the treatment of pancreatitis[79] and high-output intestinal fistulas.[80–82] As previously noted, the therapeutic potential of specific components of formulas, such as glutamine and soluble fiber, has also been described,[72, 73] although the experience is very limited in children.

## Constituents of Defined Formula Diets

### *Fat*

Because caloric intake is commonly the limiting nutrient in pediatric patients, the intake of calorically dense fat is very important. Triglycerides composed of glycerol esterified to long-chain fatty acids yield approximately 9 calories per gram when they are oxidized. The major considerations with regard to choosing the amount or type of dietary fat include (1) the use and absorption of long-chain triglycerides; (2) the use and absorption of synthetic medium-chain triglycerides; and (3) the requirements for essential fatty acids. Dietary fat consists of predominantly long-chain triglycerides. The process of digestion and absorption of long-chain triglycerides is reviewed elsewhere (see Chapter 22). The assimilation of long-chain fat is disrupted in several clinical situations: (1) pancreatic insufficiency resulting in decreased lipases, (2) bile duct obstruction or hepatitis resulting in decreased bile flow to the intestine and thereby decreased micelle formation, (3) gastrointestinal mucosal damage resulting in decreased surface area for the absorption of fatty acids, (4) metabolic derangements inhibiting the formation of chylomicrons, and (5) diseases or obstruction of the lymphatics inhibiting the transport of lymph back into the circulation. In many cases of fat malabsorption, fat intake should not be restricted, to take advantage of the energy provided by the fat that is absorbed. If steatorrhea presents as severe diarrhea, or other unacceptable circumstances, fat restrictions or modifications should be considered.

Medium-chain triglycerides are synthetic fats that contain a glycerol backbone esterified to fatty acids that are 8 to 10 carbons in length. Medium-chain triglycerides yield 8.3 calories/g on oxidation and are therefore essentially as useful as long-chain fat from an energy point of view. They are hydrolyzed more rapidly than long-chain fats in the small intestine when pancreatic lipases are present and are converted almost exclusively into free fatty acids and glycerol. If no pancreatic lipase is present, the medium-chain triglyceride can be found in the intestinal mucosa mainly as unhydrolyzed triglyceride.[83, 84] Thus, even in the absence of pancreatic lipase and bile salts, medium-chain triglycerides are transported through the intestinal lumen and through the brush border into the enterocyte intact. The unusual behavior of medium-chain triglyceride in the intestinal lumen and its absorption characteristics are due to the greater water solubility of medium-chain triglyceride and its products.

The exact mechanism and the rate-limiting step in the absorption of these different fats are unknown. The relatively high solubility of intact medium-chain triglycerides enhances their diffusion to the brush border of the enterocyte. The triglyceride and the medium-chain free fatty acids are readily taken up into the enterocyte. Within the enterocyte, the triglyceride is acted on by intracellular lipases, and the resulting free fatty acids are released directly into the portal circulation. The clinical indications for the use of medium-chain triglycerides are based on these characteristics (Table 59–15).

There are circumstances under which one, the other, or both types of fat become highly desirable as constituents of the prescribed diet. It has been demonstrated[85, 86] that the maximum absorption of long-chain fat is decreased when medium-chain triglycerides are added. The total triglyceride absorbed when both are present, however, is greater than the maximum absorption of either alone. Absorption of medium-chain triglycerides from the rat cecum[87] and the dog colon[88] has been reported. The importance of this phenomenon and whether it has any implications for the human are unclear.

If there are no specific defects in fat absorption demonstrated or anticipated, the fat of choice for a defined formula diet is regular, long-chain (dietary) fat. The use of medium-chain triglycerides in patients who have intact mechanisms for the normal digestion of fat can lead to osmotic diarrhea from the rapid lipolysis of medium-chain triglycerides to glycerol (and medium-chain free fatty acids). This diarrhea may potentiate the symptoms for which the formula was prescribed. Patients who require increased calories may conceivably be helped by a mixture of both medium-chain triglycerides and long-chain triglycerides. However, medium-chain triglyceride oil does not mix well with water-based formulas (as opposed to Microlipid emulsion, which goes into and stays in solution relatively easily), tends to adhere to plastic and other surfaces, and has a taste some find objectionable. Thus, although medium-chain triglyceride oil may seem theoretically indicated, it is not very practical to use.

**TABLE 59–15. Potential Indications for Replacement of Some or All of Dietary Long-Chain Fats with Medium-Chain Triglyceride**

- Cholestasis, including
  - Cholestatic jaundice secondary to total parenteral nutrition or medications
  - Hepatitis (any type)
  - Bile duct obstruction
  - Biliary atresia
- Bile salt depletion
  - Terminal ileal dysfunction or disease
  - Prematurity
  - Congenital deficiency of bile salts
- Pancreatic insufficiency, including
  - Cystic fibrosis
- Interruption of lymph drainage, including
  - Congenital lymphangiectasia
  - Chylothorax
  - Chylous ascites
- Descreased villous surface area, including
  - Severe enteritis
  - Short gut syndrome
- Metabolic derangements of long-chain fat assimilation, including
  - Abetalipoproteinemia

*Note:* Replacement of long-chain triglyceride with medium-chain triglyceride may lead to or even contribute to essential fatty acid deficiency.

Essential fatty acids are all long-chain fatty acids and therefore absent in medium-chain triglycerides. Because the administration of medium-chain triglycerides may decrease the absorption of long-chain triglycerides, the addition of small amounts of linoleic acid to a medium-chain triglyceride formula may be insufficient to prevent essential fatty acid insufficiency.

Cases of essential fatty acid deficiency have been reported when children with fat malabsorption received a medium-chain triglyceride–predominant formula.[89, 90] If long-chain fat absorption is severely compromised, the parenteral administration of lipid emulsions containing essential fats may be considered. Transdermal application and subsequent absorption of topical linoleic-rich vegetable oil has also prevented essential fatty acid deficiency in some cases.[91–93]

### *Carbohydrates*

Complex carbohydrates are broken down to individual monosaccharides by the brush border oligosaccharidases. The individual monosaccharides are then absorbed into the enterocytes by means of specific transport oligosaccharidases.[94] Three are clinically significant enzymes: (1) maltase (glucoamylase); (2) sucrase-isomaltase (sucra a-dextrinase); and (3) lactase.

All of the levels of these disaccharidases may be expected to be depressed when there is mucosal disease of the small intestine. Lactase appears to be the most sensitive to injury and the last of the disaccharidases to recover full activity after mucosal damage.[94–96]

Because the disaccharidases are present in older enterocytes, any process that causes rapid intestinal regeneration and therefore repopulation of the intestinal villi with young cells (i.e., recovery from acute gastroenteritis) will cause a period of relative disaccharidase deficiency for the patient. Additionally, starvation alone may be sufficient to lower disaccharidase activity because it results in decreased cell turnover, mucosal hypotrophy, and therefore decreased surface area. It may therefore be important to limit dietary sources of lactose in the malnourished child or in the child recuperating from gastrointestinal insult for a short period of time. Restriction beyond a brief period necessary to demonstrate mucosal recovery is, however, not warranted. Breath hydrogen testing may provide useful information suggesting disaccharidase activity.

In selecting a source of carbohydrate, it is important to note that the use of glucose significantly increases the osmotic concentration of a formula. A disaccharide will provide, on a gram-for-gram basis, one half of the osmotic load of a monosaccharide. The use of synthetic glucose polymers may contribute as little as one fifth to the total osmotic load of a similar amount of glucose. Many defined formula diets therefore use glucose polymers and long-chain starches as their carbohydrate source. Although it has been shown that sucrose or fructose feedings may cause increases in the intestinal level of sucrase and maltase,[97, 98] no such dietary effect on lactase activity has ever been demonstrated.

### *Protein*

A child's protein requirements may be met by using intact proteins, protein hydrolysates, individual amino acids, or a combination of these. Patients who have no known deficiency of exocrine pancreatic function and no suspected major absorptive defect or protein allergy should receive high-quality intact protein. Intact protein is considerably less expensive than other dietary forms, is much more palatable, and does not contribute significantly to a formula's osmolarity. Within a given volume and osmolarity, the formula containing intact protein will allow for significantly greater nutrient density. Patients who are unable to tolerate intact protein because of protein allergy, exocrine pancreatic deficiency, or severe intestinal mucosal disease should receive a protein hydrolysate or a synthetic amino acid formula.

The absorption of small peptides, especially dipeptides, has been shown to play a significant role in the digestion of protein.[99–101] Perhaps one fourth of absorbed protein in health is absorbed in the form of oligopeptides.[102] The oligopeptides, especially dipeptides, are absorbed and then hydrolyzed by brush border and cytoplasmic hydrolases to free amino acids.[103] The mechanisms of transport of the individual amino acids have been shown to be energy dependent and active and in many cases dependent on true carrier proteins with some degree of specificity for neutral, basic, and acidic amino acids. A lack of competition between amino acid uptake and the uptake of peptides suggests that separate carriers for absorption are present. This suggests that a formula containing a mixture of oligopeptides and free amino acids may be best to use with patients with damaged intestinal mucosa.

The use of oligopeptides (protein hydrolysates) and formulas that are mixtures of oligopeptides and free amino acids is usually adequate for the enteral support of most patients who cannot tolerate intact proteins. In rare cases of severe protein allergy, free amino acid formulas may be required.

## Enteral Energy and Protein Requirements

In most clinical situations, energy requirements for children are estimated from the age, gender, and size of the child. Actual energy requirements may vary widely among healthy individuals and are even more variable in disease. For the healthy individual, energy requirements may be estimated from the RDAs[104] (Table 59–16).

Although these numbers are based on studies of "normal intake," actual energy intakes very widely in this range. It is also worth noting that a child's caloric intake may vary significantly over the short term but is remarkably consistent over the longer term.[105] When determinations of energy requirement are crucial to the management of a particular patient, or the needs of a child seem to be significantly altered, actual energy requirements should be measured. If such assessment is not possible, the clinical response to feeding (appropriate weight gain or loss or change over time in objective measurements of body composition such as skinfold thickness) is the most valuable indicator of caloric adequacy. Conditions preventing adequate delivery of calories (e.g., vomiting, malabsorption, or excessive caloric requirements) should be considered if an appropriate response to the feedings is not demonstrated. Assessing REE in such

**TABLE 59–16. Median Heights and Weights and Recommended Energy Intake**

| CATEGORY | AGE (yr) OR CONDITION | WEIGHT (kg) | WEIGHT (lb) | HEIGHT (cm) | HEIGHT (in) | REE* (kcal/day) | AVERAGE ENERGY ALLOWANCE (kcal)† Multiples of REE | Per kg | Per day‡ |
|---|---|---|---|---|---|---|---|---|---|
| Infants | 0.0–0.5 | 6 | 13 | 60 | 24 | 320 | | 108 | 650 |
| | 0.5–1.0 | 9 | 20 | 71 | 28 | 500 | | 98 | 850 |
| Children | 1–3 | 13 | 29 | 90 | 35 | 740 | | 102 | 1300 |
| | 4–6 | 20 | 44 | 112 | 44 | 950 | | 90 | 1800 |
| | 7–10 | 28 | 62 | 132 | 52 | 1130 | | 70 | 2000 |
| Males | 11–14 | 45 | 99 | 157 | 62 | 1440 | 1.70 | 55 | 2500 |
| | 15–18 | 66 | 145 | 176 | 69 | 1760 | 1.67 | 45 | 3000 |
| | 19–24 | 72 | 160 | 177 | 70 | 1780 | 1.67 | 40 | 2900 |
| | 25–50 | 79 | 174 | 176 | 70 | 1800 | 1.60 | 37 | 2900 |
| | 51+ | 77 | 170 | 173 | 68 | 1530 | 1.50 | 30 | 2300 |
| Females | 11–14 | 46 | 101 | 157 | 62 | 1310 | 1.67 | 47 | 2200 |
| | 15–18 | 55 | 120 | 163 | 64 | 1370 | 1.60 | 40 | 2200 |
| | 19–24 | 58 | 128 | 164 | 65 | 1350 | 1.60 | 38 | 2200 |
| | 25–50 | 63 | 138 | 163 | 64 | 1380 | 1.55 | 36 | 2200 |
| | 51+ | 65 | 143 | 160 | 63 | 1280 | 1.50 | 30 | 1900 |
| Pregnant | 1st trimester | | | | | | | | +0 |
| | 2nd trimester | | | | | | | | +300 |
| | 3rd trimester | | | | | | | | +300 |
| Lactating | 1st 6 mo | | | | | | | | +500 |
| | 2nd 6 mo | | | | | | | | +500 |

*Calculation based on Food and Agriculture Organization of the United Nations (FAO) equations, then rounded.
†In the range of light-to-moderate activity, the coefficient of variation is ±20%.
‡Figure is rounded.
From National Research Council: Recommended Dietary Allowances, 10th ed. Washington, DC, National Academy Press, 1989, with permission.

cases may provide important therapeutic and diagnostic information.

The present RDAs for protein are an estimate of the "safe level of intake" (average requirement plus two standard deviations). This is in contrast to estimates of energy requirements that represent the mean for a group of normal, healthy individuals. However, even with this safety factor, the RDAs for protein intake are still intended only for healthy individuals whose energy intake is adequate.

## Vitamins and Minerals

Vitamin and mineral requirements for the pediatric population are listed in the RDAs[104] (see Table 59–7). Children in the general population commonly ingest less than the RDAs for some nutrients, such as zinc and calcium.[106] In addition, children with such conditions as fat malabsorption, short bowel syndrome, or chronic drug therapy with potential drug/nutrient interactions may be at risk for vitamin or mineral deficiencies despite an intake greater than or near the RDAs.

## Preterm Infants

The nutritional requirements of preterm, small-for-gestational-age, and low-birth-weight infants are usually higher per kilogram of body weight than those of normal-weight full-term infants. The goal of nutrition in this high-risk group has been to approximate the growth in utero of a normal fetus at the postconception age.[107]

The estimated requirements of protein are based on the net fetal accretion rate of protein: 3.5 to 4.0 g/kg/day (Table 59–17). Care must be taken to avoid increasing the protein content of the preterm diet, because excessive protein can potentially be harmful. This is due to the immaturity of the preterm infant's metabolic and excretory functions.[108]

Selected vitamin and mineral requirements for the preterm infant are outlined in Table 59–17. Requirements are based on body weight/gestational age (800 to 1200 g versus 1200 to 1800 g) and are based on rates of retention of individual nutrients and minerals.

## Administration of Special Diets

Some patients' nutritional requirements may be met by manipulating their regular diet. Others may require supplements to provide the needed nutrition. When utilizing supplements, the palatability, osmolality, and tolerance of the supplement must be considered. In addition, for children receiving enteral feedings but who are also partially dependent on PN, it may be better to provide the special supplements via the PN (e.g., phosphorus supplements, iron supplements) to maximize the tolerance and absorption of the enteral feedings. If the patient is either unable or unwilling to take adequate nutrition through the normal oral route, one of the alternatives (nasogastric, gastrostomy, nasojejunal, gastrojejunal, or jejunostomy feeding) must be used. Nasogastric tubes are usually the best initial approach to delivering nonoral enteral supplements and are usually well tolerated. If a prolonged requirement for enteral tube feedings is expected, more permanent tube placement should be considered. In most cases, it is recommended that tolerance of the feeding regimen be demonstrated with a temporary tube before a permanent tube is placed. An obvious exception is the child undergoing significant bowel resection resulting in

**TABLE 59–17. Estimated Requirements and Advisable Intakes for Preterm Infants for Protein and Major Minerals**

| BODY WEIGHT | REQUIREMENT | TISSUE INCREMENT (per day) | ESTIMATED REQUIREMENT (per day) | ADVISABLE INTAKE Per day | Per kg* | Per 100 kcal† |
|---|---|---|---|---|---|---|
| 800 to 1,200 g (26–28 weeks' gestational age) | Protein (g) | 2.32 | 3.64 | 4.0 | 4.0 | 3.1 |
| | Sodium (mEq) | 1.63 | 3.22 | 3.5 | 3.5 | 2.7 |
| | Chloride (mEq) | 1.23 | 2.79 | 3.1 | 3.1 | 2.4 |
| | Potassium (mEq) | 0.87 | 2.52 | 2.5 | 2.5 | 1.9 |
| | Calcium (mg) | 116.0 | 188.0 | 210.0 | 210.0 | 160.0 |
| | Phosphorus (mg) | 75.0 | 126.0 | 140.0 | 140.0 | 108.0 |
| | Magnesium (mg) | 3.2 | 8.7 | 10.0 | 10.0 | 7.5 |
| 1,200 to 1,800 g (29–31 weeks' gestational age) | Protein (g) | 3.01 | 4.78 | 5.2 | 3.5 | 2.7 |
| | Sodium (mEq) | 1.77 | 4.08 | 4.5 | 3.0 | 2.3 |
| | Chloride (mEq) | 1.30 | 3.47 | 3.8 | 2.5 | 2.0 |
| | Potassium (mEq) | 1.03 | 3.45 | 3.4 | 2.3 | 1.8 |
| | Calcium (mg) | 154.0 | 251.0 | 280.0 | 185.0 | 140.0 |
| | Phosphorus (mg) | 98.0 | 171.0 | 185.0 | 123.0 | 95.0 |
| | Magnesium (mg) | 4.0 | 11.7 | 13 | 8.5 | 6.5 |

*Assuming body weight of 1,000 and 1,500 g for the 800- to 1,200- and 1,200- to 1,800-g infants.
†Assuming calorie intake of 130 kcal/kg/day.
Adapted from Ziegler EE, Biga RL, Fomon SJ: Nutritional requirements of the preterm infant. In Suskind RM (ed): Textbook of Pediatric Nutrition. New York, Raven Press, 1981, p 32, with permission.

short bowel syndrome, who should probably have a gastrostomy tube placed at the time of the bowel resection. Percutaneous placement of gastrostomy tubes is gaining popularity and minimizes the hospital stay required for tube placement. Low-profile ostomy devices allow for permanent ostomy access with minimal public awareness for the self-conscious child or adolescent.

As the use of postpyloric tube feedings bypasses the important digestive and control mechanisms of the stomach, jejunal feedings of high-osmolality formulas or of complex, intact protein or long-chain triglyceride formulas or bolus feeds may not be well tolerated. Pain, nausea and vomiting, distention, and diarrhea may occur. In such cases, using a less calorically dense formula or a continuous infusion of the formula should be considered. Despite these concerns, jejunal enteral feedings can usually be undertaken without utilizing specialized formulas.

## Starting the Feeding

Formula infusion by any of the previously mentioned routes may be either intermittent or continuous. Continuously infused feedings are usually better tolerated than bolus feedings. Furthermore, the amount of calories that can be administered to a patient is greater when the formula is infused continuously than intermittently.[109] The attempted use of bolus feedings in the sick child may delay the delivery of adequate nutrition.

Continuous feedings should be instituted at a relatively slow rate. One milliliter per hour may be appropriate for an infant, whereas initial rates of 10 to 20 mL/hr may be appropriate for the older child and adolescent. Many physicians start with a dilute formula, although this is probably only indicated for the child with significant bowel dysfunction (e.g., short bowel syndrome, significant mucosal atrophy). Once initial tolerance is demonstrated, feedings may be advanced to full caloric support over 1 or 2 days with children with relatively intact gastrointestinal function. At the other end of the spectrum, an infant with significant malabsorption related to short bowel syndrome may only tolerate increases of 1 to 2 mL/hr every few days.

When first initiating enteral tube feedings or when advancing the volume or rate of the tube feedings, it is not unusual for the child to experience a few episodes of vomiting over the first few days, especially for children with compromised gastrointestinal function. Vomiting is also relatively common early in the morning for children receiving overnight tube feedings. This is especially true for those children who are also receiving PN overnight. The presence of a pathologic process underlying the vomiting must be considered. If none is found, the cost of the continuation of the tube feedings (e.g., loss of vomited nutrients and fluids, psychological impact on the child and family) must be balanced against the benefits, and an appropriate balance reached. After tube feedings have been initiated, the child should be regularly monitored. Tube feedings are now commonly done in the home with appropriate family education and professional support.

*Acknowledgment*

Portions of this chapter were revised from the chapter: LeLeiko N, Burke P, Chao C: Enteral nutrition. In Wyllie R, Hyams JS (eds): Pediatric Gastrointestinal Disease. Philadelphia, WB Saunders, 1993.

## REFERENCES

1. Heird WC: Parenteral nutrition. In Grand RJ, Sutphen JL, Dietz WH (eds): Pediatric Nutrition: Theory and Practice. Stoneham, MA, Butterworth Publishers, 1987, pp 747–761.
2. Klein S, Kinney J, Jeejeebhoy K, et al: Nutrition support in clinical practice: Review of published data and recommendations for future research directions. JPEN J Parenter Enteral Nutr 1997;21:133–156.
3. Everitt NJ, McMahon MJ: Peripheral intravenous nutrition. Nutrition 1994;10:49–57.

4. Moukarzel AA, Haddad ME, Ament ME, et al: Two hundred and thirty patient years of experience with long-term parenteral nutrition in childhood: natural history and life of central venous catheters. J Pediatr Surg 1994;29:1324.
5. Hickman RO, Buchner CD, Clift RA, et al: A modified right atrial catheter for access to the venous system in marrow transplant recipients. Surg Gynecol Obstet 1979;166:295–301.
6. Denny DF: Placement and management of long-term central venous access catheters and ports. Am J Radiol 1993;161:385–393.
7. Gullo SM: Implanted ports: technological advances and nursing care issues. Nursing Clin North Am 1993;28:859–871.
8. Intradialytic parenteral nutrition administration during outpatient hemodialysis. Dialys Transplant 1987;16:495–496.
9. Gardiner K, Barbul A: Amino acids as specific therapy in human disease. In Torosian M (ed): Nutrition for the Hospitalized Patient: Basic Science and Principles of Practice. New York, Marcel Decker, 1995, pp 183–205.
10. Heird WC: Amino acid needs and energy needs of pediatric patients receiving parenteral nutrition. Pediatr Clin North Am 1995;42:765–789.
11. Van Goudoever JB, Colen T, Wattimena JLD, et al: Immediate commencement of amino acid supplementation in preterm infants: effect on serum amino acid concentrations and protein kinetics on the first day of life. J Pediatr 1995;127:456–465.
12. Lacey JM, Wilmore DW: Is glutamine a conditionally essential amino acid? Nutr Rev 1990;48:297–309.
13. Byrne TA, Persinger RL, Young LS, et al: A new treatment for patients with short bowel syndrome. Ann Surg 1995;222:243–255.
14. Acey JM, Crouch JB, Benfell K, et al: The effects of glutamine-supplemented parenteral nutrition in premature infants. JPEN J Parenter Enteral Nutr 1996;20:74–79.
15. Tanphaichitr V, Leelahagul P: Carnitine metabolism and human carnitine deficiency. Nutrition 1993;9:246–254.
16. Bonner CM, DeBrie KL, Hug G, et al: Effects of parenteral L-carnitine supplementation on fat metabolism and nutrition in premature neonates. J Pediatr 1995;126:287–292.
17. Jones MO, Pierro A, Hammond P, et al: Glucose utilization in the surgical newborn receiving TPN. J Pediatr Surg 1993;8:1121–1125.
18. Nordenstrom J, Thorne A: Comparative studies on a new concentrated fat emulsion: Intralipid 30% vs. 20%. Clin Nutr 1993;12:160–167.
19. Haumont D, Deckelbaum RJ, Richelle M, et al: Plasma lipid and plasma lipoprotein concentrations in low birth weight infants given parenteral nutrition with twenty or ten percent lipid emulsion. J Pediatr 1989;115:787–793.
20. Haumont D, Richelle M, Deckelbaum RJ, et al: Effect of liposomal content of lipid emulsions on plasma lipid concentrations in low birth weight infants receiving parenteral nutrition. J Pediatr 1992;121:759–763.
21. Dahn MS: Structured lipids: an alternative energy source. Nutr Clin Prac 1995;10:89–90.
22. Hyltander A, Sandstrom R, Lundholm K: Metabolic effects of structured triglycerides in humans. Nutr Clin Prac 1995;10:91–97.
23. Bell SJ, Mascioli EA, Bistrian BR, et al: Alternative lipid sources for enteral and parenteral nutrition: Long- and medium-chain triglycerides, structured triglycerides, and fish oils. Persp Pract 1991;91:74–78.
24. Sandstorm R, Hyltander A, Korner U, Lundholm K: Structured triglycerides to postoperative patients: a safety and tolerance study. JPEN J Parenter Enteral Nutr 1993;17:153–157.
25. Bresson JL, Narcy P, Sachs C, et al: Energy substrate competition: comparative study of LCT and MCT utilization during continuous TPN in infants. Clin Nutr 1986;5(suppl):54(A).
26. Goulet O, De Potter S, Postaire M, et al. Long term TPN in children: utilization of medium chain triglycerides. Nutrition 1992;8:333–337.
27. Greene HL, Hambidge M, Schanler R, Tsang RC: Guidelines for the use of vitamins, trace elements, calcium, magnesium, and phosphorus in infants and children receiving total parenteral nutrition: report of the subcommittee on pediatric parenteral nutrient requirements from the Committee on Clinical Practice Issues of the American Society for Clinical Nutrition. Am J Clin Nutr 1988;48:1324–1342.
28. Multivitamin preparations for parenteral use: a statement by the nutrition advisory group. JPEN J Parenter Enteral Nutr 1975;3:258–262.
29. Driscoll DF: Total nutrient admixtures: theory and practice. Nutr Clin Prac 1995;10:114–119.
30. Hill SE, Heldman LS, Goo EDH, et al: Fatal microvascular pulmonary emboli from precipitation of total nutrient admixure solution. JPEN J Parenter Nutr Enterol 1996;20(1):81–87.
31. McKinnon BT: FDA safety alert: hazards of precipitation associated with parenteral nutrition. Nutr Clin Prac 1996;11(2):59–65.
32. World Health Organization: Energy and protein requirements. Technical Report Series #724. Geneva, World Health Organization, 1985.
33. Kaplan AS, Zemel BS, Neiswender KM, Stallings VA: Resting energy expenditure in clinical pediatrics: measured versus prediction equations. J Pediatr 1995;127:200–205.
34. Liggett SB, St. John RE, Lefrak SS: Determination of resting energy expenditure utilizing the thermodilution pulmonary artery catheter. Chest 1987;91(4):562–566.
35. Krzywda EA, Andris DA, Whipple JK, et al: Glucose response to abrupt initiation and discontinuation of total parenteral nutrition. JPEN J Parenter Enteral Nutr 1992;17:64–67.
36. Bendorf K, Friesen CA, Roberts CC: Glucose response to discontinuation of parenteral nutrition in pediatrics less than 3 years of age. JPEN J Parenter Enteral Nutr 1996;20(2):120–122.
37. Collier S, Crouch J, Hendricks K, Cacallero B: Use of cyclic parenteral nutrition in infants less than 6 months of age. Nutr Clin Prac 1994;9:65–68.
38. Collins E, Lawson L, Lau M, et al: Care of central venous catheters for total parenteral nutrition. Nutr Clin Prac 1996;11(3):109–114.
39. Bilodeau J, Poon C, Mascarenhas MR: Parenteral nutrition/care of central lines. In Altschuler SM, Liacouras CA (eds): Pediatric Gastroenterology. London, Churchill Livingstone, 1998.
40. Dollery CM, Sullivan ID, Bauraind O, et al: Thrombosis and embolism in long-term central venous access for parenteral nutrition. Lancet 1994;344:1043–1045.
41. Hospital Infection Control Practices Advisory Committee. Guideline for prevention of intravascular device-related infections: I. Intravascular device-related infections: an overview. Am J Infect Control 1996;24:262–293
42. Christenson ML, Hancock ML, Gattuso J, et al: Parenteral nutrition associated with increased infection rate in children with cancer. Cancer 1993;72:2732–2738.
43. Mulloy RH, Jadavji T, Russell ML: Tunneled central venous catheter sepsis: risk factors in a pediatric hospital. JPEN J Parenter Enteral Nutr 1991;15:460–463.
44. Nahata MC, King DR, Powell DA, et al: Management of catheter-related infections in pediatric patients. JPEN J Parenter Enteral Nutr 1988;12:58–59.
45. Centers for Disease Control and Prevention: Guidelines for prevention of intravascular device-related infections. Am J Infect Control 1996;24:262–293
46. Ament ME, Misra S, Vargas J, Reyen L: Complications of total parenteral nutrition and long-term outcome. Ann Nestle 1996;54(2):61–69.
47. Verhage AH, Cheong WK, Allard JP, Jeejeebhoy KN: Increase in lumbar spine bone mineral content in patients on long-term parenteral nutrition without vitamin D supplementation. JPEN J Parenter Enteral Nutr 1995;19:431–436.
48. Koo WWK: Parenteral nutrition-related bone disease. JPEN J Parenter Enteral Nutr 1992;16:386–394.
49. Hurley DL, McMahon MM: Long-term parenteral nutrition and metabolic bone disease. Endocrinol Metabol Clin North Am 1990;19:113–131.
50. Klein GL, Ament ME, Bluestone R, et al: Bone disease associated with total parenteral nutrition. Lancet 1980;2:1041–1044.
51. Weinsier RL, Krumdieck CL: Death resulting from overzealous total parenteral nutrition: the refeeding syndrome revisited. Am J Clin Nutr 1981;34:393–399.
52. Solomon SM, Kirby DF: The refeeding syndrome: a review. JPEN J Parenter Enteral Nutr 1990;14:90–97.
53. Merritt RJ: Cholestasis associated with total parenteral nutrition. J Pediatr Gastroenterol Nutr 1986;5:9–22.
54. Quigley EMM, Marsh MN, Shaffer JL, Markin RS: Hepatobiliary complications of total parenteral nutrition. Gastroenterology 1993;104:286–301.
55. Ament ME, Misra S, Vargas J, Reyen L: Home parenteral nutrition. Ann Nestle 1996;54:70–78.
56. Altmann GG: Demonstration of a morphological control mechanism in the small intestine: role of pancreatic secretions and bile. In Dowling RH, Riecken EO (eds): Intestinal Adaptation. New York, Schattauer Verlag, 1974, pp 33–46.
57. Dworkin LD, Levine GM: Oral intake maintains small intestinal mass, in part, by factors other than direct contact with the small bowel. Clin Res 1975;23:567A.

58. Feldman EJ, Dowling RH, McNaughton J, Peters TJ: Effects of oral versus intravenous nutrition on intestinal adaptation after small bowel resection in the dog. Gastroenterology 1976;70:712.
59. Johnson LR, Copeland EM, Dudrick SJ, et al: Structural and hormonal alterations in the gastrointestinal tract of parenterally fed rats. Gastroenterology 1975;68:1177.
60. Johnson LR: The trophic action of gastrointestinal hormones. Gastroenterology 1976;70:728.
61. Dworkin LD, Levine GM, Farber NJ, Spector MH: Small intestinal mass of the rat is partially determined by direct effects of intraluminal nutrition. Gastroenterology 1976;71:626.
62. Eastwood GL: Small bowel morphology and epithelial proliferation in intravenously alimented rabbits. Surgery 1977;82:613.
63. Wahren J, Felig P, Hagenfeldt L: Effect of protein ingestion on splanchnic and leg metabolism in normal man and in patients with diabetes mellitus. J Clin Invest 1976;57:978–999.
64. Moore FA, Moore EE, Jones TN, et al: TEN versus TPN following major torso trauma—reduced septic morbidity. J Trauma 1989;29:916–923.
65. Saito H, Trocki O, Alexander JW, et al: The effect of route of nutrient administration on the nutritional state, catabolic hormone secretion, and gut mucosal integrity after burn injury. JPEN J Parenter Enteral Nutr 1987;11:1–7.
66. LeLeiko NS, Bronstein A, Baliga BS, Munro HN: De novo purine nucleotide synthesis in the rat small and large intestine: effect of dietary protein and purines. J Pediatr Gastroenterol Nutr 1983;2:313–319.
67. LeLeiko NS, Martin BA, Walsh MJ, et al: Tissue specific gene expression results from a purine and pyrimidine-free diet and 6-mercaptopurine in the rat small intestine and colon. Gastroenterology 1987;93:1014–1020.
68. LeLeiko NS, Baliga BS, Wilkins D, et al: Comparison of purine biosynthetic pathways in the small and large bowel (abstract). Gastroenterology 1978;74:1054.
69. LeLeiko NS, Bronstein A, Munro HN: Effect of dietary purines on de novo synthesis of purine nucleotides in the small intestinal mucosa (abstract). Pediatr Res 1979;13:403.
70. Walsh MJ, Sanchez-Pozo A, LeLeiko NS: A regulatory element is characterized by purine-mediated and cell-type specific gene transcription. Mol Cell Biol 1990;10:4356–4364.
71. Harig JM, Soergel KH, Komorowski RA, Wood CM: Treatment of diversion colitis with short-chain fatty acid irrigation. N Engl J Med 1989;320:23–38.
72. Byrne TA, Morrissey TB, Nattakom TV, et al: Growth hormone, glutamine, and a modified diet enhance nutrient absorption in patients with severe short bowel syndrome. JPEN J Parenter Enteral Nutr 1995;19:296–302.
73. Byrne TA, Persinger RL, Young LS, et al: A new treatment for patients with short-bowel syndrome. Ann Surg 1995;222:243–255.
74. Seidman E, LeLeiko NS, Ament M, et al: Nutritional issues in pediatric inflammatory bowel disease. J Pediatr Gastroenterol Nutr 1991;12:424–438.
75. Meeroff JC, Phillips SF: Control of gastric emptying by osmolality of duodenal contents. Gastroenterology 1975;68:1144.
76. Saint Hilaire S, Lavers M, Kennedy J, Code C: Gastric acid secretory value of different foods. Gastroenterology 1960;39:1.
77. Elwin CE: Gastric acid responses to antral application of some amino acids, peptides, and isolated fractions of a protein hydrolysate. Scand J Gastroenterol 1974;9:239.
78. Ragins H, Levenson SM, Signer R, et al: Intrajejunal administration of an elemental diet at neutral pH avoids pancreatic stimulation: studies in dog and man. Am J Surg 1978;126:606.
79. Voitk AJ, Brown RA, McArdle AH, et al: Use of an elemental diet in the treatment of complicated pancreatitis. Am J Surg 1973;125:223.
80. Bury KD, Stevens RV, Randall HT: Use of a chemically defined, liquid elemental diet in nutritional management of fistulas of the alimentary tract. Am J Surg 1971;121:174.
81. Porter JM, Snowe RJ, Sliver D: Tuberculous enteritis with perforation and abscess formation in childhood. Surgery 1972;71:254.
82. Voitk AJ, Brown RA, McArdle AH, et al: Clinical uses of an elemental diet—preliminary studies. Can Med Assoc J 1972;107:123.
83. Clark SB, Holt PR: Inhibition of steady-state absorption of long chain triglyceride by medium-chain triglyceride on the unanesthetized rat. Gastroenterology 1969;56:214.
84. Greenberger NJ, Rodgers JB, Isselbacher KJ: Absorption of medium and long chain triglycerides: Factors influencing the hydrolysis and transport. J Clin Invest 1966;45:217.
85. Playoust MC, Isselbacher KJ: Studies on the intestinal absorption and intramucosal lipolysis of a medium chain triglyceride. J Clin Invest 1964;43:878.
86. Clark SB, Holt PR: Rate-limiting steps in steady-state intestinal absorption of trioctanoin-1-14C. J Clin Invest 1968;47:612.
87. Valdivieso VD, Schwabe AD: Absorption of medium-chain lipids from the rat cecum. Am J Dig Dis 1966;11:474.
88. Pihl BG, Glotozor DJ, Patterson JF: Absorption of medium-chain fatty acids by the dog colon. J Appl Physiol 1966;21:1059.
89. Kaufman SS, Scrivner DJ, Murray ND, Vanderhoof JA, Hart MH, Antonson DL: Influence of Portagen and Pregestimil on essential fatty acid status in infantile liver disease. Pediatrics 1992;89:151–154.
90. Pettei MJ, Daftary S, Levine JL: Essential fatty acid deficiency associated with the use of a medium-chain-triglyceride infant formula in pediatric hepatobiliary disease. Am J Clin Nutr 1991;53:1217–1221.
91. Miller DG, Williams SK, Palombo JD, et al: Cutaneous application of safflower oil in preventing essential fatty acid deficiency in patients on home parenteral nutrition. Am J Clin Nutr 1987;46:419–423.
92. Shapiro M, Rosen GH: Topical oil applications in essential fatty acid deficiency. Nutr Clin Prac 1989;4:140–144.
93. Sacks GS, Brown RO, Collier P, Kudsk KA: Failure of topical vegetable oils to prevent essential fatty acid deficiency in a critically ill patient receiving long-term parenteral nutrition. JPEN J Parenter Enteral Nutr 1994;18:274–277.
94. Van Dyke RW: Mechanisms of digestion and absorption of food. In Sleisenger MH, Fordtran JS (eds): Gastrointestinal Disease, 4th ed, Vol 2. Philadelphia, WB Saunders, 1989, pp 1062–1088.
95. Plotkin GR, Isselbacher KJ: Secondary disaccharidase deficiency in adult celiac disease (nontropical sprue) and other malabsorption states. N Engl J Med 1964;271:1033.
96. Wels JD, Zschiesche OM, Anderson J, Walker A: Intestinal disaccharidase activity in celiac sprue (gluten-sensitive enteropathy). Arch Intern Med 1969;123:33.
97. Rosensweig NS, Herman RH: Time response of jejunal sucrase and maltase activity to a high sucrase diet in normal man. Gastroenterology 1969;56:500.
98. Rosensweig NS, Herman RH: Control of jejunal sucrase and maltase activity by dietary sucrose and fructose in man. J Clin Invest 1968;47:2253.
99. Adibi SA, Soleimanpour M: Functional characterization of dipeptide transport system in human jejunum. J Clin Invest 1974;53:1368.
100. Zaloga GP: Physiologic effects of peptide-based enteral formulas. Nutr Clin Prac 1990;5:231–237.
101. Brinson RR, Hanumanthu SK, Pitts WM: A reappraisal of the peptide-based enteral formulas: clinical applications. Nutr Clin Prac 1989;4:211–217.
102. Alpers D: Digestion and absorption of carbohydrates and proteins. In Johnson L (ed): Physiology of the Gastrointestinal Tract, 2nd ed. New York, Raven Press, 1987, pp 1469–1487.
103. Kim YS, Birtwhistle W, Kim YW: Peptide hydrolases in the brush border and soluble fractions of small intestinal mucosa of rat and man. J Clin Invest 1972;51:1419.
104. National Research Council: Recommended Dietary Allowances, 10th ed. Washington, DC, National Academy Press, 1989.
105. Birch LL, Johnson SL, Andresen G, et al: The variability of young children's energy intake. N Engl J Med 1991;324:232–235.
106. Albertson AM, Tobelmann RC, Engstrom A, Asp E: Nutrient intakes of 2- to 10-year-old American children: 10-year trends. J Am Diet Assoc 1992;92:1492–1496.
107. Kleinman RE: Pediatric Nutrition, 4th ed. Elk Grove Village, IL, American Academy of Pediatrics, 1998.
108. Raiha NCR, Heinonen K, Rassin DK, et al: Milk protein quantity and quality in low-birth weight infants: I. Metabolic responses and effects on growth. Pediatrics 1976;57:659–674.
109. Parker P, Stroop S, Greene H: A controlled comparison of continuous versus intermittent feeding in the treatment of infants with intestinal disease. J Pediatr 1981;99:360.

# Chapter 60

# Management of Diarrhea

*Robert H. Squires, Jr.*

Diarrhea is an important cause of morbidity and mortality among children and the elderly in the United States and throughout the world.[1–4] An estimated 3.5 million children die worldwide each year as a consequence of diarrhea.[3] In the United States, 16.5 million children younger than 5 years of age experience 21 million episodes of diarrhea per year, which lead to an estimated 2.1 million physician visits, 210,000 hospitalizations, and 500 deaths.[1,2] Outpatient costs, which include the office visit, laboratory tests, medications, rehydration solutions, travel, additional daycare arrangements, and days missed from work, approach $289 per episode, or $1 billion dollars annually in the United States.[5]

The management of diarrhea has changed dramatically since the 1970s. We have moved away from low-sodium, high-carbohydrate "clear liquids" and withholding enteral nutrition toward defined oral electrolyte solutions and early reintroduction or continuation of formula and solid or pureed foods. This transition was driven by the desperate needs of children who have no access to intravenous fluids or adequate nutrition. Although most problematic in developing countries, similar circumstances exist for children in developed countries. Providing inexpensive, portable, effective hydration therapy and maximizing enteral nutrition to support ill, malnourished children are critical in reducing morbidity and mortality associated with childhood diarrhea.

## MECHANISMS OF DIARRHEA

Diarrhea is characterized by an increase in number and decrease in consistency of daily stools accompanied by an increase in stool volume. Approximately 98% of the endogenous and exogenous fluid that passes through the intestinal tract is normally retained by the small bowel and colon. When an individual consumes a regular diet for age, residual stool averages 200 to 225 g/day in adults and 10 g/kg/day in infants and children. Diarrhea results when intestinal solute transport mechanisms are disrupted, causing either increased secretion or decreased absorption of solutes with excess loss of salt and water in the stool[6,7] (see Chapter 3).

A primary mechanism for diarrhea has been identified in a number of clinical conditions (Table 60–1). However, for many patients the cause is multifactorial. An example would be the patient infected with rotavirus, which attacks mature villus tip cells. Loss of these cells that contain important solute transport proteins and disaccharidases reduces the absorptive surface and increases luminal osmolality created by undigested lactose. In addition, inflammatory mediators increase mucosal permeability and decrease intestinal transit time. Each of these factors contributes to the development of diarrhea.

## TREATMENT STRATEGIES

Because most childhood diarrhea is acute and self-limited, the primary treatment goals are to prevent dehydration, minimize the nutritional consequences of the mucosal injury, and identify a potentially treatable condition (Table 60–2). Oral rehydration therapy (ORT) is an effective intervention to replace salt and water loss and maintain hydration during an acute episode of viral gastroenteritis. Early introduction of enteral nutrition in conjunction with ORT minimizes the deleterious effects of starvation on intestinal mucosa. Treatable conditions should be sought if the clinical setting suggests these. Patients with particular clinical conditions (e.g., short-bowel syndrome, ileal resection, pancreatic insufficiency, hormone-secreting tumor) may respond to therapeutic interventions that reduce luminal or circulating factors that promote diarrhea. Pharmacologic agents should be restricted to specific clinical conditions and even then used with great caution.

This chapter focuses on the management of acute gastroenteritis with ORT and early reintroduction of enteral feeding. Pharmacologic therapy and preventive strategies are also reviewed.

## ORAL REHYDRATION THERAPY

### History

ORT was introduced in the United States in the early 1950s, well before our current understanding of solute absorption across the intestinal mucosal surface.[8] Harrison and colleagues reasoned that an appropriate oral solution would be one that would replace solutes lost in the stool. Their initial oral solution contained 60 mmol (60 mEq) of sodium per liter, 20 mmol (20 mEq) of potassium per liter, 54 mmol (54 mEq) of chloride per liter, and 33 mmol (33 mEq) of

**TABLE 60–1. Mechanisms of Diarrhea**

| MECHANISM | EXAMPLE |
|---|---|
| Active anion secretion | Toxigenic *Escherichia coli* |
| Reduced absorptive function | Celiac disease |
| Increased luminal osmolality | Lactase deficiency |
| Increased permeability | Malnutrition |
| Increased hydrostatic pressure | Constrictive pericarditis |
| Altered motility | Secondary to inflammatory mediators |

lactate per liter.[9] Later, they added 3.3 g of glucose per deciliter to the solute solution, based on data that indicated glucose would spare protein loss. Unfortunately, the first commercial solution contained 8 g of glucose per deciliter and had a higher osmolality than Harrison's solution. An outbreak of hypernatremia in the United States in the mid-1950s was linked to the sodium content and not the excessive carbohydrate concentration and created the misconception that sodium-containing oral electrolyte solutions were harmful.[10, 11]

The identification and characterization of coupled sodium and glucose transport was critical to the development of effective oral rehydration.[3, 12, 13] This basic knowledge was taken to the bedside in 1964 when Phillips confirmed that solutions containing glucose and sodium resulted in net absorption of salt and water from the intestinal musosa to the bloodstream in patients with cholera.[14] Subsequent studies have identified a host of sugars, amino acids, hormones, and neurotransmitters originating from a variety of mesenchymal cells and enteric neurons that affect the absorption and secretion of ions.[7] Our enhanced knowledge of intestinal solute transport provides an opportunity to explore new approaches to ORT.

**TABLE 60–2. Treatment Strategies for Acute Diarrhea**

- Rehydration
  - Oral rehydration solution
- Maintain hydration
  - Oral maintenance solution
- Improve nutrition
  - Early introduction of enteral feeding
- Identify a treatable condition
  - Enteric infection or infestation (e.g., *Giardia, Clostridium difficile*)
  - Cystic fibrosis
  - Celiac disease
  - Hormone-mediated diarrhea (e.g., VIPoma)
- Reduce luminal secretagogues
  - Lactose-free diet for primary or secondary lactase deficiency
  - Cholestyramine for bile acid–induced diarrhea (e.g., ileal resection)
  - Pancreatic enzymes for pancreatic insufficiency
- Pharmacologic agents
  - Oral rehydration solution
  - Bismuth compounds
  - Opiates
  - Probiotic bacteria
- Prevention
  - Safe water supply
  - Breast feeding
  - Vaccine development

## Development of Oral Rehydration Solution

The driving force in the development of oral rehydration solution (ORS) was an effort to find an inexpensive, effective means to treat patients with cholera where access to intravenous fluid was unavailable. Initial solutions contained up to 110 mEq of sodium per liter based on measurement of stool electrolytes in these patients.[15] However, after further studies,[16] a consensus conference in the mid-1970s sponsored by the World Health Organization (WHO) concluded that the WHO ORS should contain the following proportion of solutes (in mmol/L): sodium 90, potassium 20, chloride 80, bicarbonate 3, and glucose 111. The bicarbonate was later changed to citrate to improve its stability. In hospitals and clinics where the solution was used appropriately, the diarrhea case fatality rate fell significantly.

The WHO ORS was first used successfully in the United States on the Fort Apache Indian Reservation to treat children with dehydration.[17] However, others voiced concerns regarding the use of a solution formulated to treat cholera in otherwise healthy children with acute viral gastroenteritis.[18] During this time, most United States physicians preferred intravenous solutions for hospitalized patients and clear liquids accompanied by delayed enteral feeding for outpatient therapy.

In the early 1980s, a number of important studies were published that were to form the basis for the American Academy of Pediatrics (AAP) recommendation to support ORT. In 1982, Santosham and associates studied 146 well-nourished children 2 months to 2 years of age from Panama and the United States with acute gastroenteritis.[19] Children were given either "standard" intravenous rehydration and maintenance fluids or one of two similar oral rehydration solutions that differed only in the concentration of sodium, either 90 mmol/L or 50 mmol/L. Diluted formula was started in the ORS group after 24 hours, and stool output was replaced mL for mL with the ORS. In this study, oral rehydration was successful in 97 of 98 children, and 87 (89%) did not require intravenous therapy. Importantly, six children with hypernatremia were successfully managed with oral therapy alone. No serious complications developed in either oral therapy group, although catheter-related problems were noted in those treated with intravenous therapy. In 1983, Pizarro and colleagues treated 94 well-nourished children from Costa Rica who suffered from either hypernatremic (n = 61) or hyponatremic (n = 33) dehydration with ORS containing 90 mmol of sodium per liter.[20] Normalization of serum sodium and morbidity (e.g., seizure) compared favorably with historical controls treated with intravenous fluids. Finally, in 1985 Santosham and coworkers published data on 140 well-nourished ambulatory children younger than 2 years of age from the United States (Baltimore, MD, and Whiteriver, AZ) with acute watery diarrhea.[21] Children were randomized to one of four ORS preparations with sodium concentrations that ranged from 30 to 90 mmol/L and glucose concentrations that ranged from 20 to 50 mmol/L, and 137 of 140 (98%) were treated successfully.

The AAP Committee on Nutrition developed detailed recommendations for the use of ORS in the treatment of children with gastrointestinal fluid loss.[22] They identified three phases of management: (1) rehydration, (2) maintenance, and (3) early reintroduction of food. To replace deficit salt and water loss, 40 to 50 mL/kg of a solution that contains between 75 and 90 mmol/L of sodium and between 110 and 140 mmol/L of glucose is given over 4 hours. The patient is then assessed to determine whether the rehydration phase should be continued or the maintenance phase initiated. The maintenance solution should contain 40 to 60 mmol/L of sodium and 110 to 140 mmol/L of glucose and offered after each bowel movement. The total volume should not exceed 150 mL/kg/24 hours. Breast milk or water is given to satisfy thirst. The AAP identified the need to individualize therapy for each patient but encouraged the reintroduction of a regular diet within 24 hours of initiating therapy.

Despite firm recommendations from the AAP and the clinical data that continued to support those recommendations, United States pediatricians were slow to accept the concept of oral rehydration therapy.[23, 24] Five years after the AAP recommendations, Snyder and colleagues conducted a survey to assess how well U.S. pediatricians in training, in academics, and in private practice incorporated ORT into their practice.[24] Surprisingly, less than 30% of those surveyed used ORS appropriately, and the majority continued to withhold feeding until the second day or later; most felt that vomiting was a contraindication to ORT. Traditional clear liquids such as apple juice and soda are still used despite their inadequate salt content and high osmolality (Table 60–3).

A number of obstacles have impeded the incorporation of ORT, many of which have been addressed with clinical studies. ORT is an effective treatment regimen in both nourished and malnourished children; an estimated 1 million child deaths have been prevented each year by ORT.[25] The failure rate of ORT is only approximately 3.6% in well-nourished U.S. children.[26] ORT can be used safely in patients with hypernatremia and hyponatremia, and patients may have a more favorable outcome in terms of weight gain and duration of diarrhea when early reintroduction of feeding is utilized properly.[26] ORT is less expensive than intravenous therapy in an outpatient setting and can be delivered safely via a nasogastric tube in the patient who is unable or unwilling to take sufficient quantities of fluid by mouth.[27–29] Efforts to improve taste by substituting sucrose for glucose resulted in impaired salt and water absorption.[30] It is likely, however, that if the child is dehydrated or salt depleted, taste is not an issue. Maintenance solutions used in U.S. children may also be effective in the rehydration phase of infants with mild to moderate dehydration.[31]

Barriers remain to the use of ORT.[32] The perception that intravenous therapy is more effective than ORT and serves as the "standard" of care is held by many parents, families, nurses, physicians, and payers. Much effort has been made to overcome this perception through the work of individuals, patient advocates, and the National ORT Project. Education of mothers, physician office personnel, and emergency room personnel is a critical component to improved access to ORT. Protocols for the use of ORT should be incorporated into every pediatric and family practice training program (Table 60–4). Improper preparation of ORS from commercially prepared packets or home-prepared formulations has led to serum electrolyte abnormalities that could be avoided with proper education of the family or access to "ready-to-feed" ORS.[33, 34] Finally, economic barriers to ORT remain that can have a fatal outcome.[35]

**TABLE 60–3. Relationship Between the Solute Content of Stool Output, Traditional Clear Liquids, and Oral Rehydration Solution (ORS)**

| | $Na^+$ | $K^+$ | $Cl^-$ | $HCO_3$ | CHO | mOSM |
|---|---|---|---|---|---|---|
| **Stool Electrolyte Content (mEq/L)** | | | | | | |
| ***Etiologic Agent*** | | | | | | |
| Rotavirus | 37 | 38 | 22 | 6 | 0 | 300 |
| Toxo *Escherichia coli* | 53 | 37 | 24 | 18 | 0 | 300 |
| Cholera | 88 | 30 | 86 | 32 | 0 | 330 |
| **Solution Electrolyte Content (mEq/L)** | | | | | | |
| ***Rehydration*** | | | | | | |
| WHO ORS | 90 | 20 | 80 | 10 | 111 | 310 |
| Rehydralyte | 75 | 20 | 65 | 10 | 140 | 305 |
| ***Maintenance*** | | | | | | |
| Pedialyte | 45 | 20 | 35 | 10 | 140 | 250 |
| Infalyte | 50 | 20 | 40 | 10 | 111 | 270 |
| ***Clear Liquids*** | | | | | | |
| Gatorade | 23 | 3 | 17 | 3 | 255 | 330 |
| Cola | 2 | 0.1 | 2 | 13 | 730 | 750 |
| Kool-Aid | 3 | 0.1 | 0 | 0 | 105 | 465 |
| Apple juice | 3 | 28 | 30 | 0 | 690 | 725 |
| Hi-C | 2 | 5 | 0 | 0 | 800 | 816 |
| Popsicle | 5 | 0.5 | 0 | 0 | 710 | 719 |
| Chicken broth | 251 | 8 | 250 | 0 | 0 | 501 |

**TABLE 60–4. Oral Rehydration Therapy Protocol**

**Rehydration Phase**
- For shock or hypotension: resuscitate with extracellular-like fluid (intravenous or interosseous).
- Solutions to use for oral rehydration:
  - 75–90 mmol/L sodium (standard)
  - 40–60 mmol/L sodium (has been used successfully in United States)
- Volume: 40–50 mL/kg given over 4 hr.
- Vomiting is not a contraindication, but assess for evidence of obstruction.
- Consider infusion with nasogastric tube for the child who refuses sufficient oral fluid.
- Reassess and repeat if resuscitation is not complete.

**Maintenance Phase**
- Solutions to use:
  - 40–60 mmol/L sodium
  - 110–140 mmol/L glucose
- Volume: 150 mL/kg/24 hr.
- Breast milk, formula, or water to satisfy thirst.
- After 24 hr, offer 10 mL/kg after each stool to replace ongoing loss.

**Introduction of Feeding**
- Breast feeding should not be stopped.
- Resume full strength formula within 24 hr.
- Formula-fed infants younger than 3 months may benefit from lactose-free formula.
- If the child takes solid foods, begin complex carbohydrates and fiber (e.g., bananas, cereal, potatoes).

## New Formulations

The physician's treatment goal for the child with acute gastroenteritis and water-loss stools is to prevent dehydration. However, the goal of the family is to stop the diarrhea. Unfortunately, the current formulations of ORS are not able to enhance repair of the mucosal injury caused by the pathogen. Efforts to reduce stool volume by altering ORS osmolality or adding starch or amino acids to the solutions have been evaluated in clinical trials but without significant clinical improvement.

Neutral amino acids such as alanine and glycine enhance sodium and water absorption independent of glucose.[13, 36, 37] When amino acid–containing solutions were used in adults with cholera, more efficient intestinal absorption of salt and water was observed, although the clinical impact was difficult to assess.[38] Sazawal and associates used an ORS that contained 90 mmol/L of alanine and glucose in well-nourished children aged 3 to 48 months with mild to moderate dehydration. They noted a decrease in the duration of diarrhea and reduction in stool output, but the differences did not reach statistical significance.[39]

Boiled rice water is a constituent of many home remedies for gastroenteritis in developing countries. The use of starch, a polymer of glucose, as the glucose source has some theoretical advantages.[40] Starch provides a larger number of glucose molecules with a lower intraluminal osmotic force. Unfortunately, starch requires intestinal glucoamylase for it to be adequately digested, and this enzyme is not fully developed in infants younger than 4 months of age. Rice water also provides small peptides and amino acids that facilitate absorption of additional sodium. The additional protein provides more calories during the acute phase of rehydration, which may accelerate mucosal healing. To capitalize on these potential advantages, studies were performed to determine whether theoretical advantages were clinically important.

In 1991, Pizarro and colleagues conducted a prospective, randomized, double-blind trial comparing standard ORS with ORS containing rice-syrup solids.[41] The study involved well-nourished male Costa Rican children 3 to 18 months of age with mild to moderate dehydration as a consequence of acute gastroenteritis. The study solution was effective in the rehydration phase, and stool output decreased initially compared with that of controls; however, the differences were not significant at 24 hours. In another study, which involved 146 male children aged 3 to 36 months from Guatemala City, no clinically significant differences in stool output were noted when the children were randomized to receive ORS containing glucose, rice dextrin, or rice flour.[42]

When glucose is absorbed, the luminal fluid becomes more hypotonic, which promotes water absorption along the paracellular pathway along with sodium and chloride—a concept known as solvent drag.[43, 44] Santosham and associates studied a reduced osmolarity ORS (311 mOsm/L versus 245 mOsm/L) in 190 well-nourished Egyptian males between 1 and 14 months of age with acute, noncholera diarrhea.[45] Stool output was 36% lower in those patients receiving reduced osmolarity ORS, but after a cereal-based diet was initiated, there were no differences between the groups.

## NUTRITIONAL THERAPY

There is a complex relationship between diarrhea, malnutrition, and intestinal integrity.[8, 46] In animal models, starvation significantly alters mucosal barrier function,[47, 48] and refeeding enhances repair of mucosal injury caused by malnutrition.[49] The clinical consequences of malnutrition are seen most vividly in children from developing countries.[22] Malnutrition leads to an increased susceptibility to additional gastrointestinal infections, which further injure and inflame the mucosal surface and result in malabsorption and malnutrition. This vicious circle kills millions of children worldwide each year, yet these clinical consequences are infrequently seen in developed nations. As a result, the initial clinical studies identifying the importance of early reintroduction of feeding were considered relevant only for children in developing countries where malnutrition was an endemic problem. However, studies in well-nourished children have confirmed the importance of early feeding in this population as well.[16, 17, 50–52] The question is no longer whether early feeding following acute gastroenteritis is important, but what is best to feed the child.

Controversy continues as to whether a lactose-containing formula is appropriate to offer a child with acute gastroenteritis.[53–57] Certainly the villus tip cells that harbor lactase are most severely affected in acute gastroenteritis, particularly that caused by rotavirus. In a meta-analysis of 25 randomized clinical trials involving 2,215 patients, only those whose initial degree of dehydration was reported as "severe" failed to respond to a lactose-containing formula.[53] Also, children younger than 3 months of age with acute gastroenteritis may not tolerate a lactose-containing formula as well as older children.[55] However, children older than 3 months of age with mild or moderate dehydration can be treated successfully with a lactose-containing formula.[16, 53, 58]

Efforts to identify an optimal protein source have been difficult.[46] Breast milk protein is the ideal source for infants and should not be discontinued. For the infant who takes only formula and is not yet on solid foods or cereal, the concerns of continuing a cow's milk–based formula include enhanced absorption of cow's milk antigens, which may evoke a local or systemic immune response and increase the risk of food sensitization. However, these theoretical concerns have not been substantiated by clinical studies.[16, 51, 52] Also, the "traditional" method of using a partial-strength formula followed by full-strength formula for a period of time during treatment for gastroenteritis appears unnecessary.[16, 17, 53] Weight gain is more rapid when full-strength formula is offered within 24 hours of initiating ORT. The choice of solid foods should be based on those available in the local community. Many cultures are resistant to the introduction of unfamiliar foods, and the taste, temperature, and mother's perception of the food likely influence its acceptability.[59] Therefore, the incorporation of traditional porridge, when appropriate, into the treatment regimen can enhance recovery of the patient.[46, 59] Otherwise, foods high in complex carbohydrates and fiber appear to be most beneficial.

## PHARMACOLOGIC THERAPY

Pharmacologic therapy for acute viral gastroenteritis is not recommenced. The decision to use antibiotic therapy for specific bacterial infections is based on the clinical circumstances. However, considerable pressure is placed on the treating physician by the family to stop or shorten the course of diarrhea. Unfortunately, there are no treatment regimens capable of improving on time and "mother nature" in an otherwise healthy child. Decreasing the frequency of stool effluent with medications that reduce intestinal transit time merely "hides" stool volume within the bowel and removes an important clinical parameter used to assess the patient. Although concerns abound regarding the use of pharmacologic agents, clinical studies continue to search for a safe, affordable, and effective agent that offers a clinically important improvement on the ORT and early refeeding.

The lay literature abounds with testimonials promoting the health benefits of probiotic bacteria such as *Lactobacillus*.[60] Mechanisms by which probiotic bacteria may alter the clinical course of enteric infections include competition with pathogens for receptor sites and nutrients, production of inhibitory substances, or alteration of the environment of the intestinal lumen (e.g., acidification) to inhibit growth of enteropathogens.[61–64] The ideal probiotic would be resistant to gastric, biliary, and pancreatic fluids.[60] Although probiotic agents such as *Lactobacillus GG*[65] and the yeast *Saccharomyces boulardii*[66] may be effective in patients with recurrent *Clostridium difficile* colitis; their clinical benefit in patients with acute gastroenteritis remains unproved.

Bismuth subsalicylate (BSS) has been shown to improve the stool pattern and clinical symptoms in patients with traveler's diarrhea.[67] Its mechanism of action is poorly understood, but possibilities include direct antimicrobial effects, anti-inflammatory effects of the salicylate, prevention of binding of bile acids or microorganisms to the intestinal mucosa, or inactivation of toxins.[68] In a study from Lima, Peru, of children aged 3 to 59 months with nonbloody diarrhea, children who received 100 to 150 mg/kg/day of BSS were noted to have a decreased duration of diarrhea, total stool output, duration of hospitalization, and intake of ORS.[69] However, there was no mention of failure rates or stool frequency. Although measurements of bismuth and salicylate levels were below concentrations considered toxic, concern over potential problems from the absorption of these constituents remains. In addition, the added cost is not insignificant when compared with ORT alone.

The use of diphenoxylate has been associated with significant morbidity and unacceptable mortality when used in children with acute diarrhea.[70–72] Loperamide acts to delay intestinal transit and increase the capacitance of the intestine to allow more time for absorption, yet does not cross into the central nervous system as easily as diphenoxylate. Initial studies using loperamide in children suggested no benefit over placebo.[73, 74] More recently, a study using a higher dose of loperamide in hospitalized children aged 6 weeks to 1 year with acute diarrhea was conducted in South Africa.[75] A decrease in the total daily stool output and duration of diarrhea was seen overall. However, duration and severity did not differ between groups in those with rotavirus. Ileus associated with vomiting and drowsiness was more frequent in the treatment group, particularly those younger than 3 months of age. Therefore, the risks of using loperamide to treat children with acute gastroenteritis seem to outweigh potential benefits.

Homeopathic medicine is a traditional method of treatment in many developing countries and is gaining popularity world wide. A published study touted a significant benefit of homeopathic medicine in the treatment of children from Nicaragua aged 6 months to 5 years.[76] A critical rebuttal offered serious concerns over the methods and conclusions of the report.[77]

## PREVENTION

Prevention of acute gastroenteritis would be the best cure. The first priority is to ensure the quality of the world's water and food supply. Clean water and proper sewage disposal make an immediate and significant difference in the health of the children. Breast feeding must be promoted, because it is associated with significant levels of protection against diarrhea due to *Vibrio cholerae,*[78] *Shigella,*[79] and rotavirus in the first year of life.[80, 81] Development of vaccines to the important pathogens holds great promise. Cost-effective vaccines against rotavirus infection[82–84] are possible as knowledge of natural immunity to the virus is better.[85] Effective cholera vaccines have been tested in adults[86] and children.[87] Interestingly, infant formula supplemented with probiotics resulted in fewer episodes of diarrhea and fewer patients shed rotavirus.[88]

### REFERENCES


1. Kilgore PE, Holman RC, Clarke MJ, Glass RI: Trends of diarrheal disease-associated mortality in US children, 1968 through 1991. JAMA 1995;274:1143–1148.
2. Glass RI, Lew JF, Gangarosa RE, LeBaron CW: Estimates of the morbidity and mortality from diarrheal diseases in American children. J Pediatr 1991;118:527–533.
3. Bern C, Martines J, de Zoysa I, Glass RI: The magnitude of the global problem of diarrhoeal disease: a ten year update. Bull World Health Organ 1992;70:705–714.
4. Lew JF, Glass RI, Gangarosa RE, et al: Diarrheal deaths in the United States, 1979 through 1987. JAMA 1991;265:3280–3284.
5. Avendano P, Matson DO, Long J, et al: Costs associated with office visits for diarrhea in infants and toddlers. Pediatr Infect Dis J 1993;12:897–902.
6. Hamilton JR: Treatment of diarrhea. Pediatr Clin North Am 1985;32:419–427.
7. Field M, Rao MC, Chang EB: Intestinal electrolyte transport and diarrheal disease—part 1. N Engl J Med 1989;321:800–806.
8. Sullivan PB, Lunn PG, Northrop-Clewes C, et al: Persistent diarrhea and malnutrition—the impact of treatment on small bowel structure and permeability. J Pediatr Gastroenterol Nutr 1992;14:208–215.
9. Harrison HE: The treatment of diarrhea in infancy. Pediatr Clin North Am 1954;1:335–348.
10. Colle E, Ayoub E, Raile R: Hypertonic dehydration (hypernatremia): the role of feedings high in solutes. Pediatrics 1958;22:5–12.
11. Franz MN, Segar WE: The association of various factors and hypernatremic diarrheal dehydration. Am J Dis Child 1959;97:298–302.
12. Schultz SG, Zalusky R: Ion transport in isolated rabit ileum. II. The interaction between active sodium and active sugar transport. J Gen Physiol 1964;47:1043–1059.
13. Schultz SG: Sodium-coupled solute transport by small intestine: a status report. Am J Physiol 1977;233:249–254.
14. Phillips RA: Water and electrolyte losses in cholera. Fed Proc 1964;23:705–712.
15. Santosham M: Status of oral rehydration therapy after 25 years of experience. In Gracey M, Walker-Smith JA (eds): Diarrheal Disease. Philadelphia, Lippincott-Raven, 1997, pp 91–108.
16. Hirschhorn N, Kinzie JL, Sachar DB, et al: Decrease in net stool output in cholera during intestinal perfusion with glucose-containing solutions. N Engl J Med 1968;279:176–181.
17. Hirschhorn N, Cash R, Woodward W, Spivey G: Oral fluid therapy of Apache children with acute infectious diarrhoea. Lancet 1972;2:15–18.
18. Nichols BL, Soriano HA: A critique of oral therapy of dehydration due to diarheal syndromes. J Clin Nutr 1977;30:1457–1472.
19. Santosham M, Daum RS, Dillman L, et al: Oral rehydration therapy

of infantile diarrhea: a controlled study of well-nourished children hospitalized in the United States and Panama. N Engl J Med 1982;306:1070–1076.
20. Pizarro D, Posada G, Villavicencio N, et al: Oral rehydration in hypernatremic and hyponatremic diarrheal dehydration: treatment with oral glucose/electrolyte solution. Am J Dis Child 1983;137:730–734.
21. Santosham M, Burns B, Nadkarini V, et al: Oral rehydration therapy for acute diarrhea in ambulatory children in the United States: a double-blind comparison of four different solutions. Pediatrics 1985;76:159–166.
22. Mauer AM, Chair, Committee on Nutrition: Use of oral fluid therapy and posttreatment feeding following enteritis in children in a developed country. Pediatrics 1985;75:358–361.
23. Avery ME, Snyder JD: Oral therapy for acute diarrhea: the underused simple solution. N Engl J Med 1990;323:891–894.
24. Snyder JD: Use and misuse of oral therapy for diarrhea: comparison of US practices with American Academy of Pediatrics recommendations. Pediatrics 1991;87:28–33.
25. The United Nations Children's Fund: The State of the World's Children. New York, Oxford University Press, 1993, p 1.
26. Gavin N, Merrick N, Davidson B: Efficacy of glucose-based oral rehydration therapy. Pediatrics 1996;98:45–51.
27. Listernick R, Zieserl E, Davis AT: Outpatient oral rehydration in the US. Am J Dis Child 1986;140:211–215.
28. Pizarro D, Castillo B, Posada G, et al: Efficacy comparison of oral rehydration solutions containing either 90 or 75 millimoles of sodium per liter. Pediatrics 1987;79:190–195.
29. Gremse DA: Effectiveness of nasogastric rehydration in hospitalized children with acute diarrhea. J Pediatr Gastroenterol Nutr 1996;21:145–148.
30. Dias JA, Thillainayagam AV, Hoekstra H, et al: Improving the palatability of oral rehydration solutions has implications for salt and water transport: a study in animal models. J Pediatr Gastroenterol Nutr 1996;23:275–279.
31. Cohen MB, Mezoff AG, Laney DW, et al: Use of a single solution for oral rehydration and maintenance therapy of infants with diarrhea and mild to moderate dehydration. Pediatrics 1995;95:639–645.
32. Reis EC, Goepp JG, Katz S, Santosham M: Barriers to use of oral rehydration therapy. Pediatrics 1994;93:708–711.
33. Fontana M, Zuin G, Paccagnini S, et al: Home-made oral rehydration solutions: variations in composition. Acta Paediatr Scand 1991;80:720–722.
34. Almroth S, Latham MC: Rational home management of diarrhoea. Lancet 1995;345:709–711.
35. Meyers A, Siegel B, Vinci R: Economic barriers to the use of oral rehydration therapy: a case report. JAMA 1991;265:1724–1725.
36. Hellier MD, Thirumalai C, Holdsworth CD: The effect of amino acids and dipeptides on sodium and water absorption in man. Gut 1989;14:41–45.
37. Rohoads JM, Macleod RJ, Hamilton JR: Alanine enhances jejunal sodium absorption in the presence of glucose: studies in piglet viral diarrhea. Pediatr Res 1986;20:879–883.
38. Patra FC, Sack DA, Islam A, et al: Oral rehydration formula containing alanine and glucose for treatment of diarrhoea: a controlled trial. Br Med J 1989;298:1353–1356.
39. Sazawal S, Bhatnager S, Bhan MK, et al: Alanine-based oral rehydration solution: assessment of efficacy in acute noncholera diarrhea among children. J Pediatr Gastroenterol Nutr 1991;12:461–468.
40. Carpenter CCJ, Greenough WB, Pierce NF: Oral-rehydration therapy—the role of polymeric substrates. N Engl J Med 1988;319:1346–1348.
41. Pizarro D, Posada G, Sandi L, Moran JR: Rice-based oral electrolyte solutions for the management of infantile diarrhea. N Engl J Med 1991;324:517–521.
42. Molina S, Vettorazzi C, Peerson JM, et al: Clinical trial of glucose-oral rehydration solution (ORS), rice dextrin-ORS, and rice flour-ORS for the management of children with acute diarrhea and mild or moderate dehydration. Pediatrics 1995;95:191–197.
43. Fordtran JS, Rector FC, Carter NW: The mechanism of sodium absorption in the human intestine. J Clin Invest 1968;47:884–900.
44. Schiller LR, Santa Ana CA, Porter J, Fordtran JS: Glucose-stimulated sodium transport by the human intestine during experimental cholera. Gastroenterology 1997;112:1529–1535.
45. Santosham M, Fayad I, Abu Zikri M, et al: A double-blind clinical trial comparing World Health Organization oral rehydration solution with a reduced osmolarity solution containing equal amounts of sodium and glucose. J Pediatr 1996;128:45–51.
46. Willumsen JF, Darling JC, Kitundu JA, et al: Dietary management of acute diarrhoea in children: effect of fermented and amylase-digested weaning foods on intestinal permeability. J Pediatr Gastroenterol Nutr 1997;24:235–241.
47. Butzner JD, Butler DG, Miniats OP: Impact of chronic protein-calorie malnutrition on small intestinal repair after acute viral enteritis: a study in gnotobiotic piglets. Pediatr Res 1985;19:476–481.
48. Rothman D, Udall JN, Pang KY, et al: The effect of short-term starvation on mucosal barrier function in the newborn rabbit. Pediatr Res 1985;19:727–731.
49. Butzner JD, Gall DG: Refeeding enhances intestinal repair during an acute enteritis in infant rabbits subjected to protein-energy malnutrition. Pediatr Res 1991;29:594–600.
50. Brown KH, Gastanaduy AS, Saavedra JM, et al: Effect of continued oral feeding on clinical and nutritional outcomes of acute diarrhea in children. J Pediatr 1988;112:191–200.
51. Isolauri E, Vesikari T, Saha P, Viander M: Milk versus no milk in rapid refeeding after acute gastroenteritis. J Pediatr Gastroenterol Nutr 1986;5:254–261.
52. Margolis PA, Litteer T, Hare N, Pichichero M: Effects of unrestricted diet on mild infantile diarrhea. Am J Dis Child 1990;144:162–164.
53. Brown KH, Peerson JM, Fontaine O: Use of nonhuman milks in the dietary management of young children with acute diarrhea: a meta-analysis of clinical trials. Pediatrics 1994;93:17–27.
54. Lifshitz F, Maggioni A: The nutritional management of acute diarrhea in young infants. J Pediatr Gastroenterol Nutr 1994;19:148–150.
55. Wall CR, Webster J, Quirk P, et al: The nutritional management of acute diarrhea in young infants: effect of carbohydrate ingested. J Pediatr Gastroenterol Nutr 1994;19:170–174.
56. Halliday K, Edmeades R, Shepherd RW: Persistent post-enteritis diarrhoea in childhood. Med J Aust 1982;1:18–20.
57. Goepp JG, Katz S, Cuervo E, et al: Comparison of two regimens of feeding and oral electrolyte solutions in infants with diarrhea. J Pediatr Gastroenterol Nutr 1997;24:374–379.
58. Walker-Smith JA, Sandhu BK, Isolauri E, et al: Recommendations for feeding in childhood gastroenteritis. J Pediatr Gastroenterol Nutr 1997;24:619–620.
59. Maulen-Radovan I, Brown KH, Acosta MA, Fernandez-Varela H: Comparison of a rice-based, mixed diet versus a lactose-free, soy-protein isolate formula for young children with acute diarrhea. J Pediatr 1994;125:699–706.
60. Fuller R: Probiotics in human medicine. Gut 1991;32:439–442.
61. Mehta AM, Patel KA, Dave PJ: Purification and properties of the inhibitory protein isolated from Lactobacillus acidophilus AC1. Microbios 1983;38:73–81.
62. Silva M, Jacobus NV, Deneke C, Groback SL: Antimicrobial substance from a human Lactobacillus strain. Antimicrob Agents Chemother 1986;31:1231–1233.
63. Yasui H, Mike A, Ohwaki M: Immunogenicity of Bifidobacterium breve and change in antibody production in Peyer's patches after oral administration. J Dairy Sci 1989;72:30–35.
64. Yasui H, Kiyoshima J, Ushihima H: Passive protection against rotavirus-induced diarrhea of mouse pups born to and nursed by dams fed Bifidobacterium breve. J Infect Dis 1995;172:403–409.
65. Biller JA, Katz AJ, Flores AF, et al: Treatment of recurrent *Clostridium difficile* colitis with *Lactobacillus* GG. J Pediatr Gastroenterol Nutr 1995;21:224–226.
66. Buts JP, Corthier G, Delmee M: Saccharomyces boulardii for Clostridium difficile-associated enteropathies in infants. J Pediatr Gastroenterol Nutr 1993;16:419–425.
67. DuPont HL, Sullivan P, Pickering LK: Symptomatic treatment of diarrhea with bismuth subsalicylate among students attending a Mexican university. Gastroenterology 1977;73:715–718.
68. Soriano-Brucher HE, Avendano P, O'Ryan M, et al: Bismuth subsalicylate in the treatment of acute diarrhea in children: a clinical study. Pediatrics 1991;87:18–27.
69. Figueroa-Quintanilla D, Salazar-Lindo E, Sack RB, et al: A controlled trial of bismuth subsalicylate in infants with acute watery diarrheal disease. N Engl J Med 1993;328:1653–1658.
70. Harries JT, Rossiter M: Fatal Lomotil poisoning (letter). Lancet 1969;1:150.
71. Bargman GJ, Gardner LI: Near fatality in an infant following "lomotil" poisoning. Pediatrics 1969;44:770–771.

72. Rosenton G, Freeman M, Standard AL, Weston N: Warning: use of Lomotil in children. Pediatrics 1973;51:132–134.
73. Kassem As, Madkour AB-S, Massoub BZ, Mehanna ZB: Loperamide in acute childhood diarrhoea: a double-blind controlled trial. J Diarrhoeal Dis Res 1983;1:10–16.
74. Owens JR, Broadhead R, Hendrickse RG, et al: Loperamide in the treatment of acute gastro-enteritis in early childhood: report on a two centre double-blind controlled clinical trial. Ann Trop Paediatr 1981;1:135–141.
75. Motala C, Hill ID, Mann MD, Bowie MD: Effect of loperamide on stool output and duration of acute infectious diarrhea in infants. J Pediatr 1990;117:467–471.
76. Jacobs J, Himenez M, Gloyd SS, et al: Treatment of acute childhood diarrhea with homeopathic medicine: a randomized clinical trial in Nicaragua. Pediatrics 1994;93:719–725.
77. Sampson W, London W: Analysis of homeopathic treatment of childhood diarrhea. Pediatrics 1995;96:961–964.
78. Clemens JD, Sack D, Harris J: Breast feeding and the risk of severe cholera in rural Bangladeshi children. Am J Epidemiol 1990;131:400–411.
79. Ahmed F, Clemens JD, Rao MR, et al: Community-based evaluation of the effect of breast feeding on the risk of microbiologically confirmed or clinically presumptive shigellosis in Bangladeshi children. Pediatrics 1992;90:406–411.
80. Weinberg RJ, Tipton G, Klish WJ, Brown MR: Effect of breast feeding on morbidity in rotavirus gastroenteritis. Pediatrics 1984;74:250–253.
81. Clemens JD, Rao MC, Ahmed F, et al: Breast-feeding and the risk of life-threatening rotavirus diarrhea: prevention or postponement? Pediatrics 1993;92:680–685.
82. Smith JC, Haddix AC, Teutsch SM, Glass RI: Cost-effectiveness analysis of a rotavirus immunization program for the United States. Pediatrics 1995;96:609–615.
83. Griffiths RI, Anderson GF, Pose NR, et al: Economic impact of immunization against rotavirus gastroenteritis. Arch Pediatr Adolesc Med 1995;149:407–414.
84. Bersntein DI, Glass RI, Rodgers G, et al: Evaluation of Rhesus rotavirus monovalent and tetravalent reassortant vaccines in US children. JAMA 1995;273:1191–1196.
85. Velazquez FR, Matson DO, Calva JJ, et al: Rotavirus infection in infants as protection against subsequent infections. N Engl J Med 1996;335:1022–1028.
86. Levine MM, Kaper JB, Herrington D, et al: Safety, immunogenicity, and efficacy of recombinant live oral cholera vaccines, CVD 103 and CVD 103-HgR. Lancet 1988;2:467–470.
87. Simanjuntak CH, O'Hanley P, Punjabi NH: Safety, immunogenicity, and transmissibility of single-dose live oral cholera vaccine strain CVD 103-HgR in 24-59-month-old Indonesian children. J Infect Dis 1993;168:1169–1176.
88. Saavedra JM, Bauman NA, Oung I: Feeding of Bifidobacterium bifidum and Streptococcus thermophilus to infants in hospital for prevention of diarrhea and shedding of rotavirus. Lancet 1994;344:1046–1049.

# Index

Note: Page numbers in *italics* refer to illustrations; page numbers followed by t refer to tables.

ISBN 0-7216-7461-5

90038

9 780721 674612